Human Anatomy & Physiology

Ninth Edition

Elaine N. Marieb, R.N., Ph.D.
Holyoke Community College

Katja Hoehn, M.D., Ph.D.
Mount Royal University

PEARSON

Boston Columbus Indianapolis New York San Francisco Upper Saddle River
Amsterdam Cape Town Dubai London Madrid Milan Munich Paris Montreal Toronto
Delhi Mexico City São Paulo Sydney Hong Kong Seoul Singapore Taipei Tokyo

Editor-in-Chief: Serina Beauparlant
Acquisitions Editor: Gretchen Puttkamer
Associate Project Editor: Shannon Cutt
Director of Development: Barbara Yien
Development Editor: Alice Fugate
Art Development Manager: Laura Southworth
Senior Managing Editor: Debbie Cogan
Production and Design Manager: Michele Mangelli
Production Supervisor: David Novak
Media Producer: Aimee Pavy
Editorial Assistant: Lisa Damerel
Text Designer: tani hasegawa
Cover Designer: Riezebos Holzbaur Design Group
Art Houses: Imagineering STA Media Services Inc. and Electronic Publishing Services Inc., NYC
Art Coordinator: Jean Lake
Photo Image Lead: Donna Kalal
Photo Researcher: Kristin Piljay
Copyeditor: Anita Wagner
Proofreader: Martha Ghent
Compositor: S4Carlisle Publishing Services
Senior Manufacturing Buyer: Stacey Weinberger
Marketing Manager: Derek Perrigo and Susan Blumenthal

Cover photo of Olympic Gold Medalist Hope Solo © Ina Fassbender/Reuters.

Credits and acknowledgments borrowed from other sources and reproduced, with permission, in this textbook appear on the appropriate page within the text or on p. C-1.

Photo and illustration credits follow the Glossary.

Library of Congress Cataloging-in-Publication Data

Marieb, Elaine Nicpon
Human anatomy & physiology / Elaine N. Marieb, Katja Hoehn.—9th ed.
p. ; cm.
ISBN-13: 978-0-321-74326-8 (student ed.)
ISBN-10: 0-321-74326-1 (student ed.)
I. Hoehn, Katja. II. Title.
[DNLM: 1. Anatomy. 2. Physiological Phenomena. QS 4]
LC classification not assigned
612—dc23 2011038702

ISBN 10: 0-13-282874-X (High School Binding)
ISBN 13: 978-0-13-282874-1 (High School Binding)
1 2 3 4 5 6 7 8 9 10—RRD—15 14 13 12 11

PEARSON

www.PearsonSchool.com/Advanced

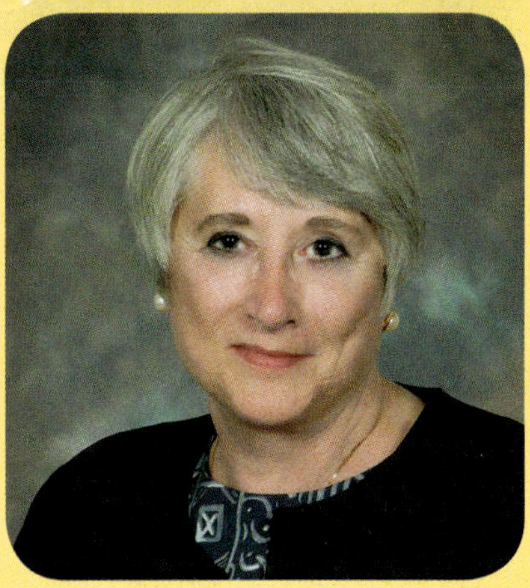

About the Authors

We dedicate this work to our students both present and past, who always inspire us to "push the envelope."

Elaine N. Marieb

For Elaine N. Marieb, taking the student's perspective into account has always been an integral part of her teaching style. Dr. Marieb began her teaching career at Springfield College, where she taught anatomy and physiology to physical education majors. She then joined the faculty of the Biological Science Division of Holyoke Community College in 1969 after receiving her Ph.D. in zoology from the University of Massachusetts at Amherst. While teaching at Holyoke Community College, where many of her students were pursuing nursing degrees, she developed a desire to better understand the relationship between the scientific study of the human body and the clinical aspects of the nursing practice. To that end, while continuing to teach full time, Dr. Marieb pursued her nursing education, which culminated in a Master of Science degree with a clinical specialization in gerontology from the University of Massachusetts. It is this experience that has informed the development of the unique perspective and accessibility for which her publications are known.

Dr. Marieb has partnered with Benjamin Cummings for over 30 years. Her first work was *Human Anatomy & Physiology Laboratory Manual* (*Cat Version*), which came out in 1981. In the years since, several other lab manual versions and study guides, as well as the softcover *Essentials of Human Anatomy & Physiology* textbook, have hit the campus bookstores. This textbook, now in its 9th edition, made its appearance in 1989 and is the latest expression of her commitment to the needs of students studying human anatomy and physiology.

Dr. Marieb has given generously to provide opportunities for students to further their education. She contributes to the New Directions, New Careers Program at Holyoke Community College by funding a staffed drop-in center and by providing several full-tuition scholarships each year for women who are returning to college after a hiatus or attending college for the first time and who would be unable to continue their studies without financial support. She funds the E. N. Marieb Science Research Awards at Mount Holyoke College, which promotes research by undergraduate science majors, and has underwritten renovation and updating of one of the biology labs in Clapp Laboratory at that college. Dr. Marieb also contributes to the University of Massachusetts at Amherst where she generously provided funding for reconstruction and instrumentation of a cutting-edge cytology research laboratory. Recognizing the severe national shortage of nursing faculty, she underwrites the Nursing Scholars of the Future Grant Program at the university.

In 1994, Dr. Marieb received the Benefactor Award from the National Council for Resource Development, American Association of Community Colleges, which recognizes her ongoing sponsorship of student scholarships, faculty teaching awards, and other academic contributions to Holyoke Community College. In May 2000, the science building at Holyoke Community College was named in her honor.

Dr. Marieb is an active member of the Human Anatomy and Physiology Society (HAPS) and the American Association for the Advancement of Science (AAAS). Additionally, while actively engaged as an author, Dr. Marieb serves as a consultant for the Benjamin Cummings *Interactive Physiology*® CD-ROM series.

When not involved in academic pursuits, Dr. Marieb is a world traveler and has vowed to visit every country on this planet. Shorter term, she serves on the scholarship committee of the Women's Resources Center and on the board of directors of several charitable institutions in Sarasota County. She is an enthusiastic supporter of the local arts and enjoys a competitive match of doubles tennis.

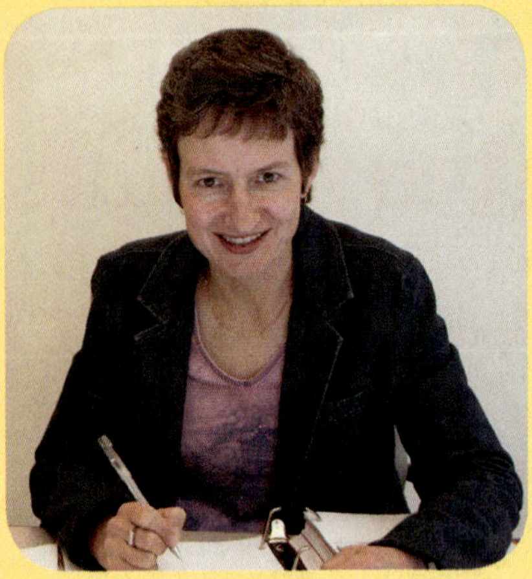

Katja Hoehn

Dr. Katja Hoehn is an associate professor in the Department of Chemical and Biological Sciences at Mount Royal University in Calgary, Canada. Dr. Hoehn's first love is teaching. Her teaching excellence has been recognized by several awards during her 17 years at Mount Royal University. These include a PanCanadian Educational Technology Faculty Award (1999), a Teaching Excellence Award from the Students' Association of Mount Royal (2001), and the Mount Royal Distinguished Faculty Teaching Award (2004).

Dr. Hoehn received her M.D. (with Distinction) from the University of Saskatchewan, and her Ph.D. in Pharmacology from Dalhousie University. In 1991, the Dalhousie Medical Research Foundation presented her with the Max Forman (Jr.) Prize for excellence in medical research. During her Ph.D. and postdoctoral studies, she also pursued her passion for teaching by presenting guest lectures to first- and second-year medical students at Dalhousie University and at the University of Calgary.

Dr. Hoehn has been a contributor to several books and has written numerous research papers in Neuroscience and Pharmacology. She oversaw a recent revision of the Benjamin Cummings *Interactive Physiology*® CD-ROM series modules, and coauthored the newest module, *The Immune System*.

Following Dr. Marieb's example, Dr. Hoehn provides financial support for students in the form of a scholarship that she established in 2006 for nursing students at Mount Royal University.

Dr. Hoehn is also actively involved in the Human Anatomy and Physiology Society (HAPS) and is a member of the American Association of Anatomists. When not teaching, she likes to spend time outdoors with her husband and two sons, compete in triathlons, and play Irish flute.

Introduce yourself to the chapter

Improved readability and navigability makes the text more accessible and easier to study.

Chapter Outlines

Chapter outlines provide a preview of the chapter and help you locate information easily.

Learning Objectives

Learning objectives are integrated into the chapter and give you a preview of what content is to come and what you are expected to learn.

Bulleted Narrative

The narrative has been bulleted wherever possible to make the text easier to read and navigate.

Check Your Understanding

Concept check questions are tied to the sections' Learning Objectives and ask you to stop, think, and check your understanding before moving on.

14

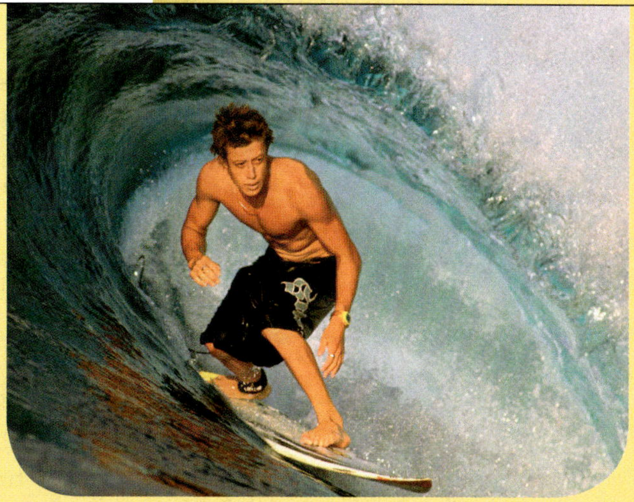

The Autonomic Nervous System

The human body is exquisitely sensitive to changes in its internal environment, and engages in a lifelong struggle to balance competing demands for resources under ever-changing conditions. Although all body systems contribute, the stability of our internal environment depends largely on the **autonomic nervous system (ANS),** the system of motor neurons that innervates smooth and cardiac muscle and glands **(Figure 14.1)**.

At every moment, signals stream from visceral organs into the CNS, and autonomic nerves make adjustments as necessary to ensure optimal support for body activities. In response to changing conditions, the ANS shunts blood to "needy" areas, speeds or slows heart rate, adjusts blood pressure and body temperature, and increases or decreases stomach secretions.

Most of this fine-tuning occurs without our awareness or attention. Can you tell when your arteries are constricting or your pupils are dilating? Probably not—but if you've ever been stuck in a checkout line, and your full bladder was contracting as if it had a mind of its own, you've been very aware of visceral activity. The ANS controls all these functions, both those we're aware of and those we're not. Indeed, as the term *autonomic* (*auto* = self; *nom* = govern) implies, this motor subdivision of the peripheral nervous system has a certain amount of functional independence. The ANS is also called the **involuntary nervous system**, which reflects its subconscious control, or the **general visceral motor system**, which indicates the location of most of its effectors.

Overview

- ✓ Define autonomic nervous system and explain its relationship to the peripheral nervous system.
- ✓ Compare the somatic and autonomic nervous systems relative to effectors, efferent pathways, and neurotransmitters released.
- ✓ Compare and contrast the functions of the parasympathetic and sympathetic divisions.

ANS Anatomy

✓ For the parasympathetic and sympathetic divisions, describe the site of CNS origin, locations of ganglia, and general fiber pathways.

Anatomically, the sympathetic and parasympathetic divisions differ in

- **Sites of origin.** Parasympathetic fibers are craniosacral—they originate in the brain (cranium) and sacral spinal cord. Sympathetic fibers are thoracolumbar—they originate in the thoracic and lumbar regions of the spinal cord.
- **Relative lengths of their fibers.** The parasympathetic division has long preganglionic and short postganglionic fibers. The sympathetic division has the opposite condition—the preganglionic fibers are short and the postganglionic fibers are long.

☑ Check Your Understanding

1. Name the three types of effectors of the autonomic nervous system.
2. Which relays instructions from the CNS to muscles more quickly, the somatic nervous system or the ANS? Explain why.
3. Which branch of the ANS would predominate if you were lying on the beach enjoying the sun and the sound of the waves? Which branch would predominate if you were on a surfboard and a shark appeared within a few feet of you?

For answers, see Appendix H.

MasteringA&P®

Reading Questions keep you on track.

Chapter 14 Chapter Test Question 5

Resources ▾ | Help | Close

Item Type: Reading Questions | **Difficulty:** 2 | **Time:** 2m | Learning Outcomes ▾ | Contact the Publisher

Manage this Item: Standard View

Chapter Test - Chapter 14 Question 5

Part A

Once a preganglionic axon reaches a trunk ganglion, one of three things can happen to the axon. Which of the following is *not* one of these three things?

- ○ The axon can ascend or descend the sympathetic trunk to synapse in another trunk ganglion.
- ○ The axon can pass through the trunk ganglion and emerge from the sympathetic trunk without synapsing.
- ○ The axon can synapse with a ganglionic neuron in the same trunk ganglion.
- ○ The axon can emerge from the sympathetic trunk to synapse in another axon.

submit | my answers | show answer | review part

Follow complex processes step by step

Focus Figures help you grasp tough topics in A&P by walking you through carefully developed step-by-step illustrations that use a big-picture layout and dramatic art to provide a context for understanding the process.

Overview

Each Overview quicky summarizes the key idea of the figure.

Big Picture Orientation

The big picture provides you with a concrete starting point for the process.

Blue Text

This text acts as the teacher's voice and explains difficult concepts. In some figures the text is broken into numbered steps to help you more easily understand difficult processes.

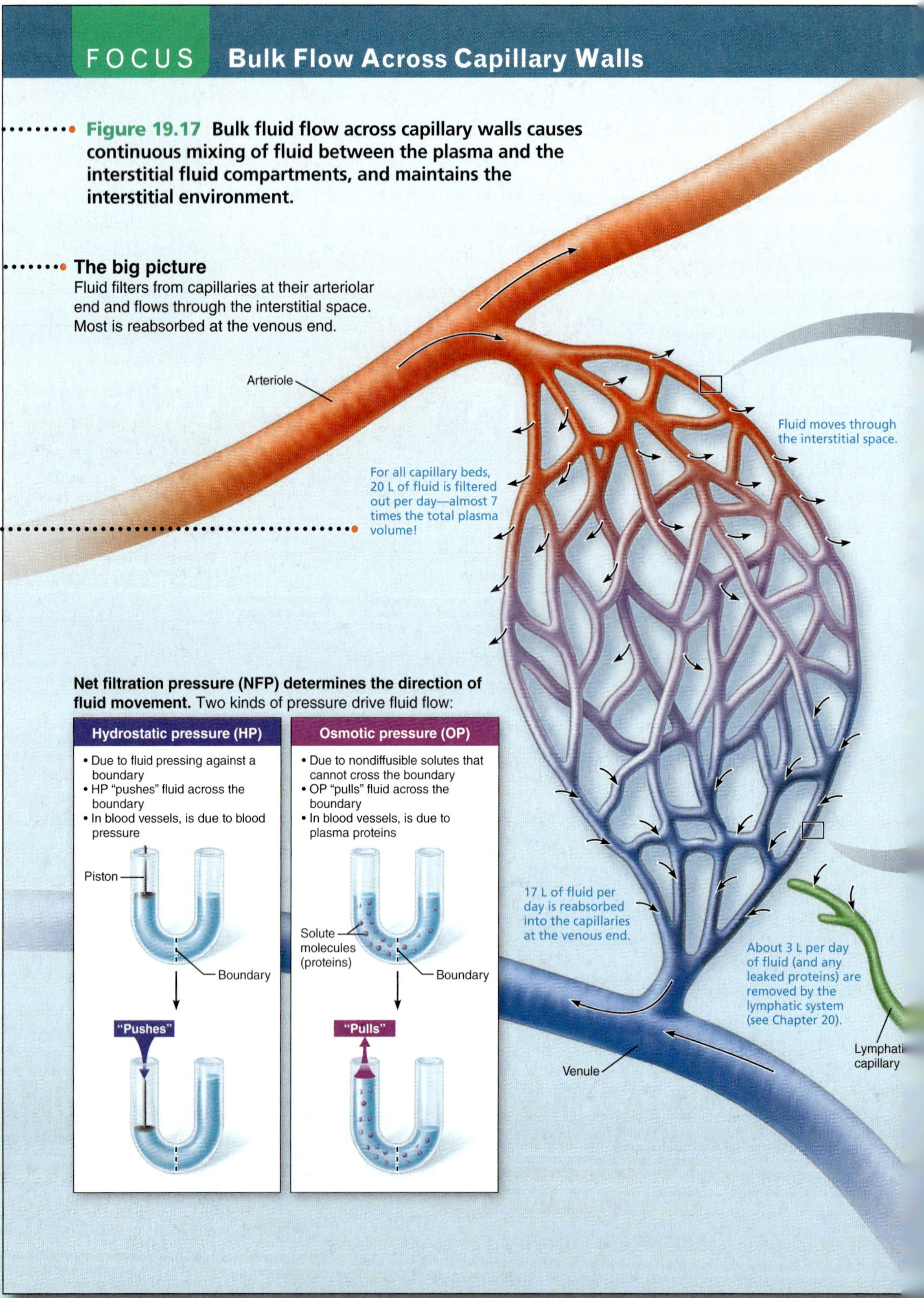

How do the pressures drive fluid flow across a capillary?

Net filtration occurs at the arteriolar end of a capillary.

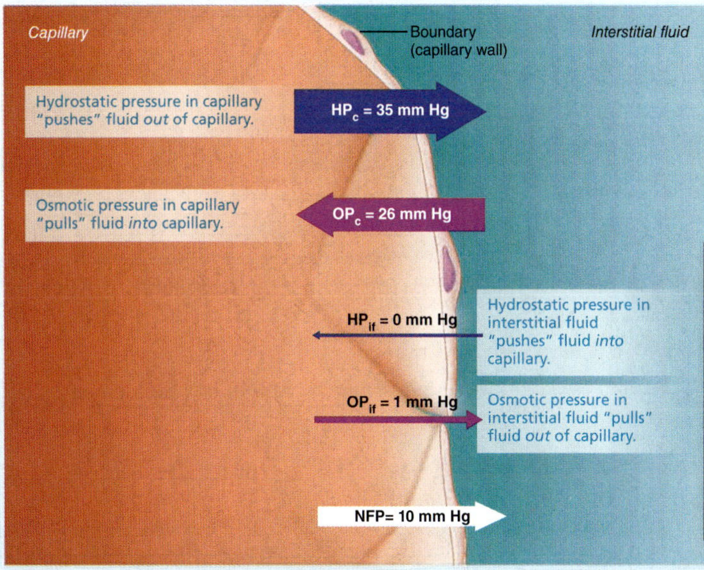

To determine the pressure driving the fluid out of the capillary at any given point, we calculate the **net filtration pressure (NFP)**—the outward pressures (HP_c and OP_{if}) minus the inward pressures (HP_{if} and OP_c). So,

$$NFP = (HP_c + OP_{if}) - (HP_{if} + OP_c)$$
$$= (35 + 1) - (0 + 26)$$
$$= 10 \text{ mm Hg (net outward pressure)}$$

As a result, fluid moves from the capillary into the interstitial space.

Net reabsorption occurs at the venous end of a capillary.

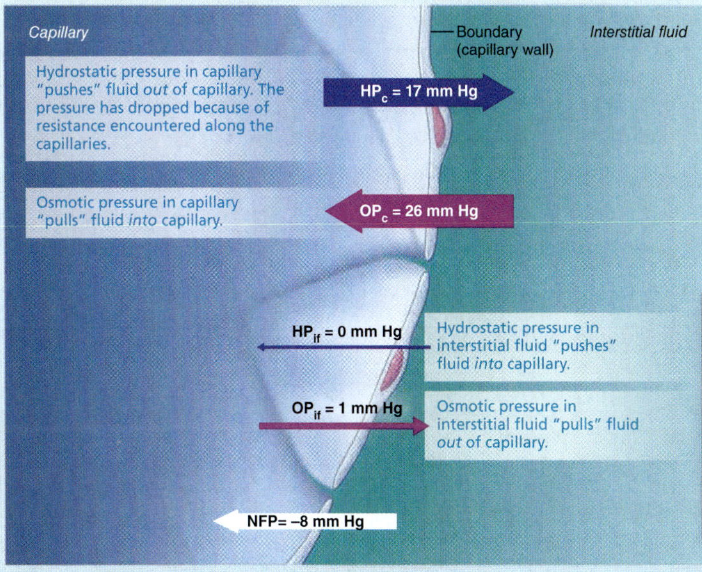

Again, we calculate the NFP:

$$NFP = (HP_c + OP_{if}) - (HP_{if} + OP_c)$$
$$= (17 + 1) - (0 + 26)$$
$$= -8 \text{ mm Hg (net inward pressure)}$$

Notice that the NFP at the venous end is a negative number. This means that reabsorption, not filtration, is occurring and so fluid moves from the interstitial space into the capillary.

MasteringA&P®

Focus Figure Tutorials

All Focus Figures have related tutorials in MasteringA&P that your teacher can assign and that will guide you through the figures step by step.

Study figures as you read the text

Select pieces of art provide more visual content and often have step-by-step text that helps you better understand structure, functions, and processes.

▾ 3-D anatomy art

Stunning 3-D anatomy art is rendered in a dramatically more dynamic, realistic style that uses vibrant, saturated colors to help you visualize key anatomical structures.

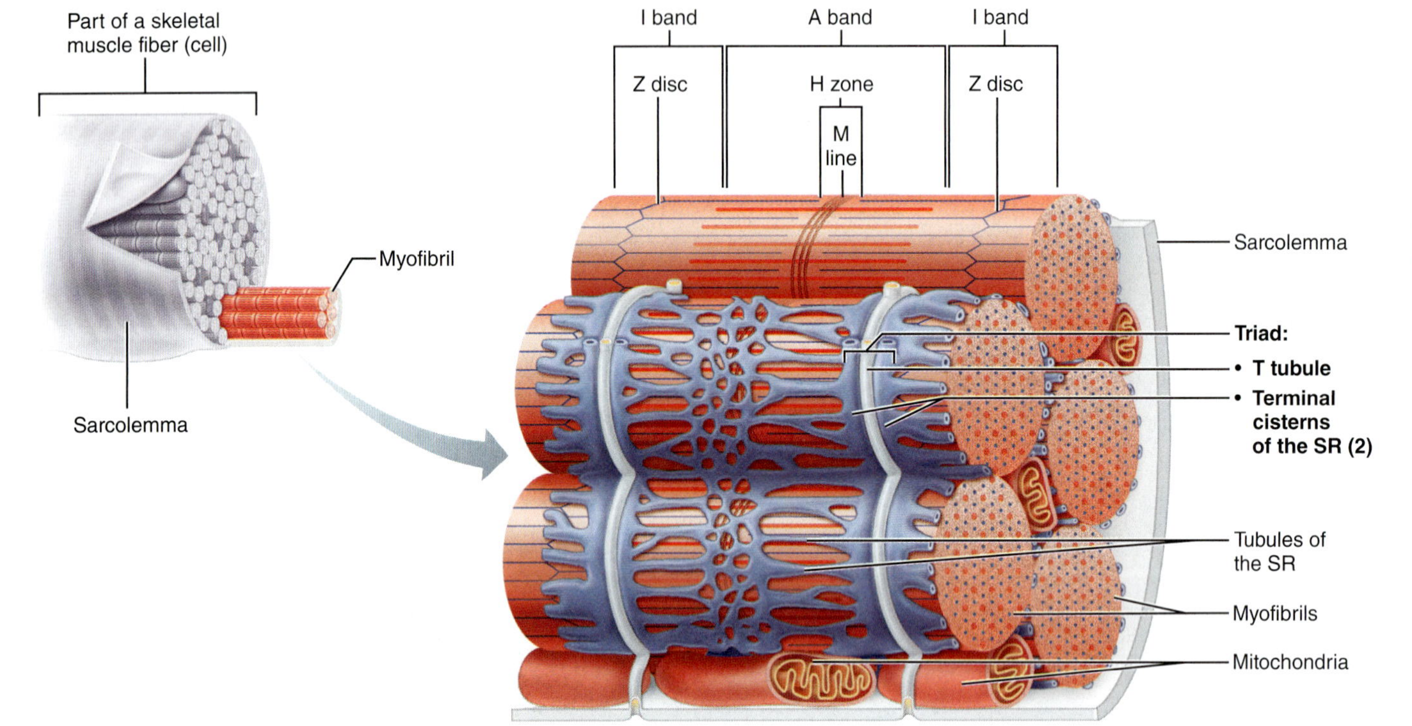

Figure 9.5 Relationship of the sarcoplasmic reticulum and T tubules to myofibrils of skeletal muscle. The tubules of the SR (blue) encircle each myofibril like a "holey" sleeve. These tubules fuse to form a net of communicating channels at the level of the H zone and saclike elements called terminal cisterns abutting the A-I junctions. The T tubules (gray) are inward invaginations of the sarcolemma that run deep into the cell between the terminal cisterns. (See detailed view in Figure 9.11, pp.290-291) Sites of close contact of these three elements (terminal cistern, T tubule, and terminal cistern) are called triads.

MasteringA&P®

NEW! Art Labeling and Ranking/Sorting Questions are drag and drop activities that allow you to assess your knowledge of terms and structures as well as the order of steps and elements involved in physiological processes.

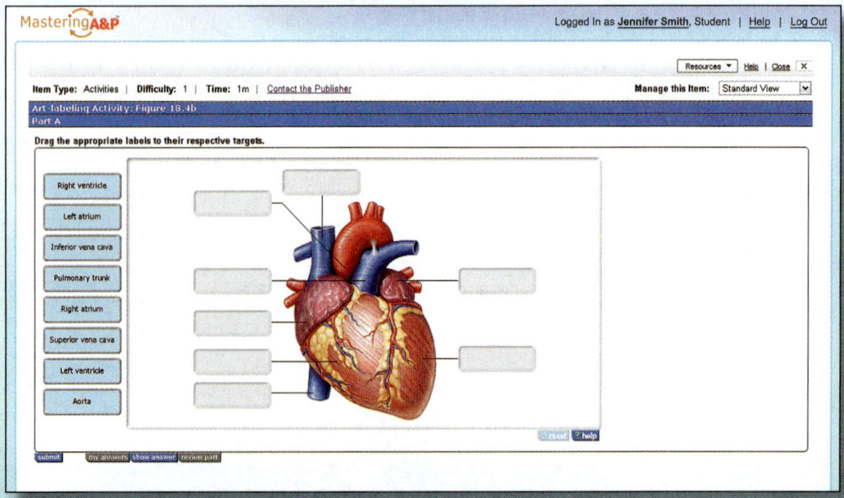

Prepare for your future career

Clinical coverage and case studies have been expanded throughout.

Homeostatic Imbalance 6.1

Minute changes from the homeostatic range for blood calcium can lead to severe neuromuscular problems ranging from hyperexcitability (when blood Ca^{2+} levels are too low) to nonresponsiveness and inability to function (with high blood Ca^{2+} levels). In addition, sustained high blood levels of Ca^{2+}, a condition known as *hypercalcemia* (hi″per-kal-se′me-ah), can lead to undesirable deposits of calcium salts in the blood vessels, kidneys, and other soft organs, which may hamper their function. ✚

Homeostatic Imbalance

Homeostatic Imbalance sections are integrated within the text and alert you to the consequences of body systems not functioning optimally. These pathological conditions are integrated with the text to clarify and illuminate normal functioning.

MasteringA&P®

NEW! Homeostatic Imbalance Clinical Questions can be assigned to you by your teacher on MasteringA&P. They help strengthen your understanding of how the body works to stay in balance and what happens when it falls out of balance.

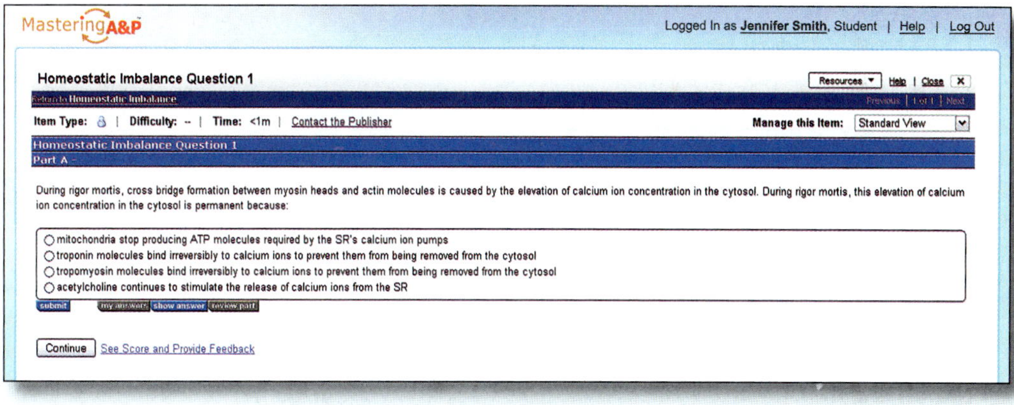

AT THE CLINIC

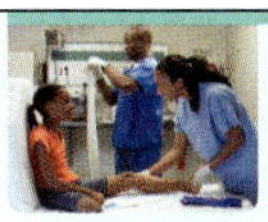

Case Study **Muscular System**

Let's continue our tale of Mrs. DeStephano's medical problems, this time looking at the notes made detailing observations of her skeletal musculature.

- Severe lacerations of the muscles of the right leg and knee
- Damage to the blood vessels serving the right leg and knee
- Transection of the sciatic nerve (the large nerve serving most of the lower limb), just above the right knee

Her physician orders daily passive range-of-motion (ROM) exercise and electrical stimulation for her right leg and a diet high in protein, carbohydrates, and vitamin C.

1. Describe the step-by-step process of wound healing that will occur in her fleshy (muscle) wounds, and note the consequences of the specific restorative process that occurs.
2. What complications in healing can be anticipated owing to vascular (blood vessel) damage in the right leg?
3. What complications in muscle structure and function result from transection of the sciatic nerve? Why are passive ROM and electrical stimulation of her right leg muscles ordered?
4. Explain the reasoning behind the dietary recommendations.

(Answers in Appendix H)

NEW! At the Clinic

End-of-chapter sections now contain an At the Clinic feature, which help you apply what you've learned. By learning related clinical terms and reading short Case Studies and answering questions, you will begin to prepare for your future career.

MasteringA&P®

NEW! Case Study Coaching Activities increase your problem-solving skills and prepare you for your future career.

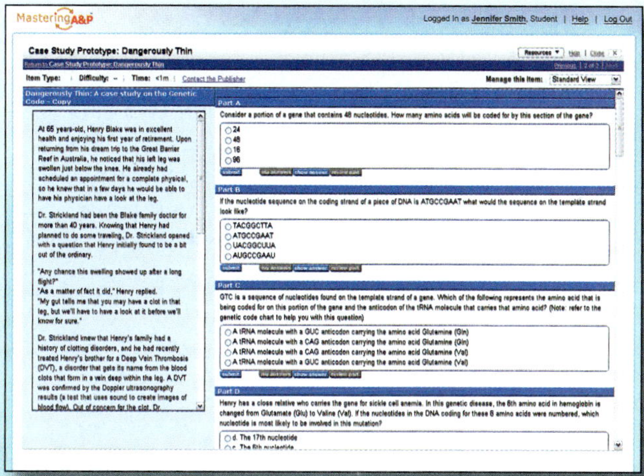

Practice what you don't understand with MasteringA&P®

MasteringA&P includes a Study Area that has many tools to help you succeed, including:

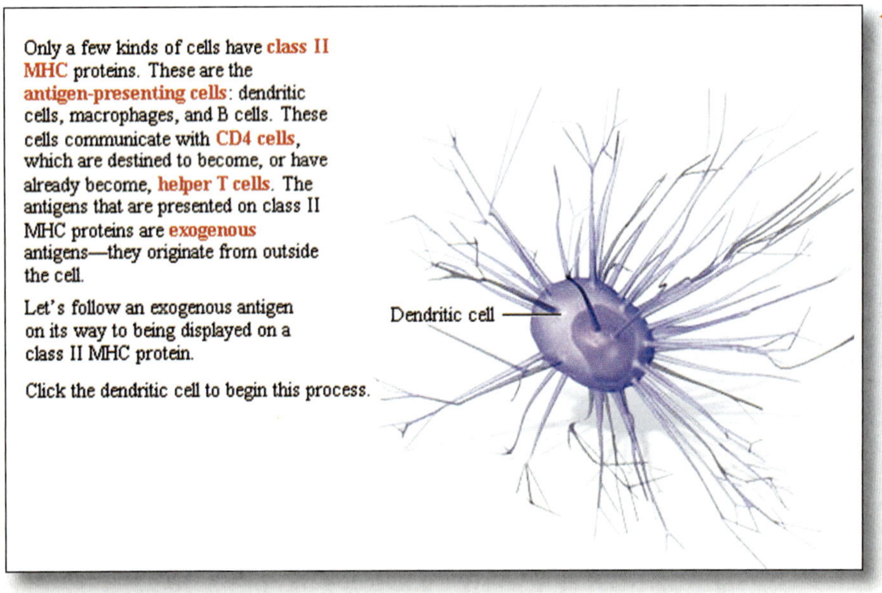

Interactive Physiology® 10-System Suite

IP helps you understand the hardest part of A&P: physiology. Fun, interactive tutorials, games, and quizzes give you additional explanations to help you grasp difficult concepts.

Modules:

- Muscular System
- Nervous System I
- Nervous System II
- Cardiovascular System
- Respiratory System
- Urinary System
- Fluids & Electrolytes
- Endocrine System
- Digestive System
- Immune System

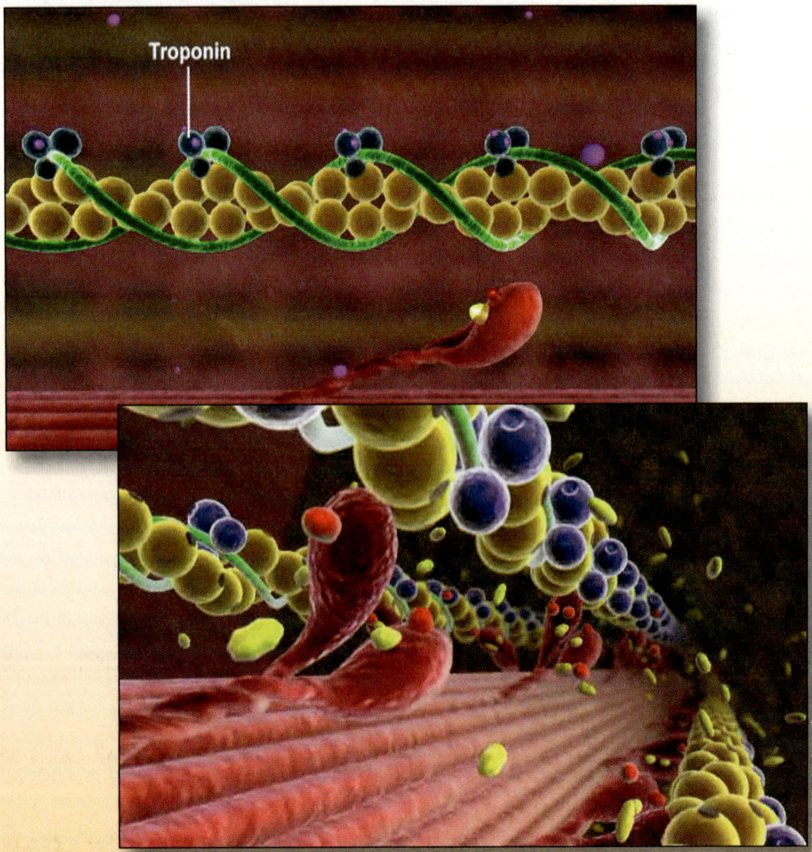

A&P Flix

A&P Flix™ are 3-D movie-quality animations with self-paced tutorials and gradable quizzes that help you master the toughest topics in A&P:

Cell Physiology
- Membrane Transport
- DNA Replication
- Mitosis
- Protein Synthesis

Muscle Physiology
- Events at the Neuromuscular Junction
- Excitation-Contraction Coupling
- Cross-Bridge Cycle

Neurophysiology
- Resting Membrane Potential
- Generation of an Action Potential
- Propagation of an Action Potential

Origins, Insertions, Actions, Innervations
- 63 animations on this topic

Group Muscle Actions & Joints
- 54 animations on this topic

MasteringA&P®

www.masteringaandp.com

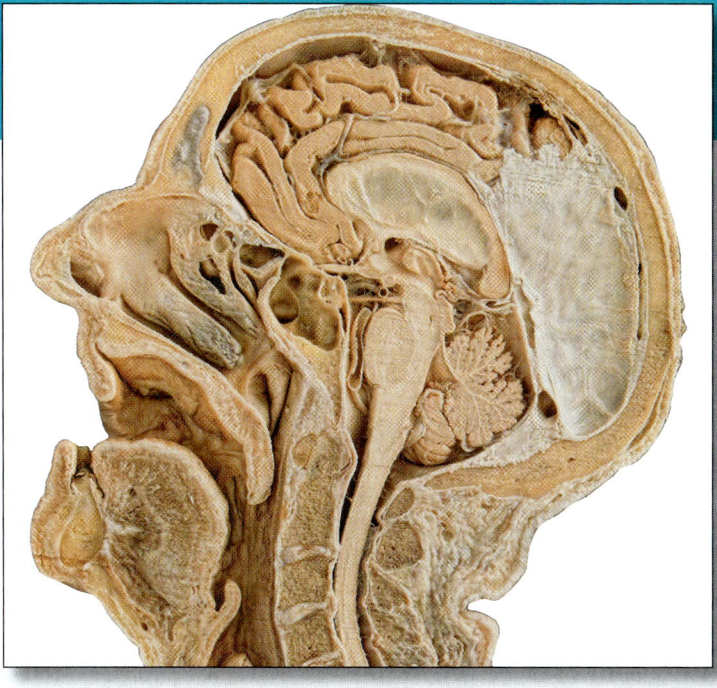

PAL | practice anatomy lab™

Practice Anatomy Lab™ (PAL™) 3.0 is a virtual anatomy study and practice tool that gives you 24/7 access to the most widely used lab specimens, including the human cadaver, anatomical models, histology, cat, and fetal pig. PAL 3.0 retains all of the key advantages of version 2.0, including ease of use, built-in audio pronunciations, rotatable bones, and simulated fill-in-the-blank lab practical exams.

Pearson eText

Pearson eText gives you access to the text whenever and wherever you can access the Internet. The eText pages look exactly like the printed text, plus you get powerful interactive and customization features.

Annotation Function
Allows you to take notes.

Google®-based
search function.

Highlight Function
Lets you highlight what you want to remember.

Zoom
Lets you zoom in and out for better viewing.

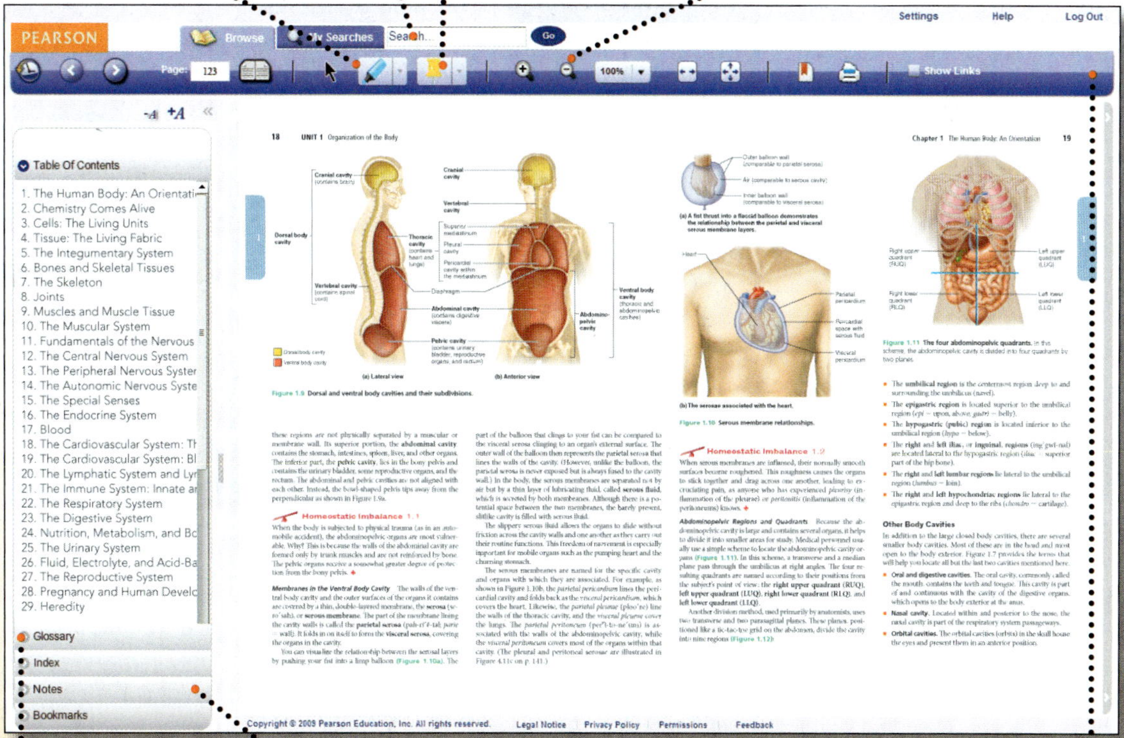

Interactive Glossary
Provides pop-up definitions and terms.

Teacher Notes
Your teacher might also share his or her notes and highlights with the class.

Hyperlinks
Links to quizzes, tests, activities, and animations.

Get 24/7 lab practice

NEW! PAL practice anatomy lab™

PAL 3.0 is an indispensable virtual anatomy study and practice tool that gives you 24/7 access to the most widely used lab specimens, including the human cadaver, anatomical models, histology, cat, and fetal pig. PAL 3.0 retains all of the key advantages of version 2.0, including ease of use, built-in audio pronunciations, rotatable bones, and simulated fill-in-the-blank lab practical exams.

NEW! Carefully prepared dissections show nerves, blood vessels, and arteries across body systems.

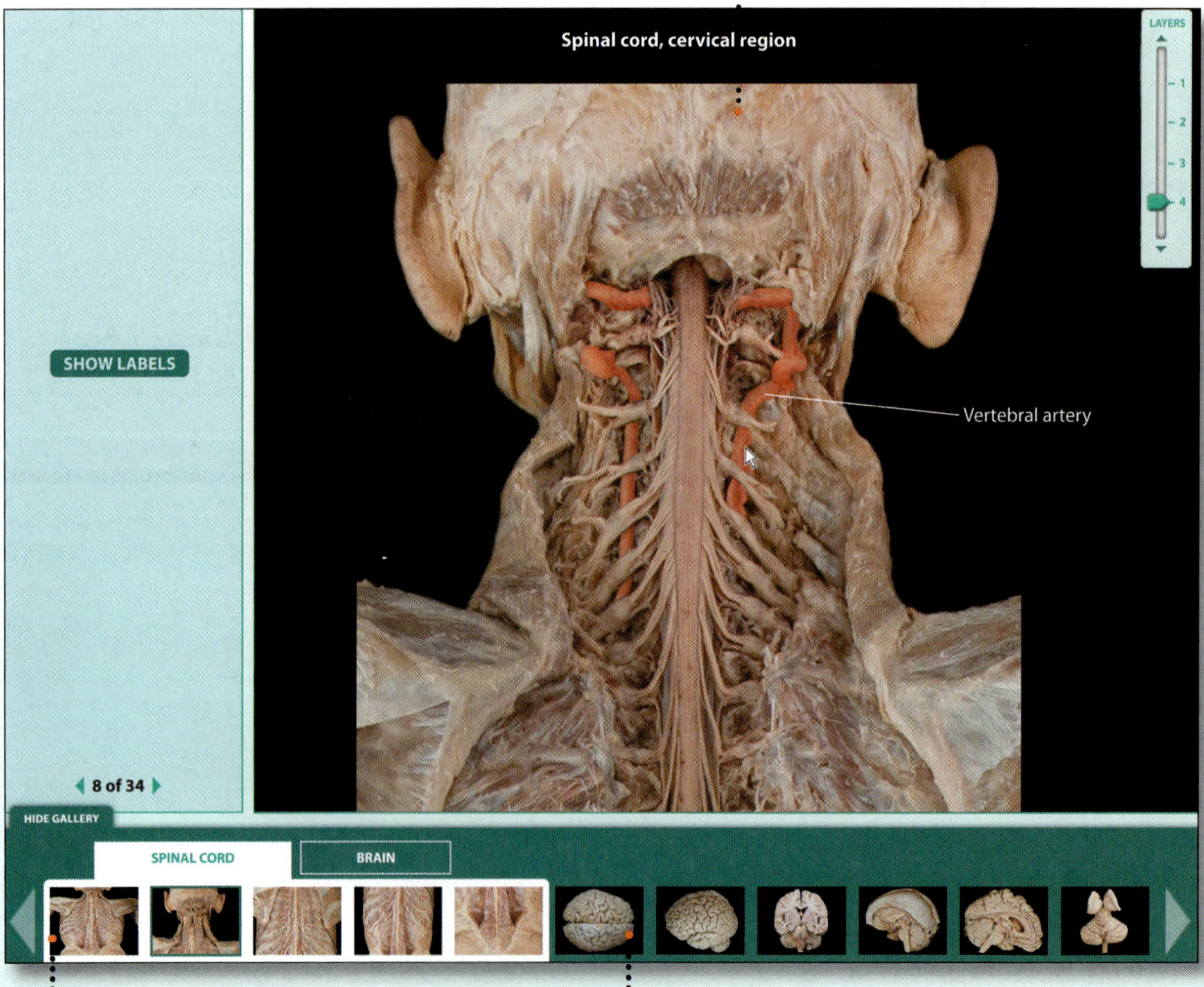

NEW! **Layering slider** allows you to peel back layers of the human cadaver and view and explore hundreds of brand-new dissections especially commissioned for 3.0.

NEW! **Photo gallery** allows you to quickly see thumbnails of images for a particular region or sub region.

PAL 3.0 is available in the **Study Area of MasteringA&P** (www.masteringaandp.com). The PAL 3.0 DVD is also available for purchase.

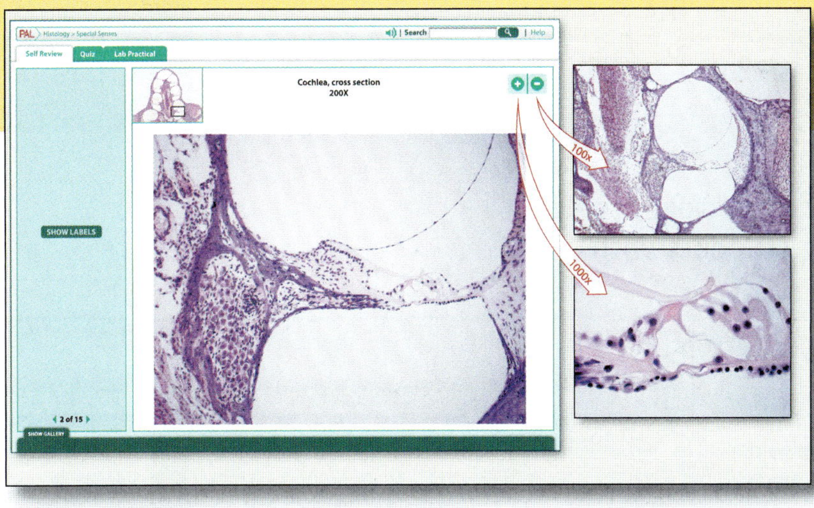

NEW! Interactive Histology

Interactive Histology module allows you to view the same tissue slide at varying magnifications, thereby helping you identify structures and their characteristics.

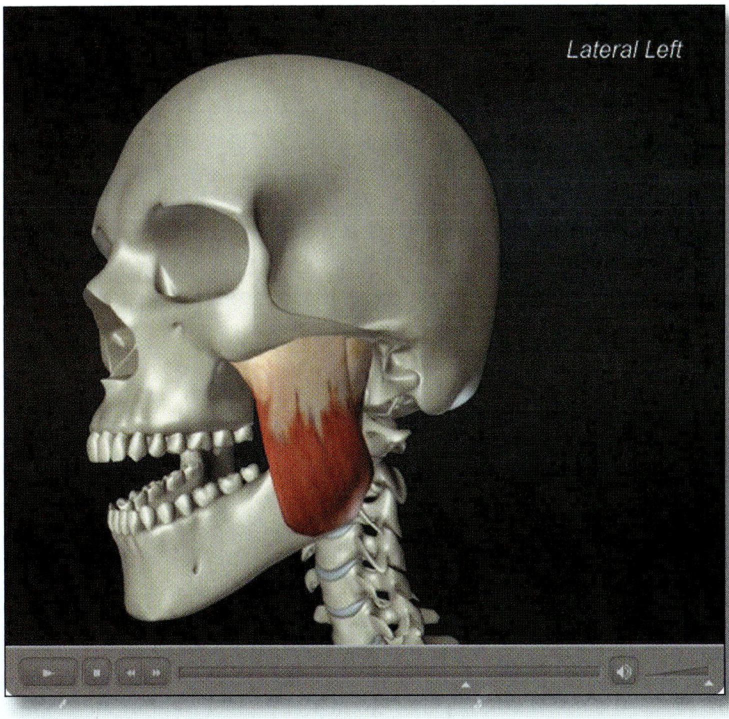

3-D Anatomy Animations

3-D Anatomy Animations of origins, insertions, actions, and innervations of over 65 muscles are now viewable in both Cadaver and Anatomical Models and modules. A new closed-captioning option provides textual presentation of narration to help you retain information.

PAL practice anatomy lab™

PAL 3.0 also includes:

- NEW! **Question randomization** feature gives you more opportunities for practice and self-assessment. Each time you retake a quiz or lab practical, a new set of questions is generated.
- NEW! **Hundreds of new images and views** are included, especially of the human cadaver, anatomical models, and histology.
- NEW! **Turn-off highlight feature** in quizzes and lab practicals gives you the option to see a structure without the highlight overlay.

physioEX™ VERSION 9

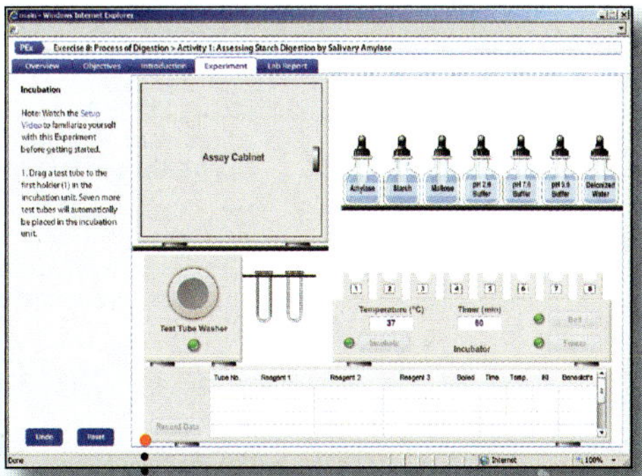

NEW! PhysioEx 9.0

PhysioEx 9.0: Laboratory Simulations in Physiology is easy-to-use laboratory simulation software with an accompanying lab manual that consists of 12 exercises containing 63 physiology lab activities. It can be used to supplement or substitute for wet labs. PhysioEx allows you to repeat labs as often as you like, perform experiments without harming live animals, and conduct experiments that are difficult to perform in a wet lab environment because of time, cost, or safety concerns.

To the Teacher: Everything from the Book is now Integrated with MasteringA&P®

All text features of *Human Anatomy & Physiology* are now assignable in MasteringA&P, providing students with unlimited opportunities to study.

NEW! Focus Figure Tutorials

Focus Figure Tutorials guide students through key parts of each Focus Figure, assessing their understanding of the major concepts through a variety of assessment tools—multiple choice questions with hints and specific wrong-answer feedback, interactive ranking and sorting exercises, and labeling activities.

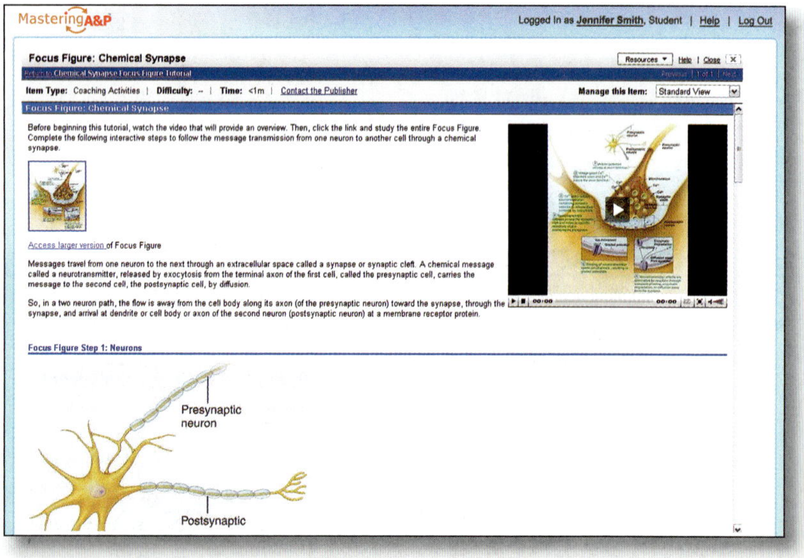

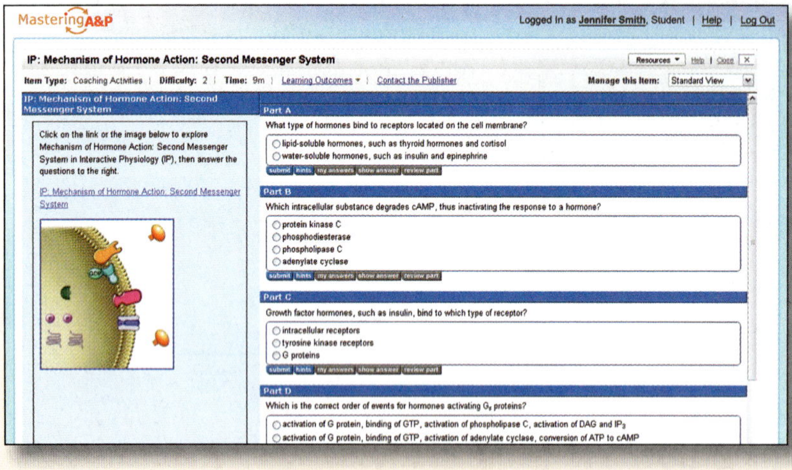

Interactive Physiology® Coaching Activities

20 new *Interactive Physiology* Coaching Activities have been added to the Item Library.

NEW! Homeostatic Imbalance Clinical Questions

Homeostatic Imbalance Clinical Questions are higher-order thinking questions that assess students on their comprehension of the Homeostatic Imbalance content in each chapter, making one of the text's hallmark features now assignable.

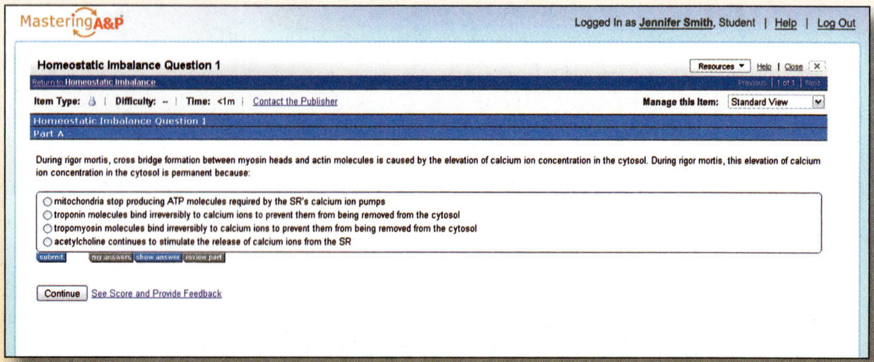

MasteringA&P®

www.masteringaandp.com

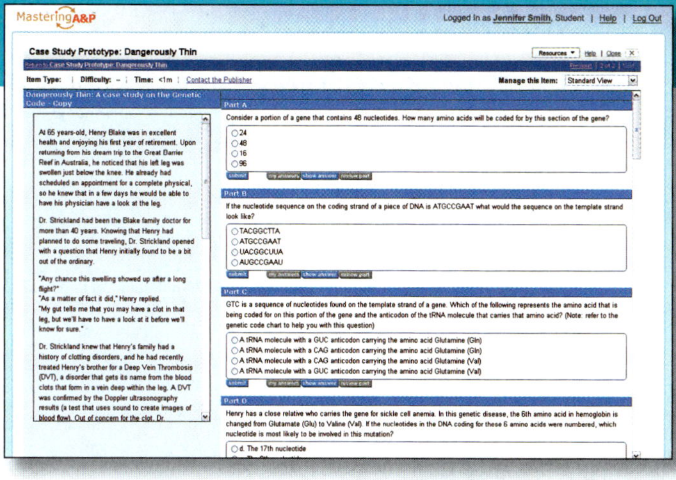

NEW! Case Study Coaching Activities

Case Study Coaching Activities increase problem-solving skills and prepare students for future careers in allied health. Corresponding Teaching Notes give teachers valuable tips on when and how to use case studies in the classroom.

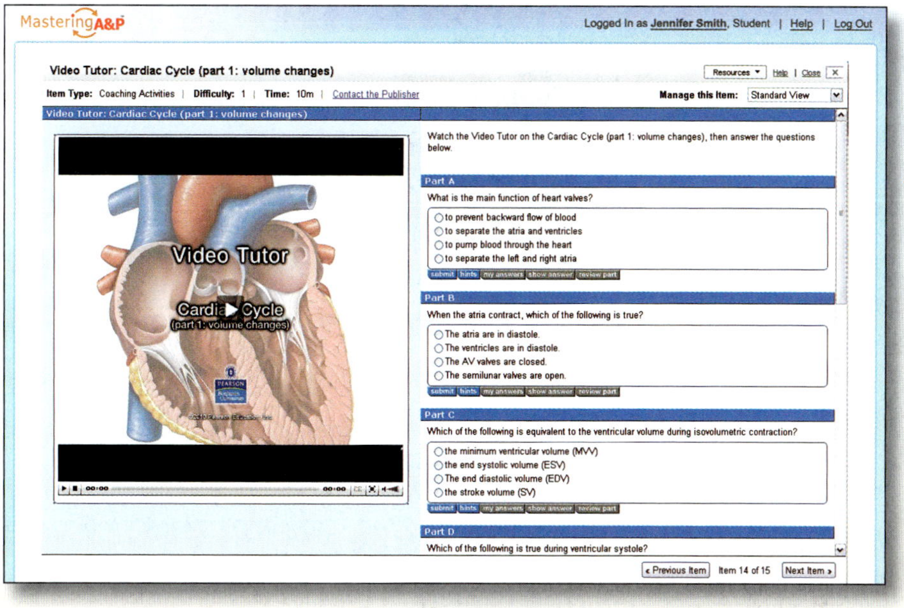

Video Tutor Coaching Activities

Video Tutors instruct and coach students on key A&P concepts using art from the book and are accompanied by questions with video hints and feedback specific to their misconceptions.

Other Text Features Now Assignable in MasteringA&P:

- **A&P Flix™** Coaching Activities offer stunning 3-D visuals of core concepts and tough physiological concepts with in-depth assessments to test student understanding. Seven new topics have been added to the Ninth Edition.
- **Art-Based Questions** are conceptual questions related to art and instruct students with wrong-answer feedback.
- **Art Labeling** and **Ranking/Sorting Questions** are drag and drop activities that allow students to assess their knowledge of terms and structures as well as the order of steps and elements involved in physiological processes.
- **PAL™ 3.0** and assessments
- **PhysioEx™ 9.0** and assessments
- **Clinical Application questions** (under Test Bank) give students the opportunity to apply their knowledge to clinical scenarios.
- **Reading Questions** keep students on track and are pre-built for easy set-up and delivery.
- **Test Bank questions** have been heavily revised with up to 600 new questions to help better assess your students.

Tools for Teachers and Students

Teacher Resources

Most of the teacher supplements and resources for this text are available electronically to qualified adopters on the Instructor Resource Center (IRC). Upon adoption or to preview, please go to www.PearsonSchool.com/Access_Request and select Option 1. Teachers will be required to complete a brief one-time registration subject to verification of educator status. Upon verification, access information and instructions will be sent to the teacher via email. Once logged into the IRC, enter the text's ISBN in the "Search our Catalog" box to locate the downloadable resources.

The following teacher resources are available:

- Instructor Resource DVD (978-0-321-80289-7 / 0-321-80289-6)
- Printed Test Bank (978-0-321-80290-3 / 0-321-80290-X)
- Transparency Acetates (978-0-321-80308-5 / 0-321-80308-6)
- Instructor Guide to Text & Media (978-0-321-79440-6 / 0-321-79440-0)
- Instructor Resource DVD for Practice Anatomy Lab 3.0 (978-0-321-74963-5 / 0-321-74963-4)
- Instructor Guide for PhysioEx™ 9.0, 1/e (978-0-321-75095-2 / 0-321-75095-0)
- Instructor Guide for Essentials of Human Anatomy & Physiology Lab Manual Lab Manual (download only) (0-321-75128-0 / 978-0-321-75128-7)

For Teachers and Students

Upon textbook purchase, students and teachers are granted access to MasteringA&P. High school teachers can obtain preview or adoption access for MasteringA&P in one of the following ways:

Preview Access
Teachers can request preview access online by visiting:
PearsonSchool.com/Access_Request
Select Option 2, and preview Access information will be sent to the teacher via email.

Adoption Access
With the purchase of this program, a Pearson Adoption Access Card, with codes and complete instructions, will be delivered with the textbook purchase. If the Access Card (ISBN: 0-13-034391-9) does not arrive with the shipment, please visit:
PearsonSchool.com/Access_Request
Select Option 3, and complete the form. Adoption access information will be sent to the teacher via email within 2 to 3 business days.

Students, ask your teacher for access.

Student Resources

The following student resources are available for purchase:

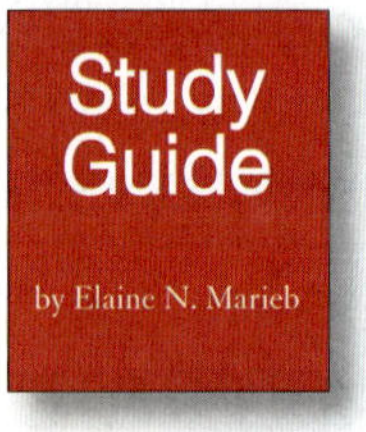

- Student Study Guide (978-0-321-79439-0 / 0-321-79439-7)

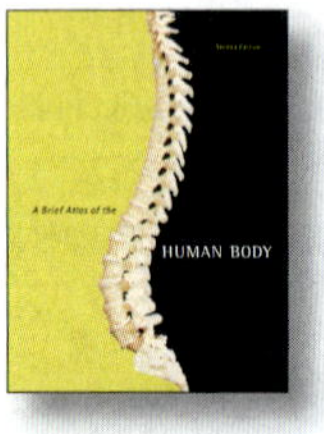

- A Brief Atlas of the Human Body 2e (978-0-321-66261-3 / 0-321-66261-X)

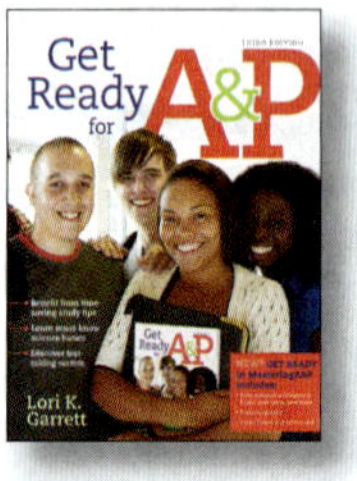

- Get Ready for A&P 3e (978-0-321-81336-7 / 0-321-81336-7

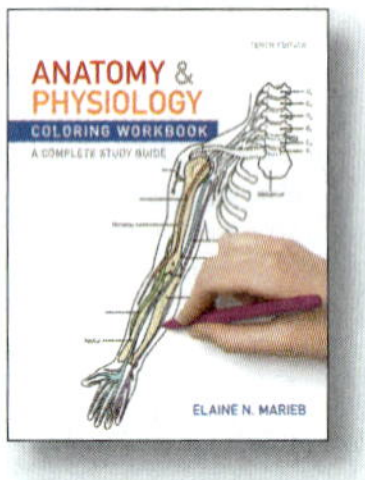

- Anatomy & Physiology Coloring Workbook: A Complete Study Guide, 10e (978-0-321-74305-3 / 0-321-74305-9)

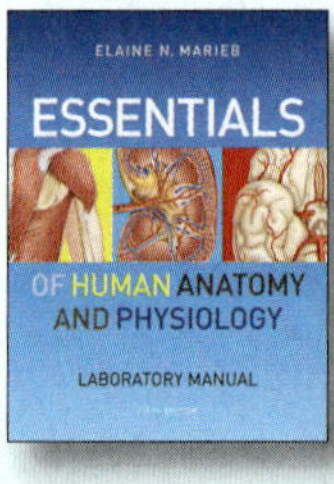

- Essentials of Human Anatomy & Physiology Lab Manual (978-0-321-75001-3 / 0-321-75001-2)

PAL practice anatomy lab

- Practice Anatomy Lab™ 3.0 CD (978-0-321-68211-6 / 0-321-68211-4)

iP

- Interactive Physiology 10 System Suite Replacement CD (0-131-36275-5 / 978-0-131-36275-8)

physioEX VERSION 9

- PhysioEx™ 9.0: Laboratory Simulations in Physiology, 1e, Workbook with DVD (978-0-321-81557-6 / 0-321-81557-2)

Preface

As educators, clinically trained individuals, and perennial students, we are continually challenged by the learning mind. What works best to help students apply new information to the world they personally understand? Our clinical backgrounds have served our teaching and writing purposes well. Perhaps even more important, our clinical experience has allowed us to see our presentations through our students' eyes and from the vantage points of their career interests.

For this edition, as for those preceding it, feedback from student and instructor reviews indicated areas of the text that needed to be revised for clarity, timeliness, and just plain reduction of verbal meatiness. Overall, feedback was positive, verifying that our approach is effective: Explaining fundamental principles and unifying themes first creates a strong base for what comes later. Backing these explanations up with comfortable analogies and familiar examples enhances students' understanding of the workings of the human body.

Unifying Themes

Three integrating themes that organized, unified, and set the tone of the first edition of this text continue to be valid and are retained in this edition. These themes are:

Interrelationships of body organ systems. The fact that nearly all regulatory mechanisms require interaction of several organ systems is continually emphasized. For example, Chapter 25, which deals with the structure and function of the urinary system, discusses the vital importance of the kidneys not only in maintaining adequate blood volume to ensure normal blood circulation, but also in continually adjusting the chemical composition of blood so that all body cells remain healthy. The unique *System Connections* feature is the culmination of this approach and should help students think of the body as a dynamic community of interdependent parts rather than as a number of isolated structural units.

Homeostasis. The normal and most desirable condition of body functioning is homeostasis. Its loss or destruction always leads to some type of pathology—temporary or permanent. Pathological conditions are integrated with the text to clarify and illuminate normal functioning, not as an end in and of themselves. For example, Chapter 19, which deals with the structure and function of blood vessels, explains how the ability of healthy arteries to expand and recoil ensures continuous blood flow and proper circulation. The chapter goes on to discuss the effects on homeostasis when arteries lose their elasticity: high blood pressure and all of its attendant problems. These homeostatic imbalances are indicated visually by a pink symbol with a fulcrum:

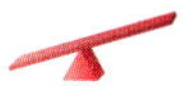

Whenever students see the imbalance symbol in text, the concept of disease as a loss of homeostasis is reinforced. Every Homeostatic Imbalance section has a new, related clinical question that is assignable in MasteringA&P. These new clinical questions help strengthen students' understanding of how the body works to stay in balance.

Complementarity of structure and function. Students are encouraged to understand the structure of an organ, a tissue, or a cell as a prerequisite to comprehending its function. Concepts of physiology are explained and related to structural characteristics that promote or allow the various functions to occur. For example, the lungs can act as a gas exchange site because the walls of their air sacs present an incredibly thin barrier between blood and air.

NEW TO THE NINTH EDITION

With every edition, our goal is powerful but simple—to make anatomy and physiology as engaging, accurate, and relevant as possible for both instructors and students. The Ninth Edition represents a monumental revision, with changes to the text and art presentation that build upon the hallmark strengths of the previous eight editions. The changes to the Ninth Edition are all driven by the needs of today's students, as we seek to make the learning of key concepts in A&P as easy as possible for them. Key concepts are important because of the overwhelming amount of material in this course. Mastering this material gives students structure for organizing this wealth of information. Below are the ways in which we've revised the Ninth Edition to make this book the one where learning happens most effectively, followed by a detailed list of specific chapter-by-chapter content changes.

An expanded art program. The drive for this revision began as a simple list. We sat down together and created a chapter-by-chapter list of the key concepts in A&P where students struggle the most. This list became the basis for our art revision plans for both the Eighth and Ninth editions. We first boiled it down to some of the toughest topics to get our list of Focus figures. These Focus figures are illustrations that use a "big picture" layout and dramatic art to walk the student through difficult physiological processes in a step-by-step way. These have been wildly popular with both instructors and students. In response to repeated requests for more, we are pleased to present 12 new Focus figures. We hope you'll be as pleased with the results of the added Focus figures in the Ninth Edition as you were in the Eighth.

All of the art in the Eighth Edition was carefully examined and reviewed by both instructors and students. Many of their suggested changes have been incorporated into this edition. As always, we have updated many figures to reflect the latest scientific findings and to improve their ability to teach important concepts. Finally, many new photos—histology, cadaver, and others—were painstakingly chosen for this edition to enhance the learning process.

Flipping through the Ninth Edition, you can see that we have built upon the dynamic, three-dimensional, and realistic art style, utilizing dramatic views and perspectives and vibrant, saturated colors.

Improved text presentation. New text features initiated in the Eighth Edition that focus students on key concepts have been retained and expanded in the Ninth Edition. In the current edition, student objectives still appear by topic throughout the chapter and some new *Check Your Understanding* questions have been added at the end of sections. These changes along with a brand-new design make the book easier than ever to study from and navigate. Our hallmark analogies and accessible, friendly style while using simpler, more concise language and shorter paragraphs make the information easier for students to manage.

Factual updates and accuracy. As authors we pride ourselves on keeping our book as up-to-date and as accurate as possible in all areas—a monumental task that requires painstaking selectivity. Although information changes even as a textbook goes to press, be assured that our intent and responsibility to update has been carried out to the best of our ability. We have incorporated current research in the field as much as possible; many of these updates are included in the chapter-by-chapter changes. A more complete list is available in the *Instructor Guide to Text and Media.*

Terminology changes. For this edition we've substantially updated the terminology to be in accordance with *Terminologia Anatomica* and *Terminologia Histologica*. Teachers can find a complete list of terminology changes detailed in the *Instructor Guide to Text and Media.*

Chapter-by-Chapter Changes

Chapter 1 The Human Body: An Orientation

- Updated information on diagnostic uses of MRI scans (*A Closer Look*).
- New MRI photo of frontal section through the torso (Figure 1.8a).
- Enhanced art showing layers of the pericardium (Figure 1.10).

Chapter 2 Chemistry Comes Alive

- Updated information on stress and aging.
- Improved art showing structure of an atom (Figure 2.1).
- New photos of blood (Figure 2.4).
- New photo of a water strider (Figure 2.10).
- Updated art for levels of protein structure (Figure 2.19).

Chapter 3 Cells: The Living Units

- New information on RNA in translation, rRNA, and tRNA.
- Revised Focus Figure 3.10: Primary Active Transport: The Na^+-K^+ Pump.
- Revised art for three types of endocytosis (Figure 3.13).
- Improved Focus Figure 3.16: G Proteins.
- New photo of smooth and rough endoplasmic reticulum (Figure 3.18).
- New TEM of lysosomes (Figure 3.21).
- Revised art and new TEM for centrioles (Figure 3.25).
- Revised Focus Figure 3.33: Mitosis.
- New Focus Figure 3.37: Translation.

Chapter 4 Tissue: The Living Fabric

- New photomicrographs of epithelium (Figure 4.3).
- New photomicrographs of connective tissues (Figure 4.8).
- New photomicrographs of muscle (Figure 4.10).
- Simplified explanation of polarity.
- Improved rendering of goblet cell (Figure 4.4), with more realistic details.
- Improved teaching effectiveness of Figure 4.11 (classes of membranes).
- Improved layout of Figure 4.12 (tissue repair).
- Added explanation to art for embryonic germ layers (Figure 4.13).

Chapter 5 The Integumentary System

- Updated information on the skin's epithelial cells and stratum corneum.
- New information on tinea versicolor ("sunspots") and friction ridges.
- Updated information on importance of the stratum corneum as a physical barrier.
- Added new term scleroderma, an autoimmune disorder characterized by hardened skin, in *At the Clinic: Related Clinical Terms.*
- New research on the role of friction ridges in the sense of touch.

Chapter 6 Bones and Skeletal Tissues

- Updated information on bone resorption and remodeling.
- New bone-related information on serotonin, glucose intolerance, and diabetes mellitus.
- Updated information on osteogenic cells and microscopic anatomy of bone cells.
- New information on osteoporosis in prostate cancer patients who receive androgen-suppressing therapy.
- New information on osteocalcin, a hormone which helps regulate bone formation and also protects against obesity, glucose intolerance, and diabetes mellitus.
- New information on the monoclonal antibody drug denosumab as a treatment for osteoporosis.

Chapter 7 The Skeleton

- New Clinical Case Study.
- New photos of the skull, temporal bone, sphenoid and ethmoid bones, mandible, and orbits (Figures 7.5–7.12).
- New photos of defects in spinal curvature (Figure 7.17).
- New photos of proximal tibia (Figure 7.33).

Chapter 8 Joints

- New Clinical Case Study.
- New Focus Figure 8.7: Types of Synovial Joints.
- Added information on meniscal transplant surgery.
- Updated information on treatment of sprains.
- Updated statistics on arthritis; updated treatment of rheumatoid arthritis.
- Updated description of sinovitis.
- Updated statistics on joint replacements in the U.S.
- Updated research aimed at future treatments of joint problems.

Chapter 9 Muscles and Muscle Tissue

- New discussion of EPOC (excess postexercise oxygen consumption).
- New photomicrograph of skeletal muscle (Figure 9.1).
- New Figure 9.9 (skeletal muscle action potentials).
- Added information of myosin head orientation in smooth muscle.
- Updated information on treatments for Duchenne muscular dystrophy.
- Streamlined discussion of muscle fatigue.
- Added skeletal muscle fibers to Figure 9.17 for better teaching effectiveness.

Chapter 10 The Muscular System

- New Focus Figure 10.1: Muscle Action.
- New Clinical Case Study.
- New photo of hip and thigh muscles (Figure 10.21).

Chapter 11 Fundamentals of the Nervous System and Nervous Tissue

- Update on multiple sclerosis risk factors and treatment.
- New information on addiction treatment and prescription drug abuse (*A Closer Look*).
- New Clinical Case Study.
- Updated discussion on neuronal transport.
- New information on gasotransmitters.
- Update on shingles and vaccination available for its prevention.
- Discuss direct and indirect neurotransmitter receptor mechanisms in two figures (Figures 11.20 and 11.21). Added relay-runner motif to G-protein linked receptor figure (Figure 11.21) to tie it to previous G-protein figure in Chapter 3.

Chapter 12 The Central Nervous System

- New Clinical Case Study.
- Updated information on premotor cortex and the role of the basal nuclei.
- New information on Alzheimer's disease and Parkinson's disease.
- Update on amyotrophic lateral sclerosis.
- Updated information on genetic causes of autism.
- New photos of brain sections (Figures 12.9, 12.10, and 12.12).
- New photo of spinal cord (Figure 12.26).

Chapter 13 The Peripheral Nervous System and Reflex Activity

- New information on vanilloid receptors, pain tolerance, and Bell's palsy.
- New SEM of nerve cross-section (Figure 13.4).
- New photos of brachial and sacral plexuses (Figures 13.10 and 13.12).
- New Clinical Case Study.

Chapter 14 The Autonomic Nervous System

- Updated information on aging and blood pressure receptors.
- Streamlined discussion of sympathetic trunks and pathways.
- More explicit statement about the "background" firing rate of neurons along sympathetic and parasympathetic axons in ANS.

Chapter 15 The Special Senses

- New Clinical Case Study.
- New information on link between vitamin C and cataract formation.
- New photos of retina (Figure 15.7), cataract (Figure 15.9), and refraction (Figure 15.11).
- New summary Table 15.1—differences between rods and cones.
- Updated discussion of olfactory processing.
- New summary Table 15.2—structures of internal ear and their functions.

Chapter 16 The Endocrine System

- New research on ghrelin and growth hormone release.
- New photo showing effects of growth hormone excess and deficiency (Figure 16.7).
- Updated information on type 1 diabetes.
- New Focus Figure 16.5: Hypothalamus and Pituitary Interactions.
- New photomicrographs of thyroid (Figure 16.8), parathyroid (Figure 16.12), adrenal gland (Figure 16.14), and pancreas (Figure 16.18).
- New flowchart of parathyroid hormone effects (Figure 16.13).

Chapter 17 Blood

- New Clinical Case Study.
- New SEMs of normal and sickled RBCs (Figure 17.8).

- New photomicrographs of leukocytes (Figure 17.10).
- Updated Figure 17.11 (leukocyte formation).
- Updated statistics on sickle cell anemia and malaria.
- Improved teaching effectiveness of Figure 17.14 (pathways of coagulation).

Chapter 18 The Cardiovascular System: The Heart

- New Clinical Case Study.
- New Focus Figure 18.9: Blood Flow Through the Heart.
- Updated information on ischemic cell death in myocardial infarction.
- New photos of the heart (Figures 18.4 and 18.6).
- Expanded overview of systemic and pulmonary circuits (in response to focus group feedback).
- Reorganized presentation of heart anatomy.
- Updated the effects of hyperkalemia and hypercalcemia on the heart.

Chapter 19 The Cardiovascular System: Blood Vessels

- Update on obesity-linked hypertension.
- New Focus Figure 19.17: Bulk Flow Across Capillary Walls.
- New photomicrograph of artery and vein (Figure 19.1).
- Added information on C-reactive protein as a marker of systemic inflammation and a predictor of future heart attacks and strokes.
- Reorganized Figure 19.15 for better teaching effectiveness.
- Reorganized section on venous return.
- Reorganized discussion of baroreceptor reflex.
- Consolidated discussion of renal regulation of blood pressure by adding material previously in Chapter 25. Moved details of renin-angiotensin-aldosterone mechanism from Figure 25.10 to Figure 19.10.
- Reorganized presentation on homeostatic imbalances of blood pressure.

Chapter 20 The Lymphatic System and Lymphoid Organs and Tissues

- New information on the spleen as a monocyte reservoir.
- New photomicrographs of thymus (Figure 20.7) and tonsil (Figure 20.8).
- Improved discussion of lymphoid cells and lymphoid tissues.
- Reorganized section on mucosa-associated lymphoid tissue (MALT).
- Updated statistics for non-Hodgkin's lymphoma.

Chapter 21 The Immune System: Innate and Adaptive Body Defenses

- Major revision of chapter to streamline presentation.
- New Clinical Case Study.
- Added coverage of lectin pathway (Figure 21.6).
- New SEM of macrophage engaged in phagocytosis (Figure 21.2).
- Two new summary tables (Tables 21.3 and 21.5).

Chapter 22 The Respiratory System

- Update on early detection of lung cancer.
- Updated discussion of cystic fibrosis.
- New Focus Figure 22.20: Oxygen-Hemoglobin Dissociation Curve.
- New photomicrograph of lung tissue (Figure 22.8).
- New SEM of pulmonary capillary casts (Figure 22.9).

Chapter 23 The Digestive System

- New photomicrograph of esophagus-stomach junction (Figure 23.12).
- New photograph of gastric ulcer (Figure 23.16).
- New photomicrograph of pancreas (Figure 23.26).
- New art on the absorption of monosaccharides (Figure 23.35).

Chapter 24 Nutrition, Metabolism, and Body Temperature Regulation

- Coverage of the USDA's new MyPlate logo (Figure 24.1) and dietary recommendations.
- New Focus Figure 24.8: Oxidative Phosphorylation.
- New Clinical Case Study.
- Updated information on obesity (*A Closer Look*).

Chapter 25 The Urinary System

- Major revision of chapter to streamline presentation.
- New Focus Figure 25.16: Medullary Osmotic Gradient.
- New information on symptoms and manifestations of renal failure.
- New Clinical Case Study.
- New SEM of nephron blood vessel casts (Figure 25.7).
- New illustration of net filtration forces (Figure 25.11).
- New illustration on tubular reabsorption and secretion (Figure 25.15).
- New photo of kidney (Figure 25.3).

Chapter 26 Fluid, Electrolyte, and Acid-Base Balance

- Updated discussion of regulation of sodium and water balance, and dehydration.
- New text and summary table (Table 26.2) contrasting extracellular fluid sodium concentration and body sodium content.

Chapter 27 The Reproductive System

- New photo of testis (Figure 27.3).
- New illustration of male perineum (Figure 27.4).
- New SEM of seminiferous tubules (Figure 27.8).
- New graph of plasma testosterone versus age (Figure 27.11).
- New photomicrograph of ovary (Figure 27.13).
- Update on circumcision and statistics on reduction in risk of HIV and other infections.

Chapter 28 Pregnancy and Human Development

- New Focus Figure 28.2: Sperm Penetration and the Cortical Reaction.
- Updated contraception methods (*A Closer Look*).
- New Clinical Case Study.
- Updated information on role of hCG.
- Updated information on assisted reproductive technologies.
- Simplified Figure 28.10 to improve teaching effectiveness.
- New photo of nursing mother (Figure 28.19).

Chapter 29 Heredity

- New Clinical Case Study.
- New photos of karyotyping (Figure 29.1).

Acknowledgments

Each new edition of this textbook holds out a promise to its authors. "You're done—the book is perfect!" Not! Although it would appear that this would be so after all the work bestowed upon it over eight editions, it still takes the better part of two years, demands our participation in many focus groups, mobilizes our library research skills, and tests our creativity once again before we finally put the last page of the new edition to rest. It never really gets easier as we grind away—the grist finer with each edition.

In all fairness, we don't work alone. Many people shared the work of this edition and deserve their proper due. Once the first draft of each chapter was complete in our estimations, it was sent off to Alice Fugate, the text developmental editor, who wielded her pen to ensure readability and consistency—factors very important to student success. Backing up Alice's work was the director of development Barbara Yien, well known for her ability to see the whole picture. After we perused and processed Alice's suggestions, the manuscript went to Shannon Cutt. Shannon, our cheery associate project editor, checked every aspect of the newly modified text before sending it on to production. Nobody escapes Shannon's ministrations—especially her amazing ability to chase down things that threaten to fall through the cracks. If we failed to meet her deadlines, a barrage of emails rained down, all asking us in the sweetest way to get the missing item in. After Shannon had assured herself that all was well, the manuscript went to Anita Wagner, our skilled copyeditor for the last several editions. Anita knows our text as well or better than we do. She checks grammar, spelling of new drugs or procedures, and verifies statistics; much of the superb accuracy of this text is to her credit as a copyeditor par excellence.

Whew! But that's not all, folks. Once the writing and editing part of the revision is complete, the manuscript goes to the production department, where the text and art come together. This business-like domain is headed by Michele Mangelli, our production manager once again. Always knowledgeable, Michele guides the production process with great skill and works seamlessly with the members of her excellent staff. She makes sure the artists are on schedule producing art with the appropriate look and accuracy, directs the industrious photo researcher Kristin Piljay, and oversees the work of David Novak (the conscientious production supervisor) and that hard-working art coordinator Jean Lake.

The last edition of this text touched every figure—making each piece of art more timely, more colorful, more accurate, or better pedagogically. The really big success in the art arena was the fabulous one- to two-page Focus figures introduced in the Eighth Edition. These new figures selected physiological concepts that students have the most difficulty with and "unpacked them." They say you never really have too much of a good thing, so this edition has 12 new Focus Figures. We hope you will like these as much as you did the last offerings. Helping to ensure that you will is Laura Southworth, the art developmental manager who worked tirelessly on these figures. She is not only the art manager but also a skilled professional artist who can illustrate just about any concept we ask for. This capability ensures that the art manuscript delivered to the talented artists of Imagineering and Electronic Publishing Services, who drew the final art, had all the information they needed to produce a quality product. Laura is truly amazing. Important in a different art arena was Lisa Lee, who supplied several of our histology photos and served as a consultant on images from other sources. Tom Fink (East Carolina University), William Karkow (Dubuque University), and Olga Malakhova and Charles Poulton (both from University of Florida College of Medicine, Gainesville) provided histology and cadaver images on an incredibly tight schedule. Thanks so much!

We also thank two people who contributed significantly to this edition: James Hewlett and William Karkow. Working on a tight schedule, James Hewlett contributed 13 new case studies, which were expertly reviewed for clinical accuracy by thoracic surgeon William Karkow.

Thanks also to Yvo Riezebos, cover designer, and tani hasegawa, text designer. Their creativity helped to produce a truly beautiful book. We are very happy that our cover photo is of the best known female goalkeeper in the world—Hope Solo. Hope won an Olympic gold medal in 2008, was named Women's Professional Soccer's Goalkeeper of the Year in 2009, and was awarded the Golden Glove at the 2011 World Cup. Sustaining the effort to produce a beautiful book all the way to press were our excellent proofreader, Martha Ghent, and S4Carlisle Publishing Services, the proficient compositor who assembled the final pages with their customary expertise.

The sponsoring editor for the last edition, Serina Beauparlant, has a jazzy new title, "Editor-in-Chief." Even with a slew of new duties, she is resolute about producing the best educational product possible—both in textbook and media. Her replacement for this edition, who took over a large number of Serina's duties, is Gretchen Puttkamer, a real go-getter. We haven't seen too much of Gretchen because she spends most of her time in the field talking to professors, students, and anyone else that will listen to her. Also contributing were several others that we rarely get to talk to, including: editorial assistants Lisa Damerel and John Maas, managing editor Debbie Cogan, Stacey Weinberger, who has been our expert manufacturing buyer for years, and our crackerjack marketing manager, Derek Perrigo, who goes the extra mile to make sure professors are enlightened about special features of the text. Kudos also to our media staff—Lauren Fogel, director of media development, Aimee Pavy, media producer, and the entire media team for PAL 3.0 and PhysioEx 9.0.

Benjamin Cummings spares no effort in its drive to publish an accurate and instructive book. Over 400 reviews were commissioned, enlisting comments and suggestions from both generalist academicians and specialists in various niches of anatomy and physiology. These reviewers' contributions have been of inestimable value in the continuing development of this text. We also want to thank the many students and colleagues who were generous with their time and comments. They did not always tell us what we wanted to hear, but assured of the sincerity of their criticism, we always listened. Input from the following reviewers resulted in the continued excellence and accuracy of this text.

Kim Aaronson, *Columbia College Chicago*
Beth Altschafl, *University of Wisconsin, Madison*
Lynne Anderson, *Meridian Community College*
Marcia Anglin, *Miami Dade College*
Peggy Arnos, *University of Toledo*
Terry Austin, *Temple College*
David Babb, *West Hills Community College*
Stephanie Baiyasi, *Delta College*
Jamal Bittar, *University of Toledo*
William Brewer, *Rochester Institute of Technology*
David Brown, *Brady School of Medicine, East Carolina University*
Bruce Butler, *Canadian University College*
Linda Canobbio, *Ocean County College*
Bob Carter, *Volunteer State Community College*
Jana Causey, *Pearl River Community College*
David Champlin, *University of Southern Maine*
Roger Choate, *Oklahoma City Community College*
Linda Costanzo, *Virginia Commonwealth University*
John Cummings, *Clemson University*
Tina Davis, *Florida State College at Jacksonville, North Campus*
Trevor Day, *Mount Royal University*
Jason Dechant, *University of Pittsburgh*
Mary Dettman, *Seminole State College of Florida*
John Druin, *Lock Haven University*
Jeff Eichold, *Oakland Community College*
Michael Ferrari, *University of Missouri, Kansas City*
Dani Frederick-Duus, *Midlands Technical College*
Sarah Gaffen, *University of Pittsburgh*
Lynn Gargan, *Tarrant County College–Northeast*
Ron Gerrits, *Milwaukee School of Engineering*
Mike Gilbert, *Fresno City College*
Lauren Gollahon, *Texas Tech University*
Cara Hampton-Sandholt, *Cosumnes River College*
William Hanna, *Massasoit Community College*
Pamela Harrison, *Mesa Community College*
Chris Harvey, *Brevard Community College–Palm Bay*
Nora Hebert, *Red Rocks Community College*
Gary Heiserman, *Salem State College*
Deb Heitzman, *Mesa Community College*
DJ Hennager, *Kirkwood Community College*
Mark Hollier, *Georgia Perimeter College*
Rodney Holmes, *Waubonsee Community College*
Mark Hubley, *Prince George's Community College*
William Karkow, *University of Dubuque*
Greg Kelly, *University of Western Ontario*
Michael Kielb, *Eastern Michigan University*
John Lepri, *University of North Carolina–Greensboro*
M. Locke, *University of Western Ontario*
Jodi Long, *Santa Fe College*
Jerri Lindsey, *Tarrant County College–Northeast Campus*
Abigail Mabe, *Walters State College*
Susan Macleod, *Fulton-Montgomery Community College*
Jane Marone, *University of Illinois at Chicago*
Laura Mastrangeo, *Hudson Valley Community College*
Alice McAfee, *University of Toledo*
Rebecca McCane, *Bluegrass Community & Technical College*
Marc McKee, *McGill University*
Marvin Merrit, *Keiser University*
Susan Mitchell, *SUNY Onondaga Community College*
Justin Moore, *American River College*
Syeda Muniam, *SUNY–Schenectady County Community College*
Mary Jane Niles, *University of San Francisco*
Lourdes Norman, *Florida State College–Jacksonville*
Justicia Opoku-Edusei, *University of Maryland*
David Osborne, *Paul L. Foster School of Medicine, Texas Tech University*
Deborah Palatinus, *Roane State Community College*
Izak Paul, *Mount Royal University*
Fred Pavalko, *Indiana University School of Medicine*
Karen Payne, *Chattanooga State Technical College*
Rafaella Pernice, *Hudson County Community College*

Sarah Pugh, *Shelton State*
Wanda Ragland, *Macomb Community College*
Terry Ravine, *University of South Alabama*
Jean Revie, *South Mountain Community College*
Mattie Roig-Watnik, *Palm Beach State College*
Sharon Schapel, *Mott Community College*
Steve Schenk, *Truckee Meadows Community College*
Michelle Stettner, *Meridian Community College*
Richard Symmons, *Cal State University–East Bay*
Bonnie Tarricone, *Ivy Tech Community College*
Carol Veil, *Anne Arundel Community College*
Delon Washo-Krupps, *Arizona State University*
Janice Webster, *Ivy Tech Community College*
Ruby White, *Eastern Michigan University*
Ruth Williams, *Oakton University*
Janice Yoder-Smith, *Tarrant County Community College*

We also want to acknowledge Katja's colleagues at Mount Royal University (Trevor Day, Janice Meeking, Izak Paul, Michael Pollock, Ruth Pickett-Seltner, Sarah Hewitt, and Kartika Tjandra) for stimulating discussions of the text; Associate Dean Tom MacAlister and Chair Tracy O'Connor for supporting Katja's involvement in this project; and Mount Royal University for providing an Internal Research Grant. We are also grateful to Katja's focus group students at Mount Royal University for their valuable and detailed feedback on the Eighth Edition's art program:

Rebecca Aje
Sarah Ankerman
Nikolina Arbutina
Sara Bird
Krizia Carlos
Darrah Crocker
Justine Hamill
Donalea Muir
Jessica Mulli
Sandra Okilj
Melissa Rowson
Robyn Shields
Sengchou Vilay-Wong
Fiona Villamar

Additionally, we would like to thank the following students at Ivy Tech Community College and Massasoit Community College, who each completed a useful and informative survey: Amanda Blevins, Jane Botelho, Paul Bowler, Erica Dupree, Elvia Garza-Sandoval, John Golbranson, Meagan Home, Joseph Madden, George Mager, Joe McManus, Ann Pavia, and Wendy Treesh.

Once again, Dr. Marieb's husband, Harvey Howell, served as a sounding board for some of her ideas, manned the copy machine, and ran the manuscript to the FedEx box daily with nary a complaint during the unbelievably busy days. Thanks also to Katja's husband, Dr. Lawrence W. Haynes, who as a fellow physiologist has provided invaluable assistance to her during the course of the revision. She also thanks her sons, Eric and Stefan Haynes, who are an inspiration and a joy.

Well, our tenure on this edition is over, but there will be another edition three years hence. We would really appreciate hearing from you concerning your opinion—suggestions and constructive criticisms—of this text. It is this type of feedback that provides the basis of each revision, and underwrites its improvement.

Elaine N. Marieb

Katja Hoehn

Elaine N. Marieb and Katja Hoehn
Anatomy and Physiology
Benjamin Cummings
1301 Sansome Street
San Francisco, CA 94111

TEACHER *to* TEACHER

I have developed a hands-on Anatomy & Physiology course that includes: observing several hours in a hospital trauma center, riding with paramedics in an ambulance, working with cadavers at two universities, and interacting with a number of speakers in the health profession. What I was lacking was a text that could bring relevance of the human body systems to everyday life. That changed when I found Elaine Marieb and Katja Hoehn's *Human Anatomy & Physiology.*

There are three unifying themes that are focused throughout the text: the Complementarity of Structure and Function, Interrelationships of Body Systems, and a greater understanding of Homeostasis and how it relates to the systems. The total integration of the themes provides a clear and consistent approach to the study of the human body.

My high school students think it is easy to read and are captivated by the System Connection segments at the end of each body system. Elaine and Katja have done an exceptional job of using real world applications backed by the latest research and clinical innovations, and have improved that feature with end-of-chapter case studies for the 9th edition. Their new Focus Figures take very difficult topics or concepts and by using beautiful step-by-step illustrations and striking 3-D artwork provide an understanding of the process unmatched by any other text, in my opinion.

The support materials include: formative and summative testing, new A&PFlix animations that bring 3-D representations of structure to life, a MasteringA&P website that includes the award-winning tutorial program called Interactive Physiology, and a new Practice Anatomy Lab. All of these features provide teachers flexibility in creating hands-on activities based on best practices, and gives students a clearer understanding of the systems.

This *Human Anatomy & Physiology* text is a very comprehensive, clinical approach that motivates and promotes student engagement in the study of the human body. Teachers will have all the tools necessary to develop a curriculum that will engage and inspire their students to become our future health care professionals.

Dewey Christensen

East High School
Sioux City, Iowa

Brief Contents

Contents

UNIT 5 Continuity

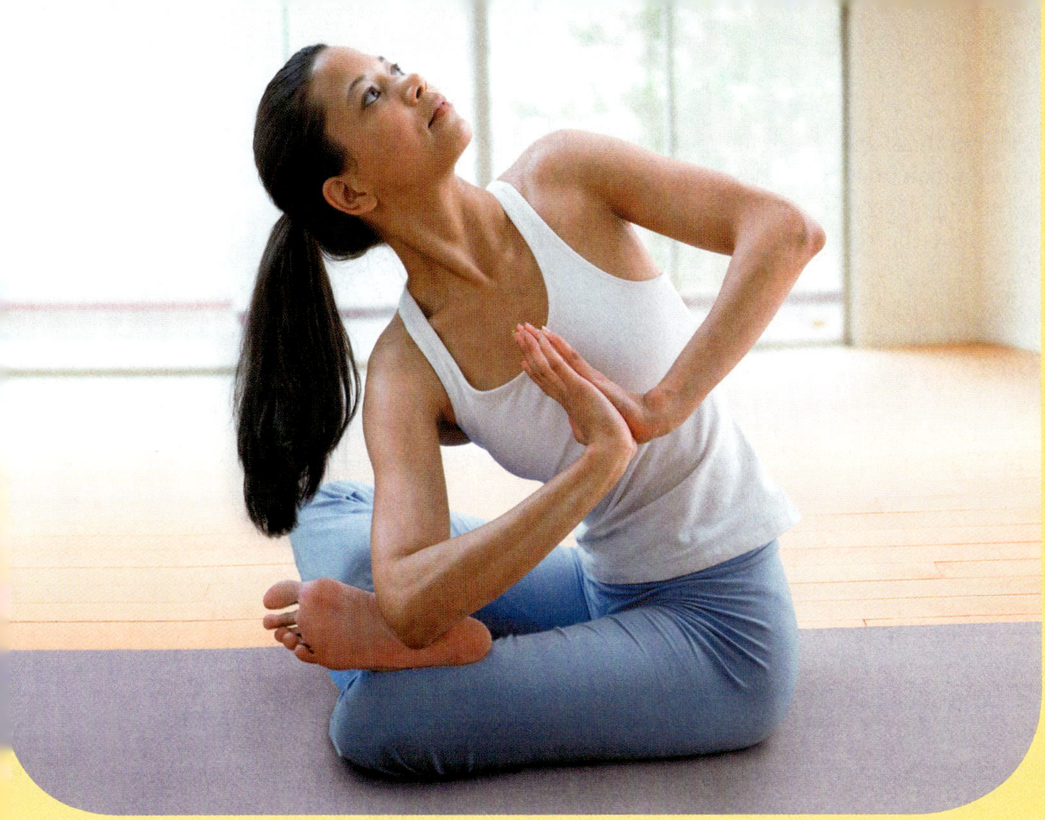

1

The Human Body: An Orientation

Welcome to the study of one of the most fascinating subjects possible—your own body. Such a study is not only highly personal, but timely as well. We get news of some medical advance almost daily. To appreciate emerging discoveries in genetic engineering, to understand new techniques for detecting and treating disease, and to make use of published facts on how to stay healthy, you'll find it helpful to learn about the workings of your body. If you are preparing for a career in the health sciences, the study of anatomy and physiology has added rewards because it provides the foundation needed to support your clinical experiences.

In this chapter we define and contrast anatomy and physiology and discuss how the human body is organized. Then we review needs and functional processes common to all living organisms. Three essential concepts—*the complementarity of structure and function, the hierarchy of structural organization,* and *homeostasis*—will unify and form the bedrock for your study of the human body. The final section of the chapter deals with the language of anatomy—terminology that anatomists use to describe the body or its parts.

An Overview of Anatomy and Physiology

✓ Define anatomy and physiology and describe their subdivisions.

✓ Explain the principle of complementarity.

Two complementary branches of science—anatomy and physiology—provide the concepts that help us to understand the human body. **Anatomy** studies the *structure* of body parts and their relationships to one another. Anatomy has a certain appeal because it is concrete. Body structures can be seen, felt, and examined closely. You don't need to imagine what they look like.

Physiology concerns the *function* of the body, in other words, how the body parts work and carry out their life-sustaining activities. When all is said and done, physiology is explainable only in terms of the underlying anatomy.

To simplify the study of the body, when we refer to body structures and/or physiological values (body temperature, heart rate, and the like), we will assume that we are talking about a healthy young (22-year-old) male weighing about 155 lb (the *reference man*) or a healthy young female weighing about 125 lb (the *reference woman*).

Topics of Anatomy

Anatomy is a broad field with many subdivisions, each providing enough information to be a course in itself. **Gross**, or **macroscopic**, **anatomy** is the study of large body structures visible to the naked eye, such as the heart, lungs, and kidneys. Indeed, the term *anatomy* (derived from the Greek words meaning "to cut apart") relates most closely to gross anatomy because in such studies preserved animals or their organs are dissected (cut up) to be examined.

Gross anatomy can be approached in different ways. In **regional anatomy**, all the structures (muscles, bones, blood vessels, nerves, etc.) in a particular region of the body, such as the abdomen or leg, are examined at the same time.

In **systemic anatomy** (sis-tem′ik),* body structure is studied system by system. For example, when studying the cardiovascular system, you would examine the heart and the blood vessels of the entire body.

Another subdivision of gross anatomy is **surface anatomy**, the study of internal structures as they relate to the overlying skin surface. You use surface anatomy when you identify the bulging muscles beneath a bodybuilder's skin, and clinicians use it to locate appropriate blood vessels in which to feel pulses and draw blood.

Microscopic anatomy deals with structures too small to be seen with the naked eye. For most such studies, exceedingly thin slices of body tissues are stained and mounted on glass slides to be examined under the microscope. Subdivisions of microscopic anatomy include **cytology** (si-tol′o-je), which considers the cells of the body, and **histology** (his-tol′o-je), the study of tissues.

Developmental anatomy traces structural changes that occur in the body throughout the life span. **Embryology** (em″bre-ol′o-je), a subdivision of developmental anatomy, concerns developmental changes that occur before birth.

Some highly specialized branches of anatomy are used primarily for medical diagnosis and scientific research. For example, *pathological anatomy* studies structural changes caused by disease. *Radiographic anatomy* studies internal structures as visualized by X-ray images or specialized scanning procedures.

Subjects of interest to anatomists range from easily seen structures down to the smallest molecule. In *molecular biology*, for example, the structure of biological molecules (chemical substances) is investigated. Molecular biology is actually a separate branch of biology, but it falls under the anatomy umbrella when we push anatomical studies to the subcellular level.

One essential tool for studying anatomy is a mastery of anatomical terminology. Others are observation, manipulation, and, in a living person, *palpation* (feeling organs with your hands) and *auscultation* (listening to organ sounds with a stethoscope). A simple example illustrates how some of these tools work together in an anatomical study.

Let's assume that your topic is freely movable joints of the body. In the laboratory, you will be able to *observe* an animal joint, noting how its parts fit together. You can work the joint (*manipulate* it) to determine its range of motion. Using *anatomical terminology*, you can name its parts and describe how they are related so that other students (and your instructor) will have no trouble understanding you. The list of word roots (at the back of the book) and the glossary will help you with this special vocabulary.

Although you will make most of your observations with the naked eye or with the help of a microscope, medical technology has developed a number of sophisticated tools that can peer into the body without disrupting it. Read about these exciting medical imaging techniques in *A Closer Look* on pp. 16–17.

Topics of Physiology

Like anatomy, physiology has many subdivisions. Most of them consider the operation of specific organ systems. For example, **renal physiology** concerns kidney function and urine production. **Neurophysiology** explains the workings of the nervous system. **Cardiovascular physiology** examines the operation of the heart and blood vessels. While

---

*For the pronunciation guide rules, see the first page of the glossary in the back of the book.

anatomy provides us with a static image of the body's architecture, physiology reveals the body's dynamic and animated workings.

Physiology often focuses on events at the cellular or molecular level. This is because the body's abilities depend on those of its individual cells, and cells' abilities ultimately depend on the chemical reactions that go on within them. Physiology also rests on principles of physics, which help to explain electrical currents, blood pressure, and the way muscles use bones to cause body movements, among other things. We present basic chemical and physical principles in Chapter 2 and throughout the book as needed to explain physiological topics.

Complementarity of Structure and Function

Although it is possible to study anatomy and physiology individually, they are really inseparable because function always reflects structure. That is, what a structure can do depends on its specific form. This key concept is called the **principle of complementarity of structure and function**.

For example, bones can support and protect body organs because they contain hard mineral deposits. Blood flows in one direction through the heart because the heart has valves that prevent backflow. Throughout this book, we accompany a description of a structure's anatomy with an explanation of its function, and we emphasize structural characteristics contributing to that function.

☑ Check Your Understanding

1. In what way does physiology depend on anatomy?
2. Would you be studying anatomy or physiology if you investigated how muscles shorten? If you explored the location of the lungs in the body?

For answers, see Appendix H.

Levels of Structural Organization

✓ Name the different levels of structural organization that make up the human body, and explain their relationships.

✓ List the 11 organ systems of the body, identify their components, and briefly explain the major function(s) of each system.

The human body has many levels of structural organization **(Figure 1.1)**. The simplest level of the structural hierarchy is the **chemical level**, which we study in Chapter 2. At this level, *atoms*, tiny building blocks of matter, combine to form *molecules* such as water and proteins. Molecules, in turn, associate in specific ways to form *organelles*, basic components of the microscopic cells. *Cells* are the smallest units of living things. We examine the **cellular level** in Chapter 3. All cells have some common functions, but individual cells vary widely in size and shape, reflecting their unique functions in the body.

The simplest living creatures are single cells, but in complex organisms such as human beings, the hierarchy continues on to the **tissue level**. *Tissues* are groups of similar cells that have a common function. The four basic tissue types in the human body are epithelium, muscle, connective tissue, and nervous tissue.

Each tissue type has a characteristic role in the body, which we explore in Chapter 4. Briefly, epithelium covers the body surface and lines its cavities. Muscle provides movement. Connective tissue supports and protects body organs. Nervous tissue provides a means of rapid internal communication by transmitting electrical impulses.

An *organ* is a discrete structure composed of at least two tissue types (four is more common) that performs a specific function for the body. The liver, the brain, and a blood vessel are very different from the stomach, but each is an organ. You can think of each organ of the body as a specialized functional center responsible for a necessary activity that no other organ can perform.

At the **organ level**, extremely complex functions become possible. Let's take the stomach for an example. Its lining is an epithelium that produces digestive juices. The bulk of its wall is muscle, which churns and mixes stomach contents (food). Its connective tissue reinforces the soft muscular walls. Its nerve fibers increase digestive activity by stimulating the muscle to contract more vigorously and the glands to secrete more digestive juices.

The next level of organization is the **organ system level**. Organs that work together to accomplish a common purpose make up an *organ system*. For example, the heart and blood vessels of the cardiovascular system circulate blood continuously to carry oxygen and nutrients to all body cells. Besides the cardiovascular system, the other organ systems of the body are the integumentary, skeletal, muscular, nervous, endocrine, lymphatic, respiratory, digestive, urinary, and reproductive systems. (Note that the immune system is closely associated with the lymphatic system.) Look ahead to Figure 1.3 on pp. 6 and 7 for an overview of the 11 organ systems, which we discuss in the next section and study in more detail in Units 2–5.

The highest level of organization is the *organism*, the living human being. The **organismal level** represents the sum total of all structural levels working together to keep us alive.

☑ Check Your Understanding

3. What level of structural organization is typical of a cytologist's field of study?
4. What is the correct structural order for the following terms: tissue, organism, organ, cell?
5. Which organ system includes the bones and cartilages? Which includes the nasal cavity, lungs, and trachea?

For answers, see Appendix H.

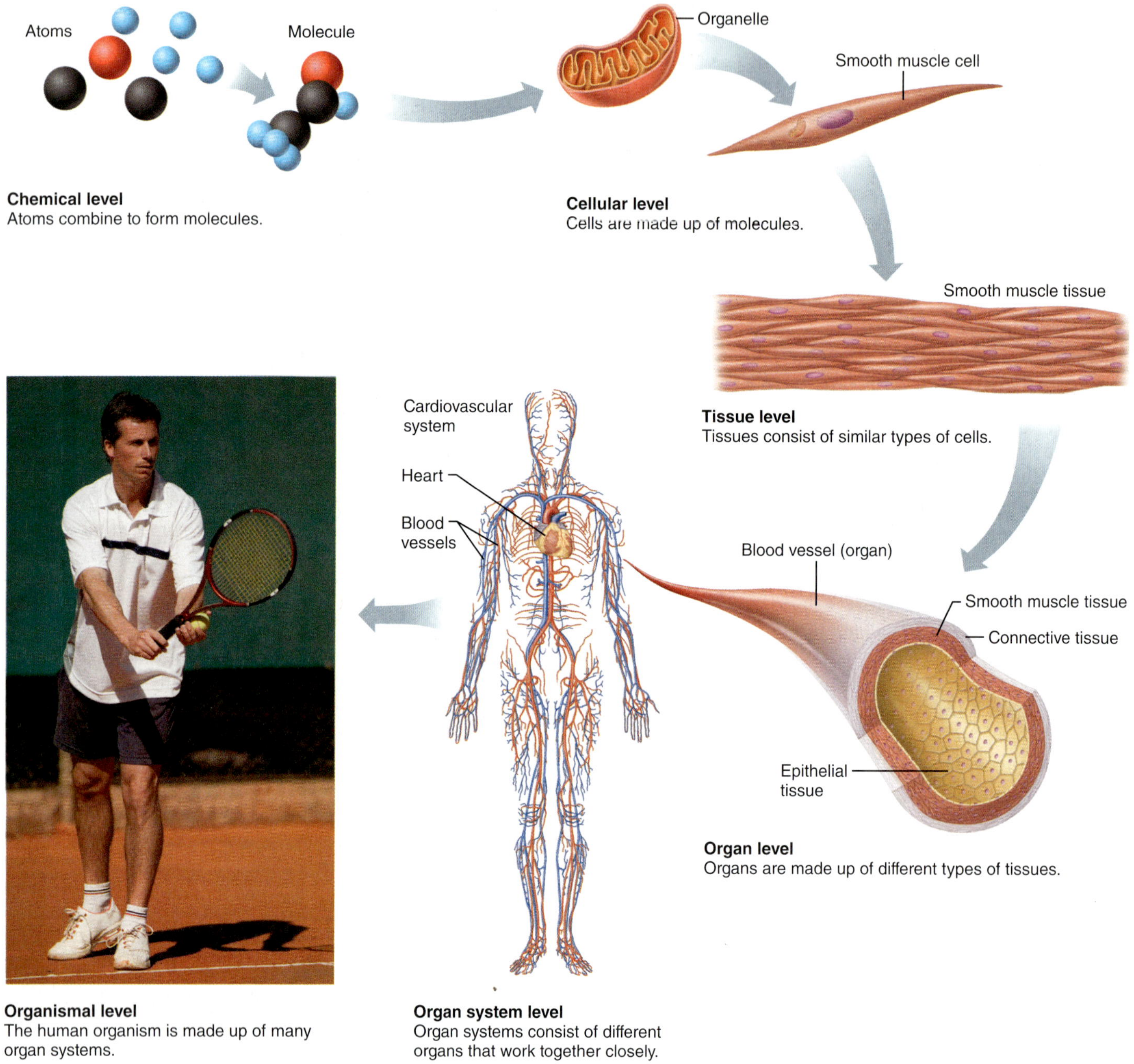

Figure 1.1 Levels of structural organization. Components of the cardiovascular system are used to illustrate the levels of structural organization in a human being.

Maintaining Life

✓ List the functional characteristics necessary to maintain life in humans.

✓ List the survival needs of the body.

Necessary Life Functions

Now that you know the structural levels of the human body, the question that naturally follows is: What does this highly organized human body do?

Like all complex animals, humans maintain their boundaries, move, respond to environmental changes, take in and digest nutrients, carry out metabolism, dispose of wastes, reproduce themselves, and grow. We will introduce these necessary life functions here and discuss them in more detail in later chapters.

We cannot emphasize too strongly that all body cells are interdependent. This interdependence is due to the fact that humans are multicellular organisms and our vital body functions are parceled out among different organ systems. Organ systems, in turn, work cooperatively to promote the well-being of the entire body. This theme is repeated throughout the book. **Figure 1.2** identifies some of the organ systems making major contributions to necessary life functions. Also, as you read this section, check **Figure 1.3** for more detailed descriptions of the body's organ systems.

Maintaining Boundaries

Every living organism must **maintain its boundaries** so that its internal environment (its inside) remains distinct from the external environment surrounding it (its outside). In single-celled organisms, the external boundary is a limiting membrane that encloses its contents and lets in needed substances while restricting entry of potentially damaging or unnecessary substances. Similarly, all the cells of our body are surrounded by a selectively permeable membrane.

Additionally, the body as a whole is enclosed and protected by the integumentary system, or skin (Figure 1.3a). This system protects our internal organs from drying out (a fatal change), bacteria, and the damaging effects of heat, sunlight, and an unbelievable number of chemicals in the external environment.

Movement

Movement includes the activities promoted by the muscular system, such as propelling ourselves from one place to another by running or swimming, and manipulating the external environment with our nimble fingers (Figure 1.3c). The skeletal system provides the bony framework that the muscles pull on as they work (Figure 1.3b). Movement also occurs when substances such as blood, foodstuffs, and urine are propelled through internal organs of the cardiovascular, digestive, and urinary systems, respectively. On the cellular level, the muscle cell's ability to move by shortening is more precisely called **contractility**.

Responsiveness

Responsiveness, or **excitability**, is the ability to sense changes (which serve as stimuli) in the environment and then respond to them. For example, if you cut your hand on broken glass, a withdrawal reflex occurs—you involuntarily pull your hand away from the painful stimulus (the broken glass). You don't have to think about it—it just happens! Likewise, when carbon dioxide in your blood rises to dangerously high levels, chemical sensors respond by sending messages to brain centers controlling respiration, and you breathe more rapidly.

Because nerve cells are highly excitable and communicate rapidly with each other via electrical impulses, the nervous system is most involved with responsiveness (Figure 1.3d). However, all body cells are excitable to some extent.

Digestion

Digestion is the breaking down of ingested foodstuffs to simple molecules that can be absorbed into the blood. The nutrient-rich blood is then distributed to all body cells by the cardiovascular system. In a simple, one-celled organism such as an amoeba,

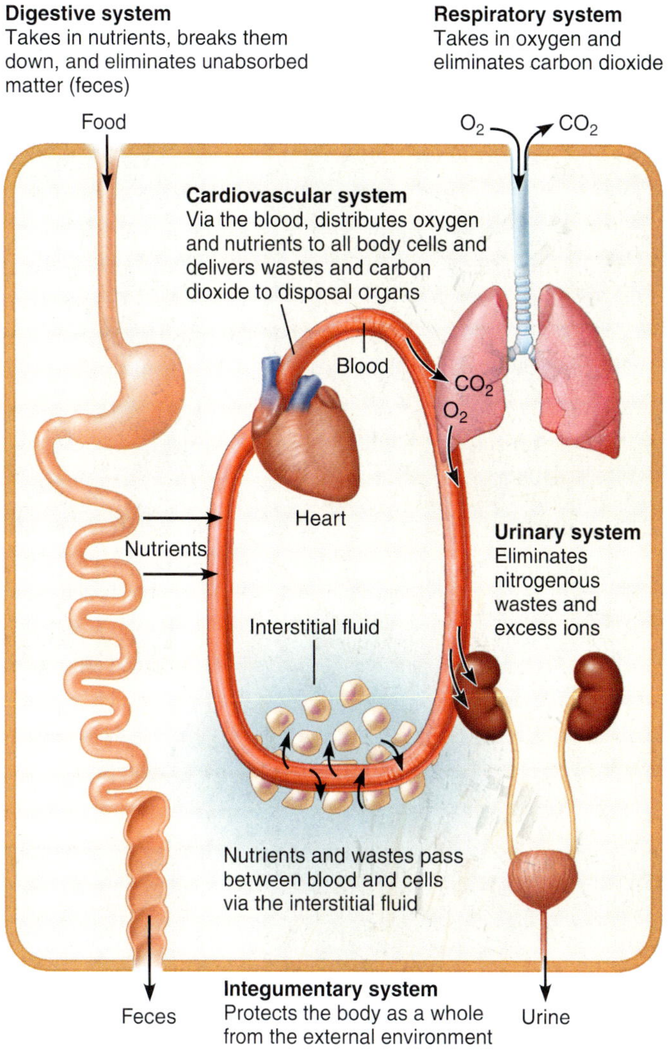

Figure 1.2 Examples of interrelationships among body organ systems.

the cell itself is the "digestion factory," but in the multicellular human body, the digestive system performs this function for the entire body (Figure 1.3i).

Metabolism

Metabolism (mĕ-tab′o-lizm; "a state of change") is a broad term that includes all chemical reactions that occur within body cells. It includes breaking down substances into their simpler building blocks (more specifically, the process of *catabolism*), synthesizing more complex cellular structures from simpler substances (*anabolism*), and using nutrients and oxygen to produce (via *cellular respiration*) ATP, the energy-rich molecules that power cellular activities. Metabolism depends on the digestive and respiratory systems to make nutrients and oxygen available to the blood and on the cardiovascular system to distribute them throughout the body (Figure 1.3i, h, and f, respectively). Metabolism is regulated largely by hormones secreted by endocrine system glands (Figure 1.3e).

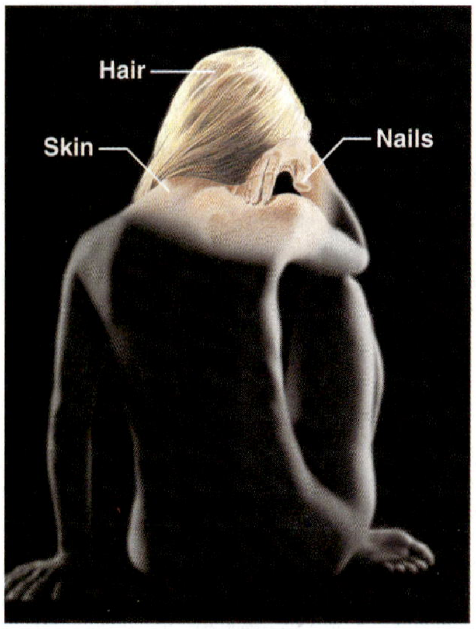

(a) Integumentary System
Forms the external body covering, and protects deeper tissues from injury. Synthesizes vitamin D, and houses cutaneous (pain, pressure, etc.) receptors and sweat and oil glands.

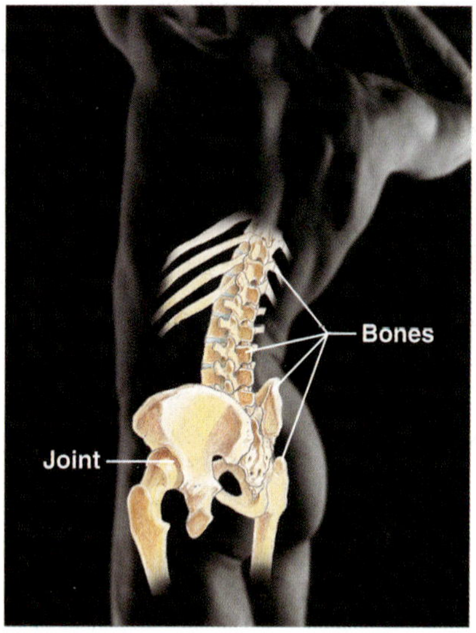

(b) Skeletal System
Protects and supports body organs, and provides a framework the muscles use to cause movement. Blood cells are formed within bones. Bones store minerals.

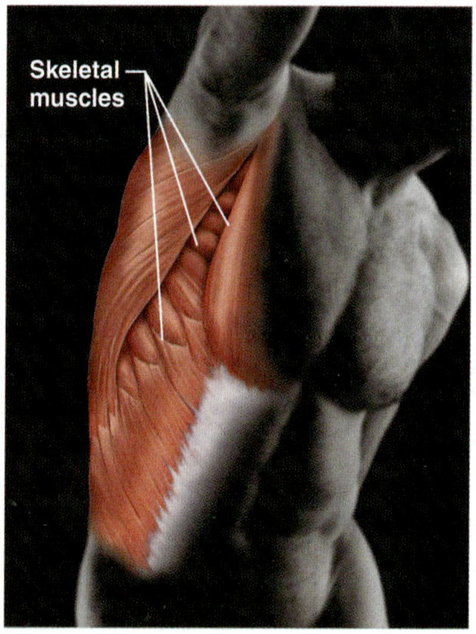

(c) Muscular System
Allows manipulation of the environment, locomotion, and facial expression. Maintains posture, and produces heat.

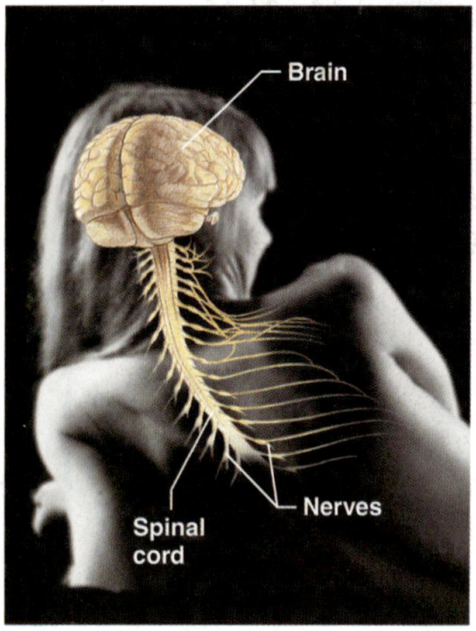

(d) Nervous System
As the fast-acting control system of the body, it responds to internal and external changes by activating appropriate muscles and glands.

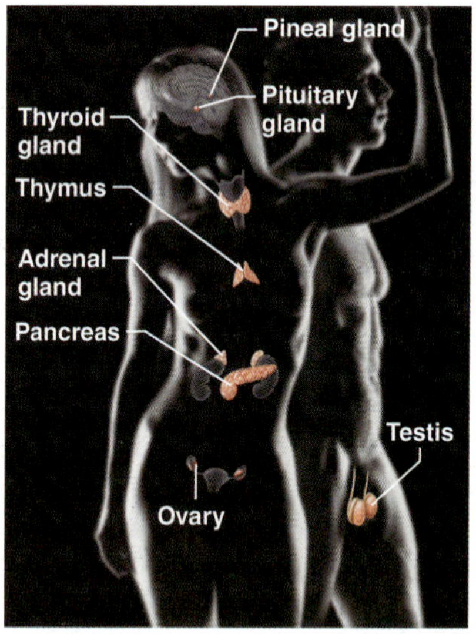

(e) Endocrine System
Glands secrete hormones that regulate processes such as growth, reproduction, and nutrient use (metabolism) by body cells.

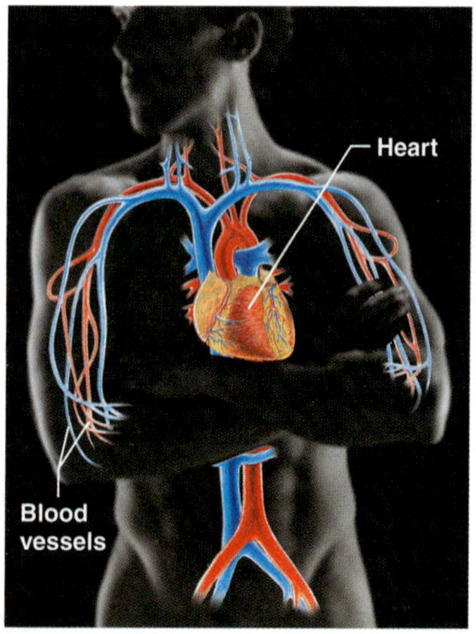

(f) Cardiovascular System
Blood vessels transport blood, which carries oxygen, carbon dioxide, nutrients, wastes, etc. The heart pumps blood.

Figure 1.3 The body's organ systems and their major functions.

Excretion

Excretion is the process of removing wastes, or *excreta* (ek-skre′tah), from the body. If the body is to operate as we expect it to, it must get rid of nonuseful substances produced during digestion and metabolism.

Several organ systems participate in excretion. For example, the digestive system rids the body of indigestible food residues in feces, and the urinary system disposes of nitrogen-containing metabolic wastes, such as urea, in urine (Figure 1.3i and j). Carbon dioxide, a by-product of cellular respiration, is carried in

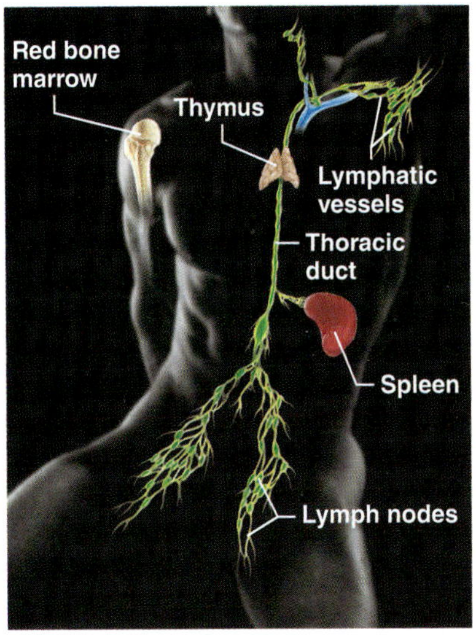

(g) Lymphatic System/Immunity
Picks up fluid leaked from blood vessels and returns it to blood. Disposes of debris in the lymphatic stream. Houses white blood cells (lymphocytes) involved in immunity. The immune response mounts the attack against foreign substances within the body.

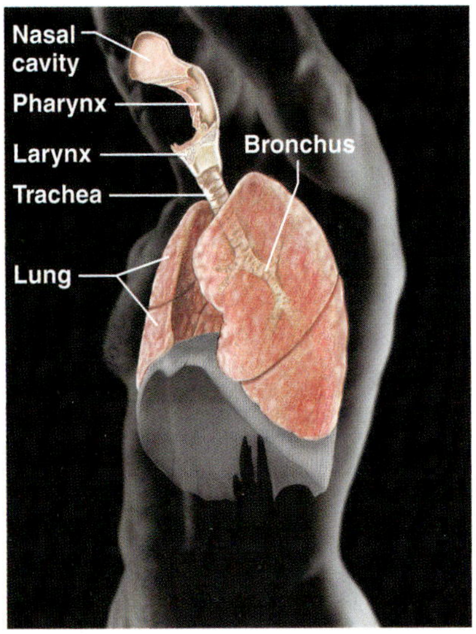

(h) Respiratory System
Keeps blood constantly supplied with oxygen and removes carbon dioxide. The gaseous exchanges occur through the walls of the air sacs of the lungs.

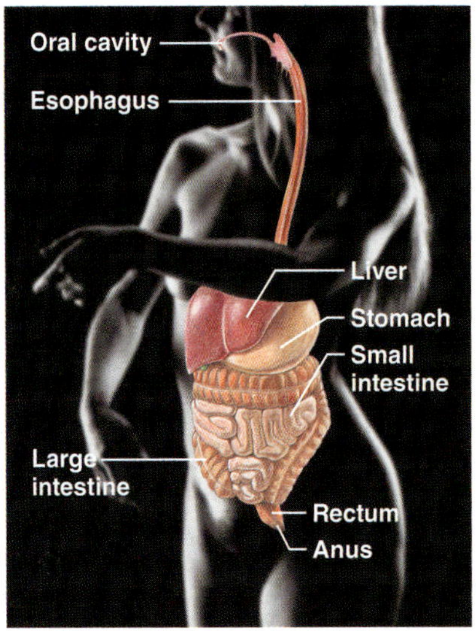

(i) Digestive System
Breaks down food into absorbable units that enter the blood for distribution to body cells. Indigestible foodstuffs are eliminated as feces.

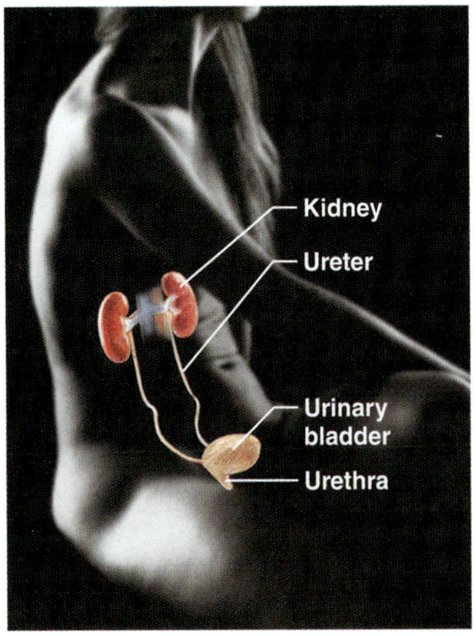

(j) Urinary System
Eliminates nitrogenous wastes from the body. Regulates water, electrolyte and acid-base balance of the blood.

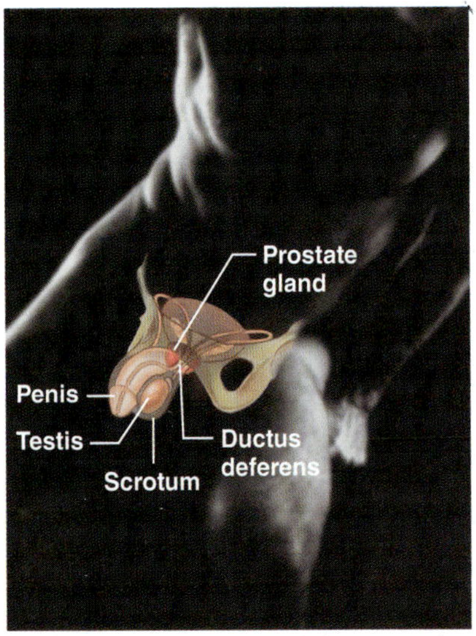

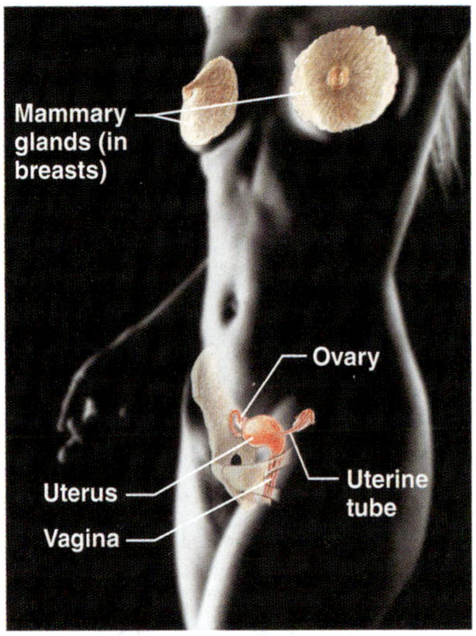

(k) Male Reproductive System **(l) Female Reproductive System**
Overall function is production of offspring. Testes produce sperm and male sex hormone, and male ducts and glands aid in delivery of sperm to the female reproductive tract. Ovaries produce eggs and female sex hormones. The remaining female structures serve as sites for fertilization and development of the fetus. Mammary glands of female breasts produce milk to nourish the newborn.

the blood to the lungs, where it leaves the body in exhaled air (Figure 1.3h).

Reproduction

Reproduction occurs at the cellular and the organismal level. In cellular reproduction, the original cell divides, producing two identical daughter cells that may then be used for body growth or repair. Reproduction of the human organism, or making a whole new person, is the major task of the reproductive system. When a sperm unites with an egg, a fertilized egg forms and develops into a baby within the mother's body. The reproductive system is directly responsible for producing offspring, but its function is exquisitely regulated by hormones of the endocrine system (Figure 1.3e).

Because males produce sperm and females produce eggs (ova), there is a division of labor in reproduction, and the reproductive organs of males and females are different (Figure 1.3k, l). Additionally, the female's reproductive structures provide the site for fertilization of eggs by sperm, and then protect and nurture the developing fetus until birth.

Growth

Growth is an increase in size of a body part or the organism as a whole. It is usually accomplished by increasing the number of cells. However, individual cells also increase in size when not dividing. For true growth to occur, constructive activities must occur at a faster rate than destructive ones.

Survival Needs

The ultimate goal of all body systems is to maintain life. However, life is extraordinarily fragile and requires several factors. These factors, which we will call *survival needs*, include nutrients (food), oxygen, water, and appropriate temperature and atmospheric pressure.

Nutrients

Nutrients, taken in via the diet, contain the chemical substances used for energy and cell building. Most plant-derived foods are rich in carbohydrates, vitamins, and minerals, whereas most animal foods are richer in proteins and fats.

Carbohydrates are the major energy fuel for body cells. Proteins, and to a lesser extent fats, are essential for building cell structures. Fats also provide a reserve of energy-rich fuel. Selected minerals and vitamins are required for the chemical reactions that go on in cells and for oxygen transport in the blood. The mineral calcium helps to make bones hard and is required for blood clotting.

Oxygen

All the nutrients in the world are useless unless **oxygen** is also available. Because the chemical reactions that release energy from foods are *oxidative* reactions that require oxygen, human cells can survive for only a few minutes without oxygen. Approximately 20% of the air we breathe is oxygen. The cooperative efforts of the respiratory and cardiovascular systems make oxygen available to the blood and body cells.

Water

Water accounts for 60–80% of our body weight and is the single most abundant chemical substance in the body. It provides the watery environment necessary for chemical reactions and the fluid base for body secretions and excretions. We obtain water chiefly from ingested foods or liquids. We lose it from the body by evaporation from the lungs and skin and in body excretions.

Normal Body Temperature

If chemical reactions are to continue at life-sustaining rates, **normal body temperature** must be maintained. As body temperature drops below 37°C (98.6°F), metabolic reactions become slower and slower, and finally stop. When body temperature is too high, chemical reactions occur at a frantic pace and body proteins lose their characteristic shape and stop functioning. At either extreme, death occurs. The activity of the muscular system generates most body heat.

Appropriate Atmospheric Pressure

Atmospheric pressure is the force that air exerts on the surface of the body. Breathing and gas exchange in the lungs depend on *appropriate* atmospheric pressure. At high altitudes, where atmospheric pressure is lower and the air is thin, gas exchange may be inadequate to support cellular metabolism.

■ ■ ■

The mere presence of these survival factors is not sufficient to sustain life. They must be present in *appropriate* amounts. Too much and too little may be equally harmful. For example, oxygen is essential, but excessive amounts are toxic to body cells. Similarly, the food we eat must be of high quality and in proper amounts. Otherwise, nutritional disease, obesity, or starvation is likely. Also, while the needs listed above are the most crucial, they do not even begin to encompass all of the body's needs. For example, we can live without gravity if we must, but the quality of life suffers.

☑ Check Your Understanding

6. What separates living beings from nonliving objects?
7. What name is given to all chemical reactions that occur within body cells?
8. Why is it necessary to be in a pressurized cabin when flying at 30,000 feet?

For answers, see Appendix H.

Homeostasis

✓ Define homeostasis and explain its significance.

✓ Describe how negative and positive feedback maintain body homeostasis.

✓ Describe the relationship between homeostatic imbalance and disease.

When you think about the fact that your body contains trillions of cells in nearly constant activity, and that remarkably little usually goes wrong with it, you begin to appreciate what a marvelous machine your body is. Walter Cannon, an American physiologist of the early twentieth century, spoke of the "wisdom of the body," and he coined the word **homeostasis** (ho″me-o-sta′sis) to describe its ability to maintain relatively stable internal conditions even though the outside world changes continuously.

Although the literal translation of homeostasis is "unchanging," the term does not really mean a static, or unchanging, state. Rather, it indicates a *dynamic* state of equilibrium, or a balance, in which internal conditions vary, but always within relatively

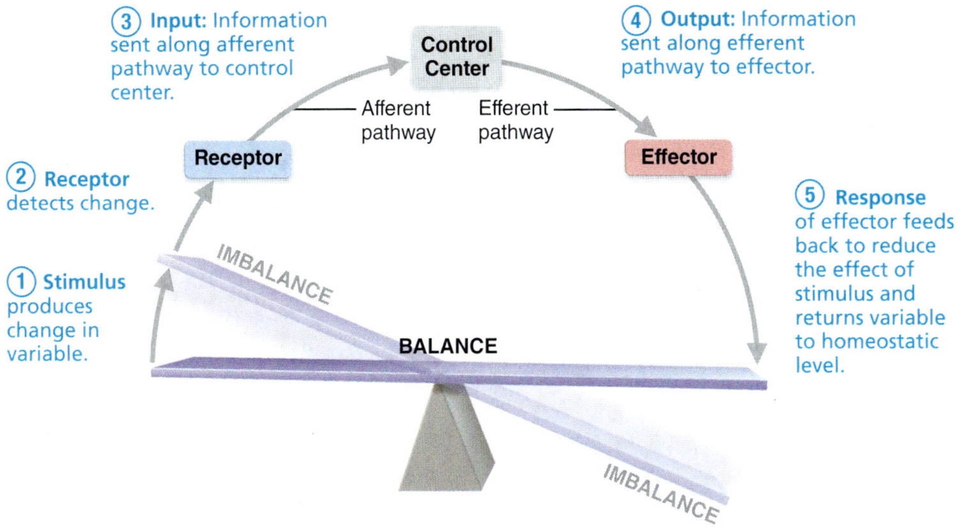

Figure 1.4 Interactions among the elements of a homeostatic control system maintain stable internal conditions.

narrow limits. In general, the body is in homeostasis when its needs are adequately met and it is functioning smoothly.

Maintaining homeostasis is more complicated than it appears at first glance. Virtually every organ system plays a role in maintaining the constancy of the internal environment. Adequate blood levels of vital nutrients must be continuously present, and heart activity and blood pressure must be constantly monitored and adjusted so that the blood is propelled to all body tissues. Also, wastes must not be allowed to accumulate, and body temperature must be precisely controlled. A wide variety of chemical, thermal, and neural factors act and interact in complex ways—sometimes helping and sometimes hindering the body as it works to maintain its "steady rudder."

Homeostatic Control

Communication within the body is essential for homeostasis. Communication is accomplished chiefly by the nervous and endocrine systems, which use neural electrical impulses or bloodborne hormones, respectively, as information carriers. We cover the details of how these two great regulating systems operate in later chapters, but here we explain the basic characteristics of control systems that promote homeostasis.

Regardless of the factor or event being regulated—the **variable**—all homeostatic control mechanisms are processes involving at least three components that work together (**Figure 1.4**). The first component, the **receptor**, is some type of sensor that monitors the environment and responds to changes, called *stimuli*, by sending information (input) to the second component, the *control center*. Input flows from the receptor to the control center along the so-called *afferent pathway*.

The **control center** determines the *set point*, which is the level or range at which a variable is to be maintained. It also analyzes the input it receives and determines the appropriate response or course of action. Information (output) then flows from the control center to the third component, the *effector*, along the *efferent pathway*. (To help you remember the difference between "afferent" and "efferent," you might note that information traveling along the afferent pathway *approaches* the control center and efferent information *exits* from the control center.)

The **effector** provides the means for the control center's response (output) to the stimulus. The results of the response then *feed back* to influence the effect of the stimulus, either reducing it (in negative feedback) so that the whole control process is shut off, or enhancing it (in positive feedback) so that the whole process continues at an even faster rate.

Negative Feedback Mechanisms

Most homeostatic control mechanisms are **negative feedback mechanisms**. In these systems, the output shuts off the original effect of the stimulus or reduces its intensity. These mechanisms cause the variable to change in a direction *opposite* to that of the initial change, returning it to its "ideal" value; thus the name "negative" feedback mechanisms.

Let's start with an example of a nonbiological negative feedback system: a home heating system connected to a temperature-sensing thermostat. The thermostat houses both the receptor (thermometer) and the control center. If the thermostat is set at 20°C (68°F), the heating system (effector) is triggered ON when the house temperature drops below that setting. As the furnace produces heat and warms the air, the temperature rises, and when it reaches 20°C or slightly higher, the thermostat triggers the furnace OFF. This process results in a cycling of "furnace-ON" and "furnace-OFF" so that the temperature in the house stays very near the desired temperature of 20°C. Your body "thermostat," located in a part of your brain called the hypothalamus, operates in a similar fashion (**Figure 1.5**).

Regulation of body temperature is only one of the many ways the nervous system maintains the constancy of the internal environment. Another type of neural control mechanism is seen in the *withdrawal reflex* mentioned earlier, in which the hand is jerked away from a painful stimulus such as broken glass.

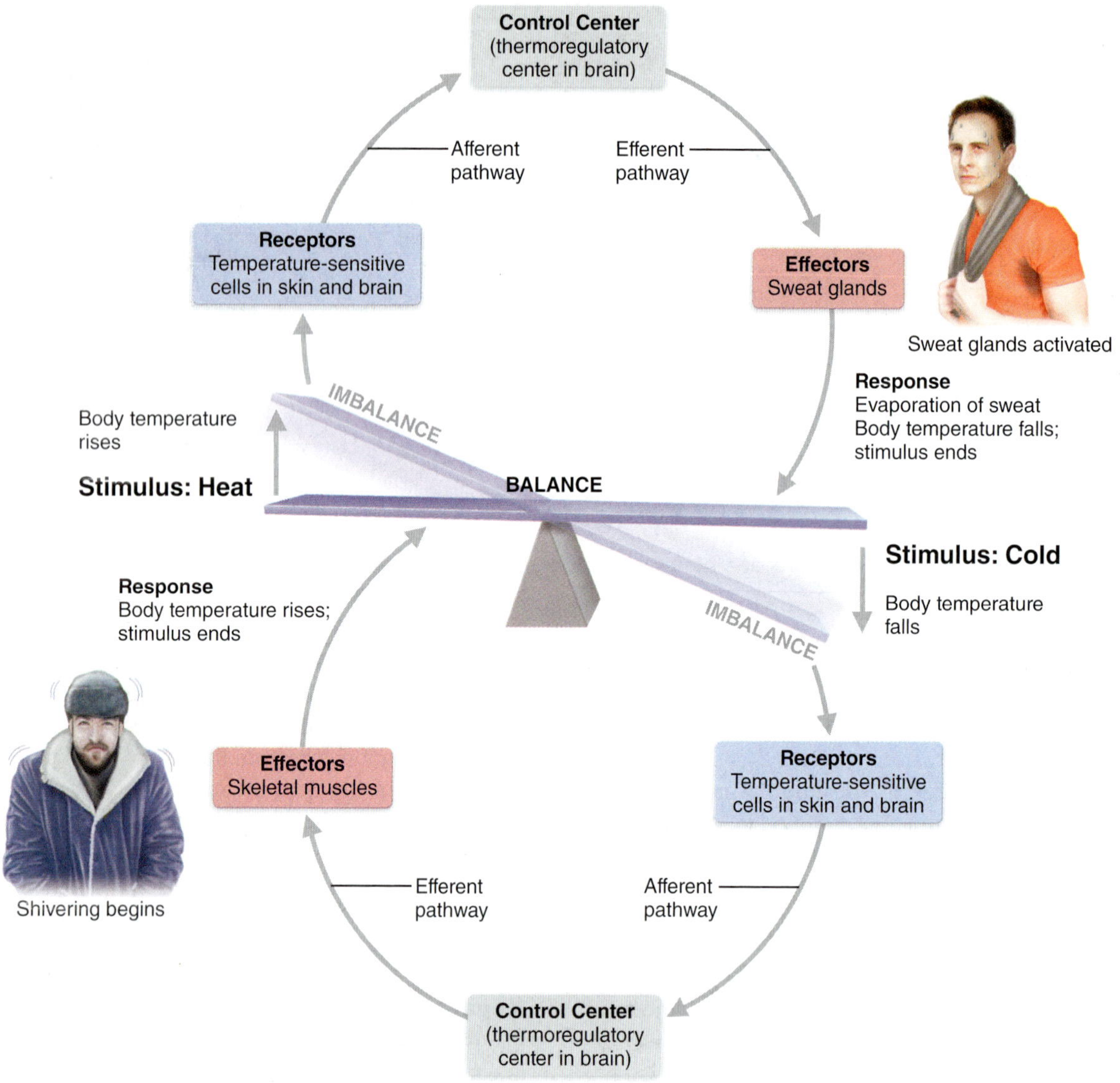

Figure 1.5 Body temperature is regulated by a negative feedback mechanism.

The endocrine system is equally important in maintaining homeostasis. A good example of a hormonal negative feedback mechanism is the control of blood sugar (glucose) by insulin. As blood sugar rises, receptors in the body sense this change, and the pancreas (the control center) secretes insulin into the blood. This change in turn prompts body cells to absorb more glucose, removing it from the bloodstream. As blood sugar falls, the stimulus for insulin release ends. The body's ability to regulate its internal environment is fundamental. All negative feedback mechanisms have the same goal: preventing sudden severe changes within the body. Body temperature and blood volume are only two of the variables that need to be regulated. There are hundreds! Other negative feedback mechanisms regulate heart rate, blood pressure, the rate and depth of breathing, and blood levels of oxygen, carbon dioxide, and minerals. Now, let's take a look at the other type of feedback control mechanism—positive feedback.

Positive Feedback Mechanisms

In **positive feedback mechanisms**, the result or response enhances the original stimulus so that the response is accelerated. This feedback mechanism is "positive" because the change that results proceeds in the *same* direction as the initial change, causing the variable to deviate further and further from its original value or range.

In contrast to negative feedback controls, which maintain some physiological function or keep blood chemicals within narrow ranges, positive feedback mechanisms usually control infrequent events that do not require continuous adjustments. Typically, they set off a series of events that may be self-perpetuating and that, once initiated, have an amplifying or waterfall effect. Because of these characteristics, positive feedback mechanisms are often referred to as *cascades* (from the Italian word meaning "to fall"). Two familiar examples of their use as homeostatic mechanisms are the enhancement of labor contractions during birth and blood clotting.

Chapter 28 describes the positive feedback mechanism in which oxytocin, a hypothalamic hormone, intensifies labor contractions during the birth of a baby (see Figure 28.17). Oxytocin causes the contractions to become both more frequent and more powerful. The increased contractions cause more oxytocin to be released, which causes more contractions, and so on until the baby is finally born. The birth ends the stimulus for oxytocin release and shuts off the positive feedback mechanism.

Blood clotting is a normal response to a break in the wall of a blood vessel and is an excellent example of an important body function controlled by positive feedback. Basically, once a vessel has been damaged, blood elements called platelets immediately begin to cling to the injured site and release chemicals that attract more platelets. This rapidly growing pileup of platelets temporarily "plugs" the tear and initiates the sequence of events that finally forms a clot **(Figure 1.6)**. Positive feedback mechanisms are likely to race out of control, so they are rarely used to promote the moment-to-moment well-being of the body. However, some positive feedback mechanisms, including this one, may have only local reach. For example, blood clotting is accelerated in injured vessels, but does not normally spread to the entire circulation.

Homeostatic Imbalance

Homeostasis is so important that most disease can be regarded as a result of its disturbance, a condition called **homeostatic imbalance**. As we age, our body's control systems become less efficient, and our internal environment becomes less and less stable. These events increase our risk for illness and produce the changes we associate with aging.

Another important source of homeostatic imbalance occurs when the usual negative feedback mechanisms are overwhelmed and destructive positive feedback mechanisms take over. Some instances of heart failure reflect this phenomenon.

Examples of homeostatic imbalance appear throughout this book to enhance your understanding of normal physiological mechanisms. This symbol introduces the homeostatic imbalance sections and alerts you to the fact that we are describing an abnormal condition. Each Homeostatic Imbalance section is numbered to correspond with critical thinking questions available in the Study Area of MasteringA&P—visit www.masteringaandp.com to find Homeostatic Imbalance questions and other helpful study tools. MAP

Check Your Understanding

9. What process allows us to adjust to either extreme heat or extreme cold?
10. When we begin to get dehydrated, we usually get thirsty, which causes us to drink fluids. Is thirst part of a negative or a positive feedback control system? Defend your choice.
11. Why is the control mechanism shown in Figure 1.6 called a positive feedback system? What event ends it?

For answers, see Appendix H.

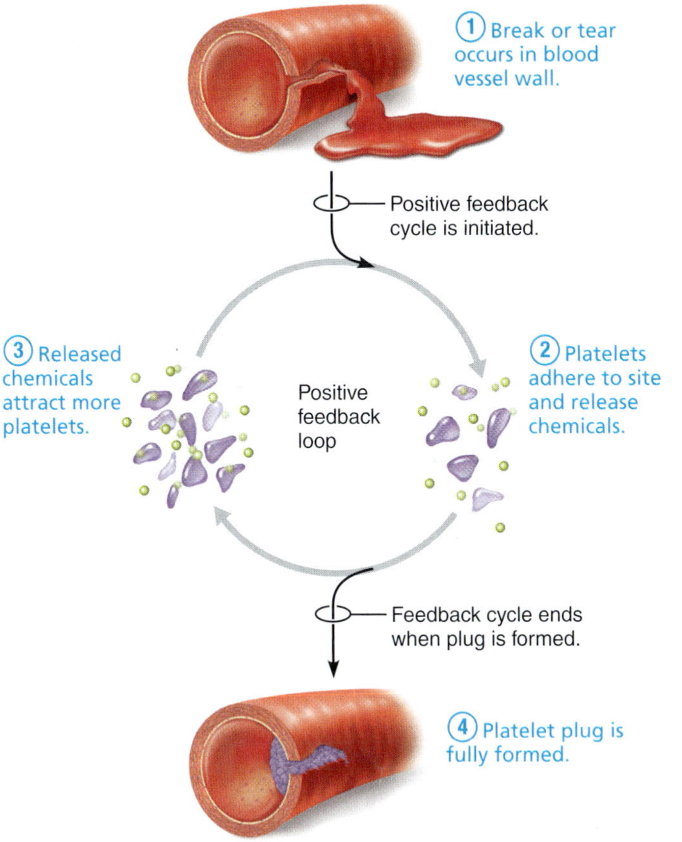

Figure 1.6 A positive feedback mechanism regulates formation of a platelet plug.

The Language of Anatomy

✓ Describe the anatomical position.

✓ Use correct anatomical terms to describe body directions, regions, and body planes or sections.

Most of us are naturally curious about our bodies, but our interest sometimes dwindles when we are confronted with the terminology of anatomy and physiology. Let's face it—you can't just pick up an anatomy and physiology book and read it as though it were a novel.

Unfortunately, confusion is likely without precise, specialized terminology. To prevent misunderstanding, anatomists use universally accepted terms to identify body structures precisely and with a minimum of words. We present and explain the language of anatomy next.

Anatomical Position and Directional Terms

To describe body parts and position accurately, we need an initial reference point, and we must indicate direction. The anatomical reference point is a standard body position called the **anatomical position**. In the anatomical position, the body is erect with feet slightly apart. This position is easy to remember because it resembles "standing at attention," except that the palms face

Table 1.1 Orientation and Directional Terms

TERM	DEFINITION	EXAMPLE
Superior (cranial)	Toward the head end or upper part of a structure or the body; above	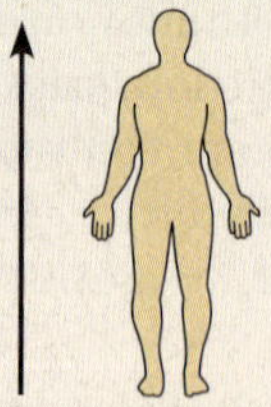 The head is superior to the abdomen.
Inferior (caudal)	Away from the head end or toward the lower part of a structure or the body; below	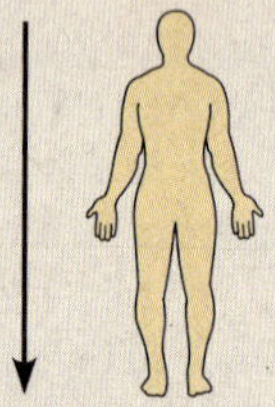 The navel is inferior to the chin.
Ventral (anterior)*	Toward or at the front of the body; in front of	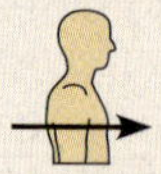 The breastbone is anterior to the spine.
Dorsal (posterior)*	Toward or at the back of the body; behind	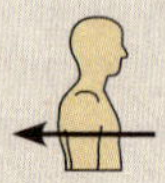 The heart is posterior to the breastbone.
Medial	Toward or at the midline of the body; on the inner side of	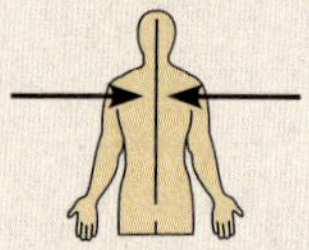 The heart is medial to the arm.
Lateral	Away from the midline of the body; on the outer side of	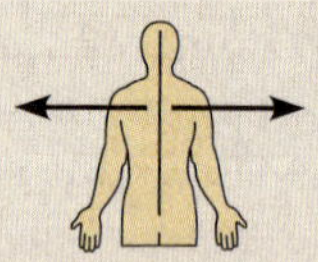 The arms are lateral to the chest.
Intermediate	Between a more medial and a more lateral structure	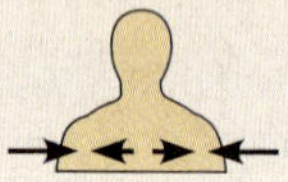 The collarbone is intermediate between the breastbone and shoulder.
Proximal	Closer to the origin of the body part or the point of attachment of a limb to the body trunk	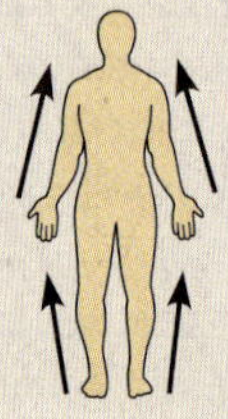 The elbow is proximal to the wrist.
Distal	Farther from the origin of a body part or the point of attachment of a limb to the body trunk	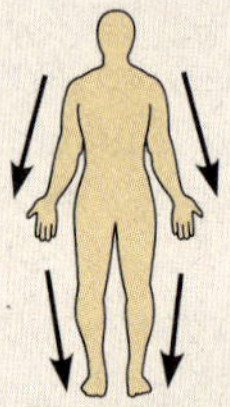 The knee is distal to the thigh.
Superficial (external)	Toward or at the body surface	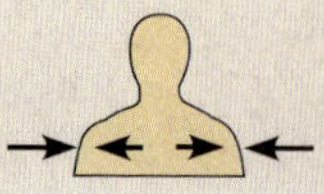 The skin is superficial to the skeletal muscles.
Deep (internal)	Away from the body surface; more internal	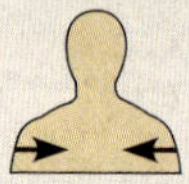 The lungs are deep to the skin.

*The terms *ventral* and *anterior* are synonymous in humans, but this is not the case in four-legged animals. *Anterior* refers to the leading portion of the body (abdominal surface in humans, head in a cat), but *ventral* specifically refers to the "belly" of a vertebrate animal, so it is the inferior surface of four-legged animals. Likewise, although the dorsal and posterior surfaces are the same in humans, the term *dorsal* specifically refers to an animal's back. Thus, the dorsal surface of four-legged animals is their superior surface.

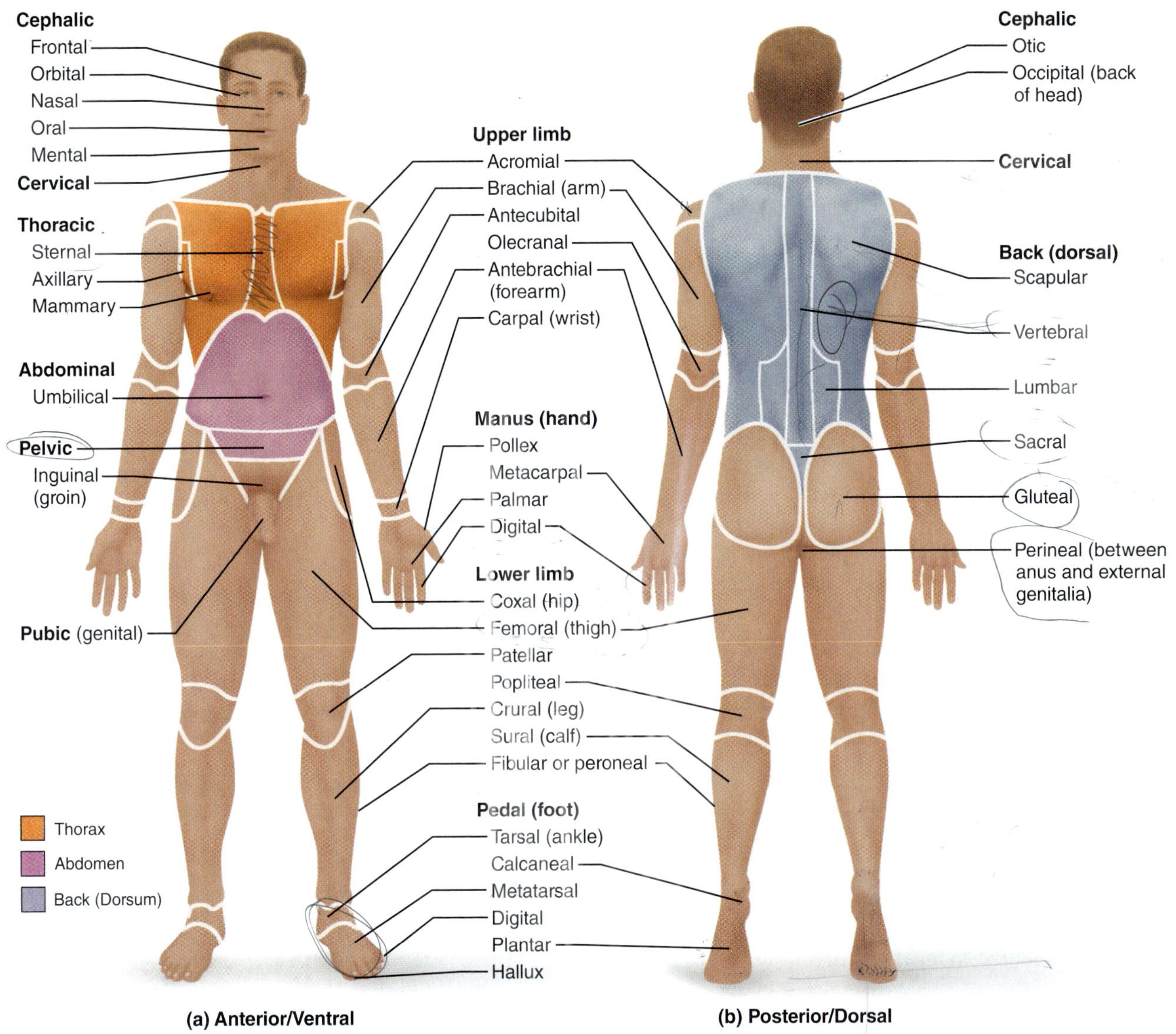

Figure 1.7 Regional terms used to designate specific body areas. (a) The anatomical position. **(b)** The heels are raised to show the plantar surface of the foot, which is actually on the inferior surface of the body.

forward and the thumbs point away from the body. You can see the anatomical position in **Table 1.1** (top) and **Figure 1.7a**.

It is essential to understand the anatomical position because most of the directional terms used in this book refer to the body *as if it were in this position, regardless of its actual position*. Another point to remember is that the terms "right" and "left" refer to those sides of the person or the cadaver (body of a deceased person) being viewed—not those of the observer.

Directional terms allow us to explain where one body structure is in relation to another. For example, we could describe the relationship between the ears and the nose informally by stating, "The ears are located on each side of the head to the right and left of the nose." Using anatomical terminology, we can condense this to "The ears are lateral to the nose." Using anatomical terms saves words and is less ambiguous.

Commonly used orientation and directional terms are defined and illustrated in Table 1.1. Many of these terms are also used in everyday conversation, but keep in mind as you study them that their anatomical meanings are very precise.

Regional Terms

The two fundamental divisions of our body are its *axial* and *appendicular* (ap″en-dik′u-lar) parts. The **axial part**, which makes up the main *axis* of our body, includes the head, neck, and trunk. The **appendicular part** consists of the *appendages*, or *limbs*, which are attached to the body's axis. **Regional terms** used to designate specific areas within these major body divisions are indicated in Figure 1.7. The common terms for a few of these body regions are given in parentheses.

Anatomical Variability

Although we use common directional and regional terms to refer to all human bodies, you know from observing the faces and body shapes of people around you that we humans differ in our external anatomy. The same kind of variability holds for internal organs as well. In some bodies, for example, a nerve or blood vessel may be somewhat out of place, or a small muscle may be missing. Nonetheless, well over 90% of all structures present in any human body match the textbook descriptions. We seldom see extreme anatomical variations because they are incompatible with life.

1

Body Planes and Sections

For anatomical studies, the body is often cut, or *sectioned*, along a flat surface called a *plane*. The most frequently used body planes are *sagittal*, *frontal*, and *transverse* planes, which lie at right angles to one another **(Figure 1.8)**. A section is named for the plane along which it is cut. Thus, a cut along a sagittal plane produces a sagittal section.

A **sagittal plane** (saj′ĭ-tal; "arrow") is a vertical plane that divides the body into right and left parts. A sagittal plane that lies exactly in the midline is the **median plane**, or **midsagittal plane** (Figure 1.8c). All other sagittal planes, offset from the midline, are **parasagittal planes** (*para* = near).

Frontal planes, like sagittal planes, lie vertically. Frontal planes, however, divide the body into anterior and posterior parts (Figure 1.8a). A frontal plane is also called a **coronal plane** (kŏ-ro′nal; "crown").

A **transverse**, or **horizontal**, **plane** runs horizontally from right to left, dividing the body into superior and inferior parts (Figure 1.8b). Of course, many different transverse planes exist, at every possible level from head to foot. A transverse section is also called a **cross section**.

Oblique sections are cuts made diagonally between the horizontal and the vertical planes. Because oblique sections are often confusing and difficult to interpret, they are seldom used.

At the bottom of Figure 1.8, you can see examples of magnetic resonance imaging (MRI) scans that correspond to the three different sections shown in the figure. Clinically, the ability to interpret sections made through the body, especially transverse sections, is important. Additionally, the new medical imaging devices (*A Closer Look*, pp. 16–17) produce sectional images rather than three-dimensional images.

It takes practice to determine or figure out an object's overall shape from sectioned material. A cross section of a banana, for example, looks like a circle and gives no indication of the whole banana's crescent shape. Likewise, sectioning the body or an organ along different planes often results in very different views. For example, a transverse section of the body trunk at the level of the kidneys would show kidney structure in cross section very nicely. A frontal section of the body trunk would show a different view of kidney anatomy, and a midsagittal section would miss the kidneys completely. With experience, you will gradually learn to relate two-dimensional sections to three-dimensional shapes.

☑ Check Your Understanding

12. What is the anatomical position? Why is it important that *you* learn this position?
13. The axillary and acromial regions are both in the general area of the shoulder. Where specifically is each located?
14. What type of cut would separate the brain into anterior and posterior parts?

For answers, see Appendix H.

Body Cavities and Membranes

✓ Locate and name the major body cavities and their subdivisions and associated membranes, and list the major organs contained within them.

✓ Name the four quadrants or nine regions of the abdominopelvic cavity and list the organs they contain.

Anatomy and physiology textbooks typically describe two sets of internal body cavities called the dorsal and ventral body cavities. These cavities are closed to the outside and provide different degrees of protection to the organs contained within them. Because these two cavities differ in their mode of embryonic development, and their lining membranes, the dorsal body cavity is not recognized as such in many anatomical references. However, the idea of two sets of internal body cavities is a useful learning concept and we use it here.

Dorsal Body Cavity

The **dorsal body cavity**, which protects the fragile nervous system organs, has two subdivisions (**Figure 1.9**, on p. 18, gold areas). The **cranial cavity**, in the skull, encases the brain. The **vertebral**, or **spinal**, **cavity**, which runs within the bony vertebral column, encloses the delicate spinal cord. The spinal cord is essentially a continuation of the brain, and the cranial and spinal cavities are continuous with one another.

Ventral Body Cavity

The more anterior and larger of the closed body cavities is the **ventral body cavity** (Figure 1.9, deep-red areas). Like the dorsal cavity, it has two major subdivisions, the *thoracic cavity* and the *abdominopelvic cavity*. The ventral body cavity houses internal organs collectively called the **viscera** (vis′er-ah; *viscus* = an organ in a body cavity), or visceral organs.

The superior subdivision, the **thoracic cavity** (tho-ras′ik), is surrounded by the ribs and muscles of the chest. The thoracic cavity is further subdivided into lateral **pleural cavities** (ploo′ral), each enveloping a lung, and the medial **mediastinum** (me″de-ah-sti′num). The mediastinum contains the **pericardial cavity** (per″ĭ-kar′de-al), which encloses the heart, and it also surrounds the remaining thoracic organs (esophagus, trachea, and others).

The thoracic cavity is separated from the more inferior **abdominopelvic cavity** (ab-dom′ĭ-no-pel′vic) by the diaphragm, a dome-shaped muscle important in breathing. The abdominopelvic cavity, as its name suggests, has two parts. However,

(Text continues on p. 18.)

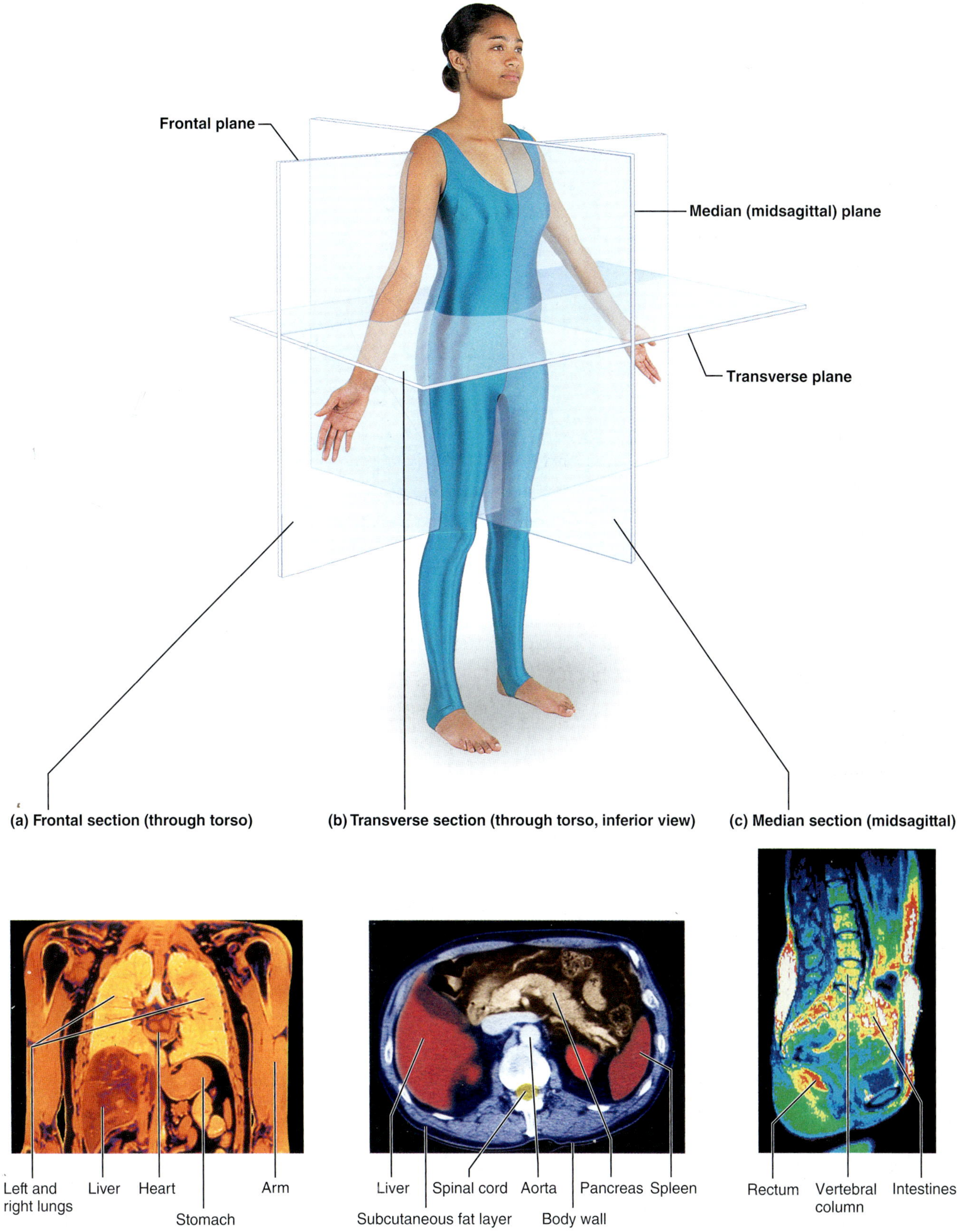

Figure 1.8 **Planes of the body with corresponding magnetic resonance imaging (MRI) scans.**

Medical Imaging: Illuminating the Body

Until 50 years ago, the **magical** but **murky** X ray was the only nonsurgical means to extract information from within a living body. Produced by directing ***X rays***, electromagnetic waves of very short wavelength, at the body, an **X ray** or **radiograph** is essentially a **shadowy negative image** of internal structures. Dense structures absorb the X rays most and so appear as light areas. Hollow air-containing organs and fat, which absorb the X rays less, show up as dark areas. What X rays do best is visualize hard, bony structures and locate abnormally dense structures (tumors, tuberculosis nodules) in the lungs.

1

The 1950s saw the advent of ultrasound and of nuclear medicine, which uses radioisotopes to scan the body to not only reveal the structure of our "insides" but also wring out information about the hidden workings of their molecules.

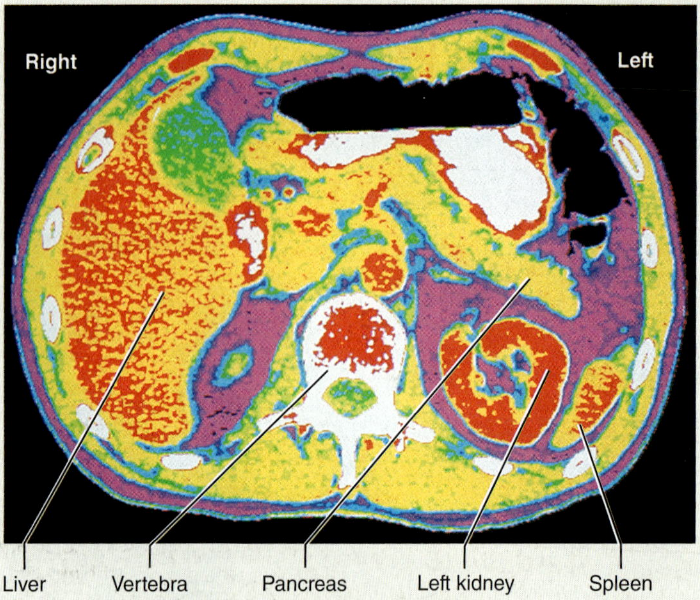

(a) A CT scan through the superior abdomen.

Computed tomography (**CT**, formerly called **computerized axial tomography**, **CAT**) uses a refined version of X-ray equipment. As the patient is slowly moved through the doughnut-shaped CT machine, its X-ray tube rotates around the body and sends beams from all directions to a specific level of the patient's body. Because at any moment its beam is confined to a "slice" of the body about as thick as a dime, CT ends the confusion resulting from overlapping structures seen in conventional X rays. The device's computer translates this information into a detailed, cross-sectional picture of each body region scanned. CT scans are at the forefront for evaluating most problems that affect the brain and abdomen. Their clarity, illustrated in photo (a), has all but eliminated exploratory surgery.

Xenon CT is a CT brain scan enhanced with radioactive xenon gas to quickly trace blood flow. Inhaled xenon rapidly enters the bloodstream and distributes to different body tissues in proportion to their blood flow. Absence of xenon from part of the brain indicates that a stroke is occurring there, information that aids treatment.

Dynamic spatial reconstruction (DSR) uses ultrafast CT scanners to provide three-dimensional images of body organs from any angle, and scrutinize their movements and changes in their internal volumes at normal speed, in slow motion, and at a specific moment. DSR's greatest value has been to visualize the heart beating and blood flowing through blood vessels. This information allows clinicians to evaluate heart defects, constricted or blocked blood vessels, and the status of coronary bypass grafts.

Another computer-assisted X-ray technique, **digital subtraction angiography (DSA)** (*angiography* = vessel pictures), provides an unobstructed view of small arteries. Conventional radiographs are taken before and after a contrast medium is injected into an artery. The computer subtracts the "before" image from the "after" image, eliminating all traces of body structures that obscure the vessel. DSA is often used to identify blockages in the arteries that supply the heart wall, as in photo (b), and in the brain.

Just as the X ray spawned related technologies, so too did nuclear medicine in the form of **positron emission tomography (PET)**. PET excels in observing *metabolic processes*. The patient is given an injection of radioisotopes tagged to biological molecules (such as glucose) and is then positioned in the PET scanner. As the radioisotopes are absorbed by the most active brain cells, high-energy gamma rays are produced. The computer analyzes the gamma-ray emission and produces a live-action picture of the brain's biochemical activity in vivid colors. PET's greatest value has been its ability to provide insights into brain activity in people affected by mental illness, stroke, Alzheimer's disease, and epilepsy. One of its most exciting uses has been to determine which areas of the healthy brain are most active during certain tasks (e.g., speaking, listening to music, or figuring out a mathematical problem), providing direct evidence of the functions of specific brain regions. Currently PET can reveal signs of trouble in those with undiagnosed Alzheimer's disease (AD) because regions of beta-amyloid accumulation (a defining characteristic of AD) show up in brilliant red and yellow, as in photo (c). PET scans can also help to predict who may develop AD in the future by identifying areas of decreased metabolism in crucial memory areas of the brain.

Sonography, or **ultrasound imaging**, has some distinct advantages over the approaches examined so far. The equipment is inexpensive, and the ultrasound used as its energy source seems to be safer than the ionizing forms of radiation used in nuclear medicine. The body is probed with pulses of sound waves that cause echoes when reflected and scattered by body tissues. A computer analyzes these echoes to construct somewhat blurry outlines of body organs. A single easy-to-use handheld device emits the sound and picks up the echoes, so sections can be scanned from many different body planes.

Because of its safety, ultrasound is the imaging technique of choice in obstetrics for determining fetal age and position and locating the placenta. However, sound waves have low penetrating power and rapidly dissipate in air, so sonography

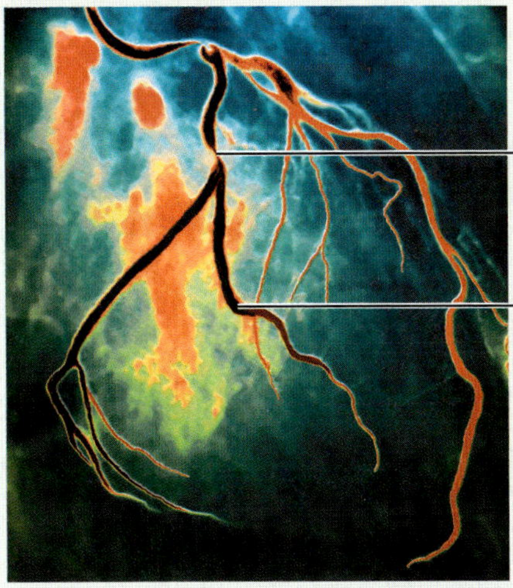

(b) A DSA image of the arteries that supply the heart.

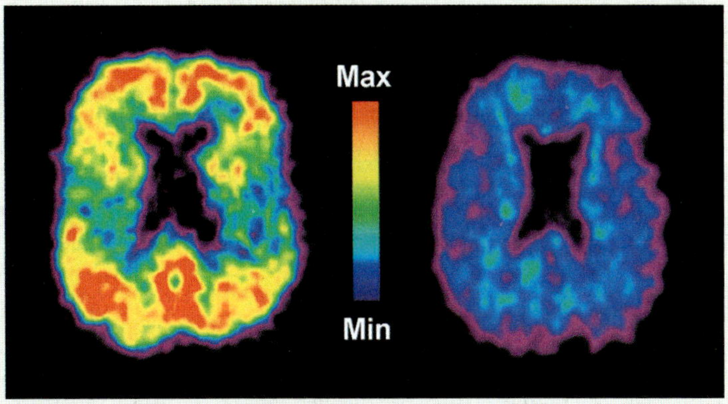

(c) In a PET scan, regions of beta-amyloid accumulation "light up" (red-yellow) in an Alzheimer's patient (*left*) but not in a healthy person (*right*).

is of little value for looking at air-filled structures (the lungs) or those surrounded by bone (the brain and spinal cord).

Magnetic resonance imaging (MRI) produces high-contrast images of our soft tissues, an area in which X rays and CT scans are weak. As initially developed, MRI primarily maps the body's content of hydrogen, most of which is in water. The technique subjects the body to magnetic fields up to 60,000 times stronger than that of the earth to pry information from the body's molecules. The patient lies in a chamber within a huge magnet. Hydrogen molecules act like tiny magnets, spinning like tops in the magnetic field. Their energy is further enhanced by radio waves, and when the radio waves are turned off, the energy released is translated into a visual image.

MRI distinguishes body tissues based on their water content, so it can differentiate between the fatty white matter and the more watery gray matter of the brain. Because dense structures do not show up at all in MRI, it peers easily into the skull and vertebral column, enabling the delicate nerve fibers of the spinal cord to be seen. MRI is also particularly good at detecting tumors and degenerative disease. Multiple sclerosis plaques do not show up well in CT scans, but are dazzlingly clear in MRI scans. MRI can also tune in on metabolic reactions, such as processes that generate energy-rich ATP molecules.

Until recently, trying to diagnose asthma and other lung problems has been off limits to MRI scans because the lungs have a low water content. However, an alternate tack—filling the lungs with a gas that can be magnetized (hyperpolarized helium-3 or xenon-129)—has yielded spectacular pictures of the lungs in just the few seconds it takes the patient to inhale, hold the breath briefly, and then exhale. This technique offers a distinct improvement over the hours required for conventional MRI and it has the additional advantage of using a magnetic field as little as one-tenth that of the conventional MRI. Lately, MRI scans have become the "diagnostic darling" in emergency rooms for their ability to accurately diagnose heart attacks or ischemic strokes—conditions that require rapid treatment to prevent fatal consequences. Also exciting are the so-called **bloodless MRIs** currently being tested in animals, which measure water flow instead of blood flow.

Newer variations of MRI include **magnetic resonance spectroscopy (MRS)**, which maps the distribution of elements other than hydrogen to reveal more about how disease changes body chemistry. Other advances in computer techniques display MRI scans in three dimensions to guide laser surgery.

The **functional MRI** tracks blood flow into the brain in real time. Prior to the 1990s, matching thoughts, deeds, and disease to brain activity was the sole domain of PET. Because functional MRI does not require injections of tracers and can pinpoint much smaller brain areas than PET, it may provide a desirable alternative and has transformed neuroscience. Clinical studies are also using functional MRI to determine if a patient in the vegetative state has conscious thought. However, some researchers worry that the brightly colored images explain little about the mechanisms of human thought—that is, it is not possible to assume a particular mental state from the activation of a particular brain region.

Despite its advantages, the powerful magnets of the clanging, claustrophobia-inducing MRI present some thorny problems. For example, they can "suck" metal objects, such as implanted pacemakers and loose tooth fillings, through the body. Moreover, although such strong magnetic fields are currently considered safe, there is no convincing evidence that they are risk free.

Although stunning, medical images other than straight X rays are abstractions assembled within the "mind" of a computer. They are artificially enhanced for sharpness and artificially colored to increase contrast (all their colors are "phony"). The images are several steps removed from direct observation.

As you can see, medical science offers remarkable diagnostic tools. Consider the **M2A Swallowable Imaging Capsule**, a tiny camera that a patient swallows like a pill, and then excretes normally 8–72 hours later. As the M2A travels through the digestive tract, it photographs the small intestine and beams the color images to a small video data recorder worn on a belt or harness. A study found the device to be 60% effective at detecting intestinal problems, compared to a 35% success rate with other imaging techniques. At present the M2A can provide images only of the small intestine because the battery gives out before it enters the large intestine.

New imaging technologies also make long-distance surgery possible. Visual images of a diseased organ travel via fiber-optic cable to surgeons at another location (even a different country), who manipulate delicate robotic instruments to remove the organ.

1

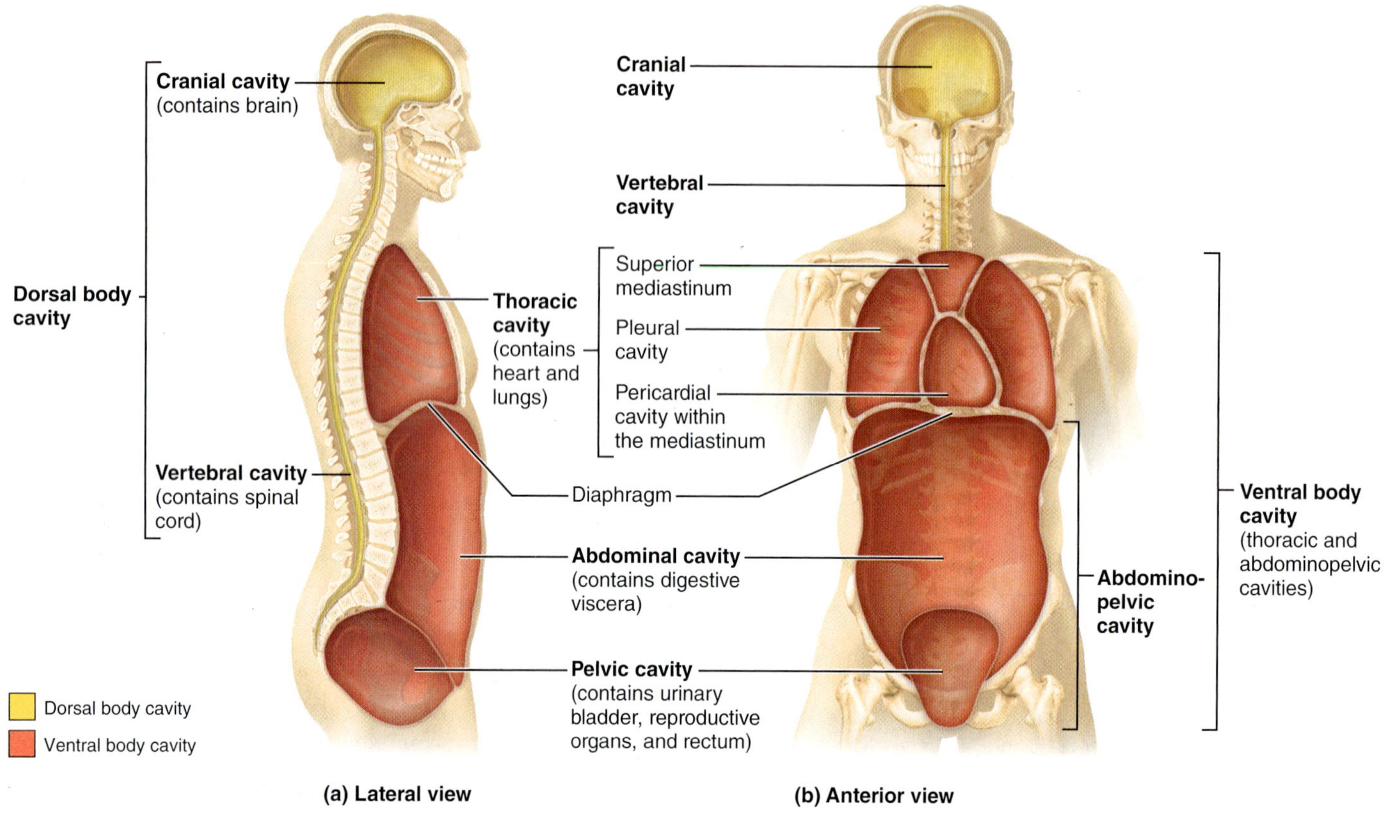

Figure 1.9 Dorsal and ventral body cavities and their subdivisions.

these regions are not physically separated by a muscular or membrane wall. Its superior portion, the **abdominal cavity**, contains the stomach, intestines, spleen, liver, and other organs. The inferior part, the **pelvic cavity**, lies in the bony pelvis and contains the urinary bladder, some reproductive organs, and the rectum. The abdominal and pelvic cavities are not aligned with each other. Instead, the bowl-shaped pelvis tips away from the perpendicular as shown in Figure 1.9a.

Homeostatic Imbalance 1.1

When the body is subjected to physical trauma (as in an automobile accident), the abdominopelvic organs are most vulnerable. Why? This is because the walls of the abdominal cavity are formed only by trunk muscles and are not reinforced by bone. The pelvic organs receive a somewhat greater degree of protection from the bony pelvis. +

Membranes in the Ventral Body Cavity The walls of the ventral body cavity and the outer surfaces of the organs it contains are covered by a thin, double-layered membrane, the **serosa** (se-ro′sah), or **serous membrane**. The part of the membrane lining the cavity walls is called the **parietal serosa** (pah-ri′ĕ-tal; *parie* = wall). It folds in on itself to form the **visceral serosa**, covering the organs in the cavity.

You can visualize the relationship between the serosal layers by pushing your fist into a limp balloon **(Figure 1.10a)**. The part of the balloon that clings to your fist can be compared to the visceral serosa clinging to an organ's external surface. The outer wall of the balloon then represents the parietal serosa that lines the walls of the cavity. (However, unlike the balloon, the parietal serosa is never exposed but is always fused to the cavity wall.) In the body, the serous membranes are separated not by air but by a thin layer of lubricating fluid, called **serous fluid**, which is secreted by both membranes. Although there is a potential space between the two membranes, the barely present, slitlike cavity is filled with serous fluid.

The slippery serous fluid allows the organs to slide without friction across the cavity walls and one another as they carry out their routine functions. This freedom of movement is especially important for mobile organs such as the pumping heart and the churning stomach.

The serous membranes are named for the specific cavity and organs with which they are associated. For example, as shown in Figure 1.10b, the *parietal pericardium* lines the pericardial cavity and folds back as the *visceral pericardium*, which covers the heart. Likewise, the *parietal pleurae* (ploo′re) line the walls of the thoracic cavity, and the *visceral pleurae* cover the lungs. The *parietal peritoneum* (per″ĭ-to-ne′um) is associated with the walls of the abdominopelvic cavity, while the *visceral peritoneum* covers most of the organs within that cavity. (The pleural and peritoneal serosae are illustrated in Figure 4.11c on p. 141.)

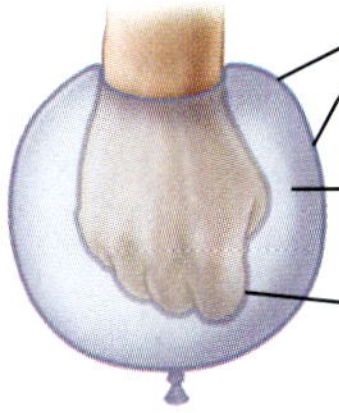

(a) A fist thrust into a flaccid balloon demonstrates the relationship between the parietal and visceral serous membrane layers.

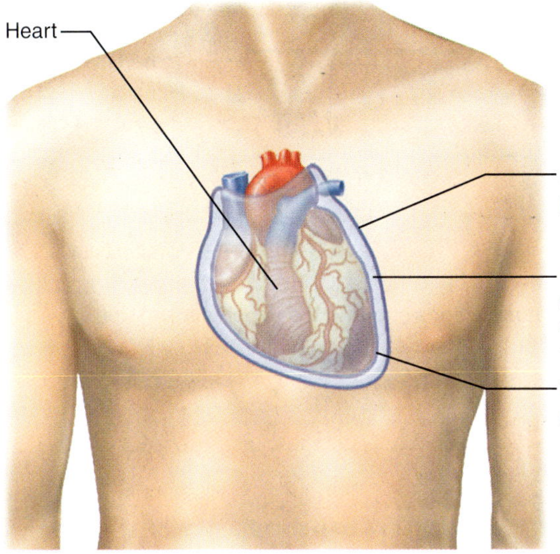

(b) The serosae associated with the heart.

Figure 1.10 Serous membrane relationships.

Homeostatic Imbalance 1.2

When serous membranes are inflamed, their normally smooth surfaces become roughened. This roughness causes the organs to stick together and drag across one another, leading to excruciating pain, as anyone who has experienced *pleurisy* (inflammation of the pleurae) or *peritonitis* (inflammation of the peritoneums) knows. ✚

Abdominopelvic Regions and Quadrants Because the abdominopelvic cavity is large and contains several organs, it helps to divide it into smaller areas for study. Medical personnel usually use a simple scheme to locate the abdominopelvic cavity organs **(Figure 1.11)**. In this scheme, a transverse and a median plane pass through the umbilicus at right angles. The four resulting quadrants are named according to their positions from the subject's point of view: the **right upper quadrant (RUQ)**, **left upper quadrant (LUQ)**, **right lower quadrant (RLQ)**, and **left lower quadrant (LLQ)**.

Another division method, used primarily by anatomists, uses two transverse and two parasagittal planes. These planes, positioned like a tic-tac-toe grid on the abdomen, divide the cavity into nine regions **(Figure 1.12)**:

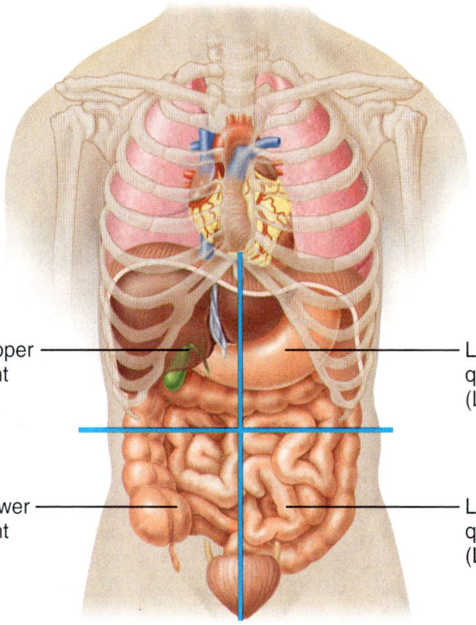

Figure 1.11 The four abdominopelvic quadrants. In this scheme, the abdominopelvic cavity is divided into four quadrants by two planes.

- The **umbilical region** is the centermost region deep to and surrounding the umbilicus (navel).
- The **epigastric region** is located superior to the umbilical region (*epi* = upon, above; *gastri* = belly).
- The **hypogastric (pubic) region** is located inferior to the umbilical region (*hypo* = below).
- The **right** and **left iliac**, or **inguinal**, **regions** (ing′gwĭ-nal) are located lateral to the hypogastric region (*iliac* = superior part of the hip bone).
- The **right** and **left lumbar regions** lie lateral to the umbilical region (*lumbus* = loin).
- The **right** and **left hypochondriac regions** lie lateral to the epigastric region and deep to the ribs (*chondro* = cartilage).

Other Body Cavities

In addition to the large closed body cavities, there are several smaller body cavities. Most of these are in the head and most open to the body exterior. Figure 1.7 provides the terms that will help you locate all but the last two cavities mentioned here.

- **Oral and digestive cavities.** The oral cavity, commonly called the mouth, contains the teeth and tongue. This cavity is part of and continuous with the cavity of the digestive organs, which opens to the body exterior at the anus.
- **Nasal cavity.** Located within and posterior to the nose, the nasal cavity is part of the respiratory system passageways.
- **Orbital cavities.** The orbital cavities (orbits) in the skull house the eyes and present them in an anterior position.

1

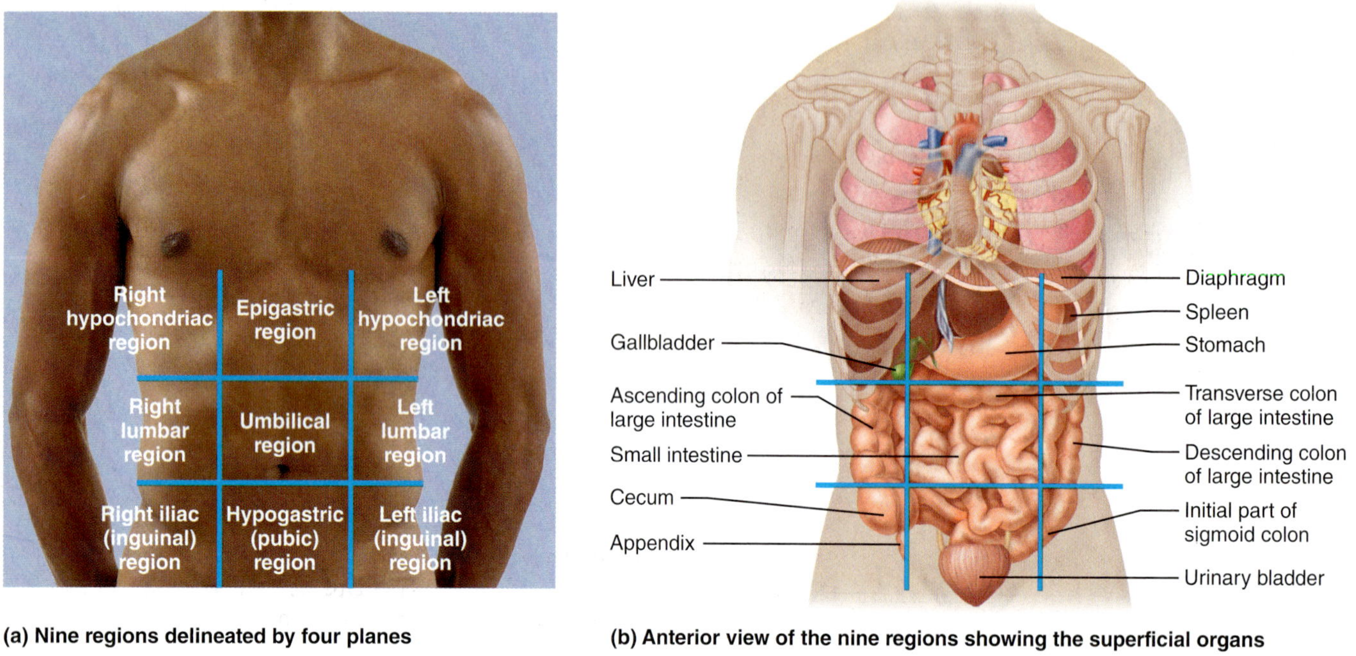

Figure 1.12 The nine abdominopelvic regions. In **(a)** the superior transverse plane is just inferior to the ribs; the inferior transverse plane is just superior to the hip bones; and the parasagittal planes lie just medial to the nipples.

- **Middle ear cavities.** The middle ear cavities in the skull lie just medial to the eardrums. These cavities contain tiny bones that transmit sound vibrations to the hearing receptors in the inner ears.
- **Synovial cavities.** Synovial (sĭ-no′ve-al) cavities are joint cavities. They are enclosed within fibrous capsules that surround freely movable joints of the body (such as the elbow and knee joints). Like the serous membranes, membranes lining synovial cavities secrete a lubricating fluid that reduces friction as the bones move across one another.

Check Your Understanding

15. Joe went to the emergency room where he complained of severe pains in the lower right quadrant of his abdomen. What might be his problem?
16. Of the uterus, small intestine, spinal cord, and heart, which is/are in the dorsal body cavity?
17. When you rub your cold hands together, the friction between them results in heat that warms your hands. Why doesn't warming friction result during movements of the heart, lungs, and digestive organs?

For answers, see Appendix H.

Chapter Summary

MAP™ For more chapter study tools, go to the Study Area of MasteringA&P at **www.masteringaandp.com**.

There you will find:

- Interactive Physiology iP
- A&PFlix A&PFlix
- Practice Anatomy Lab PAL
- PhysioEx PEx
- Videos, Practice Quizzes and Tests, MP3 Tutor Sessions, Case Studies, and much more!

An Overview of Anatomy and Physiology (pp. 2–3)

1. Anatomy is the study of body structures and their relationships. Physiology is the science of how body parts function.

Topics of Anatomy (p. 2)

2. Major subdivisions of anatomy include gross anatomy, microscopic anatomy, and developmental anatomy.

Topics of Physiology (pp. 2–3)

3. Typically, physiology concerns the functioning of specific organs or organ systems. Examples include cardiac physiology, renal physiology, and muscle physiology.
4. Physiology is explained by chemical and physical principles.

Complementarity of Structure and Function (p. 3)

5. Anatomy and physiology are inseparable: What a body can do depends on the unique architecture of its parts. This principle is called the complementarity of structure and function.

Levels of Structural Organization (pp. 3–4)

1. The levels of structural organization of the body, from simplest to most complex, are: chemical, cellular, tissue, organ, organ system, and organismal.
2. The 11 organ systems of the body are the integumentary, skeletal, muscular, nervous, endocrine, cardiovascular, lymphatic, respiratory, digestive, urinary, and reproductive systems. The immune system is a functional system closely associated with the lymphatic system. (For functions of these systems see pp. 6–7.)

Maintaining Life (pp. 4–8)

Necessary Life Functions (pp. 4–8)

1. All living organisms carry out certain vital functional activities necessary for life, including maintenance of boundaries, movement, responsiveness, digestion, metabolism, excretion, reproduction, and growth.

Survival Needs (p. 8)

2. Survival needs include nutrients, water, oxygen, and appropriate temperature and atmospheric pressure.

Homeostasis (pp. 8–11)

1. Homeostasis is a dynamic equilibrium of the internal environment. All body systems contribute to homeostasis, but the nervous and endocrine systems are most important. Homeostasis is necessary for health.

Homeostatic Control (pp. 9–11)

2. Control mechanisms of the body contain at least three elements that work together: receptor(s), control center, and effector(s).
3. Negative feedback mechanisms reduce the effect of the original stimulus, and are essential for maintaining homeostasis. Body temperature, heart rate, breathing rate and depth, and blood levels of glucose and certain ions are regulated by negative feedback mechanisms.
4. Positive feedback mechanisms intensify the initial stimulus, leading to an enhancement of the response. They rarely contribute to homeostasis, but blood clotting and labor contractions are regulated by such mechanisms.

Homeostatic Imbalance (p. 11)

5. With age, the efficiency of negative feedback mechanisms declines, and positive feedback mechanisms occur more frequently. These changes underlie certain disease conditions.

The Language of Anatomy (pp. 11–20)

Anatomical Position and Directional Terms (pp. 11–13)

1. In the anatomical position, the body is erect, facing forward, feet slightly apart, arms at sides with palms forward.
2. Directional terms allow body parts to be located precisely. Terms that describe body directions and orientation include: superior/inferior; anterior/posterior; ventral/dorsal; medial/lateral; intermediate; proximal/distal; and superficial/deep.

Regional Terms (p. 13)

3. Regional terms are used to designate specific areas of the body (see Figure 1.7).

Anatomical Variability (p. 14)

4. People vary internally as well as externally, but extreme variations are rare.

Body Planes and Sections (p. 14)

5. The body or its organs may be cut along planes, or imaginary lines, to produce different types of sections. Frequently used planes are sagittal, frontal, and transverse.

Body Cavities and Membranes (pp. 14–20)

6. The body contains two major closed cavities. The dorsal cavity, subdivided into the cranial and spinal cavities, contains the brain and spinal cord. The ventral cavity is subdivided into the thoracic cavity, which houses the heart and lungs, and the abdominopelvic cavity, which contains the liver, digestive organs, and reproductive structures.
7. The walls of the ventral cavity and the surfaces of the organs it contains are covered with thin membranes, the parietal and visceral serosae, respectively. The serosae produce a thin fluid that decreases friction during organ functioning.
8. The abdominopelvic cavity may be divided by four planes into nine abdominopelvic regions (epigastric, umbilical, hypogastric, right and left iliac, right and left lumbar, and right and left hypochondriac), or by two planes into four quadrants. (For boundaries and organs contained, see Figures 1.11 and 1.12.)
9. There are several smaller body cavities. Most of these are in the head and open to the exterior.

1

Review Questions

Multiple Choice/Matching

(Some questions have more than one correct answer. Select the best answer or answers from the choices given.)

1. The correct sequence of levels forming the structural hierarchy is **(a)** organ, organ system, cellular, chemical, tissue, organismal; **(b)** chemical, cellular, tissue, organismal, organ, organ system; **(c)** chemical, cellular, tissue, organ, organ system, organismal; **(d)** organismal, organ system, organ, tissue, cellular, chemical.
2. The structural and functional unit of life is **(a)** a cell, **(b)** an organ, **(c)** the organism, **(d)** a molecule.
3. Which of the following is a *major* functional characteristic of all organisms? **(a)** movement, **(b)** growth, **(c)** metabolism, **(d)** responsiveness, **(e)** all of these.
4. Two of these organ systems bear the *major* responsibility for ensuring homeostasis of the internal environment. Which two? **(a)** nervous system, **(b)** digestive system, **(c)** cardiovascular system, **(d)** endocrine system, **(e)** reproductive system.
5. In (a)–(e), a directional term [e.g., distal in (a)] is followed by terms indicating different body structures or locations (e.g., the

elbow/the wrist). In each case, choose the structure or organ that matches the given directional term.
(a) distal: the elbow/the wrist
(b) lateral: the hip bone/the umbilicus
(c) superior: the nose/the chin
(d) anterior: the toes/the heel
(e) superficial: the scalp/the skull

6. Assume that the body has been sectioned along three planes: **(1)** a median plane, **(2)** a frontal plane, and **(3)** a transverse plane made at the level of each of the organs listed below. Which organs would be visible in only one or two of these three cases?
(a) urinary bladder, **(b)** brain, **(c)** lungs, **(d)** kidneys, **(e)** small intestine, **(f)** heart.

7. Relate each of the following conditions or statements to either the dorsal body cavity or the ventral body cavity.
(a)surrounded by the bony skull and the vertebral column
(b) includes the thoracic and abdominopelvic cavities
(c) contains the brain and spinal cord
(d) contains the heart, lungs, and digestive organs

8. Which of the following relationships is *incorrect*?
(a) visceral peritoneum/outer surface of small intestine
(b) parietal pericardium/outer surface of heart
(c) parietal pleura/wall of thoracic cavity

9. Which ventral cavity subdivision has no bony protection?
(a) thoracic cavity, **(b)** abdominal cavity, **(c)** pelvic cavity.

10. Terms that apply to the backside of the body in the anatomical position include:
(a) ventral; anterior
(b) back; rear
(c) posterior; dorsal
(d) medial; lateral

Short Answer Essay Questions

11. According to the principle of complementarity, how does anatomy relate to physiology?

12. Construct a table that lists the 11 systems of the body, names two organs of each system (if appropriate), and describes the overall or major function of each system.

13. List and describe briefly five external factors that must be present or provided to sustain life.

14. Define homeostasis.

15. Compare and contrast the operation of negative and positive feedback mechanisms in maintaining homeostasis. Provide two examples of variables controlled by negative feedback mechanisms and one example of a process regulated by a positive feedback mechanism.

16. Why is an understanding of the anatomical position important?

17. Define plane and section.

18. Provide the anatomical term that correctly names each of the following body regions: (a) arm, (b) thigh, (c) chest, (d) fingers and toes, (e) anterior aspect of the knee.

19. Use as many directional terms as you can to describe the relationship between the elbow's olecranal region and your palm.

20. (a) Make a diagram showing the nine abdominopelvic regions, and name each region. Name two organs (or parts of organs) that could be located in each of the named regions. (b) Make a similar sketch illustrating how the abdominopelvic cavity may be divided into quadrants, and name each quadrant.

Critical Thinking and Clinical Application Questions

1. John has been suffering agonizing pain with each breath and has been informed by the physician that he has pleurisy. (a) Specifically, what membranes are involved in this condition? (b) What is their usual role in the body? (c) Explain why John's condition is so painful.

2. At the clinic, Harry was told that blood would be drawn from his antecubital region. What body part was Harry asked to hold out? Later, the nurse came in and gave Harry a shot of penicillin in the area just distal to his acromial region. Did Harry take off his shirt or drop his pants to receive the injection? Before Harry left, the nurse noticed that Harry had a nasty bruise on his gluteal region. What part of his body was black and blue?

3. A man is behaving abnormally, and his physician suspects that he has a brain tumor. Which of the following medical imaging techniques would best localize the tumor in the man's brain (and why)? Conventional X ray, DSA, PET, sonography, MRI.

4. Calcium levels in Mr. Gallariani's blood are dropping to dangerously low levels. The hormone PTH is released and soon blood calcium levels begin to rise. Shortly after, PTH release slows. Is this an example of a positive or negative feedback mechanism? What is the initial stimulus? What is the result?

5. Mr. Harvey, a computer programmer, has been complaining of numbness and pain in his right hand. The nurse practitioner diagnosed his problem as carpal tunnel syndrome and prescribed use of a splint. Where will Mr. Harvey apply the splint?

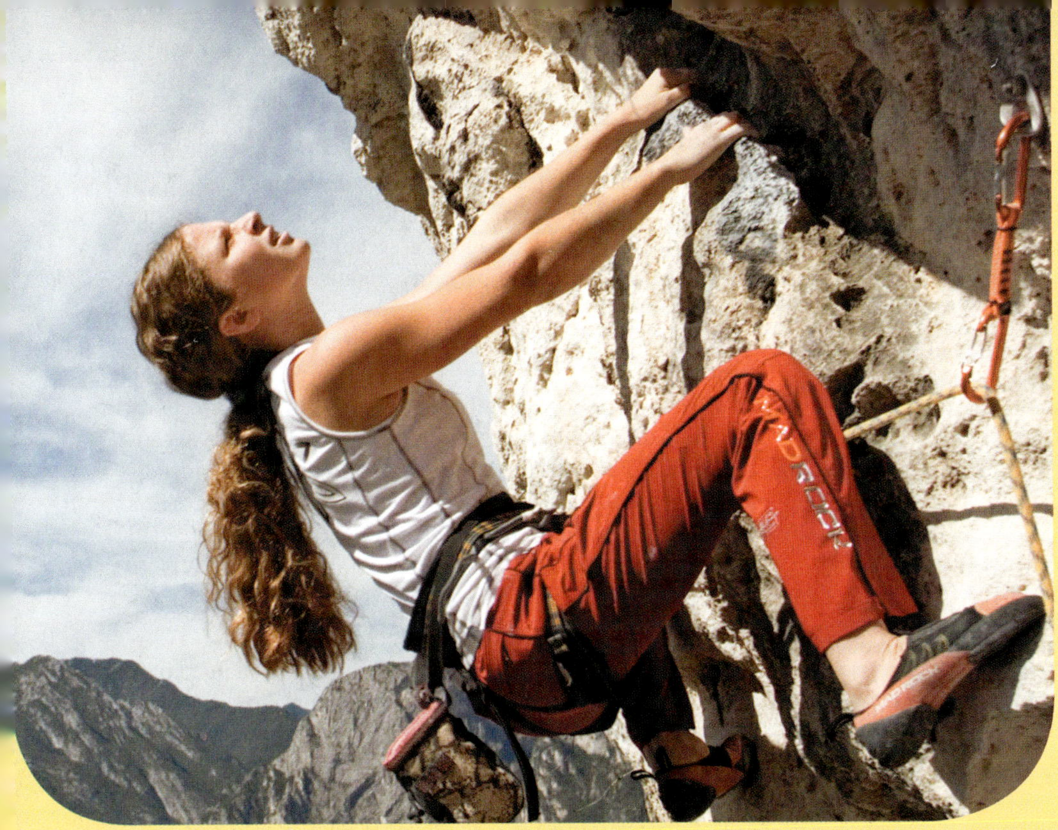

2

Chemistry Comes Alive

Why study chemistry in an anatomy and physiology course? The answer is simple. Your entire body is made up of chemicals, thousands of them, continuously interacting with one another at an incredible pace. Although it is possible to study anatomy without much reference to chemistry, chemical reactions underlie all physiological processes—movement, digestion, the pumping of your heart, and even your thoughts. This chapter presents the basic chemistry and biochemistry (the chemistry of living material) you need to understand body functions.

PART 1
Basic Chemistry

Definition of Concepts: Matter and Energy

✓ Differentiate between matter and energy and between potential energy and kinetic energy.

✓ Describe the major energy forms.

2

Matter

Matter is the "stuff" of the universe. More precisely, **matter** is anything that occupies space and has mass. With some exceptions, it can be seen, smelled, and felt.

For all practical purposes, we can consider mass to be the same as weight. However, this statement is not quite accurate. The *mass* of an object is equal to the actual amount of matter in the object, and it remains constant wherever the object is. In contrast, weight varies with gravity. So while your mass is the same at sea level and on a mountaintop, you weigh just slightly less on that mountaintop. The science of chemistry studies the nature of matter, especially how its building blocks are put together and interact.

States of Matter

Matter exists in *solid*, *liquid*, and *gaseous states*. Examples of each state are found in the human body. Solids, like bones and teeth, have a definite shape and volume. Liquids such as blood plasma have a definite volume, but they conform to the shape of their container. Gases have neither a definite shape nor a definite volume. The air we breathe is a gas.

Energy

Compared with matter, energy is less tangible. It has no mass, does not take up space, and we can measure it only by its effects on matter. **Energy** is defined as the capacity to do work, or to put matter into motion. The greater the work done, the more energy is used doing it. A baseball player who has just hit the ball over the fence uses much more energy than a batter who bunts the ball back to the pitcher.

Kinetic Versus Potential Energy

Energy exists in two forms, or work capacities, and each can be transformed to the other. **Kinetic energy** (ki-net′ik) is energy in action. We see evidence of kinetic energy in the constant movement of the tiniest particles of matter (atoms) as well as in larger objects (a bouncing ball). Kinetic energy does work by moving objects, which in turn can do work by moving or pushing on other objects. For example, a push on a swinging door sets it into motion.

Potential energy is stored energy, that is, inactive energy that has the *potential*, or capability, to do work but is not presently doing so. The batteries in an unused toy have potential energy, as does water confined behind a dam. Your leg muscles have potential energy when you sit still on the couch. When potential energy is released, it becomes kinetic energy and so is capable of doing work. For example, dammed water becomes a rushing torrent when the dam is opened, and that rushing torrent can move a turbine at a hydroelectric plant, or charge a battery.

Actually, energy is a topic of physics, but matter and energy are inseparable. Matter is the substance, and energy is the mover of the substance. All living things are composed of matter and they all require energy to grow and function. The release and use of energy by living systems gives us the elusive quality we call life. Now let's consider the forms of energy used by the body as it does its work.

Forms of Energy

- **Chemical energy** is the form stored in the bonds of chemical substances. When chemical reactions occur that rearrange the atoms of the chemicals in a certain way, the potential energy is unleashed and becomes kinetic energy, or energy in action.

  For example, some of the energy in the foods you eat is eventually converted into the kinetic energy of your moving arm. However, food fuels cannot be used to energize body activities directly. Instead, some of the food energy is captured temporarily in the bonds of a chemical called *adenosine triphosphate* (*ATP*) (ah-den′o-sēn tri″fos′fāt). Later, ATP's bonds are broken and the stored energy is released as needed to do cellular work. Chemical energy in the form of ATP is the most useful form of energy in living systems because it is used to run almost all functional processes.
- **Electrical energy** results from the movement of charged particles. In your home, electrical energy is found in the flow of electrons along the household wiring. In your body, electrical currents are generated when charged particles called *ions* move along or across cell membranes. The nervous system uses electrical currents, called *nerve impulses*, to transmit messages from one part of the body to another. Electrical currents traveling across the heart stimulate it to contract (beat) and pump blood. (This is why a strong electrical shock, which interferes with such currents, can cause death.)
- **Mechanical energy** is energy *directly* involved in moving matter. When you ride a bicycle, your legs provide the mechanical energy that moves the pedals.
- **Radiant energy**, or **electromagnetic energy** (e-lek″tro-mag-net′ik), is energy that travels in waves. These waves, which vary in length, are collectively called the *electromagnetic spectrum*. They include visible light, infrared waves, radio waves, ultraviolet waves, and X rays. Light energy, which stimulates the retinas of our eyes, is important in vision. Ultraviolet waves cause sunburn, but they also stimulate your body to make vitamin D.

Energy Form Conversions

With few exceptions, energy is easily converted from one form to another. For example, the chemical energy (in gasoline) that powers the motor of a speedboat is converted into the mechanical energy of the whirling propeller that makes the boat skim across the water.

Energy conversions are quite inefficient. Some of the initial energy supply is always "lost" to the environment as heat. (It is not really lost because energy cannot be created or destroyed, but that portion given off as heat is at least partly *unusable*.) It is easy to demonstrate this principle. Electrical energy is converted into light energy in a lightbulb. But if you touch a lit bulb, you will soon discover that some of the electrical energy is producing heat instead.

Likewise, all energy conversions in the body liberate heat. This heat helps to maintain our relatively high body temperature, which influences body functioning. For example, when matter is heated, the kinetic energy of its particles increases and they begin to move more quickly. The higher the temperature, the faster the body's chemical reactions occur. We will learn more about this later.

☑ Check Your Understanding

1. What form of energy is found in the food we eat?
2. What form of energy is used to transmit messages from one part of the body to another?
3. What type of energy is available when we are still? When we are exercising?

For answers, see Appendix H.

Composition of Matter: Atoms and Elements

✓ Define chemical element and list the four elements that form the bulk of body matter.

✓ Define atom. List the subatomic particles, and describe their relative masses, charges, and positions in the atom.

✓ Define atomic number, atomic mass, atomic weight, isotope, and radioisotope.

All matter is composed of **elements**, unique substances that cannot be broken down into simpler substances by ordinary chemical methods. Among the well-known elements are oxygen, carbon, gold, silver, copper, and iron.

At present, 118 elements are recognized. Of these, 92 occur in nature. The rest are made artificially in particle accelerator devices.

Four elements—carbon, oxygen, hydrogen, and nitrogen—make up about 96% of body weight, and 20 others are present in the body, some in trace amounts. Table 2.1 on p. 26 lists the elements contributing to body mass and gives their importance. In Appendix E, an oddly shaped checkerboard called the **periodic table** provides a more complete listing of the known elements and helps to explain the properties of each element that make it react as it does with other elements.

Each element is composed of more or less identical particles or building blocks, called **atoms**. The smallest atoms are less than 0.1 nanometer (nm) in diameter, and the largest are only about five times as large. [1 nm = 0.0000001 (or 10^{-7}) centimeter (cm), or 40 billionths of an inch!]

Every element's atoms differ from those of all other elements and give the element its unique physical and chemical properties. *Physical properties* are those we can detect with our senses (such as color and texture) or measure (such as boiling point and freezing point). *Chemical properties* pertain to the way atoms interact with other atoms (bonding behavior) and account for the facts that iron rusts, animals can digest their food, and so on.

We designate each element by a one- or two-letter chemical shorthand called an **atomic symbol**, usually the first letter(s) of the element's name. For example, C stands for carbon, O for oxygen, and Ca for calcium. In a few cases, the atomic symbol is taken from the Latin name for the element. For example, sodium is indicated by Na, from the Latin word *natrium*.

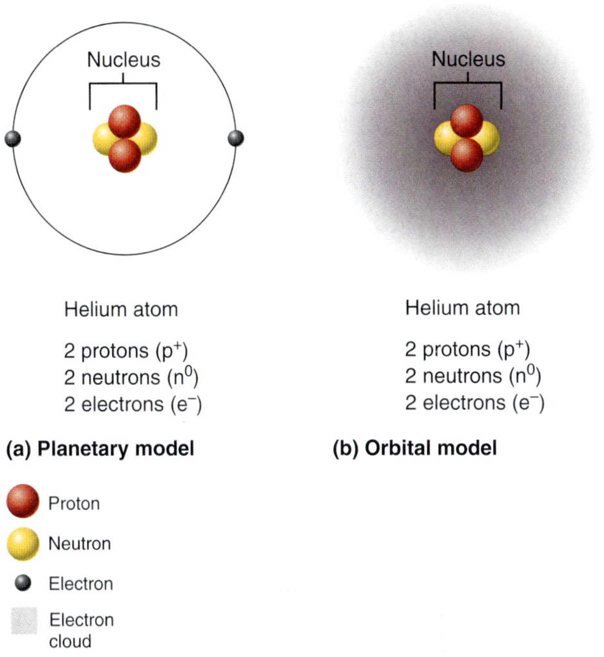

Figure 2.1 Two models of the structure of an atom.

Atomic Structure

The word *atom* comes from the Greek word meaning "indivisible." However, we now know that atoms are clusters of even smaller particles called protons, neutrons, and electrons and that even those subatomic particles can be subdivided with high-technology tools. Still, the old idea of atomic indivisibility is useful because an atom loses the unique properties of its element when it is split into its subatomic particles.

An atom's subatomic particles differ in mass, electrical charge, and position in the atom. An atom has a central **nucleus** containing protons and neutrons tightly bound together. The nucleus, in turn, is surrounded by orbiting electrons (Figure 2.1). **Protons** (p^+) bear a positive electrical charge, and **neutrons** (n^0) are neutral, so the nucleus is positively charged overall. Protons and neutrons are heavy particles and have approximately the same mass, arbitrarily designated as 1 **atomic mass unit** (1 amu). Since all of the heavy subatomic particles are concentrated in the nucleus, the nucleus is fantastically dense. It accounts for nearly the entire mass (99.9%) of the atom.

The tiny **electrons** (e^-) bear a negative charge equal in strength to the positive charge of the proton. However, an electron has only about 1/2000 the mass of a proton, and the mass of an electron is usually designated as 0 amu.

All atoms are electrically neutral because the number of protons in an atom is precisely balanced by its number of electrons (the + and − charges will then cancel the effect of each other). For example, hydrogen has one proton and one electron, and iron has 26 protons and 26 electrons. For any atom, the number of protons and electrons is always equal.

2

Table 2.1 Common Elements Composing the Human Body*

ELEMENT	ATOMIC SYMBOL	APPROX. % BODY MASS†	FUNCTIONS
Major (96.1%)			
Oxygen	O	65.0	A major component of both organic (carbon-containing) and inorganic (non-carbon-containing) molecules. As a gas, it is needed for the production of cellular energy (ATP).
Carbon	C	18.5	A primary component of all organic molecules, which include carbohydrates, lipids (fats), proteins, and nucleic acids.
Hydrogen	H	9.5	A component of all organic molecules. As an ion (proton), it influences the pH of body fluids.
Nitrogen	N	3.2	A component of proteins and nucleic acids (genetic material).
Lesser (3.9%)			
Calcium	Ca	1.5	Found as a salt in bones and teeth. Its ionic (Ca^{2+}) form is required for muscle contraction, conduction of nerve impulses, and blood clotting.
Phosphorus	P	1.0	Part of calcium phosphate salts in bones and teeth. Also present in nucleic acids, and part of ATP.
Potassium	K	0.4	Its ion (K^+) is the major positive ion (cation) in cells. Necessary for conduction of nerve impulses and muscle contraction.
Sulfur	S	0.3	Component of proteins, particularly muscle proteins.
Sodium	Na	0.2	As an ion (Na^+), sodium is the major positive ion found in extracellular fluids (fluids outside of cells). Important for water balance, conduction of nerve impulses, and muscle contraction.
Chlorine	Cl	0.2	Its ion (chloride, Cl^-) is the most abundant negative ion (anion) in extracellular fluids.
Magnesium	Mg	0.1	Present in bone. Also an important cofactor in a number of metabolic reactions.
Iodine	I	0.1	Needed to make functional thyroid hormones.
Iron	Fe	0.1	Component of hemoglobin (which transports oxygen within red blood cells) and some enzymes.
Trace (less than 0.01%)			
Chromium (Cr); cobalt (Co); copper (Cu); fluorine (F); manganese (Mn); molybdenum (Mo); selenium (Se); silicon (Si); tin (Sn); vanadium (V); zinc (Zn)			
These elements are referred to as *trace elements* because they are required in very minute amounts; many are found as part of enzymes or are required for enzyme activation.			

*A listing of the elements by ascending order of atomic number appears in the periodic table, Appendix E.

†Percentage of "wet" body mass; includes water.

The **planetary model** of the atom, illustrated in Figure 2.1a, is a simplified (and now outdated) model of atomic structure. As you can see, it depicts electrons moving around the nucleus in fixed, generally circular orbits. But we can never determine the exact location of electrons at a particular time because they jump around following unknown trajectories. So, instead of speaking of specific orbits, chemists talk about **orbitals**—regions around the nucleus in which a given electron or electron pair is likely to be found most of the time. This more modern model of atomic structure, called the **orbital model**, is more useful for predicting the chemical behavior of atoms. As illustrated in Figure 2.1b, the orbital model depicts *probable* regions of greatest electron density by denser shading (this haze is called the *electron cloud*). However, the planetary model is simpler to depict, so we will use that model in most illustrations of atomic structure in this text.

Hydrogen, with just one proton and one electron, is the simplest atom. You can visualize the spatial relationships in the hydrogen atom by imagining it as a sphere enlarged until its diameter equals the length of a football field. In that case, the nucleus could be represented by a lead ball the size of a gumdrop in the exact center of the sphere. Its lone electron could be pictured as a fly buzzing about unpredictably within the sphere. Though not completely accurate, this mental image demonstrates that most of the volume of an atom is empty space, and nearly all of its mass is concentrated in the central nucleus.

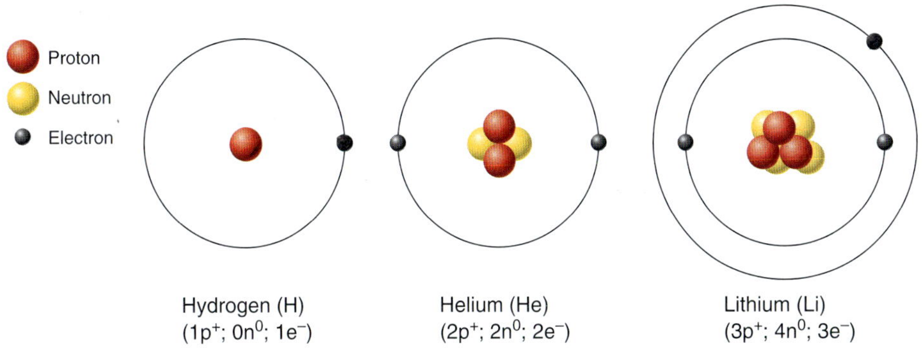

Figure 2.2 Atomic structure of the three smallest atoms.

Identifying Elements

All protons are alike, regardless of the atom considered. The same is true of all neutrons and all electrons. So what determines the unique properties of each element? The answer is that atoms of different elements are composed of *different numbers* of protons, neutrons, and electrons.

The simplest and smallest atom, hydrogen, has one proton, one electron, and no neutrons **(Figure 2.2)**. Next in size is the helium atom, with two protons, two neutrons, and two orbiting electrons. Lithium follows with three protons, four neutrons, and three electrons. If we continued this step-by-step progression, we would get a graded series of atoms containing from 1 to 112 protons, an equal number of electrons, and a slightly larger number of neutrons at each step.

All we really need to know to identify a particular element, however, are its atomic number, mass number, and atomic weight. Taken together, these provide a fairly complete picture of each element.

Atomic Number

The **atomic number** of any atom is equal to the number of protons in its nucleus and is written as a subscript to the left of its atomic symbol. Hydrogen, with one proton, has an atomic number of 1 ($_1$H). Helium, with two protons, has an atomic number of 2 ($_2$He), and so on. The number of protons is always equal to the number of electrons in an atom, so the atomic number *indirectly* tells us the number of electrons in the atom as well. As we will see shortly, this information is important indeed, because electrons determine the chemical behavior of atoms.

Mass Number and Isotopes

The **mass number** of an atom is the sum of the masses of its protons and neutrons. The mass of the electrons is so small that it is ignored. Recall that protons and neutrons have a mass of 1 amu. Hydrogen has only one proton in its nucleus, so its atomic and mass numbers are the same: 1. Helium, with two protons and two neutrons, has a mass number of 4.

The mass number is usually indicated by a superscript to the left of the atomic symbol. For example, helium is $^4_2$He. This simple notation allows us to deduce the total number and kinds of subatomic particles in any atom because it indicates the number of protons (the atomic number), the number of electrons (equal to the atomic number), and the number of neutrons (mass number minus atomic number). In our example, we can do the subtraction to find that $^4_2$He has two neutrons.

From what we have said so far, it may appear as if each element has one, and only one, type of atom representing it. This is not the case. Nearly all known elements have two or more structural variations called **isotopes** (iso-tōps), which have the same number of protons (and electrons), but differ in the number of neutrons they contain. Earlier, when we said that hydrogen has a mass number of 1, we were speaking of ^{1}H, its most abundant isotope. Some hydrogen atoms have a mass of 2 or 3 amu (atomic mass units), which means that they have one proton and, respectively, one or two neutrons **(Figure 2.3)**.

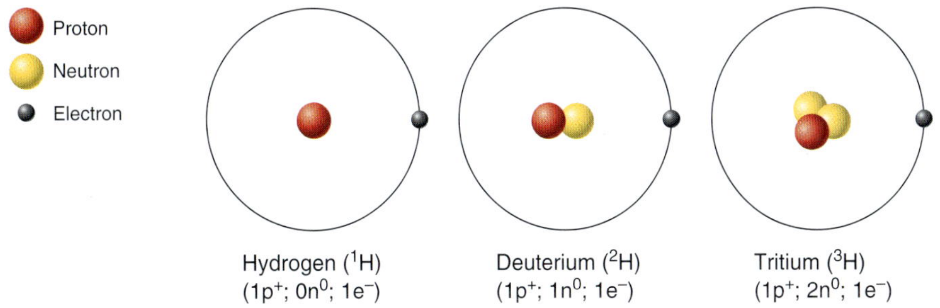

Figure 2.3 Isotopes of hydrogen.

Carbon has several isotopes. The most abundant of these are ^{12}C, ^{13}C, and ^{14}C. Each of the carbon isotopes has six protons (otherwise it would not be carbon), but ^{12}C has six neutrons, ^{13}C has seven, and ^{14}C has eight. Isotopes can also be written with the mass number following the symbol: C-14, for example.

2

Atomic Weight

You might think that atomic weight should be the same as atomic mass, and this would be so if atomic weight referred to the weight of a single atom. However, **atomic weight** is an average of the relative weights (mass numbers) of *all* the isotopes of an element, taking into account their relative abundance in nature. As a rule, the atomic weight of an element is approximately equal to the mass number of its most abundant isotope. For example, the atomic weight of hydrogen is 1.008, which reveals that its lightest isotope (^{1}H) is present in much greater amounts in our world than its ^{2}H or ^{3}H forms.

Radioisotopes

The heavier isotopes of many elements are unstable, and their atoms decompose spontaneously into more stable forms. This process of atomic decay is called *radioactivity*, and isotopes that exhibit this behavior are called **radioisotopes** (ra″de-o-i′so-tōps). The disintegration of a radioactive nucleus may be compared to a tiny explosion. It occurs when subatomic *alpha* (α) *particles* (packets of 2p + 2n), *beta* (β) *particles* (electron-like negative particles), or *gamma* (γ) *rays* (electromagnetic energy) are ejected from the atomic nucleus.

Why does this happen? The answer is complex, but for our purposes, the important point to know is that the dense nuclear particles are composed of even smaller particles called *quarks* that associate in one way to form protons and in another way to form neutrons. Apparently, the "glue" that holds these nuclear particles together is weaker in the heavier isotopes. When radioisotopes disintegrate, the element may transform to a different element.

Because we can detect radioactivity with scanners, and radioactive isotopes share the same chemistry as their more stable isotopes, radioisotopes are valuable tools for biological research and medicine. Most radioisotopes used in the clinical setting are used for diagnosis, that is, to localize and illuminate damaged or cancerous tissues. For example, iodine-131 is used to determine the size and activity of the thyroid gland and to detect thyroid cancer. The sophisticated PET scans described in *A Closer Look* in Chapter 1 use radioisotopes to probe the workings of molecules deep within our bodies. All radioisotopes, regardless of the purpose for which they are used, damage living tissue, and all radioisotopes gradually lose their radioactive behavior. The time required for a radioisotope to lose one-half of its activity is called its *half-life*. The half-lives of radioisotopes vary dramatically from hours to thousands of years.

Alpha emission is easily blocked outside the body but if absorbed causes considerable damage. For this reason, inhaled alpha particles from decaying radon are second only to smoking as a cause of lung cancer. (Radon results naturally from decay of uranium in the ground.) Gamma emission has the greatest penetrating power. Radium-226, cobalt-60, and certain other radioisotopes that decay by gamma emission are used to destroy localized cancers.

Contrary to what some believe, ionizing radiation does not damage organic molecules directly. Instead, it knocks electrons out of other atoms and sends them flying, like bowling balls smashing through pins all along their path. It is the electron energy and the unstable molecules left behind that do the damage.

☑ Check Your Understanding

4. What two elements besides H and N make up the bulk of living matter?
5. An element has a mass of 207 and has 125 neutrons in its nucleus. How many protons and electrons does it have and where are they located?
6. How do the terms atomic mass and atomic weight differ?

For answers, see Appendix H.

How Matter Is Combined: Molecules and Mixtures

✓ Define molecule, and distinguish between a compound and a mixture.

✓ Compare solutions, colloids, and suspensions.

Molecules and Compounds

Most atoms do not exist in the free state, but instead are chemically combined with other atoms. Such a combination of two or more atoms held together by chemical bonds is called a **molecule**.

If two or more atoms of the *same* element combine, the resulting substance is called a *molecule of that element*. When two hydrogen atoms bond, the product is a molecule of hydrogen gas and is written as H_2. Similarly, when two oxygen atoms combine, a molecule of oxygen gas (O_2) is formed. Sulfur atoms commonly combine to form sulfur molecules containing eight sulfur atoms (S_8).

When two or more *different* kinds of atoms bind, they form molecules of a **compound**. Two hydrogen atoms combine with one oxygen atom to form the compound water (H_2O). Four hydrogen atoms combine with one carbon atom to form the compound methane (CH_4). Notice again that molecules of methane and water are compounds, but molecules of hydrogen gas are not, because compounds always contain atoms of at least two different elements.

Compounds are chemically pure, and all of their molecules are identical. So, just as an atom is the smallest particle of an element that still has the properties of the element, a molecule is the smallest particle of a compound that still has the specific

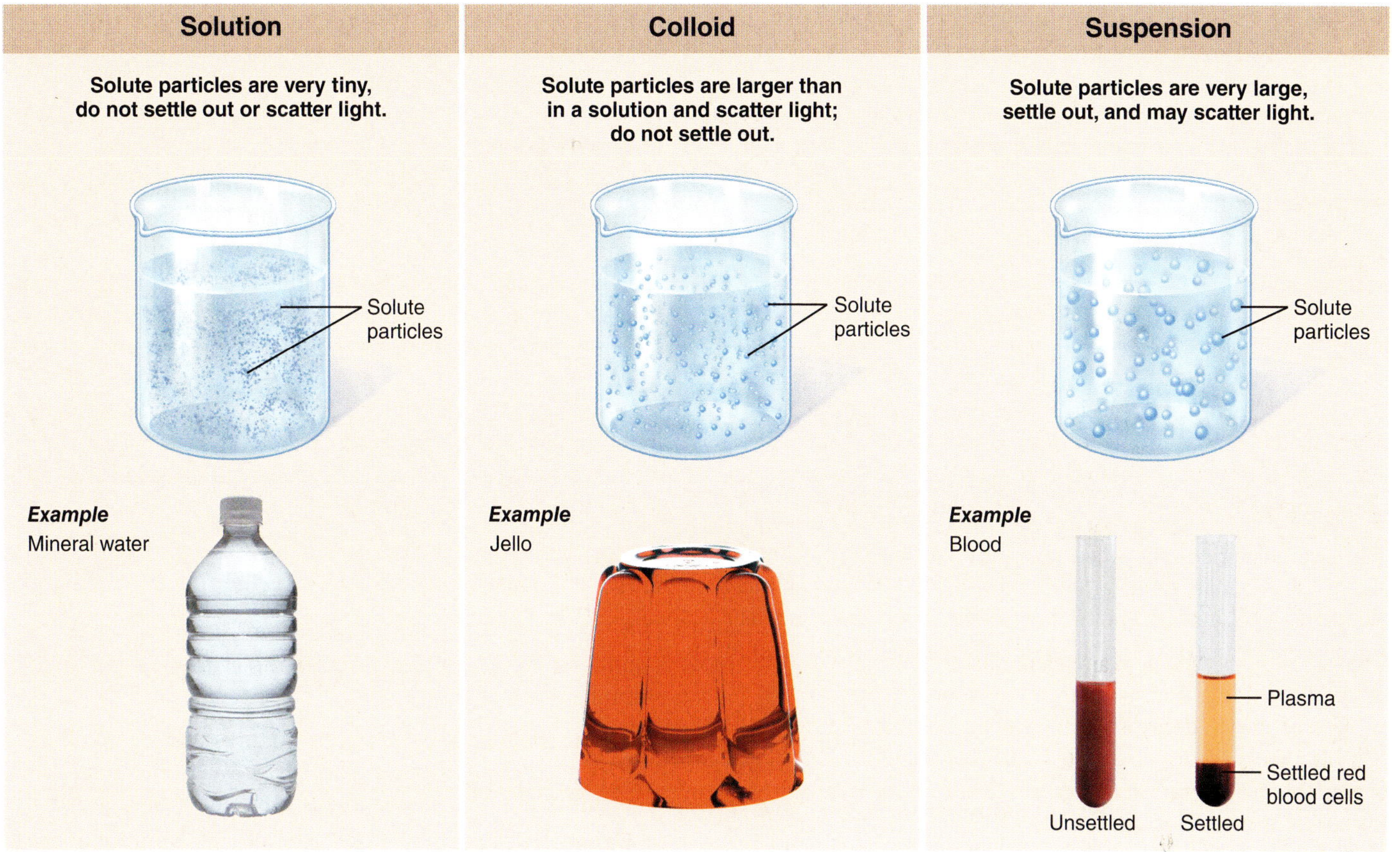

Figure 2.4 **The three basic types of mixtures.**

characteristics of the compound. This concept is important because the properties of compounds are usually very different from those of the atoms they contain. Water, for example, is very different from the elements hydrogen and oxygen. Indeed, it is next to impossible to tell what atoms are in a compound without analyzing it chemically.

Mixtures

Mixtures are substances composed of two or more components *physically intermixed*. Most matter in nature exists in the form of mixtures, but there are only three basic types: *solutions*, *colloids*, and *suspensions* **(Figure 2.4)**.

Solutions

Solutions are homogeneous mixtures of components that may be gases, liquids, or solids. *Homogeneous* means that the mixture has exactly the same composition or makeup throughout—a sample taken from any part of the mixture has the same composition (in terms of the atoms or molecules it contains) as a sample taken from any other part of the mixture. Examples include the air we breathe (a mixture of gases) and seawater (a mixture of salts, which are solids, and water). The substance present in the greatest amount is called the **solvent** (or dissolving medium). Solvents are usually liquids. Substances present in smaller amounts are called **solutes**.

Water is the body's chief solvent. Most solutions in the body are *true solutions* containing gases, liquids, or solids dissolved in water. True solutions are usually transparent. Examples are saline solution [table salt (NaCl) and water], a mixture of glucose and water, and mineral water. The solutes of true solutions are minute, usually in the form of individual atoms and molecules. Consequently, they are not visible to the naked eye, do not settle out, and do not scatter light. In other words, if a beam of light is passed through a true solution, you will not see the path of light.

Concentration of Solutions We describe true solutions in terms of their *concentration*, which may be indicated in various ways. Solutions used in a college laboratory or a hospital are often described in terms of the **percent** (parts per 100 parts) of the solute in the total solution. This designation always refers to the solute percentage, and unless otherwise noted, water is assumed to be the solvent.

Milligrams per deciliter (*mg/dl*) is another common concentration measurement. (A deciliter is 100 milliliters or 0.1 liter.)

Still another way to express the concentration of a solution is in terms of its **molarity** (mo-lar′ĭ-te), or moles per liter, indicated by *M*. This method is more complicated but much more useful. To understand molarity, you must understand what a mole is. A **mole** of any element or compound is equal to its atomic weight or **molecular weight** (sum of the atomic weights) weighed out in grams. This concept is easier than it seems, as illustrated by the following example.

Glucose is $C_6H_{12}O_6$, which indicates that it has 6 carbon atoms, 12 hydrogen atoms, and 6 oxygen atoms. To compute the molecular weight of glucose, you would look up the atomic weight of each of its atoms in the periodic table (see Appendix E) and compute its molecular weight as follows:

Atom	Number of Atoms		Atomic Weight		Total Atomic Weight
C	6	×	12.011	=	72.066
H	12	×	1.008	=	12.096
O	6	×	15.999	=	95.994
					180.156

Then, to make a *one-molar* solution of glucose, you would weigh out 180.156 grams (g), called a *gram molecular weight*, of glucose and add enough water to make 1 liter (L) of solution. In short, a one-molar solution (abbreviated 1.0 *M*) of a chemical substance is one gram molecular weight of the substance (or one gram atomic weight in the case of elemental substances) in 1 L (1000 milliliters) of solution.

The beauty of using the mole as the basis of preparing solutions is its precision. One mole of any substance always contains exactly the same number of solute particles, that is, 6.02×10^{23}. This number is called **Avogadro's number** (av″o-gad′rōz). So whether you weigh out 1 mole of glucose (180 g) or 1 mole of water (18 g) or 1 mole of methane (16 g), in each case you will have 6.02×10^{23} molecules of that substance.* This allows almost mind-boggling precision to be achieved.

Because solute concentrations in body fluids tend to be quite low, those values are usually reported in terms of millimoles (m*M*; 1/1000 mole).

Colloids

Colloids (kol′oidz), also called *emulsions*, are *heterogeneous* mixtures, which means that their composition is dissimilar in different areas of the mixture. Colloids often appear translucent or milky and although the solute particles are larger than those in true solutions, they still do not settle out. However, they do scatter light, so the path of a light beam shining through a colloidal mixture is visible.

Colloids have many unique properties, including the ability of some to undergo **sol-gel transformations**, that is, to change reversibly from a fluid (sol) state to a more solid (gel) state. Jell-O, or any gelatin product (Figure 2.4), is a familiar example of a nonliving colloid that changes from a sol to a gel when refrigerated (and that gel will liquefy again if placed in the sun). Cytosol, the semifluid material in living cells, is also a colloid, largely because of its dispersed proteins. Its sol-gel transformations underlie many important cell activities, such as cell division and changes in cell shape.

Suspensions

Suspensions are *heterogeneous* mixtures with large, often visible solutes that tend to settle out. An example of a suspension is a mixture of sand and water. So is blood, in which the living blood cells are suspended in the fluid portion of blood (blood plasma). If left to stand, the suspended cells will settle out unless some means—mixing, shaking, or circulation in the body—keeps them in suspension.

As you can see, all three types of mixtures are found in both living and nonliving systems. In fact, living material is the most complex mixture of all, since it contains all three kinds of mixtures interacting with one another.

Distinguishing Mixtures from Compounds

Now let's zero in on how to distinguish mixtures and compounds from one another. Mixtures differ from compounds in several important ways:

- The chief difference between mixtures and compounds is that no chemical bonding occurs between the components of a mixture. The properties of atoms and molecules are not changed when they become part of a mixture. Remember they are only physically intermixed.
- Depending on the mixture, its components can be separated by physical means—straining, filtering, evaporation, and so on. Compounds, by contrast, can be separated into their constituent atoms only by chemical means (breaking bonds).
- Some mixtures are homogeneous, whereas others are heterogeneous. A bar of 100% pure (elemental) iron is homogeneous, as are all compounds. As already mentioned, heterogeneous substances vary in their makeup from place to place. For example, iron ore is a heterogeneous mixture that contains iron and many other elements.

☑ Check Your Understanding

7. What is the meaning of the term "molecule"?
8. Why is sodium chloride (NaCl) considered a compound, but oxygen gas is not?
9. Blood contains a liquid component and living cells. Would it be classified as a compound or a mixture? Why?

For answers, see Appendix H.

Chemical Bonds

✓ Explain the role of electrons in chemical bonding and in relation to the octet rule.

✓ Differentiate among ionic, covalent, and hydrogen bonds.

✓ Compare and contrast polar and nonpolar compounds.

*The important exception to this rule concerns molecules that ionize and break up into charged particles (ions) in water, such as salts, acids, and bases (see p. 39). For example, simple table salt (sodium chloride) breaks up into two types of charged particles. Therefore, in a 1.0 *M* solution of sodium chloride, 2 *moles* of solute particles are actually in solution.

As noted earlier, when atoms combine with other atoms, they are held together by **chemical bonds**. A chemical bond is not a physical structure like a pair of handcuffs linking two people together. Instead, it is an energy relationship between the electrons of the reacting atoms, and it is made or broken in less than a trillionth of a second.

The Role of Electrons in Chemical Bonding

Electrons forming the electron cloud around the nucleus of an atom occupy regions of space called **electron shells** that consecutively surround the atomic nucleus. The atoms known so far can have electrons in seven shells (numbered 1 to 7 from the nucleus outward), but the actual number of electron shells occupied in a given atom depends on the number of electrons that atom has. Each electron shell contains one or more orbitals. (Recall from our earlier discussion that *orbitals* are regions around the nucleus in which a given electron is likely to be found most of the time.)

It is important to understand that each electron shell represents a different **energy level**, because this prompts you to think of electrons as particles with a certain amount of potential energy. In general, the terms *electron shell* and *energy level* are used interchangeably.

How much potential energy does an electron have? The answer depends on the energy level that it occupies. The attraction between the positively charged nucleus and negatively charged electrons is greatest when electrons are closest to the nucleus and falls off with increasing distance. This statement explains why electrons farthest from the nucleus (1) have the greatest potential energy (it takes more energy for them to overcome the nuclear attraction and reach the more distant energy levels) and (2) are most likely to interact chemically with other atoms. (They are the least tightly held by their own atomic nucleus and the most easily influenced by other atoms and molecules.)

Each electron shell can hold a specific number of electrons. Shell 1, the shell immediately surrounding the nucleus, accommodates only 2 electrons. Shell 2 holds a maximum of 8, and shell 3 has room for 18. Subsequent shells hold larger and larger numbers of electrons, and the shells tend to be filled with electrons consecutively. For example, shell 1 fills completely before any electrons appear in shell 2.

Which electrons are involved in chemical bonding? When we consider bonding behavior, the only electrons that are important are those in the atom's outermost energy level. Inner electrons usually do not take part in bonding because they are more tightly held by the atomic nucleus.

When the outermost energy level of an atom is filled to capacity or contains eight electrons, the atom is stable. Such atoms are *chemically inert*, that is, unreactive. A group of elements called the *noble gases*, which include helium and neon, typify this condition **(Figure 2.5a)**. On the other hand, atoms in which the outermost energy level contains fewer than eight electrons tend to gain, lose, or share electrons with other atoms to achieve stability (Figure 2.5b).

What about atoms that have more than 20 electrons, in which the energy levels beyond shell 2 can contain *more* than eight electrons? The number of electrons that can participate in bonding is still limited to a total of eight. The term **valence shell** (va′lens) specifically indicates an atom's outermost energy level *or that portion of it* containing the electrons that are chemically reactive. Hence, the key to chemical reactivity is the **octet rule** (ok-tet′), or **rule of eights**. Except for shell 1, which is full when it has two electrons, atoms tend to interact in such a way that they have eight electrons in their valence shell.

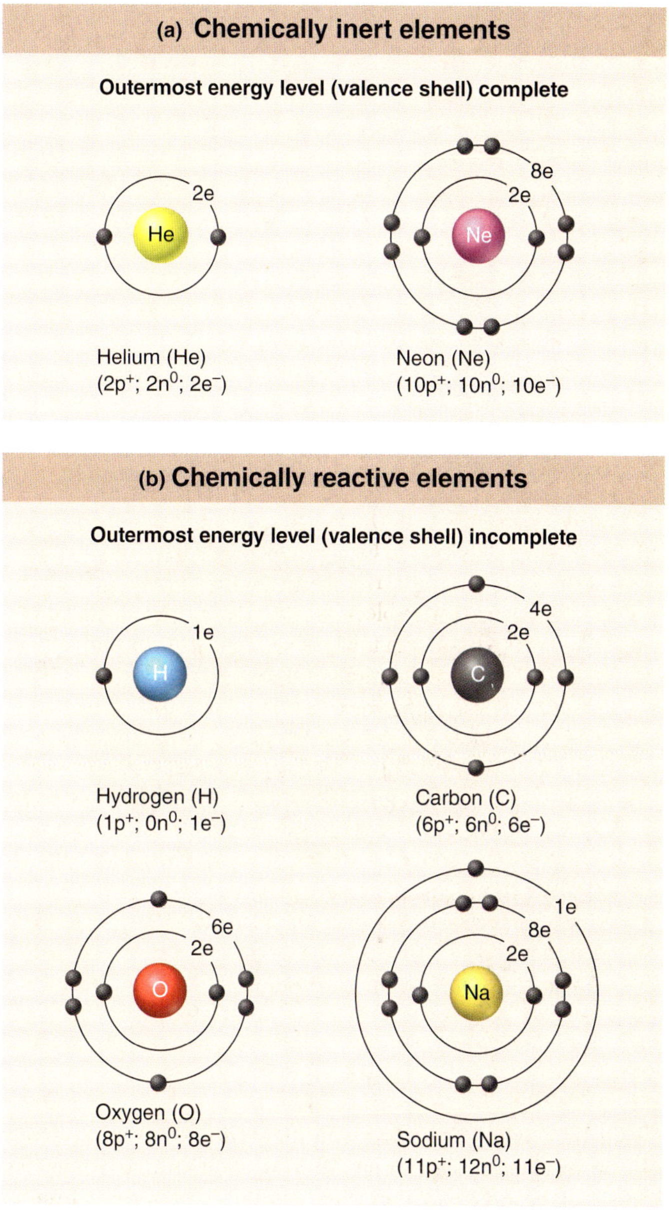

Figure 2.5 Chemically inert and reactive elements. (*Note*: For simplicity, each atomic nucleus is shown as a sphere with the atom's symbol; individual protons and neutrons are not shown.)

Types of Chemical Bonds

Three major types of chemical bonds—*ionic*, *covalent*, and *hydrogen bonds*—result from attractive forces between atoms.

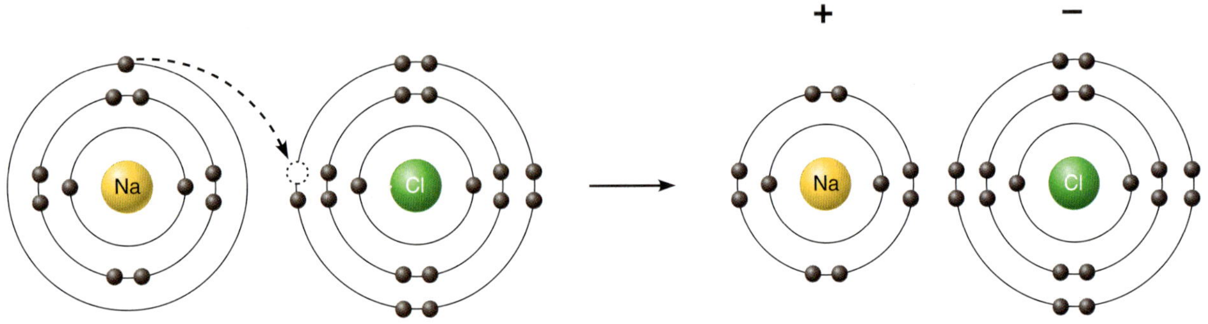

(a) Sodium gains stability by losing one electron, and chlorine becomes stable by gaining one electron.

(b) After electron transfer, the oppositely charged ions formed attract each other.

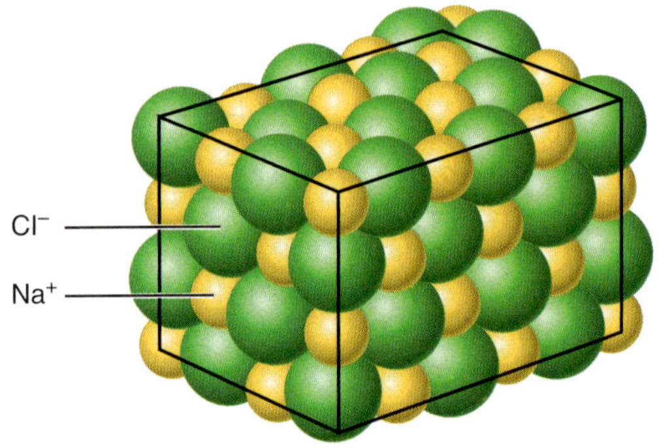

(c) Large numbers of Na^+ and Cl^- ions associate to form salt (NaCl) crystals.

Figure 2.6 Formation of an ionic bond.

Ionic Bonds

Recall that atoms are electrically neutral. However, electrons can be transferred from one atom to another, and when this happens, the precise balance of + and − charges is lost so that charged particles called **ions** are formed. An **ionic bond** (i-on′ik) is a chemical bond between atoms formed by the transfer of one or more electrons from one atom to the other. The atom that gains one or more electrons is the *electron acceptor*. It acquires a net negative charge and is called an **anion** (an′i-on). The atom that loses electrons is the *electron donor*. It acquires a net positive charge and is called a **cation** (kat′i-on). (To remember this term, think of the "t" in "cation" as a + sign.) Both anions and cations are formed whenever electron transfer between atoms occurs. Because opposite charges attract, these ions tend to stay close together, resulting in an ionic bond.

One example of ionic bonding is the formation of table salt, or sodium chloride (NaCl), by interaction of sodium and chlorine atoms **(Figure 2.6)**. Sodium, with an atomic number of 11, has only one electron in its valence shell. It would be very difficult to attempt to fill this shell by adding seven more. However, if this single electron is lost, shell 2 with eight electrons becomes the valence shell (outermost energy level containing electrons) and is full. Thus, by losing the lone electron in its third energy level, sodium achieves stability and becomes a cation (Na^+). On the other hand, chlorine, atomic number 17, needs only one electron to fill its valence shell. By accepting an electron, chlorine achieves stability and becomes an anion.

When sodium and chlorine atoms interact, this is exactly what happens. Sodium donates an electron to chlorine (Figure 2.6a), and the oppositely charged ions created in this exchange attract each other, forming sodium chloride (Figure 2.6b). Ionic bonds are commonly formed between atoms with one or two valence shell electrons (the metallic elements, such as sodium, calcium, and potassium) and atoms with seven valence shell electrons (such as chlorine, fluorine, and iodine).

Most ionic compounds fall in the chemical category called *salts*. In the dry state, salts such as sodium chloride do not exist as individual molecules. Instead, they form **crystals**, large arrays of cations and anions held together by ionic bonds (Figure 2.6c).

Sodium chloride is an excellent example of the difference in properties between a compound and its constituent atoms. Sodium is a silvery white metal, and chlorine in its molecular state is a poisonous green gas used to make bleach. However, sodium chloride is a white crystalline solid that we sprinkle on our food.

Covalent Bonds

Electrons do not have to be completely transferred for atoms to achieve stability. Instead, they may be *shared* so that each atom is able to fill its outer electron shell at least part of the time. Electron sharing produces molecules in which the shared electrons occupy a single orbital common to both atoms, which constitutes a **covalent bond** (ko-va′lent).

Hydrogen with its single electron can fill its only shell (shell 1) by sharing a pair of electrons with another atom. When it shares with another hydrogen atom, a molecule of hydrogen gas is formed. The shared electron pair orbits around the molecule as a whole, satisfying the stability needs of each atom.

Hydrogen can also share an electron pair with different kinds of atoms to form a compound **(Figure 2.7a)**. Carbon has four electrons in its outermost shell, but needs eight to achieve stability. Hydrogen has one electron, but needs two. When a methane

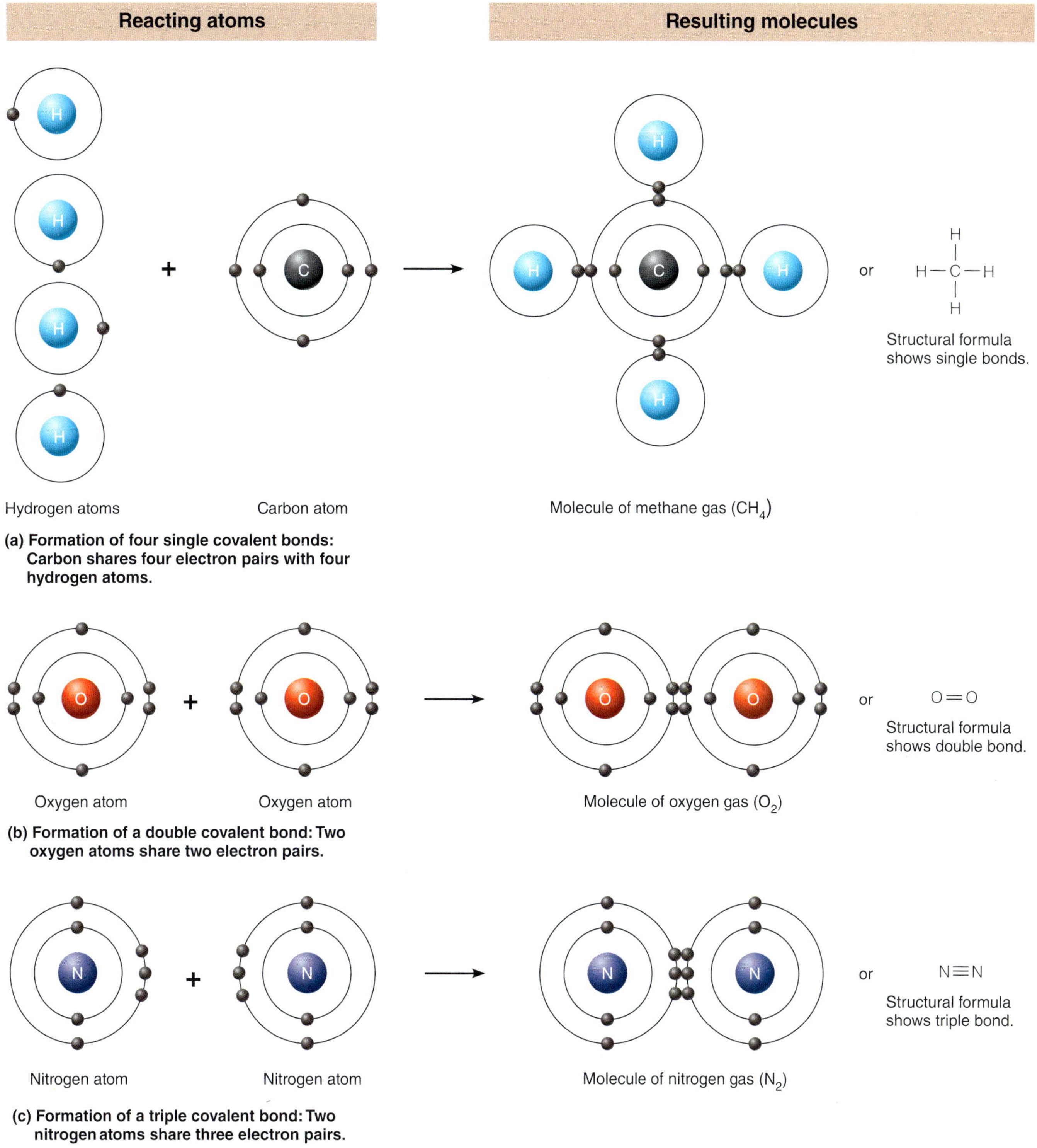

Figure 2.7 Formation of covalent bonds.

molecule (CH_4) is formed, carbon shares four pairs of electrons with four hydrogen atoms (one pair with each hydrogen). Again, the shared electrons orbit and "belong to" the whole molecule, ensuring the stability of each atom.

When two atoms share one pair of electrons, a single covalent bond is formed (indicated by a single line connecting the atoms, such as H—H). In some cases, atoms share two or three electron pairs, resulting in *double* or *triple covalent bonds* (Figure 2.7b and c). (These bonds are indicated by double or triple connecting lines such as O=O or N≡N.)

Polar and Nonpolar Molecules In the covalent bonds we have discussed, the shared electrons are shared equally between the atoms of the molecule for the most part. The molecules formed

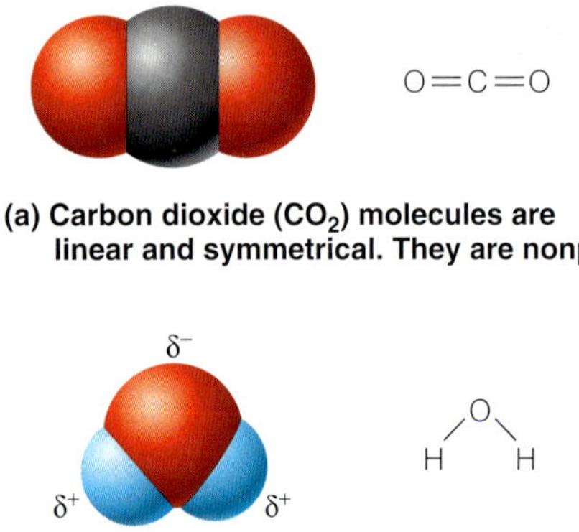

(a) Carbon dioxide (CO_2) molecules are linear and symmetrical. They are nonpolar.

(b) V-shaped water (H_2O) molecules have two poles of charge—a slightly more negative oxygen end (δ^-) and a slightly more positive hydrogen end (δ^+).

Figure 2.8 Carbon dioxide and water molecules have different shapes, as illustrated by molecular models.

Ionic bond	Polar covalent bond	Nonpolar covalent bond
Complete transfer of electrons	Unequal sharing of electrons	Equal sharing of electrons
Separate ions (charged particles) form	Slight negative charge (δ^-) at one end of molecule, slight positive charge (δ^+) at other end	Charge balanced among atoms
Na^+ Cl^-	δ^- O, H H, δ^+ δ^+	O=C=O
Sodium chloride	Water	Carbon dioxide

Figure 2.9 Ionic, polar covalent, and nonpolar covalent bonds compared along a continuum.

are electrically balanced and are called **nonpolar molecules** (because they do not have separate + and − poles of charge).

Such electrical balance is not always the case. When covalent bonds are formed, the resulting molecule always has a specific three-dimensional shape, with the bonds formed at definite angles. A molecule's shape helps determine what other molecules or atoms it can interact with. It may also result in unequal electron pair sharing, creating a **polar molecule**, especially in nonsymmetrical molecules containing atoms with different electron-attracting abilities.

In general, *small* atoms with six or seven valence shell electrons, such as oxygen, nitrogen, and chlorine, are electron-hungry and attract electrons very strongly, a capability called **electronegativity**. On the other hand, most atoms with only one or two valence shell electrons tend to be **electropositive**. In other words, their electron-attracting ability is so low that they usually lose *their* valence shell electrons to other atoms. Potassium and sodium, each with one valence shell electron, are good examples of electropositive atoms.

Carbon dioxide and water illustrate how molecular shape and the relative electron-attracting abilities of atoms determine whether a covalently bonded molecule is nonpolar or polar. In carbon dioxide (CO_2), carbon shares four electron pairs with two oxygen atoms (two pairs are shared with each oxygen). Oxygen is very electronegative and so attracts the shared electrons much more strongly than does carbon. However, because the carbon dioxide molecule is linear and symmetrical **(Figure 2.8a)**, the electron-pulling ability of one oxygen atom offsets that of the other, like a standoff between equally strong teams in a game of tug-of-war. As a result, the shared electrons orbit the entire molecule and carbon dioxide is a nonpolar compound.

In contrast, a water molecule (H_2O) is bent, or V shaped (Figure 2.8b). The two electropositive hydrogen atoms are located at the same end of the molecule, and the very electronegative oxygen is at the opposite end. This arrangement allows oxygen to pull the shared electrons toward itself and away from the two hydrogen atoms. In this case, the electron pairs are *not* shared equally, but spend more time in the vicinity of oxygen. Because electrons are negatively charged, the oxygen end of the molecule is slightly more negative (the charge is indicated with a delta and minus as δ^-) and the hydrogen end slightly more positive (indicated by δ^+). Because water has two poles of charge, it is a *polar molecule*, or **dipole** (di′pōl).

Polar molecules orient themselves toward other dipoles or toward charged particles (such as ions and some proteins), and they play essential roles in chemical reactions in body cells. The polarity of water is particularly significant, as you will see later in this chapter.

Different molecules exhibit different degrees of polarity, and we can see a gradual change from ionic to nonpolar covalent bonding as summarized in **Figure 2.9**. Ionic bonds (complete electron transfer) and nonpolar covalent bonds (equal electron sharing) are the extremes of a continuum, with various degrees of unequal electron sharing in between.

Hydrogen Bonds

Unlike the stronger ionic and covalent bonds, hydrogen bonds are more like attractions than true bonds. Hydrogen bonds form when a hydrogen atom, already covalently linked to one electronegative atom (usually nitrogen or oxygen), is attracted by another electron-hungry atom, so that a "bridge" forms between them.

Hydrogen bonding is common between dipoles such as water molecules, because the slightly negative oxygen atoms of one molecule attract the slightly positive hydrogen atoms of other molecules **(Figure 2.10a)**. Hydrogen bonding is responsible for the tendency of water molecules to cling together and form films, referred to as *surface tension*. This tendency helps explain why water beads up into spheres when it sits on a hard surface and why water striders can walk on a pond's surface (Figure 2.10b).

Although hydrogen bonds are too weak to bind atoms together to form molecules, they are important *intramolecular bonds* (literally, bonds within molecules), which hold different parts of a single large molecule in a specific three-dimensional shape. Some large biological molecules, such as proteins and DNA, have numerous hydrogen bonds that help maintain and stabilize their structures.

Check Your Understanding

10. What kinds of bonds form between water molecules?
11. Oxygen ($_8O$) and argon ($_{18}A$) are both gases. Oxygen combines readily with other elements, but argon does not. What accounts for this difference?
12. Assume imaginary compound XY has a polar covalent bond. How does its charge distribution differ from that of XX molecules?

For answers, see Appendix H.

Chemical Reactions

- ✓ Define the three major types of chemical reactions: synthesis, decomposition, and exchange. Comment on the nature of oxidation-reduction reactions and their importance.
- ✓ Explain why chemical reactions in the body are often irreversible.
- ✓ Describe factors that affect chemical reaction rates.

As we noted earlier, all particles of matter are in constant motion because of their kinetic energy. Movement of atoms or molecules in a solid is usually limited to vibration because the particles are united by fairly rigid bonds. But in liquids or gases, particles dart about randomly, sometimes colliding with one another and interacting to undergo chemical reactions. A **chemical reaction** occurs whenever chemical bonds are formed, rearranged, or broken.

Chemical Equations

We can write chemical reactions in symbolic form as chemical equations. For example, we indicate the joining of two hydrogen atoms to form hydrogen gas as

$$H + H \rightarrow H_2 \text{ (hydrogen gas)}$$

reactants   product

and the combining of four hydrogen atoms and one carbon atom to form methane as

$$4H + C \rightarrow CH_4 \text{ (methane)}$$

reactants   product

Notice that in equations, a number written as a *subscript* indicates that the atoms are joined by chemical bonds. But a number written as a *prefix* denotes the number of *unjoined* atoms or molecules. For example, CH_4 reveals that four hydrogen atoms are bonded together with carbon to form the methane molecule, but 4H signifies four unjoined hydrogen atoms.

A chemical equation is like a sentence describing what happens in a reaction. It contains the following information: the number and kinds of reacting substances, or **reactants**; the chemical composition of the **product(s)**; and in balanced equations, the relative proportion of each reactant and product.

In the equations above, the reactants are atoms, as indicated by their atomic symbols (H, C). The product in each case is a

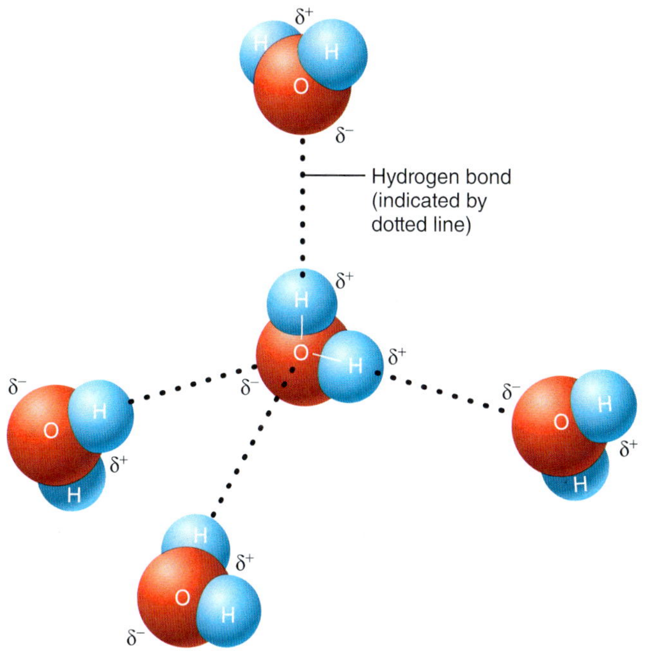

(a) The slightly positive ends (δ+) of the water molecules become aligned with the slightly negative ends (δ−) of other water molecules.

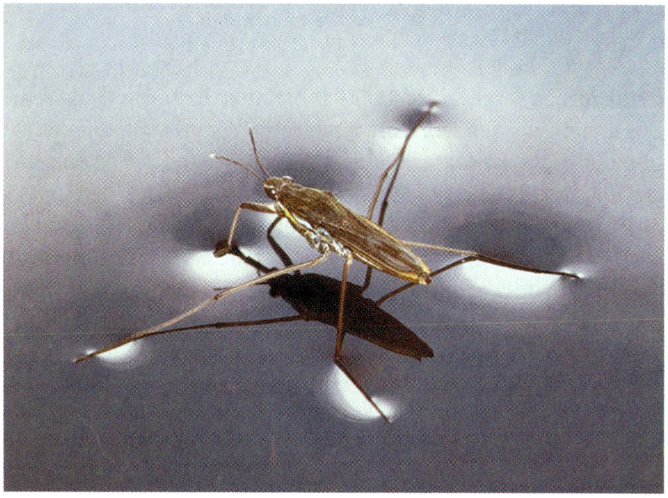

(b) A water strider can walk on a pond because of the high surface tension of water, a result of the combined strength of its hydrogen bonds.

Figure 2.10 Hydrogen bonding between polar water molecules.

2

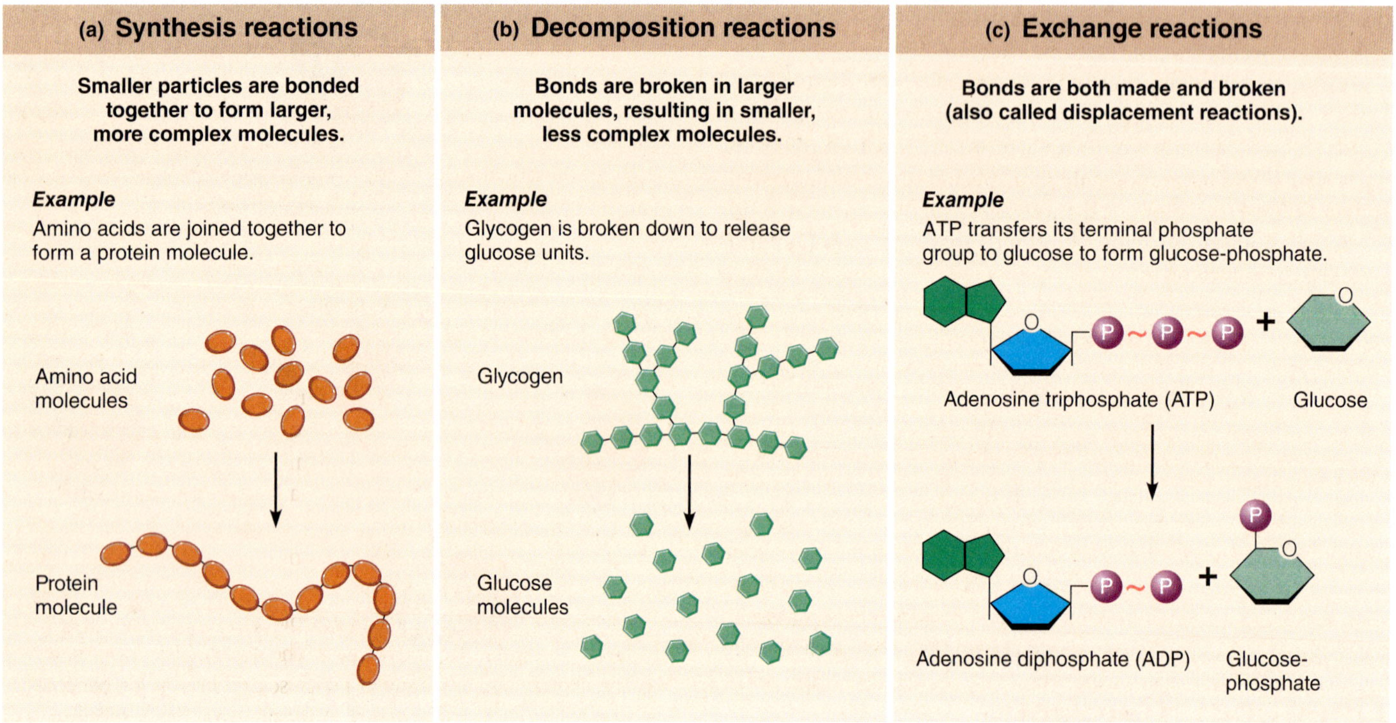

Figure 2.11 Patterns of chemical reactions.

molecule, as represented by its **molecular formula** (H_2, CH_4). The equation for the formation of methane may be read in terms of molecules or moles—as *either* "four hydrogen atoms plus one carbon atom yield one molecule of methane" *or* "four moles of hydrogen atoms plus one mole of carbon yield one mole of methane." Using moles is more practical because it is impossible to measure out one atom or one molecule of anything!

Patterns of Chemical Reactions

Most chemical reactions exhibit one of three recognizable patterns: They are either *synthesis*, *decomposition*, or *exchange reactions.*

When atoms or molecules combine to form a larger, more complex molecule, the process is a **synthesis**, or **combination, reaction**. A synthesis reaction always involves bond formation. It can be represented (using arbitrary letters) as

$$A + B \rightarrow AB$$

Synthesis reactions are the basis of constructive, or **anabolic**, activities in body cells, such as joining small molecules called amino acids into large protein molecules **(Figure 2.11a)**. Synthesis reactions are conspicuous in rapidly growing tissues.

A **decomposition reaction** occurs when a molecule is broken down into smaller molecules or its constituent atoms:

$$AB \rightarrow A + B$$

Essentially, decomposition reactions are reverse synthesis reactions: Bonds are broken. Decomposition reactions underlie all degradative, or **catabolic**, processes in body cells. For example, the bonds of glycogen molecules are broken to release simpler molecules of glucose sugar (Figure 2.11b).

Exchange, or **displacement**, **reactions** involve both synthesis and decomposition. Bonds are both made and broken. In an exchange reaction, parts of the reactant molecules change partners, so to speak, producing different product molecules:

$$AB + C \rightarrow AC + B \quad \text{and} \quad AB + CD \rightarrow AD + CB$$

An exchange reaction occurs when ATP reacts with glucose and transfers its end phosphate group (indicated by a circled P in Figure 2.11c) to glucose, forming glucose-phosphate. At the same time, the ATP becomes ADP. This important reaction occurs whenever glucose enters a body cell, and it effectively traps the glucose fuel molecule inside the cell.

Another group of important chemical reactions in living systems is **oxidation-reduction reactions**, called **redox reactions** for short. Oxidation-reduction reactions are decomposition reactions in that they are the basis of all reactions in which food fuels are broken down for energy (that is, in which ATP is produced). They are also a special type of exchange reaction because electrons are exchanged between the reactants. The reactant losing the electrons is referred to as the *electron donor* and is said to be **oxidized**. The reactant taking up the transferred electrons is called the *electron acceptor* and is said to become **reduced**.

Redox reactions also occur when ionic compounds are formed. Recall that in the formation of NaCl (see Figure 2.6), sodium loses an electron to chlorine. Consequently, sodium is oxidized and becomes a sodium ion, and chlorine is reduced and becomes a chloride ion. However, not all oxidation-reduction reactions involve *complete transfer* of electrons—some simply change the pattern of electron sharing in covalent bonds. For example, a substance is oxidized both by losing hydrogen atoms and by combining with oxygen. The common factor in these events is that electrons that formerly "belonged" to the reactant molecule are lost. The electrons are lost either entirely (as when hydrogen is removed and takes its electron with it) or relatively (as the shared electrons spend more time in the vicinity of the very electronegative oxygen atom).

To understand the importance of oxidation-reduction reactions in living systems, take a look at the overall equation for *cellular respiration*, which represents the major pathway by which glucose is broken down for energy in body cells:

$$\underset{\text{glucose}}{C_6H_{12}O_6} + \underset{\text{oxygen}}{6O_2} \rightarrow \underset{\text{carbon dioxide}}{6CO_2} + \underset{\text{water}}{6H_2O} + \underset{\text{cellular energy}}{ATP}$$

As you can see, it is an oxidation-reduction reaction. Consider what happens to the hydrogen atoms (and their electrons). Glucose is oxidized to carbon dioxide as it loses hydrogen atoms, and oxygen is reduced to water as it accepts the hydrogen atoms. This reaction is described in detail in Chapter 24, along with other topics of cellular metabolism.

Energy Flow in Chemical Reactions

Because all chemical bonds represent stored chemical energy, all chemical reactions ultimately result in net absorption or release of energy. Reactions that release energy are called **exergonic reactions**. These reactions yield products with less energy than the initial reactants, along with energy that can be harvested for other uses. With a few exceptions, catabolic and oxidative reactions are exergonic.

In contrast, the products of energy-absorbing, or **endergonic**, reactions contain more potential energy in their chemical bonds than did the reactants. Anabolic reactions are typically energy-absorbing endergonic reactions. Essentially this is a case of "one hand washing the other"—the energy released when fuel molecules are broken down (oxidized) is captured in ATP molecules and then used to synthesize the complex biological molecules the body needs to sustain life.

Reversibility of Chemical Reactions

All chemical reactions are theoretically reversible. If chemical bonds can be made, they can be broken, and vice versa. Reversibility is indicated by a double arrow. When the arrows differ in length, the longer arrow indicates the major direction in which the reaction proceeds:

$$A + B \rightleftharpoons AB$$

In this example, the forward reaction (reaction going to the right) predominates. Over time, the product (AB) accumulates and the reactants (A and B) decrease in amount.

When the arrows are of equal length, as in

$$A + B \rightleftharpoons AB$$

neither the forward reaction nor the reverse reaction is dominant. In other words, for each molecule of product (AB) formed, one product molecule breaks down, releasing the reactants A and B. Such a chemical reaction is said to be in a state of **chemical equilibrium**.

Once chemical equilibrium is reached, there is no further *net change* in the amounts of reactants and products unless more of either are added to the mix. Product molecules are still formed and broken down, but the balance established when equilibrium was reached (such as greater numbers of product molecules) remains unchanged.

Chemical equilibrium is analogous to the admission scheme used by many large museums in which tickets are sold according to time of entry. If 300 tickets are issued for the 9 AM admission, 300 people will be admitted when the doors open. Thereafter, when 6 people leave, 6 are admitted, and when another 15 people leave, 15 more are allowed in. There is a continual turnover, but the museum contains about 300 art lovers throughout the day.

All chemical reactions are reversible, but many biological reactions show so little tendency to go in the reverse direction that they are irreversible for all practical purposes. Chemical reactions that release energy will not go in the opposite direction unless energy is put back into the system. For example, when our cells break down glucose via the reactions of cellular respiration to yield carbon dioxide and water, some of the energy released is trapped in the bonds of ATP. Because the cells then use ATP's energy for various functions (and more glucose will be along with the next meal), this particular reaction is never reversed in our cells. Furthermore, if a product of a reaction is continuously removed from the reaction site, it is unavailable to take part in the reverse reaction. This situation occurs when the carbon dioxide that is released during glucose breakdown leaves the cell, enters the blood, and is eventually removed from the body by the lungs.

Factors Influencing the Rate of Chemical Reactions

What influences how quickly chemical reactions go? For atoms and molecules to react chemically in the first place, they must *collide* with enough force to overcome the repulsion between their electrons. Interactions between valence shell electrons—the basis of bond making and breaking—cannot occur long distance. The force of collisions depends on how fast the particles are moving. Solid, forceful collisions between rapidly moving particles in which valence shells overlap are much more likely to cause reactions than are collisions in which the particles graze each other lightly.

Temperature Increasing the temperature of a substance increases the kinetic energy of its particles and the force of their collisions. For this reason, chemical reactions proceed more quickly at higher temperatures.

Concentration Chemical reactions progress most rapidly when the reacting particles are present in high numbers, because the chance of successful collisions is greater. As the concentration of the reactants declines, the reaction slows. Chemical equilibrium eventually occurs unless additional reactants are added or products are removed from the reaction site.

Particle Size Smaller particles move faster than larger ones (at the same temperature) and tend to collide more frequently and more forcefully. Hence, the smaller the reacting particles, the faster a chemical reaction goes at a given temperature and concentration.

Catalysts Many chemical reactions in nonliving systems can be speeded up simply by heating, but drastic increases in body temperature are life threatening because important biological molecules are destroyed. Still, at normal body temperatures, most chemical reactions would proceed far too slowly to maintain life were it not for the presence of catalysts. **Catalysts** (kat′ah-lists) are substances that increase the rate of chemical reactions without themselves becoming chemically changed or part of the product. Biological catalysts are called *enzymes* (en′zīmz). Later in this chapter we describe how enzymes work.

☑ Check Your Understanding

13. Which reaction type—synthesis, decomposition, or exchange—occurs when fats are digested in your small intestine?
14. Why are many reactions that occur in living systems irreversible for all intents and purposes?
15. What specific name is given to decomposition reactions in which food fuels are broken down for energy?

For answers, see Appendix H.

PART 2
Biochemistry

Biochemistry is the study of the chemical composition and reactions of living matter. All chemicals in the body fall into one of two major classes: organic or inorganic compounds. **Organic compounds** contain carbon. All organic compounds are covalently bonded molecules, and many are large.

All other chemicals in the body are considered **inorganic compounds**. These include water, salts, and many acids and bases. Organic and inorganic compounds are equally essential for life. Trying to decide which is more valuable is like trying to decide whether the ignition system or the engine is more essential to run your car!

Inorganic Compounds

✓ Explain the importance of water and salts to body homeostasis.

✓ Define acid and base, and explain the concept of pH.

Water

Water is the most abundant and important inorganic compound in living material. It makes up 60–80% of the volume of most living cells. What makes water so vital to life? The answer lies in several properties:

- **High heat capacity.** Water has a high heat capacity. In other words, it absorbs and releases large amounts of heat before changing appreciably in temperature itself. This property of water prevents sudden changes in temperature caused by external factors, such as sun or wind exposure, or by internal conditions that release heat rapidly, such as vigorous muscle activity. As part of blood, water redistributes heat among body tissues, ensuring temperature homeostasis.
- **High heat of vaporization.** When water evaporates, or vaporizes, it changes from a liquid to a gas (water vapor). This transformation requires that large amounts of heat be absorbed to break the hydrogen bonds that hold water molecules together. This property is extremely beneficial when we sweat. As perspiration (mostly water) evaporates from our skin, large amounts of heat are removed from the body, providing efficient cooling.
- **Polar solvent properties.** Water is an unparalleled solvent. Indeed, it is often called the **universal solvent**. Biochemistry is "wet chemistry." Biological molecules do not react chemically unless they are in solution, and virtually all chemical reactions occurring in the body depend on water's solvent properties.

  Because water molecules are polar, they orient themselves with their slightly negative ends toward the positive ends of the solutes, and vice versa, first attracting the solute molecules, and then surrounding them. This polarity of water explains why ionic compounds and other small reactive molecules (such as acids and bases) *dissociate* in water, their ions separating from each other and becoming evenly scattered in the water, forming true solutions **(Figure 2.12)**.

  Water also forms layers of water molecules, called **hydration layers**, around large charged molecules such as proteins, shielding them from the effects of other charged substances in the vicinity and preventing them from settling out of solution. Such protein-water mixtures are *biological colloids*. Blood plasma and cerebrospinal fluid (which surrounds the brain and spinal cord) are examples of colloids.

  Water is the body's major transport medium because it is such an excellent solvent. Nutrients, respiratory gases, and metabolic wastes carried throughout the body are dissolved in blood plasma, and many metabolic wastes are excreted from the body in urine, another watery fluid. Specialized molecules that lubricate the body (e.g., mucus) also use water as their dissolving medium.
- **Reactivity.** Water is an important *reactant* in many chemical reactions. For example, foods are digested to their building blocks by adding a water molecule to each bond to be broken. Such decomposition reactions are more specifically called **hydrolysis reactions** (hi-drol′ĭ-sis; "water splitting"). Conversely, when large carbohydrate or protein molecules are synthesized from smaller molecules, a water molecule is removed for every bond formed, a reaction called **dehydration synthesis**.
- **Cushioning.** By forming a resilient cushion around certain body organs, water helps protect them from physical trauma.

The cerebrospinal fluid surrounding the brain exemplifies water's cushioning role.

Salts

A **salt** is an ionic compound containing cations other than H^+ and anions other than the hydroxyl ion (OH^-). As already noted, when salts are dissolved in water, they dissociate into their component ions (Figure 2.12). For example, sodium sulfate (Na_2SO_4) dissociates into two Na^+ ions and one SO_4^{2-} ion. It dissociates easily because the ions are already formed. All that remains is for water to overcome the attraction between the oppositely charged ions.

All ions are **electrolytes** (e-lek′tro-līts), substances that conduct an electrical current in solution. (Note that groups of atoms that bear an overall charge, such as sulfate, are called *polyatomic ions.*)

Salts commonly found in the body include NaCl, $CaCO_3$ (calcium carbonate), and KCl (potassium chloride). However, the most plentiful salts are the calcium phosphates that make bones and teeth hard. In their ionized form, salts play vital roles in body function. For instance, the electrolyte properties of sodium and potassium ions are essential for nerve impulse transmission and muscle contraction. Ionic iron forms part of the hemoglobin molecules that transport oxygen within red blood cells, and zinc and copper ions are important to the activity of some enzymes. Other important functions of the elements found in body salts are summarized in Table 2.1 on p. 26.

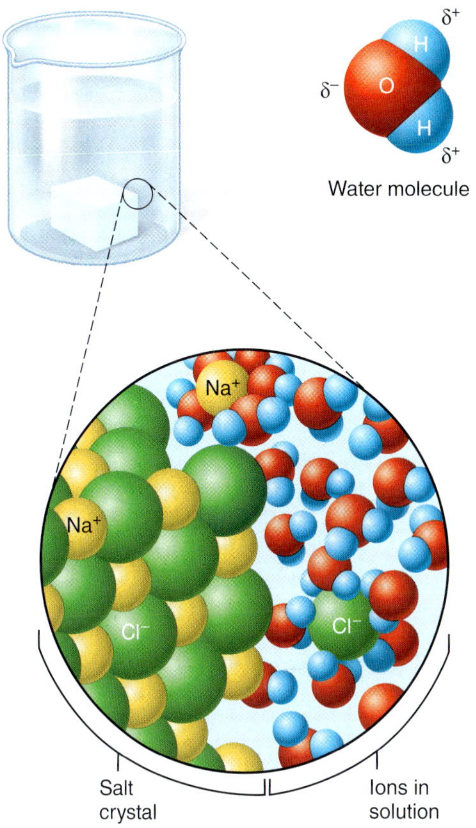

Figure 2.12 Dissociation of salt in water.

Homeostatic Imbalance 2.1

Maintaining proper ionic balance in our body fluids is one of the most crucial homeostatic roles of the kidneys. When this balance is severely disturbed, virtually nothing in the body works. All the physiological activities listed above and thousands of others are disrupted and grind to a stop. ✚

Acids and Bases

Like salts, acids and bases are electrolytes. They ionize and dissociate in water and can then conduct an electrical current.

Acids

Acids have a sour taste, can react with (dissolve) many metals, and "burn" a hole in your rug. But for our purposes the most useful definition of an acid is a substance that releases **hydrogen ions** (H^+) in detectable amounts. Because a hydrogen ion is just a hydrogen nucleus, or "naked" proton, acids are also defined as **proton donors**.

When acids dissolve in water, they release hydrogen ions (protons) and anions. It is the concentration of protons that determines the acidity of a solution. The anions have little or no effect on acidity. For example, hydrochloric acid (HCl), an acid produced by stomach cells that aids digestion, dissociates into a proton and a chloride ion:

$$HCl \rightarrow \underset{\text{proton}}{H^+} + \underset{\text{anion}}{Cl^-}$$

Other acids found or produced in the body include acetic acid ($HC_2H_3O_2$, commonly abbreviated as HAc), which is the acidic portion of vinegar; and carbonic acid (H_2CO_3). The molecular formula for an acid is easy to recognize because the hydrogen is written first.

Bases

Bases have a bitter taste, feel slippery, and are **proton acceptors**—that is, they take up hydrogen ions (H^+) in detectable amounts. Common inorganic bases include the *hydroxides* (hi-drok′sīds), such as magnesium hydroxide (milk of magnesia) and sodium hydroxide (lye). Like acids, hydroxides dissociate when dissolved in water, but in this case **hydroxyl ions (OH^-)** (hi-drok′sil) and cations are liberated. For example, ionization of sodium hydroxide (NaOH) produces a hydroxyl ion and a sodium ion, and the hydroxyl ion then binds to (accepts) a proton present in the solution. This reaction produces water and simultaneously reduces the acidity (hydrogen ion concentration) of the solution:

$$NaOH \rightarrow \underset{\text{cation}}{Na^+} + \underset{\text{hydroxyl ion}}{OH^-}$$

and then

$$OH^- + H^+ \rightarrow \underset{\text{water}}{H_2O}$$

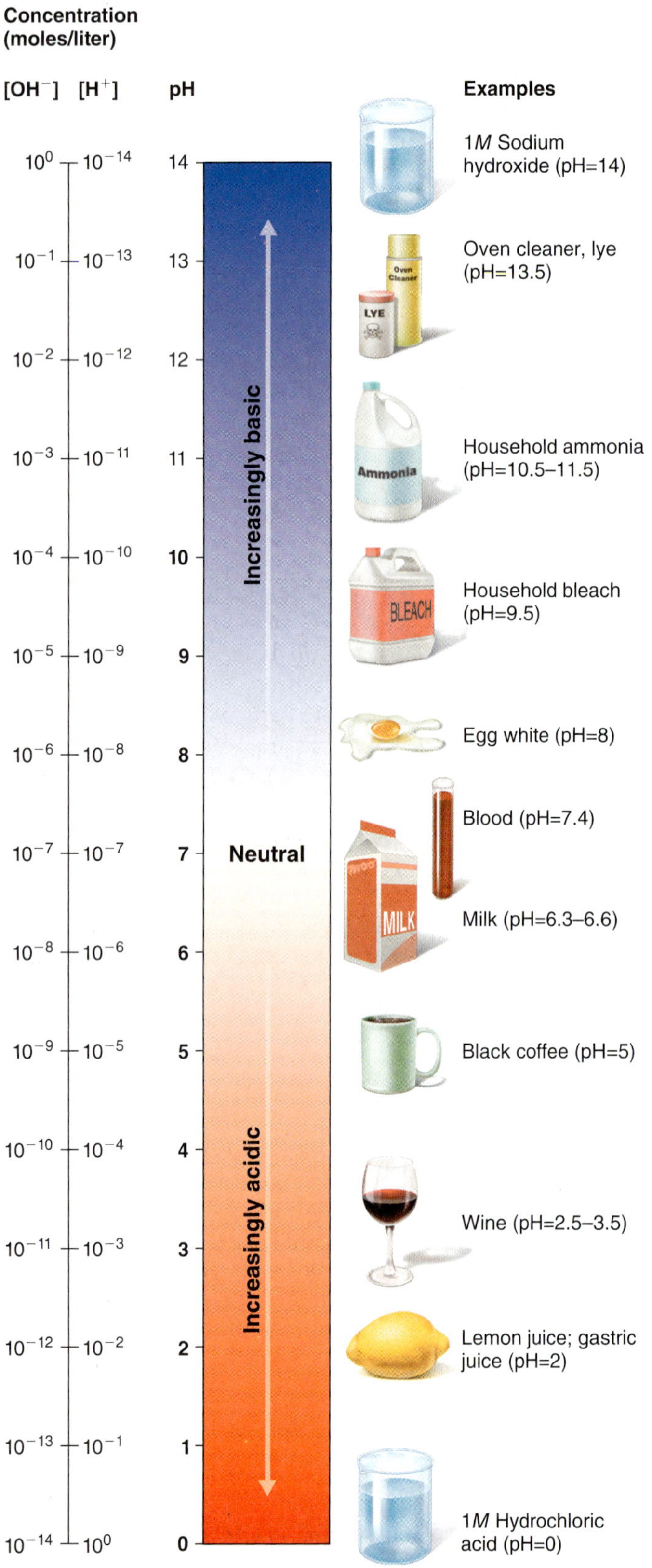

Figure 2.13 The pH scale and pH values of representative substances. The pH scale is based on the number of hydrogen ions in solution. The actual concentrations of hydrogen ions, [H⁺], and hydroxyl ions, [OH⁻], in moles per liter are indicated for each pH value noted. At a pH of 7, [H⁺] = [OH⁻] and the solution is neutral.

Bicarbonate ion (HCO_3^-), an important base in the body, is particularly abundant in blood. **Ammonia (NH_3)**, a common waste product of protein breakdown in the body, is also a base. It has one pair of unshared electrons that strongly attracts protons. By accepting a proton, ammonia becomes an ammonium ion:

$$NH_3 + H^+ \rightarrow \underset{\text{ammonium ion}}{NH_4^+}$$

pH: Acid-Base Concentration

The more hydrogen ions in a solution, the more acidic the solution is. Conversely, the greater the concentration of hydroxyl ions (the lower the concentration of H^+), the more basic, or *alkaline* (al′kuh-līn), the solution becomes. The relative concentration of hydrogen ions in various body fluids is measured in concentration units called **pH units** (pe-āch′).

The idea for a pH scale was devised by a Danish biochemist and part-time beer brewer named Sören Sörensen in 1909. He was searching for a convenient means of checking the acidity of his alcoholic product to prevent its spoilage by bacterial action. (Acidic conditions inhibit many bacteria.) The pH scale that resulted is based on the concentration of hydrogen ions in a solution, expressed in terms of moles per liter, or molarity. The pH scale runs from 0 to 14 and is *logarithmic*. In other words, each successive change of one pH unit represents a tenfold change in hydrogen ion concentration (**Figure 2.13**). The pH of a solution is thus defined as the negative logarithm of the hydrogen ion concentration $[H^+]$ in moles per liter, or $-\log[H^+]$. (Note that brackets [ ] indicate concentration of a substance.)

At a pH of 7 (at which $[H^+]$ is 10^{-7} *M*), the solution is *neutral*—neither acidic nor basic. The number of hydrogen ions exactly equals the number of hydroxyl ions (pH = pOH). Absolutely pure (distilled) water has a pH of 7.

Solutions with a pH below 7 are acidic—the hydrogen ions outnumber the hydroxyl ions. The lower the pH, the more acidic the solution. A solution with a pH of 6 has ten times as many hydrogen ions as a solution with a pH of 7.

Solutions with a pH higher than 7 are alkaline, and the relative concentration of hydrogen ions decreases by a factor of 10 with each higher pH unit. Thus, solutions with pH values of 8 and 12 have, respectively, 1/10 and 1/100,000 (1/10 × 1/10 × 1/10 × 1/10 × 1/10) as many hydrogen ions as a solution of pH 7.

The approximate pH of several body fluids and of a number of common substances appears in Figure 2.13. Notice that as the hydrogen ion concentration decreases, the hydroxyl ion concentration rises, and vice versa.

Neutralization

What happens when acids and bases are mixed? They react with each other in displacement reactions to form water and a salt. For example, when hydrochloric acid and sodium hydroxide interact, sodium chloride (a salt) and water are formed.

$$\underset{\text{acid}}{HCl} + \underset{\text{base}}{NaOH} \rightarrow \underset{\text{salt}}{NaCl} + \underset{\text{water}}{H_2O}$$

This type of reaction is called a **neutralization reaction**, because the joining of H^+ and OH^- to form water neutralizes the solution. Although the salt produced is written in molecular form (NaCl), remember that it actually exists as dissociated sodium and chloride ions when dissolved in water.

Buffers

Living cells are extraordinarily sensitive to even slight changes in the pH of the environment. In high concentrations, acids and bases are extremely damaging to living tissue. Imagine what would happen to all those hydrogen bonds in biological molecules with large numbers of free H^+ running around. (Can't you just hear those molecules saying "Why share hydrogen when I can have my own?")

Homeostasis of acid-base balance is carefully regulated by the kidneys and lungs and by chemical systems (proteins and other types of molecules) called **buffers**. Buffers resist abrupt and large swings in the pH of body fluids by releasing hydrogen ions (acting as acids) when the pH begins to rise and by binding hydrogen ions (acting as bases) when the pH drops. Because blood comes into close contact with nearly every body cell, regulating its pH is particularly critical. Normally, blood pH varies within a very narrow range (7.35 to 7.45). If blood pH varies from these limits by more than a few tenths of a unit, it may be fatal.

To comprehend how chemical buffer systems operate, you must thoroughly understand strong and weak acids and bases. The first important concept is that the acidity of a solution reflects *only* the free hydrogen ions, not those still bound to anions. Consequently, acids that dissociate completely and irreversibly in water are called **strong acids**, because they can dramatically change the pH of a solution. Examples are hydrochloric acid and sulfuric acid. If we could count out 100 hydrochloric acid molecules and place them in 1 milliliter (ml) of water, we could expect to end up with 100 H^+, 100 Cl^-, and no undissociated hydrochloric acid molecules in that solution.

Acids that do not dissociate completely, like carbonic acid (H_2CO_3) and acetic acid (HAc), are **weak acids**. If we were to place 100 acetic acid molecules in 1 ml of water, the reaction would be something like this:

$$100\ \text{HAc} \rightarrow 90\ \text{HAc} + 10\ \text{H}^+ + 10\ \text{Ac}^-$$

Because undissociated acids do not affect pH, the acetic acid solution is much less acidic than the HCl solution. Weak acids dissociate in a predictable way, and molecules of the intact acid are in dynamic equilibrium with the dissociated ions. Consequently, the dissociation of acetic acid may also be written as

$$\text{HAc} \rightleftharpoons \text{H}^+ + \text{Ac}^-$$

This viewpoint allows us to see that if H^+ (released by a strong acid) is added to the acetic acid solution, the equilibrium will shift to the left and some H^+ and Ac^- will recombine to form HAc. On the other hand, if a strong base is added and the pH begins to rise, the equilibrium shifts to the right and more HAc molecules dissociate to release H^+. This characteristic of weak acids allows them to play important roles in the chemical buffer systems of the body.

The concept of strong and weak bases is more easily explained. Remember that bases are proton acceptors. Thus, **strong bases** are those, like hydroxides, that dissociate easily in water and quickly tie up H^+. On the other hand, sodium bicarbonate (commonly known as baking soda) ionizes incompletely and reversibly. Because it accepts relatively few protons, its released bicarbonate ion is considered a **weak base**.

Now let's examine how one buffer system helps to maintain pH homeostasis of the blood. Although there are other chemical blood buffers, the **carbonic acid–bicarbonate system** is a major one. Carbonic acid (H_2CO_3) dissociates reversibly, releasing bicarbonate ions (HCO_3^-) and protons (H^+):

$$\text{H}_2\text{CO}_3 \underset{\text{Response to drop in pH}}{\overset{\text{Response to rise in pH}}{\rightleftharpoons}} \text{HCO}_3^- + \text{H}^+$$

H^+ donor (weak acid) | H^+ acceptor (weak base) | proton

The chemical equilibrium between carbonic acid (a weak acid) and bicarbonate ion (a weak base) resists changes in blood pH by shifting to the right or left as H^+ ions are added to or removed from the blood. As blood pH rises (becomes more alkaline due to the addition of a strong base), the equilibrium shifts to the right, forcing more carbonic acid to dissociate. Similarly, as blood pH begins to drop (becomes more acidic due to the addition of a strong acid), the equilibrium shifts to the left as more bicarbonate ions begin to bind with protons. As you can see, strong bases are replaced by a weak base (bicarbonate ion) and protons released by strong acids are tied up in a weak one (carbonic acid). In either case, the blood pH changes much less than it would in the absence of the buffering system. We discuss acid-base balance and buffers in more detail in Chapter 26.

Check Your Understanding

16. Water makes up 60–80% of living matter. What property makes it an excellent solvent?
17. Salts are electrolytes. What does that mean?
18. Which ion is responsible for increased acidity?
19. To minimize the sharp pH shift that occurs when a strong acid is added to a solution, is it better to add a weak base or a strong base? Why?

For answers, see Appendix H.

Organic Compounds

- ✓ Describe and compare the building blocks, general structures, and biological functions of carbohydrates and lipids.
- ✓ Explain the role of dehydration synthesis and hydrolysis in forming and breaking down organic molecules.

Molecules unique to living systems—carbohydrates, lipids (fats), proteins, and nucleic acids—all contain carbon and hence are organic compounds. Organic compounds are generally distinguished by the fact that they contain carbon, and inorganic

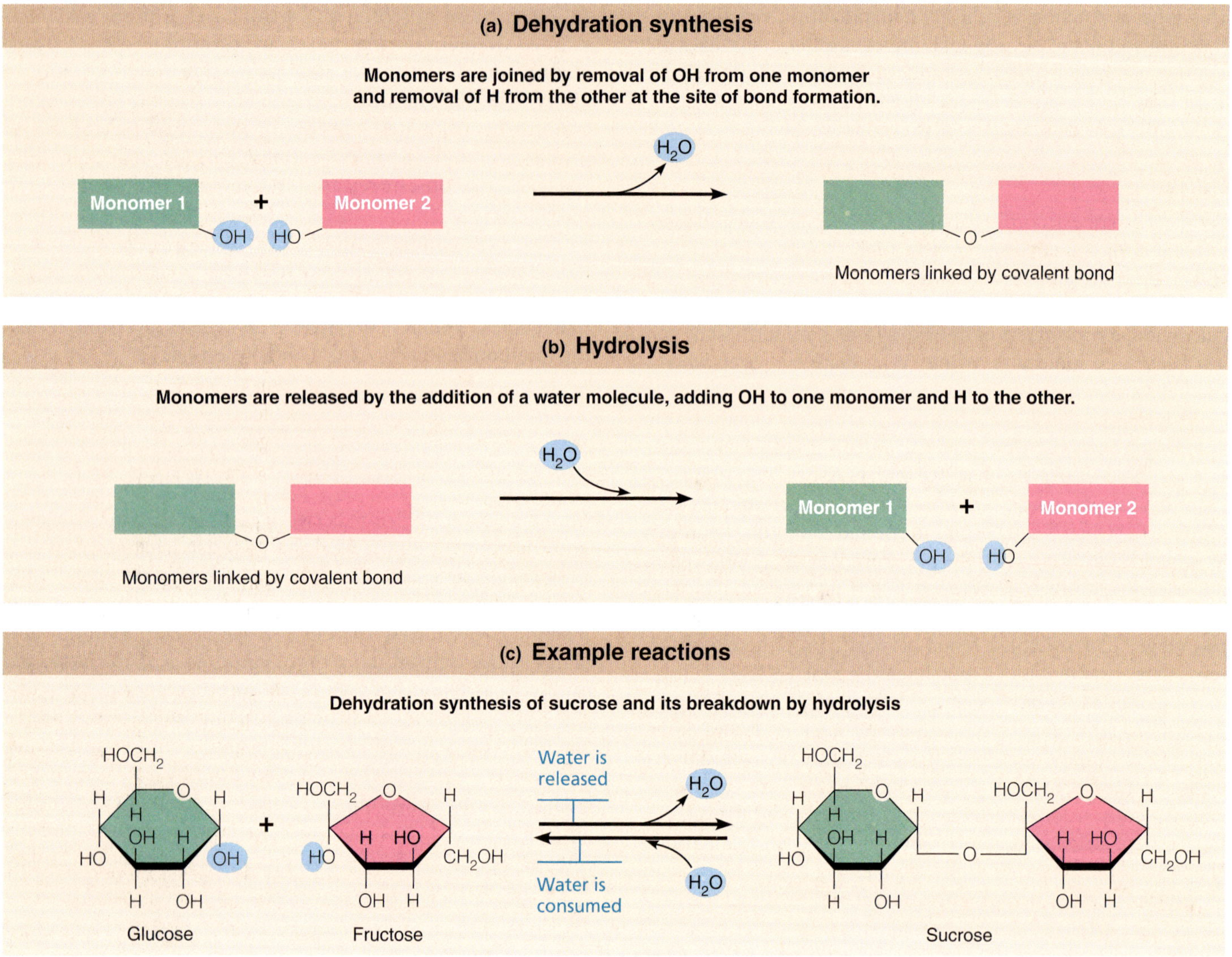

Figure 2.14 Dehydration synthesis and hydrolysis. Biological molecules are formed from their monomers, or units, by dehydration synthesis and broken down to the monomers by hydrolysis reactions.

compounds are defined as compounds that lack carbon. You should be aware of a few irrational exceptions to this generalization: Carbon dioxide and carbon monoxide, for example, contain carbon but are considered inorganic compounds.

For the most part, organic molecules are very large molecules, but their interactions with other molecules typically involve only small, reactive parts of their structure called *functional groups* (acid groups, amines, and others). The most important functional groups involved in biochemical reactions are illustrated in Appendix B.

What makes carbon so special that "living" chemistry depends on its presence? To begin with, no other *small* atom is so precisely **electroneutral**. The consequence of its electroneutrality is that carbon never loses or gains electrons. Instead, it always shares them. Furthermore, with four valence shell electrons, carbon forms four covalent bonds with other elements, as well as with other carbon atoms. As a result, carbon can help form long, chainlike molecules (common in fats), ring structures (typical of carbohydrates and steroids), and many other structures that are uniquely suited for specific roles in the body.

As you will see shortly, many biological molecules (carbohydrates and proteins for example) are polymers. **Polymers** are chainlike molecules made of many similar or repeating units (**monomers**), which are joined together by dehydration synthesis (**Figure 2.14**). During dehydration synthesis, a hydrogen atom is removed from one monomer and a hydroxyl group is removed from the monomer it is to be joined with. As a covalent bond unites the monomers, a water molecule is released. This removal of a water molecule at the bond site occurs each time a monomer is added to the growing polymer chain.

Carbohydrates

Carbohydrates, a group of molecules that includes sugars and starches, represent 1–2% of cell mass. Carbohydrates contain carbon, hydrogen, and oxygen, and generally the hydrogen and oxygen atoms occur in the same 2:1 ratio as in water. This ratio is reflected in the word *carbohydrate* ("hydrated carbon").

A carbohydrate can be classified according to size and solubility as a monosaccharide ("one sugar"), disaccharide ("two sugars"), or polysaccharide ("many sugars"). Monosaccharides are the monomers, or building blocks, of the other carbohydrates. In general, the larger the carbohydrate molecule, the less soluble it is in water.

Monosaccharides

Monosaccharides (mon″o-sak′ah-rīdz), or *simple sugars*, are single-chain or single-ring structures containing from three to seven carbon atoms **(Figure 2.15a)**. Usually the carbon, hydrogen, and oxygen atoms occur in the ratio 1:2:1, so a general formula for a monosaccharide is $(CH_2O)_n$, where *n* is the number of carbons in the sugar. Glucose, for example, has six carbon atoms, and its molecular formula is $C_6H_{12}O_6$. Ribose, with five carbons, is $C_5H_{10}O_5$.

Monosaccharides are named generically according to the number of carbon atoms they contain. Most important in the body are the pentose (five-carbon) and hexose (six-carbon) sugars. For example, the pentose *deoxyribose* (de-ok″sĭ-ri′bōs) is part of DNA, and *glucose*, a hexose, is blood sugar.

Two other hexoses, *galactose* and *fructose*, are **isomers** (ī′so-mers) of glucose. That is, they have the same molecular formula ($C_6H_{12}O_6$), but as you can see in Figure 2.15a, their atoms are arranged differently, giving them different chemical properties.

Disaccharides

A **disaccharide** (di-sak′ah-rīd), or *double sugar*, is formed when two monosaccharides are joined by *dehydration synthesis* (Figure 2.14a, c). In this synthesis reaction, a water molecule is lost as the bond is made, as illustrated by the synthesis of sucrose (soo′krōs):

$$\underset{\text{glucose + fructose}}{2C_6H_{12}O_6} \rightarrow \underset{\text{sucrose}}{C_{12}H_{22}O_{11}} + \underset{\text{water}}{H_2O}$$

Notice that the molecular formula for sucrose contains two hydrogen atoms and one oxygen atom less than the total number of hydrogen and oxygen atoms in glucose and fructose, because a water molecule is released during bond formation.

Important disaccharides in the diet are *sucrose* (glucose + fructose), which is cane or table sugar; *lactose* (glucose + galactose), found in milk; and *maltose* (glucose + glucose), also called malt sugar (Figure 2.15b). Disaccharides are too large to pass through cell membranes, so they must be digested to their simple sugar units to be absorbed from the digestive tract into the blood. This decomposition process is *hydrolysis*, essentially the reverse of dehydration synthesis (Figure 2.14a, b). A water molecule is added to each bond, breaking the bonds and releasing the simple sugar units.

Polysaccharides

Polysaccharides (pol″e-sak′ah-rīdz) are polymers of simple sugars linked together by dehydration synthesis. Because polysaccharides are large, fairly insoluble molecules, they are ideal storage products. Another consequence of their large size is that they lack the sweetness of the simple and double sugars.

Only two polysaccharides are of major importance to the body: starch and glycogen. Both are polymers of glucose. Only their degree of branching differs.

Starch is the storage carbohydrate formed by plants. The number of glucose units composing a starch molecule is high and variable. When we eat starchy foods such as grain products and potatoes, the starch must be digested for its glucose units to be absorbed. We are unable to digest *cellulose*, another polysaccharide found in all plant products. However, it is important in providing the *bulk* (one form of fiber) that helps move feces through the colon.

Glycogen (gli′ko-jen), the storage carbohydrate of animal tissues, is stored primarily in skeletal muscle and liver cells. Like starch, it is highly branched and is a very large molecule (Figure 2.15c). When blood sugar levels drop sharply, liver cells break down glycogen and release its glucose units to the blood. Since there are many branch endings from which glucose can be released simultaneously, body cells have almost instant access to glucose fuel.

Carbohydrate Functions

The major function of carbohydrates in the body is to provide a ready, easily used source of cellular fuel. Most cells can use only a few types of simple sugars, and glucose is at the top of the "cellular menu." As described in our earlier discussion of oxidation-reduction reactions (pp. 36–37), glucose is broken down and oxidized within cells. During these chemical reactions, electrons are transferred. This relocation of electrons releases the bond energy stored in glucose, and this energy is used to synthesize ATP. When ATP supplies are sufficient, dietary carbohydrates are converted to glycogen or fat and stored. Those of us who have gained weight from eating too many carbohydrate-rich snacks have personal experience with this conversion process!

Only small amounts of carbohydrates are used for structural purposes. For example, some sugars are found in our genes. Others are attached to the external surfaces of cells where they act as "road signs" to guide cellular interactions.

Lipids

Lipids are insoluble in water but dissolve readily in other lipids and in organic solvents such as alcohol and ether. Like carbohydrates, all lipids contain carbon, hydrogen, and oxygen, but the proportion of oxygen in lipids is much lower. In addition, phosphorus is found in some of the more complex lipids. Lipids include *triglycerides*, *phospholipids* (fos″fo-lip′idz), *steroids* (stě′roidz), and a number of other lipoid substances. **Table 2.2** on p. 46 gives the locations and functions of some lipids found in the body.

2

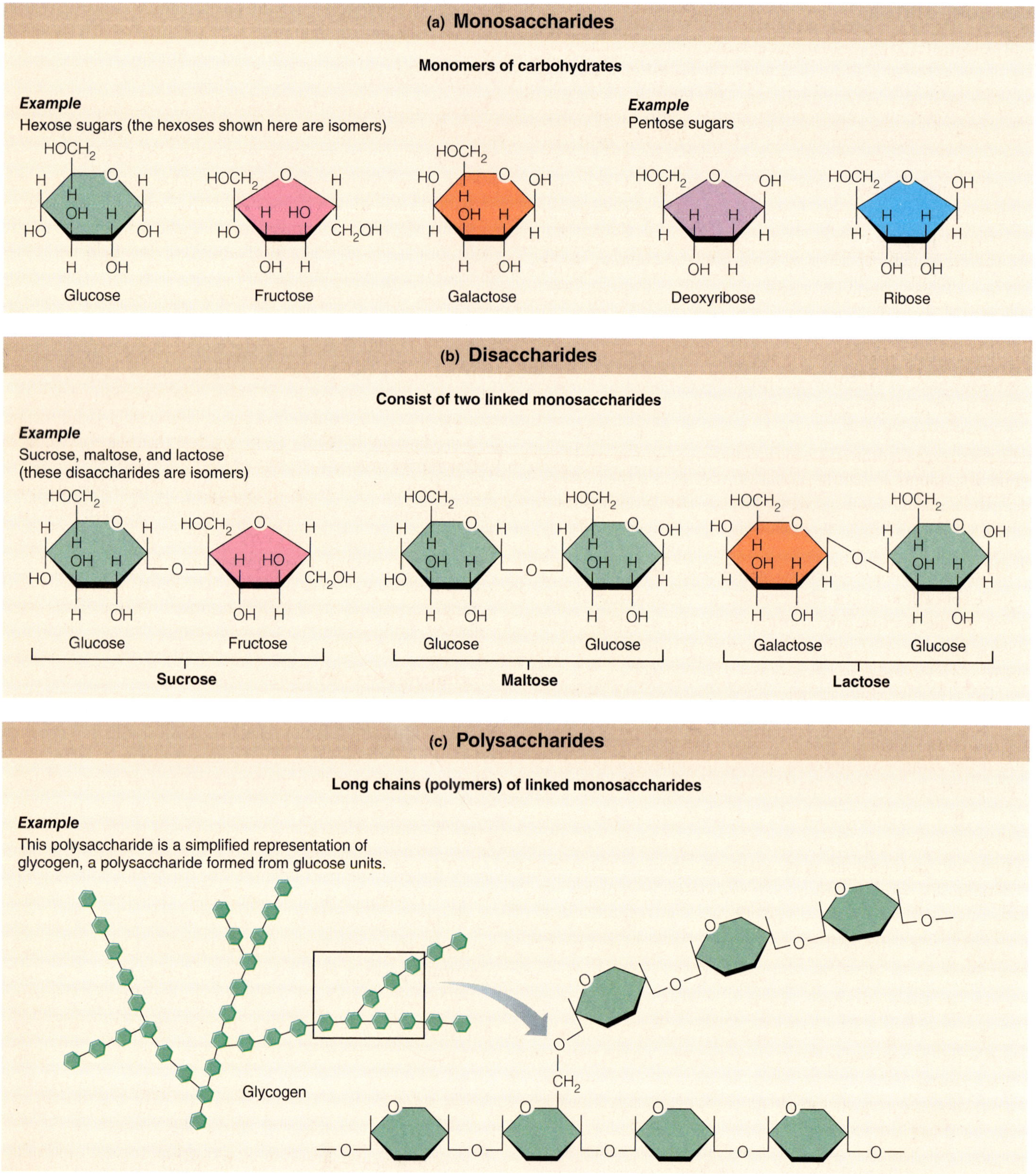

Figure 2.15 Carbohydrate molecules important to the body.*

*Notice that in Figure 2.15 the carbon (C) atoms present at the angles of the carbohydrate ring structures are not illustrated and in Figure 2.15c only the oxygen atoms and one CH_2 group are shown. The illustrations at right give an example of this shorthand style: The full structure of glucose is on the left and the shorthand structure on the right. This style is used for nearly all organic ringlike structures illustrated in this chapter.

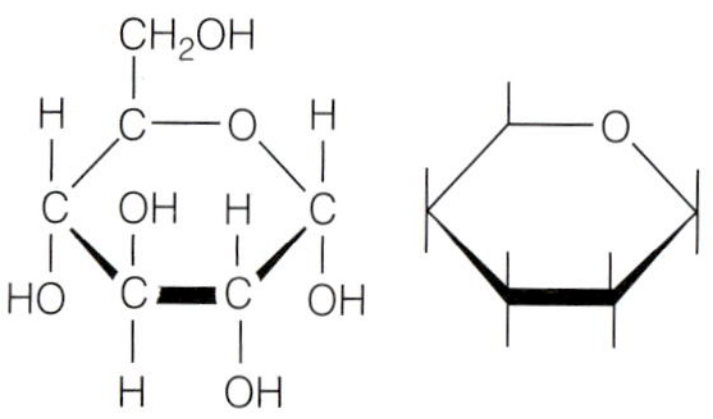

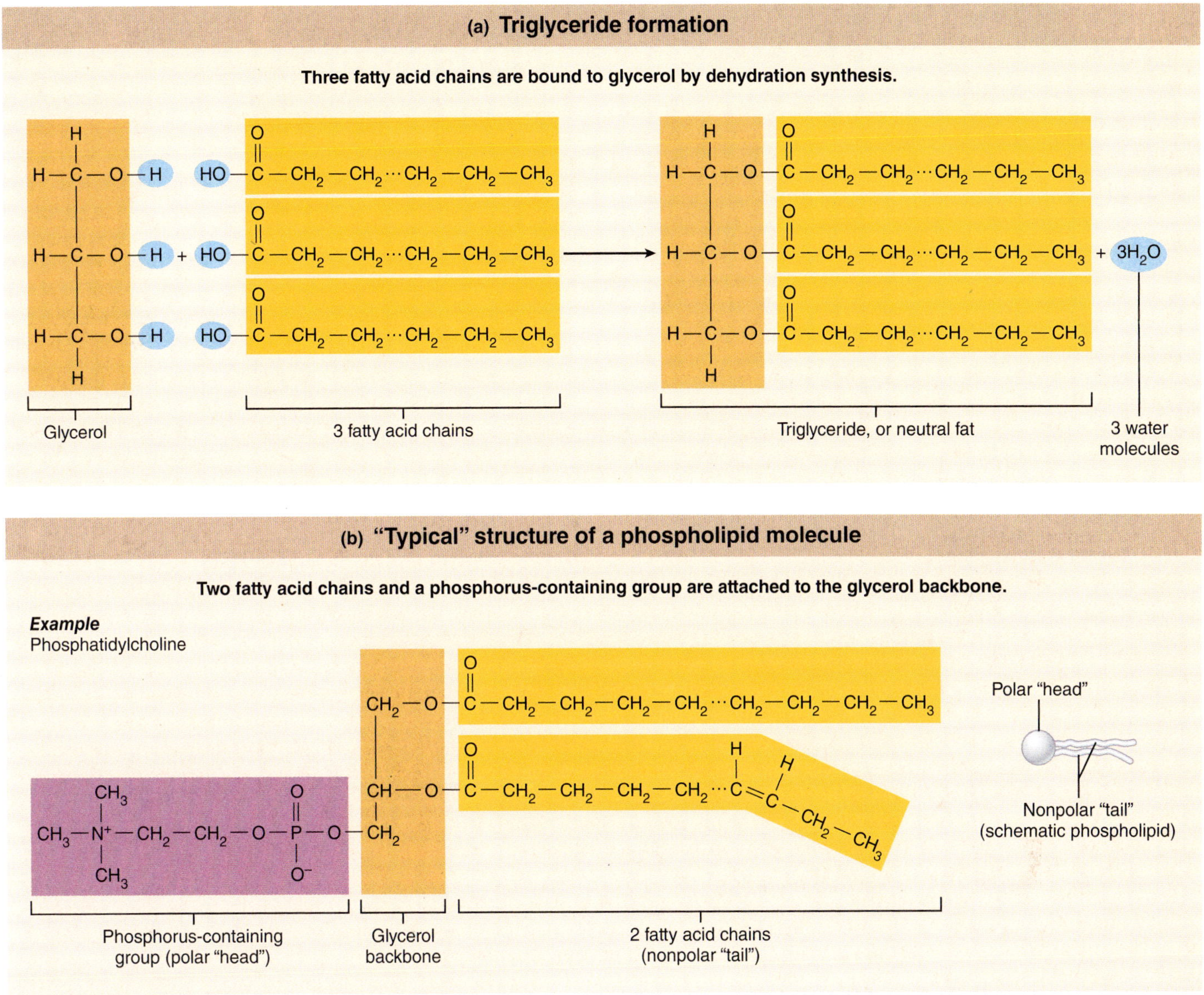

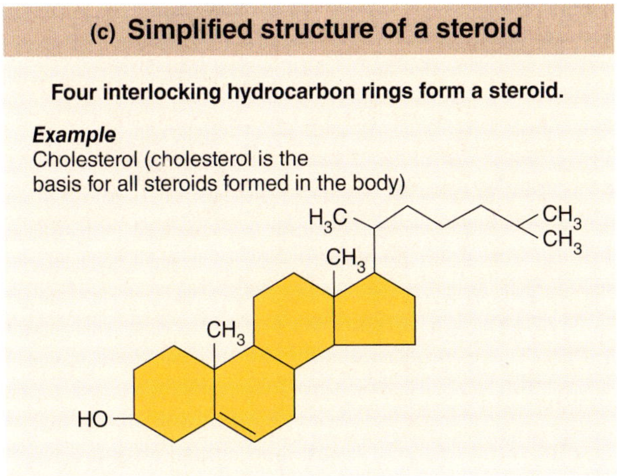

Figure 2.16 Lipids. The general structure of **(a)** triglycerides, or neutral fats, **(b)** phospholipids, and **(c)** cholesterol.

Triglycerides (Neutral Fats)

Triglycerides (tri-glis′er-īdz), also called **neutral fats**, are commonly known as *fats* when solid or *oils* when liquid. A triglyceride is composed of two types of building blocks, **fatty acids** and **glycerol** (glis′er-ol), in a 3:1 ratio of fatty acids to glycerol **(Figure 2.16a)**. Fatty acids are linear chains of carbon and hydrogen atoms (hydrocarbon chains) with an organic acid group (—COOH) at one end. Glycerol is a modified simple sugar (a sugar alcohol).

Fat synthesis involves attaching three fatty acid chains to a single glycerol molecule by dehydration synthesis. The result is an E-shaped molecule. The glycerol backbone is the same in all triglycerides, but the fatty acid chains vary, resulting in different kinds of fats and oils.

These are large molecules, often consisting of hundreds of atoms, and ingested fats and oils must be broken down to their building blocks before they can be absorbed. Their hydrocarbon chains make the triglycerides nonpolar molecules. Because polar and nonpolar molecules do not interact, oil (or fats) and water do not mix. Consequently, triglycerides provide the body's

2

Table 2.2 Representative Lipids Found in the Body

LIPID TYPE	LOCATION/FUNCTION
Triglycerides (Neutral Fats)	
	Fat deposits (in subcutaneous tissue and around organs) protect and insulate body organs, and are the major source of *stored* energy in the body.
Phospholipids (phosphatidylcholine; cephalin; others)	
	Chief components of cell membranes. Participate in the transport of lipids in plasma. Prevalent in nervous tissue.
Steroids	
Cholesterol	The structural basis for manufacture of all body steroids. A component of cell membranes.
Bile salts	These breakdown products of cholesterol are released by the liver into the digestive tract, where they aid fat digestion and absorption.
Vitamin D	A fat-soluble vitamin produced in the skin on exposure to UV radiation. Necessary for normal bone growth and function.
Sex hormones	Estrogen and progesterone (female hormones) and testosterone (a male hormone) are produced in the gonads. Necessary for normal reproductive function.
Adrenocortical hormones	Cortisol, a glucocorticoid, is a metabolic hormone necessary for maintaining normal blood glucose levels. Aldosterone helps to regulate salt and water balance of the body by targeting the kidneys.
Other Lipoid Substances	
Fat-soluble vitamins:	
A	Ingested in orange-pigmented vegetables and fruits. Converted in the retina to retinal, a part of the photoreceptor pigment involved in vision.
E	Ingested in plant products such as wheat germ and green leafy vegetables. Claims have been made (but not proved in humans) that it promotes wound healing, contributes to fertility, and may help to neutralize highly reactive particles called free radicals believed to be involved in triggering some types of cancer.
K	Made available to humans largely by the action of intestinal bacteria. Also prevalent in a wide variety of foods. Necessary for proper clotting of blood.
Eicosanoids (prostaglandins; leukotrienes; thromboxanes)	Group of molecules derived from fatty acids found in all cell membranes. The potent prostaglandins have diverse effects, including stimulation of uterine contractions, regulation of blood pressure, control of gastrointestinal tract motility, and secretory activity. Both prostaglandins and leukotrienes are involved in inflammation. Thromboxanes are powerful vasoconstrictors.
Lipoproteins	Lipoid and protein-based substances that transport fatty acids and cholesterol in the bloodstream. Major varieties are high-density lipoproteins (HDLs) and low-density lipoproteins (LDLs).

most efficient and compact form of stored energy, and when they are oxidized, they yield large amounts of energy.

Triglycerides are found mainly beneath the skin, where they insulate the deeper body tissues from heat loss and protect them from mechanical trauma. For example, women are usually more successful English Channel swimmers than men. Their success is due partly to their thicker subcutaneous fatty layer, which helps insulate them from the bitterly cold water of the Channel.

The length of a triglyceride's fatty acid chains and their degree of *saturation* with H atoms determine how solid the molecule is at a given temperature. Fatty acid chains with only single covalent bonds between carbon atoms are referred to as **saturated**. Their fatty acid chains are straight and, at room temperature, the molecules of a saturated fat are packed closely together, forming a solid. Fatty acids that contain one or more double bonds between carbon atoms are said to be **unsaturated** (**monounsaturated** and **polyunsaturated**, respectively). The double bonds cause the fatty acid chains to kink so that they cannot be packed closely enough to solidify. Hence, triglycerides with short fatty acid chains or unsaturated fatty acids are oils (liquid at room temperature) and are typical of plant lipids. Examples include olive and peanut oils (rich in monounsaturated fats) and corn, soybean, and safflower oils, which contain a high percentage of polyunsaturated fatty acids. Longer fatty acid chains and more saturated fatty acids are common in animal fats such as butterfat and the fat of meats, which are solid at room temperature. Of the two types of fatty acids, the unsaturated variety, especially olive oil, is said to be more "heart healthy."

Trans fats, common in many margarines and baked products, are oils that have been solidified by addition of H atoms at sites of carbon double bonds. They have recently been branded as increasing the risk of heart disease even more than the solid animal fats. Conversely, the **omega-3 fatty acids**, found naturally in cold-water fish, appear to decrease the risk of heart disease and some inflammatory diseases.

Phospholipids

Phospholipids are modified triglycerides. Specifically, they are diglycerides with a phosphorus-containing group and two, rather than three, fatty acid chains (Figure 2.16b). The phosphorus-containing group gives phospholipids their distinctive chemical properties. Although the hydrocarbon portion (the "tail") of the molecule is nonpolar and interacts only with nonpolar molecules, the phosphorus-containing part (the "head") is polar and attracts other polar or charged particles, such as water or ions. This unique characteristic of phospholipids allows them to be used as the chief material for building cellular membranes. Some biologically important phospholipids and their functions are listed in Table 2.2.

Steroids

Structurally, steroids differ quite a bit from fats and oils. **Steroids** are basically flat molecules made of four interlocking hydrocarbon rings. Like triglycerides, steroids are fat soluble and contain little oxygen. The single most important molecule in our steroid chemistry is *cholesterol* (ko-les′ter-ol) (Figure 2.16c). We ingest cholesterol in animal products such as eggs, meat, and cheese, and our liver produces some.

Cholesterol has earned bad press because of its role in atherosclerosis, but it is essential for human life. Cholesterol is found in cell membranes and is the raw material for synthesis of vitamin D, steroid hormones, and bile salts. Although steroid hormones are present in the body in only small quantities, they are vital to homeostasis. Without sex hormones, reproduction would be impossible, and a total lack of the corticosteroids produced by the adrenal glands is fatal.

Eicosanoids

The **eicosanoids** (i-ko′sah-noyds) are diverse lipids chiefly derived from a 20-carbon fatty acid (arachidonic acid) found in all cell membranes. Most important of these are the *prostaglandins* and their relatives, which play roles in various body processes including blood clotting, regulation of blood pressure, inflammation, and labor contractions (Table 2.2). Their synthesis and inflammatory actions are blocked by NSAIDs (nonsteroidal anti-inflammatory drugs) and the newer COX inhibitors.

☑ Check Your Understanding

20. What are the monomers of carbohydrates called? Which monomer is blood sugar?
21. What is the animal form of stored carbohydrate called?
22. How do triglycerides differ from phospholipids in body function and location?
23. What is the result of hydrolysis reactions and how are these reactions accomplished in the body?

For answers, see Appendix H.

Proteins

✓ Describe the four levels of protein structure.
✓ Indicate the function of molecular chaperones.
✓ Describe enzyme action.

The full set of proteins made by the body, called the *proteome*, and the way those proteins network in the body or change with disease, is a matter of intense biotech research.

Protein composes 10–30% of cell mass and is the basic structural material of the body. However, not all proteins are construction materials. Many play vital roles in cell function. Proteins, which include enzymes (biological catalysts), hemoglobin of the blood, and contractile proteins of muscle, have the most varied functions of any molecules in the body. All proteins contain carbon, oxygen, hydrogen, and nitrogen, and many contain sulfur as well.

Amino Acids and Peptide Bonds

The building blocks of proteins are molecules called **amino acids**, of which there are 20 common types (see Appendix C). All amino acids have two important functional groups: a basic group called an *amine* (ah′mēn) *group* ($—NH_2$), and an organic *acid group* ($—COOH$). An amino acid may therefore act either as a base (proton acceptor) or an acid (proton donor). All amino acids are identical except for a single group of atoms called their *R group*. Hence, it is differences in the R group that make each amino acid chemically unique, as the examples in **Figure 2.17** show.

Proteins are long chains of amino acids joined together by dehydration synthesis, with the amine end of one amino acid linked to the acid end of the next. The resulting bond produces a characteristic arrangement of linked atoms called a **peptide bond** **(Figure 2.18)**. Two united amino acids form a *dipeptide*, three a *tripeptide*, and ten or more a *polypeptide*. Although polypeptides containing more than 50 amino acids are called proteins, most proteins are **macromolecules**, large, complex molecules containing from 100 to over 10,000 amino acids.

Because each type of amino acid has distinct properties, the sequence in which they are bound together produces proteins that vary widely in both structure and function. We can think of the 20 amino acids as a 20-letter "alphabet" used in specific combinations to form "words" (proteins). Just as a change in one letter can produce a word with an entirely different meaning (flour → floor) or that is nonsensical (flour → flocr), changes in the kinds or positions of amino acids can yield proteins with different functions or proteins that are nonfunctional. Nevertheless, there are thousands of different proteins in the body, each with distinct functional properties, and all constructed from different combinations of the 20 common amino acids.

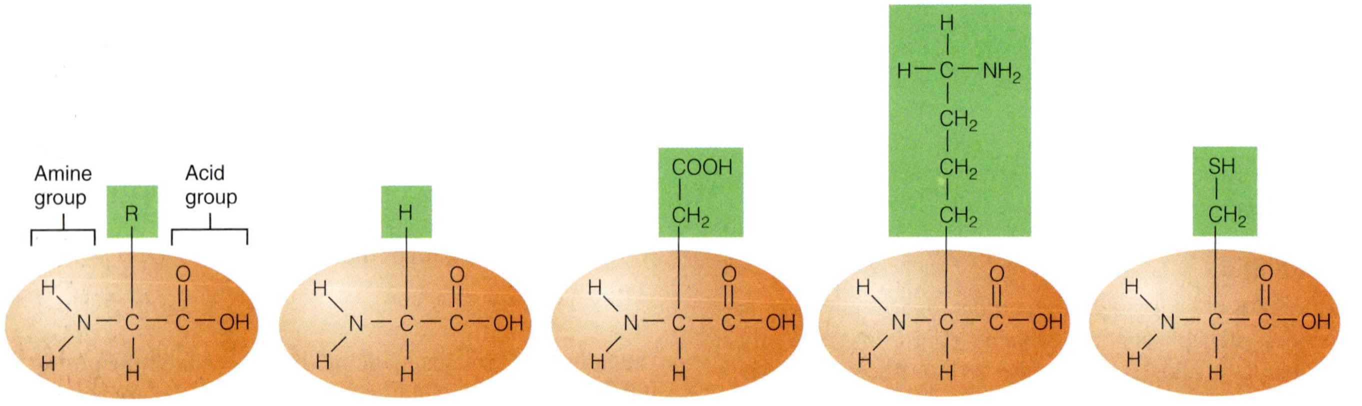

(a) Generalized structure of all amino acids.

(b) Glycine is the simplest amino acid.

(c) Aspartic acid (an acidic amino acid) has an acid group (—COOH) in the R group.

(d) Lysine (a basic amino acid) has an amine group ($—NH_2$) in the R group.

(e) Cysteine (a basic amino acid) has a sulfhydryl (—SH) group in the R group, which suggests that this amino acid is likely to participate in intramolecular bonding.

Figure 2.17 Amino acid structures. All amino acids have both an amine group ($—NH_2$) and an acid group (—COOH). They differ only in their R groups (green). Differences in their R groups allow them to function differently in the body.

Structural Levels of Proteins

Proteins can be described in terms of four structural levels. The linear sequence of amino acids composing the polypeptide chain is called the *primary structure* of a protein. This structure, which resembles a strand of amino acid "beads," is the backbone of the protein molecule **(Figure 2.19a)**.

Proteins do not normally exist as simple, linear chains of amino acids. Instead, they twist or bend upon themselves to form a more complex *secondary structure*. The most common type of secondary structure is the **alpha (α)-helix**, which resembles a Slinky toy or the coils of a telephone cord (Figure 2.19b). The α-helix is formed by coiling of the primary chain and is stabilized by hydrogen bonds formed between NH and CO groups in amino acids in the primary chain which are approximately four amino acids apart. Hydrogen bonds in α-helices always link different parts of the *same* chain together.

In another type of secondary structure, the **beta (β)-pleated sheet**, the primary polypeptide chains do not coil, but are linked side by side by hydrogen bonds to form a pleated, ribbonlike structure that resembles an accordion's bellows (Figure 2.19b). Notice that in this type of secondary structure, the hydrogen bonds may link together *different polypeptide chains* as well as *different parts* of the same chain that has folded back on itself. A single polypeptide chain may exhibit both types of secondary structure at various places along its length.

Many proteins have *tertiary structure* (ter′she-a″re), the next higher level of complexity, which is superimposed on secondary structure. Tertiary structure is achieved when α-helical or

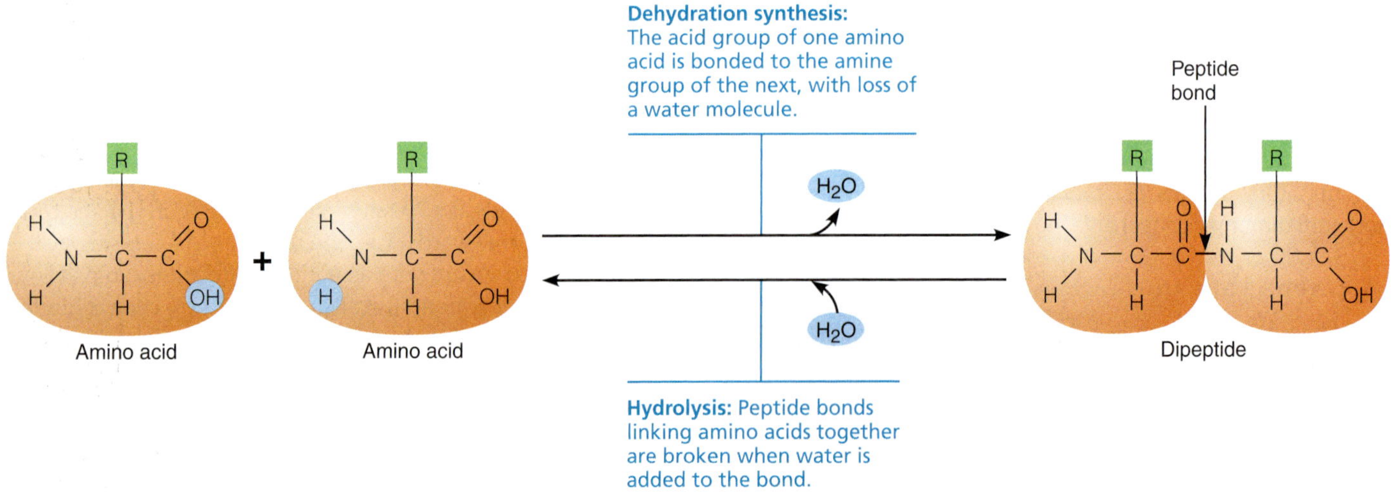

Figure 2.18 Amino acids are linked together by peptide bonds. Peptide bonds are formed by dehydration synthesis and broken by hydrolysis reactions.

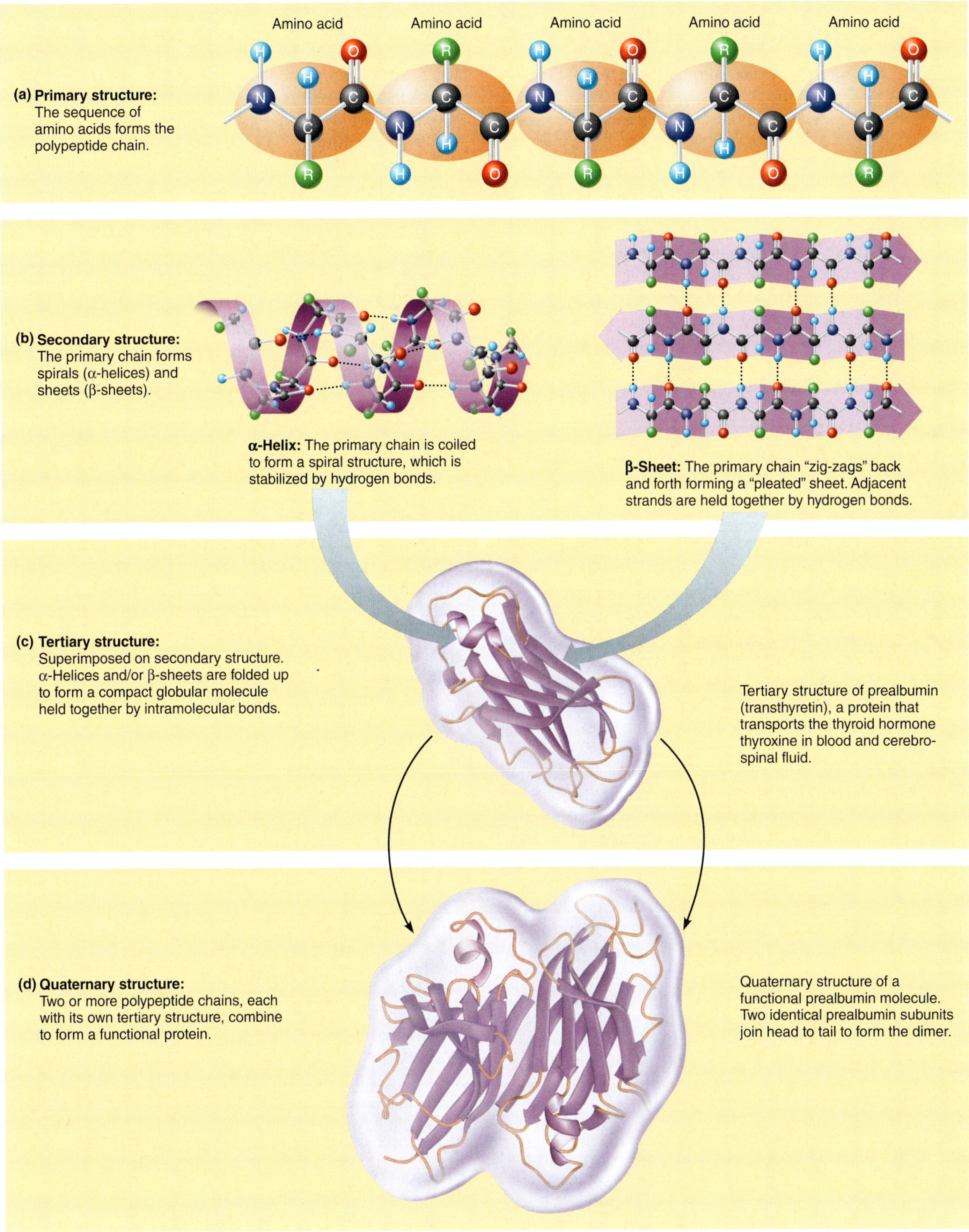

Figure 2.19 Levels of protein structure.

β-pleated regions of the polypeptide chain fold upon one another to produce a compact ball-like, or *globular*, molecule (Figure 2.19c). The unique structure is maintained by both covalent and hydrogen bonds between amino acids that are often far apart in the primary chain.

When two or more polypeptide chains aggregate in a regular manner to form a complex protein, the protein has *quaternary structure* (kwah′ter-na″re). Prealbumin, a protein that transports thyroid hormone in the blood, exhibits this structural level (Figure 2.19d).

How do these different levels of structure arise? Although a protein with tertiary or quaternary structure looks a bit like a clump of congealed pasta, the ultimate overall structure of any protein is very specific and is dictated by its primary structure. In other words, the types and relative positions of amino acids in the protein backbone determine where bonds can form to produce the complex coiled or folded structures that keep water-loving amino acids near the surface and water-fleeing amino acids buried in the protein's core. In addition, cells decorate many proteins by attaching sugars or fatty acids to them in ways that are difficult to imagine or predict.

Fibrous and Globular Proteins

The overall structure of a protein determines its biological function. In general, proteins are classified according to their overall appearance and shape as either fibrous or globular.

Fibrous proteins are extended and strandlike. Some exhibit only secondary structure, but most have tertiary or even quaternary structure as well. For example, *collagen* (kol′ah-jen) is a composite of the helical tropocollagen molecules packed together side by side to form a strong ropelike structure. Fibrous proteins are insoluble in water, and very stable—qualities ideal for providing mechanical support and tensile strength to the body's tissues. Besides collagen, which is the single most abundant protein in the body, the fibrous proteins include keratin, elastin, and certain contractile proteins of muscle (Table 2.3). Because fibrous proteins are the chief building materials of the body, they are also known as **structural proteins**.

Globular proteins are compact, spherical proteins that have at least tertiary structure. Some also exhibit quaternary structure. The globular proteins are water-soluble, chemically active molecules, and they play crucial roles in virtually all biological processes. Consequently, this group is also called **functional proteins**. Some (antibodies) help to provide immunity, others (protein-based hormones) regulate growth and development, and still others (enzymes) are catalysts that oversee just about every chemical reaction in the body. The roles of these and selected other proteins found in the body are summarized in Table 2.3.

Protein Denaturation

Fibrous proteins are stable, but globular proteins are quite the opposite. The activity of a protein depends on its specific three-dimensional structure, and intramolecular bonds, particularly hydrogen bonds, are important in maintaining that structure. However, hydrogen bonds are fragile and easily broken by many chemical and physical factors, such as excessive acidity or temperature. Although individual proteins vary in their sensitivity to environmental conditions, hydrogen bonds begin to break when the pH drops or the temperature rises above normal (physiological) levels, causing proteins to unfold and lose their specific three-dimensional shape. In this condition, a protein is said to be **denatured**.

Fortunately, the disruption is reversible in most cases, and the "scrambled" protein regains its native structure when desirable conditions are restored. However, if the temperature or pH change is so extreme that protein structure is damaged beyond repair, the protein is *irreversibly denatured*. The coagulation of egg white (primarily albumin protein) that occurs when you boil or fry an egg is an example of irreversible protein denaturation. There is no way to restore the white, rubbery protein to its original translucent form.

When globular proteins are denatured, they can no longer perform their physiological roles because their function depends on the presence of specific arrangements of atoms, called **active sites**, on their surfaces. The active sites are regions that fit and interact chemically with other molecules of complementary shape and charge. Because atoms contributing to an active site may actually be far apart in the primary chain, disruption of intramolecular bonds separates them and destroys the active site. For example, hemoglobin becomes totally unable to bind and transport oxygen when blood pH is too acidic, because the structure needed for its function has been destroyed.

We will describe most types of body proteins in conjunction with the organ systems or functional processes to which they are closely related. However, two groups of proteins—*molecular chaperones* and *enzymes*—are intimately involved in the normal functioning of all cells, so we will consider these incredibly complex molecules here.

☑ Check Your Understanding

24. What does the name "amino acid" tell you about the structure of this molecule?

25. What is the primary structure of proteins?

26. What are the two types of secondary structure in proteins?

For answers, see Appendix H.

Molecular Chaperones

In addition to enzymes, all cells contain a class of unrelated globular proteins called **molecular chaperones** which, among other things, help proteins to achieve their functional three-dimensional structure. Although its amino acid sequence determines the precise way a protein folds, the folding process also requires the help of molecular chaperones to ensure that the folding is quick and accurate. Molecular chaperones can associate with a broad range of "client" proteins, allowing them to perform a dizzying array of jobs. For example, specific molecular chaperones

- Prevent accidental, premature, or incorrect folding of polypeptide chains or their association with other polypeptides
- Aid the desired folding and association process

Table 2.3 Representative Types of Proteins in the Body

CLASSIFICATION ACCORDING TO: OVERALL STRUCTURE	GENERAL FUNCTION	EXAMPLES FROM THE BODY
Fibrous		
	Structural framework/ mechanical support	*Collagen*, found in all connective tissues, is the single most abundant protein in the body. It is responsible for the tensile strength of bones, tendons, and ligaments.
		Keratin is the structural protein of hair and nails and a water-resistant material of skin.
		Elastin is found, along with collagen, where durability and flexibility are needed, such as in the ligaments that bind bones together.
		Spectrin internally reinforces and stabilizes the surface membrane of some cells, particularly red blood cells. *Dystrophin* reinforces and stabilizes the surface membrane of muscle cells. *Titin* helps organize the intracellular structure of muscle cells and accounts for the elasticity of skeletal muscles.
	Movement	*Actin* and *myosin*, contractile proteins, are found in substantial amounts in muscle cells, where they cause muscle cell shortening (contraction); they also function in cell division in all cell types. Actin is important in intracellular transport, particularly in nerve cells.
Globular		
	Catalysis	Protein enzymes are essential to virtually every biochemical reaction in the body; they increase the rates of chemical reactions by at least a millionfold. Examples include *salivary amylase* (in saliva), which catalyzes the breakdown of starch, and *oxidase enzymes*, which act to oxidize food fuels.
	Transport	*Hemoglobin* transports oxygen in blood, and *lipoproteins* transport lipids and cholesterol. Other transport proteins in the blood carry iron, hormones, or other substances. Some globular proteins in plasma membranes are involved in membrane transport (as carriers or channels).
	Regulation of pH	Many plasma proteins, such as *albumin*, function reversibly as acids or bases, thus acting as buffers to prevent wide swings in blood pH.
	Regulation of metabolism	*Peptide* and *protein hormones* help to regulate metabolic activity, growth, and development. For example, *growth hormone* is an anabolic hormone necessary for optimal growth; *insulin* helps regulate blood sugar levels.
	Body defense	*Antibodies* (immunoglobulins) are specialized proteins released by immune cells that recognize and inactivate foreign substances (bacteria, toxins, some viruses).
		Complement proteins, which circulate in blood, enhance both immune and inflammatory responses.
	Protein management	*Molecular chaperones* aid folding of new proteins in both healthy and damaged cells and transport of metal ions into and within the cell. They also promote breakdown of damaged proteins.

- Help to translocate proteins and certain metal ions (copper, iron, zinc) across cell membranes
- Promote the breakdown of damaged or denatured proteins
- Interact with immune cells to trigger the immune response to diseased cells in the body

The first such proteins discovered were called *heat shock proteins* (*hsp*) because they seemed to protect cells from the destructive effects of heat. It was later found that these proteins are produced in response to a variety of traumatizing stimuli—for example, in the oxygen-deprived cells of a heart attack patient—and the name *stress proteins* replaced hsp for that particular group of molecular chaperones. It is now clear that these proteins are vitally important to cell function in all types of stressful circumstances. Although a lot of environmental stress can turn your hair gray or cause cardiac problems, it seems that a little stress can delay aging. As part of the heat shock response, special protein repair molecules patch up damaged proteins and refold them correctly, helping to hold off the grim reaper and prolong life.

Enzymes and Enzyme Activity

Enzymes are globular proteins that act as biological catalysts. *Catalysts* are substances that regulate and accelerate the rate of biochemical reactions but are not used up or changed in those

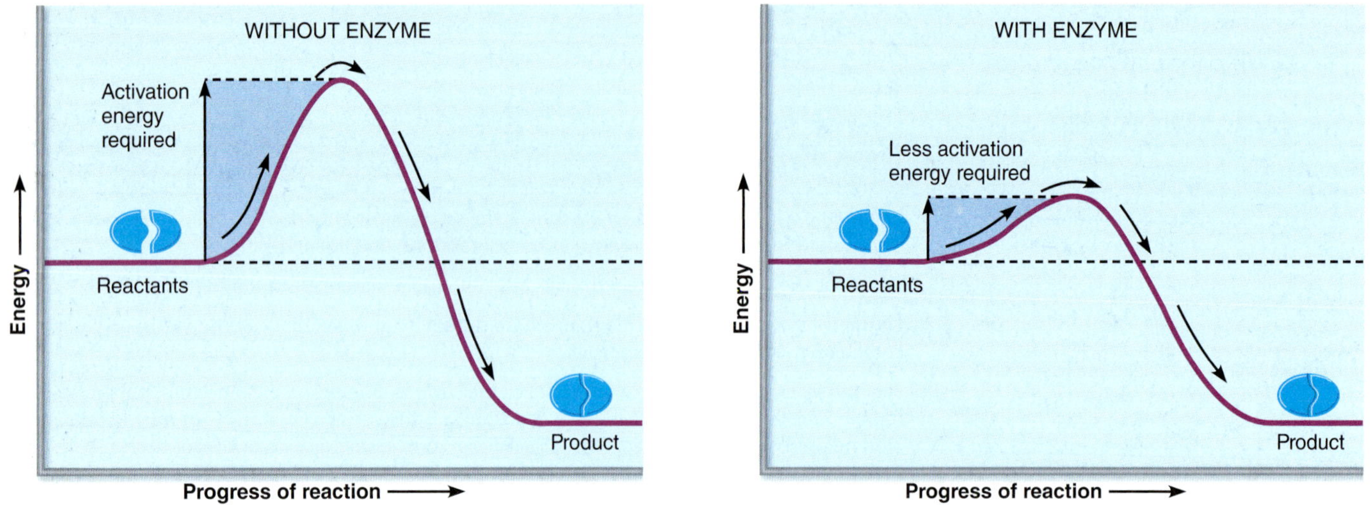

Figure 2.20 Enzymes lower the activation energy required for a reaction.

reactions. More specifically, enzymes can be thought of as chemical traffic cops that keep our metabolic pathways flowing. Enzymes cannot force chemical reactions to occur between molecules that would not otherwise react. They can only increase the speed of reaction, and they do so by staggering amounts—from 100,000 to over 1 billion times the rate of an uncatalyzed reaction. Without enzymes, biochemical reactions proceed so slowly that for practical purposes they do not occur at all.

Characteristics of Enzymes Some enzymes are purely protein. In other cases, the functional enzyme consists of two parts, collectively called a **holoenzyme**: an **apoenzyme** (the protein portion) and a **cofactor**. Depending on the enzyme, the cofactor may be an ion of a metal element such as copper or iron, or an organic molecule needed to assist the reaction in some particular way. Most organic cofactors are derived from vitamins (especially the B complex vitamins). This type of cofactor is more precisely called a **coenzyme**.

Each enzyme is chemically specific. Some enzymes control only a single chemical reaction. Others exhibit a broader specificity in that they can bind with molecules that differ slightly and thus regulate a small group of related reactions. The substance on which an enzyme acts is called a **substrate**.

The presence of specific enzymes determines not only which reactions will be speeded up, but also which reactions will occur—no enzyme, no reaction. This also means that unwanted or unnecessary chemical reactions do not occur.

Most enzymes are named for the type of reaction they catalyze. *Hydrolases* (hi′druh-lās-es) add water during hydrolysis reactions, *oxidases* (ok′sĭ-dās-es) oxidize reactants by adding oxygen or removing hydrogen, and so on. You can recognize most enzyme names by the suffix *-ase*.

In many cases, enzymes are part of cellular membranes in a bucket-brigade type of arrangement. The product of one enzyme-catalyzed reaction becomes the substrate of the neighboring enzyme, and so on. Some enzymes are produced in an inactive form and must be activated in some way before they can function, often by a change in the pH of their surroundings. For example, digestive enzymes produced in the pancreas are activated in the small intestine, where they actually do their work. If they were produced in active form, the pancreas would digest itself.

Sometimes, enzymes are inactivated immediately after they have performed their catalytic function. This is true of enzymes that promote blood clot formation when the wall of a blood vessel is damaged. Once clotting is triggered, those enzymes are inactivated. Otherwise, you would have blood vessels full of solid blood instead of one protective clot. (Eek!)

Enzyme Action How do enzymes perform their catalytic role? Every chemical reaction requires that a certain amount of energy, called **activation energy**, be absorbed to prime the reaction. The activation energy is the amount of energy needed to break the bonds of the reactants so that they can rearrange themselves and become the product. It is present when kinetic energy pushes the reactants to an energy level where their random collisions are forceful enough to ensure interaction. Activation energy is needed regardless of whether the overall reaction is ultimately energy absorbing or energy releasing.

One way to increase kinetic energy is to increase the temperature, but higher temperatures denature proteins. (This is why a high fever can be a serious event.) Enzymes allow reactions to occur at normal body temperature by decreasing the amount of activation energy required **(Figure 2.20)**.

Exactly how do enzymes accomplish this remarkable feat? The answer is not fully understood. However, we know that, due to structural and electrostatic factors, they decrease the randomness of reactions by binding to the reacting molecules temporarily and presenting them to each other in the proper position for chemical interaction (bond making or breaking) to occur.

Three basic steps appear to be involved in enzyme action **(Figure 2.21)**.

1. **Substrate(s) bind to the enzyme's active site, temporarily forming an enzyme-substrate complex.** Substrate binding causes the active site to change shape so that the substrate and the active site fit together precisely, and in an orientation that favors reaction. Whether the shape of the substrate

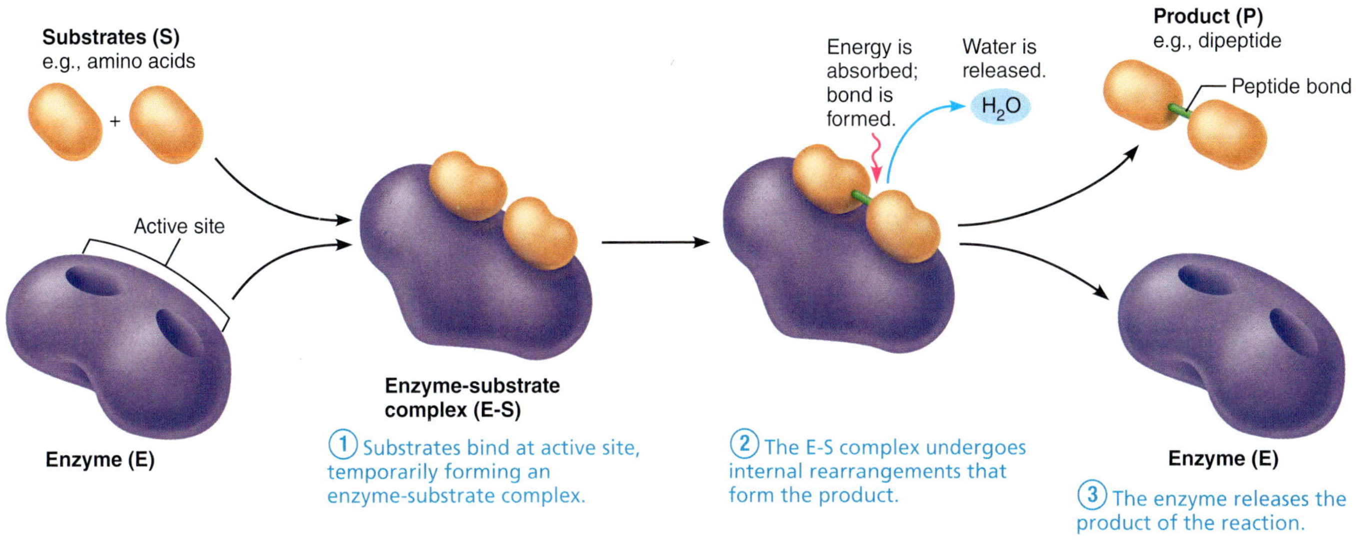

Figure 2.21 Mechanism of enzyme action. In this example, the enzyme catalyzes the formation of a dipeptide from specific amino acids. *Summary*: E + S → E-S → P + E

forces the enzyme to wiggle into a complementary shape or whether the enzyme wiggles around trying several different conformations until one finally fits the substrate is still a question. Although enzymes are specific for particular substrates, other (nonsubstrate) molecules may act as *enzyme inhibitors* if their structure is similar enough to occupy or block the enzyme's active site.

② **The enzyme-substrate complex undergoes internal rearrangements that form the product(s).** This step shows the catalytic role of an enzyme.

③ **The enzyme releases the product(s) of the reaction.** If the enzyme became part of the product, it would be a reactant and not a catalyst. The enzyme is not changed and returns to its original shape, available to catalyze another reaction.

Because enzymes are unchanged by their catalytic role and can act again and again, cells need only small amounts of each enzyme. Catalysis occurs with incredible speed. Most enzymes can catalyze millions of reactions per minute.

☑ Check Your Understanding

27. What is the main event that molecular chaperones prevent?
28. How do enzymes reduce the amount of activation energy needed to make a chemical reaction go?

For answers, see Appendix H.

Nucleic Acids (DNA and RNA)

✓ Compare and contrast DNA and RNA.

The **nucleic acids** (nu-kle′ic), composed of carbon, oxygen, hydrogen, nitrogen, and phosphorus, are the largest molecules in the body. The nucleic acids include two major classes of molecules, **deoxyribonucleic acid (DNA)** (de-ok″sĭ-ri″bo-nu-kle′ik) and **ribonucleic acid (RNA)**.

The structural units of nucleic acids, called **nucleotides**, are quite complex. Each nucleotide consists of three components: a nitrogen-containing base, a pentose sugar, and a phosphate group (Figure 2.22a). Five major varieties of nitrogen-containing bases can contribute to nucleotide structure: **adenine**, abbreviated **A** (ad′ĕ-nēn); **guanine**, **G** (gwan′ēn); **cytosine**, **C** (si′to-sēn); **thymine**, **T** (thi′mēn); and **uracil**, **U** (u′rah-sil). Adenine and guanine are large, two-ring bases (called purines), whereas cytosine, thymine, and uracil are smaller, single-ring bases (called pyrimidines).

The stepwise synthesis of a nucleotide involves the attachment of a base to the pentose sugar to form first a *nucleoside*, named for the nitrogenous base it contains. The nucleotide is formed when a phosphate group is bonded to the sugar of the nucleoside.

Although DNA and RNA are both composed of nucleotides, they differ in many respects, as summarized in Table 2.4 on p. 55. Typically, DNA is found in the nucleus (control center) of the cell, where it constitutes the *genetic material*, also called the *genes*, or more recently the *genome*. DNA has two fundamental roles: It replicates (reproduces) itself before a cell divides, ensuring that the genetic information in the descendant cells is identical, and it provides the basic instructions for building every protein in the body. Although we have said that enzymes govern all chemical reactions, remember that enzymes, too, are proteins formed at the direction of DNA.

By providing the information for protein synthesis, DNA determines what type of organism you will be—frog, human, oak tree—and directs your growth and development. It also accounts for your uniqueness. A technique called DNA fingerprinting can help solve forensic mysteries (for example, verify one's presence at a crime scene), identify badly burned or mangled bodies at a disaster scene, and establish or disprove paternity. DNA fingerprinting analyzes tiny samples of DNA taken from blood, semen, or other body tissues and shows the results as a "genetic barcode" that distinguishes each of us from all others.

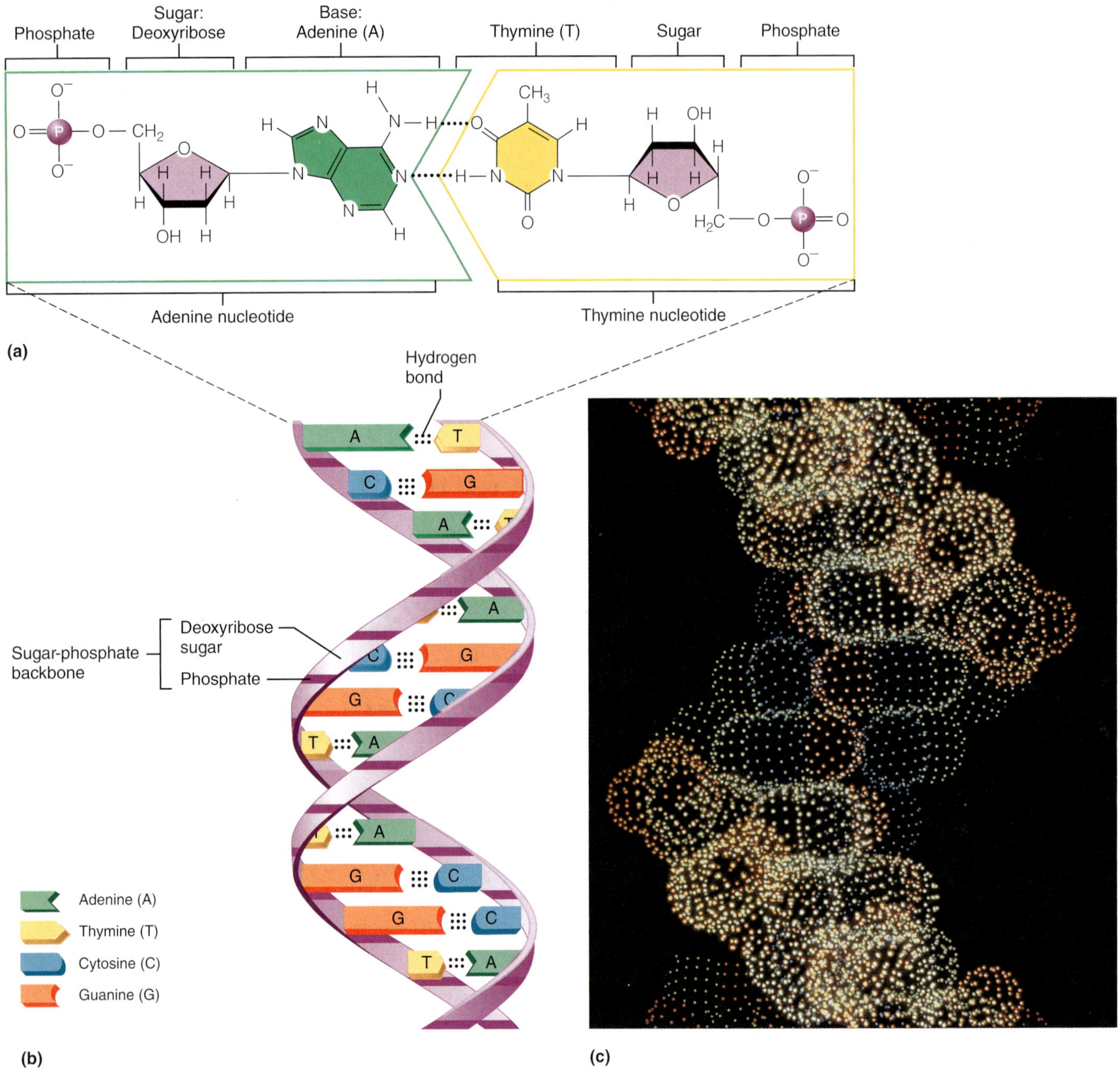

Figure 2.22 Structure of DNA. (a) The unit of DNA is the nucleotide, which is composed of a deoxyribose sugar molecule linked to a phosphate group, with a base attached to the sugar. Two nucleotides, linked by hydrogen bonds between their complementary bases, are illustrated. **(b)** DNA is a coiled double polymer of nucleotides (a double helix). The backbones of the ladderlike molecule are formed by alternating sugar and phosphate units. The rungs are formed by the binding together of complementary bases (A-T and G-C) by hydrogen bonds (shown by dotted lines). **(c)** Computer-generated image of a DNA molecule.

DNA is a long, double-stranded polymer—a double chain of nucleotides (Figure 2.22b and c). The bases in DNA are A, G, C, and T, and its pentose sugar is *deoxyribose* (as reflected in its name). Its two nucleotide chains are held together by hydrogen bonds between the bases, so that a ladderlike molecule is formed. Alternating sugar and phosphate components of each chain form the *backbones* or "uprights" of the "ladder," and the joined bases form the "rungs." The whole molecule is coiled into a spiral staircase–like structure called a **double helix**.

Bonding of the bases is very specific: A always bonds to T, and G always bonds to C. A and T are therefore called **complementary bases**, as are C and G. According to these base-pairing rules, ATGA on one DNA nucleotide strand would necessarily be bonded to TACT (a complementary base sequence) on the other strand.

Table 2.4 Comparison of DNA and RNA

CHARACTERISTIC	DNA	RNA
Major cellular site	Nucleus	Cytoplasm (cell area outside the nucleus)
Major functions	Is the genetic material; directs protein synthesis; replicates itself before cell division	Carries out the genetic instructions for protein synthesis
Sugar	Deoxyribose	Ribose
Bases	Adenine, guanine, cytosine, thymine	Adenine, guanine, cytosine, uracil
Structure	Double strand coiled into a double helix	Single strand, straight or folded

RNA is located chiefly outside the nucleus and can be considered a "molecular slave" of DNA. That is, RNA carries out the orders for protein synthesis issued by DNA. [Viruses in which RNA (rather than DNA) is the genetic material are an exception to this generalization.]

RNA molecules are single strands of nucleotides. RNA bases include A, G, C, and U (U replaces the T found in DNA), and its sugar is *ribose* instead of deoxyribose. The three major varieties of RNA (messenger RNA, ribosomal RNA, and transfer RNA) are distinguished by their relative size and shape, and each has a specific role to play in carrying out DNA's instructions for protein synthesis. In addition to these three RNAs, small RNA molecules called *microRNAs* (*miRNAs*) appear to control genetic expression by shutting down genes or altering their expression. We discuss DNA replication and the relative roles of DNA and RNA in protein synthesis in Chapter 3.

Check Your Understanding

29. How do DNA and RNA differ in the bases and sugars they contain?
30. What are two important roles of DNA?

For answers, see Appendix H.

Adenosine Triphosphate (ATP)

✓ Explain the role of ATP in cell metabolism.

Glucose is the most important cellular fuel, but none of the chemical energy contained in its bonds is used directly to power cellular work. Instead, energy released during glucose catabolism is coupled to the synthesis of **adenosine triphosphate (ATP)**. In other words, some of this energy is captured and stored as small packets of energy in the bonds of ATP. ATP is the primary energy-transferring molecule in cells and it provides a form of energy that is immediately usable by all body cells.

Structurally, ATP is an adenine-containing RNA nucleotide to which two additional phosphate groups have been added (Figure 2.23). Chemically, the triphosphate tail of ATP can be compared to a tightly coiled spring ready to uncoil with tremendous energy when the catch is released. Actually, ATP is a very unstable energy-storing molecule because its three negatively charged phosphate groups are closely packed and repel each other. When its terminal high-energy phosphate bonds are broken (hydrolyzed), the chemical "spring" relaxes and the molecule as a whole becomes more stable.

Cells tap ATP's bond energy during coupled reactions by using enzymes to transfer the terminal phosphate groups from ATP to other compounds. These newly *phosphorylated* molecules are said to be "primed" and temporarily become more energetic and capable of performing some type of cellular work. In the process of doing their work, they lose the phosphate group. The amount of energy released and transferred during ATP hydrolysis corresponds closely to that needed to drive most biochemical reactions. As a result, cells are protected from excessive energy release that might be damaging, and energy squandering is kept to a minimum.

Cleaving the terminal phosphate bond of ATP yields a molecule with two phosphate groups—*adenosine diphosphate*

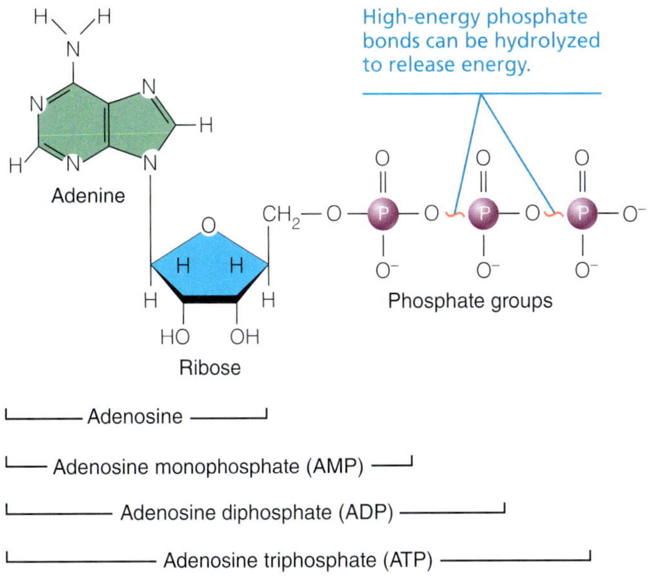

Figure 2.23 Structure of ATP (adenosine triphosphate). ATP is an adenine nucleotide to which two additional phosphate groups have been attached during breakdown of food fuels. When the terminal phosphate group is cleaved off, energy is released to do useful work and ADP (adenosine diphosphate) is formed. When the terminal phosphate group is cleaved off ADP, a similar amount of energy is released and AMP (adenosine monophosphate) is formed.

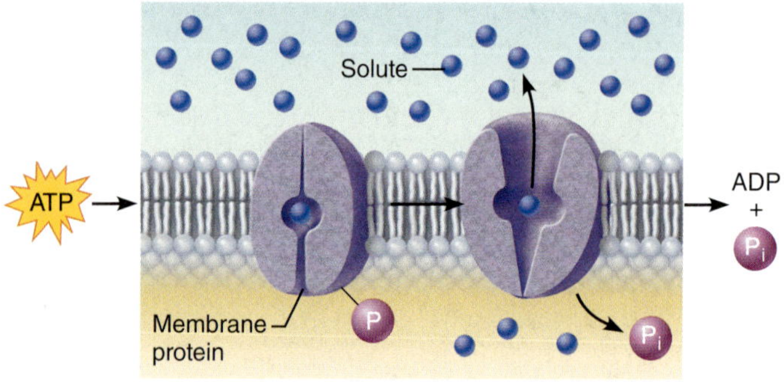

(a) Transport work: ATP phosphorylates transport proteins, activating them to transport solutes (ions, for example) across cell membranes.

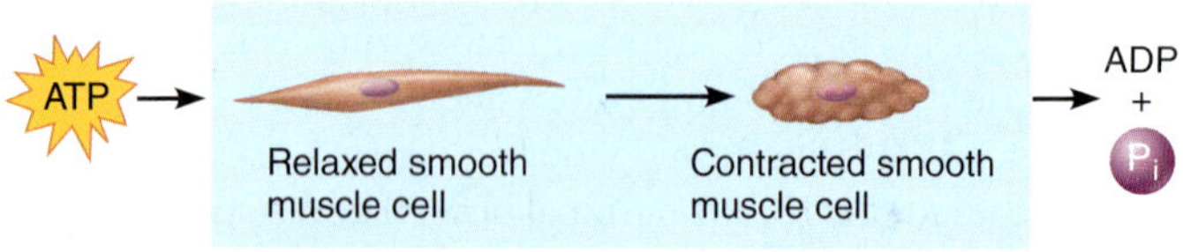

(b) Mechanical work: ATP phosphorylates contractile proteins in muscle cells so the cells can shorten.

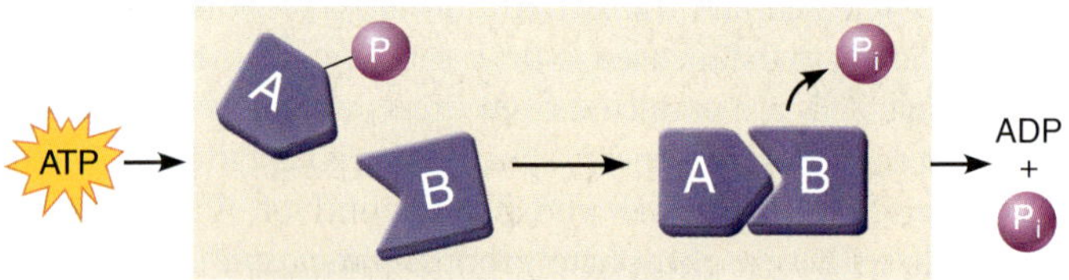

(c) Chemical work: ATP phosphorylates key reactants, providing energy to drive energy-absorbing chemical reactions.

Figure 2.24 Three examples of cellular work driven by energy from ATP.

(*ADP*)—and an inorganic phosphate group, indicated by P_i, accompanied by a transfer of energy:

$$\text{ATP} \underset{H_2O}{\overset{H_2O}{\rightleftharpoons}} \text{ADP} + P_i + \text{energy}$$

As ATP is hydrolyzed to provide energy for cellular needs, ADP accumulates. Cleavage of the terminal phosphate bond of ADP liberates a similar amount of energy and produces adenosine monophosphate (AMP).

The cell's ATP supplies are replenished as glucose and other fuel molecules are oxidized and their bond energy is released. The same amount of energy that is liberated when ATP's terminal phosphates are cleaved off must be captured and used to reverse the reaction to reattach phosphates and re-form the energy-transferring phosphate bonds. Without ATP, molecules cannot be made or degraded, cells cannot transport substances across their membrane boundaries, muscles cannot shorten to tug on other structures, and life processes cease **(Figure 2.24)**.

Check Your Understanding

31. Glucose is an energy-rich molecule. So why do body cells need ATP?
32. What change occurs in ATP when it releases energy?

For answers, see Appendix H.

Chapter Summary

PART 1 Basic Chemistry

Definition of Concepts: Matter and Energy (pp. 23–25)

Matter (p. 24)

1. Matter is anything that takes up space and has mass.

Energy (pp. 24–25)

2. Energy is the capacity to do work or put matter into motion.
3. Energy exists as potential energy (stored energy or energy of position) and kinetic energy (active or working energy).
4. Forms of energy involved in body functioning are chemical, electrical, radiant, and mechanical. Of these, chemical (bond) energy is most important.
5. Energy may be converted from one form to another, but some energy is always unusable (lost as heat) in such transformations.

Composition of Matter: Atoms and Elements (pp. 25–28)

1. Elements are unique substances that cannot be decomposed into simpler substances by ordinary chemical methods. Four elements (carbon, hydrogen, oxygen, and nitrogen) make up 96% of body weight.

Atomic Structure (pp. 25–26)

2. The building blocks of elements are atoms.
3. Atoms are composed of positively charged protons, negatively charged electrons, and uncharged neutrons. Protons and neutrons are located in the atomic nucleus, constituting essentially the atom's total mass. Electrons are outside the nucleus in the electron shells. In any atom, the number of electrons equals the number of protons.

Identifying Elements (pp. 27–28)

4. Atoms may be identified by their atomic number (p^+) and mass number ($p^+ + n^0$). The notation ^4_2He means that helium (He) has an atomic number of 2 and a mass number of 4.
5. Isotopes of an element differ in the number of neutrons they contain. The atomic weight of any element is approximately equal to the mass number of its most abundant isotope.

Radioisotopes (p. 28)

6. Many heavy isotopes are unstable (radioactive). These so-called radioisotopes decompose to more stable forms by emitting alpha or beta particles or gamma rays. Radioisotopes are useful in medical diagnosis and treatment and in biochemical research.

How Matter Is Combined: Molecules and Mixtures (pp. 28–30)

Molecules and Compounds (pp. 28–29)

1. A molecule is the smallest unit resulting from the chemical bonding of two or more atoms. If the atoms are different, they form a molecule of a compound.

Mixtures (pp. 29–30)

2. Mixtures are physical combinations of solutes in a solvent. Mixture components retain their individual properties.
3. The types of mixtures, in order of increasing solute size, are solutions, colloids, and suspensions.
4. Solution concentrations are typically designated in terms of percent or molarity.

Distinguishing Mixtures from Compounds (p. 30)

5. Compounds are homogeneous; their elements are chemically bonded. Mixtures may be homogeneous or heterogeneous; their components are physically combined and separable.

Chemical Bonds (pp. 30–35)

The Role of Electrons in Chemical Bonding (p. 31)

1. Electrons of an atom occupy areas of space called electron shells or energy levels. Electrons in the shell farthest from the nucleus (valence shell) are most energetic.
2. Chemical bonds are energy relationships between valence shell electrons of the reacting atoms. Atoms with a full valence shell or eight valence shell electrons are chemically unreactive (inert). Those with an incomplete valence shell interact with other atoms to achieve stability.

Types of Chemical Bonds (pp. 31–35)

3. Ionic bonds are formed when valence shell electrons are completely transferred from one atom to another.
4. Covalent bonds are formed when atoms share electron pairs. If the electron pairs are shared equally, the molecule is nonpolar. If they are shared unequally, it is polar (a dipole).
5. Hydrogen bonds are weak bonds formed between one hydrogen atom, already covalently linked to an electronegative atom, and another electronegative atom (such as nitrogen or oxygen). They bind together different molecules (e.g., water molecules) or different parts of the same molecule (as in protein molecules).

Chemical Reactions (pp. 35–38)

Chemical Equations (pp. 35–36)

1. Chemical reactions involve the formation, breaking, or rearrangement of chemical bonds.

Patterns of Chemical Reactions (pp. 36–37)

2. Chemical reactions are either anabolic (constructive) or catabolic (destructive). They include synthesis, decomposition, and exchange reactions. Oxidation-reduction reactions may be considered a special type of exchange (or decomposition) reaction.

Energy Flow in Chemical Reactions (p. 37)

3. Bonds are energy relationships and there is a net loss or gain of energy in every chemical reaction.
4. In exergonic reactions, energy is liberated. In endergonic reactions, energy is absorbed.

Reversibility of Chemical Reactions (p. 37)

5. If reaction conditions remain unchanged, all chemical reactions eventually reach a state of chemical equilibrium in which the reaction proceeds in both directions at the same rate.
6. All chemical reactions are theoretically reversible, but many biological reactions go in only one direction because of energy requirements or the removal of reaction products.

Factors Influencing the Rate of Chemical Reactions (pp. 37–38)

7. Chemical reactions occur only when particles collide and valence shell electrons interact.
8. The smaller the reacting particles, the greater their kinetic energy and the faster the reaction rate. Higher temperature or reactant concentration, as well as the presence of catalysts, increases chemical reaction rates.

PART 2 Biochemistry

Inorganic Compounds (pp. 38–41)

1. Most inorganic compounds do not contain carbon. Those found in the body include water, salts, and inorganic acids and bases.

Water (pp. 38–39)

2. Water is the single most abundant compound in the body. It absorbs and releases heat slowly, acts as a universal solvent, participates in chemical reactions, and cushions body organs.

Salts (p. 39)

3. Salts are ionic compounds that dissolve in water and act as electrolytes. Calcium and phosphorus salts contribute to the hardness of bones and teeth. Ions of salts are involved in many physiological processes.

Acids and Bases (pp. 39–41)

4. Acids are proton donors; in water, they ionize and dissociate, releasing hydrogen ions (which account for their properties) and anions.

iP Fluid, Electrolyte and Acid/Base Balance; Topic: Acid Base Homeostasis, pp. 1–12, 16, 17.

5. Bases are proton acceptors. The most common inorganic bases are the hydroxides; bicarbonate ion and ammonia are important bases in the body.
6. pH is a measure of hydrogen ion concentration of a solution (in moles per liter). A pH of 7 is neutral; a higher pH is alkaline, and a lower pH is acidic. Normal blood pH is 7.35–7.45. Buffers help to prevent excessive changes in the pH of body fluids.

iP Fluid, Electrolyte and Acid/Base Balance; Topic: Introduction to Body Fluids, pp. 1–8.

2

Organic Compounds (pp. 41–56)

1. Organic compounds contain carbon. Those found in the body include carbohydrates, lipids, proteins, and nucleic acids, all of which are synthesized by dehydration synthesis and digested by hydrolysis. All of these biological molecules contain C, H, and O. Proteins and nucleic acids also contain N.

Carbohydrates (p. 43)

2. Carbohydrate building blocks are monosaccharides, the most important of which are hexoses (glucose, fructose, galactose) and pentoses (ribose, deoxyribose).
3. Disaccharides (sucrose, lactose, maltose) and polysaccharides (starch, glycogen) are composed of linked monosaccharide units.
4. Carbohydrates, particularly glucose, are the major energy fuel for forming ATP. Excess carbohydrates are stored as glycogen or converted to fat for storage.

Lipids (pp. 43–47)

5. Lipids dissolve in fats or organic solvents, but not in water.
6. Triglycerides are composed of fatty acid chains and glycerol. They are found chiefly in fatty tissue where they provide insulation and reserve body fuel. Unsaturated fatty acid chains produce oils. Saturated fatty acids produce solid fats typical of animal fats.
7. Phospholipids are modified phosphorus-containing triglycerides that have polar and nonpolar portions. They are found in all plasma membranes.
8. The steroid cholesterol is found in cell membranes and is the basis of steroid hormones, bile salts, and vitamin D.

Proteins (pp. 47–53)

9. The unit of proteins is the amino acid, and 20 common amino acids are found in the body.
10. Many amino acids joined by peptide bonds form a polypeptide. A protein (one or more polypeptides) is distinguished by the number and sequence of amino acids in its chain(s) and by the complexity of its three-dimensional structure.
11. Fibrous proteins, such as keratin and collagen, have secondary (α-helix or β-pleated sheet) and perhaps tertiary and quaternary structure. Fibrous proteins are used as structural materials.
12. Globular proteins achieve tertiary and sometimes quaternary structure and are generally spherical, soluble molecules. Globular proteins (e.g., enzymes, some hormones, antibodies, hemoglobin) perform special functional roles for the cell (e.g., catalysis, molecule transport).
13. Proteins are denatured by extremes of temperature or pH. Denatured globular proteins are unable to perform their usual function.
14. Molecular chaperones assist in folding proteins into their functional 3-D shape. They are synthesized in greater amounts when cells are stressed by environmental factors.
15. Enzymes are biological catalysts. They increase the rate of chemical reactions by decreasing the amount of activation energy needed. They do this by combining with the reactants and holding them in the proper position to interact. Many enzymes require cofactors to function.

Nucleic Acids (DNA and RNA) (pp. 53–55)

16. Nucleic acids include deoxyribonucleic acid (DNA) and ribonucleic acid (RNA). The structural unit of nucleic acids is the nucleotide, which consists of a nitrogenous base (adenine, guanine, cytosine, thymine, or uracil), a sugar (ribose or deoxyribose), and a phosphate group.
17. DNA is a double-stranded helix. It contains deoxyribose and the bases A, G, C, and T. DNA specifies protein structure and replicates itself exactly before cell division.
18. RNA is single stranded. It contains ribose and the bases A, G, C, and U. RNAs involved in carrying out DNA's instructions for protein synthesis include messenger, ribosomal, and transfer RNA.

Adenosine Triphosphate (ATP) (pp. 55–56)

19. ATP is the universal energy compound of body cells. Some of the energy liberated by the breakdown of glucose and other food fuels is captured in the bonds of ATP molecules and transferred via coupled reactions to energy-consuming reactions.

Review Questions

Multiple Choice/Matching

(Some questions have more than one correct answer. Select the best answer or answers from the choices given.)

1. Which of the following forms of energy is the stimulus for vision? **(a)** chemical, **(b)** electrical, **(c)** mechanical, **(d)** radiant.
2. All of the following are examples of the four major elements contributing to body mass except **(a)** hydrogen, **(b)** carbon, **(c)** nitrogen, **(d)** sodium, **(e)** oxygen.
3. The mass number of an atom is **(a)** equal to the number of protons it contains, **(b)** the sum of its protons and neutrons, **(c)** the sum of all of its subatomic particles, **(d)** the average of the mass numbers of all of its isotopes.
4. A deficiency in this element can be expected to reduce the hemoglobin content of blood: **(a)** Fe, **(b)** I, **(c)** F, **(d)** Ca, **(e)** K.
5. Which set of terms best describes a proton? **(a)** negative charge, massless, in the orbital; **(b)** positive charge, 1 amu, in the nucleus; **(c)** uncharged, 1 amu, in the nucleus.
6. The subatomic particles responsible for the chemical behavior of atoms are **(a)** electrons, **(b)** ions, **(c)** neutrons, **(d)** protons.
7. In the body, carbohydrates are stored in the form of **(a)** glycogen, **(b)** starch, **(c)** cholesterol, **(d)** polypeptides.

8. Which of the following does *not* describe a mixture? **(a)** properties of its components are retained, **(b)** chemical bonds are formed, **(c)** components can be separated physically, **(d)** includes both heterogeneous and homogeneous examples.
9. In a beaker of water, the water-water bonds can properly be called **(a)** ionic bonds, **(b)** polar covalent bonds, **(c)** nonpolar covalent bonds, **(d)** hydrogen bonds.
10. When a pair of electrons is shared between two atoms, the bond formed is called **(a)** a single covalent bond, **(b)** a double covalent bond, **(c)** a triple covalent bond, **(d)** an ionic bond.
11. Molecules formed when electrons are shared unequally are **(a)** salts, **(b)** polar molecules, **(c)** nonpolar molecules.
12. Which of the following covalently bonded molecules are polar?

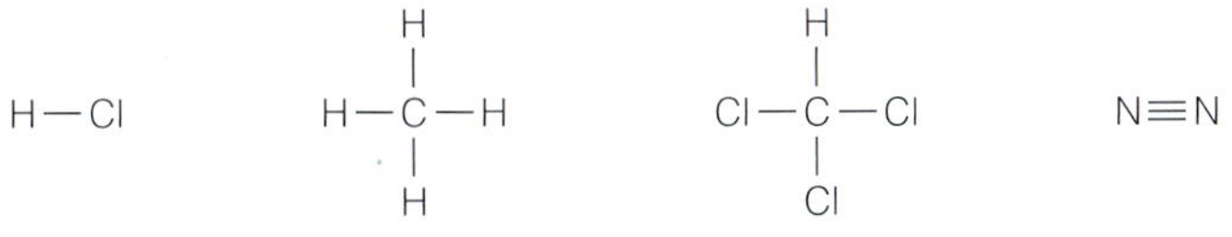

(a) **(b)** **(c)** **(d)**

13. Identify each reaction as one of the following: **(a)** a synthesis reaction, **(b)** a decomposition reaction, **(c)** an exchange reaction.
    ______________ (1) $2Hg + O_2 \rightarrow 2HgO$
    ______________ (2) $HCl + NaOH \rightarrow NaCl + H_2O$
14. Factors that accelerate the rate of chemical reactions include all but **(a)** the presence of catalysts, **(b)** increasing the temperature, **(c)** increasing the particle size, **(d)** increasing the concentration of the reactants.
15. Which of the following molecules is an inorganic molecule? **(a)** sucrose, **(b)** cholesterol, **(c)** collagen, **(d)** sodium chloride.
16. Water's importance to living systems reflects **(a)** its polarity and solvent properties, **(b)** its high heat capacity, **(c)** its high heat of vaporization, **(d)** its chemical reactivity, **(e)** all of these.
17. Acids **(a)** release hydroxyl ions when dissolved in water, **(b)** are proton acceptors, **(c)** cause the pH of a solution to rise, **(d)** release protons when dissolved in water.
18. A chemist, during the course of an analysis, runs across a chemical composed of carbon, hydrogen, and oxygen in the proportion 1:2:1 and having a six-sided molecular shape. It is probably **(a)** a pentose, **(b)** an amino acid, **(c)** a fatty acid, **(d)** a monosaccharide, **(e)** a nucleic acid.
19. A triglyceride consists of **(a)** glycerol plus three fatty acids, **(b)** a sugar-phosphate backbone to which two amino groups are attached, **(c)** two to several hexoses, **(d)** amino acids that have been thoroughly saturated with hydrogen.
20. A chemical has an amine group and an organic acid group. It does not, however, have any peptide bonds. It is **(a)** a monosaccharide, **(b)** an amino acid, **(c)** a protein, **(d)** a fat.
21. The lipid(s) used as the basis of vitamin D, sex hormones, and bile salts is/are **(a)** triglycerides, **(b)** cholesterol, **(c)** phospholipids, **(d)** prostaglandin.
22. Enzymes are organic catalysts that **(a)** alter the direction in which a chemical reaction proceeds, **(b)** determine the nature of the products of a reaction, **(c)** increase the speed of a chemical reaction, **(d)** are essential raw materials for a chemical reaction that are converted into some of its products.

Short Answer Essay Questions

23. Define or describe energy, and explain the relationship between potential and kinetic energy.
24. Some energy is lost in every energy conversion. Explain the meaning of this statement. (Direct your response to answering the question: Is it really lost? If not, what then?)
25. Provide the atomic symbol for each of the following elements: (a) calcium, (b) carbon, (c) hydrogen, (d) iron, (e) nitrogen, (f) oxygen, (g) potassium, (h) sodium.
26. Consider the following information about three atoms:

    $^{12}_{6}C \quad ^{13}_{6}C \quad ^{14}_{6}C$

    (a) How are they similar to one another? (b) How do they differ from one another? (c) What are the members of such a group of atoms called? (d) Using the planetary model, draw the atomic configuration of $^{12}_{6}C$ showing the relative position and numbers of its subatomic particles.
27. How many moles of aspirin, $C_9H_8O_4$, are in a bottle containing 450 g by weight? (*Note*: The approximate atomic weights of its atoms are $C = 12$, $H = 1$, and $O = 16$.)
28. Given the following types of atoms, decide which type of bonding, ionic or covalent, is most likely to occur: (a) two oxygen atoms; (b) four hydrogen atoms and one carbon atom; (c) a potassium atom ($^{39}_{19}K$) and a fluorine atom ($^{19}_{9}F$).
29. What are hydrogen bonds and how are they important in the body?
30. The following equation, which represents the oxidative breakdown of glucose by body cells, is a reversible reaction.

    Glucose + oxygen $\rightarrow$ carbon dioxide + water + ATP

    (a) How can you indicate that the reaction is reversible? (b) How can you indicate that the reaction is in chemical equilibrium? (c) Define chemical equilibrium.
31. Differentiate clearly between primary, secondary, and tertiary protein structure.
32. Dehydration and hydrolysis reactions are essentially opposite reactions. How are they related to the synthesis and degradation (breakdown) of biological molecules?
33. Describe the mechanism of enzyme action.
34. Explain the importance of molecular chaperones.
35. Explain why, if you pour water into a glass very carefully, you can "stack" the water slightly above the rim of the glass.

Critical Thinking and Clinical Application Questions

1. As Ben jumped on his bike and headed for the freshwater lake, his mother called after him, "Don't swim if we have an electrical storm—it looks threatening." This was a valid request. Why?
2. Some antibiotics act by binding to certain essential enzymes in the target bacteria. (a) How might these antibiotics influence the chemical reactions controlled by the enzymes? (b) What is the anticipated effect on the bacteria? On the person taking the antibiotic prescription?
3. Mrs. Roberts, in a diabetic coma, has just been admitted to Noble Hospital. Her blood pH indicates that she is in severe acidosis, and measures are quickly instituted to bring her blood pH back within normal limits. (a) Define pH and note the normal pH of blood. (b) Why is severe acidosis a problem?
4. Jimmy, a 12-year-old boy, was awakened suddenly by a loud crash. As he sat up in bed, straining to listen, his fright was revealed by his rapid breathing (hyperventilation), a breathing pattern effective in ridding the blood of CO_2. At this point, was his blood pH rising or falling?
5. After you eat a protein bar, which chemical reactions introduced in this chapter must occur for the amino acids in the protein bar to be converted into proteins in your body cells?

AT THE CLINIC

Related Clinical Terms

Acidosis (as″ĭ-do′sis; *acid* = sour, sharp) A condition of acidity or low pH (below 7.35) of the blood; high hydrogen ion concentration.

Alkalosis (al″kah-lo′sis) A condition of basicity or high pH (above 7.45) of the blood; low hydrogen ion concentration.

2

Heavy metals Metals with toxic effects on the body, including arsenic, mercury, and lead. Iron, also included in this group, is toxic in high concentrations.

Ionizing radiation Radiation that causes atoms to ionize; for example, radioisotope emissions and X rays.

Ketosis (ke-to′sis) A condition resulting from excessive ketones (breakdown products of fats) in the blood; common during starvation and acute attacks of diabetes mellitus.

Radiation sickness Disease resulting from exposure of the body to radioactivity; digestive system organs are most affected.

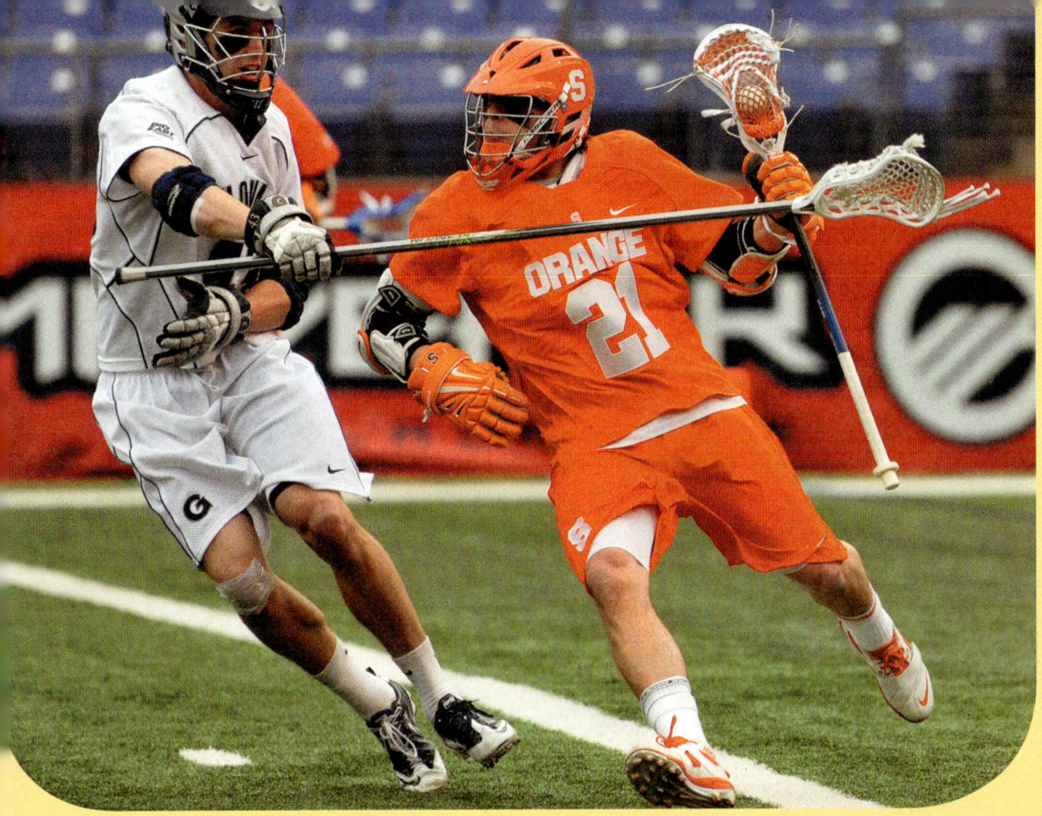

3 Cells: The Living Units

Just as bricks and timbers are the structural units of a house, **cells** are the structural units of all living things, from one-celled "generalists" like amoebas to complex multicellular organisms such as humans, dogs, and trees. The human body has 50 to 100 trillion of these tiny building blocks.

This chapter focuses on structures and functions shared by all cells. We address specialized cells and their unique functions in later chapters.

The Cellular Basis of Life

✓ Define cell.

✓ List the three major regions of a generalized cell and their functions.

The English scientist Robert Hooke first observed plant cells with a crude microscope in the late 1600s. Then, in the 1830s two German scientists, Matthias Schleiden and Theodor Schwann, proposed that all living things are composed of cells. German pathologist Rudolf Virchow extended this idea by contending that cells arise only from other cells.

Since the late 1800s, cell research has been exceptionally fruitful and provided us with four concepts collectively known as the **cell theory**:

- A *cell* is the basic structural and functional unit of living organisms. When you define cell properties, you define the properties of life.
- The activity of an organism depends on both the individual and the collective activities of its cells.
- According to the *principle of complementarity of structure and function*, the biochemical activities of cells are dictated by their shapes or forms, and by the relative number of their specific subcellular structures.
- Continuity of life from one generation to another has a cellular basis.

We will expand on all of these concepts as we progress. Let us begin with the idea that the cell is the smallest living unit. Whatever its form, however it behaves, the cell is the microscopic package that contains all the parts necessary to survive in an ever-changing world. It follows then that loss of cellular homeostasis underlies virtually every disease.

The trillions of cells in the human body include over 200 different cell types that vary greatly in shape, size, and function **(Figure 3.1)**. The disc-shaped red blood cells, branching nerve cells, and cubelike cells of kidney tubules are just a few examples of the shapes cells take. Cells also vary in length—ranging from 2 micrometers (1/12,000 of an inch) in the smallest cells to over a meter in the nerve cells that cause you to wiggle your toes. A cell's shape reflects its function. For example, the flat, tilelike epithelial cells that line the inside of your cheek fit closely together, forming a living barrier that protects underlying tissues from bacterial invasion.

Regardless of type, all cells are composed chiefly of carbon, hydrogen, nitrogen, oxygen, and trace amounts of several other elements. In addition, all cells have the same basic parts and some common functions. For this reason, it is possible to speak of a **generalized**, or **composite**, **cell** **(Figure 3.2)**.

A human cell has three main parts:

- The *plasma membrane*: the outer boundary of the cell.
- The *cytoplasm* (si′to-plazm): the intracellular fluid packed with *organelles*, small structures that perform specific cell functions.
- The *nucleus* (nu′kle-us): an organelle that controls cellular activities. Typically the nucleus lies near the cell's center.

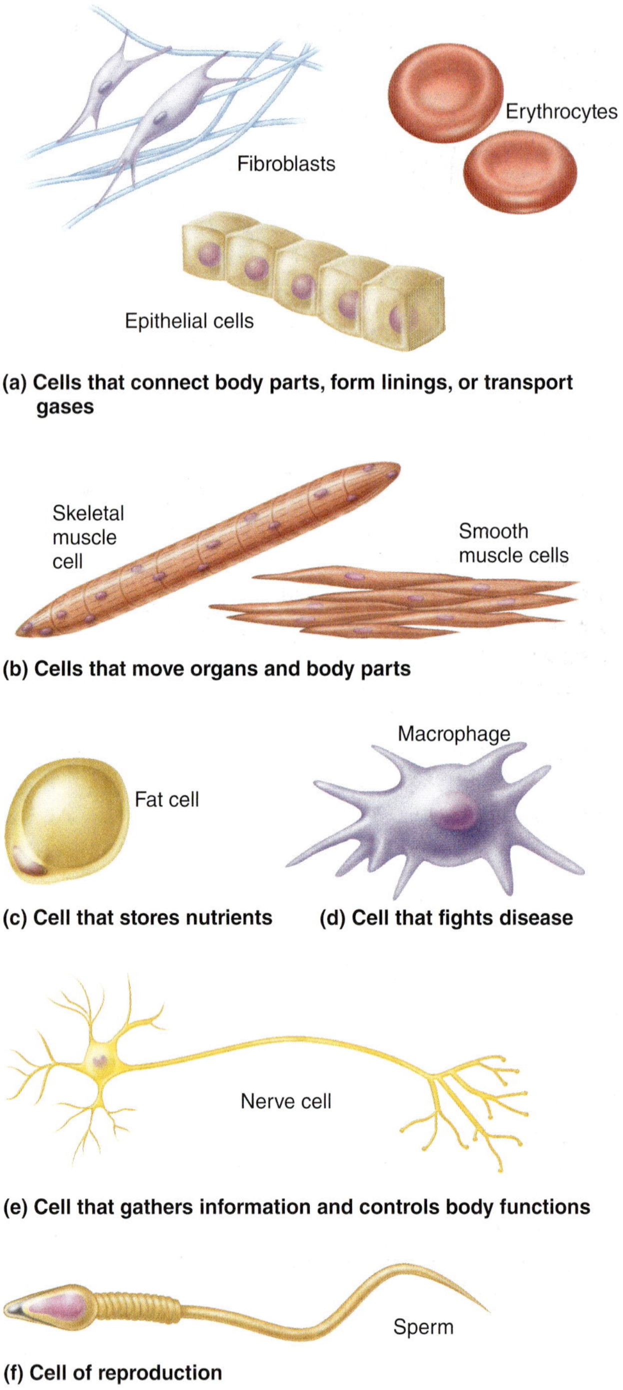

Figure 3.1 Cell diversity. (Note that cells are not drawn to the same scale.)

☑ Check Your Understanding

1. Summarize the four key points of the cell theory.
2. How would you explain the meaning of a "generalized cell" to a classmate?

For answers, see Appendix H.

Next, let's examine the three main parts of the cell in greater detail.

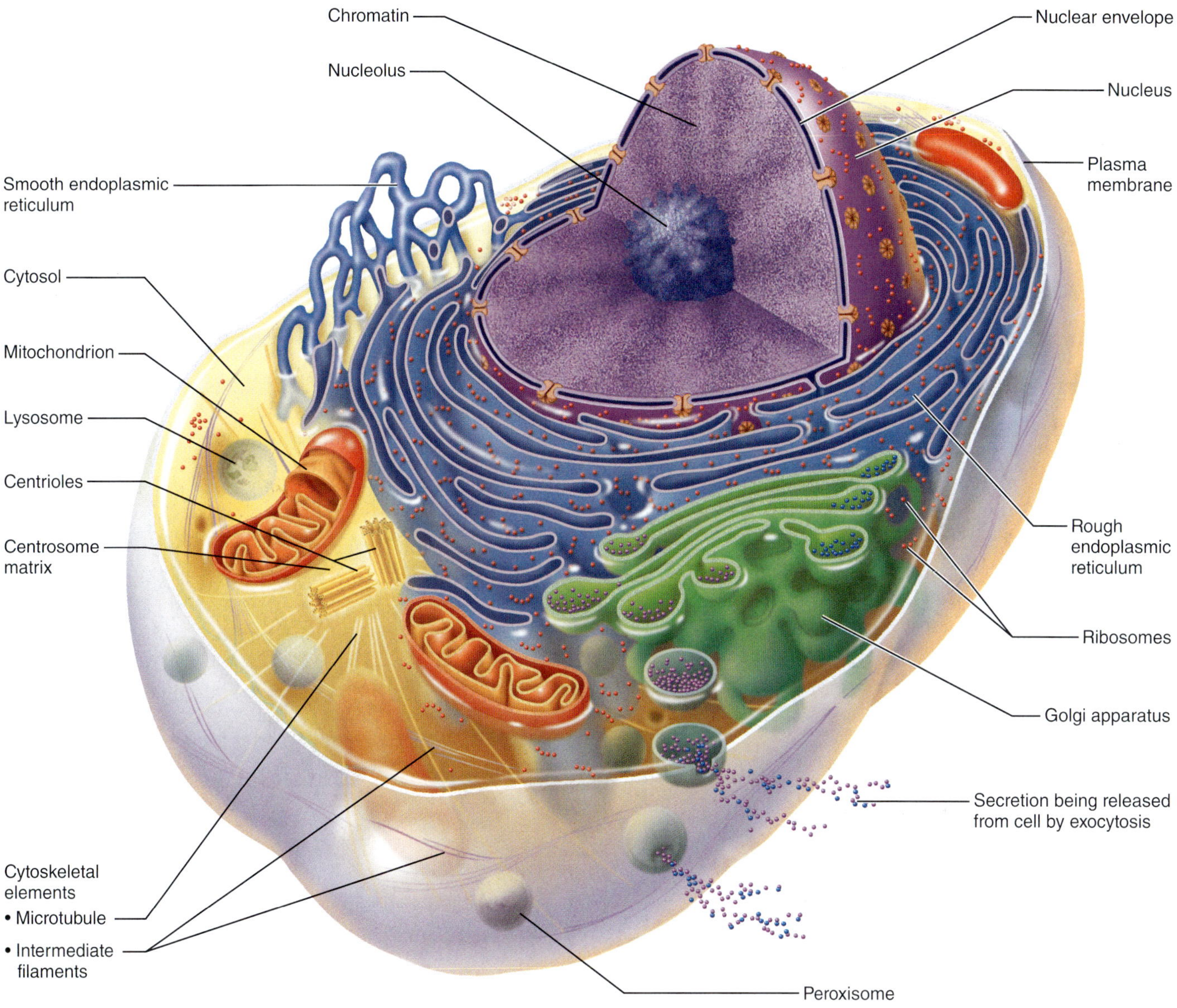

Figure 3.2 Structure of the generalized cell. No cell is exactly like this one, but this composite illustrates features common to many human cells. Note that not all of the organelles are drawn to the same scale in this illustration.

The Plasma Membrane: Structure

✓ Describe the chemical composition of the plasma membrane and relate it to membrane functions.

✓ Compare the structure and function of tight junctions, desmosomes, and gap junctions.

The flexible **plasma membrane** defines the extent of a cell, thereby separating two of the body's major fluid compartments—the *intracellular* fluid within cells and the *extracellular* fluid (ECF) outside cells. The term *cell membrane* is commonly used as a synonym for plasma membrane, but because nearly all cellular organelles are enclosed in a membrane, in this book we will always refer to the cell's surface, or outer limiting membrane, as the plasma membrane. The plasma membrane is much more than a passive envelope. As you will see, its unique structure allows it to play a dynamic role in cellular activities.

The Fluid Mosaic Model

The **fluid mosaic model** of membrane structure depicts the plasma membrane as an exceedingly thin (7–10 nm) structure composed of a double layer, or bilayer, of lipid molecules with protein molecules "plugged into" or dispersed in it **(Figure 3.3)**. The proteins, many of which float in the fluid *lipid bilayer*, form a constantly changing mosaic pattern. The model is named for this characteristic.

Membrane Lipids

The lipid bilayer forms the basic "fabric" of the membrane. It is constructed largely of *phospholipids*, with smaller amounts of *glycolipids*, *cholesterol*, and areas called *lipid rafts*.

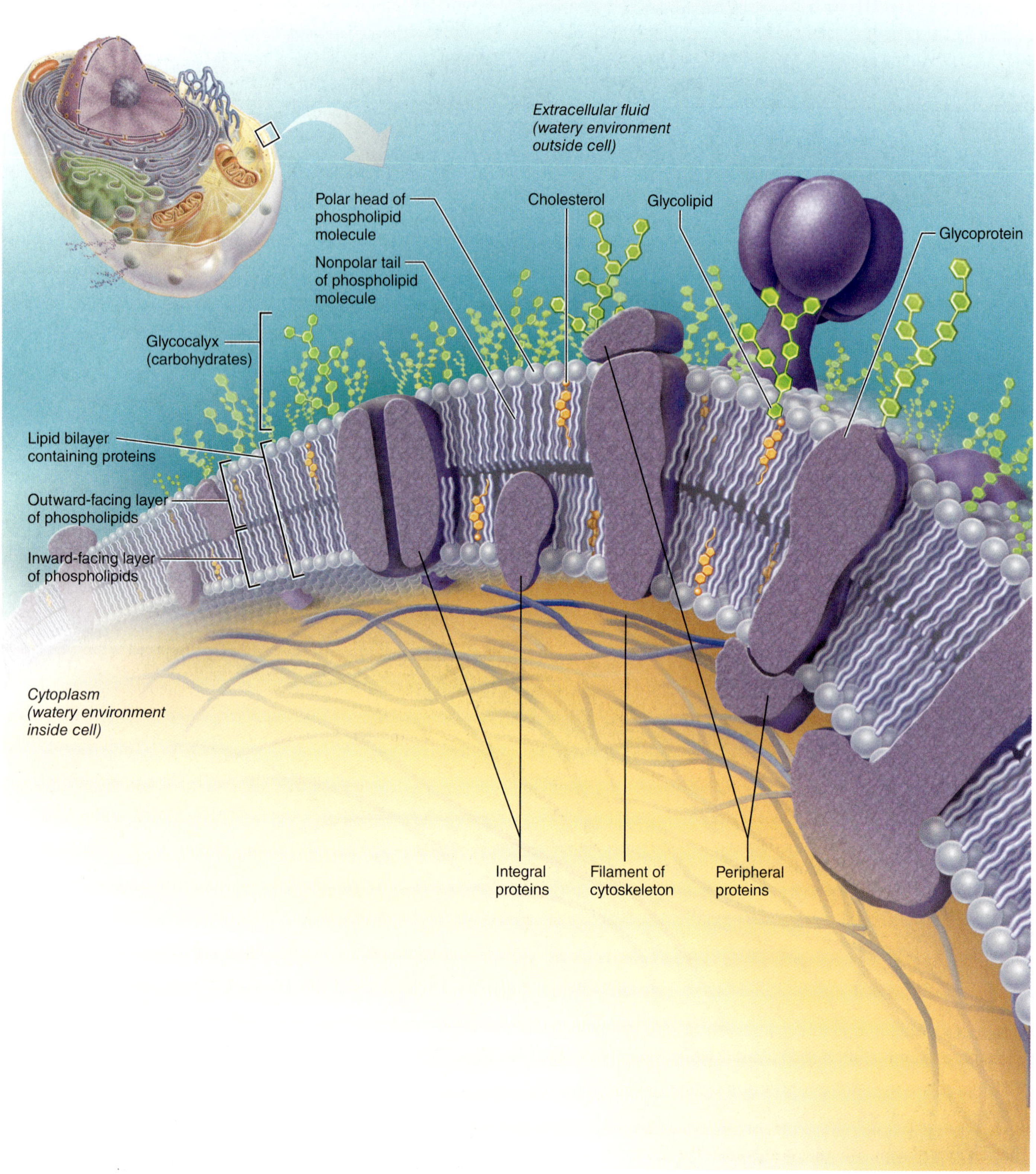

Figure 3.3 The plasma membrane. The lipid bilayer forms the basic structure of the membrane. The associated proteins are involved in membrane functions such as membrane transport, catalysis, and cell-to-cell recognition.

Phosphlipids Each lollipop-shaped phospholipid molecule has a polar "head" that is charged and is **hydrophilic** (*hydro* = water, *philic* = loving), and an uncharged, nonpolar "tail" that is made of two fatty acid chains and is **hydrophobic** (*phobia* = fear). The polar heads are attracted to water—the main constituent of both the intracellular and extracellular fluids—and so they lie on both the inner and outer surfaces of the membrane. The nonpolar tails, being hydrophobic, avoid water and line up in the center of the membrane.

The result is that all plasma membranes, indeed all biological membranes, share a sandwich-like structure: They are composed of two parallel sheets of phospholipid molecules lying tail to tail, with their polar heads exposed to water on either side of the membrane or organelle. This self-orienting property of phospholipids encourages biological membranes to self-assemble into closed, generally spherical, structures and to reseal themselves when torn.

With a consistency similar to olive oil, the plasma membrane is a dynamic fluid structure in constant flux. Its lipid molecules move freely from side to side, parallel to the membrane surface, but their polar-nonpolar interactions prevent them from flip-flopping or moving from one half of the bilayer to the other half. The inward-facing and outward-facing surfaces of the plasma membrane differ in the kinds and amounts of lipids they contain, and these variations are important in determining local membrane structure and function. Most membrane phospholipids are unsaturated, a condition which kinks their tails (increasing the space between them) and increases membrane fluidity. (See the illustration of phosphatidylcholine in Figure 2.16b, p. 45.)

Glycolipids **Glycolipids** (gli″ko-lip′idz) are lipids with attached sugar groups. Found only on the outer plasma membrane surface, glycolipids account for about 5% of total membrane lipids. Their sugar groups, like the phosphate-containing groups of phospholipids, make that end of the glycolipid molecule polar, whereas the fatty acid tails are nonpolar.

Cholesterol Some 20% of membrane lipid is cholesterol. Like phospholipids, cholesterol has a polar region (its hydroxyl group) and a nonpolar region (its fused ring system). It wedges its platelike hydrocarbon rings between the phospholipid tails, stabilizing the membrane, while decreasing the mobility of the phospholipids and the fluidity of the membrane.

Membrane Proteins

A cell's plasma membrane bristles with proteins that allow it to communicate with its environment. Proteins make up about half of the plasma membrane by mass and are responsible for most of the specialized membrane functions. Some membrane proteins float freely. Others are "tethered" to intracellular structures that make up the *cytoskeleton* and are restricted in their movement.

There are two distinct populations of membrane proteins, integral and peripheral (Figure 3.3).

Integral Proteins **Integral proteins** are firmly inserted into the lipid bilayer. Some protrude from one membrane face only, but most are *transmembrane proteins* that span the entire membrane and protrude on both sides. Whether transmembrane or not, all integral proteins have both hydrophobic and hydrophilic regions. This structural feature allows them to interact with both the nonpolar lipid tails buried in the membrane and the water inside and outside the cell.

Some transmembrane proteins are involved in transport, and cluster together to form *channels*, or pores, through which small, water-soluble molecules or ions can move, thus bypassing the lipid part of the membrane. Others act as *carriers* that bind to a substance and then move it through the membrane **(Figure 3.4a)**. Some transmembrane proteins are enzymes (Figure 3.4d). Still others are receptors for hormones or other chemical messengers and relay messages to the cell interior—a process called *signal transduction* (Figure 3.4b).

Peripheral Proteins Unlike integral proteins, **peripheral proteins** (Figure 3.3) are not embedded in the lipid bilayer. Instead, they attach loosely to integral proteins and are easily removed without disrupting the membrane. Peripheral proteins include a network of filaments that helps support the membrane from its cytoplasmic side (Figure 3.4c). Some peripheral proteins are enzymes. Others are motor proteins involved in mechanical functions, such as changing cell shape during cell division and muscle cell contraction. Still others link cells together.

Lipid Rafts

About 20% of the outer membrane surface contains **lipid rafts**, dynamic assemblies of saturated phospholipids (which pack together tightly) associated with unique lipids called sphingolipids and lots of cholesterol. The quiltlike lipid rafts are more stable and less fluid than the rest of the membrane, and they can include or exclude specific proteins to various extents. Because of these qualities, lipid rafts are assumed to be concentrating platforms for certain receptor molecules or for protein molecules needed for cell signaling (discussed on p. 81), membrane invagination (see endocytosis, p. 77), or other functions.

The Glycocalyx

Many of the proteins that abut the extracellular fluid are glycoproteins with branching sugar groups. The term **glycocalyx** (gli″ko-kal′iks; "sugar covering") describes the fuzzy, sticky, carbohydrate-rich area at the cell surface. Quite honestly, you can think of your cells as sugar-coated. The glycocalyx on each cell's surface is enriched both by glycolipids and by glycoproteins secreted by the cell.

Because every cell type has a different pattern of sugars in its glycocalyx, the glycocalyx provides highly specific biological markers by which approaching cells recognize each other (Figure 3.4f). For example, a sperm recognizes an ovum (egg cell) by the ovum's unique glycocalyx. Cells of the immune system identify a bacterium by binding to certain membrane glycoproteins in the bacterial glycocalyx.

3

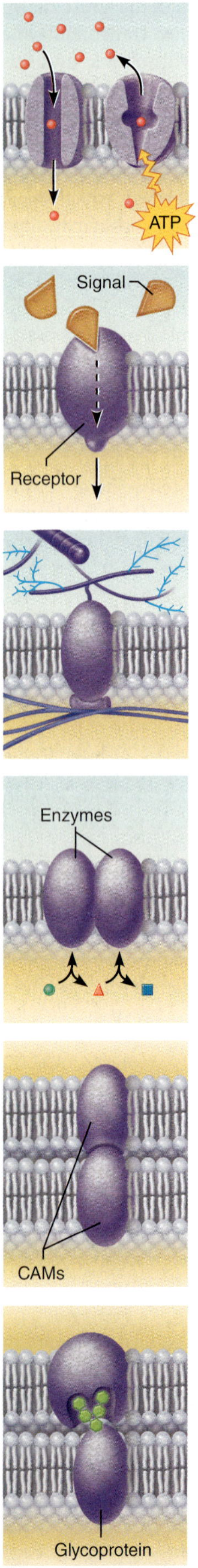

(a) Transport

- A protein (left) that spans the membrane may provide a hydrophilic channel across the membrane that is selective for a particular solute.
- Some transport proteins (right) hydrolyze ATP as an energy source to actively pump substances across the membrane.

(b) Receptors for signal transduction

- A membrane protein exposed to the outside of the cell may have a binding site that fits the shape of a specific chemical messenger, such as a hormone.
- When bound, the chemical messenger may cause a change in shape in the protein that initiates a chain of chemical reactions in the cell.

(c) Attachment to the cytoskeleton and extracellular matrix

- Elements of the cytoskeleton (cell's internal supports) and the extracellular matrix (fibers and other substances outside the cell) may anchor to membrane proteins, which helps maintain cell shape and fix the location of certain membrane proteins.
- Others play a role in cell movement or bind adjacent cells together.

(d) Enzymatic activity

- A membrane protein may be an enzyme with its active site exposed to substances in the adjacent solution.
- A team of several enzymes in a membrane may catalyze sequential steps of a metabolic pathway as indicated (left to right) here.

(e) Intercellular joining

- Membrane proteins of adjacent cells may be hooked together in various kinds of intercellular junctions.
- Some membrane proteins (cell adhesion molecules or CAMs) of this group provide temporary binding sites that guide cell migration and other cell-to-cell interactions.

(f) Cell-cell recognition

- Some glycoproteins (proteins bonded to short chains of sugars) serve as identification tags that are specifically recognized by other cells.

Figure 3.4 Membrane proteins perform many tasks. A single protein may perform a combination of these functions.

Homeostatic Imbalance 3.1

Definite changes occur in the glycocalyx of a cell that is becoming cancerous. In fact, a cancer cell's glycocalyx may change almost continuously, allowing it to keep ahead of immune system recognition mechanisms and avoid destruction. (Cancer is discussed on pp. 145–146.) ✚

☑ Check Your Understanding

3. What basic structure do all cellular membranes share?
4. Why do phospholipids, which form the greater part of membranes, organize into a bilayer—tail-to-tail—in a watery environment?
5. What is the importance of the glycocalyx in cell interactions?

For answers, see Appendix H.

Cell Junctions

Although certain cell types—blood cells, sperm cells, and some immune system cells—are "footloose" in the body, many other types are knit into tight communities. Typically, three factors act to bind cells together:

- Glycoproteins in the glycocalyx act as an adhesive.
- Wavy contours of the membranes of adjacent cells fit together in a tongue-and-groove fashion.
- Special cell junctions form **(Figure 3.5)**.

Because junctions are the most important factor securing cells together, let's look more closely at the various types.

Tight Junctions

In a **tight junction**, a series of integral protein molecules in the plasma membranes of adjacent cells fuse together, forming an *impermeable junction* that encircles the cell (Figure 3.5a). Tight junctions help prevent molecules from passing through the extracellular space between adjacent cells. For example, tight junctions between epithelial cells lining the digestive tract keep digestive enzymes and microorganisms in the intestine from seeping into the bloodstream. (Although called "impermeable" junctions, some tight junctions are leaky and may allow certain ions to pass.)

Desmosomes

Desmosomes (des′muh-sōmz; "binding bodies") are *anchoring junctions*—mechanical couplings scattered like rivets along the sides of abutting cells to prevent their separation (Figure 3.5b). On the cytoplasmic face of each plasma membrane is a buttonlike thickening called a *plaque*. Adjacent cells are held together by thin linker protein filaments (cadherins) that extend from the plaques and fit together like the teeth of a zipper in the intercellular space. Thicker keratin filaments (intermediate filaments, which form part of the cytoskeleton) extend from the cytoplasmic side of the plaque across the width of the cell to anchor to the plaque on the cell's opposite side. In this way, desmosomes bind neighboring cells together and also contribute to a continuous internal network of strong "guy-wires."

This arrangement distributes tension throughout a cellular sheet and reduces the chance of tearing when it is subjected to

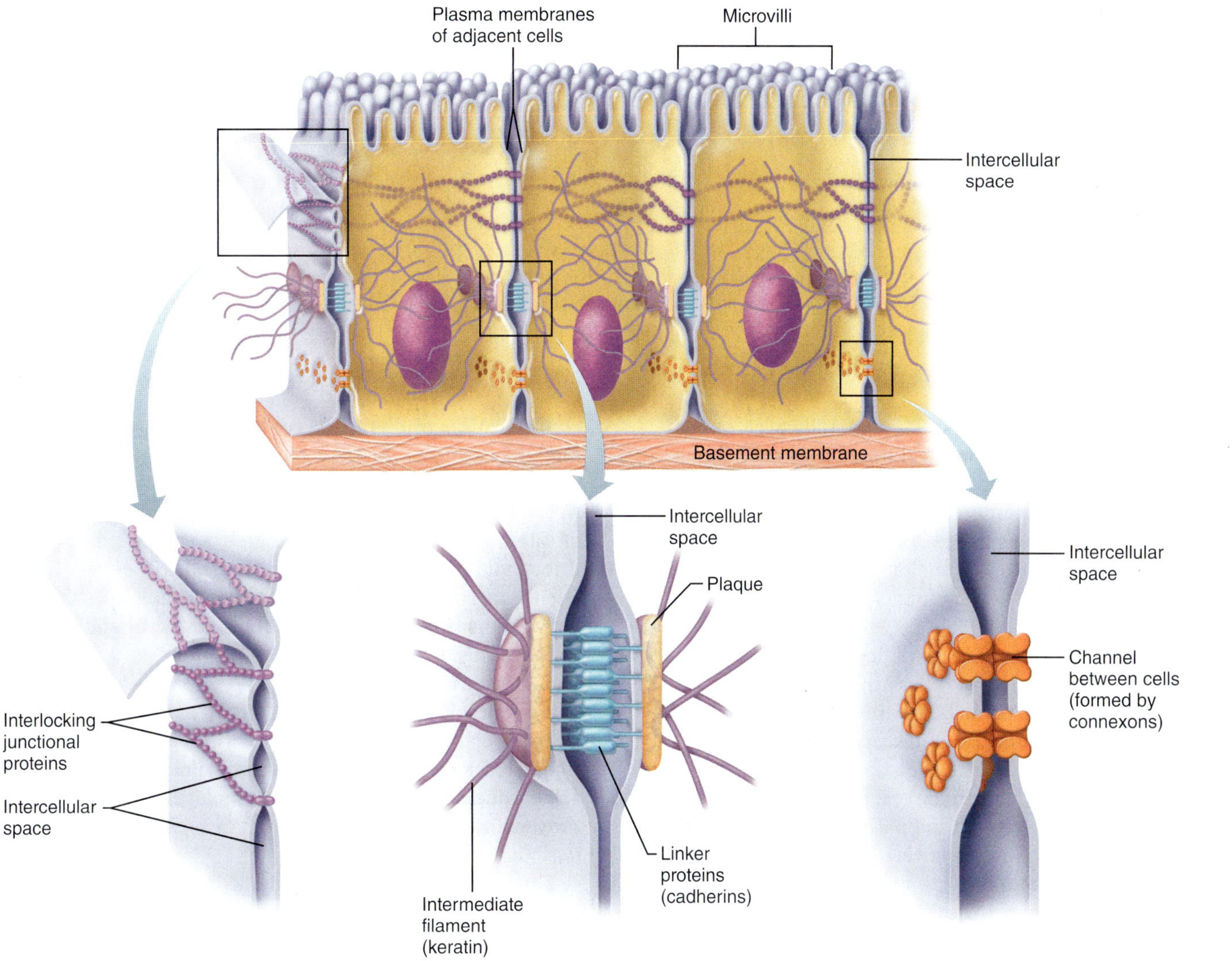

(a) Tight junctions: Impermeable junctions prevent molecules from passing through the intercellular space.

(b) Desmosomes: Anchoring junctions bind adjacent cells together like a molecular "Velcro" and help form an internal tension-reducing network of fibers.

(c) Gap junctions: Communicating junctions allow ions and small molecules to pass for intercellular communication.

Figure 3.5 Cell junctions. An epithelial cell is shown joined to adjacent cells by three common types of cell junctions. (Note: Except for epithelia, it is unlikely that a single cell will have all three junction types.)

pulling forces. Desmosomes are abundant in tissues subjected to great mechanical stress, such as skin and heart muscle.

Gap Junctions

A **gap junction**, or *nexus* (nek′sus; "bond"), is a communicating junction between adjacent cells. At gap junctions the adjacent plasma membranes are very close, and the cells are connected by hollow cylinders called *connexons* (kŏ-nek′sonz), composed of transmembrane proteins. The many different types of connexon proteins vary the selectivity of the gap junction channels. Ions, simple sugars, and other small molecules pass through these water-filled channels from one cell to the next (Figure 3.5c).

Gap junctions are present in electrically excitable tissues, such as the heart and smooth muscle, where ion passage from cell to cell helps synchronize their electrical activity and contraction.

Check Your Understanding

6. Which two types of cell junctions would you expect to find between muscle cells of the heart?

For answer, see Appendix H.

The Plasma Membrane: Membrane Transport

- ✓ Relate plasma membrane structure to active and passive transport processes.
- ✓ Compare and contrast simple diffusion, facilitated diffusion, and osmosis relative to substances transported, direction, and mechanism.

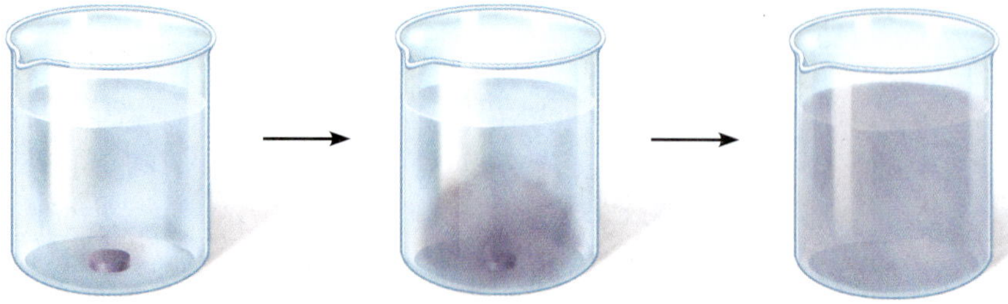

3

Figure 3.6 Diffusion. Molecules in solution move continuously and collide constantly with other molecules, causing them to move away from areas of their highest concentration and become evenly distributed. From left to right, molecules from a dye pellet diffuse into the surrounding water down their concentration gradient.

Our cells are bathed in an extracellular fluid called **interstitial fluid** (in″ter-stish′al) that is derived from the blood. Like a rich, nutritious "soup," interstitial fluid contains thousands of ingredients, including amino acids, sugars, fatty acids, vitamins, regulatory substances such as hormones and neurotransmitters, salts, and waste products. To remain healthy, each cell must extract from this mix the exact amounts of the substances it needs at specific times.

Although there is continuous traffic across the plasma membrane, it is a **selectively**, or **differentially**, **permeable** barrier: It allows some substances to pass while excluding others. It allows nutrients to enter the cell, but keeps many undesirable substances out. At the same time, it keeps valuable cell proteins and other necessary substances in the cell, but allows wastes to exit.

Substances move through the plasma membrane in essentially two ways—passively or actively. In **passive processes**, substances cross the membrane without any energy input from the cell. In **active processes**, the cell provides the metabolic energy (usually ATP) needed to move substances across the membrane. Table 3.1 on p. 72 summarizes passive transport processes, and Table 3.2 on p. 78 summarizes active transport.

Homeostatic Imbalance 3.2

Selective permeability is a characteristic of healthy, intact cells. When a cell (or its plasma membrane) is severely damaged, the membrane becomes permeable to virtually everything, and substances flow into and out of the cell freely. This phenomenon is evident when someone has been severely burned. Precious fluids, proteins, and ions "weep" from the damaged cells. +

Passive Processes

The two main types of passive transport are *diffusion* (dĭ-fu′zhun) and *filtration*. Diffusion is an important means of passive membrane transport for every cell of the body. Because filtration generally occurs only across capillary walls, we will discuss it later in conjunction with capillary transport.

Diffusion

Diffusion is the tendency of molecules or ions to move from an area where they are in higher concentration to an area where they are in lower concentration, that is, down or along their **concentration gradient**. The constant random and high-speed motion of molecules and ions (a result of their intrinsic kinetic energy) results in collisions. With each collision, the particles ricochet off one another and change direction. The overall effect of this erratic movement is to scatter or disperse the particles throughout the environment **(Figure 3.6)**. The greater the difference in concentration of the diffusing molecules and ions between the two areas, the more collisions occur and the faster the net diffusion of the particles.

Because the driving force for diffusion is the kinetic energy of the molecules themselves, the speed of diffusion is influenced by molecular *size* (the smaller, the faster) and by *temperature* (the warmer, the faster). In a closed container, diffusion eventually produces a uniform mixture of molecules. In other words, the system reaches equilibrium, with molecules moving equally in all directions (no *net* movement).

Diffusion is immensely important in physiological systems and it occurs rapidly because the distances molecules are moving are very short, perhaps 1/1000 (or less) the thickness of this page! Examples include the movement of ions across cell membranes and the movement of neurotransmitters between two nerve cells.

The plasma membrane is a physical barrier to free diffusion because of its hydrophobic core. However, a molecule or ion *will* diffuse through the membrane if the molecule is (1) lipid soluble, (2) small enough to pass through membrane channels, or (3) assisted by a carrier molecule.

The unassisted diffusion of lipid-soluble or very small particles is called *simple diffusion*. Assisted diffusion is known as *facilitated diffusion*. A special name, *osmosis*, is given to the diffusion of a solvent (usually water) through a membrane.

Simple Diffusion In **simple diffusion**, nonpolar and lipid-soluble substances diffuse directly through the lipid bilayer **(Figure 3.7a)**. Such substances include oxygen, carbon dioxide, and fat-soluble vitamins. Because oxygen concentration is always higher in the blood than in tissue cells, oxygen continuously diffuses from the blood into the cells. Carbon dioxide, on the other hand, is in higher concentration within the cells, so it diffuses from tissue cells into the blood.

Facilitated Diffusion Certain molecules, notably glucose and other sugars, some amino acids, and ions are transported

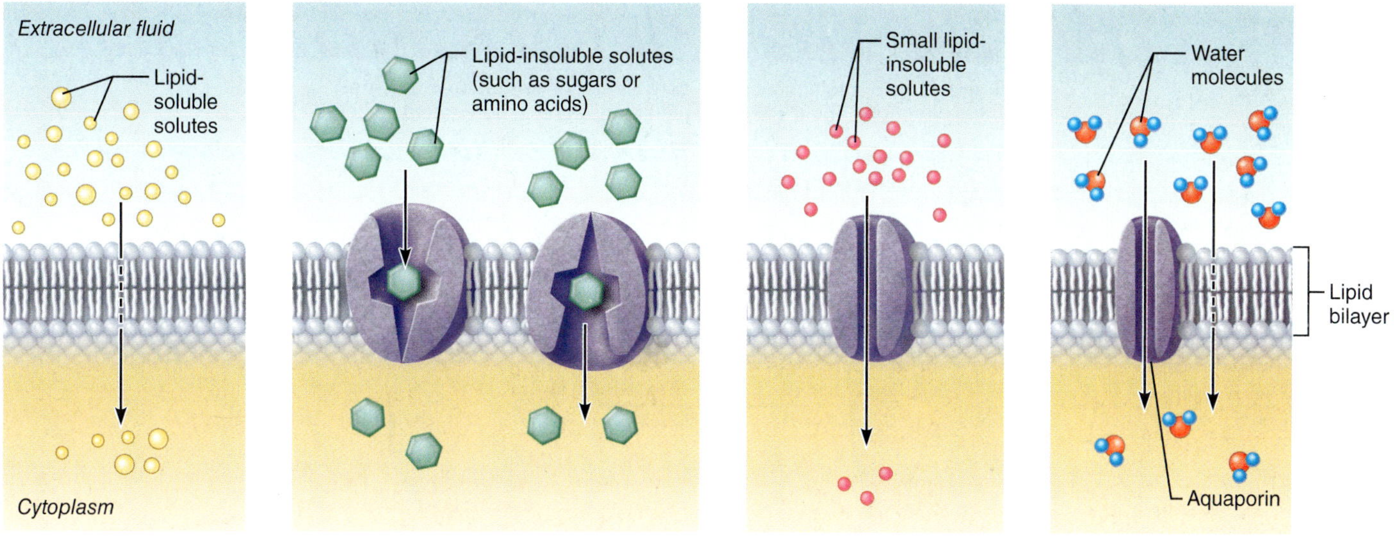

(a) Simple diffusion of fat-soluble molecules directly through the phospholipid bilayer

(b) Carrier-mediated facilitated diffusion via protein carrier specific for one chemical; binding of substrate causes transport protein to change shape

(c) Channel-mediated facilitated diffusion through a channel protein; mostly ions selected on basis of size and charge

(d) Osmosis, diffusion of a solvent such as water through a specific channel protein (aquaporin) or through the lipid bilayer

Figure 3.7 Diffusion through the plasma membrane.

passively even though they are unable to pass through the lipid bilayer. Instead they move through the membrane by a passive transport process called **facilitated diffusion** in which the transported substance either (1) binds to protein carriers in the membrane and is ferried across or (2) moves through water-filled protein channels.

- **Carrier-mediated facilitated diffusion. Carriers** are transmembrane integral proteins that are specific for transporting certain polar molecules or classes of molecules, such as sugars and amino acids, that are too large to pass through membrane channels. Alterations in the shape of the carrier allow it to first envelop and then release the transported substance, shielding it en route from the nonpolar regions of the membrane. Essentially, changes in the conformation of the carrier protein move the binding site from one face of the membrane to the other (Figure 3.7b and Table 3.1).

  Note that a substance transported by carrier-mediated facilitated diffusion, such as glucose, moves down its concentration gradient, just as in simple diffusion. Glucose is normally in higher concentrations in the blood than in the cells, where it is rapidly used for ATP synthesis. So, glucose transport within the body is *typically* unidirectional—into the cells. However, carrier-mediated transport is limited by the number of protein carriers present. For example, when all the glucose carriers are "engaged," they are said to be *saturated*, and glucose transport is occurring at its maximum rate.

- **Channel-mediated facilitated diffusion. Channels** are transmembrane proteins that transport substances, usually ions or water, through aqueous channels from one side of the membrane to the other (Figure 3.7c and d). Channels are selective due to pore size and the charges of the amino acids lining the channel. *Leakage channels* are always open and simply allow ions or water to move according to concentration gradients. *Gated channels* are controlled (opened or closed) by chemical or electrical signals.

  Like carriers, many channels can be inhibited by certain molecules, show saturation, and tend to be specific. Substances moving through them also follow the concentration gradient (always moving down the gradient). When a substance crosses the membrane by simple diffusion, the rate of diffusion is not controllable because the lipid solubility of the membrane is not immediately changeable. By contrast, the rate of facilitated diffusion *is* controllable because the permeability of the membrane can be altered by regulating the activity or number of individual carriers or channels.

Oxygen, water, glucose, and various ions are vitally important to cellular homeostasis. Their passive transport by diffusion (either simple or facilitated) represents a tremendous saving of cellular energy. Indeed, if these substances had to be transported actively, cell expenditures of ATP would increase exponentially!

Osmosis The diffusion of a solvent, such as water, through a selectively permeable membrane is **osmosis** (oz-mo′sis; *osmos* = pushing). Even though water is highly polar, it passes via osmosis through the lipid bilayer (Figure 3.7d). This is surprising because you'd expect water to be repelled by the hydrophobic lipid tails. One hypothesis is that random movements of the membrane lipids open small gaps between their wiggling tails, allowing water to slip and slide its way through the membrane by moving from gap to gap.

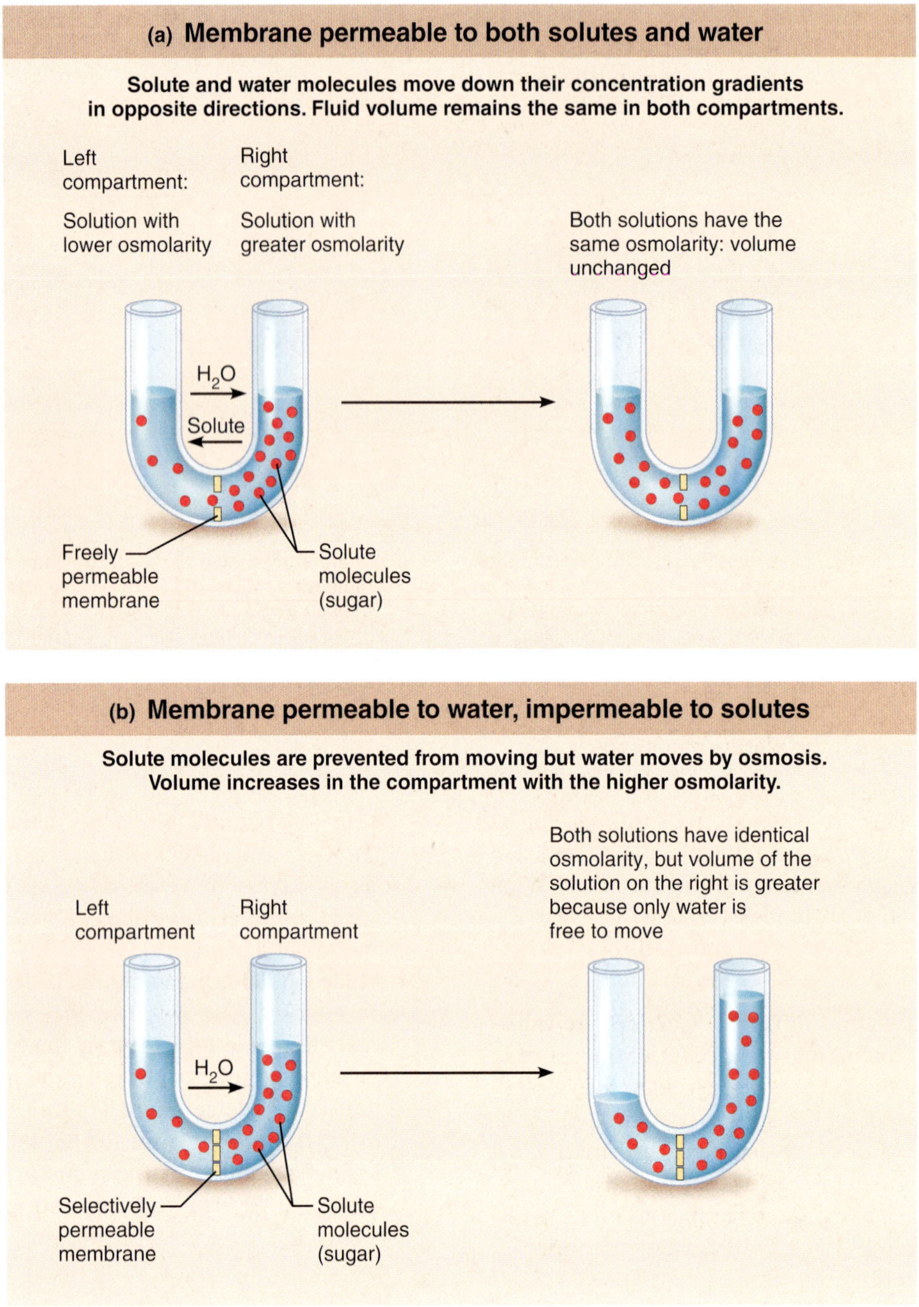

Figure 3.8 **Influence of membrane permeability on diffusion and osmosis.**

Water also moves freely and reversibly through water-specific channels constructed by transmembrane proteins called **aquaporins (AQPs)**, which allow single-file diffusion of water molecules. Although water-filled aquaporin channels are believed to be present in all cell types, they are particularly abundant in red blood cells and in cells involved in water balance such as kidney tubule cells.

Osmosis occurs whenever the water concentration differs on the two sides of a membrane. If distilled water is present on both sides of a selectively permeable membrane, no *net* osmosis occurs, even though water molecules move in both directions through the membrane. If the solute concentration on the two sides of the membrane differs, water concentration differs as well (as solute concentration increases, water concentration decreases).

The extent to which solutes decrease water's concentration depends on the *number*—not the *type*—of solute particles, because one molecule or one ion of solute (theoretically) displaces one water molecule. The total concentration of all solute particles in a solution is referred to as the solution's **osmolarity** (oz″mo-lar′ĭ-te). When equal volumes of aqueous solutions of different osmolarity are separated by a membrane that is *permeable to all molecules* in the system, net diffusion of both solute

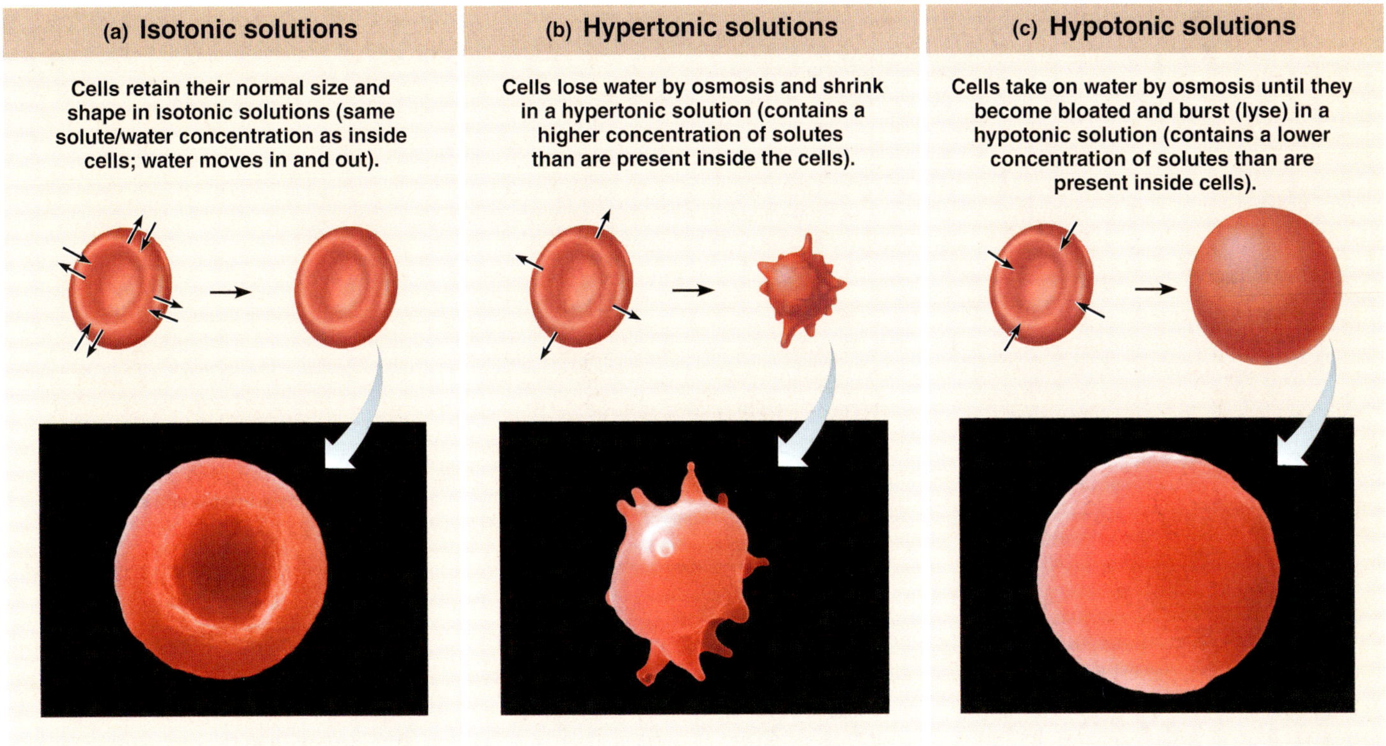

Figure 3.9 The effect of solutions of varying tonicities on living red blood cells.

and water occurs, each moving down its own concentration gradient. Equilibrium is reached when the water (and solute) concentration on both sides of the membrane is the same **(Figure 3.8a)**.

If we consider the same system, but make the membrane *impermeable to solute particles*, we see quite a different result (Figure 3.8b). Water quickly diffuses from the left to the right compartment and continues to do so until its concentration is the same on the two sides of the membrane. Notice that in this case equilibrium results from the movement of water alone (the solutes are prevented from moving). Notice also that the movement of water leads to dramatic changes in the volumes of the two compartments.

The last situation mimics osmosis across plasma membranes of living cells, with one major difference. In our examples, the volumes of the compartments are infinitely expandable and the effect of pressure exerted by the added weight of the higher fluid column is not considered. In living plant cells, which have rigid cell walls external to their plasma membranes, this is not the case. As water diffuses into the cell, the point is finally reached where the **hydrostatic pressure** (the back pressure exerted by water against the membrane) within the cell is equal to its **osmotic pressure** (the tendency of water to move into the cell by osmosis). At this point, there is no further (net) water entry. As a rule, the higher the amount of nondiffusible, or *nonpenetrating*, solutes in a cell, the higher the osmotic pressure and the greater the hydrostatic pressure must be to resist further net water entry. In our plant cell, hydrostatic pressure is pushing water out, and osmotic pressure is pulling water in; therefore, you could think of the osmotic pressure as an osmotic "suck."

However, such major changes in hydrostatic (and osmotic) pressures do not occur in living animal cells, which lack rigid cell walls. Osmotic imbalances cause animal cells to swell or shrink (due to net water gain or loss) until either (1) the solute concentration is the same on both sides of the plasma membrane, or (2) the membrane stretches to its breaking point.

Tonicity Such changes in animal cells lead us to the important concept of *tonicity* (to-nis′ĭ-te). As noted, many solutes, particularly intracellular proteins and selected ions, cannot diffuse through the plasma membrane. Consequently, any change in their concentration alters the water concentration on the two sides of the membrane and results in a net loss or gain of water by the cell.

Tonicity refers to the ability of a solution to change the shape or tone of cells by altering the cells' internal water volume (*tono* = tension).

- **Isotonic** ("the same tonicity") **solutions** have the same concentrations of nonpenetrating solutes as those found in cells (0.9% saline or 5% glucose). Cells exposed to isotonic solutions retain their normal shape, and exhibit no net loss or gain of water **(Figure 3.9a)**. As you might expect, the body's extracellular fluids and most intravenous solutions (solutions infused into the body via a vein) are isotonic.
- **Hypertonic solutions** have a higher concentration of nonpenetrating solutes than seen in the cell (for example, a strong saline solution). Cells immersed in hypertonic solutions lose water and shrink, or *crenate* (kre′nat) (Figure 3.9b).

3

Table 3.1 Passive Membrane Transport Processes

PROCESS	ENERGY SOURCE	DESCRIPTION	EXAMPLES
Diffusion			
Simple diffusion	Kinetic energy	Net movement of molecules from an area of their higher concentration to an area of their lower concentration, that is, along their concentration gradient	Fats, oxygen, carbon dioxide move through the lipid bilayer of the membrane
Facilitated diffusion	Kinetic energy	Same as simple diffusion, but the diffusing substance is attached to a lipid-soluble membrane carrier protein (carrier-mediated facilitated diffusion) or moves through a membrane channel (channel-mediated facilitated diffusion)	Glucose and some ions move into cells
Osmosis	Kinetic energy	Diffusion of water through a selectively permeable membrane	Movement of water into and out of cells directly through the lipid bilayer of the membrane or via membrane channels (aquaporins)

- **Hypotonic solutions** are more dilute (contain a lower concentration of nonpenetrating solutes) than cells. Cells placed in a hypotonic solution plump up rapidly as water rushes into them (Figure 3.9c). Distilled water represents the most extreme example of hypotonicity. Because it contains *no* solutes, water continues to enter cells until they finally burst, or *lyse.*

Notice that osmolarity and tonicity are not the same. A solution's osmolarity is based solely on its total solute concentration. In contrast, its tonicity is based on how the solution affects cell volume, which depends on (1) solute concentration and (2) solute permeability of the plasma membrane. Osmolarity is expressed as osmoles per liter (osmol/L) where 1 osmol is equal to 1 mole of nonionizing molecules.* A 0.3 osmol/L solution of NaCl is isotonic because sodium ions are usually prevented from diffusing through the plasma membrane. But if the cell is immersed in a 0.3 osmol/L solution of a penetrating solute, the solute will enter the cell and water will follow. The cell will swell and burst, just as if it had been placed in pure water.

Osmosis is extremely important in determining distribution of water in the various fluid-containing compartments of the body (cells, blood, and so on). In general, osmosis continues until osmotic and hydrostatic pressures acting at the membrane are equal. For example, the hydrostatic pressure of blood against the capillary wall forces water out of capillary blood, but the solutes in blood that are too large to cross the capillary membrane draw water back into the bloodstream. As a result, very little net loss of plasma fluid occurs.

Simple diffusion and osmosis occurring directly through the plasma membrane are not selective processes. In those processes, whether a molecule can pass through the membrane depends chiefly on its size or its solubility in lipid, not on its structure. Facilitated diffusion, on the other hand, is often highly selective. The carrier for glucose, for example, combines specifically with glucose, in much the same way an enzyme binds to its specific substrate and ion channels allow only selected ions to pass.

Homeostatic Imbalance 3.3

Hypertonic solutions are sometimes infused intravenously into the bloodstream of patients who are edematous (swollen because their tissues retain water). This is done to draw excess water out of the extracellular space and move it into the bloodstream so the kidneys can eliminate it. Hypotonic solutions may be used (with care) to rehydrate the tissues of extremely dehydrated patients. In mild cases of dehydration, drinking hypotonic fluids (such as apple juice and sports drinks) usually does the trick. +

Table 3.1 summarizes passive membrane transport processes.

Check Your Understanding

7. What is the energy source for all types of diffusion?
8. What determines the direction of any diffusion process?
9. What are the two types of facilitated diffusion and how do they differ?

For answers, see Appendix H.

Active Processes

- ✓ Differentiate between primary and secondary active transport.
- ✓ Compare and contrast endocytosis and exocytosis in terms of function and direction.
- ✓ Compare and contrast pinocytosis, phagocytosis, and receptor-mediated endocytosis.

*Osmolarity (Osm) is determined by multiplying molarity (moles per liter, or *M*) by the number of particles resulting from ionization. For example, since NaCl ionizes to $Na^+ + Cl^-$, a 1 *M* solution of NaCl is a 2 Osm solution. For substances that do not ionize (e.g., glucose), molarity and osmolarity are the same. More precisely, the term *osmolality* is used, which is equal to the number of particles mixed into a kilogram of water.

Whenever a cell uses energy to move solutes across the membrane, the process is referred to as *active*. Substances moved actively across the plasma membrane are usually unable to pass in the necessary direction by passive transport processes. The substance may be too large to pass through the channels, incapable of dissolving in the lipid bilayer, or unable to move down its concentration gradient.

There are two major means of active membrane transport: active transport and vesicular transport.

Active Transport

Like carrier-mediated facilitated diffusion, **active transport** requires carrier proteins that combine *specifically* and *reversibly* with the transported substances. However, facilitated diffusion always follows concentration gradients because its driving force is kinetic energy. In contrast, active transporters or **solute pumps** move solutes, most importantly ions, "uphill" *against* a concentration gradient. To do this work, cells must expend energy.

Active transport processes are distinguished according to their source of energy:

- In *primary active transport*, the energy to do work comes *directly from hydrolysis of ATP*.
- In *secondary active transport*, transport is driven indirectly *by energy stored in ionic gradients* created by primary active transport pumps. Secondary active transport systems are all *coupled systems*; that is, they move more than one substance at a time.

  In a **symport system,** the two transported substances move in the same direction (*sym* = same). In an **antiport system** (*anti* = opposite, against), the transported substances "wave to each other" as they cross the membrane in opposite directions.

Primary Active Transport In **primary active transport**, hydrolysis of ATP results in the phosphorylation of the transport protein. This step causes the protein to change its shape in such a manner that it "pumps" the bound solute across the membrane.

Primary active transport systems include calcium and hydrogen pumps, but the most investigated example of a primary active transport system is the **sodium-potassium pump**, for which the carrier, or "pump," is an enzyme called **Na^+-K^+ ATPase**. In the body, the concentration of K^+ inside the cell is some 10 times higher than that outside, and the reverse is true of Na^+. These ionic concentration differences are essential for excitable cells like muscle and nerve cells to function normally and for all body cells to maintain their normal fluid volume. Because Na^+ and K^+ leak slowly but continuously through leakage channels in the plasma membrane along their concentration gradient (and cross more rapidly in stimulated muscle and nerve cells), the Na^+-K^+ pump operates almost continuously as an antiporter. It simultaneously drives Na^+ out of the cell against a steep concentration gradient and pumps K^+ back in.

Earlier we said that solutes diffuse down their concentration gradients. This is true for uncharged solutes, but only partially true for ions. The negatively and positively charged faces of the plasma membrane can help or hinder diffusion of ions driven by a concentration gradient. It is more correct to say that ions diffuse according to **electrochemical gradients**, thereby recognizing the effect of both electrical and concentration (chemical) forces. Hence, the electrochemical gradients maintained by the Na^+-K^+ pump underlie most secondary active transport of nutrients and ions, and are crucial for cardiac, skeletal muscle, and neuron function.

Figure 3.10 on p. 74, *Focus on Primary Active Transport: The Na^+-K^+ Pump*, describes the operation of the Na^+-K^+pump. Make sure you understand this process thoroughly before moving on to the topic of secondary active transport.

Secondary Active Transport A single ATP-powered pump, such as the Na^+-K^+ pump, can indirectly drive the **secondary active transport** of several other solutes. By moving sodium across the plasma membrane against its concentration gradient, the pump stores energy (in the ion gradient). Then, just as water pumped uphill can do work as it flows back down (to turn a water wheel, for instance), a substance pumped across a membrane can do work as it leaks back, propelled "downhill" along its concentration gradient. In this way, as sodium moves back into the cell with the help of a carrier protein, other substances are "dragged along," or cotransported, by the same carrier protein **(Figure 3.11)**. This is a symport system.

For example, some sugars, amino acids, and many ions are cotransported via secondary active transport into cells lining the small intestine. Because the energy for this type of transport is the concentration gradient of the ion (in this case Na^+), Na^+ has to be pumped back out of the cell to maintain its diffusion gradient. Ion gradients can also drive antiport systems such as those that help regulate intracellular pH by using the sodium gradient to expel hydrogen ions.

Regardless of whether the energy is provided directly (primary active transport) or indirectly (secondary active transport), each membrane pump or cotransporter transports only specific substances. Active transport systems provide a way for the cell to be very selective in cases where substances cannot pass by diffusion. No pump—no transport.

Vesicular Transport

In **vesicular transport**, fluids containing large particles and macromolecules are transported across cellular membranes inside membranous sacs called *vesicles*. Like active transport, vesicular transport moves substances into the cell (endocytosis) and out of the cell (exocytosis). It is also used for combination processes such as *transcytosis*, moving substances into, across, and then out of the cell, and *vesicular trafficking*, moving substances from one area (or membranous organelle) in the cell to another. Vesicular transport processes are energized by ATP (or in some cases another energy-rich compound, *GTP*—guanosine triphosphate).

Endocytosis, Transcytosis, and Vesicular Trafficking Virtually all forms of vesicular transport involve an assortment of protein-coated vesicles of three types and, with some exceptions, all are mediated by membrane receptors. Before we get specific about each type of coated vesicular transport, let's look at the general scheme of endocytosis.

Figure 3.10 **Primary active transport is the process in which solutes are moved across cell membranes against electrochemical gradients using energy supplied directly by ATP. The action of the Na^+–K^+ pump is an important example of primary active transport.** A&PFlix *Available at www.masteringaandp.com*

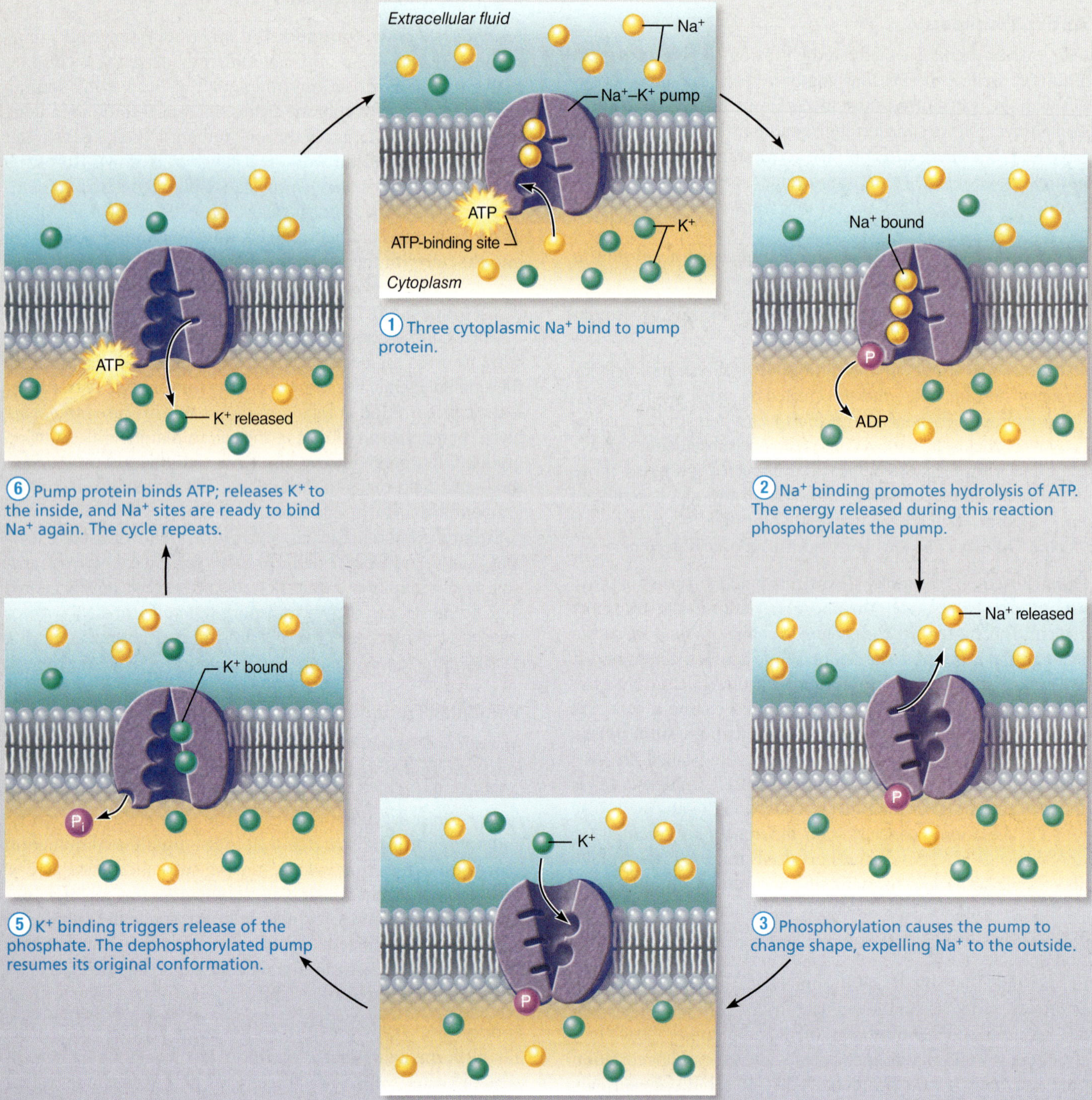

(1) Three cytoplasmic Na^+ bind to pump protein.

(2) Na^+ binding promotes hydrolysis of ATP. The energy released during this reaction phosphorylates the pump.

(3) Phosphorylation causes the pump to change shape, expelling Na^+ to the outside.

(4) Two extracellular K^+ bind to pump.

(5) K^+ binding triggers release of the phosphate. The dephosphorylated pump resumes its original conformation.

(6) Pump protein binds ATP; releases K^+ to the inside, and Na^+ sites are ready to bind Na^+ again. The cycle repeats.

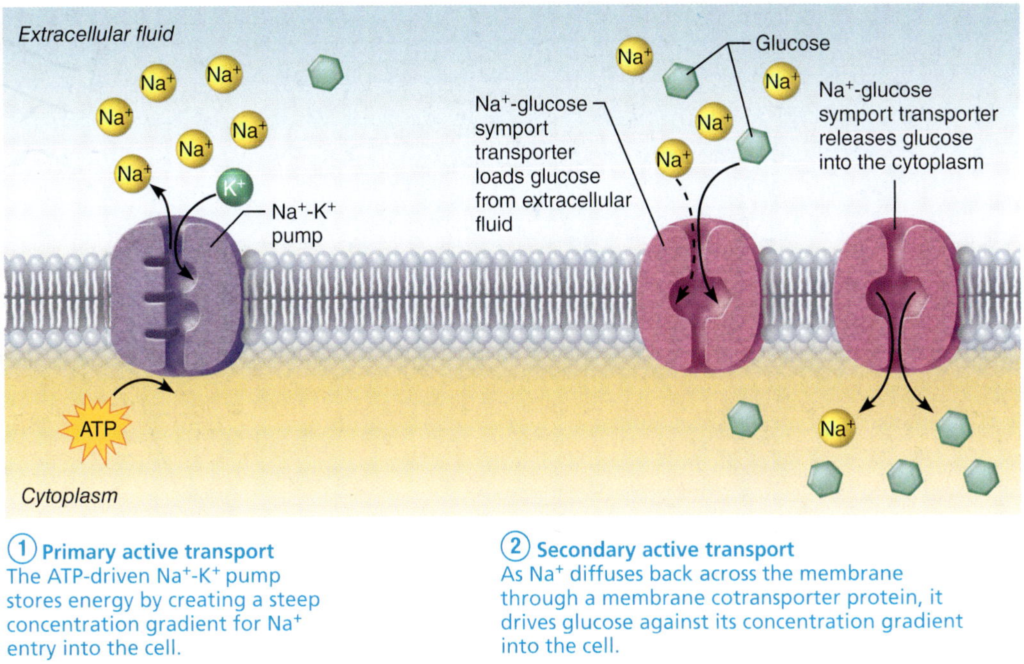

Figure 3.11 Secondary active transport is driven by the concentration gradient created by primary active transport.

Protein-coated vesicles provide the main route for endocytosis and transcytosis of bulk solids, most macromolecules, and fluids. On occasion, these vesicles are also hijacked by pathogens seeking entry into a cell.

Figure 3.12 shows the basic steps in endocytosis and transcytosis. (1) An infolding portion of the plasma membrane, called a *coated pit*, progressively encloses the substance to be taken into the cell. The coating found on the cytoplasmic face of the pit is most often the bristlelike protein **clathrin** (klă′thrin; "lattice clad"). The clathrin coat (clathrin and some accessory proteins) acts in both selecting the cargo and deforming the membrane to produce the vesicle. (2) The vesicle detaches, and (3) the coat proteins are recycled back to the plasma membrane.

(4) The uncoated vesicle then typically fuses with a sorting vesicle called an *endosome*. (5) Some membrane components and receptors of the fused vesicle may be recycled back to the plasma membrane in a transport vesicle. (6) The remaining contents of the vesicle may (a) combine with a *lysosome* (li′so-sōm), a specialized cell structure containing digestive enzymes, where the ingested substance is degraded or released (if iron or cholesterol), or (b) be transported completely across the cell and released by exocytosis on the opposite side (*transcytosis*). Transcytosis is common in the endothelial cells lining blood vessels because it provides a quick means to get substances from the blood to the interstitial fluid.

Based on the nature and quantity of material taken up and the means of uptake, three types of endocytosis that use clathrin-coated vesicles are recognized: phagocytosis, pinocytosis, and receptor-mediated endocytosis.

- **Phagocytosis.** In **phagocytosis** (fag″o-si-to′sis; "cell eating"), the cell engulfs some relatively large or solid material, such as a clump of bacteria, cell debris, or inanimate particles (asbestos fibers or glass, for example) **(Figure 3.13a)**. When a particle binds to receptors on the cell's surface, cytoplasmic extensions called pseudopods (soo′do-pahdz; *pseudo* = false, *pod* = foot) form and flow around the particle. This forms an endocytotic vesicle called a **phagosome** (fag′o-sōm; "eaten body"). In most cases, the phagosome then fuses with a lysosome and its contents are digested. Any indigestible contents are ejected from the cell by exocytosis.

  In the human body, only macrophages and certain white blood cells are "experts" at phagocytosis. Commonly referred to as *phagocytes*, these cells help protect the body by ingesting and disposing of bacteria, other foreign substances, and dead tissue cells. The disposal of dying cells is crucial, because dead cell remnants trigger inflammation in the surrounding area or may stimulate an undesirable immune response. Most phagocytes move about by **amoeboid motion** (ah-me′boyd; "changing shape"); that is, the flowing of their cytoplasm into temporary extensions allows them to creep along.

- **Pinocytosis.** In **pinocytosis** ("cell drinking"), also called **fluid-phase endocytosis**, a bit of infolding plasma membrane (which begins as a protein-coated pit) surrounds a very small volume of extracellular fluid containing dissolved molecules (Figure 3.13b). This droplet enters the cell and fuses with an endosome. Unlike phagocytosis, pinocytosis is a routine activity of most cells, affording them a nonselective way of sampling the extracellular fluid. It is particularly important in cells that absorb nutrients, such as cells that line the intestines.

  As mentioned, bits of the plasma membrane are removed when the membranous sacs are internalized. However, these membranes are recycled back to the plasma membrane by exocytosis as described shortly, so the surface area of the plasma membrane remains remarkably constant.

3

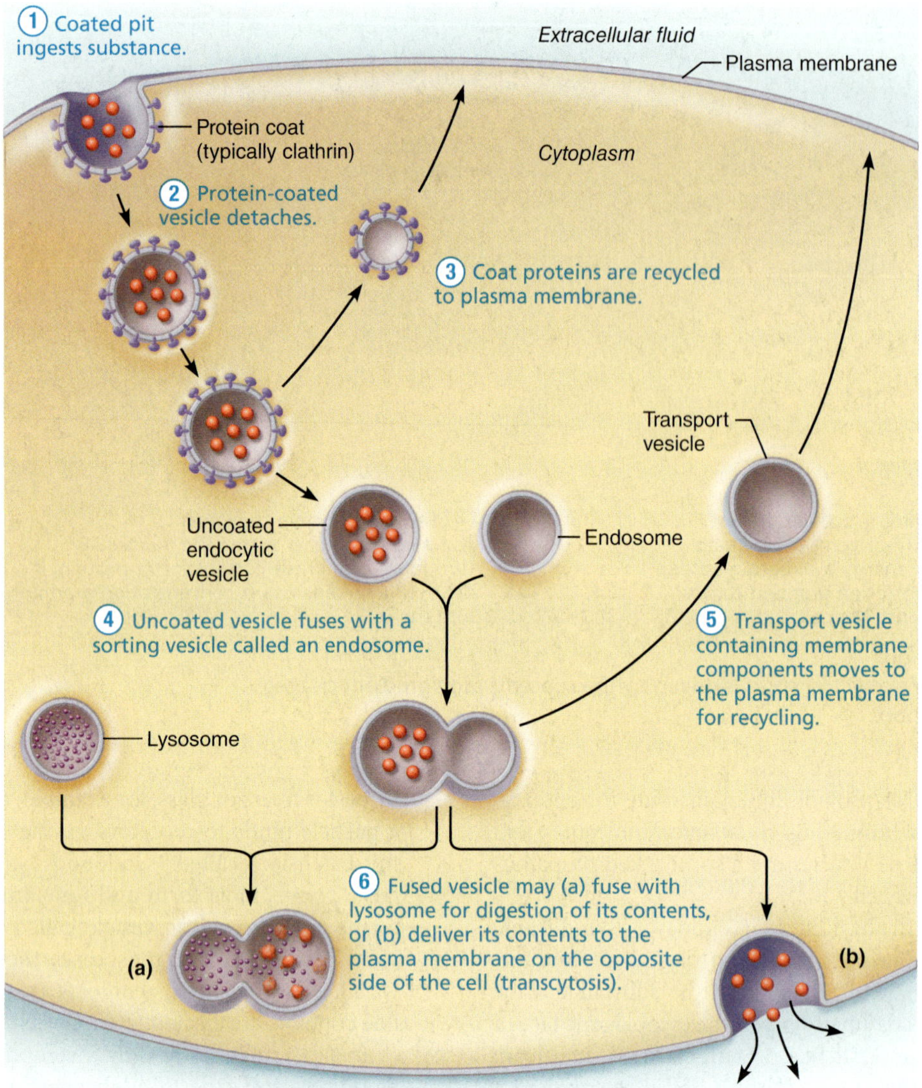

Figure 3.12 Events of endocytosis mediated by protein-coated pits. Note the three possible fates for a vesicle and its contents, shown in (5) and (6).

- **Receptor-mediated endocytosis.** The main mechanism for the *specific* endocytosis and transcytosis of most macromolecules by body cells is **receptor-mediated endocytosis** (Figure 3.13c). This exquisitely selective mechanism allows cells to concentrate material that is present only in small amounts in the extracellular fluid. The receptors for this process are plasma membrane proteins that bind only certain substances. Both the receptors and attached molecules are internalized in a clathrin-coated pit and then dealt with in one of the ways discussed above. Substances taken up by receptor-mediated endocytosis include enzymes, insulin (and some other hormones), low-density lipoproteins (such as cholesterol attached to a transport protein), and iron. Unfortunately, flu viruses, diphtheria, and cholera toxins also use this route to enter our cells.

Different coat proteins are used for certain other types of vesicular transport. For example, **caveolae** (ka″ve-o′le; "little caves"), tubular or flask-shaped inpocketings of the plasma membrane seen in many cell types, are involved in a unique kind of receptor-mediated endocytosis. Like clathrin-coated pits, caveolae capture specific molecules (folic acid, tetanus toxin) from the extracellular fluid in coated vesicles and participate in some forms of transcytosis. However, caveolae are smaller than clathrin-coated vesicles. Additionally, their cage-like protein coat is thinner.

Caveolae are closely associated with lipid rafts that are platforms for G proteins, receptors for hormones (for example, insulin), and enzymes involved in cell regulation. These vesicles appear to provide sites for cell signaling and cross talk between signaling pathways. Their precise role in the cell is still being worked out.

Vesicles coated with still another coat protein (coatomer) function in most types of intracellular vesicular trafficking. Perhaps the most important thing to remember about the coat

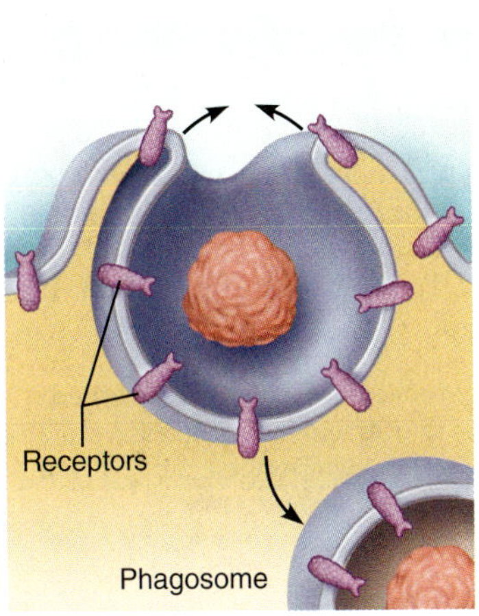

(a) Phagocytosis
The cell engulfs a large particle by forming projecting pseudopods ("false feet") around it and enclosing it within a membrane sac called a phagosome. The phagosome is combined with a lysosome. Undigested contents remain in the vesicle (now called a residual body) or are ejected by exocytosis. Vesicle may or may not be protein-coated but has receptors capable of binding to microorganisms or solid particles.

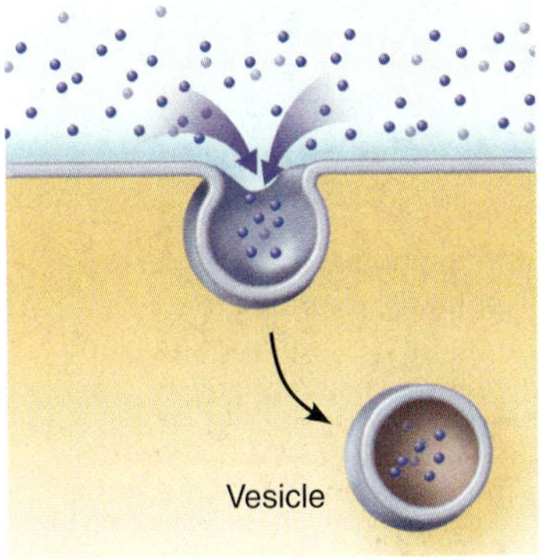

(b) Pinocytosis
The cell "gulps" a drop of extracellular fluid containing solutes into tiny vesicles. No receptors are used, so the process is nonspecific. Most vesicles are protein-coated.

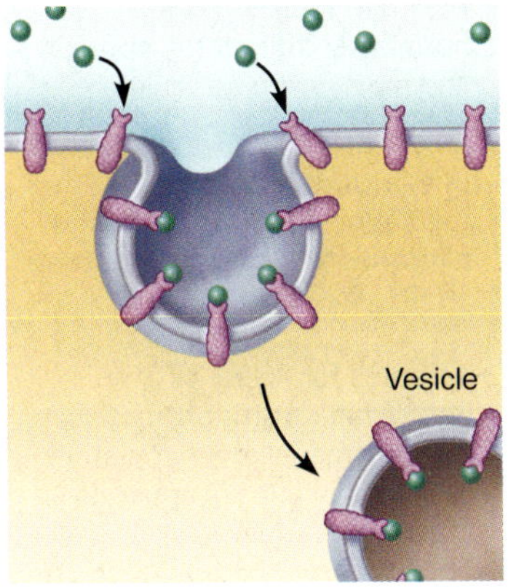

(c) Receptor-mediated endocytosis
Extracellular substances bind to specific receptor proteins, enabling the cell to ingest and concentrate specific substances (ligands) in protein-coated vesicles. Ligands may simply be released inside the cell, or combined with a lysosome to digest contents. Receptors are recycled to the plasma membrane in vesicles.

Figure 3.13 Comparison of three types of endocytosis.

proteins in general is that they play a significant role in all forms of endocytosis.

Exocytosis Vesicular transport processes that eject substances from the cell interior into the extracellular fluid are called **exocytosis** (ek″so-si-to′sis; "out of the cell"). Typically stimulated by a cell-surface signal such as binding of a hormone to a membrane receptor or a change in membrane voltage, exocytosis accounts for hormone secretion, neurotransmitter release, mucus secretion, and in some cases, ejection of wastes. The substance to be removed from the cell is first enclosed in a protein-coated membranous sac called a *secretory vesicle*. In most cases, the vesicle migrates to the plasma membrane, fuses with it, and then ruptures, spilling the sac contents out of the cell **(Figure 3.14)**.

(a) The process of exocytosis

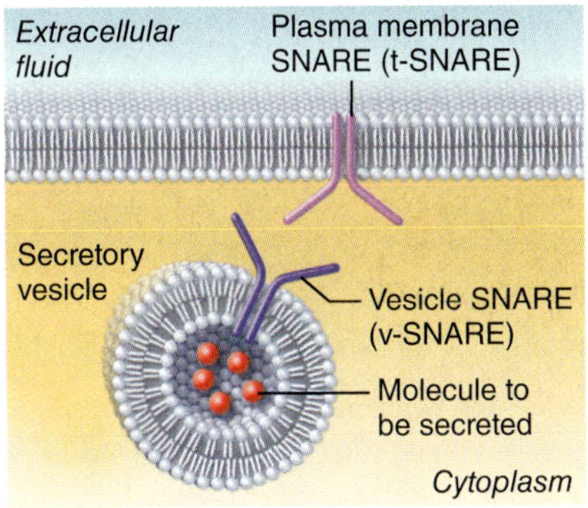

① The membrane-bound vesicle migrates to the plasma membrane.

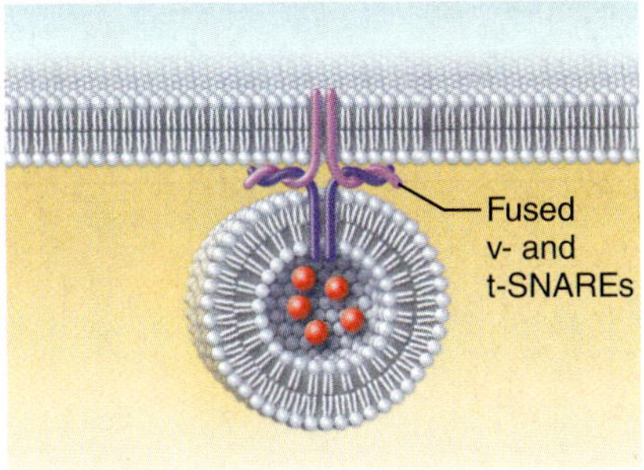

② There, proteins at the vesicle surface (v-SNAREs) bind with t-SNAREs (plasma membrane proteins).

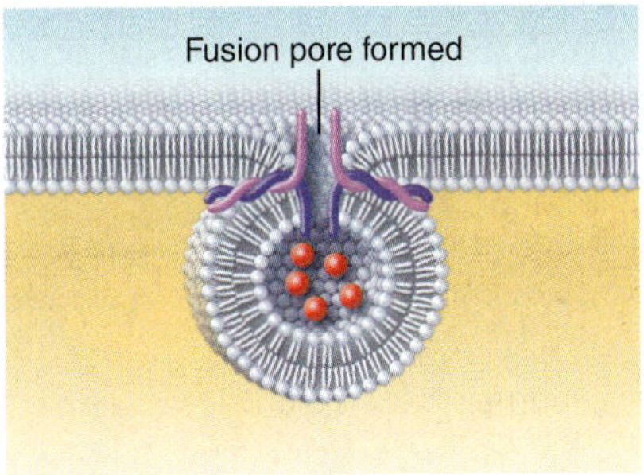

③ The vesicle and plasma membrane fuse and a pore opens up.

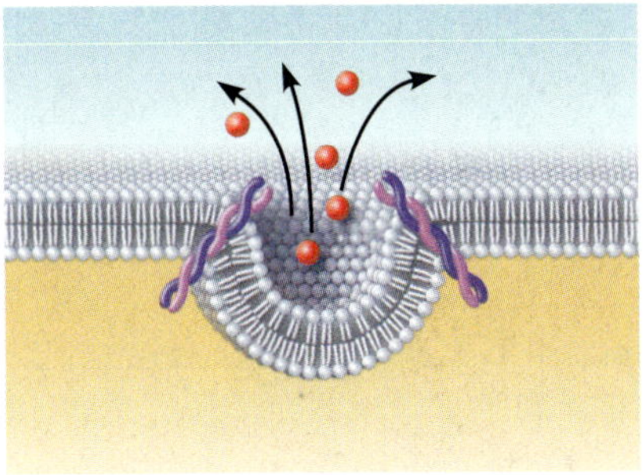

④ Vesicle contents are released to the cell exterior.

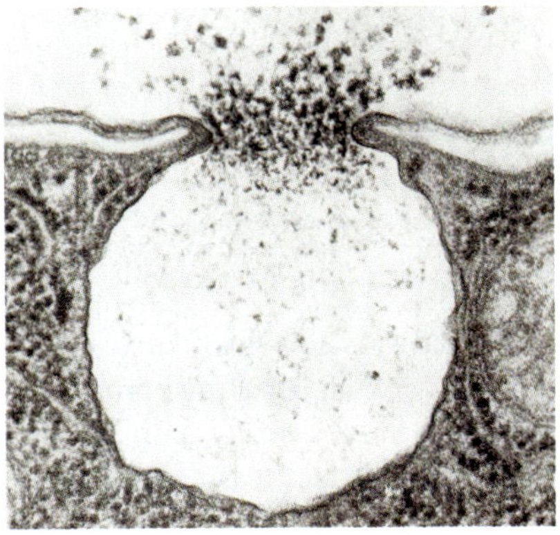

(b) Photomicrograph of a secretory vesicle releasing its contents by exocytosis (100,000×)

Figure 3.14 Exocytosis.

3

3

Table 3.2 Active Membrane Transport Processes

PROCESS	ENERGY SOURCE	DESCRIPTION	EXAMPLES
Active Transport			
Primary active transport	ATP	Transport of substances against a concentration (or electrochemical) gradient. Performed across the plasma membrane by a solute pump, directly using energy of ATP hydrolysis.	Ions (Na^+, K^+, H^+, Ca^{2+}, and others)
Secondary active transport	Ion concentration gradient maintained with ATP	Cotransport (coupled transport) of two solutes across the membrane. Energy is supplied indirectly by the ion gradient created by primary active transport. Symporters move the transported substances in the same direction; antiporters move transported substances in opposite directions across the membrane.	Movement of polar or charged solutes, e.g., amino acids (into cell by symporters); Ca^{2+}, H^+ (out of cells via antiporters)
Vesicular Transport			
Endocytosis			
▪ Via clathrin-coated vesicles			
Phagocytosis	ATP	"Cell eating": A large external particle (proteins, bacteria, dead cell debris) is surrounded by a "seizing foot" and becomes enclosed in a vesicle (phagosome).	In the human body, occurs primarily in protective phagocytes (some white blood cells and macrophages)
Pinocytosis (fluid-phase endocytosis)	ATP	Plasma membrane sinks beneath an external fluid droplet containing small solutes. Membrane edges fuse, forming a fluid-filled vesicle.	Occurs in most cells; important for taking in dissolved solutes by absorptive cells of the kidney and intestine
Receptor-mediated endocytosis	ATP	Selective endocytosis and transcytosis. External substance binds to membrane receptors.	Means of intake of some hormones, cholesterol, iron, and most macromolecules
▪ Via caveolin-coated vesicles (caveolae)	ATP	Selective endocytosis (and transcytosis). External substance binds to membrane receptors (often associated with lipid rafts).	Roles not fully known; proposed roles include cholesterol regulation and trafficking, and platforms for signal transduction
Vesicular trafficking			
▪ Via coatomer-coated vesicles	ATP	Vesicles pinch off from organelles and travel to other organelles to deliver their cargo.	Accounts for nearly all intracellular trafficking between certain organelles (endoplasmic reticulum and Golgi apparatus). Exceptions include vesicles budding from the trans face of the Golgi apparatus, which are clathrin-coated.
Exocytosis	ATP	Secretion or ejection of substances from a cell. The substance is enclosed in a membranous vesicle, which fuses with the plasma membrane and ruptures, releasing the substance to the exterior.	Secretion of neurotransmitters, hormones, mucus, etc.; ejection of cell wastes

Exocytosis, like other mechanisms in which vesicles are targeted to their destinations, involves a "docking" process in which transmembrane proteins on the vesicles, fancifully called v-SNAREs (*v* for vesicle), recognize certain plasma membrane proteins, called t-SNAREs (*t* for target), and bind with them. This binding causes the membranes to "corkscrew" together and fuse, rearranging the lipid monolayers without mixing them (Figure 3.14a). As described, membrane material added by exocytosis is removed by endocytosis—the reverse process.

Table 3.2 summarizes active membrane transport processes.

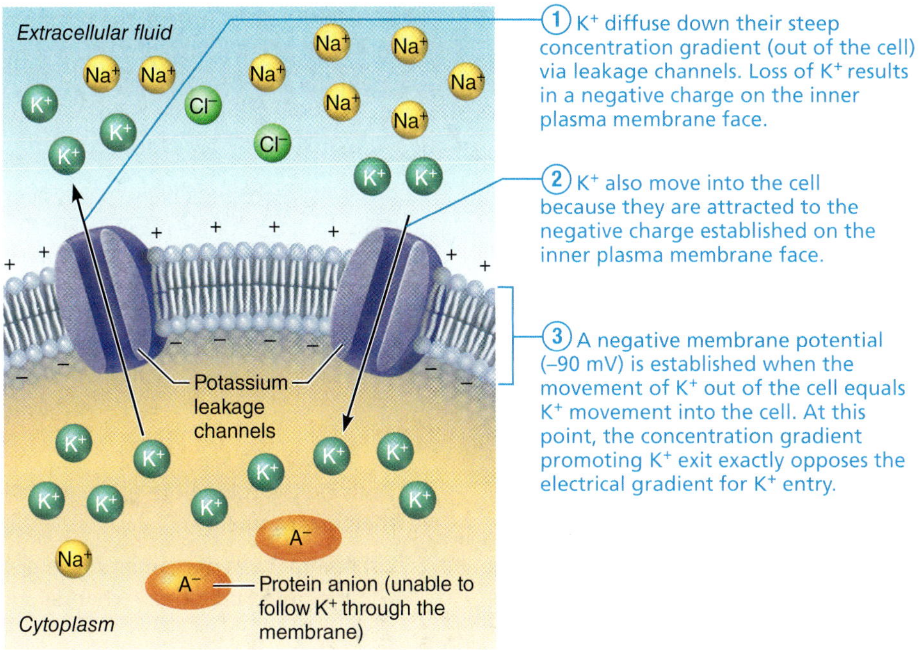

Figure 3.15 The key role of K^+ in generating the resting membrane potential. The resting membrane potential is largely determined by K^+ because at rest, the membrane is much more permeable to K^+ than Na^+. The active transport of sodium and potassium ions (in a ratio of 3:2) by the Na^+-K^+ pump maintains these conditions.

Check Your Understanding

10. What happens when the Na^+-K^+ pump is phosphorylated? When K^+ binds to the pump protein?
11. As a cell grows, its plasma membrane expands. Does this membrane expansion involve endocytosis or exocytosis?
12. Phagocytic cells gather in the lungs, particularly in the lungs of smokers. What is the connection?
13. Which vesicular transport process allows a cell to take in cholesterol from the extracellular fluid?

For answers, see Appendix H.

The Plasma Membrane: Generation of a Resting Membrane Potential

✓ Define membrane potential and explain how the resting membrane potential is established and maintained.

As you're now aware, the selective permeability of the plasma membrane can lead to dramatic osmotic flows, but that is not its only consequence. An equally important result is the generation of a **membrane potential**, or voltage, across the membrane. A *voltage* is electrical potential energy resulting from the separation of oppositely charged particles. In cells, the oppositely charged particles are ions, and the barrier that keeps them apart is the plasma membrane.

In their resting state, all body plasma membranes exhibit a **resting membrane potential** that typically ranges from −50 to −100 millivolts (mV), depending on cell type. For this reason, all cells are said to be **polarized.** The minus sign before the voltage indicates that the *inside* of the cell is negative compared to its outside. This voltage (or charge separation) exists *only at the membrane*. If we added up all the negative and positive charges in the cytoplasm, we would find that the cell interior is electrically neutral. Likewise, the positive and negative charges in the extracellular fluid balance each other exactly.

So how does the resting membrane potential come about, and how is it maintained? The short answer is that diffusion causes ionic imbalances that polarize the membrane, and active transport processes *maintain* that membrane potential. First, let's look at how diffusion polarizes the membrane.

Selective Diffusion Establishes Membrane Potential

Many kinds of ions are found both inside cells and in the extracellular fluid, but the resting membrane potential is determined mainly by the concentration gradient of potassium (K^+) and by the differential permeability of the plasma membrane to K^+ and other ions **(Figure 3.15)**. Recall that K^+ and protein anions predominate inside body cells, and the extracellular fluid contains relatively more Na^+, which is largely balanced by Cl^-. The unstimulated plasma membrane is somewhat permeable to K^+ because of leakage channels, but impermeable to the protein anions. Consequently, K^+ diffuses out of the cell along its concentration gradient but the protein anions are unable to follow, and this loss of positive charges makes the membrane interior more negative (Figure 3.15 (1)).

As more and more K^+ leaves the cell, the negativity of the inner membrane face becomes great enough to attract K^+ back toward and even into the cell (Figure 3.15 ②). At a membrane voltage of -90 mV, potassium's concentration gradient is exactly balanced by the electrical gradient (membrane potential), and one K^+ enters the cell as one leaves (Figure 3.15 ③).

In many cells, sodium (Na^+) also contributes to the resting membrane potential. Sodium is strongly attracted to the cell interior by its concentration gradient, bringing the resting membrane potential to -70 mV. However, potassium still largely determines the resting membrane potential because the membrane is much more permeable to K^+ than to Na^+. Even though the membrane is permeable to Cl^-, in most cells Cl^- does not contribute to the resting membrane potential, because its concentration and electrical gradients exactly balance each other.

We may be tempted to believe that massive flows of K^+ ions are needed to generate the resting potential, but this is not the case. Surprisingly, the number of ions producing the membrane potential is so small that it does not change ion concentrations in any significant way.

In a cell at rest, very few ions cross its plasma membrane. However, Na^+ and K^+ are not at equilibrium and there is some net movement of K^+ out of the cell and of Na^+ into the cell. Na^+ is strongly pulled into the cell by both its concentration gradient and the interior negative charge. If only passive forces were at work, these ion concentrations would eventually become equal inside and outside the cell.

Active Transport Maintains Electrochemical Gradients

Now let's look at how active transport processes maintain the membrane potential that diffusion has established, with the result that the cell exhibits a *steady state*. The rate of active transport is equal to, and depends on, the rate of Na^+ diffusion into the cell. If more Na^+ enters, more is pumped out. (This is like being in a leaky boat. The more water that comes in, the faster you bail!) The Na^+-K^+ pump couples sodium and potassium transport and, on average, each "turn" of the pump ejects $3Na^+$ out of the cell and carries $2K^+$ back in (see Figure 3.10). Because the membrane is always 50 to 100 times more permeable to K^+, the ATP-dependent Na^+-K^+ pump maintains both the membrane potential (the charge separation) and the osmotic balance. Indeed, if Na^+ was not continuously removed from cells, so much would accumulate intracellularly that the osmotic gradient would draw water into the cells, causing them to burst.

As we described on p. 73, diffusion of charged particles across the membrane is affected not only by concentration gradients, but by the electrical charge on the inner and outer faces of the membrane. Together these gradients make up the *electrochemical gradient*. The diffusion of K^+ across the plasma membrane is aided by the membrane's greater permeability to it and by the ion's concentration gradient, but the negative charges on the cell interior resist K^+ diffusion. In contrast, a steep electrochemical gradient draws Na^+ into the cell, but the membrane's relative impermeability to it limits Na^+ diffusion.

The transient opening of gated Na^+ and K^+ channels in the plasma membrane "upsets" the resting membrane potential. As we describe in later chapters, this is a normal means of activating neurons and muscle cells.

☑ Check Your Understanding

14. What process establishes the resting membrane potential?
15. Is the inside of the plasma membrane negative or positive relative to its outside in a polarized membrane?

For answers, see Appendix H.

The Plasma Membrane: Cell-Environment Interactions

✓ Describe the role of the glycocalyx when cells interact with their environment.

✓ List several roles of membrane receptors and that of voltage-gated membrane channel proteins.

Cells are biological minifactories and, like other factories, they receive and send orders from and to the outside community. But *how* does a cell interact with its environment, and *what* activates it to carry out its homeostatic functions?

Sometimes cells interact directly with other cells. However, in many cases cells respond to extracellular chemicals, such as hormones and neurotransmitters distributed in body fluids. Cells also interact with extracellular molecules that act as signposts to guide cell migration during development and repair.

Whether cells interact directly or indirectly, however, the glycocalyx is always involved. The best-understood glycocalyx molecules fall into two large families—cell adhesion molecules and plasma membrane receptors (see Figure 3.4, p. 66). Another group of membrane proteins, voltage-gated channel proteins, are important in cells that respond to electrical signals.

Roles of Cell Adhesion Molecules (CAMs)

Thousands of **cell adhesion molecules (CAMs)** are found on almost every cell in the body. CAMs play key roles in embryonic development and wound repair (situations where cell mobility is important) and in immunity. These sticky glycoproteins (*cadherins* and *integrins*) act as

- The molecular "Velcro" that cells use to anchor themselves to molecules in the extracellular space and to each other (see desmosome discussion on pp. 66–67)
- The "arms" that migrating cells use to haul themselves past one another
- SOS signals sticking out from the blood vessel lining that rally protective white blood cells to a nearby infected or injured area
- Mechanical sensors that respond to changes in local tension or fluid movement at the cell surface by stimulating synthesis or degradation of adhesive membrane (tight) junctions
- Transmitters of intracellular signals that direct cell migration, proliferation, and specialization

Roles of Plasma Membrane Receptors

A huge and diverse group of integral proteins and glycoproteins that serve as binding sites are collectively known as **membrane receptors**. Some function in contact signaling, and others in chemical signaling. Let's take a look.

Contact Signaling

Contact signaling, in which cells come together and touch, is the means by which cells recognize one another. It is particularly important for normal development and immunity. Some bacteria and other infectious agents use contact signaling to identify their "preferred" target tissues.

Chemical Signaling

Most plasma membrane receptors are involved in *chemical signaling*. **Ligands** are chemicals that bind specifically to plasma membrane receptors. Ligands include most *neurotransmitters* (nervous system signals), *hormones* (endocrine system signals), and *paracrines* (chemicals that act locally and are rapidly destroyed).

Different cells respond in different ways to the same ligand. Acetylcholine, for instance, stimulates skeletal muscle cells to contract, but inhibits heart muscle. Why do different cells respond so differently? The reason is that a target cell's response depends on the internal machinery that the receptor is linked to, not the specific ligand that binds to it.

Though cell responses to receptor binding vary widely, there is a fundamental similarity: When a ligand binds to a membrane receptor, the receptor's structure changes, and cell proteins are altered in some way. For example:

- *Catalytic receptor proteins* are membrane proteins that respond to ligands by becoming activated enzymes.
- *Chemically gated channel-linked receptors*, common in muscle and nerve cells, respond by transiently opening or closing ion gates, which in turn changes the excitability of the cell.
- **G protein–linked receptors** exert their effect indirectly through a **G protein**, a regulatory molecule that acts as a middleman or relay to activate (or inactivate) a membrane-bound enzyme or ion channel. This in turn generates one or more intracellular chemical signals, commonly called **second messengers**, which connect plasma membrane events to the internal metabolic machinery of the cell. Two important second messengers are **cyclic AMP** and ionic calcium, both of which typically activate *protein kinase enzymes*, which transfer phosphate groups from ATP to other proteins. In this way, the protein kinases can activate a whole series of enzymes that bring about the desired cellular activity. Because a single enzyme can catalyze hundreds of reactions, the amplification effect of such a chain of events is tremendous, much like that stirred up by a chain letter. *Focus on G Proteins* **(Figure 3.16)** on p. 82 describes a G protein signaling system. Take a moment to study this carefully because this key signaling pathway is involved in neurotransmission, smell, vision, and hormone action (Chapters 11, 15, and 16).

Nitric oxide (*NO*) is an important signaling molecule even though it doesn't act in any of the ways we have already described. One of nature's simplest molecules, NO is made of a single atom of nitrogen and one of oxygen. It is also an environmental pollutant and the first gas known to act as a biological messenger. Because of its tiny size, it slips into and out of cells easily. Its unpaired electron makes it highly reactive and it reacts with head-spinning speed with other key molecules to spur cells into a broad array of activities. You will hear more about NO in the neural, cardiovascular, and immune system chapters.

Role of Voltage-Gated Membrane Channel Proteins: Electrical Signaling

In *electrical signaling*, certain plasma membrane proteins are channel proteins that respond to changes in membrane potential by opening or closing the channel. Such voltage-gated channels are common in excitable tissues like neural and muscle tissues, and are crucial to their normal function.

☑ Check Your Understanding

16. What term is used to indicate signaling chemicals that bind to membrane receptors? Which type of membrane receptor is most important in directing intracellular events by promoting formation of second messengers?

For answer, see Appendix H.

The Cytoplasm

- ✓ Describe the composition of the cytosol.
- ✓ Discuss the structure and function of mitochondria.
- ✓ Discuss the structure and function of ribosomes, the endoplasmic reticulum, and the Golgi apparatus, including functional interrelationships among these organelles.
- ✓ Compare the functions of lysosomes and peroxisomes.

Cytoplasm ("cell-forming material"), the cellular material between the plasma membrane and the nucleus, is the site of most cellular activities. Although early microscopists thought that the cytoplasm was a structureless gel, the electron microscope reveals that it consists of three major elements: the cytosol, organelles, and inclusions.

The **cytosol** (si′to-sol) is the viscous, semitransparent fluid in which the other cytoplasmic elements are suspended. It is a complex mixture with properties of both a colloid and a true solution. Dissolved in the cytosol, which is largely water, are proteins, salts, sugars, and a variety of other solutes.

The **organelles** are the metabolic machinery of the cell. Each type of organelle carries out a specific function for the cell—some synthesize proteins, others package those proteins, and so on.

Inclusions are chemical substances that may or may not be present, depending on cell type. Examples include stored nutrients, such as the glycogen granules in liver and muscle cells; lipid droplets in fat cells; pigment (melanin) granules in certain skin and hair cells; and crystals of various types.

FOCUS G Proteins

Figure 3.16 G proteins act as middlemen or relays between extracellular first messengers and intracellular second messengers that cause responses within the cell.

The sequence described here is like a molecular relay race. Instead of a baton passed from runner to runner, the message (a shape change) is passed from molecule to molecule as it makes its way across the cell membrane from outside to inside the cell.

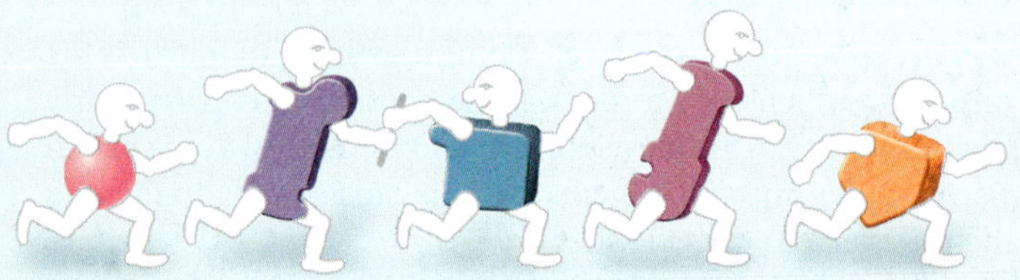

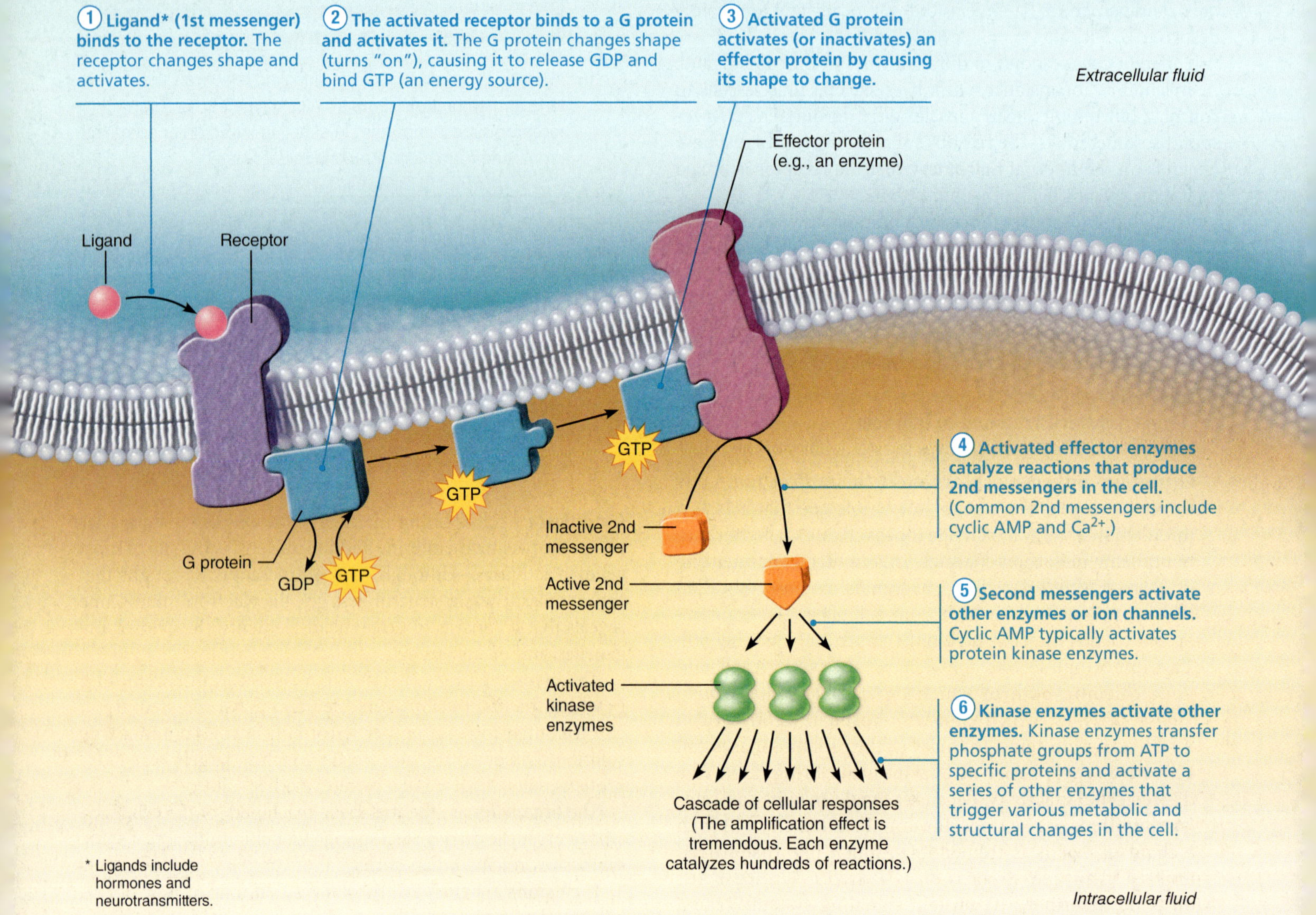

* Ligands include hormones and neurotransmitters.

Cytoplasmic Organelles

The organelles ("little organs") are specialized cellular compartments or structures, each performing its own job to maintain the life of the cell. Some organelles, the *nonmembranous organelles*, lack membranes. Examples are the cytoskeleton, centrioles, and ribosomes.

Most organelles, however, are bounded by a membrane similar in composition to the plasma membrane. This membrane enables the *membranous organelles* (such as peroxisomes, lysosomes, endoplasmic reticulum, and Golgi apparatus) to maintain an internal environment different from that of the surrounding cytosol. This compartmentalization is crucial to cell functioning. Without it, thousands of enzymes would be randomly mixed and biochemical activity would be chaotic. Besides providing splendid isolation for an organelle, its membrane often unites it with the rest of an interactive intracellular system called the *endomembrane system* (see p. 87), and the lipid and protein makeup of the membrane allows it to recognize and interact with other organelles. Now let's consider what goes on in each of the workshops of our cellular factory.

Mitochondria

Mitochondria (mi″to-kon′dre-ah) are threadlike (*mitos* = thread) or lozenge-shaped membranous organelles. In living cells they squirm, elongate, and change shape almost continuously. They are the power plants of a cell, providing most of its ATP supply. The density of mitochondria in a particular cell reflects that cell's energy requirements, and mitochondria generally cluster where the action is. Busy cells like kidney and liver cells have hundreds of mitochondria, whereas relatively inactive cells (such as unchallenged lymphocytes) have just a few.

A mitochondrion is enclosed by *two* membranes, each with the general structure of the plasma membrane **(Figure 3.17)**. The *outer membrane* is smooth and featureless, but the *inner membrane* folds inward, forming shelflike **cristae** (krĭ′ste; "crests") that protrude into the *matrix*, the gel-like substance within the mitochondrion. Intermediate products of food fuels (glucose and others) are broken down to water and carbon dioxide by teams of enzymes, some dissolved in the mitochondrial matrix and others forming part of the crista membrane.

As the metabolites are broken down and oxidized, some of the energy released is captured and used to attach phosphate groups to ADP molecules to form ATP. This multistep mitochondrial process (described in Chapter 24) is called *aerobic cellular respiration* (a-er-o′bik) because it requires oxygen.

Mitochondria are complex organelles: They contain their own DNA, RNA, and ribosomes and are able to reproduce themselves. Mitochondrial genes (some 37 of them) direct the synthesis of 1% of the proteins required for mitochondrial function, and the DNA of the cell's nucleus encodes the remaining proteins needed to carry out cellular respiration. When cellular requirements for ATP increase, the mitochondria synthesize more cristae or simply pinch in half (a process called *fission*) to increase their number, then grow to their former size.

Intriguingly, mitochondria are similar to bacteria in the purple bacteria phylum, and mitochondrial DNA is bacteria-like.

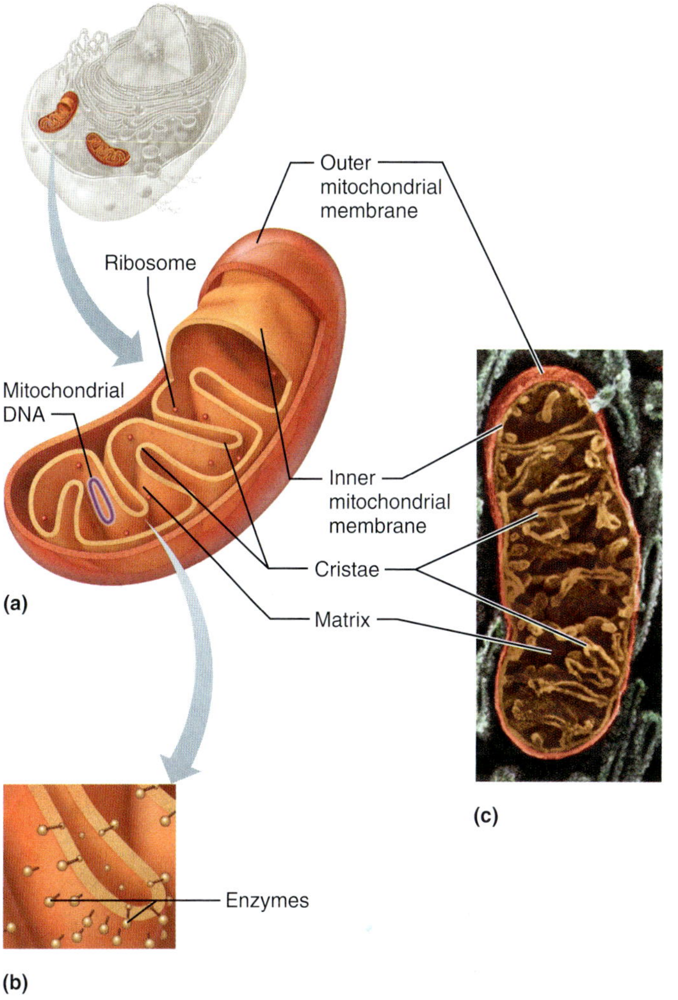

Figure 3.17 Mitochondrion. (a) Diagram of a longitudinally sectioned mitochondrion. **(b)** Close-up of a crista showing enzymes (stalked particles). **(c)** Electron micrograph of a mitochondrion (50,000×).

It is widely believed that mitochondria arose from bacteria that invaded the ancient ancestors of plant and animal cells, and that this unique merger gave rise to all complex cells.

Ribosomes

Ribosomes (ri′bo-sōmz) are small, dark-staining granules composed of proteins and a variety of RNAs called *ribosomal RNAs*. Each ribosome has two globular subunits that fit together like the body and cap of an acorn. Ribosomes are sites of protein synthesis, a function we discuss in detail later in this chapter.

Some ribosomes float freely in the cytoplasm. Others are attached to membranes, forming a complex called the *rough endoplasmic reticulum* (see p. 84). These two ribosomal populations appear to divide the chore of protein synthesis.

- *Free ribosomes* float freely in the cytoplasm. They make soluble proteins that function in the cytosol, as well as those imported into mitochondria and some other organelles.

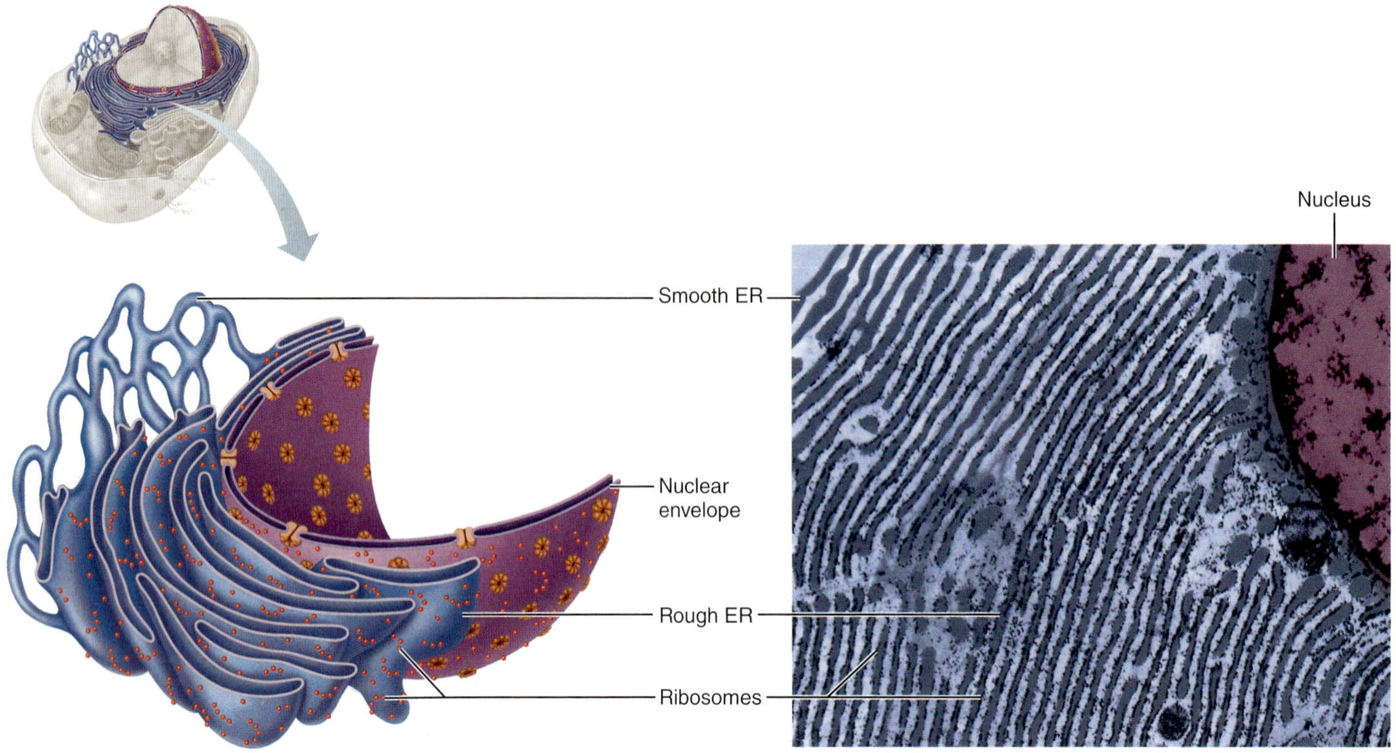

(a) Diagrammatic view of smooth and rough ER

(b) Electron micrograph of smooth and rough ER (25,000×)

Figure 3.18 The endoplasmic reticulum.

- *Membrane-bound ribosomes* are attached to membranes, forming a complex called the *rough endoplasmic reticulum* **(Figure 3.18)**. They synthesize proteins destined either for incorporation into cell membranes or lysosomes, or for export from the cell.

Ribosome subunits can switch back and forth between these two functions, attaching to and detaching from the membranes of the endoplasmic reticulum, according to the type of protein they are making at a given time.

Endoplasmic Reticulum (ER)

The **endoplasmic reticulum (ER)** (en″do-plaz′mik rĕ-tik′u-lum; "network within the cytoplasm") is an extensive system of interconnected tubes and parallel membranes enclosing fluid-filled cavities, or **cisterns** (sis-ternz) as shown in Figure 3.18. Coiling and twisting through the cytosol, the ER is continuous with the outer nuclear membrane and accounts for about half of the cell's membranes. There are two distinct varieties: rough ER and smooth ER.

Rough Endoplasmic Reticulum The external surface of the **rough ER** is studded with ribosomes, hence the name "rough" (see Figures 3.2 and 3.18a, b). Proteins assembled on these ribosomes thread their way into the fluid-filled interior of the ER cisterns (as described on pp. 105 and 108). When complete, the newly made proteins are enclosed in vesicles for their journey to the Golgi apparatus where they undergo further processing.

The rough ER has several functions. Its ribosomes manufacture all proteins secreted from cells. For this reason, the rough ER is particularly abundant and well developed in most secretory cells, antibody-producing plasma cells, and liver cells, which produce most blood proteins. It is also the cell's "membrane factory" where integral proteins and phospholipids that form part of all cellular membranes are manufactured. The enzymes needed to catalyze lipid synthesis have their active sites on the external (cytosolic) face of the ER membrane, where the needed substrates are readily available.

Smooth Endoplasmic Reticulum The **smooth ER** (see Figures 3.2 and 3.18) is continuous with the rough ER and consists of tubules arranged in a looping network. Its enzymes (all integral proteins forming part of its membranes) play no role in protein synthesis. Instead, the enzymes catalyze reactions involved with the following tasks:

- Metabolize lipids, synthesize cholesterol, and synthesize the lipid components of lipoproteins (in liver cells)
- Synthesize steroid-based hormones such as sex hormones (testosterone-synthesizing cells of the testes are full of smooth ER)
- Absorb, synthesize, and transport fats (in intestinal cells)
- Detoxify drugs, certain pesticides, and cancer-causing chemicals (in liver and kidneys)
- Break down stored glycogen to form free glucose (in liver cells especially)

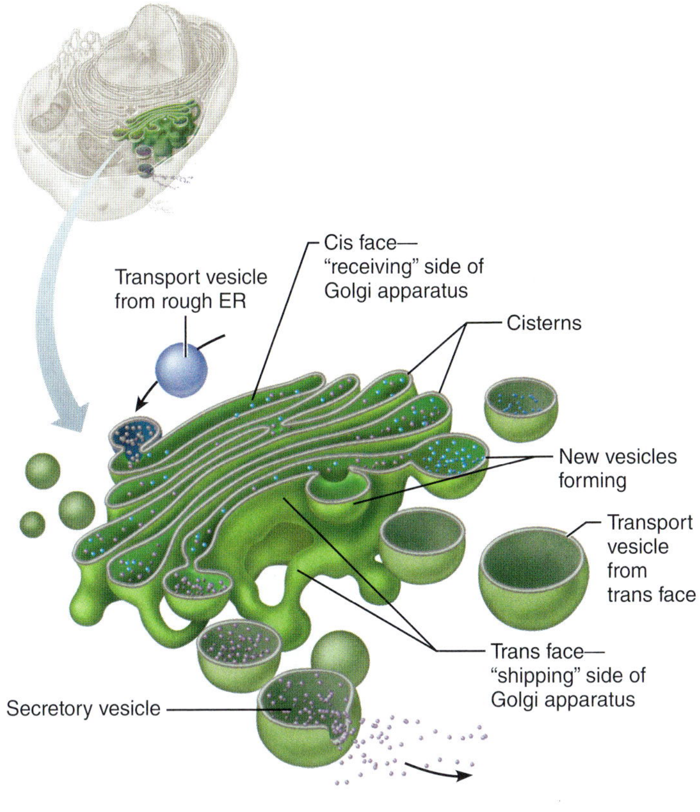

(a) Many vesicles in the process of pinching off from the Golgi apparatus.

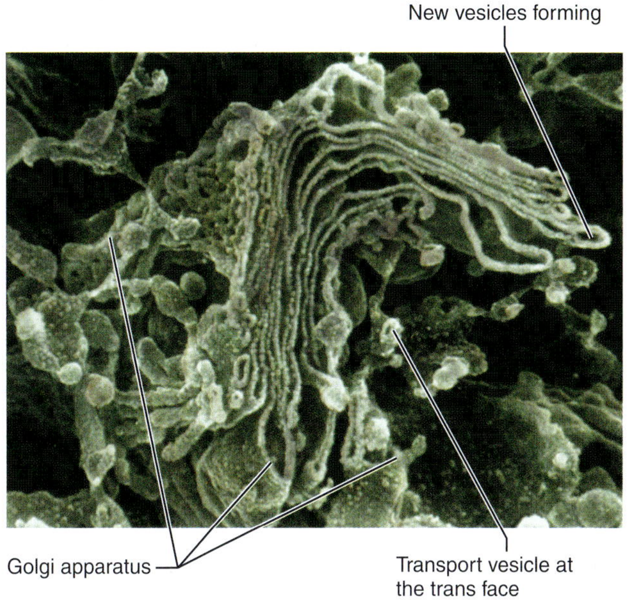

(b) Electron micrograph of the Golgi apparatus (90,000×)

Figure 3.19 Golgi apparatus. Note: In (a), the vesicles shown in the process of pinching off from the membranous Golgi apparatus would have a protein coating on their external surfaces. The diagram omits these proteins for simplicity.

Additionally, skeletal and cardiac muscle cells have an elaborate smooth ER (called the sarcoplasmic reticulum) that plays an important role in storing and releasing calcium ions during muscle contraction. Except for the examples given above, most body cells contain relatively little, if any, smooth ER.

Golgi Apparatus

The **Golgi apparatus** (gol′je) consists of stacked and flattened membranous sacs, shaped like hollow dinner plates, associated with swarms of tiny membranous vesicles **(Figure 3.19)**. The Golgi apparatus is the principal "traffic director" for cellular proteins. Its major function is to modify, concentrate, and package the proteins and lipids made at the rough ER and destined for export from the cell.

The Golgi's odd shape is a side effect of its job. A protein complex pulls membranous sacs containing newly synthesized proteins off the Golgi and in the process, the membranes are flattened like rubber bands. Transport vesicles that bud off from the rough ER move to and fuse with the membranes at the convex *cis face,* the "receiving" side, of the Golgi apparatus. Inside the apparatus, the proteins are modified: Some sugar groups are trimmed while others are added, and in some cases, phosphate groups are added.

The various proteins are "tagged" for delivery to a specific address, sorted, and packaged in at least three types of vesicles that bud from the concave *trans face* (the "shipping" side) of the Golgi stack:

- Vesicles containing proteins destined for export pinch off from the trans face as **secretory vesicles, or granules**, which migrate to the plasma membrane and discharge their contents from the cell by exocytosis (**Figure 3.20**, pathway A). Specialized secretory cells, such as the enzyme-producing cells of the pancreas, have a prominent Golgi apparatus.
- The Golgi apparatus pinches off other vesicles containing lipids and transmembrane proteins destined for the plasma membrane (Figure 3.20, pathway B) or for other membranous organelles.
- The Golgi apparatus also packages digestive enzymes into membranous lysosomes that remain in the cell (Figure 3.20, pathway C), as discussed shortly.

Peroxisomes

Peroxisomes (pĕ-roks′ĭ-sōmz; "peroxide bodies") are spherical membranous sacs containing a variety of powerful enzymes, the most important of which are oxidases and catalases.

Oxidases use molecular oxygen (O_2) to detoxify harmful substances, including alcohol and formaldehyde. Their most important function is to neutralize **free radicals**, highly reactive

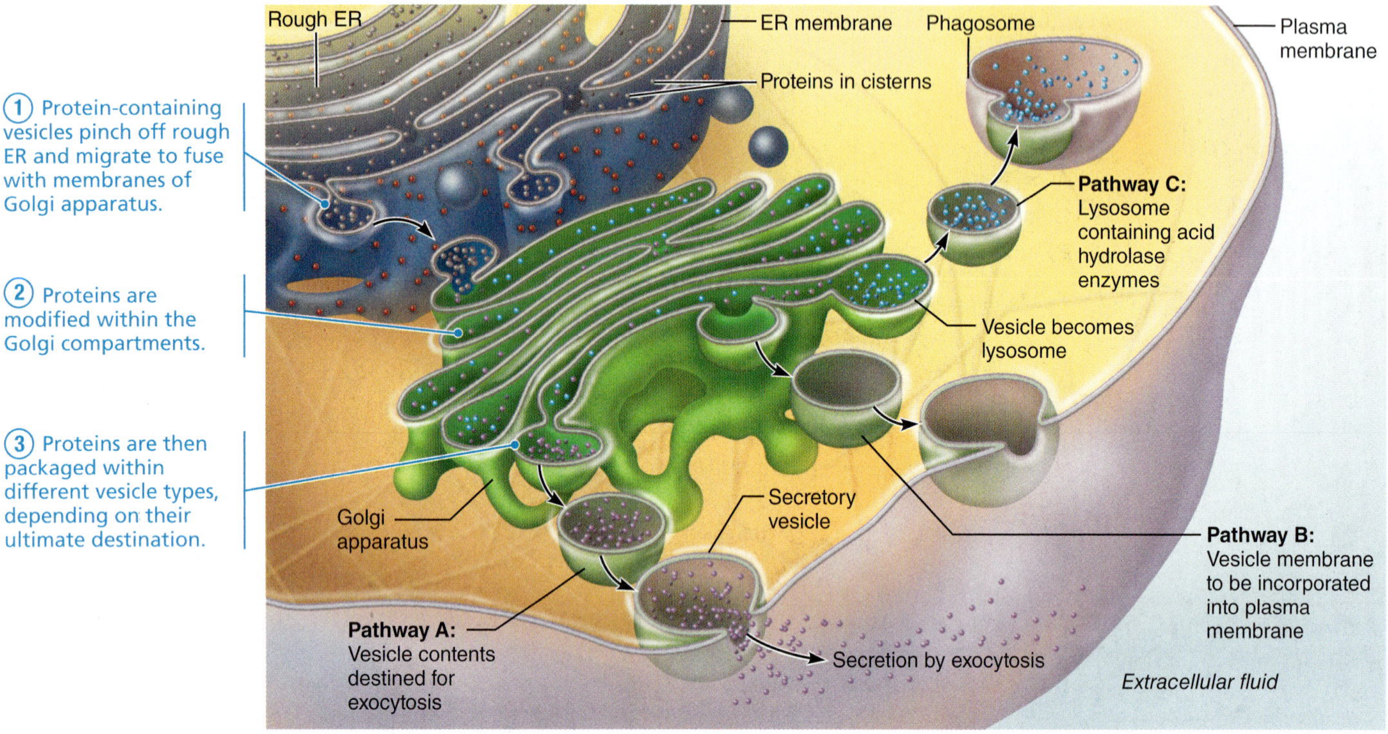

Figure 3.20 The sequence of events from protein synthesis on the rough ER to the final distribution of those proteins. The protein coats on the transport vesicles are not illustrated.

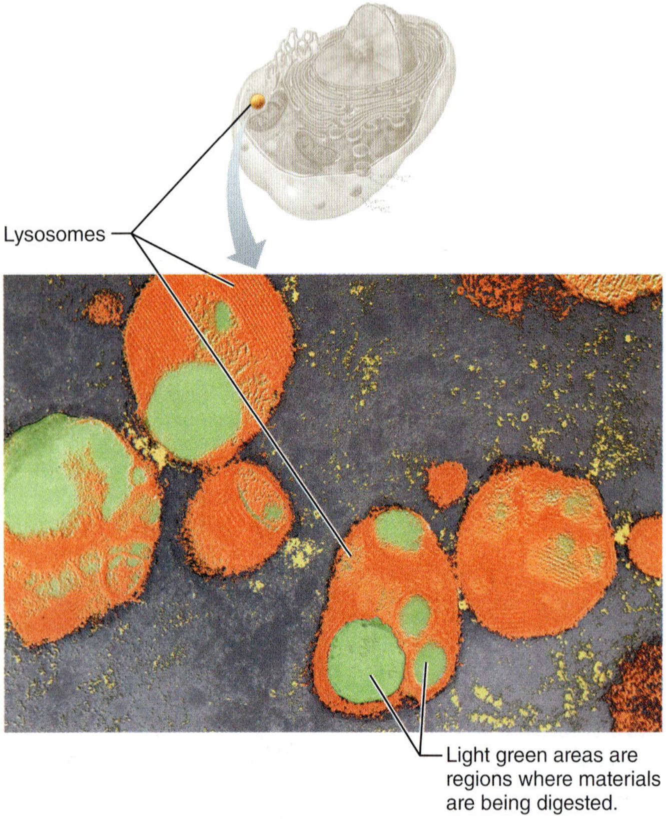

Figure 3.21 Electron micrograph of lysosomes (20,000×).

chemicals with unpaired electrons that can scramble the structure of biological molecules. Oxidases convert free radicals to hydrogen peroxide, which is also reactive and dangerous but which the catalases quickly convert to water. Free radicals and hydrogen peroxide are normal by-products of cellular metabolism, but they have devastating effects on cells if allowed to accumulate.

Peroxisomes are especially numerous in liver and kidney cells, which are very active in detoxification. They also play a role in energy metabolism by breaking down and synthesizing fatty acids. Peroxisomes look like small lysosomes (see Figure 3.2), and for many years it was thought that they were self-replicating organelles formed when existing peroxisomes simply pinch in half. Recent evidence, however, suggests that most new peroxisomes form by budding off of the endoplasmic reticulum via a special ER machinery that differs from that used for vesicles destined for modification in the Golgi apparatus.

Lysosomes

Born as endosomes which contain inactive enzymes, **lysosomes** ("disintegrator bodies") are spherical membranous organelles containing activated digestive enzymes **(Figure 3.21)**. As you might guess, lysosomes are large and abundant in phagocytes, the cells that dispose of invading bacteria and cell debris. Lysosomal enzymes can digest almost all kinds of biological molecules. They work best in acidic conditions and so are called *acid hydrolases*.

The lysosomal membrane is adapted to serve lysosomal functions in two important ways. First, it contains H^+ (proton) "pumps," which are ATPases that gather hydrogen ions from the surrounding cytosol to maintain the organelle's acidic pH. Second, it retains the dangerous acid hydrolases while permitting the final products of digestion to escape so that they can be used by the cell or excreted. In this way, lysosomes provide sites where digestion can proceed *safely* within a cell.

Lysosomes function as a cell's "demolition crew" by

- Digesting particles taken in by endocytosis, particularly ingested bacteria, viruses, and toxins
- Degrading worn-out or nonfunctional organelles
- Performing metabolic functions, such as glycogen breakdown and release
- Breaking down nonuseful tissues, such as the webs between the fingers and toes of a developing fetus and the uterine lining during menstruation
- Breaking down bone to release calcium ions into the blood

The lysosomal membrane is ordinarily quite stable, but it becomes fragile when the cell is injured or deprived of oxygen and when excessive amounts of vitamin A are present. When lysosomes rupture, the cell digests itself, a process called **autolysis** (aw″tol′ĭ-sis). Autolysis is the basis for desirable destruction of cells, as in the fourth list item above.

Homeostatic Imbalance 3.4

Lysosomes degrade glycogen and certain lipids in the brain at a relatively constant rate. In *Tay-Sachs disease*, an inherited condition seen mostly in Jews from Central Europe, the lysosomes lack an enzyme needed to break down a glycolipid abundant in nerve cell membranes. As a result, the nerve cell lysosomes swell with undigested lipids, which interfere with nervous system functioning. Affected infants typically have doll-like features and pink translucent skin. At 3 to 6 months of age, the first signs of disease appear (listlessness, motor weakness). These symptoms progress to mental retardation, seizures, blindness, and ultimately death within 18 months. ✚

The Endomembrane System

The **endomembrane system** is a system of organelles (most described above) that work together mainly to (1) produce, degrade, store, and export biological molecules, and (2) degrade potentially harmful substances. It includes the ER, Golgi apparatus, secretory vesicles, and lysosomes, as well as the nuclear membrane—that is, all of the membranous organelles or elements that are either structurally continuous or arise via forming or fusing transport vesicles **(Figure 3.22)**. There are continuities between the nuclear envelope (itself an extension of the rough ER) and the rough and smooth ER (Figure 3.18). The plasma membrane, though not actually an *endo*membrane, is also functionally part of this system.

Besides these direct structural relationships, a wide variety of indirect interactions (indicated by arrows in Figure 3.22) occur among the members of the system. Some of the vesicles "born" in the ER migrate to and fuse with the Golgi apparatus or the plasma membrane, and vesicles arising from the Golgi

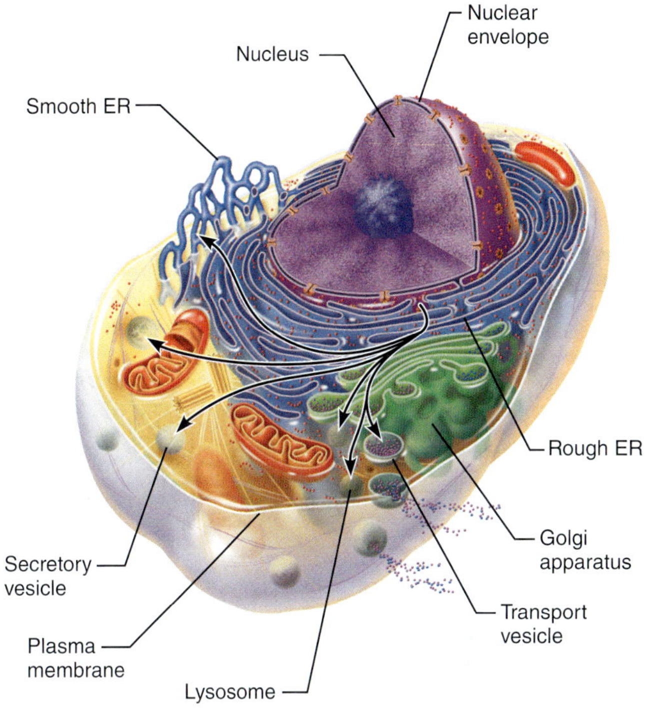

Figure 3.22 The endomembrane system.

apparatus can become part of the plasma membrane, secretory vesicles, or lysosomes.

☑ Check Your Understanding

17. Which organelle is the major site of ATP synthesis?
18. What are three organelles involved in protein synthesis and how do these organelles interact in that process?
19. Compare the functions of lysosomes and peroxisomes.

For answers, see Appendix H.

Cytoskeleton

✓ Name and describe the structure and function of cytoskeletal elements.

The **cytoskeleton**, literally, "cell skeleton," is an elaborate network of rods running through the cytosol and hundreds of accessory proteins that link these rods to other cell structures. It acts as a cell's "bones," "muscles," and "ligaments" by supporting cellular structures and providing the machinery to generate various cell movements. The three types of rods in the cytoskeleton are *microfilaments*, *intermediate filaments*, and *microtubules*. None of these is membrane covered.

Microfilaments The thinnest elements of the cytoskeleton, **microfilaments** (mi″kro-fil′ah-ments), are semiflexible strands of the protein *actin* ("ray") **(Figure 3.23a)**. Each cell has its own unique arrangement of microfilaments, so no two cells are alike. However, nearly all cells have a fairly dense cross-linked network of microfilaments, called the *terminal web*, attached to

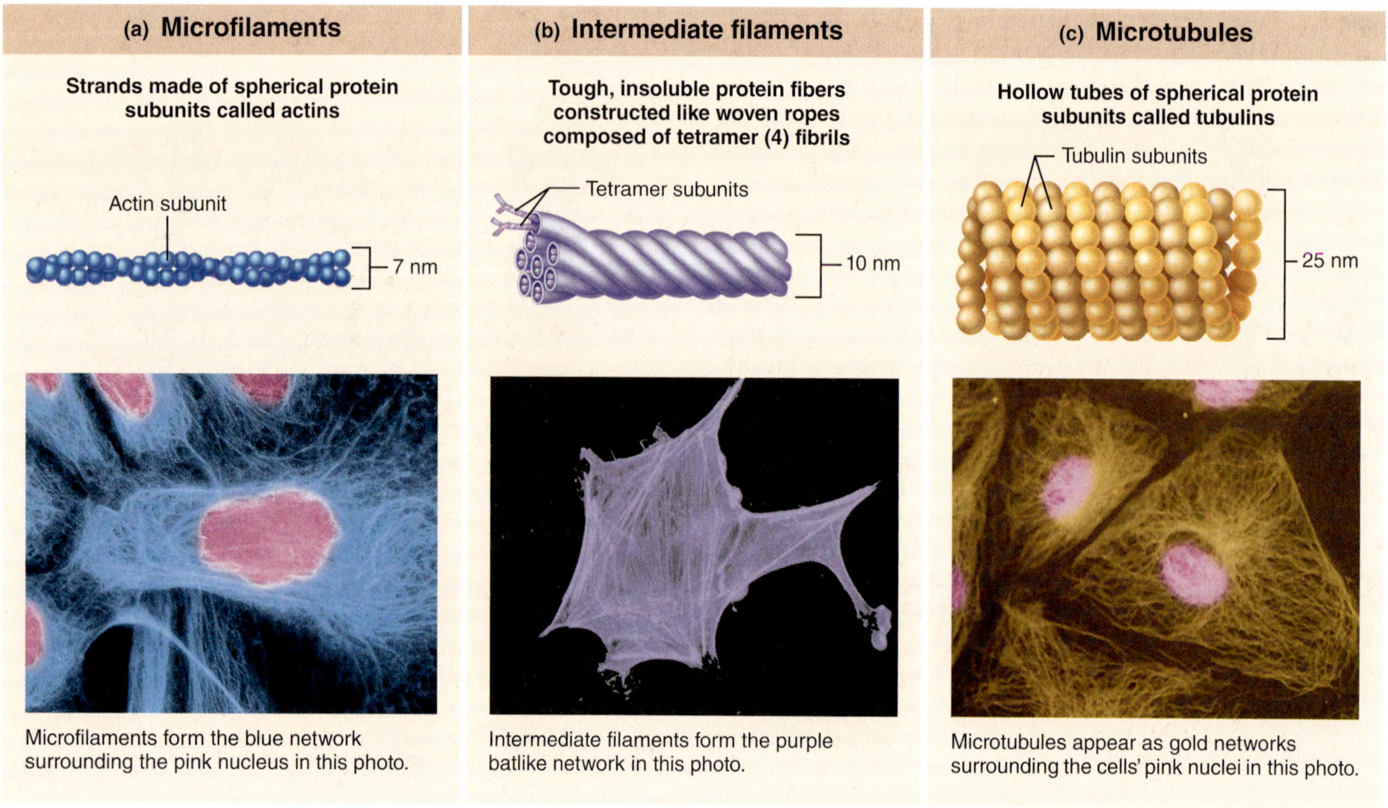

Figure 3.23 Cytoskeletal elements support the cell and help to generate movement. Diagrams (above) and photos (below). The photos are of fibroblasts treated to fluorescently tag the structure of interest.

the cytoplasmic side of their plasma membrane (see Figure 3.28 on p. 91). The web strengthens the cell surface, resists compression, and transmits force during cellular movements and shape changes.

Most microfilaments are involved in cell motility (movement) or changes in cell shape. You could say that cells move "when they get their act(in) together." For example, actin filaments interact with another protein, *unconventional myosin* (mi′o-sin), to generate contractile forces in a cell **(Figure 3.24b)**. This interaction also forms the cleavage furrow that pinches one cell into two during cell division. Microfilaments attached to cell adhesion molecules (see Figure 3.4e) are responsible for the crawling movements of amoeboid motion, and for the membrane changes that accompany endocytosis and exocytosis. Except in muscle cells, where they are highly developed, stable, and long-lived, actin filaments are constantly breaking down and re-forming from smaller subunits whenever and wherever their services are needed.

Intermediate Filaments **Intermediate filaments** are tough, insoluble protein fibers that resemble woven ropes. Made of twisted units of *tetramer* (4) *fibrils*, they have a diameter between those of microfilaments and microtubules (Figure 3.23b). Intermediate filaments are the most stable and permanent of the cytoskeletal elements and have high tensile strength. They attach to desmosomes, and their main job is to act as internal guy-wires to resist pulling forces exerted on the cell. Because the protein composition of intermediate filaments varies in different cell types, there are numerous names for these cytoskeletal elements—for example, they are called neurofilaments in nerve cells and keratin filaments in epithelial cells.

Microtubules The elements with the largest diameter, **microtubules** (mi″kro-tu′būlz), are hollow tubes made of spherical protein subunits called *tubulins* (Figure 3.23c). Most microtubules radiate from a small region of cytoplasm near the nucleus called the *centrosome* or *cell center* (see Figures 3.2, 3.25). Microtubules are remarkably dynamic organelles, constantly growing out from the centrosome, disassembling, and then reassembling at the same or different sites. The stiff but bendable microtubules determine the overall shape of the cell, as well as the distribution of cellular organelles.

Mitochondria, lysosomes, and secretory vesicles attach to the microtubules like ornaments hanging from tree branches. Tiny protein machines called **motor proteins** (*kinesins*, *dyneins*, and others) continually move and reposition the organelles along the microtubules.

Motor proteins work by changing their shapes. Powered by ATP, some motor proteins appear to act like train engines moving substances along on the microtubular "railroad tracks."

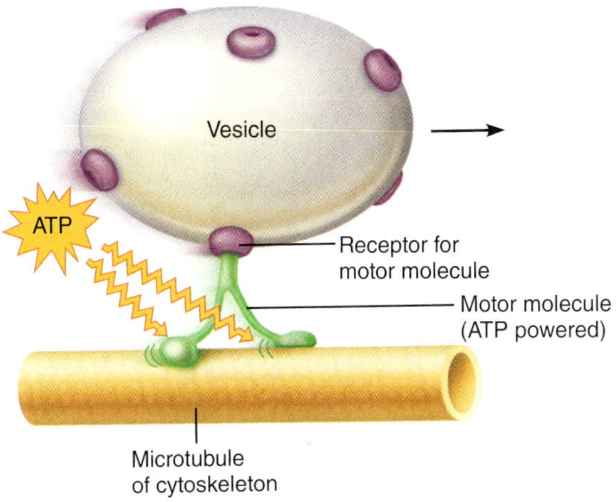

(a) Motor molecules can attach to receptors on vesicles or organelles, and carry the organelles along the microtubule "tracks" of the cytoskeleton.

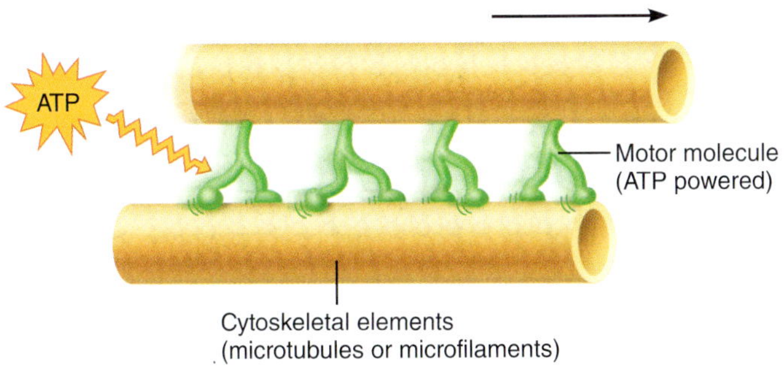

(b) In some types of cell motility, motor molecules attached to one element of the cytoskeleton can cause it to slide over another element, which the motor molecules grip, release, and grip at a new site. Muscle contraction and cilia movement work this way.

Figure 3.24 Microtubules and microfilaments function in cell motility by interacting with motor molecules powered by ATP.

Others move "hand over hand" somewhat like an orangutan—gripping, releasing, and then gripping again at a new site further along the microtubule (Figure 3.24).

Centrosome and Centrioles

✓ Describe the roles of centrioles in cell division and in formation of cilia and flagella.

As mentioned, microtubules are anchored at one end in an inconspicuous region near the nucleus called the **centrosome** or *cell center*. The centrosome acts as a *microtubule organizing center*. It has few distinguishing marks other than a granular-looking *matrix* that contains paired **centrioles**, small, barrel-shaped organelles oriented at right angles to each other **(Figure 3.25)**. The centrosome matrix is best known for generating microtubules and organizing the mitotic spindle in cell division (see Figure 3.33). Each centriole consists of a pinwheel array of nine *triplets* of microtubules, each connected to the next by nontubulin proteins and arranged to form a hollow tube. Centrioles also form the bases of cilia and flagella, our next topics.

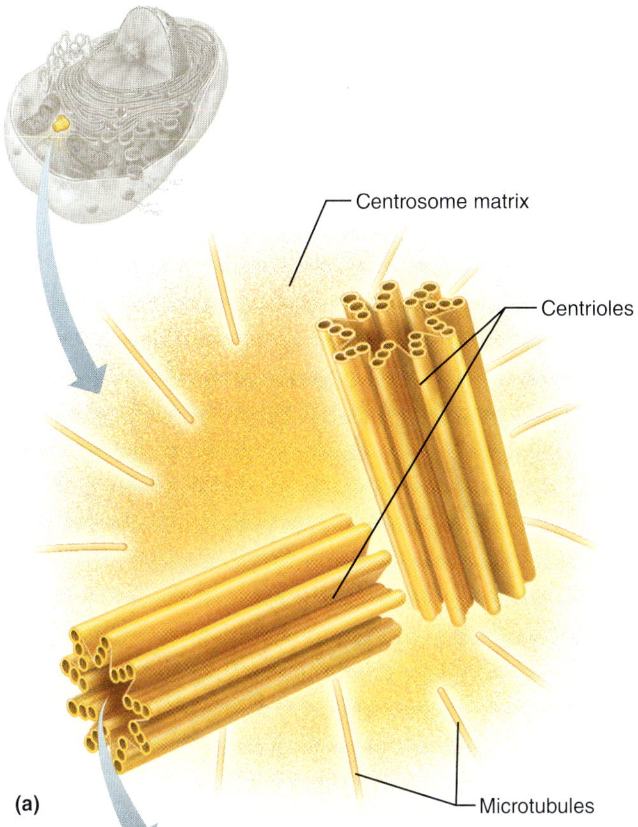

(a)

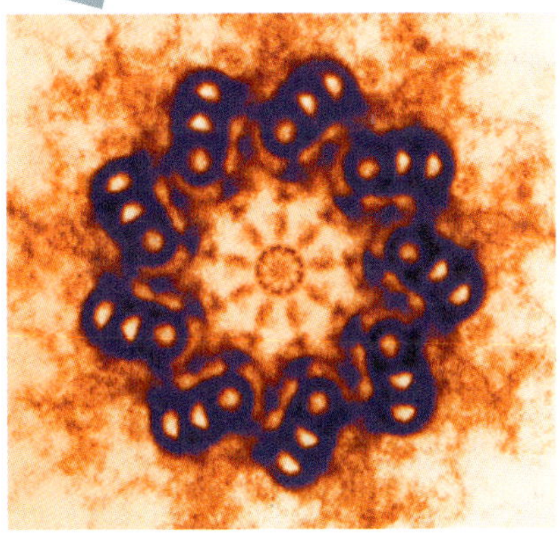

(b)

Figure 3.25 Centrioles. (a) Three-dimensional view of a centriole pair oriented at right angles, as they are usually seen in the cell. The centrioles are located in an inconspicuous region to one side of the nucleus called the centrosome, or cell center. **(b)** An electron micrograph showing a cross section of a centriole (190,000×). Notice that it is composed of nine microtubule triplets.

Cellular Extensions

✓ Describe how the two main types of cell extensions, cilia and microvilli, differ in structure and function.

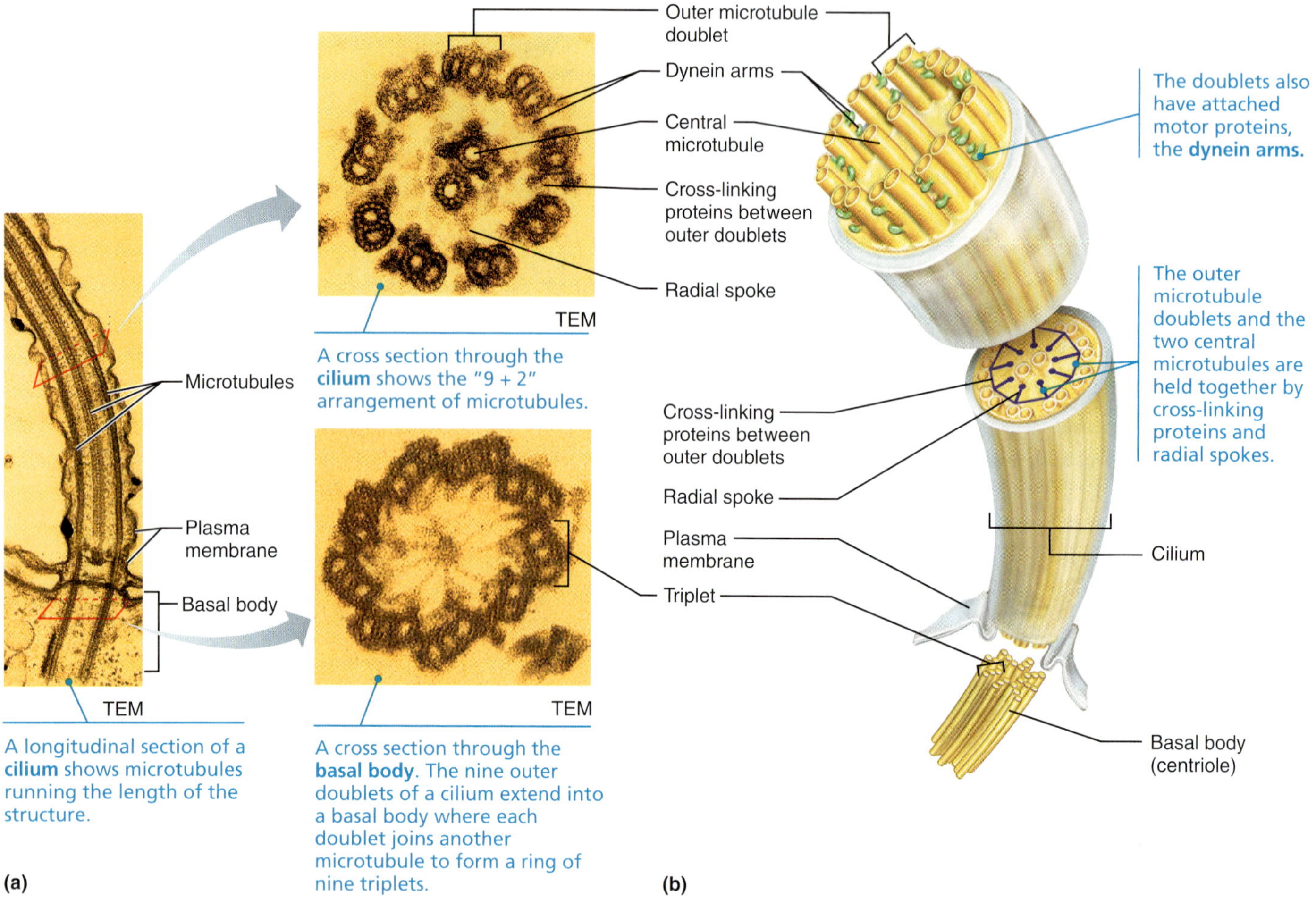

Figure 3.26 Structure of a cilium. (TEM = transmission electron micrograph.)

Cilia and Flagella

Cilia (sil′e-ah; "eyelashes") are whiplike, motile cellular extensions **(Figure 3.26)** that occur, typically in large numbers, on the exposed surfaces of certain cells. Ciliary action moves substances in one direction across cell surfaces. For example, ciliated cells that line the respiratory tract propel mucus laden with dust particles and bacteria upward away from the lungs.

When a cell is about to form cilia, the centrioles multiply and line up beneath the plasma membrane at the cell's free (exposed) surface. Microtubules then "sprout" from each centriole, forming the ciliary projections by exerting pressure on the plasma membrane.

Flagella (flah-jel′ah) are also projections formed by centrioles, but are substantially longer than cilia. The only flagellated cell in the human body is a sperm, which has one propulsive flagellum, commonly called a tail. Notice that cilia *propel other substances* across a cell's surface, whereas a flagellum *propels the cell itself.*

Centrioles forming the bases of cilia and flagella are commonly referred to as **basal bodies** (ba′sal) (Figure 3.26a). The "9 + 2" pattern of microtubules in the cilium or flagellum itself (nine *doublets*, or pairs, of microtubules encircling one central pair) differs slightly from that of a centriole (nine microtubule *triplets*). Additionally, the cilium has flexible "wagon wheels" of cross-linking proteins (purple in Figure 3.26b), and motor proteins (green dynein arms in Figure 3.26b) that promote movement of the cilium or flagellum.

Just how ciliary activity is coordinated is not fully understood, but microtubules are definitely involved. Extending from the microtubule doublets are arms composed of the motor protein dynein (Figure 3.26). The dynein side arms of one doublet grip the adjacent doublet, and powered by ATP, push it up, release, and then grip again. Because the doublets are physically restricted by other proteins, they cannot slide far and instead are forced to bend. The collective bending action of all the doublets causes the cilium to bend.

As a cilium moves, it alternates rhythmically between a propulsive *power stroke*, when it is nearly straight and moves in an arc, and a *recovery stroke*, when it bends and returns to its initial position **(Figure 3.27a)**. With these two strokes, the cilium produces a pushing motion in a single direction that repeats some 10 to 20 times per second. The bending of one cilium is quickly followed by the bending of the next and then the next, creating a current at the cell surface that brings to mind the traveling waves that pass across a field of grass on a windy day (Figure 3.27b).

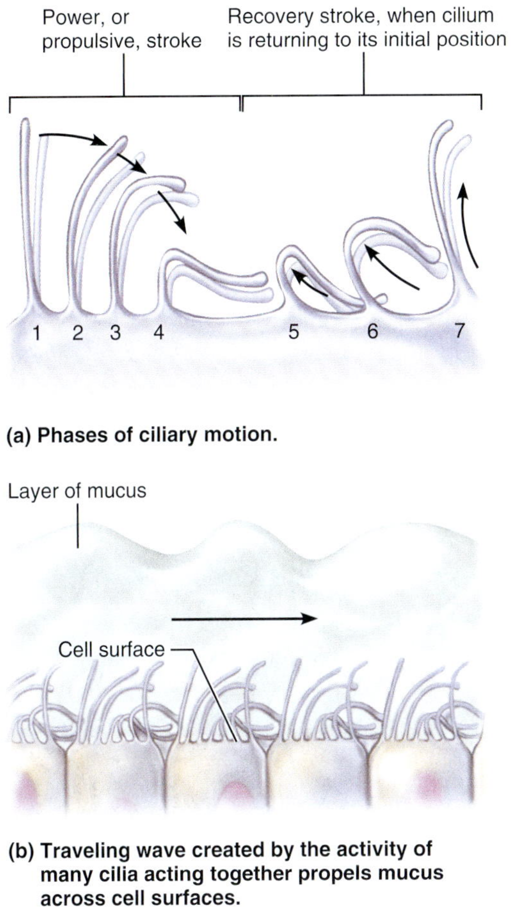

Figure 3.27 Ciliary function.

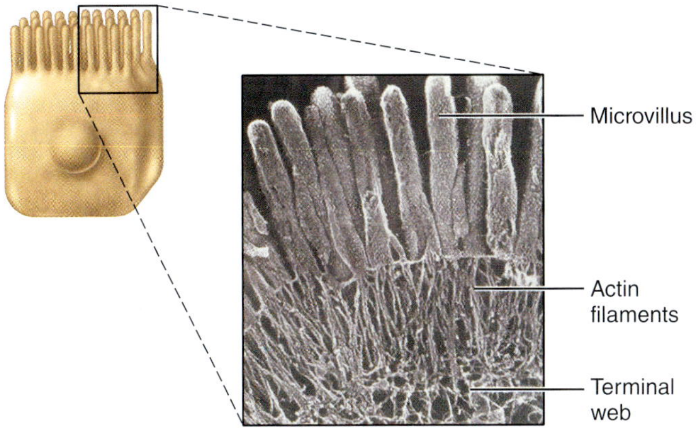

Figure 3.28 Microvilli.

The motile cilia just discussed are familiar to most biology students, but many have not heard of *primary cilia*, their nonmotile cousins. Present as a single cilium on the surface of most body cells, primary cilia function as antennae that probe the external environment for molecules their receptors can recognize. Because of this ability, primary cilia can coordinate several intracellular pathways that regulate embryonic development and maintain healthy tissues later in life.

Microvilli

Microvilli (mi″kro-vil′i; "little shaggy hairs") are minute, fingerlike extensions of the plasma membrane that project from an exposed cell surface (Figure 3.5 top and **Figure 3.28**). They increase the plasma membrane surface area tremendously and are most often found on the surface of absorptive cells such as intestinal and kidney tubule cells. Microvilli have a core of bundled actin filaments that extend into the so-called *terminal web* of the cytoskeleton of the cell. Actin is sometimes a contractile protein, but in microvilli it appears to function as a mechanical "stiffener."

☑ Check Your Understanding

20. How are microtubules and microfilaments related functionally?
21. Of microfilaments, microtubules, or intermediate filaments, which is most important in maintaining cell shape?
22. The major function of cilia is to move substances across the free cell surface. What is the major role of microvilli?

For answers, see Appendix H.

The Nucleus

✓ Outline the structure and function of the nuclear envelope, nucleolus, and chromatin.

Anything that works, works best when it is controlled. For cells, the control center is the gene-containing **nucleus** (*nucle* = pit, kernel). The nucleus can be compared to a computer, design department, construction boss, and board of directors—all rolled into one. As the genetic library, it contains the instructions needed to build nearly all the body's proteins. Additionally, it dictates the kinds and amounts of proteins to be synthesized at any one time in response to signals acting on the cell.

Most cells have only one nucleus, but some, including skeletal muscle cells, bone destruction cells, and some liver cells, are **multinucleate** (mul″tĭ-nu′kle-āt), that is, they have many nuclei. The presence of more than one nucleus usually signifies that a larger-than-usual cytoplasmic mass must be regulated.

Except for mature red blood cells, whose nuclei are ejected before the cells enter the bloodstream, all of our body cells are nucleated. **Anucleate** (a-nu′kle-āt; *a* = without) cells cannot reproduce and therefore live in the bloodstream for only three to four months before they deteriorate. Without a nucleus, a cell cannot produce mRNA to make proteins, and when its enzymes and cell structures start to break down (as all eventually do), they cannot be replaced.

The nucleus, averaging 5 μm in diameter, is larger than any of the cytoplasmic organelles. Although most often spherical or oval, its shape usually conforms to the shape of the cell. The nucleus has three recognizable regions or structures: the *nuclear envelope* (*membrane*), *nucleoli*, and *chromatin* **(Figure 3.29a)**.

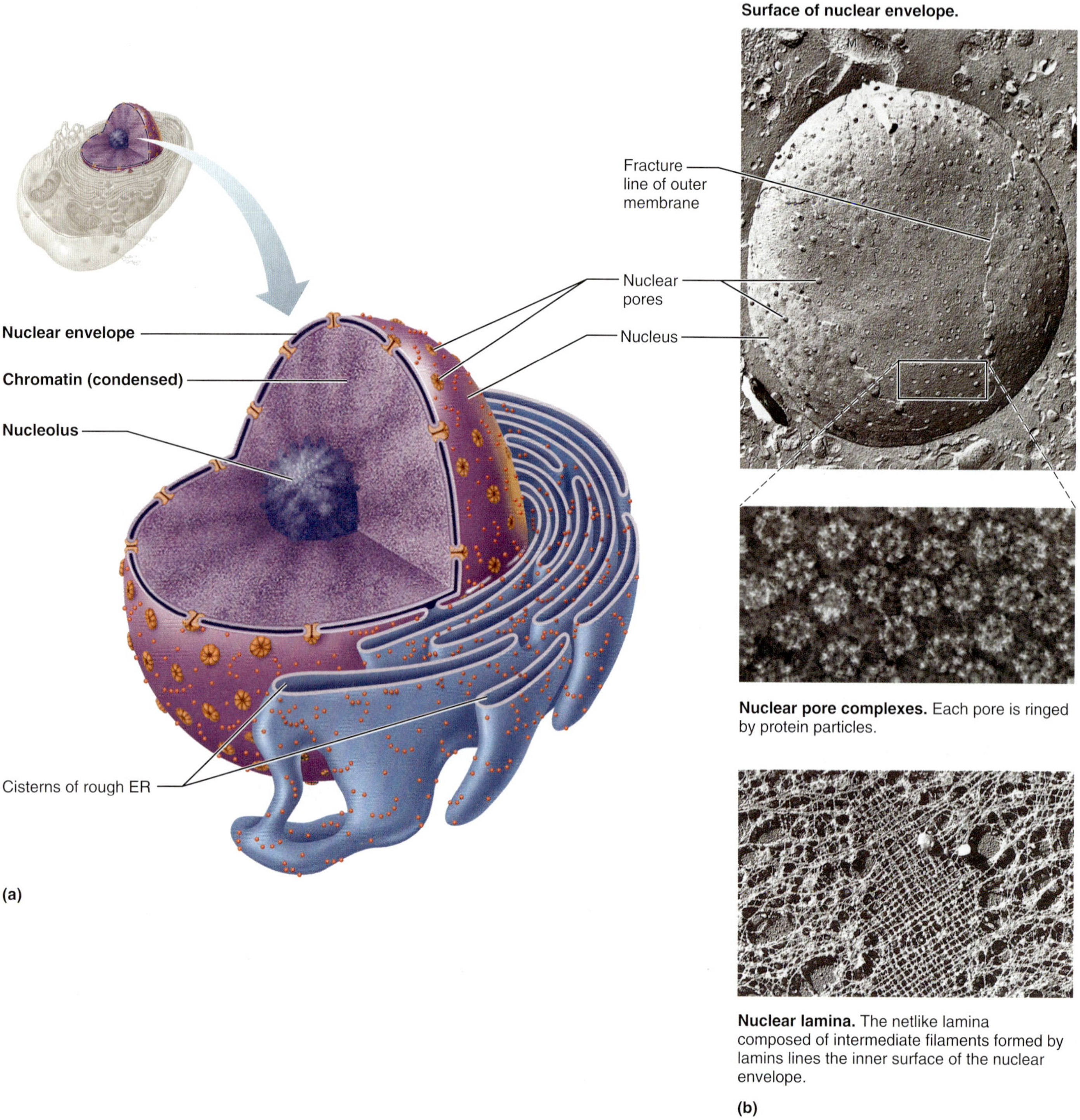

Figure 3.29 The nucleus. (a) Three-dimensional diagram of the nucleus, showing the continuity of its double membrane with the ER. **(b)** Freeze-fracture transmission electron micrographs (TEMs).

The Nuclear Envelope

The nucleus is bounded by the **nuclear envelope**, a *double* membrane barrier separated by a fluid-filled space (similar to the mitochondrial membrane). The outer nuclear membrane is continuous with the rough ER of the cytoplasm and is studded with ribosomes on its external face. The inner nuclear membrane is lined by the *nuclear lamina*, a network of *lamins* (rod-shaped proteins that assemble to form intermediate filaments) that maintains the shape of the nucleus and acts as a scaffold to organize DNA in the nucleus (Figure 3.29b, bottom).

At various points, the nuclear envelope is punctuated by **nuclear pores**. An intricate complex of proteins, called a *nuclear pore complex*, lines each pore, forming an aqueous transport channel and regulating entry and exit of molecules (e.g., mRNAs) and large particles into and out of the nucleus (Figure 3.29b, middle).

Like other cell membranes, the nuclear envelope is selectively permeable, but here substances pass much more freely than elsewhere. Small molecules pass through the relatively large nuclear pore complexes unhindered. Protein molecules imported from the cytoplasm and RNA molecules exported from the nucleus are transported through the central channel of the pores in an energy-dependent process by soluble transport proteins (importins and others). Such large molecules must display specific signals to enter or exit the nucleus.

The nuclear envelope encloses a jellylike fluid called *nucleoplasm* (nu′kle-o-plazm) in which other nuclear elements are suspended. Like the cytosol, the nucleoplasm contains dissolved salts, nutrients, and other essential solutes.

Nucleoli

Nucleoli (nu-kle′o-li; "little nuclei") are the dark-staining spherical bodies found within the nucleus where ribosomal subunits are assembled. They are not membrane bounded. Typically, there are one or two nucleoli per nucleus, but there may be more. Nucleoli are usually large in growing cells that are making large amounts of tissue proteins.

Nucleoli are associated with *nucleolar organizer regions*, which contain the DNA that issues genetic instructions for synthesizing ribosomal RNA (rRNA). As molecules of rRNA are synthesized, they are combined with proteins to form the two kinds of ribosomal subunits. (The proteins are manufactured on ribosomes in the cytoplasm and "imported" into the nucleus.) Most of these subunits leave the nucleus through the nuclear pores and enter the cytoplasm, where they join to form functional ribosomes.

Chromatin

Seen through a light microscope, **chromatin** (kro′mah-tin) appears as a fine, unevenly stained network, but special techniques reveal it as a system of bumpy threads weaving through the nucleoplasm. Chromatin is composed of approximately

- 30% **DNA**, our genetic material
- 60% globular **histone proteins** (his′tōn), which package and regulate the DNA
- 10% RNA chains, newly formed or forming

The fundamental units of chromatin are **nucleosomes** (nu′kle-o-sōmz; "nuclear bodies"), which consist of flattened disc-shaped cores or clusters of eight histone proteins connected like beads on a string by a DNA molecule. The DNA winds (like a ribbon of Velcro) twice around each nucleosome and continues on to the next cluster via *linker* DNA segments (**Figure 3.30** ① and ②).

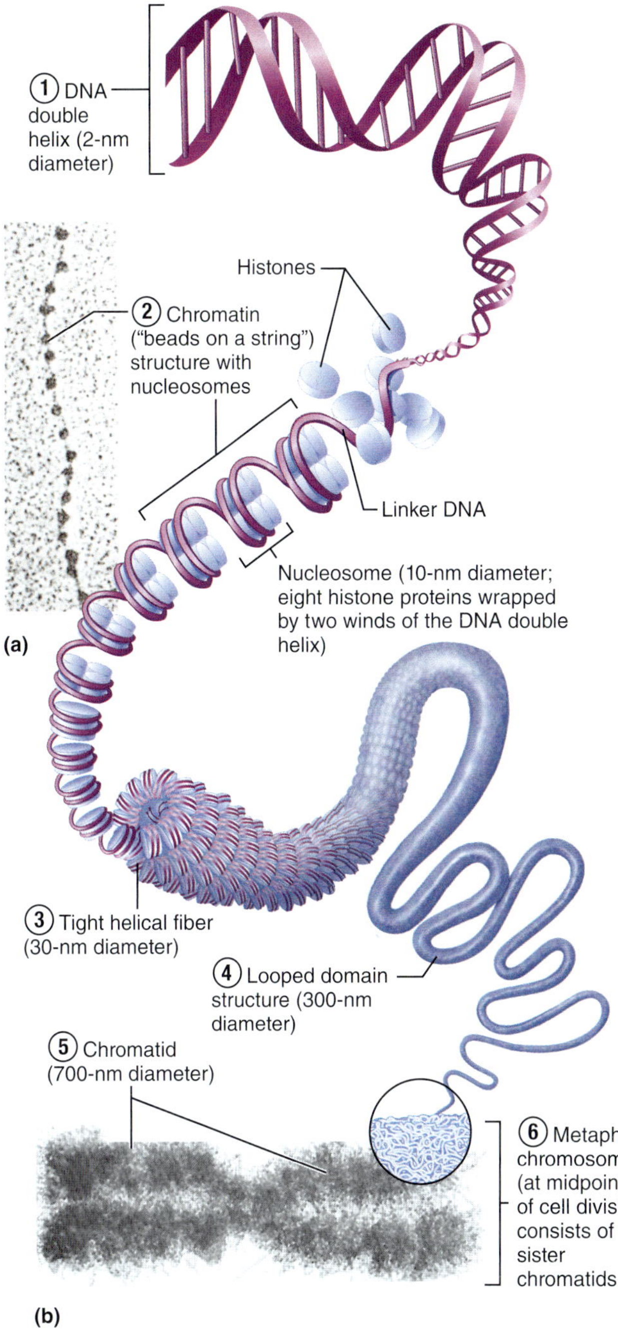

Figure 3.30 Chromatin and chromosome structure. **(a)** Electron micrograph of chromatin fiber (125,000×). **(b)** DNA packed in a chromosome. The levels of increasing structural complexity (coiling) from the DNA helix to the metaphase chromosome are indicated in order from the smallest (① DNA double helix) to the largest and most complex (⑥ chromosome).

Histones provide a physical means for packing the very long DNA molecules (some 2 meters' worth per cell) in a compact, orderly way, but they also play an important role in gene regulation. In a nondividing cell, for example, the presence of methyl groups on histone proteins shuts down the nearby DNA, and attachment of a phosphate group to a particular histone protein

(Text continues on p. 96)

Table 3.3 Parts of the Cell: Structure and Function

CELL PART*	STRUCTURE	FUNCTIONS
Plasma Membrane (Figure 3.3)		
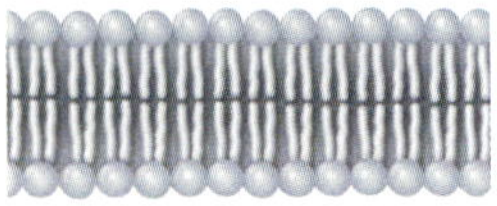	Membrane made of a double layer of lipids (phospholipids, cholesterol, and so on) within which proteins are embedded. Proteins may extend entirely through the lipid bilayer or protrude on only one face. Most externally facing proteins and some lipids have attached sugar groups.	Serves as an external cell barrier, and acts in transport of substances into or out of the cell. Maintains a resting potential that is essential for functioning of excitable cells. Externally facing proteins act as receptors (for hormones, neurotransmitters, and so on), transport proteins, and in cell-to-cell recognition.
Cytoplasm		
	Cellular region between the nuclear and plasma membranes. Consists of fluid **cytosol** containing dissolved solutes, **organelles** (the metabolic machinery of the cytoplasm), and **inclusions** (stored nutrients, secretory products, pigment granules).	
Organelles		
▪ Mitochondria (Figure 3.17) 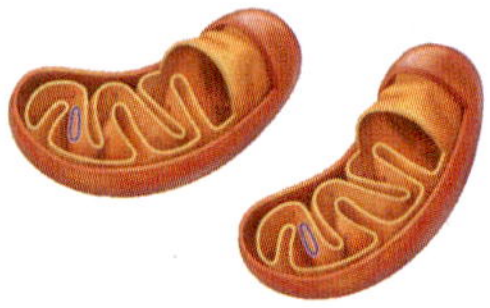	Rodlike, double-membrane structures; inner membrane folded into projections called cristae.	Site of ATP synthesis; powerhouse of the cell.
▪ Ribosomes (Figures 3.18, 3.37–3.39) 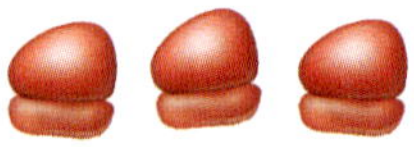	Dense particles consisting of two subunits, each composed of ribosomal RNA and protein. Free or attached to rough endoplasmic reticulum.	The sites of protein synthesis.
▪ Rough endoplasmic reticulum (Figures 3.18, 3.39) 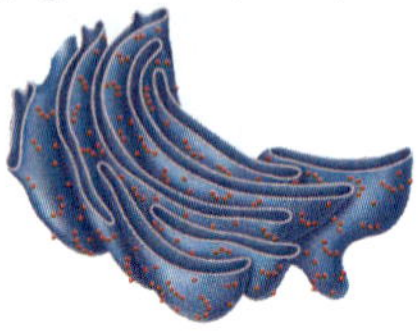	Membranous system enclosing a cavity, the cistern, and coiling through the cytoplasm. Externally studded with ribosomes.	Sugar groups are attached to proteins within the cisterns. Proteins are bound in vesicles for transport to the Golgi apparatus and other sites. External face synthesizes phospholipids.
▪ Smooth endoplasmic reticulum (Figure 3.18) 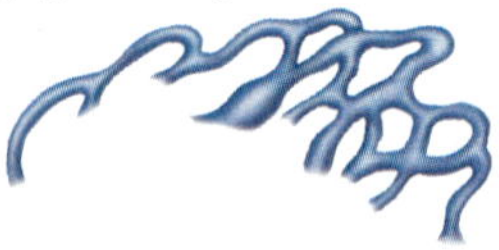	Membranous system of sacs and tubules; free of ribosomes.	Site of lipid and steroid (cholesterol) synthesis, lipid metabolism, and drug detoxification.
▪ Golgi apparatus (Figures 3.19, 3.20) 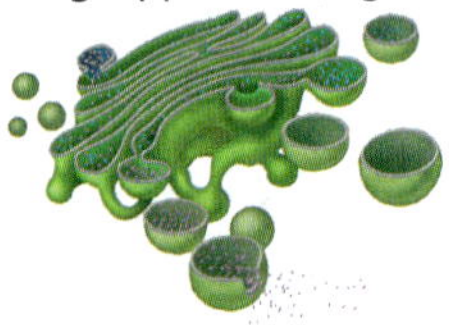	A stack of flattened membranes and associated vesicles close to the nucleus.	Packages, modifies, and segregates proteins for secretion from the cell, inclusion in lysosomes, and incorporation into the plasma membrane.
▪ Peroxisomes (Figure 3.2) 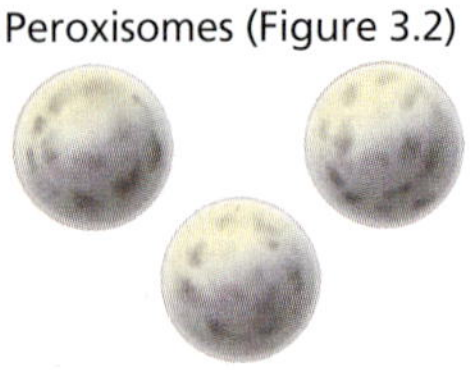	Membranous sacs of catalase and oxidase enzymes.	The enzymes detoxify a number of toxic substances. The most important enzyme, catalase, breaks down hydrogen peroxide.

* Individual cellular structures are not drawn to scale.

Table 3.3 *(continued)*

CELL PART*	STRUCTURE	FUNCTIONS
Cytoplasm		
▪ Lysosomes (Figure 3.21) 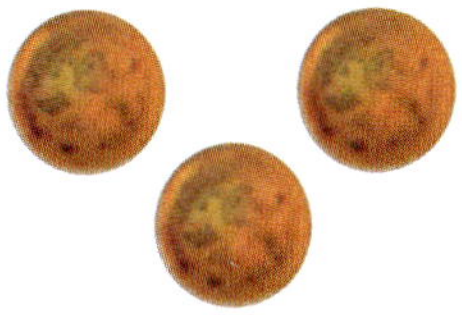	Membranous sacs containing acid hydrolases.	Sites of intracellular digestion.
▪ Microtubules (Figures 3.23–3.25) 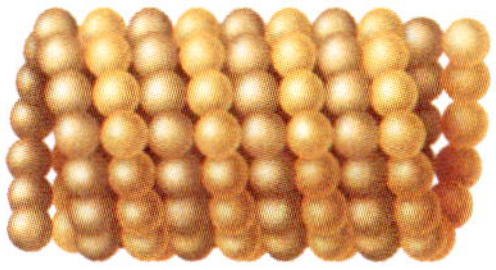	Cylindrical structures made of tubulin proteins.	Support the cell and give it shape. Involved in intracellular and cellular movements. Form centrioles and cilia and flagella, if present.
▪ Microfilaments (Figures 3.23, 3.24) 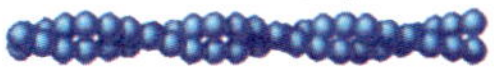	Fine filaments composed of the protein actin.	Involved in muscle contraction and other types of intracellular movement, help form the cell's cytoskeleton.
▪ Intermediate filaments (Figure 3.23) 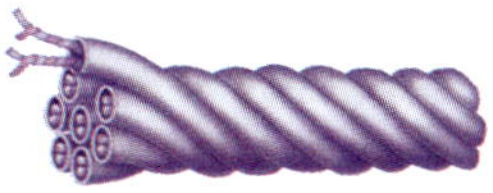	Protein fibers; composition varies.	The stable cytoskeletal elements; resist mechanical forces acting on the cell.
▪ Centrioles (Figure 3.25) 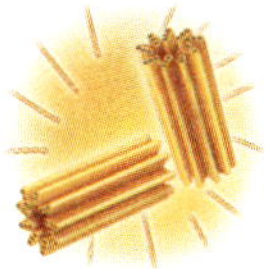	Paired cylindrical bodies, each composed of nine triplets of microtubules.	Organize a microtubule network during mitosis (cell division) to form the spindle and asters. Form the bases of cilia and flagella.
Inclusions	Varied; includes stored nutrients such as lipid droplets and glycogen granules, protein crystals, pigment granules.	Storage for nutrients, wastes, and cell products.
Cellular Extensions		
▪ Cilia (Figures 3.26, 3.27) 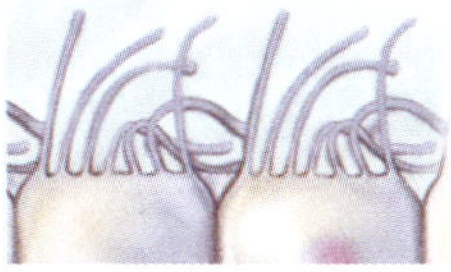	Short cell-surface projections; each cilium composed of nine pairs of microtubules surrounding a central pair.	Coordinated movement creates a unidirectional current that propels substances across cell surfaces.
▪ Flagellum 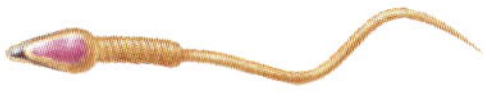	Like a cilium, but longer; only example in humans is the sperm tail.	Propels the cell.
▪ Microvilli (Figure 3.28) 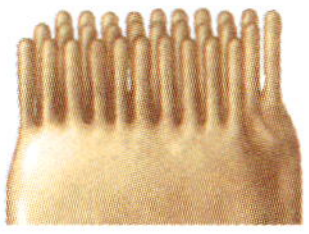	Tubular extensions of the plasma membrane; contain a bundle of actin filaments.	Increase surface area for absorption.
Nucleus (Figures 3.2, 3.29)		
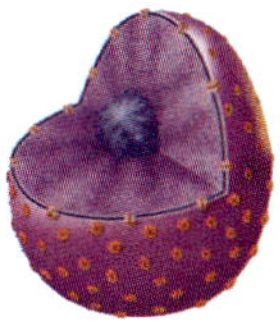	Largest organelle. Surrounded by the nuclear envelope; contains fluid nucleoplasm, nucleoli, and chromatin.	Control center of the cell; responsible for transmitting genetic information and providing the instructions for protein synthesis.

Table 3.3 Parts of the Cell: Structure and Function *(continued)*

CELL PART*	STRUCTURE	FUNCTIONS
Nucleus (Figures 3.2, 3.29)		
▪ Nuclear envelope (Figure 3.29) 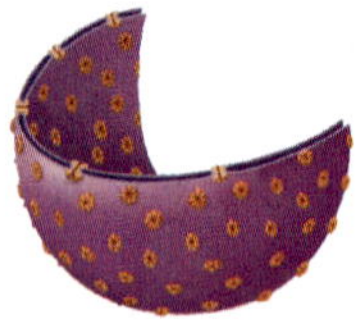	Double-membrane structure pierced by pores. Outer membrane continuous with the endoplasmic reticulum.	Separates the nucleoplasm from the cytoplasm and regulates passage of substances to and from the nucleus.
▪ Nucleolus (Figure 3.29) 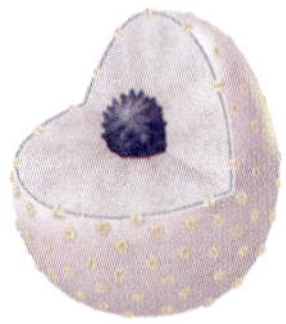	Dense spherical (non-membrane-bounded) bodies, composed of ribosomal RNA and proteins.	Site of ribosome subunit manufacture.
▪ Chromatin (Figure 3.30) 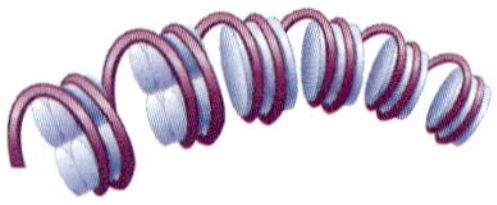	Granular, threadlike material composed of DNA and histone proteins.	DNA constitutes the genes.

may indicate that the cell is about to commit suicide. On the other hand, addition of acetyl groups to histone exposes different DNA segments, or genes, so that they can dictate the specifications for synthesizing proteins or various RNA species. Such active chromatin segments, referred to as *extended chromatin*, are not usually visible under the light microscope. The generally inactive *condensed chromatin* segments are darker staining and more easily detected. Understandably, the most active body cells have much larger amounts of extended chromatin.

Interestingly, particular chromatin strands occupy discrete regions in the nucleus called *chromosome territories*. Depending on the specific genes contained, and the cell and tissue type, the chromosome territory patterns change during development. At the simplest level, active and inactive genetic regions can be separated from each other, which in turn would enhance or repress genetic expression.

When a cell is preparing to divide, the chromatin threads coil and condense enormously to form short, barlike bodies called **chromosomes** ("colored bodies") (Figure 3.30 (5) and (6)). Chromosome compactness prevents the delicate chromatin strands from tangling and breaking during the movements that occur during cell division. Next, we describe the functions of DNA and the events of cell division.

Table 3.3 summarizes the parts of the cell beginning on p. 94.

Check Your Understanding

23. If a cell ejects or loses its nucleus, what is its fate and why?
24. What is the role of nucleoli?
25. What is the importance of the histone proteins present in the nucleus?

For answers, see Appendix H.

Cell Growth and Reproduction

The Cell Cycle

✓ List the phases of the cell cycle and describe the key events of each phase.

✓ Describe the process of DNA replication.

The **cell cycle** is the series of changes a cell goes through from the time it is formed until it reproduces. The outer ring of Figure 3.31 shows the two major periods of the cell cycle:

- *Interphase* (in green), in which the cell grows and carries on its usual activities
- *Cell division* or the *mitotic phase* (in yellow), during which it divides into two cells

Interphase

Interphase is the period from cell formation to cell division. Early cytologists, unaware of the constant molecular activity in cells and impressed by the obvious movements of cell division, called interphase the resting phase of the cell cycle. (The term *interphase* reflects this idea of a stage *between* cell divisions.) However, this image is misleading because during interphase a cell is carrying out all its routine activities and is "resting" only from dividing. Perhaps a more accurate name for this phase would be *metabolic phase* or *growth phase*.

Subphases In addition to carrying on its life-sustaining reactions, an interphase cell prepares for the next cell division. Interphase is divided into G_1, S, and G_2 subphases (the Gs stand for *gaps* before and after the S phase, and S is for *synthetic*). In all three subphases, the cell grows by producing proteins and organelles, but chromatin is reproduced only during the S subphase.

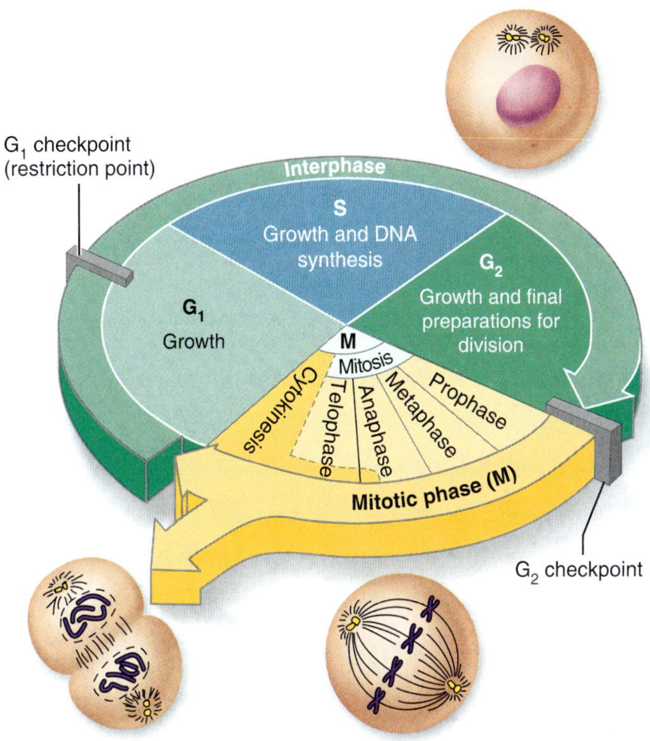

Figure 3.31 The cell cycle. During G_1, cells grow rapidly and carry out their routine functions. The S phase is the period of DNA synthesis. In G_2, materials needed for cell division are synthesized and growth continues. During the M phase (cell division), mitosis and cytokinesis occur, producing two daughter cells. Important checkpoints at which mitosis may be prevented from occurring are found throughout interphase; the diagram shows two.

- **G_1 (gap 1 subphase):** The cell is metabolically active, synthesizing proteins rapidly and growing vigorously (Figure 3.31, light green area). This is the most variable phase in terms of length. In cells that divide rapidly, G_1 typically lasts several minutes to hours, but in those that divide slowly, G_1 may last for days or even years. Cells that permanently cease dividing are said to be in the **G_0 phase**. For most of G_1, virtually no activities directly related to cell division occur. However, as G_1 ends, the centrioles start to replicate in preparation for cell division.
- **S phase:** DNA is replicated, ensuring that the two future cells being created will receive identical copies of the genetic material (Figure 3.31, blue area). New histones are made and assembled into chromatin. One thing is sure, without a proper S phase, there can be no correct mitotic phase. (We will describe DNA replication next.)
- **G_2 (gap 2 subphase):** The final phase of interphase is brief (Figure 3.31, dark green area). Enzymes and other proteins needed for division are synthesized and moved to their proper sites. By the end of G_2, centriole replication (begun in G_1) is complete. The cell is now ready to divide. Throughout S and G_2, the cell continues to grow and carries on with business as usual.

DNA Replication Before a cell can divide, its DNA must be replicated exactly, so that identical copies of the cell's genes can be passed to each of its offspring. During the S phase, replication begins simultaneously on several chromatin threads and continues until all the DNA has been replicated.

Human DNA molecules are very long. Replication of a DNA molecule begins at several *origins of replication* along its length that have a specific nucleotide sequence, a strategy that greatly increases the speed of replication.

Replication is still being studied but appears to involve several events:

1. Enzymes attach to origins of replication and separate the DNA strands so that *replication bubbles* form. At each end of a replication bubble is a Y-shaped area, a *replication fork*, where the helical parental DNA strands are being unwound **(Figure 3.32)**.
2. Once the bubbles are formed, the parental DNA strands are ready to serve as templates for making complementary DNA strands from free DNA precursors dissolved in the nucleoplasm (Figure 3.32). However, there is a problem here because the *polymerase enzymes* that synthesize DNA cannot start a new DNA strand from scratch. They can only add new nucleotides to a strand that already exists. This problem is solved by formation of a short, complementary **RNA primer**, about 10 bases long, by a *primase enzyme*.
3. Continuing from the primer, the enzyme **DNA polymerase** positions complementary nucleotides along the template strand and then covalently links them together. DNA polymerase works only in one direction. Consequently, one strand, the **leading strand**, is synthesized continuously once primed, following the movement of the replication fork. The other strand, called the **lagging strand**, is constructed in segments in the opposite direction and requires that a primer initiate replication of each segment.
4. Ligase enzymes splice the short segments of DNA together. Eventually DNA polymerases replace the primers with DNA nucleotides.

The end result is that two DNA molecules are formed from the original DNA helix (the template strands) and are identical to it. Because each new molecule consists of one old and one new nucleotide strand, this mechanism of DNA replication is called **semiconservative replication** (Figure 3.32).

As soon as replication ends, histones (synthesized in the cytoplasm and imported into the nucleus) associate with the DNA, completing the formation of two new chromatin strands. The chromatin strands, united by a buttonlike centromere (a stretch of repetitive DNA), remain held together by the centromere and a protein complex called *cohesin*, until the cell enters the anaphase stage of mitotic cell division (see p. 101). They are then distributed to the daughter cells as described next, ensuring that each cell has identical genetic information.

The progression from DNA replication into cell division presumes that the newly synthesized DNA is not damaged in any way. If damage occurs, the cell cycle stops until the DNA repair mechanism has fixed the problem.

3

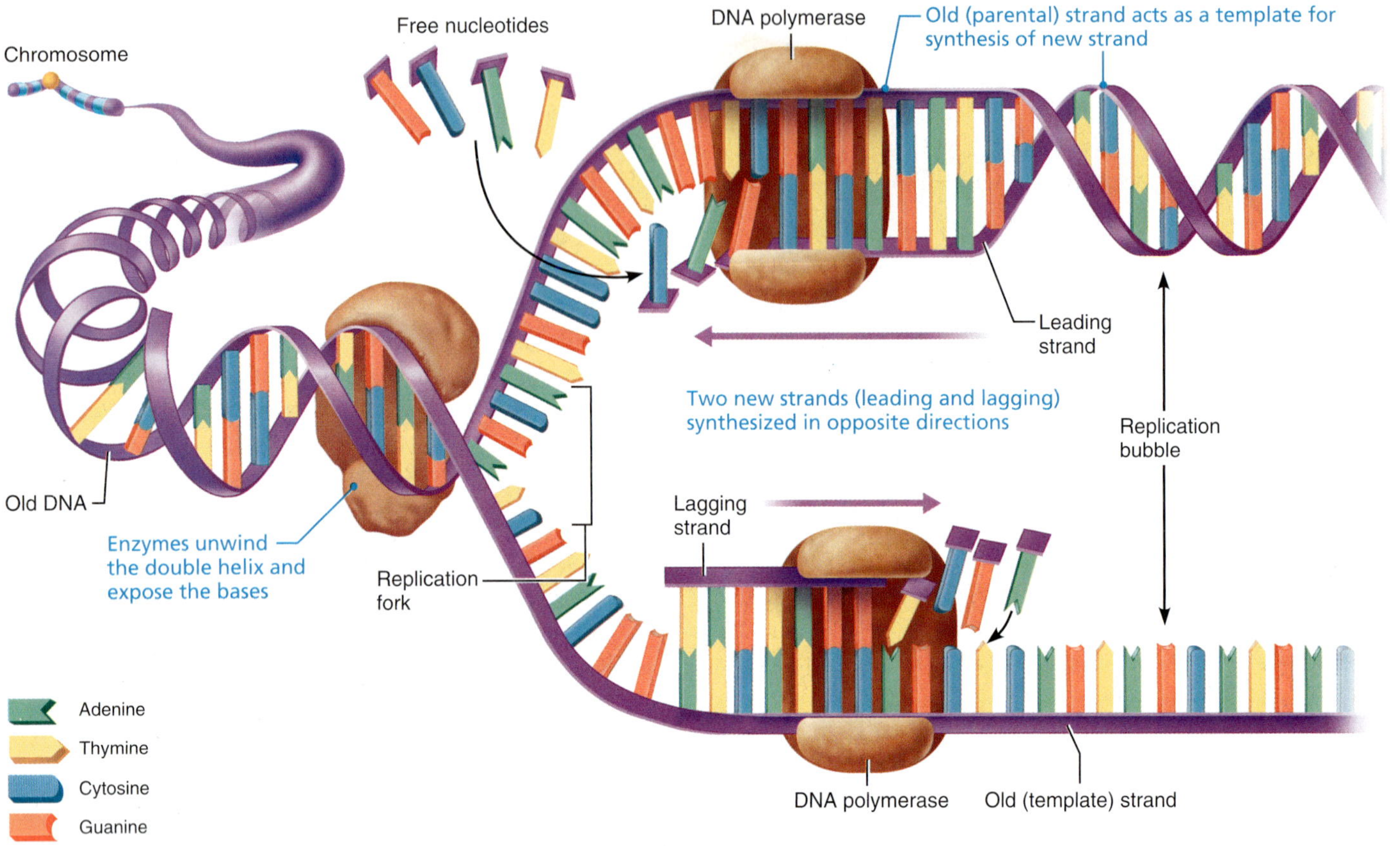

Figure 3.32 Replication of DNA: summary. Once the DNA helix is uncoiled, and the hydrogen bonds between its base pairs are broken, each nucleotide strand of the DNA acts as a template for constructing a complementary strand, as illustrated on the right-hand side of the diagram. (The step in which RNA primers are formed to start the process at replication bubbles is not shown.) DNA polymerases work in one direction only, so the two new strands (leading and lagging) are synthesized in opposite directions. (The DNA ligase enzymes that join the DNA fragments on the lagging strand are not illustrated.) Each DNA molecule formed consists of one old (template) strand and one newly assembled strand and constitutes a chromatid of a chromosome.

Cell Division

Cell division is essential for body growth and tissue repair. Cells that continually wear away, such as cells of the skin and intestinal lining, reproduce themselves almost continuously. Others, such as liver cells, divide more slowly (to maintain the size of the organ they compose) but retain the ability to reproduce quickly if the organ is damaged. Most cells of nervous tissue, skeletal muscle, and heart muscle lose their ability to divide when they are fully mature, and repairs are made with scar tissue (a fibrous type of connective tissue).

Events of Cell Division In most body cells, cell division, which is called the **M (mitotic) phase** of the cell cycle, involves two distinct events (Figure 3.31, yellow area):

- **Mitosis** (mi-to′sis; *mit* = thread; *osis* = process), the division of the nucleus
- **Cytokinesis** (si-to-kĭ-ne′sis; *kines* = movement), the division of the cytoplasm

A different process of nuclear division called *meiosis* (mi-o′sis) produces sex cells (ova and sperm) with only half the number of genes found in other body cells. We discuss the details of meiosis in Chapter 27. Here we concentrate on mitotic cell division.

Mitosis Mitosis is the series of events that parcels out the replicated DNA of the mother cell to two daughter cells. Described as four phases—**prophase**, **metaphase**, **anaphase**, and **telophase**—mitosis is actually a continuous process, with one phase merging smoothly into the next. Its duration varies according to cell type, but in human cells it typically lasts about an hour or less. *Focus on Mitosis* **(Figure 3.33)**, pp. 100–101, describes the phases of mitosis in detail.

Cytokinesis Cytokinesis, or the division of the cytoplasm, begins during late anaphase and is completed after mitosis ends. A *contractile ring* made of actin filaments (Figure 3.33) draws the plasma membrane inward to form a **cleavage furrow** over the center of the cell. The furrow deepens until it pinches the cytoplasmic mass into two parts, yielding two daughter cells. Each is smaller and has less cytoplasm than the mother cell, but is genetically identical to it. The daughter cells then enter the interphase portion of the life cycle until it is their turn to divide.

Control of Cell Division The signals that prod cells to divide are incompletely understood, but we know that the ratio of cell surface area to cell volume is important. The amount of nutrients a growing cell requires is directly related to its volume. Volume increases with the cube of cell radius, whereas surface area increases more slowly with the square of the radius.

For example, a 64-fold (4^3) increase in cell volume is accompanied by only a 16-fold (4^2) increase in surface area. Consequently, the surface area of the plasma membrane becomes inadequate for nutrient and waste exchange when a cell reaches a certain critical size. Cell division solves this problem because the smaller daughter cells have a favorable ratio of surface area to volume. These surface-volume relationships help explain why most cells are microscopic in size.

Two other factors that influence when cells divide are chemical signals (growth factors, hormones, and others) released by other cells and the availability of space. Normal cells stop proliferating when they begin touching, a phenomenon called *contact inhibition*. The system that controls the cell cycle has been compared to the timer on a washing machine. Like that timer, the control system for the cell cycle is driven by a built-in clock. However, just as the washer's cycle is subject to adjustments (by regulating the flow from the faucet, say, or by an internal water-level sensor), the cell cycle is regulated by both internal and external factors.

Two groups of proteins are crucial to the ability of a cell to accomplish the S phase and enter mitosis:

- **Cyclins**, regulatory proteins whose levels rise and fall during each cell cycle
- **Cdks (cyclin-dependent kinases)**, which are present in a constant concentration in the cell and are activated by binding to particular cyclins

A new batch of cyclins accumulates during each interphase. Subsequent joining of specific Cdk and cyclin proteins initiates enzymatic cascades that phosphorylate histones and other proteins needed for cell division. At the end of mitosis, enzymes destroy the cyclins.

A number of "switches" and crucial checkpoints for cell division occur throughout interphase. These built-in stop signals halt the cell cycle until overridden by internal or external go-ahead signals. In many cells, a G_1 checkpoint, called the *restriction point*, seems to be most important (see Figure 3.31). If the cell is prevented from progressing past this checkpoint, it enters the nondividing state (G_0). Another important checkpoint, and the first to be understood, occurs late in G_2, when a threshold amount of a protein complex called **MPF (M-phase promoting factor)** is required to give the okay signal to pass the G_2 checkpoint and enter M phase. Later in M phase, MPF is inactivated.

Besides these "go" signals, there are a number of so-called repressor genes that inhibit cell division. One example is the *p53* gene that initiates a series of enzymatic events that produce growth-inhibiting factors. Roughly half of all cancers have abnormal *p53* genes. Contact with other cells does not inhibit these cancerous cells and they divide wildly, making them dangerous to their host.

☑ Check Your Understanding

26. If one of the DNA strands being replicated "reads" CGAATG, what will be the base sequence of the corresponding DNA strand?
27. During what phase of the cell cycle is DNA synthesized?
28. What are three events occurring in prophase that are undone in telophase?

For answers, see Appendix H.

3

Protein Synthesis

✓ Define gene and genetic code and explain the function of genes.

✓ Name the two phases of protein synthesis and describe the roles of DNA, mRNA, tRNA, and rRNA in each phase.

✓ Contrast triplets, codons, and anticodons.

In addition to directing its own replication, DNA serves as the master blueprint for protein synthesis. Although cells also make lipids and carbohydrates, DNA does not dictate their structure. Historically, DNA is said to specify *only* the structure of protein molecules, including the enzymes that catalyze the synthesis of all classes of biological molecules.

Much of the metabolic machinery of the cell is concerned in some way with protein synthesis. This is not surprising, seeing as structural proteins constitute most of the dry cell material, and functional proteins direct almost all cellular activities. Essentially, cells are miniature protein factories that synthesize the huge variety of proteins that determine the chemical and physical nature of cells—and therefore of the whole body.

Recall from Chapter 2 that proteins are composed of polypeptide chains, which in turn are made up of amino acids. For purposes of this discussion, we define a **gene** as a segment of a DNA molecule that carries instructions for creating one polypeptide chain. Supposedly we humans have an estimated 25,000 protein coding genes. (Note, however, that some genes specify the structure of certain varieties of RNA as their final product.)

The four nucleotide bases (A, G, T, and C) are the "letters" used in the genetic alphabet, and the information of DNA is found in the sequence of these bases. Each sequence of three bases, called a **triplet**, can be thought of as a "word" that specifies a particular amino acid. For example, the triplet AAA calls for the amino acid phenylalanine, and CCT calls for glycine. The sequence of triplets in each gene forms a "sentence" that tells exactly how a particular polypeptide is to be made: It specifies the number, kinds, and order of amino acids needed to build a particular polypeptide.

Variations in the arrangement of A, T, C, and G allow our cells to make all the different kinds of proteins needed. Even a "small" gene has an estimated 210 base pairs in sequence. The ratio between DNA bases in the gene and amino acids in the polypeptide is 3:1 (because each triplet stands for one amino acid), so we would expect the polypeptide specified by such a gene to contain 70 amino acids.

(Text continues on p. 102.)

FOCUS Mitosis

Figure 3.33 Mitosis is the process of nuclear division in which the chromosomes are distributed to two daughter nuclei. Together with cytokinesis, it produces two identical daughter cells. A&PFlix *Available at www.masteringaandp.com*

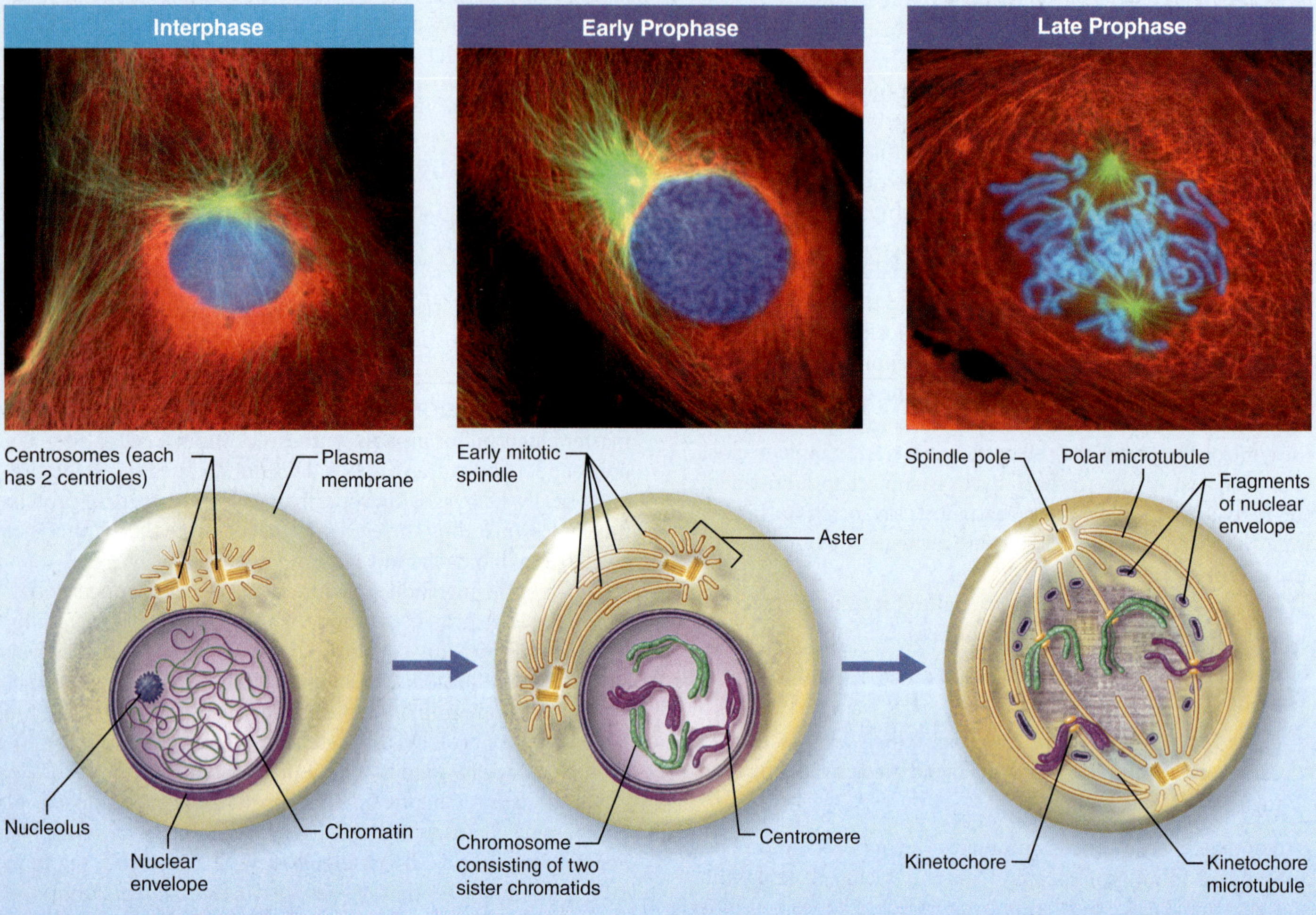

Interphase

Interphase
Interphase is the period of a cell's life when it carries out its normal metabolic activities and grows. Interphase is not part of mitosis.

- During interphase, the DNA-containing material is in the form of chromatin. The nuclear envelope and one or more nucleoli are intact and visible.
- There are three distinct periods of interphase:
  G_1: The centrioles begin replicating.
  S: DNA is replicated.
  G_2: Final preparations for mitosis are completed and centrioles finish replicating.

The light micrographs show dividing lung cells from a newt. The chromosomes appear blue and the microtubules green. (The red fibers are intermediate filaments.) The schematic drawings show details not visible in the micrographs. For simplicity, only four chromosomes are drawn.

Prophase—first phase of mitosis

Early Prophase

- The chromatin condenses, forming barlike *chromosomes*.
- Each duplicated chromosome consists of two identical threads, called *sister chromatids*, held together at the *centromere*. (Later when the chromatids separate, each will be a new chromosome.)
- As the chromosomes appear, the nucleoli disappear, and the two centrosomes separate from one another.
- The centrosomes act as focal points for growth of a microtubule assembly called the *mitotic spindle*. As the microtubules lengthen, they propel the centrosomes toward opposite ends (poles) of the cell.
- Microtubule arrays called *asters* ("stars") extend from the centrosome matrix.

Late Prophase

- The nuclear envelope breaks up, allowing the spindle to interact with the chromosomes.
- Some of the growing spindle microtubules attach to *kinetochores* (ki-ne´ to-korz), special protein structures at each chromosome's centromere. Such microtubules are called *kinetochore microtubules*.
- The remaining spindle microtubules (not attached to any chromosomes) are called *polar microtubules*. The microtubules slide past each other, forcing the poles apart.
- The kinetochore microtubules pull on each chromosome from both poles in a tug-of-war that ultimately draws the chromosomes to the center, or equator, of the cell.

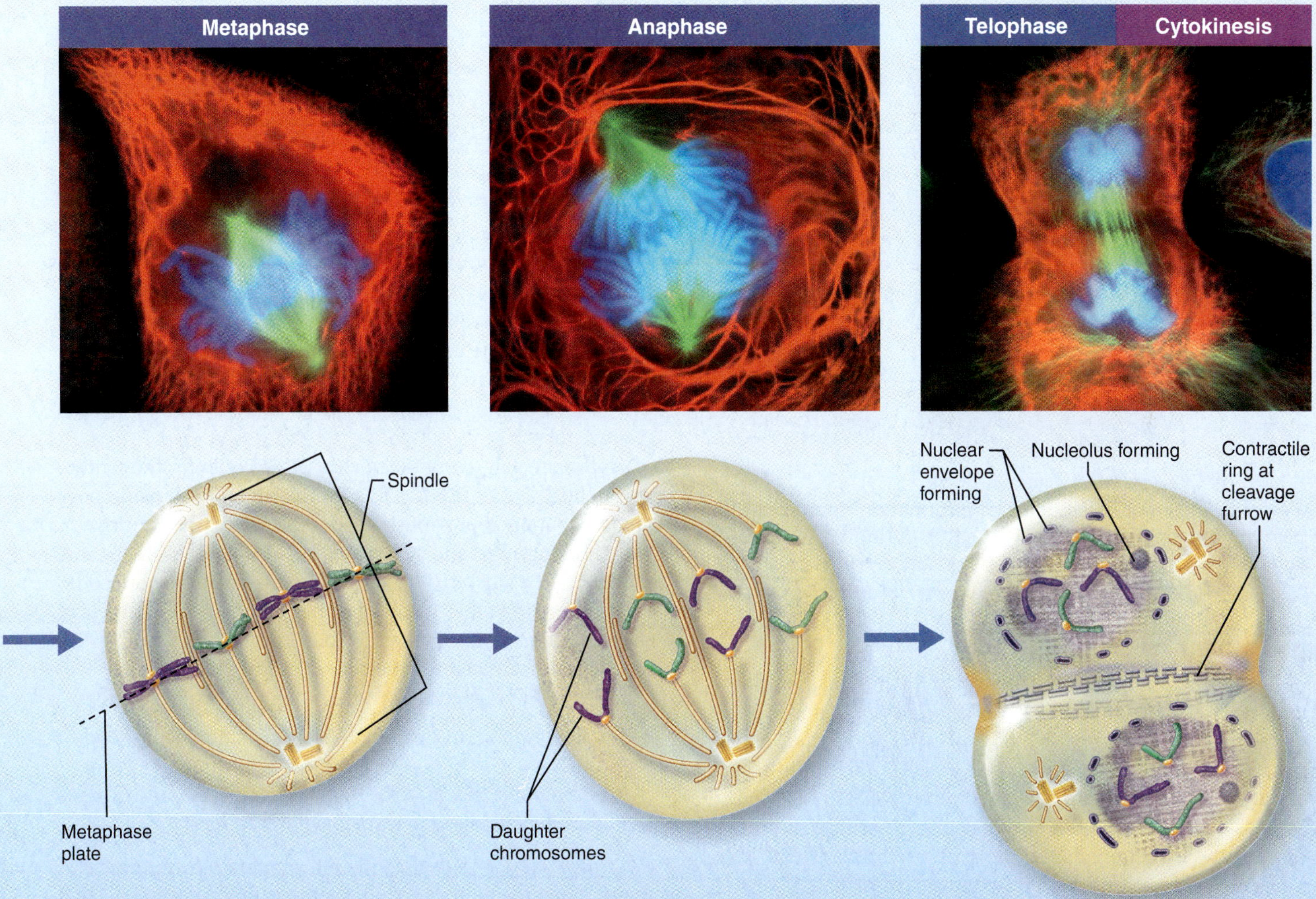

Metaphase—second phase of mitosis

- The two centrosomes are at opposite poles of the cell.
- The chromosomes cluster at the midline of the cell, with their centromeres precisely aligned at the *equator* of the spindle. This imaginary plane midway between the poles is called the *metaphase plate*.
- Enzymes act to separate the chromatids from each other.

Anaphase—third phase of mitosis

The shortest phase of mitosis, anaphase begins abruptly as the centromeres of the chromosomes split simultaneously. Each chromatid now becomes a chromosome in its own right.

- The kinetochore microtubules, moved along by motor proteins in the kinetochores, gradually pull each chromosome toward the pole it faces.
- At the same time, the polar microtubules slide past each other, lengthen, and push the two poles of the cell apart.
- The moving chromosomes look V shaped. The centromeres lead the way, and the chromosomal "arms" dangle behind them.
- Moving and separating the chromosomes is helped by the fact that the chromosomes are short, compact bodies. Diffuse threads of chromatin would trail, tangle, and break, resulting in imprecise "parceling out" to the daughter cells.

Telophase—final phase of mitosis

Telophase

Telophase begins as soon as chromosomal movement stops. This final phase is like prophase in reverse.

- The identical sets of chromosomes at the opposite poles of the cell uncoil and resume their threadlike chromatin form.
- A new nuclear envelope forms around each chromatin mass, nucleoli reappear within the nuclei, and the spindle breaks down and disappears.
- Mitosis is now ended. The cell, for just a brief period, is binucleate (has two nuclei) and each new nucleus is identical to the original mother nucleus.

Cytokinesis—division of cytoplasm

Cytokinesis begins during late anaphase and continues through and beyond telophase. A contractile ring of actin microfilaments forms the *cleavage furrow* and pinches the cell apart.

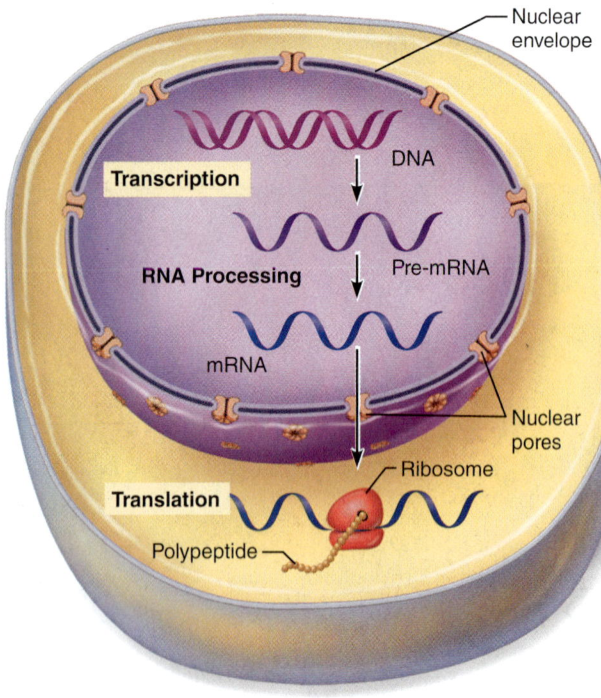

Figure 3.34 Simplified scheme of information flow from the DNA gene to mRNA to protein structure during transcription and translation. (Note that mRNA is first synthesized as pre-mRNA, which is processed by enzymes before leaving the nucleus.)

Most genes of higher organisms contain **exons**, which are amino acid–specifying informational sequences. Exons are often separated by **introns**, which are noncoding, often repetitive, segments that range from 60 to 100,000 nucleotides. Once considered a type of "junk DNA," intron DNA is believed to serve as a reservoir or scrapyard of ready-to-use DNA segments for genome evolution, as well as a rich source of small RNA molecules. The rest of the DNA (indeed, most of it) is essentially "dark matter" whose function is still a mystery. It is in these regions that *pseudogenes* (false genes) are found. Pseudogenes are genetic fossils that are the remains of damaged genes. They "look like" real genes but have deficits that render them functionless.

The Role of RNA

By itself, DNA is like a CD recording: The information it contains cannot be used without a decoding mechanism (a CD player). Furthermore, most polypeptides are manufactured at ribosomes in the cytoplasm, but in interphase cells, DNA never leaves the nucleus. So, DNA requires not only a decoder, but a messenger as well. The decoding and messenger functions are carried out by RNA, the second type of nucleic acid.

As you learned in Chapter 2, RNA differs from DNA: RNA is single stranded, and it has the sugar ribose instead of deoxyribose, and the base uracil (U) instead of thymine (T). Three forms of RNA typically act together to carry out DNA's instructions for polypeptide synthesis:

- **Messenger RNA (mRNA)**, relatively long nucleotide strands resembling "half-DNA" molecules (one of the two strands of a DNA molecule coding for protein structure). mRNA carries a transcript of the code to the cytoplasm, where protein synthesis occurs.
- **Ribosomal RNA (rRNA)**, along with proteins, forms the ribosomes, which consist of two subunits—one large and one small. The two subunit types combine to form functional ribosomes, which are the sites of protein synthesis.
- **Transfer RNA (tRNA)**, small, roughly L-shaped molecules that ferry amino acids to the ribosomes. There they decode mRNA's message for amino acid sequence in the polypeptide to be built.

All types of RNA are formed on the DNA in the nucleus in much the same way as DNA replicates itself: The DNA helix separates and one of its strands serves as a template for synthesizing a complementary RNA strand. Once formed, the RNA molecule is released from the DNA template and migrates into the cytoplasm. Its job done, the DNA recoils into its helical, inactive form.

Approximately 2% of the nuclear DNA codes for the synthesis of short-lived mRNA. DNA in the nucleolar organizer regions (mentioned previously) codes for the synthesis of rRNA, which is long-lived and stable, as is tRNA coded by other DNA sequences. Because rRNA and tRNA do not transport codes for synthesizing other molecules, they are the final products of the genes that code for them. Ribosomal RNA and tRNA act together to "translate" the message carried by mRNA.

Essentially, polypeptide synthesis involves two major steps:

1. *Transcription*, in which DNA's information is encoded in mRNA
2. *Translation*, in which the information carried by mRNA is decoded and used to assemble polypeptides

Figure 3.34 summarizes the information flow in these two major steps. The figure also indicates the "RNA processing" that removes introns from mRNA before this molecule leaves the nucleus and moves into the cytoplasm.

Transcription

A transcriptionist converts a message from a recording or shorthand notes into a written copy. In other words, information is transferred from one form or format to another.

In cells, **transcription** transfers information from a DNA base sequence to the complementary base sequence of an mRNA molecule. The form is different, but the same information is being conveyed. Once the mRNA molecule is made, it detaches and leaves the nucleus via a nuclear pore, and heads for the protein synthesis machinery, the ribosome.

Transcription cannot begin until gene-activating chemicals called *transcription factors* stimulate histones at the site-to-be of gene transcription to loosen. The transcription factors then bind to the promoter. The **promoter** is a special DNA sequence that contains the *start point* (beginning of the gene to be transcribed). It specifies where mRNA synthesis starts and which DNA strand is going to serve as the *template strand* (Figure 3.35,

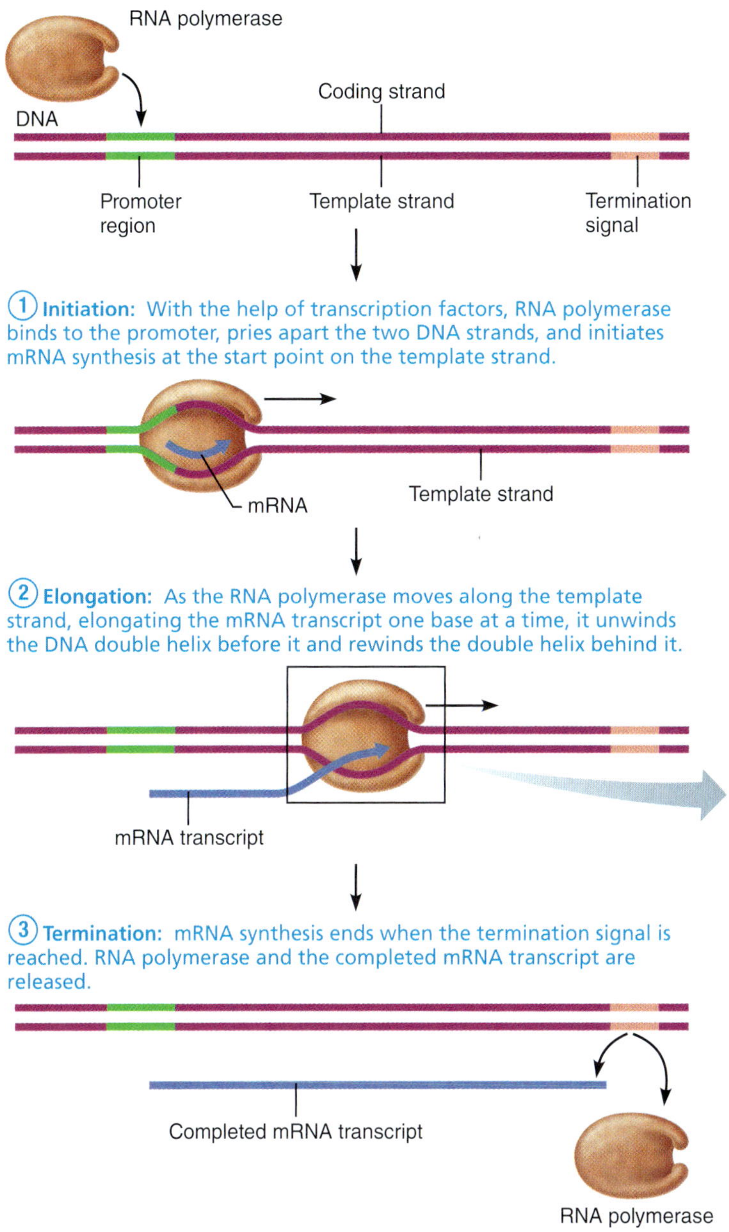

Figure 3.35 Overview of stages of transcription.

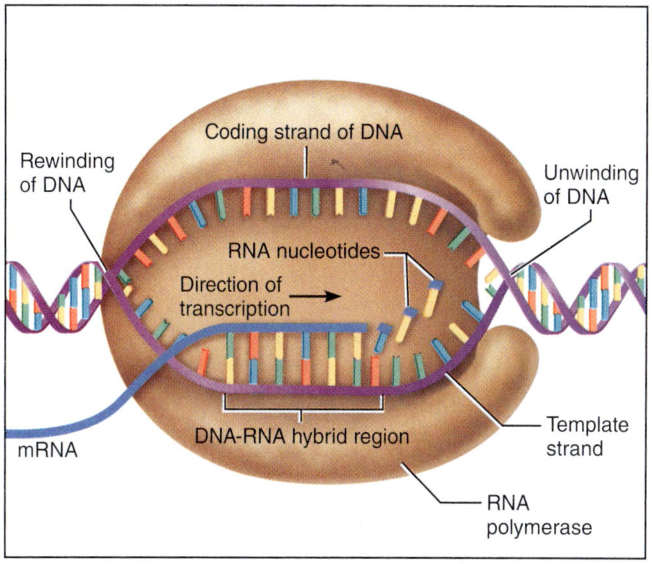

The DNA-RNA hybrid: At any given moment, 16–18 base pairs of DNA are unwound and the most recently made RNA is still bound to DNA. This small region is called the DNA-RNA hybrid.

top). The uncoiled DNA strand not used as a template is called the *coding strand* because it has the same (coded) sequence as the mRNA to be built (except for the U in mRNA in place of T in DNA). The transcription factors also help position **RNA polymerase**, the enzyme that oversees the synthesis of mRNA, correctly at the promoter. Once these preparations are made, RNA polymerase can initiate transcription.

Transcription involves three basic phases: initiation, elongation, and termination **(Figure 3.35)**.

① **Initiation.** Once properly positioned, RNA polymerase pulls apart the strands of the DNA double helix so transcription can begin at the start point in the promoter.

② **Elongation.** Using incoming RNA nucleotides as substrates, the RNA polymerase aligns them with complementary DNA bases on the template strand and then links them together. As RNA polymerase elongates the mRNA strand one base at a time, it unwinds the DNA helix in front of it, and rewinds the helix behind it. At any given moment, 16 to 18 base pairs of DNA are unwound and the most recently made mRNA is still hydrogen-bonded (H-bonded) to the template DNA. This small region—called the **DNA-RNA hybrid**—is up to 12 base pairs long.

③ **Termination.** When the polymerase reaches a special base sequence called a **termination signal**, transcription ends and the newly formed mRNA separates from the DNA template.

Processing of mRNA Before translation can begin, editing and further processing are needed to clean up the mRNA transcript. Recall that mammalian DNA like ours has coding regions (exons) separated by non-protein-coding regions (introns). Because the DNA is transcribed sequentially, the mRNA initially made, called *pre-mRNA* or *primary transcript*, is still

First base	Second base: U	Second base: C	Second base: A	Second base: G	Third base
U	UUU, UUC — Phe UUA, UUG — Leu	UCU, UCC, UCA, UCG — Ser	UAU, UAC — Tyr UAA Stop UAG Stop	UGU, UGC — Cys UGA Stop UGG Trp	U C A G
C	CUU, CUC, CUA, CUG — Leu	CCU, CCC, CCA, CCG — Pro	CAU, CAC — His CAA, CAG — Gln	CGU, CGC, CGA, CGG — Arg	U C A G
A	AUU, AUC, AUA — Ile AUG Met or Start	ACU, ACC, ACA, ACG — Thr	AAU, AAC — Asn AAA, AAG — Lys	AGU, AGC — Ser AGA, AGG — Arg	U C A G
G	GUU, GUC, GUA, GUG — Val	GCU, GCC, GCA, GCG — Ala	GAU, GAC — Asp GAA, GAG — Glu	GGU, GGC, GGA, GGG — Gly	U C A G

Figure 3.36 The genetic code. The three bases in an mRNA codon are designated as the first, second, and third. Each set of three specifies a particular amino acid, represented here by an abbreviation (see list below). The codon AUG (which specifies the amino acid methionine) is the usual start signal for protein synthesis. The word *stop* indicates the codons that serve as signals to terminate protein synthesis.

Abb.*	Amino acid	Abb.*	Amino acid
Ala	alanine	Leu	leucine
Arg	arginine	Lys	lysine
Asn	asparagine	Met	methionine
Asp	aspartic acid	Phe	phenylalanine
Cys	cysteine	Pro	proline
Glu	glutamic acid	Ser	serine
Gln	glutamine	Thr	threonine
Gly	glycine	Trp	tryptophan
His	histidine	Tyr	tyrosine
Ile	isoleucine	Val	valine

*Abbreviation for the amino acid

littered with introns. Before the newly formed RNA can be used as a messenger, it must be processed, or edited—that is, sections corresponding to introns must be removed. Large RNA-protein complexes called *spliceosomes* snip out the introns and splice together the remaining exon-coded sections in the order in which they occurred in the DNA, producing functional mRNA.

Although many introns degrade naturally, some contain active segments (such as microRNAs) that can function to control, interfere with, or silence other genes. Additionally, a number of specific RNA-binding proteins, called *mRNA complex proteins*, must become associated with the edited mRNA. These mRNA complex proteins guide the export of mRNA from the nucleus, determine its localization, translation, and stability, and check it for premature termination codons.

Translation

A translator takes a message in one language and restates it in another. In the **translation** step of protein synthesis, the language of nucleic acids (base sequence) is translated into the language of proteins (amino acid sequence).

Genetic Code The rules by which the base sequence of a gene is translated into an amino acid sequence are called the **genetic code**. For each triplet, or three-base sequence on DNA, the corresponding three-base sequence on mRNA is called a **codon**. Since there are four kinds of RNA (or DNA) nucleotides, there are 4^3, or 64, possible codons. Three of these 64 codons are "stop signs" that call for termination of polypeptide synthesis. All the rest code for amino acids.

Because there are only about 20 amino acids, some are specified by more than one codon. This redundancy in the genetic code helps protect against problems due to transcription (and translation) errors. **Figure 3.36** shows the genetic code and a complete codon list.

Role of tRNA Translation involves the mRNAs, tRNAs, and rRNAs mentioned above. Before we get into the actual details of the translation process, let's look at how the tRNAs are so well suited for their roles in translation.

Shaped like a handheld drill, tRNA is well suited to its dual function of binding to both an amino acid and an mRNA codon. The amino acid (picked up from the cytoplasmic pool) is bound to one end of tRNA, at a region called the stem. At the other end, the head, is its **anticodon** (an″ti-ko′don), a three-base sequence complementary to the mRNA codon calling for the amino acid carried by that particular tRNA. Because anticodons form hydrogen bonds with complementary codons, tRNA is the link between the language of nucleic acids and the language of proteins. For example, if the mRNA codon is AUA, which specifies isoleucine, the tRNAs carrying isoleucine will have the anticodon UAU, which can bind to the AUA codons.

There are approximately 45 types of tRNA, each capable of binding with a specific amino acid. The attachment process is controlled by an aminoacyl-tRNA synthetase enzyme and is activated by ATP. Once its amino acid is loaded, the tRNA (now called an *aminoacyl-tRNA* because of its amino acid cargo) migrates to the ribosome, where its amino acid is maneuvered into the proper position, as specified by the mRNA codons and described below. The ribosome is more than just a passive attachment site for mRNA and tRNA. Like a vise, the ribosome holds the tRNA and mRNA close together to coordinate the coupling of codons and anticodons, and positions the next (incoming) amino acid for addition to the growing polypeptide chain. To do its job, the ribosome has a binding site for mRNA and three binding sites for tRNA: an A (aminoacyl) site for an incoming aminoacyl-tRNA, a P (peptidyl) site for the tRNA holding the growing polypeptide chain, and an E (exit) site for an outgoing tRNA, as illustrated in *Focus on Translation* (**Figure 3.37**, on pp. 106–107). Now we are ready to put the parts together—so let's go!

Sequence of Events in Translation Translation entails a now familiar sequence of named events—*initiation, elongation*, and *termination*—which occur in the cytoplasm. Each of these phases requires energy in the form of ATP and a specific set of protein factors and enzymes. Figure 3.37 summarizes these events.

① **Initiation.** A small ribosomal subunit binds to a special methionine-carrying **initiator tRNA**, and then to the "new" mRNA to be decoded. With the initiator tRNA still in tow, the small ribosomal subunit scans along the mRNA until it encounters the *start codon*—the first AUG triplet it meets. When the initiator tRNA's UAC anticodon "recognizes" and binds to the start codon, a large ribosomal subunit unites with the small one, forming a functional ribosome.

At the end of this phase the mRNA is firmly positioned in the groove between the ribosomal subunits, the initiator tRNA is sitting in the P site, and the A site is vacant, ready for the next aminoacyl tRNA to deliver its cargo. The next phase, elongation of the polypeptide, now begins.

② **Elongation.** During the three-step cycle of elongation, the mRNA is moved through the ribosome in one direction and one amino acid at a time is added to the growing polypeptide (Figure 3.37).

(2a) **Codon recognition.** The incoming aminoacyl-tRNA binds to a complementary codon in the A site of a ribosome.

(2b) **Peptide bond formation.** Once the accuracy of the codon-anticodon binding is checked, an enzymatic component in the large ribosomal subunit catalyzes peptide bond formation between the amino acid of the tRNA in the P site to that of the tRNA in the A site.

(2a) **Translocation.** This step translocates, or moves, the tRNA in the A site to the P site. The unloaded (vacant) tRNA is transferred to the E site, from which it is released and ready to be recharged with an amino acid from the cytoplasmic pool.

This orderly "musical chairs" process continues: the peptidyl-tRNAs transfer their polypeptide cargo to the aminoacyl-tRNAs, and then the P-site-to-E-site and A-site-to-P-site movements of the tRNAs occur (Figure 3.37). As the ribosome "chugs" along the mRNA track and the mRNA is progressively read, its initial portion passes through the ribosome and may become attached successively to several other ribosomes, all reading the same message simultaneously and sequentially. This multiple ribosome–mRNA complex, a *polyribosome*, efficiently produces multiple copies of the same protein (**Figure 3.38**, on p. 108).

③ **Termination.** The mRNA strand continues to be read sequentially until its last codon, the *stop codon* (one UGA, UAA, or UAG) enters the A site. The stop codon is the "period" at the end of the mRNA sentence—it tells the ribosome that translation of that mRNA is finished. As a result, a *protein release factor* binds to the stop codon at the A site and directs the addition of water (instead of an amino acid) to the polypeptide chain. This hydrolyzes (breaks) the bond between the polypeptide and the tRNA in the P site. The completed polypeptide chain is then released from the ribosome, and the ribosome separates into its two subunits (Figure 3.38a). The released protein may undergo processing before it folds into its complex 3-D structure and floats off, ready to work. When the message of the mRNA that directed its formation is no longer needed, it is degraded.

Processing in the Rough ER As noted earlier in the chapter, ribosomes attach to and detach from the rough ER. When a short "leader" peptide called an ER **signal sequence** is present in a protein being synthesized, the associated ribosome attaches to the membrane of the rough ER. This signal sequence, with its attached cargo of a ribosome and mRNA, is guided to appropriate receptor sites on the ER membrane by a signal recognition particle (SRP), a protein chaperone that cycles between the ER and the cytosol. **Figure 3.39** on p.108 details the subsequent events occurring at the ER.

Summary: From DNA to Proteins The genetic information of a cell is translated into the production of proteins via a sequence of information transfer that is completely directed by complementary base pairing. The transfer of information goes from DNA base sequence (triplets) to the complementary base sequence of mRNA (codons) and then to the tRNA base sequence (anticodons), which is identical to the template DNA sequence except for the substitution of uracil (U) for thymine (T) (**Figure 3.40**, on p. 109).

Other Roles of DNA

The story of DNA doesn't end with the production of proteins encoded by exons. Scientists are finding that intron DNA actually codes for a surprising variety of active RNA species, including the following:

- **Antisense RNAs**, made on the DNA strand complementary to the template strand for mRNA, can intercept and bind to the protein-coding mRNA strand and prevent it from being translated into protein.
- **MicroRNAs** are small RNAs that can use RNA interference machinery to interfere with and suppress mRNAs made by certain exons, thus effectively silencing them.
- **Riboswitches** are folded RNAs that code, like mRNA, for a particular protein. What sets them apart from other mRNAs is a region that acts as a switch to turn protein synthesis on or off in response to metabolic changes in their immediate environment, such as shifting concentrations of amino acids or other small molecules in the cell. When it senses these changes, the riboswitch changes shape, thereby stopping or starting production of the protein it specifies.

Beyond the discussion here and in Chapter 29, we still have much to learn about these versatile RNA species that arise from intron DNA and appear to play a role in heredity. Another area of research focuses on the multitasking of DNA segments.

(Text continues on p. 109)

Figure 3.37 Translation is the process in which genetic information carried by an mRNA is decoded in the ribosome to form a particular polypeptide. The "translators" are tRNA molecules that can recognize and bind specifically both to a codon and an amino acid. A&P Flix *Available at www.masteringaandp.com*

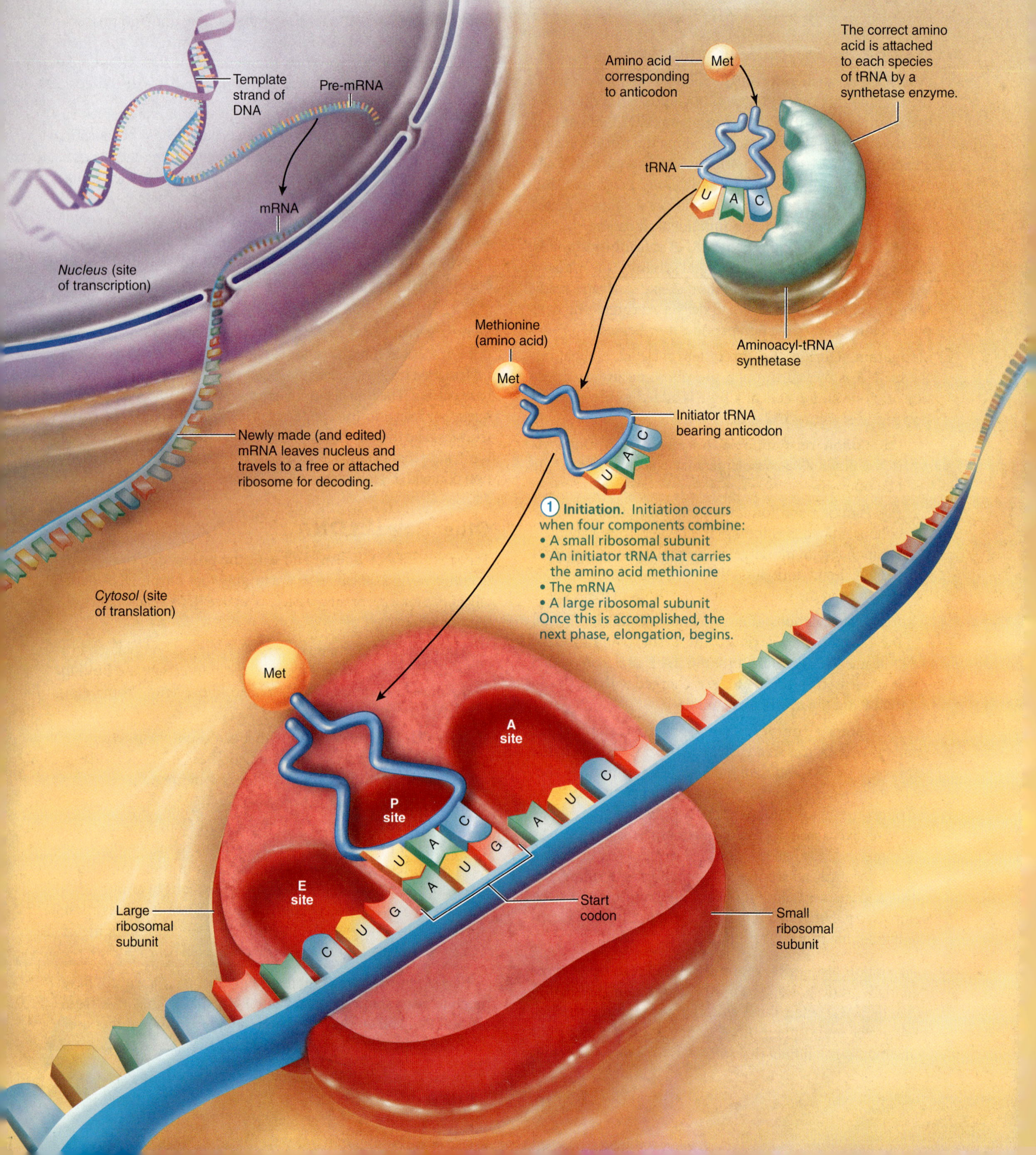

2 Elongation. Amino acids are added one at a time to the growing peptide chain via a process that has three repeating steps.

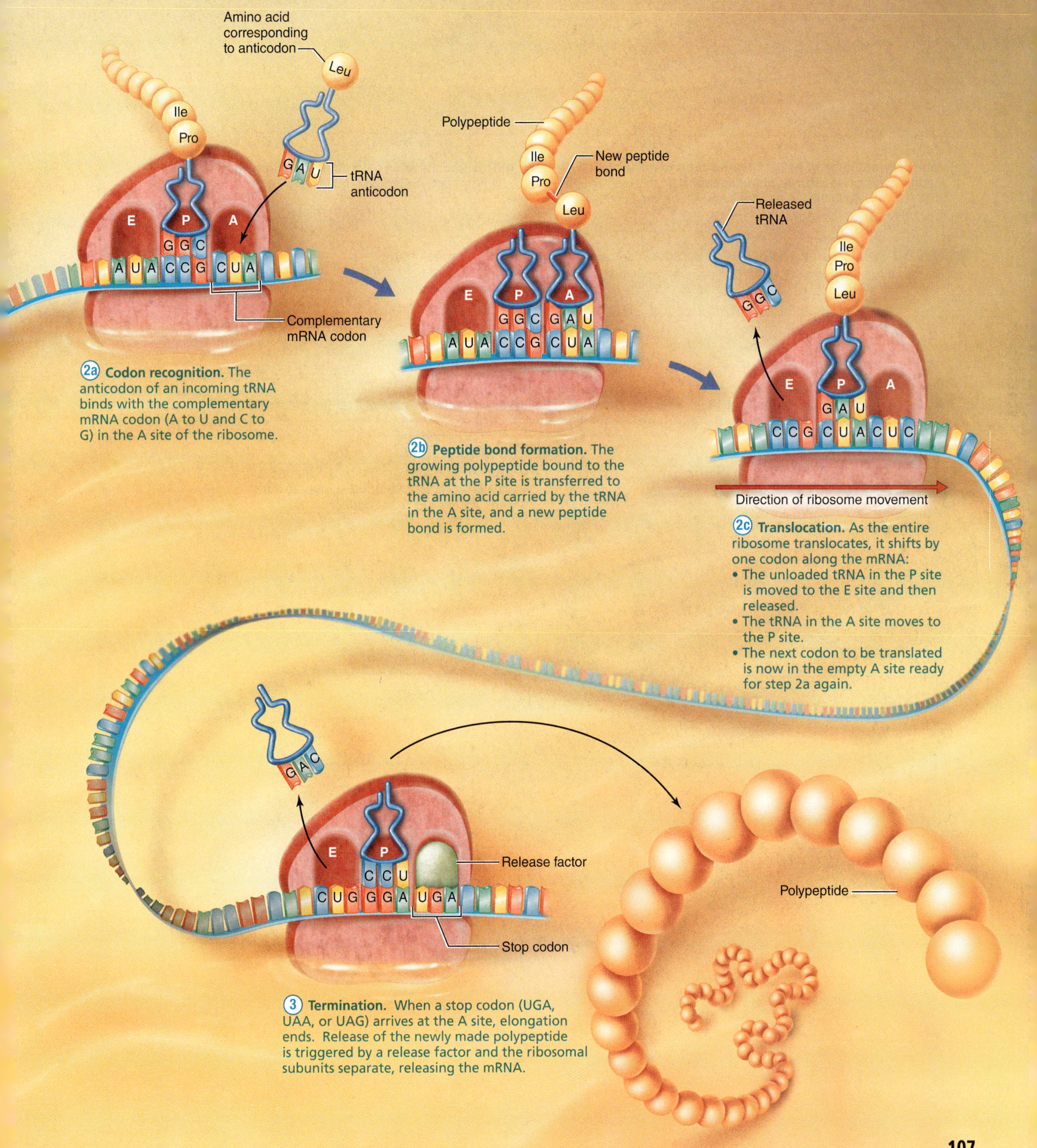

2a Codon recognition. The anticodon of an incoming tRNA binds with the complementary mRNA codon (A to U and C to G) in the A site of the ribosome.

2b Peptide bond formation. The growing polypeptide bound to the tRNA at the P site is transferred to the amino acid carried by the tRNA in the A site, and a new peptide bond is formed.

2c Translocation. As the entire ribosome translocates, it shifts by one codon along the mRNA:

- The unloaded tRNA in the P site is moved to the E site and then released.
- The tRNA in the A site moves to the P site.
- The next codon to be translated is now in the empty A site ready for step 2a again.

3 Termination. When a stop codon (UGA, UAA, or UAG) arrives at the A site, elongation ends. Release of the newly made polypeptide is triggered by a release factor and the ribosomal subunits separate, releasing the mRNA.

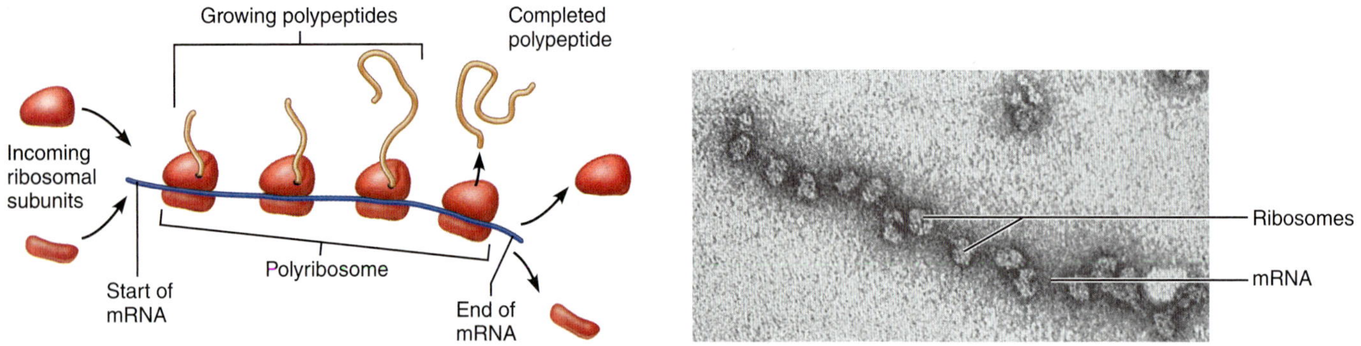

(a) Each polyribosome consists of one strand of mRNA being read by several ribosomes simultaneously. In this diagram, the mRNA is moving to the left and the "oldest" functional ribosome is farthest to the right.

(b) This transmission electron micrograph shows a large polyribosome (400,000×).

Figure 3.38 Polyribosome arrays. Polyribosome arrays allow a single strand of mRNA to be translated into hundreds of the same polypeptide molecules in a short time.

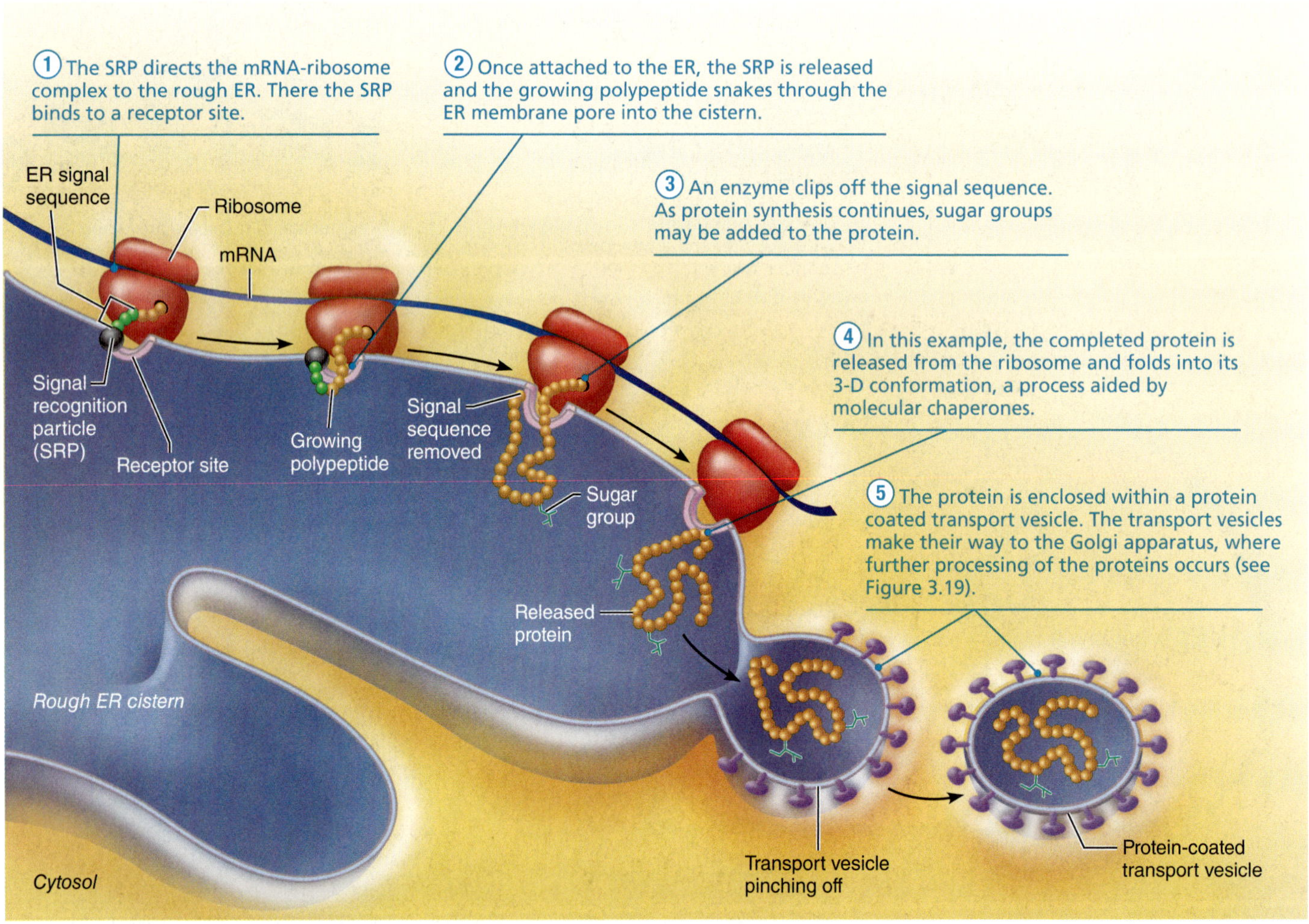

Figure 3.39 Rough ER processing of proteins. An endoplasmic reticulum (ER) signal sequence in a newly forming protein causes the signal recognition particle (SRP) to direct the mRNA-ribosome complex to the rough ER.

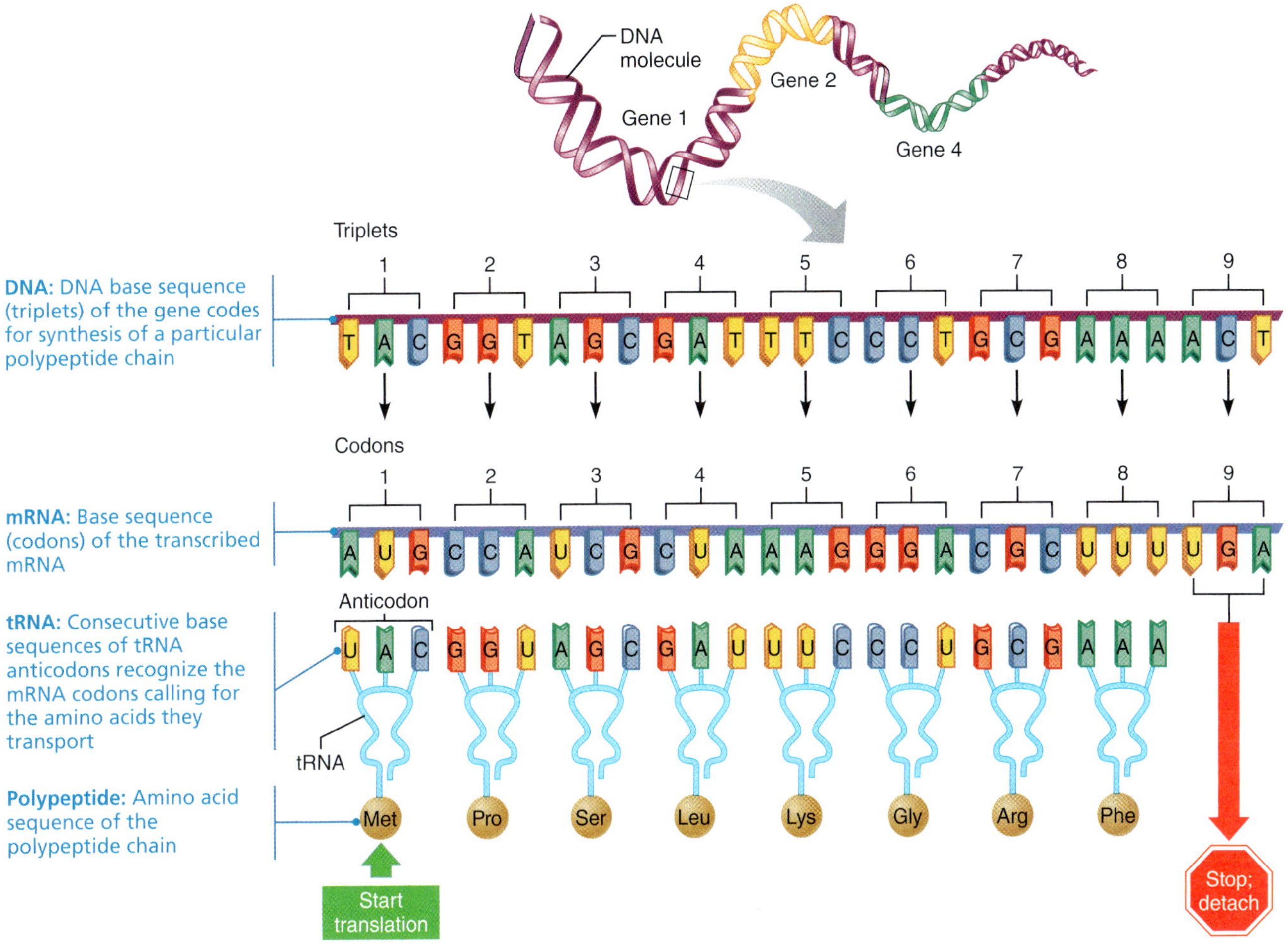

Figure 3.40 Information transfer from DNA to RNA to polypeptide. Information is transferred from the DNA of the gene to the complementary messenger RNA molecule, whose codons are then "read" (translated) by transfer RNA anticodons. Notice that the "reading" of the mRNA by tRNA anticodons reestablishes the base (triplet) sequence of the DNA genetic code (except that T is replaced by U).

Check Your Understanding

29. Codons and anticodons are both three-base sequences. How do they differ?
30. How do the A, P, and E ribosomal sites differ functionally during protein synthesis?
31. What is the role of DNA in transcription?

For answers, see Appendix H.

Degradation of Organelles and Cytosolic Proteins

✓ Define autophagy and indicate its major cellular function.

✓ Describe the importance of ubiquitin-dependent degradation of soluble proteins.

The workings of the cytoplasm are complex and seemingly unending. Without some system to get rid of malfunctioning or obsolete organelles, cells would soon become gummed up with debris.

Not to worry. The process called *autophagy* ("self-eating") sweeps up bits of cytoplasm and excess organelles into double-membrane vesicles called *autophagosomes*. They are then delivered to lysosomes for digestion of the contents to amino acids, fatty acids, and the like, which the cell reuses.

Autophagy may have evolved as a response to cell starvation and it speeds up in response to several kinds of stress, such as low oxygen, high temperature, or lack of growth factors. However, autophagosomes are busy continuously. Although autophagy can lead to programmed cell death (see apoptosis, p. 110), it makes a greater contribution to cell survival and provides a fail-safe system against complete self-destruction when such a dire response is not necessary.

Autophagy is exactly what the doctor ordered for disposal of large cytoplasmic structures and protein aggregates. But lysosomal enzymes do not have access to soluble proteins that are misfolded, damaged, or unneeded and need to be disposed of. Examples of unneeded proteins include some that are used only in cell division and must be degraded at precise points in the cell cycle, and short-lived transcription factors.

So how does the cell prevent such proteins from accumulating while stopping the cytosolic enzymes from destroying virtually all soluble proteins? It seems that the cell has a different strategy for destroying such proteins.

3

Proteins called **ubiquitins** (u-bĭ′kwĭ-tinz) mark doomed proteins for attack (proteolysis) by attaching to them in an ATP-dependent reaction. The tagged proteins are then hydrolyzed to small peptides by soluble enzymes or by **proteasomes**, giant "waste disposal" complexes composed of protein-digesting enzymes, and the ubiquitin is recycled. Proteasome activity is critical during starvation when these complexes degrade preexisting proteins to provide amino acids for synthesis of new and needed proteins.

Extracellular Materials

✓ Name and describe the composition of extracellular materials.

Extracellular materials are any substances contributing to body mass that are found outside the cells. Classes of extracellular materials include

- *Body fluids*, mainly interstitial fluid, blood plasma, and cerebrospinal fluid. These fluids are important transport and dissolving media.
- *Cellular secretions*, such as substances that aid in digestion (intestinal and gastric fluids) and some that act as lubricants (saliva, mucus, and serous fluids).
- The *extracellular matrix*, the most abundant extracellular material. Most body cells are in contact with a jellylike substance composed of proteins and polysaccharides. Secreted by the cells, these molecules self-assemble into an organized mesh in the extracellular space, where they serve as a universal "cell glue" that helps to hold body cells together. As described in Chapter 4, the extracellular matrix is particularly abundant in connective tissues—in some cases so abundant that it (rather than living cells) accounts for the bulk of that tissue type. Depending on the structure to be formed, the extracellular matrix in connective tissue ranges from soft to rock-hard.

☑ Check Your Understanding

32. What is the importance of ubiquitin in the life of a cell?
33. What are two body fluids that inhabit the extracellular space and what role does each play in the body?

For answers, see Appendix H.

Developmental Aspects of Cells

✓ Discuss some theories of cell differentiation and aging.

✓ Indicate the value of apoptosis to the body.

We all begin life as a single cell, the fertilized egg, and all the cells of our body arise from it. Very early in development, cells begin to specialize, some becoming liver cells, some nerve cells, and so on. All our cells carry the same genes, so how can one cell become so different from another? This is a fascinating question.

Apparently, cells in various regions of the embryo are exposed to different chemical signals that channel them into specific pathways of development. When the embryo consists of just a few cells, the major signals may be nothing more than slight differences in oxygen and carbon dioxide concentrations between the more superficial and the deeper cells. But as development continues, cells release chemicals that influence development of neighboring cells by triggering processes that switch some genes "off" and others "on." Some genes are active in all cells. For example, genes for rRNA and ATP synthesis are "on" in all cells, but genes for synthesizing the enzymes needed to produce thyroxine are "on" only in cells that are going to be part of the thyroid gland. Hence, the story of cell specialization lies in the kinds of proteins made and reflects the activation of different genes in different cell types.

Cell specialization leads to *structural* variation—different organelles come to predominate in different cells. For example, muscle cells make large amounts of actin and myosin, and their cytoplasm fills with microfilaments. Liver and phagocytic cells produce more lysosomes. The development of specific and distinctive features in cells is called **cell differentiation**.

Apoptosis and Modified Rates of Cell Division

During early development, cell death and destruction are normal events. Nature takes few chances. More cells than needed are produced, and excesses are eliminated later in a type of programmed cell death called **apoptosis** (ap″o-to′sis; "falling away"). Apoptosis is particularly common in the developing nervous system. It is also responsible for "carving out" fingers and toes from their embryonic webbed precursors. This process of controlled cellular suicide also eliminates cells that are stressed, no longer needed, injured, or aged.

How does apoptosis work? In response to internal cellular damage or to some extracellular signal, mitochondrial membranes become permeable, allowing cytochrome c and other factors to leak into the cytosol. These chemicals trigger apoptosis by activating intracellular enzymes called *caspases*. The activated caspases unleash a torrent of digestive activity within the cell, destroying the cell's DNA, cytoskeleton, and so on, producing a quick, neat death. The apoptotic cell shrinks without leaking its contents into the surrounding tissue, detaches from other cells, and rounds up. Because the dying cell releases a chemical that attracts macrophages, and sprouts "eat me" signals, it is immediately phagocytized.

Most organs are well formed and functional long before birth, but the body continues to grow and enlarge by forming new cells throughout childhood and adolescence. Once we reach adult size, cell division is important mainly to replace short-lived cells and repair wounds.

During young adulthood, cell numbers remain fairly constant. However, local changes in the rate of cell division are common. For example, when a person is anemic, his or her bone marrow undergoes **hyperplasia** (hi″per-pla′ze-ah), or accelerated growth (*hyper* = over; *plas* = grow), to produce red blood cells at a faster rate. If the anemia is remedied, the excessive marrow activity ceases. **Atrophy** (at′ro-fe), a decrease in size of an organ or body tissue, can result from loss of normal stimulation or from diseases like muscular dystrophy. Muscles that lose their nerve supply atrophy and waste away, and lack of exercise leads to thinned, brittle bones.

Cell Aging

Cell aging is a complicated process with many causes, but to be perfectly frank, the precise reason an otherwise healthy person grows old and dies is still a mystery.

The *wear-and-tear theory* attributes aging to little chemical insults and formation of free radicals, both of which have cumulative effects. For example, environmental toxins such as pesticides, alcohol, and bacterial toxins may damage cell membranes, poison enzyme systems, or cause "mistakes" in DNA replication. Temporary lack of oxygen, which occurs increasingly with age as our blood vessels clog with fatty materials, accelerates rates of cell death throughout the body.

According to the *mitochondrial theory of aging*, free radicals deserve most of the blame. Most free radicals are produced in the mitochondria, because these organelles have the highest metabolic rate. This finding implies that diminished energy production by radical-damaged mitochondria, due perhaps to an increasing burden of mutations in mitochondrial DNA, weakens (and ages) cells. X rays and other types of radiation, and some chemicals, also generate huge numbers of free radicals, which can overwhelm the peroxisomal enzymes. Vitamins C and E act as antioxidants in the body and may help to absorb or defuse free radicals. With age, glucose (blood sugar) becomes party to cross-linking proteins together, a condition that severely disrupts protein function and accelerates the course of atherosclerosis.

Another theory attributes cell aging to progressive disorders in the immune system. According to this theory, cell damage results from (1) autoimmune responses, which means the immune system turns against one's own tissues, and (2) a progressive weakening of the immune response, so that the body is less able to get rid of cell-damaging pathogens.

The idea that cell aging and chronic illnesses result from inflammation (and an overactive immune system) has been kicking around since the 1800s. In the 1990s evidence did in fact emerge to link inflammation to aging. C-reactive protein, a protein that indicates acute inflammation, is elevated in heart disease and is an amazingly accurate predictor of future heart attacks. It seems that as we age, acute episodes of inflammation tend to become chronic.

Perhaps the most widely accepted theory of cell aging is the *genetic theory*, which suggests that cessation of mitosis and cell aging are "programmed into our genes." One interesting notion here is that a *telomere clock* determines the number of times a cell can divide. **Telomeres** (*telo* = end; *mer* = piece) are nonsensical strings of nucleotides that cap the ends of chromosomes and provide protection from fraying, fusing with other chromosomes, inappropriate repair, and losing important genetic information, much like plastic caps preserve the ends of shoelaces. In human telomeres, the base sequence TTAGGG is repeated a thousand times or more (like a DNA stutter). Though telomeres carry no genes, they appear to be vital for chromosomal survival, because each time DNA is replicated, 100 to 200 of the end nucleotides are lost and the telomeres get a bit shorter. When telomeres reach a certain minimum length, it is thought that the stop-division signal is given.

The idea that cell longevity depends on telomere integrity was supported by the discovery of *telomerase*, an enzyme that lengthens the previously shortened telomeres. Pegged as the "immortality enzyme," telomerase is found in germ line cells (cells that give rise to sperm and ova), but it is absent or barely detectable in other adult cell types.

☑ Check Your Understanding

34. What is apoptosis and what is its importance in the body?
35. What is the wear-and-tear theory of aging?

For answers, see Appendix H.

In this chapter we have described the structure and function of the generalized cell. One of the wonders of the cell is the disparity between its minute size and its extraordinary activity, which reflects the diversity of its organelles. The evidence for division of labor and functional specialization among organelles is inescapable. Only ribosomes synthesize proteins, while protein packaging is the bailiwick of the Golgi apparatus. Membranes compartmentalize most organelles, allowing them to work without hindering or being hindered by other cell activities, and the plasma membrane regulates molecular traffic across the cell's boundary. Now that you know what cells have in common, you are ready to explore how they differ in the various body tissues, the topic of Chapter 4.

Chapter Summary

For more chapter study tools, go to the Study Area of MasteringA&P at **www.masteringaandp.com**.
There you will find:

- Interactive Physiology iP
- A&PFlix
- Practice Anatomy Lab PAL
- PhysioEx PEx
- Videos, Practice Quizzes and Tests, MP3 Tutor Sessions, Case Studies, and much more!

The Cellular Basis of Life (p. 62)

1. All living organisms are composed of cells—the basic structural and functional units of life. Cells vary widely in both shape and size.
2. The principle of complementarity states that the biochemical activity of cells reflects the operation of their organelles.
3. The generalized cell is a concept that typifies all cells. The generalized cell has three major regions—the nucleus, cytoplasm, and plasma membrane.

3

The Plasma Membrane: Structure (pp. 63–67)

1. The plasma membrane encloses cell contents, mediates exchanges with the extracellular environment, and plays a role in cellular communication.

The Fluid Mosaic Model (pp. 63–65)

2. The plasma membrane is a fluid bilayer of lipids (phospholipids, cholesterol, and glycolipids) within which proteins are inserted.
3. The lipids have both hydrophilic and hydrophobic regions that organize their aggregation and self-repair. The lipids form the structural part of the plasma membrane.
4. Most proteins are integral transmembrane proteins that extend entirely through the membrane. Some, appended to the integral proteins, are peripheral proteins.
5. Proteins are responsible for most specialized membrane functions: Some are enzymes, some are receptors, and others mediate membrane transport functions.

The Glycocalyx (pp. 65–66)

6. Externally facing glycoproteins contribute to the glycocalyx.

Cell Junctions (pp. 66–67)

7. Cell junctions join cells together and may aid or inhibit movement of molecules between or past cells.
8. Tight junctions are impermeable junctions. Desmosomes mechanically couple cells into a functional community. Gap junctions allow joined cells to communicate.

The Plasma Membrane: Membrane Transport (pp. 67–69)

1. The plasma membrane acts as a selectively permeable barrier. Substances move across the plasma membrane by passive processes, which depend on the kinetic energy of molecules, and by active processes, which depend on the use of cellular energy (ATP).

Passive Processes (pp. 68–72)

2. Diffusion is the movement of molecules (driven by kinetic energy) down a concentration gradient. Fat-soluble solutes can diffuse directly through the membrane by dissolving in the lipid.
3. Facilitated diffusion is the passive movement of certain solutes across the membrane either by their binding with a membrane carrier protein or by their moving through a membrane channel. As with other diffusion processes, it is driven by kinetic energy, but the carriers and channels are selective.
4. Osmosis is the diffusion of a solvent, such as water, through a selectively permeable membrane. Water diffuses through membrane channels (aquaporins) or directly through the lipid portion of the membrane from a solution of lesser osmolarity (total concentration of all solute particles) to a solution of greater osmolarity.
5. The presence of solutes unable to permeate the plasma membrane leads to changes in cell tone that may cause the cell to swell or shrink. Net osmosis ceases when the solute concentration on both sides of the plasma membrane reaches equilibrium.
6. Solutions that cause a net loss of water from cells are hypertonic. Those causing net water gain are hypotonic. Those causing neither gain nor loss of water are isotonic.

Active Processes (pp. 72–79)

7. Active transport (solute pumping) depends on a carrier protein and energy. Substances transported move against concentration or electrical gradients. In primary active transport, such as that provided by the Na^+-K^+ pump, ATP directly provides the energy.
8. In secondary active transport, the energy of an ion gradient (produced by a primary active transport process) is used to transport a substance passively. Many active transport systems are coupled, and cotransported substances move in either the same (symport) or opposite (antiport) directions across the membrane.
9. Vesicular transport also requires that energy be provided. Endocytosis brings substances into the cell, typically in protein-coated vesicles. If the substance is relatively large particles, the process is called phagocytosis. If the substance is dissolved molecules, the process is pinocytosis. Receptor-mediated endocytosis is selective: Engulfed molecules attach to receptors on the membrane before endocytosis occurs. Exocytosis, which uses SNAREs to anchor the vesicles to the plasma membrane, ejects substances (hormones, wastes, secretions) from the cell.
10. Most endocytosis (and transcytosis) is mediated by clathrin-coated vesicles. Other types of protein coating are found in caveolae and vesicles involved in vesicular trafficking. Caveolae appear to be important as sites that accumulate receptors involved in cell signaling.

The Plasma Membrane: Generation of a Resting Membrane Potential (pp. 79–80)

1. All cells in the resting stage exhibit a voltage across their membrane, called the resting membrane potential. Because of the membrane potential, both concentration and electrical gradients determine the ease of an ion's diffusion.

Selective Diffusion Establishes Membrane Potential (pp. 79–80)

2. The resting membrane potential is generated by concentration gradients of ions and the differential permeability of the plasma membrane to ions, particularly potassium ions. Sodium is in high extracellular concentration and low intracellular concentration, and the membrane is poorly permeable to it. Potassium is in high concentration in the cell and low concentration in the extracellular fluid. The membrane is more permeable to potassium than to sodium. Protein anions in the cell are too large to cross the membrane and Cl^-, the main anion in extracellular fluid, is repelled by the negative charge on the inner membrane face.

Active Transport Maintains Electrochemical Gradients (p. 80)

3. Essentially, a negative membrane potential is established when the movement of K^+ out of the cell equals K^+ movement into the cell. Na^+ movements across the membrane contribute minimally to establishing the membrane potential. The greater outward diffusion of potassium (than inward diffusion of sodium) leads to a charge separation at the membrane (inside negative). This charge separation is maintained by the operation of the sodium-potassium pump.

iP Nervous System I; Topics: Ion Channels, pp. 3, 8, 9; The Membrane Potential, pp. 1–17.

The Plasma Membrane: Cell-Environment Interactions (pp. 80–81)

1. Cells interact directly and indirectly with other cells. Indirect interactions involve extracellular chemicals carried in body fluids or forming part of the extracellular matrix.
2. Molecules of the glycocalyx are intimately involved in cell-environment interactions. Most are cell adhesion molecules or membrane receptors.
3. Activated membrane receptors act as catalysts, regulate channels, or, like G protein–linked receptors, act through second messengers such as cyclic AMP and Ca^{2+}. Ligand

binding results in changes in protein structure or function within the targeted cell.

The Cytoplasm (pp. 81–91)

1. The cytoplasm, the cellular region between the nuclear and plasma membranes, consists of the cytosol (fluid cytoplasmic environment), inclusions (nonliving nutrient stores, pigment granules, crystals, etc.), and cytoplasmic organelles.

Cytoplasmic Organelles (pp. 83–89)

2. The cytoplasm is the major functional area of the cell. These functions are mediated by organelles.
3. Mitochondria, organelles limited by a double membrane, are sites of ATP formation. Their internal enzymes carry out the oxidative reactions of cellular respiration.
4. Ribosomes, composed of two subunits containing ribosomal RNA and proteins, are the sites of protein synthesis. They may be free or attached to membranes.
5. The rough endoplasmic reticulum is a ribosome-studded membrane system. Its cisterns act as sites for protein modification. Its external face acts in phospholipid synthesis. Vesicles pinched off from the ER transport the proteins to other cell sites.
6. The smooth endoplasmic reticulum synthesizes lipid and steroid molecules. It also acts in fat metabolism and in drug detoxification. In muscle cells, it is a calcium ion depot.
7. The Golgi apparatus is a membranous system close to the nucleus that packages protein secretions for export, packages enzymes into lysosomes for cellular use, and modifies proteins destined to become part of cellular membranes.
8. Lysosomes are membranous sacs of acid hydrolases packaged by the Golgi apparatus. Sites of intracellular digestion, they degrade worn-out organelles and tissues that are no longer useful, and they release ionic calcium from bone.
9. Peroxisomes are membranous sacs containing oxidase enzymes that protect the cell from the destructive effects of free radicals and other toxic substances by converting them first to hydrogen peroxide and then water.
10. The cytoskeleton includes microtubules, intermediate filaments, and microfilaments. Microtubules organize the cytoskeleton and are important in intracellular transport. Microfilaments are important in cell motility or movement of cell parts. Motility functions involve motor proteins. Intermediate filaments help cells resist mechanical stress and connect other elements.

Cellular Extensions (pp. 89–91)

11. Centrioles organize the mitotic spindle and are the bases of cilia and flagella.
12. Microvilli are extensions of the plasma membrane that increase its surface area for absorption.

The Nucleus (pp. 91–96)

1. The nucleus is the control center of the cell. Most cells have a single nucleus. Without a nucleus, a cell cannot divide or synthesize more proteins, and is destined to die.
2. The nucleus is surrounded by the nuclear envelope, a double membrane penetrated by fairly large pores.
3. Nucleoli are nuclear sites of ribosome subunit synthesis.
4. Chromatin is a complex network of slender threads containing histone proteins and DNA. The chromatin units are called nucleosomes. When a cell begins to divide, the chromatin coils and condenses, forming chromosomes.

Cell Growth and Reproduction (pp. 96–110)

The Cell Cycle (pp. 96–99)

1. The cell cycle is the series of changes that a cell goes through from the time it is formed until it divides.
2. Interphase is the nondividing phase of the cell cycle. Interphase consists of G_1, S, and G_2 subphases. During G_1, the cell grows and centriole replication begins. During the S phase, DNA replicates. During G_2, the final preparations for division are made. Many checkpoints occur during interphase at which the cell gets the go-ahead signal to go through mitosis or is prevented from continuing to mitosis.
3. DNA replication occurs before cell division, ensuring that both daughter cells have identical genes. The DNA helix uncoils, and each DNA nucleotide strand acts as a template for the formation of a complementary strand. Base pairing provides the guide for the proper positioning of nucleotides.
4. The semiconservative replication of a DNA molecule produces two DNA molecules identical to the parent molecule, each formed of one "old" and one "new" strand.
5. Cell division, essential for body growth and repair, occurs during the M phase. Cell division consists of two distinct phases: mitosis (nuclear division) and cytokinesis (division of the cytoplasm).
6. Mitosis, consisting of prophase, metaphase, anaphase, and telophase, parcels out the replicated chromosomes to two daughter nuclei, each genetically identical to the mother nucleus. Cytokinesis, which begins late in mitosis, divides the cytoplasmic mass into two parts.
7. Cell division is stimulated by certain chemicals (including growth factors and some hormones) and increasing cell size. Lack of space and inhibitory chemicals deter cell division. Cyclin-Cdk complexes regulate cell division.

Protein Synthesis (pp. 99–105)

8. A gene is defined as a DNA segment that provides the instructions to synthesize one polypeptide chain. Since the major structural materials of the body are proteins, and all enzymes are proteins, this amply covers the synthesis of all biological molecules.
9. The base sequence of exon DNA provides the information for protein structure. Each three-base sequence (triplet) calls for a particular amino acid to be built into a polypeptide chain.
10. The RNA molecules acting in protein synthesis are synthesized on single strands of the DNA template. RNA nucleotides are joined according to base-pairing rules.
11. Instructions for making a polypeptide chain are carried from the DNA to the ribosomes via messenger RNA. Ribosomal RNA forms part of the protein synthesis sites. A transfer RNA ferries each amino acid to the ribosome and binds to a codon on the mRNA strand specifying its amino acid.
12. Protein synthesis involves (a) transcription, synthesis of a complementary mRNA, and (b) translation, "reading" of the mRNA by tRNA and peptide bonding of the amino acids into the polypeptide chain. Ribosomes coordinate translation.

Other Roles of DNA (pp. 105–109)

13. Introns and other DNA sequences encode many RNA species that may interfere with or promote the function of specific genes.

Degradation of Organelles and Cytosolic Proteins (pp. 109–110)

14. Organelles and large protein aggregates are picked up by autosomes and delivered to lysosomes for digestion. This process, autophagy, is very important for keeping the cytoplasm free of deteriorating organelles and other debris.

3

15. Soluble proteins that are damaged or no longer needed are targeted for destruction by attachment of ubiquitin. Cytosolic enzymes or proteasomes then degrade these proteins.

Extracellular Materials (p. 110)

1. Extracellular materials are substances found outside the cells. They include body fluids, cellular secretions, and extracellular matrix. Extracellular matrix is particularly abundant in connective tissues.

Developmental Aspects of Cells (pp. 110–111)

1. The first cell of an organism is the fertilized egg. Early in development, cell specialization begins and reflects differential gene activation.

Apoptosis and Modified Rates of Cell Division (p. 110)

2. Apoptosis is programmed cell death. Its function is to dispose of damaged or unnecessary cells.
3. During adulthood, cell numbers remain fairly constant. Cell division occurs primarily to replace lost cells.

Cell Aging (p. 111)

4. Cellular aging may reflect chemical insults, progressive disorders of immunity, or a genetically programmed decline in the rate of cell division with age.

Review Questions

Multiple Choice/Matching

(Some questions have more than one correct answer. Select the best answer or answers from the choices given.)

1. The smallest unit capable of life by itself is **(a)** the organ, **(b)** the organelle, **(c)** the tissue, **(d)** the cell, **(e)** the nucleus.
2. The major types of lipid found in the plasma membranes are (choose two) **(a)** cholesterol, **(b)** triglycerides, **(c)** phospholipids, **(d)** fat-soluble vitamins.
3. Membrane junctions that allow nutrients or ions to flow from cell to cell are **(a)** desmosomes, **(b)** gap junctions, **(c)** tight junctions, **(d)** all of these.
4. The term used to describe the type of solution in which cells will lose water to their environment is **(a)** isotonic, **(b)** hypertonic, **(c)** hypotonic, **(d)** catatonic.
5. Osmosis always involves **(a)** a selectively permeable membrane, **(b)** a difference in solvent concentration, **(c)** diffusion, **(d)** active transport, **(e)** a, b, and c.
6. A physiologist observes that the concentration of sodium inside a cell is decidedly lower than that outside the cell. Sodium diffuses easily across the plasma membrane of such cells when they are dead, but *not* when they are alive. What cellular function that is lacking in dead cells explains the difference? **(a)** osmosis, **(b)** diffusion, **(c)** active transport (solute pumping), **(d)** dialysis.
7. The solute-pumping type of active transport is accomplished by **(a)** exocytosis, **(b)** phagocytosis, **(c)** electrical forces in the cell membrane, **(d)** changes in shape and position of carrier molecules in the plasma membrane.
8. The endocytotic process in which a sampling of particulate matter is engulfed and brought into the cell is called **(a)** phagocytosis, **(b)** pinocytosis, **(c)** exocytosis.
9. Which is *not* true of centrioles? **(a)** They start to duplicate in G_1, **(b)** they lie in the centrosome, **(c)** they are made of microtubules, **(d)** they are membrane-walled barrels lying parallel to each other.
10. The nuclear substance composed of histone proteins and DNA is **(a)** chromatin, **(b)** the nucleolus, **(c)** nuclear sap, or nucleoplasm, **(d)** nuclear pores.
11. The information sequence that determines the nature of a protein is the **(a)** nucleotide, **(b)** gene, **(c)** triplet, **(d)** codon.
12. Mutations may be caused by **(a)** X rays, **(b)** certain chemicals, **(c)** radiation from ionizing radioisotopes, **(d)** all of these.
13. The phase of mitosis during which centrioles reach the poles and chromosomes attach to the spindle is **(a)** anaphase, **(b)** metaphase, **(c)** prophase, **(d)** telophase.
14. Final preparations for cell division are made during the life cycle subphase called **(a)** G_1, **(b)** G_2, **(c)** M, **(d)** S.
15. The RNA synthesized on one of the DNA strands is **(a)** mRNA, **(b)** tRNA, **(c)** rRNA, **(d)** all of these.
16. The RNA species that travels from the nucleus to the cytoplasm carrying the coded message specifying the sequence of amino acids in the protein to be made is **(a)** mRNA, **(b)** tRNA, **(c)** rRNA, **(d)** all of these.
17. If DNA has a sequence of AAA, then a segment of mRNA synthesized on it will have a sequence of **(a)** TTT, **(b)** UUU, **(c)** GGG, **(d)** CCC.
18. A nerve cell and a lymphocyte are presumed to differ in their **(a)** specialized structure, **(b)** suppressed genes and embryonic history, **(c)** genetic information, **(d)** a and b, **(e)** a and c.
19. A pancreas cell makes proteins (enzymes) that it releases to the small intestine. Which of the following best describes the path of these proteins from synthesis to exocytosis at the pancreatic cell's plasma membrane (PM)? **(a)** Golgi → rough ER → PM, **(b)** smooth ER → Golgi → lysosome → PM, **(c)** rough ER → Golgi → PM, **(d)** nucleus → Golgi → PM.

Short Answer Essay Questions

20. Which organelle is responsible for a newborn having distinctive toes and fingers instead of webbed digits?
21. Explain why mitosis can be thought of as cellular immortality.
22. Contrast the roles of ER-bound ribosomes with those free in the cytosol.
23. Cells lining the trachea have whiplike motile extensions on their free surfaces. What are these extensions, what is their source, and what is their function?
24. Name the three phases of interphase and describe an activity unique to each phase.
25. Comment on the role of the sodium-potassium pump in maintaining a cell's resting membrane potential.
26. Differentiate between primary and secondary active transport processes.
27. Cell division typically yields two daughter cells, each with one nucleus. How is the occasional binucleate condition of liver cells explained?

Critical Thinking and Clinical Application Questions

1. Explain why limp celery becomes crisp and the skin of your fingertips wrinkles when placed in tap water. (The principle is exactly the same.)
2. A "red-hot" bacterial infection of the intestinal tract irritates the intestinal cells and interferes with digestion. Such a condition is often accompanied by diarrhea, which causes loss of body water. On the basis of what you have learned about osmotic water flows, explain why diarrhea may occur.
3. Two examples of chemotherapeutic drugs (drugs used to treat cancer) and their cellular actions are listed below. Explain why each drug could be fatal to a cell.
   - Vincristine (brand name Oncovin): damages the mitotic spindle
   - Doxorubicin (Adriamycin): binds to DNA and blocks mRNA synthesis
4. The normal function of one tumor suppressor gene is to prevent cells with damaged chromosomes and DNA from "progressing from G_1 to S," whereas another tumor suppressor gene prevents "passage from G_2 to M." When these tumor suppressor genes fail to work, cancer can result. Explain what the phrases in quotations mean.
5. In their anatomy lab, many students are exposed to the chemical preservatives phenol, formaldehyde, and alcohol. Our cells break down these toxins very effectively. What cellular organelle is responsible for this?
6. Dynein is missing from the cilia and flagella of individuals with a specific inherited disorder. These individuals have severe respiratory problems and, if males, are sterile. What is the structural connection between these two symptoms?
7. Explain why alcoholics are likely to have much more smooth ER than teetotalers.
8. Fresh water is a precious natural resource in Florida and it is said that supplies are dwindling. Desalinizing (removing salt from) ocean water has been recommended as a solution to the problem. Why shouldn't we drink salt water?

AT THE CLINIC

Related Clinical Terms

Anaplasia (an′ah-pla′ze-ah; *an* = without, not; *plas* = to grow) Abnormalities in cell structure and loss of differentiation; for example, cancer cells typically lose the appearance of the parent cells and come to resemble undifferentiated or embryonic cells.

Dysplasia (dis-pla′ze-ah; *dys* = abnormal) A change in cell size, shape, or arrangement due to chronic irritation or inflammation (infections, etc.).

Hypertrophy (hi-per′tro-fe) Growth of an organ or tissue due to an increase in the size of its cells. Hypertrophy is a normal response of skeletal muscle cells when they are challenged to lift excessive weight; differs from hyperplasia, which is an increase in size due to an increase in cell number.

Liposomes (lip′o-sōmz) Hollow microscopic sacs formed of phospholipids that can be filled with a variety of drugs. Serve as multipurpose vehicles for drugs, genetic material, and cosmetics.

Mutation A change in DNA base sequence that may lead to incorporation of incorrect amino acids in particular positions in the resulting protein; the affected protein may remain unimpaired or may function abnormally or not at all, leading to disease.

Necrosis (nĕ-kro′sis; *necros* = death; *osis* = process) Death of a cell or group of cells due to injury or disease. Acute injury causes the cells to swell and burst, and induces the inflammatory response. (This is uncontrolled cell death, in contrast to apoptosis described in the text.)

4

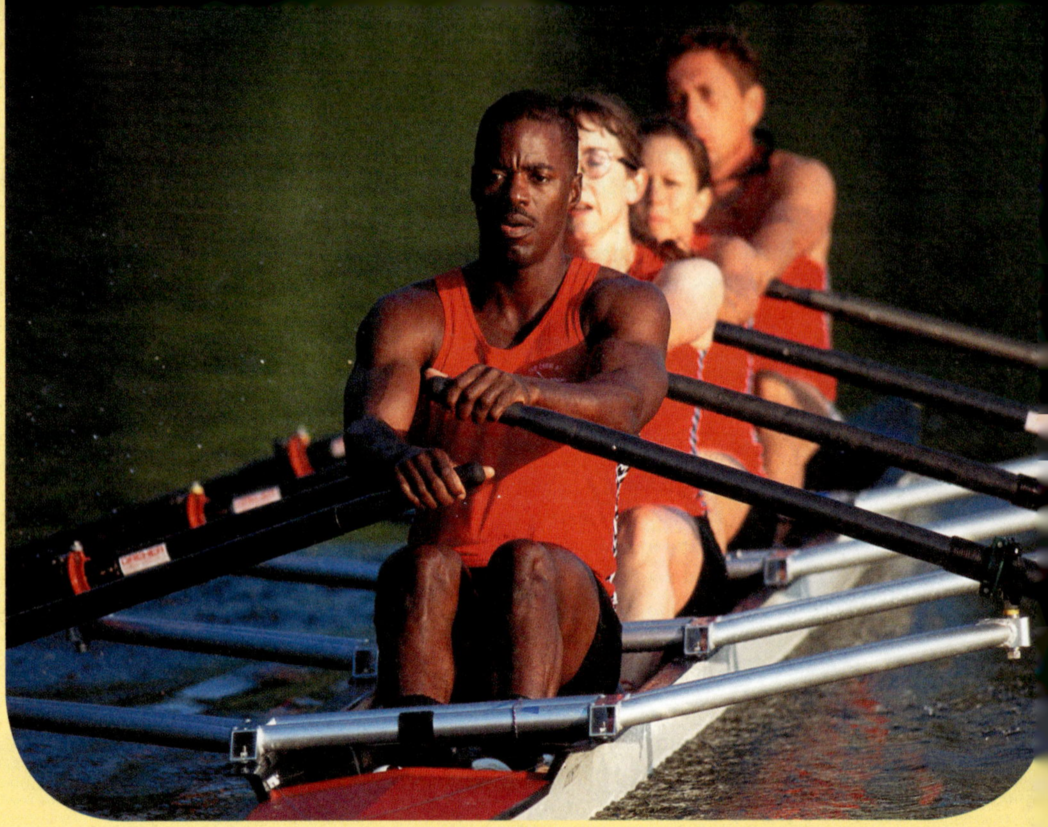

Tissue: The Living Fabric

Unicellular (one-cell) organisms are rugged individualists. Each cell alone obtains and digests its food, ejects its wastes, and carries out all the other activities necessary to keep itself alive and "buzzin' around on all cylinders." But in the multicellular human body, cells do not operate independently. Instead, they form tight cell communities that live and work together.

Individual body cells are specialized, with each type performing specific functions that help maintain homeostasis and benefit the body as a whole. Cell specialization is obvious: Muscle cells look and act differently from skin cells, which in turn are easy to distinguish from brain cells. Cell specialization allows the body to function in sophisticated ways, but division of labor has certain hazards. When a particular group of cells is indispensable, its injury or loss can disable or even destroy the body.

Tissues (*tissu* = woven) are groups of cells that are similar in structure and perform a common or related function. Four primary tissue types interweave to form

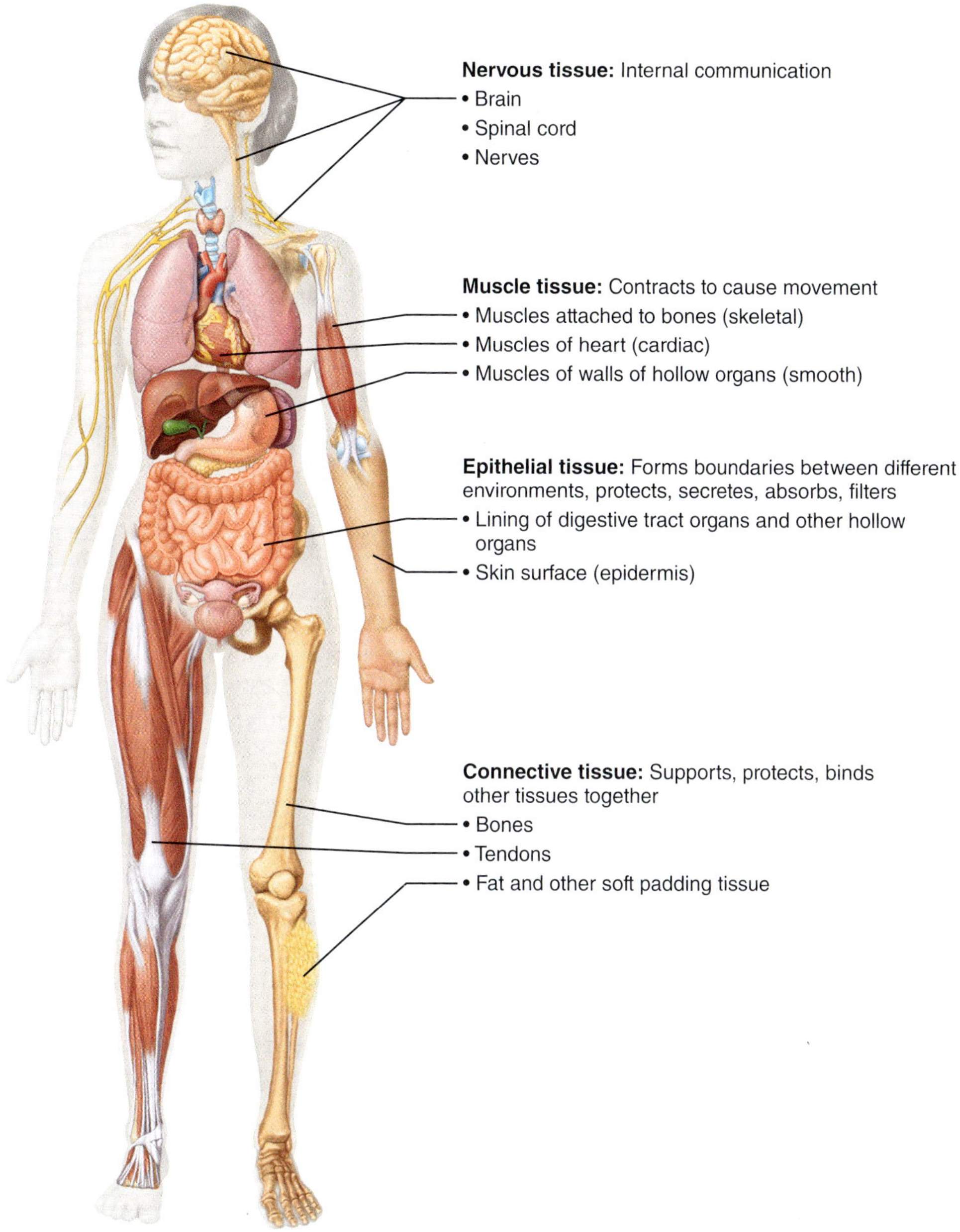

Figure 4.1 Overview of four basic tissue types: epithelial, connective, muscle, and nervous tissues.

the "fabric" of the body. These basic tissues are epithelial, connective, nervous, and muscle tissue.

If we summarized the role of each primary tissue in a single word, we could say that epithelial tissue *covers*, connective tissue *supports*, nervous tissue *controls*, and muscle tissue *produces movement.* However, these words reveal only a fraction of what each tissue does **(Figure 4.1)**.

As we explained in Chapter 1, tissues are organized into organs such as the kidneys and heart. Most organs contain all four tissue types, and their arrangement determines the organ's structure and capabilities. The study of tissues, or **histology**, complements the study of gross anatomy. Together they provide the structural basis for understanding organ physiology.

Preparing Human Tissue for Microscopy

✓ List the steps involved in preparing animal tissue for microscopic viewing.

Microscopy allows us to study tissue structure. Before a specimen can be viewed through a microscope, it must be **fixed** (preserved) and then cut into **sections** (slices) thin enough to transmit light or electrons. Finally, the specimen must be **stained** to enhance contrast.

The stains used in light microscopy are beautifully colored organic dyes, most of which were originally developed by clothing manufacturers in the mid-1800s. Many dyes consist of negatively charged molecules (acidic stains) or positively charged molecules (basic stains) that bind within the tissue to macromolecules of the opposite charge. Different parts of cells and tissues take up different dyes, distinguishing different anatomical structures.

For transmission electron microscopy (TEM), tissue sections are "stained" with heavy metal salts. These metals deflect electrons in the beam to different extents, providing contrast. Electron-microscope images are in shades of gray because color is a property of light, not of electron waves, but the image may be artificially colored to enhance contrast. Another kind of electron microscopy, scanning electron microscopy (SEM), provides three-dimensional pictures of an unsectioned tissue surface.

Preserved tissue we see under the microscope has been exposed to many procedures that alter its original condition and introduce minor distortions called **artifacts**. For this reason, most microscopic structures we view are not exactly like those in living tissue.

Check Your Understanding

1. What is the purpose of fixing tissue for microscopic viewing?
2. What types of stains are used to stain tissues to be viewed with an electron microscope?

For answers, see Appendix H.

Epithelial Tissue

✓ List several structural and functional characteristics of epithelial tissue.

✓ Name, classify, and describe the various types of epithelia, and indicate their chief function(s) and location(s).

Epithelial tissue (ep″ĭ-the′le-ul), or an **epithelium** (plural: epithelia), is a sheet of cells that covers a body surface or lines a body cavity (*epithe* = laid on, covering). Two forms occur in the body:

- *Covering and lining epithelium,* which forms the outer layer of the skin; dips into and lines the open cavities of the urogenital, digestive, and respiratory systems; and covers the walls and organs of the closed ventral body cavity
- *Glandular epithelium,* which fashions the glands of the body

Epithelia form boundaries between different environments, and nearly all substances received or given off by the body must pass through an epithelium. For example, the epidermis of the skin lies between the inside and the outside of the body. Epithelium lining the urinary bladder separates underlying cells of the bladder wall from urine.

In its role as an interface tissue, epithelium accomplishes many functions, including (1) protection, (2) absorption, (3) filtration, (4) excretion, (5) secretion, and (6) sensory reception, all of which will be touched upon later in this chapter.

Special Characteristics of Epithelium

Epithelial tissues have five distinguishing characteristics: polarity, specialized contacts, supported by connective tissues, being avascular but innervated, and having the ability to regenerate.

Polarity

All epithelia have an **apical surface**, an upper free surface exposed to the body exterior or the cavity of an internal organ, and a lower attached **basal surface**. The two surfaces differ in both structure and function. For this reason, we say that epithelia exhibit *apical-basal polarity.*

Although some apical surfaces are smooth and slick, most have **microvilli**, fingerlike extensions of the plasma membrane. Microvilli tremendously increase the exposed surface area. In epithelia that absorb or secrete (export) substances (those lining the intestine or kidney tubules, for instance), the microvilli are often so dense that the cell apices have a fuzzy appearance called a *brush border*. Some epithelia, such as that lining the trachea (windpipe), have motile **cilia** (tiny hairlike projections) that propel substances along their free surface.

Adjacent to the basal surface of an epithelium is a thin supporting sheet called the **basal lamina** (lam′ĭ-nah; "sheet"). This noncellular, adhesive sheet consists largely of glycoproteins secreted by the epithelial cells plus some fine collagen fibers. The basal lamina acts as a selective filter that determines which molecules diffusing from the underlying connective tissue are allowed to enter the epithelium. The basal lamina also acts as scaffolding along which epithelial cells can migrate to repair a wound.

Specialized Contacts

Except for glandular epithelia (discussed on pp. 124–125), epithelial cells fit closely together to form continuous sheets. Lateral contacts, including *tight junctions* and *desmosomes*, bind adjacent cells together at many points (these junctions are described in Chapter 3). The tight junctions help keep proteins in the apical region of the plasma membrane from diffusing into the basal region, and thus help to maintain epithelial polarity.

Supported by Connective Tissue

All epithelial sheets rest upon and are supported by connective tissue. Just deep to the basal lamina is the **reticular lamina**, a layer of extracellular material containing a fine network of collagen protein fibers that "belongs to" the underlying connective tissue. The two laminae form the **basement membrane**, which reinforces the epithelial sheet, helps it resist stretching and tearing, and defines the epithelial boundary.

Homeostatic Imbalance 4.1

An important characteristic of cancerous epithelial cells is their failure to respect the basement membrane boundary, which they penetrate to invade the tissues beneath. +

Avascular but Innervated

Although epithelium is *avascular* (contains no blood vessels), it is *innervated* (supplied by nerve fibers). Epithelial cells are nourished by substances diffusing from blood vessels in the underlying connective tissue.

Regeneration

Epithelium has a high regenerative capacity. Some epithelia are exposed to friction and their surface cells rub off. Others are damaged by hostile substances in the external environment (bacteria, acids, smoke). If and when their apical-basal polarity and lateral contacts are destroyed, epithelial cells begin to reproduce themselves rapidly. As long as epithelial cells receive adequate nutrition, they can replace lost cells by cell division.

☑ Check Your Understanding

3. Epithelial tissue is the only tissue type that has polarity, that is, an apical and a basal surface. Why is this important?
4. Which of the following properties apply to epithelial tissue? Has blood vessels, can repair itself (regenerate), cells joined by lateral contacts.

For answers, see Appendix H.

Classification of Epithelia

Each epithelium has two names. The first name indicates the number of cell layers present, and the second describes the shape of its cells. Based on the number of cell layers, there are simple and stratified epithelia **(Figure 4.2a)**.

- **Simple epithelia** consist of a single cell layer. They are typically found where absorption, secretion, and filtration occur and a thin epithelial barrier is desirable.
- **Stratified epithelia**, composed of two or more cell layers stacked on top of each other, are common in high-abrasion areas where protection is important, such as the skin surface and the lining of the mouth.

In cross section, all epithelial cells have six (somewhat irregular) sides, and an apical surface view of an epithelial sheet looks like a honeycomb. This polyhedral shape allows the cells to be closely packed. However, epithelial cells vary in height, and on that basis, there are three common shapes of epithelial cells (Figure 4.2b):

- **Squamous cells** (skwa′mus) are flattened and scalelike (*squam* = scale).
- **Cuboidal cells** (ku-boi′dahl) are boxlike, approximately as tall as they are wide.
- **Columnar cells** (kŏ-lum′nar) are tall and column shaped.

In each case, the shape of the nucleus conforms to that of the cell. The nucleus of a squamous cell is a flattened disc; that of a cuboidal cell is spherical; and a columnar cell nucleus is elongated from top to bottom and usually located closer to the cell base. Keep nuclear shape in mind when you attempt to identify epithelial types.

Simple epithelia are easy to classify by cell shape because the cells usually have the same shape. In stratified epithelia, however, cell shape differs in the different layers. To avoid ambiguity, stratified epithelia are named according to the shape of the cells in the *apical* layer. This naming system will become clearer as we explore the specific epithelial types.

As you read about the epithelial classes, study **Figure 4.3**. Try to pick out the individual cells within each epithelium. This is not always easy, because the boundaries between epithelial cells often are indistinct. Furthermore, the nucleus of a particular cell may or may not be visible, depending on the plane of the cut made to prepare the tissue slides.

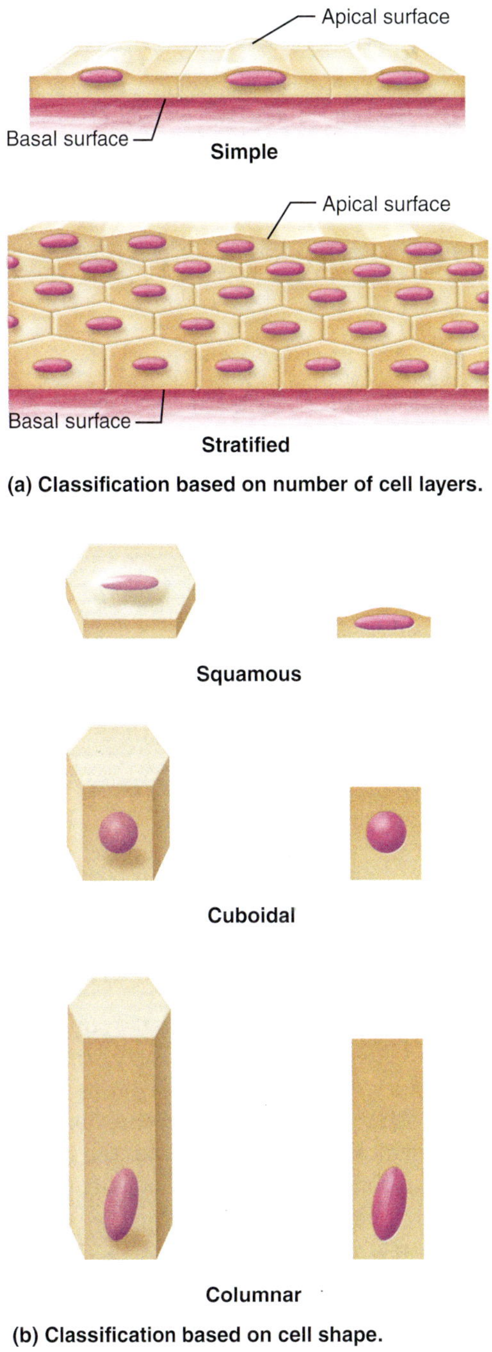

Figure 4.2 Classification of epithelia. Note that cell shape influences the shape of the nucleus.

Simple Epithelia

The simple epithelia are most concerned with absorption, secretion, and filtration. Because they consist of a single cell layer and are usually very thin, protection is not one of their specialties.

(a) Simple squamous epithelium

Description: Single layer of flattened cells with disc-shaped central nuclei and sparse cytoplasm; the simplest of the epithelia.

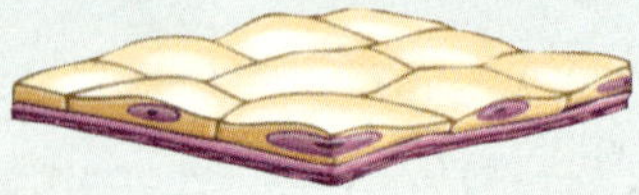

Function: Allows materials to pass by diffusion and filtration in sites where protection is not important; secretes lubricating substances in serosae.

Location: Kidney glomeruli; air sacs of lungs; lining of heart, blood vessels, and lymphatic vessels; lining of ventral body cavity (serosae).

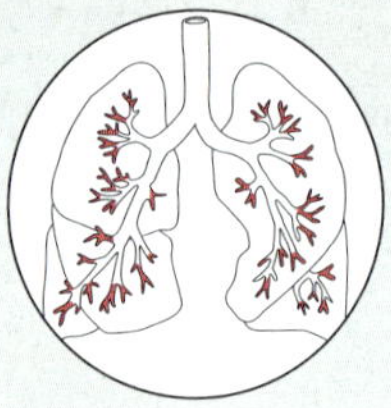

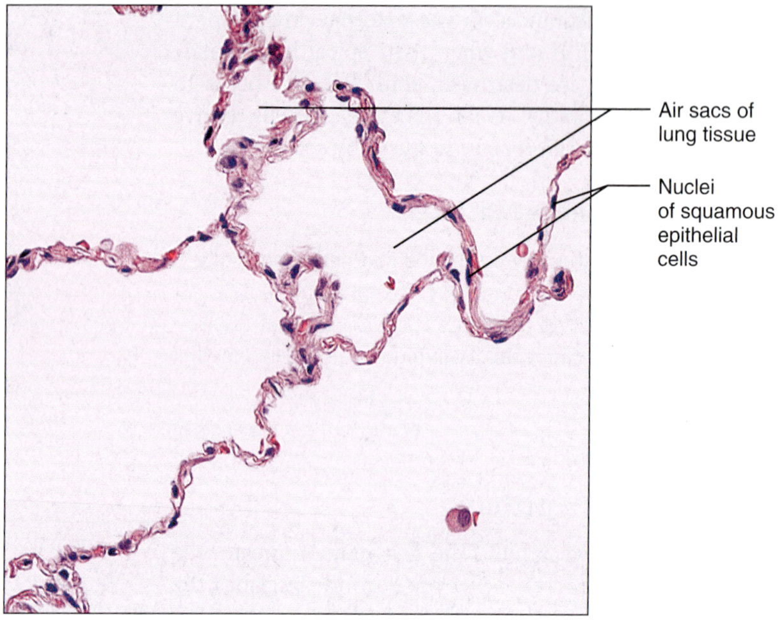

Photomicrograph: Simple squamous epithelium forming part of the alveolar (air sac) walls (140×).

Figure 4.3 Epithelial tissues. (a) Simple epithelium. (For related images, see *A Brief Atlas of the Human Body*, Plates 1 and 2.)

Simple Squamous Epithelium The cells of a **simple squamous epithelium** are flattened laterally, and their cytoplasm is sparse (Figure 4.3a). In a surface view, the close-fitting cells resemble a tiled floor. When the cells are cut perpendicular to their free surface, they resemble fried eggs seen from the side, with their cytoplasm wisping out from the slightly bulging nucleus.

Thin and often permeable, simple squamous epithelium is found where filtration or the exchange of substances by rapid diffusion is a priority. In the kidneys, it forms part of the filtration membrane. In the lungs, it forms the walls of the air sacs across which gas exchange occurs (Figure 4.3a).

Two simple squamous epithelia in the body have special names that reflect their location.

- **Endothelium** (en″do-the′le-um; "inner covering") provides a slick, friction-reducing lining in lymphatic vessels and in all hollow organs of the cardiovascular system—blood vessels and the heart. Capillaries consist exclusively of endothelium, and its exceptional thinness encourages the efficient exchange of nutrients and wastes between the bloodstream and surrounding tissue cells.
- **Mesothelium** (mez″o-the′le-um; "middle covering") is the epithelium found in serous membranes, the membranes lining the ventral body cavity and covering its organs.

Simple Cuboidal Epithelium **Simple cuboidal epithelium** consists of a single layer of cells as tall as they are wide (Figure 4.3b). The spherical nuclei stain darkly, causing the cell layer to look like a string of beads when viewed microscopically. Important functions of simple cuboidal epithelium are secretion and absorption. This epithelium forms the walls of the smallest ducts of glands and of many kidney tubules.

Simple Columnar Epithelium **Simple columnar epithelium** is a single layer of tall, closely packed cells, aligned like soldiers in a row (Figure 4.3c). It lines the digestive tract from the stomach through the rectum. Columnar cells are mostly associated with absorption and secretion, and the digestive tract lining has two distinct modifications that make it ideal for that dual function:

- Dense microvilli on the apical surface of absorptive cells
- Tubular glands made primarily of cells that secrete mucus-containing intestinal juice

Additionally, some simple columnar epithelia display cilia on their free surfaces, which help move substances or cells through an internal passageway.

Pseudostratified Columnar Epithelium The cells of **pseudostratified columnar epithelium** (soo″do-stră′tĭ-fīd) vary in height (Figure 4.3d). All of its cells rest on the basement membrane, but only the tallest reach the free surface of the epithelium. Because the cell nuclei lie at different levels above the basement membrane, the tissue gives the false (pseudo) impression that

(b) Simple cuboidal epithelium

Description: Single layer of cubelike cells with large, spherical central nuclei.

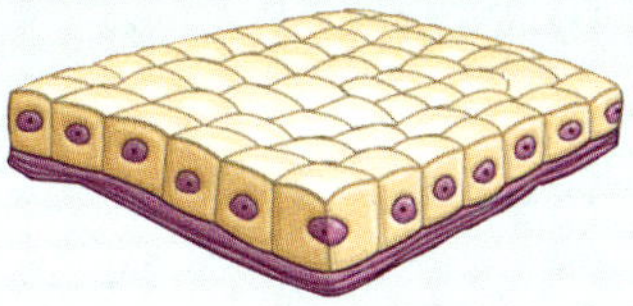

Function: Secretion and absorption.

Location: Kidney tubules; ducts and secretory portions of small glands; ovary surface.

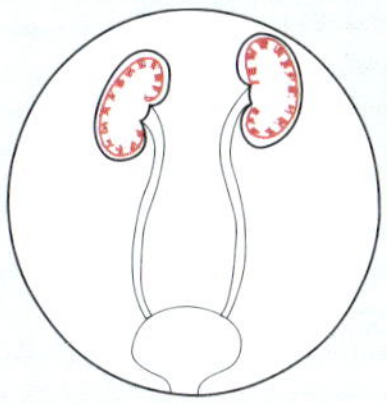

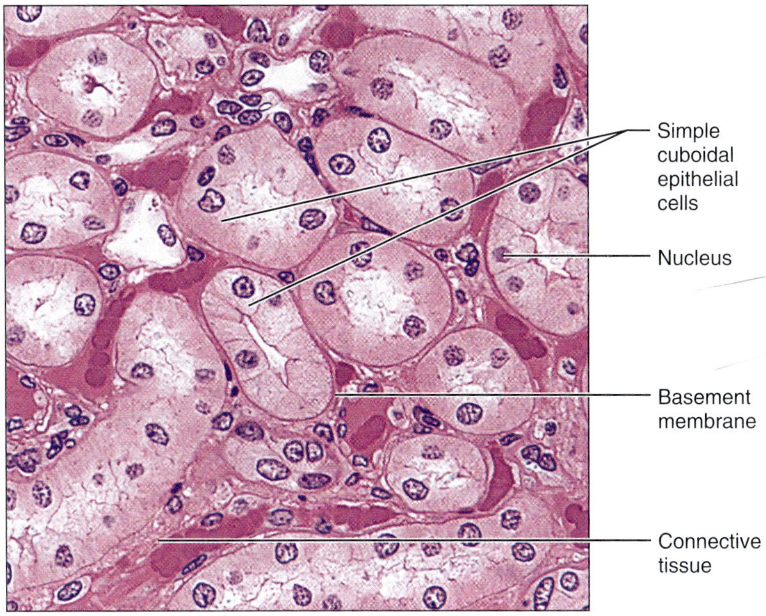

Photomicrograph: Simple cuboidal epithelium in kidney tubules (430×).

(c) Simple columnar epithelium

Description: Single layer of tall cells with *round* to *oval* nuclei; some cells bear cilia; layer may contain mucus-secreting unicellular glands (goblet cells).

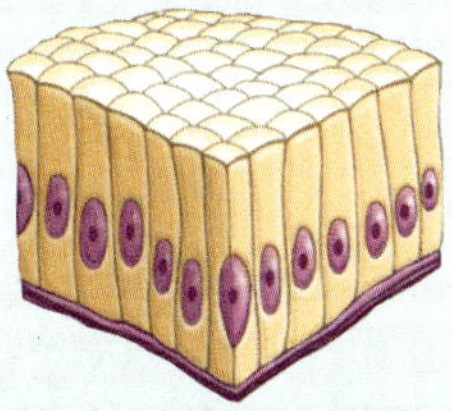

Function: Absorption; secretion of mucus, enzymes, and other substances; ciliated type propels mucus (or reproductive cells) by ciliary action.

Location: Nonciliated type lines most of the digestive tract (stomach to rectum), gallbladder, and excretory ducts of some glands; ciliated variety lines small bronchi, uterine tubes, and some regions of the uterus.

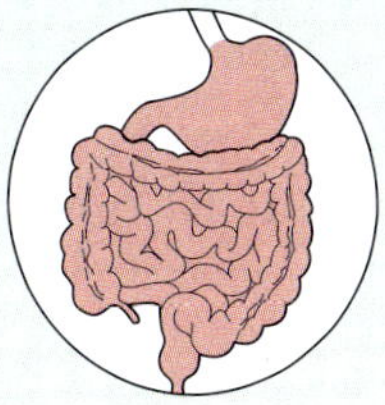

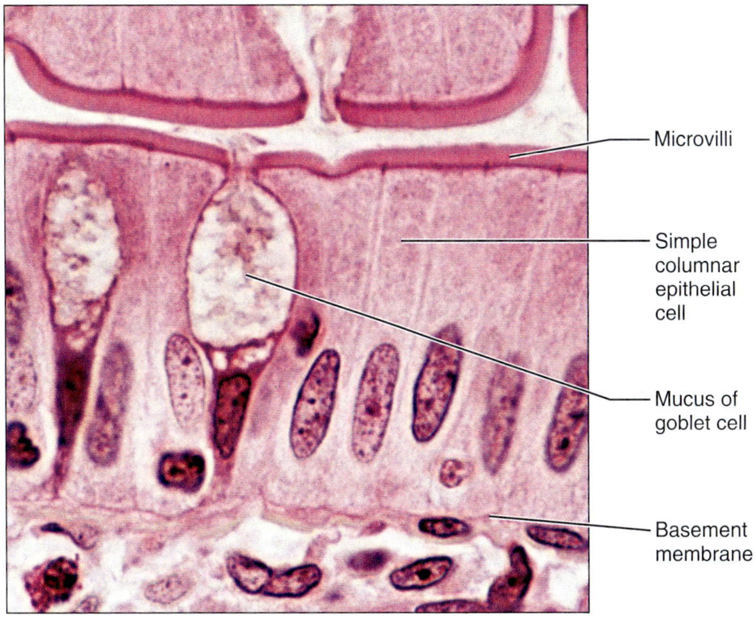

Photomicrograph: Simple columnar epithelium of the small intestine mucosa (660×).

Figure 4.3 *(continued)* **(b)** and **(c)** Simple epithelium. (For related images, see *A Brief Atlas of the Human Body*, Plates 3, 4, and 5.)

(d) Pseudostratified columnar epithelium

Description: Single layer of cells of differing heights, some not reaching the free surface; nuclei seen at different levels; may contain mucus-secreting cells and bear cilia.

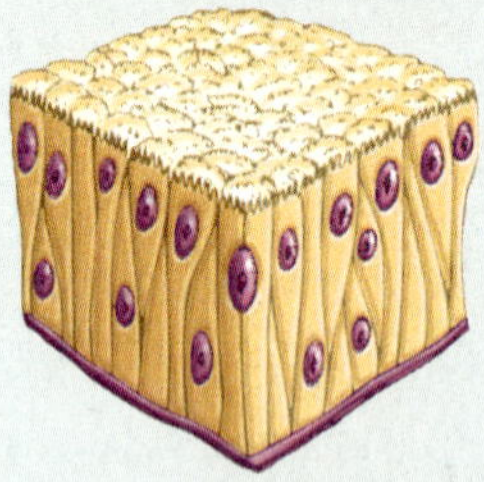

Function: Secrete substances, particularly mucus; propulsion of mucus by ciliary action.

Location: Nonciliated type in male's sperm-carrying ducts and ducts of large glands; ciliated variety lines the trachea, most of the upper respiratory tract.

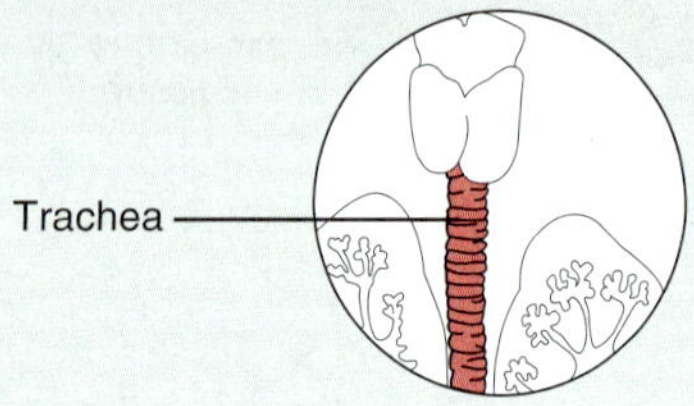

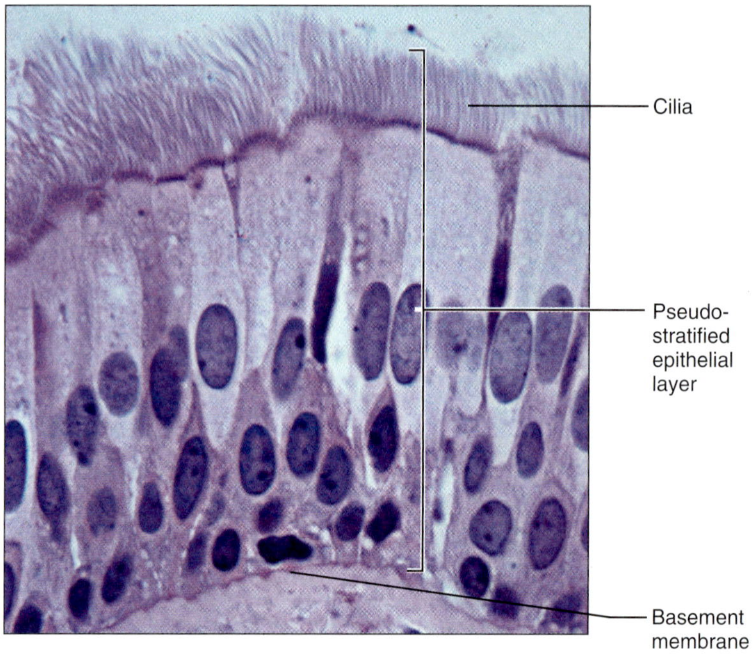

Photomicrograph: Pseudostratified ciliated columnar epithelium lining the human trachea (800×).

Figure 4.3 *(continued)* **Epithelial tissues. (d)** Simple epithelium. (For a related image, see *A Brief Atlas of the Human Body*, Plate 6.)

several cell layers are present; hence "pseudostratified." The short cells are relatively unspecialized and give rise to the taller cells. This epithelium, like the simple columnar variety, secretes or absorbs substances. A ciliated version containing mucus-secreting cells lines most of the respiratory tract. Here the motile cilia propel sheets of dust-trapping mucus superiorly away from the lungs.

Stratified Epithelia

Stratified epithelia contain two or more cell layers. They regenerate from below; that is, the basal cells divide and push apically to replace the older surface cells. Stratified epithelia are considerably more durable than simple epithelia, and protection is their major (but not their only) role.

Stratified Squamous Epithelium **Stratified squamous epithelium** is the most widespread of the stratified epithelia (Figure 4.3e). Composed of several layers, it is thick and well suited for its protective role in the body. Its free surface cells are squamous, and cells of the deeper layers are cuboidal or columnar. This epithelium is found in areas subjected to wear and tear, and its surface cells are constantly being rubbed away and replaced by division of its basal cells. Because epithelium depends on nutrients diffusing from deeper connective tissue, the epithelial cells farther from the basement membrane are less viable and those at the apical surface are often flattened and atrophied.

To avoid memorizing all its locations, simply remember that this epithelium forms the external part of the skin and extends a short distance into every body opening that is directly continuous with the skin. The outer layer, or epidermis, of the skin is *keratinized* (ker′ah-tin″īzd), meaning its surface cells contain *keratin*, a tough protective protein. (We discuss the epidermis in Chapter 5.) The other stratified squamous epithelia of the body are *nonkeratinized.*

Stratified Cuboidal and Columnar Epithelia **Stratified cuboidal epithelium** is quite rare in the body, mostly found in the ducts of some of the larger glands (sweat glands, mammary glands). It typically has two layers of cuboidal cells.

Stratified columnar epithelium also has a limited distribution in the body. Small amounts are found in the pharynx, the male urethra, and lining some glandular ducts. This epithelium also occurs at transition areas or junctions between two other types of epithelia. Only its apical layer of cells is columnar. Because of their relative scarcity in the body, Figure 4.3 does not illustrate these two stratified epithelia (but see *A Brief Atlas of the Human Body*, Plates 8 and 9).

Transitional Epithelium **Transitional epithelium** forms the lining of hollow urinary organs, which stretch as they fill with urine (Figure 4.3f). Cells of its basal layer are cuboidal or columnar. The apical cells vary in appearance, depending on the degree of distension (stretching) of the organ. When the organ is distended with urine, the transitional epithelium thins from about six cell layers to three, and its domelike apical cells flatten

(e) Stratified squamous epithelium

Description: Thick membrane composed of several cell layers; basal cells are cuboidal or columnar and metabolically active; surface cells are flattened (squamous); in the keratinized type, the surface cells are full of keratin and dead; basal cells are active in mitosis and produce the cells of the more superficial layers.

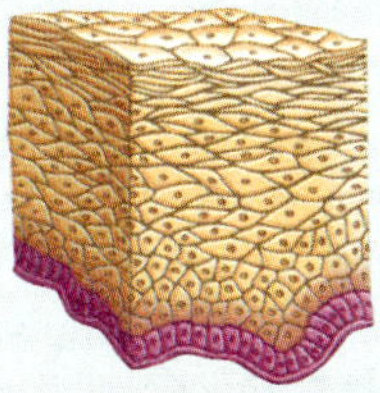

Function: Protects underlying tissues in areas subjected to abrasion.

Location: Nonkeratinized type forms the moist linings of the esophagus, mouth, and vagina; keratinized variety forms the epidermis of the skin, a dry membrane.

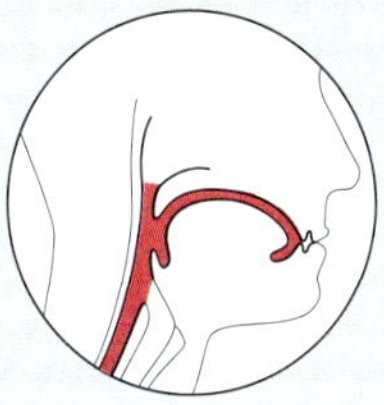

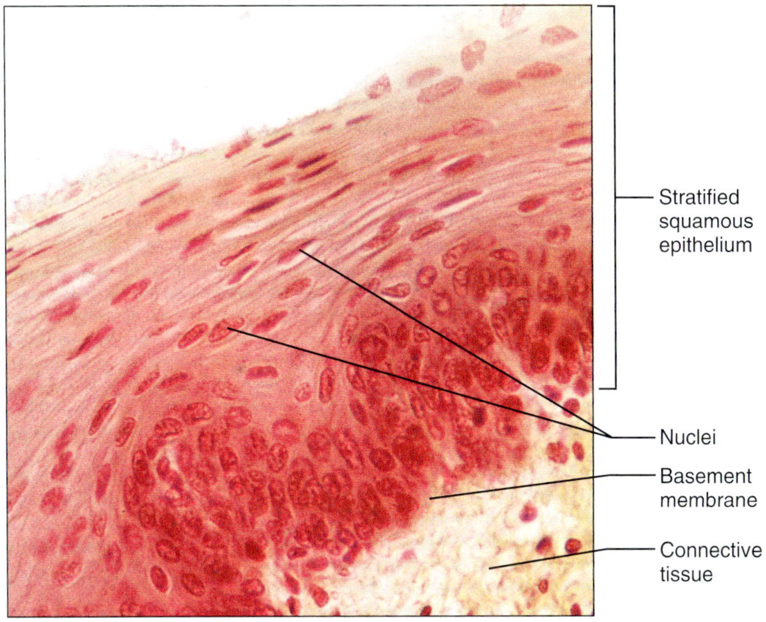

Photomicrograph: Stratified squamous epithelium lining the esophagus (285×).

(f) Transitional epithelium

Description: Resembles both stratified squamous and stratified cuboidal; basal cells cuboidal or columnar; surface cells dome shaped or squamouslike, depending on degree of organ stretch.

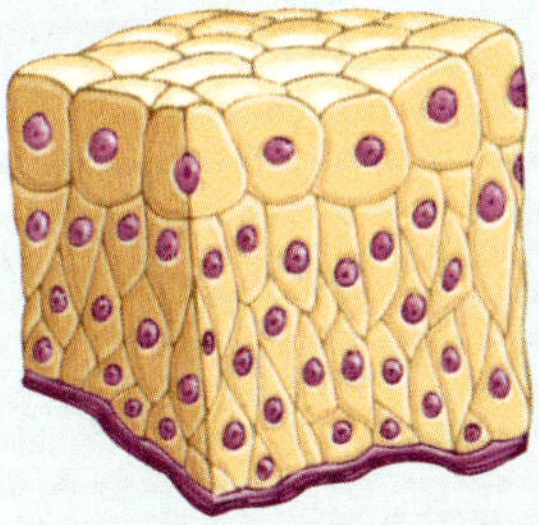

Function: Stretches readily, permits stored urine to distend urinary organ.

Location: Lines the ureters, bladder, and part of the urethra.

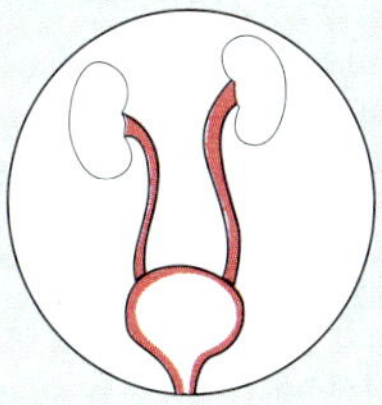

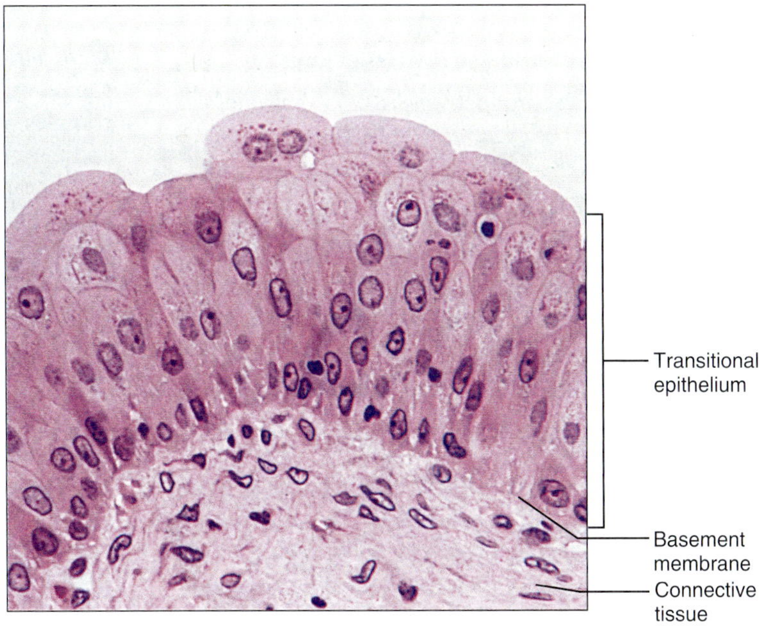

Photomicrograph: Transitional epithelium lining the bladder, relaxed state (360×); note the bulbous, or rounded, appearance of the cells at the surface; these cells flatten and elongate when the bladder fills with urine.

Figure 4.3 *(continued)* **(e)** and **(f)** Stratified epithelium. (For related images, see *A Brief Atlas of the Human Body*, Plates 7 and 10.)

and become squamouslike. The ability of transitional cells to change their shape (undergo "transitions") allows a greater volume of urine to flow through a tubelike organ. In the bladder, it allows more urine to be stored.

Check Your Understanding

5. Stratified epithelia are "built" for protection or to resist abrasion. What are the simple epithelia better at?
6. Some epithelia are pseudostratified. What does this mean?
7. Where is transitional epithelium found and what is its importance at those sites?

For answers, see Appendix H.

Glandular Epithelia

- ✓ Define gland.
- ✓ Differentiate between exocrine and endocrine glands, and between multicellular and unicellular glands.
- ✓ Describe how multicellular exocrine glands are classified structurally and functionally.

A **gland** consists of one or more cells that make and secrete a particular product. This product, called a **secretion**, is an aqueous (water-based) fluid that usually contains proteins, but there is variation. For example, some glands release a lipid- or steroid-rich secretion.

Secretion is an active process. Glandular cells obtain needed substances from the blood and transform them chemically into a product that is then discharged from the cell. Notice that the term *secretion* can refer to both the gland's *product* and the *process* of making and releasing that product.

Glands are classified according to two sets of traits:

- Where they release their product—glands may be *endocrine* ("internally secreting") or *exocrine* ("externally secreting")
- Relative cell number—glands may be *unicellular* ("one-celled") or *multicellular* ("many-celled")

Unicellular glands are scattered within epithelial sheets. By contrast, most multicellular epithelial glands form by invagination (inward growth) of an epithelial sheet into the underlying connective tissue. At least initially, most have *ducts*, tubelike connections to the epithelial sheets.

Endocrine Glands

Because **endocrine glands** eventually lose their ducts, they are often called *ductless glands*. They produce **hormones**, messenger chemicals that they secrete by exocytosis directly into the extracellular space. From there the hormones enter the blood or lymphatic fluid and travel to specific target organs. Each hormone prompts its target organ(s) to respond in some characteristic way. For example, hormones produced by certain intestinal cells cause the pancreas to release enzymes that help digest food in the digestive tract.

Endocrine glands are structurally diverse, so one description does not fit all. Most are compact multicellular organs, but some individual hormone-producing cells are scattered in the digestive tract lining (mucosa) and in the brain, giving rise to their collective description as the *diffuse endocrine system*. Endocrine secretions are also varied, ranging from modified amino acids to peptides, glycoproteins, and steroids. Since not all endocrine glands are epithelial derivatives, we defer consideration of their structure and function to Chapter 16.

Exocrine Glands

All **exocrine glands** secrete their products onto body surfaces (skin) or into body cavities. The unicellular glands do so directly (by exocytosis), whereas the multicellular glands do so via an epithelium-walled duct that transports the secretion to the epithelial surface. Exocrine glands are a diverse lot and many of their products are familiar. They include mucous, sweat, oil, and salivary glands, the liver (which secretes bile), the pancreas (which synthesizes digestive enzymes), and many others.

Unicellular Exocrine Glands The only important examples of **unicellular** (or one-celled) glands are *mucous cells* and *goblet cells*. Unicellular glands are sprinkled in the epithelial linings of the intestinal and respiratory tracts amid columnar cells with other functions (see Figure 4.3c).

In humans, all such glands produce **mucin** (mu′sin), a complex glycoprotein that dissolves in water when secreted. Once dissolved, mucin forms mucus, a slimy coating that protects and lubricates surfaces. In **goblet cells** the cuplike accumulation of mucin distends the top of the cell, making the cells look like a glass with a stem (thus "goblet" cell, **Figure 4.4**). This distortion does not occur in **mucous cells**.

Multicellular Exocrine Glands Compared to the unicellular glands, **multicellular exocrine glands** are structurally more complex. They have two basic parts: an epithelium-derived *duct* and a *secretory unit* (*acinus*) consisting of secretory cells. In all but the simplest glands, *supportive connective tissue* surrounds the secretory unit and supplies it with blood vessels and nerve fibers, and forms a *fibrous capsule* that extends into the gland and divides it into *lobes.*

Multicellular exocrine glands can be classified by structure and by type of secretion.

- **Structural classification.** On the basis of their duct structures, multicellular exocrine glands are either simple or compound **(Figure 4.5)**. **Simple glands** have an unbranched duct, whereas **compound glands** have a branched duct. The glands are further categorized by their secretory units as (1) **tubular** if the secretory cells form tubes; (2) **alveolar** (al-ve′o-lar) if the secretory cells form small, flasklike sacs (*alveolus* = "small hollow cavity"); or (3) **tubuloalveolar** if they have both types of secretory units. Note that the term **acinar** (as′ĭ-nar; "berrylike") is used interchangeably with alveolar.
- **Modes of secretion.** Multicellular exocrine glands secrete their products in different ways, so they can also be

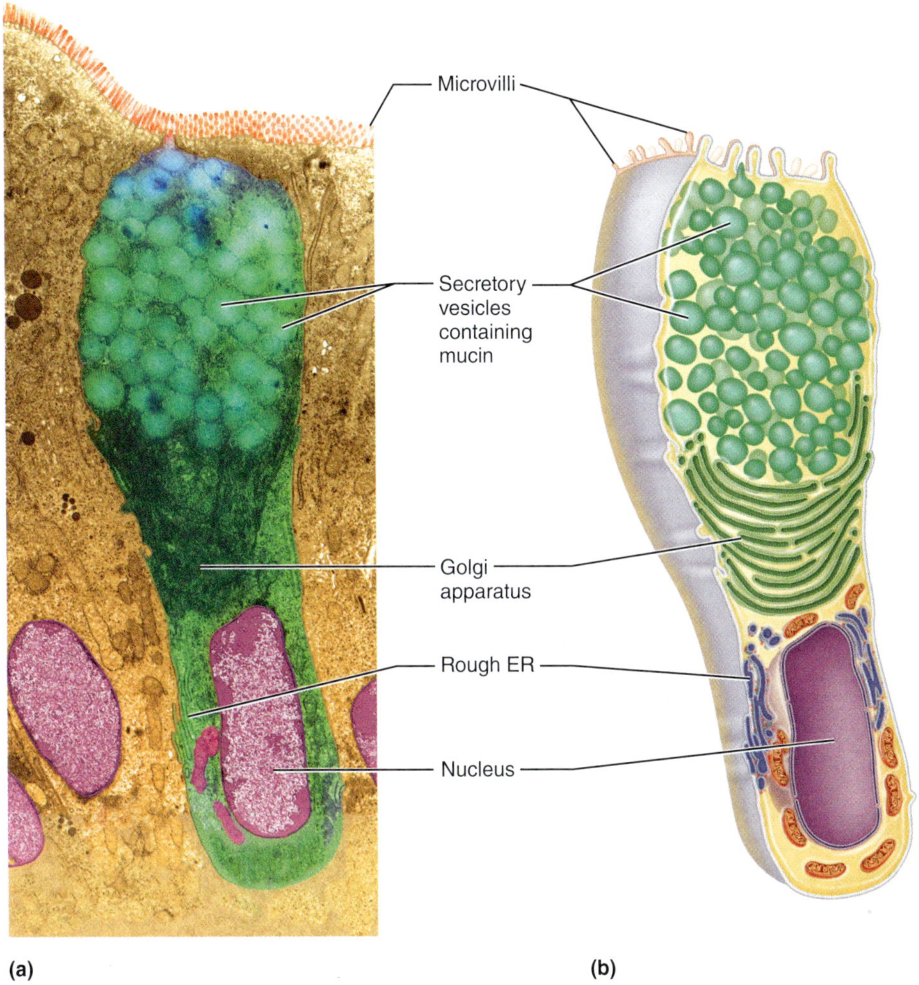

Figure 4.4 Goblet cell (unicellular exocrine gland). (a) Photomicrograph of a goblet cell in the simple columnar epithelium lining the small intestine (1640×). **(b)** Corresponding diagram. Notice the secretory vesicles and well-developed rough ER and Golgi apparatus.

described functionally as *merocrine*, *holocrine*, or *apocrine* glands. Most are **merocrine glands** (mer′o-krin), which secrete their products by exocytosis as they are produced. The secretory cells are not altered in any way (so think "merely secrete" to remember their mode of secretion). The pancreas, most sweat glands, and salivary glands belong to this class **(Figure 4.6a)**.

Secretory cells of **holocrine glands** (hol′o-krin) accumulate their products within them until they rupture. (They are replaced by the division of underlying cells.) Because holocrine gland secretions include the synthesized product plus dead cell fragments (*holo* = whole, all), you could say that their cells "die for their cause." Sebaceous (oil) glands of the skin are the only true example of holocrine glands (Figure 4.6b).

Although *apocrine glands* (ap′o-krin) are present in other animals, there is some controversy over whether humans have this third gland type. Like holocrine glands, apocrine glands accumulate their products, but in this case only just beneath the free surface. Eventually, the apex of the cell pinches off (*apo* = from, off), releasing the secretory granules and a small amount of cytoplasm. The cell repairs its damage and the process repeats again and again. The best possibility in humans is the release of lipid droplets by lactating mammary glands, but most histologists classify mammary glands as merocrine glands because this is the means by which milk proteins are secreted.

☑ Check Your Understanding

8. What common secretion do all unicellular exocrine glands produce?
9. How are multicellular exocrine glands classified?
10. Which gland type—merocrine or holocrine—would you expect to have the highest rate of cell division? Why?

For answers, see Appendix H.

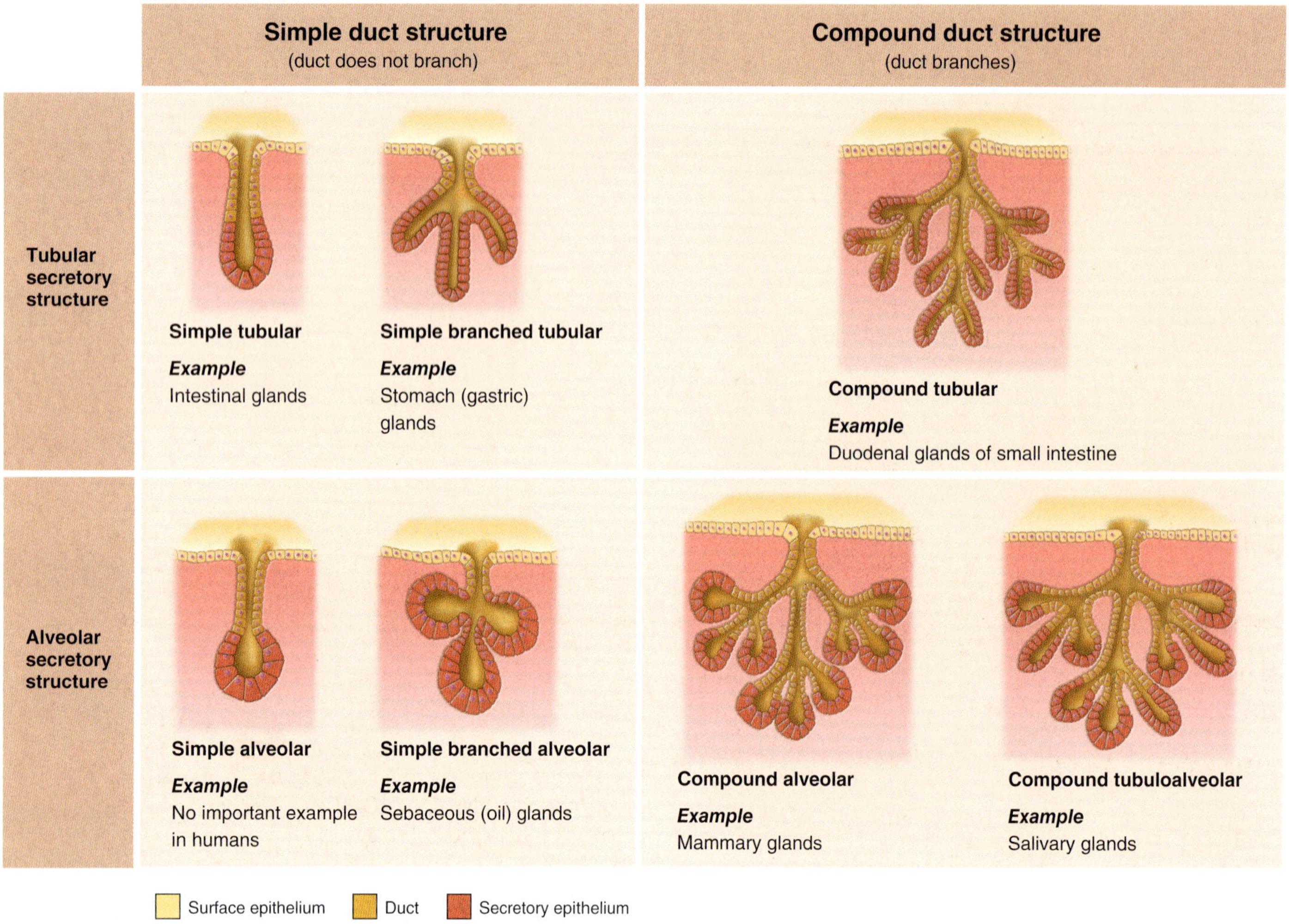

Figure 4.5 Types of multicellular exocrine glands. Multicellular glands are classified according to duct type (simple or compound) and the structure of their secretory units (tubular, alveolar, or tubuloalveolar).

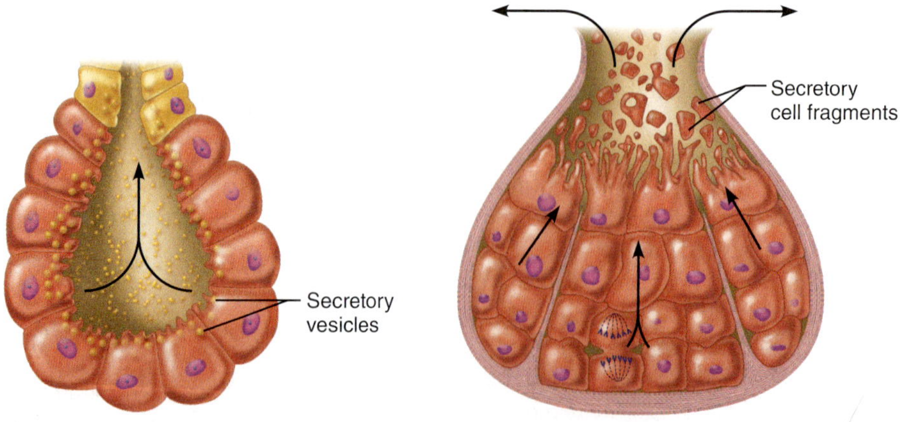

(a) Merocrine glands secrete their products by exocytosis.

(b) In holocrine glands, the entire secretory cell ruptures, releasing secretions and dead cell fragments.

Figure 4.6 Chief modes of secretion in human exocrine glands.

Connective Tissue

✓ Indicate common characteristics of connective tissue, and list and describe its structural elements.

Connective tissue is the most abundant and widely distributed of the primary tissues, but its amount in particular organs varies. For example, skin consists primarily of connective tissue, while the brain contains very little.

There are four main classes of connective tissue and several subclasses (**Table 4.1** on p. 129). The main classes are (1) *connective tissue proper* (which includes fat and the fibrous tissue of ligaments), (2) *cartilage*, (3) *bone*, and (4) *blood*.

Connective tissue does much more than just *connect* body parts. Its major functions include (1) *binding and supporting*, (2) *protecting*, (3) *insulating*, (4) *storing* reserve fuel, and (5) *transporting* substances within the body. For example, bone and cartilage support and protect body organs by providing the hard underpinnings of the skeleton. Fat insulates and protects body organs and provides a fuel reserve. Blood transports substances inside the body.

Common Characteristics of Connective Tissue

Connective tissues share three characteristics that set them apart from other primary tissues:

- **Common origin.** All connective tissues arise from *mesenchyme* (an embryonic tissue).
- **Degrees of vascularity.** Connective tissues run the gamut of vascularity. Cartilage is avascular. Dense connective tissue is poorly vascularized, and the other types of connective tissue have a rich supply of blood vessels.
- **Extracellular matrix.** All other primary tissues are composed mainly of cells, but connective tissues are largely nonliving **extracellular matrix** (ma′triks; "womb"), which separates, often widely, the living cells of the tissue. Because of its matrix, connective tissue can bear weight, withstand great tension, and endure abuses, such as physical trauma and abrasion that no other tissue can tolerate.

Structural Elements of Connective Tissue

Connective tissues have three main elements: *ground substance*, *fibers*, and *cells* (Table 4.1). Together ground substance and fibers make up the extracellular matrix. (Note that some authors use the term *matrix* to indicate the ground substance only.)

The composition and arrangement of these three elements vary tremendously. The result is an amazing diversity of connective tissues, each adapted to perform a specific function in the body. For example, the matrix can be delicate and fragile to form a soft "packing" around an organ, or it can form "ropes" (tendons and ligaments) of incredible strength. Nonetheless, connective tissues have a common structural plan, and we use *areolar connective tissue* (ah-re′o-lar) as our *prototype*, or model (**Figure 4.7** and Figure 4.8a). All other subclasses are simply variants of this plan.

Ground Substance

Ground substance is the unstructured material that fills the space between the cells and contains the fibers. It is composed of *interstitial (tissue) fluid, cell adhesion proteins*, and *proteoglycans* (pro″te-o-gli′kanz). Cell adhesion proteins (*fibronectin, laminin*, and others) serve mainly as a connective tissue glue that allows connective tissue cells to attach to matrix elements. The proteoglycans consist of a protein core to which *glycosaminoglycans* (GAGs) (gli″kos-ah-me″no-gli′kanz) are attached. The strand-like GAGs, most importantly *chondroitin sulfate* and *hyaluronic acid* (hi″ah-lu-ron′ik), are large, negatively charged polysaccharides that stick out from the core protein like the fibers of a bottle brush. The proteoglycans tend to form huge aggregates in which the GAGs intertwine and trap water, forming a substance that varies from a fluid to a viscous gel. The higher the GAG content, the more viscous the ground substance.

The ground substance consists of large amounts of fluid and functions as a molecular sieve, or medium, through which nutrients and other dissolved substances can diffuse between the blood capillaries and the cells. The fibers embedded in the ground substance make it less pliable and hinder diffusion somewhat.

Connective Tissue Fibers

The fibers of connective tissue provide support. Three types of fibers are found in connective tissue matrix: collagen, elastic, and reticular fibers. Of these, collagen fibers are by far the strongest and most abundant.

Collagen fibers are constructed primarily of the fibrous protein *collagen*. Collagen molecules are secreted into the extracellular space, where they assemble spontaneously into cross-linked fibrils, which in turn are bundled together into the thick collagen fibers seen with a microscope. Because their fibrils cross-link, collagen fibers are extremely tough and provide high tensile strength (that is, the ability to resist being pulled apart) to the matrix. Indeed, stress tests show that collagen fibers are stronger than steel fibers of the same size!

Elastic fibers are long, thin fibers that form branching networks in the extracellular matrix. These fibers contain a rubber-like protein, *elastin*, that allows them to stretch and recoil like rubber bands. Connective tissue can stretch only so much before its thick, ropelike collagen fibers become taut. Then, when the tension lets up, elastic fibers snap the connective tissue back to its normal length and shape. Elastic fibers are found where greater elasticity is needed, for example, in the skin, lungs, and blood vessel walls.

Reticular fibers are short, fine, collagenous fibers with a slightly different chemistry and form. They are continuous with collagen fibers, and they branch extensively, forming delicate networks (*reticul* = network) that surround small blood vessels and support the soft tissue of organs. They are particularly abundant where connective tissue abuts other tissue types, for example, in the basement membrane of epithelial tissues, and around capillaries, where they form fuzzy "nets" that allow more "give" than the larger collagen fibers.

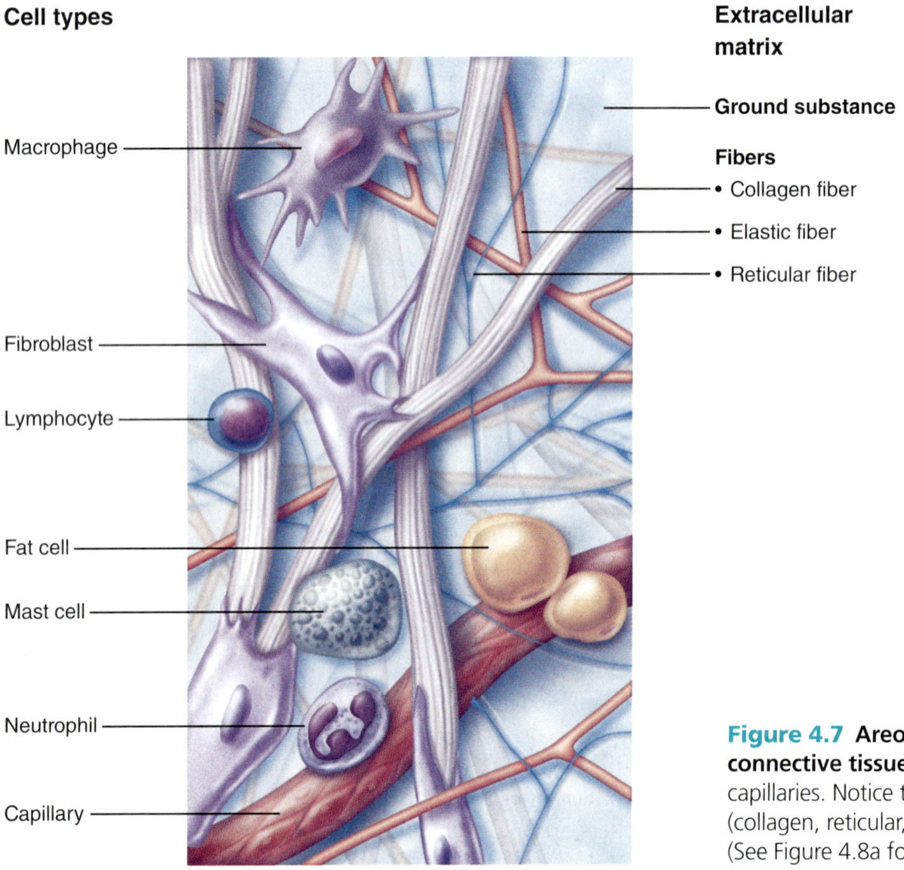

Figure 4.7 Areolar connective tissue: A prototype (model) connective tissue. This tissue underlies epithelia and surrounds capillaries. Notice the various cell types and three classes of fibers (collagen, reticular, elastic) embedded in the ground substance. (See Figure 4.8a for a less idealized version.)

Connective Tissue Cells

Each major class of connective tissue has a resident cell type that exists in immature and mature forms (see Table 4.1). The immature (undifferentiated) cells, indicated by the suffix *blast* (literally, "bud" or "sprout," but the suffix means "forming"), are actively mitotic cells that secrete the ground substance and the fibers characteristic of their particular matrix. As listed in the third column of Table 4.1, the primary blast cell types by connective tissue class are (1) connective tissue proper: **fibroblast**; (2) cartilage: **chondroblast** (kon′dro-blast″); and (3) bone: **osteoblast** (os′te-o-blast″). The **hematopoietic stem cell** (hem″ah-to-poy-et′ik), which is the undifferentiated blast cell that produces blood cells, is not included in Table 4.1 because it is not located in "its" tissue (blood) and does not make the fluid matrix (plasma) of that tissue. Blood formation is considered in Chapter 17.

Once they synthesize the matrix, the blast cells assume their mature, less active mode, indicated by the suffix *cyte* (Table 4.1, third column). The mature cells maintain the health of the matrix. However, if the matrix is injured, they can easily revert to their more active state to repair and regenerate the matrix. (The blood-forming stem cells are always actively mitotic.)

Additionally, connective tissue is home to an assortment of other cell types, such as

- **Fat cells**, which store nutrients.
- **White blood cells** (neutrophils, eosinophils, lymphocytes), and other cell types that are concerned with tissue response to injury.
- **Mast cells**, which typically cluster along blood vessels. These oval cells detect foreign microorganisms (e.g., bacteria, fungi) and initiate local inflammatory responses against them. In mast cell cytoplasm are secretory granules (*mast* = stuffed full of granules) containing chemicals that mediate inflammation, especially in severe allergies. These chemicals include
  - *Heparin* (hep′ah-rin), an anticoagulant chemical that prevents blood clotting when free in the bloodstream (but in human mast cells it appears to regulate the action of other mast cell chemicals)
  - *Histamine* (his′tah-mēn), a substance that makes capillaries leaky
  - *Proteases* (protein-degrading enzymes)
  - Various other enzymes
- **Macrophages** (mak′ro-fāj″-es; *macro* = large; *phago* = eat), large, irregularly shaped cells that avidly phagocytize a broad variety of foreign materials, ranging from foreign molecules to entire bacteria to dust particles. These "big eaters" also dispose of dead tissue cells, and they are central actors in the immune system. Macrophages, which are peppered throughout loose connective tissue, bone marrow, and lymphatic tissue, may be attached to connective tissue fibers (fixed) or may migrate freely through the matrix. Some macrophages have

Table 4.1 Comparison of Classes of Connective Tissues

TISSUE CLASS AND EXAMPLE	SUBCLASSES	COMPONENTS: CELLS	COMPONENTS: MATRIX	GENERAL FEATURES
Connective Tissue Proper 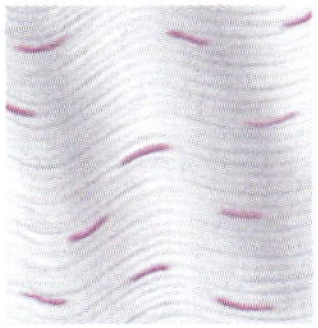 *Dense regular connective tissue*	1. Loose connective tissue ▪ Areolar ▪ Adipose ▪ Reticular 2. Dense connective tissue ▪ Regular ▪ Irregular ▪ Elastic	Fibroblasts Fibrocytes Defense cells Adipocytes	Gel-like ground substance All three fiber types: collagen, reticular, elastic	Six different types; vary in density and types of fibers Functions as a binding tissue Resists mechanical stress, particulary tension Provides reservoir for water and salts Nutrient (fat) storage
Cartilage 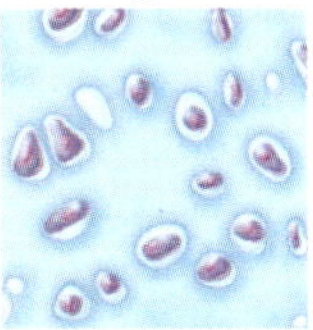 *Hyaline cartilage*	1. Hyaline cartilage 2. Elastic cartilage 3. Fibrocartilage	Chondroblasts found in growing cartilage Chondrocytes	Gel-like ground substance Fibers: collagen, elastic fibers in some	Resists compression because of the large amounts of water held in the matrix Functions to cushion and support body structures
Bone Tissue 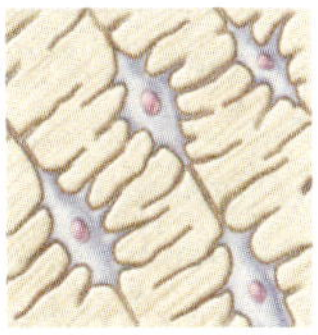 *Compact bone*	1. Compact bone 2. Spongy bone	Osteoblasts Osteocytes	Gel-like ground substance calcified with inorganic salts Fibers: collagen	Hard tissue that resists both compression and tension Functions in support
Blood 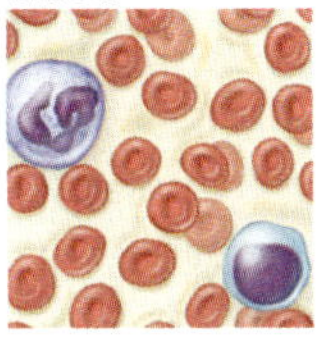	See Chapter 17 for details on blood cell formation and differentiation.	Erythrocytes (RBC) Leukocytes (WBC) Platelets	Plasma No fibers	A fluid tissue Functions to carry O_2, CO_2, nutrients, wastes, and other substances (hormones, for example)

selective appetites. For example, those of the spleen primarily dispose of aging red blood cells, but they will not turn down other "delicacies" that come their way.

☑ Check Your Understanding

11. What are four functions of connective tissue?
12. What are the three types of fibers found in connective tissues?

For answers, see Appendix H.

Types of Connective Tissue

✓ Describe the types of connective tissue found in the body, and indicate their characteristic functions.

As noted, all classes of connective tissue consist of living cells surrounded by a matrix. Their major differences reflect cell type, and types and relative amounts of fibers, as summarized in Table 4.1.

As mentioned earlier, mature connective tissues arise from a common embryonic tissue, called **mesenchyme** (meh′zin-kīm). Mesenchyme has a fluid ground substance containing fine sparse fibers and star-shaped *mesenchymal cells*. It arises during the early weeks of embryonic development and eventually differentiates (specializes) into all other connective tissue cells. However, some mesenchymal cells remain and provide a source of new cells in mature connective tissues.

Figure 4.8 illustrates the connective tissues that we describe in the next sections. Study this figure as you read along.

Connective Tissue Proper—Loose Connective Tissues

Connective tissue proper has two subclasses: **loose connective tissues** (areolar, adipose, and reticular) and **dense connective tissues** (dense regular, dense irregular, and elastic). Except for bone, cartilage, and blood, all mature connective tissues are connective tissue proper.

Areolar Connective Tissue The functions of **areolar connective tissue** (Figure 4.8a) include:

- Supporting and binding other tissues (the job of the fibers)
- Holding body fluids (the ground substance's role)
- Defending against infection (via the activity of white blood cells and macrophages)
- Storing nutrients as fat (in fat cells)

Fibroblasts, flat branching cells that appear spindle shaped in profile, predominate, but numerous macrophages are also seen and present a formidable barrier to invading microorganisms. Fat cells appear singly or in clusters, and occasional mast cells are identified easily by the large, darkly stained cytoplasmic granules that often obscure their nuclei. Other cell types are scattered throughout.

The most obvious structural feature of this tissue is the loose arrangement of its fibers. The rest of the matrix, occupied by ground substance, appears to be empty space when viewed through the microscope, and in fact, the Latin term *areola* means "a small open space." Because of its loose nature, areolar connective tissue provides a reservoir of water and salts for surrounding body tissues, always holding approximately as much fluid as there is in the entire bloodstream. Essentially all body cells obtain their nutrients from and release their wastes into this "tissue fluid."

The high content of hyaluronic acid makes its ground substance viscous, like molasses, which may hinder the movement of cells through it. Some white blood cells, which protect the body from disease-causing microorganisms, secrete the enzyme hyaluronidase to liquefy the ground substance and ease their passage. (Unhappily, some harmful bacteria have the same ability.) When a body region is inflamed, the areolar tissue in the area soaks up excess fluids like a sponge, and the affected area swells and becomes puffy, a condition called **edema** (ĕ-de′mah).

Areolar connective tissue is the most widely distributed connective tissue in the body, and it serves as a universal packing material between other tissues. It binds body parts together while allowing them to move freely over one another; wraps small blood vessels and nerves; surrounds glands; and forms the subcutaneous tissue, which cushions and attaches the skin to underlying structures. It is the connective tissue that most epithelia rest on and is present in all mucous membranes as the *lamina propria*. (Mucous membranes line body cavities open to the exterior.)

Adipose (Fat) Tissue **Adipose tissue** (ad′ĭ-pōs) is similar to areolar tissue in structure and function, but its nutrient-storing ability is much greater. Consequently, **adipocytes** (ad′ĭ-po-sītz), commonly called *adipose* or *fat cells*, account for 90% of this tissue's mass. The matrix is scanty and the cells are packed closely together, giving a chicken-wire appearance to the tissue. A glistening oil droplet (almost pure triglyceride) occupies most of a fat cell's volume and displaces the nucleus to one side (Figure 4.8b). Mature adipocytes are among the largest cells in the body. As they take up or release fat, they become plumper or more wrinkled, respectively.

Adipose tissue is richly vascularized, indicating its high metabolic activity. Without the fat stores in our adipose tissue, we could not live for more than a few days without eating. Adipose tissue is certainly abundant: It constitutes 18% of an average person's body weight, and a chubby person's body can be 50% fat without being considered morbidly obese.

Adipose tissue may develop almost anywhere areolar tissue is plentiful, but it usually accumulates in subcutaneous tissue, where it acts as a shock absorber, as insulation, and as an energy storage site. Because fat is a poor conductor of heat, it helps prevent heat loss from the body. Other sites where fat accumulates include surrounding the kidneys, behind the eyeballs, and at genetically determined fat depots such as the abdomen and hips.

The abundant fat beneath the skin serves the general nutrient needs of the entire body, and smaller depots of fat serve the local nutrient needs of highly active organs. Such depots occur around the hard-working heart and around lymph nodes (where cells of the immune system are furiously fighting infection), within some muscles, and as individual fat cells in the bone marrow, where new blood cells are produced at a rapid rate. Many of these local depots are highly enriched in special lipids.

The adipose tissue just described is sometimes called *white fat*, or *white adipose tissue*, to distinguish it from **brown fat**, or **brown adipose tissue**. White fat stores nutrients (mainly for other cells), but brown fat contains abundant mitochondria, which use the lipid fuels to heat the bloodstream to warm the body (rather than to produce ATP molecules). The richly vascular brown fat occurs mainly on the back of babies who (as yet) lack the ability to produce body heat by shivering. Scant deposits occur in adults, mostly above the collar bones, on the neck and abdomen, and around the spine.

Reticular Connective Tissue **Reticular connective tissue** resembles areolar connective tissue, but the only fibers in its matrix are reticular fibers, which form a delicate network along which fibroblasts called **reticular cells** (Figure 4.8c) are scattered. Although reticular *fibers* are widely distributed in the body, reticular tissue is limited to certain sites. It forms a labyrinth-like **stroma** (literally, "bed" or "mattress"), or internal framework, that can support many free blood cells (mostly lymphocytes) in lymph nodes, the spleen, and bone marrow.

Connective Tissue Proper—Dense Connective Tissues

The three varieties of dense connective tissue are dense regular, dense irregular, and elastic. Since all three have fibers as their prominent element, dense connective tissues are often called **fibrous connective tissues**.

Dense Regular Connective Tissue **Dense regular connective tissue** contains closely packed bundles of collagen fibers running in the same direction, parallel to the direction of pull (Figure 4.8d). This arrangement results in white, flexible structures

(a) Connective tissue proper: loose connective tissue, areolar

Description: Gel-like matrix with all three fiber types; cells: fibroblasts, macrophages, mast cells, and some white blood cells.

Function: Wraps and cushions organs; its macrophages phagocytize bacteria; plays important role in inflammation; holds and conveys tissue fluid.

Location: Widely distributed under epithelia of body, e.g., forms lamina propria of mucous membranes; packages organs; surrounds capillaries.

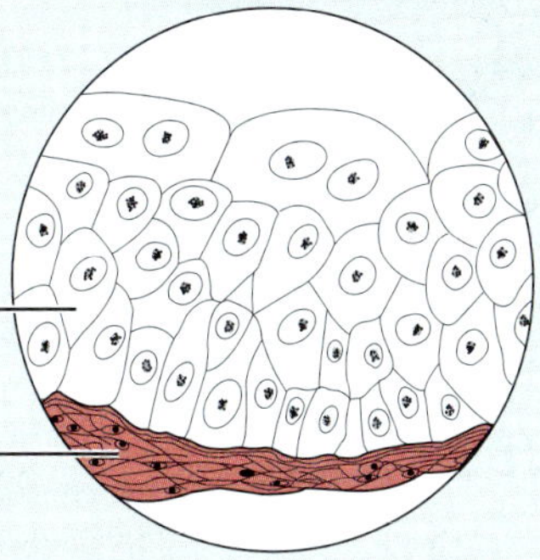

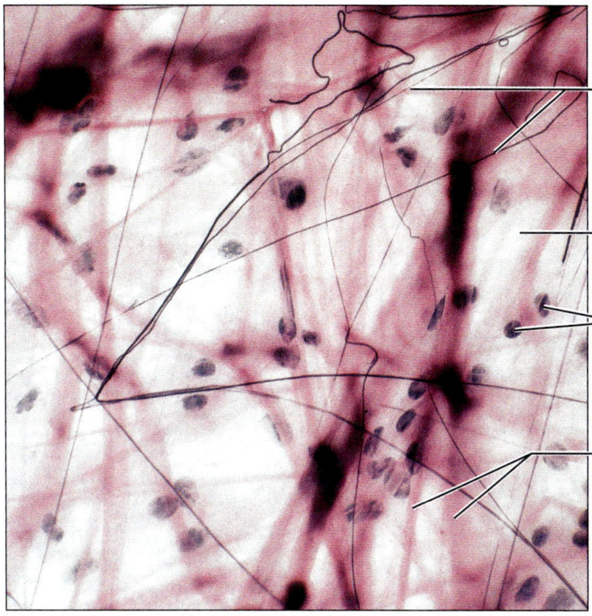

Photomicrograph: Areolar connective tissue, a soft packaging tissue of the body (340×).

(b) Connective tissue proper: loose connective tissue, adipose

Description: Matrix as in areolar, but very sparse; closely packed adipocytes, or fat cells, have nucleus pushed to the side by large fat droplet.

Function: Provides reserve food fuel; insulates against heat loss; supports and protects organs.

Location: Under skin in subcutaneous tissue; around kidneys and eyeballs; within abdomen; in breasts.

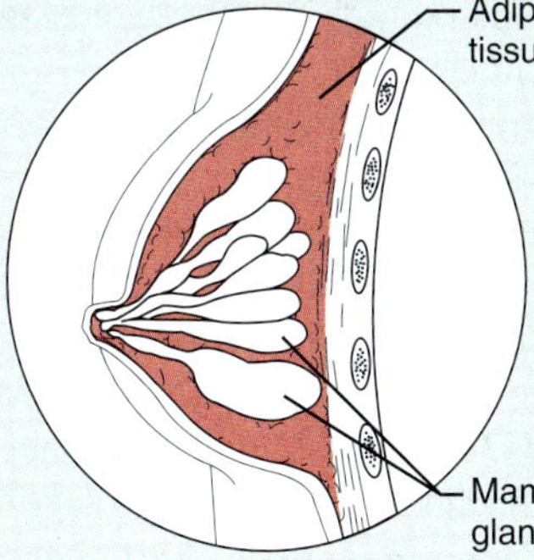

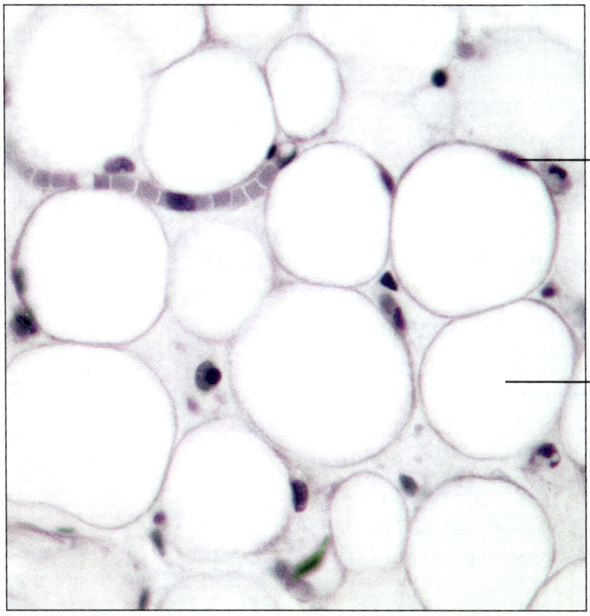

Photomicrograph: Adipose tissue from the subcutaneous layer under the skin (350×).

Figure 4.8 Connective tissues. (a) and **(b)** Connective tissue proper. (For related images, see *A Brief Atlas of the Human Body*, Plates 11 and 12.)

(c) Connective tissue proper: loose connective tissue, reticular

Description: Network of reticular fibers in a typical loose ground substance; reticular cells lie on the network.

Function: Fibers form a soft internal skeleton (stroma) that supports other cell types including white blood cells, mast cells, and macrophages.

Location: Lymphoid organs (lymph nodes, bone marrow, and spleen).

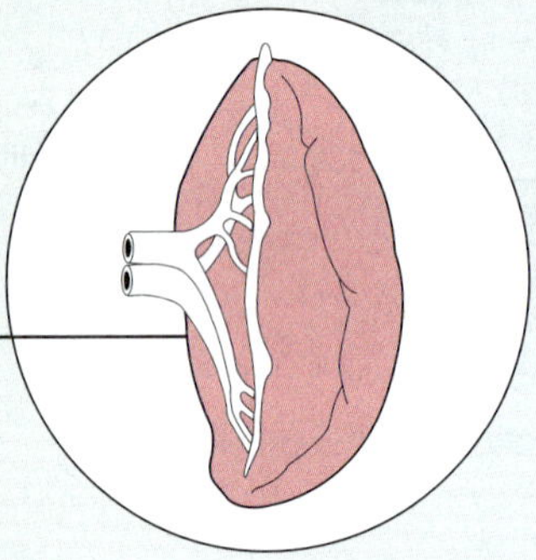

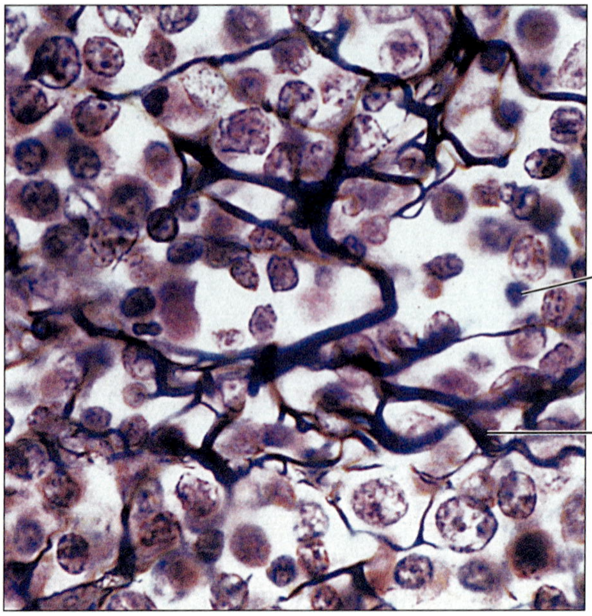

Photomicrograph: Dark-staining network of reticular connective tissue fibers forming the internal skeleton of the spleen (350×).

Figure 4.8 *(continued)* **Connective tissues. (c)** Connective tissue proper. (For a related image, see *A Brief Atlas of the Human Body*, Plate 13.)

with great resistance to tension (pulling forces) where the tension is exerted in a single direction. Crowded between the collagen fibers are rows of fibroblasts that continuously manufacture the fibers and scant ground substance.

Collagen fibers are slightly wavy (see Figure 4.8d). This allows the tissue to stretch a little, but once the fibers straighten out, there is no further "give" to this tissue. Unlike our model (areolar) connective tissue, this tissue has few cells other than fibroblasts and is poorly vascularized.

With its enormous tensile strength, dense regular connective tissue forms *tendons*, which are cords that attach muscles to bones; flat, sheetlike tendons called *aponeuroses* (ap″o-nu-ro′sēz) that attach muscles to other muscles or to bones; and the *ligaments* that bind bones together at joints. Ligaments contain more elastic fibers than tendons and are slightly more stretchy. Dense regular connective tissue also forms fascia (fash′e-ah; "a bond"), a fibrous membrane that wraps around muscles, groups of muscles, blood vessels, and nerves, binding them together like plastic sandwich wrap.

Dense Irregular Connective Tissue **Dense irregular connective tissue** has the same structural elements as the regular variety. However, the bundles of collagen fibers are much thicker and they are arranged irregularly; that is, they run in more than one plane (Figure 4.8e). This type of tissue forms sheets in body areas where tension is exerted from many different directions. It is found in the skin as the leathery *dermis*, and it forms fibrous joint capsules and the fibrous coverings that surround some organs (kidneys, bones, cartilages, muscles, and nerves).

Elastic Connective Tissue A few ligaments, such as those connecting adjacent vertebrae, are very elastic. The dense regular connective tissue in those structures is called **elastic connective tissue** (Figure 4.8f). Additionally, many of the larger arteries have stretchy sheets of elastic connective tissue in their walls.

Cartilage

Cartilage (kar′tĭ-lij), which stands up to both tension *and* compression, has qualities intermediate between dense connective tissue and bone. It is tough but flexible, providing a resilient rigidity to the structures it supports.

Cartilage lacks nerve fibers and is avascular. It receives its nutrients by diffusion from blood vessels located in the connective tissue membrane (perichondrium) surrounding it. Its ground substance contains large amounts of the GAGs chondroitin sulfate and hyaluronic acid, firmly bound collagen fibers (and in some cases elastic fibers), and is quite firm. Cartilage matrix also contains an exceptional amount of tissue fluid. In fact, cartilage is up to 80% water! The movement of tissue fluid in its matrix enables cartilage to rebound after being compressed and also helps to nourish the cartilage cells.

(d) Connective tissue proper: dense connective tissue, dense regular

Description: Primarily parallel collagen fibers; a few elastic fibers; major cell type is the fibroblast.

Function: Attaches muscles to bones or to muscles; attaches bones to bones; withstands great tensile stress when pulling force is applied in one direction.

Location: Tendons, most ligaments, aponeuroses.

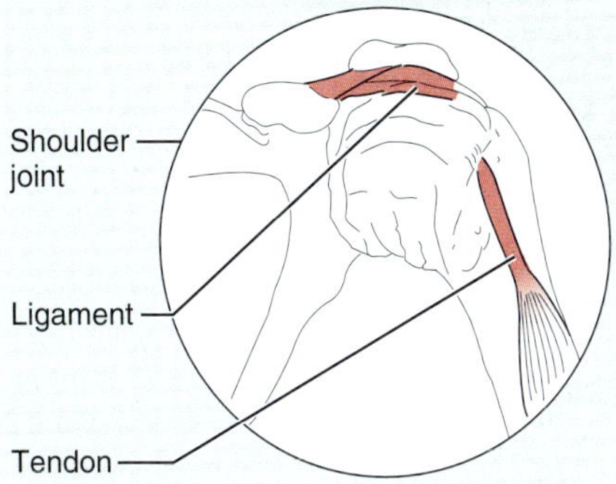

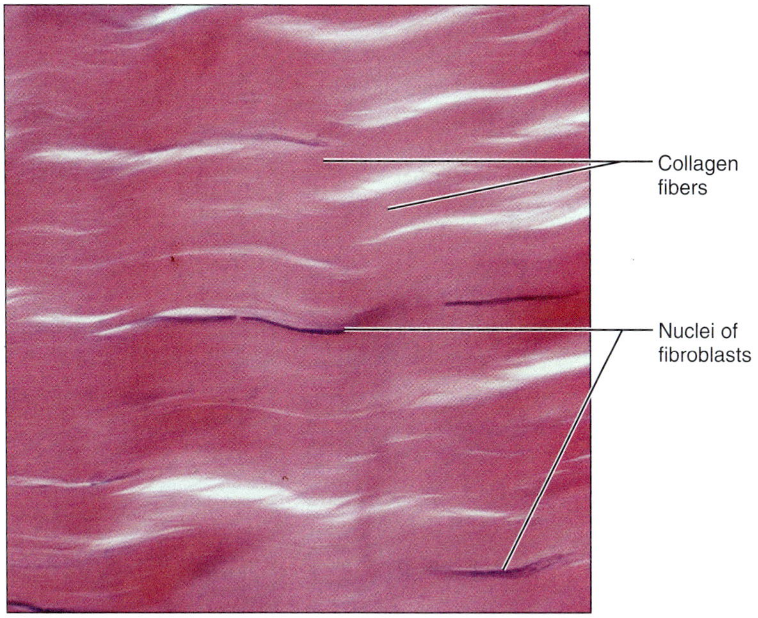

Photomicrograph: Dense regular connective tissue from a tendon (430×).

(e) Connective tissue proper: dense connective tissue, dense irregular

Description: Primarily irregularly arranged collagen fibers; some elastic fibers; fibroblast is the major cell type.

Function: Withstands tension exerted in many directions; provides structural strength.

Location: Fibrous capsules of organs and of joints; dermis of the skin; submucosa of digestive tract.

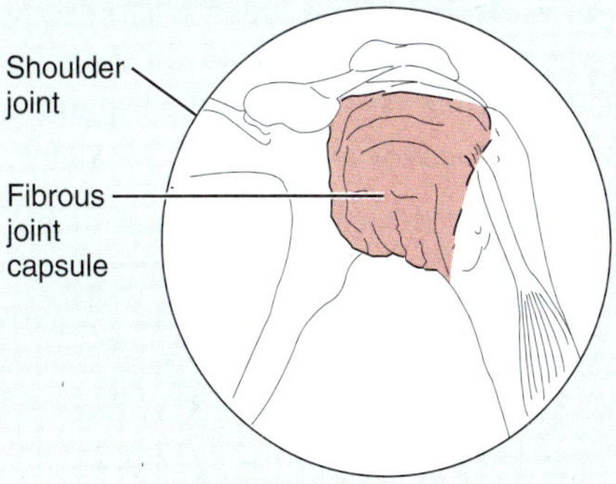

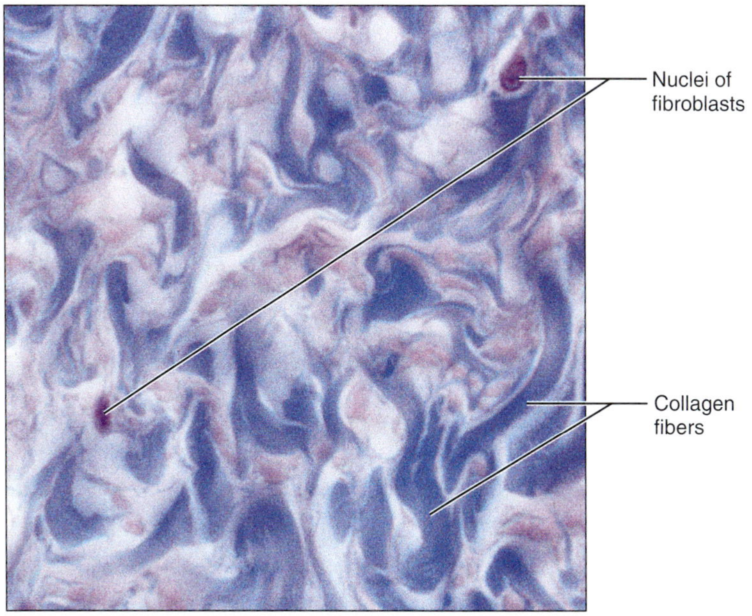

Photomicrograph: Dense irregular connective tissue from the fibrous capsule of a joint (430×).

Figure 4.8 *(continued)* **(d)** and **(e)** Connective tissue proper. (For related images, see *A Brief Atlas of the Human Body*, Plates 14 and 15.)

(f) Connective tissue proper: dense connective tissue, elastic

Description: Dense regular connective tissue containing a high proportion of elastic fibers.

Function: Allows tissue to recoil after stretching; maintains pulsatile flow of blood through arteries; aids passive recoil of lungs following inspiration.

Location: Walls of large arteries; within certain ligaments associated with the vertebral column; within the walls of the bronchial tubes.

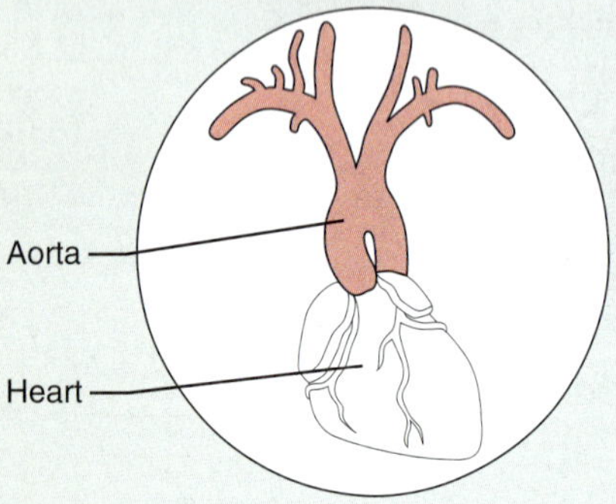

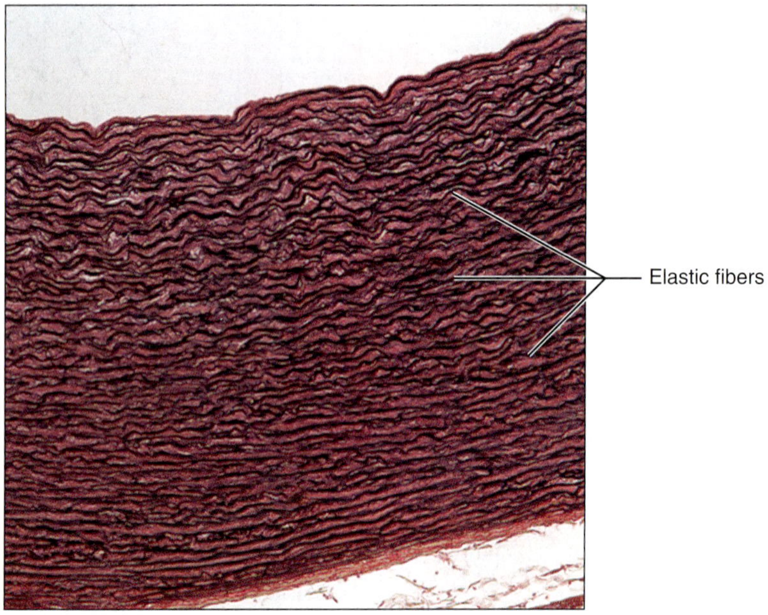

Photomicrograph: Elastic connective tissue in the wall of the aorta (250×).

Figure 4.8 *(continued)* **Connective tissues. (f)** Connective tissue proper. (For a related image, see *A Brief Atlas of the Human Body*, Plate 16.)

Chondroblasts, the predominant cell type in growing cartilage, produce new matrix until the skeleton stops growing at the end of adolescence. The firmness of the cartilage matrix prevents the cells from becoming widely separated, so **chondrocytes**, or mature cartilage cells, are typically found in small groups within cavities called *lacunae* (lah-ku′ne; "pits").

Homeostatic Imbalance 4.2

Because cartilage is avascular and aging cartilage cells lose their ability to divide, injured cartilages heal slowly. This phenomenon is excruciatingly familiar to those who have experienced sports injuries. During later life, cartilages tend to calcify or even ossify (become bony). In such cases, the chondrocytes are poorly nourished and die. ✚

There are three varieties of cartilage: *hyaline cartilage*, *elastic cartilage*, and *fibrocartilage*, each dominated by a particular fiber type.

Hyaline Cartilage **Hyaline cartilage** (hi′ah-līn), or *gristle*, is the most abundant cartilage in the body. Although it contains large numbers of collagen fibers, they are not apparent and the matrix appears glassy (*hyal* = glass, transparent) blue-white when viewed by the unaided eye. Chondrocytes account for only 1–10% of the cartilage volume (Figure 4.8g).

Hyaline cartilage provides firm support with some pliability. It covers the ends of long bones as *articular cartilage*, providing springy pads that absorb compression at joints. Hyaline cartilage also supports the tip of the nose, connects the ribs to the sternum, and supports most of the respiratory system passages. Most of the embryonic skeleton consists of hyaline cartilage before bone forms. Skeletal hyaline cartilage persists during childhood as the *epiphyseal plates* (e″pĭ-fis′e-ul), actively growing regions near the ends of long bones.

Elastic Cartilage Histologically, **elastic cartilage** (Figure 4.8h) is nearly identical to hyaline cartilage. However, elastic cartilage has many more elastic fibers. Found where strength and exceptional stretchability are needed, elastic cartilage forms the "skeletons" of the external ear (the pinna) and the epiglottis (the flap that covers the opening to the respiratory passageway when we swallow).

Fibrocartilage Structurally, **fibrocartilage** is intermediate between hyaline cartilage and dense regular connective tissues. Its rows of chondrocytes (a cartilage feature) alternate with rows of thick collagen fibers (characteristic of dense regular connective tissue) (Figure 4.8i). Because it is compressible and resists tension well, fibrocartilage is found where strong support and the ability to withstand heavy pressure are required: for example, the intervertebral discs (resilient cushions between the bony vertebrae) and the spongy cartilages of the knee (menisci) (see Figure 6.1, p. 175).

(g) Cartilage: hyaline

Description: Amorphous but firm matrix; collagen fibers form an imperceptible network; chondroblasts produce the matrix and when mature (chondrocytes) lie in lacunae.

Function: Supports and reinforces; serves as resilient cushion; resists compressive stress.

Location: Forms most of the embryonic skeleton; covers the ends of long bones in joint cavities; forms costal cartilages of the ribs; cartilages of the nose, trachea, and larynx.

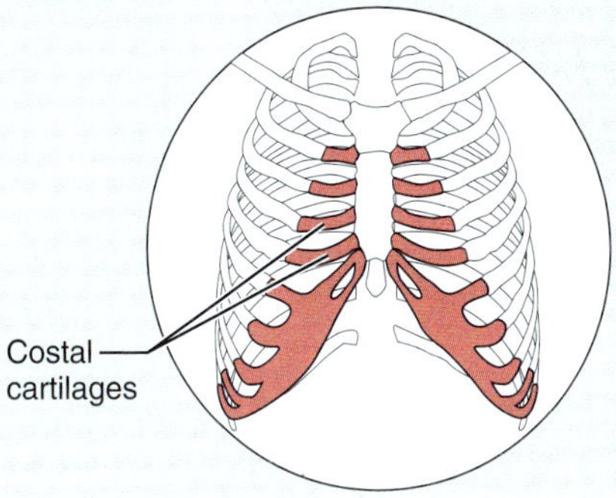

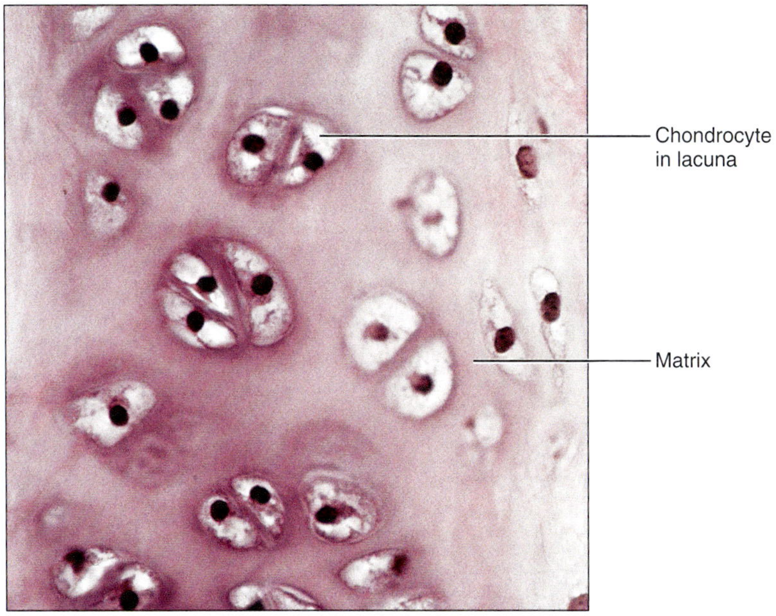

Photomicrograph: Hyaline cartilage from a costal cartilage of a rib (470×).

(h) Cartilage: elastic

Description: Similar to hyaline cartilage, but more elastic fibers in matrix.

Function: Maintains the shape of a structure while allowing great flexibility.

Location: Supports the external ear (pinna); epiglottis.

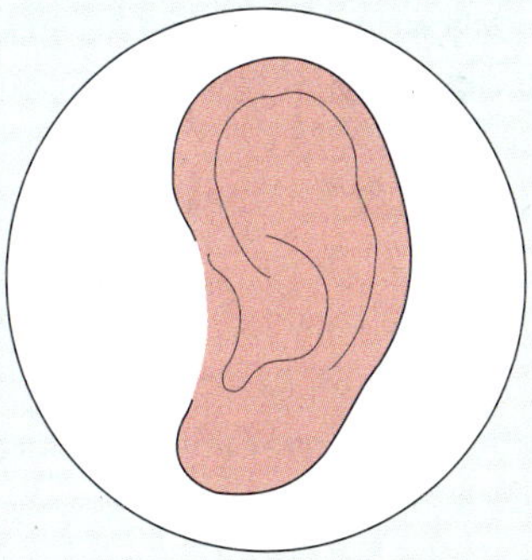

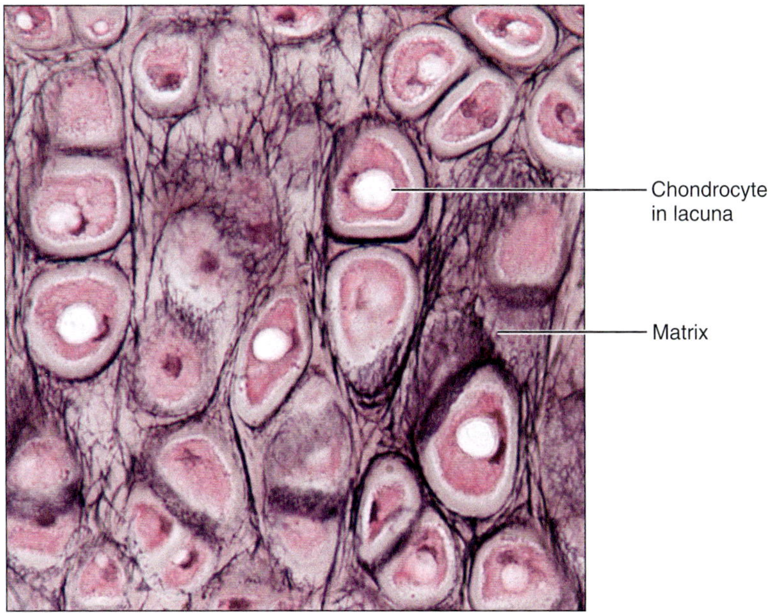

Photomicrograph: Elastic cartilage from the human ear pinna; forms the flexible skeleton of the ear (800×).

Figure 4.8 *(continued)* **(g)** and **(h)** Cartilage. (For related images, see *A Brief Atlas of the Human Body*, Plates 17 and 18.)

(i) Cartilage: fibrocartilage

Description: Matrix similar to but less firm than that in hyaline cartilage; thick collagen fibers predominate.

Function: Tensile strength allows it to absorb compressive shock.

Location: Intervertebral discs; pubic symphysis; discs of knee joint.

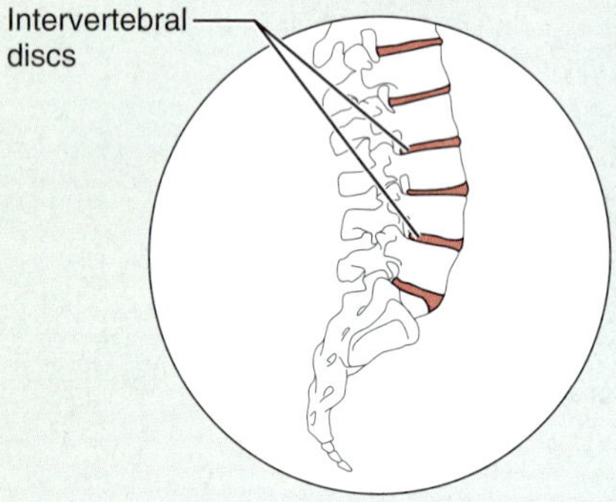

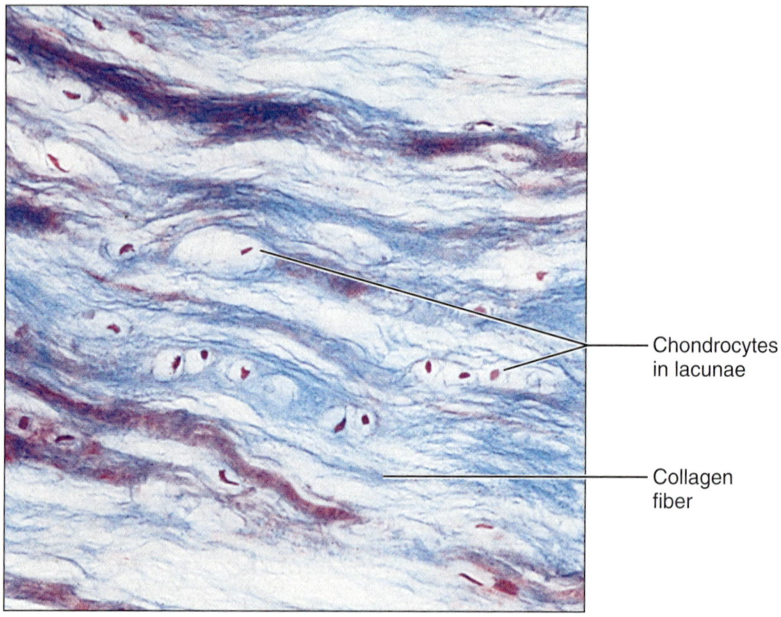

Photomicrograph: Fibrocartilage of an intervertebral disc (125×). Special staining produced the blue color seen.

Figure 4.8 *(continued)* **Connective tissues. (i)** Cartilage. (For a related image, see *A Brief Atlas of the Human Body*, Plate 19.)

Bone (Osseous Tissue)

Because of its rocklike hardness, **bone**, or **osseous tissue** (os′e-us), has an exceptional ability to support and protect body structures. Bones of the skeleton also provide cavities for storing fat and synthesizing blood cells. Bone matrix is similar to that of cartilage but is harder and more rigid because, in addition to its more abundant collagen fibers, bone has an added matrix element—inorganic calcium salts (bone salts).

Osteoblasts produce the organic portion of the matrix, and then bone salts are deposited on and between the fibers. Mature bone cells, or **osteocytes**, reside in the lacunae within the matrix they have made (Figure 4.8j). A cross section of bone tissue reveals closely packed structural units called *osteons* formed of concentric rings of bony matrix (lamellae) surrounding central canals containing the blood vessels and nerves serving the bone. Unlike cartilage, the next firmest connective tissue, bone is well supplied by invading blood vessels.

Blood

Blood, the fluid within blood vessels, is the most atypical connective tissue. It does *not* connect things or give mechanical support. It is classified as a connective tissue because it develops from mesenchyme and consists of *blood cells*, surrounded by a nonliving fluid matrix called *blood plasma* (Figure 4.8k).

The vast majority of blood cells are red blood cells, or erythrocytes, but scattered white blood cells and platelets (needed for blood clotting) are also seen. The "fibers" of blood are soluble protein molecules that precipitate, forming visible fiberlike structures during blood clotting. Blood functions as the transport vehicle for the cardiovascular system, carrying nutrients, wastes, respiratory gases, and many other substances throughout the body.

☑ Check Your Understanding

13. Which connective tissue has a soft weblike matrix capable of serving as a fluid reservoir?
14. What type of connective tissue is damaged when you cut your index finger tendon?
15. John wants to become a professional basketball player. Unfortunately he is short for his age and his epiphyseal plates have already fused. What type of connective tissue forms the epiphyseal plates?

For answers, see Appendix H.

Muscle Tissue

✓ Compare and contrast the structures and body locations of the three types of muscle tissue.

Muscle tissues are highly cellular, well-vascularized tissues that are responsible for most types of body movement. Muscle cells possess **myofilaments**, elaborate versions of the *actin* and *myosin* filaments that bring about movement or contraction in all

(j) Others: bone (osseous tissue)

Description: Hard, calcified matrix containing many collagen fibers; osteocytes lie in lacunae. Very well vascularized.

Function: Supports and protects (by enclosing); provides levers for the muscles to act on; stores calcium and other minerals and fat; marrow inside bones is the site for blood cell formation (hematopoiesis).

Location: Bones

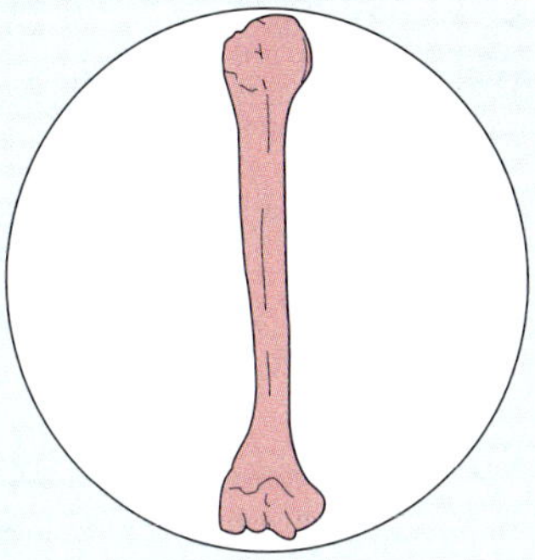

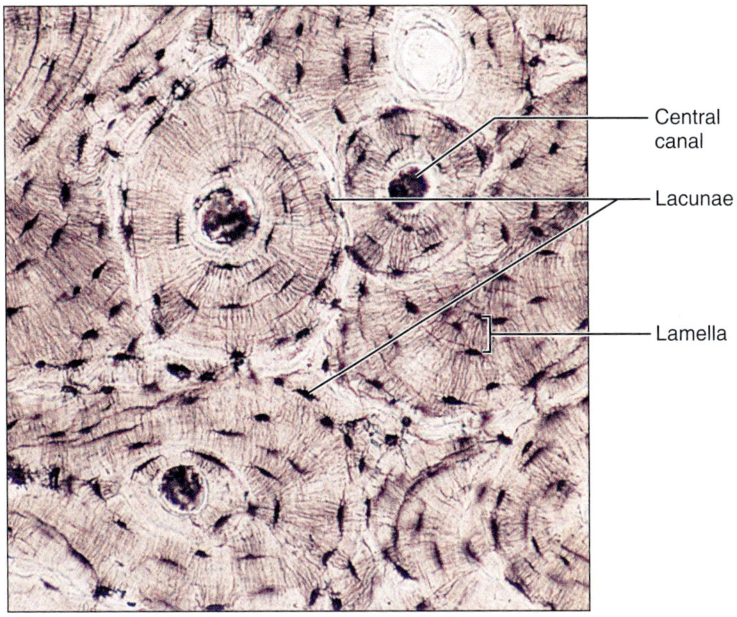

Photomicrograph: Cross-sectional view of bone (125×).

(k) Connective tissue: blood

Description: Red and white blood cells in a fluid matrix (plasma).

Function: Transport respiratory gases, nutrients, wastes, and other substances.

Location: Contained within blood vessels.

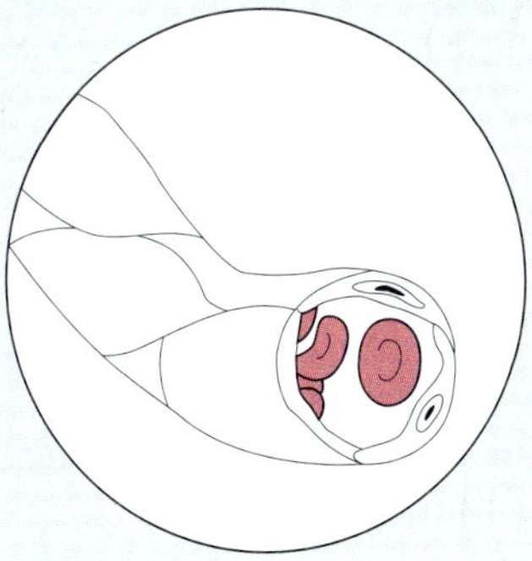

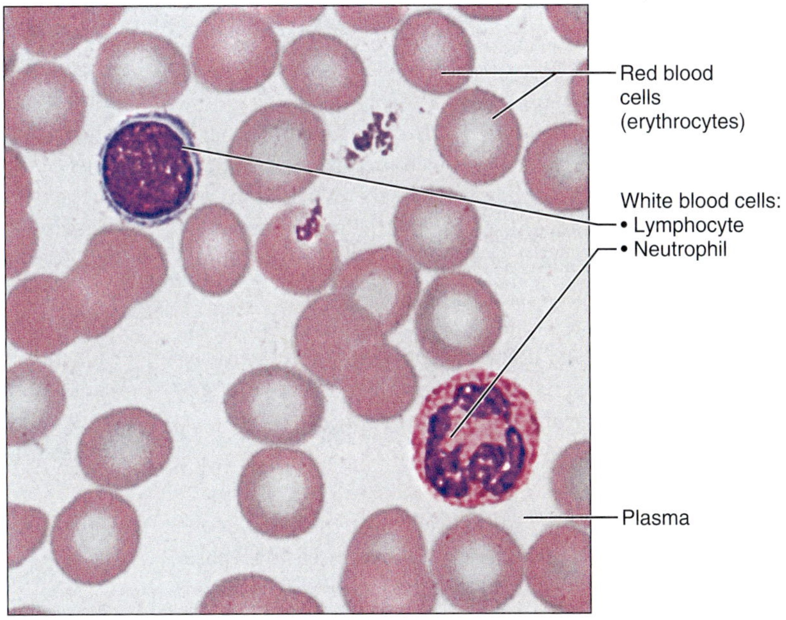

Photomicrograph: Smear of human blood (1670×); shows two white blood cells surrounded by red blood cells.

Figure 4.8 *(continued)* **(j)** Bone. (For a related image, see *A Brief Atlas of the Human Body*, Plate 20.) **(k)** Blood. (For related images, see *A Brief Atlas of the Human Body*, Plates 22–27.)

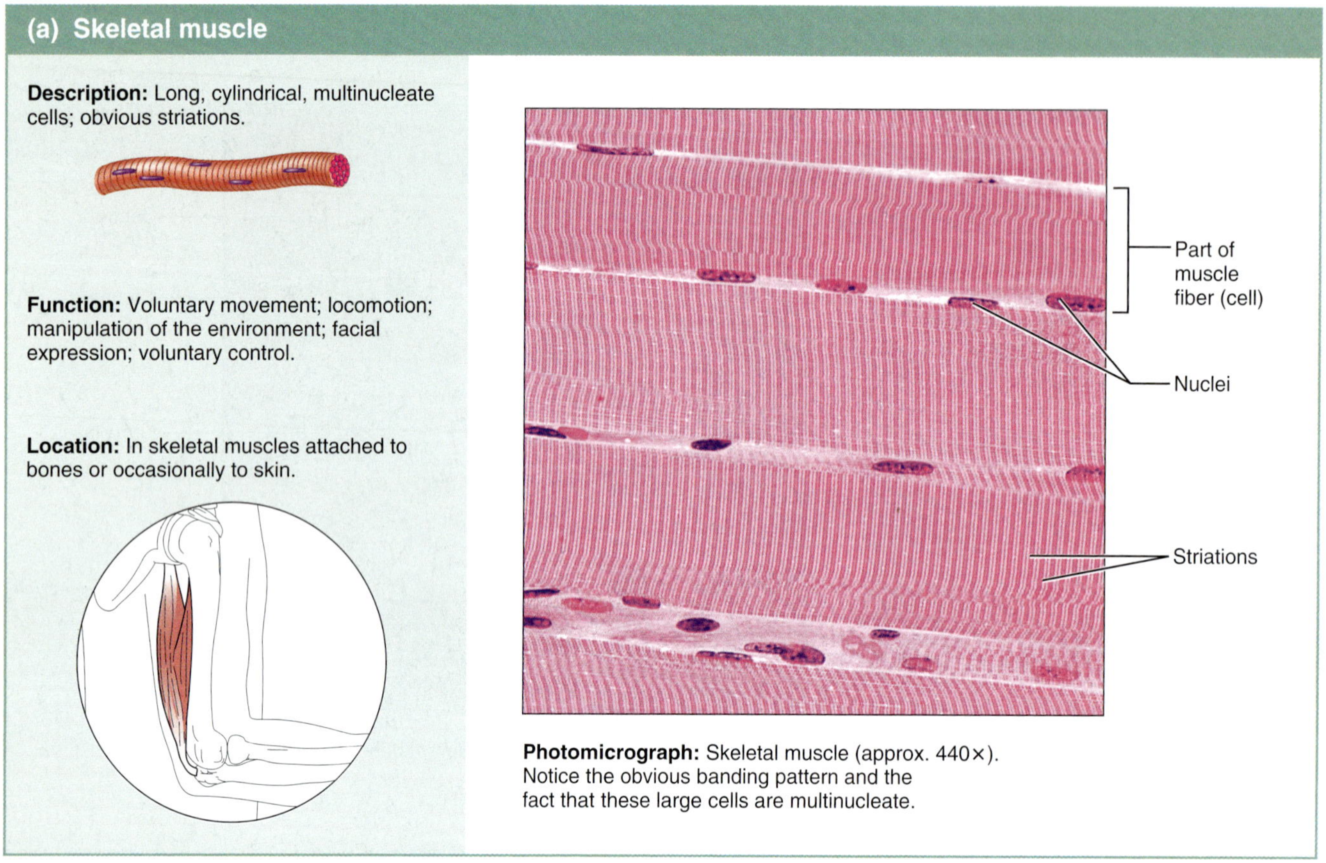

Figure 4.9 Muscle tissues. (a) Skeletal muscle tissue. (For a related image, see *A Brief Atlas of the Human Body*, Plate 28.)

cell types. There are three kinds of muscle tissue: skeletal, cardiac, and smooth.

Skeletal Muscle

Skeletal muscle tissue is packaged by connective tissue sheets into organs called *skeletal muscles* that are attached to the bones of the skeleton. These muscles form the flesh of the body, and as they contract they pull on bones or skin, causing body movements.

Skeletal muscle cells, also called **muscle fibers**, are long, cylindrical cells that contain many peripherally located nuclei. Their obvious banded, or striated, appearance reflects the precise alignment of their myofilaments **(Figure 4.9a)**.

Cardiac Muscle

Cardiac muscle is found only in the walls of the heart. Its contractions help propel blood through the blood vessels to all parts of the body. Like skeletal muscle cells, cardiac muscle cells are striated. However, cardiac cells differ structurally in that they are

- Generally uninucleate (one nucleus) with the nucleus situated centrally
- Branching cells that fit together tightly at unique junctions called **intercalated discs** (in-ter′kah-la″ted) (Figure 4.9b)

Smooth Muscle

Smooth muscle is so named because its cells have no visible striations. Individual smooth muscle cells are spindle shaped and contain one centrally located nucleus (Figure 4.9c). Smooth muscle is found mainly in the walls of hollow organs other than the heart (digestive and urinary tract organs, uterus, and blood vessels). It squeezes substances through these organs by alternately contracting and relaxing.

Because skeletal muscle contraction is under our conscious control, skeletal muscle is often referred to as **voluntary muscle**, and the other two types are called **involuntary muscle** because we do not consciously control them. We describe skeletal muscle and smooth muscle in detail in Chapter 9, and cardiac muscle in Chapter 18.

☑ Check Your Understanding

16. You are looking at muscle tissue through the microscope and you see striped branching cells that connect with one another. What type of muscle are you viewing?
17. Which muscle type(s) is voluntary? Which is injured when you pull a muscle while exercising?

For answers, see Appendix H.

(b) Cardiac muscle

Description: Branching, striated, generally uninucleate cells that interdigitate at specialized junctions (intercalated discs).

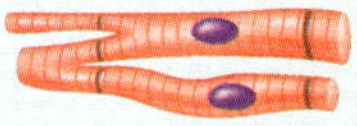

Function: As it contracts, it propels blood into the circulation; involuntary control.

Location: The walls of the heart.

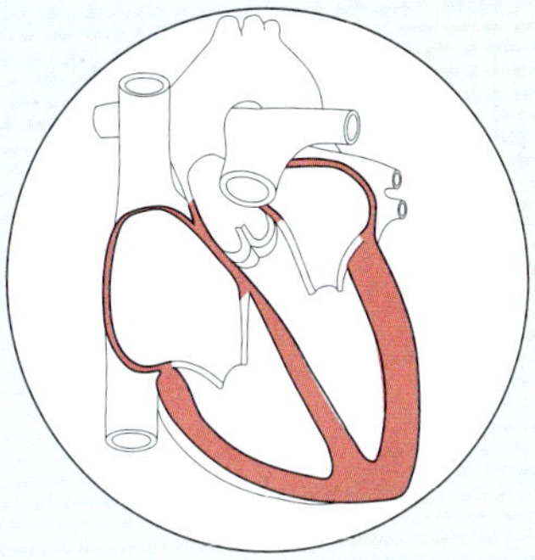

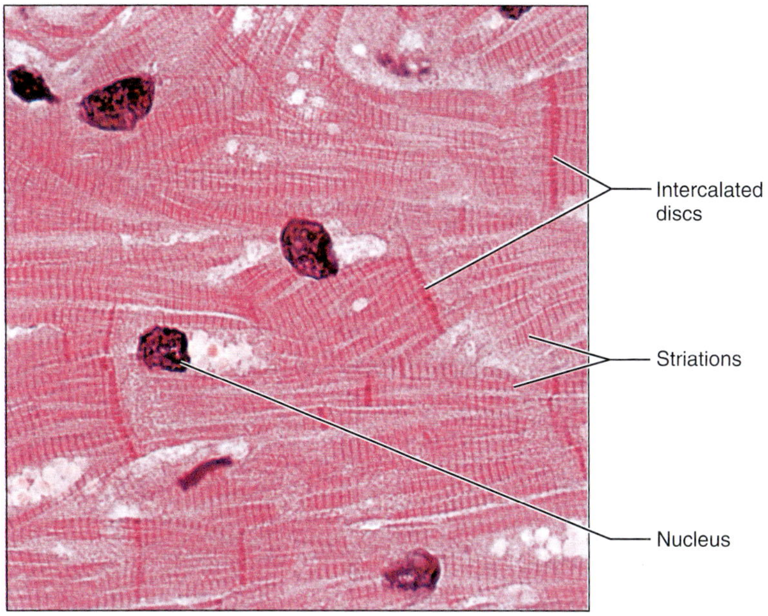

Photomicrograph: Cardiac muscle (900×); notice the striations, branching of cells, and the intercalated discs.

(c) Smooth muscle

Description: Spindle-shaped cells with central nuclei; no striations; cells arranged closely to form sheets.

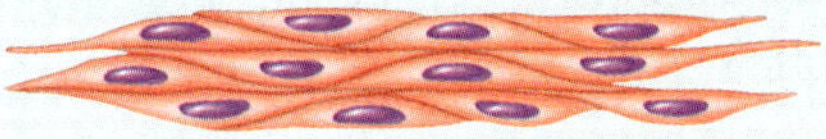

Function: Propels substances or objects (foodstuffs, urine, a baby) along internal passageways; involuntary control.

Location: Mostly in the walls of hollow organs.

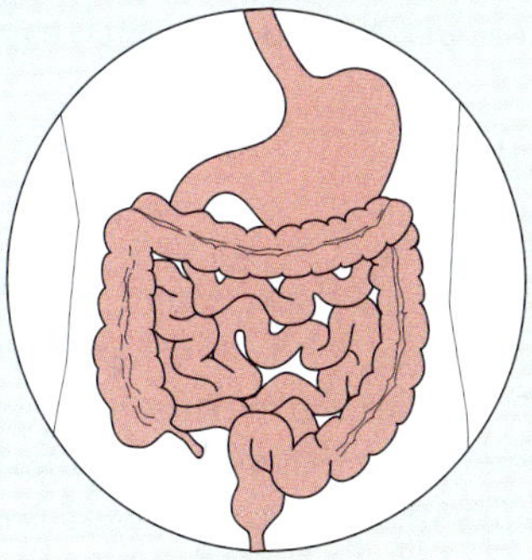

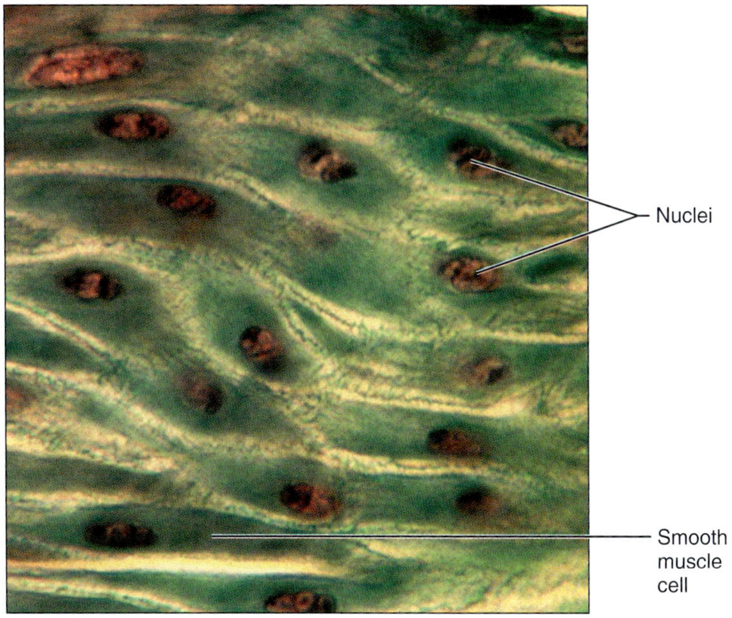

Photomicrograph: Sheet of smooth muscle (720×).

Figure 4.9 *(continued)* **(b)** Cardiac muscle tissue. (For a related image, see *A Brief Atlas of the Human Body*, Plate 31.) **(c)** Smooth muscle tissue. (For a related image, see *A Brief Atlas of the Human Body*, Plate 32.

Nervous tissue

Description: Neurons are branching cells; cell processes that may be quite long extend from the nucleus-containing cell body; also contributing to nervous tissue are nonexcitable supporting cells.

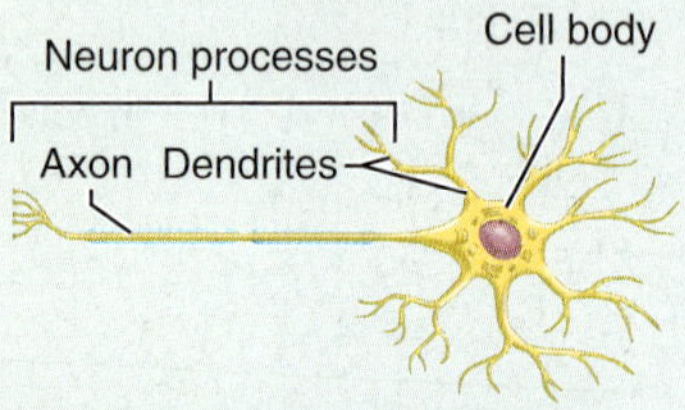

Function: Neurons transmit electrical signals from sensory receptors and to effectors (muscles and glands) which control their activity; supporting cells support and protect neurons.

Location: Brain, spinal cord, and nerves.

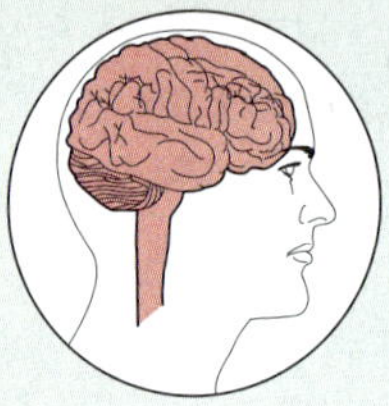

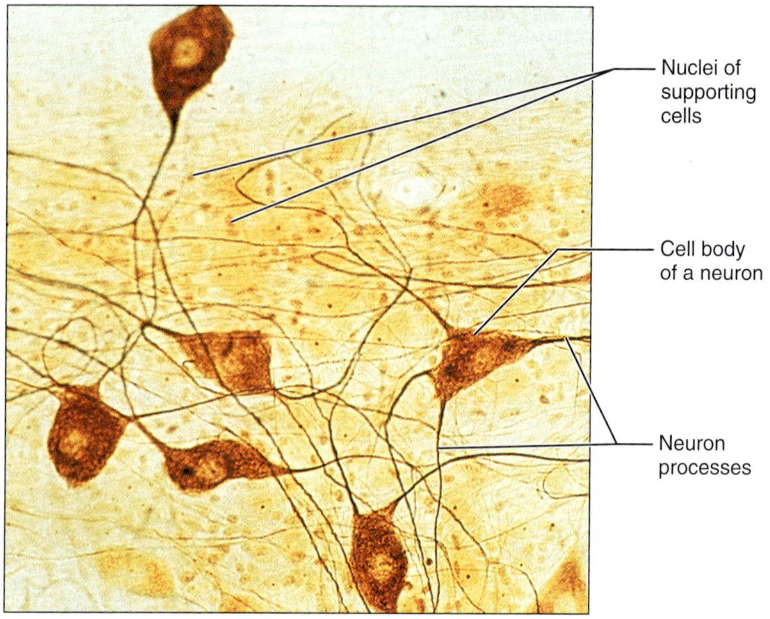

Photomicrograph: Neurons (350×)

Figure 4.10 Nervous tissue. (For a related image, see *A Brief Atlas of the Human Body*, Plate 33.)

Nervous Tissue

✓ Indicate the general characteristics of nervous tissue.

Nervous tissue is the main component of the nervous system—the brain, spinal cord, and nerves—which regulates and controls body functions. It contains two major cell types: neurons and supporting cells.

Neurons are highly specialized nerve cells that generate and conduct nerve impulses **(Figure 4.10)**. Typically, they are branching cells with cytoplasmic extensions or processes that enable them to

- Respond to stimuli (via processes called *dendrites*)
- Transmit electrical impulses over substantial distances within the body (via processes called *axons*)

Supporting cells are nonconducting cells that support, insulate, and protect the delicate neurons. Chapter 11 presents a more complete discussion of nervous tissue.

Check Your Understanding

18. How does the extended length of a neuron's processes aid its function in the body?

For answers, see Appendix H.

Covering and Lining Membranes

✓ Describe the structure and function of cutaneous, mucous, and serous membranes.

Now that we have described all four primary tissues, we can consider the body's membranes that incorporate more than one type of tissue. The covering and lining membranes are of three types: *cutaneous, mucous,* or *serous.* Essentially they all are continuous multicellular sheets composed of at least two primary tissue types: an epithelium bound to an underlying layer of connective tissue proper. Hence, these membranes are simple organs. We describe the *synovial membranes,* which line joint cavities and consist of connective tissue only, in Chapter 8.

Cutaneous Membrane

The **cutaneous membrane** (ku-ta′ne-us; *cutis* = skin) is your skin **(Figure 4.11a)**. It is an organ system consisting of a keratinized stratified squamous epithelium (epidermis) firmly attached to a thick layer of connective tissue (dermis). Unlike other epithelial membranes, the cutaneous membrane is exposed to the air and is a dry membrane. Chapter 5 is devoted to this unique organ system.

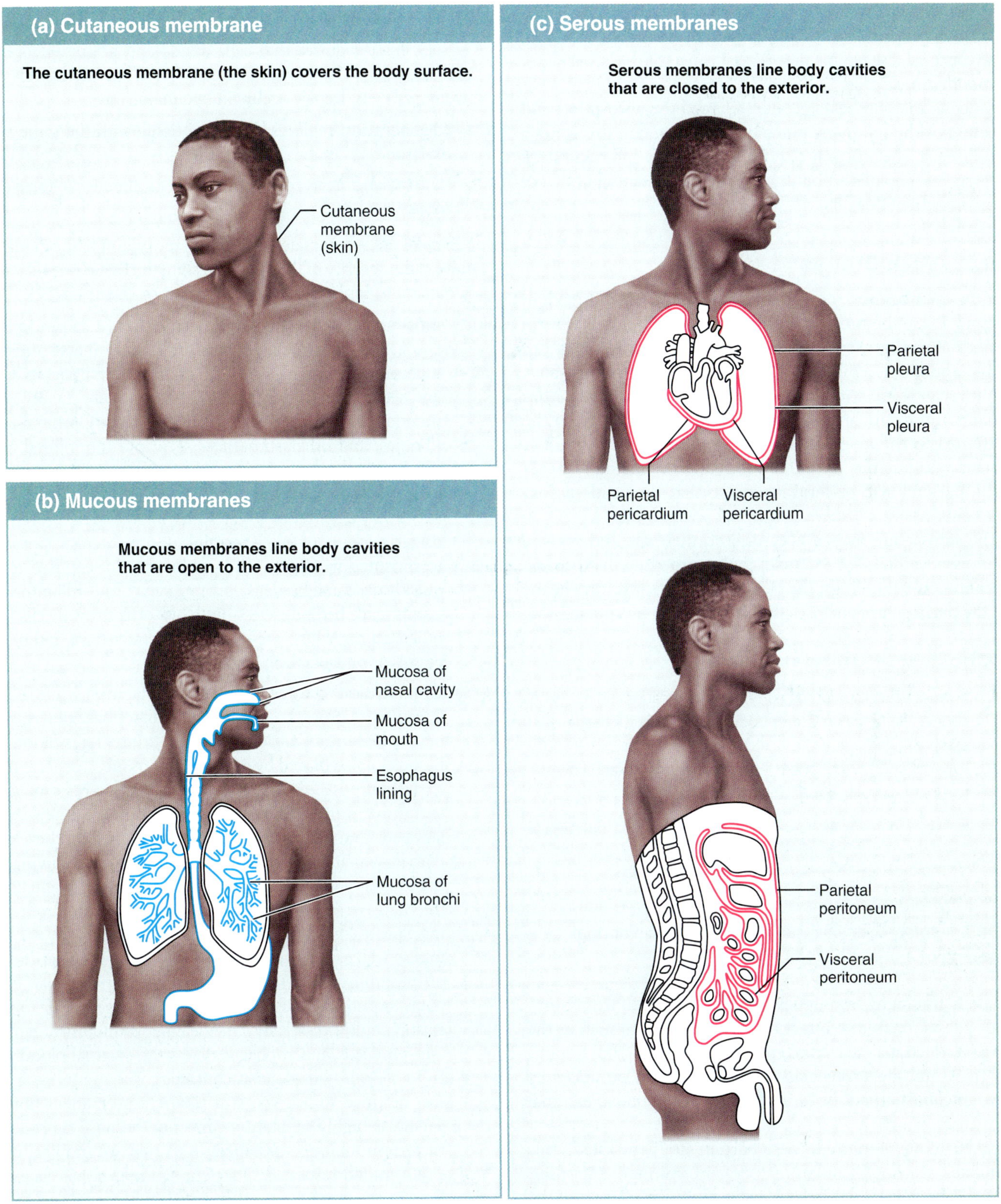

Figure 4.11 Classes of membranes.

Mucous Membranes

Mucous membranes, or **mucosae** (mu-ko′se), line all body cavities that open to the outside of the body, such as the hollow organs of the digestive, respiratory, and urogenital tracts (Figure 4.11b). In all cases, they are "wet," or moist, membranes bathed by secretions or, in the case of the urinary mucosa, urine. Notice that the term *mucosa* refers to the location of the membrane, *not* its cell composition, which varies. However, most mucosae contain either stratified squamous or simple columnar epithelia. The epithelial sheet lies directly over a layer of loose connective tissue called the **lamina propria** (lam′ĭ-nah pro′pre-ah; "one's own layer"). In some mucosae, the lamina propria rests on a third (deeper) layer of smooth muscle cells.

Mucous membranes are often adapted for absorption and secretion. Although many mucosae secrete mucus, this is not a requirement. The mucosae of both the digestive and respiratory tracts secrete copious amounts of lubricating mucus, but that of the urinary tract does not.

4

Serous Membranes

Serous membranes, or **serosae** (se-ro′se), introduced in Chapter 1, are the moist membranes found in closed ventral body cavities (Figure 4.11c). A serous membrane consists of simple squamous epithelium (a mesothelium) resting on a thin layer of loose connective (areolar) tissue. The mesothelial cells add hyaluronic acid to the fluid that filters from the capillaries in the associated connective tissue. The result is the thin, clear *serous fluid* that lubricates the facing surfaces of the parietal and visceral layers, so that they slide across each other easily.

The serosae are named according to their site and specific organ associations. For example, the **pleurae** line the thoracic wall and cover the lungs; the **pericardium** encloses the heart; and the **peritoneum** encloses the abdominopelvic viscera.

☑ Check Your Understanding

19. What type of membrane consists of epithelium and connective tissue, and lines body cavities open to the exterior?
20. What type of membrane lines the thoracic walls and covers the lungs, and what is it called?

For answers, see Appendix H.

Tissue Repair

✓ Outline the process of tissue repair involved in normal healing of a superficial wound.

The body has many techniques for protecting itself from uninvited "guests" or injury. Intact mechanical barriers such as the skin and mucosae, the cilia of epithelial cells lining the respiratory tract, and the strong acid (chemical barrier) produced by stomach glands represent three defenses at the body's external boundaries.

When tissue is injured, these barriers are penetrated. This stimulates the body's inflammatory and immune responses, which wage their battles largely in the connective tissues of the body. The *inflammatory response* is a relatively nonspecific reaction that develops quickly wherever tissues are injured, while the *immune response* is extremely specific, but takes longer to swing into action. We consider the inflammatory and immune responses in detail in Chapter 21.

Steps of Tissue Repair

Tissue repair requires that cells divide and migrate, activities that are initiated by growth factors (wound hormones) released by injured cells. Repair occurs in two major ways:

- **Regeneration** replaces destroyed tissue with the same kind of tissue.
- In **fibrosis**, fibrous connective tissue proliferates to form **scar tissue**.

Which of these occurs depends on (1) the type of tissue damaged and (2) the severity of the injury. In skin, the tissue we will use as our example, repair involves both activities (**Figure 4.12**).

① **Inflammation sets the stage.** Tissue trauma causes injured tissue cells, macrophages, mast cells, and others to release inflammatory chemicals, which cause the capillaries to dilate and become very permeable. White blood cells (neutrophils, monocytes) and plasma fluid rich in clotting proteins, antibodies, and other substances seep into the injured area. The leaked clotting proteins construct a clot, which stops the loss of blood, holds the edges of the wound together, and effectively walls in, or isolates, the injured area, preventing bacteria, toxins, or other harmful substances from spreading to surrounding tissues. The part of the clot exposed to air quickly dries and hardens, forming a *scab*. The inflammatory events leave behind excess fluid, bits of destroyed cells, and other debris, which are eventually removed via lymphatic vessels or phagocytized by macrophages.

② **Organization restores the blood supply.** Even while the inflammatory process is going on, the first phase of tissue repair, called **organization**, begins. During organization the blood clot is replaced by **granulation tissue**, a delicate pink tissue composed of several elements. It contains capillaries that grow in from nearby areas and lay down a new capillary bed. Granulation tissue is actually named for these capillaries, which protrude nublike from its surface, giving it a granular appearance. These capillaries are fragile and bleed freely, as we see when someone picks at a scab. Proliferating fibroblasts in granulation tissue produce growth factors as well as new collagen fibers to bridge the gap. Some of these fibroblasts have contractile properties that allow them to pull the margins of the wound together or to pull existing blood vessels into the healing wound. As organization proceeds, macrophages digest the original blood clot and collagen fiber deposit continues. The granulation tissue, destined to become scar tissue (a permanent fibrous patch), is highly resistant to infection because it produces bacteria-inhibiting substances. As a rule, wound healing is a self-limited response. Once enough matrix has accumulated in the injured area, the fibroblasts either revert to the resting stage or undergo apoptosis.

③ **Regeneration and fibrosis effect permanent repair.** During organization, the surface epithelium begins to *regenerate*, growing under the scab, which soon detaches. As the fibrous tissue beneath matures and contracts, the regenerating

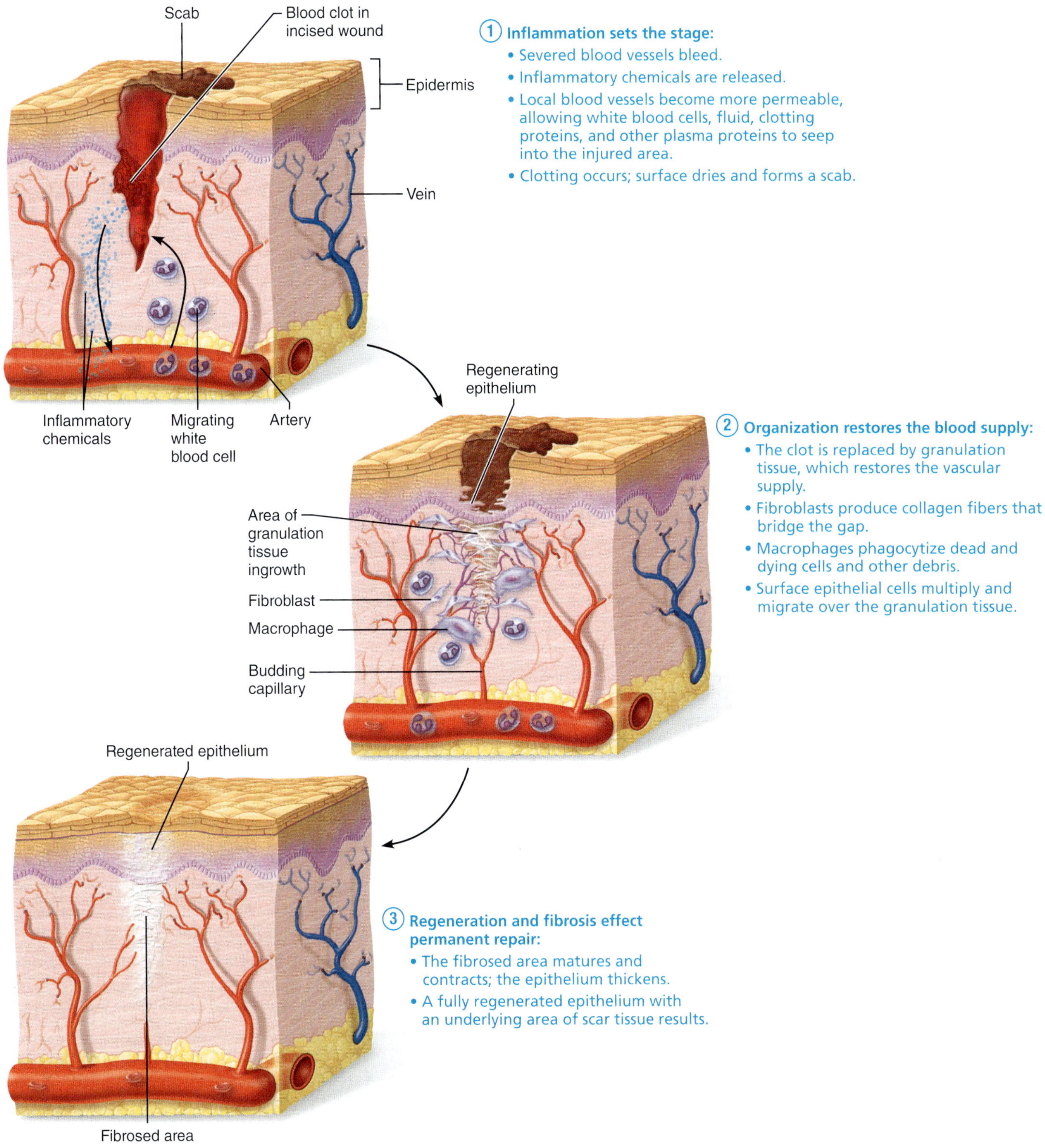

Figure 4.12 Tissue repair of a nonextensive skin wound: regeneration and fibrosis.

epithelium thickens until it finally resembles the adjacent skin. The end result is a fully regenerated epithelium, and an underlying area of scar tissue. The scar may be invisible, or visible as a thin white line, depending on the severity of the wound.

The repair process that we have just described follows healing of a wound (cut, scrape, puncture) that breaches an epithelial barrier. In simple *infections* (a pimple or sore throat), healing is solely by regeneration. Only severe (destructive) infections lead to clot formation or scarring.

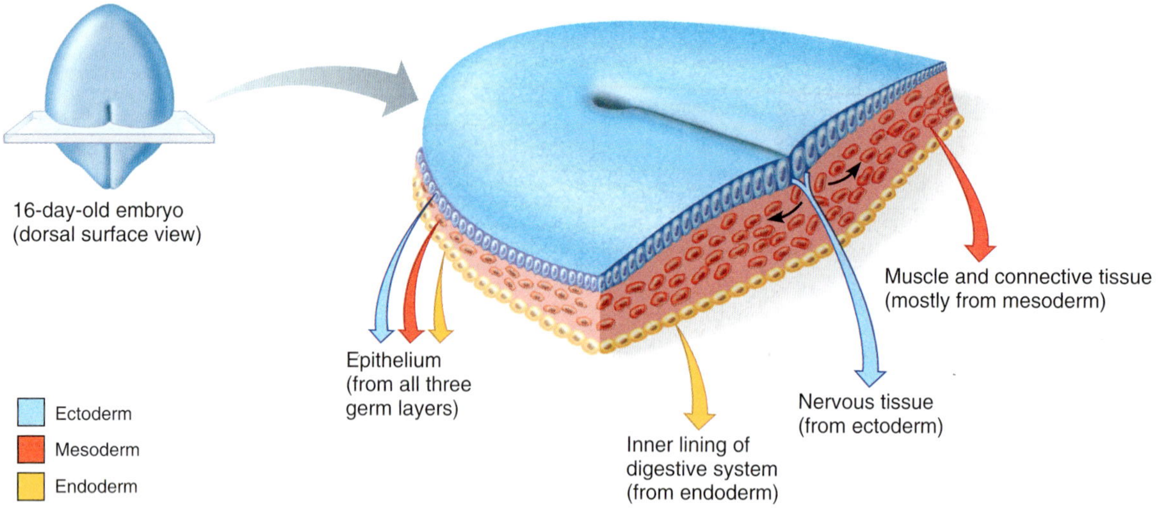

Figure 4.13 Embryonic germ layers and the primary tissue types they produce. The three embryonic layers collectively form the very early embryonic body.

Regenerative Capacity of Different Tissues

Tissues vary widely in their capacity for regeneration. Epithelial tissues, bone, areolar connective tissue, dense irregular connective tissue, and blood-forming tissue regenerate extremely well. Smooth muscle and dense regular connective tissue have a moderate capacity for regeneration, but skeletal muscle and cartilage have a weak regenerative capacity. Cardiac muscle and the nervous tissue in the brain and spinal cord have virtually no *functional* regenerative capacity, and they are routinely replaced by scar tissue. However, recent studies show that some unexpected (and highly selective) cellular division occurs in both these tissues after damage, and efforts are under way to coax them to regenerate better.

In nonregenerating tissues and in exceptionally severe wounds, fibrosis totally replaces the lost tissue. Over a period of months, the fibrous mass shrinks and becomes more and more compact. The resulting scar appears as a pale, often shiny area composed mostly of collagen fibers. Scar tissue is strong, but it lacks the flexibility and elasticity of most normal tissues. Also, it cannot perform the normal functions of the tissue it has replaced.

Homeostatic Imbalance 4.3

Scar tissue that forms in the wall of the urinary bladder, heart, or other muscular organ may severely hamper the organ's function. The normal shrinking of the scar reduces the internal volume and may hinder or even block substances from moving through a hollow organ. Scar tissue hampers muscle's ability to contract and may interfere with its normal excitation by the nervous system. In the heart, these problems may lead to progressive heart failure. In irritated visceral organs, particularly following abdominal surgery, *adhesions* may form as the newly forming scar tissue connects adjacent organs together. Such adhesions can prevent the normal shifting about (churning) of loops of the intestine, dangerously obstructing the flow of foodstuffs. Adhesions can also restrict heart movements and immobilize joints. +

☑ Check Your Understanding

21. What are the three main steps of tissue repair?
22. Why does a deep injury to the skin result in abundant scar tissue?

For answers, see Appendix H.

Developmental Aspects of Tissues

✓ Indicate the embryonic origin of each tissue class.

✓ Briefly describe tissue changes that occur with age.

One of the first events of embryonic development is the formation of the three **primary germ layers**, which lie one atop the next like a three-layered cellular pancake. From superficial to deep, these layers are the **ectoderm**, **mesoderm** (mez′o-derm), and **endoderm** **(Figure 4.13)**. These primary germ layers then specialize to form the four primary tissues—epithelium, nervous tissue, muscle, and connective tissues—that make up all body organs.

By the end of the second month of development, the primary tissues have appeared, and all major organs are in place. In general, tissue cells remain mitotic and produce the rapid growth that occurs before birth. The division of nerve cells, however, stops or nearly stops during the fetal period. After birth, the cells of most other tissues continue to divide until adult body size is achieved. Cellular division then slows greatly, although many tissues retain some ability to regenerate.

In adults, only epithelia and blood-forming tissues are highly mitotic. Some tissues that regenerate through life, such as the glandular cells of the liver, do so through division of their mature (specialized) cells. Others, like the epidermis of the skin and cells lining the intestine, have abundant *stem cells*, relatively undifferentiated cells that divide as necessary to produce new cells.

Cancer—The Intimate Enemy

The word **cancer** elicits **dread** in everyone. Why does cancer strike some and not others?

Although once perceived as disorganized cell growth, this disease is now known to be a logical, coordinated process in which a precise sequence of **tiny alterations** changes a normal cell into a **killer**.

When cells fail to follow normal controls of cell division and multiply excessively, an abnormal mass of proliferating cells called a **neoplasm** (ne'o-plazm, "new growth") results. Neoplasms are classified as **benign** ("kindly") or **malignant** ("bad"). A benign neoplasm is strictly a local affair. Its cells remain compacted, are often encapsulated, tend to grow slowly, and seldom kill their hosts if removed before they compress vital organs.

In contrast, cancers are malignant neoplasms, nonencapsulated masses that grow relentlessly. Their cells resemble immature cells, and they invade their surroundings rather than pushing them aside, as reflected in the name *cancer*, from the Latin word for "crab." Whereas normal cells become fatally "homesick" and die when they lose contact with the surrounding matrix, malignant cells tend to break away from the parent mass—the primary tumor—and travel via blood or lymph to other body organs, where they form *secondary cancer masses*.

This capability for traveling to other parts of the body, called **metastasis** (mĕ-tas'tah-sis), probably has a lot to do with signaling molecules and the cell-surface glycoproteins the cancer cells bear. Metastasis and invasiveness distinguish cancer cells from the cells of benign neoplasms. Cancer cells consume an exceptional amount of the body's nutrients, leading to weight loss and tissue wasting that contribute to death.

Carcinogenesis

Autopsies on individuals aged 50–70 who died of another cause have revealed that most of us have microscopic (but dormant) in situ (confined to origin site) neoplasms. So what changes a normal cell into a cancerous one? Some physical factors (radiation, mechanical trauma), certain viral infections, chronic inflammations, and many chemicals (tobacco tars, saccharine, some natural food chemicals).

All these factors cause *mutations*—changes in DNA that alter the expression of certain genes. However, not all carcinogens do damage because most are eliminated by peroxisomal or lysosomal enzymes or by the immune system. Furthermore, one mutation usually isn't enough. It takes several genetic changes to transform (convert) a normal cell into a cancerous cell.

The discovery of **oncogenes** (Greek *onco* = tumor), or cancer-causing genes, in rapidly spreading cancers provided a clue to the role of genes in cancer. **Proto-oncogenes**, benign forms of oncogenes in normal cells, were discovered later. Proto-oncogenes code for proteins that are essential for cell division, growth, and cellular adhesion, among other things. Many proto-oncogenes have fragile sites that break when exposed to carcinogens, converting them to oncogenes. Failure to code for certain proteins may lead to loss of an enzyme that controls an important metabolic process. Oncogenes may also "switch on" dormant genes that allow cells to become invasive and metastasize. Known oncogenes now number over 100.

Oncogenes have been detected in only 15–20% of human cancers, so investigators were not too surprised by the discovery of **tumor suppressor genes**, or **anti-oncogenes**, which suppress cancer by inactivating carcinogens, aiding DNA repair, or enhancing the immune system's counterattack. In fact, over half of all cancers involve malfunction or loss of just 2 of the 15 identified tumor suppressor genes—*p53* and *p16*. This is not surprising when you learn that *p53* prompts most cells to make proteins that stop cell division in stressed cells by promoting apoptosis or cell cycle arrest.

Furthermore, although each type of cancer is genetically distinct, human cancers appear to share a master set of genes—an activated group of 67 genes—and almost all cancer cells have gained or lost entire chromosomes. Whatever genetic factors are at work, the "seeds" of cancer appear to be in our own genes. Cancer is an intimate enemy indeed.

Let's look at the carcinogenesis of colorectal cancer, one of the best-understood human cancers. As with most cancers, a metastasis develops gradually. One of the first signs is a polyp (see photo on p. 146), a small benign growth consisting of apparently normal mucosa cells. As cell division continues, the polyp enlarges, becoming an adenoma (a term for any neoplasm of glandular epithelium). As various tumor suppressor genes are inactivated and the *K-ras* oncogene is mobilized, the mutations pile up and the adenoma becomes increasingly abnormal. The final consequence is colon carcinoma, a form of cancer that metastasizes quickly.

Cancer Prevalence

Almost half of all Americans develop cancer in their lifetime and a fifth of us will die of it. Cancer can arise from almost any cell type, but the most common cancers originate in the skin, lung, colon, breast, and prostate. Although stomach and colon cancer incidence is down, skin and lymphoid cancer rates are up.

Many cancers are preceded by observable lumps or other structural changes in tissue—for instance, *leukoplakia*, white patches in the mouth caused by the chronic irritation of ill-fitting dentures or heavy smoking. Although these lesions sometimes progress to cancer, in many cases they remain stable or even revert to normal if the environmental irritant is removed.

Diagnosis and Staging

Screening procedures are vital for early detection. Examples include *mammography* (X-ray examination of the breasts), examining breasts or testicles for lumps, examining the blood for cancer markers, and checking fecal samples for blood.

Unfortunately, most cancers are diagnosed only after symptoms have already appeared. In this case diagnosis is usually by **biopsy**: removing a tissue sample surgically and examining it microscopically for malignant cells. Increasingly, diagnosis includes chemical or genetic analysis of the sample—typing cancer cells by which genes are switched on or off, a technique described below.

Physical and histological examinations, lab tests, and imaging techniques (MRI, CT) can determine the extent of the disease (size of the neoplasm, degree of metastasis, etc.). Then, the cancer is assigned a **stage** from 1 to 4 according to the probability of cure. Stage 1 has the best probability of cure, stage 4 the worst.

4

Cancer Treatments

Most cancers are removed surgically if possible. To destroy metastasized cells, surgery is commonly followed by X irradiation and/or treatment with radioisotopes and chemotherapy (treatment with cytotoxic drugs). Recently, some oncologists have been using heat therapy (a slight upward temperature change) to make cancer cells more vulnerable to chemotherapy or radiation.

Chemotherapy is beset with the problem of resistance. Some cancer cells can eject the drugs in tiny bubbles or flattened vesicles dubbed exosomes, and these cells proliferate, forming new tumors that are resistant to chemotherapy. Furthermore, anticancer drugs have unpleasant side effects—nausea, vomiting, hair loss—because they kill *all* rapidly dividing cells, including normal tissue cells. The anticancer drugs also can damage the brain, producing a phenomenon called chemobrain—mental fuzziness and memory loss reported by many cancer patients. X rays also have side effects because, in passing through the body, they destroy healthy tissue as well as cancer cells.

Promising New Therapies

Traditional cancer treatments—"cut, burn, and poison"—are widely recognized as crude and painful. Promising new therapies focus on

- *Interrupting the signaling pathways that fuel cancer growth.* Imatinib (brand name Gleevec) incapacitates a mutated enzyme that triggers uncontrolled division of cells in two rare blood and digestive system cancers. Trastuzumab (Herceptin) is used to treat breast cancer. These drugs can provide a few extra weeks of life, before their protective effects wear off and the disease progresses again.
- *Delivering treatments more precisely to the cancer while sparing normal tissue.* One approach is to inject the patient with tiny drug-coated metal beads; then a powerful magnet positioned over the cancer guides the beads to the tumor. Or, a patient might take light-sensitive drugs that are drawn naturally into rapidly dividing cancer cells. Then, exposure to certain frequencies of laser light sets off reactions that kill the malignant cells. Proton therapy delivers highly targeted killing doses of protons (radiation) with incredible precision and effectiveness. Unlike X rays, which pass through the cancer and onward through the patient's body, protons can be slowed down and even directed to stop in the neoplasm.
- *Using genetically modified immune cells to target cancer cells.* One promising technique harvests a patient's most aggressive cancer-killing immune cells (T lymphocytes), inserts modified genes into them that make them even more efficient, multiplies the cells in the lab, and infuses them back into the patient.
- *Testing genotypes.* A few major cancer centers are beginning to genotype (test for genetic markers) every patient's tumor. The hope is to match personalized markers with drugs tailored to go after the tumor's genetic weak spot. For example, taxol, quite successful in treating breast and ovarian cancer, works only against tumors with a specific genetic makeup.

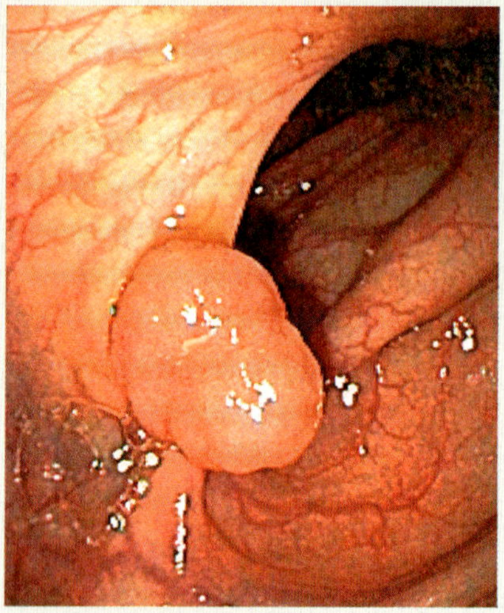

A polyp in the colon

Other experimental treatments seek to starve cancer cells by cutting off their blood supply, fix defective tumor suppressor genes and oncogenes, destroy cancer cells with viruses, or signal cancer cells to commit suicide by apoptosis. A cancer vaccine (TRICOM) contains genetically engineered viruses carrying genes for a cancer protein called carcinoembryonic antigen (CEA). When CEA proteins are delivered into the patient's body, they stimulate an immune response that orchestrates an attack on all CEA-bearing cancer cells.

At present, about half of all cancer cases are cured. Although average survival rates have not increased, cancer patients' quality of life has improved in the last decade. We can offer better treatments for cancer-associated pain, and antinausea drugs and other helpful medicines can soothe the side effects of chemotherapy.

Given good nutrition, good circulation, and relatively infrequent wounds and infections, our tissues normally function efficiently through youth and middle age. But with increasing age, epithelia thin and are more easily breached. Tissue repair is less efficient, and bone, muscle, and nervous tissues begin to atrophy, particularly when a person is not physically active. These events are due partly to decreased circulatory efficiency, which reduces delivery of nutrients to the tissues, but in some cases, diet is a contributing factor. As income declines or as chewing becomes more difficult, older people tend to eat soft foods, which may be low in protein and vitamins. As a result, tissue health suffers.

Another problem of aging tissues is the likelihood of DNA mutations in the most actively mitotic cells, which increases the risk of cancer (see *A Closer Look* on p. 145).

☑ Check Your Understanding

23. What are the names of the three embryonic germ layers?
24. Which germ layer gives rise to the nervous system?
25. Which two tissue types remain highly mitotic throughout life?

For answers, see Appendix H.

As we have seen, body cells combine to form four discrete tissue types: epithelial, connective, nervous, and muscle tissues. The cells making up each of these tissues share certain features but are by no means identical. They "belong" together because they have basic functional similarities. The important concept to carry away with you is that tissues, despite their unique abilities, cooperate to keep the body safe, healthy, and whole.

Chapter Summary

MAP™ For more chapter study tools, go to the Study Area of MasteringA&P at **www.masteringaandp.com**.
There you will find:

- Interactive Physiology iP
- A&PFlix A&PFlix
- Practice Anatomy Lab PAL
- PhysioEx PEx
- Videos, Practice Quizzes and Tests, MP3 Tutor Sessions, Case Studies, and much more!

Tissues are collections of structurally similar cells with related functions. The four primary tissues are epithelial, connective, nervous, and muscle tissues.

Preparing Human Tissue for Microscopy (pp. 117–118)

1. Preparation of tissues for microscopic examination involves cutting thin sections of the tissue and using dyes to stain the tissue. Minor distortions called artifacts can be introduced by the tissue preparation process.

Epithelial Tissue (pp. 118–126)

1. Epithelial tissue is the covering, lining, and glandular tissue of the body. Its functions include protection, absorption, excretion, filtration, secretion, and sensory reception.

Special Characteristics of Epithelium (pp. 118–119)

2. Epithelial tissues exhibit specialized contacts, polarity, avascularity, support from connective tissue, and high regenerative capacity.

Classification of Epithelia (pp. 119–124)

3. Epithelium is classified by arrangement as simple (one layer) or stratified (more than one layer) and by cell shape as squamous, cuboidal, or columnar. The terms denoting cell shape and arrangement are combined to describe the epithelium fully.
4. Simple squamous epithelium is a single layer of squamous cells. Highly adapted for filtration and exchange of substances, it forms walls of air sacs of the lungs and lines blood vessels. It contributes to serosae as mesothelium and lines all hollow circulatory system organs as endothelium.
5. Simple cuboidal epithelium, commonly active in secretion and absorption, is found in glands and in kidney tubules.
6. Simple columnar epithelium, specialized for secretion and absorption, consists of a single layer of tall columnar cells that exhibit microvilli and often mucus-producing cells. It lines most of the digestive tract.
7. Pseudostratified columnar epithelium is a simple columnar epithelium that appears stratified. Its ciliated variety, rich in mucus-secreting cells, lines most of the upper respiratory passages.
8. Stratified squamous epithelium is multilayered; cells at the free surface are squamous. It is adapted to resist abrasion. It lines the esophagus and vagina; its keratinized variety forms the skin epidermis.
9. Stratified cuboidal epithelia are rare in the body, and are found chiefly in ducts of large glands. Stratified columnar epithelium has a very limited distribution, found mainly in the male urethra and at transition areas between other epithelia types.
10. Transitional epithelium is a modified stratified squamous epithelium, adapted for responding to stretch. It lines hollow urinary system organs.

Glandular Epithelia (pp. 124–126)

11. A gland is one or more cells specialized to secrete a product.
12. On the basis of site of product release, glands are classified as exocrine or endocrine. Glands are classified structurally as multicellular or unicellular.
13. Unicellular glands, typified by goblet cells and mucous cells, are mucus-secreting single-celled glands.
14. Multicellular exocrine glands are classified according to duct structure as simple or compound, and according to the structure of their secretory parts as tubular, alveolar, or tubuloalveolar.
15. Multicellular exocrine glands of humans are classified functionally as merocrine or holocrine.

Connective Tissue (pp. 127–136)

1. Connective tissue is the most abundant and widely distributed tissue of the body. Its functions include binding and support, protection, insulation, fat storage, and transportation (blood).

Common Characteristics of Connective Tissue (p. 127)

2. Connective tissues originate from embryonic mesenchyme and have a matrix. Depending on type, a connective tissue may be well vascularized (most), poorly vascularized (dense connective tissue), or avascular (cartilage).

Structural Elements of Connective Tissue (pp. 127–129)

3. The structural elements of all connective tissues are extracellular matrix and cells.
4. The extracellular matrix consists of ground substance and fibers (collagen, elastic, and reticular). It may be fluid, gel-like, or firm.
5. Each connective tissue type has a primary cell type that can exist as a mitotic, matrix-secreting cell (blast) or as a mature cell (cyte) responsible for maintaining the matrix. The undifferentiated cell type of connective tissue proper is the fibroblast; that of cartilage is the chondroblast; that of bone is the osteoblast; and that of blood-forming tissue is the hematopoietic stem cell (see Chapter 17).

Types of Connective Tissue (pp. 129–136)

6. Embryonic connective tissue is called mesenchyme.
7. Connective tissue proper consists of loose and dense varieties. The loose connective tissues are
   - Areolar: gel-like ground substance; all three fiber types loosely interwoven; a variety of cells; forms the lamina propria and soft packing around body organs; the prototype.
   - Adipose: consists largely of adipocytes; scant matrix; insulates and protects body organs; provides reserve energy fuel. Brown fat is more important for generating body heat.
   - Reticular: finely woven reticular fibers in soft ground substance; the stroma of lymphoid organs and bone marrow.
8. Dense connective tissue proper includes
   - Dense regular: dense parallel bundles of collagen fibers; few cells, little ground substance; high tensile strength; forms tendons, ligaments, aponeuroses; in cases where this tissue also contains numerous elastic fibers it is called elastic connective tissue.
   - Dense irregular: like regular variety, but fibers are arranged in different planes; resists tension exerted from many

different directions; forms the dermis of the skin and organ capsules.

9. Cartilage exists as
   - Hyaline: firm ground substance containing collagen fibers; resists compression well; found in fetal skeleton, at articulating surfaces of bones, and trachea; most abundant type.
   - Elastic cartilage: elastic fibers predominate; provides flexible support of the external ear and epiglottis.
   - Fibrocartilage: parallel collagen fibers; provides support with compressibility; forms intervertebral discs and knee cartilages.
10. Bone (osseous tissue) consists of a hard, collagen-containing matrix embedded with calcium salts; forms the bony skeleton.
11. Blood consists of blood cells in a fluid matrix (plasma).

4

Muscle Tissue (pp. 136–139)

1. Muscle tissue consists of elongated cells specialized to contract and cause movement.
2. Based on structure and function, the muscle tissues are
   - Skeletal muscle: attached to and moves the bony skeleton; cells are cylindrical and striated.
   - Cardiac muscle: forms the walls of the heart; pumps blood; cells are branched and striated.
   - Smooth muscle: in the walls of hollow organs; propels substances through the organs; cells are spindle shaped and lack striations.

Nervous Tissue (p. 140)

1. Nervous tissue forms organs of the nervous system. It is composed of neurons and supporting cells.
2. Neurons are branching cells that receive and transmit electrical impulses. They are involved in body regulation. Supporting cells support and protect neurons.

iP Nervous System I; Topic: Anatomy Review, pp. 1, 3.

Covering and Lining Membranes (pp. 140–142)

1. Membranes are simple organs, consisting of an epithelium bound to an underlying connective tissue layer. They include mucosae, serosae, and the cutaneous membrane.

Tissue Repair (pp. 142–144)

1. Inflammation is the body's response to injury. Tissue repair begins during the inflammatory process. It may lead to regeneration, fibrosis, or both.
2. Tissue repair begins with organization, during which the blood clot is replaced by granulation tissue. If the wound is small and the damaged tissue is actively mitotic, the tissue will regenerate and cover the fibrous tissue. When a wound is extensive or the damaged tissue amitotic, it is repaired only by fibrous connective (scar) tissue.

Developmental Aspects of Tissues (pp. 144–146)

1. Epithelium arises from all three primary germ layers (ectoderm, mesoderm, endoderm); muscle and connective tissue from mesoderm; and nervous tissue from ectoderm.
2. The decrease in mass and viability seen in most tissues during old age often reflects circulatory deficits or poor nutrition.

Review Questions

Multiple Choice/Matching

(Some questions have more than one correct answer. Select the best answer or answers from the choices given.)

1. Use the key to classify each of the following described tissue types into one of the four major tissue categories.

   Key: **(a)** connective tissue **(c)** muscle
   (b) epithelium **(d)** nervous tissue

   ____ **(1)** Tissue type composed largely of nonliving extracellular matrix; important in protection and support
   ____ **(2)** The tissue immediately responsible for body movement
   ____ **(3)** The tissue that enables us to be aware of the external environment and to react to it
   ____ **(4)** The tissue that lines body cavities and covers surfaces
2. An epithelium that has several layers, with an apical layer of flattened cells, is called (choose all that apply): **(a)** ciliated, **(b)** columnar, **(c)** stratified, **(d)** simple, **(e)** squamous.
3. Match the epithelial types named in column B with the appropriate description(s) in column A.

Column A	Column B
____ **(1)** Lines most of the digestive tract	**(a)** pseudostratified ciliated columnar
____ **(2)** Lines the esophagus	**(b)** simple columnar
____ **(3)** Lines much of the respiratory tract	**(c)** simple cuboidal
____ **(4)** Forms the walls of the air sacs of the lungs	**(d)** simple squamous
____ **(5)** Found in urinary tract organs	**(e)** stratified columnar
____ **(6)** Endothelium and mesothelium	**(f)** stratified squamous
	(g) transitional

4. The gland type that secretes products such as milk, saliva, bile, or sweat through a duct is **(a)** an endocrine gland, **(b)** an exocrine gland.
5. The membrane which lines body cavities that open to the exterior is a(n) **(a)** endothelium, **(b)** cutaneous membrane, **(c)** mucous membrane, **(d)** serous membrane.
6. Scar tissue is a variety of **(a)** epithelium, **(b)** connective tissue, **(c)** muscle tissue, **(d)** nervous tissue, **(e)** all of these.

Short Answer Essay Questions

7. Define tissue.
8. Name four important functions of epithelial tissue and provide at least one example of a tissue that exemplifies each function.
9. Describe the criteria used to classify covering and lining epithelia.
10. Explain the functional classification of multicellular exocrine glands and supply an example for each class.
11. Provide examples from the body that illustrate four of the major functions of connective tissue.
12. Name the primary cell type in connective tissue proper; in cartilage; in bone.
13. Name the two major components of matrix and, if applicable, subclasses of each component.
14. Matrix is extracellular. How does the matrix get to its characteristic position?

15. Name the specific connective tissue type found in the following body locations: (a) forming the soft packing around organs, (b) supporting the ear pinna, (c) forming "stretchy" ligaments, (d) first connective tissue in the embryo, (e) forming the intervertebral discs, (f) covering the ends of bones at joint surfaces, (g) main component of subcutaneous tissue.
16. What is the function of macrophages?
17. Differentiate between the roles of neurons and the supporting cells of nervous tissue.
18. Compare and contrast skeletal, cardiac, and smooth muscle tissue relative to structure, body location, and specific function.
19. Describe the process of tissue repair, making sure you indicate factors that influence this process.
20. Indicate which primary tissue classes derive from each embryonic germ layer.
21. In what ways are adipose tissue and bone similar? How are they different?

Critical Thinking and Clinical Application Questions

1. John sustained a severe injury during football practice and is told that he has a torn knee cartilage. Can he expect a quick, uneventful recovery? Explain your response.
2. The epidermis (epithelium of the cutaneous membrane or skin) is a keratinized stratified squamous epithelium. Explain why that epithelium is much better suited for protecting the body's external surface than a mucosa consisting of a simple columnar epithelium would be.
3. Your friend is trying to convince you that if the ligaments binding the bones together at your freely movable joints (such as your knee, shoulder, and hip joints) contained more elastic fibers, you would be much more flexible. Although there is some truth to this statement, such a condition would present serious problems. Why?
4. In adults, over 90% of all cancers are either adenomas (adenocarcinomas) or carcinomas. (See Related Clinical Terms for this chapter.) In fact, cancers of the skin, lung, colon, breast, and prostate are all in these categories. Which one of the four basic tissue types gives rise to most cancers? Why do you think this is so?
5. Cindy, an overweight high school student, is overheard telling her friend that she's going to research how she can transform some of her white fat to brown fat. What is her rationale here (assuming it is possible)?
6. Mrs. Delancy went to the local meat market and bought a beef tenderloin (cut from the loin, the region along the steer's vertebral column) and some tripe (cow's stomach). What type of muscle was she preparing to eat in each case?

AT THE CLINIC

Related Clinical Terms

Adenoma (ad″ĕ-no′mah; *aden* = gland, *oma* = tumor) Any neoplasm of glandular epithelium, benign or malignant. The malignant type is more specifically called adenocarcinoma.

Autopsy (aw′top-se) Examination of the body, its organs, and its tissues after death to determine the actual cause of death; also called postmortem examination and necropsy.

Carcinoma (kar″sĭ-no′mah; *karkinos* = crab, cancer) Cancer arising in an epithelium; accounts for 90% of human cancers.

Healing by first intention The simplest type of healing; occurs when the edges of the wound are brought together by sutures, staples, or other means used to close surgical incisions. Only small amounts of granulation tissue need be formed.

Healing by second intention The wound edges remain separated, and relatively large amounts of granulation tissue bridge the gap; the manner in which unattended wounds heal. Healing is slower than in wounds in which the edges are brought together, and larger scars result.

Keloid (ke′loid) Abnormal proliferation of connective tissue during healing of skin wounds; results in large, unsightly mass of scar tissue at the skin surface.

Lesion (le′zhun; "wound") Any injury, wound, or infection that affects tissue over an area of a definite size (as opposed to being widely spread throughout the body).

Marfan's syndrome Genetic disease resulting in abnormalities of connective tissues due to a defect in fibrillin, a protein that is associated with elastin in elastic fibers. Clinical signs include loose-jointedness, long limbs and spiderlike fingers and toes, visual problems, and weakened blood vessels (especially the aorta) due to poor connective tissue reinforcement.

Osteogenesis imperfecta (brittle bone disease) An inherited condition that causes defective collagen production. Because collagen reinforces many body structures including bones, the result is weak bones that break easily. It is not unusual for its victims to have 30 or more fractures during their lifetime. Occurs in 1 out of 20,000 births. Misdiagnosis results in many infants coming to the ER with multiple fractures being treated as battered babies.

Pathology (pah-thol′o-je) Scientific study of changes in organs and tissues produced by disease.

Pus A collection of tissue fluid, bacteria, dead and dying tissue cells, white blood cells, and macrophages in an inflamed area.

Sarcoma (sar-ko′mah; *sarkos* = flesh; *oma* = tumor) Cancer arising in the mesenchyme-derived tissues, that is, in connective tissues and muscle.

Scurvy A nutritional deficiency caused by lack of adequate vitamin C needed to synthesize collagen; signs and symptoms include blood vessel disruption, delay in wound healing, weakness of scar tissue, and loosening of teeth.

VAC (vacuum-assisted closure) Innovative healing process for open-skin wounds and skin ulcers. Often induces healing when all other methods fail. Involves covering the wound with a special sponge, and then applying suction through the sponge. In response to the subsequent skin stretching, fibroblasts in the wound form more collagen tissue and new blood vessels proliferate, bringing more blood into the injured area, which also promotes healing.

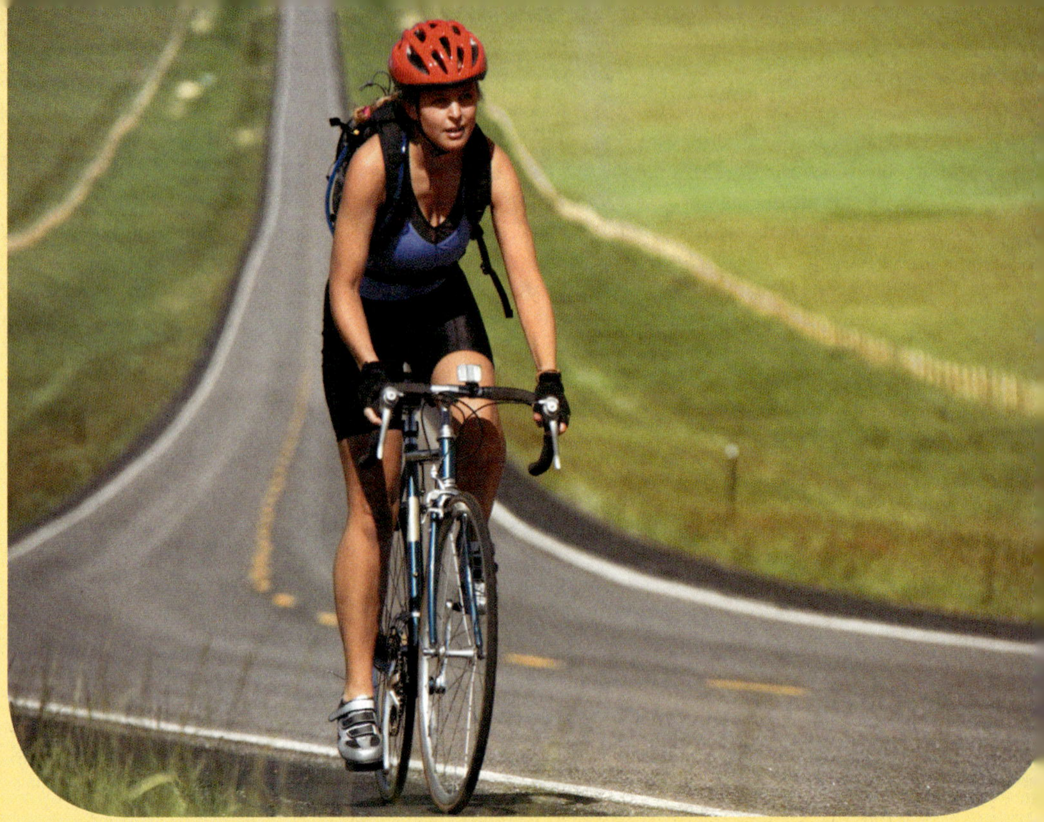

5 The Integumentary System

Would you be enticed by an ad for a coat that is waterproof, stretchable, washable, and permanent-press, that automatically repairs small cuts, rips, and burns? How about one that's guaranteed to last a lifetime? Sounds too good to be true, but you already have such a coat—your skin.

The skin and its derivatives (sweat and oil glands, hairs, and nails) make up a complex set of organs that serves several functions, mostly protective. Together, these organs form the **integumentary system** (in-teg″u-men′tar-e).

The Skin

✓ Name the tissue types composing the epidermis and dermis. List the major layers of each and describe the functions of each layer.

✓ Describe the factors that normally contribute to skin color. Briefly describe how changes in skin color may be used as clinical signs of certain disease states.

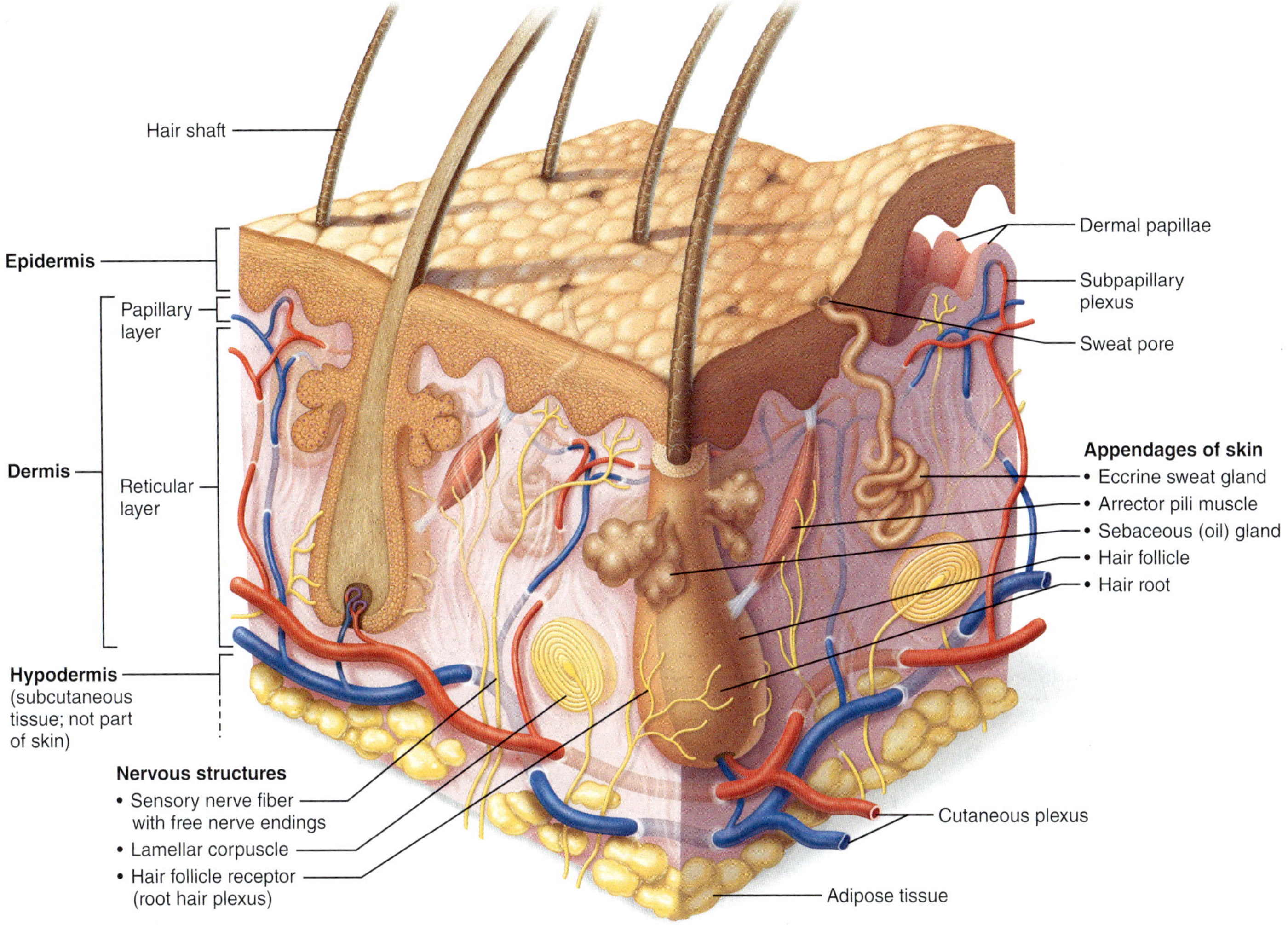

Figure 5.1 Skin structure. Three-dimensional view of the skin and underlying subcutaneous tissue. The epidermal and dermal layers have been pulled apart at the right corner to reveal the dermal papillae.

The skin receives little respect from its inhabitants, but architecturally it is a marvel. It covers the entire body, has a surface area of 1.2 to 2.2 square meters, weighs 4 to 5 kilograms (4–5 kg = 9–11 lb), and accounts for about 7% of total body weight in the average adult. Also called the integument ("covering"), the skin multitasks. Its functions go well beyond serving as a bag for body contents. Pliable yet tough, it takes constant punishment from external agents. Without our skin, we would quickly fall prey to bacteria and perish from water and heat loss.

Varying in thickness from 1.5 to 4.0 millimeters (mm) or more in different parts of the body, the skin is composed of two distinct regions **(Figure 5.1)**:

- The *epidermis* (ep″ĭ-der′mis), composed of epithelial cells, is the outermost protective shield of the body (*epi* = upon).
- The underlying *dermis,* making up the bulk of the skin, is a tough, leathery layer composed mostly of fibrous connective tissue.

Only the dermis is vascularized. Nutrients reach the epidermis by diffusing through the tissue fluid from blood vessels in the dermis.

The subcutaneous tissue just deep to the skin is known as the **hypodermis** (Figure 5.1). Strictly speaking, the hypodermis is not part of the skin, but it shares some of the skin's protective functions. The hypodermis, also called **superficial fascia** because it is superficial to the tough connective tissue wrapping (fascia) of the skeletal muscles, consists mostly of adipose tissue.

Besides storing fat, the hypodermis anchors the skin to the underlying structures (mostly to muscles), but loosely enough that the skin can slide relatively freely over those structures. Sliding skin protects us by ensuring that many blows just glance off our bodies. Because of its fatty composition, the hypodermis also acts as a shock absorber and an insulator that reduces heat loss. The hypodermis thickens markedly when a person gains weight. In females, this "extra" subcutaneous fat accumulates first in the thighs and breasts, but in males it first collects in the anterior abdomen (as a "beer belly").

Epidermis

Structurally, the **epidermis** is a keratinized stratified squamous epithelium consisting of four distinct cell types and four or five distinct layers.

Cells of the Epidermis

The cells populating the epidermis include *keratinocytes, melanocytes, dendritic cells,* and *tactile cells.*

Keratinocytes The chief role of **keratinocytes** (kĕ-rat′ĭ-no-sītz″; "keratin cells") is to produce **keratin**, the fibrous protein that helps give the epidermis its protective properties (Greek *kera* = horn) (**Figure 5.2b**, orange cells). Most epidermal cells are keratinocytes.

Tightly connected to one another by desmosomes, the keratinocytes arise in the deepest part of the epidermis from a cell layer called the stratum basale. These cells undergo almost continuous mitosis in response to prompting by epidermal growth factor, a peptide produced by various cells throughout the body. As these cells are pushed upward by the production of new cells beneath them, they make the keratin that eventually dominates their cell contents. By the time the keratinocytes reach the skin surface, they are dead, scalelike structures that are little more than keratin-filled plasma membranes.

5

Millions of dead keratinocytes rub off every day, giving us a totally new epidermis every 25 to 45 days, but cell production and keratin formation is accelerated in body areas regularly subjected to friction, such as the hands and feet. Persistent friction (from a poorly fitting shoe, for example) causes a thickening of the epidermis called a *callus*.

Melanocytes **Melanocytes** (mel′ah-no-sītz), the spider-shaped epithelial cells that synthesize the pigment **melanin** (mel′ah-nin; *melan* = black), are found in the deepest layer of the epidermis (Figure 5.2b, gray cells). As melanin is made, it accumulates in membrane-bound granules called *melanosomes* that motor proteins move along actin filaments to the ends of the melanocyte's processes (the "spider arms"). From there they are transferred to a number of nearby keratinocytes (4 to 10 depending on body area). The melanin granules accumulate on the superficial, or "sunny," side of the keratinocyte nucleus, forming a pigment shield that protects the nucleus from the damaging effects of ultraviolet (UV) radiation in sunlight.

Dendritic Cells The star-shaped **dendritic cells** arise from bone marrow and migrate to the epidermis. Also called **Langerhans cells** (lahng′er-hanz) after a German anatomist, they ingest foreign substances and are key activators of our immune system, as described later in this chapter. Their slender processes extend among the surrounding keratinocytes, forming a more or less continuous network (Figure 5.2b, purple cell).

Tactile Cells Occasional **tactile (Merkel) cells** are present at the epidermal-dermal junction. Shaped like a spiky hemisphere (Figure 5.2b, blue cell), each tactile cell is intimately associated with a disclike sensory nerve ending. The combination, called a *tactile* or *Merkel disc*, functions as a sensory receptor for touch.

Layers of the Epidermis

Variation in epidermal thickness determines if skin is *thick* or *thin.* In **thick skin**, which covers areas subject to abrasion—the palms, fingertips, and soles of the feet—the epidermis consists of five layers, or strata (stra′tah; "bed sheets"). From deep to superficial, these layers are stratum basale, stratum spinosum, stratum granulosum, stratum lucidum, and stratum corneum. In thin skin, which covers the rest of the body, the stratum lucidum appears to be absent and the other strata are thinner (Figure 5.2a, b).

Note that the terms "thick skin" and "thin skin" are really misnomers because they refer to the epidermis only. Indeed, the thickest skin in the body is on the upper back.

Stratum Basale (Basal Layer) The **stratum basale** (stra′tum bah-sa′le), the deepest epidermal layer, is attached to the underlying dermis along a wavy borderline that reminds one of corrugated cardboard. For the most part, it consists of a single row of stem cells—a continually renewing cell population—representing the youngest keratinocytes. The many mitotic nuclei seen in this layer reflect the rapid division of these cells and account for its alternate name, **stratum germinativum** (jer′mĭ-nă″tiv-um; "germinating layer"). Each time one of these basal cells divides, one daughter cell is pushed into the cell layer just above to begin its specialization into a mature keratinocyte. The other daughter cell remains in the basal layer to continue the process of producing new keratinocytes.

Some 10–25% of the cells in the stratum basale are melanocytes, and their branching processes extend among the surrounding cells, reaching well into the more superficial stratum spinosum layer. Occasional tactile cells also occur in this stratum.

Stratum Spinosum (Prickly Layer) The **stratum spinosum** (spi′no-sum; "prickly") is several cell layers thick. These cells contain a weblike system of intermediate filaments, mainly tension-resisting bundles of pre-keratin filaments, which span their cytosol to attach to desmosomes. Looking like tiny versions of the spiked iron balls used in medieval warfare, the keratinocytes in this layer appear to have spines, causing them to be called *prickle cells.* The spines do not exist in the living cells; they are artifacts that arise during tissue preparation when these cells shrink but their numerous desmosomes hold tight. Scattered among the keratinocytes are melanin granules and dendritic cells, which are most abundant in this epidermal layer.

Stratum Granulosum (Granular Layer) The thin **stratum granulosum** (gran″u-lo′sum) consists of four to six cell layers in which keratinocyte appearance changes drastically, and the process of **keratinization** (in which the cells fill with the protein keratin) begins. These cells flatten, their nuclei and organelles begin to disintegrate, and they accumulate two types of granules. The *keratohyaline granules* (ker″ah-to-hi′ah-lin) help to form keratin in the upper layers, as we will see.

The *lamellar granules* (lam′el-ar; "a small plate") contain a water-resistant glycolipid that is spewed into the extracellular space and is a major factor in slowing water loss across the epidermis. The plasma membranes of these cells thicken as cytosol proteins bind to the inner membrane face and lipids released by the lamellar granules coat their external surfaces. These events produce an epidermal water barrier and make the cells more resistant to destruction. So, you might say that keratinocytes "toughen up" to make the outer strata the strongest skin region.

Like all epithelia, the epidermis relies on capillaries in the underlying connective tissue (the dermis in this case) for its nutrients. Above the stratum granulosum, the epidermal cells are

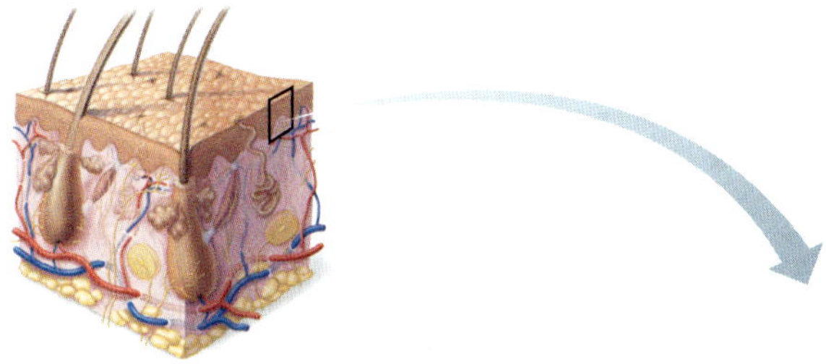

Figure 5.2 The main structural features of the skin epidermis. **(a)** Photomicrograph of the four major epidermal layers (200×). **(b)** Diagram showing these four layers and the distribution of different cell types. The four cell types are keratinocytes (orange), melanocytes (gray), dendritic cells (purple), and tactile cells (blue). A sensory nerve ending (yellow), extending from the dermis (pink), is shown associated with the tactile cell forming a tactile disc (touch receptor). Notice that numerous desmosomes join the keratinocytes together. The stratum lucidum, found only in thick skin, is not illustrated here.

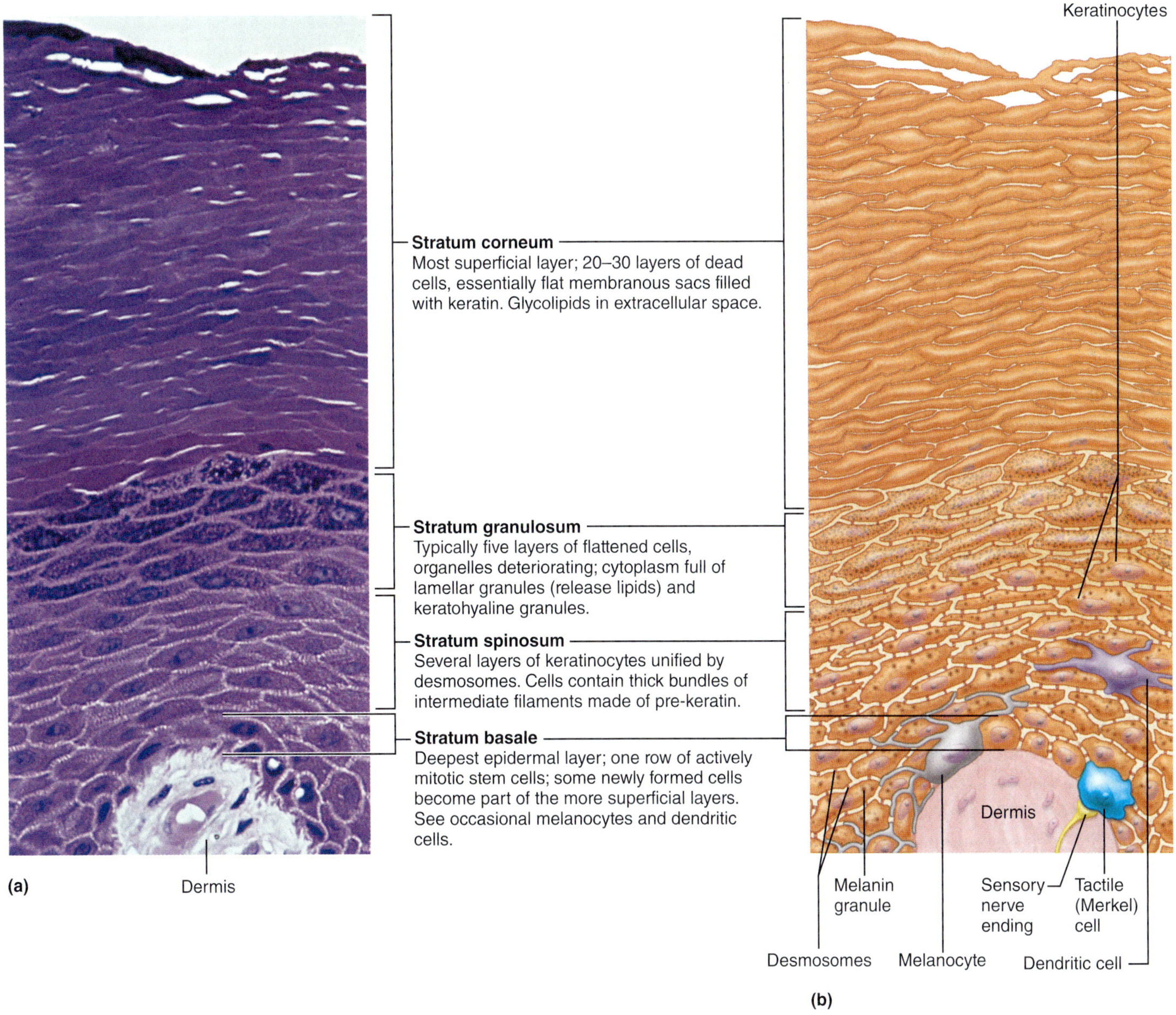

too far from the dermal capillaries and the glycolipids coating their external surfaces cut them off from nutrients, so they die. This is a normal sequence of events.

Stratum Lucidum (Clear Layer) Through the light microscope, the **stratum lucidum** (loo′sid-um; "light"), visible only in thick skin, is a thin translucent band just above the stratum granulosum. Considered by some to be a subdivision of the superficial stratum corneum, it consists of two or three rows of clear, flat, dead keratinocytes with indistinct boundaries. Here, or in the stratum corneum above, the gummy substance of the keratohyaline granules clings to the keratin filaments in the cells, causing them to aggregate in large, cable-like, parallel arrays of intermediate filaments called *tonofilaments*.

Stratum Corneum (Horny Layer) An abrupt transition occurs between the nucleated cells of the stratum granulosum and the flattened anucleate cells of the **stratum corneum** (kor′ne-um). This outermost epidermal layer is a broad zone 20 to 30 cell layers thick that accounts for up to three-quarters of the epidermal thickness. Keratin and the thickened plasma membranes of cells in this stratum protect the skin against abrasion and penetration, and the glycolipid between its cells nearly waterproofs this layer. For these reasons, the stratum corneum provides a durable "overcoat" for the body, protecting deeper cells from the hostile external environment (air) and from water loss, and rendering the body relatively insensitive to biological, chemical, and physical assaults. It is amazing that even dead cells can still play so many roles.

The differentiation from basal cells to those typical of the stratum corneum is a specialized form of apoptosis in which the nucleus and other organelles break down and the plasma membrane thickens. So, the terminal cells do not fragment, but instead eventually slough off the skin surface. The shingle-like cell remnants of the stratum corneum are referred to as *cornified,* or *horny, cells* (*cornu* = horn). They are familiar to everyone as dandruff, shed from the scalp, and dander, the loose flakes that slough off dry skin.

The average person's skin sheds some 50,000 dead cells every minute and 18 kg (40 lb) of these skin flakes in a lifetime, providing a lot of fodder for the dust mites that inhabit our homes and bed linens. The saying "Beauty is only skin deep" is especially interesting in light of the fact that nearly everything we see when we look at someone is dead!

Check Your Understanding

1. While walking barefoot in a barn, Jeremy stepped on a rusty nail that penetrated the epidermis on the sole of his foot. Name the layers the nail pierced from the superficial skin surface to the junction with the dermis.
2. The stratum basale is also called the stratum germinativum, a name that refers to its major function. What is that function?
3. Why are the desmosomes connecting the keratinocytes so important?
4. Given that epithelia are avascular, which layer would you expect to have the best-nourished cells?

For answers, see Appendix H.

Dermis

The **dermis** (*derm* = skin), the second major skin region, is strong, flexible connective tissue. Its cells are typical of those found in any connective tissue proper: fibroblasts, macrophages, and occasional mast cells and white blood cells. Its semifluid matrix, embedded with fibers, binds the entire body together like a body stocking. It is your "hide" and corresponds exactly to animal hides used to make leather.

The dermis has a rich supply of nerve fibers, blood vessels, and lymphatic vessels. The major portions of hair follicles, as well as oil and sweat glands, derive from epidermal tissue but reside in the dermis.

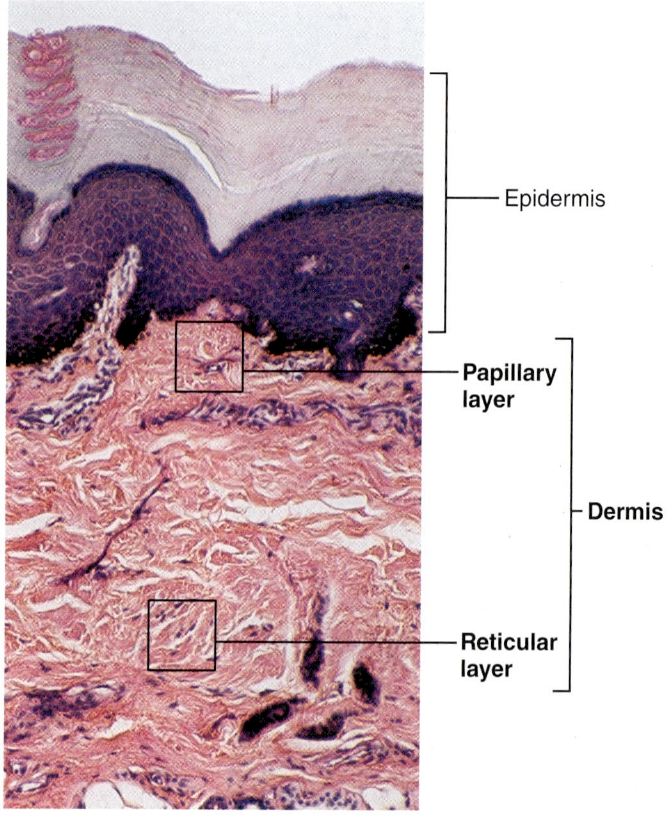

Figure 5.3 Light micrograph of the dermis identifying the papillary layer composed of areolar connective tissue and the reticular layer of dense irregular connective tissue (110×).

The dermis has two layers, the papillary and reticular, which abut one another along an indistinct boundary **(Figure 5.3)**.

Papillary Layer The thin superficial **papillary layer** (pap′il-er-e) is areolar connective tissue in which fine interlacing collagen and elastic fibers form a loosely woven mat that is heavily invested with small blood vessels. The looseness of this connective tissue allows phagocytes and other defensive cells to wander freely as they patrol the area for bacteria that have breached the skin.

Peglike projections from its surface, called **dermal papillae** (pah-pil′e; *papill* = nipple), indent the overlying epidermis (see Figure 5.1). Many dermal papillae contain capillary loops. Others house free nerve endings (pain receptors) and touch receptors called *tactile* or *Meissner's corpuscles* (mīs′nerz kor′pus-lz). Note that tactile cells and tactile corpuscles are different structures. (We consider them in more detail in Chapter 13.) In thick skin, such as the palms of the hands and soles of the feet, these papillae lie atop larger mounds called *dermal ridges,* which in turn cause the overlying epidermis to form *epidermal ridges* **(Figure 5.4a)**. Collectively, these skin ridges, referred to as **friction ridges**, are assumed to enhance the gripping ability of the fingers and feet like tire treads help grip the road. Recent studies indicate that they also contribute to our sense of touch by amplifying vibrations detected by the large lamellar corpuscles (receptors) in the dermis.

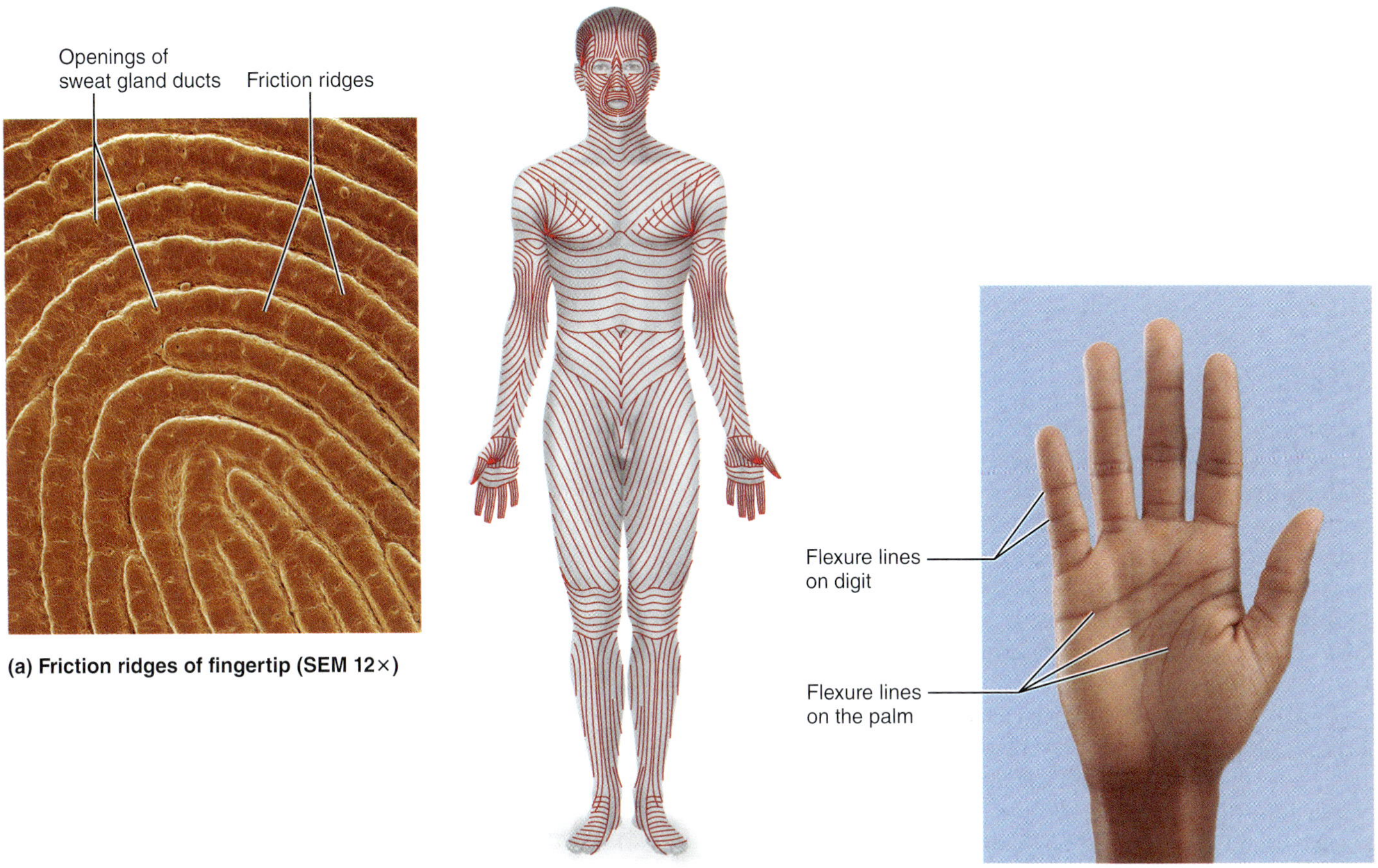

(a) Friction ridges of fingertip (SEM 12×)

(b) Cleavage lines in the reticular dermis

(c) Flexure lines of the hand

Figure 5.4 Dermal modifications result in characteristic skin markings. **(a)** Scanning electron micrograph of friction ridges (epidermal ridges topping the deeper dermal papillary ridges). Notice the sweat duct openings along the crests of the ridges, which are responsible for fingerprints. **(b)** Cleavage (tension) lines represent separations between underlying collagen fiber bundles in the reticular region of the dermis. They tend to run circularly around the trunk and longitudinally in the limbs. **(c)** Flexure lines form where the dermis is closely attached to the underlying fascia.

Friction ridge patterns are genetically determined and unique to each of us. Because sweat pores open along their crests, our fingertips leave identifying films of sweat called *fingerprints* on almost anything we touch.

Reticular Layer The deeper **reticular layer**, accounting for about 80% of the thickness of the dermis, is coarse, irregularly arranged, dense fibrous connective tissue (Figure 5.3). The network of blood vessels that nourishes this layer, the *cutaneous plexus*, lies between this layer and the hypodermis. Its extracellular matrix contains pockets of adipose cells and thick bundles of interlacing collagen fibers. The collagen fibers run in various planes, but most run parallel to the skin surface. Separations, or less dense regions, between these bundles form **cleavage (tension) lines** in the skin. These externally invisible lines tend to run longitudinally in the skin of the head and limbs and in circular patterns around the neck and trunk (Figure 5.4b).

Cleavage lines are important to surgeons because when an incision is made *parallel* to these lines, the skin gapes less and heals more readily. The collagen fibers of the dermis give skin strength and resiliency that prevent most jabs and scrapes from penetrating the dermis. In addition, collagen binds water, helping to keep skin hydrated. Elastic fibers provide the stretch-recoil properties of skin.

Flexure lines, a third type of skin marking, are dermal folds that occur at or near joints, where the dermis is tightly secured to deeper structures. (Notice the deep creases on your palms.) Since the skin cannot slide easily to accommodate joint movement in such regions, the dermis folds and deep skin creases form (Figure 5.4c). Flexure lines are also visible on the wrists, fingers, soles, and toes.

Homeostatic Imbalance 5.1

Extreme stretching of the skin, such as during pregnancy, can tear the dermis, leaving silvery white scars called *striae* (stri′e; "streaks"), commonly called "stretch marks." Short-term but acute trauma (as from a burn or wielding a hoe) can cause a *blister*, a fluid-filled pocket that separates the epidermal and dermal layers. ✚

☑ Check Your Understanding

5. Which layer of the dermis is responsible for producing fingerprint patterns?
6. Which tissue of the hypodermis makes it a good shock absorber?
7. You have just gotten a paper cut. It is very painful, but it doesn't bleed. Has the cut penetrated into the dermis or just the epidermis?

For answers, see Appendix H.

Skin Color

Three pigments contribute to skin color: melanin, carotene, and hemoglobin. Of these, only melanin is made in the skin.

Melanin is a polymer made of tyrosine amino acids. Its two forms range in color from reddish yellow to brownish black. Its synthesis depends on an enzyme in melanocytes called tyrosinase (ti-ro′sĭ-nās) and, as noted earlier, it passes from melanocytes to the basal keratinocytes. Eventually, lysosomes break down the melanosomes, so melanin pigment is found only in the deeper layers of the epidermis.

Human skin comes in different colors. However, distribution of those colors is not random—populations of darker-skinned people tend to be found nearer the equator (where greater protection from the sun is needed), and those with the lightest skin are found closer to the poles. Since all humans have the same relative number of melanocytes, differences in skin coloring reflect the kind and amount of melanin made and retained. Melanocytes of black- and brown-skinned people produce many more and darker melanosomes than those of fair-skinned individuals, and their keratinocytes retain it longer. *Freckles* and *pigmented nevi* (moles) are local accumulations of melanin.

When we expose our skin to sunlight, keratinocytes secrete chemicals that stimulate melanocytes. Prolonged sun exposure causes a substantial melanin buildup, which helps protect the DNA of viable skin cells from UV radiation by absorbing the rays and dissipating the energy as heat. Indeed, the initial signal for speeding up melanin synthesis seems to be a faster repair rate of DNA that has suffered photodamage (*photo* = light). In all but the darkest people, this defensive response causes skin to darken visibly (tanning occurs).

Homeostatic Imbalance 5.2

Despite melanin's protective effects, excessive sun exposure eventually damages the skin. It causes elastic fibers to clump, which results in leathery skin; temporarily depresses the immune system; and can alter the DNA of skin cells leading to skin cancer. The fact that dark-skinned people get skin cancer less often than fair-skinned people and get it in areas with less pigment—the soles of the feet and nail beds—attests to melanin's effectiveness as a natural sunscreen.

Ultraviolet radiation has other consequences as well, such as destroying the body's folic acid stores necessary for DNA synthesis. This can have serious consequences, particularly in pregnant women because the deficit may impair the development of the embryo's nervous system.

One condition sun exposure does not cause, regardless of its name, is *sunspots*, small circular white spots on the skin that stand out like a sore thumb in tanned skin. Actually a fungus infection, this condition—more accurately called *tinea versicolor* (*vers* = change)—occurs mainly on the arms, legs, upper chest, and back. Largely a cosmetic problem, its growth is encouraged by oily, sweaty skin. Antifungal medication works, but it takes a long time for the white patches to become pigmented again.

Many chemicals induce photosensitivity; that is, they heighten the skin's sensitivity to UV radiation and can cause an unsightly skin rash. Such substances include some antibiotic and antihistamine drugs, and many chemicals in perfumes and detergents. Small, itchy blisters erupt all over the body. Then the peeling begins—in sheets! ✚

Carotene (kar′o-tēn) is a yellow to orange pigment found in certain plant products such as carrots. It tends to accumulate in the stratum corneum and in fatty tissue of the hypodermis. Its color is most obvious in the palms and soles, where the stratum corneum is thickest, and most intense when large amounts of carotene-rich foods are eaten. However, the yellowish tinge of the skin of some Asian peoples is due to variations in melanin, as well as to carotene. In the body, carotene can be converted to vitamin A, a vitamin that is essential for normal vision, as well as for epidermal health.

The pinkish hue of fair skin reflects the crimson color of the oxygenated pigment **hemoglobin** (he′mo-glo″bin) in the red blood cells circulating through the dermal capillaries. Because Caucasian skin contains only small amounts of melanin, the epidermis is nearly transparent and allows hemoglobin's color to show through.

Homeostatic Imbalance 5.3

When hemoglobin is poorly oxygenated, both the blood and the skin of Caucasians appear blue, a condition called *cyanosis* (si″ah-no′sis; *cyan* = dark blue). Skin often becomes cyanotic during heart failure and severe respiratory disorders. In dark-skinned individuals, the skin does not appear cyanotic because of the masking effects of melanin, but cyanosis is apparent in their mucous membranes and nail beds (the same sites where the red cast of oxygenated blood is normally visible).

Many alterations in skin color signal certain disease states or even emotional states:

- *Redness*, or *erythema* (er″ĭ-the′mah): Reddened skin may indicate embarrassment (blushing), fever, hypertension, inflammation, or allergy.
- *Pallor*, or *blanching*: During fear, anger, and certain other types of emotional stress, some people become pale. Pale skin may also signify anemia or low blood pressure.
- *Jaundice* (jawn′dis), or *yellow cast*: An abnormal yellow skin tone usually signifies a liver disorder, in which yellow bile pigments accumulate in the blood and are deposited in body tissues. [Normally, the liver cells secrete the bile pigments (bilirubin) as a component of bile.]

- *Bronzing*: A bronze, almost metallic appearance of the skin is a sign of Addison's disease, in which the adrenal cortex produces inadequate amounts of its steroid hormones; or a sign of pituitary gland tumors that inappropriately secrete melanocyte-stimulating hormone (MSH).
- *Black-and-blue marks*, or *bruises*: Black-and-blue marks reveal where blood escaped from the circulation and clotted beneath the skin. Such clotted blood masses are called hematomas (he″mah-to′mah; "blood swelling"). +

Check Your Understanding

8. Melanin and carotene are two pigments that contribute to skin color. What is the third and where is it found?
9. What is cyanosis and what does it indicate?
10. Which alteration in skin color may indicate a liver disorder?

For answers, see Appendix H.

Appendages of the Skin

- ✓ List the parts of a hair follicle and explain the function of each part. Also describe the functional relationship of arrector pili muscles to the hair follicles.
- ✓ Name the regions of a hair and explain the basis of hair color. Describe the distribution, growth, replacement, and changing nature of hair during the life span.
- ✓ Describe the structure of nails.
- ✓ Compare the structure and locations of sweat and oil glands. Also compare the composition and functions of their secretions.
- ✓ Compare and contrast eccrine and apocrine glands.

Along with the skin itself, the integumentary system includes several derivatives of the epidermis. These **skin appendages** include hair and hair follicles, nails, sweat glands, and sebaceous (oil) glands. Each plays a unique role in maintaining body homeostasis.

A key step in beginning to form any of the skin's appendages is formation of an epithelial bud. This process is stimulated by a reduced production of cell adhesion factor (cadherin). Once the cell-to-cell attractions are broken, the cells can move about and rearrange themselves, allowing an epithelial bud to form.

Hairs and Hair Follicles

Hair is an important part of our body image—consider, for example, the spiky hair style of punk rockers and the flowing, glossy manes of some high-fashion models. Millions of hairs are distributed over our entire skin surface except our palms, soles, lips, nipples, and parts of the external genitalia (the head of the penis, for instance). Although hair helps to keep other mammals warm, our sparse body hair is far less luxuriant and useful. Its main function in humans is to sense insects on the skin before they bite or sting us. Hair on the scalp guards the head against physical trauma, heat loss, and sunlight. (Pity the bald man.) Eyelashes shield the eyes, and nose hairs filter large particles like lint and insects from the air we inhale.

Structure of a Hair

Hairs, or **pili** (pi′li), are flexible strands produced by hair follicles and consist largely of dead, keratinized cells. The *hard keratin* that dominates hairs and nails has two advantages over the *soft keratin* found in typical epidermal cells: (1) It is tougher and more durable, and (2) its individual cells do not flake off.

The chief regions of a hair are the *shaft*, the portion in which keratinization is complete, and the *root*, where keratinization is still ongoing. The shaft, which projects from the skin, extends about halfway down the portion of the hair embedded in the skin **(Figure 5.5)**. The root is the remainder of the hair deep within the follicle. If the shaft is flat and ribbonlike in cross section, the hair is kinky; if it is oval, the hair is silky and wavy; if it is perfectly round, the hair is straight and tends to be coarse.

A hair has three concentric layers of keratinized cells: the medulla, cortex, and cuticle (Figure 5.5a, b).

- The *medulla* (mĕ-dul′ah; "middle"), its central core, consists of large cells and air spaces. The medulla, which is the only part of the hair that contains soft keratin, is absent in fine hairs.
- The *cortex*, a bulky layer surrounding the medulla, consists of several layers of flattened cells.
- The outermost **cuticle** is formed from a single layer of cells overlapping one another like shingles on a roof. This arrangement helps separate neighboring hairs so the hair does not mat. (Hair conditioners smooth out the rough surface of the cuticle and make our hair look shiny.) The most heavily keratinized part of the hair, the cuticle provides strength and helps keep the inner layers tightly compacted.

  Because it is subjected to the most abrasion, the cuticle tends to wear away at the tip of the hair shaft, allowing keratin fibrils in the cortex and medulla to frizz out, creating "split ends."

Hair pigment is made by melanocytes at the base of the hair follicle and transferred to the cortical cells. Various proportions of melanins of different colors (yellow, rust, brown, and black) combine to produce hair color from blond to pitch black. Additionally, red hair is colored by the iron-containing pigment *trichosiderin*. When melanin production decreases (mediated by delayed-action genes) and air bubbles replace melanin in the hair shaft, hair turns gray or white.

Structure of a Hair Follicle

Hair follicles (*folli* = bag) fold down from the epidermal surface into the dermis. In the scalp, they may even extend into the hypodermis. The deep end of the follicle, located about 4 mm (1/6 in.) below the skin surface, expands to form a **hair bulb** (Figure 5.5c, d). A knot of sensory nerve endings called a **hair follicle receptor**, or **root hair plexus**, wraps around each hair bulb (see Figure 5.1). Bending the hair stimulates these endings. Consequently, our hairs act as sensitive touch receptors.

- Feel the tickle as you run your hand over the hairs on your forearm.

5

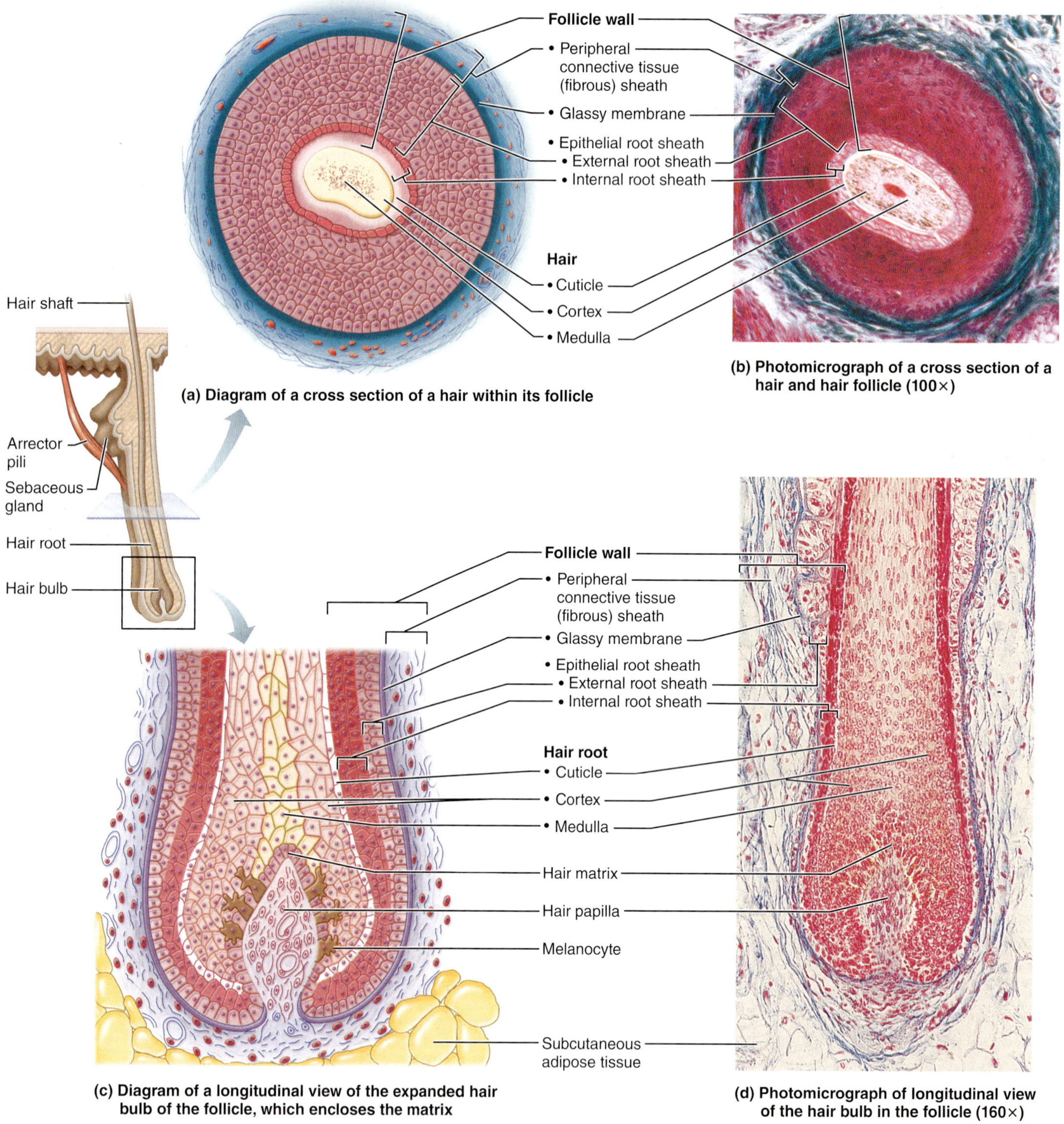

Figure 5.5 Skin appendages: Structure of a hair and hair follicle.

A *hair papilla*, a nipple-like bit of dermal tissue, protrudes into the hair bulb. This papilla contains a knot of capillaries that supplies nutrients to the growing hair and signals it to grow. Except for its location, this papilla is similar to the dermal papillae underlying other epidermal regions.

The wall of a hair follicle is composed of an outer **peripheral connective tissue sheath** (or *fibrous sheath*), derived from the dermis; a thickened basal lamina called the *glassy membrane*; and an inner **epithelial root sheath**, derived mainly from an invagination of the epidermis (Figure 5.5). The epithelial root sheath, which has external and internal parts, thins as it approaches the hair bulb, so that only a single layer of epithelial cells covers the papilla.

The cells that compose the **hair matrix**, or actively dividing area of the hair bulb that produces the hair, originate in a region called the *hair bulge* located a fraction of a millimeter above the hair bulb. When chemical signals diffusing from the hair papilla reach the hair bulge, some of its cells migrate toward the papilla, where they divide to produce the hair cells. As the matrix produces new hair cells, the older part of the hair is pushed upward, and its fused cells become increasingly keratinized and die.

Associated with each hair follicle is a bundle of smooth muscle cells called an **arrector pili** (ah-rek′tor pi′li; "raiser of hair") muscle. As you can see in Figure 5.1, most hair follicles approach the skin surface at a slight angle. The arrector pili muscle is attached in such a way that its contraction pulls the hair follicle upright and dimples the skin surface to produce goose bumps in response to cold temperatures or fear. This "hair-raising" response is not very useful to humans, with our short sparse hairs, but it is an important way for other animals to retain heat and protect themselves. Furry animals stay warmer by trapping a layer of insulating air in their fur; and a scared animal with its hair on end looks larger and more formidable to its enemy. The more important role of the arrector pili in humans is that its contractions force sebum out of hair follicles to the skin surface where it acts as a skin lubricant.

Types and Growth of Hair

Hairs come in various sizes and shapes, but as a rule they can be classified as vellus or terminal. The body hair of children and adult females is pale, fine **vellus hair** (vel′us; *vell* = wool, fleece). The coarser, longer hair of the eyebrows and scalp is **terminal hair**, which may also be darker.

At puberty, terminal hairs appear in the axillary and pubic regions of both sexes and on the face and chest (and typically the arms and legs) of males. These terminal hairs grow in response to the stimulating effects of androgens (of which *testosterone* is the most important), and when male hormones are present in large amounts, terminal hair growth is luxuriant.

Many factors influence hair growth and density, especially nutrition and hormones. Poor nutrition means poor hair growth, whereas conditions that increase local dermal blood flow (such as chronic physical irritation or inflammation) may enhance local hair growth. Many old-time bricklayers who carried their hod on one shoulder all the time developed one hairy shoulder. Undesirable hair growth (such as on a woman's upper lip) may be arrested by *electrolysis* or laser treatments, which use electricity or light energy, respectively, to destroy the hair roots.

Homeostatic Imbalance 5.4

In women, both the ovaries and the adrenal glands normally produce small amounts of androgens. Excessive hairiness, or **hirsutism** (her′soot-izm; *hirsut* = hairy), as well as other signs of masculinization, may result from an adrenal gland or ovarian tumor that secretes abnormally large amounts of androgens. Since few women want a beard or hairy chest, such tumors are surgically removed as soon as possible. ✚

The rate of hair growth varies from one body region to another and with sex and age, but it averages 2.5 mm per week. Each follicle goes through *growth cycles*. In each cycle, an active growth phase, ranging from weeks to years, is followed by a regressive phase. During the regressive phase, the hair matrix cells die and the follicle base and hair bulb shrivel somewhat, dragging the hair papilla upward to abut the region of the follicle that does not regress. The follicle then enters a resting phase for one to three months. After the resting phase, the cycling part of the follicle regenerates and activated bulge cells migrate toward the papilla. As a result, the matrix proliferates again and forms a new hair to replace the old one that has fallen out or will be pushed out by the new hair.

The life span of hairs varies and appears to be controlled by a slew of proteins. The follicles of the scalp remain active for six to ten years before becoming inactive for a few months. Because only a small percentage of the hair is shed at any one time, we lose an average of 90 scalp hairs daily. The follicles of the eyebrow hairs remain active for only three to four months, which explains why your eyebrows are never as long as the hairs on your head.

Hair Thinning and Baldness

A follicle has only a limited number of cycles in it. Given ideal conditions, hair grows fastest from the teen years to the 40s, and then its growth slows. The fact that hairs are shed faster than they are replaced leads to hair thinning and some degree of baldness, or **alopecia** (al″o-pe′she-ah), in both sexes. By age 35, noticeable hair loss occurs in 40% of men, and by age 60 that number jumps to 85%. Much less dramatic in women, the process usually begins at the anterior hairline and progresses posteriorly. Coarse terminal hairs are replaced by vellus hairs, and the hair becomes increasingly wispy.

True, or *frank*, *baldness* is a different story entirely. The most common type, **male pattern baldness**, is a genetically determined, sex-influenced condition. It is thought to be caused by a delayed-action gene that "switches on" in adulthood and changes the response of the hair follicles to DHT (dihydrotestosterone), a metabolite of testosterone. As a result, the follicular growth cycles become so short that many hairs never even emerge from their follicles before shedding, and those that do are fine vellus hairs that look like peach fuzz in the "bald" area.

Until recently, the only cure for male pattern baldness was drugs that inhibit testosterone production, but they also cause loss of sex drive—a trade-off few men would choose. Quite by accident, it was discovered that minoxidil (Rogaine), a drug used to reduce high blood pressure, has the interesting side effect in some bald men (and balding women) of stimulating hair regrowth. Although its results are variable, minoxidil is available over the counter in dropper bottles or spray form for application to the scalp. Finasteride (better known as Propecia), according to some the most promising cure for male pattern baldness, has had moderate success. Available only by prescription in once-a-day pill form, it must be taken for the rest of a person's life. Once the patient stops taking it, all of the new growth falls out.

Homeostatic Imbalance 5.5

Hair thinning can be induced by a number of factors that upset the normal balance between hair loss and replacement. Outstanding examples are acutely high fever, surgery, severe emotional trauma, and certain drugs (excessive vitamin A, some antidepressants and blood thinners, anabolic steroids, and most chemotherapy drugs). Protein-deficient diets and lactation lead to hair thinning because new hair growth stops when protein needed for keratin synthesis is not available or is being used for milk production. In all of these cases, hair regrows if the cause is removed or corrected.

In the rare condition *alopecia areata*, the immune system attacks the follicles and the hair falls out in patches. But again, the follicles survive. Hair loss due to severe burns, excessive radiation, or other factors that eliminate the follicles is permanent. ✚

☑ Check Your Understanding

11. What are the concentric regions of a hair shaft, from the outside in?
12. Why is having your hair cut painless?
13. What is the role of an arrector pili muscle?
14. What is the function of the hair papilla?

For answers, see Appendix H.

Nails

A **nail** is a scalelike modification of the epidermis that forms a clear protective covering on the dorsal surface of the distal part of a finger or toe **(Figure 5.6)**. Nails, which correspond to the hooves or claws of other animals, are useful as "tools" to help pick up small objects or scratch an itch.

In contrast to *soft keratin* of the epidermis, nails (like hairs) contain *hard keratin*. Each nail has a *free edge*, a *nail plate* or *body* (visible attached portion), and a proximal *root* (embedded in the skin). The deeper layers of the epidermis extend beneath the nail as the *nail bed*, and the nail itself corresponds to the superficial keratinized layers. The thickened proximal portion of the nail bed, called the **nail matrix**, is responsible for nail growth. As the nail cells produced by the matrix become heavily keratinized, the nail body slides distally over the nail bed.

Nails normally appear pink because of the rich bed of capillaries in the underlying dermis. However, the region that lies over the thick nail matrix appears as a white crescent called the *lunule* (lu′nool; "little moon"). The proximal and lateral borders of the nail are overlapped by skin folds, called **nail folds**. The proximal nail fold projects onto the nail body as the **cuticle** or **eponychium** (ep″o-nik′e-um; "on the nail"). The thickened region beneath the free edge of the nail where dirt and debris tend to accumulate is the **hyponychium** ("below nail"), informally called the quick. It secures the free edge of the nail plate at the fingertip.

Changes in nail appearance can help diagnose certain conditions. For example, yellow-tinged nails may indicate a respiratory or thyroid gland disorder, while thickened yellow nails may signal a fungus infection. An outward concavity of the nail (spoon nail) may signal an iron deficiency, and horizontal lines (Beau's lines) across the nails may hint of malnutrition.

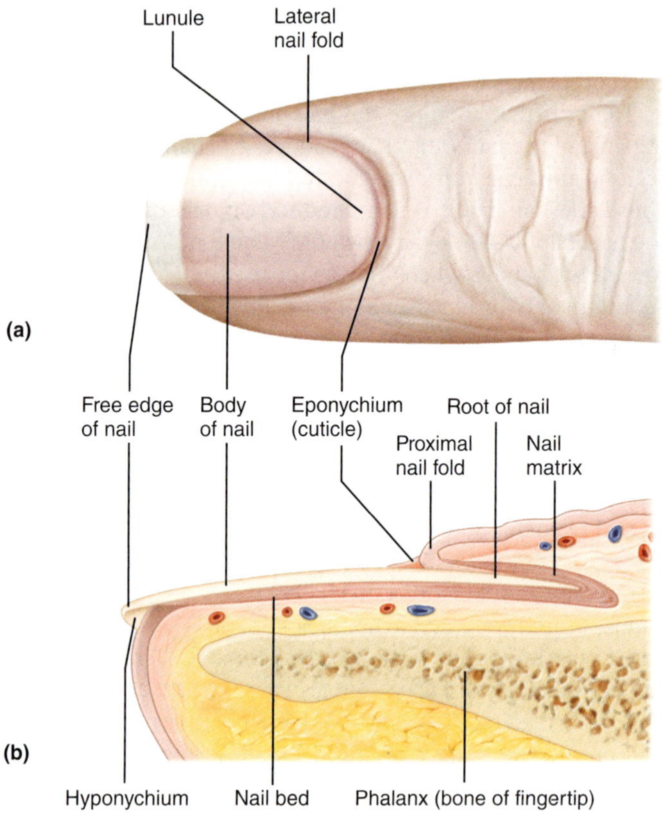

Figure 5.6 Skin appendages: Structure of a nail. (a) Surface view of the distal part of a finger. **(b)** Sagittal section of the fingertip. The nail matrix that forms the nail lies beneath the lunule.

☑ Check Your Understanding

15. Why is the lunule of a nail white instead of pink like the rest of the nail?
16. Why are nails so hard?

For answers, see Appendix H.

Sweat (Sudoriferous) Glands

Sweat glands, also called **sudoriferous glands** (su″do-rif′er-us; *sudor* = sweat), are distributed over the entire skin surface except the nipples and parts of the external genitalia. Their number is staggering—up to 3 million per person.

We have two types of sweat glands: eccrine and apocrine. In both types, the secretory cells are associated with myoepithelial cells, specialized cells that contract when stimulated by the nervous system. Their contraction forces the sweat into and through the gland's duct system to the skin surface.

Eccrine (Merocrine) Sweat Glands

Eccrine sweat glands (ek′rin; "secreting"), also called **merocrine sweat glands**, are far more numerous and are particularly abundant on the palms, soles of the feet, and forehead. Each is a simple, coiled, tubular gland. The secretory part lies coiled in the dermis, and the duct extends to open in a funnel-shaped *pore* (*por* = channel) at the skin surface **(Figure 5.7b)**.

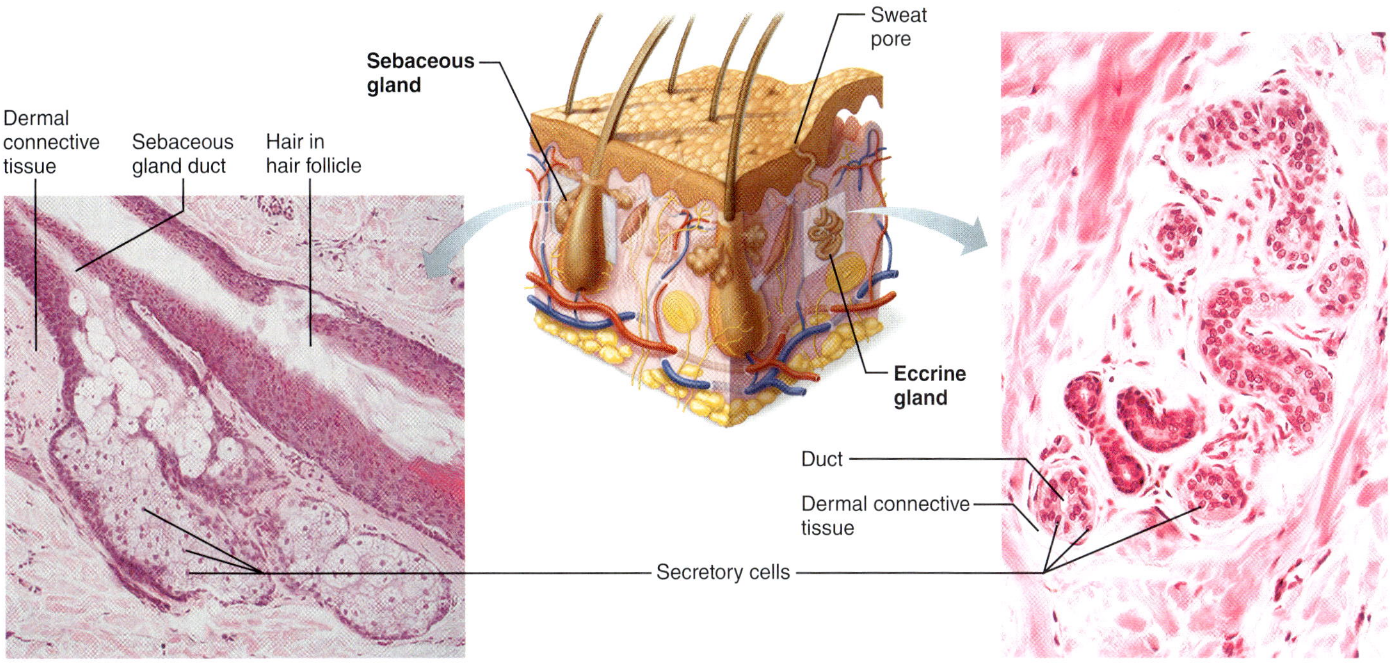

(a) Photomicrograph of a sectioned sebaceous gland (90×)

(b) Photomicrograph of a sectioned eccrine gland (140×)

Figure 5.7 Skin appendages: Cutaneous glands.

(These sweat pores are different from the so-called pores of a person's complexion, which are actually the external outlets of hair follicles.)

Eccrine gland secretion, commonly called sweat, is a hypotonic filtrate of the blood that passes through the secretory cells of the sweat glands and is released by exocytosis. It is 99% water, with some salts (mostly sodium chloride), vitamin C, antibodies, a microbe-killing peptide dubbed *dermcidin*, and traces of metabolic wastes (urea, uric acid, and ammonia). The exact composition depends on heredity and diet. Small amounts of ingested drugs may also be excreted by this route. Normally, sweat is acidic with a pH between 4 and 6.

The sympathetic division of the autonomic nervous system, over which we have little control, regulates sweating. Its major role is to prevent the body from overheating. Heat-induced sweating begins on the forehead and spreads inferiorly over the remainder of the body. Emotionally induced sweating—the so-called "cold sweat" brought on by fright or nervousness—begins on the palms, soles, and axillae (armpits) and then spreads to other body areas.

Apocrine Sweat Glands

Apocrine sweat glands (ap′o-krin), approximately 2000 of them, are largely confined to the axillary and anogenital areas. In spite of their name, they are merocrine glands, which release their product by exocytosis like the eccrine sweat glands. Larger than eccrine glands, they lie deeper in the dermis or even in the hypodermis, and their ducts empty into hair follicles.

Apocrine secretion contains the same basic components as true sweat, plus fatty substances and proteins. Consequently, it is viscous and sometimes has a milky or yellowish color. The secretion is odorless, but when bacteria on the skin decompose its organic molecules, it takes on a musky and generally unpleasant odor, the basis of body odor.

Apocrine glands begin functioning at puberty under the influence of the male sex hormones (*androgens*) and play little role in maintaining a constant body temperature. Their precise function is not yet known, but they are activated by sympathetic nerve fibers during pain and stress. Because sexual foreplay increases their activity, and they enlarge and recede with the phases of a woman's menstrual cycle, they may be the human equivalent of other animals' sexual scent glands.

Ceruminous glands (sĕ-roo′mĭ-nus; *cera* = wax) are modified apocrine glands found in the lining of the external ear canal. Their secretion mixes with sebum produced by nearby sebaceous glands to form a sticky, bitter substance called *cerumen*, or earwax, that is thought to deter insects and block entry of foreign material.

Mammary glands, another variety of specialized sweat glands, secrete milk. Although they are properly part of the integumentary system, we will consider the mammary glands in Chapter 27 with female reproductive organs.

Sebaceous (Oil) Glands

The **sebaceous glands** (se-ba′shus; "greasy"), or **oil glands** (Figure 5.7a), are simple branched alveolar glands that are found all over the body except in the thick skin of the palms and soles. They are small on the body trunk and limbs, but quite large on the face, neck, and upper chest. These glands secrete an oily substance called **sebum** (se′bum). The central cells of the alveoli accumulate oily lipids until they become so engorged that they burst, so functionally these glands are *holocrine glands* (see p. 125). The accumulated lipids and cell fragments constitute sebum.

Most, but not all, sebaceous glands develop as outgrowths of hair follicles and secrete sebum into a hair follicle, or occasionally to a pore on the skin surface. Arrector pili contractions force sebum out of the hair follicles to the skin surface. Sebum softens and lubricates the hair and skin, prevents hair from becoming brittle, and slows water loss from the skin when external humidity is low. Perhaps even more important is its *bactericidal* (bacterium-killing) action.

Hormones, especially androgens, stimulate the secretion of sebum. Sebaceous glands are relatively inactive during childhood but are activated in both sexes during puberty, when androgen production begins to rise.

5

Homeostatic Imbalance 5.6

If accumulated sebum blocks a sebaceous gland duct, a *whitehead* appears on the skin surface. If the material oxidizes and dries, it darkens to form a *blackhead*. *Acne* is an active inflammation of the sebaceous glands accompanied by "pimples" (pustules or cysts) on the skin. It is usually caused by bacterial infection, particularly by staphylococcus, and can range from mild to severe, leading to permanent scarring.

Overactive sebaceous glands can cause *seborrhea* (seb″o-re′ah; "fast-flowing sebum"), known as "cradle cap" in infants. Seborrhea begins on the scalp as pink, raised lesions that gradually become yellow to brown and begin to slough off oily scales. ✚

Check Your Understanding

17. Which cutaneous glands are associated with hair follicles?
18. When Anthony returned home from a run in 85°F weather, his face was dripping with sweat. Why?
19. What is the difference between heat-induced sweating and a "cold sweat," and which variety of sweat gland is involved?
20. Sebaceous glands are not found in thick skin. Why is their absence in those body regions desirable?

For answers, see Appendix H.

Functions of the Integumentary System

✓ Describe how the skin accomplishes at least five different functions.

First and foremost, our skin is a barrier. Like the skin of a grape, it keeps its contents juicy and whole. The skin is also a master at self (wound) repair, and interacts immediately with other body systems by making potent molecules, all the while protecting deeper tissues from damaging external agents. Even this short list hints that the skin and its derivatives perform a variety of functions, including: protection, body temperature regulation, cutaneous sensation, metabolic functions, blood reservoir, and excretion.

Protection

Given its superficial location, the skin is our most vulnerable organ system, exposed to microorganisms, abrasion, temperature extremes, and harmful chemicals. The skin constitutes at least three types of barriers: chemical, physical, and biological.

Chemical Barriers

Chemical barriers include skin secretions and melanin. Although the skin's surface teems with bacteria, the low pH of skin secretions—the so-called **acid mantle**—retards their multiplication. In addition, dermcidin in sweat and bactericidal substances in sebum kill many bacteria outright. Skin cells also secrete natural antibiotics called *defensins* that literally punch holes in bacteria, making them look like sieves. Wounded skin releases large quantities of protective peptides called *cathelicidins* that are particularly effective in preventing infection by group A streptococcus bacteria.

As discussed earlier, melanin provides a chemical pigment shield to prevent UV damage to skin cells.

Physical Barriers

The continuity of skin and the hardness of its keratinized cells provide physical barriers. As a physical barrier, the skin is a remarkable compromise. A thicker epidermis would be more impenetrable, but we would pay the price in loss of suppleness and agility.

The outstanding barrier capacity of the skin arises from the structure of its stratum corneum, which has been compared to bricks and mortar. Multiple layers of dead flat cells are the bricks and the glycolipids surrounding them are the mortar. Epidermal continuity works hand in hand with the acid mantle and certain chemicals in skin secretions to ward off bacterial invasion. The water-resistant glycolipids of the epidermis block most diffusion of water and water-soluble substances between cells, preventing both their loss from and entry into the body through the skin. However, there is a continual small loss of water through the epidermis, and if immersed in water (other than salt water), the skin will take in some water and swell slightly.

Substances that *do* penetrate the skin in limited amounts include

- *Lipid-soluble substances*, such as oxygen, carbon dioxide, fat-soluble vitamins (A, D, E, and K), and steroids (estrogens)
- *Oleoresins* (o″le-o-rez′inz) of certain plants, such as poison ivy and poison oak
- *Organic solvents*, such as acetone, dry-cleaning fluid, and paint thinner, which dissolve the cell lipids
- *Salts of heavy metals*, such as lead and mercury
- Selected drugs (nitroglycerine, nicotine, seasickness medications)

- Drug agents called *penetration enhancers* that help ferry other drugs into the body

Alcoholic drinks dramatically enhance skin permeability for at least 24 hours after their ingestion.

Homeostatic Imbalance 5.7

Organic solvents and heavy metals are devastating to the body and can be lethal. Passage of organic solvents through the skin into the blood can shut down the kidneys and also cause brain damage. Absorption of lead results in anemia and neurological defects. These substances should never be handled with bare hands. ✚

Biological Barriers

Biological barriers include the dendritic cells of the epidermis, macrophages in the dermis, and DNA itself.

Dendritic cells are active elements of the immune system. To activate the immune response, the foreign substances, or *antigens*, must be presented to specialized white blood cells called lymphocytes. In the epidermis, the dendritic cells play this role.

Dermal macrophages constitute a second line of defense to dispose of viruses and bacteria that manage to penetrate the epidermis. They, too, act as antigen "presenters."

Although melanin provides a fairly good chemical sunscreen, DNA itself is a remarkably effective biologically based sunscreen. Electrons in DNA molecules absorb UV radiation and transfer it to the atomic nuclei, which heat up and vibrate vigorously. Since the heat dissipates to surrounding water molecules instantaneously, the DNA converts potentially destructive radiation into harmless heat.

Body Temperature Regulation

The body works best when its temperature remains within homeostatic limits. Like car engines, we need to get rid of the heat generated by our internal reactions. As long as the external temperature is lower than body temperature, the skin surface loses heat to the air and to cooler objects in its environment, just as a car radiator loses heat to the air and other nearby parts.

Under normal resting conditions, and as long as the environmental temperature is below 31–32°C (88–90°F), sweat glands secrete about 500 ml (0.5 L) of sweat per day. This routine and unnoticeable sweating is called *insensible perspiration*. When body temperature rises, the nervous system stimulates dermal blood vessels to dilate and the sweat glands into vigorous secretory activity. Indeed, on a hot day, sweat becomes noticeable and can account for the loss of up to 12 L (about 3 gallons) of body water in one day. This visible output of sweat is called *sensible perspiration*. Evaporation of sweat from the skin surface dissipates body heat and efficiently cools the body, preventing overheating.

When the external environment is cold, dermal blood vessels constrict. Their constriction causes the warm blood to bypass the skin temporarily and allows skin temperature to drop to that of the external environment. This slows passive heat loss from the body, conserving body heat. Chapter 24 discusses body temperature regulation.

Cutaneous Sensation

The skin is richly supplied with **cutaneous sensory receptors**, which are actually part of the nervous system. The cutaneous receptors are classified as *exteroceptors* (ek″ster-o-sep′torz) because they respond to stimuli arising outside the body. For example, tactile (Meissner's) corpuscles (in the dermal papillae) and tactile discs allow us to become aware of a caress or the feel of our clothing against our skin, whereas lamellar (also called Pacinian) corpuscles (in the deeper dermis or hypodermis) alert us to bumps or contacts involving deep pressure. Hair follicle receptors report on wind blowing through our hair and a playful tug on a pigtail. Free nerve endings that meander throughout the skin sense painful stimuli (irritating chemicals, extreme heat or cold, and others). We defer detailed discussion of these cutaneous receptors to Chapter 13.

Figure 5.1 illustrates all the cutaneous receptors mentioned above except for tactile corpuscles, which are found only in skin that lacks hairs, and tactile cells, shown in Figure 5.2b.

Metabolic Functions

The skin is a chemical factory, fueled in part by the sun's rays. When sunlight bombards the skin, modified cholesterol molecules are converted to a vitamin D precursor, which is transported via the blood to other body areas to be ultimately converted to vitamin D, which plays various roles in calcium metabolism. For example, calcium cannot be absorbed from the digestive tract without vitamin D.

Among its other metabolic functions, the epidermis makes chemical conversions that supplement those of the liver. For example, keratinocyte enzymes can

- "Disarm" many cancer-causing chemicals that penetrate the epidermis
- Convert some harmless chemicals into carcinogens
- Activate some steroid hormones—for instance, they can transform cortisone applied to irritated skin into hydrocortisone, a potent anti-inflammatory drug

Skin cells also make several biologically important proteins, including collagenase, an enzyme that aids the natural turnover of collagen (and deters wrinkles).

Blood Reservoir

The dermal vascular supply is extensive and can hold about 5% of the body's entire blood volume. When other body organs, such as vigorously working muscles, need a greater blood supply, the nervous system constricts the dermal blood vessels. This constriction shunts more blood into the general circulation, making it available to the muscles and other body organs.

Excretion

The body eliminates limited amounts of nitrogen-containing wastes (ammonia, urea, and uric acid) in sweat, although most such wastes are excreted in urine. Profuse sweating is an important avenue for water and salt (sodium chloride) loss.

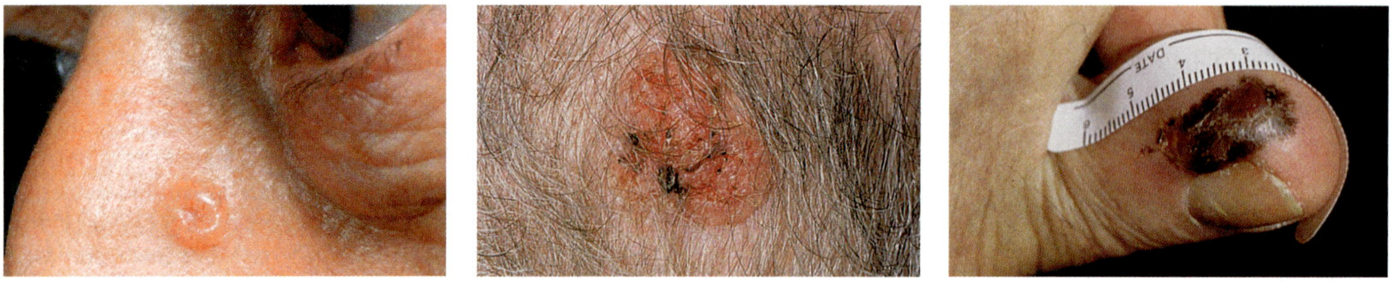

(a) Basal cell carcinoma (b) Squamous cell carcinoma (c) Melanoma

Figure 5.8 Photographs of skin cancers.

☑ Check Your Understanding

21. What chemicals produced in the skin help provide barriers to bacteria? List at least three and explain how the chemicals are protective.
22. Which epidermal cells play a role in body immunity?
23. How is sunlight important to bone health?
24. How does the skin contribute to body metabolism?

For answers, see Appendix H.

Homeostatic Imbalances of Skin

✓ Summarize the characteristics of the three major types of skin cancers.

✓ Explain why serious burns are life threatening. Describe how to determine the extent of a burn and differentiate first-, second-, and third-degree burns.

Loss of homeostasis in body cells and organs reveals itself on the skin, sometimes in startling ways. The skin can develop more than 1000 different conditions and ailments. The most common skin disorders are bacterial, viral, or yeast infections. Related Clinical Terms on pp. 171–172 summarizes a number of these. Less common, but far more damaging to body well-being, are skin cancer and burns, considered next.

Skin Cancer

One in five Americans develops skin cancer at some point. Most tumors that arise in the skin are benign and do not spread (metastasize) to other body areas. (A wart, a neoplasm caused by a virus, is one example.) However, some skin tumors are malignant, or cancerous, and invade other body areas.

The single most important risk factor for skin cancer is overexposure to the UV radiation in sunlight, which damages DNA bases. Adjacent pyrimidine bases often respond by fusing, forming lesions called *dimers*. UV radiation also appears to disable a tumor suppressor gene [*p53* or the patched (*ptc*) gene]. In limited numbers of cases, however, frequent irritation of the skin by infections, chemicals, or physical trauma seems to be a predisposing factor.

Interestingly, sunburned skin accelerates its production of Fas, a protein that causes genetically damaged skin cells to commit suicide, reducing the risk of mutations that will cause sun-linked skin cancer. The death of these gene-damaged cells causes the skin to peel after a sunburn.

There is no such thing as a "healthy tan," but the good news for sun worshippers is the newly developed skin lotions that can fix damaged DNA before the involved cells become cancerous. These lotions contain tiny oily vesicles (liposomes) filled with enzymes that initiate repair of the DNA mutations most commonly caused by sunlight. The liposomes penetrate the epidermis and enter the keratinocytes, ultimately making their way into the nuclei to bind to specific sites where two DNA bases have fused. There, by selectively cutting the DNA strands, they begin a DNA repair process that is completed by cellular enzymes.

The three major forms of skin cancer are basal cell carcinoma, squamous cell carcinoma, and melanoma.

Basal Cell Carcinoma

Basal cell carcinoma (kar″sĭ-no′mah), the least malignant and most common, accounts for nearly 80% of cases. Stratum basale cells proliferate, invading the dermis and hypodermis. The cancer lesions occur most often on sun-exposed areas of the face and appear as shiny, dome-shaped nodules that later develop a central ulcer with a pearly, beaded edge (**Figure 5.8a**). Basal cell carcinoma is relatively slow-growing, and metastasis seldom occurs before it is noticed. Full cure by surgical excision is the rule in 99% of cases.

Squamous Cell Carcinoma

Squamous cell carcinoma, the second most common skin cancer, arises from the keratinocytes of the stratum spinosum. The lesion appears as a scaly reddened papule (small, rounded elevation) that arises most often on the head (scalp, ears, and lower lip), and hands (Figure 5.8b). It tends to grow rapidly and metastasize if not removed. If it is caught early and removed surgically or by radiation therapy, the chance of complete cure is good.

Melanoma

Melanoma (mel″ah-no′mah), cancer of melanocytes, is the most dangerous skin cancer because it is highly metastatic and resistant to chemotherapy. It accounts for only 2–3% of skin cancers, but its incidence is increasing rapidly (by 3–8% per year in the United States). Melanoma can begin wherever there is pigment. Most such cancers appear spontaneously, and about one-third develop from preexisting moles. It usually appears as a spreading brown to black patch (Figure 5.8c) that metastasizes rapidly to surrounding lymph and blood vessels.

The key to surviving melanoma is early detection. The chance of survival is poor if the lesion is over 4 mm thick. The usual therapy for melanoma is wide surgical excision accompanied by immunotherapy (immunizing the body against its cancer cells).

The American Cancer Society suggests that we regularly examine our skin for new moles or pigmented spots. Apply the **ABCD rule** for recognizing melanoma:

Asymmetry: The two sides of the pigmented spot or mole do not match.

Border irregularity: The borders of the lesion exhibit indentations.

Color: The pigmented spot contains several colors (blacks, browns, tans, and sometimes blues and reds).

Diameter: The spot is larger than 6 mm in diameter (the size of a pencil eraser).

Some experts add an E, for elevation above the skin surface.

Burns

Burns are a devastating threat to the body primarily because of their effects on the skin. A **burn** is tissue damage inflicted by intense heat, electricity, radiation, or certain chemicals, all of which denature cell proteins and kill cells in the affected areas.

The immediate threat to life resulting from severe burns is a catastrophic loss of body fluids containing proteins and electrolytes. This leads to dehydration and electrolyte imbalance, and then renal failure (kidney shutdown) and circulatory shock (inadequate blood circulation due to reduced blood volume). To save the patient, the lost fluids must be replaced immediately via the intravenous (IV) route.

Evaluating Burns

In adults, the volume of fluid lost can be estimated by computing the percentage of body surface burned using the **rule of nines**. This method divides the body into 11 areas, each accounting for 9% of total body area, plus an additional area surrounding the genitals accounting for 1% of body surface area **(Figure 5.9)**. The rule of nines is only approximate, so special tables are used when greater accuracy is desired.

Burn patients also need thousands of extra food calories daily to replace lost proteins and allow tissue repair. No one can eat enough food to provide these calories, so burn patients are given supplementary nutrients through gastric tubes and IV lines. After the initial crisis has passed, infection becomes the main threat and sepsis (widespread bacterial infection) is the leading cause of death in burn victims. Burned skin is sterile for about 24 hours. Thereafter, bacteria, fungi, and other pathogens easily invade areas where the skin barrier is destroyed, and they multiply rapidly in the nutrient-rich environment of dead tissues. Adding to this problem is the fact that the immune system becomes deficient within one to two days after severe burn injury.

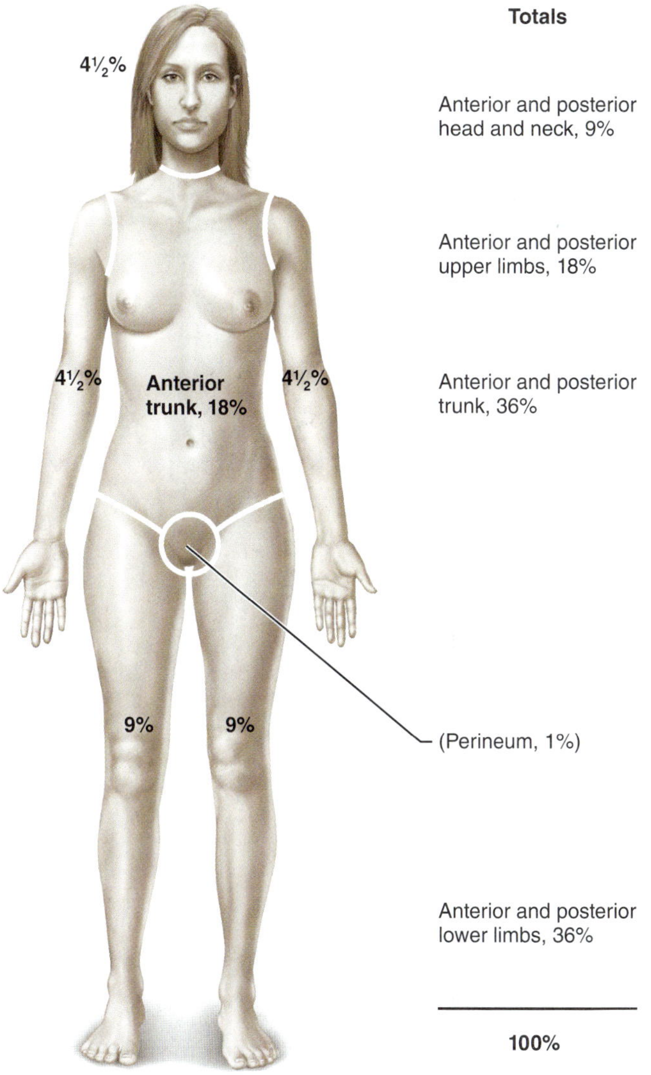

Figure 5.9 Estimating the extent and severity of burns using the rule of nines. Surface area values for the anterior body surface are indicated on the human figure. Total surface area (anterior and posterior body surfaces) for each body region is indicated to the right of the figure.

Burns are classified according to their severity (depth) as first-, second-, or third-degree burns. In **first-degree burns**, only the epidermis is damaged. Symptoms include localized redness, swelling, and pain. First-degree burns tend to heal in two to three days without special attention. Sunburn is usually a first-degree burn.

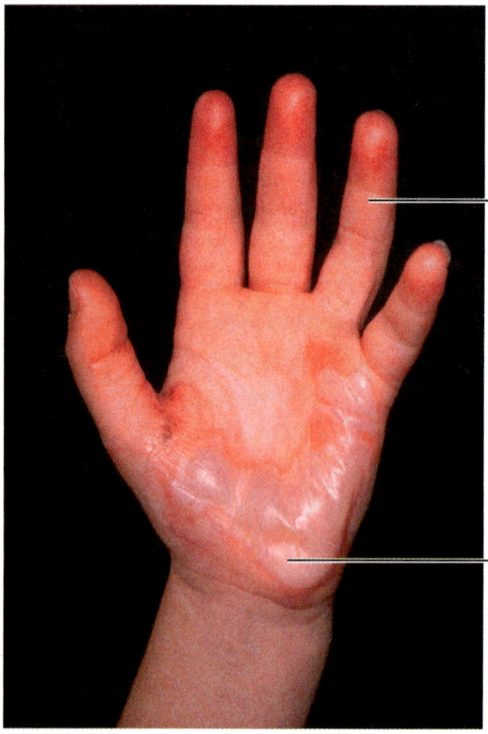

(a) Skin bearing partial thickness burn (1st- and 2nd-degree burns)

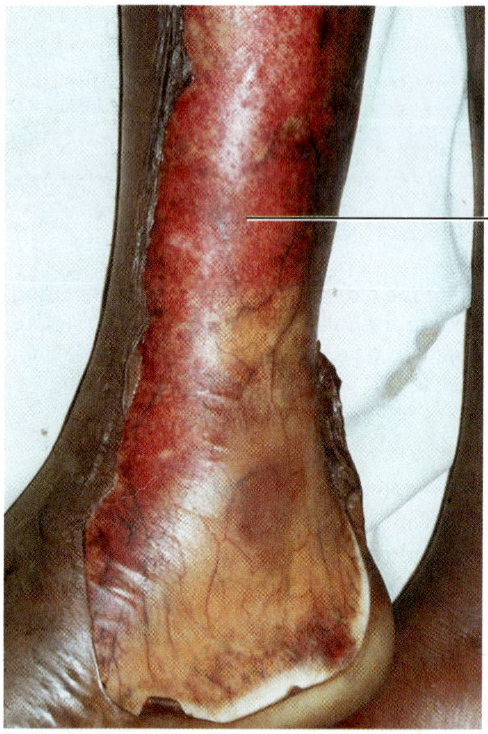

(b) Skin bearing full thickness burn (3rd-degree burn)

Figure 5.10 Partial thickness and full thickness burns.

Second-degree burns injure the epidermis and the upper region of the dermis. Symptoms mimic those of first-degree burns, but blisters also appear. The burned area is red and painful, but skin regeneration occurs with little or no scarring within three to four weeks if care is taken to prevent infection. First- and second-degree burns are referred to as *partial-thickness burns* **(Figure 5.10a)**.

Third-degree burns are *full-thickness burns*, involving the entire thickness of the skin (Figure 5.10b). The burned area appears gray-white, cherry red, or blackened, and initially there is little or no edema. Since the nerve endings have been destroyed, the burned area is not painful. Although skin might eventually regenerate by proliferating epithelial cells at the edges of the burn or stem cells in hair follicles, it is usually impossible to wait that long because of fluid loss and infection. Skin grafting is advised.

In general, burns are considered critical if any of the following conditions exists:

- Over 25% of the body has second-degree burns
- Over 10% of the body has third-degree burns
- There are third-degree burns of the face, hands, or feet

Facial burns introduce the possibility of burned respiratory passageways, which can swell and cause suffocation. Burns at joints are also troublesome because scar tissue can severely limit joint mobility.

Treating Burns

To prepare a burned area for a skin graft, the *eschar* (es′kar), or burned skin, must first be debrided (removed). To prevent infection and fluid loss, the area is then flooded with antibiotics and covered temporarily with a synthetic membrane, animal (pig) skin, cadaver skin, or "living bandage" made from the thin amniotic sac membrane that surrounds a fetus. Then healthy skin is transplanted to the burned site. Unless the graft is taken from the patient (an autograft), however, there is a good chance that the patient's immune system will reject it (see p. 790 in Chapter 21). Even if the graft "takes," extensive scar tissue often forms in the burned areas.

An exciting technique eliminates many of the traditional problems of skin grafting and rejection. Synthetic skin—a silicone "epidermis" bound to a spongy "dermal" layer composed of collagen and ground cartilage—is applied to the debrided area. In time, the patient's own dermal tissue absorbs and replaces the artificial one. Then the silicone sheet is peeled off and replaced with a network of epidermal cells cultured from the patient's own skin. The body does not reject this artificial skin, which saves lives and results in minimal scarring. However, it is more likely to become infected than is an autograft.

☑ Check Your Understanding

25. Which type of skin cancer develops from the youngest epidermal cells?
26. What name is given to the rule for recognizing the signs of melanoma?

27. The healing of burns and epidermal regeneration is usually uneventful unless the burn is a third-degree burn. What accounts for this difference?
28. Although the anterior head and face represent only a small percentage of the body surface, burns to this area are often more serious than those to the body trunk. Why?

For answers, see Appendix H.

Developmental Aspects of the Integumentary System

✓ Describe and attempt to explain the causes of changes that occur in the skin from birth to old age.

The epidermis develops from the embryonic ectoderm, and the dermis and hypodermis develop from mesoderm. By the end of the fourth month of development, the skin is fairly well formed. The epidermis has all its strata, dermal papillae are obvious, fingerprints have developed, and rudimentary epidermal derivatives have formed by downward projections of cells from the basal layer. During the fifth and sixth months, the fetus is covered with a downy coat of delicate colorless hairs called the *lanugo coat* (lah-nu′go; "wool"). This hairy cloak is shed by the seventh month, and vellus hairs appear.

From Infancy to Adulthood

When a baby is born, its skin is covered with *vernix caseosa* (ver′niks kă-se-o′sah; "varnish of cheese"), a white, cheesy-looking substance produced by the sebaceous glands that protects the fetus's skin within the water-filled amnion. The newborn's skin is very thin and often has accumulations in the sebaceous glands on the forehead and nose that appear as small white spots called *milia* (mil′e-ah). These normally disappear by the third week after birth.

During infancy and childhood, the skin thickens, and more subcutaneous fat is deposited. Although we all have approximately the same number of sweat glands, the number that function increases in the first two years after birth and is determined by climate. For this reason, people who grow up in hot climates have more active sweat glands than those raised in cooler areas of the world.

During adolescence, the skin and hair become oilier as sebaceous glands are activated, and acne may appear. Acne generally subsides in early adulthood, and skin reaches its optimal appearance when we reach our 20s and 30s. Thereafter, the skin starts to show the effects of cumulative environmental assaults (abrasion, wind, sun, chemicals). Scaling and various kinds of skin inflammation, or **dermatitis** (der″mah-ti′tis), become more common.

Aging Skin

As old age approaches, the rate of epidermal cell replacement slows, the skin thins, and its susceptibility to bruises and other injuries increases. The lubricating substances produced by the skin glands that make young skin so soft become deficient. Skin becomes dry and itchy, although people with naturally oily skin seem to postpone this dryness until later in life. Elastic fibers clump, and collagen fibers become fewer and stiffer. The subcutaneous fat layer diminishes, leading to the intolerance to cold so common in elderly people. Additionally, declining levels of sex hormones result in similar fat distribution in elderly men and women.

The decreasing elasticity of the skin, along with the loss of subcutaneous tissue, inevitably leads to wrinkling. Decreasing numbers of melanocytes and dendritic cells enhance the risk and incidence of skin cancer in this age group. As a rule, redheads and fair-skinned individuals, who have less melanin to begin with, show age-related changes more rapidly than do those with darker skin and hair.

By age 50, the number of active hair follicles has declined by two-thirds and continues to fall, resulting in hair thinning. Hair loses its luster in old age, and the delayed-action genes responsible for graying and male pattern baldness become active.

Although there is no known way to avoid skin aging, one of the best ways to slow the process is to shield your skin from both the UVA (aging rays) and UVB (rays that burn) of the sun. Aged skin that has been protected from the sun, while it grows thinner and loses some elasticity, still remains unwrinkled and unmarked. Wear protective clothing and apply sunscreens or sunblocks with a sun protection factor (SPF) of 15 or higher. Remember, the same sunlight that produces that fashionable tan also causes the sagging, blotchy, wrinkled skin of old age complete with pigmented "liver spots." Much of this havoc is due to UVA activation of enzymes called matrix metalloproteinases, which degrade collagen and other dermal components. A drug called tretinoin, related to vitamin A, inhibits these enzymes and is used in some skin creams to slow photo-aging. Good nutrition, plenty of fluids, and cleanliness may also delay the process.

☑ Check Your Understanding

29. What is the source of vernix caseosa that covers the skin of the newborn baby?
30. What change in the skin leads to cold intolerance in the elderly?
31. How does UV radiation contribute to skin wrinkles?

For answers, see Appendix H.

The skin is only about as thick as a paper towel—not too impressive as organ systems go. Yet, when it is severely damaged, nearly every body system reacts. Metabolism accelerates or may be impaired, immune system changes occur, bones may soften, the cardiovascular system may fail—the list goes on and on. On the other hand, when the skin is intact and performing its functions, the body as a whole benefits. *System Connections* on p. 168 summarizes homeostatic interrelationships between the integumentary system and other organ systems.

Homeostatic Interrelationships Between the Integumentary System and Other Body Systems

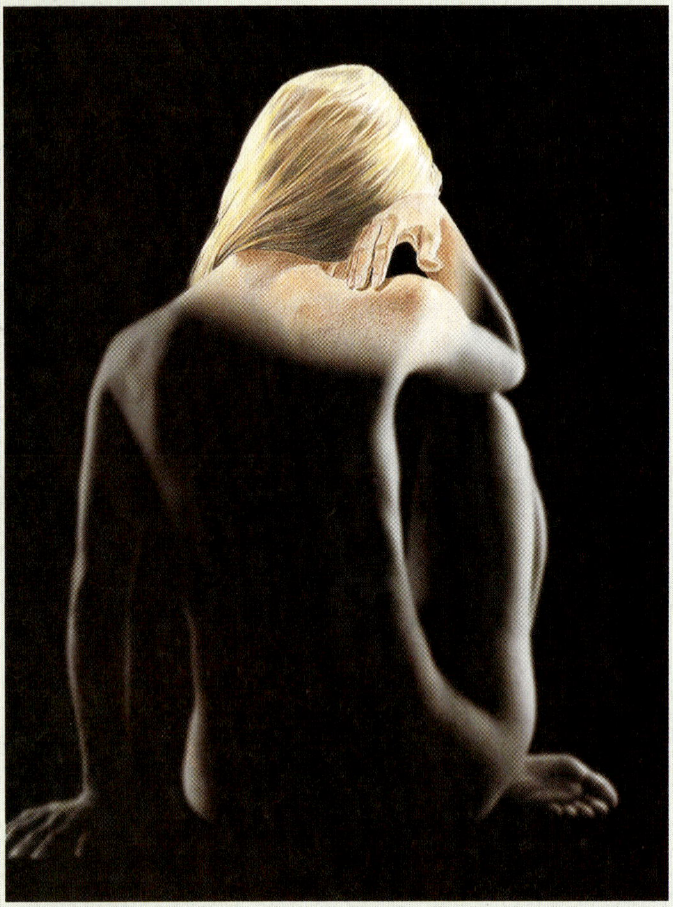

Skeletal System Chapters 6–8

- Skin protects bones; skin synthesizes a vitamin D precursor needed for normal calcium absorption and deposit of bone (calcium) salts, which make bones hard
- Skeletal system provides support for skin

Muscular System Chapters 9–10

- Skin protects muscles
- Active muscles generate large amounts of heat, which increases blood flow to the skin and may activate sweat glands in skin

Nervous System Chapters 11–15

- Skin protects nervous system organs; cutaneous sensory receptors for touch, pressure, pain, and temperature located in skin (see Figure 5.1)
- Nervous system regulates diameter of blood vessels in skin; activates sweat glands, contributing to thermoregulation; interprets cutaneous sensation; activates arrector pili muscles

Endocrine System Chapter 16

- Skin protects endocrine organs; converts some hormones to their active forms; synthesizes a vitamin D precursor
- Androgens produced by the endocrine system activate sebaceous glands and are involved in regulating hair growth

Cardiovascular System Chapters 17–19

- Skin protects cardiovascular organs; prevents fluid loss from body; serves as blood reservoir
- Cardiovascular system transports oxygen and nutrients to skin and removes wastes from skin; provides substances needed by skin glands to make their secretions

Lymphatic System/Immunity Chapters 20–21

- Skin protects lymphatic organs; prevents pathogen invasion; dendritic cells and macrophages help activate the immune system
- Lymphatic system prevents edema by picking up excessive leaked fluid; immune system protects skin cells

Respiratory System Chapter 22

- Skin protects respiratory organs; hairs in nose help filter out dust from inhaled air
- Respiratory system furnishes oxygen to skin cells and removes carbon dioxide via gas exchange with blood

Digestive System Chapter 23

- Skin protects digestive organs; provides vitamin D needed for calcium absorption; performs some of the same chemical conversions as liver cells
- Digestive system provides needed nutrients to the skin

Urinary System Chapters 25–26

- Skin protects urinary organs; excretes salts and some nitrogenous wastes in sweat
- Urinary system activates vitamin D precursor made by keratinocytes; disposes of nitrogenous wastes of skin metabolism

Reproductive System Chapter 27

- Skin protects reproductive organs; cutaneous receptors respond to erotic stimuli; highly modified sweat glands (mammary glands) produce milk
- During pregnancy, skin stretches to accommodate growing fetus; changes in skin pigmentation may occur

Chapter Summary

The Skin (pp. 150–157)

1. The skin, or integument, is composed of two discrete tissue layers, an outer epidermis and a deeper dermis, resting on subcutaneous tissue, the hypodermis.

Epidermis (pp. 151–154)

2. The epidermis is an avascular, keratinized sheet of stratified squamous epithelium. Most epidermal cells are keratinocytes. Scattered among the keratinocytes in the deepest epidermal layers are melanocytes, dendritic cells, and tactile cells.
3. From deep to superficial, the strata, or layers of the epidermis, are the basale, spinosum, granulosum, lucidum, and corneum. The stratum lucidum is absent in thin skin. The mitotically active stratum basale is the source of new cells for epidermal growth. The most superficial layers are increasingly keratinized and less viable.

Dermis (pp. 154–156)

4. The dermis, composed mainly of dense, irregular connective tissue, is well supplied with blood vessels, lymphatic vessels, and nerves. Cutaneous receptors, glands, and hair follicles reside within the dermis.
5. The more superficial papillary layer exhibits dermal papillae that protrude into the epidermis above, as well as dermal ridges. Dermal ridges and epidermal ridges together form the friction ridges that produce fingerprints.
6. In the deeper, thicker reticular layer, the connective tissue fibers are much more densely interwoven. Less dense regions between the collagen bundles produce cleavage, or tension, lines in the skin. Points of tight dermal attachment to the hypodermis produce dermal folds, or flexure lines.

Skin Color (pp. 156–157)

7. Skin color reflects the amount of pigments (melanin and carotene) in the skin and the oxygenation level of hemoglobin in blood.
8. Melanin production is stimulated by exposure to ultraviolet radiation in sunlight. Melanin, produced by melanocytes and transferred to keratinocytes, protects the keratinocyte nuclei from the damaging effects of UV radiation.
9. Skin color is affected by emotional state. Alterations in normal skin color (jaundice, bronzing, erythema, and others) may indicate certain disease states.

Appendages of the Skin (pp. 157–162)

1. Skin appendages, which derive from the epidermis, include hairs and hair follicles, nails, and glands (sweat and sebaceous).

Hairs and Hair Follicles (pp. 157–160)

2. A hair, produced by a hair follicle, consists of heavily keratinized cells. A typical hair has a central medulla, a cortex, and an outer cuticle and root and shaft portions. Hair color reflects the amount and kind of melanin present.
3. A hair follicle consists of an inner epithelial root sheath and an outer peripheral connective tissue sheath derived from the dermis. The base of the hair follicle is a hair bulb with a matrix that produces the hair. A hair follicle is richly vascularized and well supplied with nerve fibers. Arrector pili muscles pull the follicles into an upright position, producing goose bumps, and propel sebum to the skin surface when they contract.
4. Except for hairs of the scalp and around the eyes, hairs formed initially are fine vellus hairs; at puberty, under the influence of androgens, coarser, darker terminal hairs appear in the axillae and the genital region.
5. The rate of hair growth varies in different body regions and with sex and age. Differences in life span of hairs account for differences in length on different body regions. Hair thinning reflects factors that lengthen follicular resting periods, age-related atrophy of hair follicles, and a delayed-action gene.

Nails (p. 160)

6. A nail is a scalelike modification of the epidermis that covers the dorsum of a finger (or toe) tip. The actively growing region is the nail matrix.

Sweat (Sudoriferous) Glands (pp. 160–161)

7. Eccrine (merocrine) sweat glands, with a few exceptions, are distributed over the entire body surface. Their primary function is thermoregulation. They are simple coiled tubular glands that secrete a salt solution containing small amounts of other solutes. Their ducts usually empty to the skin surface via pores.
8. Apocrine sweat glands, which may function as scent glands, are found primarily in the axillary and anogenital areas. Their secretion is similar to eccrine secretion, but it also contains proteins and fatty substances on which bacteria thrive.

Sebaceous (Oil) Glands (pp. 161–162)

9. Sebaceous glands occur all over the body surface except for the palms and soles. They are simple alveolar glands; their oily holocrine secretion is called sebum. Sebaceous gland ducts usually empty into hair follicles.
10. Sebum lubricates the skin and hair, prevents water loss from the skin, and acts as a bactericidal agent. Sebaceous glands are activated (at puberty) and controlled by androgens.

Functions of the Integumentary System (pp. 162–164)

1. Protection. The skin protects by chemical barriers (the antibacterial nature of sebum, defensins, cathelicidins, the acid mantle, and the UV shield of melanin), physical barriers (the hardened keratinized and lipid-rich surface), and biological barriers (dendritic cells, macrophages, and DNA).
2. Body temperature regulation. The skin vasculature and sweat glands, regulated by the nervous system, play an important role in maintaining body temperature homeostasis.
3. Cutaneous sensation. Cutaneous sensory receptors respond to temperature, touch, pressure, and pain stimuli.

4. Metabolic functions. A vitamin D precursor is synthesized from cholesterol by epidermal cells. Skin cells also play a role in some chemical conversions.
5. Blood reservoir. The extensive vascular supply of the dermis allows the skin to act as a blood reservoir.
6. Excretion. Sweat contains small amounts of nitrogenous wastes and plays a minor role in excretion.

Homeostatic Imbalances of Skin (pp. 164–167)

1. The most common skin disorders result from infections.

Skin Cancer (pp. 164–165)

2. The most common cause of skin cancer is exposure to ultraviolet radiation.
3. Basal cell carcinoma and squamous cell carcinoma are cured if they are removed before metastasis. Melanoma, a cancer of melanocytes, is less common but more dangerous.

Burns (pp. 165–166)

4. In severe burns, the initial threat is loss of protein- and electrolyte-rich body fluids, which may lead to circulatory collapse. The second threat is overwhelming bacterial infection.
5. The extent of a burn may be evaluated by using the rule of nines. The severity of burns is indicated by the terms first degree, second degree, and third degree. Third-degree burns are full-thickness burns that require grafting for successful recovery.

Developmental Aspects of the Integumentary System (p. 167)

1. The epidermis develops from embryonic ectoderm; the dermis (and hypodermis) develops from mesoderm.
2. The fetus exhibits a downy lanugo coat. Fetal sebaceous glands produce vernix caseosa, which helps protect the fetus's skin from its watery environment.

From Infancy to Adulthood (p. 167)

3. A newborn's skin is thin. During childhood the skin thickens and more subcutaneous fat is deposited. At puberty, sebaceous glands are activated and terminal hairs appear in greater numbers.

Aging Skin (p. 167)

4. In old age, the rate of epidermal cell replacement declines and the skin and hair thin. Skin glands become less active. Loss of collagen and elastic fibers and subcutaneous fat leads to wrinkling; delayed-action genes cause graying and balding. Photodamage is a major cause of skin aging.

5

Review Questions

Multiple Choice/Matching

(Some questions have more than one correct answer. Select the best answer or answers from the choices given.)

1. Which epidermal cell type is most numerous? **(a)** keratinocyte, **(b)** melanocyte, **(c)** dendritic cell, **(d)** tactile cell.
2. Which cell functions as part of the immune system? **(a)** keratinocyte, **(b)** melanocyte, **(c)** dendritic cell, **(d)** tactile cell.
3. The epidermis provides a physical barrier due largely to the presence of **(a)** melanin, **(b)** carotene, **(c)** collagen, **(d)** keratin.
4. Skin color is determined by **(a)** the amount of blood, **(b)** pigments, **(c)** oxygenation level of the blood, **(d)** all of these.
5. The sensations of touch and pressure are picked up by receptors located in **(a)** the stratum spinosum, **(b)** the dermis, **(c)** the hypodermis, **(d)** the stratum corneum.
6. Which is not a true statement about the papillary layer of the dermis? **(a)** it is largely areolar connective tissue, **(b)** it is most responsible for the toughness of the skin, **(c)** it contains nerve endings that respond to stimuli, **(d)** it is highly vascular.
7. Skin surface markings that reflect points of tight dermal attachment to underlying tissues are called **(a)** tension lines, **(b)** papillary ridges, **(c)** flexure lines, **(d)** dermal papillae.
8. Which of the following is not an epidermal derivative? **(a)** hair, **(b)** sweat gland, **(c)** sensory receptor, **(d)** sebaceous gland.
9. An arrector pili muscle **(a)** is associated with each sweat gland, **(b)** can cause a hair to stand up straight, **(c)** enables each hair to be stretched when wet, **(d)** provides new cells for continued growth of its associated hair.
10. The product of this type of sweat gland includes protein and lipid substances that become odoriferous as a result of bacterial action: **(a)** apocrine gland, **(b)** eccrine gland, **(c)** sebaceous gland, **(d)** pancreatic gland.
11. Sebum **(a)** lubricates the surface of the skin and hair, **(b)** consists of cell fragments and fatty substances, **(c)** in excess may cause seborrhea, **(d)** all of these.
12. The rule of nines is helpful clinically in **(a)** diagnosing skin cancer, **(b)** estimating the extent of a burn, **(c)** estimating how serious a cancer is, **(d)** preventing acne.

Short Answer Essay Questions

13. Which epidermal cells are also called prickle cells? Which contain keratohyaline and lamellar granules?
14. Is a bald man really hairless? Explain.
15. You go to the beach to swim on an extremely hot, sunny summer afternoon. Describe two ways in which your integumentary system acts to preserve homeostasis during your outing.
16. Distinguish clearly between first-, second-, and third-degree burns.
17. Describe the process of hair formation, and list several factors that may influence (a) growth cycles and (b) hair texture.
18. What color does carotene impart to the skin?
19. Why does skin wrinkle and what factors accelerate the wrinkling process?
20. Explain each of these familiar phenomena in terms of what you learned in this chapter: (a) pimples, (b) dandruff, (c) greasy hair and "shiny nose," (d) stretch marks from gaining weight, (e) freckles.
21. Count Dracula, the most famous vampire, rumored to have killed at least 200,000 people, was based on a real person who lived in eastern Europe about 600 years ago. He was indeed a "monster," although he was not a real vampire. The historical Count Dracula may have suffered from which of the following? (Hint: See Related Clinical Terms.) (a) porphyria, (b) EB, (c) halitosis, (d) vitiligo. Explain your answer.

22. Why are there no skin cancers that originate from stratum corneum cells?
23. A man got his finger caught in a machine at the factory. The damage was less serious than expected, but the entire nail was torn off his right index finger. The parts lost were the body, root, bed, matrix, and eponychium of the nail. First, define each of these parts. Then, tell if this nail is likely to grow back.
24. On an outline diagram of the human body, mark off various regions according to the rule of nines. What percentage of the total body surface is affected if the skin over the following body parts is burned? (a) the entire posterior trunk and buttocks, (b) an entire lower limb, (c) the entire front of the left upper limb.
25. A common belief is that having your hair cut makes it become thicker. Explain why this belief is not true.

Critical Thinking and Clinical Application Questions

1. Dean, a 40-year-old aging beach boy, is complaining to you that although his suntan made him popular when he was young, now his face is all wrinkled, and he has several darkly pigmented moles that are growing rapidly and are as big as large coins. He shows you the moles, and immediately you think "ABCD." What does that mean and why should he be concerned?
2. Victims of third-degree burns demonstrate the loss of vital functions performed by the skin. What are the two most important problems encountered clinically with such patients? Explain each in terms of the absence of skin.
3. Thelma, a 30-year-old resident of a mental hospital, has an abnormal growth of hair on the dorsum of her right index finger. The orderly comments that she gnaws on that finger continuously. What do you think is the relationship between Thelma's gnawing activity and her hairy finger?
4. A model is concerned about a new scar on her abdomen. She tells her surgeon that there is practically no scar from the appendix operation done when she was 16, but this new gallbladder scar is "gross." Her appendectomy scar is small, obliquely located on the inferior abdominal surface, and very indistinct. By contrast, the gallbladder scar is large, lumpy, and runs at right angles to the central axis of the body trunk. Can you explain why the scars are so different?
5. Osteomalacia, a condition of soft bones, is prevalent in Muslim countries that decree that their women wear the burka, a garment that covers all but their eyes. What is the cause and effect here?
6. Mrs. Gaucher received second-degree burns on her abdomen when she dropped a kettle of boiling water. She asked her doctor (worriedly) if she would need a skin graft. What do you think he told her?

AT THE CLINIC

Related Clinical Terms

Albinism (al′bĭ-nizm; *alb* = white) Inherited condition in which melanocytes do not synthesize melanin owing to a lack of tyrosinase. An albino's skin is pink, the hair pale or white, and the irises of the eyes unpigmented or poorly so.

Boils and carbuncles (kar′bung-klz; "little glowing embers") Inflammation of hair follicles and sebaceous glands in which an infection has spread to the underlying hypodermis; common on the dorsal neck. Carbuncles are composite boils. A common cause is bacterial infection.

Cold sores (fever blisters) Small fluid-filled blisters that itch and smart; usually occur around the lips and in the mucosa of the mouth; caused by a herpes simplex infection. The virus localizes in a cutaneous nerve, where it remains dormant until activated by emotional upset, fever, or UV radiation.

Contact dermatitis Itching, redness, and swelling, progressing to blister formation; caused by exposure of the skin to chemicals (e.g., poison ivy oleoresin) that provoke an allergic response in sensitive individuals.

Decubitus ulcer (de-ku′bĭ-tus) Localized breakdown and ulceration of skin due to interference with its blood supply. Usually occurs over a bony prominence, such as the hip or heel, that is subjected to continuous pressure; also called a bedsore.

Dermatology The branch of medicine that studies and treats disorders of the skin.

Eczema (ek′ze-mah) A skin rash characterized by itching, blistering, oozing, and scaling of the skin. A common allergic reaction in children, but also occurs (typically in a more severe form) in adults. Frequent causes include allergic reactions to certain foods (fish, eggs, and others) or to inhaled dust or pollen. Treated by methods used for other allergic disorders.

Epidermolysis bullosa (EB) A group of hereditary disorders characterized by inadequate or faulty synthesis of keratin, collagen, and/or basement membrane "cement" that results in lack of cohesion between layers of the skin and mucosa. A simple touch causes layers to separate and blister. For this reason, EB victims are called "touch-me-nots." In severe cases fatal blistering occurs in major vital organs. Because the blisters rupture easily, victims suffer frequent infections. Treatments are aimed at relieving the symptoms and preventing infection.

Impetigo (im″pĕ-ti′go; *impet* = an attack) Pink, fluid-filled, raised lesions (common around the mouth and nose) that develop a yellow crust and eventually rupture. Caused by staphylococcus infection, it is contagious, and common in school-age children.

Porphyria (por-fer′e-ah; "purple") An inherited condition in which certain enzymes needed to form the heme of hemoglobin of blood are lacking. Without these enzymes, metabolic intermediates of the heme pathway called porphyrins build up, spill into the circulation, and eventually cause lesions throughout the body, especially when exposed to sunlight. The skin becomes lesioned and scarred; fingers, toes, and nose are disfigured; gums degenerate and teeth become prominent. Believed to be the basis of folklore about vampires.

Psoriasis (so-ri′ah-sis) A chronic autoimmune condition characterized by raised, reddened epidermal patches covered with silvery scales that itch or burn, crack, and sometimes bleed or become infected. When severe, it may be disfiguring and

Related Clinical Terms *(continued)*

debilitating. Trauma, infection, hormonal changes, or stress often trigger the autoimmune attacks. Cortisone-containing topicals (medications applied to the skin surface) may control mild cases. For more severe cases, self-injected drugs called biologicals and/or phototherapy with UV light in conjunction with chemotherapeutic drugs provides some relief.

Rosacea (ro-za′she-ah) A chronic skin eruption produced by dilated small blood vessels of the face, particularly the nose and cheeks. Papules and acne-like pustules may or may not occur. More common in women, but tends to be more severe when it occurs in men. Cause is unknown, but stress, some endocrine disorders, and anything that produces flushing (hot beverages, alcohol, sunlight, etc.) can aggravate this condition.

Vitiligo (vit″ĭ-li′go; *viti* = a vine, winding) The most prevalent skin pigmentation disorder, characterized by a loss of melanocytes and uneven dispersal of melanin, so that unpigmented skin regions (light spots) are surrounded by normally pigmented areas. An autoimmune disorder.

Scleroderma (*scler* = hard) An autoimmune disorder characterized by stiff, hardened skin due to abnormal amounts of collagen in the dermis that severely limit joint movements and facial expressions. A classic sign of the disorder is Raynaud disease in which the fingers and toes become white and painful because of poor blood flow to those areas. The fibrosis that occurs in systemic cases may affect a variety of organs including the lungs, eventually leading to suffocation, and the kidneys, leading to renal hypertension because of blood vessel constriction and occlusion. Environmental factors including organic solvents, asbestos, and even silicone breast implants have all been suspect scleroderma triggers.

5

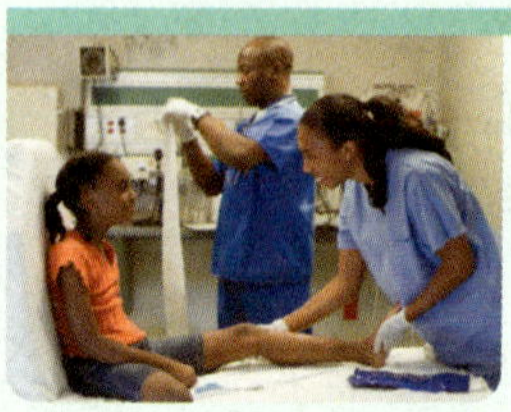

Case Study Integumentary System

A terrible collision between a trailer truck and a bus has occurred on Route 91. Several of the passengers are rushed to area hospitals for treatment. We will follow a few of these people in clinical case studies that will continue through the book from one organ system to the next.

Examination of Mrs. DeStephano, a 45-year-old woman, reveals several impairments of homeostasis. Relative to her integumentary system, the following comments are noted on her chart:

- Epidermal abrasions of the right arm and shoulder
- Severe lacerations of the right cheek and temple
- Cyanosis apparent

The lacerated areas are cleaned, sutured (stitched), and bandaged by the emergency room (ER) personnel, and Mrs. DeStephano is admitted for further tests.

Relative to her signs:

1. What protective mechanisms are impaired or deficient in the abraded areas?
2. Assuming that bacteria are penetrating the dermis in these areas, what remaining skin defenses might act to prevent further bacterial invasion?
3. What benefit is conferred by suturing the lacerations? (Hint: See Chapter 4, p. 149, Related Clinical Terms, healing by first intention.)
4. Mrs. DeStephano's cyanotic skin may hint at what additional problem (and impairment of what body systems or functions)?

(Answers in Appendix H)

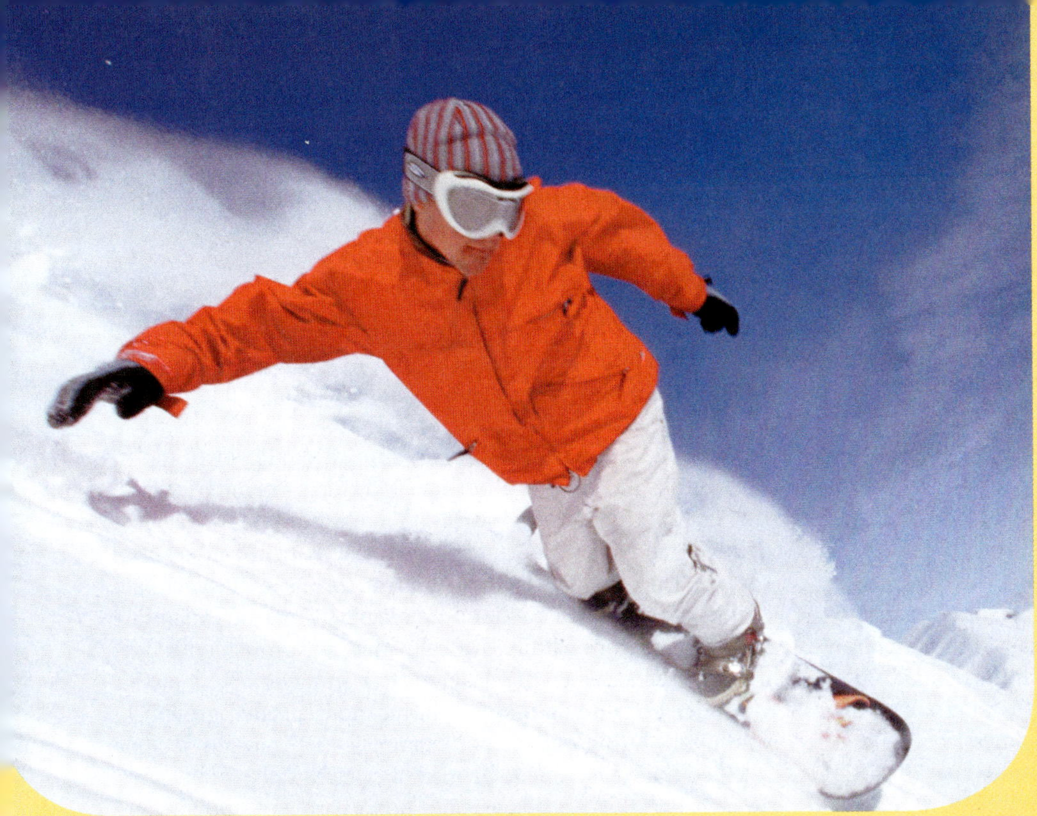

6

Bones and Skeletal Tissues

All of us have heard the expressions "bone tired" and "bag of bones"—rather unflattering and inaccurate images of one of our most phenomenal tissues and our main skeletal elements. Our brains, not our bones, convey feelings of fatigue. As for "bag of bones," they are indeed more prominent in some of us, but without bones to form our internal supporting skeleton we would all creep along the ground like slugs, lacking any definite shape or form. Along with its bones, the skeleton contains resilient cartilages, which we briefly discuss in this chapter. However, our major focus is the structure and function of bone tissue and the dynamics of its formation and remodeling throughout life.

Skeletal Cartilages

✓ Describe the functional properties of the three types of cartilage tissue.

✓ Locate the major cartilages of the adult skeleton.

✓ Explain how cartilage grows.

The human skeleton is initially made up of cartilages and fibrous membranes, but bone soon replaces most of these early supports. The few cartilages that remain in adults are found mainly in regions where flexible skeletal tissue is needed.

Basic Structure, Types, and Locations

A **skeletal cartilage** is made of some variety of *cartilage tissue* molded to fit its body location and function. Cartilage consists primarily of water, which accounts for its resilience, that is, its ability to spring back to its original shape after being compressed.

The cartilage, which contains no nerves or blood vessels, is surrounded by a layer of dense irregular connective tissue, the *perichondrium* (per″ĭ-kon′dre-um; "around the cartilage"). The perichondrium acts like a girdle to resist outward expansion when the cartilage is compressed. Additionally, the perichondrium contains the blood vessels from which nutrients diffuse through the matrix to reach the cartilage cells internally. This mode of nutrient delivery limits cartilage thickness.

As we described in Chapter 4, there are three types of cartilage tissue in the body: hyaline, elastic, and fibrocartilage. The skeletal cartilages include examples from all three. All three types have the same basic components—cells called *chondrocytes*, encased in small cavities (lacunae) within an *extracellular matrix* containing a jellylike ground substance and fibers.

Hyaline Cartilages

Hyaline cartilages, which look like frosted glass when freshly exposed, provide support with flexibility and resilience. They are the most abundant skeletal cartilages. Their chondrocytes are spherical (see Figure 4.8g), and the only fiber type in their matrix is fine collagen fibers (which are undetectable microscopically). Colored blue in **Figure 6.1**, skeletal hyaline cartilages include

- *Articular cartilages*, which cover the ends of most bones at movable joints
- *Costal cartilages*, which connect the ribs to the sternum (breastbone)
- *Respiratory cartilages*, which form the skeleton of the *larynx* (*voicebox*) and reinforce other respiratory passageways
- *Nasal cartilages*, which support the external nose

Elastic Cartilages

Elastic cartilages resemble hyaline cartilages (see Figure 4.8h), but they contain more stretchy elastic fibers and so are better able to stand up to repeated bending. They are found in only two skeletal locations, shown in green in Figure 6.1—the external ear and the epiglottis (the flap that bends to cover the opening of the larynx each time we swallow).

Fibrocartilages

Highly compressible with great tensile strength, **fibrocartilages** consist of roughly parallel rows of chondrocytes alternating with thick collagen fibers (see Figure 4.8i). Fibrocartilages occur in sites that are subjected to both pressure and stretch, such as the padlike cartilages (menisci) of the knee and the discs between vertebrae, colored red in Figure 6.1.

Growth of Cartilage

Unlike bone, which has a hard matrix, cartilage has a flexible matrix which can accommodate mitosis. It is the ideal tissue to use to rapidly lay down the embryonic skeleton and to provide for new skeletal growth.

Cartilage grows in two ways. In **appositional growth** (ap″o-zish′un-al; "growth from outside"), cartilage-forming cells in the surrounding perichondrium secrete new matrix against the external face of the existing cartilage tissue. In **interstitial growth** (in″ter-stish′al; "growth from inside"), the lacunae-bound chondrocytes divide and secrete new matrix, expanding the cartilage from within. Typically, cartilage growth ends during adolescence when the skeleton stops growing.

Under certain conditions—during normal bone growth in youth and during old age, for example—cartilage can become calcified (hardened due to deposit of calcium salts). Note, however, that calcified cartilage is not bone; cartilage and bone are always distinct tissues.

☑ Check Your Understanding

1. Which type of cartilage is most plentiful in the adult body?
2. What two body structures contain flexible elastic cartilage?
3. Cartilage grows by interstitial growth. What does this mean?

For answers, see Appendix H.

Classification of Bones

✓ Name the major regions of the skeleton and describe their relative functions.

✓ Compare and contrast the four bone classes and provide examples of each class.

The 206 named bones of the human skeleton are divided into two groups: axial and appendicular.

The **axial skeleton** forms the long axis of the body and includes the bones of the skull, vertebral column, and rib cage, shown in orange in Figure 6.1. Generally speaking these bones protect, support, or carry other body parts.

The **appendicular skeleton** (ap″en-dik′u-lar) consists of the bones of the upper and lower limbs and the girdles (shoulder bones and hip bones) that attach the limbs to the axial skeleton (colored gold in Figure 6.1). Bones of the limbs help us move from place to place (locomotion) and manipulate our environment.

Bones come in many sizes and shapes. For example, the pisiform bone of the wrist is the size and shape of a pea, whereas the femur (thigh bone) is nearly 2 feet long in some people and has a large, ball-shaped head. The unique shape of each bone fulfills a particular need. The femur, for example, withstands great pressure, and its hollow-cylinder design provides maximum strength with minimum weight to accommodate our upright posture.

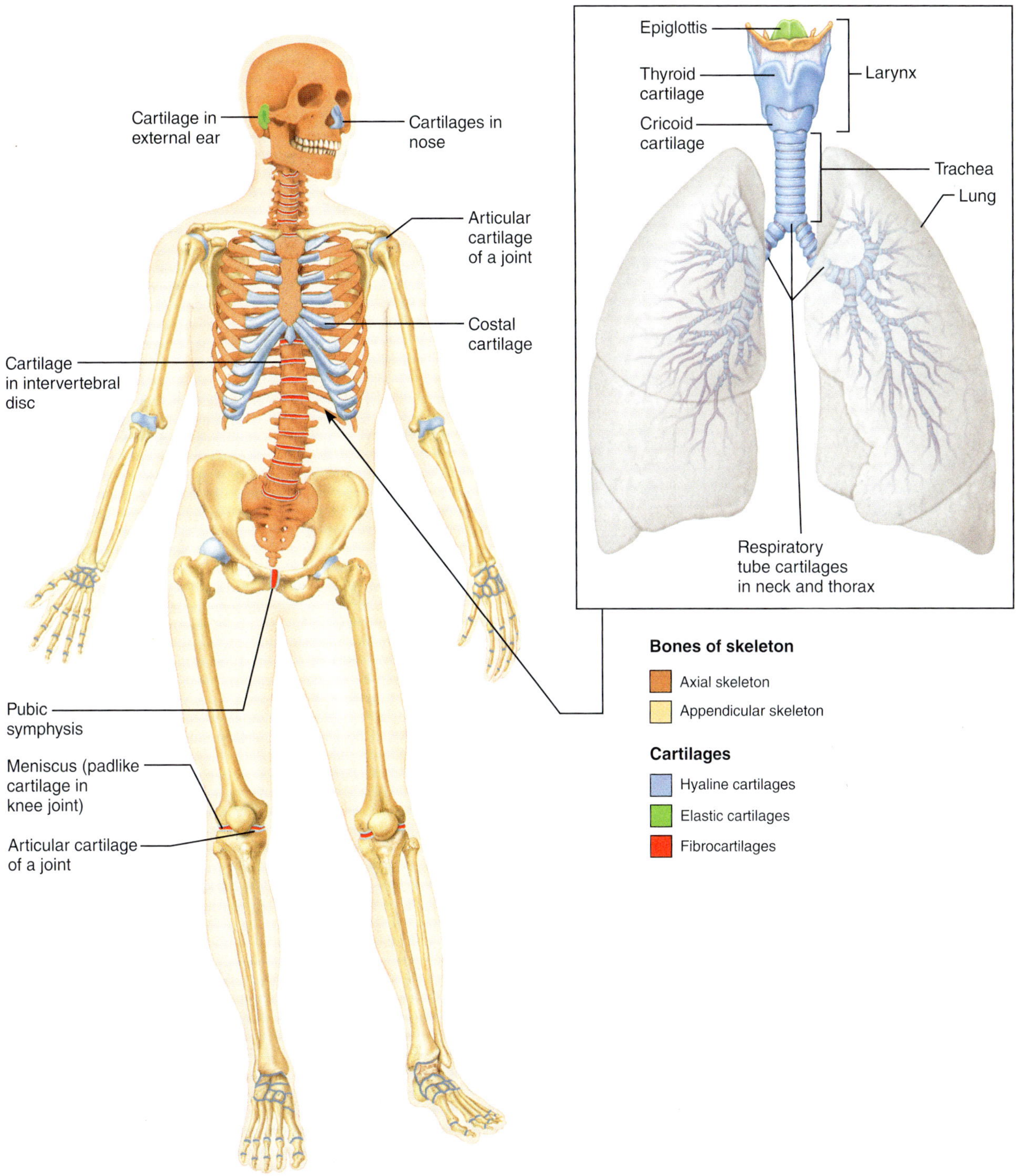

Figure 6.1 The bones and cartilages of the human skeleton. The cartilages that support the respiratory tubes and larynx are drawn separately at the right.

Generally, bones are classified by their shape as long, short, flat, or irregular **(Figure 6.2)**.

- **Long bones**, as their name suggests, are considerably longer than they are wide (Figure 6.2a). A long bone has a shaft plus two ends which are often expanded. All limb bones except the patella (kneecap) and the wrist and ankle bones are long bones. Notice that these bones are named for their elongated shape, *not* their overall size. The three bones in each of your fingers are long bones, even though they are small.
- **Short bones** are roughly cube shaped. The bones of the wrist and ankle are examples (Figure 6.2d). **Sesamoid bones** (ses′ah-moid; "shaped like a sesame seed") are a special type of short bone that form in a tendon (for example, the patella). They vary in size and number in different individuals. Some

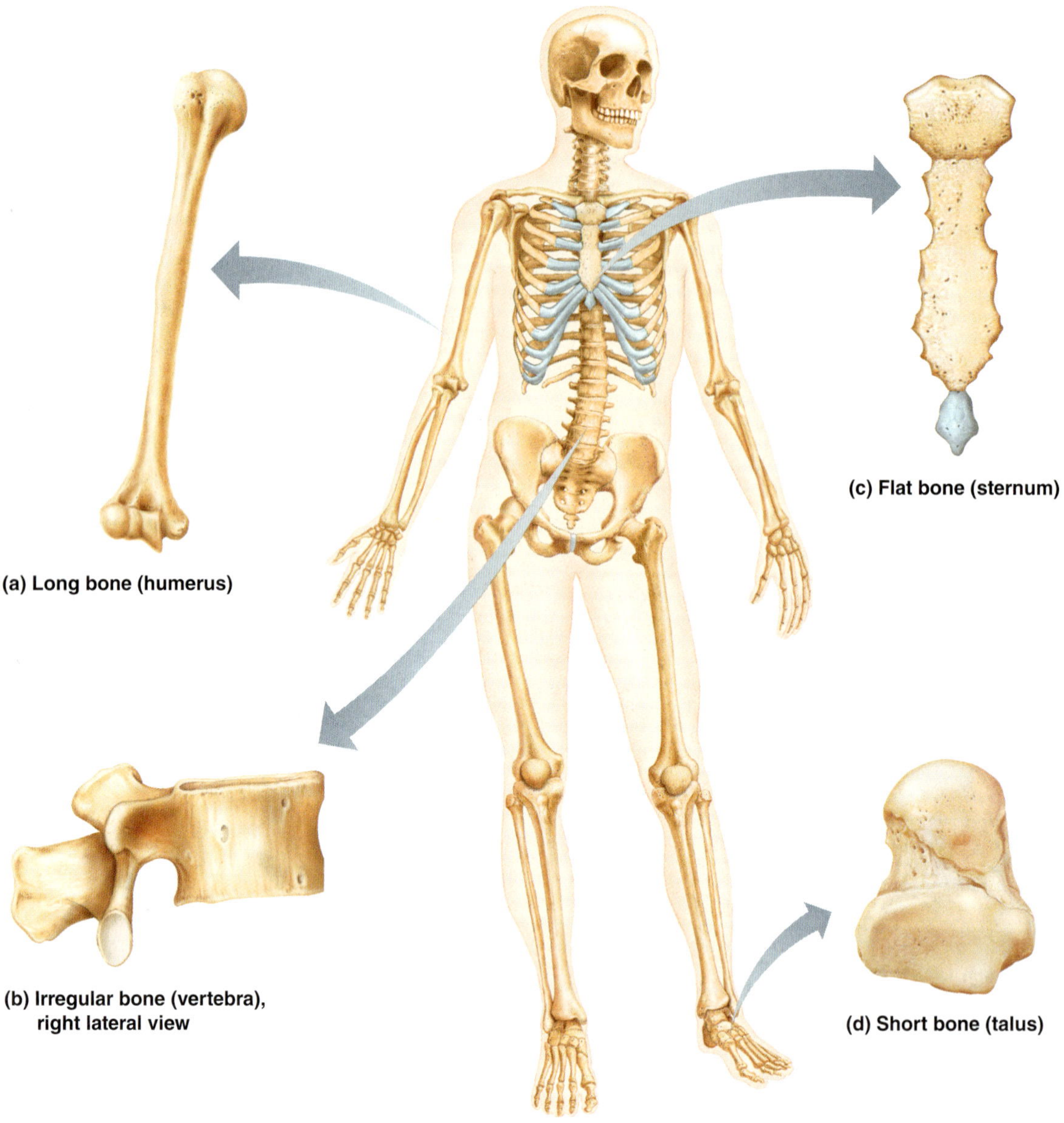

Figure 6.2 Classification of bones on the basis of shape.

sesamoid bones act to alter the direction of pull of a tendon. The function of others is not known.

- **Flat bones** are thin, flattened, and usually a bit curved. The sternum (breastbone), scapulae (shoulder blades), ribs, and most skull bones are flat bones (Figure 6.2c).
- **Irregular bones** have complicated shapes that fit none of the preceding classes. Examples include the vertebrae and the hip bones (Figure 6.2b).

Check Your Understanding

4. What are the components of the axial skeleton?
5. Contrast the general function of the axial skeleton to that of the appendicular skeleton.
6. What bone class do the ribs and skull bones fall into?

For answers, see Appendix H.

Functions of Bones

✓ List and describe seven important functions of bones.

Our bones perform seven important functions:

- **Support.** Bones provide a framework that supports the body and cradles its soft organs. For example, bones of lower limbs act as pillars to support the body trunk when we stand, and the rib cage supports the thoracic wall.
- **Protection.** The fused bones of the skull protect the brain. The vertebrae surround the spinal cord, and the rib cage helps protect the vital organs of the thorax.
- **Movement.** Skeletal muscles, which attach to bones by tendons, use bones as levers to move the body and its parts. As a result, we can walk, grasp objects, and breathe. The design of joints determines the types of movement possible.

- **Mineral and growth factor storage.** Bone is a reservoir for minerals, most importantly calcium and phosphate. The stored minerals are released into the bloodstream in their ionic form as needed for distribution to all parts of the body. Indeed, "deposits" and "withdrawals" of minerals to and from the bones go on almost continuously. Additionally, mineralized bone matrix stores important growth factors.
- **Blood cell formation.** Most blood cell formation, or **hematopoiesis** (hem″ah-to-poi-e′sis), occurs in the red marrow cavities of certain bones.
- **Triglyceride (fat) storage.** Fat, a source of energy for the body, is stored in bone cavities.
- **Hormone production.** Bones produce osteocalcin, a hormone which not only helps regulate bone formation, but also protects against obesity, glucose intolerance, and diabetes mellitus. (Osteocalcin is discussed further in Chapter 16.)

Check Your Understanding

7. What is the functional relationship between skeletal muscles and bones?
8. What two types of substances are stored in bone matrix?
9. Describe two functions of a bone's marrow cavities.

For answers, see Appendix H.

Bone Structure

- ✓ Describe the gross anatomy of a typical flat bone and a long bone. Indicate the locations and functions of red and yellow marrow, articular cartilage, periosteum, and endosteum.
- ✓ Indicate the functional importance of bone markings.
- ✓ Describe the histology of compact and spongy bone.
- ✓ Discuss the chemical composition of bone and the advantages conferred by its organic and inorganic components.

Because they contain different types of tissue, bones are organs. (Recall that an organ contains several different tissues.) Although bone (osseous) tissue dominates bones, they also contain nervous tissue in their nerves, cartilage in their articular cartilages, fibrous connective tissue lining their cavities, and muscle and epithelial tissues in their blood vessels. We will consider bone structure at three levels: gross, microscopic, and chemical.

Gross Anatomy

Bone Textures: Compact and Spongy Bone

Every bone has a dense outer layer that looks smooth and solid to the naked eye. This external layer is **compact bone** (Figures 6.3 and 6.4). Internal to this is **spongy bone** (also called *trabecular bone*), a honeycomb of small needle-like or flat pieces called **trabeculae** (trah-bek′u-le; "little beams"). In living bones the open spaces between trabeculae are filled with red or yellow bone marrow.

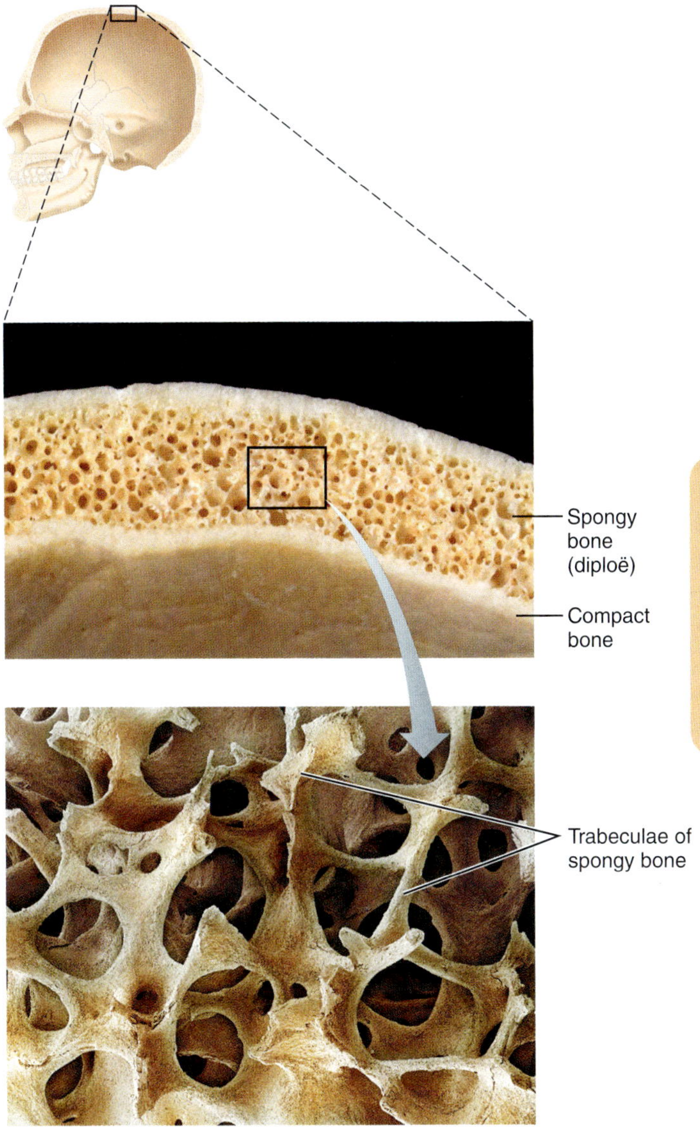

Figure 6.3 Flat bones consist of a layer of spongy bone sandwiched between two thin layers of compact bone. (Photomicrograph at bottom, 25×)

Structure of Short, Irregular, and Flat Bones

Short, irregular, and flat bones share a simple design: They all consist of thin plates of spongy bone covered by compact bone. These plates are covered outside and inside by connective tissue membranes, respectively the periosteum and endosteum (described on pp. 178–179). However, these bones are not cylindrical and so they have no shaft or epiphyses. They contain bone marrow (between their trabeculae), but no well-defined marrow cavity. Where they form movable joints with their neighbors, hyaline cartilage covers their surfaces.

Figure 6.3 shows a typical flat bone of the skull. In flat bones, the spongy bone is called the **diploë** (dip′lo-e; "folded") and the whole arrangement resembles a stiffened sandwich.

Structure of a Typical Long Bone

With few exceptions, all long bones have the same general structure: a shaft, bone ends, and membranes **(Figure 6.4)**.

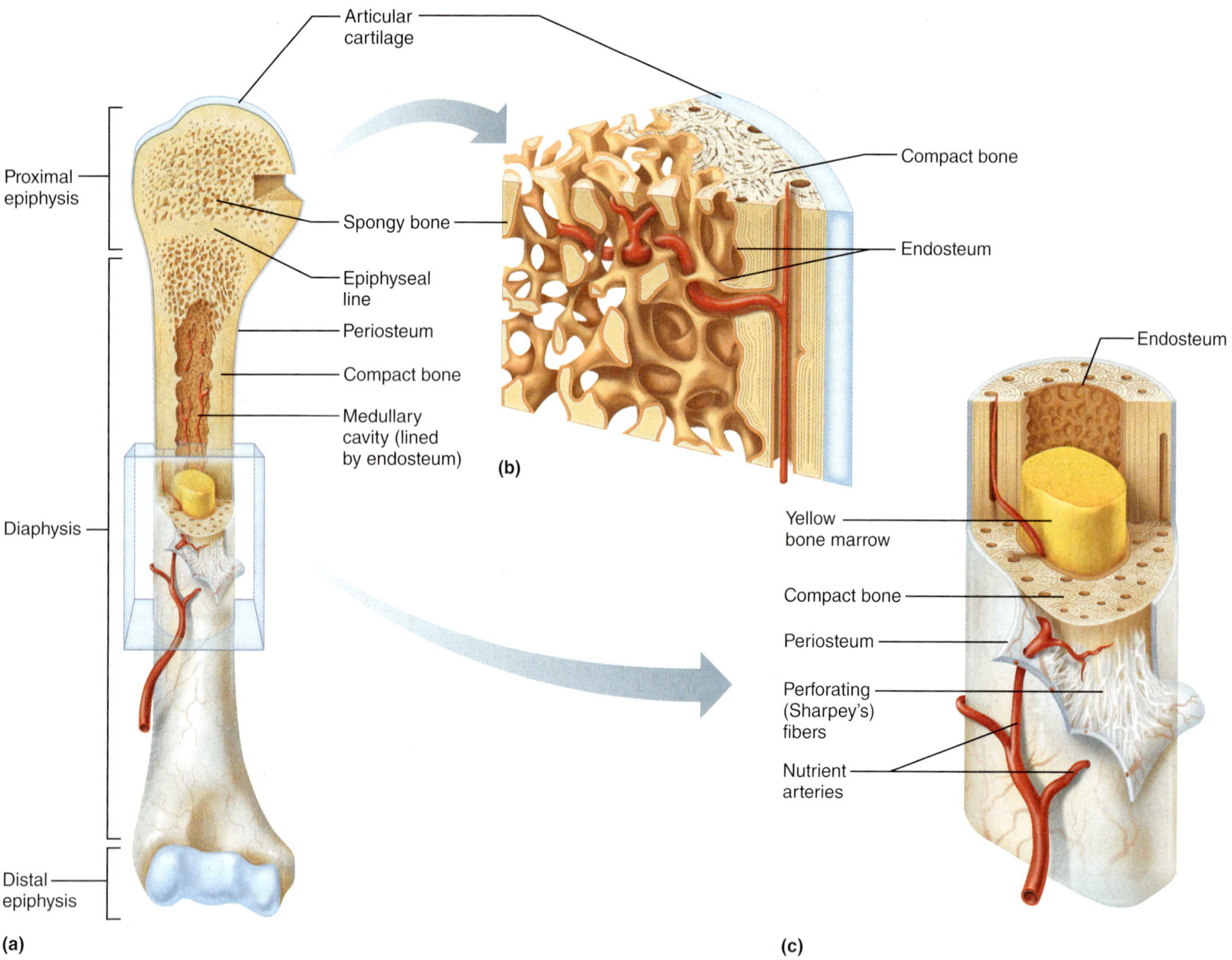

Figure 6.4 The structure of a long bone (humerus of arm). (a) Anterior view with bone sectioned frontally to show the interior at the proximal end. **(b)** Enlarged view of spongy bone and compact bone of the epiphysis of (a). (For related images, see *A Brief Atlas of the Human Body*, Plates 20 and 21.) **(c)** Enlarged cross-sectional view of the shaft (diaphysis) of (a). Note that the external surface of the diaphysis is covered by periosteum, but the articular surface of the epiphysis is covered with hyaline cartilage.

Diaphysis A tubular **diaphysis** (di-af′ĭ-sis; *dia* = through, *physis* = growth), or shaft, forms the long axis of the bone. It is constructed of a relatively thick *collar* of compact bone that surrounds a central **medullary cavity** (med′u-lar-e; "middle"), or *marrow cavity*. In adults, the medullary cavity contains fat (yellow marrow) and is called the **yellow marrow cavity**.

Epiphyses The **epiphyses** (e-pif′ĭ-sēz; singular: epiphysis) are the bone ends (*epi* = upon). In many cases, they are broader than the diaphysis. An outer shell of compact bone forms the epiphysis exterior and their interior contains spongy bone. A thin layer of articular (hyaline) cartilage covers the joint surface of each epiphysis, cushioning the opposing bone ends during movement and absorbing stress.

Between the diaphysis and each epiphysis of an adult long bone is an **epiphyseal line**, a remnant of the **epiphyseal plate**, a disc of hyaline cartilage that grows during childhood to lengthen the bone. The flared portion of the bone where the diaphysis and epiphysis meet, whether it is the epiphyseal plate or line, is sometimes called the *metaphysis* (*meta* = between).

Membranes A glistening white, double-layered membrane called the **periosteum** (per″e-os′te-um; *peri* = around, *osteo* = bone) covers the external surface of the entire bone except the joint surfaces. The outer *fibrous layer* of the periosteum is dense irregular connective tissue. The inner *osteogenic layer*, abutting the bone surface, consists primarily of primitive stem cells, *osteogenic cells*, that give rise to all bone cells except bone-destroying cells. These cell types are described shortly.

The periosteum is richly supplied with nerve fibers and blood vessels, which pass through the shaft to enter the marrow cavity via **nutrient foramina** (fo-ra′me-nah; "openings"). *Perforating (Sharpey's) fibers*—tufts of collagen fibers that extend from its fibrous layer into the bone matrix—secure the periosteum to the underlying bone (Figure 6.4). The periosteum also provides anchoring points for tendons and ligaments. At these points the perforating fibers are exceptionally dense.

A delicate connective tissue membrane called the **endosteum** (en-dos′te-um; "within the bone") covers internal bone surfaces (Figure 6.4). The endosteum covers the trabeculae of spongy bone and lines the canals that pass through the compact bone. Like the periosteum, the endosteum contains osteogenic cells that can differentiate into other bone cells.

Location of Hematopoietic Tissue in Bones

Hematopoietic tissue, **red marrow**, is typically found within the trabecular cavities of spongy bone of long bones and in the diploë of flat bones. For this reason, both these cavities are often called **red marrow cavities**. In newborn infants, the medullary cavity of the diaphysis and all areas of spongy bone contain red bone marrow. In most adult long bones, the fat-containing medullary cavity extends well into the epiphysis, and little red marrow is present in the spongy bone cavities. For this reason, blood cell production in adult long bones routinely occurs only in the heads of the femur and humerus (the long bone of the arm).

The red marrow found in the diploë of flat bones (such as the sternum) and in some irregular bones (such as the hip bone) is much more active in hematopoiesis. When clinicians suspect problems with the blood-forming tissue, they obtain red marrow samples from these sites. However, yellow marrow in the medullary cavity can revert to red marrow if a person becomes very anemic and needs more red blood cells.

Bone Markings

The external surfaces of bones are rarely smooth and featureless. Instead, they display projections, depressions, and openings. These **bone markings** serve as sites of muscle, ligament, and tendon attachment, as joint surfaces, or as conduits for blood vessels and nerves.

Projections—bone markings that bulge outward from the surface—include heads, trochanters, spines, and others. Each has distinguishing features and functions. In most cases, bone projections indicate the stresses created by muscles attached to and pulling on them or are modified surfaces where bones meet and form joints.

Bone markings that are depressions and openings include fossae (singular: fossa), sinuses, foramina (singular: foramen), and grooves. They usually allow nerves and blood vessels to pass. **Table 6.1** describes the most important types of bone markings. Familiarize yourself with these terms because you will meet them again as identifying marks of the individual bones studied in the lab.

Microscopic Anatomy of Bone

Cells of Bone Tissue

Five major cell types populate bone tissue: osteogenic cells, osteoblasts, osteocytes, bone lining cells, and osteoclasts. All of these except for the osteoclasts originate from mesenchymal cells. Each cell type is essentially a specialized form of the same basic cell type that transforms to a mature or functional form that serves bone growth in some specific way **(Figure 6.5)**. Bone cells, like other connective tissue cells, are surrounded by an extracellular matrix of their making.

Osteogenic Cells **Osteogenic cells**, also called **osteoprogenitor cells**, are mitotically active stem cells found in the membranous periosteum and endosteum. In growing bones they are flattened or squamous cells. When stimulated, these cells differentiate into osteoblasts or bone lining cells (see below), while others persist as osteogenic cells.

Osteoblasts **Osteoblasts** are bone-forming cells that secrete the bone matrix. Like their close relatives, the fibroblasts and chondroblasts, they are actively mitotic. The unmineralized bone matrix they secrete includes collagen (90% of bone protein) and calcium-binding proteins that make up the initial unmineralized bone, or *osteoid*. As described later, osteoblasts also play a role in matrix calcification.

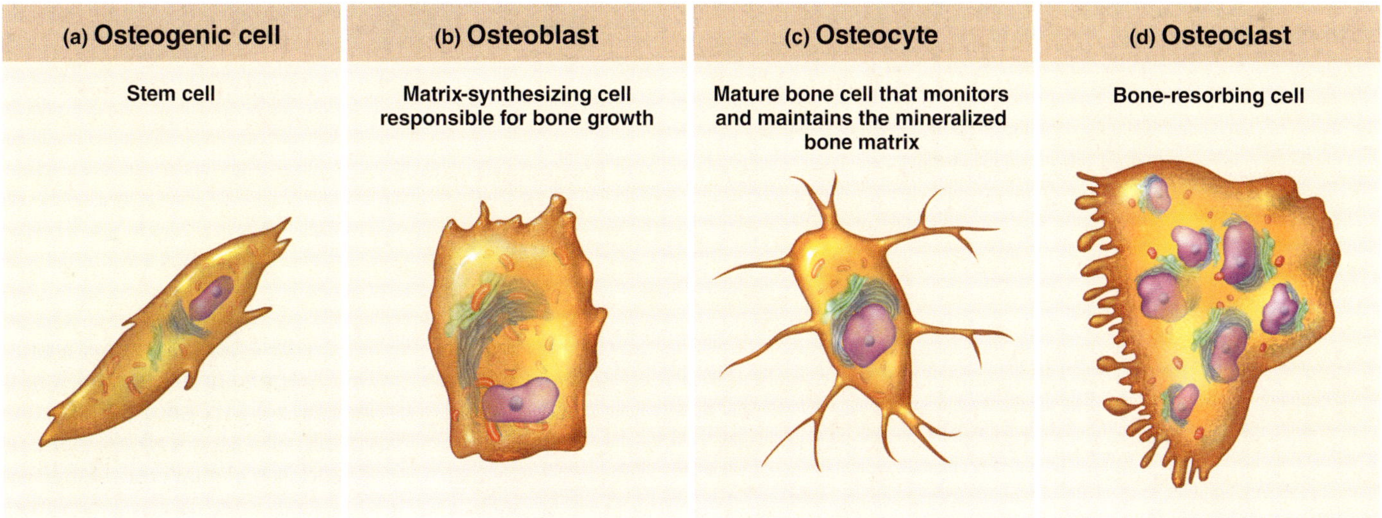

Figure 6.5 Comparison of different types of bone cells. The bone lining cell, similar in appearance to the osteogenic cell and similar to the osteocyte in function, is not illustrated.

6

Table 6.1 Bone Markings

NAME OF BONE MARKING	DESCRIPTION
Projections That Are Sites of Muscle and Ligament Attachment	
Tuberosity (too″bĕ-ros′ĭ-te)	Large rounded projection; may be roughened
Crest	Narrow ridge of bone; usually prominent
Trochanter (tro-kan′ter)	Very large, blunt, irregularly shaped process (the only examples are on the femur)
Line	Narrow ridge of bone; less prominent than a crest
Tubercle (too′ber-kl)	Small rounded projection or process
Epicondyle (ep″ĭ-kon′dīl)	Raised area on or above a condyle
Spine	Sharp, slender, often pointed projection
Process	Any bony prominence

ILLUSTRATIONS

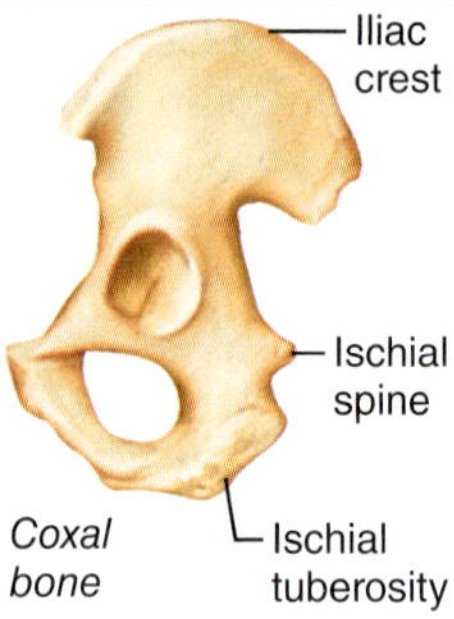

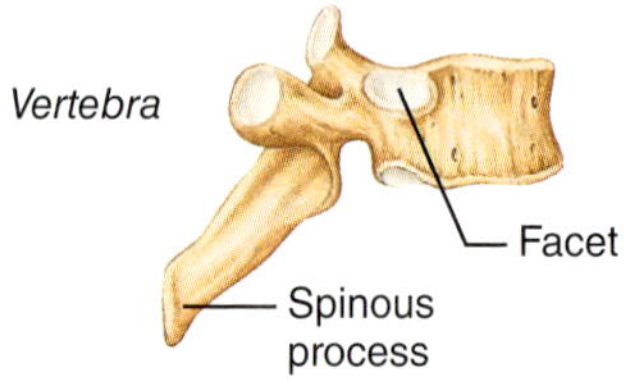

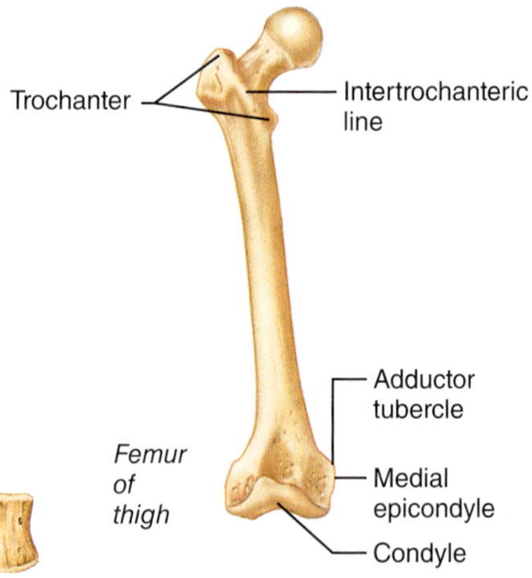

NAME OF BONE MARKING	DESCRIPTION
Projections That Help to Form Joints	
Head	Bony expansion carried on a narrow neck
Facet	Smooth, nearly flat articular surface
Condyle (kon′dīl)	Rounded articular projection
Ramus (ra′mus)	Armlike bar of bone

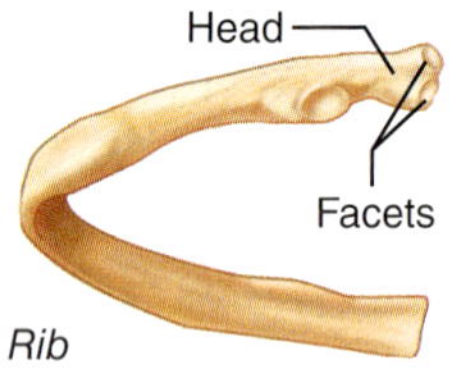

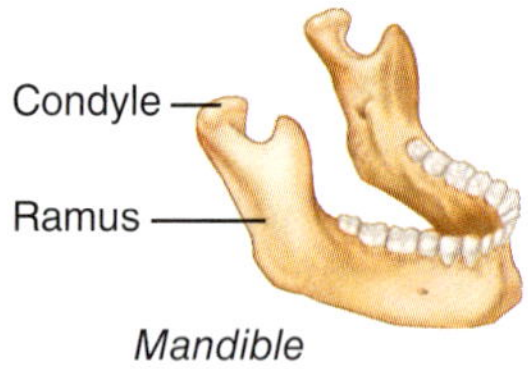

NAME OF BONE MARKING	DESCRIPTION
Depressions and Openings	
For Passage of Blood Vessels and Nerves	
Groove	Furrow
Fissure	Narrow, slitlike opening
Foramen (fo-ra′men)	Round or oval opening through a bone
Notch	Indentation at the edge of a structure
Others	
Meatus (me-a′tus)	Canal-like passageway
Sinus	Cavity within a bone, filled with air and lined with mucous membrane
Fossa (fos′ah)	Shallow, basinlike depression in a bone, often serving as an articular surface

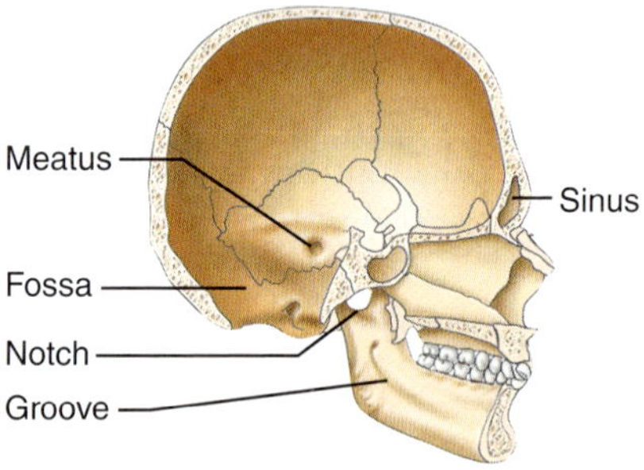

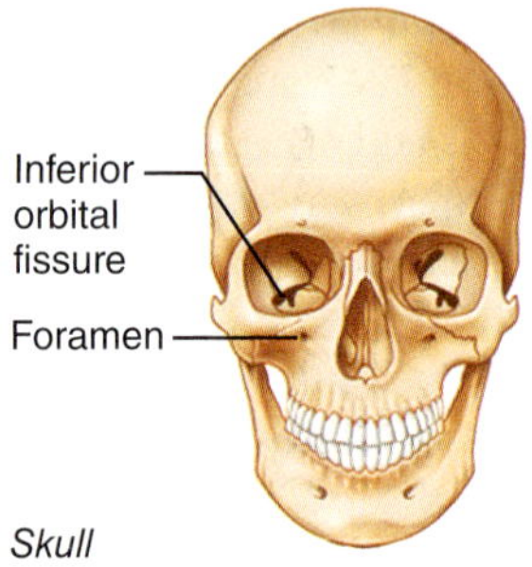

When actively depositing matrix, osteoblasts are cube shaped. When inactive, they resemble the flattened osteogenic cells or may differentiate into bone lining cells. When the osteoblasts become completely surrounded by the matrix being secreted, they become osteocytes.

Osteocytes The spidery **osteocytes** (Figure 6.5) are mature bone cells that occupy spaces (lacunae) that conform to their shape. Osteocytes monitor and maintain the bone matrix. If they die, the surrounding matrix is resorbed. Osteocytes also act as stress or strain "sensors" and respond to mechanical stimuli (bone loading, bone deformation, weightlessness). They communicate this information to the cells responsible for bone remodeling (osteoblasts and osteoclasts) so that bone matrix can be made or degraded as necessary to preserve calcium homeostasis. We discuss the bone-destroying *osteoclast* on p. 187 when we explore bone remodeling.

Bone Lining Cells **Bone lining cells** are flat cells found on bone surfaces where bone remodeling is not going on. Like osteocytes, they are thought to help maintain the matrix. Bone lining cells on the external bone surface are also called *periosteal cells*, whereas those lining internal surfaces are called *endosteal cells*.

Osteoclasts Derived from the same hematopoietic stem cells that differentiate into macrophages, **osteoclasts** are giant multinucleate cells located at sites of bone resorption. When actively resorbing (breaking down) bone, the osteoclasts rest in a shallow depression called a *resorption bay* and exhibit a distinctive *ruffled border* which directly contacts the bone. The deep plasma membrane infoldings of the ruffled border tremendously increase the surface area for enzymatically degrading the bones and seal off that area from the surrounding matrix.

Compact Bone

Although compact bone looks solid, a microscope reveals that it is riddled with passageways that serve as conduits for nerves and blood vessels (see Figure 6.7).

Osteon (Haversian System) The structural unit of compact bone is called either the **osteon** (os′te-on) or the **Haversian system** (ha-ver′zhen). Each osteon is an elongated cylinder oriented parallel to the long axis of the bone. Functionally, osteons are tiny weight-bearing pillars.

As shown in the "exploded" view in **Figure 6.6**, an osteon is a group of hollow tubes of bone matrix, one placed outside the next like the growth rings of a tree trunk. Each matrix tube is a **lamella** (lah-mel′ah; "little plate"), and for this reason compact bone is often called **lamellar bone**. Although all of the collagen fibers in a particular lamella run in a single direction, the collagen fibers in adjacent lamellae always run in different directions. This alternating pattern is beautifully designed to withstand torsion stresses—the adjacent lamellae reinforce one another to resist twisting. You can think of the osteon's design as a "twister resister."

Collagen fibers are not the only part of bone lamellae that are beautifully ordered. The tiny crystals of bone salts align between the collagen fibrils and thus also alternate their direction in adjacent lamellae.

Canals and Canaliculi Running through the core of each osteon is the **central canal**, or **Haversian canal**, containing small blood vessels and nerve fibers that serve the osteon's cells. Canals of a second type called **perforating canals**, or **Volkmann's canals** (folk′mahnz), lie at right angles to the long axis of the bone and connect the blood and nerve supply of the periosteum to those in the central canals and the medullary cavity **(Figure 6.7a)**. Unlike the central canals of osteons, the perforating canals are not surrounded by concentric lamellae, but like all other internal bone cavities, these canals are lined with endosteum.

Spider-shaped osteocytes (Figures 6.5c and 6.7b) occupy **lacunae** (*lac* = hollow; *una* = little) at the junctions of the lamellae. Hairlike canals called *canaliculi* (kan″ah-lik′u-li) connect the lacunae to each other and to the central canal.

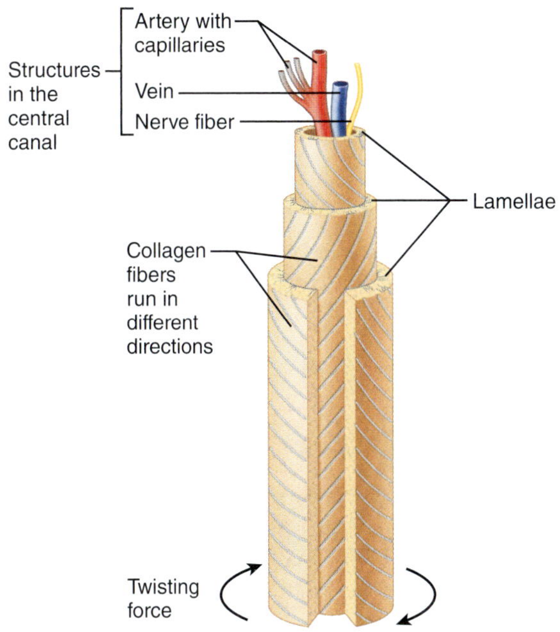

Figure 6.6 A single osteon. The osteon is drawn as if pulled out like a telescope to illustrate the individual lamellae.

The manner in which canaliculi are formed is interesting. When bone is forming, the osteoblasts secreting bone matrix surround blood vessels and maintain contact with one another and local osteocytes by tentacle-like projections containing gap junctions. Then, as the newly secreted matrix hardens and the maturing cells become trapped within it, a system of tiny canals—the *canaliculi* filled with tissue fluid and containing the osteocyte extensions—is formed. The canaliculi tie all the osteocytes in a mature osteon together, allowing them to communicate and permitting nutrients and wastes to be relayed from one osteocyte to the next throughout the osteon. Although bone matrix is hard and impermeable to nutrients, its canaliculi and cell-to-cell relays (via gap junctions) allow bone cells to be well nourished.

Interstitial and Circumferential Lamellae Not all the lamellae in compact bone are part of complete osteons. Lying between intact osteons are incomplete lamellae called **interstitial lamellae** (in″ter-stish′al) (Figure 6.7c, right photomicrograph). They either fill the gaps between forming osteons or are remnants of osteons that have been cut through by bone remodeling (discussed later). **Circumferential lamellae**, located just deep to the periosteum and just superficial to the endosteum, extend around the entire circumference of the diaphysis (Figure 6.7a) and effectively resist twisting of the long bone.

Spongy Bone

In contrast to compact bone, spongy bone looks like a poorly organized, even haphazard, tissue (see Figure 6.4 and Figure 6.3b). However, the trabeculae in spongy bone align precisely along lines of stress and help the bone resist stress. These tiny bone struts are as carefully positioned as the cables on a suspension bridge.

6

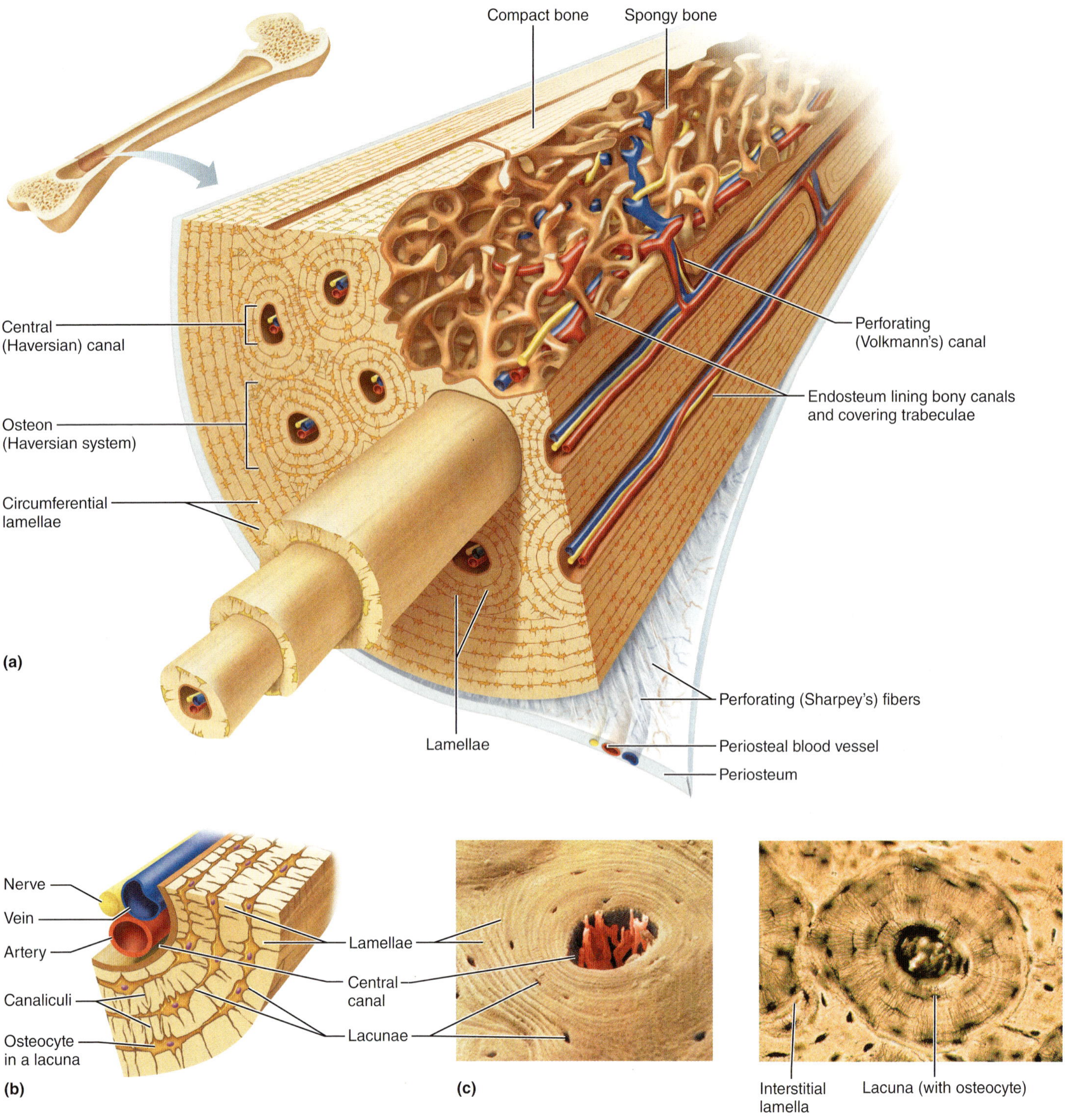

Figure 6.7 Microscopic anatomy of compact bone. (a) Diagram of a pie-shaped segment of compact bone. **(b)** Close-up of a portion of one osteon. Note the position of osteocytes in the lacunae. **(c)** SEM (left) of cross-sectional view of an osteon (410×). Light photomicrograph (right) of a cross-sectional view of an osteon (410×).

Only a few cells thick, trabeculae contain irregularly arranged lamellae and osteocytes interconnected by canaliculi. No osteons are present. Nutrients reach the osteocytes of spongy bone by diffusing through the canaliculi from capillaries in the endosteum surrounding the trabeculae.

Chemical Composition of Bone

Bone contains both organic and inorganic substances. *Organic components* include bone cells and osteoid. Its *inorganic components* are mineral salts.

Organic Components

The organic components of bone include its cells (osteogenic cells, osteoblasts, osteocytes, bone-lining cells, and osteoclasts) and **osteoid** (os′te-oid), the organic part of the matrix. Osteoid, which makes up approximately one-third of the matrix, includes ground substance (composed of proteoglycans and glycoproteins) and collagen fibers, both of which are made and secreted by osteoblasts. These organic substances, particularly collagen, contribute both to a bone's structure and to the flexibility and tensile strength that allow it to resist stretch and twisting.

Bone's resilience is thought to come from *sacrificial bonds* in or between collagen molecules. These bonds stretch and break easily on impact, dissipating energy to prevent the force from rising to a fracture value. In the absence of continued or additional trauma, most of the sacrificial bonds re-form.

Inorganic Components

The balance of bone tissue (65% by mass) consists of inorganic *hydroxyapatites* (hi-drok″se-ap′ah-tītz), or *mineral salts*, largely calcium phosphates present as tiny, tightly packed, needle-like crystals in and around collagen fibers in the extracellular matrix. The crystals account for the most notable characteristic of bone—its exceptional hardness, which allows it to resist compression.

The proper combination of organic and inorganic matrix elements makes bone exceedingly durable and strong without being brittle. Healthy bone is half as strong as steel in resisting compression and fully as strong as steel in resisting tension.

Because of the mineral salts they contain, bones last long after death and provide an enduring "monument." In fact, skeletal remains many centuries old can still reveal the shapes and sizes of ancient peoples, the kinds of work they did, and many of the ailments they suffered, such as arthritis. *Growth arrest lines*, horizontal lines on long bones, provide visible proof of illness when the body uses nutrients to fight disease and the bones stop growing.

☑ Check Your Understanding

10. Are crests, tubercles, and spines bony projections or depressions?
11. How does the structure of compact bone differ from that of spongy bone when viewed with the naked eye?
12. Which membrane lines the internal canals and covers the trabeculae of a bone?
13. Which component of bone—organic or inorganic—makes it hard?
14. Which cell has a ruffled border and acts to break down bone matrix?

For answers, see Appendix H.

Bone Development

✓ Compare and contrast intramembranous ossification and endochondral ossification.

✓ Describe the process of long bone growth that occurs at the epiphyseal plates.

Ossification and **osteogenesis** (os″te-o-jen′ĕ-sis) are synonyms meaning the process of bone formation (*os* = bone, *genesis* = beginning). In embryos this process leads to the formation of the bony skeleton. Later another form of ossification known as *bone growth* goes on until early adulthood as the body increases in size. Bones are capable of growing thicker throughout life. However, ossification in adults serves mainly for bone *remodeling* and repair.

Formation of the Bony Skeleton

Before week 8, the skeleton of a human embryo is constructed entirely from fibrous membranes and hyaline cartilage. Bone tissue begins to develop at about this time and eventually replaces most of the existing fibrous or cartilage structures.

- In *endochondral ossification* (*endo* = within, *chondro* = cartilage), a bone develops by replacing hyaline cartilage. The resulting bone is called a **cartilage**, or **endochondral**, **bone**.
- In *intramembranous ossification*, a bone develops from a fibrous membrane and the bone is called a **membrane bone**.

The beauty of using flexible structures (membranes and cartilages) to fashion the embryonic skeleton is that they can accommodate mitosis. Were the early skeleton composed of calcified bone tissue from the outset, growth would be much more difficult.

Endochondral Ossification

Except for the clavicles, essentially all bones below the base of the skull form by **endochondral ossification** (en″do-kon′dral). Beginning late in the second month of development, this process uses hyaline cartilage "bones" formed earlier as models, or patterns, for bone construction. It is more complex than intramembranous ossification because the hyaline cartilage must be broken down as ossification proceeds.

For example, the formation of a long bone typically begins in the center of the hyaline cartilage shaft at a region called the **primary ossification center**. First, blood vessels infiltrate the perichondrium covering the hyaline cartilage "bone," converting it to a vascularized periosteum. As a result of this change in nutrition, the underlying mesenchymal cells specialize into osteoblasts. The stage is now set for ossification to begin **(Figure 6.8)**:

① **A bone collar forms around the diaphysis of the hyaline cartilage model.** Osteoblasts of the newly converted periosteum secrete osteoid against the hyaline cartilage diaphysis, encasing it in a cuff or collar of bone called the *periosteal bone collar.*

② **Cartilage in the center of the diaphysis calcifies and then develops cavities.** As the bone collar forms, chondrocytes within the shaft hypertrophy (enlarge) and signal the surrounding cartilage matrix to calcify. Then, because calcified cartilage matrix is impermeable to diffusing nutrients, the chondrocytes die and the matrix begins to deteriorate. This deterioration opens up cavities, but the bone collar stabilizes the hyaline cartilage model. Elsewhere, the cartilage remains healthy and continues to grow briskly, causing the cartilage model to elongate.

6

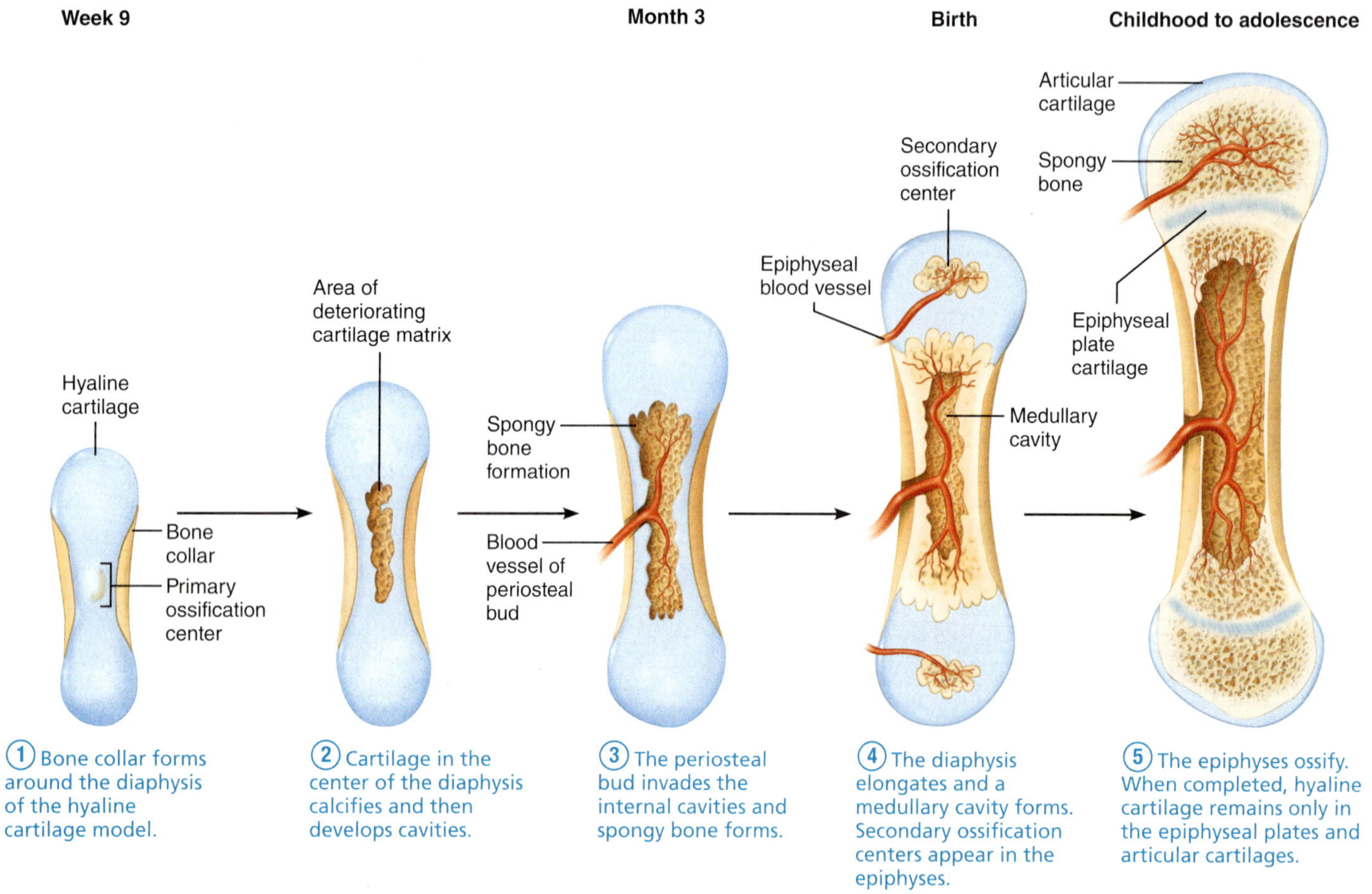

Figure 6.8 Endochondral ossification in a long bone.

③ **The periosteal bud invades the internal cavities and spongy bone forms.** In month 3, the forming cavities are invaded by a collection of elements called the **periosteal bud**, which contains a nutrient artery and vein, nerve fibers, red marrow elements, osteogenic cells, and osteoclasts. The entering osteoclasts partially erode the calcified cartilage matrix, and the osteogenic cells become osteoblasts and secrete osteoid around the remaining calcified fragments of hyaline cartilage, forming bone-covered cartilage trabeculae. In this way, the earliest version of spongy bone forms in a developing long bone.

④ **The diaphysis elongates and a medullary cavity forms.** As the primary ossification center enlarges, osteoclasts break down the newly formed spongy bone and open up a medullary cavity in the center of the diaphysis. Throughout the fetal period (week 9 until birth), the rapidly growing epiphyses consist only of cartilage, and the hyaline cartilage models continue to elongate by division of viable cartilage cells at the epiphyses. Ossification "chases" cartilage formation along the length of the shaft as cartilage calcifies, erodes, and then is replaced by bony spicules on the epiphyseal surfaces facing the medullary cavity.

⑤ **The epiphyses ossify.** At birth, most of our long bones have a bony diaphysis surrounding remnants of spongy bone, a widening medullary cavity, and two cartilaginous epiphyses. Shortly before or after birth, **secondary ossification centers** appear in one or both epiphyses, and the epiphyses gain bony tissue. (Typically, the large long bones form secondary centers in both epiphyses, whereas the small long bones form only one secondary ossification center.) The cartilage in the center of the epiphysis calcifies and deteriorates, opening up cavities that allow a periosteal bud to enter. Then bone trabeculae appear, just as they did earlier in the primary ossification center.

In short bones, only the primary ossification center is formed. Most irregular bones develop from several distinct ossification centers.

Secondary ossification reproduces almost exactly the events of primary ossification, except that the spongy bone in the interior is retained and no medullary cavity forms in the epiphyses. When secondary ossification is complete, hyaline cartilage remains only at two places:

- On the epiphyseal surfaces, as the *articular cartilages*
- At the junction of the diaphysis and epiphysis, where it forms the *epiphyseal plates*

Intramembranous Ossification

Intramembranous ossification forms the cranial bones of the skull (frontal, parietal, occipital, and temporal bones) and the clavicles. Most bones formed by this process are flat bones. At about week 8 of development, ossification begins within fibrous connective tissue membranes formed by *mesenchymal cells.* This process involves four major steps, depicted in **Figure 6.9**.

Postnatal Bone Growth

During infancy and youth, long bones lengthen entirely by interstitial growth of the epiphyseal plate cartilage and its replacement by bone, and all bones grow in thickness by appositional growth. Most bones stop growing during adolescence. However, some facial bones, such as those of the nose and lower jaw, continue to grow almost imperceptibly throughout life.

Growth in Length of Long Bones

Longitudinal bone growth mimics many of the events of endochondral ossification and depends on the presence of epiphyseal cartilage. The cartilage is relatively inactive on the side of the epiphyseal plate facing the epiphysis, a region called the *resting* or *quiescent zone.* But the epiphyseal plate cartilage abutting the diaphysis organizes into a pattern that allows fast, efficient growth. The cartilage cells here form tall columns, like coins in a stack. The cells at the "top" (epiphysis-facing) side of the stack abutting the resting zone comprise the *proliferation* or *growth zone* **(Figure 6.10)**. These cells divide quickly, pushing the epiphysis away from the diaphysis and lengthening the entire long bone.

Meanwhile, the older chondrocytes in the stack, which are closer to the diaphysis (*hypertrophic zone* in Figure 6.10), hypertrophy, and their lacunae erode and enlarge, leaving large interconnecting spaces. Subsequently, the surrounding cartilage matrix calcifies and these chondrocytes die and deteriorate, producing the *calcification zone.*

This leaves long slender spicules of calcified cartilage at the epiphysis-diaphysis junction, which look like stalactites hanging from the roof of a cave. These calcified spicules ultimately become part of the *ossification* or *osteogenic zone*, and are invaded by marrow elements from the medullary cavity. Osteoclasts partly erode the cartilage spicules, then osteoblasts quickly cover them with new bone, and ultimately spongy bone replaces them. Eventually as osteoclasts digest the spicule tips, the medullary cavity also lengthens. During growth, the epiphyseal plate maintains a constant thickness because the rate of cartilage growth on its epiphysis-facing side is balanced by its replacement with bony tissue on its diaphysis-facing side.

Longitudinal growth is accompanied by almost continuous remodeling of the epiphyseal ends to maintain the proportion between the diaphysis and epiphyses. Bone remodeling involves both new bone formation and bone resorption **(Figure 6.11)**.

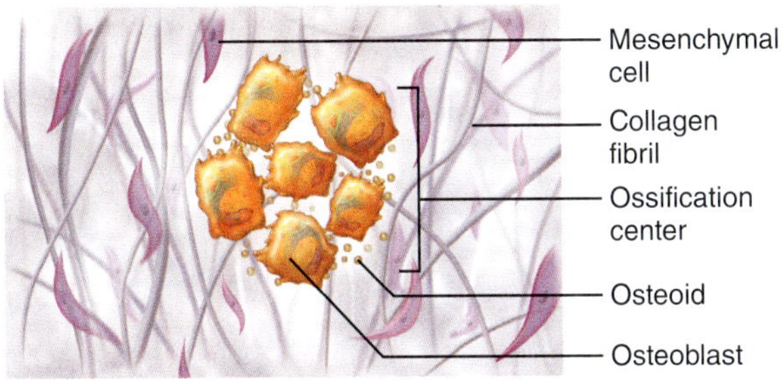

(1) Ossification centers appear in the fibrous connective tissue membrane.
- Selected centrally located mesenchymal cells cluster and differentiate into osteoblasts, forming an ossification center that produces the first trabeculae of spongy bone.

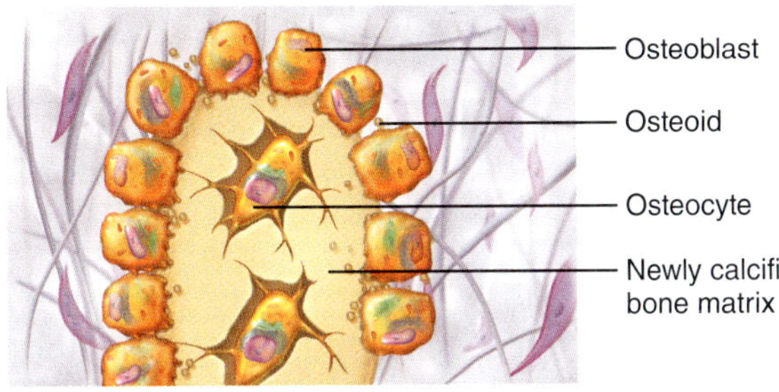

(2) Osteoid is secreted within the fibrous membrane and calcifies.
- Osteoblasts begin to secrete osteoid, which calcifies in a few days.
- Trapped osteoblasts become osteocytes.

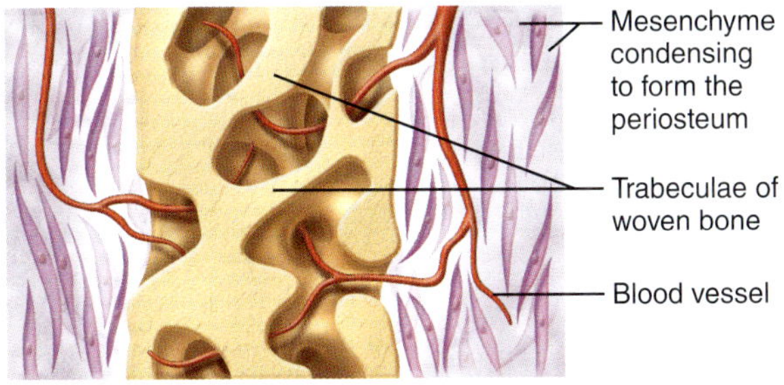

(3) Woven bone and periosteum form.
- Accumulating osteoid is laid down between embryonic blood vessels in a manner that results in a network (instead of concentric lamellae) of trabeculae called woven bone.
- Vascularized mesenchyme condenses on the external face of the woven bone and becomes the periosteum.

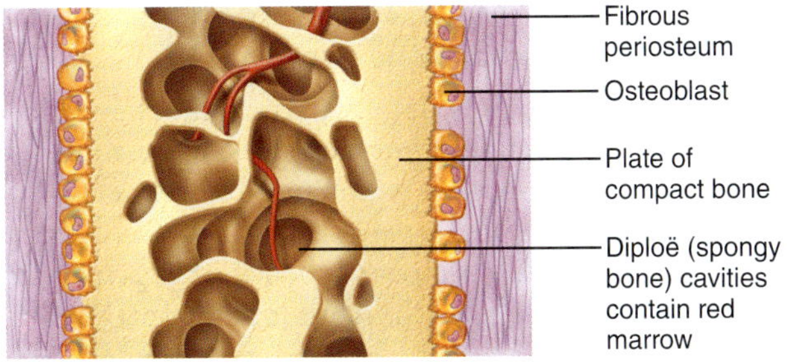

(4) Lamellar bone replaces woven bone, just deep to the periosteum. Red marrow appears.
- Trabeculae just deep to the periosteum thicken. Mature lamellar bone replaces them, forming compact bone plates.
- Spongy bone (diploë), consisting of distinct trabeculae, persists internally and its vascular tissue becomes red marrow.

Figure 6.9 Intramembranous ossification. Diagrams (3) and (4) represent much lower magnification than diagrams (1) and (2).

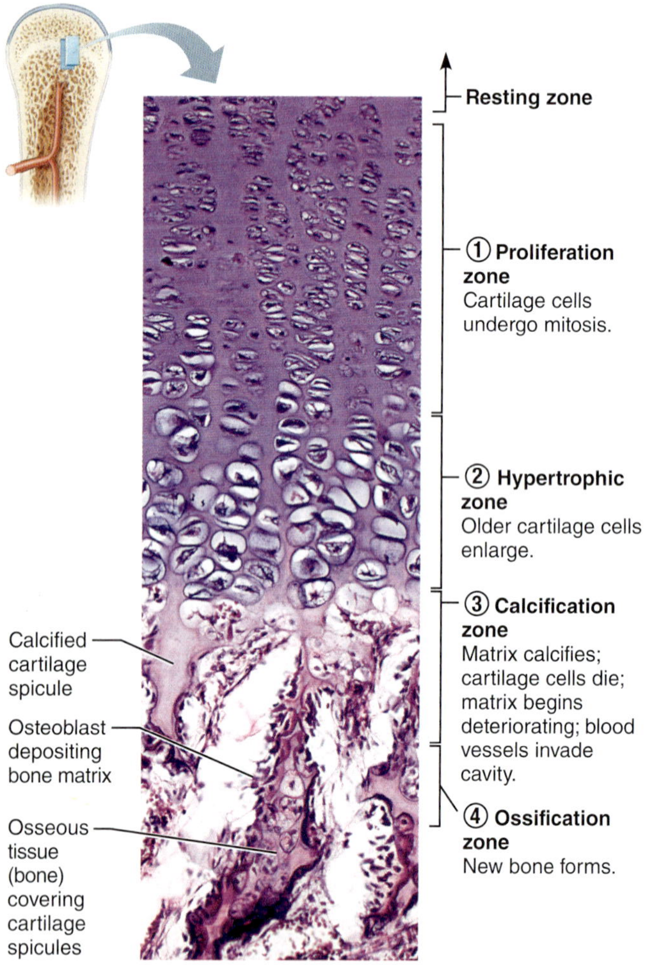

Figure 6.10 Growth in length of a long bone occurs at the epiphyseal plate. The side of the epiphyseal plate facing the epiphysis contains resting cartilage cells. The cells of the epiphyseal plate proximal to the resting cartilage area are arranged in four zones—proliferation, hypertrophic, calcification, and ossification—from the region of the earliest stage of growth ① to the region where bone is replacing the cartilage ④ (115×).

We describe it in more detail later in conjunction with the changes that occur in adult bones.

As adolescence ends, the chondroblasts of the epiphyseal plates divide less often and the plates become thinner and thinner until they are entirely replaced by bone tissue. Longitudinal bone growth ends when the bone of the epiphysis and diaphysis fuses. This process, called *epiphyseal plate closure*, happens at about 18 years of age in females and 21 years of age in males. Once this has occurred, only the articular cartilage remains in bones. However, as noted earlier, an adult bone can still widen by appositional growth if stressed by excessive muscle activity or body weight.

Growth in Width (Thickness)

Growing bones widen as they lengthen. As with cartilages, bones increase in thickness or, in the case of long bones, diameter, by appositional growth. Osteoblasts beneath the periosteum secrete bone matrix on the external bone surface as osteoclasts on the endosteal surface of the diaphysis remove bone (Figure 6.11). However, normally there is slightly more building up than breaking down. This unequal process produces a thicker, stronger bone but prevents it from becoming too heavy.

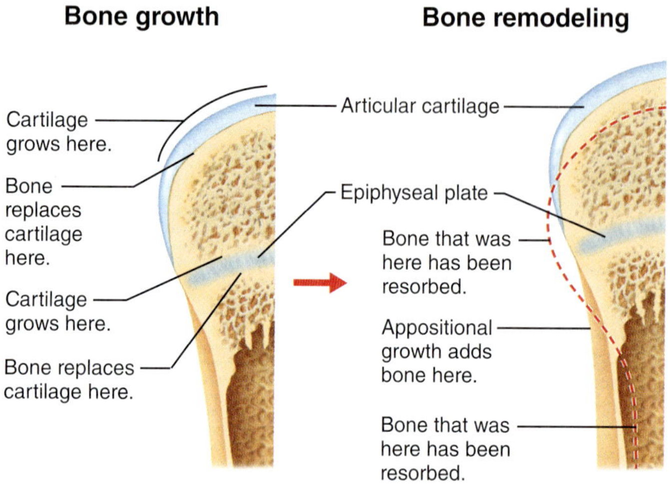

Figure 6.11 Long bone growth and remodeling during youth. The events at the left depict endochondral ossification that occurs at the articular cartilages and epiphyseal plates as the bone lengthens. Events at the right show bone remodeling during long bone growth to maintain proper bone proportions. The dashed red outline matches the view on the left.

☑ Check Your Understanding

15. Bones don't begin with bone tissue. What do they begin with?
16. When describing endochondral ossification, some say "bone chases cartilage." What does that mean?
17. Where is the primary ossification center located in a long bone? Where is (are) the secondary ossification center(s) located?
18. As a long bone grows in length, what is happening in the hypertrophic zone of the epiphyseal plate?

For answers, see Appendix H.

Hormonal Regulation of Bone Growth

The bone growth that occurs until young adulthood is exquisitely controlled by a symphony of hormones. During infancy and childhood, the single most important stimulus of epiphyseal plate activity is *growth hormone* released by the anterior pituitary gland. Thyroid hormones modulate the activity of growth hormone, ensuring that the skeleton has proper proportions as it grows.

At puberty, male and female sex hormones (testosterone and estrogens, respectively) are released in increasing amounts. Initially these sex hormones promote the growth spurt typical of adolescence, as well as the masculinization or feminization of specific parts of the skeleton. Later the hormones induce epiphyseal closure, ending longitudinal bone growth.

Excesses or deficits of any of these hormones can result in abnormal skeletal growth. For example, hypersecretion of growth hormone in children results in excessive height (gigantism), and deficits of growth hormone or thyroid hormone produce characteristic types of dwarfism.

Bone Homeostasis: Remodeling and Repair

- ✓ Compare the locations and remodeling functions of the osteoblasts, osteocytes, and osteoclasts.
- ✓ Explain how hormones and physical stress regulate bone remodeling.
- ✓ Describe the steps of fracture repair.

Bones appear to be the most lifeless of body organs, and may even summon images of a graveyard. But as you have just learned, bone is a dynamic and active tissue, and small-scale changes in bone architecture occur continually. Every week we recycle 5–7% of our bone mass, and as much as half a gram of calcium may enter or leave the adult skeleton each day! Spongy bone is replaced every three to four years; compact bone, every ten years or so. This is fortunate because when bone remains in place for long periods more of the calcium salts crystallize (see description below) and the bone becomes more brittle—ripe conditions for fracture.

When we break bones—the most common disorder of bone homeostasis—they undergo a remarkable process of self-repair.

Bone Remodeling

In the adult skeleton, bone deposit and bone resorption occur at the surfaces of both the periosteum and the endosteum. Together, the two processes constitute **bone remodeling**. "Packets" of adjacent osteoblasts and osteoclasts called *remodeling units* coordinate bone remodeling (with help from the stress-sensing osteocytes).

In healthy young adults, total bone mass remains constant, an indication that the rates of bone deposit and resorption are essentially equal. Remodeling does not occur uniformly, however. For example, the distal part of the femur, or thigh bone, is fully replaced every five to six months, whereas its shaft is altered much more slowly.

Bone Deposit

An *osteoid seam*—an unmineralized band of gauzy-looking bone matrix 10–12 micrometers (μm) wide—marks areas of new matrix deposits by osteoblasts. Between the osteoid seam and the older mineralized bone, there is an abrupt transition called the *calcification front*. Because the osteoid seam is always of constant width and the change from unmineralized to mineralized matrix is sudden, it seems that the osteoid must mature for about a week before it can calcify.

The precise trigger for calcification is still controversial, but mechanical signals are definitely involved. One critical factor is the product of the local concentrations of calcium and phosphate (P_i) ions (the $Ca^{2+} \cdot P_i$ product) in the endosteal cavity. When the $Ca^{2+} \cdot P_i$ product reaches a certain level, tiny crystals of hydroxyapatite form spontaneously and catalyze further crystallization of calcium salts in the area. Other factors involved are matrix proteins that bind and concentrate calcium, and the enzyme *alkaline phosphatase* (shed in *matrix vesicles* by the osteoblasts), which is essential for mineralization. Once proper conditions are present, calcium salts are deposited all at once and with great precision throughout the "matured" matrix.

Bone Resorption

As noted earlier, the giant **osteoclasts** accomplish **bone resorption**. Osteoclasts move along a bone surface, digging depressions or grooves as they break down the bone matrix. The ruffled border of the osteoclast clings tightly to the bone, sealing off the area of bone destruction and secreting *lysosomal enzymes* that digest the organic matrix and *protons* (H^+). The resulting acidic brew in the resorption bay converts the calcium salts into soluble forms that pass easily into solution. Osteoclasts may also phagocytize the demineralized matrix and dead osteocytes. The digested matrix end products, growth factors, and dissolved minerals are then endocytosed, transported across the osteoclast (by transcytosis), and released at the opposite side. There they enter the interstitial fluid and then the blood.

When resorption of a given area of bone is completed, the osteoclasts undergo apoptosis. There is much to learn about osteoclast activation, but PTH and proteins secreted by T cells of the immune system appear to be important.

Control of Remodeling

Remodeling goes on continuously in the skeleton, regulated by genetic factors and two control loops that serve different "masters." One is a negative feedback hormonal loop that maintains Ca^{2+} homeostasis in the blood. The other involves responses to mechanical and gravitational forces acting on the skeleton.

The hormonal feedback becomes much more meaningful when you understand calcium's importance in the body. Ionic calcium is necessary for an amazing number of physiological processes, including transmission of nerve impulses, muscle contraction, blood coagulation, secretion by glands and nerve cells, and cell division.

The human body contains 1200–1400 g of calcium, more than 99% present as bone minerals. Most of the remainder is in body cells. Less than 1.5 g is present in blood, and the hormonal control loop normally maintains blood Ca^{2+} within the narrow range of 9–11 mg per dl (100 ml) of blood. Calcium is absorbed from the intestine under the control of vitamin D metabolites. The daily dietary calcium requirement is 400–800 mg from birth until age 10, and 1200–1500 mg from ages 11 to 24.

Hormonal Controls The hormonal controls primarily involve **parathyroid hormone (PTH)**, produced by the parathyroid glands. To a much lesser extent **calcitonin** (kal″sĭ-to′nin), produced by parafollicular cells (C cells) of the thyroid gland, may be involved.

6

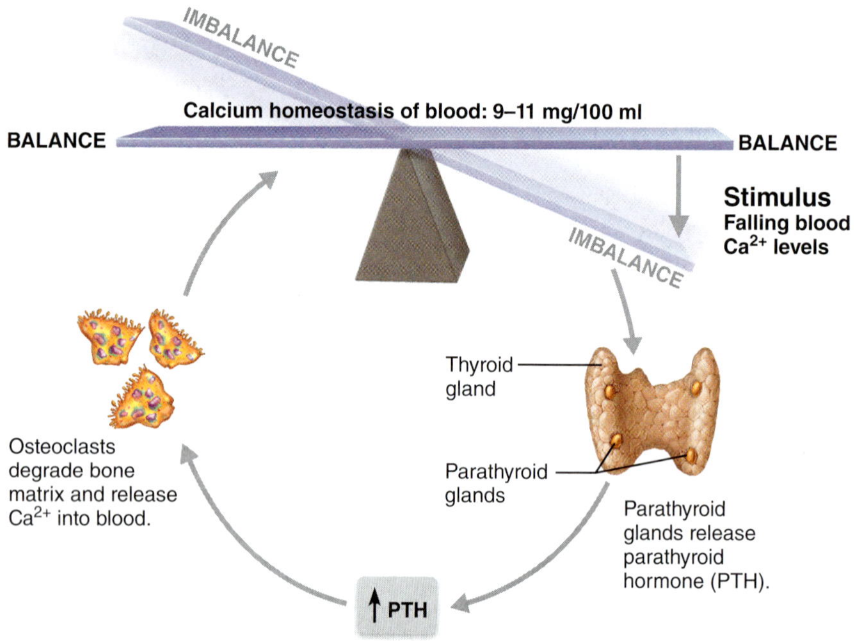

Figure 6.12 Parathyroid hormone (PTH) control of blood calcium levels.

When blood levels of ionic calcium decline, PTH is released **(Figure 6.12)**. The increased PTH level stimulates osteoclasts to resorb bone, releasing calcium into blood. Osteoclasts are no respecters of matrix age: When activated, they break down both old and new matrix. As blood concentrations of calcium rise, the stimulus for PTH release ends. The decline of PTH reverses its effects and causes blood Ca^{2+} levels to fall.

In humans, calcitonin appears to be a hormone in search of a function because its effects on calcium homeostasis are negligible. When administered at pharmacological (abnormally high) doses, it does lower blood calcium levels temporarily.

These hormonal controls act to preserve blood calcium homeostasis, not the skeleton's strength or well-being. In fact, if blood calcium levels are low for an extended time, the bones become so demineralized that they develop large, punched-out-looking holes. Thus, the bones serve as a storehouse from which ionic calcium is drawn as needed.

Homeostatic Imbalance 6.1

Minute changes from the homeostatic range for blood calcium can lead to severe neuromuscular problems ranging from hyperexcitability (when blood Ca^{2+} levels are too low) to nonresponsiveness and inability to function (with high blood Ca^{2+} levels). In addition, sustained high blood levels of Ca^{2+}, a condition known as *hypercalcemia* (hi″per-kal-se′me-ah), can lead to undesirable deposits of calcium salts in the blood vessels, kidneys, and other soft organs, which may hamper their function. ✚

Other hormones are also involved in modifying bone density and bone turnover. For example, *leptin*, a hormone released by adipose tissue, plays a role in regulating bone density. Best known for its effects on weight and energy balance (see pp. 940–941), in animal studies leptin appears to inhibit osteoblasts. It does so through an additional pathway mediated by the hypothalamus, which activates sympathetic nerves serving bones. However, the full scope of leptin's bone-modifying activity in humans is still being worked out.

It is also evident that the brain, intestine, and skeleton have ongoing conversations that help regulate the balance between bone formation and destruction, with serotonin serving as a hormonal go-between. *Serotonin* is better known as a neurotransmitter that regulates mood and sleep, but most of the body's serotonin is made in the gut (intestine) and the blood-brain barrier (see Chapter 12) bars it from entering the brain. The role of gut serotonin is still poorly understood. What is known is that when we eat, serotonin is secreted and circulated via the blood to the bones where it interferes with osteoblast activity. Reduction of bone turnover after eating may lock calcium in bone when new calcium is flooding into the bloodstream.

This is a troubling finding for those taking Prozac and other antidepressant drugs that inhibit serotonin uptake, making it more available to bone cells. Such patients have lower bone density and suffer more fractures than people not taking these drugs.

Response to Mechanical Stress The second set of controls regulating bone remodeling, bone's response to mechanical stress (muscle pull) and gravity, keeps the bones strong where stressors are acting.

Wolff's law holds that a bone grows or remodels in response to the demands placed on it. The first thing to understand is that a bone's anatomy reflects the common stresses it encounters. For example, a bone is loaded (stressed) whenever weight bears down on it or muscles pull on it. This loading is usually off center and tends to bend the bone. Bending compresses the bone on one side and subjects it to tension (stretching) on the other **(Figure 6.13)**.

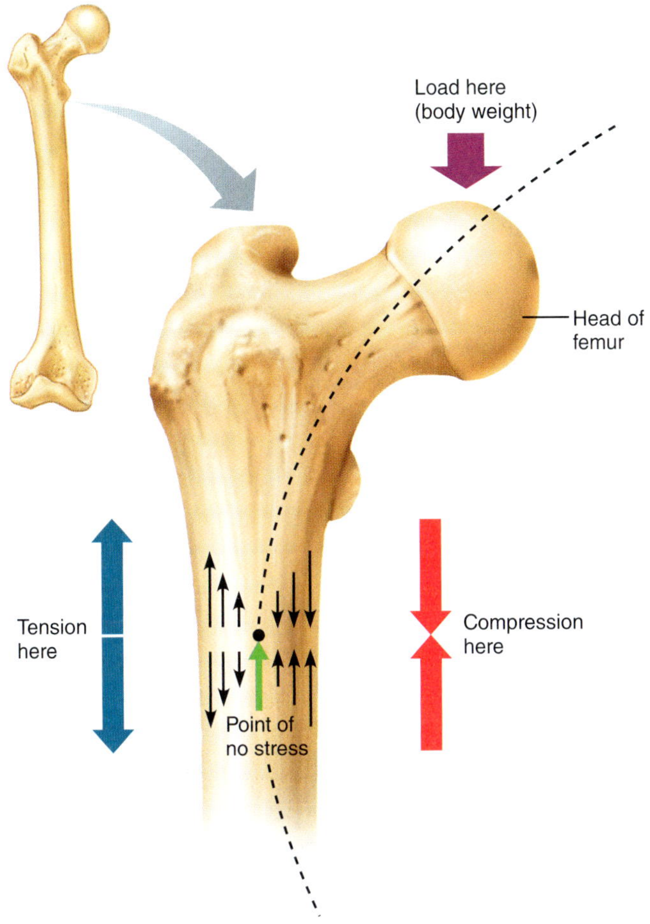

Figure 6.13 Bone anatomy and bending stress. Body weight transmitted to the head of the femur (thigh bone) threatens to bend the bone along the indicated arc, compressing it on one side (converging arrows on right) and stretching it on the other side (diverging arrows on left). Because these two forces cancel each other internally, much less bone material is needed internally than superficially.

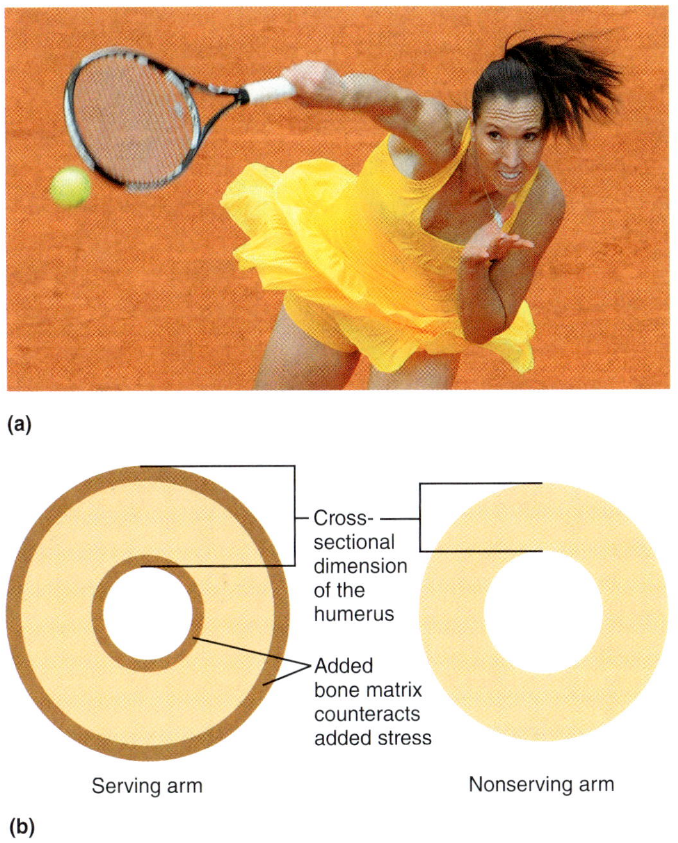

Figure 6.14 Vigorous exercise can strengthen bone. The brown rings in (b) represent differences in the cross-sectional areas of the serving and nonserving arms of a professional tennis player. Average increases in bone rigidity and strength of 62% and 45%, respectively, were recorded in the serving arms. The structural changes were more pronounced in those who began training at an early age. *Source:* C. B. Ruff, "Gracilization of the Modern Human Skeleton," *American Scientist* 94(6): p. 513, Nov–Dec 2006.

As a result of these mechanical stressors, long bones are thickest midway along the diaphysis, exactly where bending stresses are greatest (bend a stick and it will split near the middle). Both compression and tension are minimal toward the center of the bone (they cancel each other out), so a bone can "hollow out" for lightness (using spongy bone instead of compact bone) without jeopardy.

Wolff's law also explains several other observations:

- Handedness (being right or left handed) results in the bones of one upper limb being thicker than those of the less-used limb. Vigorous exercise of the most-used limb leads to large increases in bone strength **(Figure 6.14)**.
- Curved bones are thickest where they are most likely to buckle.
- The trabeculae of spongy bone form trusses, or struts, along lines of compression.
- Large, bony projections occur where heavy, active muscles attach. The bones of weight lifters have enormous thickenings at the attachment sites of the most-used muscles.

Wolff's law also explains the featureless bones of the fetus and the atrophied bones of bedridden people—situations in which bones are not stressed.

How do mechanical forces communicate with the cells responsible for remodeling? Deforming a bone produces an electrical current. Because compressed and stretched regions are oppositely charged, it has been suggested that electrical signals direct remodeling. This principle underlies some of the devices used to speed bone repair and heal fractures. Fluid flows within the canaliculi also appear to provide stimuli that direct the remodeling process.

The skeleton is continuously subjected to both hormonal influences and mechanical forces. At the risk of constructing too large a building on too small a foundation, we can speculate that:

- Hormonal controls determine *whether* and *when* remodeling occurs in response to changing blood calcium levels.
- Mechanical stress determines *where* remodeling occurs.

For example, when bone must be broken down to increase blood calcium levels, PTH is released and targets the osteoclasts.

Table 6.2 Common Types of Fractures

FRACTURE TYPE	DESCRIPTION AND COMMENTS	FRACTURE TYPE	DESCRIPTION AND COMMENTS
Comminuted	Bone fragments into three or more pieces. Particularly common in the aged, whose bones are more brittle 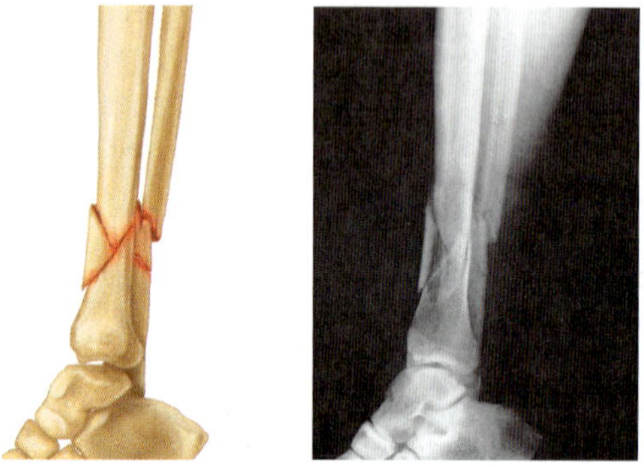	**Compression**	Bone is crushed. Common in porous bones (i.e., osteoporotic bones) subjected to extreme trauma, as in a fall 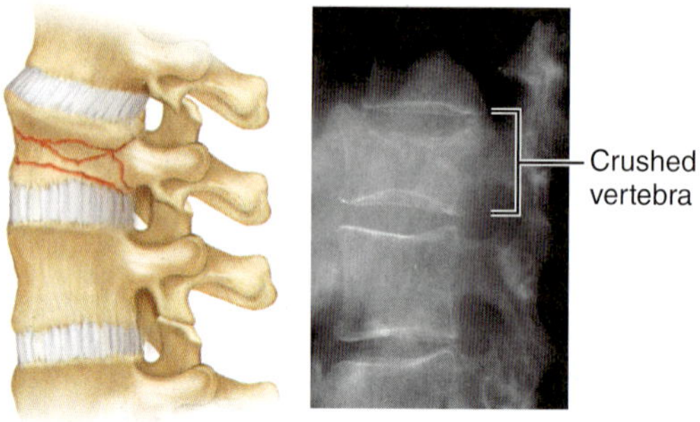
Spiral	Ragged break occurs when excessive twisting forces are applied to a bone. Common sports fracture 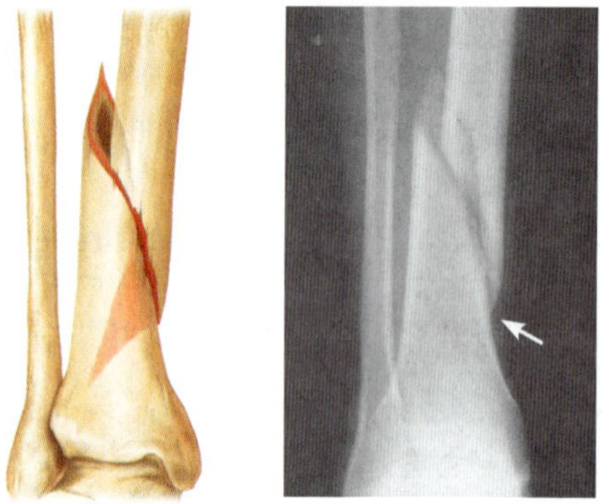	**Epiphyseal**	Epiphysis separates from the diaphysis along the epiphyseal plate. Tends to occur where cartilage cells are dying and calcification of the matrix is occurring 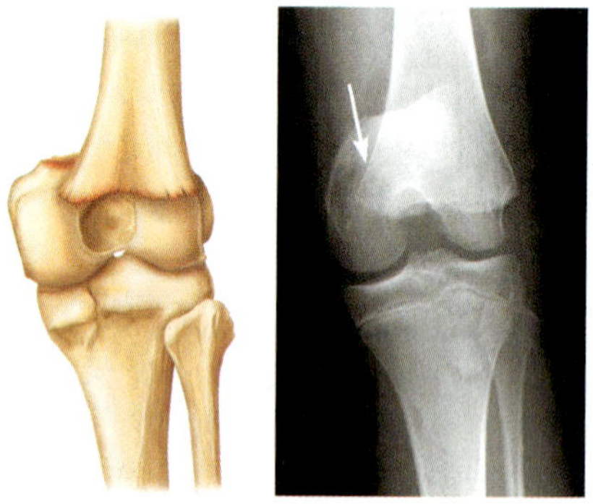
Depressed	Broken bone portion is pressed inward. Typical of skull fracture 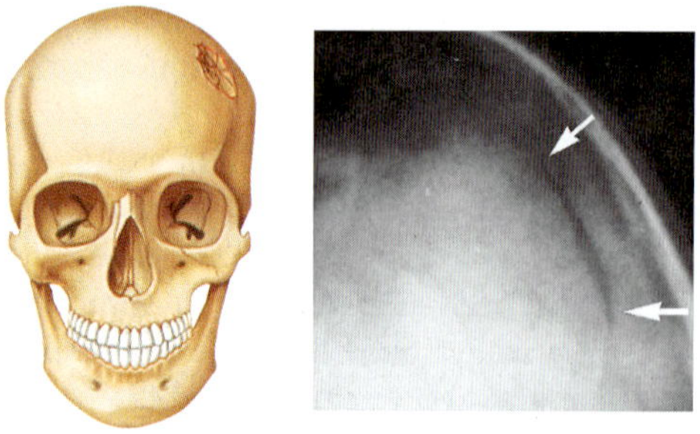	**Greenstick**	Bone breaks incompletely, much in the way a green twig breaks. Only one side of the shaft breaks; the other side bends. Common in children, whose bones have relatively more organic matrix and are more flexible than those of adults 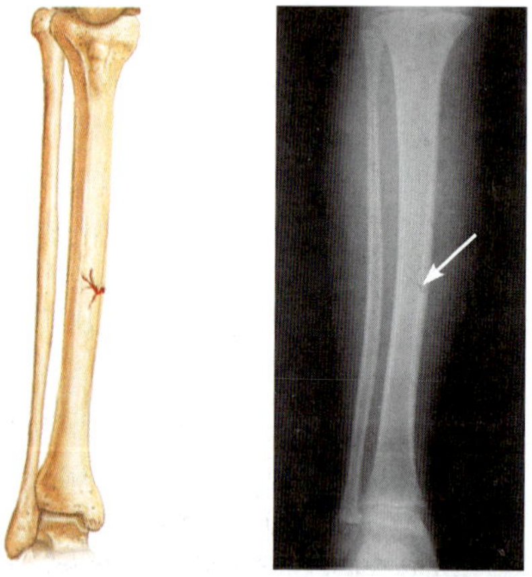

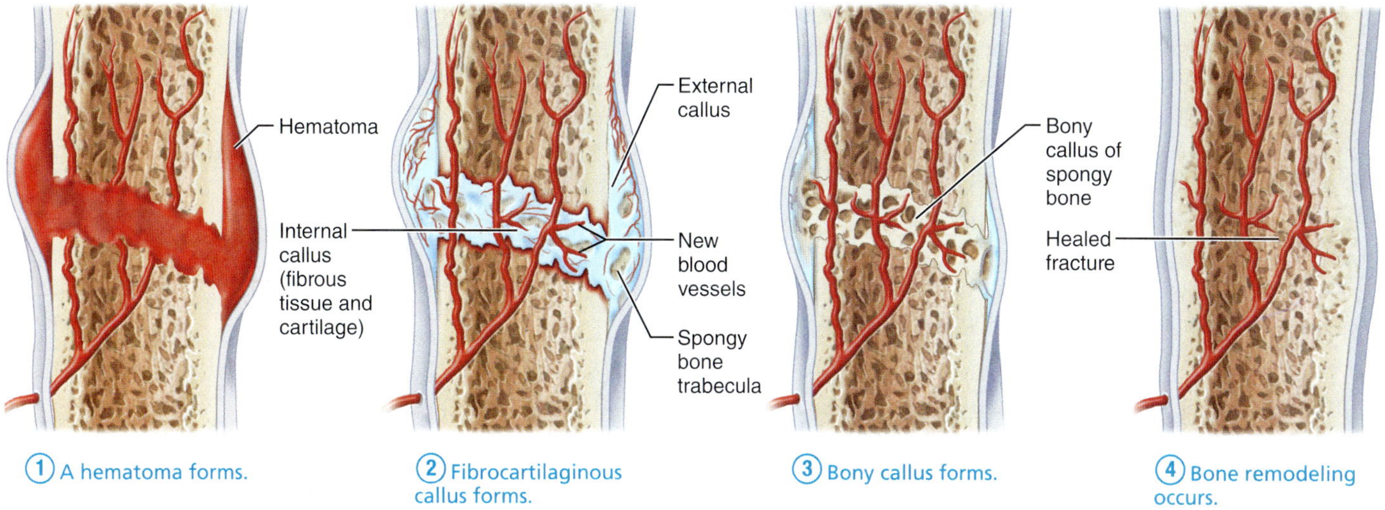

Figure 6.15 Stages in the healing of a bone fracture.

However, mechanical forces determine which osteoclasts are most sensitive to PTH stimulation, so that bone in the least stressed areas (which is temporarily dispensable) is broken down.

Bone Repair

Despite their remarkable strength, bones are susceptible to **fractures**, or breaks. During youth, most fractures result from exceptional trauma that twists or smashes the bones (sports injuries, automobile accidents, and falls, for example). In old age, most fractures occur as bones thin and weaken.

Fracture Classification

Fractures may be classified by

- Position of the bone ends after fracture: In *nondisplaced fractures*, the bone ends retain their normal position. In *displaced fractures*, the bone ends are out of normal alignment.
- Completeness of the break: If the bone is broken through, the fracture is a *complete fracture*. If not, it is an *incomplete fracture*.
- Whether the bone ends penetrate the skin: If so, the fracture is an *open* (*compound*) *fracture*. If not, it is a *closed* (*simple*) *fracture*.

In addition to these three either-or classifications, all fractures can be described in terms of the location of the fracture, its external appearance, and/or the nature of the break (Table 6.2).

Fracture Treatment and Repair

Treatment involves *reduction*, the realignment of the broken bone ends. In *closed* (*external*) *reduction*, the physician's hands coax the bone ends into position. In *open* (*internal*) *reduction*, the bone ends are secured together surgically with pins or wires.

After the broken bone is reduced, it is immobilized either by a cast or traction to allow healing. A simple fracture of small or medium-sized bones in young adults heals in six to eight weeks, but it takes much longer for large, weight-bearing bones and for bones of elderly people (because of their poorer circulation).

Repair in a simple fracture involves four major stages (Figure 6.15):

1. **A hematoma forms.** When a bone breaks, blood vessels in the bone and periosteum, and perhaps in surrounding tissues, are torn and hemorrhage. As a result, a **hematoma** (he″mah-to′mah), a mass of clotted blood, forms at the fracture site. Soon, bone cells deprived of nutrition die, and the tissue at the site becomes swollen, painful, and inflamed.
2. **Fibrocartilaginous callus forms.** Within a few days, several events lead to the formation of soft *granulation tissue*, also called the *soft callus* (kal′us; "hard skin"). Capillaries grow into the hematoma and phagocytic cells invade the area and begin cleaning up the debris. Meanwhile, fibroblasts and cartilage and osteogenic cells invade the fracture site from the nearby periosteum and endosteum and begin reconstructing the bone. The fibroblasts produce collagen fibers that span the break and connect the broken bone ends. Some precursor cells differentiate into chondroblasts that secrete cartilage matrix. Within this mass of repair tissue, osteoblasts begin forming spongy bone. The cartilage cells farthest from the capillaries secrete an externally bulging cartilaginous matrix that later calcifies. This entire mass of repair tissue, now called the **fibrocartilaginous callus**, splints the broken bone.
3. **Bony callus forms.** Within a week, new bone trabeculae appear in the fibrocartilaginous callus and gradually convert it to a **bony (hard) callus** of spongy bone. Bony callus formation continues until a firm union forms about two months later. This process generally repeats the events of endochondral ossification.
4. **Bone remodeling occurs.** Beginning during bony callus formation and continuing for several months after, the bony callus is remodeled. The excess material on the diaphysis exterior and within the medullary cavity is removed, and

compact bone is laid down to reconstruct the shaft walls. The final structure of the remodeled area resembles the original unbroken bony region because it responds to the same set of mechanical stressors.

☑ Check Your Understanding

19. If osteoclasts in a long bone are more active than osteoblasts, how will bone mass change?
20. Which stimulus—PTH (a hormone) or mechanical forces acting on the skeleton—is more important in maintaining homeostatic blood calcium levels?
21. How does an open fracture differ from a closed fracture?
22. How do bone growth and bone remodeling differ?

For answers, see Appendix H.

Homeostatic Imbalances of Bone

✓ Contrast the disorders of bone remodeling seen in osteoporosis, osteomalacia, and Paget's disease.

Imbalances between bone deposit and bone resorption underlie nearly every disease that affects the human skeleton.

Osteomalacia and Rickets

Osteomalacia (os″te-o-mah-la′she-ah; "soft bones") includes a number of disorders in which the bones are poorly mineralized. Osteoid is produced, but calcium salts are not adequately deposited, so bones are soft and weak. The main symptom is pain when weight is put on the affected bones.

Rickets is the analogous disease in children. Because young bones are still growing rapidly, rickets is much more severe than adult osteomalacia. Bowed legs and deformities of the pelvis, skull, and rib cage are common. Because the epiphyseal plates cannot calcify, they continue to widen, and the ends of long bones become visibly enlarged and abnormally long.

Osteomalacia and rickets are caused by insufficient calcium in the diet or by a vitamin D deficiency. Drinking vitamin D–fortified milk and exposing the skin to sunlight (which spurs the body to form vitamin D) usually cure these disorders. Although the seeming elimination of rickets in the United States has been heralded as a public health success, rickets still rears its head in isolated situations. For example, if a mother who breast-feeds her infant becomes vitamin D deficient because of sun-deprivation or dreary winter weather, the infant too will be vitamin D deficient and will develop rickets.

Osteoporosis

For most of us, the phrase "bone problems of the elderly" brings to mind the stereotype of a victim of osteoporosis—a hunched-over old woman shuffling behind her walker. **Osteoporosis** (os″te-o-po-ro′sis) refers to a group of diseases in which bone resorption outpaces bone deposit. The bones become so fragile that something as simple as a hearty sneeze or stepping off a curb can cause them to break. The composition of the matrix remains normal but bone mass declines, and the bones become porous and light (**Figure 6.16**).

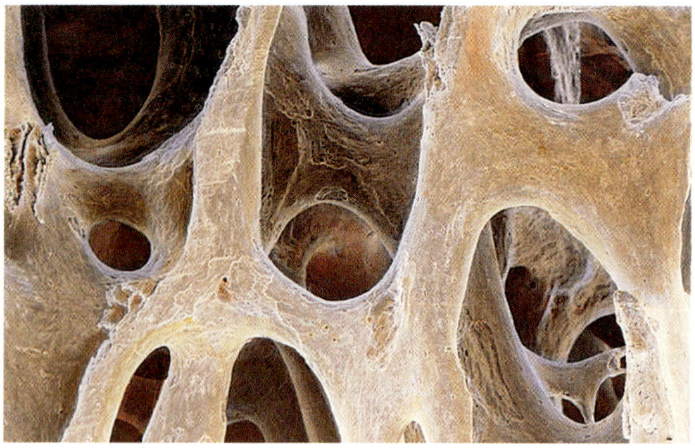

(a) Normal bone

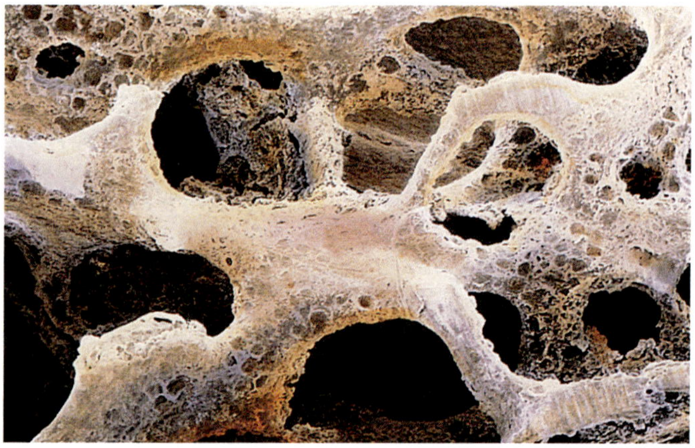

(b) Osteoporotic bone

Figure 6.16 The contrasting architecture of normal versus osteoporotic bone. Scanning electron micrographs, 300×.

Even though osteoporosis affects the entire skeleton, the spongy bone of the spine is most vulnerable, and compression fractures of the vertebrae are common. The femur, particularly its neck, is also very susceptible to fracture (a *broken hip*) in people with osteoporosis.

Risk Factors for Osteoporosis

Osteoporosis occurs most often in the aged, particularly in postmenopausal women. Although men develop it to a lesser degree, 30% of American women between the ages of 60 and 70 have osteoporosis, and 70% have it by age 80. Moreover, 30% of all Caucasian women (the most susceptible group) will experience a bone fracture due to osteoporosis.

Sex hormones—androgens in males and estrogens in females—help maintain the health and normal density of the skeleton by restraining osteoclasts and promoting deposit of new bone. After menopause, however, estrogen secretion wanes, and estrogen deficiency is strongly implicated in osteoporosis in older women.

Several other factors can contribute to osteoporosis:

- Petite body form
- Insufficient exercise to stress the bones
- A diet poor in calcium and protein
- Abnormal vitamin D receptors
- Smoking (which reduces estrogen levels)
- Hormone-related conditions such as hyperthyroidism, low blood levels of thyroid-stimulating hormone, and diabetes mellitus

Osteoporosis can develop at any age as a result of immobility. It can also occur in males with prostate cancer who are being treated with androgen-suppressing drugs.

Treating Osteoporosis

Osteoporosis has traditionally been treated with calcium and vitamin D supplements, weight-bearing exercise, and *hormone (estrogen) replacement therapy (HRT)*. Frustratingly, HRT slows the loss of bone but does not reverse it. Additionally, because of the increased risk of heart attack, stroke, and breast cancer associated with estrogen replacement therapy, it is a controversial treatment these days. Although not a substitute for HRT, estrogenic compounds in soy products (principally the isoflavones daidzein and genistein) offer a good addition or adjunct for some patients.

Newer drugs are available. Bisphosphonates decrease osteoclast activity and number, and partially reverse osteoporosis in the spine. Selective estrogen receptor modulators (SERMs), such as raloxifene, dubbed "estrogen light," mimic estrogen's beneficial bone-sparing properties without targeting the uterus or breast. Additionally, *statins*, drugs used to lower cholesterol levels, have an unexpected side effect of increasing bone mineral density up to 8% over four years. The monoclonal antibody drug *denosumab* significantly reduces fractures in men fighting prostate cancer and improves bone density in the elderly.

Preventing Osteoporosis

How can osteoporosis be prevented (or at least delayed)? The first requirement is to get enough calcium while your bones are still increasing in density (bones reach their peak density during early adulthood). Second, keep in mind that excessive intake of carbonated beverages and alcohol leaches minerals from bone and decreases bone density. Finally, get plenty of weight-bearing exercise (walking, jogging, tennis, etc.) throughout life. This will increase bone mass above normal values and provide a greater buffer against age-related bone loss.

Paget's Disease

Often discovered by accident when X rays are taken for some other reason, **Paget's disease** (paj′ets) is characterized by excessive and haphazard bone deposit and resorption. The newly formed bone, called *Pagetic bone*, is hastily made and has an abnormally high ratio of spongy bone to compact bone. This, along with reduced mineralization, causes a spotty weakening of the bones. Late in the disease, osteoclast activity wanes, but osteoblasts continue to work, often forming irregular bone thickenings or filling the marrow cavity with Pagetic bone.

Paget's disease may affect any part of the skeleton, but it is usually a localized condition. The spine, pelvis, femur, and skull are most often involved and become increasingly deformed and painful. It rarely occurs before age 40, and it affects about 3% of North American elderly people. Its cause is unknown, but a virus may trigger it. Drug therapies include calcitonin (administered by a nasal inhaler), and the newer bisphosphonates, which have shown success in preventing bone breakdown.

Check Your Understanding

23. Which bone disorder is characterized by excessive deposit of weak, poorly mineralized bone?
24. What are three measures that may help to maintain healthy bone density?
25. What name is given to "adult rickets"?

For answers, see Appendix H.

Developmental Aspects of Bones: Timing of Events

✓ Describe the timing and cause of changes in bone architecture and bone mass throughout life.

Bones are on a precise schedule from the time they form until death. The mesoderm germ layer gives rise to embryonic mesenchymal cells, which in turn produce the membranes and cartilages that form the embryonic skeleton. These structures then ossify according to an amazingly predictable timetable that allows fetal age to be determined easily from either X rays or sonograms. Although each bone has its own developmental schedule, most long bones begin ossifying by 8 weeks after conception and have well-developed primary ossification centers by 12 weeks **(Figure 6.17)**.

Birth to Young Adulthood

At birth, most long bones of the skeleton are well ossified except for their epiphyses. After birth, secondary ossification centers develop in a predictable sequence. The epiphyseal plates persist and provide for long bone growth all through childhood and the sex hormone–mediated growth spurt at adolescence. By age 25, nearly all bones are completely ossified and skeletal growth ceases.

Age-Related Changes in Bone

In children and adolescents, bone formation exceeds bone resorption. In young adults, these processes are in balance, and in old age, resorption predominates. Despite the environmental factors (discussed earlier) that influence bone density, genetics still plays the major role in determining how much a person's bone density will change over a lifetime. A single gene that codes for vitamin D's cellular docking site helps determine both

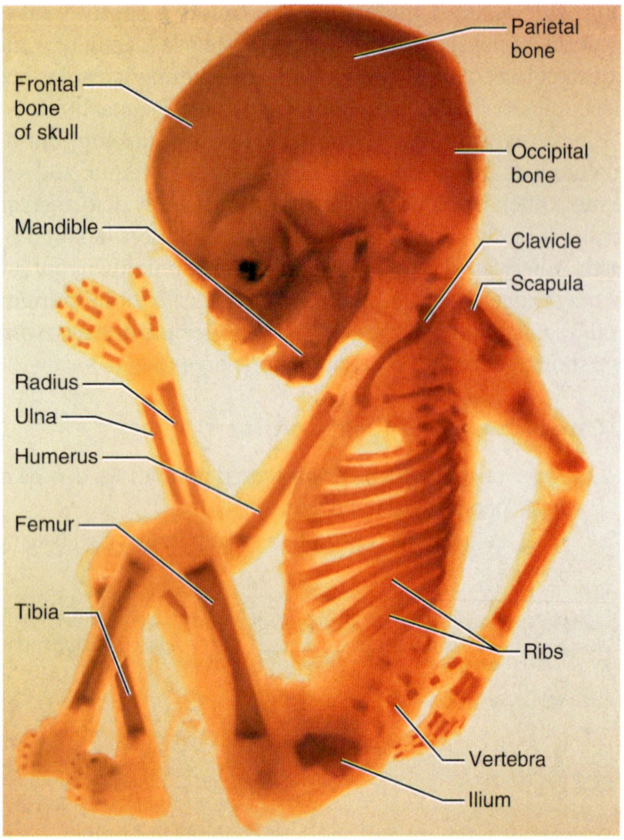

Figure 6.17 Fetal primary ossification centers at 12 weeks. The darker areas indicate primary ossification centers in the skeleton of a 12-week-old fetus.

the tendency to accumulate bone mass during early life and a person's risk of osteoporosis later in life.

Beginning in the fourth decade of life, bone mass decreases with age. The only exception appears to be in bones of the skull. Among young adults, skeletal mass is generally greater in males than in females. Age-related bone loss is faster in whites than in blacks (who have greater bone density to begin with) and faster in females than in males.

Qualitative changes also occur: More osteons remain incompletely formed, mineralization is less complete, and the amount of nonviable bone increases, reflecting a diminished blood supply to the bones in old age. These age-related changes are also bad news because fractures heal more slowly in old people.

Electrical stimulation of fracture sites and daily ultrasound treatments hasten repair and healing. Presumably electrical fields inhibit PTH stimulation of osteoclasts and induce formation of growth factors that stimulate osteoblasts.

Check Your Understanding

26. What is the status of bone structure at birth?
27. The decrease in bone mass that begins in the fourth decade of life affects nearly all bones. What are the exceptions?

For answers, see Appendix H.

This chapter has examined skeletal cartilages and bones—their architecture, composition, and dynamic nature. We have also discussed the role of bones in maintaining overall body homeostasis, as summarized in *System Connections*. Now we are ready to look at the individual bones of the skeleton and how they contribute to its functions, both collectively and individually.

Chapter Summary

For more chapter study tools, go to the Study Area of MasteringA&P at **www.masteringaandp.com.**

There you will find:

- Interactive Physiology iP
- A&PFlix A&PFlix
- Practice Anatomy Lab PAL
- PhysioEx PEx
- Videos, Practice Quizzes and Tests, MP3 Tutor Sessions, Case Studies, and much more!

Skeletal Cartilages (pp. 173–174)

Basic Structure, Types, and Locations (p. 174)

1. A skeletal cartilage exhibits chondrocytes housed in lacunae (cavities) within the extracellular matrix (ground substance and fibers). It contains large amounts of water (which accounts for its resilience), lacks nerve fibers, is avascular, and is surrounded by a fibrous perichondrium that resists expansion.
2. Hyaline cartilages appear glassy; the fibers are collagenous. They provide support with flexibility and resilience and are the most abundant skeletal cartilages, accounting for the articular, costal, respiratory, and nasal cartilages.
3. Elastic cartilages contain abundant elastic fibers, in addition to collagen fibers, and are more flexible than hyaline cartilages. They support the outer ear and epiglottis.
4. Fibrocartilages, which contain thick collagen fibers, are the most compressible cartilages and resist stretching. They form intervertebral discs and knee joint cartilages.

Growth of Cartilage (p. 174)

5. Cartilages grow from within (interstitial growth) and by adding new cartilage tissue at the periphery (appositional growth).

Classification of Bones (pp. 174–176)

1. Bones are classified as long, short, flat, or irregular on the basis of their shape and their proportion of compact or spongy bone.

Functions of Bones (pp. 176–177)

1. Bones give the body shape; protect and support body organs; provide levers for muscles to pull on; store calcium and other minerals; store growth factors and triglyceride; and are the site of blood cell and osteocalcin production.

Homeostatic Interrelationships Between the Skeletal System and Other Body Systems

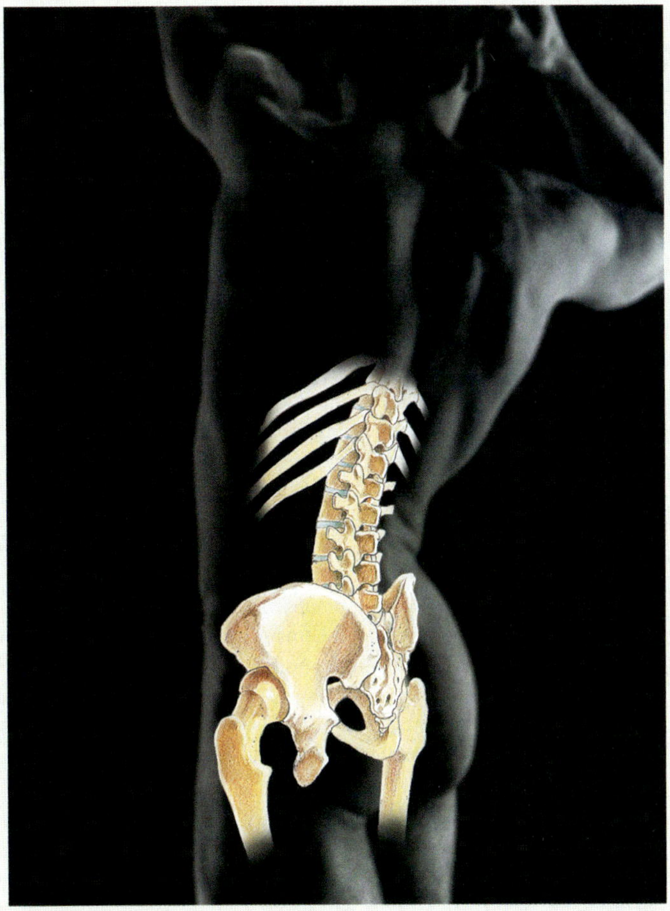

Integumentary System Chapter 5

- Skeletal system provides support for body organs including the skin
- Skin provides vitamin D needed for proper calcium absorption and use

Muscular System Chapters 9–10

- Skeletal system provides levers plus ionic calcium for muscle activity
- Muscle pull on bones increases bone strength and viability; helps determine bone shape

Nervous System Chapters 11–15

- Skeletal system protects brain and spinal cord; provides depot for calcium ions needed for neural function
- Nerves innervate bone and joint capsules, providing for pain and joint sense

Endocrine System Chapter 16

- Skeletal system provides some bony protection; stores calcium needed for second-messenger signaling mechanisms
- Hormones regulate uptake and release of calcium from bone; promote long bone growth and maturation

Cardiovascular System Chapters 17–19

- Bone marrow cavities provide site for blood cell formation; matrix stores calcium needed for cardiac muscle activity
- Cardiovascular system delivers nutrients and oxygen to bones; carries away wastes

Lymphatic System/Immunity Chapters 20–21

- Skeletal system provides some protection to lymphatic organs; bone marrow is site of origin for lymphocytes involved in immune response
- Lymphatic system drains leaked tissue fluids; immune cells protect against pathogens

Respiratory System Chapter 22

- Skeletal system protects lungs by enclosure (rib cage)
- Respiratory system provides oxygen; disposes of carbon dioxide

Digestive System Chapter 23

- Skeletal system provides some bony protection to intestines, pelvic organs, and liver
- Digestive system provides nutrients needed for bone health and growth

Urinary System Chapters 25–26

- Skeletal system protects pelvic organs (urinary bladder, etc.)
- Urinary system activates vitamin D; disposes of nitrogenous wastes

Reproductive System Chapter 27

- Skeletal system protects some reproductive organs by enclosure
- Gonads produce hormones that influence the form of the skeleton and epiphyseal closure

Bone Structure (pp. 177–183)

Gross Anatomy (pp. 177–179)

1. Flat bones consist of two thin plates of compact bone enclosing a diploë (spongy bone layer). Short and irregular bones resemble flat bones structurally.
2. A long bone is composed of a diaphysis (shaft) and epiphyses (ends). The medullary cavity of the diaphysis contains yellow marrow; the epiphyses contain spongy bone. The epiphyseal line is the remnant of the epiphyseal plate. Periosteum covers the diaphysis; endosteum lines inner bone cavities. Hyaline cartilage covers joint surfaces.
3. In adults, hematopoietic tissue (red marrow) is found within the diploë of flat bones and occasionally within the epiphyses of long bones. In infants, red marrow is also found in the medullary cavity.
4. Bone markings are important anatomical landmarks that reveal sites of muscle attachment, points of articulation, and sites of blood vessel and nerve passage.

Microscopic Anatomy of Bone (pp. 179–182)

5. There are five types of bone cells—osteogenic cells (bone stem cells), osteoblasts (matrix-synthesizing cells), osteocytes (bone matrix maintenance cells), bone lining cells (line surfaces where no bone activity is ongoing), and osteoclasts (bone destruction cells).
6. The structural unit of compact bone, the osteon, consists of a central canal surrounded by concentric lamellae of bone matrix. Osteocytes, embedded in lacunae, are connected to each other and the central canal by canaliculi.
7. Spongy bone has slender trabeculae containing irregular lamellae, which enclose red marrow–filled cavities.

Chemical Composition of Bone (pp. 182–183)

8. Bone is composed of living cells and matrix. The extracellular matrix includes osteoid, organic substances that are secreted by osteoblasts and give the bone tensile strength. Its inorganic (mineral) components, the hydroxyapatites (calcium salts), make bone hard.

Bone Development (pp. 183–187)

Formation of the Bony Skeleton (pp. 183–185)

1. Intramembranous ossification forms the clavicles and most skull bones. The ground substance of the bone matrix is deposited between collagen fibers within the fibrous membrane to form bone. Eventually, compact bone plates enclose the diploë.
2. Most bones are formed by endochondral ossification of a hyaline cartilage model. Osteoblasts beneath the periosteum secrete bone matrix on the cartilage model, forming the bone collar. As the cartilage model deteriorates, internal cavities open up, allowing periosteal bud entry. Bone matrix is deposited around the cartilage remnants but is later broken down.

Postnatal Bone Growth (pp. 185–187)

3. Long bones increase in length by interstitial growth of the epiphyseal plate cartilage and its replacement by bone.
4. Appositional growth increases bone diameter/thickness.

Bone Homeostasis: Remodeling and Repair (pp. 187–192)

Bone Remodeling (pp. 187–191)

1. Bone is continually deposited and resorbed in response to hormonal and mechanical stimuli. Together these processes constitute bone remodeling.
2. An unmineralized osteoid seam appears at areas of new bone deposit; calcium salts are deposited a few days later.
3. Osteoclasts release lysosomal enzymes and acids on bone surfaces to be resorbed. The dissolved products are transcytosed to the opposite face of the osteoclast for release to the extracellular fluid.
4. The hormonal controls of bone remodeling serve blood calcium homeostasis. When blood calcium levels decline, PTH is released and stimulates osteoclasts to digest bone matrix, releasing ionic calcium. As blood calcium levels rise, PTH secretion declines.
5. Mechanical stress and gravity acting on the skeleton help maintain skeletal strength. Bones thicken, develop heavier prominences, or rearrange their trabeculae in sites where stressed.

Bone Repair (pp. 191–192)

6. Fractures are treated by open or closed reduction. The healing process involves formation of a hematoma, a fibrocartilaginous callus, a bony callus, and bone remodeling, in succession.

Homeostatic Imbalances of Bone (pp. 192–193)

1. Imbalances between bone formation and resorption underlie all skeletal disorders.
2. Osteomalacia and rickets occur when bones are inadequately mineralized. The bones become soft and deformed. The most frequent cause is inadequate vitamin D.
3. Osteoporosis is any condition in which bone breakdown outpaces bone formation, causing bones to become weak and porous. Postmenopausal women are particularly susceptible.
4. Paget's disease is characterized by excessive and abnormal bone remodeling.

Developmental Aspects of Bones: Timing of Events (pp. 193–194)

1. Osteogenesis is predictable and precisely timed.
2. Longitudinal long bone growth continues until the end of adolescence. Skeletal mass increases dramatically during puberty and adolescence, when formation exceeds resorption.
3. Bone mass is fairly constant in young adulthood, but beginning in the 40s, bone resorption exceeds formation.

Review Questions

Multiple Choice/Matching

(Some questions have more than one correct answer. Select the best answer or answers from the choices given.)

1. Which is a function of the skeletal system? **(a)** support, **(b)** hematopoietic site, **(c)** storage, **(d)** providing levers for muscle activity, **(e)** all of these.
2. A bone with approximately the same width, length, and height is most likely **(a)** a long bone, **(b)** a short bone, **(c)** a flat bone, **(d)** an irregular bone.
3. The shaft of a long bone is properly called the **(a)** epiphysis, **(b)** periosteum, **(c)** diaphysis, **(d)** compact bone.
4. Sites of hematopoiesis include all but **(a)** red marrow cavities of spongy bone, **(b)** the diploë of flat bones, **(c)** medullary cavities in bones of infants, **(d)** medullary cavities in bones of a healthy adult.

5. An osteon has **(a)** a central canal carrying blood vessels, **(b)** concentric lamellae, **(c)** osteocytes in lacunae, **(d)** canaliculi that connect lacunae to the central canal, **(e)** all of these.
6. The organic portion of matrix is important in providing all but **(a)** tensile strength, **(b)** hardness, **(c)** ability to resist stretch, **(d)** flexibility.
7. The flat bones of the skull develop from **(a)** areolar tissue, **(b)** hyaline cartilage, **(c)** fibrous connective tissue, **(d)** compact bone.
8. The remodeling of bone is a function of which cells? **(a)** chondrocytes and osteocytes, **(b)** osteoblasts and osteoclasts, **(c)** chondroblasts and osteoclasts, **(d)** osteoblasts and osteocytes.
9. Bone remodeling in adults is regulated and directed mainly by **(a)** growth hormone, **(b)** thyroid hormones, **(c)** sex hormones, **(d)** mechanical stress, **(e)** PTH.
10. Where within the epiphyseal plate are the dividing cartilage cells located? **(a)** nearest the shaft, **(b)** in the marrow cavity, **(c)** farthest from the shaft, **(d)** in the primary ossification center.
11. Wolff's law is concerned with **(a)** calcium homeostasis of the blood, **(b)** the shape of a bone being determined by mechanical stresses placed on it, **(c)** the electrical charge on bone surfaces.
12. Formation of the bony callus in fracture repair is followed by **(a)** hematoma formation, **(b)** fibrocartilaginous callus formation, **(c)** bone remodeling, **(d)** formation of granulation tissue.
13. The fracture type in which the bone ends are incompletely separated is **(a)** greenstick, **(b)** compound, **(c)** simple, **(d)** comminuted, **(e)** compression.
14. The disorder in which bones are porous and thin but bone composition is normal is **(a)** osteomalacia, **(b)** osteoporosis, **(c)** Paget's disease.

Short Answer Essay Questions

15. Compare bone to cartilage tissue relative to its resilience, speed of regeneration, and access to nutrients.
16. Describe in proper sequence the events of endochondral ossification.
17. Osteocytes residing in lacunae of osteons of healthy compact bone are located quite a distance from the blood vessels in the central canals, yet they are well nourished. How can this be explained?
18. As we grow, our long bones increase in diameter, but the thickness of the compact bone of the shaft remains relatively constant. Explain this phenomenon.
19. Describe the process of new bone formation in an adult bone. Use the terms osteoid seam and calcification front in your discussion.
20. Compare and contrast controls of bone remodeling exerted by hormones and by mechanical and gravitational forces, including the actual purpose of each control system and changes in bone architecture that might occur.
21. (a) During what period of life does skeletal mass increase dramatically? Begin to decline? (b) Why are fractures most common in elderly individuals? (c) Why are greenstick fractures most common in children?
22. Yolanda is asked to review a bone slide that her professor has set up under the microscope. She sees concentric layers surrounding a central cavity. Is this bone section taken from the diaphysis or the epiphyseal plate of the specimen?

Critical Thinking and Clinical Application Questions

1. Following a motorcycle accident, a 22-year-old man was rushed to the emergency room. X rays revealed a spiral fracture of his right tibia (main bone of the leg). Two months later, X rays revealed good bony callus formation. What is bony callus?
2. Mrs. Abbruzzo brought her 4-year-old daughter to the doctor, complaining that she didn't "look right." The child's forehead was enlarged, her rib cage was knobby, and her lower limbs were bent and deformed. X rays revealed very thick epiphyseal plates. Mrs. Abbruzzo was advised to increase dietary amounts of vitamin D and milk and to "shoo" the girl outside to play in the sun. Considering the child's signs and symptoms, what disease do you think she has? Explain the doctor's instructions.
3. You overhear some anatomy students imagining out loud what their bones would look like if they had compact bone on the inside and spongy bone on the outside, instead of the other way around. You tell them that such imaginary bones would be poorly designed mechanically and would break easily. Explain your reason for saying this.
4. What would a long bone look like at the end of adolescence if bone remodeling did not occur?
5. Why do you think wheelchair-bound people with paralyzed lower limbs have thin, weak bones of the leg and thigh?
6. Jay Beckenstein went to weight-lifting camp in the summer between seventh and eighth grade. He noticed that the camp trainer put tremendous pressure on him and his friends to improve their strength. After an especially vigorous workout, Jay's arm felt extremely sore and weak around the elbow. He went to the camp doctor, who took X rays and then told him that the injury was serious, for the "end of his upper arm bone was starting to twist off." What had happened? Could the same thing happen to Jay's 23-year-old sister, Trixie, who was also starting a program of weight lifting? Why or why not?
7. Old Norse stories tell of a famous Viking named Egil, who lived around 900 AD. His skull was greatly enlarged and misshapen, and the cranial bones were thickened (6 cm, more than 2 inches, thick). After he died, his skull was dug up and it withstood the blow of an ax without damage. In life, he had headaches from the pressure exerted by enlarged vertebrae on his spinal cord. So much blood was diverted to his bones to support their extensive remodeling that his fingers and toes always felt cold and his heart was damaged through overexertion. What bone disorder did Egil probably have?

AT THE CLINIC

Related Clinical Terms

Achondroplasia (a-kon″dro-pla′ze-ah; *a* = without; *chondro* = cartilage; *plasi* = mold, shape) A congenital condition involving defective cartilage and endochondral bone growth so that the limbs are too short but the membrane bones are of normal size; a type of dwarfism.

Bony spur Abnormal projection from a bone due to bony overgrowth; common in aging bones.

Ostealgia (os″te-al′je-ah; *algia* = pain) Pain in a bone.

Osteitis (os″te-i′tis; *itis* = inflammation) Inflammation of bony tissue.

Related Clinical Terms *(continued)*

Osteogenesis imperfecta Also called brittle bone disease, a disorder in which the bone matrix contains inadequate collagen, putting it at risk for shattering.

Osteomyelitis (os″te-o-mi″ĕ-li′tis) Inflammation of bone and bone marrow caused by pus-forming bacteria that enter the body via a wound (e.g., compound bone fracture), or spread from an infection near the bone. Commonly affects the long bones, causing acute pain and fever. May result in joint stiffness, bone destruction, and shortening of a limb. Treatment involves antibiotics, draining any abscesses (local collections of pus), and removing dead bone fragments (which prevent healing).

Osteosarcoma (os″te-o-sar-ko′mah) A form of bone cancer typically arising in a long bone of a limb and most often in those 10–25 years of age. Grows aggressively, painfully eroding the bone; tends to metastasize to the lungs and cause secondary lung tumors. Usual treatment is amputation of the affected bone or limb, followed by chemotherapy and surgical removal of any metastases. Survival rate is about 50% if detected early.

Pathologic fracture Fracture in a diseased bone involving slight (coughing or a quick turn) or no physical trauma. For example, a hip bone weakened by osteoporosis may break and cause the person to fall, rather than breaking because of the fall.

Traction ("pulling") Placing sustained tension on a body region to keep the parts of a fractured bone in proper alignment. Also prevents spasms of skeletal muscles, which would separate the fractured bone ends or crush the spinal cord in the case of vertebral column fractures.

6

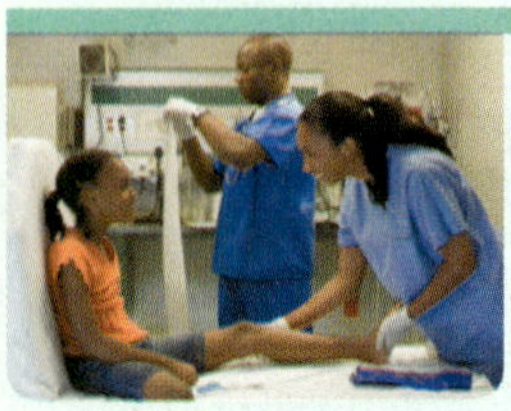

Case Study Skeletal System

Remember Mrs. DeStephano? When we last heard about her she was being admitted for further studies. Relative to her skeletal system, the following notes have been added to her chart.

- Fracture of superior right tibia (shinbone of leg); skin lacerated; area cleaned and protruding bone fragments subjected to internal (open) reduction and casted
- Nutrient artery of tibia damaged
- Medial meniscus (fibrocartilage disc) of right knee joint crushed; knee joint inflamed and painful

Relative to these notes:

1. What type of fracture does Mrs. DeStephano have?
2. What problems can be predicted with such fractures and how are they treated?
3. What is internal reduction? Why was a cast applied?
4. Given an uncomplicated recovery, approximately how long should it take before Mrs. DeStephano has a good solid bony callus?
5. What complications might be predicted by the fact that the nutrient artery is damaged?
6. What new techniques might be used to enhance fracture repair if healing is delayed or impaired?
7. How likely is it that Mrs. DeStephano's knee cartilage will regenerate? Why?

(Answers in Appendix H)

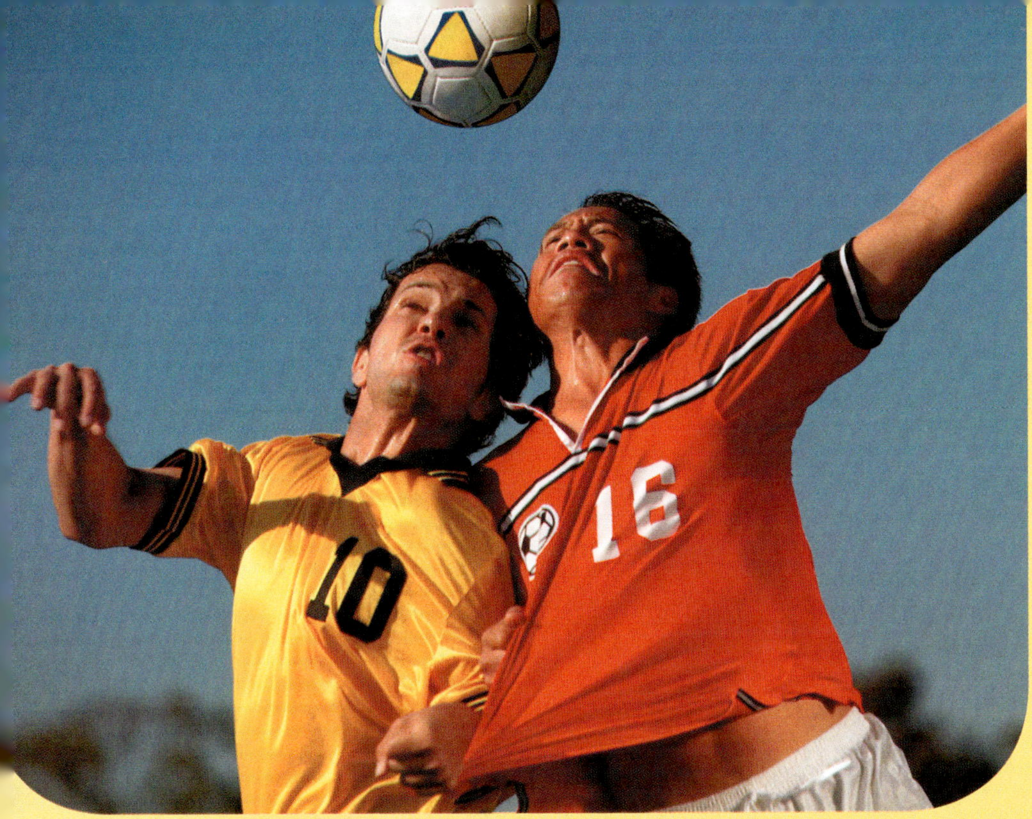

7 The Skeleton

The word *skeleton* comes from the Greek word meaning "dried-up body" or "mummy," a rather unflattering description. Nonetheless, the human skeleton is a triumph of design and engineering that puts most skyscrapers to shame. It is strong, yet light, and almost perfectly adapted for the protective, locomotor, and manipulative functions it performs.

The **skeleton**, or **skeletal system**, composed of bones, cartilages, joints, and ligaments, accounts for about 20% of body mass (about 30 pounds in a 160-pound person). Bones make up most of the skeleton. Cartilages occur only in isolated areas, such as the nose, parts of the ribs, and the joints. Ligaments connect bones and reinforce joints, allowing required movements while restricting motions in other directions. Joints, the junctions between bones, provide for the remarkable mobility of the skeleton. We discuss joints and ligaments separately in Chapter 8.

PART 1
The Axial Skeleton

✓ Name the major parts of the axial and appendicular skeletons and describe their relative functions.

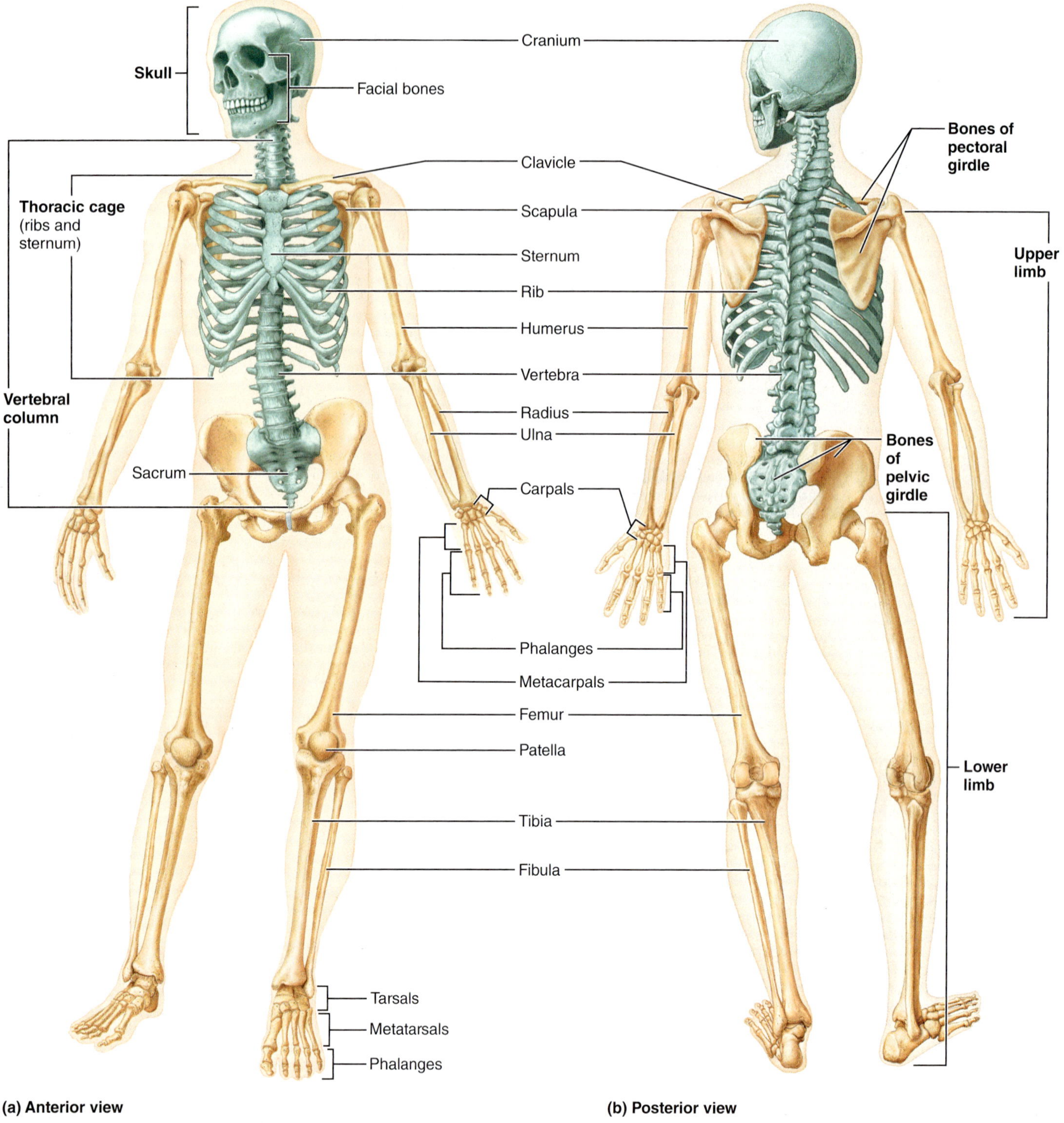

Figure 7.1 The human skeleton. Bones of the axial skeleton are colored green. Bones of the appendicular skeleton are gold.

As described in Chapter 6, the skeleton is divided into *axial* and *appendicular* portions (see Figures 6.1 and 7.1). The **axial skeleton** is structured from 80 bones segregated into three major regions: the *skull*, *vertebral column*, and *thoracic cage* **(Figure 7.1)**. This part of the skeleton (1) forms the longitudinal axis of the body, (2) supports the head, neck, and trunk, and (3) protects the brain, spinal cord, and the organs in the thorax. As we will see later in this chapter, the bones of the appendicular skeleton, which allow us to interact with and manipulate our environment, are appended to the axial skeleton.

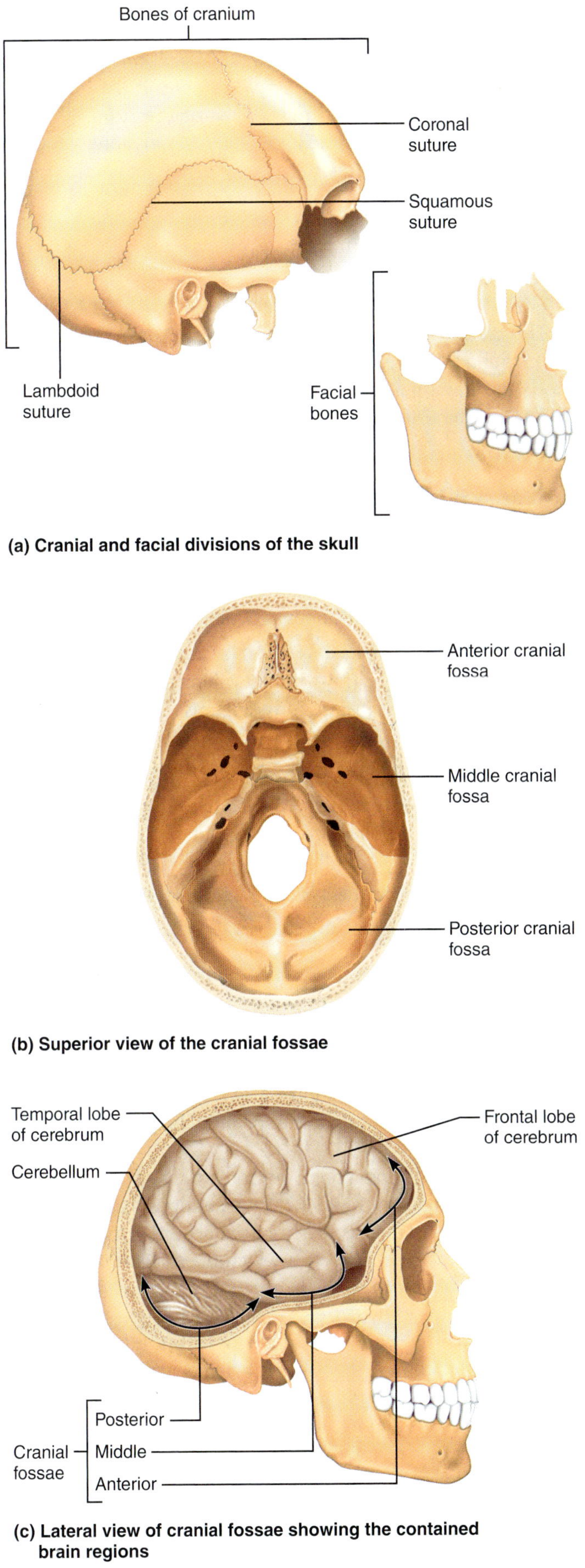

Figure 7.2 The skull: Cranial and facial divisions and fossae.

Check Your Understanding

1. What are the three main parts of the axial skeleton?
2. Which part of the skeleton—axial or appendicular—is important in protecting internal organs?

For answers, see Appendix H.

The Skull

✓ Name, describe, and identify the skull bones. Identify their important markings.

✓ Compare and contrast the major functions of the cranium and the facial skeleton.

The **skull** is the body's most complex bony structure. It is formed by *cranial* and *facial bones*, 22 in all. The cranial bones, or **cranium** (kra′ne-um), enclose and protect the fragile brain and furnish attachment sites for head and neck muscles. The facial bones (1) form the framework of the face, (2) contain cavities for the special sense organs of sight, taste, and smell, (3) provide openings for air and food passage, (4) secure the teeth, and (5) anchor the facial muscles of expression, which we use to show our feelings. As you will see, the individual skull bones are well suited to their assignments.

Most skull bones are flat bones. Except for the mandible, which is connected to the rest of the skull by freely movable joints, all bones of the adult skull are firmly united by interlocking joints called **sutures** (soo′cherz). The suture lines have a saw-toothed or serrated appearance.

The major skull sutures, the *coronal*, *sagittal*, *squamous*, and *lambdoid sutures*, connect cranial bones (Figures 7.2a, 7.4b, and 7.5a). Most other skull sutures connect facial bones and are named according to the specific bones they connect.

Overview of Skull Geography

It is worth surveying basic skull "geography" before describing the individual bones. With the lower jaw removed, the skull resembles a lopsided, hollow, bony sphere. The facial bones form its anterior aspect, and the cranium forms the rest of the skull **(Figure 7.2a)**.

The cranium can be divided into a vault and a base. The *cranial vault*, also called the *calvaria* (kal-va′re-ah; "bald part of skull"), forms the superior, lateral, and posterior aspects of the skull, as well as the forehead. The *cranial base* forms the skull's inferior aspect. Internally, prominent bony ridges divide the base into three distinct "steps" or fossae—the *anterior*, *middle*, and *posterior cranial fossae* (Figure 7.2b and c). The brain sits snugly in these cranial fossae, completely enclosed by the cranial vault. Overall, the brain is said to occupy the *cranial cavity*.

In addition to the large cranial cavity, the skull has many smaller cavities. These include the middle and internal ear cavities (carved into the lateral side of its base) and, anteriorly, the

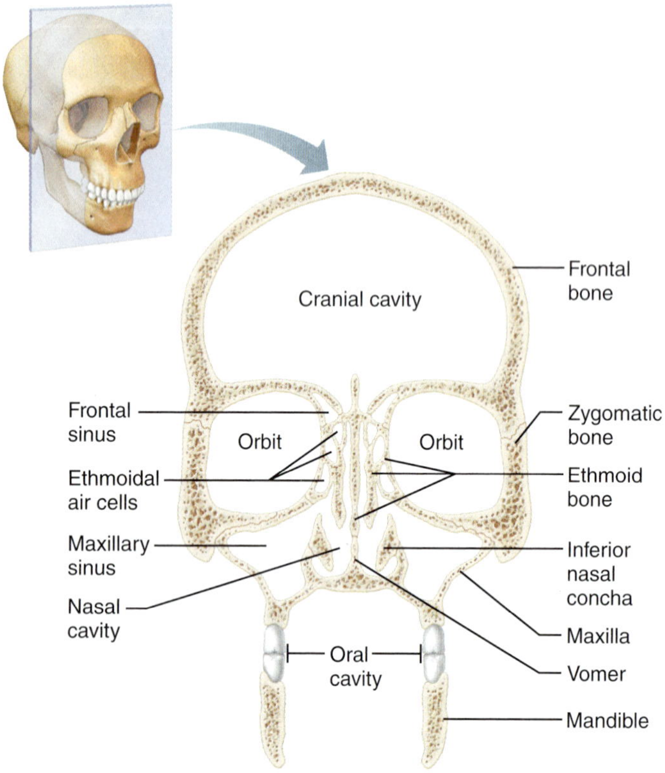

Figure 7.3 Major cavities of the skull, frontal section.

nasal cavity and the orbits **(Figure 7.3)**. The *orbits* house the eyeballs. Several bones of the skull contain air-filled sinuses, which lighten the skull.

The skull also has about 85 named openings (foramina, canals, fissures, etc.). The most important of these provide passageways for the spinal cord, the major blood vessels serving the brain, and the 12 pairs of cranial nerves (numbered I through XII), which transmit information to and from the brain.

As you read about the bones of the skull, locate each bone on the different skull views in **Figures 7.4**, **7.5**, and **7.6**. The skull bones and their important markings are also summarized in **Table 7.1** (pp. 216–217). The color-coded boxes before a bone's name in the text and in Table 7.1 correspond to the color of that bone in the figures. For example, note the color of the frontal bone in Table 7.1 and see how you can easily find it in Figures 7.4 and 7.5.

Cranium

The eight cranial bones are the paired parietal and temporal bones and the unpaired frontal, occipital, sphenoid, and ethmoid bones. Together, these construct the brain's protective bony "helmet." Because its superior aspect is curved, the cranium is self-bracing. This allows the bones to be thin, and, like an eggshell, the cranium is remarkably strong for its weight.

Frontal Bone

The shell-shaped **frontal bone** (Figures 7.4a, 7.5, and 7.7) forms the anterior cranium. It articulates posteriorly with the paired parietal bones via the prominent *coronal suture.*

The most anterior part of the frontal bone is the vertical *squamous part*, commonly called the *forehead.* The frontal squamous region ends inferiorly at the **supraorbital margins**, the thickened superior margins of the orbits that lie under the eyebrows. From here, the frontal bone extends posteriorly, forming the superior wall of the *orbits* and most of the **anterior cranial fossa (Figure 7.7a and b)**. This fossa supports the frontal lobes of the brain. Each supraorbital margin is pierced by a **supraorbital foramen (notch)**, which allows the supraorbital artery and nerve to pass to the forehead (Figure 7.4a).

The smooth portion of the frontal bone between the orbits is the **glabella** (glah-bel′ah). Just inferior to this the frontal bone meets the nasal bones at the *frontonasal suture* (Figure 7.4a). The areas lateral to the glabella are riddled internally with sinuses, called the **frontal sinuses** (Figures 7.5c and 7.3).

Parietal Bones and the Major Sutures

The two large **parietal bones** are curved, rectangular bones that form most of the superior and lateral aspects of the skull; hence they form the bulk of the cranial vault. The four largest sutures occur where the parietal bones articulate (form a joint) with other cranial bones:

- The **coronal suture** (kŏ-ro′nul), where the parietal bones meet the frontal bone anteriorly (Figures 7.2a and 7.5)
- The **sagittal suture**, where the parietal bones meet superiorly at the cranial midline (Figure 7.4b)
- The **lambdoid suture** (lam′doid), where the parietal bones meet the occipital bone posteriorly (Figures 7.2a, 7.4b, and 7.5)
- The **squamous suture** (one on each side), where a parietal and temporal bone meet on the lateral aspect of the skull (Figures 7.2a and 7.5)

Occipital Bone

The **occipital bone** (ok-sip′ĭ-tal) forms most of the skull's posterior wall and base. It articulates anteriorly with the paired parietal and temporal bones via the *lambdoid* and *occipitomastoid sutures*, respectively (Figure 7.5). The basilar part of the occipital bone also joins with the sphenoid bone in the cranial base (Figure 7.6a).

Internally, the occipital bone forms the walls of the **posterior cranial fossa** (Figures 7.7 and 7.2c), which supports the cerebellum of the brain. In the base of the occipital bone is the **foramen magnum** ("large hole") through which the inferior part of the brain connects with the spinal cord. The foramen magnum is flanked laterally by two occipital condyles (Figure 7.6). The rockerlike **occipital condyles** articulate with the first vertebra of the spinal column in a way that permits a nodding ("yes") motion of the head. Hidden medially and superiorly to each occipital condyle is a **hypoglossal canal** (Figure 7.7a), through which a cranial nerve (XII) passes.

Just superior to the foramen magnum is a median protrusion called the **external occipital protuberance** (Figures 7.4b, 7.5, and 7.6). You can feel this knoblike projection just below

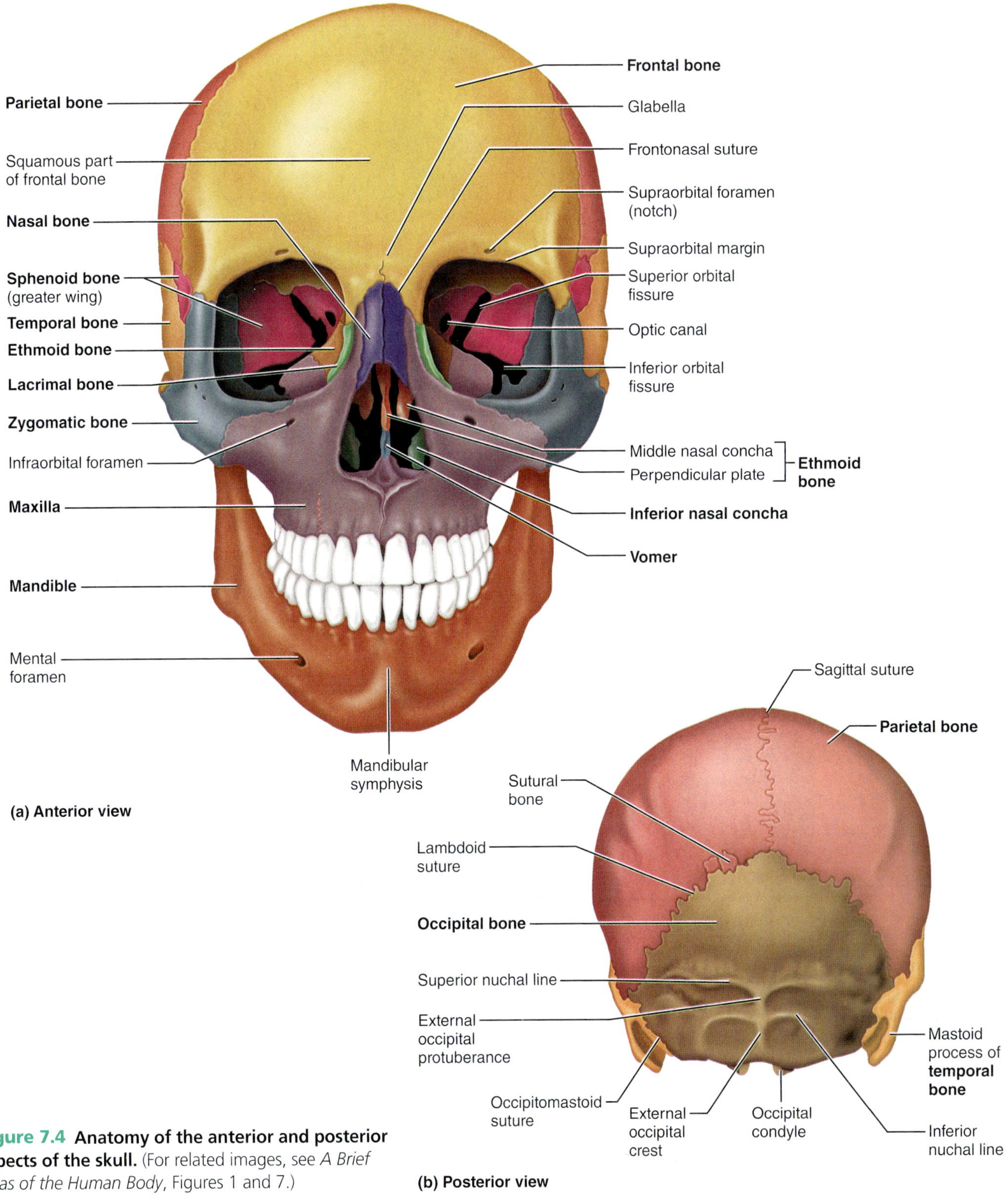

Figure 7.4 Anatomy of the anterior and posterior aspects of the skull. (For related images, see *A Brief Atlas of the Human Body*, Figures 1 and 7.)

the most bulging part of your posterior skull. A number of inconspicuous ridges, the *external occipital crest* and the *superior* and *inferior nuchal lines* (nu′kal), mark the occipital bone near the foramen magnum. The external occipital crest secures the *ligamentum nuchae* (lig″ah-men′tum noo′ke; *nucha* = back of the neck), a sheetlike elastic ligament that connects the vertebrae of the neck to the skull. The nuchal lines, and the bony regions between them, anchor many neck and back muscles. The superior nuchal line marks the upper limit of the neck.

(Text continues on p. 208.)

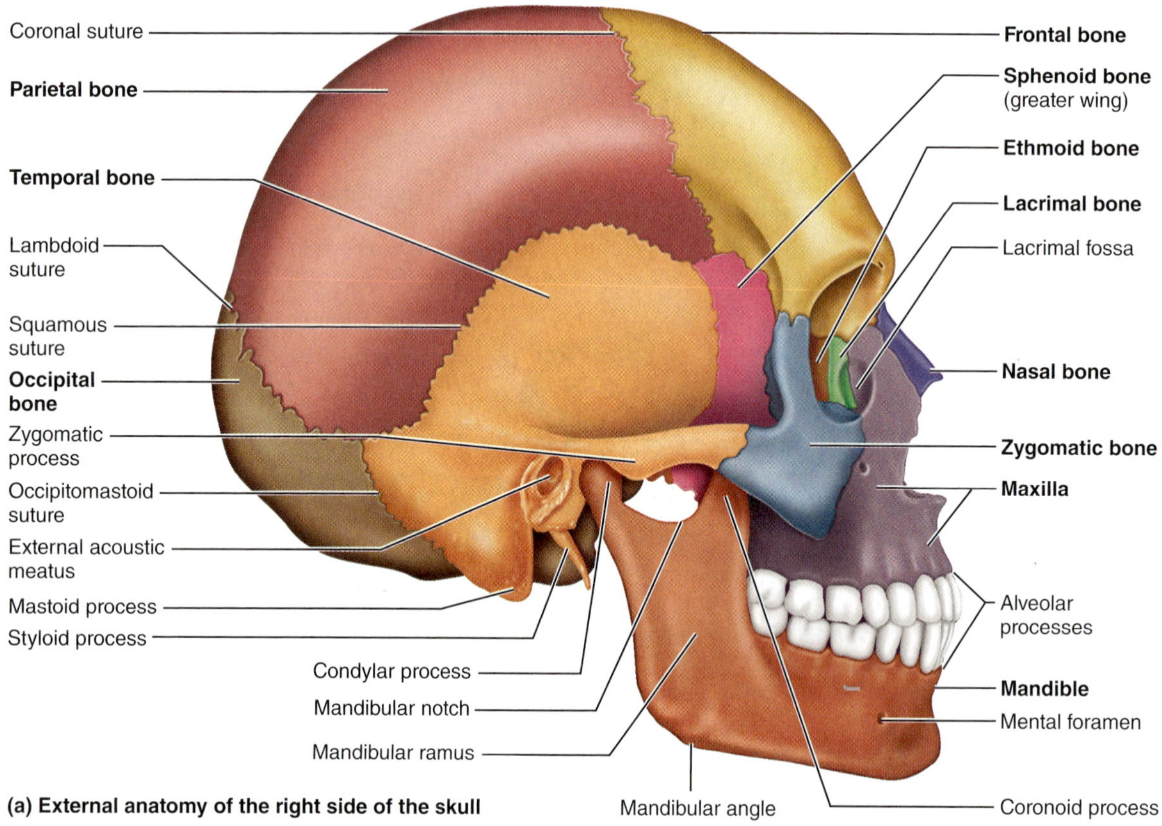

(a) External anatomy of the right side of the skull

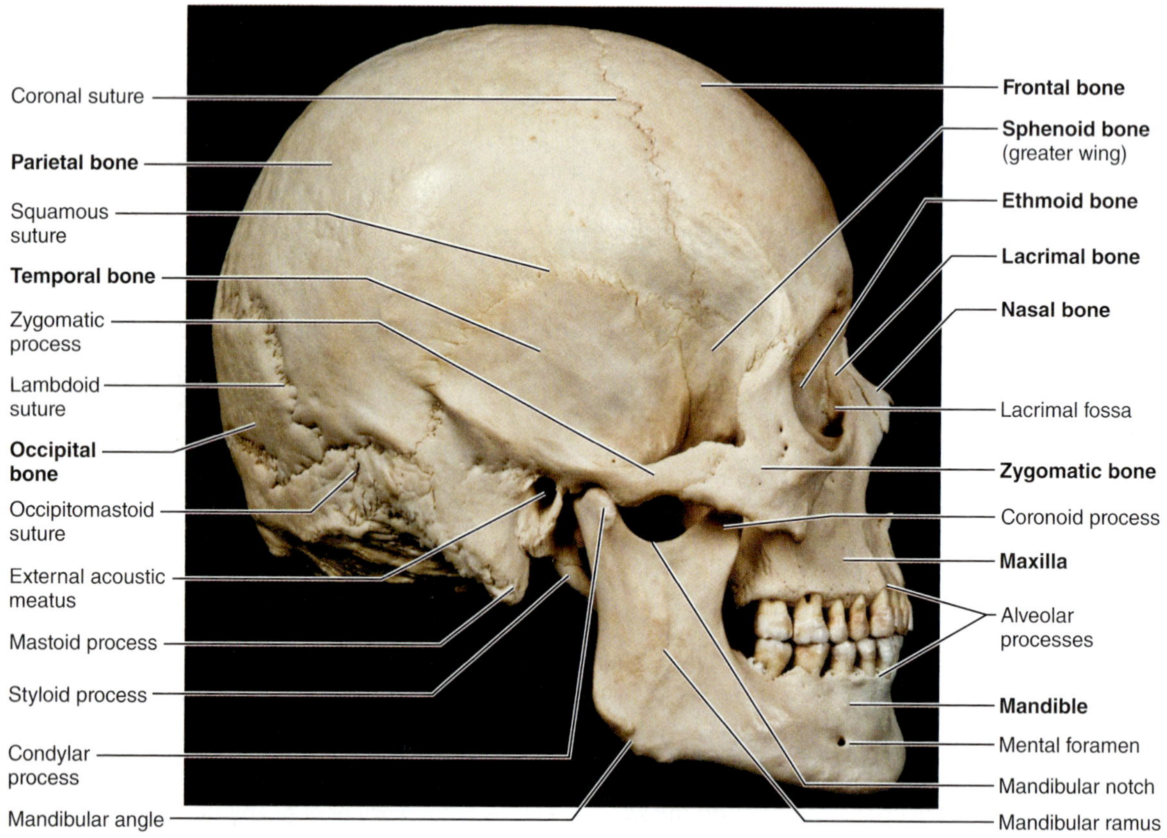

(b) Photograph of right side of skull

Figure 7.5 Bones of the lateral aspect of the skull, external and internal views. (For related images, see *A Brief Atlas of the Human Body*, Figures 2 and 3.)

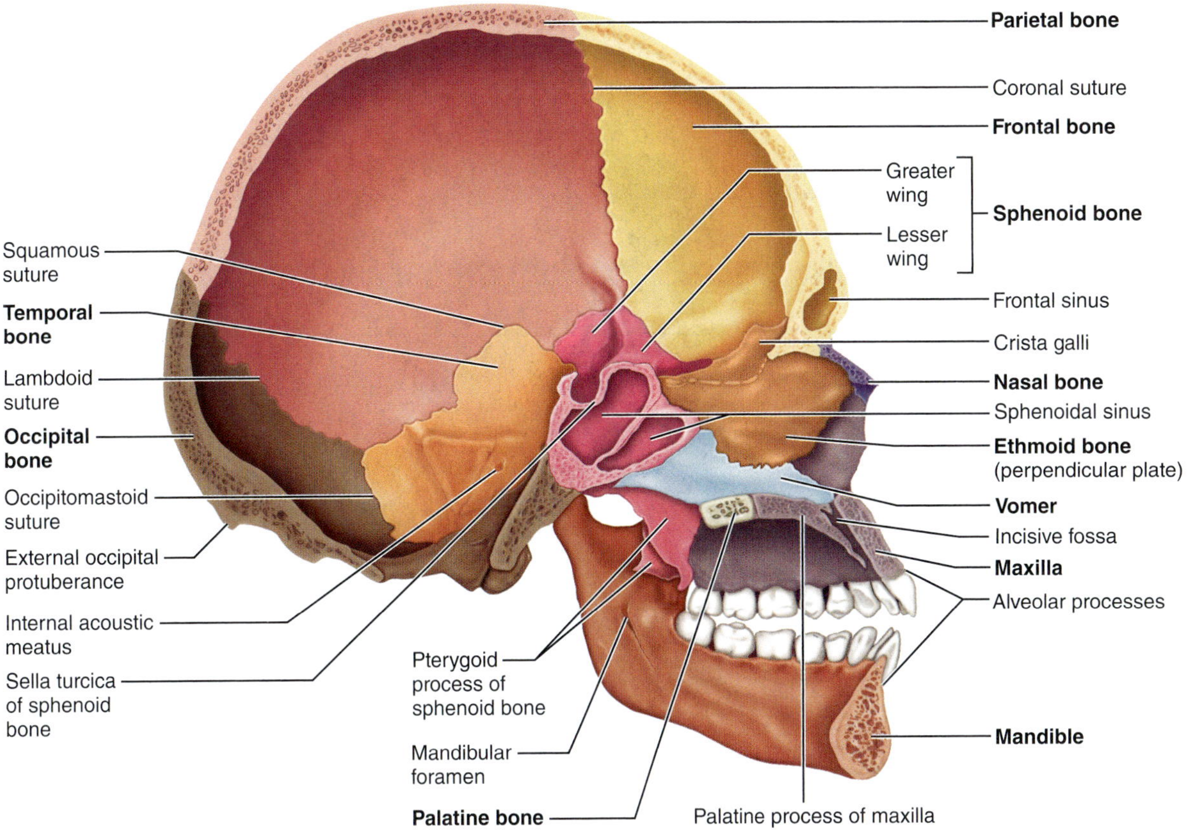

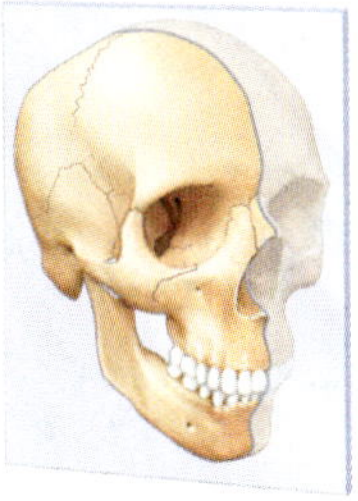

(c) Midsagittal section showing the internal anatomy of the left half of skull

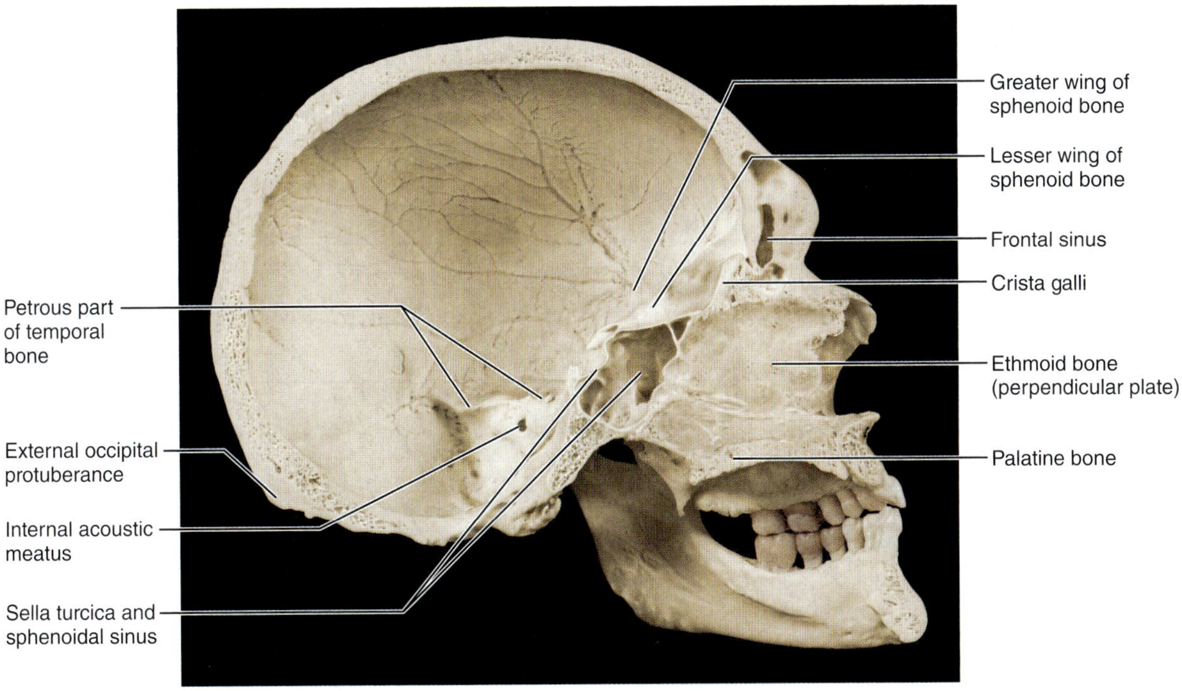

(d) Photo of skull cut through the midline, same view as in (c)

Figure 7.5 *(continued)*

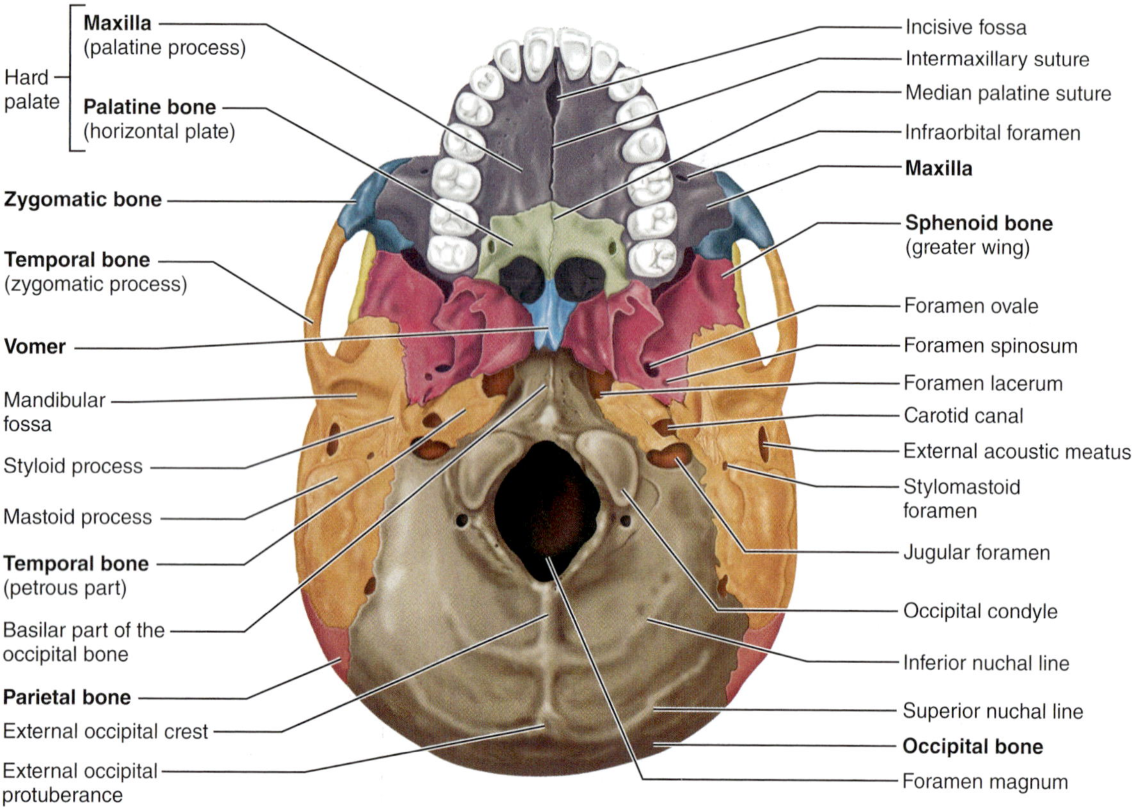

(a) Inferior view of the skull (mandible removed)

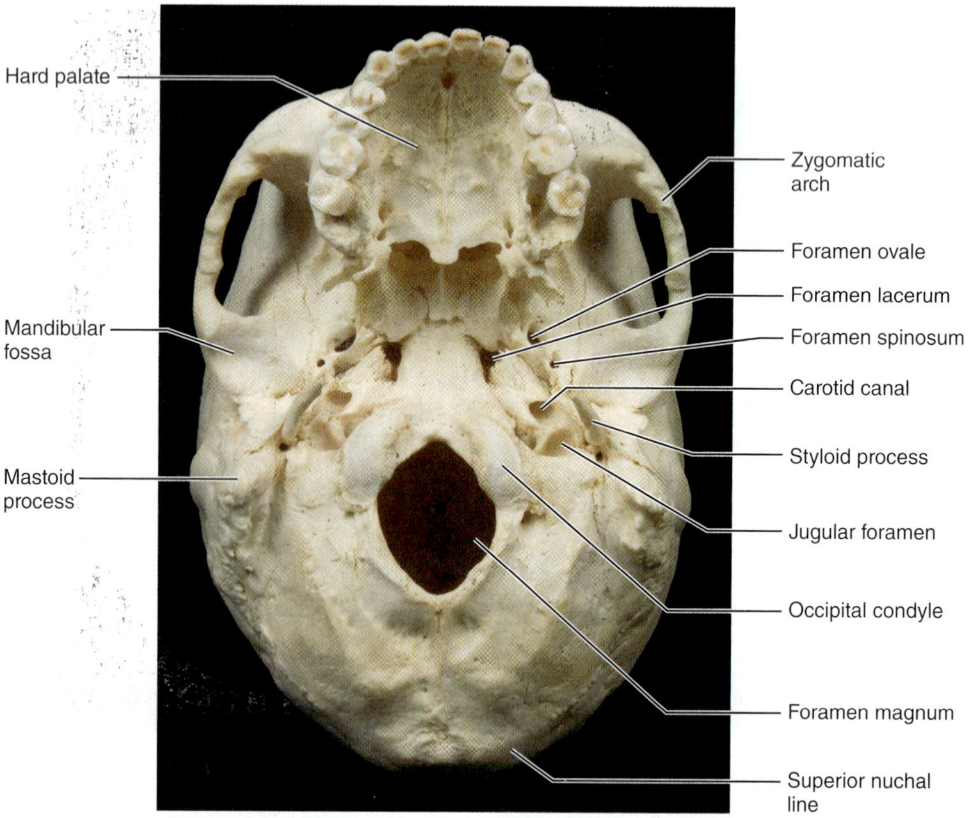

(b) Photo of inferior view of the skull

Figure 7.6 Inferior aspect of the skull, mandible removed. (For related images, see *A Brief Atlas of the Human Body*, Figure 4.)

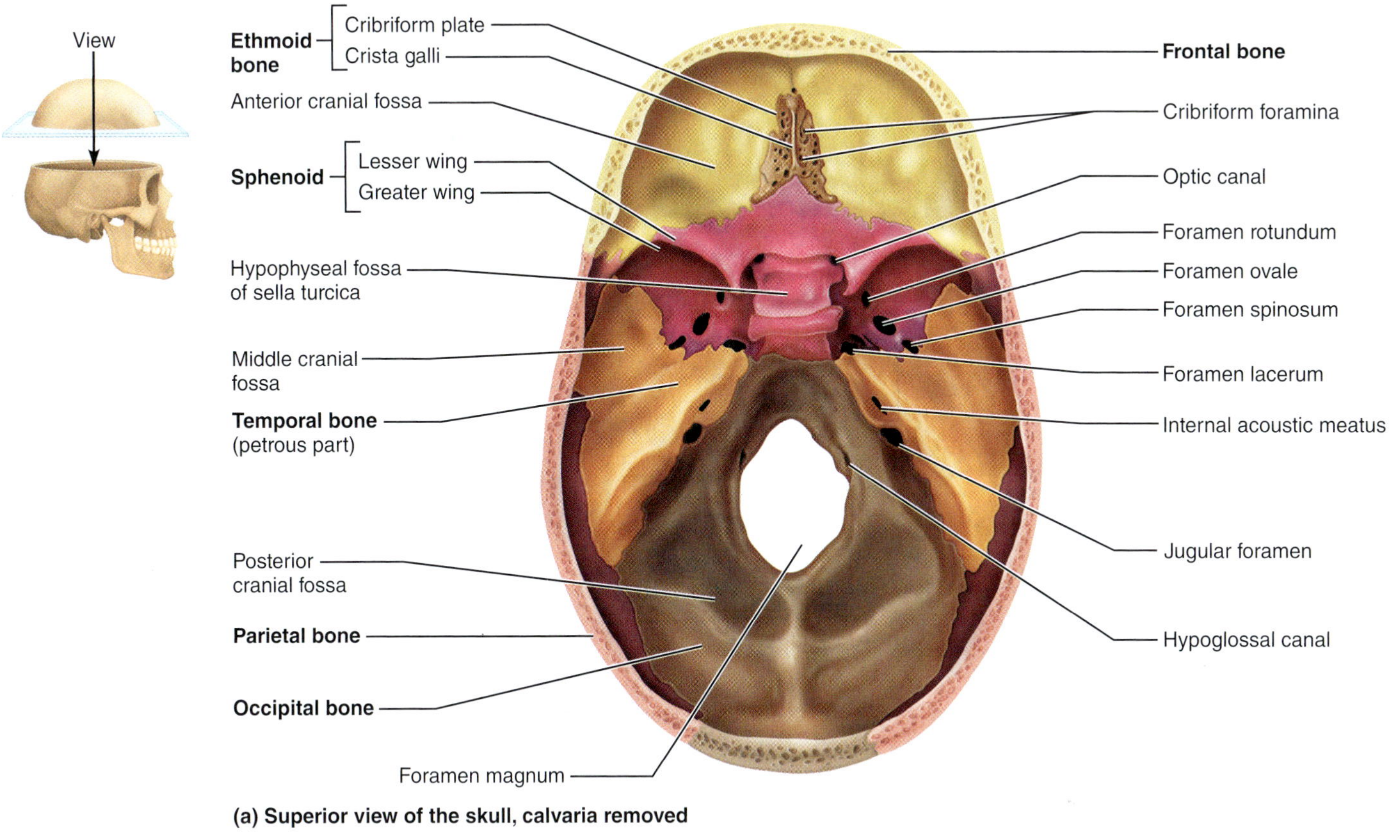

(a) Superior view of the skull, calvaria removed

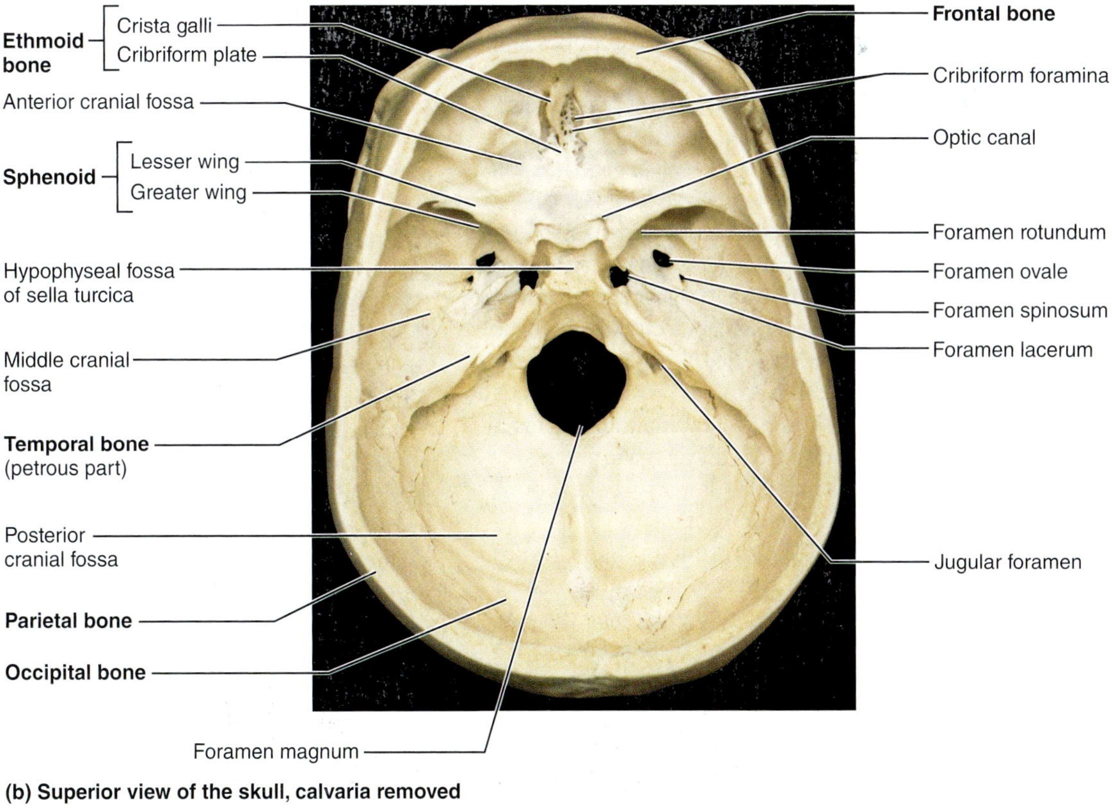

(b) Superior view of the skull, calvaria removed

Figure 7.7 The base of the cranial cavity. (For related images, see *A Brief Atlas of the Human Body*, Figure 5.)

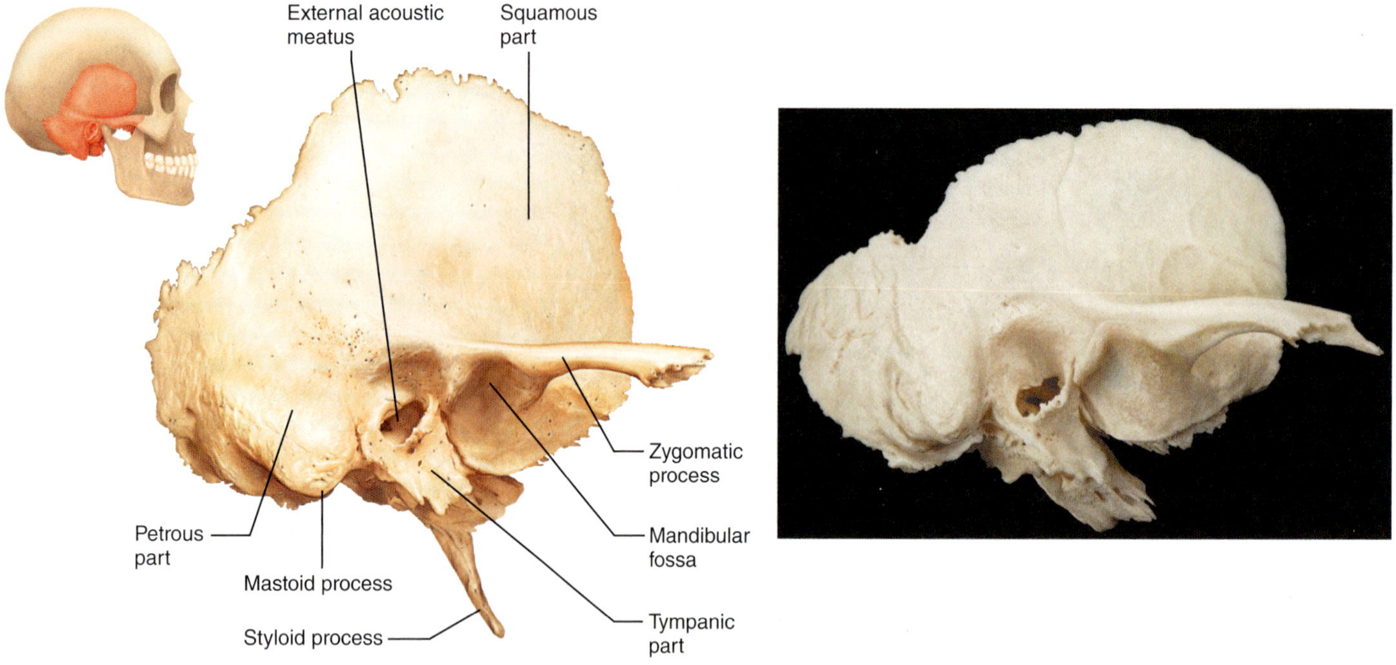

Figure 7.8 The temporal bone. Right lateral view. (For related images, see *A Brief Atlas of the Human Body*, Figures 2 and 8.)

Temporal Bones

The two **temporal bones** are best viewed on the lateral skull surface (Figure 7.5). They lie inferior to the parietal bones and meet them at the squamous sutures. The temporal bones form the inferolateral aspects of the skull and parts of the cranial base. The use of the terms *temple* and *temporal*, from the Latin word *temporum*, meaning "time," came about because gray hairs, a sign of time's passing, usually appear first at the temples.

Each temporal bone has a complicated shape **(Figure 7.8)** and is described in terms of its three major parts, the *squamous*, *tympanic*, and *petrous parts*. The flaring **squamous part** abuts the squamous suture. It has a barlike **zygomatic process** that meets the zygomatic bone of the face anteriorly. Together, these two bony structures form the **zygomatic arch**, which you can feel as the projection of your cheek (*zygoma* = cheekbone). The small, oval **mandibular fossa** (man-dib′u-lar) on the inferior surface of the zygomatic process receives the condylar process of the mandible (lower jawbone), forming the freely movable *temporomandibular joint*.

The **tympanic part** (tim-pan′ik; "eardrum") (Figure 7.8) of the temporal bone surrounds the **external acoustic meatus**, or external ear canal, through which sound enters the ear. The external acoustic meatus and the eardrum at its deep end are part of the *external ear*. In a dried skull, the eardrum has been removed and part of the middle ear cavity deep to the external meatus can also be seen.

The thick **petrous part** (pet′rus) of the temporal bone houses the *middle* and *internal ear cavities*, which contain sensory receptors for hearing and balance. Extending from the occipital bone posteriorly to the sphenoid bone anteriorly, it contributes to the cranial base (Figures 7.6 and 7.7). In the floor of the cranial cavity, the petrous part of the temporal bone looks like a miniature mountain ridge (*petrous* = rocky). The posterior slope of this ridge lies in the posterior cranial fossa; the anterior slope is in the middle cranial fossa. Together, the sphenoid bone and the petrous portions of the temporal bones construct the **middle cranial fossa** (Figures 7.7 and 7.2b), which supports the temporal lobes of the brain.

Several foramina penetrate the bone of the petrous region (Figure 7.6). The large **jugular foramen** at the junction of the occipital and petrous temporal bones allows passage of the internal jugular vein and three cranial nerves (IX, X, and XI). The **carotid canal** (kar-rot′id), just anterior to the jugular foramen, transmits the internal carotid artery into the cranial cavity. The two internal carotid arteries supply blood to over 80% of the cerebral hemispheres of the brain; their closeness to the internal ear cavities explains why, during excitement or exertion, we sometimes hear our rapid pulse as a thundering sound in the head. The **foramen lacerum** (la′ser-um) is a jagged opening (*lacerum* = torn or lacerated) between the petrous temporal bone and the sphenoid bone. It is almost completely closed by cartilage in a living person, but it is conspicuous in a dried skull, and students usually ask its name. The **internal acoustic meatus**, positioned superolateral to the jugular foramen (Figures 7.5c and d, and 7.7), transmits cranial nerves VII and VIII.

A conspicuous feature of the petrous part of the temporal bone is the **mastoid process** (mas′toid; "breast"), which acts as an anchoring site for some neck muscles (Figures 7.5, 7.6, and 7.8). This process can be felt as a lump just posterior to the ear. The needle-like **styloid process** (sti′loid; "stakelike") is an attachment point for several tongue and neck muscles and for a ligament that secures the hyoid bone of the neck to the skull (see Figure 7.15). The **stylomastoid foramen**, between the styloid and mastoid processes, allows cranial nerve VII (the facial nerve) to leave the skull (Figure 7.6).

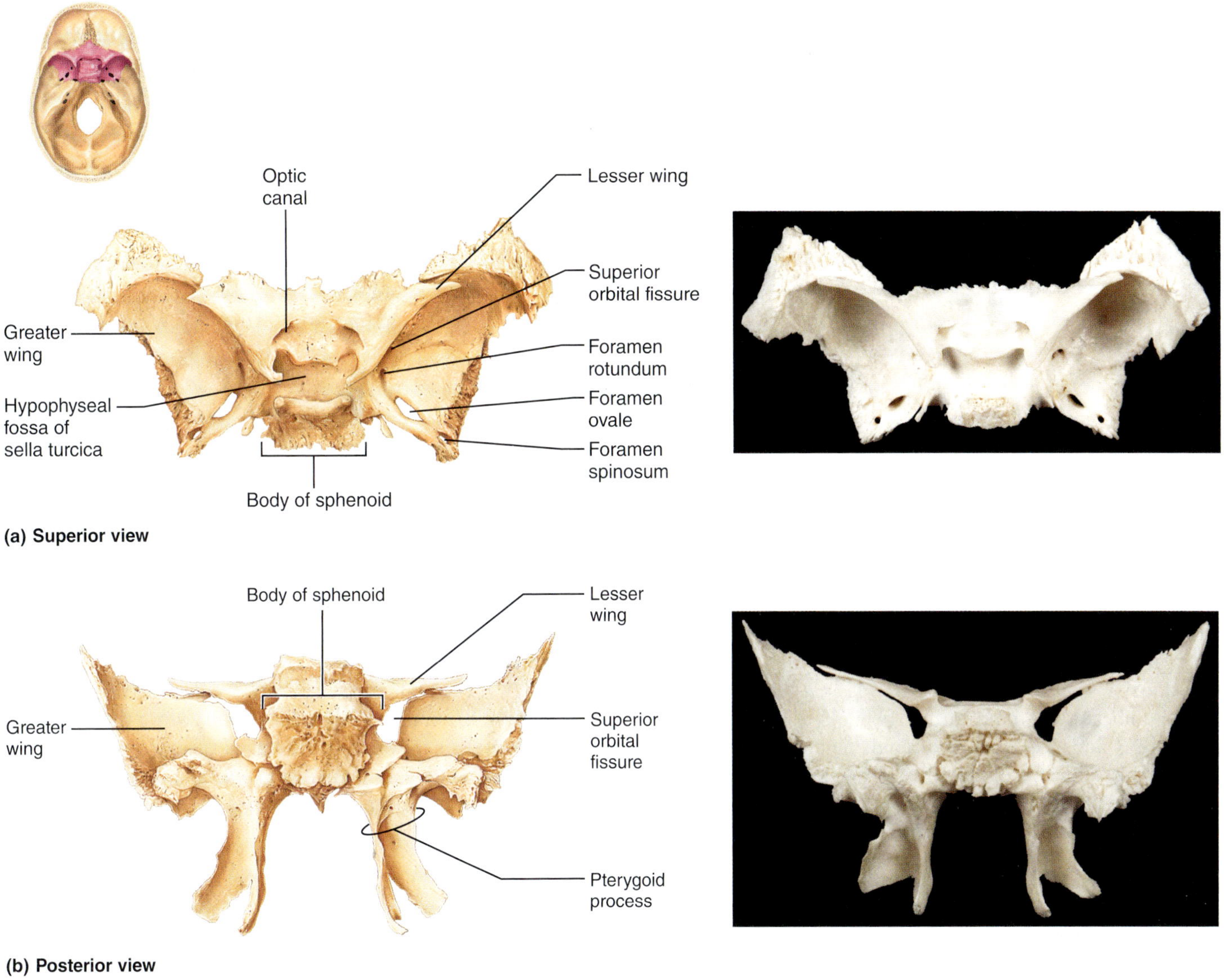

Figure 7.9 The sphenoid bone. (For related images, see *A Brief Atlas of the Human Body*, Figures 5 and 9).

Homeostatic Imbalance 7.1

The mastoid process is full of air cavities (sinuses) called **mastoid air cells**. Their position adjacent to the middle ear cavity (a high-risk area for infections spreading from the throat) puts them at risk for infection themselves. A mastoid sinus infection, or *mastoiditis*, is notoriously difficult to treat. Because the mastoid air cells are separated from the brain by only a very thin bony plate, mastoid infections may spread to the brain as well. Surgical removal of the mastoid process was once the best way to prevent life-threatening brain inflammations in people susceptible to repeated bouts of mastoiditis. Today, antibiotic therapy is the treatment of choice. ✚

Sphenoid Bone

The bat-shaped **sphenoid bone** (sfe′noid; *sphen* = wedge) spans the width of the middle cranial fossa (Figure 7.7). The sphenoid is considered the keystone of the cranium because it forms a central wedge that articulates with all other cranial bones. It is a challenging bone to study because of its complex shape. As shown in **Figure 7.9**, it consists of a central body and three pairs of processes: the greater wings, lesser wings, and pterygoid processes (ter′ĭ-goid). Within the **body** of the sphenoid are the paired **sphenoidal sinuses** (see Figures 7.5c and d, and 7.14).

The superior surface of the body bears a saddle-shaped prominence, the **sella turcica** (sel′ah ter′sĭ-kah), meaning "Turk's saddle." The seat of this saddle, called the **hypophyseal fossa**, forms a snug enclosure for the pituitary gland (hypophysis).

The **greater wings** project laterally from the sphenoid body, forming parts of (1) the middle cranial fossa (Figures 7.7 and 7.2b), (2) the posterior walls of the orbits (Figure 7.4a), and (3) the external wall of the skull, where they are seen as flag-shaped, bony areas medial to the zygomatic arch (Figure 7.5). The hornlike **lesser wings** form part of the floor of the anterior cranial fossa (Figure 7.7) and part of the medial walls of the orbits. The trough-shaped **pterygoid processes** project inferiorly

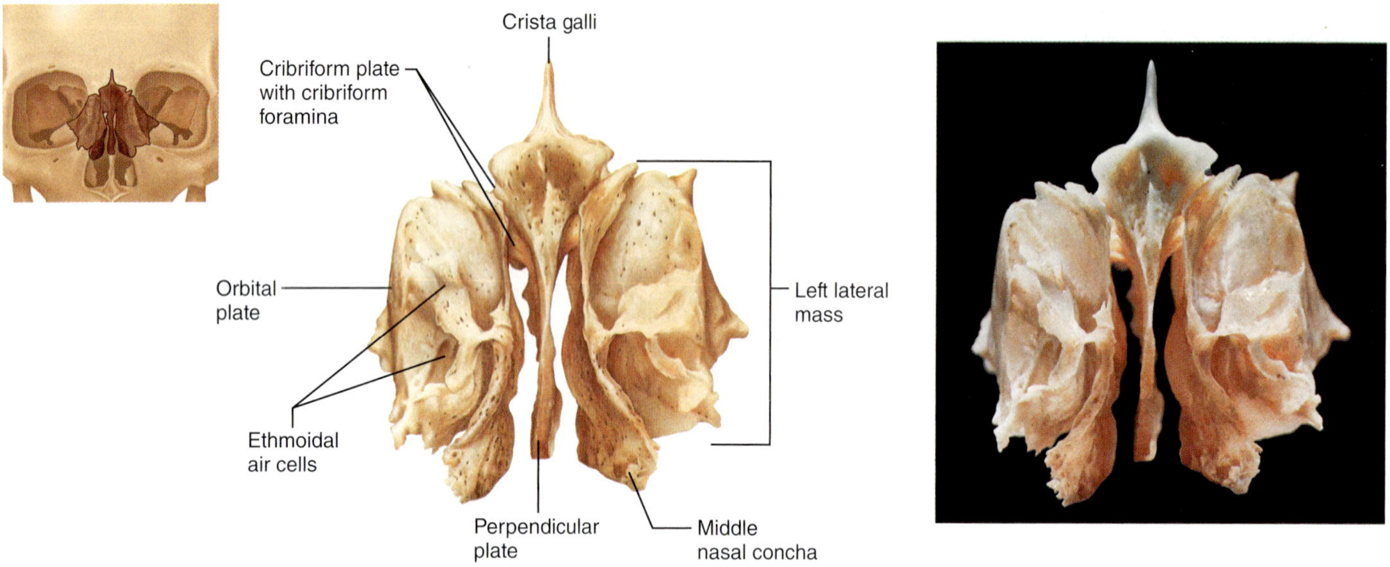

Figure 7.10 The ethmoid bone. Anterior view. (For related images, see *A Brief Atlas of the Human Body*, Figures 3 and 10.)

from the junction of the body and greater wings (Figure 7.9b). They anchor the pterygoid muscles, which are important in chewing.

A number of openings in the sphenoid bone are visible in Figures 7.7 and 7.9. The **optic canals** lie anterior to the sella turcica; they allow the optic nerves (cranial nerves II) to pass to the eyes. On each side of the sphenoid body is a crescent-shaped row of four openings. The anteriormost of these, the **superior orbital fissure**, is a long slit between the greater and lesser wings. It allows cranial nerves that control eye movements (III, IV, VI) to enter the orbit. This fissure is most obvious in an anterior view of the skull (Figure 7.4; see also Figure 7.9b). The **foramen rotundum** and **foramen ovale** (o-va′le) provide passageways for branches of cranial nerve V (the maxillary and mandibular nerves, respectively) to reach the face (Figure 7.7). The foramen rotundum is in the medial part of the greater wing and is usually oval, despite its name meaning "round opening." The foramen ovale, a large, oval foramen posterior to the foramen rotundum, is also visible in an inferior view of the skull (Figure 7.6). Posterolateral to the foramen ovale is the small **foramen spinosum** (Figure 7.7); it transmits the *middle meningeal artery*, which serves the internal faces of some cranial bones.

Ethmoid Bone

Like the temporal and sphenoid bones, the delicate **ethmoid bone** has a complex shape **(Figure 7.10)**. Lying between the sphenoid and the nasal bones of the face, it is the most deeply situated bone of the skull. It forms most of the bony area between the nasal cavity and the orbits.

The superior surface of the ethmoid is formed by the paired horizontal **cribriform plates** (krib′rĭ-form) (see also Figure 7.7), which help form the roof of the nasal cavities and the floor of the anterior cranial fossa. The cribriform plates are punctured by tiny holes (*cribr* = sieve) called *cribriform foramina* that allow the filaments of the olfactory nerves to pass from the smell receptors in the nasal cavities to the brain. Projecting superiorly between the cribriform plates is a triangular process called the **crista galli** (kris′tah gah′le; "rooster's comb"). The outermost covering of the brain (the dura mater) attaches to the crista galli and helps secure the brain in the cranial cavity.

The **perpendicular plate** of the ethmoid bone projects inferiorly in the median plane and forms the superior part of the nasal septum, which divides the nasal cavity into right and left halves (Figure 7.5c and d). Flanking the perpendicular plate on each side is a **lateral mass** riddled with sinuses called **ethmoidal air cells** (Figures 7.10 and 7.14), for which the bone itself is named (*ethmos* = sieve). Extending medially from the lateral masses, the delicately coiled **superior** and **middle nasal conchae** (kong′ke; *concha* = shell), named after the conch shells found on warm ocean beaches, protrude into the nasal cavity (Figures 7.10 and 7.13a). The lateral surfaces of the ethmoid's lateral masses are called **orbital plates** because they contribute to the medial walls of the orbits.

Sutural Bones

Sutural bones are tiny, irregularly shaped bones or bone clusters that occur within sutures, most often in the lambdoid suture (Figure 7.4b). Structurally unimportant, their number varies, and not all skulls exhibit them. The significance of these tiny bones is unknown.

Check Your Understanding

3. Look at Figure 7.4. Which of the skull bones illustrated in view (a) are cranial bones?
4. Which bone forms the crista galli?
5. Which skull bones house the external ear canals?
6. What bones abut one another at the sagittal suture? At the lambdoid suture?

For answers, see Appendix H.

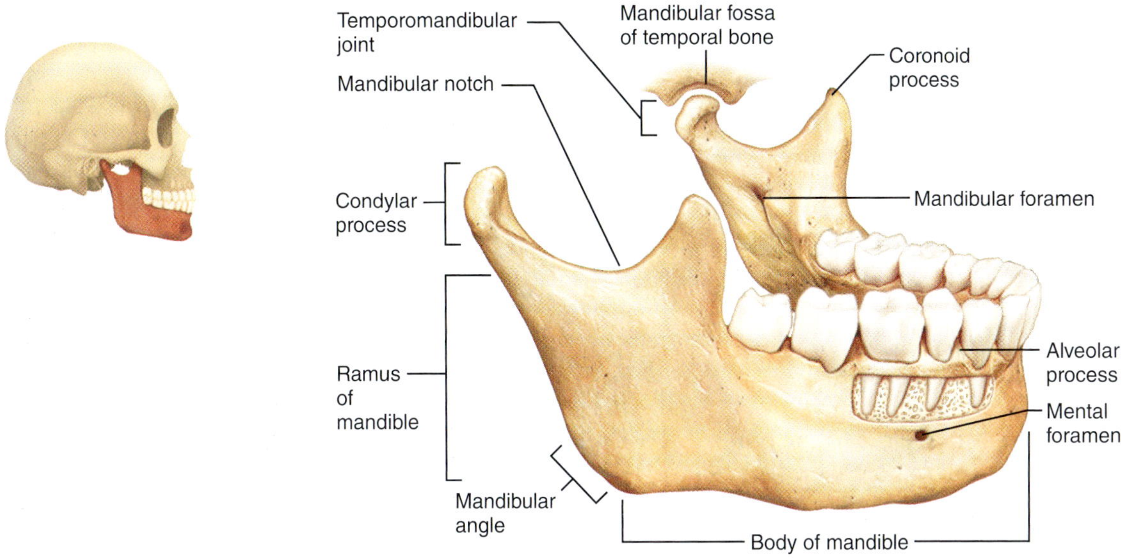

(a) Mandible, right lateral view

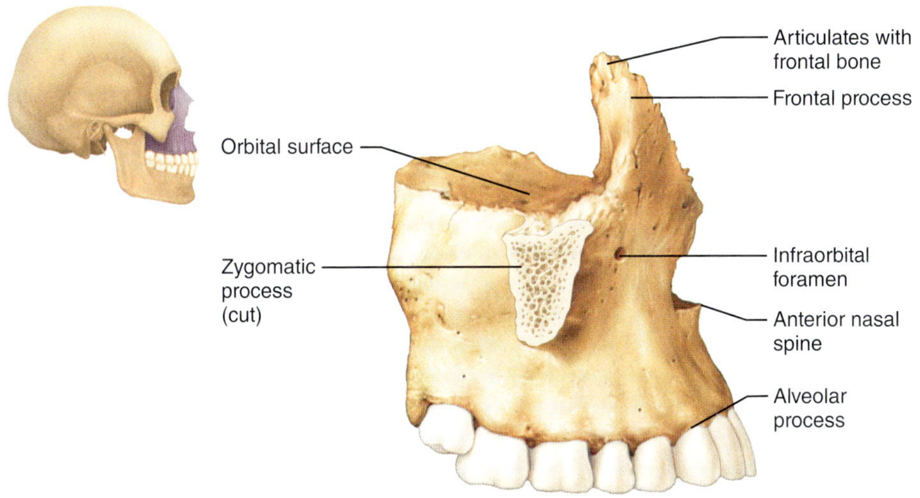

(b) Maxilla, right lateral view

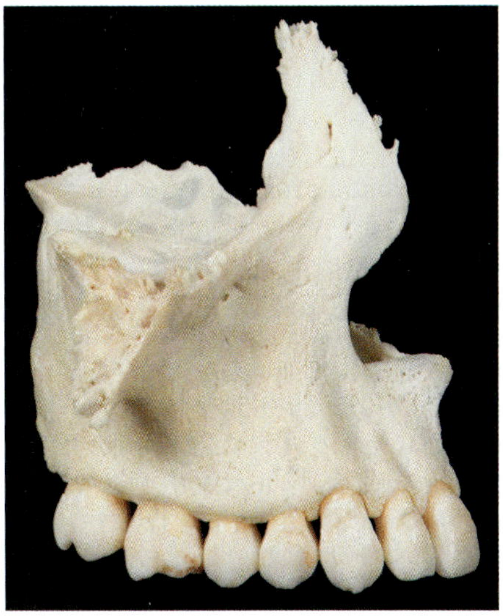

(c) Maxilla, photo of right lateral view

Figure 7.11 Detailed anatomy of the mandible and the maxilla. (For related images, see *A Brief Atlas of the Human Body,* Figures 11 and 12.)

Facial Bones

The facial skeleton is made up of 14 bones (see Figures 7.4a and 7.5a), of which only the mandible and the vomer are unpaired. The maxillae, zygomatics, nasals, lacrimals, palatines, and inferior nasal conchae are paired bones. As a rule, the facial skeleton of men is more elongated than that of women. Women's faces tend to be rounder and less angular.

Mandible

The U-shaped **mandible** (man′dĭ-bl), or lower jawbone (Figures 7.4a and 7.5, and **Figure 7.11a**), is the largest, strongest bone of the face. It has a body, which forms the chin, and two upright *rami* (*rami* = branches). Each ramus meets the body posteriorly at a **mandibular angle**. At the superior margin of each ramus are two processes separated by the **mandibular notch**. The anterior **coronoid process** (kor′o-noid; "crown-shaped") is an insertion point for the large temporalis muscle that elevates the lower jaw during chewing. The posterior **condylar process** articulates with the mandibular fossa of the temporal bone, forming the *temporomandibular joint* on the same side.

The mandibular **body** anchors the lower teeth. Its superior border, called the **alveolar process** (al-ve′o-lar), contains the sockets (*dental alveoli*) in which the teeth are embedded. In the midline of the mandibular body is a slight ridge, the **mandibular symphysis** (sim′fih-sis), indicating where the two mandibular bones fused during infancy (Figure 7.4a).

Large **mandibular foramina**, one on the medial surface of each ramus, permit the nerves responsible for tooth sensation to pass to the teeth in the lower jaw. Dentists inject lidocaine into these foramina to prevent pain while working on the lower teeth. The **mental foramina**, openings on the lateral aspects of the mandibular body, allow blood vessels and nerves to pass to the skin of the chin (*ment* = chin) and lower lip.

Maxillary Bones

The **maxillary bones**, or **maxillae** (mak-sil′le; "jaws") (Figures 7.4 to 7.6 and 7.11b and c), are fused medially. They form the upper jaw and the central portion of the facial skeleton. All facial bones except the mandible articulate with the maxillae. Hence, the maxillae are considered the keystone bones of the facial skeleton.

The maxillae carry the upper teeth in their **alveolar processes**. Just inferior to the nose the maxillae meet medially, forming the pointed **anterior nasal spine** at their junction. The **palatine processes** (pă′lah-tīn) of the maxillae project posteriorly from the alveolar processes and fuse medially at the *intermaxillary suture*, forming the anterior two-thirds of the hard palate, or bony roof of the mouth (Figures 7.5c and d and 7.6). Just posterior to the teeth is a midline foramen, called the **incisive fossa**, which serves as a passageway for blood vessels and nerves.

The **frontal processes** extend superiorly to the frontal bone, forming part of the lateral aspects of the bridge of the nose (Figures 7.4a and 7.11b). The regions that flank the nasal cavity laterally contain the **maxillary sinuses** (see Figure 7.14), the largest of the paranasal sinuses. They extend from the orbits to the roots of the upper teeth. Laterally, the maxillae articulate with the zygomatic bones via their **zygomatic processes**.

The **inferior orbital fissure** is located deep within the orbit (Figure 7.4a) at the junction of the maxilla with the greater wing of the sphenoid. It permits the zygomatic nerve, the maxillary nerve (a branch of cranial nerve V), and blood vessels to pass to the face. Just below the eye socket on each side is an **infraorbital foramen** that allows the infraorbital nerve (a continuation of the maxillary nerve) and artery to reach the face.

Zygomatic Bones

The irregularly shaped **zygomatic bones** (Figures 7.4a, 7.5a, and 7.6) are commonly called the cheekbones (*zygoma* = cheekbone). They articulate with the zygomatic processes of the temporal bones posteriorly, the zygomatic processes of the frontal bone superiorly, and with the zygomatic processes of the maxillae anteriorly. The zygomatic bones form the prominences of the cheeks and part of the inferolateral margins of the orbits.

Nasal Bones

The thin, basically rectangular **nasal bones** (na′zal) are fused medially, forming the bridge of the nose (Figures 7.4a and 7.5a). They articulate with the frontal bone superiorly, the maxillary bones laterally, and the perpendicular plate of the ethmoid bone posteriorly. Inferiorly they attach to the cartilages that form most of the skeleton of the external nose.

Lacrimal Bones

The delicate, fingernail-shaped **lacrimal bones** (lak′rĭ-mal) contribute to the medial walls of each orbit (Figures 7.4a and 7.5a). They articulate with the frontal bone superiorly, the ethmoid bone posteriorly, and the maxillae anteriorly. Each lacrimal bone contains a deep groove that helps form a **lacrimal fossa**. The lacrimal fossa houses the *lacrimal sac*, part of the passageway that allows tears to drain from the eye surface into the nasal cavity (*lacrima* = tears).

Palatine Bones

Each L-shaped **palatine bone** is fashioned from two bony plates, the *horizontal* and *perpendicular* (see Figures 7.13a and 7.6a), and has three important articular processes, the *pyramidal, sphenoidal*, and *orbital*. The **horizontal plates**, joined at the median palatine suture, complete the posterior portion of the hard palate. The superiorly projecting **perpendicular (vertical) plates** form part of the posterolateral walls of the nasal cavity and a small part of the orbits.

Vomer

The slender, plow-shaped **vomer** (vo′mer; "plow") lies in the nasal cavity, where it forms part of the nasal septum (see Figures 7.4a and 7.13b). It is described below in connection with the nasal cavity.

Inferior Nasal Conchae

The paired **inferior nasal conchae** are thin, curved bones in the nasal cavity. They project medially from the lateral walls of the nasal cavity, just inferior to the middle nasal conchae of the ethmoid bone (see Figures 7.4a and 7.13a). They are the largest of the three pairs of conchae and, like the others, they form part of the lateral walls of the nasal cavity.

☑ Check Your Understanding

7. Women with prominent (high) cheekbones are often considered beautiful by the modeling industry. What bones are the "cheekbones"?
8. Johnny was vigorously exercising the only joints in the skull that are freely movable. What would you guess he was doing?
9. What bones are the keystone bones of the facial skeleton?

For answers, see Appendix H.

Special Characteristics of the Orbits and Nasal Cavity

✓ Define the bony boundaries of the orbits, nasal cavity, and paranasal sinuses.

Two restricted skull regions, the orbits and the nasal cavity, are formed from an amazing number of bones. Even though we have already described the individual bones forming these structures, we give a brief summary here to pull the parts together.

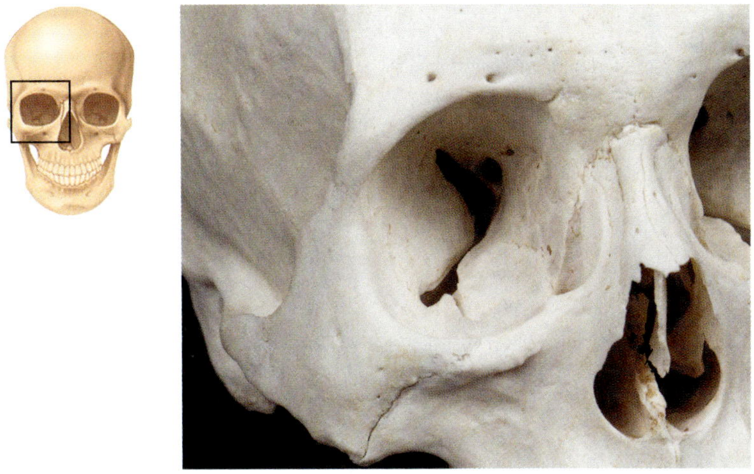

(a) Photograph, right orbit

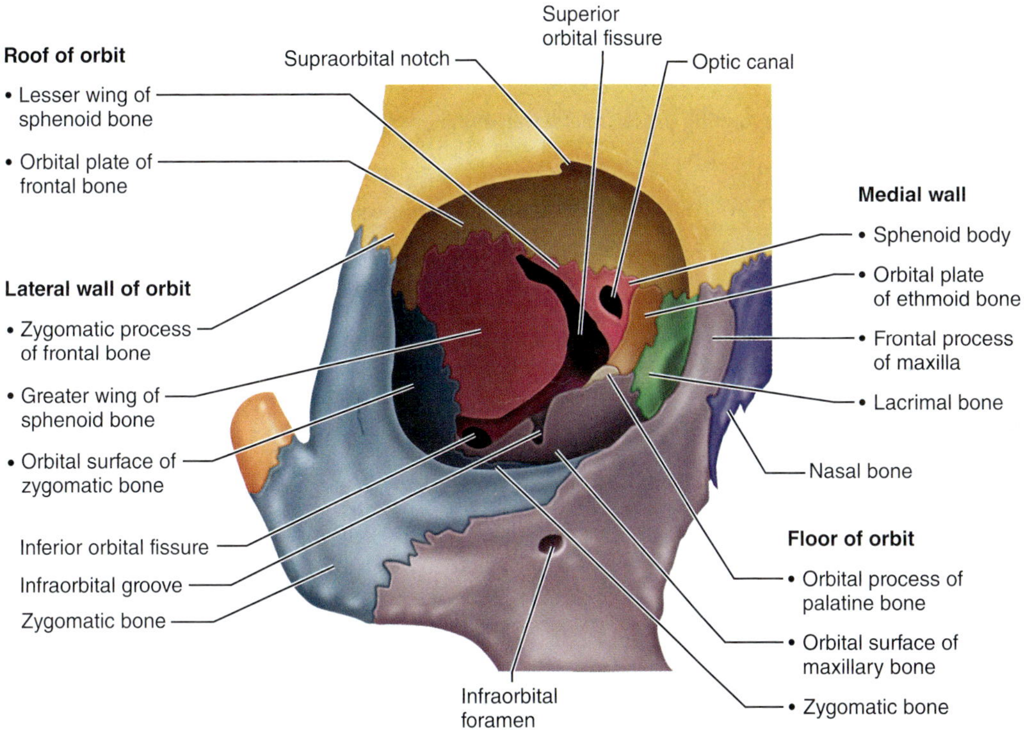

(b) Contribution of each of the seven bones forming the right orbit

Figure 7.12 Bones that form the orbits. (For a related image, see *A Brief Atlas of the Human Body,* Figure 14.)

The Orbits

The cone-shaped **orbits** are bony cavities in which the eyes are firmly encased and cushioned by fatty tissue. The muscles that move the eyes and the tear-producing lacrimal glands are also housed in the orbits. The walls of each orbit are formed by parts of seven bones—the frontal, sphenoid, zygomatic, maxilla, palatine, lacrimal, and ethmoid bones. Their relationships are shown in **Figure 7.12**. Also seen in the orbits are the superior and inferior orbital fissures and the optic canals, described earlier.

The Nasal Cavity

The **nasal cavity** is constructed of bone and hyaline cartilage **(Figure 7.13)**. The *roof* of the nasal cavity is formed by the cribriform plates of the ethmoid. The *lateral walls* are largely shaped by the superior and middle conchae of the ethmoid bone, the perpendicular plates of the palatine bones, and the inferior nasal conchae. The depressions under cover of the conchae on the lateral walls are called *meatuses* (*meatus* = passage), so there are superior, middle, and inferior meatuses. The *floor* of the nasal cavity is formed by the palatine processes of the

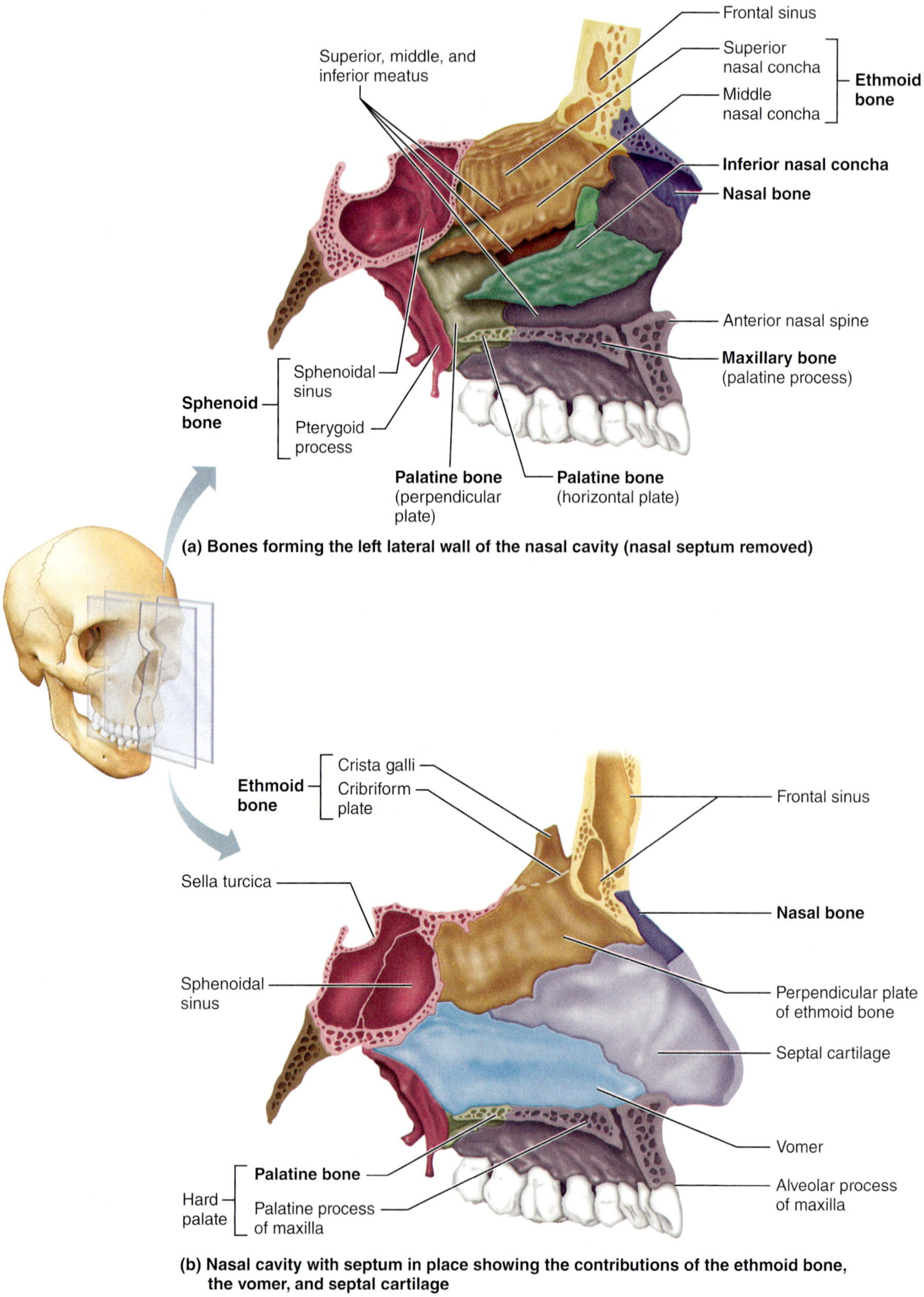

Figure 7.13 Bones of the nasal cavity. (For a related image, see *A Brief Atlas of the Human Body*, Figure 15.)

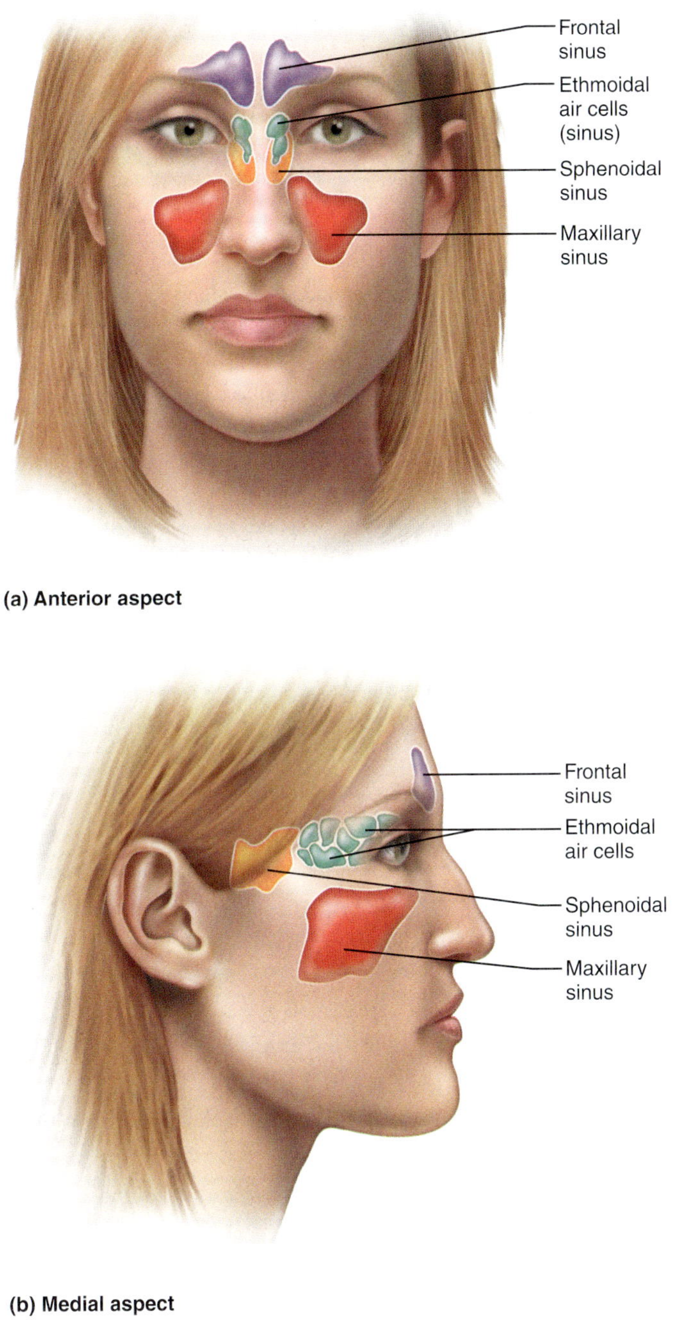

Figure 7.14 **Paranasal sinuses.**

maxillae and the palatine bones. The nasal cavity is divided into right and left parts by the *nasal septum*. The bony portion of the septum is formed by the vomer inferiorly and the perpendicular plate of the ethmoid bone superiorly (Figure 7.13b). A sheet of cartilage called the *septal cartilage* completes the septum anteriorly.

The nasal septum and conchae are covered with a mucus-secreting mucosa that moistens and warms the entering air and helps cleanse it of debris. The scroll-shaped conchae increase the turbulence of air flowing through the nasal cavity. This swirling forces more of the inhaled air into contact with the warm, damp mucosa and encourages trapping of airborne particles (dust, pollen, bacteria) in the sticky mucus.

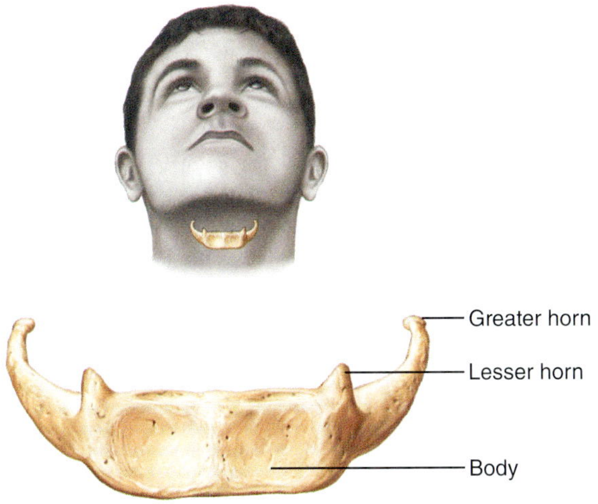

Figure 7.15 **The hyoid bone, anterior view.**

Paranasal Sinuses

Five skull bones—the frontal, sphenoid, ethmoid, and paired maxillary bones—contain mucosa-lined, air-filled sinuses that give them a rather moth-eaten appearance in an X-ray image. These particular sinuses are called **paranasal sinuses** because they cluster around the nasal cavity **(Figure 7.14)**.

Small openings connect the sinuses to the nasal cavity and act as "two-way streets": Air enters the sinuses from the nasal cavity, and mucus formed by the sinus mucosae drains into the nasal cavity. The mucosa of the sinuses also helps to warm and humidify inspired air. The paranasal sinuses lighten the skull and enhance the resonance of the voice.

☑ Check Your Understanding

10. What bones contain the paranasal sinuses?
11. The perpendicular plates of the palatine bones and the superior and middle conchae of the ethmoid bone form a substantial part of the nasal cavity walls. Which bone forms the roof of that cavity?
12. What bone forms the bulk of the orbit floor and what sense organ is found in the orbit of a living person?

For answers, see Appendix H.

The Hyoid Bone

Though not really part of the skull, the **hyoid bone** (hi′oid; "U-shaped") lies just inferior to the mandible in the anterior neck, and looks like a miniature version of it **(Figure 7.15)**. The hyoid bone is unique in that it is the only bone of the body that does not articulate directly with any other bone. Instead, it is anchored by the narrow *stylohyoid ligaments* to the styloid processes of the temporal bones. Horseshoe-shaped, with a body and two pairs of *horns*, or *cornua*, the hyoid bone acts as a movable base for the tongue. Its body and greater horns are attachment points for neck muscles that raise and lower the larynx during swallowing and speech.

(Text continues on p. 218.)

Table 7.1 Bones of the Skull

BONE COLOR CODE*	COMMENTS	IMPORTANT MARKINGS
Cranial Bones		
Frontal (1) (Figures 7.4a, 7.5, and 7.7)	Forms forehead, superior part of orbits, and most of the anterior cranial fossa; contains sinuses	**Supraorbital foramina (notches):** allow the supraorbital arteries and nerves to pass
Parietal (2) (Figures 7.4 and 7.5)	Form most of the superior and lateral aspects of the skull	
Occipital (1) (Figures 7.4b, 7.5, 7.6, and 7.7)	Forms posterior aspect and most of the base of the skull	**Foramen magnum:** allows passage of the spinal cord from the brain stem to the vertebral canal **Hypoglossal canals:** allow passage of the hypoglossal nerves (cranial nerve XII) **Occipital condyles:** articulate with the atlas (first vertebra) **External occipital protuberance** and **nuchal lines:** sites of muscle attachment **External occipital crest:** attachment site of ligamentum nuchae
Temporal (2) (Figures 7.5, 7.6, 7.7, and 7.8)	Form inferolateral aspects of the skull and contribute to the middle cranial fossa; have squamous, tympanic, and petrous parts	**Zygomatic process:** helps to form the zygomatic arch, which forms the prominence of the cheek **Mandibular fossa:** articular point of the condylar process of the mandible **External acoustic meatus:** canal leading from the external ear to the eardrum **Styloid process:** attachment site for several neck muscles and for a ligament to the hyoid bone **Mastoid process:** attachment site for several neck and tongue muscles **Stylomastoid foramen:** allows cranial nerve VII (facial nerve) to pass **Jugular foramen:** allows passage of the internal jugular vein and cranial nerves IX, X, and XI **Carotid canal:** allows passage of the internal carotid artery
Sphenoid (1) (Figures 7.4a, 7.5, 7.6, 7.7, and 7.9)	Keystone of the cranium; contributes to the middle cranial fossa and orbits; main parts are the body, greater wings, lesser wings, and pterygoid processes	**Sella turcica:** hypophyseal fossa portion is the seat of the pituitary gland **Optic canals:** allow passage of optic nerves (cranial nerves II) and the ophthalmic arteries **Superior orbital fissures:** allow passage of cranial nerves III, IV, VI, part of V (ophthalmic division), and ophthalmic vein **Foramen rotundum (2):** allows passage of the maxillary division of cranial nerve V **Foramen ovale (2):** allows passage of the mandibular division of cranial nerve V **Foramen spinosum (2):** allows passage of the middle meningeal artery

Table 7.1 *(continued)*

BONE COLOR CODE*	COMMENTS	IMPORTANT MARKINGS
Ethmoid (1) (Figures 7.4a, 7.5, 7.7, 7.10, and 7.14)	Helps to form the anterior cranial fossa; forms part of the nasal septum and the lateral walls and roof of the nasal cavity; contributes to the medial wall of the orbit	**Crista galli:** attachment point for the falx cerebri, a dural membrane fold **Cribriform plates:** allow passage of filaments of the olfactory nerves (cranial nerve I) **Superior** and **middle nasal conchae:** form part of lateral walls of nasal cavity; increase turbulence of air flow
Auditory ossicles (malleus, incus, and stapes) (2 each)	Found in middle ear cavity; involved in sound transmission; see Figure 15.24b, p. 571	
Facial Bones		
Mandible (1) (Figures 7.4a, 7.5, and 7.11a)	The lower jaw	**Coronoid processes:** insertion points for the temporalis muscles **Condylar processes:** articulate with the temporal bones in the temporomandibular joints of the jaw **Mandibular symphysis:** medial fusion point of the mandibular bones **Dental alveoli:** sockets for the teeth **Mandibular foramina:** permit the inferior alveolar nerves to pass **Mental foramina:** allow blood vessels and nerves to pass to the chin and lower lip
Maxilla (2) (Figures 7.4a, 7.5, 7.6, and 7.11b)	Keystone bones of the face; form the upper jaw and parts of the hard palate, orbits, and nasal cavity walls	**Dental alveoli:** sockets for teeth **Zygomatic processes:** help form the zygomatic arches **Palatine processes:** form the anterior hard palate; meet medially in intermaxillary suture **Frontal process:** forms part of lateral aspect of bridge of nose **Incisive fossa:** permits blood vessels and nerves to pass through anterior hard palate (fused palatine processes) **Inferior orbital fissure:** permits maxillary branch of cranial nerve V, the zygomatic nerve, and blood vessels to pass **Infraorbital foramen:** allows passage of infraorbital nerve to skin of face
Zygomatic (2) (Figures 7.4a, 7.5a, and 7.6a)	Form the cheeks and part of the orbits	
Nasal (2) (Figures 7.4a and 7.5)	Form the bridge of the nose	
Lacrimal (2) (Figures 7.4a and 7.5a)	Form part of the medial orbit walls	**Lacrimal fossa:** houses the lacrimal sac, which helps to drain tears into the nasal cavity
Palatine (2) (Figures 7.5c, 7.6a, and 7.13)	Form posterior part of the hard palate and a small part of nasal cavity and orbit walls	**Median palatine suture:** medial fusion point of the horizontal plates of the palatine bones, which form the posterior part of the hard palate
Vomer (1) (Figures 7.4a and 7.13b)	Inferior part of the nasal septum	
Inferior nasal concha (2) (Figures 7.4a and 7.13a)	Form part of the lateral walls of the nasal cavity	

*The color code beside each bone name corresponds to the bone's color in Figures 7.4 to 7.13. The number in parentheses ( ) following the bone name indicates the total number of such bones in the body.

The Vertebral Column

General Characteristics

- ✓ Describe the structure of the vertebral column, list its components, and describe its curvatures.
- ✓ Indicate a common function of the spinal curvatures and the intervertebral discs.

Some people think of the **vertebral column** as a rigid supporting rod, but this is inaccurate. Also called the **spine** or **spinal column**, the vertebral column consists of 26 irregular bones connected in such a way that a flexible, curved structure results **(Figure 7.16)**.

Serving as the axial support of the trunk, the spine extends from the skull to the pelvis, where it transmits the weight of the trunk to the lower limbs. It also surrounds and protects the delicate spinal cord and provides attachment points for the ribs and for the muscles of the back and neck.

In the fetus and infant, the vertebral column consists of 33 separate bones, or **vertebrae** (ver′tě-bre). Inferiorly, nine of these eventually fuse to form two composite bones, the sacrum and the tiny coccyx. The remaining 24 bones persist as individual vertebrae separated by intervertebral discs.

Regions and Curvatures

The vertebral column is about 70 cm (28 inches) long in an average adult and has five major regions (Figure 7.16). The seven vertebrae of the neck are the **cervical vertebrae** (ser′vĭ-kal), the next 12 are the **thoracic vertebrae** (tho-ras′ik), and the five supporting the lower back are the **lumbar vertebrae** (lum′bar). Remembering common meal times—7 AM, 12 noon, and 5 PM—will help you recall the number of bones in these three regions of the spine. The vertebrae become progressively larger from the cervical to the lumbar region, as they must support greater and greater weight.

Inferior to the lumbar vertebrae is the **sacrum** (sa′krum), which articulates with the hip bones of the pelvis. The terminus of the vertebral column is the tiny **coccyx** (kok′siks).

All of us have the same number of cervical vertebrae. Variations in numbers of vertebrae in other regions occur in about 5% of people.

When you view the vertebral column from the side, you can see the four curvatures that give it its S, or sinusoid, shape. The **cervical** and **lumbar curvatures** are concave posteriorly; the **thoracic** and **sacral curvatures** are convex posteriorly. These curvatures increase the resilience and flexibility of the spine, allowing it to function like a spring rather than a rigid rod.

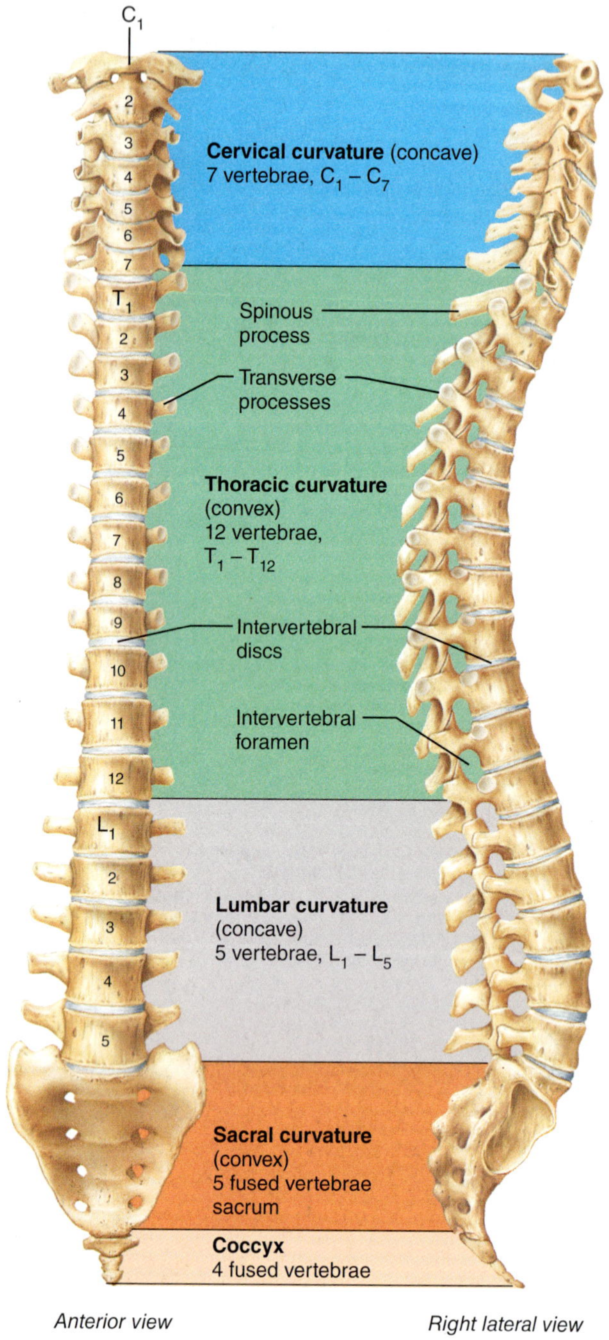

Figure 7.16 The vertebral column. Notice the curvatures in the lateral view. (The terms convex and concave refer to the curvature of the posterior aspect of the vertebral column.) (For a related image, see *A Brief Atlas of the Human Body*, Figure 17.)

Homeostatic Imbalance 7.2

There are several types of abnormal spinal curvatures **(Figure 7.17)**. Some are congenital (present at birth); others result from disease, poor posture, or unequal muscle pull on the spine. *Scoliosis* (sko″le-o′sis), literally, "twisted disease," is an abnormal *lateral* curvature that occurs most often in the thoracic region. It is quite common during late childhood, particularly in girls, for some unknown reason. Other, more severe cases result from abnormal vertebral structure, lower limbs of unequal length, or muscle paralysis. If muscles on one side of the body are nonfunctional, those of the opposite side exert an unopposed pull on the spine and force it out of alignment. Scoliosis is treated (with body braces or surgically) before growth ends to prevent permanent deformity and breathing difficulties due to a compressed lung.

Kyphosis (ki-fo′sis), or hunchback, is a *dorsally* exaggerated *thoracic* curvature. It is particularly common in elderly people because of osteoporosis, but may also reflect tuberculosis of the spine, rickets, or osteomalacia.

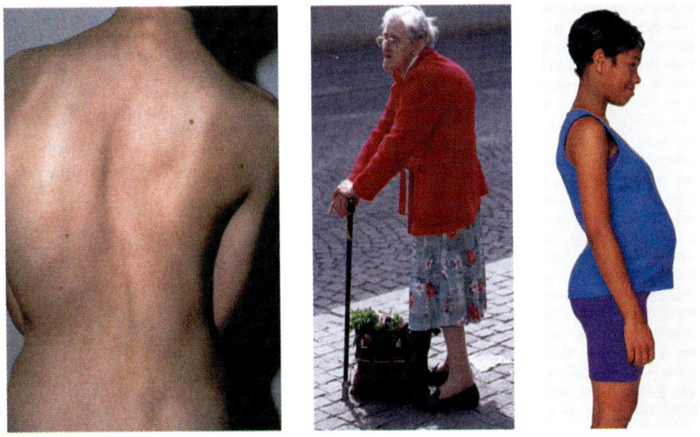

(a) Scoliosis (b) Kyphosis (c) Lordosis

Figure 7.17 Abnormal spinal curvatures.

Lordosis, or swayback, is an accentuated *lumbar* curvature. It, too, can result from spinal tuberculosis or osteomalacia. Temporary lordosis is common in those carrying a large load up front, such as men with "potbellies" and pregnant women. In an attempt to preserve their center of gravity, these individuals automatically throw back their shoulders, accentuating their lumbar curvature. +

Ligaments

Like a tall, tremulous TV transmitting tower, the vertebral column cannot possibly stand upright by itself. It must be held in place by an elaborate system of cable-like supports. In the case of the vertebral column, straplike ligaments and the trunk muscles assume this role.

The major supporting ligaments are the **anterior** and **posterior longitudinal ligaments** (Figure 7.18). These run as continuous bands down the front and back surfaces of the vertebrae from the neck to the sacrum. The broad anterior ligament is strongly attached to both the bony vertebrae and the discs. Along with its supporting role, it prevents hyperextension of the spine (bending too far backward). The posterior ligament, which resists hyperflexion of the spine (bending too sharply forward), is narrow and relatively weak. It attaches only to the discs. However, the **ligamentum flavum**, which connects adjacent vertebrae, contains elastic connective tissue and is especially strong. It stretches as we bend forward and then recoils when we resume an erect posture. Short ligaments connect each vertebra to those immediately above and below.

Intervertebral Discs

Each **intervertebral disc** is a cushionlike pad composed of two parts. The inner gelatinous **nucleus pulposus** (pul-po′sus; "pulp") acts like a rubber ball, giving the disc its elasticity and compressibility. Surrounding the nucleus pulposus is a strong collar composed of collagen fibers superficially and fibrocartilage internally, the **anulus fibrosus** (an′u-lus fi-bro′sus; "ring of fibers") (Figure 7.18a, c). The anulus fibrosus limits the expansion of the nucleus pulposus when the spine is compressed. It also acts like a woven strap to bind successive vertebrae together, withstands twisting forces, and resists tension in the spine.

Sandwiched between the bodies of neighboring vertebrae, the intervertebral discs act as shock absorbers during walking, jumping, and running. They allow the spine to flex and extend, and to a lesser extent to bend laterally. At points of compression, the discs flatten and bulge out a bit between the vertebrae. The discs are thickest in the lumbar and cervical regions, which enhances the flexibility of these regions.

Collectively the discs account for about 25% of the height of the vertebral column. They flatten somewhat during the course of the day, so we are always a few millimeters shorter at night than when we awake in the morning.

Homeostatic Imbalance 7.3

Severe or sudden physical trauma to the spine—for example, from bending forward while lifting a heavy object—may result in herniation of one or more discs. A **herniated** (**prolapsed**)

7

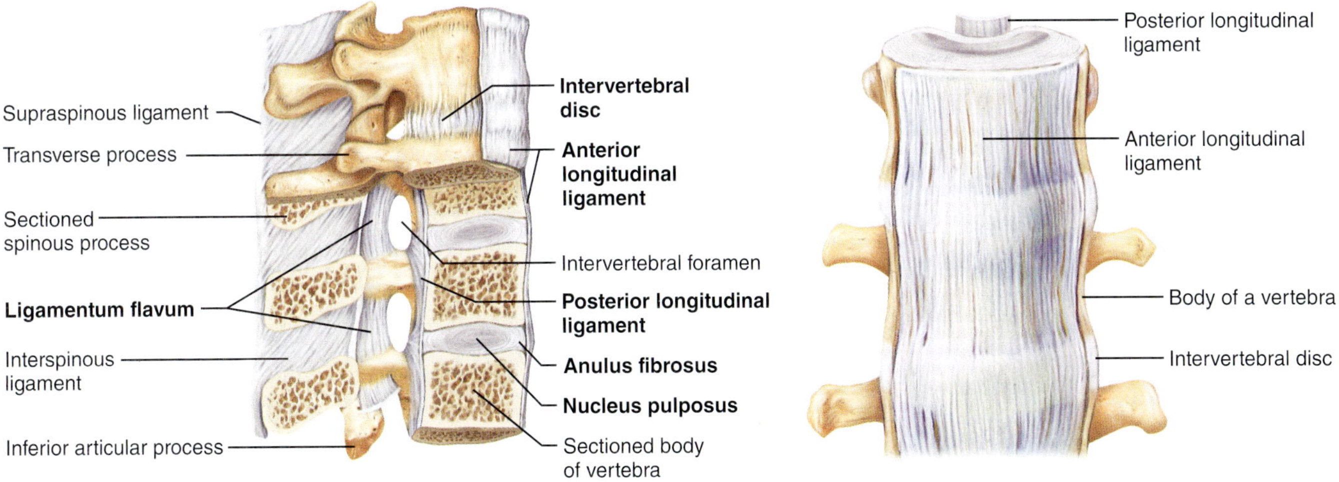

(a) Median section of three vertebrae, illustrating the composition of the discs and the ligaments

(b) Anterior view of part of the spinal column, showing the anterior longitudinal ligament

Figure 7.18 Ligaments and fibrocartilage discs uniting the vertebrae.

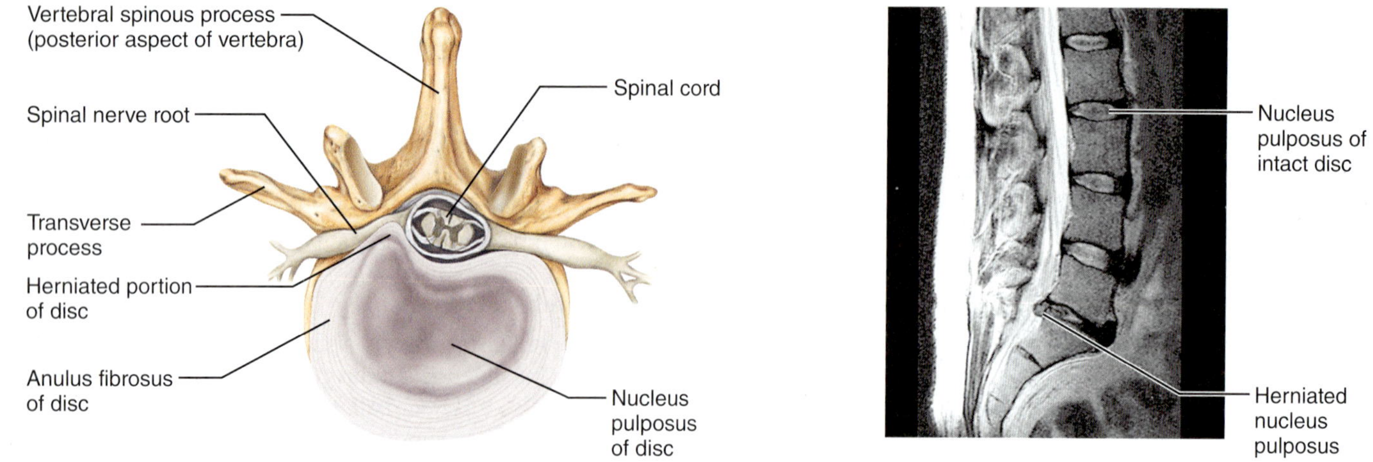

(c) Superior view of a herniated intervertebral disc

(d) MRI of lumbar region of vertebral column in sagittal section showing herniated disc

Figure 7.18 *(continued)* **Ligaments and fibrocartilage discs uniting the vertebrae.**

disc (commonly called a *slipped disc*) usually involves rupture of the anulus fibrosus followed by protrusion of the spongy nucleus pulposus through the anulus (Figure 7.18c, d). If the protrusion presses on the spinal cord or on spinal nerves exiting from the cord, numbness or excruciating pain may result.

Herniated discs are generally treated with moderate exercise, massage, heat therapy, and painkillers. If this fails, the protruding disc may have to be removed surgically and a bone graft done to fuse the adjoining vertebrae. For those preferring to avoid general anesthesia, part of the disc can be vaporized with a laser in an outpatient procedure called percutaneous laser disc decompression that takes only 30 to 40 minutes. If necessary, tears in the anulus can be sealed by electrothermal means at the same time. The patient leaves with only an adhesive bandage to mark the spot. ✚

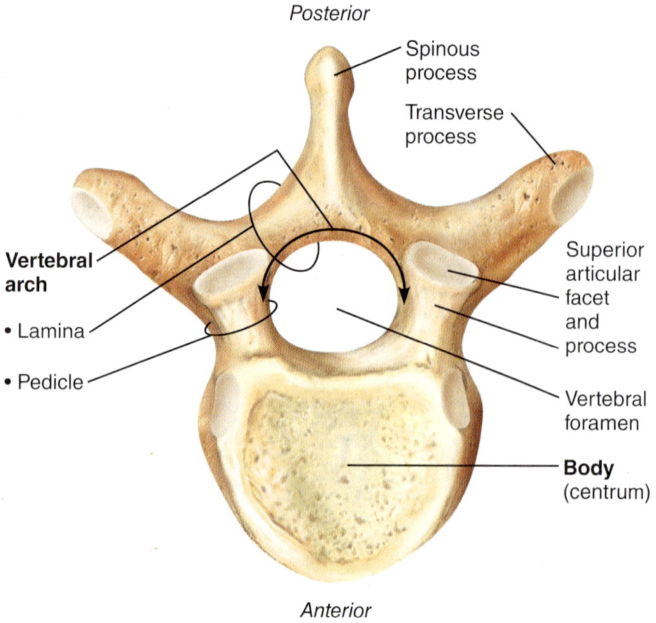

Figure 7.19 Typical vertebral structures. Superior view of a thoracic vertebra. Only bone features are illustrated in this and subsequent bone figures in this chapter. Articular cartilage is not depicted.

☑ Check Your Understanding

13. What are the five major regions of the vertebral column?
14. In which two of these regions is the vertebral column concave posteriorly?
15. Besides the spinal curvatures, which skeletal elements help to make the vertebral column flexible?

For answers, see Appendix H.

General Structure of Vertebrae

✓ Discuss the structure of a typical vertebra and describe regional features of cervical, thoracic, and lumbar vertebrae.

All vertebrae have a common structural pattern **(Figure 7.19)**. Each vertebra consists of a **body**, or **centrum**, anteriorly and a **vertebral arch** posteriorly. The disc-shaped body is the weight-bearing region. Together, the body and vertebral arch enclose an opening called the **vertebral foramen**. Successive vertebral foramina of the articulated vertebrae form the long **vertebral canal**, through which the spinal cord passes.

The vertebral arch is a composite structure formed by two pedicles and two laminae. The **pedicles** (ped′ĭ-kelz; "little feet"), short bony pillars projecting posteriorly from the vertebral body, form the sides of the arch. The **laminae** (lam′ĭ-ne), flattened plates that fuse in the median plane, complete the arch posteriorly. The pedicles have notches on their superior and inferior borders, providing lateral openings between adjacent vertebrae called **intervertebral foramina** (see Figure 7.16). The spinal nerves issuing from the spinal cord pass through these foramina.

Seven processes project from the vertebral arch. The **spinous process** is a median posterior projection arising at the junction of the two laminae. A **transverse process** extends laterally from each side of the vertebral arch. The spinous and transverse processes are attachment sites for muscles that move the vertebral column and for ligaments that stabilize it. The paired **superior** and **inferior articular processes** protrude superiorly and inferiorly,

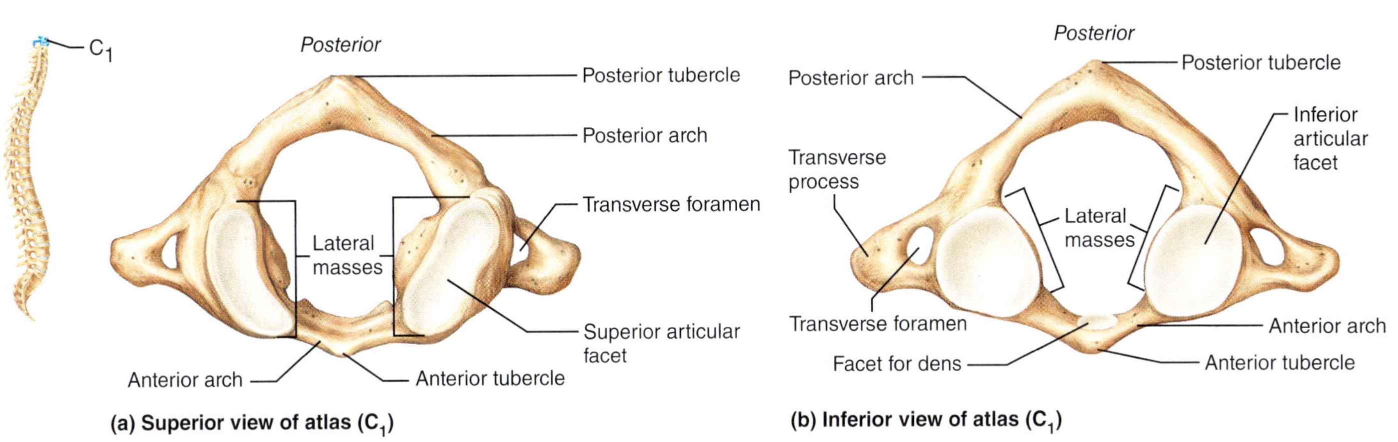

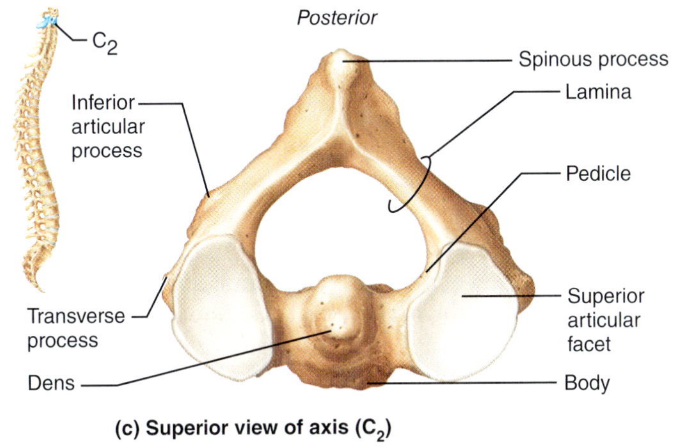

Figure 7.20 The first and second cervical vertebrae. (For a related image, see *A Brief Atlas of the Human Body*, Figure 18.)

respectively, from the pedicle-lamina junctions. The smooth joint surfaces of the articular processes, called *facets* ("little faces"), are covered with hyaline cartilage. The inferior articular processes of each vertebra form movable joints with the superior articular processes of the vertebra immediately below. Thus, successive vertebrae join both at their bodies and at their articular processes.

Regional Vertebral Characteristics

Beyond their common structural features, vertebrae exhibit variations that allow different regions of the spine to perform slightly different functions and movements. In general, movements that can occur between vertebrae are (1) flexion and extension (anterior bending and posterior straightening of the spine), (2) lateral flexion (bending the *upper body* to the right or left), and (3) rotation (in which vertebrae rotate on one another in the longitudinal axis of the spine). The regional vertebral characteristics described in this section are illustrated and summarized in **Table 7.2** on p. 223.

Cervical Vertebrae

The seven cervical vertebrae, identified as C_1–C_7, are the smallest, lightest vertebrae (see Figure 7.16). The first two (C_1 and C_2) are unusual and we will skip them for the moment. The "typical" cervical vertebrae (C_3–C_7) have the following distinguishing features (see Figure 7.21 and Table 7.2):

- The body is oval—wider from side to side than in the anteroposterior dimension.
- Except in C_7, the spinous process is short, projects directly back, and is *bifid* (bi′fid), or split at its tip.
- The vertebral foramen is large and generally triangular.
- Each transverse process contains a **transverse foramen** through which the vertebral arteries pass to service the brain.

The spinous process of C_7 is not bifid and is much larger than those of the other cervical vertebrae (see Figure 7.21a). Because its spinous process is palpable through the skin, C_7 can be used as a landmark for counting the vertebrae and is called the **vertebra prominens** ("prominent vertebra").

The first two cervical vertebrae, the atlas and the axis, are somewhat more robust than the typical cervical vertebra. They have no intervertebral disc between them, and they are highly modified, reflecting their special functions. The **atlas** (C_1) has no body and no spinous process **(Figure 7.20a and b)**. Essentially, it is a ring of bone consisting of *anterior* and *posterior arches* and a *lateral mass* on each side. Each lateral mass has articular facets on both its superior and inferior surfaces. The superior articular facets receive the occipital condyles of the skull—they "carry" the skull, just as Atlas supported the heavens in Greek mythology. These joints allow you to nod "yes." The inferior articular facets form joints with the axis (C_2) below.

The **axis**, which has a body and the other typical vertebral processes, is not as specialized as the atlas. In fact, its only unusual feature is the knoblike **dens** (denz; "tooth") projecting superiorly from its body. The dens is actually the "missing" body of the atlas, which fuses with the axis during embryonic development. Cradled in the anterior arch of the atlas by the transverse ligament **(Figure 7.21a)**, the dens acts as a pivot for the rotation of the atlas. Hence, this joint allows you to rotate your head from side to side to indicate "no."

Thoracic Vertebrae

The 12 thoracic vertebrae (T_1–T_{12}) all articulate with the ribs (see Table 7.2, Figure 7.16, and Figure 7.21b). The first looks much like C_7, and the last four show a progression toward

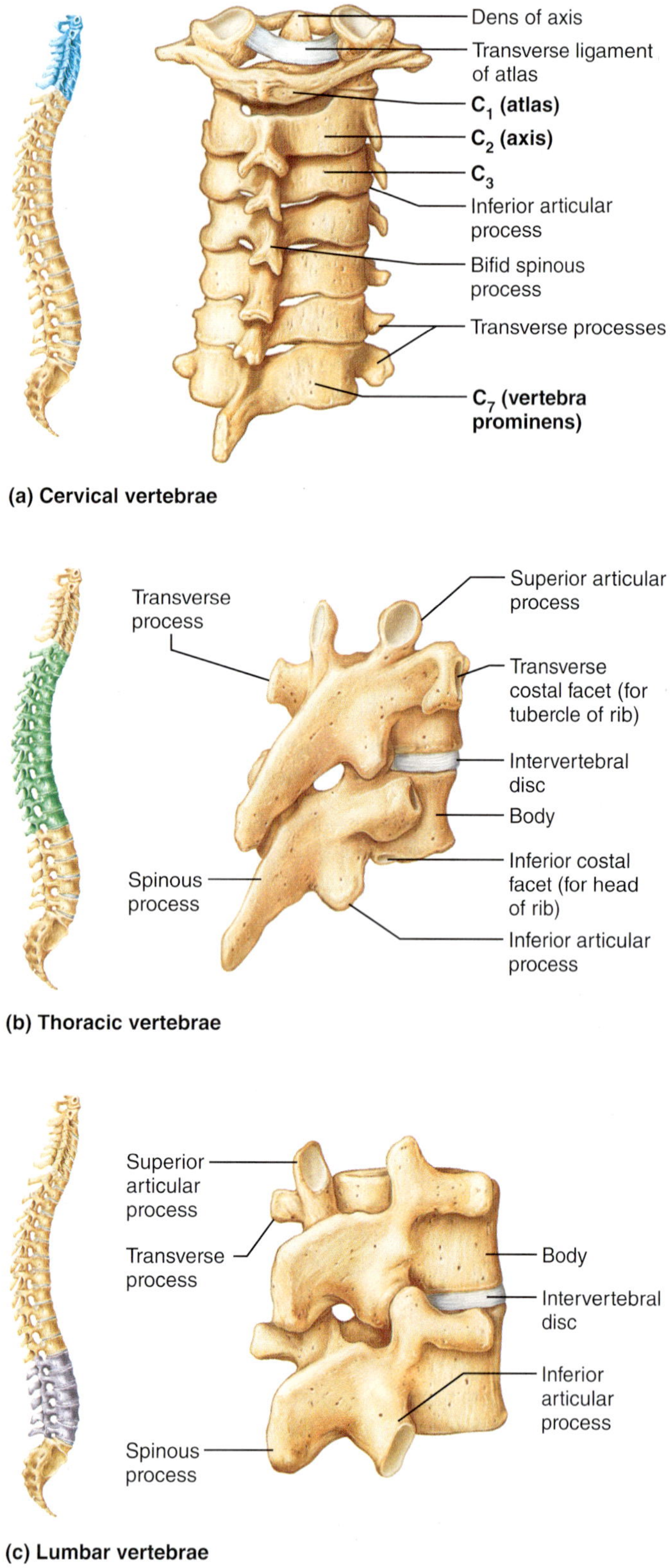

Figure 7.21 Posterolateral views of articulated vertebrae. Notice the bulbous tip on the spinous process of C_7, the vertebra prominens. (For a related image, see *A Brief Atlas of the Human Body*, Figures 19, 20, and 21.)

lumbar vertebral structure. The thoracic vertebrae increase in size from the first to the last. Unique characteristics of these vertebrae include the following:

- The body is roughly heart shaped. It typically bears two small facets, commonly called *demifacets* (half-facets), on each side, one at the superior edge (the *superior costal facet*) and the other at the inferior edge (the *inferior costal facet*). The demifacets receive the heads of the ribs. (The bodies of T_{10}–T_{12} vary from this pattern by having only a single facet to receive their respective ribs.)
- The vertebral foramen is circular.
- The spinous process is long and points sharply downward.
- With the exception of T_{11} and T_{12}, the transverse processes have facets, the *transverse costal facets*, that articulate with the tubercles of the ribs.
- The superior and inferior articular facets lie mainly in the frontal plane, a situation that prevents flexion and extension, but which allows this region of the spine to rotate. Lateral flexion, though possible, is restricted by the ribs.

Lumbar Vertebrae

The lumbar region of the vertebral column, commonly referred to as the small of the back, receives the most stress. The enhanced weight-bearing function of the five lumbar vertebrae (L_1–L_5) is reflected in their sturdier structure. Their bodies are massive and kidney shaped in a superior view (see Table 7.2, Figure 7.16, and Figure 7.21). Other characteristics typical of these vertebrae:

- The pedicles and laminae are shorter and thicker than those of other vertebrae.
- The spinous processes are short, flat, and hatchet shaped and are easily seen when a person bends forward. These processes are robust and project directly backward, adaptations for the attachment of the large back muscles.
- The vertebral foramen is triangular.
- The orientation of the facets of the articular processes of the lumbar vertebrae differs substantially from that of the other vertebra types (see Table 7.2). These modifications lock the lumbar vertebrae together and provide stability by preventing rotation of the lumbar spine. Flexion and extension are possible (as when you do sit-ups), as is lateral flexion.

Sacrum

The triangular sacrum, which shapes the posterior wall of the pelvis, is formed by five fused vertebrae (S_1–S_5) in adults (**Figure 7.22**, and see Figure 7.16). It articulates superiorly (via its **superior articular processes**) with L_5 and inferiorly with the coccyx. Laterally, the sacrum articulates, via its **auricular surfaces**, with the two hip bones to form the **sacroiliac joints** (sa″kro-il′e-ak) of the pelvis.

The **sacral promontory** (prom′on-tor″e; "high point of land projecting into the sea"), the anterosuperior margin of the first sacral vertebra, bulges anteriorly into the pelvic cavity. The body's center of gravity lies about 1 cm posterior to this

Table 7.2 Regional Characteristics of Cervical, Thoracic, and Lumbar Vertebrae

CHARACTERISTIC	CERVICAL (3–7)	THORACIC	LUMBAR
Body	Small, wide side to side	Larger than cervical; heart shaped; bears two costal facets	Massive; kidney shaped
Spinous process	Short; bifid; projects directly posterior	Long; sharp; projects inferiorly	Short; blunt; rectangular; projects directly posteriorly
Vertebral foramen	Triangular	Circular	Triangular
Transverse processes	Contain foramina	Bear facets for ribs (except T_{11} and T_{12})	Thin and tapered
Superior and inferior articular processes	Superior facets directed superoposteriorly	Superior facets directed posteriorly	Superior facets directed posteromedially (or medially)
	Inferior facets directed inferoanteriorly	Inferior facets directed anteriorly	Inferior facets directed anterolaterally (or laterally)
Movements allowed	Flexion and extension; lateral flexion; rotation; the spine region with the greatest range of movement	Rotation; lateral flexion possible but restricted by ribs; flexion and extension limited	Flexion and extension; some lateral flexion; rotation prevented

Superior View

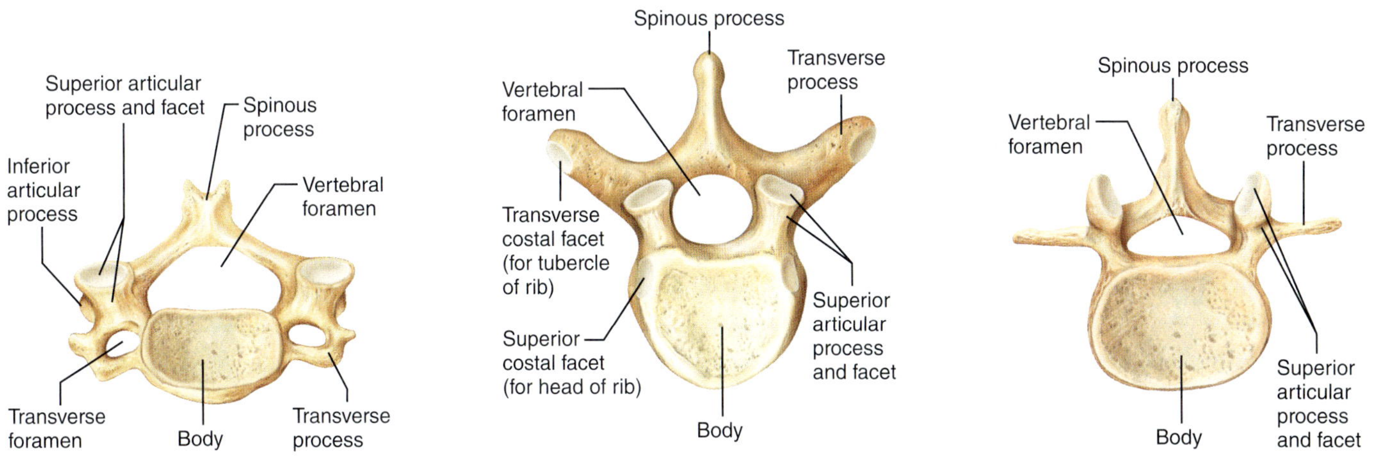

(a) Cervical **(b) Thoracic** **(c) Lumbar**

Right Lateral View

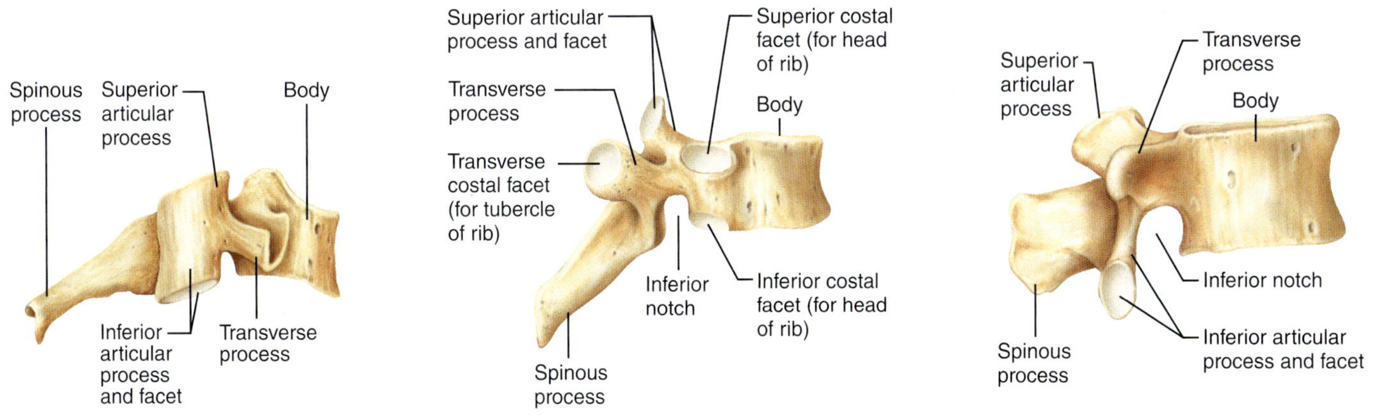

(a) Cervical **(b) Thoracic** **(c) Lumbar**

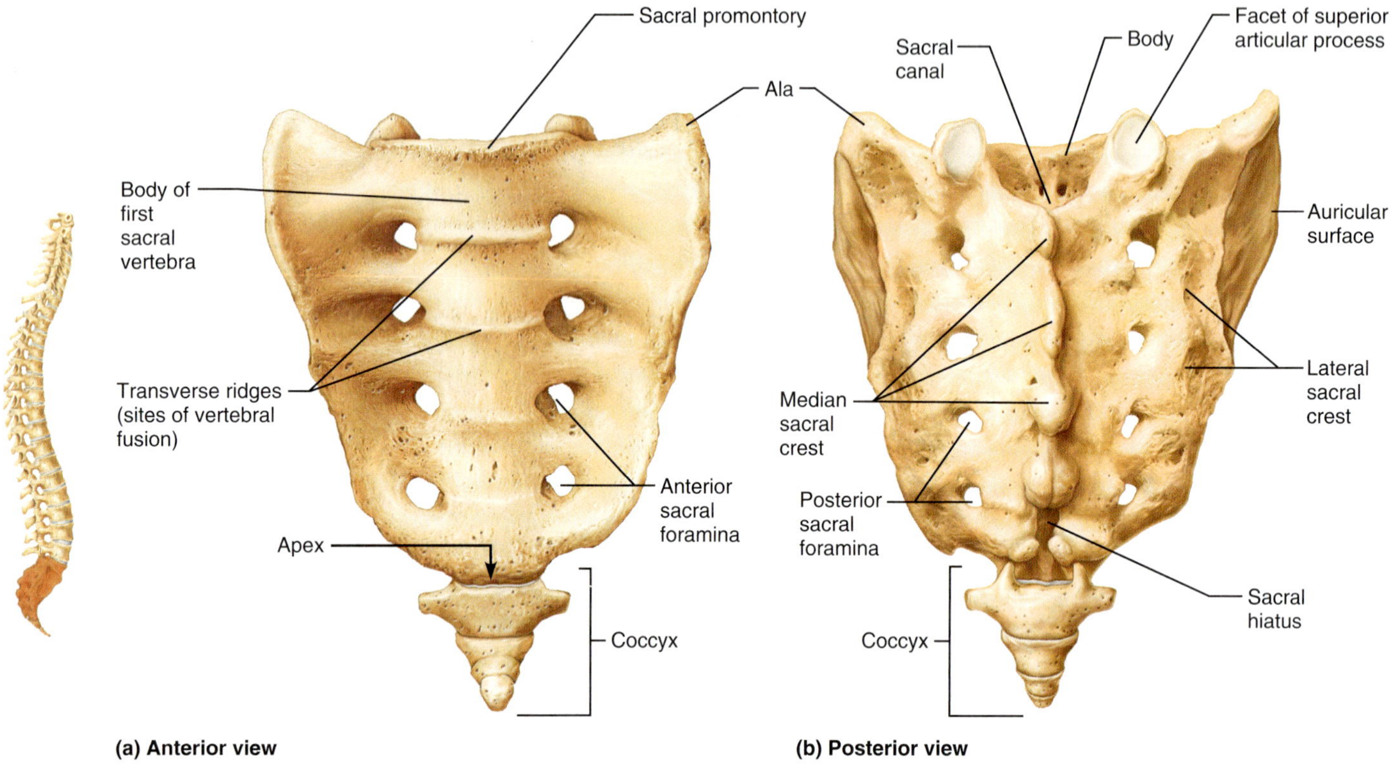

Figure 7.22 The sacrum and coccyx. (For a related image, see *A Brief Atlas of the Human Body*, Figure 22.)

landmark. Four ridges, the **transverse ridges**, cross its concave anterior aspect, marking the lines of fusion of the sacral vertebrae. The **anterior sacral foramina** lie at the lateral ends of these ridges and transmit blood vessels and anterior rami of the sacral spinal nerves. The regions lateral to these foramina expand superiorly as the winglike **alae**.

In its posterior midline the sacral surface is roughened by the **median sacral crest** (the fused spinous processes of the sacral vertebrae). This is flanked laterally by the **posterior sacral foramina**, which transmit the posterior rami of the sacral spinal nerves, and then the **lateral sacral crests** (remnants of the transverse processes of S_1–S_5).

The vertebral canal continues inside the sacrum as the **sacral canal**. Since the laminae of the fifth (and sometimes the fourth) sacral vertebrae fail to fuse medially, an enlarged external opening called the **sacral hiatus** (hi-a′tus; "gap") is obvious at the inferior end of the sacral canal.

Coccyx

The coccyx, our tailbone, is a small triangular bone (Figure 7.22, and see Figure 7.16). It consists of four (or in some cases three or five) vertebrae fused together. The coccyx articulates superiorly with the sacrum. (The name *coccyx* is from the Greek word meaning "cuckoo" and was so named because of its fancied resemblance to a bird's beak.) Except for the slight support the coccyx affords the pelvic organs, it is a nearly useless bone. Occasionally, a baby is born with an unusually long coccyx, which may need to be removed surgically.

■ ■ ■

The characteristics of the regional vertebrae are summarized in Table 7.2.

☑ Check Your Understanding

16. What is the normal number of cervical vertebrae? Of thoracic vertebrae?
17. How would a complete fracture of the dens affect the mobility of the vertebral column?
18. How can you distinguish a lumbar vertebra from a thoracic vertebra?

For answers, see Appendix H.

The Thoracic Cage

✓ Name and describe the bones of the thoracic cage (bony thorax).

✓ Differentiate true from false ribs.

Anatomically, the thorax is the chest, and its bony underpinnings are called the **thoracic cage** or *bony thorax*. Elements of the thoracic cage include the thoracic vertebrae posteriorly, the ribs laterally, and the sternum and costal cartilages anteriorly. The costal cartilages secure the ribs to the sternum **(Figure 7.23a)**.

Roughly cone shaped with its broad dimension positioned inferiorly, the bony thorax forms a protective cage around the vital organs of the thoracic cavity (heart, lungs, and great blood vessels), supports the shoulder girdles and upper limbs, and provides

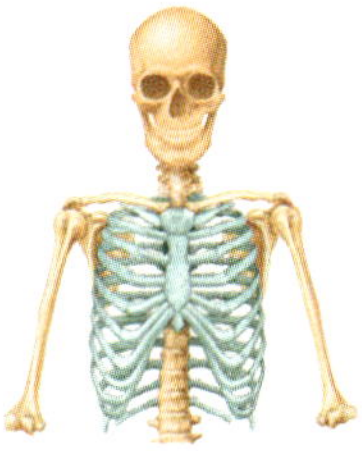

Figure 7.23 The thoracic cage. (For a related image, see *A Brief Atlas of the Human Body*, Figure 23a–d.)

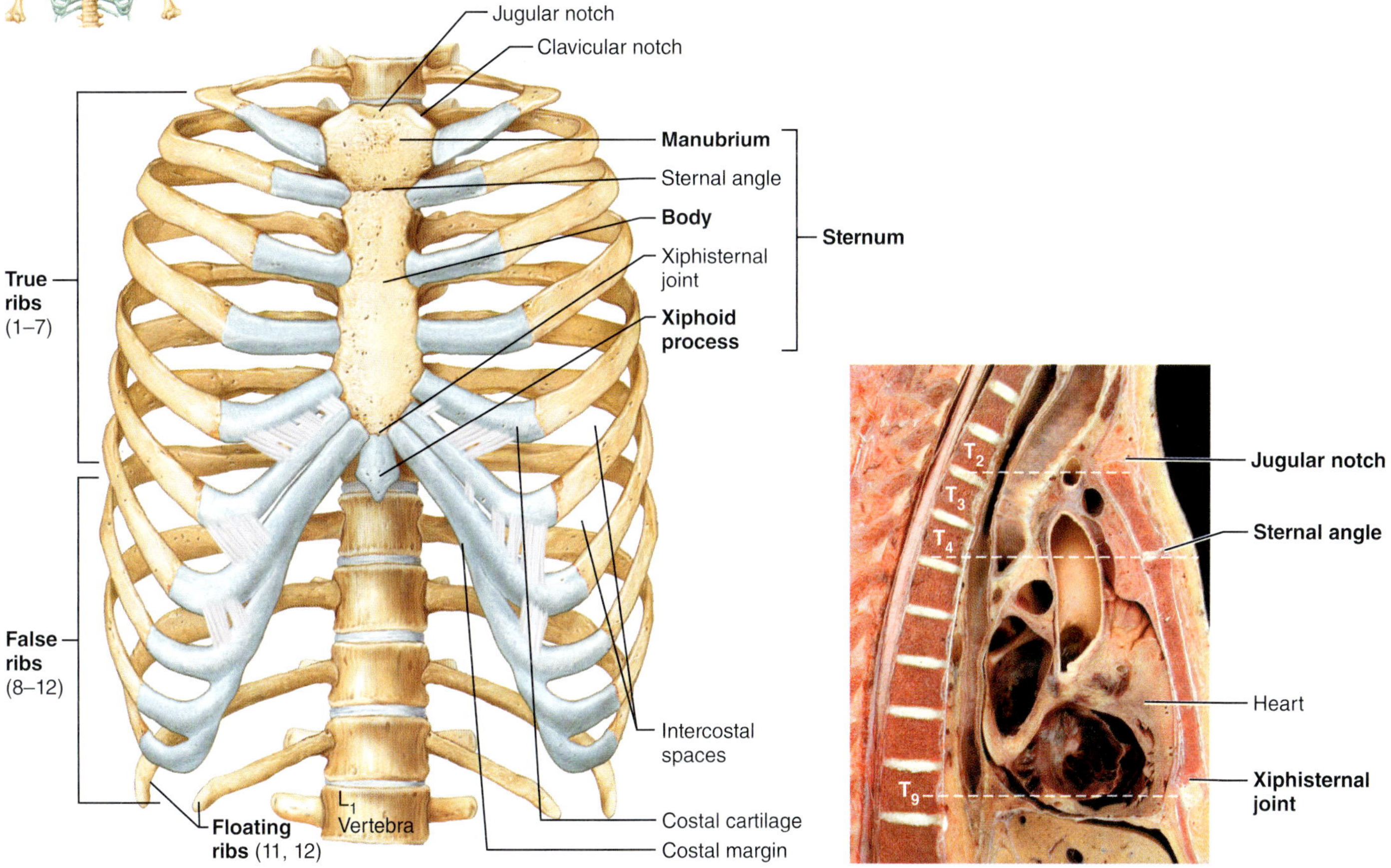

(a) Skeleton of the thoracic cage, anterior view

(b) Midsagittal section through the thorax, showing the relationship of surface anatomical landmarks of the thorax to the vertebral column

attachment points for many muscles of the neck, back, chest, and shoulders. The *intercostal spaces* between the ribs are occupied by the intercostal muscles, which lift and then depress the thorax during breathing.

Sternum

The **sternum** (breastbone) lies in the anterior midline of the thorax. Vaguely resembling a dagger, it is a flat bone approximately 15 cm (6 inches) long, resulting from the fusion of three bones: the manubrium, the body, and the xiphoid process. The *manubrium* (mah-nu′bre-um; "knife handle") is the superior portion, which is shaped like the knot in a necktie. The manubrium articulates via its **clavicular notches** (klah-vik′u-lar) with the clavicles (collarbones) laterally, and just below this, it also articulates with the first two pairs of ribs. The *body*, or midportion, forms the bulk of the sternum. The sides of the body are notched where it articulates with the costal cartilages of the second to seventh ribs. The *xiphoid process* (zif′oid; "swordlike") forms the inferior end of the sternum. This small, variably shaped process is a plate of hyaline cartilage in youth, but it is usually ossified in adults over the age of 40. The xiphoid process articulates only with the sternal body and serves as an attachment point for some abdominal muscles.

Homeostatic Imbalance 7.4

In some people, the xiphoid process projects posteriorly. In such cases, blows to the chest can push the xiphoid into the underlying heart or liver, causing massive hemorrhage. +

The sternum has three important anatomical landmarks: the jugular notch, the sternal angle, and the xiphisternal joint (Figure 7.23). The easily palpated **jugular** (*suprasternal*) **notch** is the central indentation in the superior border of the manubrium. If you slide your finger down the anterior surface of your neck, it will land in the jugular notch. The jugular notch is generally in line with the disc between the second and third thoracic vertebrae and the point where the left common carotid artery issues from the aorta (Figure 7.23b).

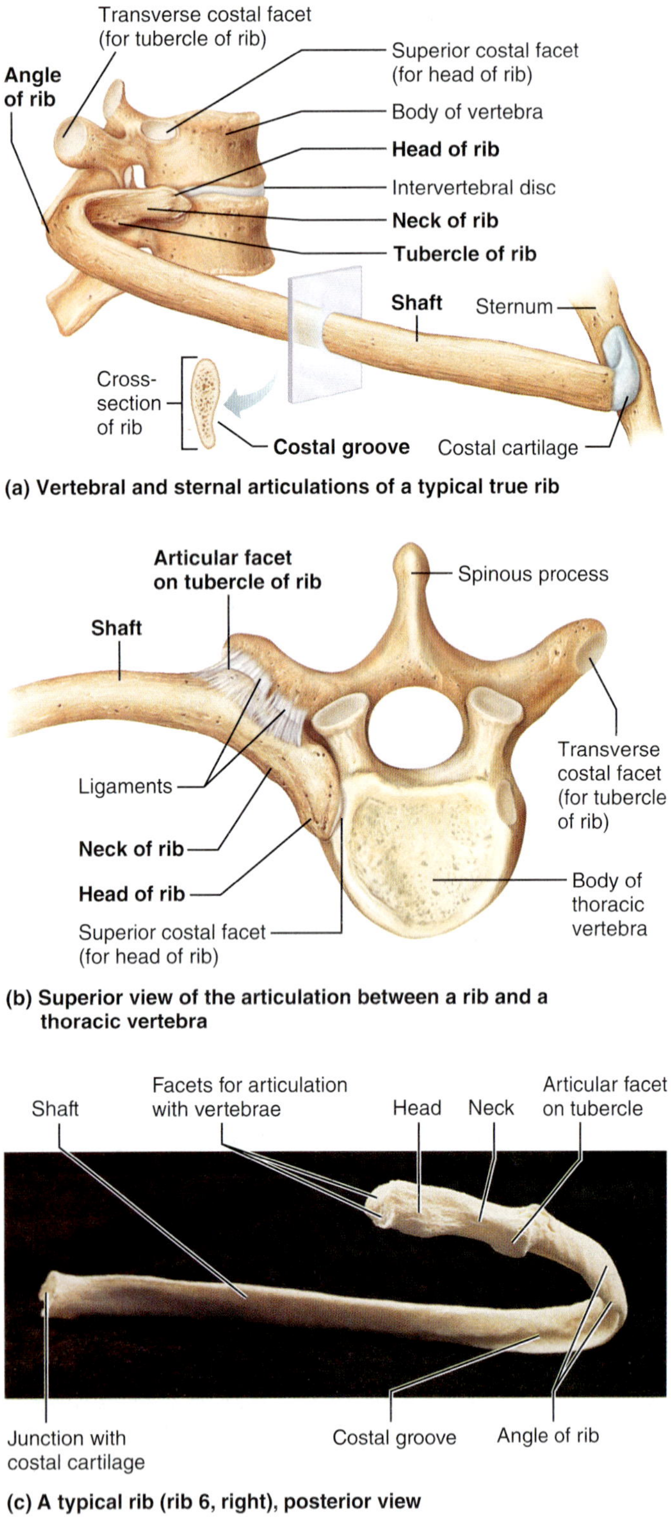

Figure 7.24 Ribs. All ribs illustrated in this figure are right ribs. (For a related image, see *A Brief Atlas of the Human Body,* Figure 23e and f.)

The **sternal angle** is felt as a horizontal ridge across the front of the sternum, where the manubrium joins the sternal body. This cartilaginous joint acts like a hinge, allowing the sternal body to swing anteriorly when we inhale. The sternal angle is in line with the disc between the fourth and fifth thoracic vertebrae and at the level of the second pair of ribs. It is a handy reference point for finding the second rib and thus for counting the ribs during a physical examination and for listening to sounds made by specific heart valves.

The **xiphisternal joint** (zif″ĭ-ster′nul) is the point where the sternal body and xiphoid process fuse. It lies at the level of the ninth thoracic vertebra. The heart lies on the diaphragm just deep to this joint.

Ribs

Twelve pairs of **ribs** form the flaring sides of the thoracic cage (Figure 7.23a). All ribs attach posteriorly to the thoracic vertebrae (bodies and transverse processes) and curve inferiorly toward the anterior body surface. The superior seven rib pairs attach directly to the sternum by individual costal cartilages (bars of hyaline cartilage). These are **true** or **vertebrosternal ribs** (ver″tĕ-bro-ster′nal). (Notice that the anatomical name indicates the two attachment points of a rib—the posterior attachment given first.)

The remaining five pairs of ribs are called **false ribs** because they either attach indirectly to the sternum or entirely lack a sternal attachment. Rib pairs 8–10 attach to the sternum indirectly, each joining the costal cartilage immediately above it. These ribs are also called **vertebrochondral ribs** (ver″tĕ-bro-kon′dral). The inferior margin of the rib cage, or **costal margin**, is formed by the costal cartilages of ribs 7–10. Rib pairs 11 and 12 are called **vertebral ribs** or **floating ribs** because they have no anterior attachments. Instead, their costal cartilages lie embedded in the muscles of the lateral body wall.

The ribs increase in length from pair 1 to pair 7, then decrease in length from pair 8 to pair 12. Except for the first rib, which lies deep to the clavicle, the ribs are easily felt in people of normal weight.

A typical rib is a bowed flat bone **(Figure 7.24)**. The bulk of a rib is simply called the *shaft*. Its superior border is smooth, but its inferior border is sharp and thin and has a *costal groove* on its inner face that lodges the intercostal nerves and blood vessels.

In addition to the shaft, each rib has a head, neck, and tubercle. The wedge-shaped *head*, the posterior end, articulates with the vertebral bodies by two facets: One joins the body of the same-numbered thoracic vertebra, the other articulates with the body of the vertebra immediately superior. The *neck* is the constricted portion of the rib just beyond the head. Lateral to this, the knoblike *tubercle* articulates with the costal facet of the transverse process of the same-numbered thoracic vertebra. Beyond the tubercle, the shaft angles sharply forward (at the angle of the rib) and then extends to attach to its costal cartilage anteriorly. The costal cartilages provide secure but flexible rib attachments to the sternum.

The first pair of ribs is quite atypical. They are flattened superiorly to inferiorly and are quite broad, forming a horizontal table that supports the subclavian blood vessels that serve the upper limbs. There are also other exceptions to the typical rib pattern. Rib 1 and ribs 10–12 articulate with only one vertebral body, and ribs 11 and 12 do not articulate with a vertebral transverse process.

Figure 7.25 The pectoral girdle and clavicle. (For a related image, see *A Brief Atlas of the Human Body*, Figure 24.)

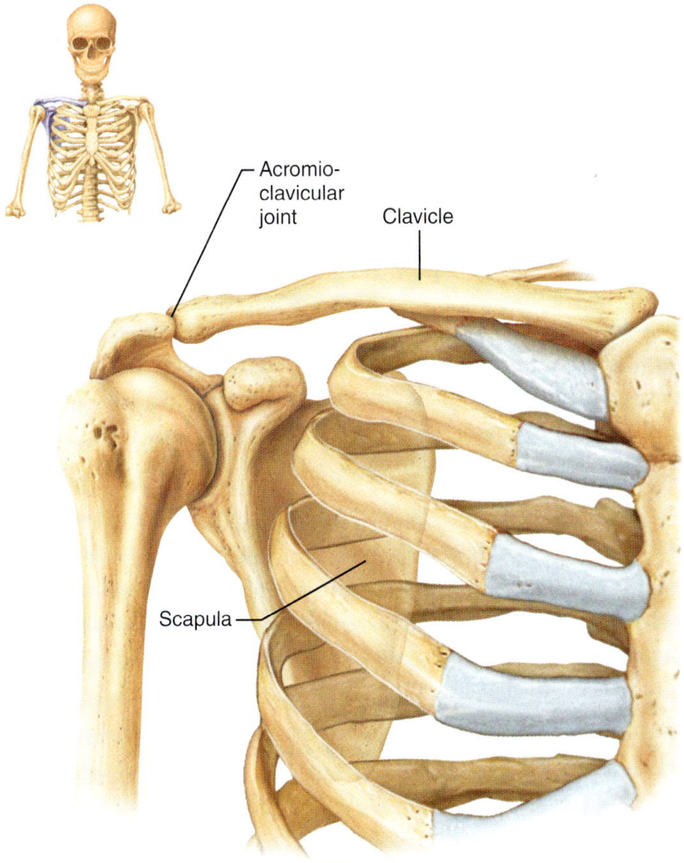

(a) Articulated pectoral girdle

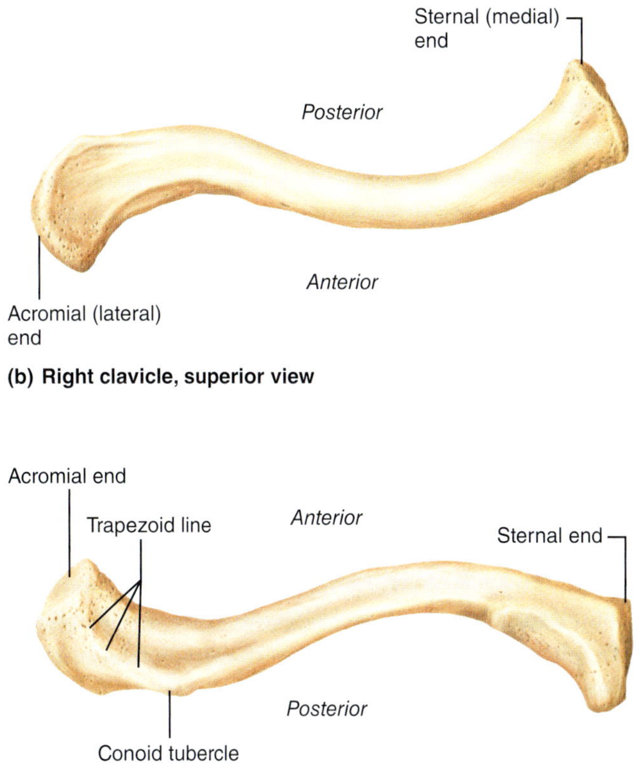

(b) Right clavicle, superior view

(c) Right clavicle, inferior view

Check Your Understanding

19. How does a true rib differ from a false rib?
20. What is the sternal angle and what is its clinical importance?
21. Besides the ribs and sternum, there is a third group of bones making up the thoracic cage. What is it?

For answers, see Appendix H.

PART 2
The Appendicular Skeleton

Bones of the limbs and their girdles are collectively called the **appendicular skeleton** because they are appended to the axial skeleton that forms the longitudinal axis of the body (see Figure 7.1). The yokelike *pectoral girdles* (pek′tor-al; "chest") attach the upper limbs to the body trunk. The more sturdy *pelvic girdle* secures the lower limbs. Although the bones of the upper and lower limbs differ in their functions and mobility, they have the same fundamental plan: Each limb is composed of three major segments connected by movable joints.

The appendicular skeleton enables us to carry out the movements typical of our freewheeling and manipulative lifestyle. Each time we take a step, throw a ball, or pop a caramel into our mouth, we are making good use of our appendicular skeleton.

The Pectoral (Shoulder) Girdle

- ✓ Identify bones forming the pectoral girdle and relate their structure and arrangement to the function of this girdle.
- ✓ Identify important bone markings on the pectoral girdle.

The **pectoral girdle**, or **shoulder girdle**, consists of the *clavicle* (klav′ĭ-kl) anteriorly and the *scapula* (skap′u-lah) posteriorly (**Figure 7.25** and Table 7.3 on p. 233). The paired pectoral girdles and their associated muscles form your shoulders. Although the term *girdle* usually signifies a beltlike structure encircling the body, a single pectoral girdle, or even the pair, does not quite satisfy this description. Anteriorly, the medial end of each clavicle joins the sternum; the distal ends of the clavicles meet the scapulae laterally. However, the scapulae fail to complete the ring posteriorly, because their medial borders do not join each other or the axial skeleton. Instead, the scapulae are attached to the thorax and vertebral column only by the muscles that clothe their surfaces.

The pectoral girdles attach the upper limbs to the axial skeleton and provide attachment points for many of the muscles that move the upper limbs. These girdles are very light and allow the upper limbs a degree of mobility not seen anywhere else in the body. This mobility is due to the following factors:

- Because only the clavicle attaches to the axial skeleton, the scapula can move quite freely across the thorax, allowing the arm to move with it.
- The socket of the shoulder joint (the scapula's glenoid cavity) is shallow and poorly reinforced, so it does not restrict the movement of the humerus (arm bone). Although this arrangement is good for flexibility, it is bad for stability: Shoulder dislocations are fairly common.

Clavicles

The **clavicles** ("little keys"), or collarbones, are slender, S-shaped bones that can be felt along their entire course as they extend horizontally across the superior thorax (Figure 7.25). Each clavicle is cone shaped at its medial **sternal end**, which attaches to the sternal manubrium, and flattened at its lateral **acromial end** (ah-kro′me-al), which articulates with the scapula. The medial two-thirds of the clavicle is convex anteriorly; its lateral third is concave anteriorly. Its superior surface is fairly smooth, but the inferior surface is ridged and grooved by ligaments and by the action of the muscles that attach to it. The *trapezoid line* and the *conoid tubercle*, for example, are anchoring points for a ligament that connects the clavicle to the scapula.

Besides anchoring many muscles, the clavicles act as braces: They hold the scapulae and arms out laterally, away from the narrower superior part of the thorax. This bracing function becomes obvious when a clavicle is fractured: The entire shoulder region collapses medially. The clavicles also transmit compression forces from the upper limbs to the axial skeleton, for example, when someone pushes a car to a gas station.

The clavicles are not very strong and are likely to fracture, for example, when a person uses outstretched arms to break a fall. The curves in the clavicle ensure that it usually fractures anteriorly (outward). If it were to collapse posteriorly (inward), bone splinters would damage the subclavian artery, which passes just deep to the clavicle to serve the upper limb. The clavicles are exceptionally sensitive to muscle pull and become noticeably larger and stronger in those who perform manual labor or athletics involving the shoulder and arm muscles.

Scapulae

The **scapulae**, or *shoulder blades*, are thin, triangular flat bones (Figure 7.25a and **Figure 7.26**). Interestingly, their name derives from a word meaning "spade" or "shovel," for ancient cultures made spades from the shoulder blades of animals. The scapulae lie on the dorsal surface of the rib cage, between ribs 2 and 7.

Each scapula has three borders. The *superior border* is the shortest, sharpest border. The *medial*, or *vertebral*, *border* parallels the vertebral column. The thick *lateral*, or *axillary*, *border* abuts the armpit and ends superiorly in a small, shallow fossa, the **glenoid cavity** (gle′noid; "pit-shaped"). This cavity articulates with the humerus of the arm, forming the shoulder joint.

Like all triangles, the scapula has three corners or *angles*. The superior scapular border meets the medial border at the *superior angle* and the lateral border at the *lateral angle*. The medial and lateral borders join at the *inferior angle*. The inferior angle moves extensively as the arm is raised and lowered, and is an important landmark for studying scapular movements.

The anterior, or costal, surface of the scapula is concave and relatively featureless. Its posterior surface bears a prominent **spine** that is easily felt through the skin. The spine ends laterally in an enlarged, roughened triangular projection called the **acromion** (ah-kro′me-on; "point of the shoulder"). The acromion articulates with the acromial end of the clavicle, forming the **acromioclavicular joint**.

Projecting anteriorly from the superior scapular border is the **coracoid process** (kor′ah-coid); *corac* means "beaklike," but this process looks more like a bent little finger. The coracoid process helps anchor the biceps muscle of the arm. It is bounded by the **suprascapular notch** (a nerve passage) medially and by the glenoid cavity laterally.

Several large fossae appear on both sides of the scapula and are named according to location. The *infraspinous* and *supraspinous fossae* are inferior and superior, respectively, to the spine. The *subscapular fossa* is the shallow concavity formed by the entire anterior scapular surface. Lying within these fossae are muscles with similar names.

☑ Check Your Understanding

22. What two bones construct each pectoral girdle?
23. Where is the single point of attachment of the pectoral girdle to the axial skeleton?
24. What is the major shortcoming of the flexibility allowed by the shoulder joint?

For answers, see Appendix H.

The Upper Limb

✓ Identify or name the bones of the upper limb and their important markings.

Thirty separate bones form the bony framework of each upper limb (see Figures 7.27 to 7.29, and **Table 7.3** on p. 233). Each of these bones may be described regionally as a bone of the arm, forearm, or hand. (Keep in mind that anatomically the "arm" is only that part of the upper limb between the shoulder and elbow.)

Arm

The **humerus** (hu′mer-us), the sole bone of the arm, is a typical long bone **(Figure 7.27)**. The largest, longest bone of the upper limb, it articulates with the scapula at the shoulder and with the radius and ulna (forearm bones) at the elbow.

At the proximal end of the humerus is its smooth, hemispherical **head**, which fits into the glenoid cavity of the scapula in a manner that allows the arm to hang freely at one's side. Immediately inferior to the head is a slight constriction, the **anatomical neck**. Just inferior to this are the lateral **greater tubercle** and the more medial **lesser tubercle**, separated by the **intertubercular sulcus**, or *bicipital groove* (bi-sip′ĭ-tal). These tubercles are sites of attachment of the rotator cuff muscles. The intertubercular sulcus guides

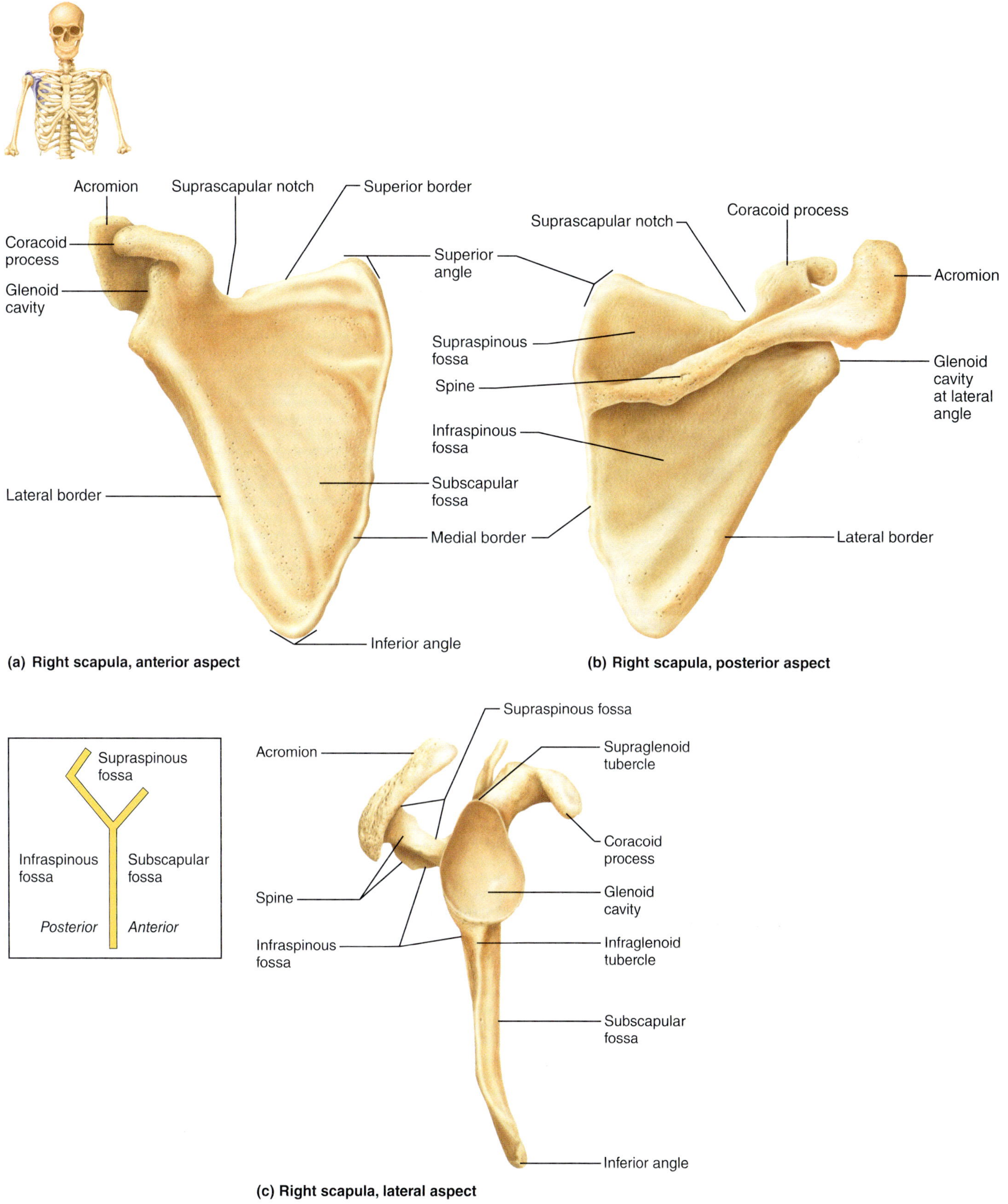

Figure 7.26 The scapula. View (c) is accompanied by a schematic representation of its orientation. (For a related image, see *A Brief Atlas of the Human Body*, Figure 24.)

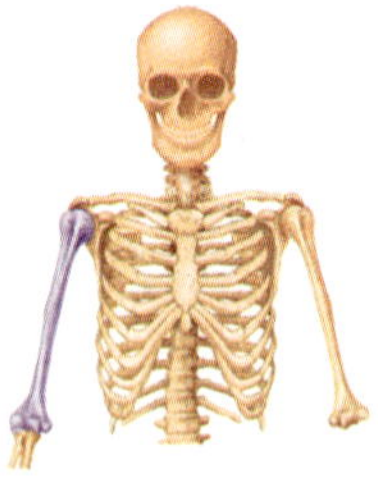

Figure 7.27 The humerus of the right arm and detailed views of articulation at the elbow. (For a related image, see *A Brief Atlas of the Human Body*, Figure 25.)

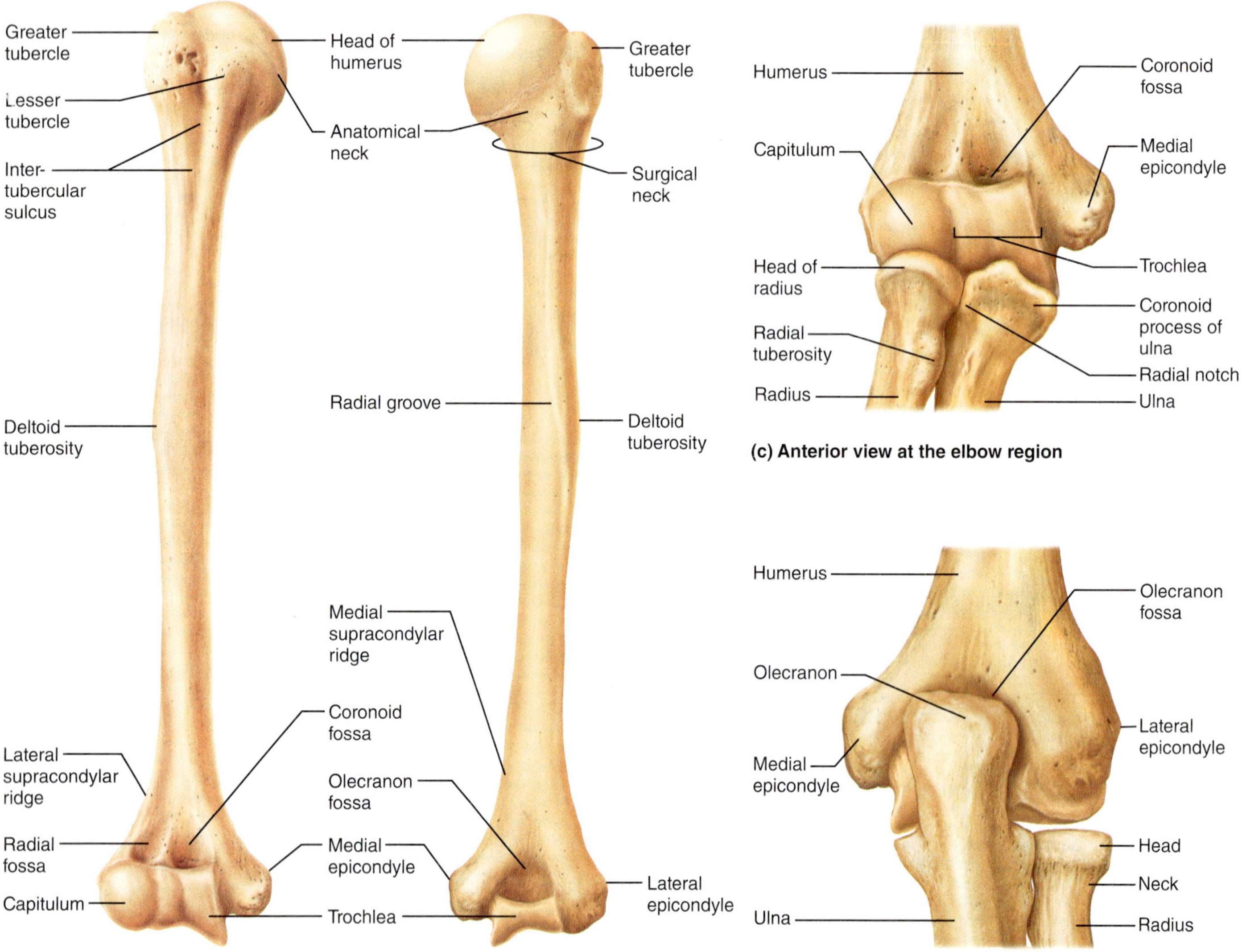

(a) Anterior view **(b) Posterior view** **(c) Anterior view at the elbow region** **(d) Posterior view of extended elbow**

a tendon of the biceps muscle of the arm to its attachment point at the rim of the glenoid cavity (the supraglenoid tubercle). Just distal to the tubercles is the **surgical neck**, so named because it is the most frequently fractured part of the humerus. About midway down the shaft on its lateral side is the V-shaped **deltoid tuberosity**, the roughened attachment site for the deltoid muscle of the shoulder. Nearby, the **radial groove** runs obliquely down the posterior aspect of the shaft, marking the course of the radial nerve, an important nerve of the upper limb.

At the distal end of the humerus are two condyles: a medial **trochlea** (trok′le-ah; "pulley"), which looks like an hourglass tipped on its side, and the lateral ball-like **capitulum** (kah-pit′u-lum). These condyles articulate with the ulna and the radius, respectively (Figure 7.27c and d). The condyle pair is flanked by the **medial** and **lateral epicondyles** (muscle attachment sites). Directly above these epicondyles are the **medial** and **lateral supracondylar ridges**. The ulnar nerve, which runs behind the medial epicondyle, is responsible for the painful, tingling sensation you experience when you hit your "funny bone."

Superior to the trochlea on the anterior surface is the **coronoid fossa**; on the posterior surface is the deeper **olecranon fossa** (o-lek′rah-non). These two depressions allow the corresponding processes of the ulna to move freely when the elbow is flexed and extended. A small **radial fossa**, lateral to the coronoid fossa, receives the head of the radius when the elbow is flexed.

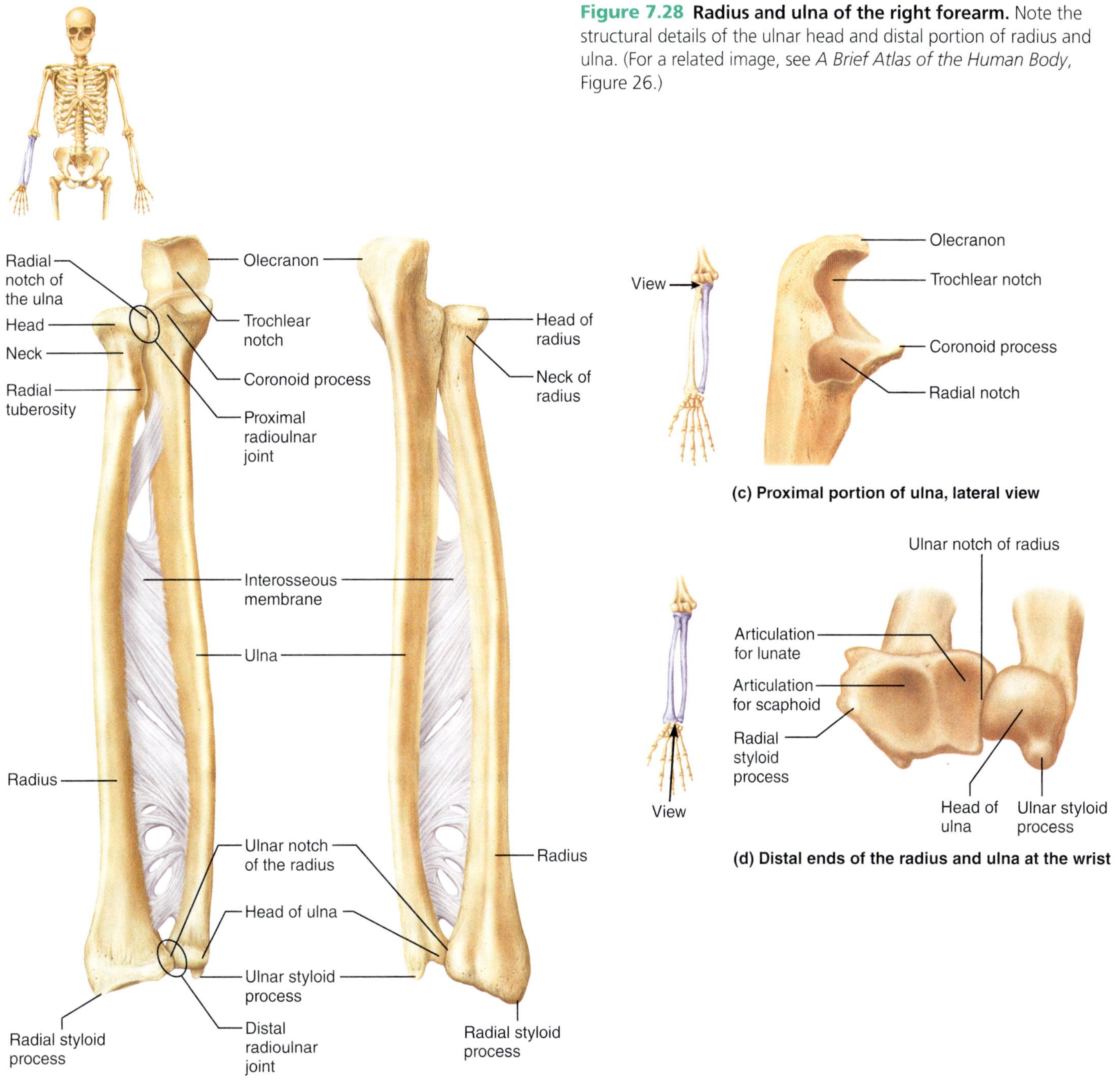

Figure 7.28 Radius and ulna of the right forearm. Note the structural details of the ulnar head and distal portion of radius and ulna. (For a related image, see *A Brief Atlas of the Human Body*, Figure 26.)

(a) Anterior view

(b) Posterior view

(c) Proximal portion of ulna, lateral view

(d) Distal ends of the radius and ulna at the wrist

Forearm

Two parallel long bones, the radius and the ulna, form the skeleton of the forearm, or *antebrachium* (an″te-bra′ke-um) **(Figure 7.28)**. Unless a person's forearm muscles are very bulky, these bones are easily palpated along their entire length. Their proximal ends articulate with the humerus; their distal ends form joints with bones of the wrist. The radius and ulna articulate with each other both proximally and distally at small **radioulnar joints** (ra″de-o-ul′nar), and they are connected along their entire length by a flat, flexible ligament, the **interosseous membrane** (in″ter-os′e-us; "between the bones").

In the anatomical position, the radius lies laterally (on the thumb side) and the ulna medially. However, when you rotate your forearm so that the palm faces posteriorly (a movement called pronation), the distal end of the radius crosses over the ulna and the two bones form an X (see Figure 8.6a, p. 259).

Ulna

The **ulna** (ul′nah; "elbow") is slightly longer than the radius. It has the main responsibility for forming the elbow joint with the humerus. Its proximal end looks like the adjustable end of a monkey wrench: It bears two prominent processes, the **olecranon** (elbow)

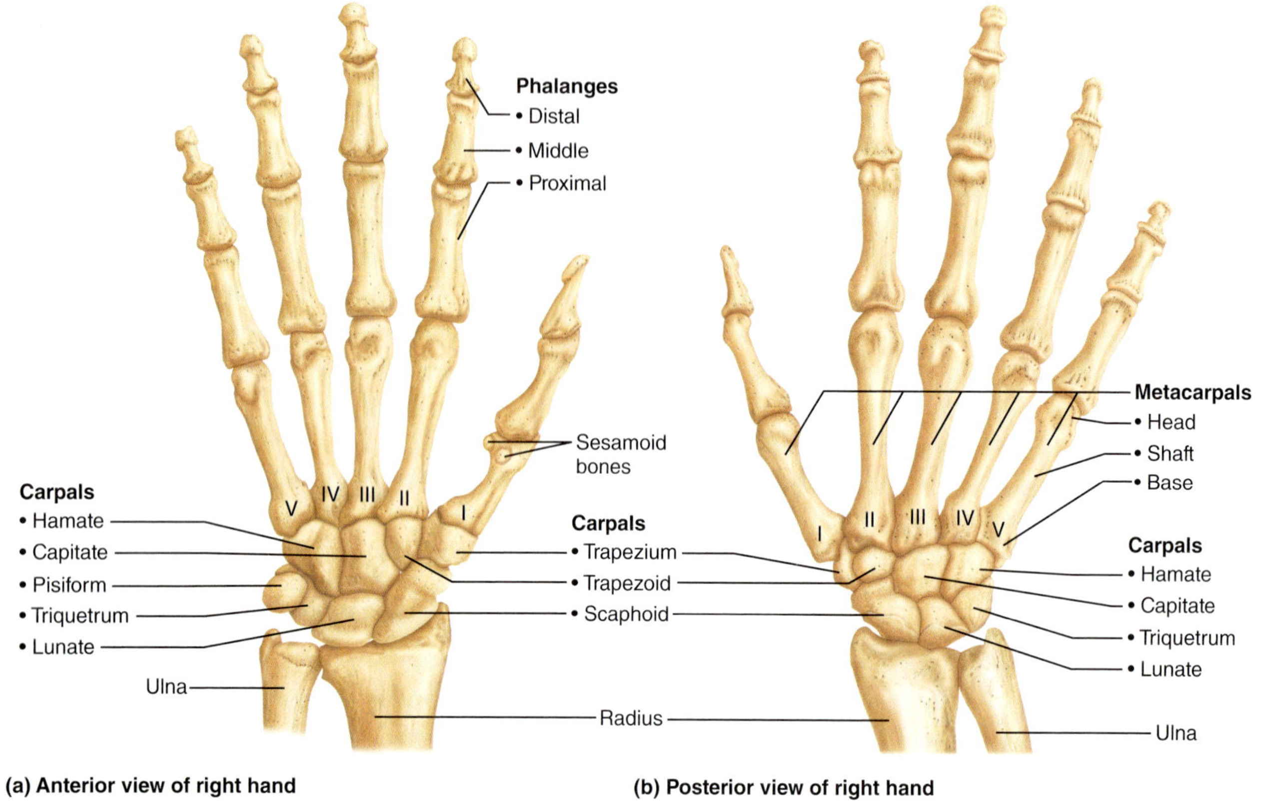

Figure 7.29 Bones of the right hand. (For a related image, see *A Brief Atlas of the Human Body*, Figure 27.)

and the **coronoid process**, separated by a deep concavity, the **trochlear notch** (Figure 7.28c). Together, these two processes grip the trochlea of the humerus, forming a hinge joint that allows the forearm to be bent upon the arm (flexed), then straightened again (extended). When the forearm is fully extended, the olecranon "locks" into the olecranon fossa (Figure 7.27d), keeping the forearm from hyperextending (moving posteriorly beyond the elbow joint). The posterior olecranon forms the angle of the elbow when the forearm is flexed and is the bony part that rests on the table when you lean on your elbows. On the lateral side of the coronoid process is a small depression, the **radial notch**, where the ulna articulates with the head of the radius.

Distally the ulnar shaft narrows and ends in a knoblike **head** (Figure 7.28d). Medial to the head is the **ulnar styloid process**, from which a ligament runs to the wrist. The ulnar head is separated from the bones of the wrist by a disc of fibrocartilage and plays little or no role in hand movements.

Radius

The **radius** ("rod") is thin at its proximal end and wide distally—the opposite of the ulna. The **head** of the radius is shaped somewhat like the head of a nail (Figure 7.28). The superior surface of this head is concave, and it articulates with the capitulum of the humerus. Medially, the head articulates with the radial notch of the ulna (Figure 7.27c). Just inferior to the head is the rough **radial tuberosity**, which anchors the biceps muscle of the arm. Distally, where the radius is expanded, it has a medial **ulnar notch** (Figure 7.28d), which articulates with the ulna, and a lateral **radial styloid process** (an anchoring site for ligaments that run to the wrist). Between these two markings, the radius is concave where it articulates with carpal bones of the wrist.

The ulna contributes more heavily to the elbow joint, and the radius is the major forearm bone contributing to the wrist joint. When the radius moves, the hand moves with it.

Homeostatic Imbalance 7.5

Colles' fracture is a break in the distal end of the radius. It is a common fracture when a falling person attempts to break his or her fall with outstretched hands. ✚

Hand

The skeleton of the hand **(Figure 7.29)** includes the bones of the *carpus* (wrist); the bones of the *metacarpus* (palm); and the *phalanges* (bones of the fingers).

Carpus (Wrist)

A "wrist" watch is actually worn on the distal forearm (over the lower ends of the radius and ulna), not on the wrist at all. The true wrist, or carpus, is the proximal part of the structure we generally call our "hand." The carpus consists of eight marble-size short bones, or **carpals** (kar′palz), closely united by ligaments. Because gliding movements occur between these bones, the carpus as a whole is quite flexible.

Table 7.3 Bones of the Appendicular Skeleton, Part 1: Pectoral Girdle and Upper Limb

BODY REGION	BONES*	ILLUSTRATION	LOCATION	MARKINGS
Pectoral girdle (Figures 7.25, 7.26)	**Clavicle** (2)		Clavicle is in superoanterior thorax; articulates medially with sternum and laterally with scapula	Acromial end; sternal end
	Scapula (2)		Scapula is in posterior thorax; forms part of the shoulder; articulates with humerus and clavicle	Glenoid cavity; spine; acromion; coracoid process; infraspinous, supraspinous, and subscapular fossae
Upper limb Arm (Figure 7.27)	**Humerus** (2)		Humerus is sole bone of arm; between scapula and elbow	Head; greater and lesser tubercles; intertubercular sulcus; radial groove; deltoid tuberosity; trochlea; capitulum; coronoid and olecranon fossae; epicondyles; radial fossa
Forearm (Figure 7.28)	**Ulna** (2)		Ulna is the medial bone of forearm between elbow and wrist; with the humerus forms elbow joint	Coronoid process; olecranon; radial notch; trochlear notch; ulnar styloid process; head
	Radius (2)		Radius is the lateral bone of forearm; articulates with carpals to form part of the wrist joint	Head; radial tuberosity; radial styloid process; ulnar notch
Hand (Figure 7.29)	8 **Carpals** (16): scaphoid, lunate, triquetrum, pisiform, trapezium, trapezoid, capitate, hamate		Carpals form a bony crescent at the wrist; arranged in two rows of four bones each	
	5 **Metacarpals** (10)		Metacarpals form the palm; one in line with each digit	
	14 **Phalanges** (28): distal, middle, proximal		Phalanges form the fingers; three in digits 2–5; two in digit 1 (the thumb)	

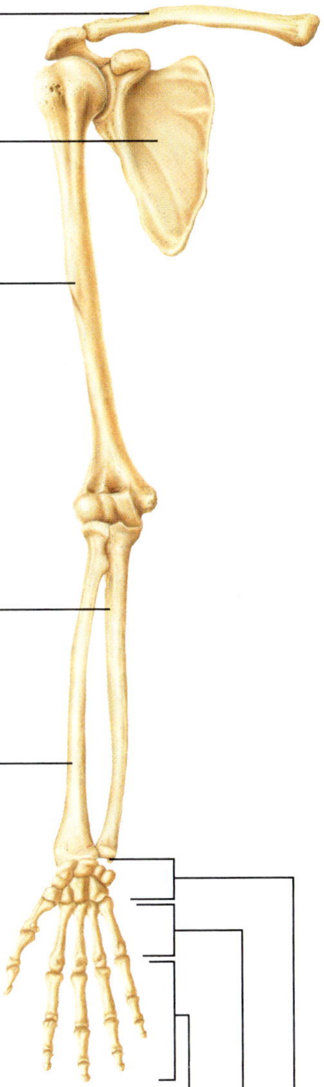

Anterior view of pectoral girdle and upper limb

*The number in parentheses ( ) following the bone name denotes the total number of such bones in the body.

The carpals are arranged in two irregular rows of four bones each (Figure 7.29). In the proximal row (lateral to medial) are the **scaphoid** (skaf′oid; "boat-shaped"), **lunate** (lu′nāt; "moon-like"), **triquetrum** (tri-kwet′rum; "triangular"), and **pisiform** (pi′sĭ-form; "pea-shaped"). Of these, all but the pisiform participate in forming the wrist joint. The carpals of the distal row (lateral to medial) are the **trapezium** (trah-pe′ze-um; "little table"), **trapezoid** (tră′peh-zoid; "four-sided"), **capitate** ("head-shaped"), and **hamate** (ham′āt; "hooked").

There are numerous memory-jogging phrases to help you recall the carpals in the order given above. If you don't have one, try: **S**ally **l**eft **t**he **p**arty **t**o **t**ake **C**indy **h**ome. As with all such memory jogs, the first letter of each word is the first letter of the term you need to remember.

7

Homeostatic Imbalance 7.6

The arrangement of its bones is such that the carpus is concave anteriorly and a ligament roofs over this concavity, forming the notorious *carpal tunnel.* Besides the median nerve (which supplies the lateral side of the hand), several long muscle tendons crowd into this tunnel. Overuse and inflammation of the tendons cause them to swell, compressing the median nerve, which causes tingling and numbness of the areas served, and movements of the thumb weaken. Pain is greatest at night. Those who repeatedly flex their wrists and fingers, such as those who work at computer keyboards all day, are particularly susceptible to this nerve impairment, called *carpal tunnel syndrome.* This condition is treated by splinting the wrist during sleep or by surgery. ✚

Metacarpus (Palm)

Five **metacarpals** radiate from the wrist like spokes to form the **metacarpus** or palm of the hand (*meta* = beyond). These small long bones are not named, but instead are numbered I to V from thumb to little finger. The **bases** of the metacarpals articulate with the carpals proximally and each other medially and laterally (Figure 7.29). Their bulbous **heads** articulate with the proximal phalanges of the fingers. When you clench your fist, the heads of the metacarpals become prominent as your *knuckles.*

Metacarpal I, associated with the thumb, is the shortest and most mobile. It occupies a more anterior position than the other metacarpals. Consequently, the joint between metacarpal I and the trapezium is a unique saddle joint that allows *opposition*, the action of touching your thumb to the tips of your other fingers.

Phalanges (Fingers)

The **fingers**, or **digits** of the upper limb, are numbered 1 to 5 beginning with the thumb, or **pollex** (pol′eks). In most people, the third finger is the longest. Each hand contains 14 miniature long bones called **phalanges** (fah-lan′jēz). Except for the thumb, each finger has three phalanges: *distal, middle*, and *proximal.* The thumb has no middle phalanx. [Phalanx (fa′langks; "a closely knit row of soldiers") is the singular term for phalanges.]

Check Your Understanding

25. Which bones play the major role in forming the elbow joint?
26. Which bones of the upper limb have a styloid process?
27. Where are carpals found and what type of bone (short, irregular, long, or flat) are they?

For answers, see Appendix H.

The Pelvic (Hip) Girdle

✓ Name the bones contributing to the os coxae, and relate the pelvic girdle's strength to its function.

✓ Describe differences in the male and female pelves and relate these to functional differences.

The **pelvic girdle**, or **hip girdle**, attaches the lower limbs to the axial skeleton, transmits the full weight of the upper body to the lower limbs, and supports the visceral organs of the pelvis (Figures 7.30 and 7.31 and **Table 7.4**, p. 237). Unlike the pectoral girdle, which is sparingly attached to the thoracic cage, the pelvic girdle is secured to the axial skeleton by some of the strongest ligaments in the body. And unlike the shallow glenoid cavity of the scapula, the corresponding sockets of the pelvic girdle are deep and cuplike and firmly secure the head of the femur in place. Thus, even though both the shoulder and hip joints are ball-and-socket joints, very few of us can wheel or swing our legs about with the same degree of freedom as our arms. The pelvic girdle lacks the mobility of the pectoral girdle but is far more stable.

The pelvic girdle is formed by the sacrum* (a part of the axial skeleton) and a pair of **hip bones**, each also called an **os coxae** (ahs kok′se), or **coxal bone** (*coxa* = hip). Each hip bone unites with its partner anteriorly and with the sacrum posteriorly **(Figure 7.30)**.

Each large, irregularly shaped hip bone consists of three separate bones during childhood: the ilium, ischium, and pubis **(Figure 7.31)**. In adults, these bones are firmly fused and their boundaries are indistinguishable. Their names are retained, however, to refer to different regions of the composite hip bone.

At the point of fusion of the ilium, ischium, and pubis is a deep hemispherical socket called the **acetabulum** (as″ĕ-tab′u-lum; "vinegar cup") on the lateral surface of the pelvis (Figure 7.31). The acetabulum receives the head of the femur, or thigh bone, at this *hip joint.*

Ilium

The **ilium** (il′e-um; "flank") is a large flaring bone that forms the superior region of a coxal bone. It consists of a **body** and a superior winglike portion called the **ala** (a′lah). When you rest your hands on your hips, you are resting them on the thickened superior margins of the alae, the **iliac crests**, to which many muscles attach. Each iliac crest ends anteriorly in the blunt **anterior superior iliac spine** and posteriorly in the sharp **posterior superior iliac spine**.

Located below these are the less prominent *anterior* and *posterior inferior iliac spines.* All of these spines are attachment points for the muscles of the trunk, hip, and thigh. The anterior

*Some authorities do not consider the sacrum part of the pelvic girdle, but here we follow the convention in *Terminologia Anatomica.*

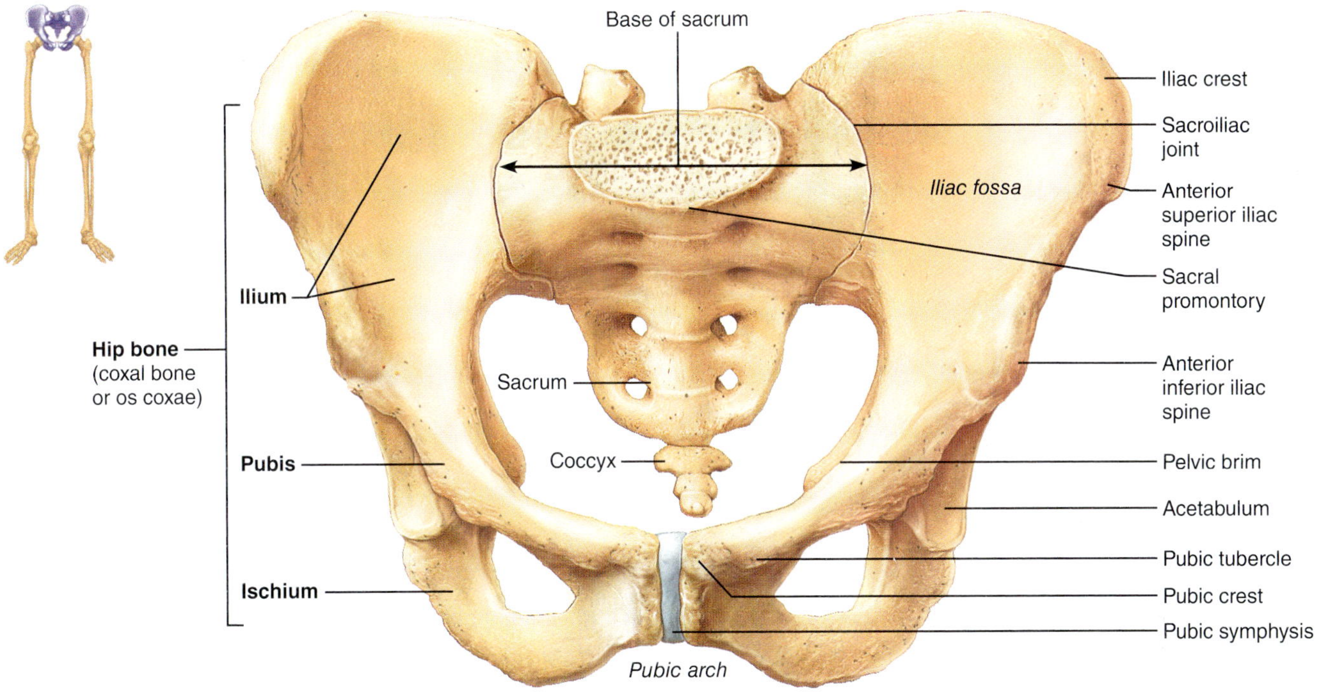

Figure 7.30 Pelvis. The pelvis consists of the two hip (coxal) bones, the sacrum, and the coccyx.

superior iliac spine is an especially important anatomical landmark. It is easily felt through the skin and is visible in thin people. The posterior superior iliac spine is difficult to palpate, but its position is revealed by a skin dimple in the sacral region.

Just inferior to the posterior inferior iliac spine, the ilium indents deeply to form the **greater sciatic notch** (si-at′ik), through which the thick cordlike sciatic nerve passes to enter the thigh. The broad posterolateral surface of the ilium, the **gluteal surface** (gloo′te-al), is crossed by three ridges, the **posterior**, **anterior**, and **inferior gluteal lines**, to which the gluteal (buttock) muscles attach.

The medial surface of the iliac ala exhibits a concavity called the **iliac fossa**. Posterior to this, the roughened **auricular surface** (aw-rik′u-lar; "ear-shaped") articulates with the same-named surface of the sacrum, forming the *sacroiliac joint* (Figure 7.30). The weight of the body is transmitted from the spine to the pelvis through the sacroiliac joints. Running inferiorly and anteriorly from the auricular surface is a robust ridge called the **arcuate line** (ar′ku-at; "bowed"). The arcuate line helps define the *pelvic brim*, the superior margin of the *true pelvis*, which we will discuss shortly. Anteriorly, the body of the ilium joins the pubis; inferiorly it joins the ischium.

Ischium

The **ischium** (is′ke-um; "hip") forms the posteroinferior part of the hip bone (Figures 7.30 and 7.31). Roughly L- or arc-shaped, it has a thicker, superior **body** adjoining the ilium and a thinner, inferior **ramus** (*ramus* = branch). The ramus joins the pubis anteriorly. The ischium has three important markings. Its **ischial spine** projects medially into the pelvic cavity and serves as a point of attachment of the *sacrospinous ligament* running from the sacrum. Just inferior to the ischial spine is the **lesser sciatic notch**. A number of nerves and blood vessels pass through this notch to supply the anogenital area. The inferior surface of the ischial body is rough and grossly thickened as the **ischial tuberosity**. When we sit, our weight is borne entirely by the ischial tuberosities, which are the strongest parts of the hip bones.

A massive ligament runs from the sacrum to each ischial tuberosity. This *sacrotuberous ligament* (not illustrated) helps hold the pelvis together. The ischial tuberosity is also a site of attachment of the large hamstring muscles of the posterior thigh.

Pubis

The **pubis** (pu′bis; "sexually mature"), or *pubic bone*, forms the anterior portion of the hip bone (Figures 7.30 and 7.31). In the anatomical position, it lies nearly horizontally and the urinary bladder rests upon it. Essentially, the pubis is V shaped with **superior** and **inferior pubic rami** issuing from its flattened medial **body**. The anterior border of the pubis is thickened to form the **pubic crest**. At the lateral end of the pubic crest is the **pubic tubercle**, one of the attachments for the *inguinal ligament*. As the two rami of the pubis run laterally to join with the body and ramus of the ischium, they define a large opening in the hip bone, the **obturator foramen** (ob″tu-ra′tor), through which a few blood vessels and nerves pass. Although the obturator foramen is large, it is nearly closed by a fibrous membrane in life (*obturator* = closed up).

The bodies of the two pubic bones are joined by a fibrocartilage disc, forming the midline **pubic symphysis** joint. Inferior to this joint, the inferior pubic rami angle laterally, forming an inverted V-shaped arch called the **pubic arch** or **subpubic angle**. The acuteness of this arch helps to differentiate the male and female pelves.

(Text continues on p. 238.)

7

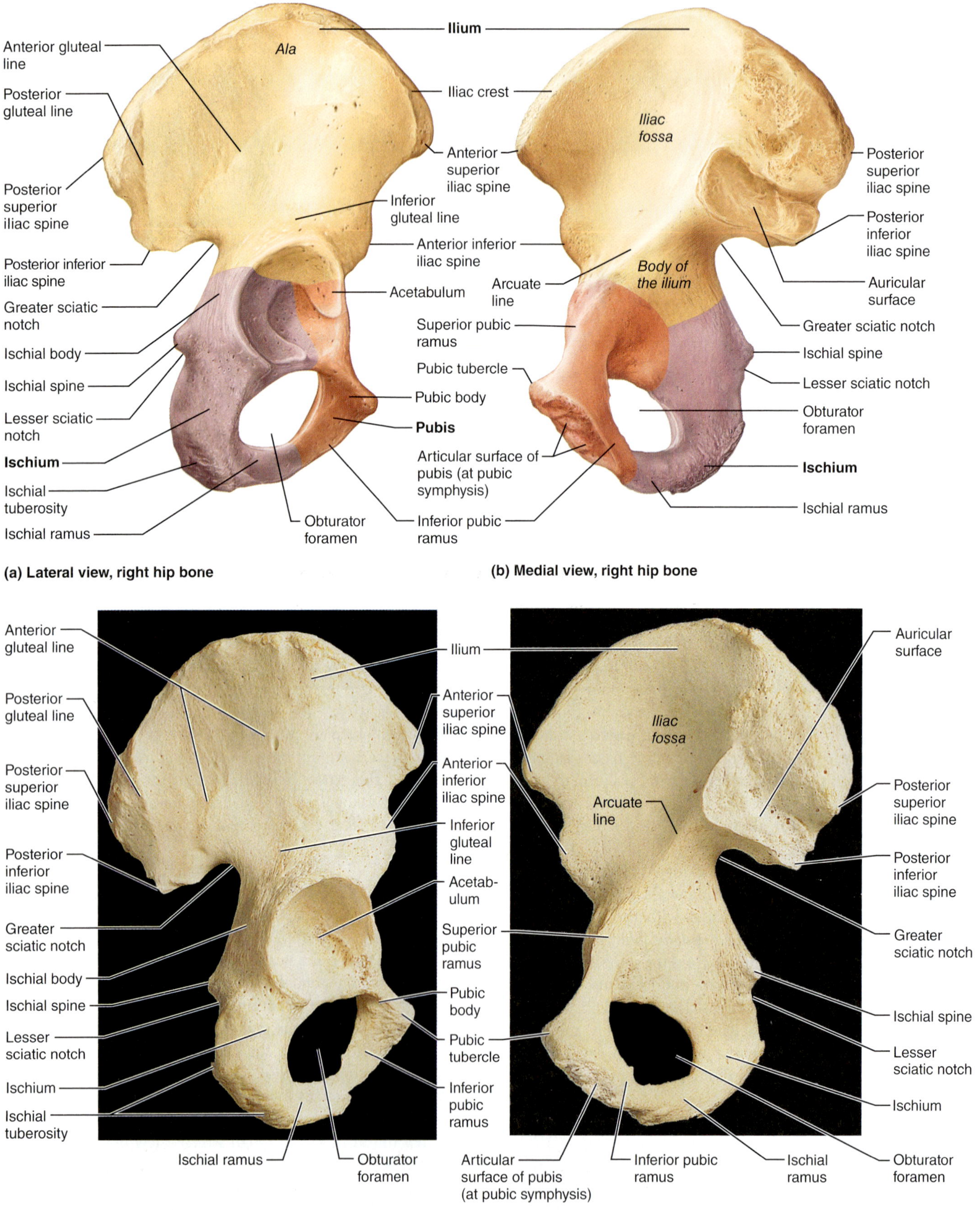

(c) Lateral view, right hip bone **(d) Medial view, right hip bone**

Figure 7.31 The hip (coxal) bones. Lateral and medial views of the right hip bone. The point of fusion of the ilium (gold), ischium (violet), and pubic (red) bones at the acetabulum is indicated in the diagrams (a, b). (For a related image, see *A Brief Atlas of the Human Body*, Figure 28.)

Table 7.4 Comparison of the Male and Female Pelves

CHARACTERISTIC	FEMALE	MALE
General structure and functional modifications	Tilted forward; adapted for childbearing; true pelvis defines the birth canal; cavity of the true pelvis is broad, shallow, and has a greater capacity	Tilted less far forward; adapted for support of a male's heavier build and stronger muscles; cavity of the true pelvis is narrow and deep
Bone thickness	Less; bones lighter, thinner, and smoother	Greater; bones heavier and thicker, and markings are more prominent
Acetabula	Smaller; farther apart	Larger; closer
Pubic angle/arch	Broader (80° to 90°); more rounded	Angle is more acute (50° to 60°)
Anterior view		

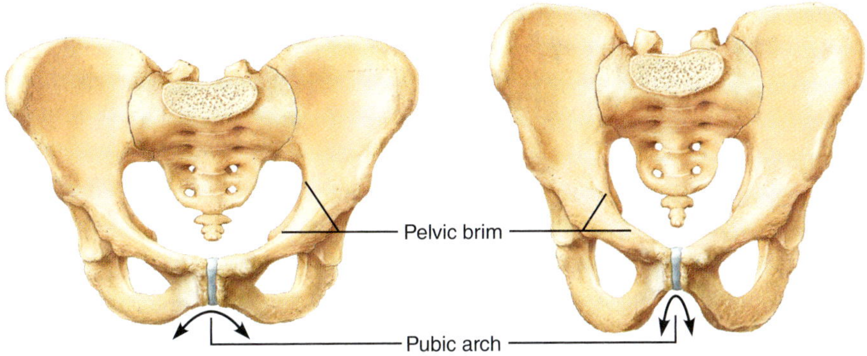

CHARACTERISTIC	FEMALE	MALE
Sacrum	Wider; shorter; sacral curvature is accentuated	Narrow; longer; sacral promontory more ventral
Coccyx	More movable; projects inferiorly	Less movable; projects anteriorly
Greater sciatic notch	Wide and shallow	Narrow and deep
Left lateral view	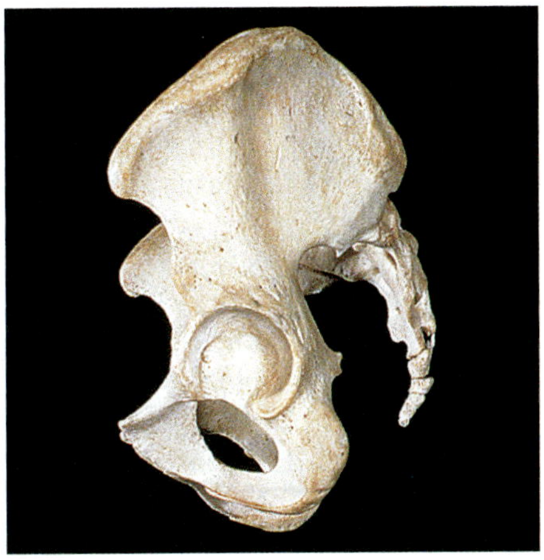	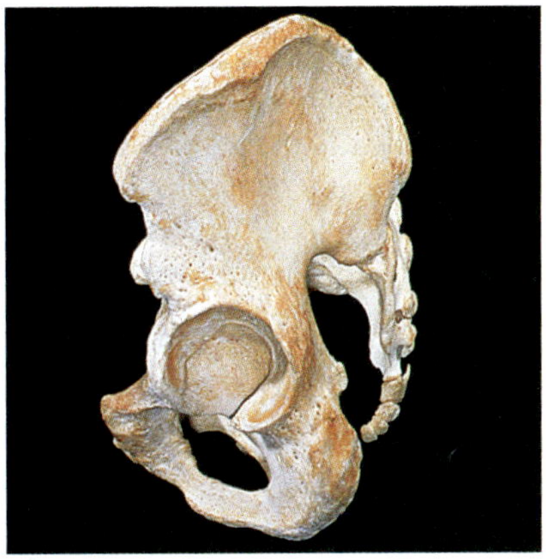

CHARACTERISTIC	FEMALE	MALE
Pelvic inlet (brim)	Wider; oval from side to side	Narrow; basically heart shaped
Pelvic outlet	Wider; ischial tuberosities shorter, farther apart and everted	Narrower; ischial tuberosities longer, sharper, and point more medially
Posteroinferior view	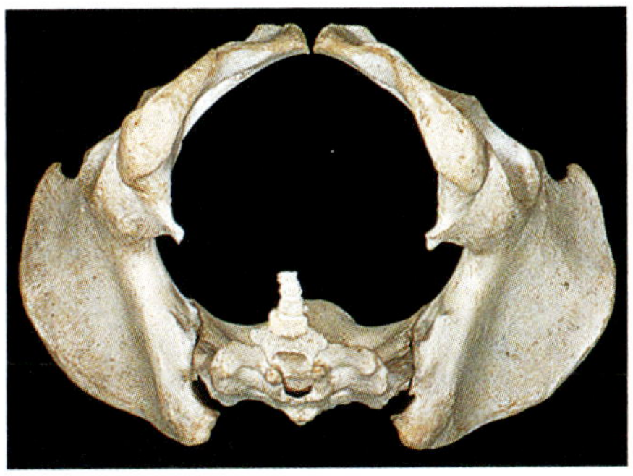	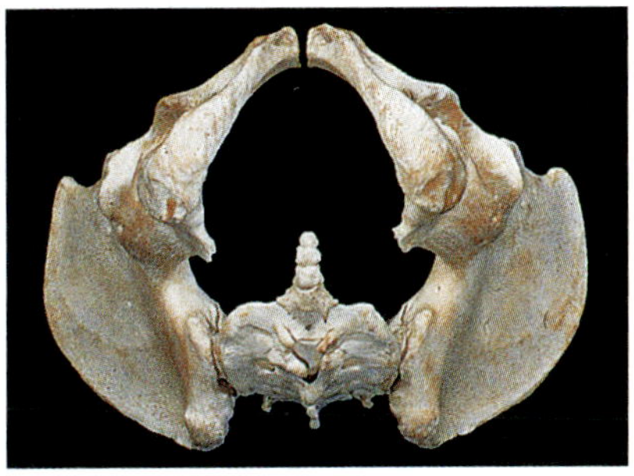

Pelvic Structure and Childbearing

The deep, basinlike structure formed by the hip bones, sacrum, and coccyx is called the **pelvis** or the *bony pelvis*. The differences between the male and female pelves are striking. The female pelvis is modified for childbearing: It tends to be wider, shallower, lighter, and rounder than that of a male. The female pelvis not only accommodates a growing fetus, but it must be large enough to allow the infant's relatively large head to exit at birth. The major differences between the typical male and female pelves are summarized and illustrated in Table 7.4.

The pelvis is said to consist of a false (greater) pelvis and a true (lesser) pelvis separated by the **pelvic brim**, a continuous oval ridge that runs from the pubic crest through the arcuate line and sacral promontory (Figure 7.30). The **false pelvis**, that portion superior to the pelvic brim, is bounded by the alae of the ilia laterally and the lumbar vertebrae posteriorly. The false pelvis is really part of the abdomen and helps support the abdominal viscera. It does not restrict childbirth in any way.

7

The **true pelvis** is the region inferior to the pelvic brim that is almost entirely surrounded by bone. It forms a deep bowl containing the pelvic organs. Its dimensions, particularly those of its *inlet* and *outlet*, are critical to the uncomplicated delivery of a baby, and they are carefully measured by an obstetrician.

The **pelvic inlet** *is* the pelvic brim, and its widest dimension is from right to left along the frontal plane. As labor begins, an infant's head typically enters the inlet with its forehead facing one ilium and its occiput facing the other. A sacral promontory that is particularly large can impair the infant's entry into the true pelvis.

The **pelvic outlet**, illustrated in the photos at the bottom of Table 7.4, is the inferior margin of the true pelvis. It is bounded anteriorly by the pubic arch, laterally by the ischia, and posteriorly by the sacrum and coccyx. Both the coccyx and the ischial spines protrude into the outlet opening, so a sharply angled coccyx or unusually large spines can interfere with delivery. The largest dimension of the outlet is the anteroposterior diameter.

Generally, after the baby's head passes through the inlet, it rotates so that the forehead faces posteriorly and the occiput anteriorly, and this is the usual position of the baby's head as it leaves the mother's body (see Figure 28.18 (2)). Thus, during birth, the infant's head makes a quarter turn to follow the widest dimensions of the true pelvis.

☑ Check Your Understanding

28. The ilium and pubis help to form the os coxae. What other bone is involved in forming the os coxae?
29. The pelvic girdle is a heavy, strong girdle. How does its structure reflect its function?
30. Which of the following terms or phrases refer to the female pelvis? Wider, shorter sacrum; cavity narrow and deep; narrow heart-shaped inlet; more movable coccyx; long ischial spines.

For answers, see Appendix H.

The Lower Limb

✓ Identify the lower limb bones and their important markings.

The lower limbs carry the entire weight of the erect body and are subjected to exceptional forces when we jump or run. Thus, it is not surprising that the bones of the lower limbs are thicker and stronger than comparable bones of the upper limbs. The three segments of each lower limb are the thigh, the leg, and the foot (see **Table 7.5** on p. 243).

Thigh

The **femur** (fe′mur; "thigh"), the single bone of the thigh **(Figure 7.32)**, is the largest, longest, strongest bone in the body. Its durable structure reflects the fact that the stress on the femur during vigorous jumping can reach 280 kg/cm^2 (about 2 tons per square inch)! The femur is clothed by bulky muscles that prevent us from palpating its course down the length of the thigh. Its length is roughly one-quarter of a person's height.

Proximally, the femur articulates with the hip bone and then courses medially as it descends toward the knee. This arrangement allows the knee joints to be closer to the body's center of gravity and provides for better balance. The medial course of the two femurs is more pronounced in women because of their wider pelvis, a situation that may contribute to the greater incidence of knee problems in female athletes.

The ball-like **head** of the femur has a small central pit called the **fovea capitis** (fo′ve-ah kă′pĭ-tis; "pit of the head"). The short *ligament of the head of the femur* runs from this pit to the acetabulum, where it helps secure the femur. The head is carried on a *neck* that angles *laterally* to join the shaft. This arrangement reflects the fact that the femur articulates with the lateral aspect (rather than the inferior region) of the pelvis. The neck is the weakest part of the femur and is often fractured, an injury commonly called a broken hip.

At the junction of the shaft and neck are the lateral **greater trochanter** (tro-kan′ter) and posteromedial **lesser trochanter**. These projections serve as sites of attachment for thigh and buttock muscles. The two trochanters are connected by the **intertrochanteric line** anteriorly and by the prominent **intertrochanteric crest** posteriorly.

Inferior to the intertrochanteric crest on the posterior shaft is the **gluteal tuberosity**, which blends into a long vertical ridge, the **linea aspera** (lin′e-ah as′per-ah; "rough line"), inferiorly. Distally, the linea aspera diverges, forming the **medial** and **lateral supracondylar lines**. All of these markings are sites of muscle attachment. Except for the linea aspera, the femur shaft is smooth and rounded.

Distally, the femur broadens and ends in the wheel-like **lateral** and **medial condyles**, which articulate with the tibia of the leg. The **medial** and **lateral epicondyles** (sites of muscle attachment) flank the condyles superiorly. On the superior part of the medial epicondyle is a bump, the **adductor tubercle**. The smooth **patellar surface**, between the condyles on the anterior femoral surface, articulates with the *patella* (pah-tel′ah), or kneecap (see Figure 7.32 and Table 7.5). Between the condyles on the posterior aspect of the femur is the deep, U-shaped

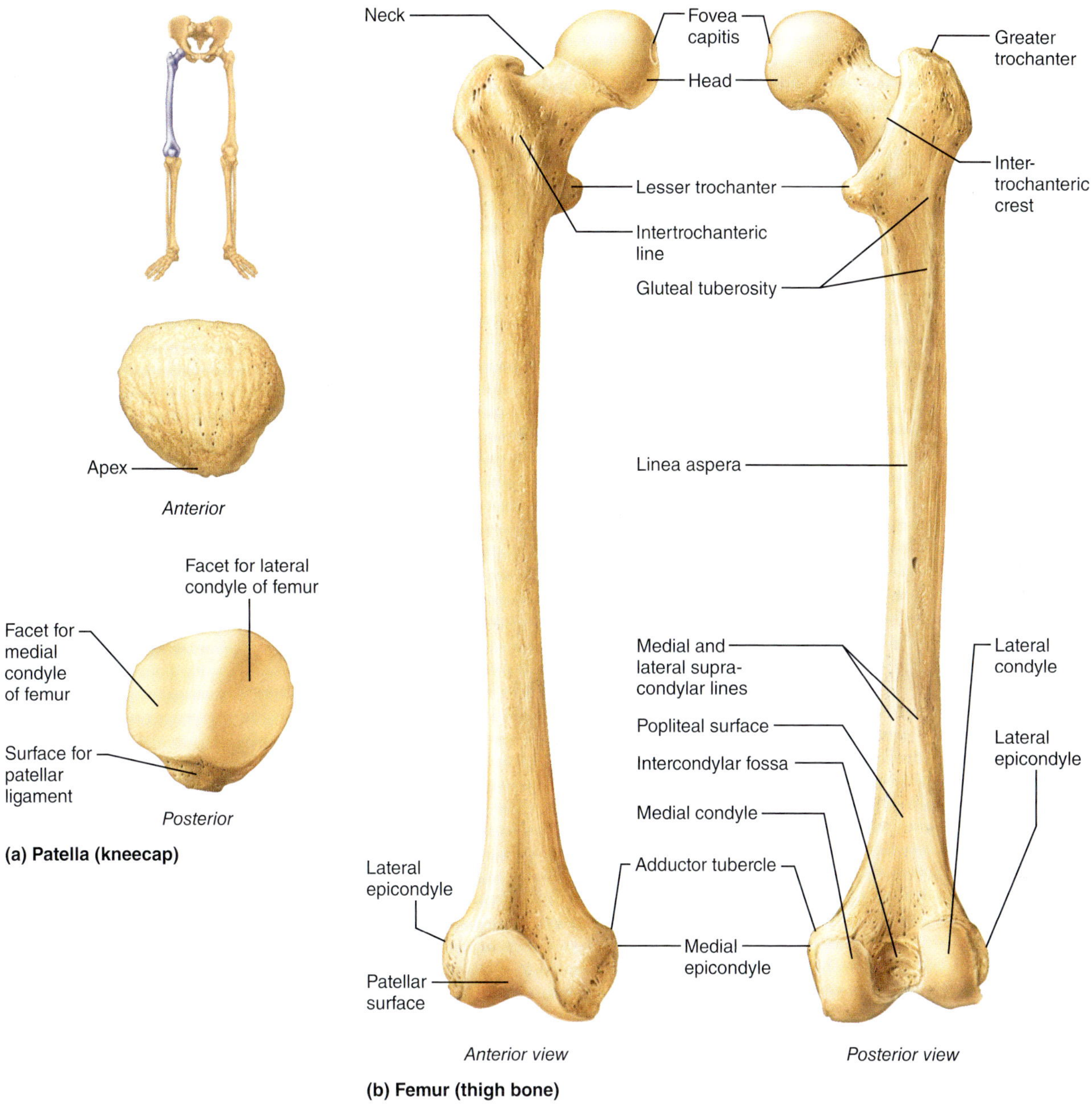

Figure 7.32 Bones of the right knee and thigh. (For a related image, see *A Brief Atlas of the Human Body*, Figure 29.)

intercondylar fossa, and superior to that on the shaft is the smooth *popliteal surface*.

The **patella** ("small pan") is a triangular sesamoid bone enclosed in the (quadriceps) tendon that secures the anterior thigh muscles to the tibia. It protects the knee joint anteriorly and improves the leverage of the thigh muscles acting across the knee.

Leg

Two parallel bones, the tibia and fibula, form the skeleton of the leg, the region of the lower limb between the knee and the ankle **(Figure 7.33)**. These two bones are connected by an *interosseous membrane* and articulate with each other both proximally and distally. Unlike the joints between the radius and ulna of the forearm, the *tibiofibular joints* (tib″e-o-fib′u-lar) of the leg allow essentially no movement. The bones of the leg thus form a less flexible but stronger and more stable limb than those of the forearm. The medial tibia articulates proximally with the femur to form the modified hinge joint of the knee and distally with the talus bone of the foot at the ankle. The fibula, by contrast, does not contribute to the knee joint and merely helps stabilize the ankle joint.

Tibia

The **tibia** (tib′e-ah; "shinbone") receives the weight of the body from the femur and transmits it to the foot. It is second only to the femur in size and strength. At its broad proximal end are the concave **medial** and **lateral condyles**, which look

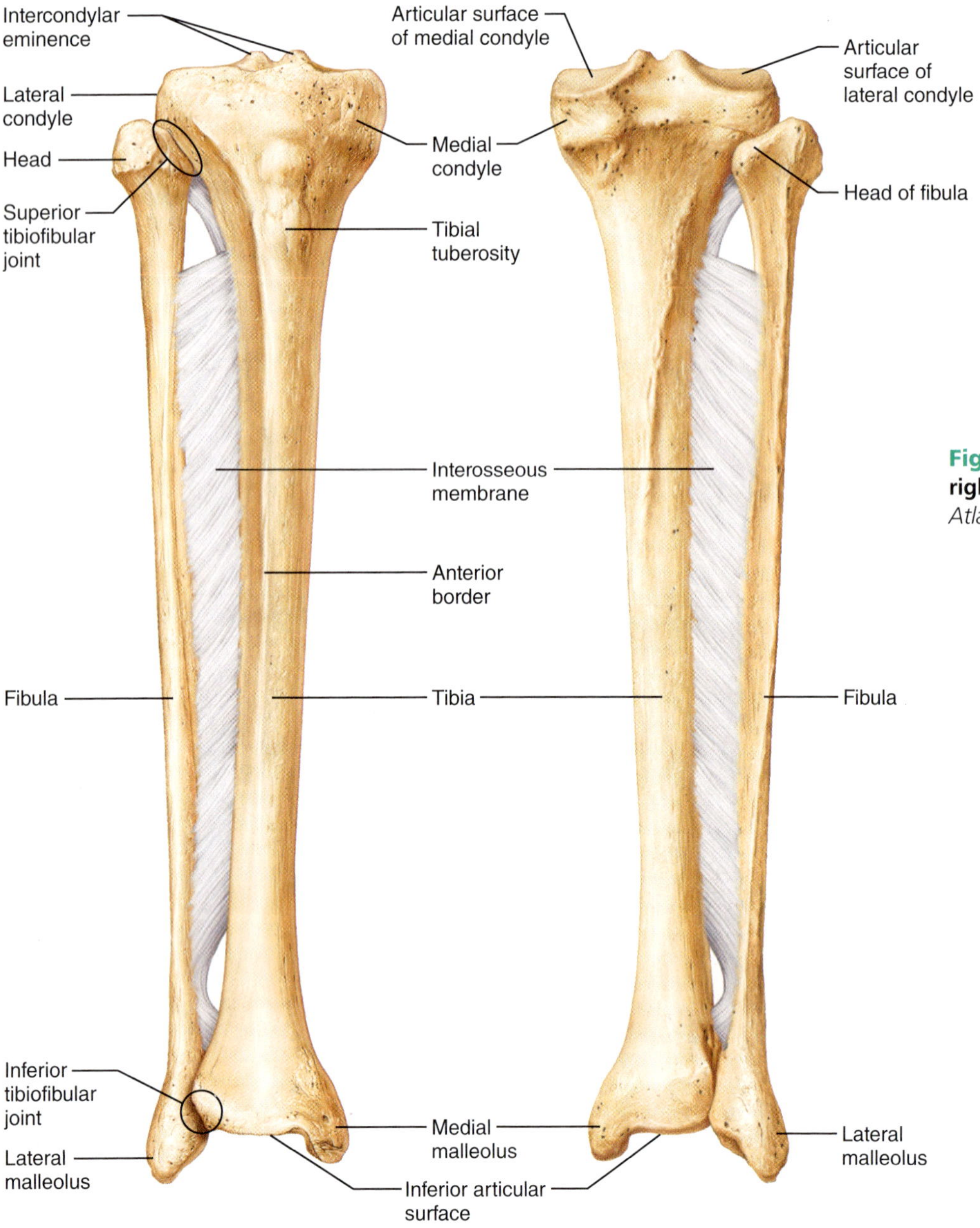

(a) Anterior view **(b) Posterior view**

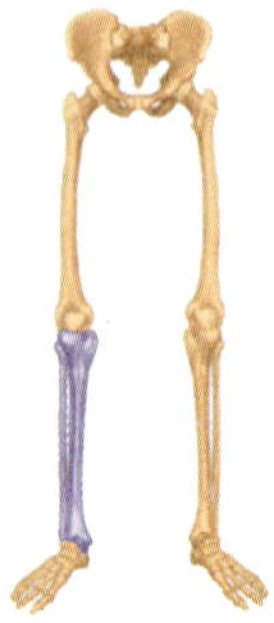

Figure 7.33 The tibia and fibula of the right leg. (For a related image, see *A Brief Atlas of the Human Body,* Figure 30.)

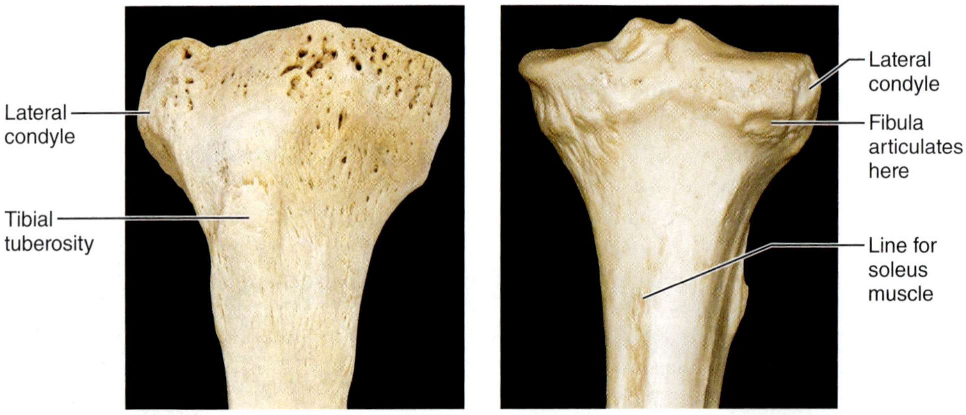

(c) Anterior view, proximal tibia **(d) Posterior view, proximal tibia**

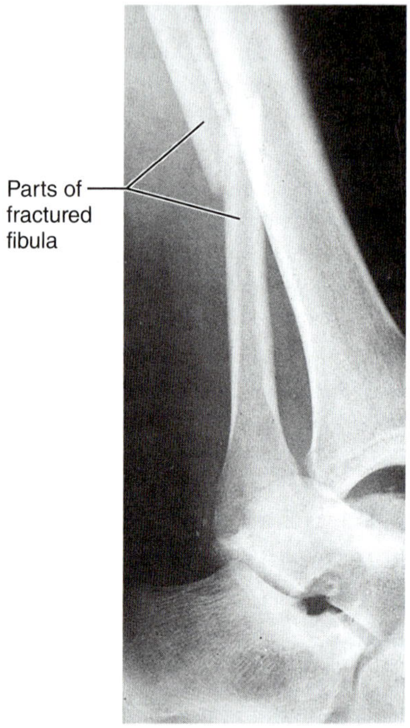

(e) X ray of Pott's fracture of the fibula

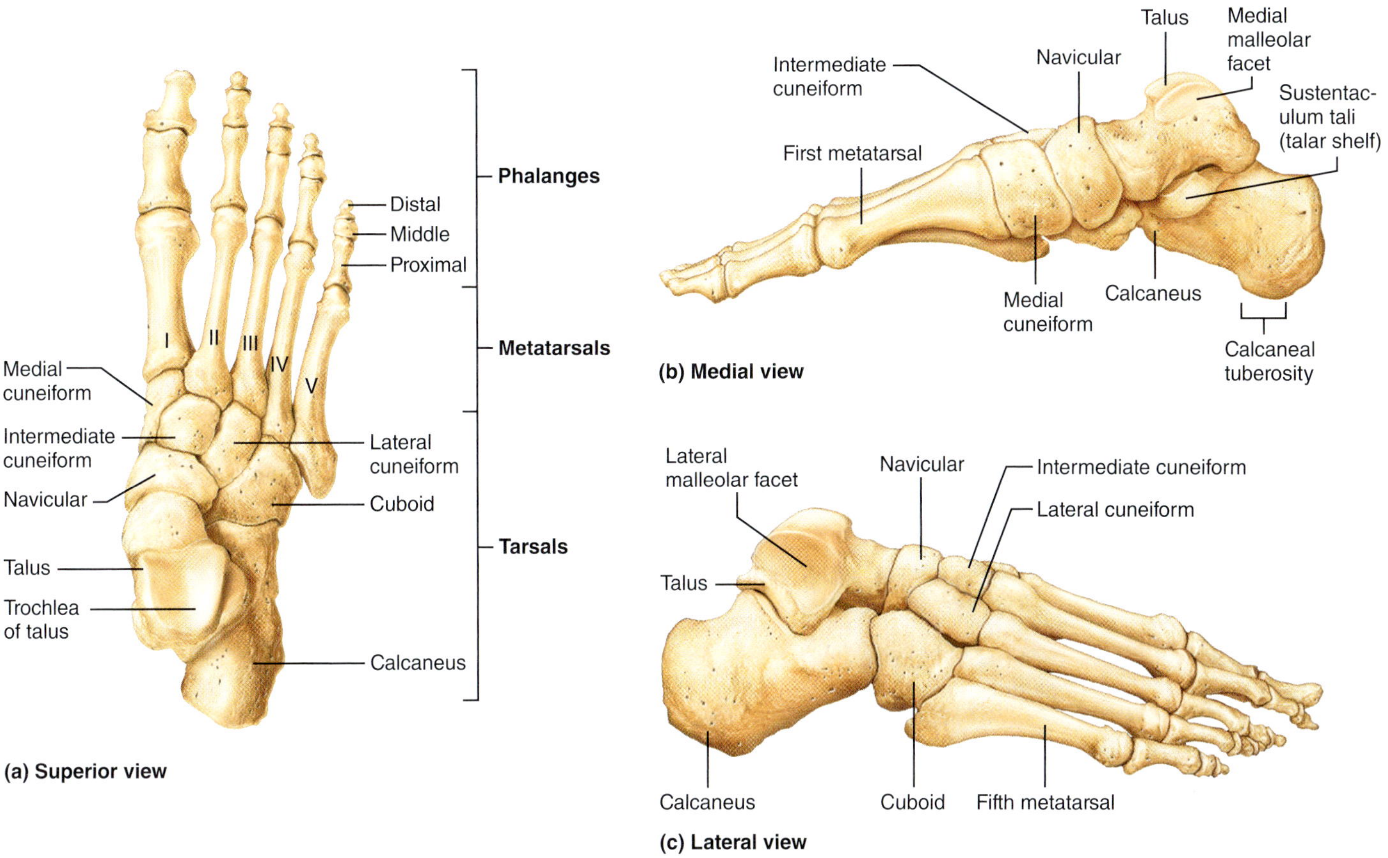

Figure 7.34 Bones of the right foot. (For a related image, see *A Brief Atlas of the Human Body*, Figure 31a, c, and d.)

like two huge checkers lying side by side. These are separated by an irregular projection, the **intercondylar eminence**. The tibial condyles articulate with the corresponding condyles of the femur. The inferior region of the lateral tibial condyle bears a facet that indicates the site of the *superior tibiofibular joint*. Just inferior to the condyles, the tibia's anterior surface displays the rough **tibial tuberosity**, to which the patellar ligament attaches.

The tibial shaft is triangular in cross section. Neither the tibia's sharp **anterior border** nor its medial surface is covered by muscles, so they can be felt just deep to the skin along their entire length. The anguish of a "bumped" shin is an experience familiar to nearly everyone. Distally the tibia is flat where it articulates with the talus bone of the foot. Medial to that joint surface is an inferior projection, the **medial malleolus** (mah-le′o-lus; "little hammer"), which forms the medial bulge of the ankle. The **fibular notch**, on the lateral surface of the tibia, participates in the *inferior tibiofibular joint*.

Fibula

The **fibula** (fib′u-lah; "pin") is a sticklike bone with slightly expanded ends. It articulates proximally and distally with the lateral aspects of the tibia. Its proximal end is its **head**; its distal end is the **lateral malleolus**. The lateral malleolus forms the conspicuous lateral ankle bulge and articulates with the talus. The fibular shaft is heavily ridged and appears to have been twisted a quarter turn. The fibula does not bear weight, but several muscles originate from it.

Homeostatic Imbalance 7.7

A *Pott's fracture* occurs at the distal end of the fibula, the tibia, or both. It is a common sports injury. (See Figure 7.33e.) ✚

☑ Check Your Understanding

31. What lower limb bone is the second largest bone in the body?
32. Where is the medial malleolus located?
33. Which of the following sites is not a site of muscle attachment? Greater trochanter, lesser trochanter, gluteal tuberosity, lateral condyle.

For answers, see Appendix H.

Foot

The skeleton of the foot includes the bones of the *tarsus*, the bones of the *metatarsus*, and the *phalanges*, or toe bones **(Figure 7.34)**. The foot has two important functions: It supports our body weight, and it acts as a lever to propel the body forward when we walk and run. A single bone could serve both purposes, but it would adapt poorly to uneven ground. Segmentation makes the foot pliable, avoiding this problem.

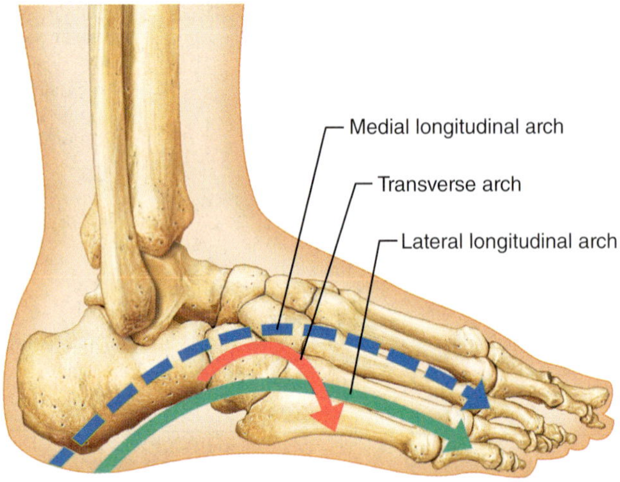

(a) Lateral aspect of right foot

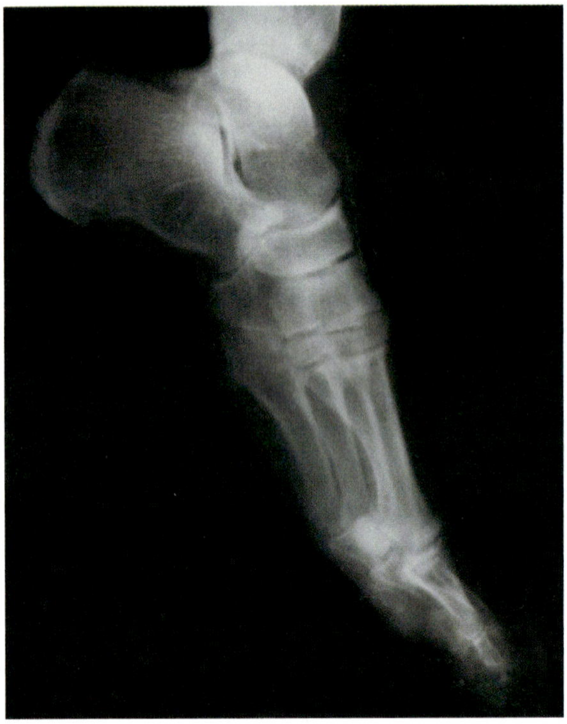

(b) X ray, medial aspect of right foot

Figure 7.35 **Arches of the foot.**

Tarsus

The **tarsus** is made up of seven bones called **tarsals** (tar′salz) that form the posterior half of the foot. It corresponds to the carpus of the hand. Body weight is carried primarily by the two largest, most posterior tarsals: the **talus** (ta′lus; "ankle"), which articulates with the tibia and fibula superiorly, and the strong **calcaneus** (kal-ka′ne-us; "heel bone"), which forms the heel of the foot and carries the talus on its superior surface. The thick *calcaneal*, or *Achilles*, *tendon* of the calf muscles attaches to the posterior surface of the calcaneus. The part of the calcaneus that touches the ground is the **calcaneal tuberosity**, and its shelflike projection that supports part of the talus is the **sustentaculum tali** (sus″ten-tak′u-lum ta′le; "supporter of the talus") or **talar shelf**. The tibia articulates with the talus at the *trochlea* of the talus. The remaining tarsals are the lateral **cuboid**, the medial **navicular** (nah-vik′u-lar), and the anterior **medial**, **intermediate**, and **lateral cuneiform bones** (ku-ne′i-form; "wedge-shaped"). The cuboid and cuneiform bones articulate with the metatarsal bones anteriorly.

Metatarsus

The **metatarsus** consists of five small, long bones called **metatarsals**. These are numbered I to V beginning on the medial (great toe) side of the foot. The first metatarsal, which plays an important role in supporting body weight, is short and thick. The arrangement of the metatarsals is more parallel than that of the metacarpals of the hands. Distally, where the metatarsals articulate with the proximal phalanges of the toes, the enlarged head of the first metatarsal forms the "ball" of the foot.

Phalanges (Toes)

The 14 phalanges of the toes are a good deal smaller than those of the fingers and so are less nimble. But their general structure and arrangement are the same. There are three phalanges in each digit except for the great toe, the **hallux**. The hallux has only two, proximal and distal.

Arches of the Foot

A segmented structure can hold up weight only if it is arched. The foot has three arches: two *longitudinal arches* (*medial* and *lateral*) and one *transverse arch* **(Figure 7.35)**, which account for its awesome strength. These arches are maintained by the interlocking shapes of the foot bones, by strong ligaments, and by the pull of some tendons during muscle activity. The ligaments and muscle tendons provide a certain amount of springiness. In general, the arches "give," or stretch slightly, when weight is applied to the foot and spring back when the weight is removed, which makes walking and running more economical in terms of energy use than would otherwise be the case.

If you examine your wet footprints, you will see that the medial margin from the heel to the head of the first metatarsal leaves no print. This is because the **medial longitudinal arch** curves well above the ground. The talus is the keystone of this arch, which originates at the calcaneus, rises toward the talus, and then descends to the three medial metatarsals.

The **lateral longitudinal arch** is very low. It elevates the lateral part of the foot just enough to redistribute some of the weight to the calcaneus and the head of the fifth metatarsal (to the ends of the arch). The cuboid is the keystone bone of this arch.

The two longitudinal arches serve as pillars for the **transverse arch**, which runs obliquely from one side of the foot to the other, following the line of the joints between the tarsals and metatarsals. Together, the arches of the foot form a half-dome that distributes about half of a person's standing and walking weight to the heel bones and half to the heads of the metatarsals.

Table 7.5 Bones of the Appendicular Skeleton, Part 2: Pelvic Girdle and Lower Limb

BODY REGION	BONES*	ILLUSTRATION	LOCATION	MARKINGS
Pelvic girdle (Figures 7.30, 7.31)	**Coxal** (2) (hip)	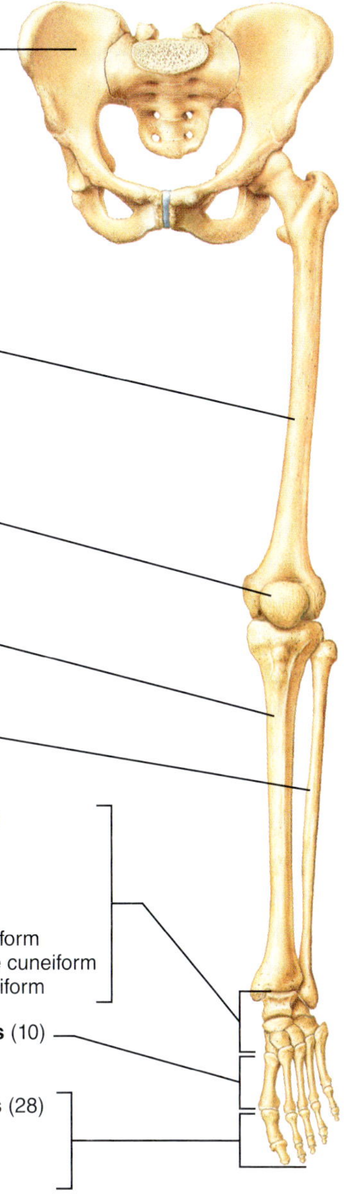	Each coxal (hip) bone is formed by the fusion of an ilium, ischium, and pubis; the coxal bones articulate anteriorly at the pubic symphysis and form sacroiliac joints with the sacrum posteriorly; girdle consisting of both coxal bones and the sacrum is basinlike	Iliac crest; anterior and posterior iliac spines; auricular surface; greater and lesser sciatic notches; obturator foramen; ischial tuberosity and spine; acetabulum; pubic arch; pubic crest; pubic tubercle
Lower limb Thigh (Figure 7.32)	**Femur** (2)		Femur is the sole bone of thigh; between hip joint and knee; largest bone of the body	Head; greater and lesser trochanters; neck; lateral and medial condyles and epicondyles; gluteal tuberosity; linea aspera
Kneecap (Figure 7.32)	**Patella** (2)		Patella is a sesamoid bone formed within the tendon of the quadriceps (anterior thigh) muscles	
Leg (Figure 7.33)	**Tibia** (2)		Tibia is the larger and more medial bone of leg; between knee and foot	Medial and lateral condyles; tibial tuberosity; anterior border; medial malleolus
	Fibula (2)		Fibula is the lateral bone of leg; sticklike	Head; lateral malleolus
Foot (Figure 7.34)	7 **Tarsals** (14) talus calcaneus navicular cuboid lateral cuneiform intermediate cuneiform medial cuneiform		Tarsals are seven bones forming the proximal part of the foot; the talus articulates with the leg bones at the ankle joint; the calcaneus, the largest tarsal, forms the heel	
	5 **Metatarsals** (10)		Metatarsals are five bones numbered I–V	
	14 **Phalanges** (28) distal middle proximal		Phalanges form the toes; three in digits 2–5, two in digit 1 (the great toe)	

* The number in parentheses ( ) following the bone name denotes the total number of such bones in the body.

Homeostatic Imbalance 7.8

Standing immobile for extended periods places excessive strain on the tendons and ligaments of the feet (because the muscles are inactive) and can result in fallen arches, or "flat feet," particularly if a person is overweight. Running on hard surfaces can also cause arches to fall unless the runner wears shoes that give proper arch support. ✚

The bones of the thigh, leg, and foot are summarized in Table 7.5.

☑ Check Your Understanding

34. Besides supporting our weight, what is a major function of the arches of the foot?
35. What are the two largest tarsal bones in each foot, and which one forms the heel of the foot?

For answers, see Appendix H.

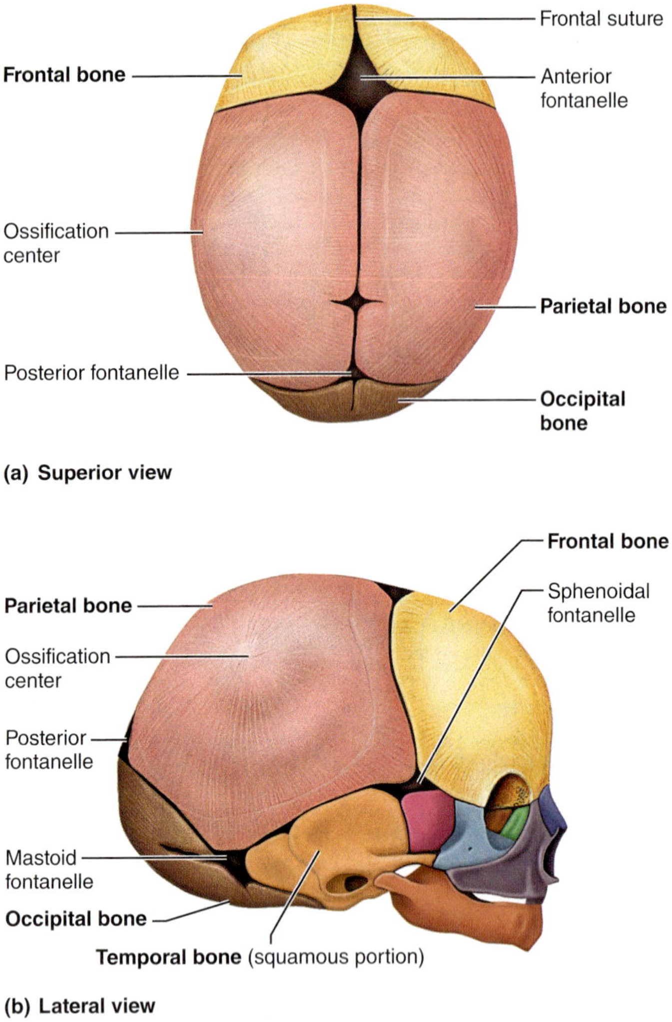

Figure 7.36 Skull of a newborn. Notice that the infant's skull has more bones than that of an adult. (For a related image, see *A Brief Atlas of the Human Body*, Figure 16.)

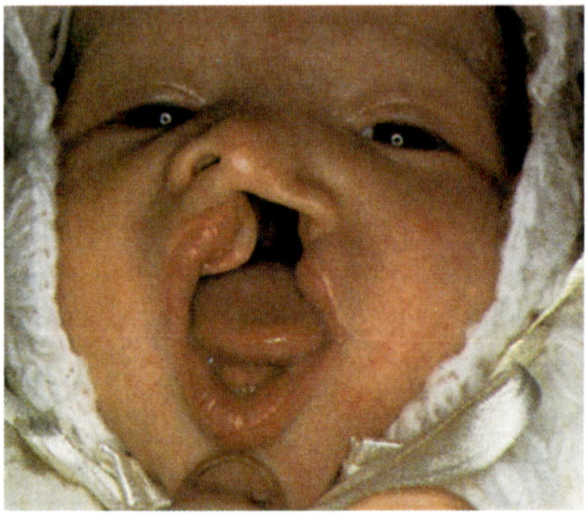

Figure 7.37 A baby born with a cleft lip and palate.

Homeostatic Imbalance 7.9

Several congenital abnormalities may distort the skull. Most common is *cleft palate*, a condition in which the right and left halves of the palate fail to fuse medially **(Figure 7.37)**. The persistent opening between the oral and nasal cavities interferes with sucking and can lead to aspiration (inhalation) of food into the lungs and *aspiration pneumonia*.✚

Developmental Aspects of the Skeleton

- ✓ Define fontanelles and indicate their significance.
- ✓ Describe how skeletal proportions change through life.
- ✓ Discuss how age-related skeletal changes may affect health.

The membrane bones of the skull start to ossify late in the second month of development. The rapid deposit of bone matrix at the ossification centers produces cone-shaped protrusions in the developing bones. At birth, the skull bones are still incomplete and are connected by as yet unossified remnants of fibrous membranes called **fontanelles** (fon″tah-nelz′) **(Figure 7.36)**. The fontanelles allow the infant's head to be compressed slightly during birth, and they accommodate brain growth in the fetus and infant. A baby's pulse can be felt surging in these "soft spots"; hence their name (*fontanelle* = little fountain). The large, diamond-shaped *anterior fontanelle* is palpable for 1½ to 2 years after birth. The others are replaced by bone by the end of the first year.

The skeleton changes throughout life, but the changes in childhood are most dramatic. At birth, the baby's cranium is huge relative to its face, and several bones are still unfused (e.g., the mandible and frontal bones). The maxillae and mandible are foreshortened, and the contours of the face are flat (Figure 7.39). By 9 months after birth, the cranium is already half of its adult size (volume) because of the rapid growth of the brain. By 8 to 9 years, the cranium has almost reached adult proportions.

Between the ages of 6 and 13, the head appears to enlarge substantially as the face literally grows out from the skull. The jaws, cheekbones, and nose become more prominent. These facial changes are correlated with the expansion of the nose and paranasal sinuses, and development of the permanent teeth. Figure 7.39 tracks how differential bone growth alters body proportions throughout life.

Only the thoracic and sacral curvatures are well developed at birth. These so-called **primary curvatures** are convex posteriorly, and an infant's spine arches, like that of a four-legged animal **(Figure 7.38)**.

The **secondary curvatures**—cervical and lumbar—are convex anteriorly and are associated with a child's development. They result from reshaping of the intervertebral discs rather than from modifications of the vertebrae. The cervical curvature is present before birth but is not pronounced until the baby starts to lift its head (at about 3 months). The lumbar curvature develops when the baby begins to walk (at about 12 months). The lumbar curvature positions the weight of the trunk over the body's center of gravity, providing optimal balance when standing.

Vertebral problems (scoliosis or lordosis; see Figure 7.17a and c) may appear during the early school years, when rapid growth of the limb bones stretches many muscles. During the

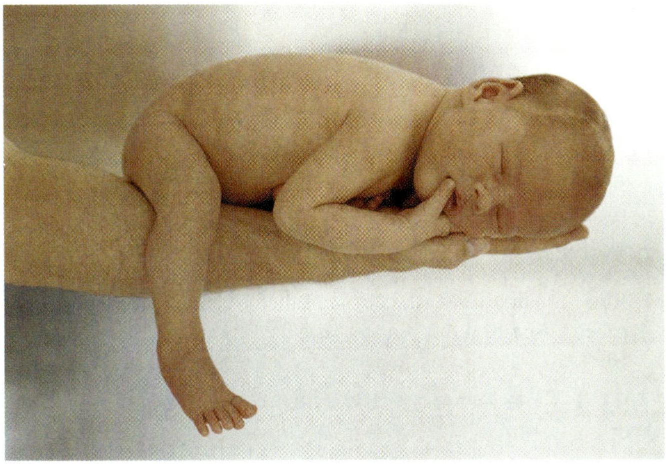

Figure 7.38 The C-shaped spine of a newborn infant.

preschool years, lordosis is often present, but this is usually rectified as the abdominal muscles become stronger and the pelvis tilts forward. The thorax grows wider, but a true "military posture" (head erect, shoulders back, abdomen in, and chest out) does not develop until adolescence.

Homeostatic Imbalance 7.10

The appendicular skeleton can also suffer from a number of congenital abnormalities. One that occurs in just over 1% of infants and is quite severe is *dysplasia of the hip* (dis-pla′ze-ah; "bad formation"). The acetabulum forms incompletely or the ligaments of the hip joint are loose, so the head of the femur slips out of its socket. Early treatment (a splint or harness to hold the femur in place or surgery to tighten hip ligaments) is essential to prevent permanent crippling. +

During youth, growth of the skeleton not only increases overall body height but also changes body proportions **(Figure 7.39)**. At birth, the head and trunk are approximately 1½ times as long as the lower limbs. The lower limbs grow more rapidly than the trunk from this time on, and by the age of 10, the head and trunk are approximately the same height as the lower limbs, a condition that persists thereafter. During puberty, the female pelvis broadens in preparation for childbearing, and the entire male skeleton becomes more robust. Once adult height is reached, a healthy skeleton changes very little until late middle age.

Old age affects many parts of the skeleton, especially the spine. As the discs become thinner, less hydrated, and less elastic, the risk of disc herniation increases. By 55 years, a loss of several centimeters in stature is common. Further shortening can be produced by osteoporosis of the spine or by kyphosis (called "dowager's hump" in the elderly; see Figure 7.17b). What was done during youth may be undone in old age as the vertebral column gradually resumes its initial arc shape.

The thorax becomes more rigid with age, largely because the costal cartilages ossify. This loss of rib cage elasticity causes shallow breathing, which leads to less efficient gas exchange.

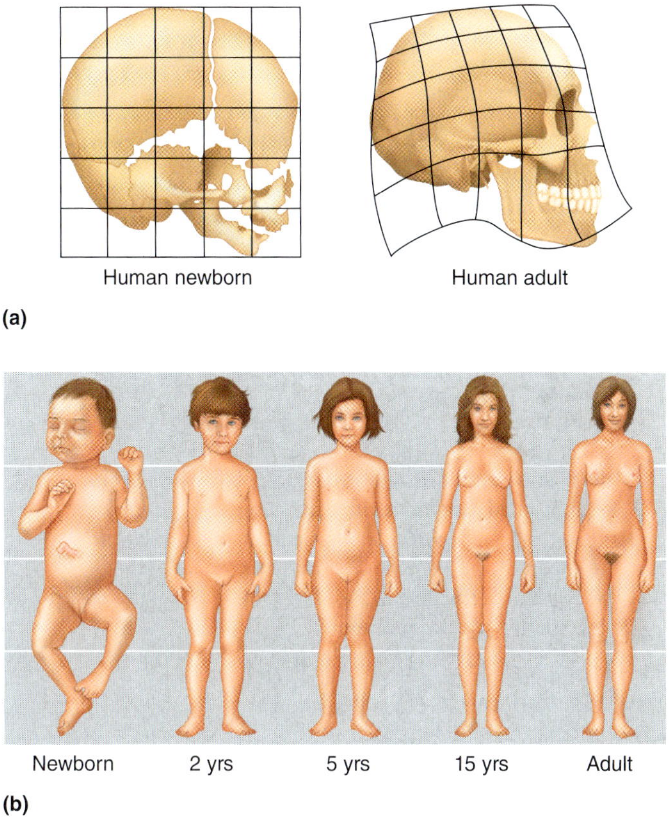

Figure 7.39 Different growth rates of body parts determine body proportions. (a) Differential growth transforms the rounded, foreshortened skull of a newborn to the sloping skull of an adult. **(b)** During growth of a human, the arms and legs grow faster than the head and trunk, as seen in this conceptualization of different-aged individuals all drawn at the same height.

All bones, you will recall, lose mass with age. Cranial bones lose less mass than most, but changes in facial contours with age are common. As the bony tissue of the jaws declines, the jaws look small and childlike once again. If the elderly person loses his or her teeth, this loss of bone from the jaws is accelerated, because the alveolar region bone is resorbed. As bones become more porous, they are more likely to fracture, especially the vertebrae and the neck of the femur.

Check Your Understanding

36. What developmental events result in a dramatic enlargement of the facial skeleton between the ages of 6 and 13?
37. Under what conditions does the lumbar curvature of the spine develop?

For answers, see Appendix H.

Our skeleton is a marvelous substructure, to be sure, but it is much more than that. It is a protector and supporter of other body systems, and without it (and the joints considered in Chapter 8), our muscles would be almost useless. The homeostatic relationships between the skeletal system and other body systems are illustrated in *System Connections* in Chapter 6 (p. 195).

Chapter Summary

1. The axial skeleton forms the longitudinal axis of the body. Its principal subdivisions are the skull, vertebral column, and thoracic cage. It provides support and protection (by enclosure).
2. The appendicular skeleton consists of the bones of the pectoral and pelvic girdles and the limbs. It allows mobility for manipulation and locomotion.

PART 1 The Axial Skeleton

The Skull (pp. 201–217)

1. The skull is formed by 22 bones. The cranium forms the vault and base of the skull, which protect the brain. The facial skeleton provides openings for the respiratory and digestive passages and attachment points for facial muscles.
2. Except for the temporomandibular joints, all bones of the adult skull are joined by immovable sutures.
3. **Cranium.** The eight bones of the cranium include the paired parietal and temporal bones and the single frontal, occipital, ethmoid, and sphenoid bones (see Table 7.1, pp. 216–217).
4. **Facial bones.** The 14 bones of the face include the paired maxillae, zygomatics, nasals, lacrimals, palatines, and inferior nasal conchae and the single mandible and vomer bones (Table 7.1).
5. **Orbits and nasal cavity.** Both the orbits and the nasal cavities are complicated bony regions formed of several bones.
6. **Paranasal sinuses.** Paranasal sinuses occur in the frontal, ethmoid, sphenoid, and maxillary bones.
7. **Hyoid bone.** The hyoid bone, supported in the neck by ligaments, serves as an attachment point for tongue and neck muscles.

The Vertebral Column (pp. 218–224)

1. **General characteristics.** The vertebral column includes 24 movable vertebrae (7 cervical, 12 thoracic, and 5 lumbar) and the sacrum and coccyx.
2. The fibrocartilage intervertebral discs act as shock absorbers and provide flexibility to the vertebral column.
3. The primary curvatures of the vertebral column are the thoracic and sacral; the secondary curvatures are the cervical and lumbar. Curvatures increase spine flexibility.
4. **General structure of vertebrae.** With the exception of C_1 and C_2, all vertebrae have a body, two transverse processes, two superior and two inferior articular processes, a spinous process, and a vertebral arch.
5. **Regional vertebral characteristics.** Special features distinguish the regional vertebrae (see Table 7.2, p. 223).

The Thoracic Cage (pp. 224–227)

1. The bones of the thoracic cage include the 12 rib pairs, the sternum, and the thoracic vertebrae. The thoracic cage protects the organs of the thoracic cavity.
2. **Sternum.** The sternum consists of the fused manubrium, body, and xiphoid process.
3. **Ribs.** The first seven rib pairs are called true ribs; the rest are called false ribs. Ribs 11 and 12 are floating ribs.

PART 2 The Appendicular Skeleton

The Pectoral (Shoulder) Girdle* (pp. 227–228)

1. Each pectoral girdle consists of one clavicle and one scapula. The pectoral girdles attach the upper limbs to the axial skeleton.
2. **Clavicles.** The clavicles hold the scapulae laterally away from the thorax. The sternoclavicular joints are the only attachment points of the pectoral girdle to the axial skeleton.
3. **Scapulae.** The scapulae articulate with the clavicles and with the humerus bones of the arms.

The Upper Limb* (pp. 228–234)

1. Each upper limb consists of 30 bones and is specialized for mobility.
2. **Arm/forearm/hand.** The skeleton of the arm is composed solely of the humerus; the skeleton of the forearm is composed of the radius and ulna; and the skeleton of the hand consists of the carpals, metacarpals, and phalanges.

The Pelvic (Hip) Girdle* (pp. 234–238)

1. The pelvic girdle, a heavy structure specialized for weight bearing, is composed of two hip bones and the sacrum. It secures the lower limbs to the axial skeleton.
2. Each hip bone consists of three fused bones: ilium, ischium, and pubis. The acetabulum occurs at the point of fusion.
3. **Ilium/ischium/pubis.** The ilium is the superior flaring portion of the hip bone. Each ilium forms a secure joint with the sacrum posteriorly. The ischium is a curved bar of bone; we sit on the ischial tuberosities. The V-shaped pubic bones articulate anteriorly at the pubic symphysis.
4. **Pelvic structure and childbearing.** The pelvis is the deep, basinlike structure formed by the hip bones, sacrum, and coccyx. The male pelvis is deep and narrow with larger, heavier bones than those of the female. The female pelvis, which forms the birth canal, is shallow and wide.

The Lower Limb* (pp. 238–243)

1. Each lower limb consists of the thigh, leg, and foot and is specialized for weight bearing and locomotion.
2. **Thigh.** The femur is the only bone of the thigh. Its ball-shaped head articulates with the acetabulum.
3. **Leg.** The bones of the leg are the tibia, which participates in forming both the knee and ankle joints, and the fibula.
4. **Foot.** The bones of the foot include the tarsals, metatarsals, and phalanges. The most important tarsals are the calcaneus (heel bone) and the talus, which articulates with the tibia superiorly.
5. The foot is supported by three arches (lateral, medial, and transverse) that distribute body weight to the heel and ball of the foot.

Developmental Aspects of the Skeleton (pp. 244–245)

1. Fontanelles, which allow brain growth and ease birth passage, are present in the skull at birth. Growth of the cranium after birth is related to brain growth. Increase in size of the facial skeleton follows tooth development and enlargement of nose and sinus cavities.
2. The vertebral column is C shaped at birth (thoracic and sacral curvatures are present); the secondary curvatures form when the baby begins to lift its head and walk.
3. Long bones continue to grow in length until late adolescence. The head and torso, initially 1½ times the length of the lower limbs, equal their length by the age of 10.
4. Changes in the female pelvis (preparatory for childbirth) occur during puberty.
5. Once at adult height, the skeleton changes little until late middle age. With old age, the intervertebral discs thin; this, along with osteoporosis, leads to a gradual loss in height and increased risk of disc herniation. Loss of bone mass increases the risk of fractures, and thoracic cage rigidity promotes breathing difficulties.

***For associated bone markings, see the pages indicated in the section heads.**

Review Questions

Multiple Choice/Matching

(Some questions have more than one correct answer. Select the best answer or answers from the choices given.)

1. Match the bones in column B with their description in column A. (Note that some descriptions require more than a single choice.)

Column A	Column B
____ (1) connected by the coronal suture	(a) ethmoid
	(b) frontal
____ (2) keystone bone of cranium	(c) mandible
	(d) maxillary
____ (3) keystone bone of the face	(e) occipital
	(f) palatine
____ (4) form the hard palate	(g) parietal
____ (5) allows the spinal cord to pass	(h) sphenoid
	(i) temporal
____ (6) forms the chin	
____ (7) contain paranasal sinuses	
____ (8) contains mastoid sinuses	

2. Match the key terms with the bone descriptions that follow.

Key:

(a) clavicle (b) ilium (c) ischium
(d) pubis (e) sacrum (f) scapula
(g) sternum

____ (1) bone of the axial skeleton to which the pectoral girdle attaches
____ (2) markings include glenoid cavity and acromion
____ (3) features include the ala, crest, and greater sciatic notch
____ (4) doubly curved; acts as a shoulder strut
____ (5) hip bone that articulates with the axial skeleton
____ (6) the "sit-down" bone
____ (7) anteriormost bone of the pelvic girdle
____ (8) part of the vertebral column

3. Use key choices to identify the bone descriptions that follow.

Key:

(a) carpals (b) femur (c) fibula
(d) humerus (e) radius (f) tarsals
(g) tibia (h) ulna

____ (1) articulates with the acetabulum and the tibia
____ (2) forms the lateral aspect of the ankle
____ (3) bone that "carries" the hand
____ (4) the wrist bones
____ (5) end shaped like a monkey wrench
____ (6) articulates with the capitulum of the humerus
____ (7) largest bone of this "group" is the calcaneus

Short Answer Essay Questions

4. Name the cranial and facial bones and compare and contrast the functions of the cranial and facial skeletons.
5. How do the relative proportions of the cranium and face of a fetus compare with those of an adult skull?
6. Name and diagram the normal vertebral curvatures. Which are primary and which are secondary curvatures?
7. List at least two specific anatomical characteristics each for typical cervical, thoracic, and lumbar vertebrae that would allow anyone to identify each type correctly.
8. What is the function of the intervertebral discs?
9. Distinguish between the anulus fibrosus and nucleus pulposus regions of a disc. Which provides durability and strength? Which provides resilience? Which part is involved in a "slipped" disc?
10. What is a true rib? A false rib?
11. The major function of the shoulder girdle is flexibility. What is the major function of the pelvic girdle? Relate these functional differences to anatomical differences seen in these girdles.
12. List three important differences between the male and female pelves.
13. Briefly describe the anatomical characteristics and impairment of function seen in cleft palate and hip dysplasia.
14. Compare a young adult skeleton to that of an extremely aged person relative to bone mass in general and the bony structure of the skull, thorax, and vertebral column in particular.
15. Peter Howell, a teaching assistant in the anatomy class, picked up a hip bone and pretended it was a telephone. He held the big hole in this bone right up to his ear and said, "Hello, obturator, obturator (operator, operator)." Name the structure he was helping the students to learn.

Critical Thinking and Clinical Application Questions

1. Justiniano worked in a poultry-packing plant where his job was cutting open chickens and stripping out their visceral organs. After work, he typed for long hours on his computer keyboard, writing a book about his work in the plant. Soon, his wrist

and hand began to hurt whenever he flexed it, and he began to awaken at night with pain and tingling on the thumb-half of his hand. What condition did he probably have?

2. Ralph had polio as a boy and was partially paralyzed in one lower limb for over a year. Although no longer paralyzed, he now has a severe lateral curvature of the lumbar spine. Explain what has happened and identify his condition.
3. Mary's grandmother slipped on a scatter rug and fell heavily to the floor. Her left lower limb was laterally rotated and noticeably shorter than the right, and when she attempted to get up, she winced with pain. Mary surmised that her grandmother might have "fractured her hip," which later proved to be true. What bone was probably fractured and at what site? Why is a "fractured hip" a common type of fracture in the elderly?
4. Mrs. Shea came up with what she considered to be a clever idea to bypass the long lines at Disney World. She had her husband rent a wheelchair and he wheeled her around from one exhibit to another for the better part of three days. As they sat on the plane, waiting to take off for Chicago, she complained to him that she had two sore spots on her buttocks. Why? What do you suppose would happen (to her buttocks) if she was wheeled around for a few more days?

AT THE CLINIC

7

Related Clinical Terms

Chiropractic (ki″ro-prak′tik) A system of treating disease by manipulating the vertebral column based on the idea that most diseases are due to pressure on nerves caused by faulty bone alignment; a specialist in this field is a chiropractor.

Clubfoot A relatively common congenital defect (one in 700 births) in which the soles of the feet face medially and the toes point inferiorly; may be genetically induced or reflect an abnormal position of the foot during fetal development.

Laminectomy Surgical removal of a vertebral lamina; most often done to relieve the symptoms of a ruptured disc.

Orthopedist (or″tho-pe′dist) or **orthopedic surgeon** A physician who specializes in restoring lost skeletal system function or repairing damage to bones and joints.

Pelvimetry Measurement of the dimensions of the inlet and outlet of the pelvis, usually to determine whether the pelvis is of adequate size to allow normal delivery of a baby.

Spina bifida (spi′nah bĭ′fĭ-dah; "cleft spine") Congenital defect of the vertebral column in which one or more of the vertebral arches are incomplete; ranges in severity from inconsequential to severe conditions that impair neural functioning and encourage nervous system infections.

Spinal fusion Surgical procedure involving insertion of bone chips (or crushed bone) to immobilize and stabilize a specific region of the vertebral column, particularly in cases of vertebral fracture and herniated discs.

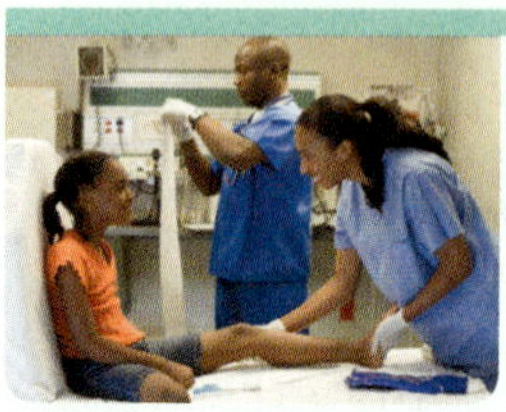

Case Study Skeleton

Kayla Tanner, a 45-year-old mother of four, was a passenger on the bus involved in an accident on Route 91. When paramedics arrived on the scene, they found Mrs. Tanner lying on her side in the aisle. Upon examination, they found that her right thigh appeared shorter than her left thigh. They also noticed that even slight hip movement caused considerable pain. Suspecting a hip dislocation, they stabilized and transported her.

In the emergency department, doctors discovered a decreased ability to sense light touch in her right foot, and she was unable to move her toes or ankle. Dislocation of her right hip was confirmed by X ray. Mrs. Tanner was sedated to relax the muscles around the hip, and then doctors placed her in the supine position and performed a closed reduction ("popped" the femur back in place).

1. Mrs. Tanner's pelvic girdle contains a hemispherical socket at the point where her femur attaches. Name this structure.
2. Name the structure on the femur that forms the "ball" that fits into the "socket" you named in question 1.
3. There are three bones in the pelvic girdle that fuse together at a point within the structure that you named in question 1. Name those three bones.
4. Mrs. Tanner suffered an injury to the hip joint, but if you were asked to rest your hands on your hips, you would not actually touch this joint. What structure in the pelvic girdle would your hands be resting on?
5. The sedation that Mrs. Tanner was given was to relax the large muscles of the thigh and buttocks that attach to the proximal end of the femur. Name the structures on the femur where these muscles attach.
6. Mrs. Tanner's injury caused damage to the sciatic nerve that passes across the hip and down into the thigh, lower leg, and foot. Name the pelvic structure that this nerve passes through as it travels into the upper thigh.

(Answers in Appendix H)

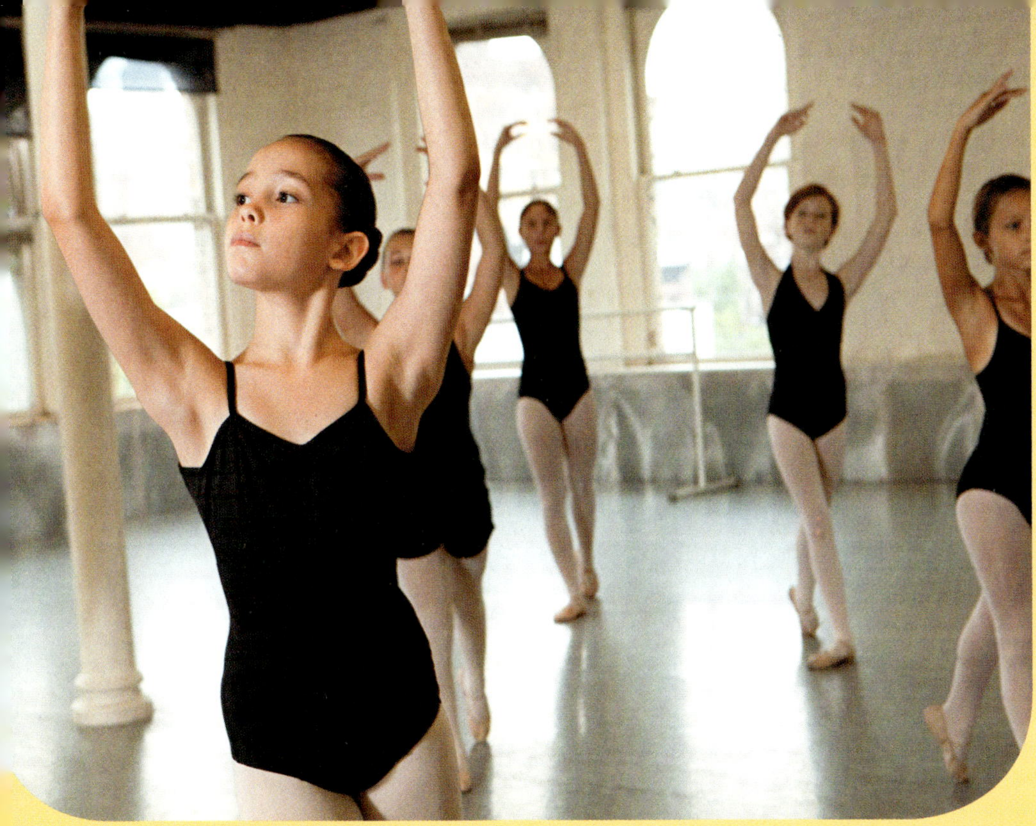

8

Joints

The graceful movements of ballet dancers and the rough-and-tumble grapplings of football players demonstrate the great variety of motion allowed by **joints**, or **articulations**—the sites where two or more bones meet. Our joints have two fundamental functions: They give our skeleton mobility, and they hold it together, sometimes playing a protective role in the process.

Joints are the weakest parts of the skeleton. Nonetheless, their structure resists various forces, such as crushing or tearing, that threaten to force them out of alignment.

Classification of Joints

✓ Define joint or articulation.

✓ Classify joints by structure and by function.

Joints are classified by structure and by function. The *structural classification* focuses on the material binding the bones together and whether or not a joint cavity is present. Structurally, there are *fibrous*, *cartilaginous*, and *synovial joints* (Table 8.1 on p. 253).

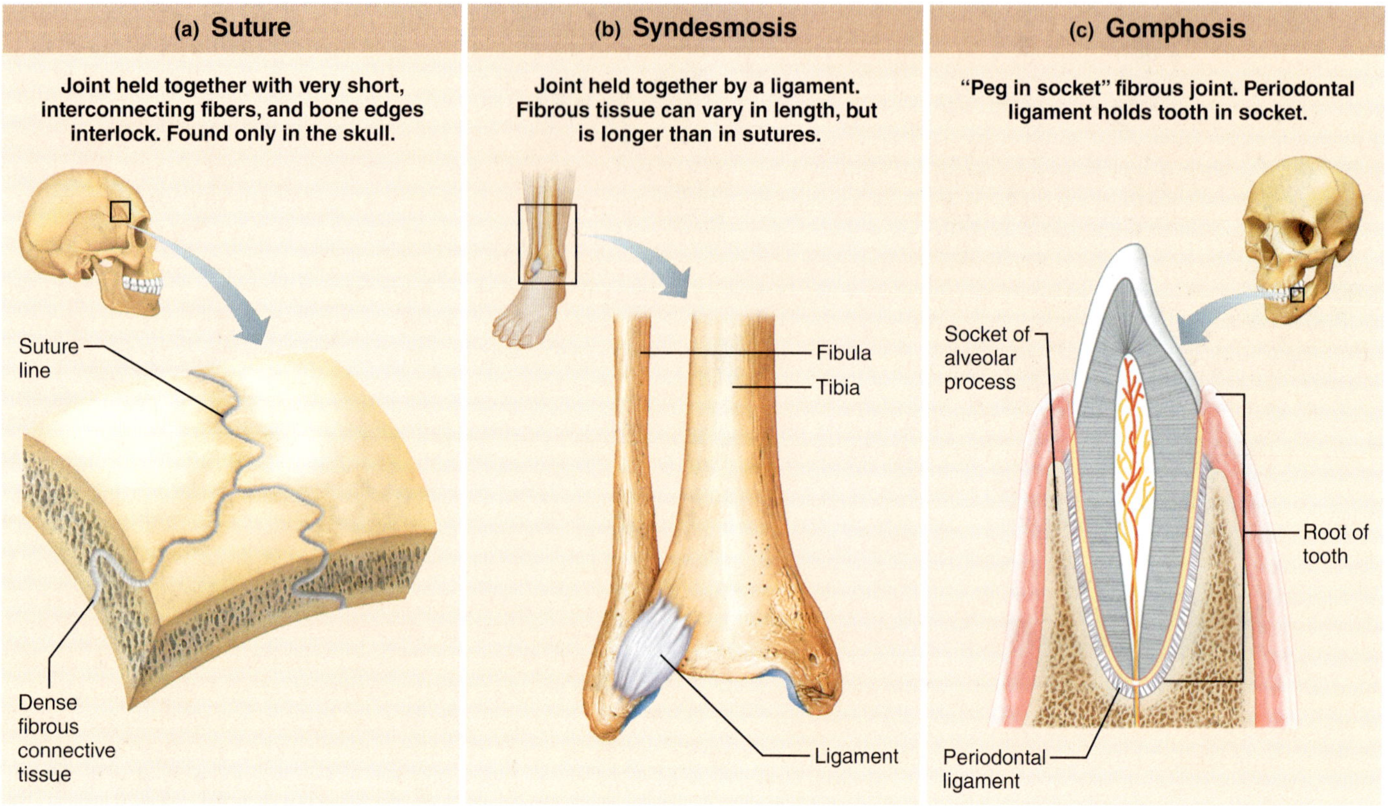

Figure 8.1 **Fibrous joints.**

The *functional classification* is based on the amount of movement allowed at the joint. On this basis, there are **synarthroses** (sin″ar-thro′sēz; *syn* = together, *arthro* = joint), which are immovable joints; **amphiarthroses** (am″fe-ar-thro′sēz; *amphi* = on both sides), slightly movable joints; and **diarthroses** (di″ar-thro′sēz; *dia* = through, apart), or freely movable joints. Freely movable joints predominate in the limbs. Immovable and slightly movable joints are largely restricted to the axial skeleton. This localization of functional joint types is understandable because the less movable the joint, the more stable it is likely to be.

In general, fibrous joints are immovable, and synovial joints are freely movable. However, cartilaginous joints have both rigid and slightly movable examples. Since the structural categories are more clear-cut, we will use the structural classification in this discussion, indicating functional properties where appropriate.

Fibrous Joints

✓ Describe the general structure of fibrous joints. Name and give an example of each of the three common types of fibrous joints.

In **fibrous joints**, the bones are joined by fibrous tissue, namely dense fibrous connective tissue, and no joint cavity is present. The amount of movement allowed depends on the length of the connective tissue fibers uniting the bones. Most fibrous joints are immovable, although a few are slightly movable. The three types of fibrous joints are *sutures*, *syndesmoses*, and *gomphoses*.

Sutures

Sutures, literally "seams," occur only between bones of the skull **(Figure 8.1a)**. The wavy articulating bone edges interlock, and the junction is completely filled by a minimal amount of very short connective tissue fibers that are continuous with the periosteum. The result is nearly rigid splices that knit the bones together, yet allow the skull to expand as the brain grows during youth. During middle age, the fibrous tissue ossifies and the skull bones fuse into a single unit. At this stage, the closed sutures are more precisely called **synostoses** (sin″os-to′sēz), literally, "bony junctions." Because movement of the cranial bones would damage the brain, the immovable nature of sutures is a protective adaptation.

Syndesmoses

In **syndesmoses** (sin″des-mo′sēz), the bones are connected exclusively by *ligaments* (*syndesmos* = ligament), cords or bands of fibrous tissue. Although the connecting fibers are always longer than those in sutures, they vary quite a bit in length.

The amount of movement allowed at a syndesmosis depends on the length of the connecting fibers. If the fibers are short (as in the ligament connecting the distal ends of the tibia and fibula, Figure 8.1b), little or no movement is allowed, a characteristic best described as "give." If the fibers are long (as in the ligament-like interosseous membrane connecting the radius and ulna, Figure 7.28, p. 231), a large amount of movement is possible.

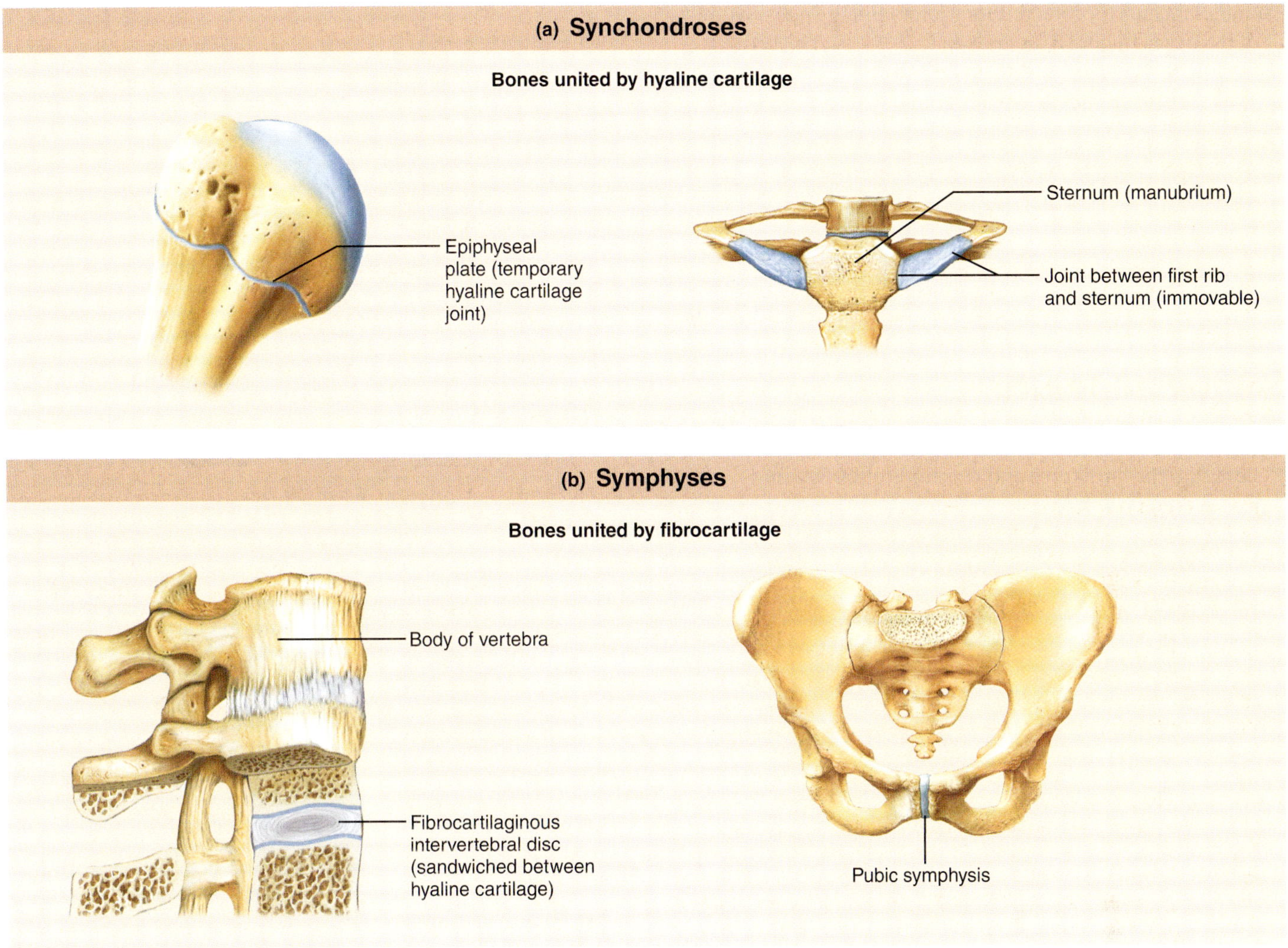

Figure 8.2 Cartilaginous joints.

Gomphoses

A **gomphosis** (gom-fo′sis) is a peg-in-socket fibrous joint (Figure 8.1c). The only example is the articulation of a tooth with its bony alveolar socket. The term *gomphosis* comes from the Greek *gompho*, meaning "nail" or "bolt," and refers to the way teeth are embedded in their sockets (as if hammered in). The fibrous connection in this case is the short **periodontal ligament** (Figure 23.11, p. 860).

Cartilaginous Joints

✓ Describe the general structure of cartilaginous joints. Name and give an example of each of the two common types of cartilaginous joints.

In **cartilaginous joints** (kar″tĭ-laj′ĭ-nus), the articulating bones are united by cartilage. Like fibrous joints, they lack a joint cavity and are not highly movable. The two types of cartilaginous joints are *synchondroses* and *symphyses*.

Synchondroses

A bar or plate of *hyaline cartilage* unites the bones at a **synchondrosis** (sin″kon-dro′sis; "junction of cartilage"). Virtually all synchondroses are synarthrotic.

The most common examples of synchondroses are the epiphyseal plates in long bones of children **(Figure 8.2a)**. Epiphyseal plates are temporary joints and eventually become synostoses. Another example of a synchondrosis is the immovable joint between the costal cartilage of the first rib and the manubrium of the sternum (Figure 8.2a).

Symphyses

A joint where *fibrocartilage* unites the bone is a **symphysis** (sim′fih-sis; "growing together"). Since fibrocartilage is compressible and resilient, it acts as a shock absorber and permits a limited amount of movement at the joint. Even though fibrocartilage is the main element of a symphysis, hyaline cartilage is also present in the form of articular cartilages on the bony surfaces. Symphyses are amphiarthrotic joints designed for strength with flexibility.

Examples include the intervertebral joints and the pubic symphysis of the pelvis (Figure 8.2b, and see **Table 8.2** on p. 254).

Check Your Understanding

1. What term is a synonym for "joint"?
2. What functional joint class contains the least-mobile joints?
3. Of sutures, symphyses, and synchondroses, which are cartilaginous joints?
4. How are joint mobility and stability related?

For answers, see Appendix H.

Synovial Joints

- ✓ Describe the structural characteristics of synovial joints.
- ✓ Compare the structures and functions of bursae and tendon sheaths.
- ✓ List three natural factors that stabilize synovial joints.

Synovial joints (si-no′ve-al; "joint eggs") are those in which the articulating bones are separated by a fluid-containing joint cavity. This arrangement permits substantial freedom of movement, and all synovial joints are freely movable diarthroses. Nearly all joints of the limbs—indeed, most joints of the body—fall into this class.

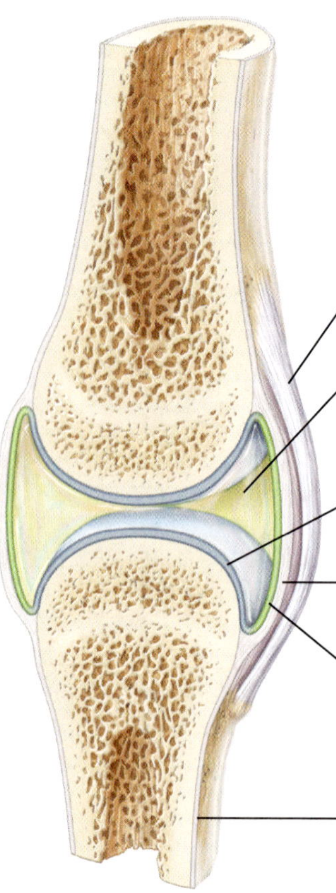

Figure 8.3 **General structure of a synovial joint.**

General Structure

Synovial joints have six distinguishing features **(Figure 8.3)**:

- **Articular cartilage.** Glassy-smooth hyaline cartilage covers the opposing bone surfaces as **articular cartilage**. These thin (1 mm or less) but spongy cushions absorb compression placed on the joint and thereby keep the bone ends from being crushed.
- **Joint (articular) cavity.** A feature unique to synovial joints, the joint cavity is really just a potential space that contains a small amount of synovial fluid.
- **Articular capsule.** The joint cavity is enclosed by a two-layered **articular capsule**, or *joint capsule*. The tough external **fibrous layer** is composed of dense irregular connective tissue that is continuous with the periostea of the articulating bones. It strengthens the joint so that the bones are not pulled apart. The inner layer of the joint capsule is a **synovial membrane** composed of loose connective tissue. Besides lining the fibrous layer internally, it covers all internal joint surfaces that are not hyaline cartilage. The synovial membrane's function is to make synovial fluid.
- **Synovial fluid.** A small amount of slippery **synovial fluid** occupies all free spaces within the joint capsule. This fluid is derived largely by filtration from blood flowing through the capillaries in the synovial membrane. Synovial fluid has a viscous, egg-white consistency (*ovum* =egg) due to hyaluronic acid secreted by cells in the synovial membrane, but it thins and becomes less viscous during joint activity.

  Synovial fluid, which is also found *within* the articular cartilages, provides a slippery, weight-bearing film that reduces friction between the cartilages. Without this lubricant, rubbing would wear away joint surfaces and excessive friction could overheat and destroy the joint tissues, essentially "cooking" them. The synovial fluid is forced from the cartilages when a joint is compressed; then as pressure on the joint is relieved, synovial fluid seeps back into the articular cartilages like water into a sponge, ready to be squeezed out again the next time the joint is loaded (put under pressure). This process, called *weeping lubrication*, lubricates the free surfaces of the cartilages and nourishes their cells. (Remember, cartilage is avascular.) Synovial fluid also contains phagocytic cells that rid the joint cavity of microbes and cellular debris.
- **Reinforcing ligaments.** Synovial joints are reinforced and strengthened by a number of bandlike **ligaments**. Most often, these are **capsular ligaments**, which are thickened parts of the fibrous layer. In other cases, they remain distinct and are found outside the capsule (as **extracapsular ligaments**) or deep to it (as **intracapsular ligaments**). Since intracapsular ligaments are covered with synovial membrane, they do not actually lie *within* the joint cavity.

  People said to be double-jointed amaze the rest of us by placing both heels behind their neck. However, they have the normal number of joints. It's just that their joint capsules and ligaments are more stretchy and loose than average.
- **Nerves and blood vessels.** Synovial joints are richly supplied with sensory nerve fibers that innervate the capsule. Some of

Table 8.1 Summary of Joint Classes

STRUCTURAL CLASS	STRUCTURAL CHARACTERISTICS	TYPES	MOBILITY
Fibrous	Bone ends/parts united by collagen fibers	Suture (short fibers)	Immobile (synarthrosis)
		Syndesmosis (longer fibers)	Slightly mobile (amphiarthrosis) and immobile
		Gomphosis (periodontal ligament)	Immobile
Cartilaginous	Bone ends/parts united by cartilage	Synchondrosis (hyaline cartilage)	Immobile
		Symphysis (fibrocartilage)	Slightly movable
Synovial	Bone ends/parts covered with articular cartilage and enclosed within an articular capsule lined with synovial membrane	1. Plane 2. Hinge 3. Pivot 4. Condylar 5. Saddle 6. Ball and socket	Freely movable (diarthrosis; movements depend on design of joint)

these fibers detect pain, as anyone who has suffered joint injury is aware, but most monitor joint position and stretch. Monitoring joint stretch is one of several ways the nervous system senses our posture and body movements (see p. 487). Synovial joints are also richly supplied with blood vessels, most of which supply the synovial membrane. There, extensive capillary beds produce the blood filtrate that is the basis of synovial fluid.

Besides the basic components described above, certain synovial joints have other structural features. Some, such as the hip and knee joints, have cushioning **fatty pads** between the fibrous layer and the synovial membrane or bone. Others have discs or wedges of fibrocartilage separating the articular surfaces. Where present, these **articular discs**, or **menisci** (mĕ-nis′ki; "crescents"), extend inward from the articular capsule and partially or completely divide the synovial cavity in two (see the menisci of the knee in Figure 8.8a, b, e, and f). Articular discs improve the fit between articulating bone ends, making the joint more stable and minimizing wear and tear on the joint surfaces. Besides the knees, articular discs occur in the jaw and a few other joints (see notations in the Structural Type column in Table 8.2).

Bursae and Tendon Sheaths

Bursae and tendon sheaths are not strictly part of synovial joints, but they are often found closely associated with them **(Figure 8.4)**. Essentially bags of lubricant, they act as "ball bearings" to reduce friction between adjacent structures during joint activity. **Bursae** (ber′se; "purse") are flattened fibrous sacs lined with synovial membrane and containing a thin film of synovial fluid. They occur where ligaments, muscles, skin, tendons, or bones rub together.

A **tendon sheath** is essentially an elongated bursa that wraps completely around a tendon subjected to friction, like a bun around a hot dog. They are common where several tendons are crowded together within narrow canals (in the wrist region, for example).

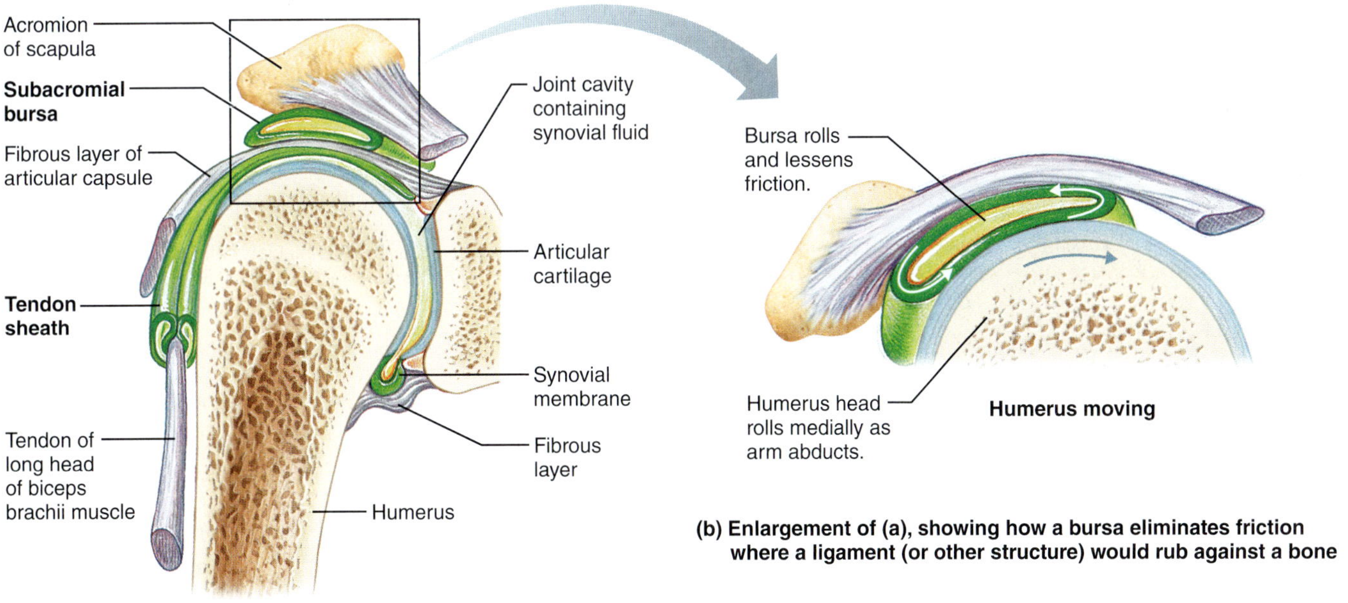

(a) Frontal section through the right shoulder joint

(b) Enlargement of (a), showing how a bursa eliminates friction where a ligament (or other structure) would rub against a bone

Figure 8.4 Bursae and tendon sheaths.

Table 8.2 Structural and Functional Characteristics of Body Joints

ILLUSTRATION	JOINT	ARTICULATING BONES	STRUCTURAL TYPE*	FUNCTIONAL TYPE; MOVEMENTS ALLOWED
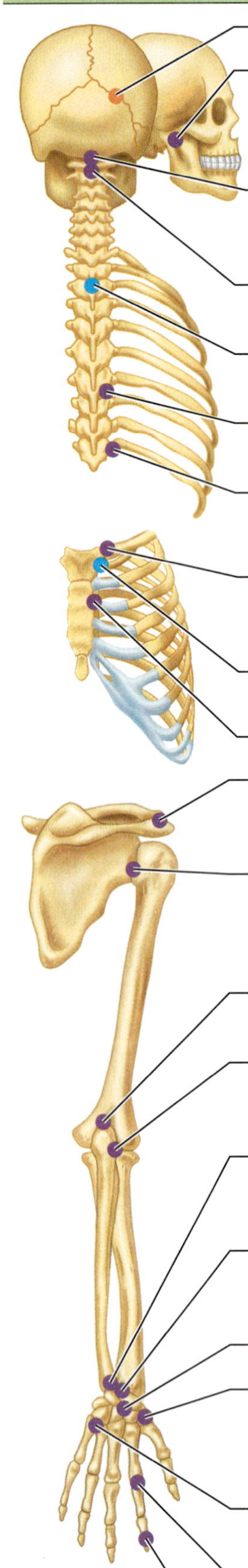	Skull	Cranial and facial bones	Fibrous; suture	Synarthrotic; no movement
	Temporo-mandibular	Temporal bone of skull and mandible	Synovial; modified hinge† (contains articular disc)	Diarthrotic; gliding and uniaxial rotation; slight lateral movement, elevation, depression, protraction, and retraction of mandible
	Atlanto-occipital	Occipital bone of skull and atlas	Synovial; condylar	Diarthrotic; biaxial; flexion, extension, lateral flexion, circumduction of head on neck
	Atlantoaxial	Atlas (C_1) and axis (C_2)	Synovial; pivot	Diarthrotic; uniaxial; rotation of the head
	Intervertebral	Between adjacent vertebral bodies	Cartilaginous; symphysis	Amphiarthrotic; slight movement
	Intervertebral	Between articular processes	Synovial; plane	Diarthrotic; gliding
	Costovertebral	Vertebrae (transverse processes or bodies) and ribs	Synovial; plane	Diarthrotic; gliding of ribs
	Sternoclavicular	Sternum and clavicle	Synovial; shallow saddle (contains articular disc)	Diarthrotic; multiaxial (allows clavicle to move in all axes)
	Sternocostal (first)	Sternum and rib 1	Cartilaginous; synchondrosis	Synarthrotic; no movement
	Sternocostal	Sternum and ribs 2–7	Synovial; double plane	Diarthrotic; gliding
	Acromio-clavicular	Acromion of scapula and clavicle	Synovial; plane (contains articular disc)	Diarthrotic; gliding and rotation of scapula on clavicle
	Shoulder (glenohumeral)	Scapula and humerus	Synovial; ball-and-socket	Diarthrotic; multiaxial; flexion, extension, abduction, adduction, circumduction, rotation of humerus
	Elbow	Ulna (and radius) with humerus	Synovial; hinge	Diarthrotic; uniaxial; flexion, extension of forearm
	Proximal radioulnar	Radius and ulna	Synovial; pivot	Diarthrotic; uniaxial; pivot (convex head of radius rotates in radial notch of ulna)
	Distal radioulnar	Radius and ulna	Synovial; pivot (contains articular disc)	Diarthrotic; uniaxial; rotation of radius around long axis of forearm to allow pronation and supination
	Wrist	Radius and proximal carpals	Synovial; condylar	Diarthrotic; biaxial; flexion, extension, abduction, adduction, circumduction of hand
	Intercarpal	Adjacent carpals	Synovial; plane	Diarthrotic; gliding
	Carpometacarpal of digit 1 (thumb)	Carpal (trapezium) and metacarpal 1	Synovial; saddle	Diarthrotic; biaxial; flexion, extension, abduction, adduction, circumduction, opposition of metacarpal I
	Carpometacarpal of digits 2–5	Carpal(s) and metacarpal(s)	Synovial; plane	Diarthrotic; gliding of metacarpals
	Metacarpo-phalangeal (knuckle)	Metacarpal and proximal phalanx	Synovial; condylar	Diarthrotic; biaxial; flexion, extension, abduction, adduction, circumduction of fingers
	Interphalangeal (finger)	Adjacent phalanges	Synovial; hinge	Diarthrotic; uniaxial; flexion, extension of fingers

Table 8.2 *(continued)*

ILLUSTRATION	JOINT	ARTICULATING BONES	STRUCTURAL TYPE*	FUNCTIONAL TYPE; MOVEMENTS ALLOWED
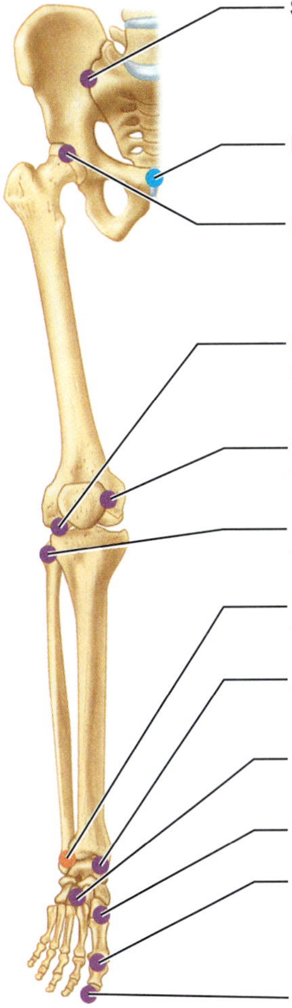	Sacroiliac	Sacrum and coxal bone	Synovial; plane in childhood, increasingly fibrous in adult	Diarthrotic in child; amphiarthrotic in adult; (more movement during pregnancy)
	Pubic symphysis	Pubic bones	Cartilaginous; symphysis	Amphiarthrotic; slight movement (enhanced during pregnancy)
	Hip (coxal)	Hip bone and femur	Synovial; ball-and-socket	Diarthrotic; multiaxial; flexion, extension, abduction, adduction, rotation, circumduction of thigh
	Knee (tibiofemoral)	Femur and tibia	Synovial; modified hinge† (contains articular discs)	Diarthrotic; biaxial; flexion, extension of leg, some rotation allowed in flexed position
	Knee (femoropatellar)	Femur and patella	Synovial; plane	Diarthrotic; gliding of patella
	Superior tibiofibular	Tibia and fibula (proximally)	Synovial; plane	Diarthrotic; gliding of fibula
	Inferior tibiofibular	Tibia and fibula (distally)	Fibrous; syndesmosis	Synarthrotic; slight "give" during dorsiflexion
	Ankle	Tibia and fibula with talus	Synovial; hinge	Diarthrotic; uniaxial; dorsiflexion, and plantar flexion of foot
	Intertarsal	Adjacent tarsals	Synovial; plane	Diarthrotic; gliding; inversion and eversion of foot
	Tarsometatarsal	Tarsal(s) and metatarsal(s)	Synovial; plane	Diarthrotic; gliding of metatarsals
	Metatarso-phalangeal	Metatarsal and proximal phalanx	Synovial; condylar	Diarthrotic; biaxial; flexion, extension, abduction, adduction, circumduction of great toe
	Interpha-langeal (toe)	Adjacent phalanges	Synovial; hinge	Diarthrotic; uniaxial; flexion; extension of toes

*__Fibrous joints__ indicated by orange circles; **cartilaginous joints** by blue circles; **synovial joints** by purple circles.
† These modified hinge joints are structurally bicondylar.

Factors Influencing the Stability of Synovial Joints

Because joints are constantly stretched and compressed, they must be stabilized so that they do not dislocate (come out of alignment). The stability of a synovial joint depends chiefly on three factors: the shapes of the articular surfaces; the number and positioning of ligaments; and muscle tone.

Articular Surfaces

The shapes of articular surfaces determine what movements are possible at a joint, but surprisingly, articular surfaces play only a minor role in joint stability. Many joints have shallow sockets or noncomplementary articulating surfaces ("misfits") that actually hinder joint stability. But when articular surfaces are large and fit snugly together, or when the socket is deep, stability is vastly improved. The ball and deep socket of the hip joint provide the best example of a joint made extremely stable by the shape of its articular surfaces.

Ligaments

The capsules and ligaments of synovial joints unite the bones and prevent excessive or undesirable motion. As a rule, the more ligaments a joint has, the stronger it is. However, when other stabilizing factors are inadequate, undue tension is placed on the ligaments and they stretch. Stretched ligaments stay stretched, like taffy, and a ligament can stretch only about 6% of its length before it snaps. Thus, when ligaments are the major means of bracing a joint, the joint is not very stable.

Muscle Tone

For most joints, the muscle tendons that cross the joint are the most important stabilizing factor. These tendons are kept taut at all times by the tone of their muscles. (*Muscle tone* is defined as low levels of contractile activity in relaxed muscles that keep the muscles healthy and ready to react to stimulation.) Muscle tone is extremely important in reinforcing the shoulder and knee joints and the arches of the foot.

Check Your Understanding

5. What are the two layers of the articular capsule?
6. How do bursae and tendon sheaths improve joint function?
7. Generally speaking, what factor is most important in stabilizing synovial joints?
8. What is the importance of weeping lubrication?

For answers, see Appendix H.

Movements Allowed by Synovial Joints

✓ Name and describe (or perform) the common body movements.

✓ Name and provide examples of the six types of synovial joints based on the movement(s) allowed.

Every skeletal muscle of the body is attached to bone or other connective tissue structures at no fewer than two points. The muscle's **origin** is attached to the immovable (or less movable) bone. Its other end, the **insertion**, is attached to the movable bone. Body movement occurs when muscles contract across joints and their insertion moves toward their origin. The movements can be described in directional terms relative to the lines, or axes, around which the body part moves and the planes of space along which the movement occurs, that is, along the transverse, frontal, or sagittal plane. (See Chapter 1 to review these planes.)

Range of motion allowed by synovial joints varies from **nonaxial movement** (slipping movements only, since there is no axis around which movement can occur) to **uniaxial movement** (movement in one plane) to **biaxial movement** (movement in two planes) to **multiaxial movement** (movement in or around all three planes of space and axes). Range of motion varies greatly in different people. In some, such as trained gymnasts or acrobats, range of joint movement may be extraordinary. The ranges of motion at the major joints are given in the far right column of Table 8.2.

There are three general types of movements: *gliding, angular movements*, and *rotation*. The most common body movements allowed by synovial joints are described next and illustrated in **Figure 8.5**.

Gliding Movements

Gliding occurs when one flat, or nearly flat, bone surface glides or slips over another (back-and-forth and side-to-side; Figure 8.5a) without appreciable angulation or rotation. Gliding occurs at the intercarpal and intertarsal joints, and between the flat articular processes of the vertebrae (Table 8.2).

Angular Movements

Angular movements (Figure 8.5b–e) increase or decrease the angle between two bones. These movements may occur in any plane of the body and include flexion, extension, hyperextension, abduction, adduction, and circumduction.

Figure 8.5 Movements allowed by synovial joints.

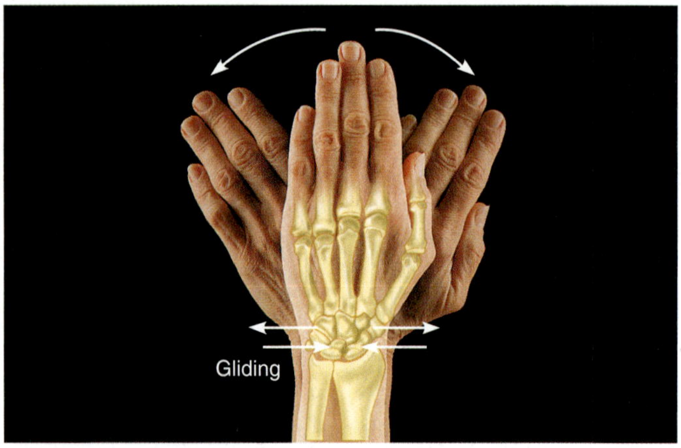

(a) Gliding movements at the wrist

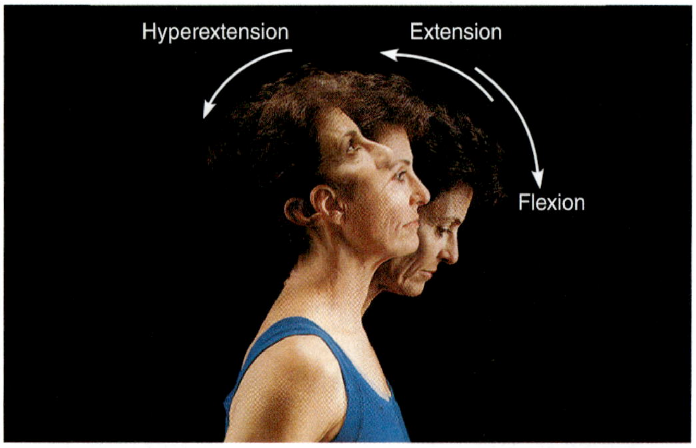

(b) Angular movements: flexion, extension, and hyperextension of the neck

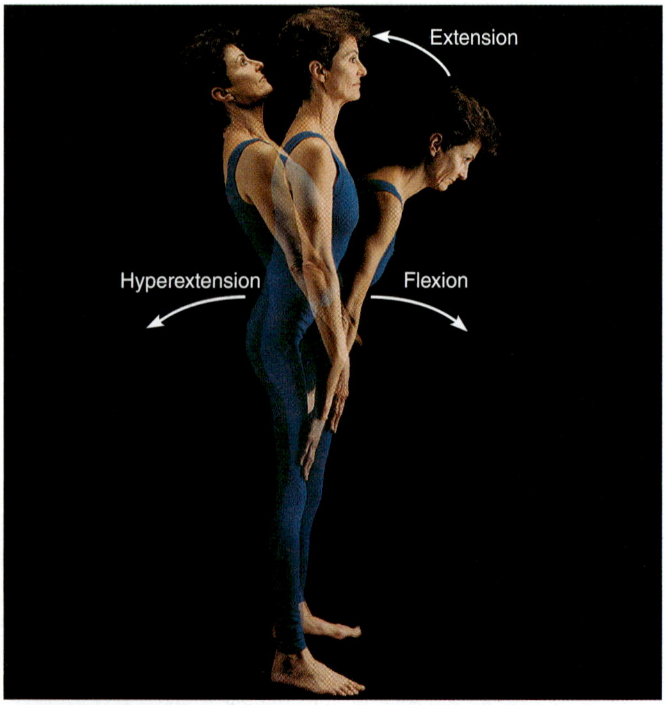

(c) Angular movements: flexion, extension, and hyperextension of the vertebral column

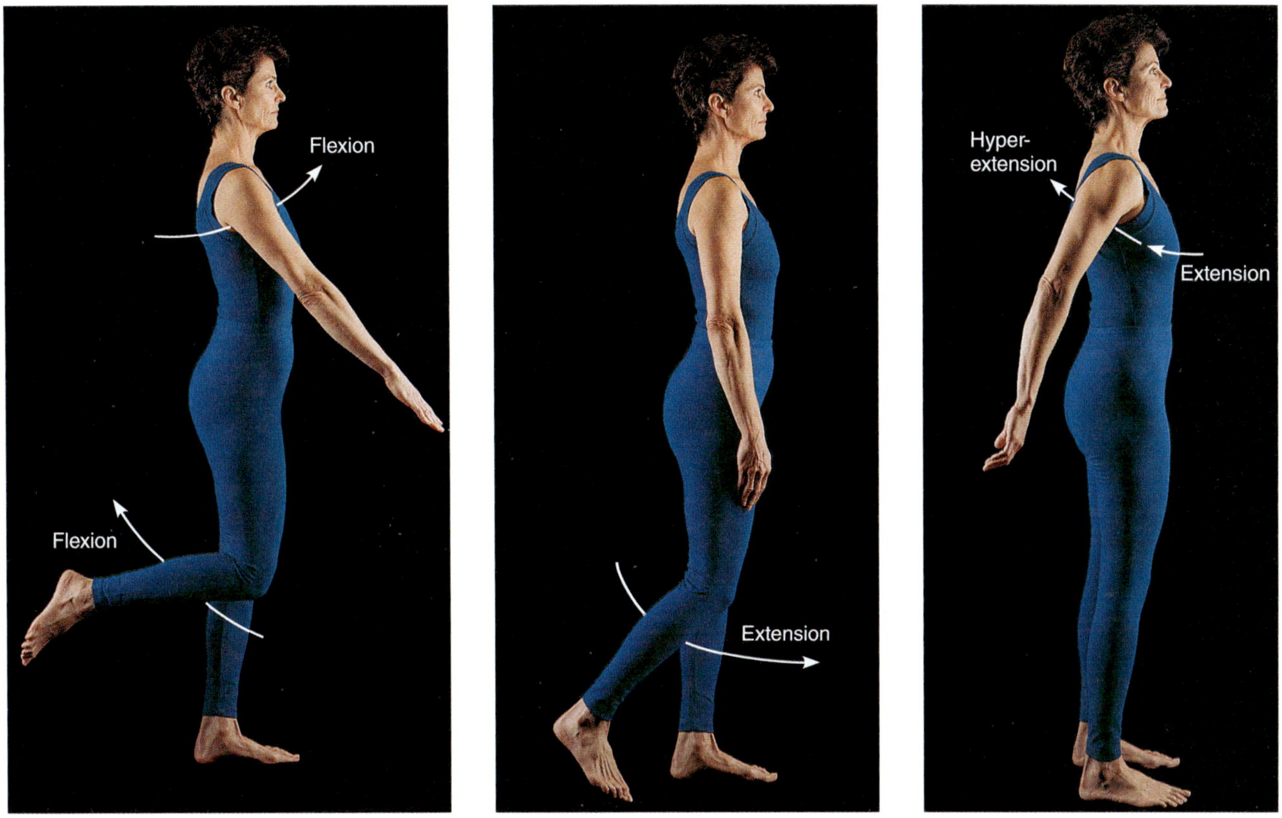

(d) Angular movements: flexion, extension, and hyperextension at the shoulder and knee

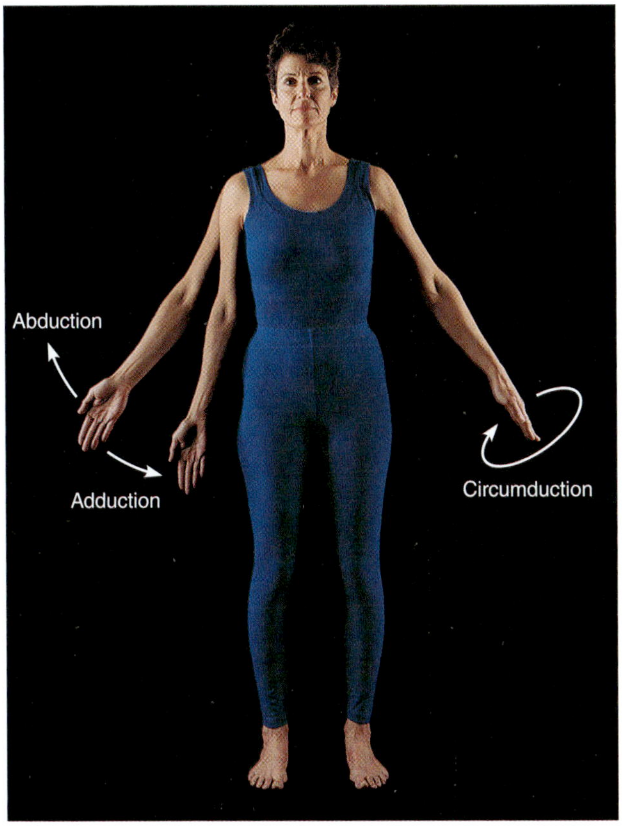

(e) Angular movements: abduction, adduction, and circumduction of the upper limb at the shoulder

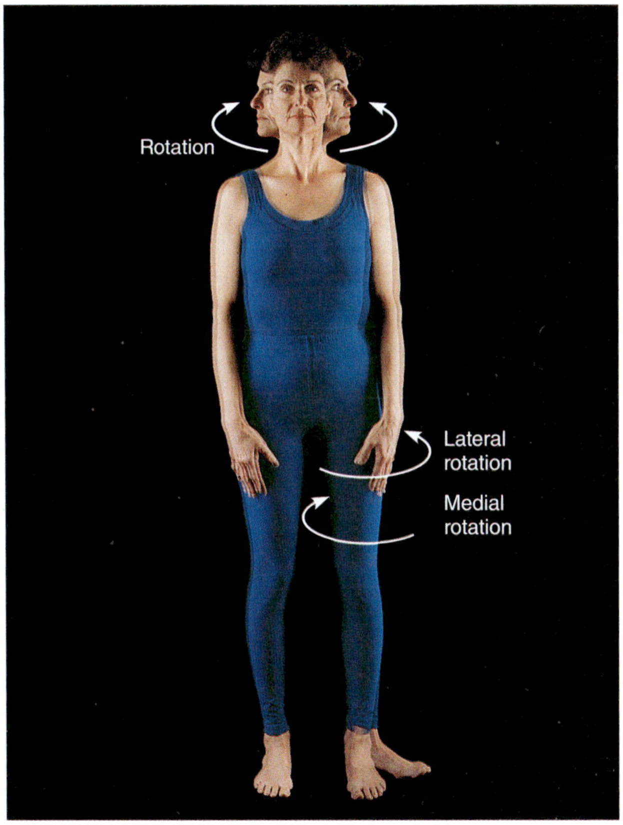

(f) Rotation of the head, neck, and lower limb

Figure 8.5 *(continued)*

Flexion **Flexion** (flek′shun) is a bending movement, usually along the sagittal plane, that *decreases the angle* of the joint and brings the articulating bones closer together. Examples include bending the head forward on the chest (Figure 8.5b) and bending the body trunk or the knee from a straight to an angled position (Figure 8.5c and d). As a less obvious example, the arm is flexed at the shoulder when the arm is lifted in an anterior direction (Figure 8.5d).

Extension **Extension** is the reverse of flexion and occurs at the same joints. It involves movement along the sagittal plane that *increases the angle* between the articulating bones and typically straightens a flexed limb or body part. Examples include straightening a flexed neck, body trunk, elbow, or knee (Figure 8.5b–d). Continuing such movements beyond the anatomical position is called **hyperextension** (literally, "superextension") (Figure 8.5b–d).

Abduction **Abduction** ("moving away") is movement of a limb *away* from the midline or median plane of the body, along the frontal plane. Raising the arm or thigh laterally is an example of abduction (Figure 8.5e). For the fingers or toes, abduction means spreading them apart. In this case "midline" is the longest digit: the third finger or second toe. Notice, however, that lateral bending of the trunk away from the body midline in the frontal plane is called lateral flexion, not abduction.

8

Adduction **Adduction** ("moving toward") is the opposite of abduction, so it is the movement of a limb *toward* the body midline or, in the case of the digits, toward the midline of the hand or foot (Figure 8.5e).

Circumduction **Circumduction** (Figure 8.5e) is moving a limb so that it describes a cone in space (*circum* = around; *duco* = to draw). The distal end of the limb moves in a circle, while the point of the cone (the shoulder or hip joint) is more or less stationary. A pitcher winding up to throw a ball is actually circumducting his or her pitching arm. Because circumduction consists of flexion, abduction, extension, and adduction performed in succession, it is the quickest way to exercise the many muscles that move the hip and shoulder ball-and-socket joints.

Rotation

Rotation is the turning of a bone around its own long axis. It is the only movement allowed between the first two cervical vertebrae and is common at the hip (Figure 8.5f) and shoulder joints. Rotation may be directed toward the midline or away from it. For example, in *medial rotation* of the thigh, the femur's anterior surface moves toward the median plane of the body; *lateral rotation* is the opposite movement.

Special Movements

Certain movements do not fit into any of the above categories and occur at only a few joints. Some of these special movements are illustrated in **Figure 8.6**.

Supination and Pronation The terms **supination** (soo″pĭ-na′shun; "turning backward") and **pronation** (pro-na′shun; "turning forward") refer to the movements of the radius around the ulna (Figure 8.6a). Rotating the forearm laterally so that the palm faces anteriorly or superiorly is supination. In the anatomical position, the hand is supinated and the radius and ulna are parallel.

In pronation, the forearm rotates medially and the palm faces posteriorly or inferiorly. Pronation moves the distal end of the radius across the ulna so that the two bones form an X. This is the forearm's position when we are standing in a relaxed manner. Pronation is a much weaker movement than supination.

A trick to help you keep these terms straight: A *pro* basketball player pronates his or her forearm to dribble the ball.

Dorsiflexion and Plantar Flexion of the Foot The up-and-down movements of the foot at the ankle are given more specific names (Figure 8.6b). Lifting the foot so that its superior surface approaches the shin is **dorsiflexion** (corresponds to wrist extension), whereas depressing the foot (pointing the toes) is **plantar flexion** (corresponds to wrist flexion).

Inversion and Eversion **Inversion** and **eversion** are special movements of the foot (Figure 8.6c). In inversion, the sole of the foot turns medially. In eversion, the sole faces laterally.

Protraction and Retraction Nonangular anterior and posterior movements in a transverse plane are called **protraction** and **retraction**, respectively (Figure 8.6d). The mandible is protracted when you jut out your jaw and retracted when you bring it back.

Elevation and Depression **Elevation** means lifting a body part superiorly (Figure 8.6e). For example, the scapulae are elevated when you shrug your shoulders. Moving the elevated part inferiorly is **depression**. During chewing, the mandible is alternately elevated and depressed.

Opposition The saddle joint between metacarpal I and the trapezium allows a movement called **opposition** of the thumb (Figure 8.6f). This movement is the action taken when you touch your thumb to the tips of the other fingers on the same hand. It is opposition that makes the human hand such a fine tool for grasping and manipulating objects.

Types of Synovial Joints

Although all synovial joints have structural features in common, they do not have a common structural plan. Based on the shape of their articular surfaces, which in turn determine the movements allowed, synovial joints can be classified further into six major categories—plane, hinge, pivot, condylar (or ellipsoid), saddle, and ball-and-socket joints. The properties of these joints are summarized in *Focus on Types of Synovial Joints* **(Figure 8.7)** on pp. 260–261.

☑ Check Your Understanding

9. John bent over to pick up a dime. What movement was occurring at his hip joint, at his knees, and between his index finger and thumb?
10. On the basis of movement allowed, which of the following joints are uniaxial? Hinge, condylar, saddle, pivot.

For answers, see Appendix H.

(Text continues on p. 262.)

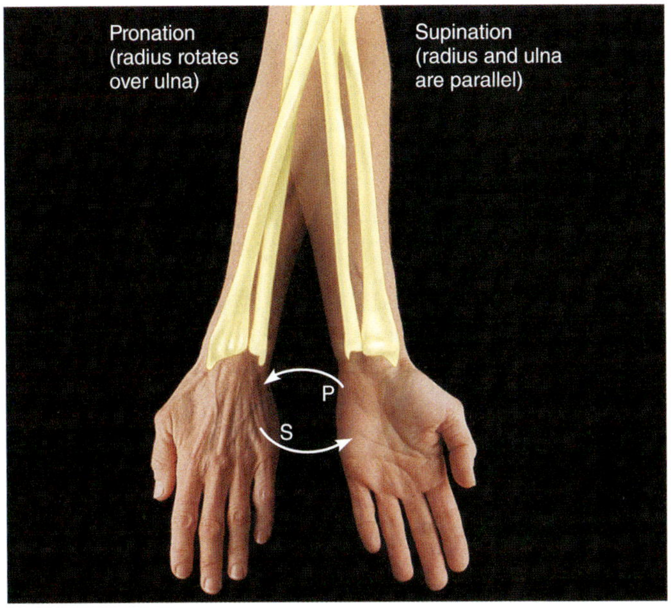

(a) Pronation (P) and supination (S)

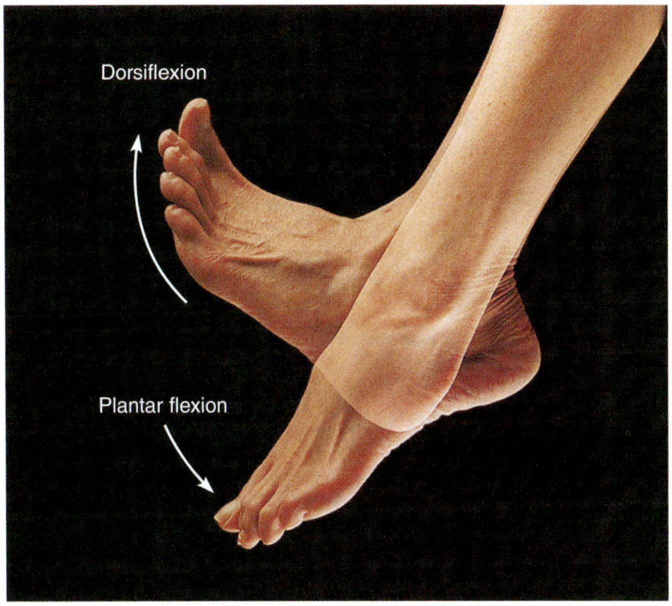

(b) Dorsiflexion and plantar flexion

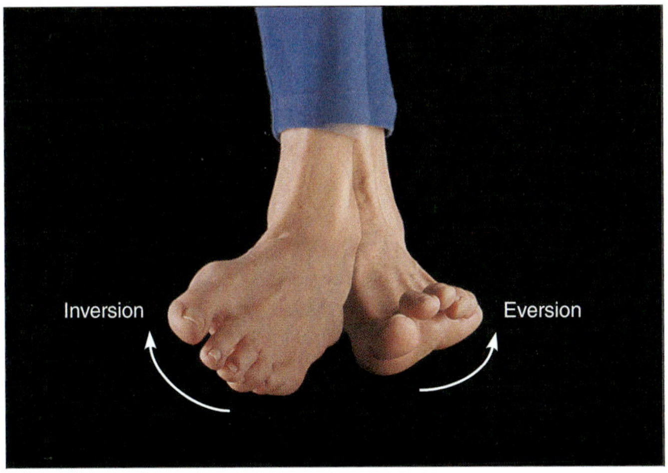

(c) Inversion and eversion

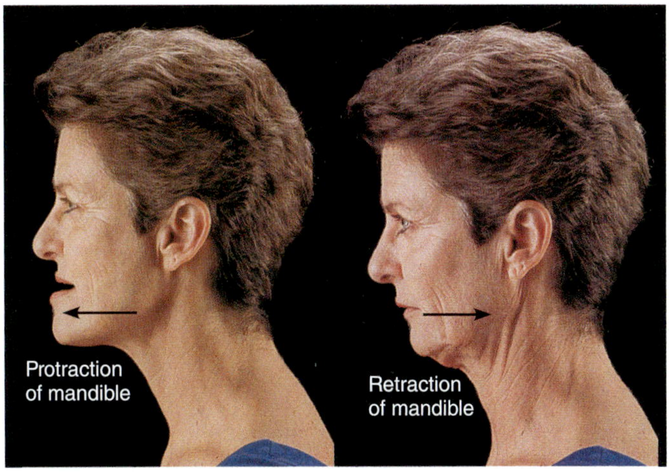

(d) Protraction and retraction

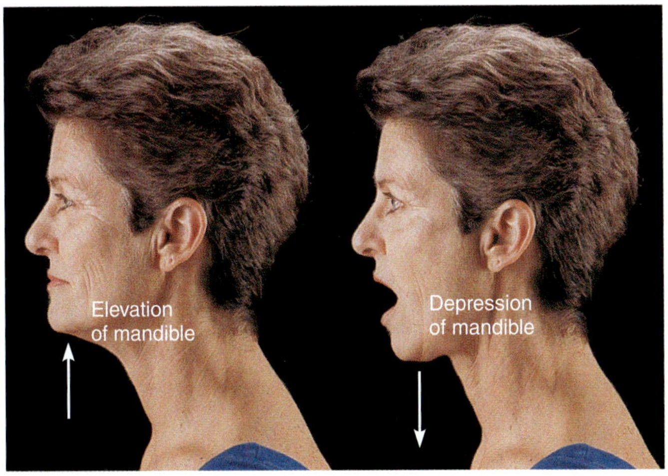

(e) Elevation and depression

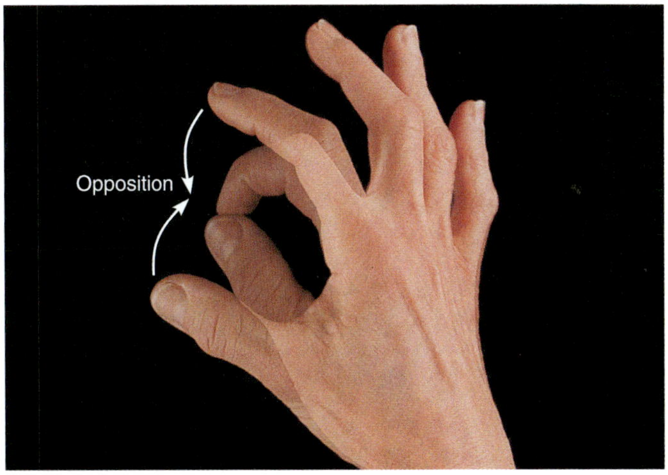

(f) Opposition

Figure 8.6 Special body movements.

Figure 8.7 The shapes of the joint surfaces define the types of movements that can occur at a synovial joint; they also determine the classification of synovial joints into six structural types.

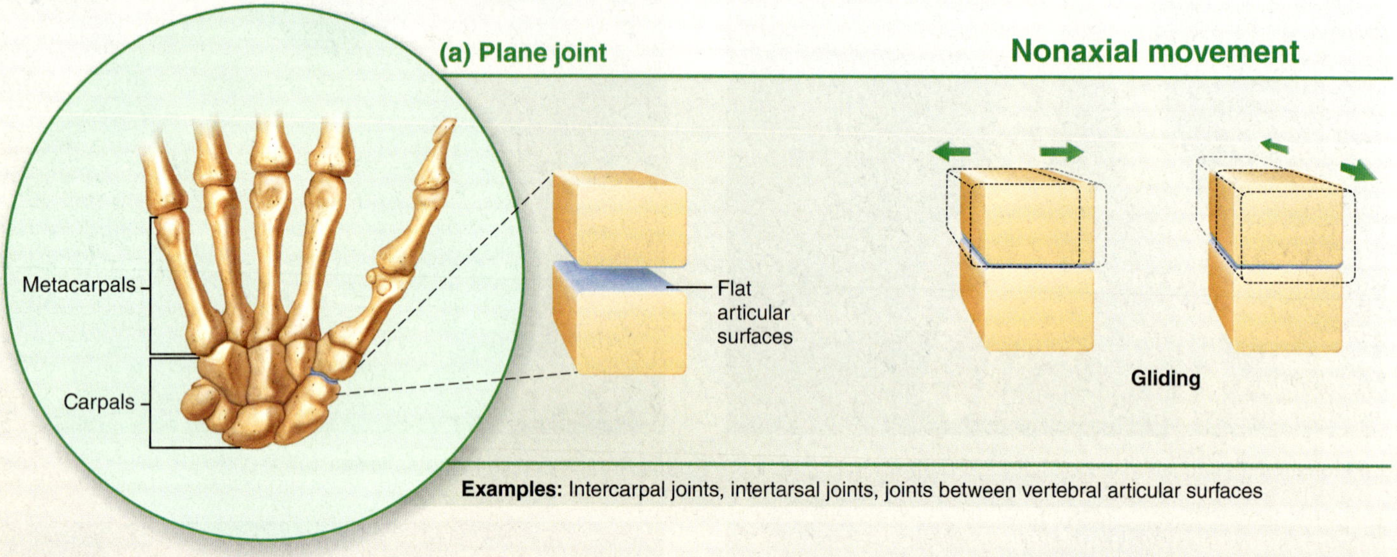

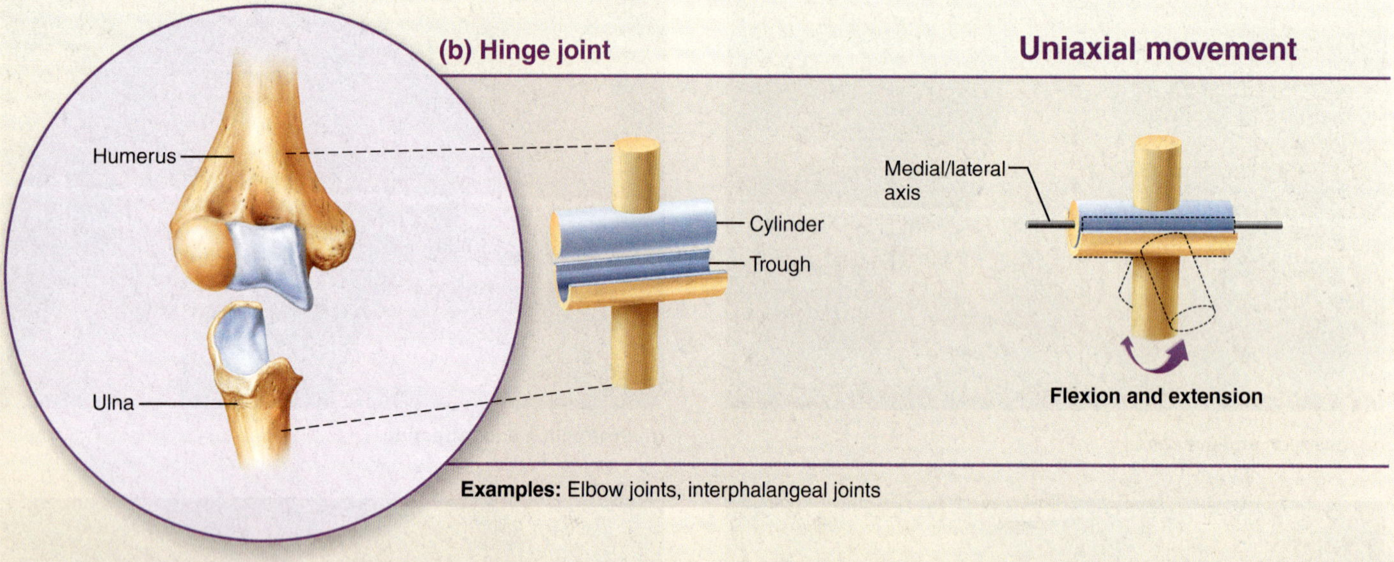

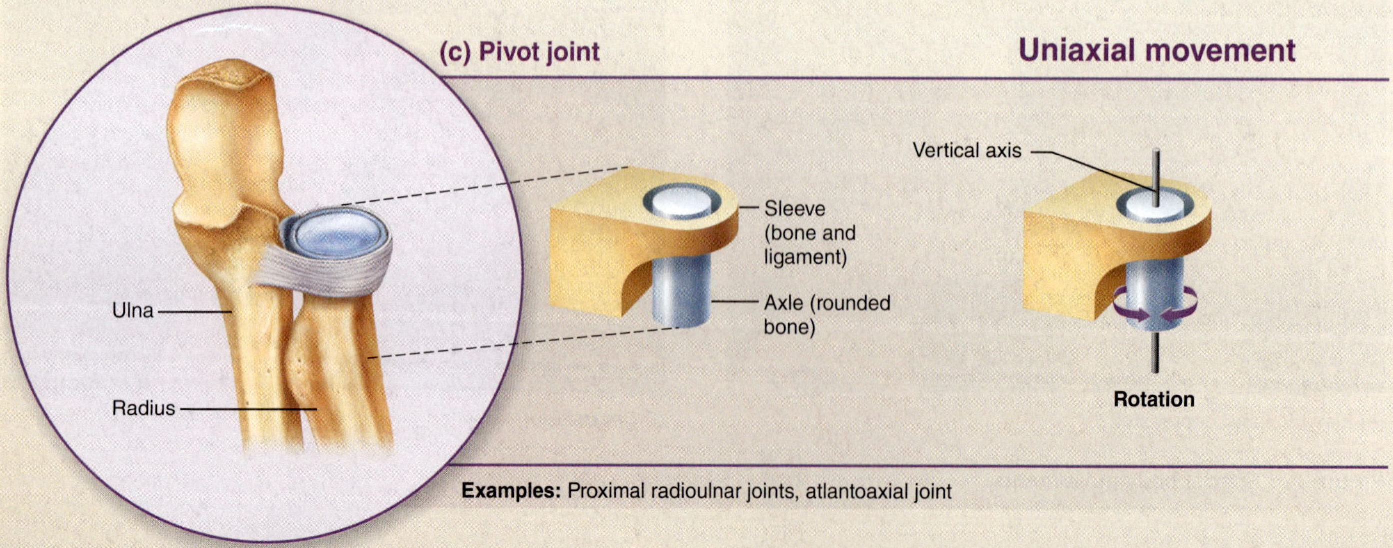

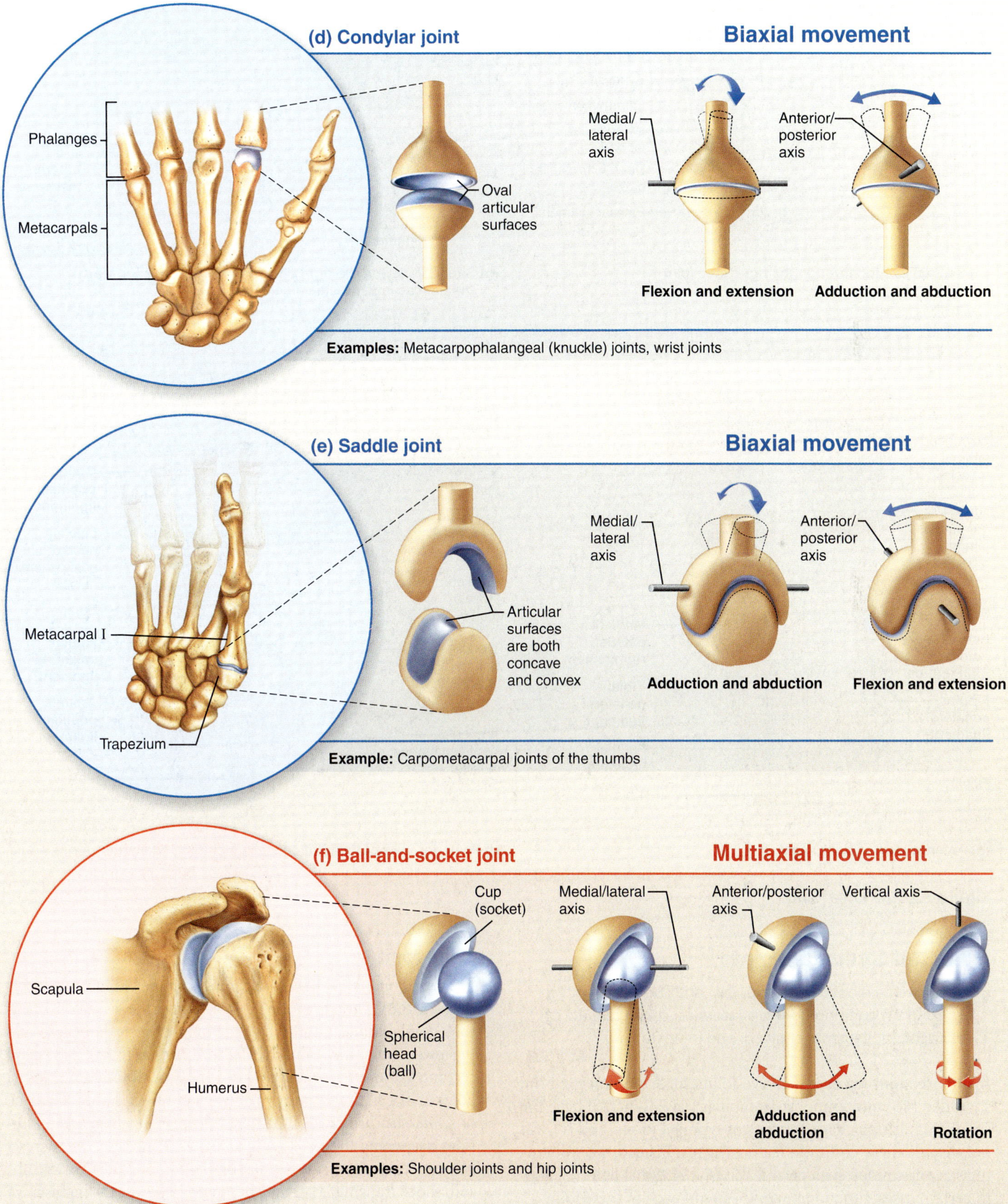
(d) Condylar joint
Biaxial movement
Phalanges
Metacarpals
Oval articular surfaces
Medial/ lateral axis
Anterior/ posterior axis
Flexion and extension
Adduction and abduction
Examples: Metacarpophalangeal (knuckle) joints, wrist joints
(e) Saddle joint
Biaxial movement
Metacarpal I
Trapezium
Articular surfaces are both concave and convex
Medial/ lateral axis
Anterior/ posterior axis
Adduction and abduction
Flexion and extension
Example: Carpometacarpal joints of the thumbs
(f) Ball-and-socket joint
Multiaxial movement
Scapula
Humerus
Cup (socket)
Spherical head (ball)
Medial/lateral axis
Anterior/posterior axis
Vertical axis
Flexion and extension
Adduction and abduction
Rotation
Examples: Shoulder joints and hip joints

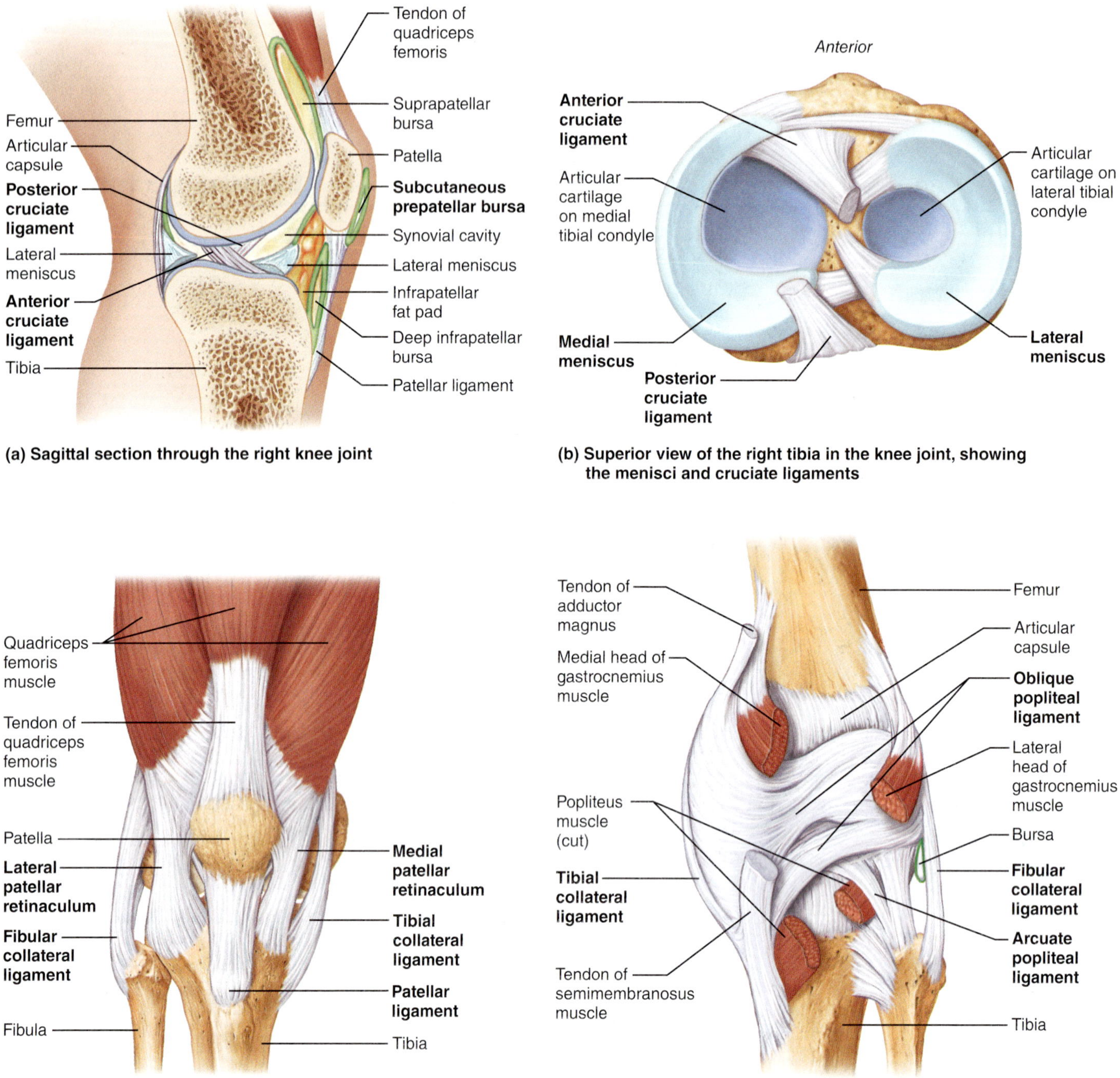

(a) Sagittal section through the right knee joint

(b) Superior view of the right tibia in the knee joint, showing the menisci and cruciate ligaments

(c) Anterior view of right knee

(d) Posterior view of the joint capsule, including ligaments

Figure 8.8 The knee joint.

Selected Synovial Joints

✓ Describe the elbow, knee, hip, jaw, and shoulder joints in terms of articulating bones, anatomical characteristics of the joint, movements allowed, and joint stability.

In this section, we examine five joints in detail: knee, elbow, shoulder, hip, and temporomandibular (jaw) joint. All have the six distinguishing characteristics of synovial joints, and we will not discuss these common features again. Instead, we will emphasize the unique structural features, functional abilities, and, in certain cases, functional weaknesses of each of these joints.

Knee Joint

The knee joint is the largest and most complex joint in the body **(Figure 8.8)**. Despite its single joint cavity, the knee consists of three joints in one: an intermediate one between the patella and the lower end of the femur (the **femoropatellar joint**), and lateral and medial joints (collectively known as the **tibiofemoral joint**) between the femoral condyles above and the C-shaped **menisci**, or *semilunar cartilages*, of the tibia below (Figure 8.8b and e). Besides deepening the shallow tibial articular surfaces, the menisci help prevent side-to-side rocking of the femur on the tibia and absorb shock transmitted to the knee joint. However, the menisci are

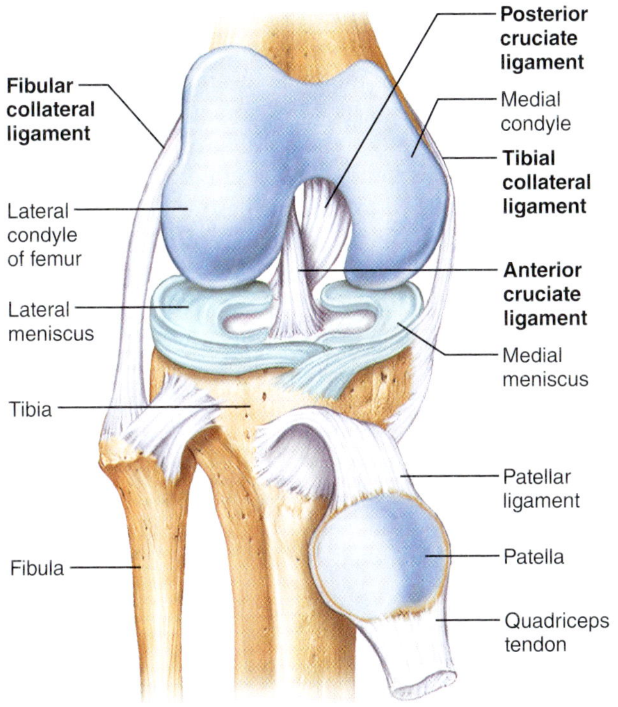

(e) Anterior view of flexed knee, showing the cruciate ligaments (articular capsule removed, and quadriceps tendon cut and reflected distally)

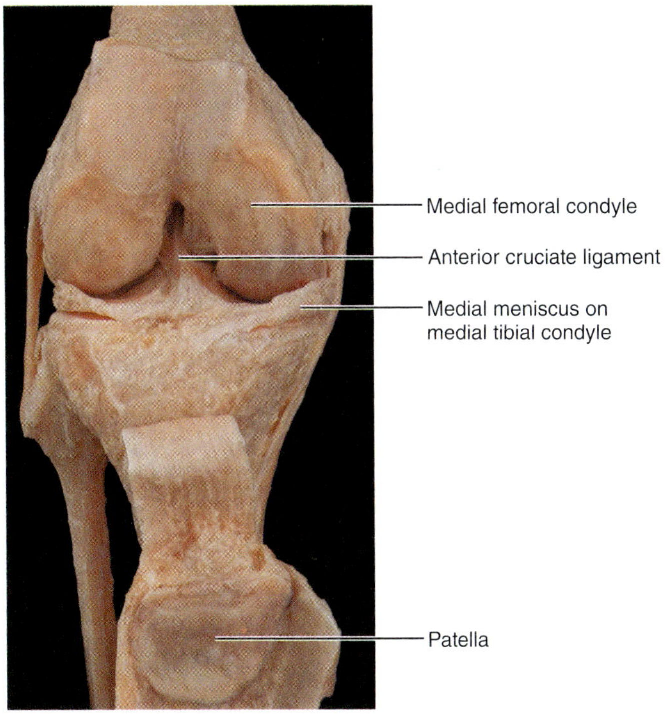

(f) Photograph of an opened knee joint; view similar to (e)

Figure 8.8 *(continued)*

attached only at their outer margins and are frequently torn free.

The tibiofemoral joint acts primarily as a hinge, permitting flexion and extension. However, structurally it is a bicondylar joint. Some rotation is possible when the knee is partly flexed, and when the knee is extending. But, when the knee is fully extended, side-to-side movements and rotation are strongly resisted by ligaments and the menisci. The femoropatellar joint is a plane joint, and the patella glides across the distal end of the femur during knee flexion.

The knee joint is unique in that its joint cavity is only partially enclosed by a capsule. The relatively thin articular capsule is present only on the sides and posterior aspects of the knee, where it covers the bulk of the femoral and tibial condyles. Anteriorly, where the capsule is absent, three broad ligaments run from the patella to the tibia below. These are the **patellar ligament** flanked by the **medial** and **lateral patellar retinacula** (ret″ĭ-nak′u-lah; "retainers"), which merge imperceptibly into the articular capsule on each side (Figure 8.8c). The patellar ligament and retinacula are actually continuations of the tendon of the bulky quadriceps muscle of the anterior thigh. Physicians tap the patellar ligament to test the knee-jerk reflex.

The synovial cavity of the knee joint has a complicated shape, with several extensions that lead into "blind alleys." At least a dozen bursae are associated with this joint, some of which are shown in Figure 8.8a. For example, notice the *subcutaneous prepatellar bursa*, which is often injured when the knee is bumped anteriorly.

All three types of joint ligaments stabilize and strengthen the capsule of the knee joint. The ligaments of two of the types, capsular and extracapsular, all act to prevent hyperextension of the knee and are stretched taut when the knee is extended. These include the following:

- The extracapsular **fibular** and **tibial collateral ligaments** are also critical in preventing lateral or medial rotation when the knee is extended. The broad, flat tibial collateral ligament runs from the medial epicondyle of the femur to the medial condyle of the tibial shaft below and is fused to the medial meniscus (Figure 8.8c–e).
- The **oblique popliteal ligament** (pop″lĭ-te′al) is actually part of the tendon of the semimembranosus muscle that fuses with the joint capsule and helps stabilize the posterior aspect of the knee joint (Figure 8.8d).
- The **arcuate popliteal ligament** arcs superiorly from the head of the fibula over the popliteus muscle and reinforces the joint capsule posteriorly (Figure 8.8d).

The knee's *intracapsular ligaments* are called *cruciate ligaments* (kroo′she-āt) because they cross each other, forming an X (*cruci* = cross) in the notch between the femoral condyles. They act as restraining straps to help prevent anterior-posterior displacement of the articular surfaces and to secure the articulating bones when we stand (Figure 8.8a, b, e). Although these ligaments are in the joint capsule, they are *outside* the synovial cavity, and synovial membrane nearly covers their surfaces. Note that the two cruciate ligaments both run superiorly to the femur and are named for their *tibial* attachment site.

The **anterior cruciate ligament** attaches to the *anterior* intercondylar area of the tibia (Figure 8.8b). From there it passes posteriorly, laterally, and upward to attach to the femur on the medial side of its lateral condyle. This ligament prevents forward sliding of the tibia on the femur and checks hyperextension of the knee. It

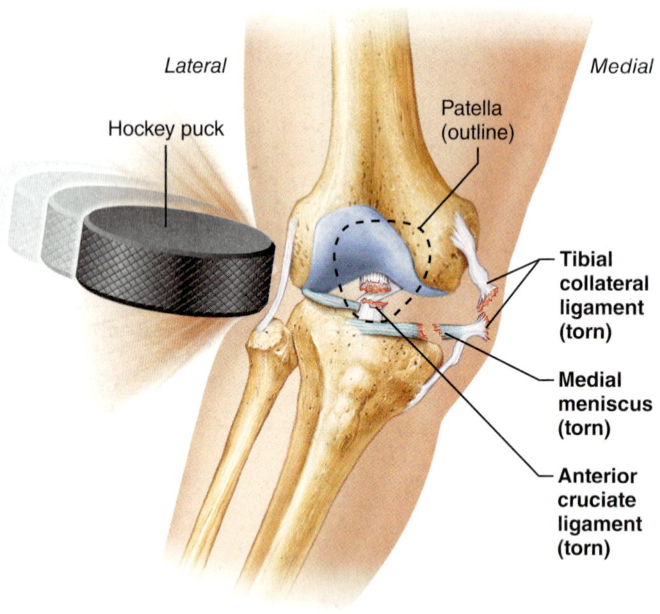

Figure 8.9 A common knee injury. Anterior view of a knee being hit by a hockey puck. Such blows to the lateral side tear both the tibial collateral ligament and the medial meniscus because the two are attached. The anterior cruciate ligament also tears.

is somewhat lax when the knee is flexed, and taut when the knee is extended.

The stronger **posterior cruciate ligament** is attached to the *posterior* intercondylar area of the tibia and passes anteriorly, medially, and superiorly to attach to the femur on the lateral side of the medial condyle (Figure 8.8a, b). This ligament prevents backward displacement of the tibia or forward sliding of the femur.

The knee capsule is heavily reinforced by muscle tendons. Most important are the strong tendons of the quadriceps muscles of the anterior thigh and the tendon of the semimembranosus muscle posteriorly (Figure 8.8c and d). The greater the strength and tone of these muscles, the less the chance of knee injury.

The knees have a built-in locking device that provides steady support for the body in the standing position. As we begin to stand up, the wheel-shaped femoral condyles roll like ball bearings across the tibial condyles and the flexed leg begins to extend at the knee. Because the lateral femoral condyle stops rolling before the medial condyle stops, the femur *spins* (rotates) medially on the tibia, until the cruciate and collateral ligaments of the knee are twisted and taut and the menisci are compressed. The tension in the ligaments effectively locks the joint into a rigid structure that cannot be flexed again until it is unlocked. This unlocking is accomplished by the popliteus muscle (see Figure 8.8d and Table 10.15, p. 370). It rotates the femur laterally on the tibia, causing the ligaments to become untwisted and slack.

Homeostatic Imbalance 8.1

Of all body joints, the knees are most susceptible to sports injuries because of their high reliance on nonarticular factors for stability and the fact that they carry the body's weight. The knee can absorb a vertical force equal to nearly seven times body weight. However, it is very vulnerable to *horizontal* blows, such as those that occur during blocking and tackling in football and in ice hockey.

When thinking of common knee injuries, remember the 3 Cs: collateral ligaments, cruciate ligaments, and cartilages (menisci). Most dangerous are *lateral blows* to the extended knee. These forces tear the tibial collateral ligament and the medial meniscus attached to it, as well as the anterior cruciate ligament **(Figure 8.9)**. It is estimated that 50% of all professional football players have serious knee injuries during their careers.

Although less devastating than the injury just described, injuries that affect only the anterior cruciate ligament (ACL) are becoming more common, particularly as women's sports become more vigorous and competitive. Most ACL injuries occur when a runner changes direction quickly, twisting a hyperextended knee. A torn ACL heals poorly, so repair usually requires a graft taken from either the patellar ligament, the hamstring tendon, or the calcaneal tendon. +

Shoulder (Glenohumeral) Joint

In the shoulder joint, stability has been sacrificed to provide the most freely moving joint of the body. The shoulder joint is a ball-and-socket joint. The large hemispherical head of the humerus fits in the small, shallow glenoid cavity of the scapula **(Figure 8.10)**, like a golf ball sitting on a tee. Although the glenoid cavity is slightly deepened by a rim of fibrocartilage, the **glenoid labrum** (*labrum* =lip), it is only about one-third the size of the humeral head and contributes little to joint stability (Figure 8.10d).

The articular capsule enclosing the joint cavity (from the margin of the glenoid cavity to the anatomical neck of the humerus) is remarkably thin and loose, qualities that contribute to this joint's freedom of movement. The few ligaments reinforcing the shoulder joint are located primarily on its anterior aspect. The superiorly located **coracohumeral ligament** (kor′ah-ko-hu′mer-ul) provides the only strong thickening of the capsule and helps support the weight of the upper limb (Figure 8.10c). Three **glenohumeral ligaments** (glĕ″no-hu′mer-ul) strengthen the front of the capsule somewhat but are weak and may even be absent (Figure 8.10c, d).

Muscle tendons that cross the shoulder joint contribute most to this joint's stability. The "superstabilizer" is the tendon of the long head of the biceps brachii muscle of the arm (Figure 8.10c). This tendon attaches to the superior margin of the glenoid labrum, travels through the joint cavity, and then runs within the intertubercular sulcus of the humerus. It secures the head of the humerus against the glenoid cavity.

Four other tendons (and the associated muscles) make up the **rotator cuff**. This cuff encircles the shoulder joint and blends with the articular capsule. The muscles include the subscapularis, supraspinatus, infraspinatus, and teres minor. (The rotator cuff muscles are illustrated in Figure 10.15, p. 351.) The rotator cuff can be severely stretched when the arm is vigorously circumducted; this is a common injury of baseball pitchers. As noted in Chapter 7, shoulder dislocations are fairly common. Because the shoulder's reinforcements are weakest anteriorly and inferiorly, the humerus tends to dislocate in the forward and downward direction.

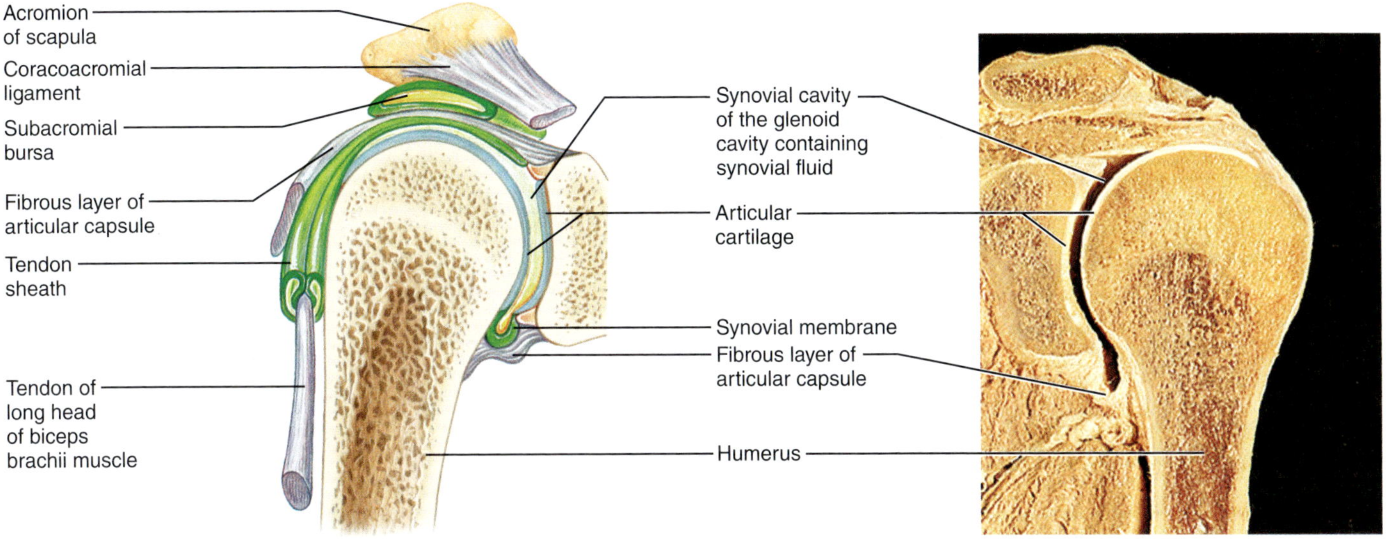

(a) Frontal section through right shoulder joint

(b) Cadaver photo corresponding to (a)

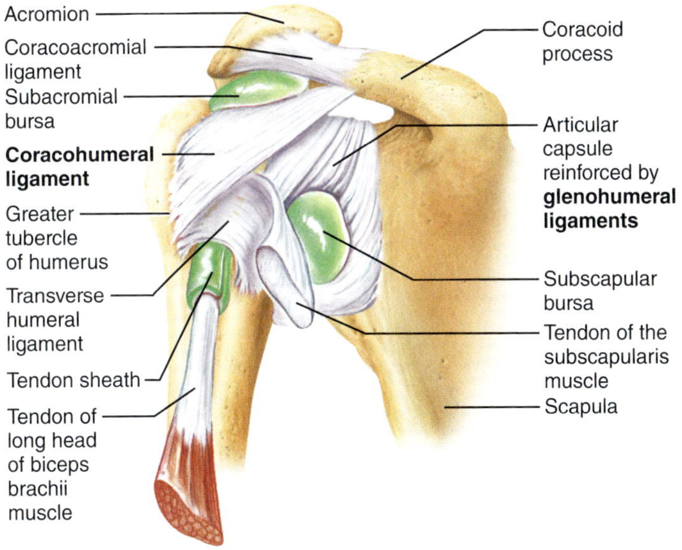

(c) Anterior view of right shoulder joint capsule

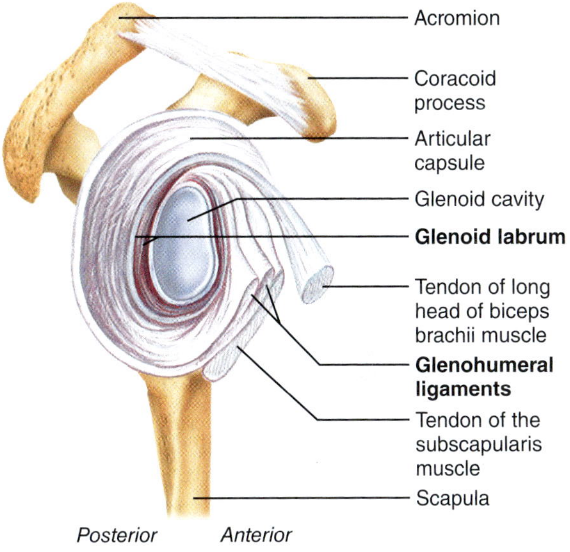

(d) Lateral view of socket of right shoulder joint, humerus removed

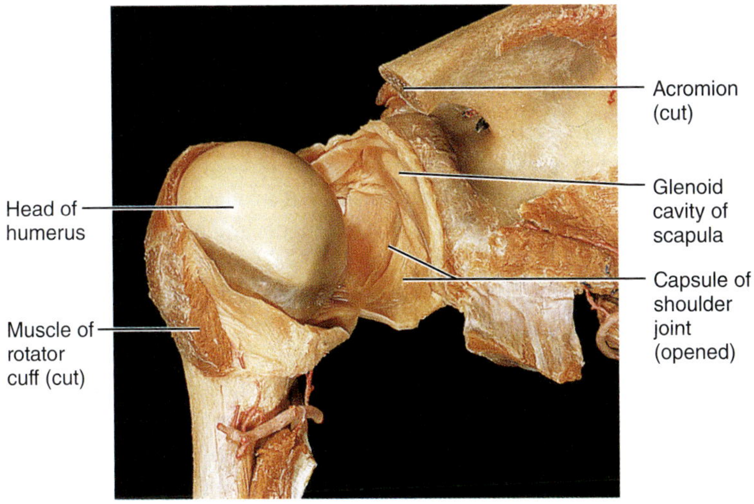

(e) Anterior view of an opened shoulder joint

Figure 8.10 The shoulder joint.

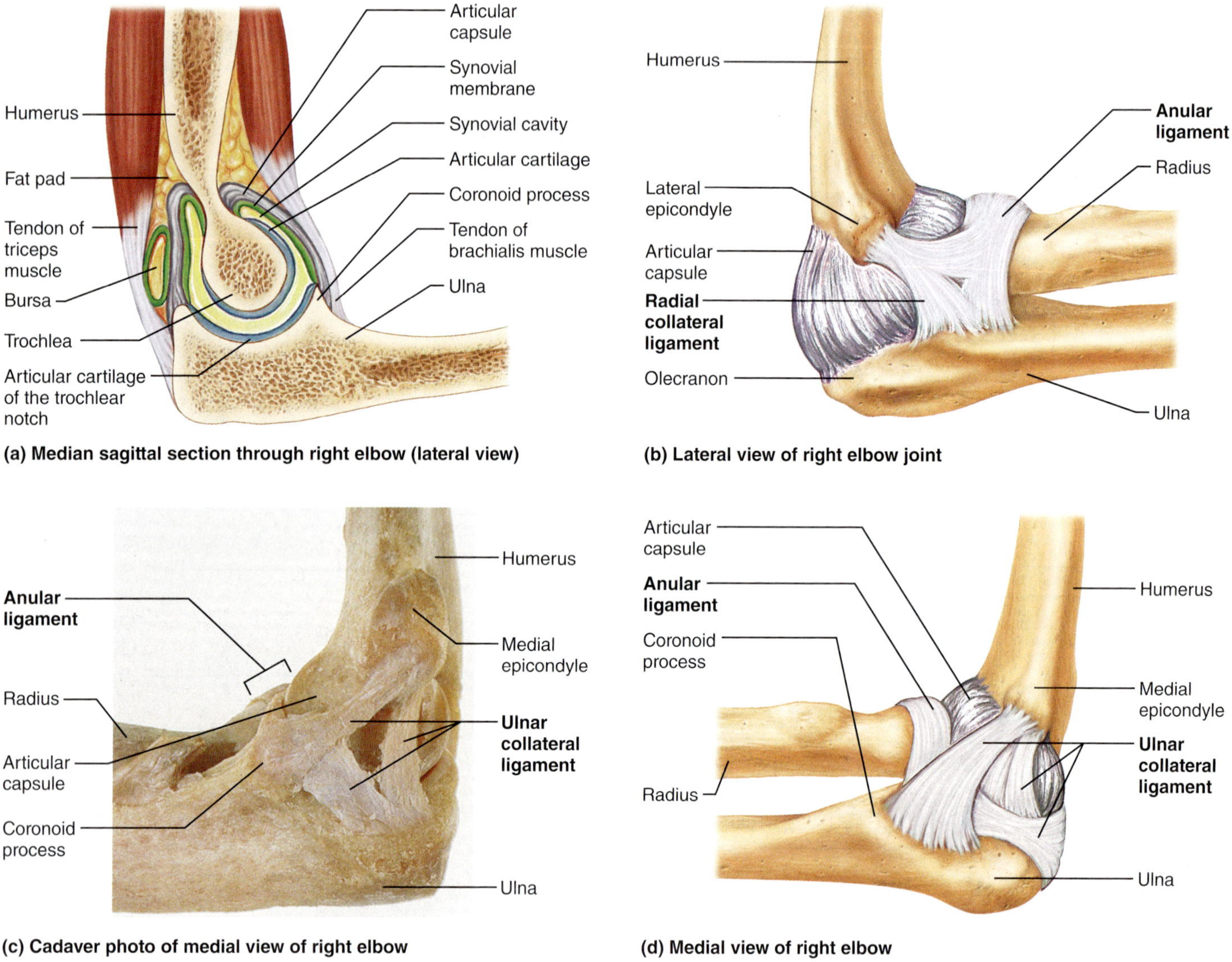

(a) Median sagittal section through right elbow (lateral view)

(b) Lateral view of right elbow joint

(c) Cadaver photo of medial view of right elbow

(d) Medial view of right elbow

Figure 8.11 The elbow joint.

Elbow Joint

Our upper limbs are flexible extensions that permit us to reach out and manipulate things in our environment. Besides the shoulder joint, the most prominent of the upper limb joints is the elbow. The elbow joint provides a stable and smoothly operating hinge that allows flexion and extension only **(Figure 8.11)**. Within the joint, both the radius and ulna articulate with the condyles of the humerus, but it is the close gripping of the trochlea by the ulna's trochlear notch that forms the "hinge" and stabilizes this joint (Figure 8.11a). A relatively lax articular capsule extends inferiorly from the humerus to the ulna and radius, and to the **anular ligament** (an′u-lar) surrounding the head of the radius (Figure 8.11b, c).

Anteriorly and posteriorly, the articular capsule is thin and allows substantial freedom for elbow flexion and extension. However, side-to-side movements are restricted by two strong capsular ligaments: the **ulnar collateral ligament** medially, and the **radial collateral ligament**, a triangular ligament on the lateral side (Figure 8.11b, c, and d). Additionally, tendons of several arm muscles, such as the biceps and triceps, cross the elbow joint and provide security.

The radius is a passive "onlooker" in the angular elbow movements. However, its head rotates within the anular ligament during supination and pronation of the forearm.

Hip Joint

The **hip** (coxal) **joint**, like the shoulder joint, is a ball-and-socket joint. It has a good range of motion, but not nearly as wide as the shoulder's range. Movements occur in all possible planes but are limited by the joint's strong ligaments and its deep socket.

The hip joint is formed by the articulation of the spherical head of the femur with the deeply cupped acetabulum of the hip bone **(Figure 8.12)**. The depth of the acetabulum is enhanced by a circular rim of fibrocartilage called the **acetabular labrum** (as″ĕ-tab′u-lar) (Figure 8.12a, b). The labrum's diameter is less than that of the head of the femur, and these articular surfaces fit snugly together, so hip joint dislocations are rare.

The thick articular capsule extends from the rim of the acetabulum to the neck of the femur and completely encloses the joint. Several strong ligaments reinforce the capsule of the hip joint.

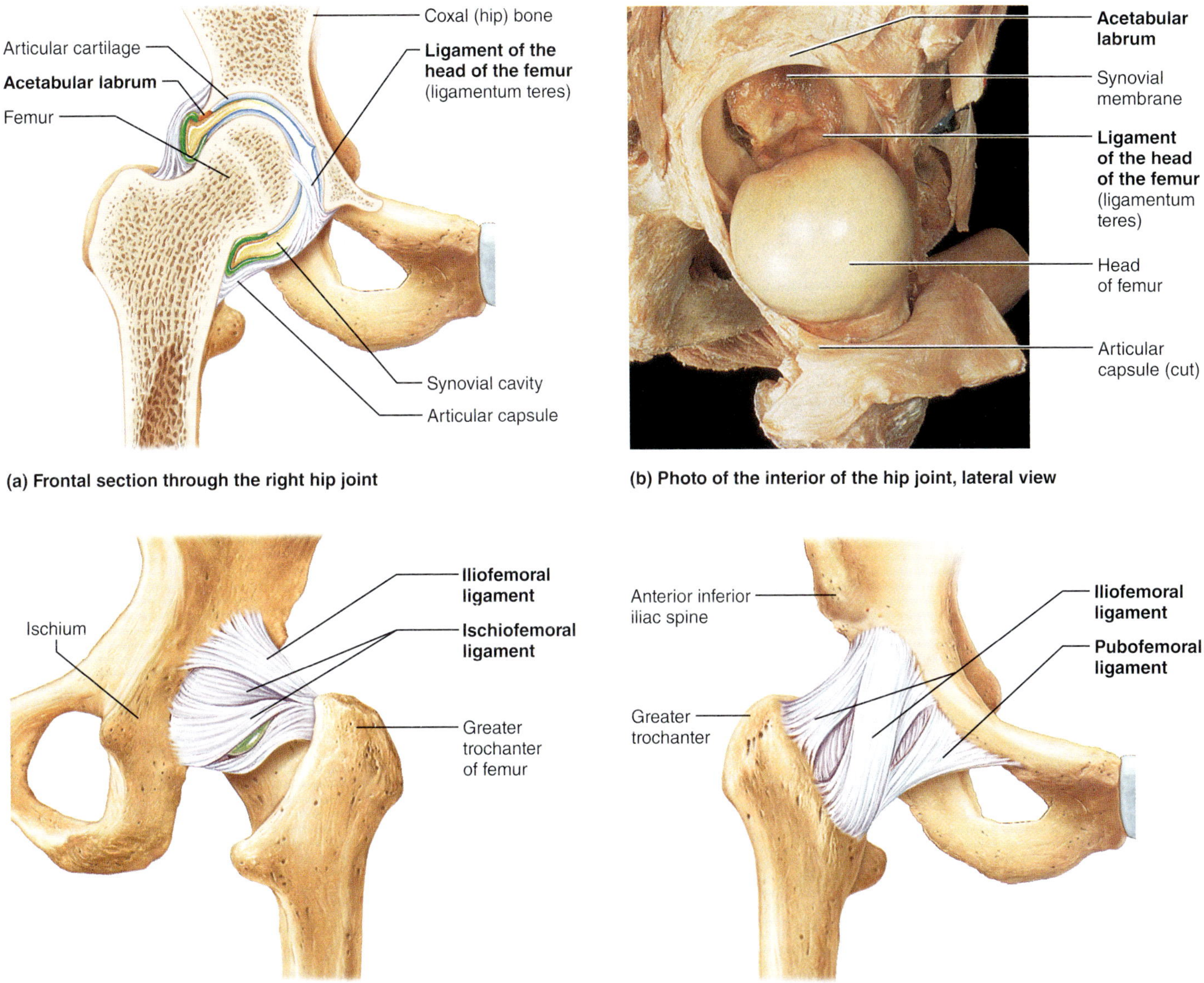

(a) Frontal section through the right hip joint

(b) Photo of the interior of the hip joint, lateral view

(c) Posterior view of right hip joint, capsule in place

(d) Anterior view of right hip joint, capsule in place

Figure 8.12 **The hip joint.**

These include the **iliofemoral ligament** (il″e-o-fem′o-ral), a strong V-shaped ligament anteriorly; the **pubofemoral ligament** (pu″bo-fem′o-ral), a triangular thickening of the inferior part of the capsule; and the **ischiofemoral ligament** (is″ke-o-fem′o-ral), a spiraling posterior ligament (Figure 8.12c, d). These ligaments are arranged in such a way that they "screw" the femur head into the acetabulum when a person stands up straight, thereby providing more stability.

The **ligament of the head of the femur**, also called the *ligamentum teres*, is a flat intracapsular band that runs from the femur head to the lower lip of the acetabulum (Figure 8.12a, b). This ligament is slack during most hip movements, so it is not important in stabilizing the joint. In fact, its mechanical function (if any) is unclear, but it does contain an artery that helps supply the head of the femur. Damage to this artery may lead to severe arthritis of the hip joint.

Muscle tendons that cross the joint and the bulky hip and thigh muscles that surround it contribute to its stability and strength. In this joint, however, stability comes chiefly from the deep socket that securely encloses the femoral head and the strong capsular ligaments.

Temporomandibular Joint

The **temporomandibular joint** (TMJ), or jaw joint, is a modified hinge joint. It lies just anterior to the ear (**Figure 8.13**). At this joint, the condylar process of the mandible articulates with the inferior surface of the squamous part of the temporal bone. The mandible's condylar process is egg shaped, whereas the articular surface of the temporal bone has a more complex shape. Posteriorly, it forms the concave **mandibular fossa**; anteriorly it forms a dense knob called the **articular tubercle**. The lateral aspect of the loose articular capsule that encloses the joint is thickened into a **lateral ligament**. Within the capsule, an articular disc divides the synovial cavity into superior and inferior compartments (Figure 8.13a, b).

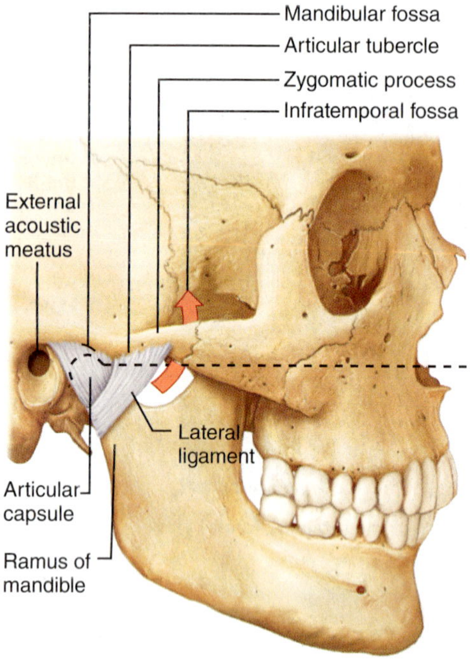

(a) Location of the joint in the skull

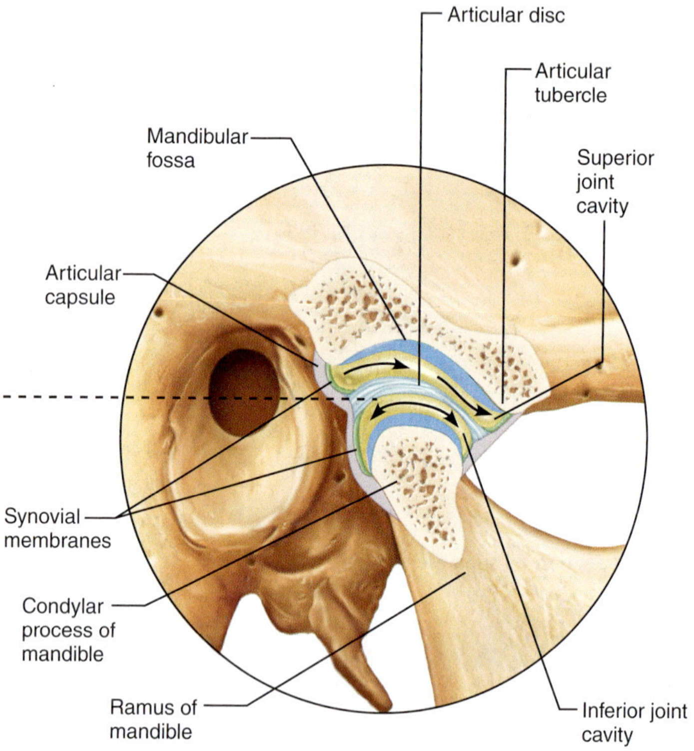

(b) Enlargement of a sagittal section through the joint

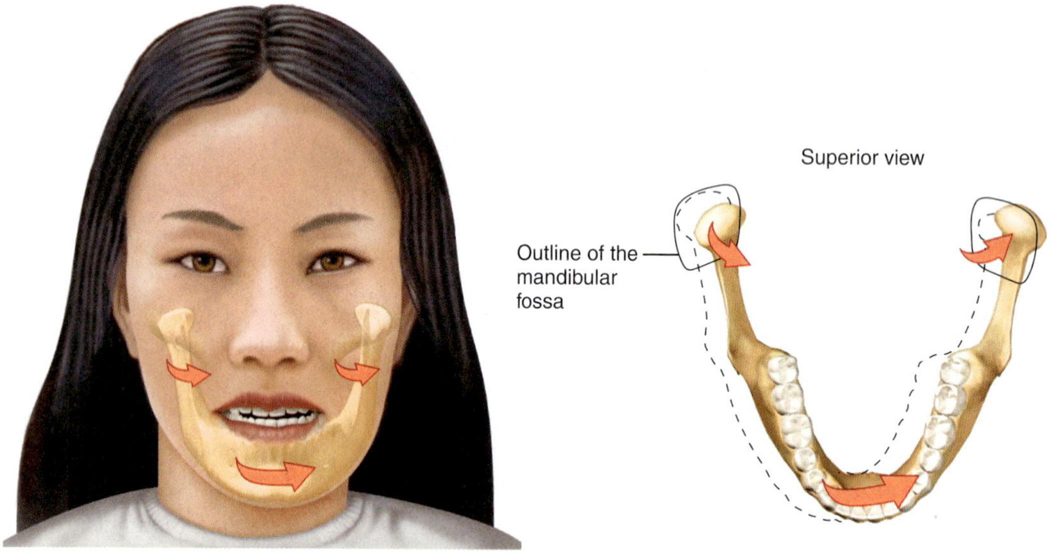

(c) Lateral excursion: lateral (side-to-side) movements of the mandible

Figure 8.13 The temporomandibular (jaw) joint. In **(b)**, note that the two parts of the joint cavity allow different movements, indicated by arrows. The inferior compartment of the joint cavity allows the condylar process of the mandible to rotate in opening and closing the mouth. The superior compartment lets the condylar process move forward to brace against the articular tubercle when the mouth opens wide, and also allows lateral excursion of this joint **(c)**.

Two distinct kinds of movement occur at the TMJ (Figure 8.13c). First, the concave inferior disc surface receives the condylar process of the mandible and allows the familiar hingelike movement of depressing and elevating the mandible while opening and closing the mouth. Second, the superior disc surface glides anteriorly along with the condylar process when the mouth is opened wide. This anterior movement braces the condylar process against the articular tubercle, so that the mandible is not forced through the thin roof of the mandibular fossa when one bites hard foods such as nuts or hard candies. The superior compartment also allows this joint to glide from side to side. As the posterior teeth are drawn into occlusion during grinding, the mandible moves with a side-to-side movement called *lateral excursion* (Figure 8.13c). This lateral jaw movement is unique to mammals and it is readily apparent in horses and cows as they chew.

Homeostatic Imbalance 8.2

Because of its shallow socket, the TMJ is the most easily dislocated joint in the body. Even a deep yawn can dislocate it. This joint almost always dislocates anteriorly, the condylar process of the mandible ending up in a skull region called the *infratemporal fossa* (Figure 8.13a). In such cases, the mouth remains wide open. To realign a dislocated TMJ, the physician places his or her thumbs in the patient's mouth between the lower molars and the cheeks, and then pushes the mandible inferiorly and posteriorly.

At least 5% of Americans suffer from painful temporomandibular disorders, the most common symptoms of which are pain in the ear and face, tenderness of the jaw muscles, popping sounds when the mouth opens, and joint stiffness. Usually caused by painful spasms of the chewing muscles, TMJ disorders often afflict people who grind their teeth; however, it can also result from jaw trauma or from poor occlusion of the teeth. Treatment usually focuses on getting the jaw muscles to relax by using massage, applying moist heat or ice, muscle-relaxant drugs, and adopting stress reduction techniques. For tooth grinders, use of a bite plate during sleep is generally recommended. +

Check Your Understanding

11. Of the five joints studied in more detail—hip, shoulder, elbow, knee, and temporomandibular—which two have menisci? Which act mainly as a uniaxial hinge? Which depend mainly on muscles and their tendons for stability?

For answers, see Appendix H.

Homeostatic Imbalances of Joints

- ✓ Name the most common joint injuries and discuss the symptoms and problems associated with each.
- ✓ Compare and contrast the common types of arthritis.
- ✓ Describe the cause and consequences of Lyme disease.

Few of us pay attention to our joints unless something goes wrong with them. Although remarkably strong, joints are more likely to be injured by forces the bony skeleton can withstand. This is the price of our flexibility. Joint pain and malfunction can be caused by a number of factors besides traumatic injury, including inflammatory conditions and degenerative processes due to friction and wear.

Common Joint Injuries

For most of us, sprains and dislocations are the most common trauma-induced joint injuries, but cartilage injuries are equally threatening to athletes.

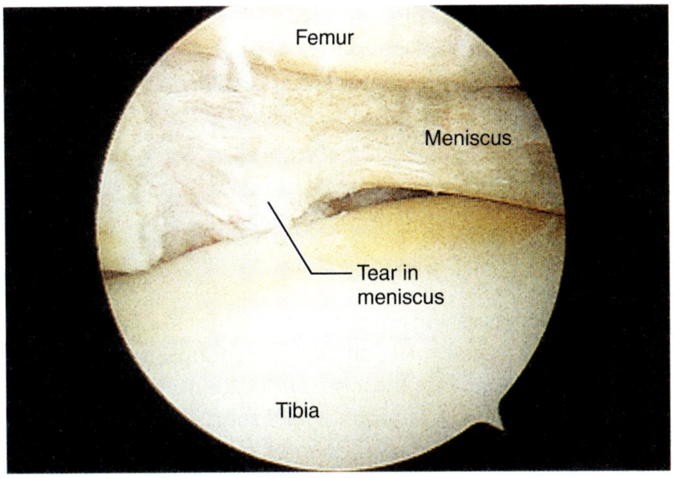

Figure 8.14 Arthroscopic photograph of a torn medial meniscus. (Courtesy of the author's tennis game.)

Cartilage Tears

Many aerobics devotees, encouraged to "feel the burn" during their workout, may feel the snap and pop of their overstressed cartilage instead. Although most cartilage injuries involve tearing of the knee menisci, tears and overuse damage to the articular cartilages of other joints is becoming increasingly common in competitive young athletes.

Cartilage tears typically occur when a meniscus is subjected to compression and shear stress at the same time. Cartilage is avascular and it rarely can obtain sufficient nourishment to repair itself, so it usually stays torn. Cartilage fragments (called loose bodies) can interfere with joint function by causing the joint to lock or bind, so most sports physicians recommend that the damaged cartilage be removed. Today, this can be done by **arthroscopic surgery** (ar-thro-skop′ik; "looking into joints"), a procedure that enables patients to be out of the hospital the same day. The arthroscope, a small instrument bearing a tiny lens and fiber-optic light source, enables the surgeon to view the joint interior, as in **Figure 8.14**. The surgeon can then repair a ligament, or remove cartilage fragments through one or more tiny slits, minimizing tissue damage and scarring. Removal of part of a meniscus does not severely impair knee joint mobility, but the joint is definitely less stable. Removal of the entire meniscus is an invitation to early onset of osteoarthritis in the joint. For younger patients a meniscal transplant may be an option to replace irreparably damaged cartilage. In the future, a tissue-engineered meniscus grown from your own stem cells may be implanted instead.

Sprains

In a **sprain**, the ligaments reinforcing a joint are stretched or torn. Common sites of sprains are the ankle, the knee, and the lumbar region of the spine. Partially torn ligaments will repair themselves, but they heal slowly because ligaments are so poorly vascularized. Sprains tend to be painful and immobilizing.

When ligaments are completely torn, there are three options:

- The torn ends of the ligament can be sewn together. This is difficult because trying to sew the hundreds of fibrous strands of a ligament together is like trying to sew two hairbrushes together.

- Certain ligaments, like the anterior cruciate ligament, are best repaired by replacing them with grafts. For example, a piece of tendon from a muscle can be attached to the articulating bones.
- For many ligaments, such as the knee's medial collateral ligament, we've come to realize that time and immobilization are just as effective as any surgical option.

Dislocations

A **dislocation (luxation)** occurs when bones are forced out of alignment. It is usually accompanied by sprains, inflammation, and difficulty in moving the joint. Dislocations may result from serious falls and are common contact sports injuries. Joints of the jaw, shoulders, fingers, and thumbs are most commonly dislocated. Like fractures, dislocations must be *reduced*; that is, the bone ends must be returned to their proper positions by a physician. *Subluxation* is a partial dislocation of a joint.

Repeat dislocations of the same joint are common because the initial dislocation stretches the joint capsule and ligaments. The resulting loose capsule provides poor reinforcement for the joint.

Inflammatory and Degenerative Conditions

Inflammatory conditions that affect joints include bursitis and tendonitis, various forms of arthritis, and Lyme disease.

Bursitis and Tendonitis

Bursitis is inflammation of a bursa and is usually caused by a blow or friction. Falling on one's knee may result in a painful bursitis of the prepatellar bursa, known as *housemaid's knee* or *water on the knee*. Prolonged leaning on one's elbows may damage the bursa close to the olecranon, producing *student's elbow*, or *olecranon bursitis*. Severe cases are treated by injecting anti-inflammatory drugs into the bursa. If excessive fluid accumulates, removing some fluid by needle aspiration may relieve the pressure.

Tendonitis is inflammation of tendon sheaths, typically caused by overuse. Its symptoms (pain and swelling) and treatment (rest, ice, and anti-inflammatory drugs) mirror those of bursitis.

Arthritis

The term **arthritis** describes over 100 different types of inflammatory or degenerative diseases that damage the joints. In all its forms, arthritis is the most widespread crippling disease in North America. One in five of us suffers its ravages. To a greater or lesser degree, all forms of arthritis have the same initial symptoms: pain, stiffness, and swelling of the joint.

Acute forms of arthritis usually result from bacterial invasion and are treated with antibiotics. Chronic forms of arthritis include osteoarthritis, rheumatoid arthritis, and gouty arthritis.

Osteoarthritis **Osteoarthritis (OA)** is the most common chronic arthritis. A chronic (long-term) degenerative condition, OA is often called "wear-and-tear arthritis." OA is most prevalent in the aged and is probably related to the normal aging process (although it is seen occasionally in younger people and some forms have a genetic basis). More women than men are affected, but nearly half of us will develop this condition by the age of 85.

Current theory holds that normal joint use prompts the release of (metalloproteinase) enzymes that break down articular cartilage, especially its collagen fibrils. In healthy individuals, this damaged cartilage is eventually replaced, but in people with OA, more cartilage is destroyed than replaced. Although its specific cause is unknown, OA may reflect the cumulative effects of years of compression and abrasion acting at joint surfaces, causing excessive amounts of the cartilage-destroying enzymes to be released. The result is softened, roughened, pitted, and eroded articular cartilages. Because this process occurs most where an uneven orientation of forces cause extensive microdamage, badly aligned or overworked joints are likely to develop OA.

As the disease progresses, the exposed bone tissue thickens and forms bony spurs (osteophytes) that enlarge the bone ends and may restrict joint movement. Patients complain of stiffness on arising that lessens somewhat with activity. The affected joints may make a crunching noise, called *crepitus* (krep′ĭ-tus), as they move and the roughened articular surfaces rub together. The joints most often affected are those of the cervical and lumbar spine and the fingers, knuckles, knees, and hips.

The course of osteoarthritis is usually slow and irreversible. In many cases, its symptoms are controllable with a mild pain reliever like aspirin or acetaminophen, along with moderate activity to keep the joints mobile. Rubbing a hot-pepper substance called capsaicin on the skin over the painful joints helps lessen the pain of OA. Glucosamine and chondroitin sulfate, nutritional supplements consisting of macromolecules normally present in cartilage, have been widely used by arthritis sufferers. However, several recent studies suggest that these supplements are no more effective than placebos. Osteoarthritis is rarely crippling, but it can be, particularly when the hip or knee joints are involved.

Rheumatoid Arthritis **Rheumatoid arthritis (RA)** (roo′mah-toid) is a chronic inflammatory disorder with an insidious onset. Though it usually arises between the ages of 30 and 50, it may occur at any age. It affects three times as many women as men. While not as common as osteoarthritis, rheumatoid arthritis affects millions, about 1% of all people.

In the early stages of RA, joint tenderness and stiffness are common. Many joints, particularly the small joints of the fingers, wrists, ankles, and feet, are afflicted at the same time and bilaterally. For example, if the right elbow is affected, most likely the left elbow is also affected. The course of RA is variable and marked by flare-ups (exacerbations) and remissions (*rheumat* =susceptible to change). Along with pain and swelling, its manifestations may include anemia, osteoporosis, muscle weakness, and cardiovascular problems.

RA is an *autoimmune disease*—a disorder in which the body's immune system attacks its own tissues. The initial trigger for this reaction is unknown, but various bacteria and viruses have been suspect. Perhaps these microorganisms bear molecules similar to some naturally present in the joints (possibly glycosaminoglycans, which are complex carbohydrates found in cartilage, joint fluid, and other connective tissues), and the immune system, once activated, attempts to destroy both.

RA begins with inflammation of the synovial membrane (*synovitis*) of the affected joints. Inflammatory cells (lymphocytes, macrophages, and others) migrate into the joint cavity from the blood and unleash a deluge of inflammatory chemicals

A CLOSER LOOK

Joints: From Knights in Shining Armor to Bionic Humans

The **technology** for fashioning **joints** in medieval suits of armor developed over centuries. The technology for creating the **prostheses** (artificial joints) used in medicine today developed, in relative terms, in a flash—less than 60 years. Unlike the joints in medieval **armor**, which was worn outside the body, today's artificial joints must function inside the body. The history of joint prostheses dates to the 1940s and 1950s, when World War II and the Korean War left large numbers of wounded who needed artificial limbs. Today, nearly 1 million Americans per year receive a total joint replacement, mostly because of the destructive effects of osteoarthritis or rheumatoid arthritis.

To produce durable, mobile joints requires substances that are strong, nontoxic, and resistant to the corrosive effects of organic acids in blood. In 1963, Sir John Charnley, an English orthopedic surgeon, revolutionized the therapy of arthritic hips with an artificial hip design that is still in use today. His device consisted of a metal ball on a stem and a cup-shaped polyethylene plastic socket anchored to the pelvis by methyl methacrylate cement. This cement proved to be exceptionally strong and relatively problem free. Hip prostheses were followed by knee prostheses, but not until 10 years later did smoothly operating total knee joint replacements become a reality. Today, the metal parts of the prostheses are strong cobalt and titanium alloys, and the number of knee replacements equals the number of hip replacements.

Replacements are now available for many other joints, including fingers, elbows, and shoulders. Total hip and knee replacements last about 10 to 15 years in elderly patients who do not excessively stress the joint. Most such operations are done to reduce pain and restore about 80% of original joint function.

Replacement joints are not yet strong or durable enough for young, active people, but making them so is a major goal. Another problem is that the prostheses work loose over time, so researchers are seeking to enhance the fit between implant and bone. One solution is to strengthen the cement that binds them (simply eliminating air bubbles from the cement increases its durability). Another solution is to use a cementless prosthesis, which allows the bone to grow into its surface, fixing it in place. In order for this to happen, a precise fit in the prosthesis and the bone must be achieved, something at which surgical robots such as ROBODOC excel.

Dramatic changes are also occurring in the way artificial joints are made. CAD/CAM (computer-aided design and computer-aided manufacturing) techniques have significantly reduced the time and cost of creating individualized joints. Fed the patient's X rays and medical information, the computer draws from a database of hundreds of normal joints and generates possible designs and modifications for a prosthesis. Once the best design is selected, the computer produces a program to direct the machines that make the prosthesis.

Joint replacement therapy is coming of age, but equally exciting are techniques that call on the ability of the patient's own tissues to regenerate.

- Bone marrow stimulation: Small holes poked through to the bone marrow allow mesenchymal stem cells from the bone marrow to migrate into the joint and produce new cartilage.
- Osteochondral grafting: Healthy bone and cartilage are removed from one part of the body and transplanted to the injured joint.
- Autologous chondrocyte implantation: Healthy chondrocytes are removed from the body and seeded onto a supporting matrix of tissue-engineered collagen. When subjected to mechanical pressure in the lab, the cells produce new cartilage, which is then implanted.
- Mesenchymal stem cell regeneration: Undifferentiated mesenchymal cells are removed from bone marrow and placed in a gel, which is packed into an area of eroded cartilage.

These techniques offer hope for younger patients, since they could stave off the need for a joint prosthesis for several years.

And so, through the centuries, the focus has shifted from jointed armor to artificial joints that can be put inside the body to restore lost function. Modern technology has accomplished what the armor designers of the Middle Ages never dreamed of.

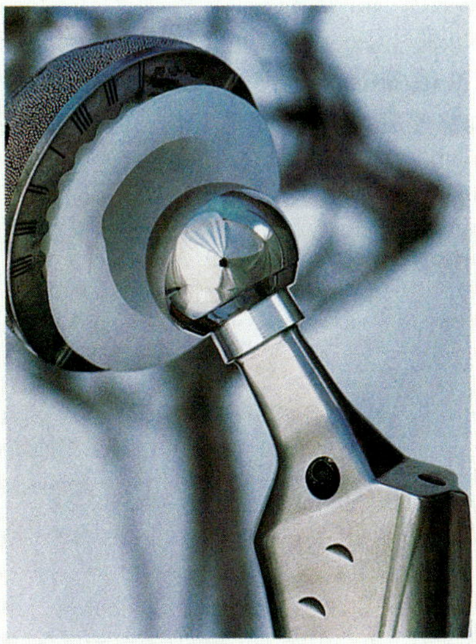

A hip prosthesis.

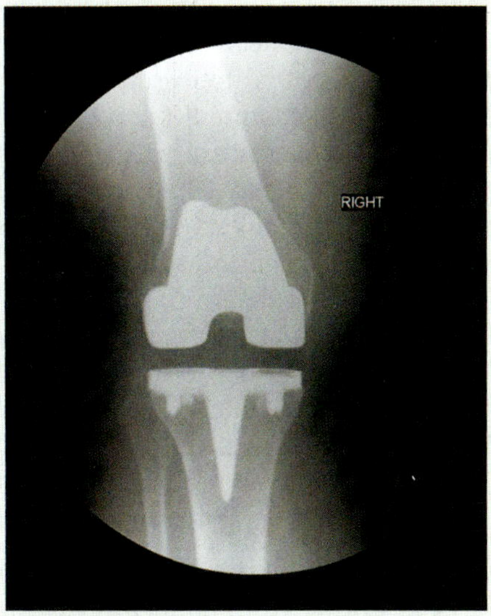

X ray of right knee showing total knee replacement prosthesis (co-designed by Kenneth Gustke, M.D., of Florida Orthopedic Institute).

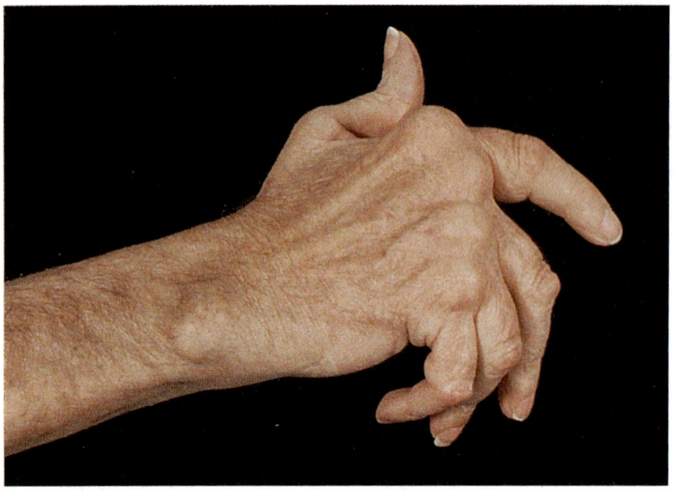

Figure 8.15 A hand deformed by rheumatoid arthritis. Inflammation has enlarged the synovial joints.

8

that destroy body tissues when released inappropriately in large amounts as in RA. Synovial fluid accumulates, causing joint swelling, and in time, the inflamed synovial membrane thickens into a **pannus** ("rag"), an abnormal tissue that clings to the articular cartilages. The pannus erodes the cartilage (and sometimes the underlying bone) and eventually scar tissue forms and connects the bone ends. Later this scar tissue ossifies and the bone ends fuse together, immobilizing the joint. This end condition, called ankylosis (ang″kĭ-lo′sis; "stiff condition"), often produces bent, deformed fingers **(Figure 8.15)**. Not all cases of RA progress to the severely crippling ankylosis stage, but all cases do involve restriction of joint movement and extreme pain.

A wonder drug for RA sufferers is still undiscovered. The goal of current RA treatment is to go beyond simply alleviating the symptoms and instead to disrupt the relentless destruction of the joints by the autoimmune processes. Steroidal and nonsteroidal anti-inflammatory drugs decrease pain and inflammation, increasing joint mobility. More powerful immune suppressants (such as methotrexate) act to slow the autoimmune reaction. Several biologic agents are available to block the action of inflammatory chemicals. An important target of many of these agents is an inflammatory chemical called *tumor necrosis factor*, an important contributor to destruction of cartilage. Together, these drugs can dramatically slow the course of RA. As a last resort, replacing the joint with a joint prosthesis (artificial joint), may be an option to restore function (see *A Closer Look*, p. 271). Indeed, some RA sufferers have over a dozen artificial joints.

Gouty Arthritis Uric acid, a normal waste product of nucleic acid metabolism, is ordinarily excreted in urine without any problems. However, when blood levels of uric acid rise excessively (due to its excessive production or slow excretion), it may be deposited as needle-shaped urate crystals in the soft tissues of joints. An inflammatory response follows, leading to an agonizingly painful attack of **gouty arthritis** (gow′te), or **gout**. The initial attack typically affects one joint, often at the base of the great toe.

Gout is far more common in men than in women because men naturally have higher blood levels of uric acid (perhaps because estrogens increase the rate of its excretion). Because gout seems to run in families, genetic factors are definitely implicated.

Untreated gout can be very destructive; the articulating bone ends fuse and immobilize the joint. Fortunately, several drugs (colchicine, nonsteroidal anti-inflammatory drugs, glucocorticoids, and others) that terminate or prevent gout attacks are available. Patients are advised to drink plenty of water and to avoid alcohol excess (which promotes uric acid overproduction), and foods high in purine-containing nucleic acids, such as liver, kidneys, and sardines.

Lyme Disease

Lyme disease is an inflammatory disease caused by spirochete bacteria transmitted by the bite of ticks that live on mice and deer. It often results in joint pain and arthritis, especially in the knees, and is characterized by a skin rash, flu-like symptoms, and foggy thinking. If untreated, neurological disorders and irregular heartbeat may ensue.

Because symptoms vary from person to person, the disease is hard to diagnose. Antibiotic therapy is the usual treatment, but it takes a long time to kill the infecting bacteria.

☑ Check Your Understanding

12. What does the term "arthritis" mean?
13. How would you determine by looking at someone suffering from arthritis if he or she has OA or RA?
14. What is the cause of Lyme disease?

For answers, see Appendix H.

Developmental Aspects of Joints

✓ Discuss factors that promote or disturb joint homeostasis.

As bones form from mesenchyme in the embryo, the joints develop in parallel. By week 8, the synovial joints resemble adult joints in form and arrangement, and synovial fluid is being secreted. During childhood, a joint's size, shape, and flexibility are modified by use. Active joints have thicker capsules and ligaments, and larger bony supports.

Injuries aside, relatively few interferences with joint function occur until late middle age. Eventually advancing years take their toll and ligaments and tendons shorten and weaken. The intervertebral discs become more likely to herniate, and osteoarthritis rears its ugly head. Many people have osteoarthritis by the time they are in their 70s. The middle years also see an increased incidence of rheumatoid arthritis.

Exercise that coaxes joints through their full range of motion, such as regular stretching and aerobics, is the key to postponing the immobilizing effects of aging on ligaments and tendons, to keeping cartilages well nourished, and to strengthening the muscles that stabilize the joints. The key word for exercising is "prudently," because excessive or abusive use of the joints guarantees early onset of osteoarthritis. The buoyancy of water relieves much of the stress on weight-bearing joints, and people who swim or exercise in a pool often retain good joint function as long as they live. As with so many medical problems, it is easier to prevent joint problems than to cure or correct them.

Check Your Understanding

15. What is the effect of regular exercise on joint health and structure?

For answers, see Appendix H.

The importance of joints is obvious: The skeleton's ability to protect other organs and to move smoothly reflects their presence. Now that we are familiar with joint structure and with the movements that joints allow, we are ready to consider how the muscles attached to the skeleton cause body movements by acting across its joints.

Chapter Summary

MAP™ For more chapter study tools, go to the Study Area of MasteringA&P at **www.masteringaandp.com**.

There you will find:

- Interactive Physiology iP
- A&PFlix *A&PFlix*
- Practice Anatomy Lab PAL
- PhysioEx PEx
- Videos, Practice Quizzes and Tests, MP3 Tutor Sessions, Case Studies, and much more!

1. Joints, or articulations, are sites where bones meet. Their functions are to hold bones together and to allow various degrees of skeletal movement.

Classification of Joints (pp. 249–250)

1. Joints are classified structurally as fibrous, cartilaginous, or synovial. They are classed functionally as synarthrotic, amphiarthrotic, or diarthrotic.

Fibrous Joints (pp. 250–251)

1. Fibrous joints occur where bones are connected by fibrous tissue; no joint cavity is present. Nearly all fibrous joints are synarthrotic.
2. **Sutures/syndesmoses/gomphoses.** The major types of fibrous joints are sutures, syndesmoses, and gomphoses.

Cartilaginous Joints (pp. 251–252)

1. In cartilaginous joints, the bones are united by cartilage; no joint cavity is present.
2. **Synchondroses/symphyses.** Cartilaginous joints include synchondroses and symphyses. Synchondroses are synarthrotic; all symphyses are amphiarthrotic.

Synovial Joints (pp. 252–269)

1. Most body joints are synovial joints, all of which are diarthrotic.

General Structure (pp. 252–253)

2. All synovial joints have a joint cavity enclosed by a fibrous layer lined with synovial membrane and reinforced by ligaments; articulating bone ends covered with articular cartilage; and synovial fluid in the joint cavity. Some (e.g., the knee) contain fibrocartilage discs that absorb shock.

Bursae and Tendon Sheaths (p. 253)

3. Bursae are fibrous sacs lined with synovial membrane and containing synovial fluid. Tendon sheaths are similar to bursae but are cylindrical structures that surround muscle tendons. Both allow adjacent structures to move smoothly over one another.

Factors Influencing the Stability of Synovial Joints (pp. 255–256)

4. Articular surfaces providing the most stability have large surfaces and deep sockets and fit snugly together.
5. Ligaments prevent undesirable movements and reinforce the joint.
6. The tone of muscles whose tendons cross the joint is the most important stabilizing factor in many joints.

Movements Allowed by Synovial Joints (pp. 256–258)

7. When a skeletal muscle contracts, the insertion (movable attachment) moves toward the origin (immovable attachment).
8. Synovial joints differ in their range of motion. Motion may be nonaxial (gliding), uniaxial (in one plane), biaxial (in two planes), or multiaxial (in all three planes).
9. Three common types of movements can occur when muscles contract across joints: (a) gliding movements, (b) angular movements (which include flexion, extension, abduction, adduction, and circumduction), and (c) rotation.
10. Special movements include supination and pronation, inversion and eversion, protraction and retraction, elevation and depression, opposition, dorsiflexion and plantar flexion.

Types of Synovial Joints (p. 258)

11. The six major categories of synovial joints are plane joints (nonaxial movement), hinge joints (uniaxial), pivot joints (uniaxial, rotation permitted), condylar joints (biaxial with angular movements in two planes), saddle joints (biaxial, like condylar joints, but with freer movement), and ball-and-socket joints (multiaxial and rotational movement).

Selected Synovial Joints (pp. 262–269)

12. The knee joint is the largest joint in the body. It is a hinge joint formed by the articulation of the tibial and femoral condyles (and anteriorly by the patella and patellar surface of the femur). Extension, flexion, and (some) rotation are allowed. Its articular surfaces are shallow and condylar. C-shaped menisci deepen the articular surfaces. The joint cavity is enclosed by a capsule only on the sides and posterior aspect. Several ligaments help prevent displacement of the joint surfaces. Muscle tone of the quadriceps and semimembranosus muscles is important in knee stability.
13. The shoulder joint is a ball-and-socket joint formed by the glenoid cavity of the scapula and the humeral head. The most freely movable joint of the body, it allows all angular and rotational movements. Its articular surfaces are shallow. Its capsule is lax and poorly reinforced by ligaments. The tendons of the biceps brachii and rotator cuff muscles help to stabilize it.
14. The elbow is a hinge joint in which the ulna (and radius) articulates with the humerus, allowing flexion and extension. Its articular surfaces are highly complementary and are the most important factor contributing to joint stability.
15. The hip joint is a ball-and-socket joint formed by the acetabulum of the hip bone and the femoral head. It is highly adapted for

weight bearing. Its articular surfaces are deep and secure. Its capsule is heavy and strongly reinforced by ligaments.

16. The temporomandibular joint is formed by (1) the condylar process of the mandible and (2) the mandibular fossa and articular tubercle of the temporal bone. This joint allows both a hingelike opening and closing of the mouth and an anterior gliding of the mandible. It often dislocates anteriorly and exhibits a number of TMJ disorders.

Homeostatic Imbalances of Joints (pp. 269–272)

Common Joint Injuries (pp. 269–270)

1. Cartilage injuries, particularly of the knee, are common in contact sports and may result from excessive compression and shear stress. The avascular cartilage is unable to repair itself.
2. Sprains involve stretching or tearing of joint ligaments. Because ligaments are poorly vascularized, healing is slow.
3. Dislocations involve displacement of the articular surfaces of bones. They must be reduced.

Inflammatory and Degenerative Conditions (pp. 270–272)

4. Bursitis and tendonitis are inflammations of a bursa and a tendon sheath, respectively.
5. Arthritis is joint inflammation or degeneration accompanied by stiffness, pain, and swelling. Acute forms generally result from bacterial infection. Chronic forms include osteoarthritis, rheumatoid arthritis, and gouty arthritis.
6. Osteoarthritis is a degenerative condition most common in the aged. Spine, knees, hips, knuckles, and fingers are most affected.
7. Rheumatoid arthritis, the most crippling arthritis, is an autoimmune disease involving severe inflammation of the joints.
8. Gouty arthritis, or gout, is joint inflammation caused by the deposit of urate salts in soft joint tissues.
9. Lyme disease is an infectious disease caused by the bite of a tick infected with spirochete bacteria.

Developmental Aspects of Joints (pp. 272–273)

1. Joints form from mesenchyme and in tandem with bone development in the embryo.
2. Excluding traumatic injury, joints usually function well until late middle age, at which time symptoms of connective tissue stiffening and osteoarthritis begin to appear. Prudent exercise delays these effects, whereas excessive exercise promotes the early onset of arthritis.

Review Questions

Multiple Choice/Matching

(Some questions have more than one correct answer. Select the best answer or answers from the choices given.)

1. Match the key terms to the appropriate descriptions.

   Key: **(a)** fibrous joints **(b)** cartilaginous joints **(c)** synovial joints

   ____ (1) exhibit a joint cavity
   ____ (2) types are sutures and syndesmoses
   ____ (3) bones connected by collagen fibers
   ____ (4) types include synchondroses and symphyses
   ____ (5) all are diarthrotic
   ____ (6) many are amphiarthrotic
   ____ (7) bones connected by a disc of hyaline cartilage or fibrocartilage
   ____ (8) nearly all are synarthrotic
   ____ (9) shoulder, hip, jaw, and elbow joints
2. Freely movable joints are **(a)** synarthroses, **(b)** diarthroses, **(c)** amphiarthroses.
3. Anatomical characteristics shared by all synovial joints include all except **(a)** articular cartilage, **(b)** a joint cavity, **(c)** an articular capsule, **(d)** presence of fibrocartilage.
4. Factors that influence the stability of a synovial joint include **(a)** shape of articular surfaces, **(b)** presence of strong reinforcing ligaments, **(c)** tone of surrounding muscles, **(d)** all of these.
5. The description "Articular surfaces deep and secure; capsule heavily reinforced by ligaments and muscle tendons; extremely stable joint" best describes **(a)** the elbow joint, **(b)** the hip joint, **(c)** the knee joint, **(d)** the shoulder joint.
6. Ankylosis means **(a)** twisting of the ankle, **(b)** tearing of ligaments, **(c)** displacement of a bone, **(d)** immobility of a joint due to fusion of its articular surfaces.
7. An autoimmune disorder in which joints are affected bilaterally and which involves pannus formation and gradual joint immobilization is **(a)** bursitis, **(b)** gout, **(c)** osteoarthritis, **(d)** rheumatoid arthritis.

Short Answer Essay Questions

8. Define joint.
9. Discuss the relative value (to body homeostasis) of immovable, slightly movable, and freely movable joints.
10. Compare the structure, function, and common body locations of bursae and tendon sheaths.
11. Joint movements may be nonaxial, uniaxial, biaxial, or multiaxial. Define what each of these terms means.
12. Compare and contrast the paired movements of flexion and extension with adduction and abduction.
13. How does rotation differ from circumduction?
14. Name two types of uniaxial, biaxial, and multiaxial joints.
15. What is the specific role of the menisci of the knee? Of the anterior and posterior cruciate ligaments?
16. The knee has been called "a beauty and a beast." Provide several reasons that might explain the negative (beast) part of this description.
17. Why are sprains and cartilage injuries a particular problem?
18. List the functions of the following elements of a synovial joint: fibrous layer of the capsule, synovial fluid, articular cartilage.

Critical Thinking and Clinical Application Questions

1. Sophie worked cleaning homes for 30 years so she could send her two children to college. Several times, she had been forced to call her employers to tell them she could not come in to work because one of her kneecaps was swollen and painful. What is Sophie's condition, and what probably caused it?

2. As Harry was running down the road, he tripped and his left ankle twisted violently to the side. When he picked himself up, he was unable to put any weight on that ankle. The diagnosis was severe dislocation and sprains of the left ankle. The orthopedic surgeon stated that she would perform a closed reduction of the dislocation and attempt ligament repair by using arthroscopy. (a) Is the ankle joint normally a stable joint? (b) What does its stability depend on? (c) What is a closed reduction? (d) Why is ligament repair necessary? (e) What does arthroscopy entail? (f) How will the use of this procedure minimize Harry's recuperation time (and suffering)?
3. Mrs. Bell, a 45-year-old woman, appeared at her physician's office complaining of unbearable pain in the interphalangeal joint of her right great toe. The joint was red and swollen. When asked about previous episodes, she recalled a similar attack two years earlier that disappeared as suddenly as it had come. Her diagnosis was arthritis. (a) What type? (b) What is the precipitating cause of this particular type of arthritis?
4. Grace heard on the evening TV news that the deer population in her state had been increasing rapidly in the past few years and it was common knowledge that deer walked the streets at night. After the program, she suddenly exclaimed, "So that's why those three boys in my son's class got Lyme disease last year." Explain what she meant by that comment.
5. Tony Bowers, an exhausted biology student, was attending a lecture. After 30 minutes or so, he lost interest and began to doze. As the lecture ended, the hubbub aroused him and he let go with a tremendous yawn. To his great distress, he couldn't close his mouth—his lower jaw was "stuck" open. What do you think had happened?

AT THE CLINIC

8

Related Clinical Terms

Ankylosing spondylitis (ang′kĭ-lōz″ing spon″dĭ-li′tis; *ankyl* = crooked, bent; *spondyl* = vertebra) A variant of rheumatoid arthritis that chiefly affects males; it usually begins in the sacroiliac joints and progresses superiorly along the spine. The vertebrae become interconnected by fibrous tissue, causing the spine to become rigid ("poker back").

Arthrology (ar-throl′o-je; *logos* = study) The study of joints.

Arthroplasty ("joint reforming") Replacing a diseased joint with an artificial joint.

Chondromalacia patellae (kon-dro-mal-a′sĭ-ah; "softening of cartilage by the patella") Damage and softening of the articular cartilages on the posterior patellar surface and the anterior surface of the distal femur; most often seen in adolescent athletes. Produces a sharp pain in the knee when the leg is extended (in climbing stairs, for example). May result when the quadriceps femoris, the main group of muscles on the anterior thigh, pulls unevenly on the patella, persistently rubbing it against the femur in the knee joint; often corrected by exercises that strengthen weakened parts of the quadriceps muscles.

Rheumatism A term used by laypeople to indicate disease involving muscle or joint pain; consequently may be used to apply to arthritis, bursitis, etc.

Synovitis (sin″o-vi′tis) Inflammation of the synovial membrane of a joint. Caused by injury, infection, or arthritis. Excess synovial fluid accumulates in the joint cavity, a condition called *effusion* that causes the joint to swell, limiting joint movement.

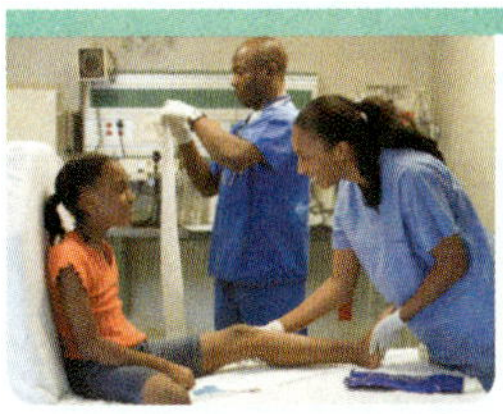

Case Study Joints

In the previous chapter, you met Kayla Tanner, a 45-year-old mother of four who suffered a dislocated right hip in the bus accident on Route 91. Prior to the closed reduction, the doctors noted that her right thigh was flexed at the hip, adducted, and medially rotated. After the reduction, the hip was put through a gentle range of motion (ROM) to assess the joint. A widened joint space in the postreduction X ray showed that the reduction was not complete, but no bone fragments were visible in the joint space. Mrs. Tanner was scheduled for immediate surgery.

The surgeons discovered that the acetabular labrum was detached from the rim of the acetabulum and was lying deep within the joint space. The detached portion of the labrum was excised, and the hip was surgically reduced. During the early healing phase (first two weeks), Mrs. Tanner was kept in traction with the hip abducted.

1. Joints can be classified by structure and by function. How would you structurally and functionally classify the joint involved in the injury in this case?
2. Name the six distinguishing features that define the structural classification of the joint involved in this injury.
3. The doctors noted that there were no bone fragments in the joint space. What is normally found in this space?
4. Surgeons had to remove a portion of Mrs. Tanner's acetabular labrum. What is this structure and what function does it supply at this joint?
5. The doctors noted that Mrs. Tanner's thigh was flexed at the hip, adducted, and medially rotated. Describe what this means in terms of the position of her leg.
6. Hip dislocations can be classified as anterior or posterior depending on which direction the head of the femur is facing after it dislocates. Based on the description you provided in question 5, which type of dislocation did Mrs. Tanner suffer?
7. In order to assess the joint as part of Mrs. Tanner's rehabilitation, clinicians would want to assess all of the movements that normally occur at the hip. List all the movements that the clinicians will need to assess.

(Answers in Appendix H)

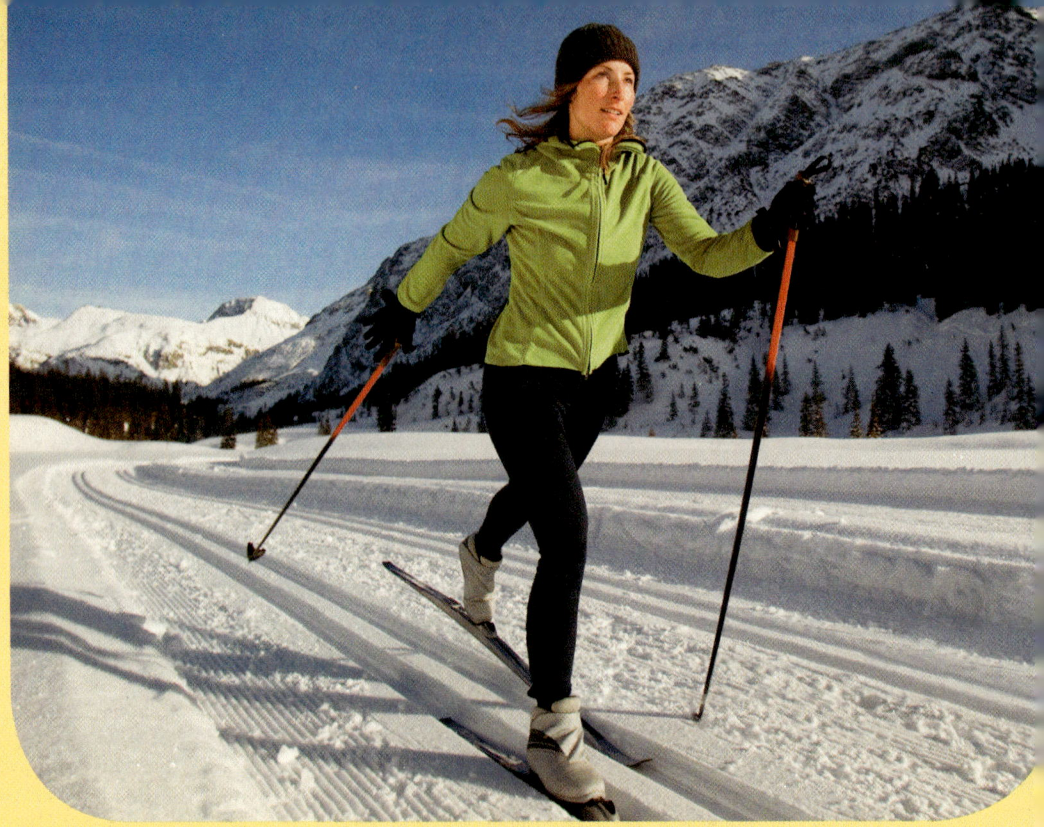

9 Muscles and Muscle Tissue

Because flexing muscles look like mice scurrying beneath the skin, some scientist long ago dubbed them *muscles*, from the Latin *mus* meaning "little mouse." Indeed, we tend to think of the rippling muscles of professional boxers or weight lifters when we hear the word *muscle*. But muscle is also the dominant tissue in the heart and in the walls of other hollow organs. In all its forms, muscle tissue makes up nearly half the body's mass.

Muscles are distinguished by their ability to transform chemical energy (ATP) into directed mechanical energy. In so doing, they become capable of exerting force.

Overview of Muscle Tissues

✓ Compare and contrast the three basic types of muscle tissue.

✓ List four important functions of muscle tissue.

Types of Muscle Tissue

Chapter 4 introduced the three types of muscle tissue—*skeletal*, *cardiac*, and *smooth*. Now we are ready to describe each type in detail, but before we do, let's introduce some terminology.

- Skeletal and smooth muscle cells (but not cardiac muscle cells) are elongated, and for this reason, they are called **muscle fibers**.
- Whenever you see the prefixes **myo** or **mys** (both are word roots meaning "muscle") or **sarco** (flesh), the reference is to muscle. For example, the plasma membrane of muscle cells is called the *sarcolemma* (sar″ko-lem′ah), literally, "muscle" (sarco) "husk" (lemma), and muscle cell cytoplasm is called *sarcoplasm*.

Okay, let's get to it.

Skeletal Muscle

Skeletal muscle tissue is packaged into the *skeletal muscles*, organs that attach to and cover the bony skeleton. Skeletal muscle fibers are the longest muscle cells and have obvious stripes called *striations* (see Figure 4.9a, p. 138). Although it is often activated by reflexes, skeletal muscle is called **voluntary muscle** because it is the only type subject to conscious control.

- When you think of skeletal muscle tissue, the key words to keep in mind are *skeletal*, *striated*, and *voluntary*.

Skeletal muscle is responsible for overall body mobility. It can contract rapidly, but it tires easily and must rest after short periods of activity. Nevertheless, it can exert tremendous power, a fact revealed by reports of people lifting cars to save their loved ones. Skeletal muscle is also remarkably adaptable. For example, your forearm muscles can exert a force of a fraction of an ounce to pick up a paper clip—or a force of about 6 pounds to pick up this book!

Cardiac Muscle

Cardiac muscle tissue occurs only in the heart (the body's blood pump), where it constitutes the bulk of the heart walls. Like skeletal muscle cells, cardiac muscle cells are striated (see Figure 4.9b, p. 139), but cardiac muscle is not voluntary. Indeed, it can and does contract without being stimulated by the nervous system. Most of us have no conscious control over how fast our heart beats.

- Key words to remember for cardiac muscle are *cardiac*, *striated*, and *involuntary*.

Cardiac muscle usually contracts at a fairly steady rate set by the heart's pacemaker, but neural controls allow the heart to speed up for brief periods, as when you race across the tennis court to make that overhead smash.

Smooth Muscle

Smooth muscle tissue is found in the walls of hollow visceral organs, such as the stomach, urinary bladder, and respiratory passages. Its role is to force fluids and other substances through internal body channels. Like skeletal muscle, smooth muscle consists of elongated cells, but smooth muscle has no striations (see Figure 4.9c, p. 139). Like cardiac muscle, smooth muscle is not subject to voluntary control. Its contractions are slow and sustained.

- We can describe smooth muscle tissue as *visceral*, *nonstriated*, and *involuntary*.

Special Characteristics of Muscle Tissue

What enables muscle tissue to perform its duties? Four special characteristics are key.

Excitability, also termed **responsiveness**, is the ability to receive and respond to a stimulus, that is, any change in the environment either inside or outside the body. In the case of muscle, the stimulus is usually a chemical—for example, a neurotransmitter released by a nerve cell, or a local change in pH. The response (sometimes separated out as an additional characteristic called conductivity) is to generate an electrical impulse that travels along the plasma membrane of the muscle cell and causes the cell to contract.

Contractility is the ability to shorten forcibly when adequately stimulated. This ability sets muscle apart from all other tissue types.

Extensibility is the ability to extend or stretch. Muscle cells shorten when contracting, but they can stretch, even beyond their resting length, when relaxed.

Elasticity is the ability of a muscle cell to recoil and resume its resting length after stretching.

Muscle Functions

Muscle performs at least four important functions for the body. It produces movement, maintains posture, stabilizes joints, generates heat, and more.

Producing Movement

Just about all movements of the human body and its parts result from muscle contraction. Skeletal muscles are responsible for all locomotion (moving from place to place) and manipulation. They enable you to respond quickly to changes in the external environment—for example, jump out of the way of a car, direct your eyes, and smile or frown.

Blood courses through your body because of the rhythmically beating cardiac muscle of your heart and the smooth muscle in the walls of your blood vessels, which helps maintain blood pressure. Smooth muscle in organs of the digestive, urinary, and reproductive tracts propels, or squeezes, substances (foodstuffs, urine, semen) through the organs and along the tract.

Maintaining Posture and Body Position

We are rarely aware of the skeletal muscles that maintain body posture. Yet these muscles function almost continuously, making one tiny adjustment after another to counteract the never-ending downward pull of gravity.

Stabilizing Joints

Even as muscles pull on bones to cause movement, they stabilize and strengthen the joints of the skeleton (Chapter 8).

Generating Heat

Muscles generate heat as they contract. This heat is vitally important in maintaining normal body temperature. Because skeletal muscle accounts for at least 40% of body mass, it is the muscle type most responsible for generating heat.

Additional Functions of Muscle

What else do muscles do? Skeletal muscles protect the more fragile internal organs (the viscera) by enclosing them. Smooth muscle forms valves to regulate the passage of substances through internal body openings, dilates and constricts the pupils of your eyes, and forms the arrector pili muscles attached to hair follicles.

■ ■ ■

9

In this chapter, we examine the structure and function of skeletal muscle. Then we consider smooth muscle more briefly, largely by comparing it with skeletal muscle. We describe cardiac muscle in detail in Chapter 18, but for easy comparison, Table 9.3 on p. 310 summarizes the characteristics of all three muscle types.

Check Your Understanding

1. When describing muscle, what does "striated" mean?
2. Harry is pondering an exam question that asks, "Which muscle type has elongated cells and is found in the walls of the urinary bladder?" How should he respond?

For answers, see Appendix H.

Skeletal Muscle

✓ Describe the gross structure of a skeletal muscle.

✓ Describe the microscopic structure and functional roles of the myofibrils, sarcoplasmic reticulum, and T tubules of skeletal muscle fibers.

✓ Describe the sliding filament model of muscle contraction.

For easy reference, **Table 9.1** on p. 283 summarizes the levels of skeletal muscle organization, gross to microscopic, that we describe in the following sections.

Gross Anatomy of a Skeletal Muscle

Each **skeletal muscle** is a discrete organ, made up of several kinds of tissues. Skeletal muscle fibers predominate, but blood vessels, nerve fibers, and substantial amounts of connective tissue are also present. We can easily examine a skeletal muscle's shape and its attachments in the body without a microscope.

Nerve and Blood Supply

In general, one nerve, one artery, and one or more veins serve each muscle. These structures all enter or exit near the central part of the muscle and branch profusely through its connective tissue sheaths (described below). Unlike cells of cardiac and smooth muscle tissues, which can contract without nerve stimulation, every skeletal muscle fiber is supplied with a nerve ending that controls its activity.

Skeletal muscle has a rich blood supply. This is understandable because contracting muscle fibers use huge amounts of energy and require almost continuous delivery of oxygen and nutrients via the arteries. Muscle cells also give off large amounts of metabolic wastes that must be removed through veins if contraction is to remain efficient. Muscle capillaries, the smallest of the body's blood vessels, are long and winding and have numerous cross-links, features that accommodate changes in muscle length. They straighten when the muscle stretches and contort when the muscle contracts.

Connective Tissue Sheaths

In an intact muscle, several different connective tissue sheaths wrap individual muscle fibers. Together these connective tissue sheaths support each cell and reinforce and hold together the muscle as a whole, preventing the bulging muscles from bursting during exceptionally strong contractions.

Let's consider these connective tissue sheaths from external to internal (see **Figure 9.1** and the top three rows of Table 9.1).

- **Epimysium.** The **epimysium** (ep″ĭ-mis′e-um; meaning "outside the muscle") is an "overcoat" of dense irregular connective tissue that surrounds the whole muscle. Sometimes it blends with the deep fascia that lies between neighboring muscles or the superficial fascia deep to the skin.
- **Perimysium and fascicles.** Within each skeletal muscle, the muscle fibers are grouped into **fascicles** (fas′ĭ-klz; "bundles") that resemble bundles of sticks. Surrounding each fascicle is a layer of fibrous connective tissue called **perimysium** (per″ĭ-mis′e-um; meaning "around the muscle [fascicles]").
- **Endomysium.** The **endomysium** (en″do-mis′e-um; meaning "within the muscle") is a wispy sheath of connective tissue that surrounds each individual muscle fiber. It consists of fine areolar connective tissue.

As shown in Figure 9.1, all of these connective tissue sheaths are continuous with one another as well as with the tendons that join muscles to bones. When muscle fibers contract, they pull on these sheaths, which transmit the pulling force to the bone to be moved. The sheaths contribute somewhat to the natural elasticity of muscle tissue, and also provide entry and exit routes for the blood vessels and nerve fibers that serve the muscle.

Attachments

Recall from Chapter 8 that most skeletal muscles span joints and attach to bones (or other structures) in at least two places. When a muscle contracts, the movable bone, the muscle's **insertion**, moves toward the immovable or less movable bone, the muscle's **origin**. In the muscles of the limbs, the origin typically lies proximal to the insertion.

Muscle attachments, whether origin or insertion, may be direct or indirect.

- In **direct**, or **fleshy**, **attachments**, the epimysium of the muscle is fused to the periosteum of a bone or perichondrium of a cartilage.

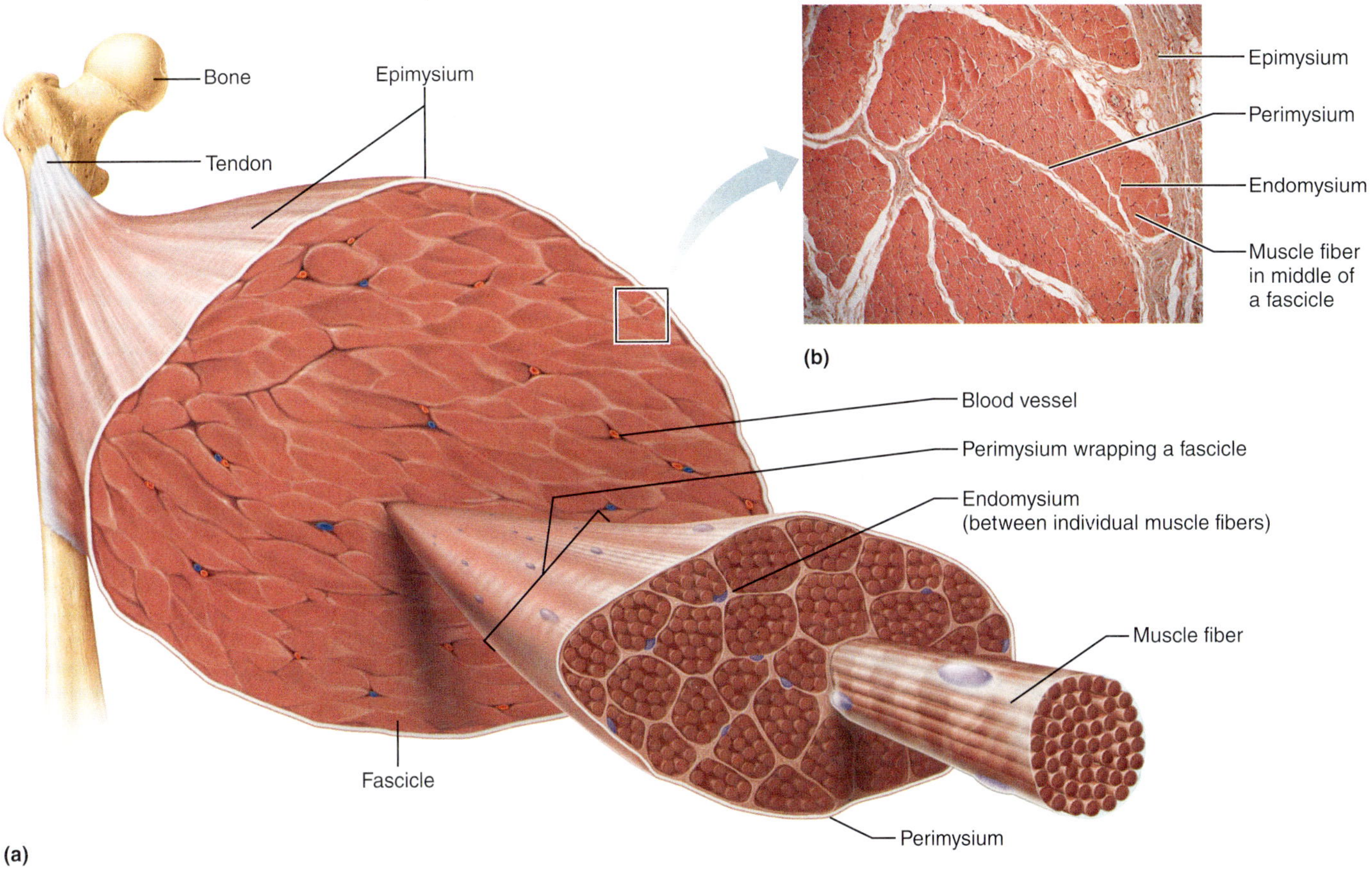

Figure 9.1 Connective tissue sheaths of skeletal muscle: epimysium, perimysium, and endomysium. (b) Photomicrograph of a cross section of part of a skeletal muscle (30×). (For a related image, see *A Brief Atlas of the Human Body*, Plate 29.)

- In **indirect attachments**, the muscle's connective tissue wrappings extend beyond the muscle either as a ropelike **tendon** (Figure 9.1a) or as a sheetlike **aponeurosis** (ap″o-nu-ro′sis). The tendon or aponeurosis anchors the muscle to the connective tissue covering of a skeletal element (bone or cartilage) or to the fascia of other muscles.

Indirect attachments are much more common because of their durability and small size. Tendons are mostly tough collagen fibers which can withstand the abrasion of rough bony projections that would tear apart the more delicate muscle tissues. Because of their relatively small size, more tendons than fleshy muscles can pass over a joint—so tendons also conserve space.

Before moving on to microscopic anatomy, you may want to review the top three rows of Table 9.1.

Microscopic Anatomy of a Skeletal Muscle Fiber

Each skeletal muscle fiber is a long cylindrical cell with multiple oval nuclei just beneath its **sarcolemma** or plasma membrane **(Figure 9.2b)**. Skeletal muscle fibers are huge cells. Their diameter typically ranges from 10 to 100 μm—up to ten times that of an average body cell—and their length is phenomenal, some up to 30 cm long. Their large size and multiple nuclei are not surprising once you learn that hundreds of embryonic cells fuse to produce each fiber.

Sarcoplasm, the cytoplasm of a muscle cell, is similar to the cytoplasm of other cells, but it contains unusually large amounts of **glycosomes** (granules of stored glycogen that provide glucose during muscle cell activity) and **myoglobin**, a red pigment that stores oxygen. Myoglobin is similar to hemoglobin, the pigment that transports oxygen in blood.

In addition to the usual organelles, a muscle cell contains three structures that are highly modified: myofibrils, sarcoplasmic reticulum, and T tubules. Let's look at these structures more closely because they play important roles in muscle contraction.

Myofibrils

A single muscle fiber contains hundreds to thousands of rodlike **myofibrils** that run parallel to its length (Figure 9.2b). The myofibrils, each 1–2 μm in diameter, are so densely packed in the fiber that mitochondria and other organelles appear to be squeezed between them. They account for about 80% of cellular volume.

(a) Photomicrograph of **portions of two isolated muscle fibers** (700×). Notice the obvious striations (alternating dark and light bands).

(b) Diagram of **part of a muscle fiber** showing the myofibrils. One **myofibril** extends from the cut end of the fiber.

(c) Small part of one **myofibril enlarged to show the myofilaments** responsible for the banding pattern. Each **sarcomere** extends from one Z disc to the next.

(d) Enlargement of one sarcomere (sectioned lengthwise). Notice the myosin heads on the thick filaments.

(e) Cross-sectional view of a sarcomere cut through in different locations.

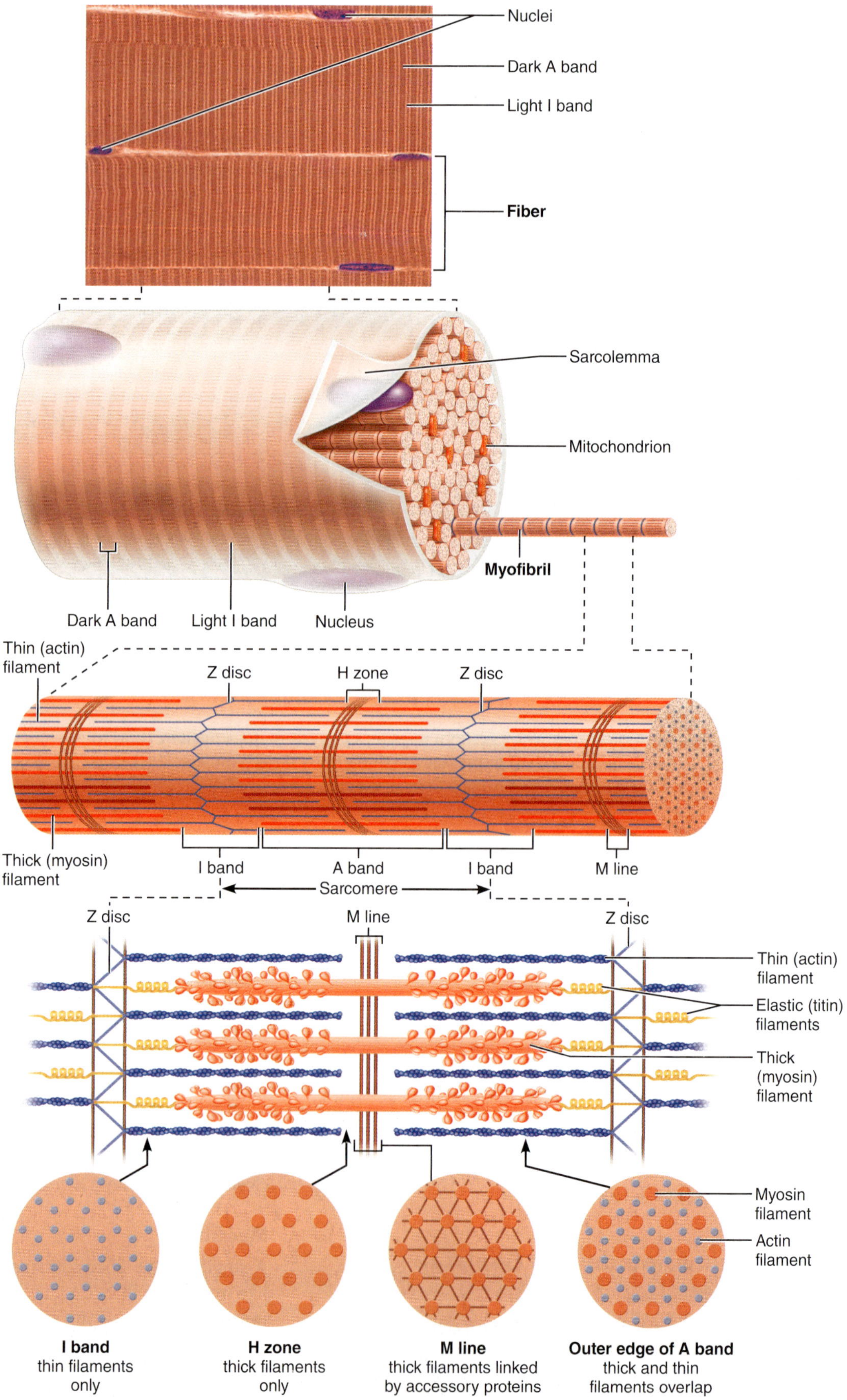

Figure 9.2 Microscopic anatomy of a skeletal muscle fiber. (For a related image, see *A Brief Atlas of the Human Body*, Plate 28.)

Myofibrils contain the contractile elements of skeletal muscle cells, the sarcomeres, which contain even smaller rodlike structures called *myofilaments*. Table 9.1 (bottom three rows; p. 283) summarizes these structures, which we discuss next.

Striations, Sarcomeres, and Myofilaments **Striations**, a repeating series of dark and light bands, are evident along the length of each myofibril. In an intact muscle fiber, the dark **A bands** and light **I bands** are nearly perfectly aligned, giving the cell its striated appearance.

As illustrated in Figure 9.2c:

- Each dark A band has a lighter region in its midsection called the **H zone** (H for *helle*; "bright").
- Each H zone is bisected vertically by a dark line called the **M line** (*M* for middle) formed by molecules of the protein myomesin.
- Each light I band also has a midline interruption, a darker area called the **Z disc** (or Z line).
- The region of a myofibril between two successive Z discs is a **sarcomere** (sar′ko-mĕr; literally, "muscle segment"). Averaging 2 μm long, a sarcomere is the smallest contractile unit of a muscle fiber—the *functional unit* of skeletal muscle. It contains an A band flanked by half an I band at each end. Within each myofibril, the sarcomeres align end to end like boxcars in a train.

If we examine the banding pattern of a myofibril at the molecular level, we see that it arises from orderly arrangement of even smaller structures within the sarcomeres. These smaller structures, the **myofilaments** or **filaments**, are the muscle equivalents of the actin- or myosin-containing microfilaments described in Chapter 3. As you will recall, the proteins actin and myosin play a role in motility and shape change in virtually every cell in the body. This property reaches its highest development in the contractile muscle fibers.

The central **thick filaments** containing myosin (red) extend the entire length of the A band (Figure 9.2c and d). They are connected in the middle of the sarcomere at the M line. The more lateral **thin filaments** containing actin (blue) extend across the I band and partway into the A band. The Z disc, a coin-shaped sheet composed largely of the protein alpha-actinin, anchors the thin filaments. We describe the third type of myofilament illustrated in Figure 9.2d, the *elastic filament*, in the next section. Intermediate (desmin) filaments (not illustrated) extend from the Z disc and connect each myofibril to the next throughout the width of the muscle cell.

Looking at the banding pattern more closely, we see that the H zone of the A band appears less dense because the thin filaments do not extend into this region. The M line in the center of the H zone is slightly darker because of the fine protein strands there that hold adjacent thick filaments together. The myofilaments are connected to the sarcolemma and held in alignment at the Z discs and the M lines.

A longitudinal view of the myofilaments (Figure 9.2d) is a bit misleading because it looks as if each thick (red) filament interdigitates with only four thin (blue) filaments. The cross section of a sarcomere on the far right in Figure 9.2e shows an area where thick and thin filaments overlap. Notice that a hexagonal arrangement of six thin filaments surrounds each thick filament, and three thick filaments enclose each thin filament.

Molecular Composition of Myofilaments Muscle contraction depends on the myosin- and actin-containing myofilaments. As noted earlier, thick filaments (about 16 nm in diameter) are composed primarily of the protein **myosin**. Each myosin molecule consists of two heavy and four light polypeptide chains, and has a rodlike tail attached by a flexible hinge to two globular *heads* **(Figure 9.3)**. The tail consists of two intertwined helical polypeptide heavy chains.

The globular heads, each associated with two light chains, are the "business end" of myosin. During contraction, they link the thick and thin filaments together, forming **cross bridges** **(Figure 9.4** on p. 284), and swivel around their point of attachment. As we will explain shortly, these cross bridges act as motors to generate force.

Each thick filament contains about 300 myosin molecules bundled together, with their tails forming the central part of the thick filament and their heads facing outward at the end of each thick filament (Figure 9.3). As a result, the central portion of a thick filament (in the H zone) is smooth, but its ends are studded with a staggered array of myosin heads. The heads bear actin and ATP-binding sites and also have intrinsic ATPase activity that splits ATP to generate energy for muscle contraction.

9

The thin filaments (7–8 nm thick) are composed chiefly of the protein **actin** (blue in Figure 9.3). Actin has kidney-shaped polypeptide subunits, called *globular actin* or *G actin*, which bear the active sites to which the myosin heads attach during contraction. In the thin filaments, G actin subunits are polymerized into long actin filaments called *filamentous*, or F, *actin*. Two intertwined actin filaments, resembling a twisted double strand of pearls, form the backbone of each thin filament (Figure 9.3).

Thin filaments also contain several regulatory proteins.

- Polypeptide strands of **tropomyosin** (tro″po-mi′o-sin), a rod-shaped protein, spiral about the actin core and help stiffen and stabilize it. Successive tropomyosin molecules are arranged end to end along the actin filaments, and in a relaxed muscle fiber, they block myosin-binding sites on actin so that myosin heads on the thick filaments cannot bind to the thin filaments.
- **Troponin** (tro′po-nin), the other major protein in thin filaments, is a globular three-polypeptide complex (Figure 9.3). One of its polypeptides (TnI) is an inhibitory subunit that binds to actin. Another (TnT) binds to tropomyosin and helps position it on actin. The third (TnC) binds calcium ions.

Both troponin and tropomyosin help control the myosin-actin interactions involved in contraction. Several other proteins help form the structure of the myofibril.

- The **elastic filament** we referred to earlier is composed of the giant protein **titin** (Figure 9.2d). Titin extends from the Z disc to the thick filament, and then runs within the thick filament (forming its core) to attach to the M line. It holds

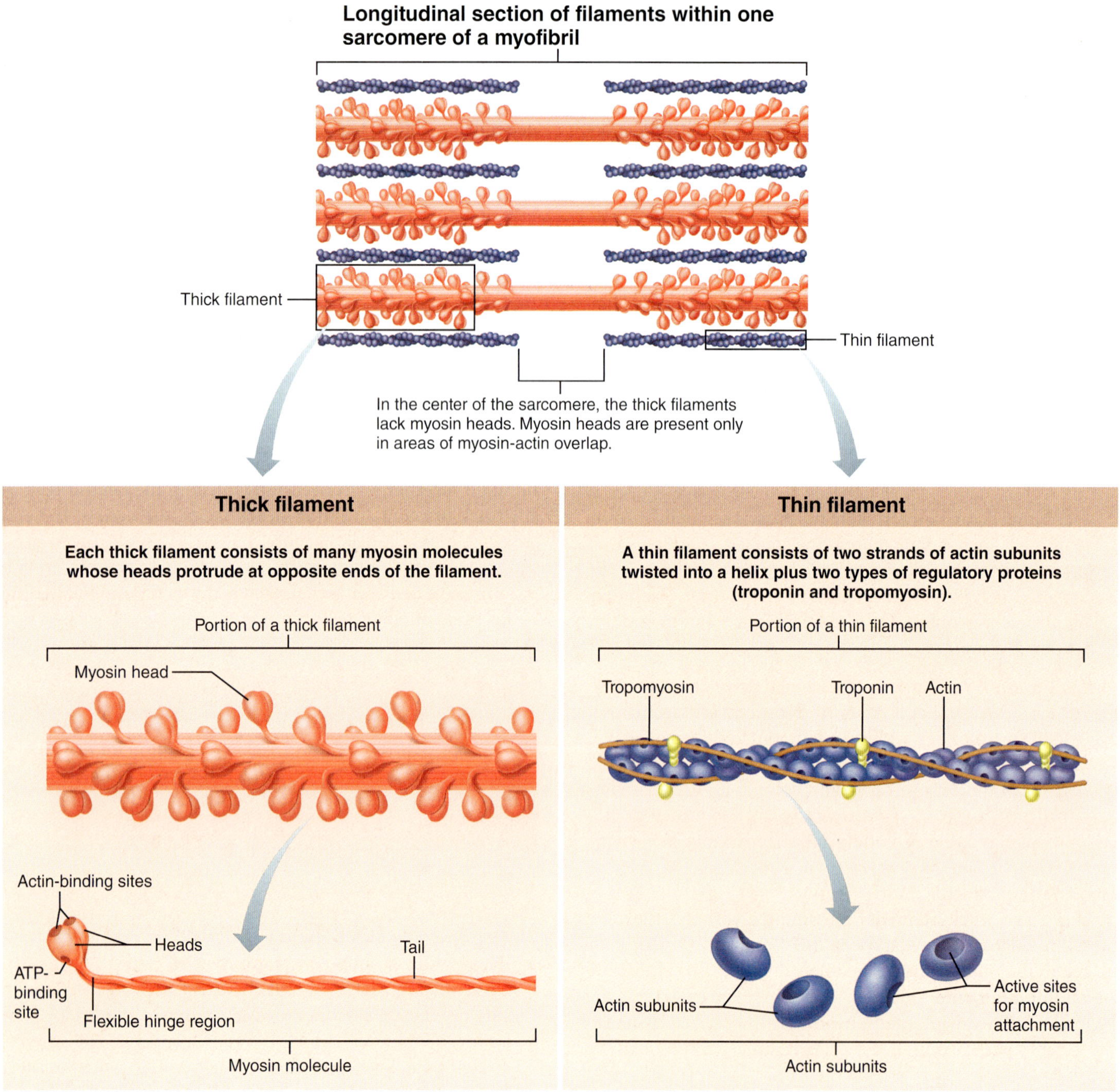

Figure 9.3 Composition of thick and thin filaments.

the thick filaments in place, thus maintaining the organization of the A band, and helps the muscle cell spring back into shape after stretching. (The part of the titin that spans the I bands is extensible, unfolding when the muscle stretches and recoiling when the tension is released.) Titin does not resist stretching in the ordinary range of extension, but it stiffens as it uncoils, helping the muscle resist excessive stretching, which might pull the sarcomeres apart.

- Another important structural protein is **dystrophin**, which links the thin filaments to the integral proteins of the sarcolemma (which in turn are anchored to the extracellular matrix).
- Other proteins that bind filaments or sarcomeres together and maintain their alignment include *nebulin*, *myomesin*, and *C proteins*.

Sarcoplasmic Reticulum and T Tubules

Skeletal muscle fibers contain two sets of intracellular tubules that help regulate muscle contraction: (1) the sarcoplasmic reticulum and (2) T tubules.

Table 9.1 Structure and Organizational Levels of Skeletal Muscle

STRUCTURE AND ORGANIZATIONAL LEVEL	DESCRIPTION	CONNECTIVE TISSUE WRAPPINGS
Muscle (organ) 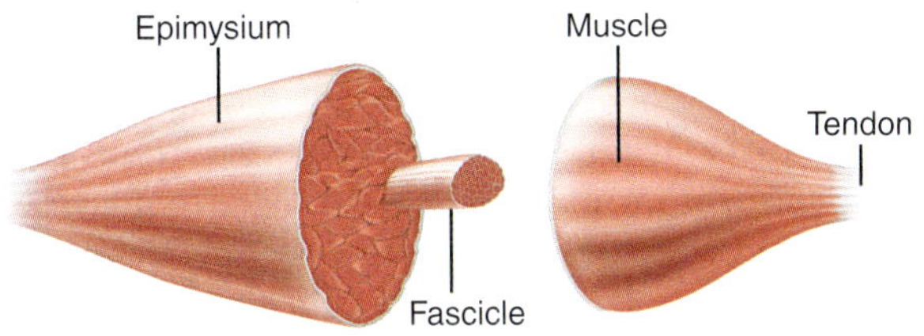	A muscle consists of hundreds to thousands of muscle cells, plus connective tissue wrappings, blood vessels, and nerve fibers.	Covered externally by the epimysium
Fascicle (a portion of the muscle) 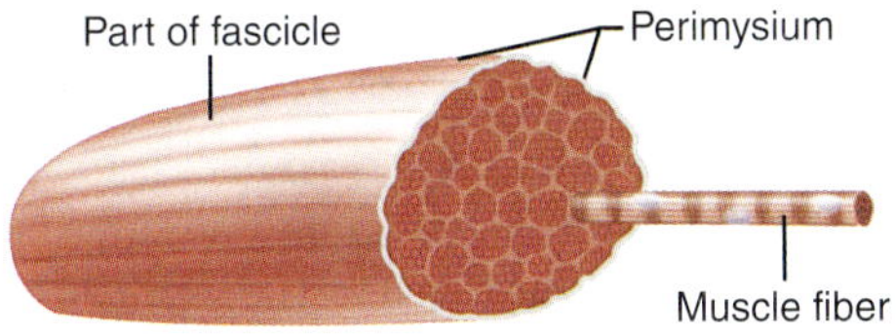	A fascicle is a discrete bundle of muscle cells, segregated from the rest of the muscle by a connective tissue sheath.	Surrounded by perimysium
Muscle Fiber (cell) 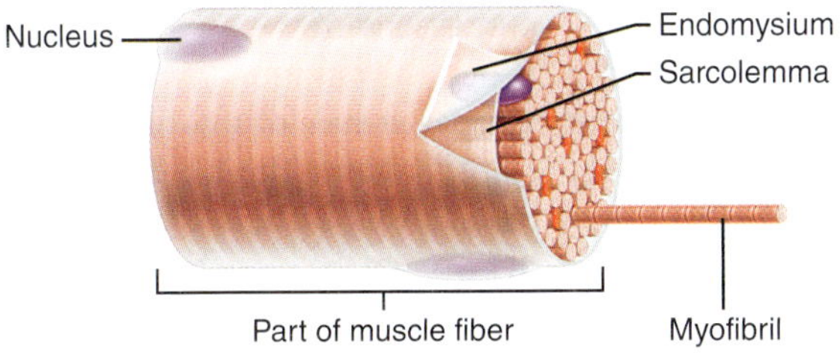	A muscle fiber is an elongated multinucleate cell; it has a banded (striated) appearance.	Surrounded by endomysium
Myofibril or Fibril (complex organelle composed of bundles of myofilaments) 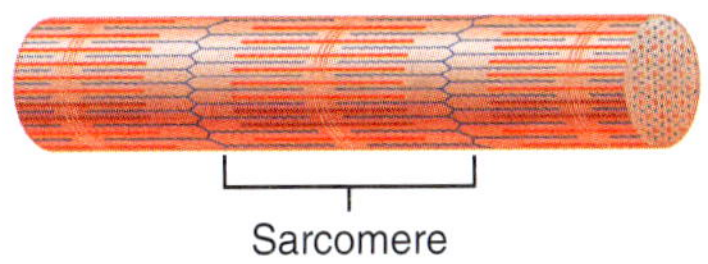	Myofibrils are rodlike contractile elements that occupy most of the muscle cell volume. Composed of sarcomeres arranged end to end, they appear banded, and bands of adjacent myofibrils are aligned.	—
Sarcomere (a segment of a myofibril) 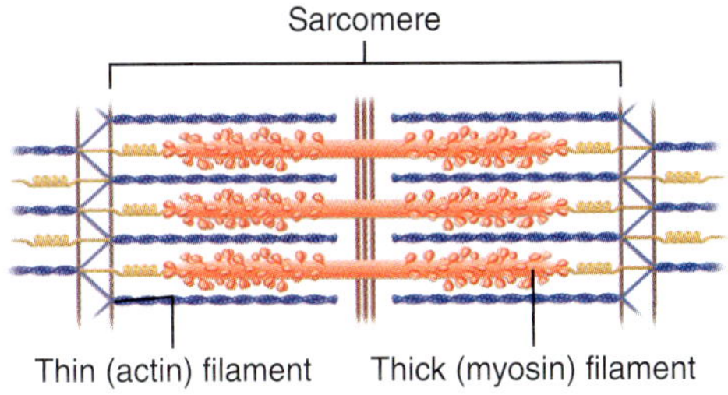	A sarcomere is the contractile unit, composed of myofilaments made up of contractile proteins.	—
Myofilament or Filament (extended macromolecular structure) 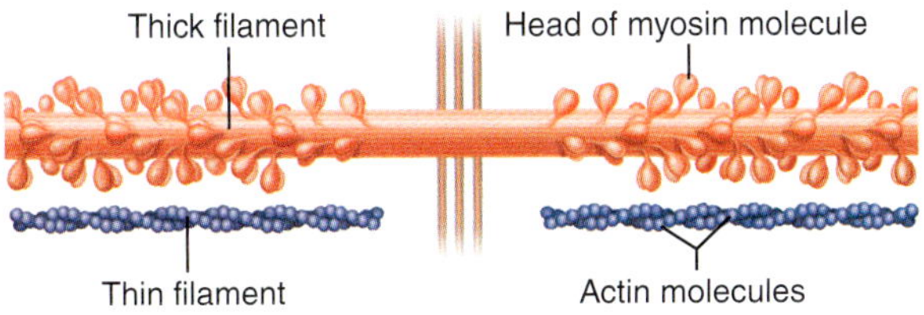	Contractile myofilaments are of two types—thick and thin. Thick filaments contain bundled myosin molecules; thin filaments contain actin molecules (plus other proteins). The sliding of the thin filaments past the thick filaments produces muscle shortening. Elastic filaments (not shown here) maintain the organization of the A band and provide elastic recoil when muscle contraction ends.	—

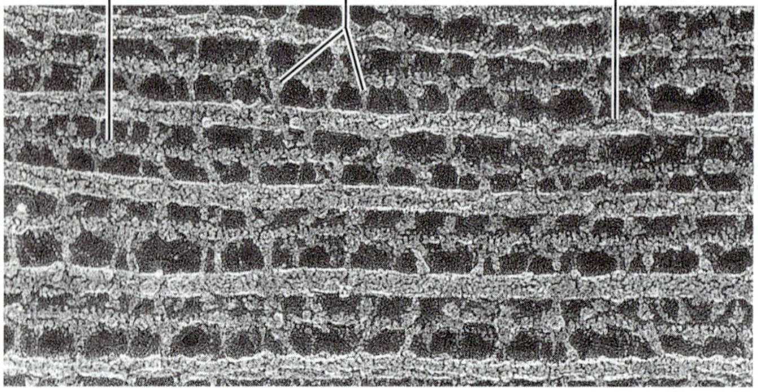

Figure 9.4 Myosin heads forming cross bridges that generate muscular contractile force. Part of a sarcomere is seen in a transmission electron micrograph (277,000×).

Sarcoplasmic Reticulum Shown in blue in **Figure 9.5**, the **sarcoplasmic reticulum (SR)** is an elaborate smooth endoplasmic reticulum. Its interconnecting tubules surround each myofibril the way the sleeve of a loosely crocheted sweater surrounds your arm.

Most SR tubules run longitudinally along the myofibril, communicating with each other at the H zone. Others called **terminal cisterns** ("end sacs") form larger, perpendicular cross channels at the A band–I band junctions and they always occur in pairs. Closely associated with the SR are large numbers of mitochondria and glycogen granules, both involved in producing the energy used during contraction.

The SR regulates intracellular levels of ionic calcium. It stores calcium and releases it on demand when the muscle fiber is stimulated to contract. As you will see, calcium provides the final "go" signal for contraction.

T Tubules At each A band–I band junction, the sarcolemma of the muscle cell protrudes deep into the cell interior, forming an elongated tube called the **T tubule** (T for "transverse"). The T tubules, shown in gray in Figure 9.5, tremendously increase the muscle fiber's surface area. Possibly the result of fusing tubelike caveolae (inpocketings of the sarcolemma), the *lumen* (cavity) of the T tubule is continuous with the extracellular space.

Along its length, each T tubule runs between the paired terminal cisterns of the SR, forming **triads**, successive groupings of the three membranous structures (terminal cistern, T tubule, and terminal cistern). As they pass from one myofibril to the next, the T tubules also encircle each sarcomere.

Muscle contraction is ultimately controlled by nerve-initiated electrical impulses that travel along the sarcolemma. Because T tubules are continuations of the sarcolemma, they conduct impulses to the deepest regions of the muscle cell and every sarcomere. These impulses signal for the release of calcium from the adjacent terminal cisterns. Think of the T tubules as a rapid telegraph system that ensures that every myofibril in the muscle fiber contracts at virtually the same time.

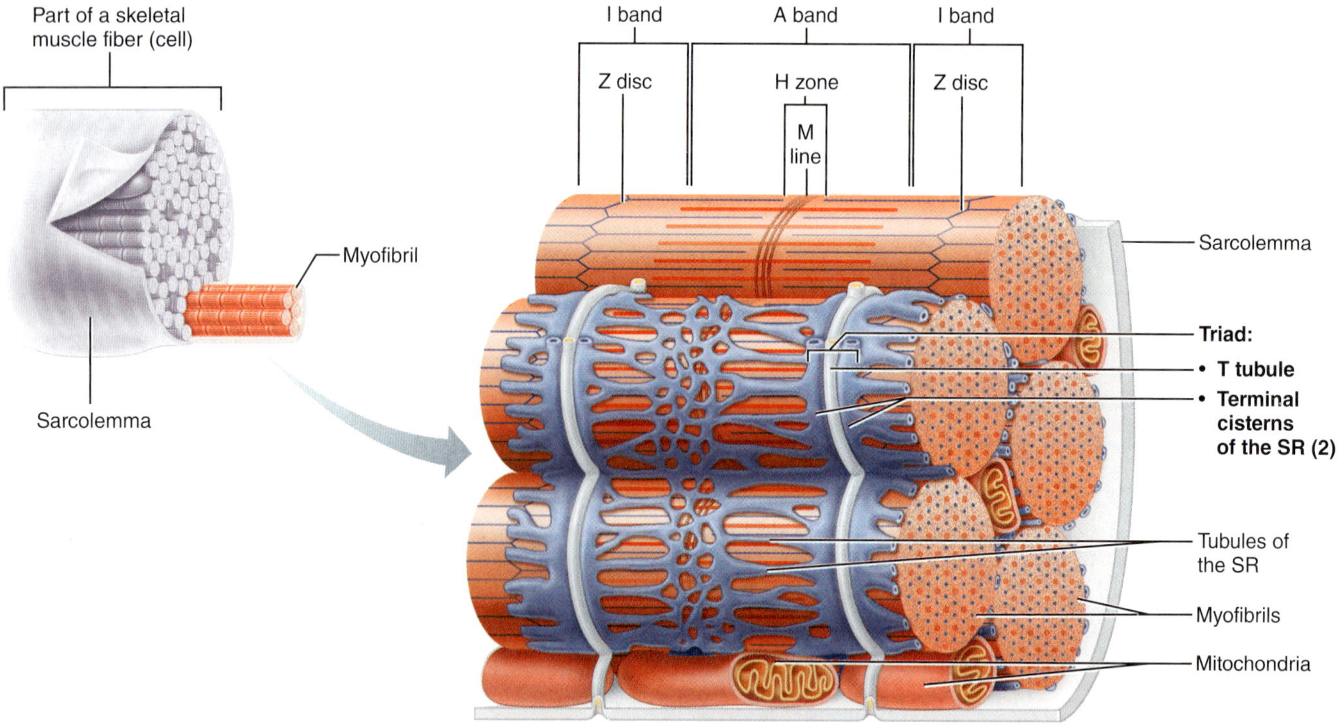

Figure 9.5 Relationship of the sarcoplasmic reticulum and T tubules to myofibrils of skeletal muscle. The tubules of the SR (blue) fuse to form a net of communicating channels at the level of the H zone and the saclike terminal cisterns abutting the A-I junctions. The T tubules (gray) are inward invaginations of the sarcolemma that run deep into the cell between the terminal cisterns. (See detailed view in Figure 9.11, pp. 290–291.) Sites of close contact of these three elements (terminal cistern, T tubule, and terminal cistern) are called triads.

Triad Relationships The roles of the T tubules and SR in providing signals for contraction are tightly linked. At the triads, where these organelles come into closest contact, integral proteins (some from the T tubule and others from the SR) protrude into the intermembrane spaces. The protruding integral proteins of the T tubule act as voltage sensors. Those of the SR form gated channels through which the terminal cisterns release Ca^{2+}. We will return to their interaction shortly.

Sliding Filament Model of Contraction

We almost always think "shortening" when we hear the word **contraction**, but to physiologists the term refers only to the activation of myosin's cross bridges, which are the force-generating sites. Shortening occurs if and when the cross bridges generate enough tension on the thin filaments to exceed the forces that oppose shortening. Contraction ends when the cross bridges become inactive, the tension declines, and then the muscle fiber relaxes.

In a relaxed muscle fiber, the thin and thick filaments overlap only at the ends of the A band (**Figure 9.6** ①). The **sliding filament model of contraction** states that during contraction the thin filaments slide past the thick ones so that the actin and myosin filaments overlap to a greater degree:

- When the nervous system stimulates muscle fibers, the myosin heads on the thick filaments latch onto myosin-binding sites on actin in the thin filaments, and the sliding begins.
- These cross bridge attachments form and break several times during a contraction, acting like tiny ratchets to generate tension and propel the thin filaments toward the center of the sarcomere.
- As this event occurs simultaneously in sarcomeres throughout the cell, the muscle cell shortens.
- Notice that as the thin filaments slide centrally, the Z discs to which they attach are pulled *toward* the M line (Figure 9.6 ②). Overall, as a muscle cell shortens: (1) the I bands shorten, (2) the distance between successive Z discs shortens, (3) the H zones disappear, and (4) the contiguous A bands move closer together but their length does not change.

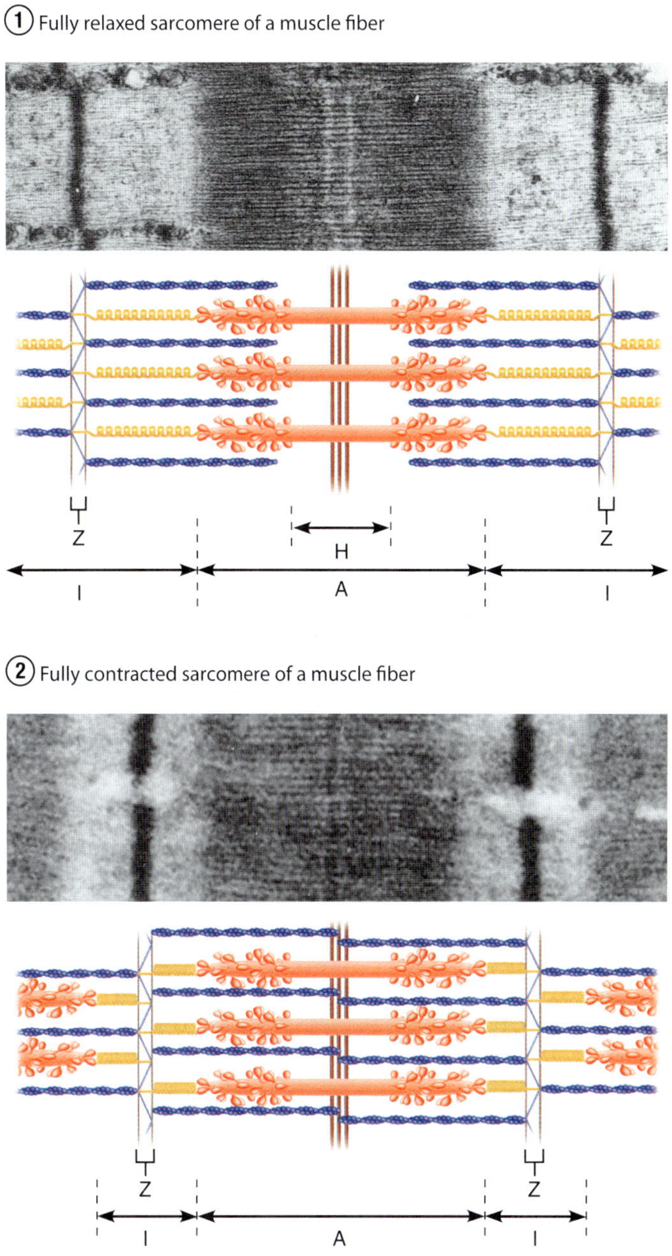

Figure 9.6 Sliding filament model of contraction. The numbers indicate events in a ① relaxed and a ② fully contracted sarcomere. At full contraction, the Z discs abut the thick filaments and the thin filaments overlap each other. The photomicrographs (top view in each case) show enlargements of 33,000×.

☑ Check Your Understanding

3. How does the term epimysium relate to the role and position of this connective tissue sheath?
4. Which myofilaments have binding sites for calcium? What specific molecule binds calcium?
5. Which region or organelle—cytosol, mitochondrion, or SR—contains the highest concentration of calcium ions in a resting muscle fiber? Which structure provides the ATP needed for muscle activity?

For answers, see Appendix H.

Physiology of Skeletal Muscle Fibers

✓ Explain how muscle fibers are stimulated to contract by describing events that occur at the neuromuscular junction.

✓ Describe how an action potential is generated.

✓ Follow the events of excitation-contraction coupling that lead to cross bridge activity.

The sliding filament model tells us how a muscle fiber contracts, but what induces it to contract in the first place? For a skeletal muscle fiber to contract:

1. The fiber must be activated, that is, stimulated by a nerve ending so that a change in membrane potential occurs.
2. Next, it must generate an electrical current, called an **action potential**, in its sarcolemma.

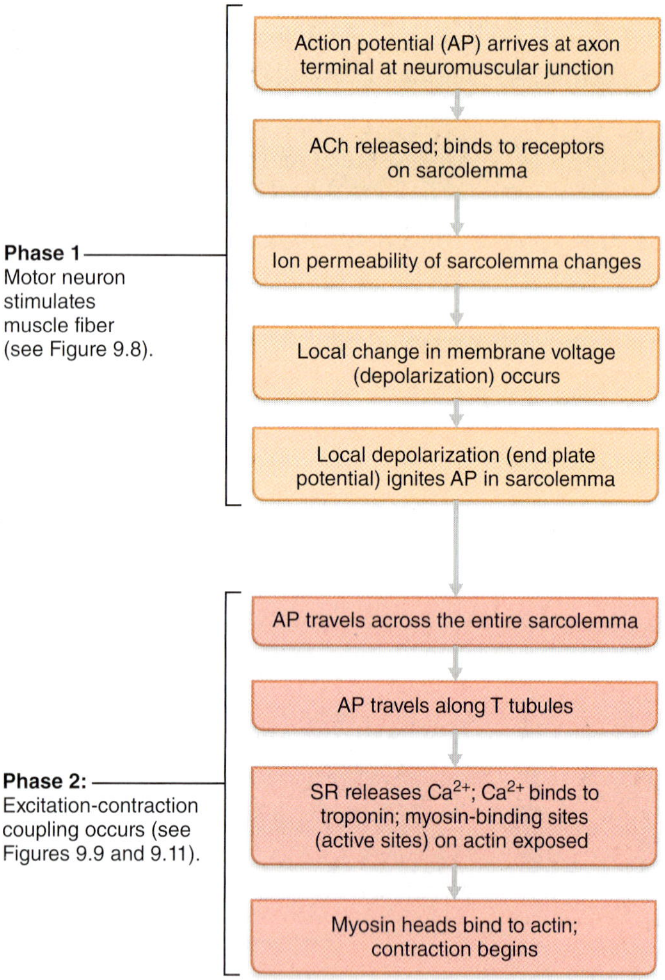

Figure 9.7 The phases leading to muscle fiber contraction.

3. The action potential is automatically propagated along the sarcolomma.
4. Then, intracellular calcium ion levels must rise briefly, providing the final trigger for contraction.

Steps 1 and 2, activation, occur at the neuromuscular junction and set the stage for the events that follow. Steps 3 and 4, which link the electrical signal to contraction, are called excitation-contraction coupling. **Figure 9.7** summarizes this series of events into two major phases, which we consider in detail below.

The Nerve Stimulus and Events at the Neuromuscular Junction

The nerve cells that activate skeletal muscle fibers are called *somatic motor neurons*, or *motor neurons of the somatic (voluntary) nervous system*. These motor neurons "reside" in the brain or spinal cord, but their long threadlike extensions called axons travel, bundled within nerves, to the muscle cells they serve.

The axon of each motor neuron divides profusely as it enters the muscle. Each axon ending gives off several short, curling branches that collectively form an elliptical **neuromuscular junction**, or **end plate**, with a single muscle fiber.

As a rule, each muscle fiber has only one neuromuscular junction, located approximately midway along its length. The axon terminal and the muscle fiber are exceedingly close (50–80 nm apart), but they remain separated by a space, the **synaptic cleft** (Figure 9.8), which is filled with a gel-like extracellular substance rich in glycoproteins and collagen fibers.

Within the moundlike axon terminal are **synaptic vesicles**, small membranous sacs containing the neurotransmitter **acetylcholine** (as″ĕ-til-ko′lēn), or **ACh**. The trough-like part of the muscle fiber's sarcolemma that helps form the neuromuscular junction is highly folded. These **junctional folds** provide a large surface area for the millions of **ACh receptors** located there. Hence, the neuromuscular junction includes the axon terminals, the synaptic cleft, and the junctional folds of the sarcolemma.

How does a motor neuron stimulate a skeletal muscle fiber? The simplest explanation is:

- When a nerve impulse reaches the end of an axon, the axon terminal releases ACh into the synaptic cleft.
- ACh diffuses across the cleft and attaches to ACh receptors on the sarcolemma of the muscle fiber.
- ACh binding triggers electrical events that ultimately generate an action potential.

Focus on Events at the Neuromuscular Junction **(Figure 9.8)** covers this process step by step. Study this figure before continuing.

After ACh binds to the ACh receptors, its effects are quickly terminated by **acetylcholinesterase** (as″ĕ-til-ko″lin-es′ter-ās), an enzyme located in the synaptic cleft. Acetylcholinesterase breaks down ACh to its building blocks, acetic acid and choline. This removal of ACh prevents continued (and most likely undesirable) muscle fiber contraction in the absence of additional nervous system stimulation.

Homeostatic Imbalance 9.1

Many toxins, drugs, and diseases interfere with events at the neuromuscular junction. For example, *myasthenia gravis* (*asthen* = weakness; *gravi* = heavy), a disease characterized by drooping upper eyelids, difficulty swallowing and talking, and generalized muscle weakness, involves a shortage of ACh receptors. Serum analysis reveals antibodies to ACh receptors, suggesting that myasthenia gravis is an autoimmune disease. Although normal numbers of receptors are initially present, they appear to be destroyed as the disease progresses. ✚

Generation of an Action Potential Across the Sarcolemma

Like the plasma membranes of all cells, a resting sarcolemma is *polarized*. That is, a voltmeter would show there is a potential difference (voltage) across the membrane and the inside is negative relative to the outer membrane face. (Chapter 3 describes the resting membrane potential.)

An action potential (AP) is the result of a predictable sequence of electrical changes. Once initiated, they occur along

Figure 9.8 **When a nerve impulse reaches a neuromuscular junction, acetylcholine (ACh) is released. Upon binding to sarcolemma receptors, ACh causes a change in sarcolemma permeability leading to a change in membrane potential.**

A&P Flix *Available at www.masteringaandp.com*

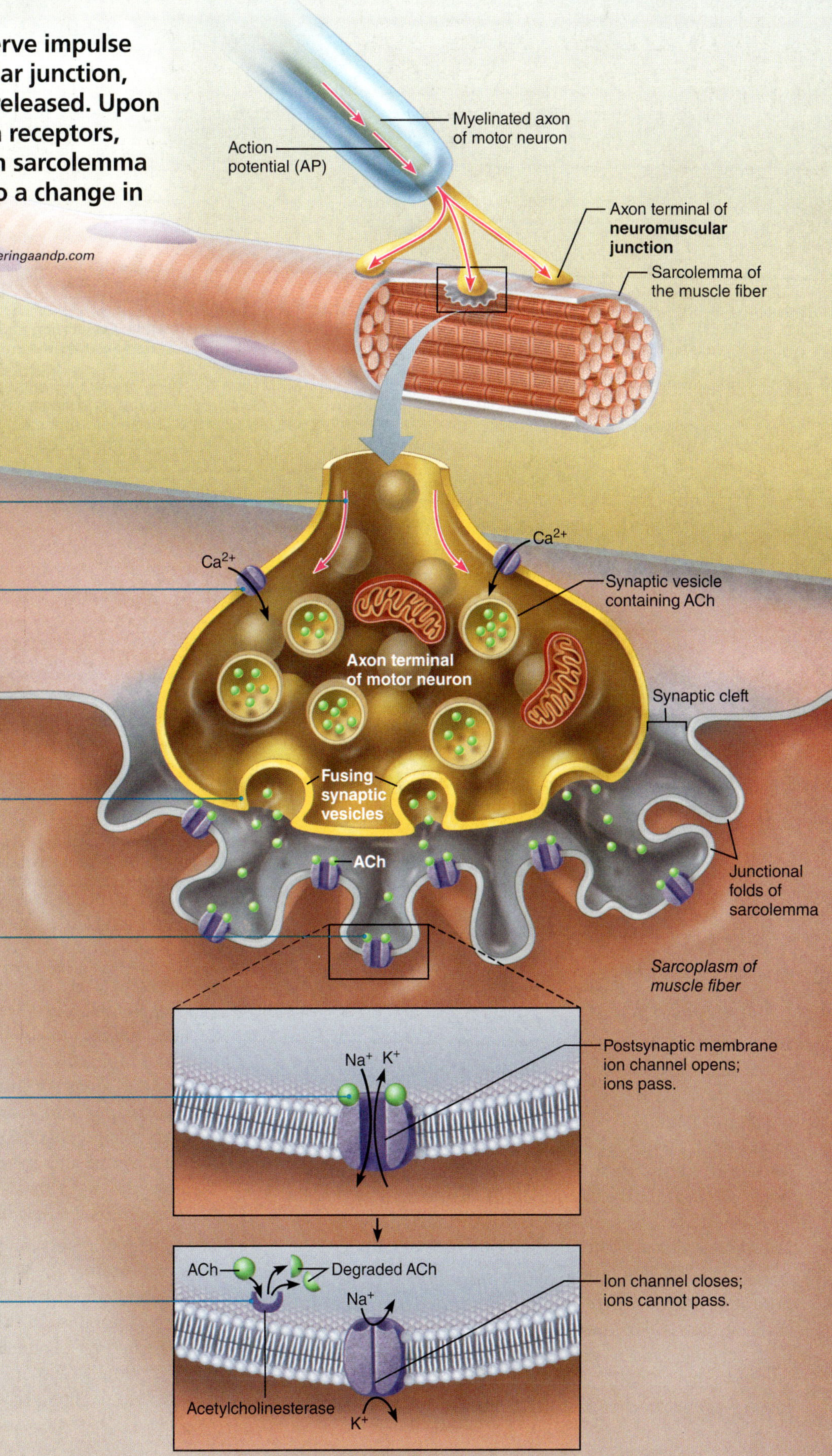

1. Action potential arrives at axon terminal of motor neuron.
2. Voltage-gated Ca^{2+} channels open. Ca^{2+} enters the axon terminal moving down its electochemical gradient.
3. Ca^{2+} entry causes ACh (a neurotransmitter) to be released by exocytosis.
4. ACh diffuses across the synaptic cleft and binds to its receptors on the sarcolemma.
5. ACh binding opens ion channels in the receptors that allow simultaneous passage of Na^+ into the muscle fiber and K^+ out of the muscle fiber. More Na^+ ions enter than K^+ ions exit, which produces a local change in the membrane potential called the end plate potential.
6. ACh effects are terminated by its breakdown in the synaptic cleft by acetylcholinesterase and diffusion away from the junction.

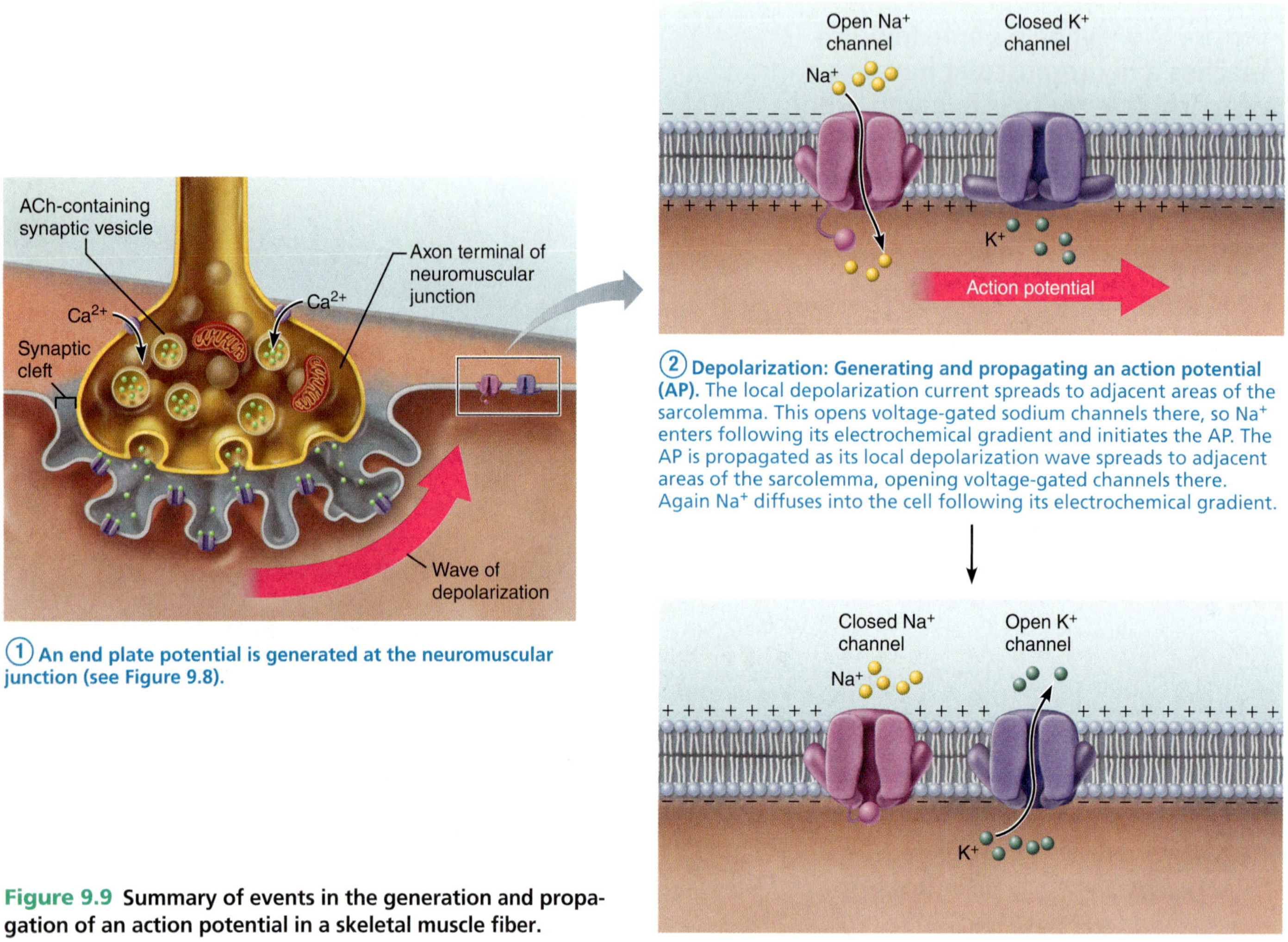

① **An end plate potential is generated at the neuromuscular junction (see Figure 9.8).**

② **Depolarization: Generating and propagating an action potential (AP).** The local depolarization current spreads to adjacent areas of the sarcolemma. This opens voltage-gated sodium channels there, so Na^+ enters following its electrochemical gradient and initiates the AP. The AP is propagated as its local depolarization wave spreads to adjacent areas of the sarcolemma, opening voltage-gated channels there. Again Na^+ diffuses into the cell following its electrochemical gradient.

③ **Repolarization: Restoring the sarcolemma to its initial polarized state (negative inside, positive outside).** Repolarization occurs as Na^+ channels close (inactivate) and voltage-gated K^+ channels open. Because K^+ concentration is substantially higher inside the cell than in the extracellular fluid, K^+ diffuses rapidly out of the muscle fiber.

Figure 9.9 Summary of events in the generation and propagation of an action potential in a skeletal muscle fiber.

the entire surface of the sarcolemma. Essentially three steps are involved **(Figure 9.9)**:

① **Generation of an end plate potential.** Binding of ACh molecules to ACh receptors at the neuromuscular junction opens *chemically (ligand) gated ion channels* that allow Na^+ and K^+ to pass (also see Figure 9.8). Because the driving force for Na^+ is greater than that for K^+, more Na^+ diffuses in than K^+ diffuses out. A transient change in membrane potential occurs as the interior of the sarcolemma becomes less negative, an event called depolarization. Initially, depolarization is a local event called an **end plate potential**.

② **Depolarization: Generation and propagation of an action potential.** The end plate potential (local depolarization at the neuromuscular junction) ignites an action potential by spreading to adjacent membrane areas and opening voltage-gated sodium channels there. Na^+ enters, following its electrochemical gradient, and once a certain membrane voltage, referred to as *threshold,* is reached, an action potential is generated (initiated).

The action potential *propagates* (moves along the length of the sarcolemma) in all directions from the neuromuscular junction, just as ripples move away from a pebble dropped into a stream. As it propagates, the local depolarization wave of the AP spreads to adjacent areas of the sarcolemma and opens voltage-gated sodium channels there. Again, Na^+, normally restricted from entering, diffuses into the cell following its electrochemical gradient.

③ **Repolarization: Restoring the sarcolemma to its initial polarized state.** The repolarization wave, like the depolarization wave, is a consequence of changes in membrane permeability. In this case, Na^+ channels close and voltage-gated K^+ channels open. Since the potassium ion concentration is substantially higher inside the cell than in the extracellular fluid, K^+ diffuses rapidly out of the muscle fiber, restoring negatively charged conditions inside (also see **Figure 9.10**).

During repolarization, a muscle fiber is said to be in a **refractory period**, because the cell cannot be stimulated again until repolarization is complete. Note that repolarization restores only the *electrical conditions* of the resting (polarized) state. The ATP-dependent Na^+-K^+ pump restores the *ionic conditions* of the resting state, but hundreds of action potentials can occur before ionic imbalances interfere with contractile activity.

Once initiated, the action potential is unstoppable. It ultimately results in contraction of the muscle fiber. Although the action potential itself lasts only a few milliseconds (ms), the contraction phase of a muscle fiber may persist for 100 ms or more and far outlasts the electrical event that triggers it.

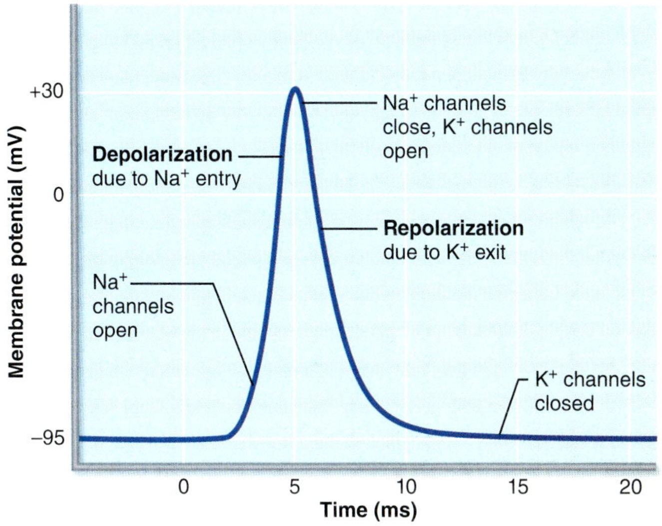

Figure 9.10 Action potential tracing indicates changes in Na^+ and K^+ ion channels.

Excitation-Contraction Coupling

Excitation-contraction (E-C) coupling is the sequence of events by which transmission of an action potential along the sarcolemma causes myofilaments to slide. The action potential is brief and ends well before any signs of contraction are obvious.

As you will see, the electrical signal does not act directly on the myofilaments. Instead, it causes the rise in intracellular levels of calcium ions, which allows the filaments to slide.

Focus on Excitation-Contraction Coupling **(Figure 9.11)** on pp. 290–291 illustrates the steps in this process. This Focus feature also reveals how the integral proteins of the T tubules and terminal cisterns in the triads interact to provide the Ca^{2+} necessary for contraction to occur. Make sure you understand this material before continuing.

Summary: Channels Involved in Initiating Muscle Contraction

So let's summarize what has to happen to excite a muscle cell, starting from the nerve ending. Essentially this process activates four sets of ion channels:

1. The process begins when the nerve impulse reaches the axon terminal and opens voltage-gated calcium channels in the axonal membrane. Calcium entry triggers release of ACh into the synaptic cleft.
2. Released ACh binds to ACh receptors in the sarcolemma, opening chemically gated Na^+-K^+ channels. Greater influx of Na^+ causes a local voltage change (the end plate potential).
3. Local depolarization opens voltage-gated sodium channels in the neighboring region of the sarcolemma. This allows more sodium to enter, which further depolarizes the sarcolemma, generating and propagating an AP.
4. Transmission of the AP along the T tubules changes the shape of voltage-sensitive proteins in the T tubules, which in turn stimulate SR calcium release channels to release Ca^{2+} into the cytosol.

Muscle Fiber Contraction: Cross Bridge Cycling

As we have noted, cross bridge formation (attachment of myosin heads to actin) requires Ca^{2+}. Let's look more closely at how calcium ions promote muscle cell contraction.

When intracellular calcium levels are low, the muscle cell is relaxed, and tropomyosin molecules physically block the active (myosin-binding) sites on actin. As Ca^{2+} levels rise, the ions bind to regulatory sites on troponin. To activate its group of seven actins, a troponin must bind two calcium ions, change shape, and then roll tropomyosin into the groove of the actin helix, away from the myosin-binding sites. In short, the tropomyosin "blockade" is removed when sufficient calcium is present. Once binding sites on actin are exposed, the events of the cross bridge cycle occur in rapid succession, as depicted in *Focus on the Cross Bridge Cycle* **(Figure 9.12)** on p. 292.

The thin filaments continue to slide as long as the calcium signal and adequate ATP are present. When nerve impulses arrive rapidly, intracellular Ca^{2+} levels soar due to successive "puffs" or rounds of Ca^{2+} released from the SR. In such cases, the muscle cells do not completely relax between successive stimuli and contraction is stronger and more sustained (within limits) until nervous stimulation ceases.

As the Ca^{2+} pumps of the SR reclaim calcium ions from the cytosol and troponin again changes shape, tropomyosin again blocks actin's myosin-binding sites. The contraction ends, and the muscle fiber relaxes.

When the cycle is ready to start again, the myosin head is in its upright high-energy configuration (see step (4) in Focus Figure 9.12), ready to take another "step" and attach to an actin site farther along the thin filament. This "walking" of the myosin heads along the adjacent thin filaments during muscle shortening is much like a centipede's gait. The thin filaments cannot slide backward as the cycle repeats again and again because some myosin heads ("legs") are always in contact with actin (the "ground"). Contracting muscles routinely shorten by 30–35% of their total resting length, so each myosin cross bridge attaches and detaches many times during a single contraction. It is likely that only half of the myosin heads of a thick filament are pulling at the same instant. The others are randomly seeking their next binding site.

(Text continues on p. 293.)

Figure 9.11 **Excitation-contraction (E-C) coupling is the sequence of events by which transmission of an action potential along the sarcolemma leads to the sliding of myofilaments.** A&P Flix *Available at www.masteringaandp.com*

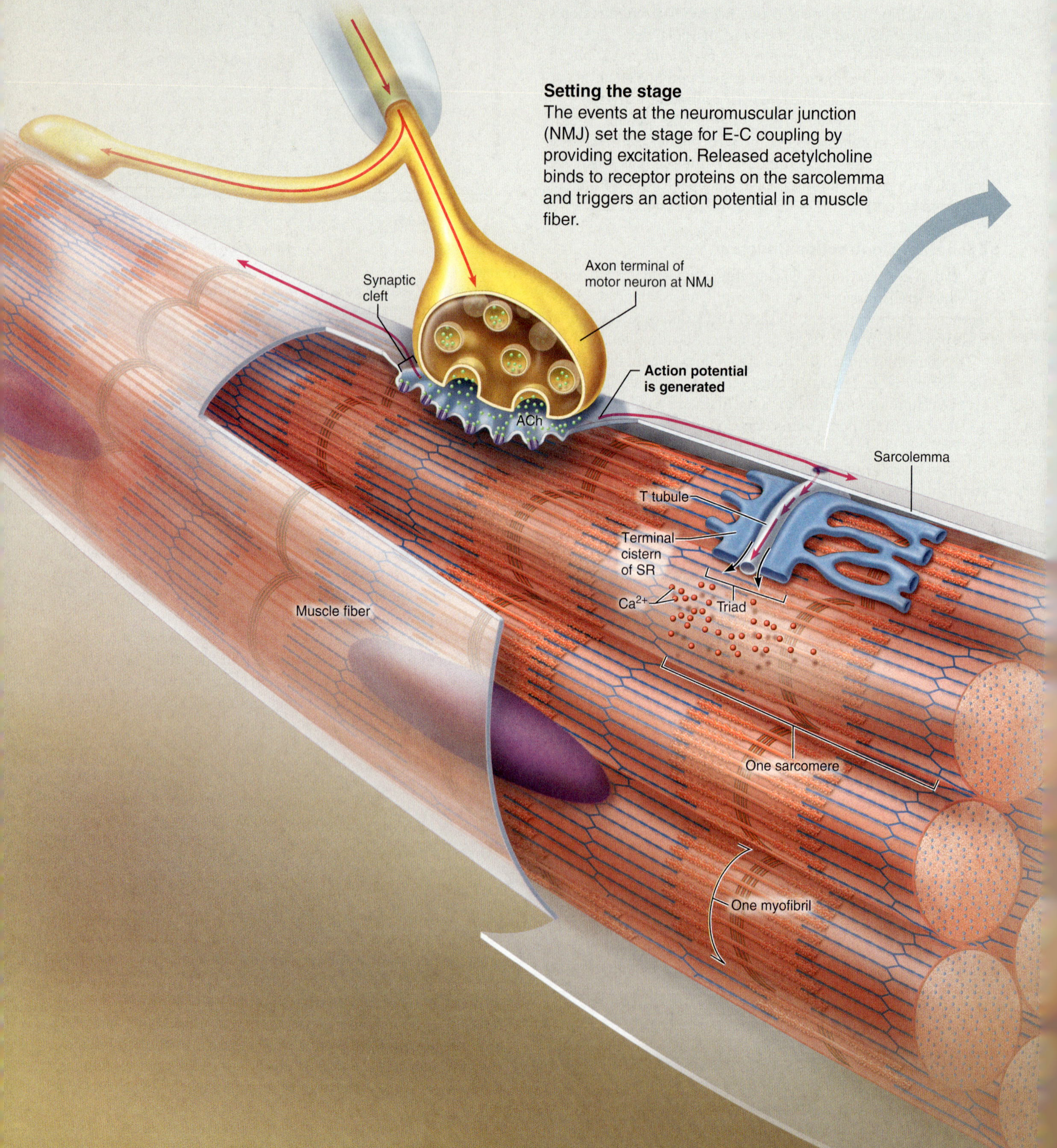

Steps in E-C Coupling:

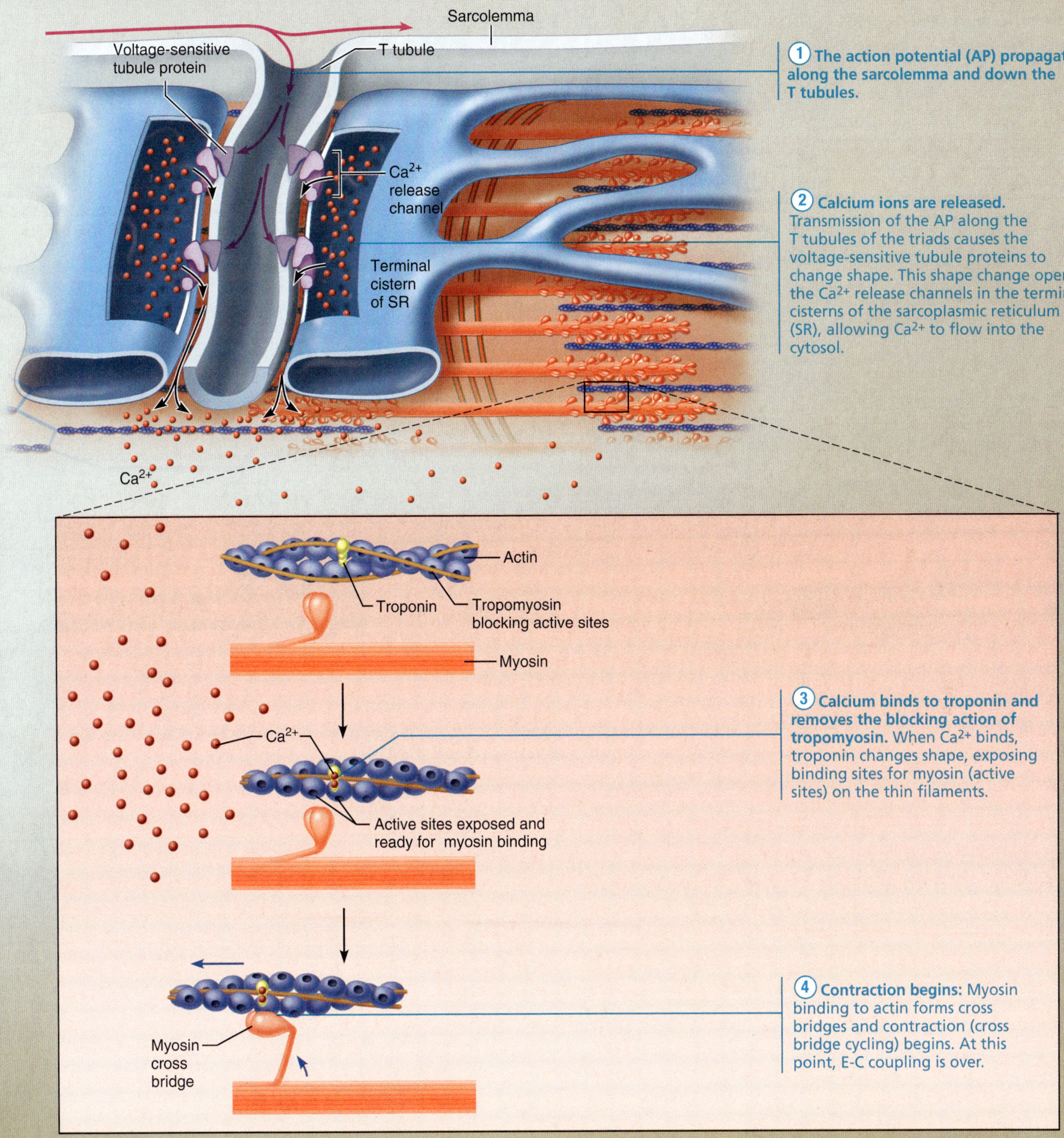

① The action potential (AP) propagates along the sarcolemma and down the T tubules.

② Calcium ions are released. Transmission of the AP along the T tubules of the triads causes the voltage-sensitive tubule proteins to change shape. This shape change opens the Ca^{2+} release channels in the terminal cisterns of the sarcoplasmic reticulum (SR), allowing Ca^{2+} to flow into the cytosol.

③ Calcium binds to troponin and removes the blocking action of tropomyosin. When Ca^{2+} binds, troponin changes shape, exposing binding sites for myosin (active sites) on the thin filaments.

④ Contraction begins: Myosin binding to actin forms cross bridges and contraction (cross bridge cycling) begins. At this point, E-C coupling is over.

The aftermath

When the muscle AP ceases, the voltage-sensitive tubule proteins return to their original shape, closing the Ca^{2+} release channels of the SR. Ca^{2+} levels in the sarcoplasm fall as Ca^{2+} is continually pumped back into the SR by active transport. Without Ca^{2+}, the blocking action of tropomyosin is restored, myosin-actin interaction is inhibited, and relaxation occurs. Each time an AP arrives at the neuromuscular junction, the sequence of E-C coupling is repeated.

Figure 9.12 The cross bridge cycle is the series of events during which myosin heads pull thin filaments toward the center of the sarcomere. A&PFlix Available at www.masteringaandp.com

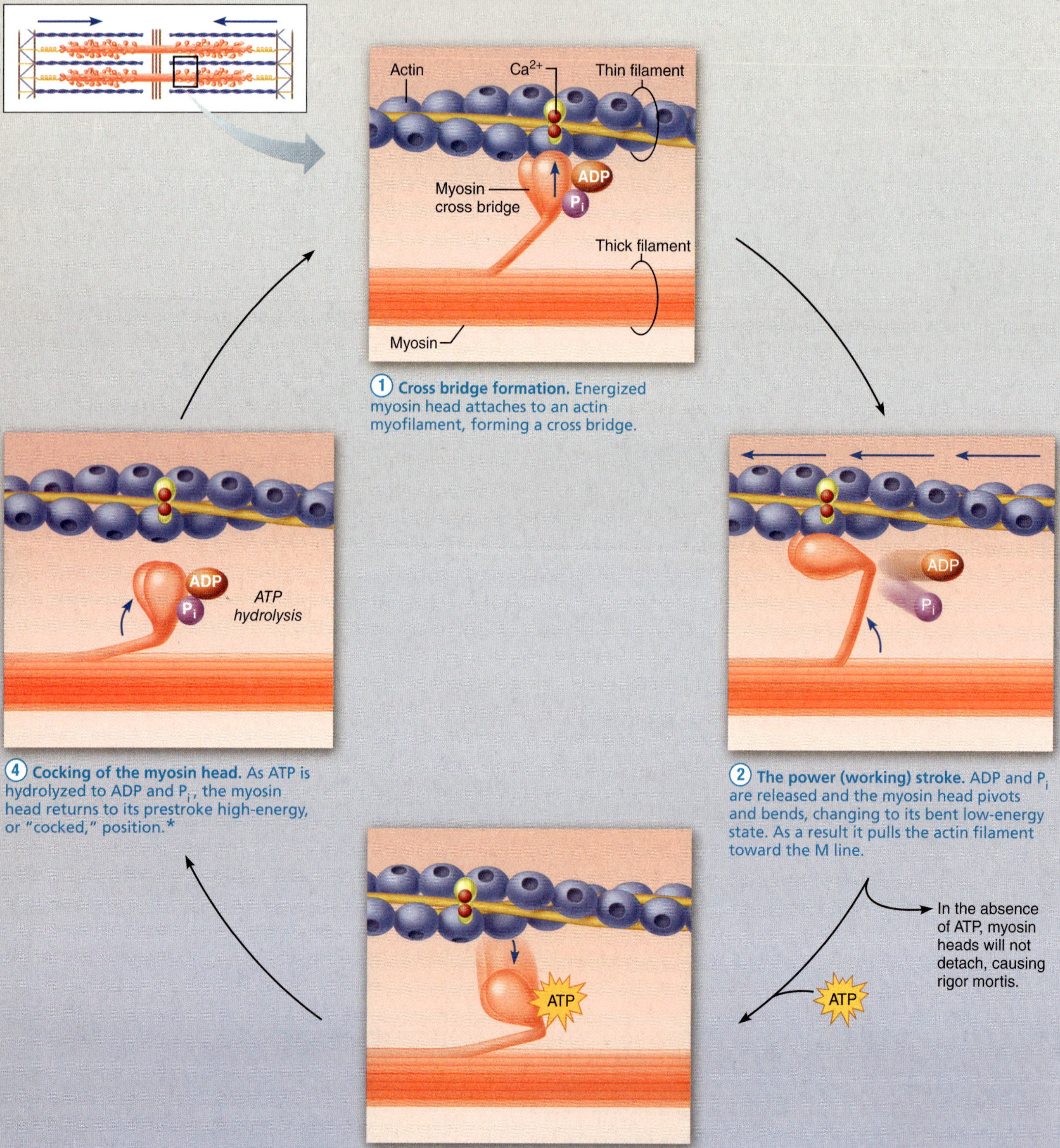

(1) **Cross bridge formation.** Energized myosin head attaches to an actin myofilament, forming a cross bridge.

(2) **The power (working) stroke.** ADP and P_i are released and the myosin head pivots and bends, changing to its bent low-energy state. As a result it pulls the actin filament toward the M line.

(3) **Cross bridge detachment.** After ATP attaches to myosin, the link between myosin and actin weakens, and the myosin head detaches (the cross bridge "breaks").

(4) **Cocking of the myosin head.** As ATP is hydrolyzed to ADP and P_i, the myosin head returns to its prestroke high-energy, or "cocked," position.*

*This cycle will continue as long as ATP is available and Ca^{2+} is bound to troponin.

Except for the brief period following muscle cell excitation, calcium ion concentrations in the cytosol are kept almost undetectably low. There is a reason for this: Sustained high calcium activates apoptosis, leading to cell death.

Homeostatic Imbalance 9.2

Rigor mortis (death rigor) illustrates the fact that cross bridge detachment is ATP driven. Most muscles begin to stiffen 3 to 4 hours after death. Peak rigidity occurs at 12 hours and then gradually dissipates over the next 48 to 60 hours. Dying cells are unable to exclude calcium (which is in higher concentration in the extracellular fluid), and the calcium influx into muscle cells promotes formation of myosin cross bridges. Shortly after breathing stops, ATP synthesis ceases, but ATP continues to be consumed and cross bridge detachment is impossible. Actin and myosin become irreversibly cross-linked, producing the stiffness of rigor mortis, which gradually disappears as muscle proteins break down after death. ✚

Check Your Understanding

6. What are the three structural components of a neuromuscular junction?
7. What is the final trigger for contraction? What is the initial trigger?
8. What prevents the filaments from sliding back to their original position each time a myosin cross bridge detaches from actin?
9. What would happen if a muscle fiber suddenly ran out of ATP when sarcomeres had only partially contracted?

For answers, see Appendix H.

Contraction of a Skeletal Muscle

✓ Define motor unit and muscle twitch, and describe the events occurring during the three phases of a muscle twitch.

✓ Explain how smooth, graded contractions of a skeletal muscle are produced.

✓ Differentiate between isometric and isotonic contractions.

In its relaxed state, a muscle is soft and unimpressive, not what you would expect of a prime mover of the body. However, within a few milliseconds, it can contract to become a hard elastic structure with dynamic characteristics that intrigue not only biologists but engineers and physicists as well.

Before we consider muscle contraction on the organ level, let's note a few principles of muscle mechanics.

- The principles governing contraction of a single muscle fiber and of a skeletal muscle consisting of a large number of fibers are pretty much the same.
- The force exerted by a contracting muscle on an object is called **muscle tension**. The opposing force exerted on the muscle by the weight of the object to be moved is called the **load**.
- A contracting muscle does not always shorten and move the load. If muscle tension develops but the load is not moved, the contraction is called *isometric* ("same measure")—think of trying to lift a 2000-lb car. If the muscle tension developed overcomes the load and muscle shortening occurs, the contraction is *isotonic* ("same tension"), as when you lift a 5-lb sack of sugar. We will describe isometric and isotonic contractions in detail, but for now the important thing to remember when reading the accompanying graphs is this: *Increasing muscle tension* is measured for isometric contractions, whereas the *amount of muscle shortening* (distance in millimeters) is measured for isotonic contractions.
- A skeletal muscle contracts with varying force and for different periods of time in response to stimuli of varying frequencies and intensities. To understand how this occurs, we must look at the nerve-muscle functional unit called a *motor unit*. This is our next topic.

The Motor Unit

Each muscle is served by at least one *motor nerve*, and each motor nerve contains axons (fibrous extensions) of up to hundreds of motor neurons. As an axon enters a muscle, it branches into a number of terminals, each of which forms a neuromuscular junction with a single muscle fiber. A **motor unit** consists of one motor neuron and all the muscle fibers it innervates, or supplies **(Figure 9.13)**. When a motor neuron fires (transmits an action potential), all the muscle fibers it innervates contract.

The number of muscle fibers per motor unit may be as high as several hundred or as few as four. Muscles that exert fine control (such as those controlling the fingers and eyes) have small motor units. By contrast, large, weight-bearing muscles, whose movements are less precise (such as the hip muscles), have large motor units. The muscle fibers in a single motor unit are not clustered together but are spread throughout the muscle. As a result, stimulation of a single motor unit causes a weak contraction of the *entire* muscle.

The Muscle Twitch

Muscle contraction is easily investigated in the laboratory using an isolated muscle. The muscle is attached to an apparatus that produces a **myogram**, a recording of contractile activity. The line recording the activity is called a *tracing*.

A **muscle twitch** is a motor unit's response to a single action potential of its motor neuron. The muscle fibers contract quickly and then relax. Every twitch myogram has three distinct phases **(Figure 9.14a)**.

1. **Latent period.** The **latent period** is the first few milliseconds following stimulation when excitation-contraction coupling is occurring. During this period, cross bridges begin to cycle but muscle tension is not yet measurable and the myogram does not show a response.
2. **Period of contraction.** During the period of contraction, cross bridges are active, from the onset to the peak of tension development, and the myogram tracing rises to a peak. This period lasts 10–100 ms. If the tension (pull) becomes great enough to overcome the resistance of the load, the muscle shortens.
3. **Period of relaxation.** This final phase, lasting 10–100 ms, is initiated by reentry of Ca^{2+} into the SR. Because contractile force is declining, muscle tension decreases to zero and

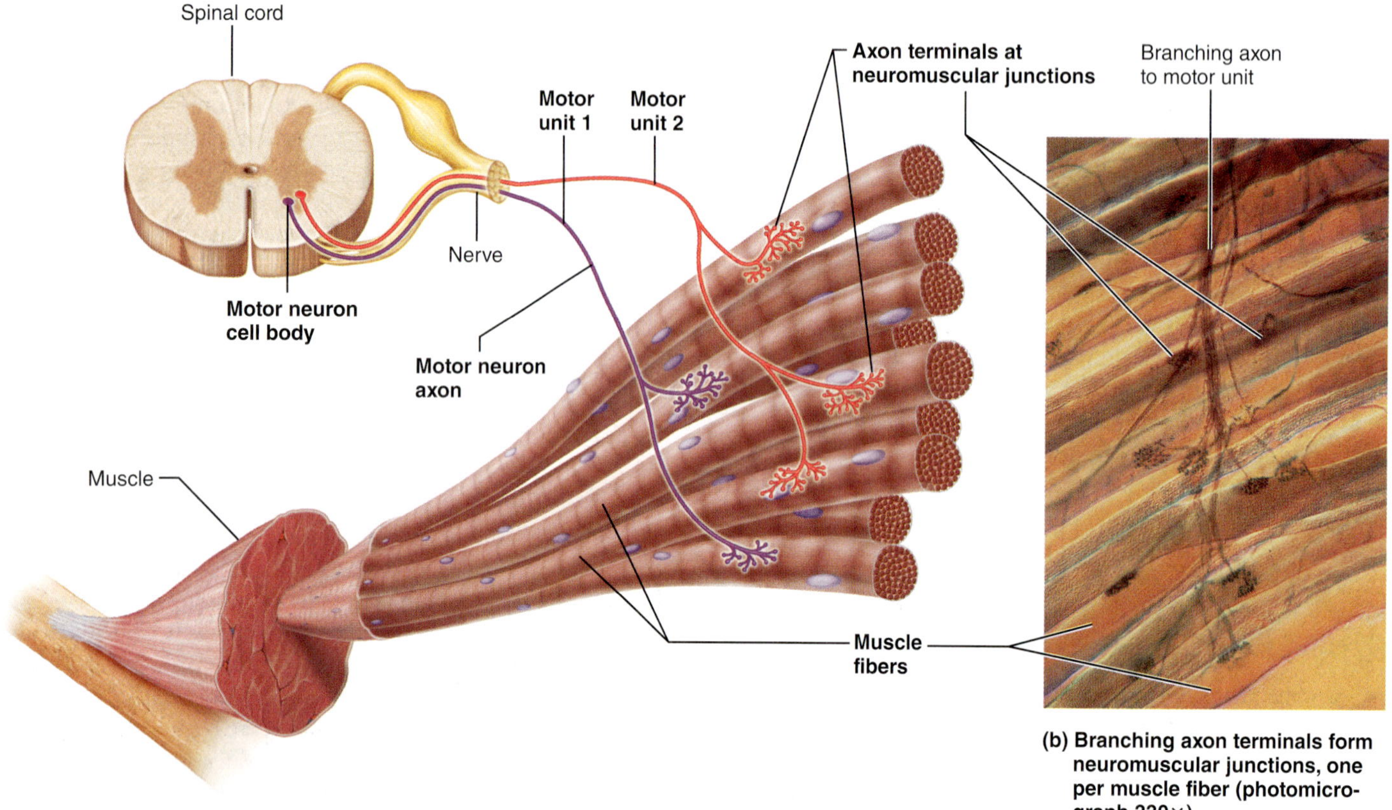

(a) Axons of motor neurons extend from the spinal cord to the muscle. There each axon divides into a number of axon terminals that form neuromuscular junctions with muscle fibers scattered throughout the muscle.

(b) Branching axon terminals form neuromuscular junctions, one per muscle fiber (photomicrograph 330×).

Figure 9.13 A motor unit consists of one motor neuron and all the muscle fibers it innervates. (For a related image, see *A Brief Atlas of the Human Body*, Plate 30.)

the tracing returns to the baseline. If the muscle shortened during contraction, it now returns to its initial length. Notice that a muscle contracts faster than it relaxes, as revealed by the asymmetric nature of the myogram tracing.

As you can see in Figure 9.14b, twitch contractions of some muscles are rapid and brief, as with the muscles controlling eye movements. In contrast, the fibers of fleshy calf muscles (gastrocnemius and soleus) contract more slowly and remain contracted for much longer periods. These differences between muscles reflect variations in enzymes and metabolic properties of the myofibrils.

Graded Muscle Responses

Muscle twitches—like those single, jerky contractions provoked in a laboratory—may result from certain neuromuscular problems, but this is *not* the way our muscles normally operate. Instead, healthy muscle contractions are relatively smooth and vary in strength as different demands are placed on them. These variations, needed for proper control of skeletal movement, are referred to as **graded muscle responses**.

In general, muscle contraction can be graded in two ways: by changing the frequency of stimulation, and by changing the strength of stimulation.

Muscle Response to Changes in Stimulus Frequency The nervous system achieves greater muscular force by increasing the firing rate of motor neurons. For example, if two identical stimuli (electrical shocks or nerve impulses) are delivered to a muscle in rapid succession, the second twitch will be stronger than the first. On a myogram the second twitch will appear to ride on the shoulders of the first **(Figure 9.15a, b)**.

This phenomenon, called **wave** or **temporal summation**, occurs because the second contraction occurs before the muscle has completely relaxed. Because the muscle is already partially contracted and more calcium is being squirted into the cytosol to replace that being reclaimed by the SR, muscle tension produced during the second contraction causes more shortening than the first. In other words, the contractions are added together. (However, the refractory period is always honored. Thus, if a second stimulus arrives before repolarization is complete, no wave summation occurs.)

If the stimulus strength is held constant and the muscle is stimulated at an increasingly faster rate: (1) the relaxation time between twitches becomes shorter and shorter, (2) the concentration of Ca^{2+} in the cytosol rises higher and higher, and (3) the degree of wave summation becomes greater and greater, progressing to a sustained but quivering contraction referred to as **unfused** or **incomplete tetanus** (Figure 9.15b).

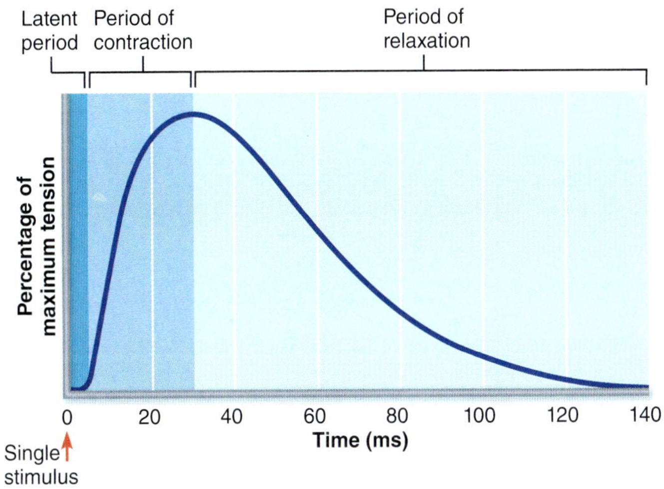

(a) Myogram showing the three phases of an isometric twitch

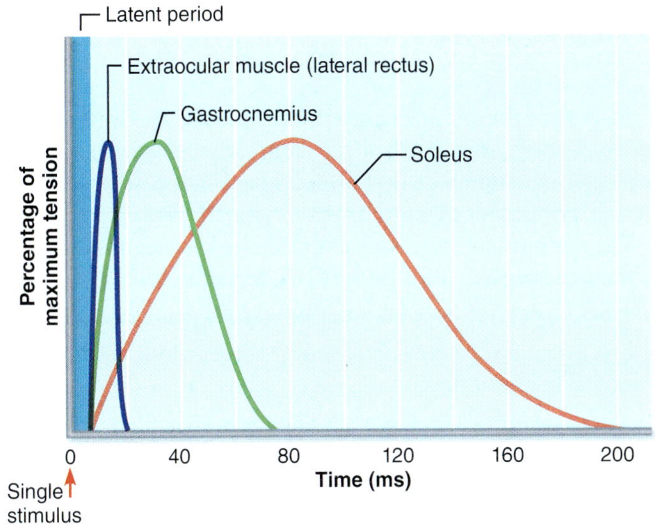

(b) Comparison of the relative duration of twitch responses of three muscles

Figure 9.14 The muscle twitch.

Finally, as the stimulation frequency continues to increase, muscle tension increases until it reaches maximal tension. At this point all evidence of muscle relaxation disappears and the contractions fuse into a smooth, sustained contraction plateau called **fused** or **complete tetanus** (tet′ah-nus; *tetan* = rigid, tense) (Figure 9.15c). (Note that this term is often confused with the bacterial disease called tetanus that causes severe involuntary contractions.) In the real world, fused tetanus happens infrequently, for example, when someone shows superhuman strength by lifting a fallen tree limb off a companion.

Vigorous muscle activity cannot continue indefinitely. Prolonged tetanus inevitably leads to muscle fatigue, a situation in which the muscle cannot contract and its tension drops to zero.

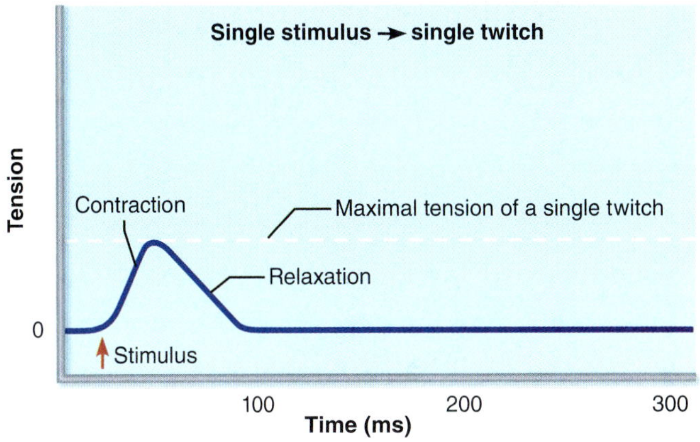

(a) A single stimulus is delivered. The muscle contracts and relaxes.

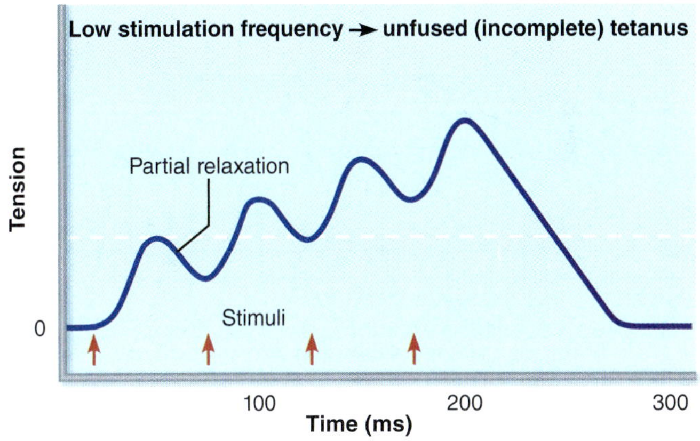

(b) If another stimulus is applied before the muscle relaxes completely, then more tension results. This is wave (or temporal) summation and results in unfused (or incomplete) tetanus.

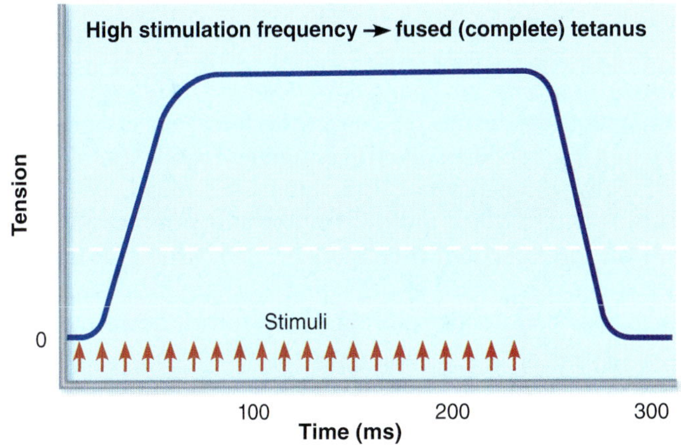

(c) At higher stimulus frequencies, there is no relaxation at all between stimuli. This is fused (complete) tetanus.

Figure 9.15 A muscle's response to changes in stimulation frequency. (Note that tension is measured in grams.)

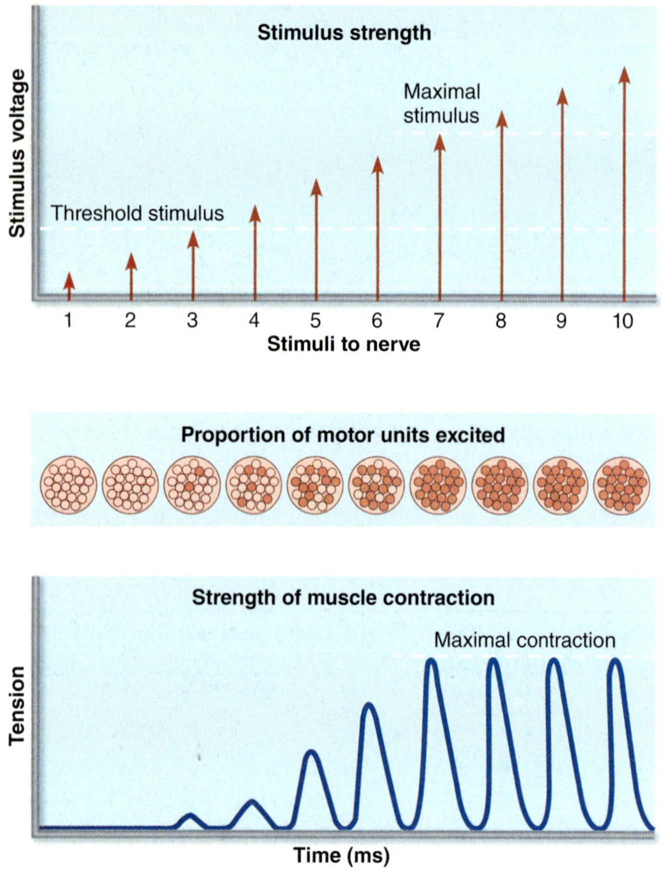

Figure 9.16 Relationship between stimulus intensity (graph at top) and muscle tension (tracing below). Below threshold voltage, the tracing shows no muscle response (stimuli 1 and 2). Once threshold (3) is reached, increases in voltage excite (recruit) more and more motor units until the maximal stimulus is reached (7). Further increases in stimulus voltage produce no further increase in contractile strength.

Muscle Response to Changes in Stimulus Strength Wave summation contributes to contractile force, but its primary function is to produce smooth, continuous muscle contractions by rapidly stimulating a specific number of muscle cells. **Recruitment**, also called **multiple motor unit summation**, controls the force of contraction more precisely. In the laboratory, recruitment is achieved by delivering shocks of increasing voltage to the muscle, calling more and more muscle fibers into play.

- Stimuli that produce no observable contractions are **subthreshold stimuli**.
- The stimulus at which the first observable contraction occurs is called the **threshold stimulus** (Figure 9.16). Beyond this point, the muscle contracts more and more vigorously as the stimulus strength increases.
- The **maximal stimulus** is the strongest stimulus that increases contractile force. It represents the point at which all the muscle's motor units are recruited.

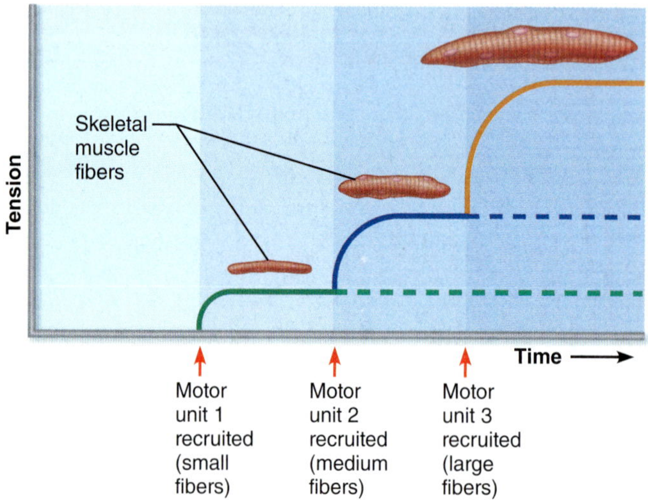

Figure 9.17 The size principle of recruitment. Recruitment of motor neurons controlling skeletal muscle fibers is orderly and follows the size principle.

Increasing the stimulus intensity beyond the maximal stimulus does not produce a stronger contraction. In the body, the same phenomenon is caused by neural activation of an increasingly large number of motor units serving the muscle.

The recruitment process is not random. Instead it is dictated by the *size principle* (Figure 9.17). In any muscle:

- The motor units with the smallest muscle fibers are activated first because they are controlled by the smallest, most highly excitable motor neurons.
- As motor units with larger and larger muscle fibers begin to be excited, contractile strength increases.
- The largest motor units, containing large, coarse muscle fibers, have as much as 50 times the contractile force of the smallest ones. They are controlled by the largest, least excitable (highest-threshold) neurons and are activated only when the most powerful contraction is necessary.

Why is the size principle important? It allows the increases in force during weak contractions (for example, those that maintain posture or slow movements) to occur in small steps, whereas gradations in muscle force are progressively greater when large amounts of force are needed for vigorous activities such as jumping or running. The size principle explains how the same hand that lightly pats your cheek can deliver a stinging slap at the volleyball during a match.

Although *all* the motor units of a muscle may be recruited simultaneously to produce an exceptionally strong contraction, motor units are more commonly activated asynchronously. At a given instant, some are in tetanus (usually unfused tetanus) while others are resting and recovering. This technique helps prolong a strong contraction by preventing or delaying fatigue. It also explains how weak contractions promoted by infrequent stimuli can remain smooth.

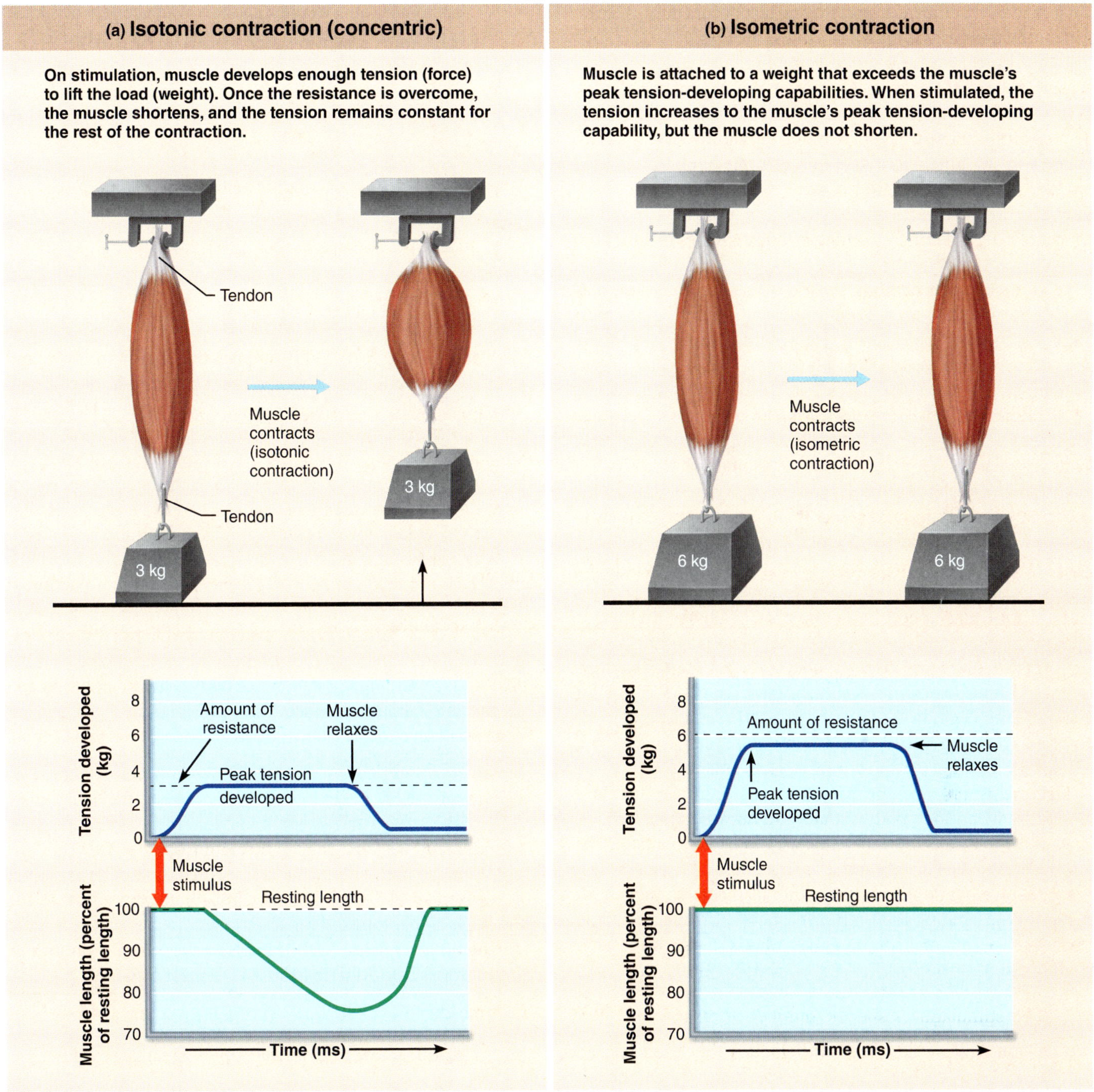

Figure 9.18 **Isotonic (concentric) and isometric contractions.**

Isotonic and Isometric Contractions

As noted earlier, there are two main categories of contractions—*isotonic* and *isometric*. In **isotonic contractions** (*iso* = same; *ton* = tension), muscle length changes and moves a load. Once sufficient tension has developed to move the load, the tension remains relatively constant through the rest of the contractile period **(Figure 9.18a)**.

Isotonic contractions come in two "flavors"—*concentric* and *eccentric*. **Concentric contractions** are those in which the muscle shortens and does work, such as picking up a book or kicking a ball. Concentric contractions are probably more familiar, but **eccentric contractions**, in which the muscle generates force as it lengthens, are equally important for coordination and purposeful movements.

Eccentric contractions occur in your calf muscle, for example, as you walk up a steep hill. Eccentric contractions are about 50% more forceful than concentric ones at the same load and more often cause delayed-onset muscle soreness. (Consider how your calf muscles *feel* the day after hiking up that hill.) The reason is unclear, but it may be that the muscle stretching that occurs during eccentric contractions causes microtears in the muscles.

Biceps curls provide a simple example of how concentric and eccentric contractions work together in our everyday activities. When you flex your elbow to raise this textbook to your shoulder, the biceps muscle in your arm is contracting concentrically. When you straighten your arm to return the book to the desktop, the isotonic contraction of your biceps is eccentric. Basically, eccentric contractions put the body in position to contract concentrically. All jumping and throwing activities involve both types of contraction.

In **isometric contractions** (*metric* = measure), tension may build to the muscle's peak tension-producing capacity, but the muscle *neither shortens nor lengthens* (Figure 9.18b). Isometric contractions occur when a muscle attempts to move a load that is greater than the force (tension) the muscle is able to develop—think of trying to lift a piano single-handedly. Muscles contract isometrically when they act primarily to maintain upright posture or to hold joints stationary while movements occur at other joints.

Consider a knee bend. When you squat for a few seconds, the quadriceps muscles of your anterior thigh contract isometrically to hold your knee in the flexed position. When you start to rise to the upright position, they continue to contract isometrically until their tension exceeds the load (weight of your upper body). At that point muscle shortening (concentric contraction) begins. So the quadriceps contractile sequence for a deep knee bend from start to finish is (1) flex knee (eccentric), (2) hold squat position (isometric), (3) extend knee (isometric, then concentric). Of course, this list does not even begin to consider the isometric contractions of the posterior thigh muscles or of the trunk muscles that maintain a relatively erect trunk posture during this movement.

Electrochemical and mechanical events occurring within a muscle are identical in both isotonic and isometric contractions. However, the results are different. In isotonic contractions, the thin filaments slide. In isometric contractions, the cross bridges generate force but do *not* move the thin filaments, so there is no change in the banding pattern from that of the resting state. (You could say that they are "spinning their wheels" on the same actin binding sites.)

Muscle Tone

Skeletal muscles are described as voluntary, but even relaxed muscles are almost always slightly contracted, a phenomenon called **muscle tone**. Muscle tone is due to spinal reflexes that activate first one group of motor units and then another in response to activated stretch receptors in the muscles. Muscle tone does not produce active movements, but it keeps the muscles firm, healthy, and ready to respond to stimulation. Skeletal muscle tone also helps stabilize joints and maintain posture.

☑ Check Your Understanding

10. What is a motor unit?
11. What is happening in the muscle during the latent period of a twitch contraction?
12. Jay is competing in a chin-up competition. What type of muscle contractions are occurring in his biceps muscles immediately after he grabs the bar? As his body begins to move upward toward the bar? When his body begins to approach the mat?

For answers, see Appendix H.

Muscle Metabolism

✓ Describe three ways in which ATP is regenerated during skeletal muscle contraction.

✓ Define EPOC and muscle fatigue. List possible causes of muscle fatigue.

Providing Energy for Contraction

As a muscle contracts, ATP supplies the energy to move and detach cross bridges, operate the calcium pump in the SR, and return Na^+ and K^+ to the cell exterior and interior respectively after excitation-contraction coupling. Surprisingly, muscles store very limited reserves of ATP—4 to 6 seconds' worth at most, just enough to get you going. Because ATP is the *only* energy source used directly for contractile activities, it must be regenerated as fast as it is broken down if contraction is to continue.

Fortunately, after ATP is hydrolyzed to ADP and inorganic phosphate in muscle fibers, it is regenerated within a fraction of a second by one or more of the three pathways summarized in **Figure 9.19**: (1) direct phosphorylation of ADP by creatine phosphate, (2) anaerobic, glycolysis, which converts glucose to lactic acid, and (3) aerobic respiration. All body cells use glycolysis and aerobic respiration to produce ATP, so we touch on them here but describe them in detail later, in Chapter 24.

Direct Phosphorylation of ADP by Creatine Phosphate (Figure 9.19a) As we begin to exercise vigorously, the demand for ATP soars and consumes the ATP stored in working muscles within a few twitches. Then **creatine phosphate (CP)** (kre′ah-tin), a unique high-energy molecule stored in muscles, is tapped to regenerate ATP while the metabolic pathways adjust to the suddenly higher demand for ATP.

Coupling CP with ADP transfers energy and a phosphate group from CP to ADP to form ATP almost instantly:

$$\text{Creatine phosphate} + \text{ADP} \xrightarrow{\text{creatine kinase}} \text{creatine} + \text{ATP}$$

Muscle cells store two to three times more CP than ATP. The CP-ADP reaction, catalyzed by the enzyme **creatine kinase**, is so efficient that the amount of ATP in muscle cells changes very little during the initial period of contraction.

Together, stored ATP and CP provide for maximum muscle power for about 15 seconds—long enough to energize a 100-meter dash (slightly longer if the activity is less vigorous). The coupled reaction is readily reversible, and to keep CP "on tap," CP reserves are replenished during periods of rest or inactivity.

Anaerobic Pathway: Glycolysis and Lactic Acid Formation (Figure 9.19b) As stored ATP and CP are exhausted, more ATP is generated by breaking down (catabolizing) glucose obtained from the blood or glycogen stored in the muscle. The initial phase of glucose breakdown is **glycolysis** (gli-kol′ĭ-sis;

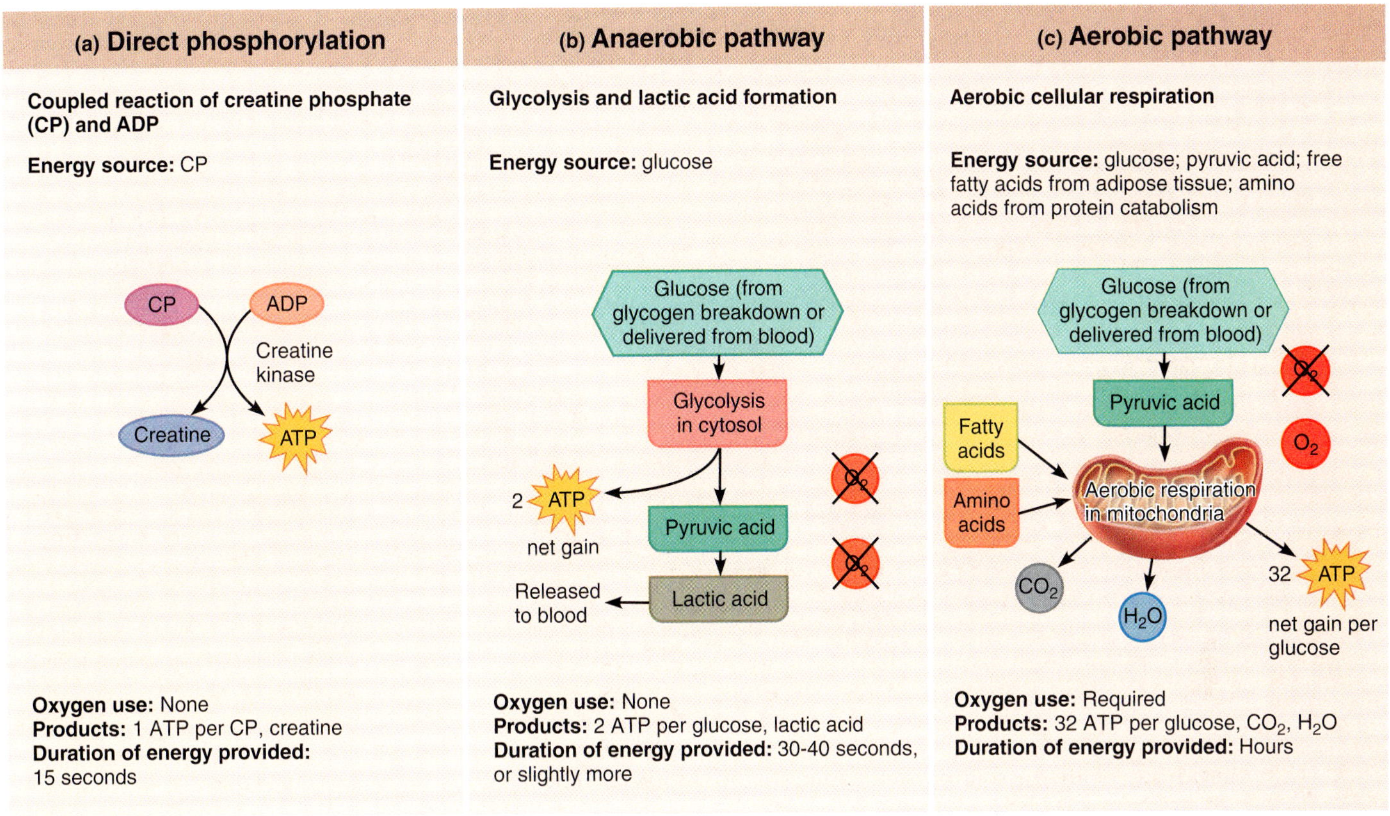

Figure 9.19 Pathways for regenerating ATP during muscle activity. The fastest pathway is direct phosphorylation **(a)**, and the slowest is aerobic respiration **(c)**.

"sugar splitting"). This pathway occurs in both the presence and the absence of oxygen, but because it does not use oxygen, it is an anaerobic (an-a′er-ōb-ik; "without oxygen") pathway. During glycolysis, glucose is broken down to two *pyruvic acid* molecules, releasing enough energy to form small amounts of ATP (2 ATP per glucose).

Ordinarily, pyruvic acid produced during glycolysis then enters the mitochondria and reacts with oxygen to produce still more ATP in the oxygen-using pathway called aerobic respiration, described shortly. But when muscles contract vigorously and contractile activity reaches about 70% of the maximum possible (for example, when you run 600 meters with maximal effort), the bulging muscles compress the blood vessels within them, impairing blood flow and oxygen delivery. Under these anaerobic conditions, most of the pyruvic acid produced during glycolysis is converted into **lactic acid**, and the overall process is referred to as **anaerobic glycolysis**. Thus, during oxygen deficit, lactic acid is the end product of cellular metabolism of glucose.

Most of the lactic acid diffuses out of the muscles into the bloodstream. Subsequently, the liver, heart, or kidney cells pick up the lactic acid and use it as an energy source. Additionally, liver cells can reconvert it to pyruvic acid or glucose and release it back into the bloodstream for muscle use, or convert it to glycogen for storage.

The anaerobic pathway harvests only about 5% as much ATP from each glucose molecule as the aerobic pathway, but it produces ATP about 2½ times faster. For this reason, when large amounts of ATP are needed for moderate periods (30–40 seconds) of strenuous muscle activity, glycolysis can provide most of the ATP needed as long as the required fuels and enzymes are available. Together, stored ATP and CP and the glycolysis–lactic acid pathway can support strenuous muscle activity for nearly a minute.

Although anaerobic glycolysis readily fuels spurts of vigorous exercise, it has shortcomings. Huge amounts of glucose are used to produce relatively small harvests of ATP, and the accumulating lactic acid is partially responsible for muscle soreness during intense exercise.

Aerobic Respiration (Figure 9.19c) Because the amount of creatine phosphate is limited, muscles must metabolize nutrients to transfer energy from foodstuffs to ATP. During rest and light to moderate exercise, even if prolonged, 95% of the ATP used for muscle activity comes from aerobic respiration. **Aerobic respiration** occurs in the mitochondria, requires oxygen, and involves a sequence of chemical reactions that break the bonds of fuel molecules and release energy to make ATP.

Aerobic respiration, which includes glycolysis and the reactions that take place in the mitochondria, breaks down glucose entirely. Water, carbon dioxide, and large amounts of ATP are its final products.

$$\text{Glucose} + \text{oxygen} \rightarrow \text{carbon dioxide} + \text{water} + \text{ATP}$$

The carbon dioxide released diffuses out of the muscle tissue into the blood, to be removed from the body by the lungs.

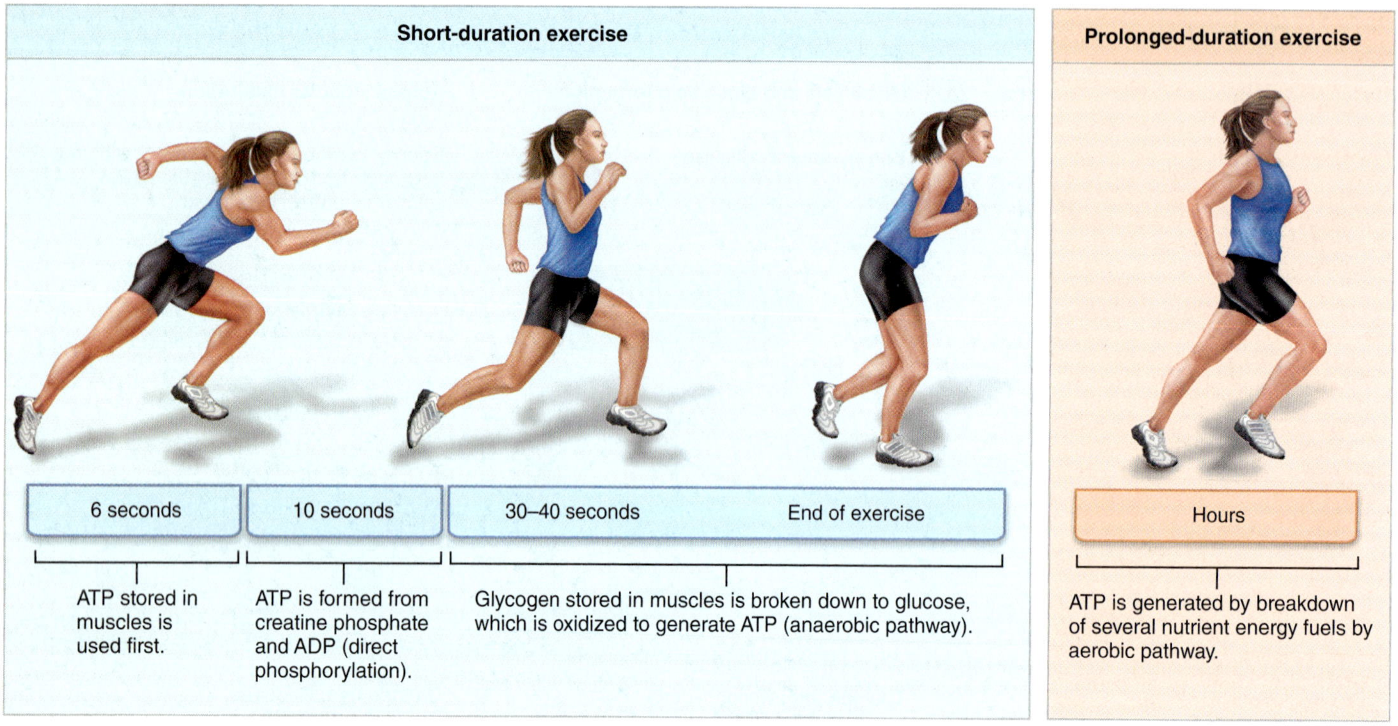

Figure 9.20 Comparison of energy sources used during short-duration exercise and prolonged-duration exercise.

As exercise begins, muscle glycogen provides most of the fuel. Shortly thereafter, bloodborne glucose, pyruvic acid from glycolysis, and free fatty acids are the major sources of fuels. After about 30 minutes, fatty acids become the major energy fuels. Aerobic respiration provides a high yield of ATP (about 32 ATP per glucose), but it is slow because of its many steps and it requires continuous delivery of oxygen and nutrient fuels to keep it going.

Energy Systems Used During Sports Which pathways predominate during exercise? As long as a muscle cell has enough oxygen, it will form ATP by the aerobic pathway. When ATP demands are within the capacity of the aerobic pathway, light to moderate muscular activity can continue for several hours in well-conditioned individuals **(Figure 9.20)**. However, when exercise demands begin to exceed the ability of the muscle cells to carry out the necessary reactions quickly enough, anaerobic pathways begin to contribute more and more of the total ATP generated. The length of time a muscle can continue to contract using aerobic pathways is called **aerobic endurance**, and the point at which muscle metabolism converts to anaerobic glycolysis is called **anaerobic threshold.**

Activities that require a surge of power but last only a few seconds, such as weight lifting, diving, and sprinting, rely entirely on ATP and CP stores. The more on-and-off or burstlike activities of tennis, soccer, and a 100-meter swim appear to be fueled almost entirely by anaerobic glycolysis (Figure 9.20). Prolonged activities such as marathon runs and jogging, where endurance rather than power is the goal, depend mainly on aerobic respiration using both glucose and fatty acids as fuels.

Levels of CP and ATP don't change much during prolonged exercise because ATP is generated at the same rate as it is used—a "pay as you go" system. Compared to anaerobic energy production, aerobic generation of ATP is relatively slow, but the ATP harvest is enormous.

Muscle Fatigue

Muscle fatigue is a state of *physiological inability to contract* even though the muscle still may be receiving stimuli. Although many factors appear to contribute to fatigue, its specific causes are not fully understood. Most experimental evidence indicates that fatigue is due to a problem in excitation-contraction coupling or, in rare cases, problems at the neuromuscular junction. Availability of ATP declines during contraction, but it is abnormal for a muscle to totally run out of ATP. So, lack of ATP is not a fatigue-producing factor in moderate exercise.

Several ionic imbalances contribute to muscle fatigue. As action potentials are transmitted, potassium is lost from the muscle cells, and accumulates in the fluids of the T tubules. This ionic change disturbs the membrane potential of the muscle cells and halts Ca^{2+} release from the SR.

Theoretically, in short-duration exercise, an accumulation of inorganic phosphate (P_i) from CP and ATP breakdown may interfere with calcium release from the SR. Alternatively, it may interfere with the release of P_i from myosin and thus hamper myosin's power strokes. Lactic acid has long been assumed to be a major cause of fatigue, and excessive intracellular accumulation of lactic acid (which causes the muscles to ache) raises the concentration of H^+ and alters contractile proteins. However, pH is normally regulated within normal limits in all but the greatest degree of exertion. Additionally, lactic acid actually counteracts high K^+ levels, which do lead to muscle fatigue (as noted above).

In general, intense exercise of short duration produces fatigue rapidly via ionic disturbances that alter E-C coupling, but recovery is also rapid. In contrast, the slow-developing fatigue of prolonged low-intensity exercise may require several hours for complete recovery. It appears that this type of exercise damages the SR, interfering with Ca^{2+} regulation and release, and therefore with muscle activation.

Excess Postexercise Oxygen Consumption (EPOC)

Whether or not fatigue occurs, vigorous exercise alters a muscle's chemistry dramatically. For a muscle to return to its resting state, all the following must occur:

- Its oxygen reserves in myoglobin must be replenished.
- The accumulated lactic acid must be reconverted to pyruvic acid.
- Glycogen stores must be replaced.
- ATP and creatine phosphate reserves must be resynthesized.

The use of these muscle stores during anaerobic exercise simply defers when the oxygen is consumed, because replacing them requires oxygen uptake and aerobic metabolism after exercise ends. Additionally, the liver must convert any lactic acid persisting in blood to glucose or glycogen. Once exercise stops, the repayment process begins.

The extra amount of oxygen that the body must take in for these restorative processes is called the **excess postexercise oxygen consumption (EPOC)**, formerly called the oxygen debt. EPOC represents the difference between the amount of oxygen needed for totally aerobic muscle activity and the amount actually used. All anaerobic sources of ATP used during muscle activity contribute to EPOC.

Heat Production During Muscle Activity

Only about 40% of the energy released during muscle contraction is converted to useful work (still, this percentage is significantly higher than that of many mechanical devices). The rest is given off as heat, which has to be dealt with to maintain body homeostasis.

When you exercise vigorously, you start to feel hot as the liberated heat warms your blood. Like a car's cooling system that dissipates heat, several homeostatic processes prevent heat in the body from building to dangerous levels. These processes include sweating and radiating heat from the skin surface.

Shivering represents the opposite side of homeostatic balance. In this case the body is too cold and muscle contractions are used to produce more heat.

Check Your Understanding

13. When Eric returned from jogging, he was breathing heavily, sweating profusely, and complained that his legs ached and felt weak. His wife poured him a sports drink and urged him to take it easy until he could "catch his breath." On the basis of what you have learned about muscle energy metabolism, respond to the following questions: Why is Eric breathing heavily? Which ATP-generating pathway have his working muscles been using that makes him breathless? What metabolic products might account for his sore muscles and muscle weakness?

For answers, see Appendix H.

Force of Muscle Contraction

✓ Describe factors that influence the force, velocity, and duration of skeletal muscle contraction.

✓ Describe three types of skeletal muscle fibers and explain the relative value of each type.

The force of muscle contraction depends on the number of myosin cross bridges that are attached. This in turn is affected by four factors **(Figure 9.21)**: (1) number of muscle fibers stimulated, (2) relative size of the fibers, (3) frequency of stimulation, and (4) degree of muscle stretch. Let's examine the role of each factor.

Number of Muscle Fibers Recruited

As already discussed, the more motor units that are recruited, the greater the muscle force.

Size of Muscle Fibers

The bulkier the muscle (the greater its cross-sectional area), the more tension it can develop and the greater its strength, but there is more to it than this. As noted earlier, the large fibers of large motor units produce the most powerful movements. Regular resistance exercise increases muscle force by causing muscle cells to *hypertrophy* (hi-per′tro-fe), or increase in size.

Frequency of Stimulation

As a muscle begins to contract, the force generated by the cross bridges—the **internal tension**—stretches the connective tissue sheaths (noncontractile components). These in turn become taut and transfer their tension, called the **external tension**, to the load

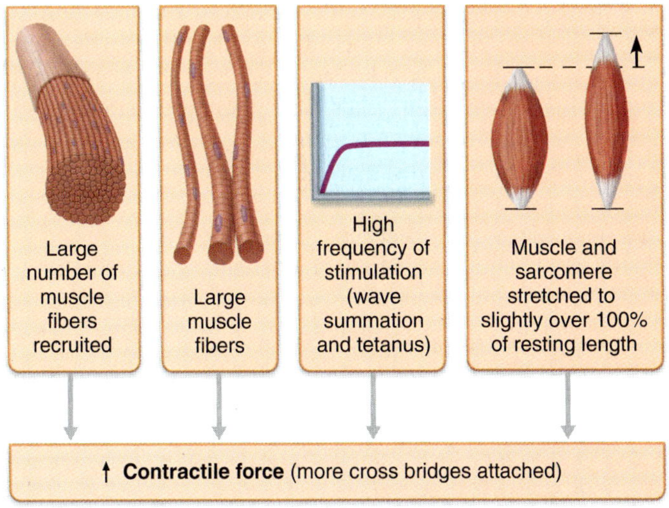

Figure 9.21 Factors that increase the force of skeletal muscle contraction.

Figure 9.22 Length-tension relationships of sarcomeres in skeletal muscles. A muscle generates maximum force when it is between 80 and 120% of its optimal resting length. Increases and decreases beyond this optimal range reduce its force and ability to generate tension.

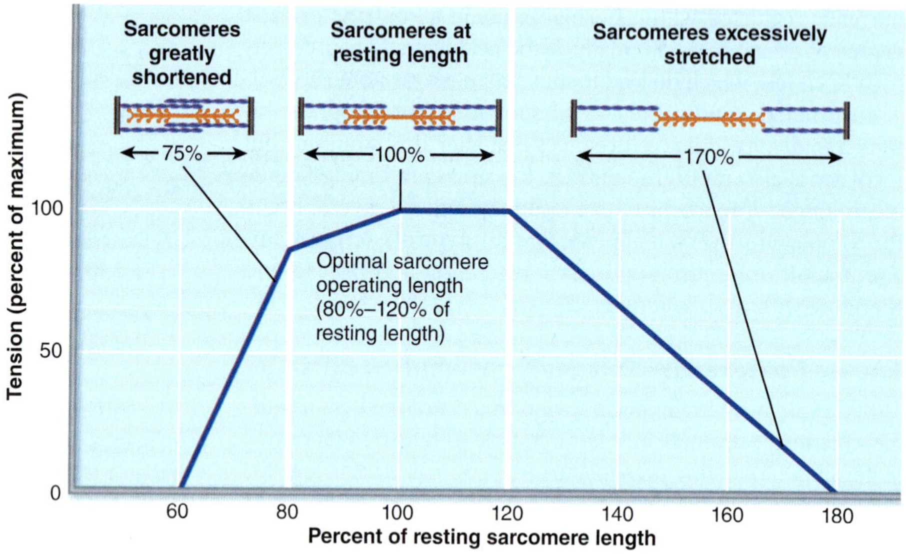

9

(muscle insertion). When the contraction ends, the noncontractile components recoil and help return the muscle to its resting length.

Time is required to take up slack and stretch the noncontractile components, and while this is happening, the internal tension is already declining. So, in brief twitch contractions, the external tension is always less than the internal tension. However, when a muscle is stimulated rapidly, contractions are summed, becoming stronger and more vigorous and ultimately producing tetanus (see Figure 9.15).

During tetanic contractions more time is available to stretch the noncontractile components, and external tension approaches the internal tension. So, the more rapidly a muscle is stimulated, the greater the force it exerts.

Degree of Muscle Stretch

The optimal operating length for a muscle fiber is the length at which it can generate maximum force (Figure 9.21 and **Figure 9.22**). Within a sarcomere, the ideal **length-tension relationship** occurs when a muscle is slightly stretched and the thin and thick filaments overlap optimally, because this relationship permits sliding along nearly the entire length of the thin filaments.

If a muscle fiber stretches so much that the filaments do not overlap, the myosin heads have nothing to attach to and cannot generate tension. Alternatively, if the sarcomeres are so compressed and cramped that the Z discs abut the thick myofilaments, and the thin filaments touch and interfere with one another, little or no further shortening can occur.

If you stretch a muscle to various extents and stimulate it tetanically, the active tension the muscle can generate varies with length (Figure 9.22). A severely stretched muscle (say one over 180% of its optimal length) cannot develop tension. Likewise, at 75% of a muscle's resting length, its ability to generate force (or shorten) is limited because the actin myofilaments in its sarcomeres overlap and the thick filaments run into the Z discs, restricting further shortening.

In the body, skeletal muscles are maintained near their optimal operating length by the way they are attached to bones. The joints normally prevent bone movements that would stretch attached muscles beyond their optimal range.

Velocity and Duration of Contraction

Muscles vary in how fast they can contract and how long they can continue to contract before they fatigue. These characteristics are influenced by muscle fiber type, load, and recruitment.

Muscle Fiber Type

There are several ways of classifying muscle fibers, but learning about these classes will be easier if you pay attention to just two functional characteristics:

- **Speed of contraction.** On the basis of speed (velocity) of fiber shortening, there are **slow fibers** and **fast fibers**. The difference reflects how fast their myosin ATPases split ATP, and the pattern of electrical activity of their motor neurons. Contraction duration also varies with fiber type and depends on how quickly Ca^{2+} moves from the cytosol into the SR.
- **Major pathways for forming ATP.** The cells that rely mostly on the oxygen-using aerobic pathways for ATP generation are **oxidative fibers**. Those that rely more on anaerobic glycolysis are **glycolytic fibers**.

Using these two criteria, we can classify skeletal muscle cells as: **slow oxidative fibers**, **fast oxidative fibers**, or **fast glycolytic fibers**.

Table 9.2 gives details about each group, but a word to the wise: Do not approach this information by rote memorization—you'll just get frustrated. Instead, start with what you know for any category and see how the characteristics listed support that.

For example, think about a *slow oxidative fiber* (Table 9.2, first column, and **Figure 9.23**, right side). We can see that it

- Contracts *slowly* because its myosin ATPases are slow (a criterion)
- Depends on *oxygen* delivery and aerobic pathways (its major pathways for forming ATP give it *high oxidative capacity*—a criterion)

- Resists fatigue and has high endurance (typical of fibers that depend on aerobic metabolism)
- Is thin (a large amount of cytoplasm impedes diffusion of O_2 and nutrients from the blood)
- Has relatively little power (a thin cell can contain only a limited number of myofibrils)
- Has many mitochondria (actual sites of oxygen use)
- Has a rich capillary supply (the better to deliver bloodborne O_2)
- Is red (its color stems from an abundant supply of myoglobin, muscle's oxygen-binding pigment that stores O_2 reserves in the cell and helps O_2 diffuse through the cell)

Add these features together and you have a muscle fiber best suited to endurance-type activities.

Now think about a *fast glycolytic fiber* (Table 9.2, third column, and Figure 9.23, left side). In contrast, it

- Contracts *rapidly* due to the activity of fast myosin ATPases
- Does not use oxygen
- Depends on plentiful *glycogen* reserves for fuel rather than on blood-delivered nutrients
- Tires quickly because glycogen reserves are short-lived and lactic acid accumulates quickly, making it a fatigable fiber
- Has a large diameter, indicating the plentiful myofilaments that allow it to contract powerfully before it "poops out"

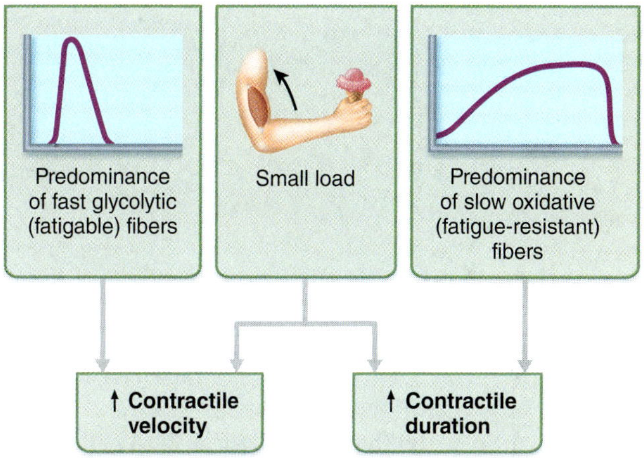

Figure 9.23 Factors influencing velocity and duration of skeletal muscle contraction.

- Has few mitochondria, little myoglobin and few capillaries (making it white), and is a much thicker cell (because it doesn't depend on continuous oxygen and nutrient diffusion from the blood)

For these reasons, a fast glycolytic fiber is best suited for short-term, rapid, intense movements (moving furniture across the room, for example).

Table 9.2 Structural and Functional Characteristics of the Three Types of Skeletal Muscle Fibers

	SLOW OXIDATIVE FIBERS	FAST OXIDATIVE FIBERS	FAST GLYCOLYTIC FIBERS
Metabolic Characteristics			
Speed of contraction	Slow	Fast	Fast
Myosin ATPase activity	Slow	Fast	Fast
Primary pathway for ATP synthesis	Aerobic	Aerobic (some anaerobic glycolysis)	Anaerobic glycolysis
Myoglobin content	High	High	Low
Glycogen stores	Low	Intermediate	High
Recruitment order	First	Second	Third
Rate of fatigue	Slow (fatigue-resistant)	Intermediate (moderately fatigue-resistant)	Fast (fatigable)
Activities Best Suited For			
	Endurance-type activities—e.g., running a marathon; maintaining posture (antigravity muscles)	Sprinting, walking	Short-term intense or powerful movements, e.g., hitting a baseball
Structural Characteristics			
Color	Red	Red to pink	White (pale)
Fiber diameter	Small	Intermediate	Large
Mitochondria	Many	Many	Few
Capillaries	Many	Many	Few

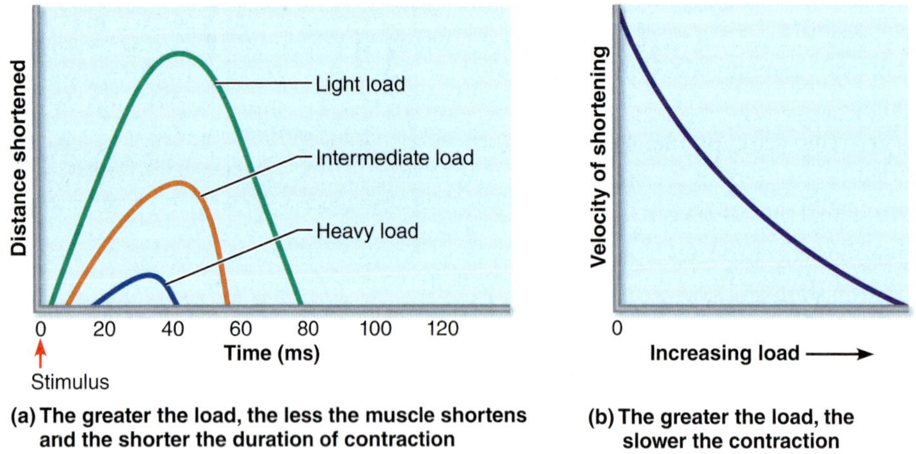

Figure 9.24 **Influence of load on duration and velocity of muscle contraction.**

Finally, consider the less common intermediate muscle fiber types, called *fast oxidative fibers* (Table 9.2, middle column). They have many characteristics intermediate between the other two types (fiber diameter and power, for example). Like fast glycolytic fibers, they contract quickly, but like slow oxidative fibers, they are oxygen dependent and have a rich supply of myoglobin and capillaries.

Some muscles have a predominance of one fiber type, but most contain a mixture of fiber types, which gives them a range of contractile speeds and fatigue resistance. For example, a calf muscle can propel us in a sprint (using its white fast glycolytic fibers) or a long-distance race (making good use of its slow and fast oxidative fibers). But, as might be expected, all muscle fibers in a particular *motor unit* are of the same type.

Although everyone's muscles contain mixtures of the three fiber types, some people have relatively more of one kind. These differences are genetically initiated, but can be modified by exercise and no doubt determine athletic capabilities, such as endurance versus strength, to a large extent. For example, muscles of marathon runners have a high percentage of slow oxidative fibers (about 80%), while those of sprinters contain a higher percentage (about 60%) of fast oxidative and glycolytic fibers. Interconversion between the "fast" fiber types occurs as a result of specific exercise regimes, as we'll describe below.

Load

Because muscles are attached to bones, they are always pitted against some resistance, or load, when they contract. As you might expect, they contract fastest when there is no added load on them. A greater load results in a longer latent period, a slower contraction, and a shorter duration of contraction **(Figure 9.24)**. If the load exceeds the muscle's maximum tension, the speed of shortening is zero and the contraction is isometric (see Figure 9.18b).

Recruitment

In the same way that many hands on a project can get a job done more quickly and also can keep working longer, the more motor units that are contracting, the faster and more prolonged the contraction.

☑ Check Your Understanding

14. List two factors that influence contractile force and two that influence velocity of contraction.
15. Jim called several friends to help him move. Would he prefer to have those with more slow oxidative muscle fibers or those with more fast glycolytic fibers as his helpers? Why?

For answers, see Appendix H.

Adaptations to Exercise

✓ Compare and contrast the effects of aerobic and resistance exercise on skeletal muscles and on other body systems.

The amount of work a muscle does is reflected in changes in the muscle itself. When used actively or strenuously, muscles may become larger or stronger, or more efficient and fatigue resistant. Inactivity, on the other hand, *always* leads to muscle weakness and wasting.

Aerobic (Endurance) Exercise

Aerobic, or **endurance**, **exercise** such as swimming, jogging, fast walking, and biking results in several recognizable changes in skeletal muscles:

- The number of capillaries surrounding the muscle fibers increases.
- The number of mitochondria within the muscle fibers also increases.
- The fibers synthesize more myoglobin.

These changes occur in all fiber types, but are most dramatic in slow oxidative fibers, which depend primarily on aerobic pathways. The changes result in more efficient muscle metabolism and in greater endurance, strength, and resistance to fatigue. Additionally, regular endurance exercise may convert fast glycolytic fibers into fast oxidative fibers.

Resistance Exercise

The moderately weak but sustained muscle activity required for endurance exercise does not promote significant skeletal muscle hypertrophy, even though the exercise may go on for hours. Muscle hypertrophy—think of the bulging biceps and chest muscles of a professional weight lifter—results mainly from high-intensity **resistance exercise** (typically under anaerobic conditions) such as weight lifting or isometric exercise, which pits muscles against high-resistance or immovable forces. Here strength, not stamina, is important, and a few minutes every other day is sufficient to allow a proverbial weakling to put on 50% more muscle within a year.

The additional muscle bulk largely reflects the increased size of individual muscle fibers (particularly the fast glycolytic variety) rather than an increased number of muscle fibers. [However, some of the bulk may result from longitudinal splitting of the fibers and subsequent growth of these "split" cells, or from the proliferation and fusion of satellite cells (see p. 312). The controversy is still raging.] Vigorously stressed muscle fibers also contain more mitochondria, form more myofilaments and myofibrils, store more glycogen, and develop more connective tissue between muscle cells.

Collectively these changes promote significant increases in muscle strength and size. Resistance activities can also convert fast oxidative fibers to fast glycolytic fibers. However, if the specific exercise routine is discontinued, the converted fibers revert to their original metabolic properties.

Resistance training can produce incredibly bulging muscles, but if done unwisely, some muscles may develop more than others. Because muscles work in antagonistic pairs or groups, opposing muscles must be equally strong to work together smoothly. When muscle training is not balanced, individuals can become *muscle-bound*, which means they lack flexibility, have a generally awkward stance, and are unable to make full use of their muscles.

A Balanced Exercise Program

Whatever the activity, exercise gains adhere to the *overload principle*. Forcing a muscle to work hard increases muscle strength and endurance. As muscles adapt to these greater demands, they must be overloaded even more to produce further gains.

However, always follow a heavy-workout day with a day of rest or an easy workout to let your muscles recover and repair themselves. Doing too much too soon, or ignoring the warning signs of muscle or joint pain, increases your risk of **overuse injuries** that may lead to lifetime disability.

Endurance and resistance exercises produce different patterns of muscular response, so it is important to know what your exercise goals are. Lifting weights will not improve your endurance for a triathlon. By the same token, jogging will do little to improve your muscle definition or enhance your strength for moving furniture. A program that alternates aerobic and anaerobic activities provides the best balance for optimal health.

Homeostatic Imbalance 9.3

To remain healthy, muscles must be active. Immobilization due to enforced bed rest or loss of neural stimulation results in *disuse atrophy* (degeneration and loss of mass), which begins almost as soon as the muscles are immobilized. Under such conditions, muscle strength can decline at the rate of 5% per day!

As noted earlier, even at rest, muscles receive weak intermittent stimuli from the nervous system. When totally deprived of neural stimulation, a paralyzed muscle may atrophy to one-quarter of its initial size. Fibrous connective tissue replaces the lost muscle tissue, making muscle rehabilitation impossible. +

Check Your Understanding

16. How do aerobic and resistance exercise differ in their effects on muscle size and function?

For answers, see Appendix H.

Smooth Muscle

- ✓ Compare the gross and microscopic anatomy of smooth muscle cells to that of skeletal muscle cells.
- ✓ Compare and contrast the contractile mechanisms and the means of activation of skeletal and smooth muscles.
- ✓ Distinguish between unitary and multi unit smooth muscle structurally and functionally.

Except for the heart, which is made of cardiac muscle, the muscle in the walls of all the body's hollow organs is almost entirely smooth muscle. The chemical and mechanical events of contraction are essentially the same in all muscle tissues, but smooth muscle is distinctive in several ways, as summarized in **Table 9.3** on p. 310.

Microscopic Structure of Smooth Muscle Fibers

Smooth muscle fibers are spindle-shaped cells of variable size, each with one centrally located nucleus **(Figure 9.25b)**. Typically, they have a diameter of 5–10 μm and are 30–200 μm long. Skeletal muscle fibers are up to 10 times wider and thousands of times longer.

Smooth muscle lacks the coarse connective tissue sheaths seen in skeletal muscle. However, a small amount of fine connective tissue (endomysium), secreted by the smooth muscles themselves and containing blood vessels and nerves, is found between smooth muscle fibers.

Most smooth muscle is organized into sheets of closely apposed fibers. These sheets occur in the walls of all but the smallest blood vessels and in the walls of hollow organs of the respiratory, digestive, urinary, and reproductive tracts. In most cases, there are two sheets of smooth muscle with their fibers oriented at right angles to each other, as in the intestine (Figure 9.25).

- In the *longitudinal layer*, the muscle fibers run parallel to the long axis of the organ. Consequently, when these fibers contract, the organ dilates and shortens.

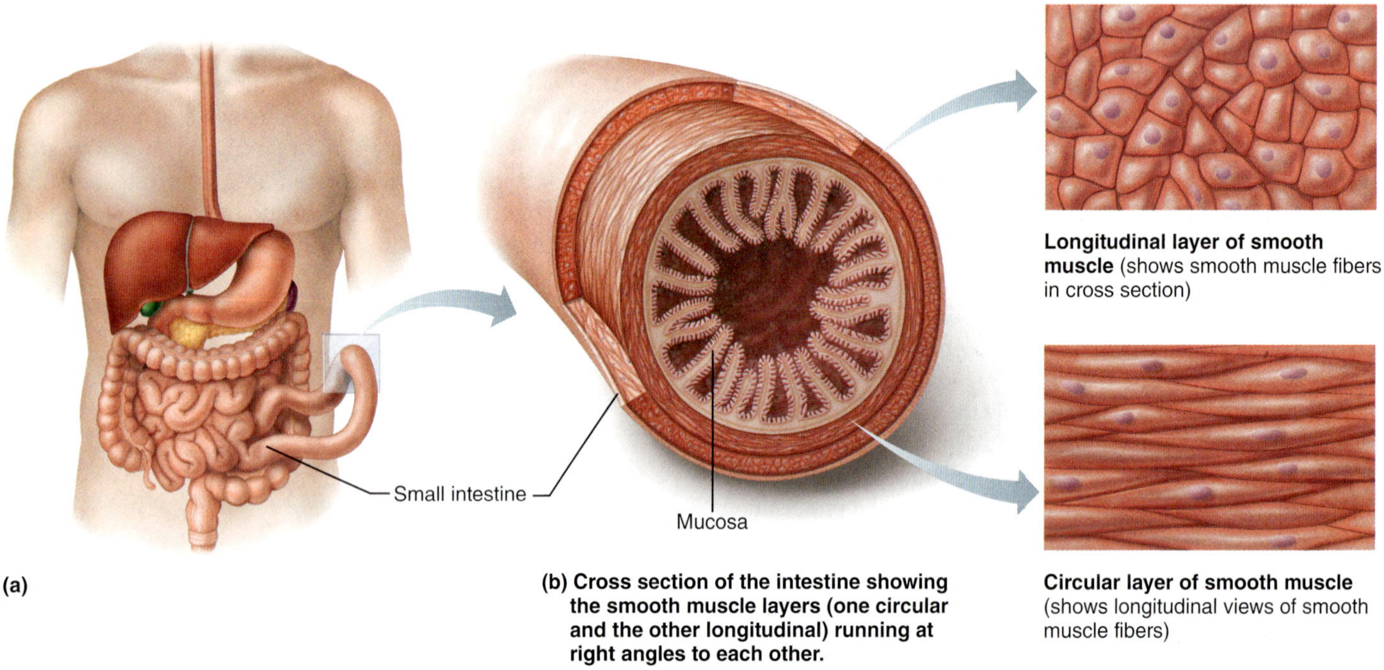

Figure 9.25 Arrangement of smooth muscle in the walls of hollow organs.

- In the *circular layer*, the fibers run around the circumference of the organ. Contraction of this layer constricts the lumen of the organ and elongates the organ.

The alternating contraction and relaxation of these layers mixes substances in the lumen and squeezes them through the organ's internal pathway. This propulsive action is called **peristalsis** (per″ĭ-stal′sis; "around contraction"). Contraction of smooth muscle in the rectum, urinary bladder, and uterus helps those organs to expel their contents. Smooth muscle contraction also accounts for the constricted breathing of asthma and for stomach cramps.

Smooth muscle lacks the highly structured neuromuscular junctions of skeletal muscle. Instead, the innervating nerve fibers, which are part of the autonomic (involuntary) nervous system, have numerous bulbous swellings, called **varicosities** (**Figure 9.26**). The varicosities release neurotransmitter into a wide synaptic cleft in the general area of the smooth muscle cells. Such junctions are called **diffuse junctions**. Comparing the neural input to skeletal and smooth muscles, you could say that skeletal muscle gets priority mail while smooth muscle gets bulk mailings.

The sarcoplasmic reticulum of smooth muscle fibers is much less developed than that of skeletal muscle and lacks a specific pattern relative to the myofilaments. Some SR tubules of smooth muscle touch the sarcolemma at several sites, forming what resembles half-triads that may couple the action potential to calcium release from the SR.

T tubules are absent, but the sarcolemma has multiple **caveolae**, pouchlike infoldings that sequester bits of extracellular fluid containing a high concentration of Ca^{2+} close to the membrane (**Figure 9.27a**). Consequently, when calcium channels in the caveolae open, Ca^{2+} influx occurs rapidly. Although the SR *does* release some of the calcium that triggers contraction, most Ca^{2+} enters through calcium channels directly from the extracellular space. This situation is quite different from what we see in skeletal muscle, which does not depend on extracellular Ca^{2+} for excitation-contraction coupling. Contraction ends when cytoplasmic calcium is actively transported into the SR and out of the cell.

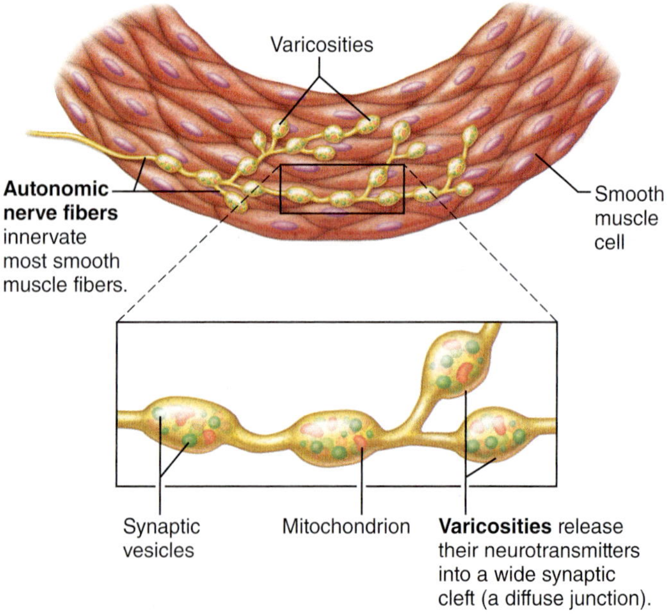

Figure 9.26 Innervation of smooth muscle.

There are no striations in smooth muscle, as its name indicates, and therefore no sarcomeres. Smooth muscle fibers do contain interdigitating thick and thin filaments, but the myosin filaments are a lot shorter than the actin filaments and the type of myosin contained differs from skeletal muscle. The proportion and organization of smooth muscle myofilaments differ from skeletal muscle in the following ways:

- **Thick filaments are fewer but have myosin heads along their entire length.** The ratio of thick to thin filaments is much lower in smooth muscle than in skeletal muscle (1:13 compared to 1:2). However, thick filaments of smooth muscle contain actin-gripping myosin heads along their *entire length,* a feature that makes smooth muscle as powerful as a skeletal muscle of the same size. Also, in smooth muscle the myosin heads are oriented in one direction on one side of the filament and in the opposite direction on the other side.
- **No troponin complex in thin filaments.** As in skeletal muscle, tropomyosin mechanically stabilizes the thin filaments, but smooth muscle has no calcium-binding troponin complex. Instead, a protein called *calmodulin* acts as the calcium-binding site.
- **Thick and thin filaments arranged diagonally.** Bundles of contractile proteins crisscross within the smooth muscle cell so they spiral down the long axis of the cell like the stripes on a barber pole. Because of this diagonal arrangement, the smooth muscle cells contract in a twisting way so that they look like tiny corkscrews (Figure 9.27b).
- **Intermediate filament–dense body network.** Smooth muscle fibers contain a lattice-like arrangement of noncontractile *intermediate filaments* that resist tension. They attach at regular intervals to cytoplasmic structures called dense bodies (Figure 9.27). The **dense bodies**, which are also tethered to the sarcolemma, act as anchoring points for thin filaments and therefore correspond to Z discs of skeletal muscle.

  The intermediate filament–dense body network forms a strong, cable-like intracellular cytoskeleton that harnesses the pull generated by the sliding of the thick and thin filaments. During contraction, areas of the sarcolemma between the dense bodies bulge outward, making the cell look puffy (Figure 9.27b). Dense bodies at the sarcolemma surface also bind the muscle cell to the connective tissue fibers outside the cell (endomysium) and to adjacent cells. This arrangement transmits the pulling force to the surrounding connective tissue and partly accounts for the synchronous contractions of most smooth muscle.

Contraction of Smooth Muscle

Mechanism of Contraction

In most cases, adjacent smooth muscle fibers exhibit slow, synchronized contractions, the whole sheet responding to a stimulus in unison. This synchronization reflects electrical coupling of smooth muscle cells by *gap junctions*, specialized cell connections described in Chapter 3. Skeletal muscle fibers are electrically isolated from one another, each stimulated to contract by its own neuromuscular junction. By contrast, gap junctions allow smooth muscles to transmit action potentials from fiber to fiber.

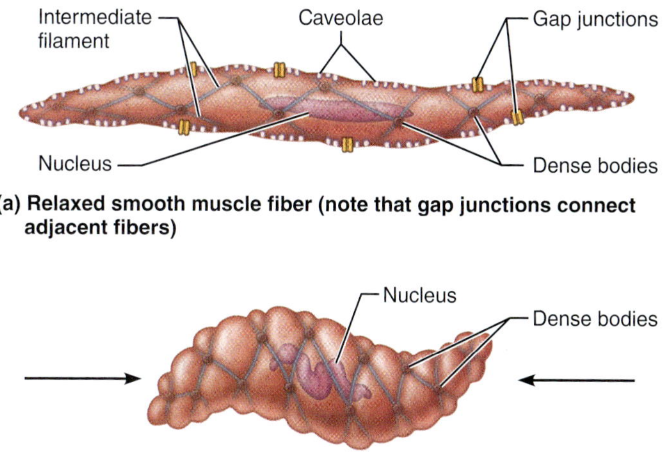

Figure 9.27 Intermediate filaments and dense bodies of smooth muscle fibers harness the pull generated by myosin cross bridges. Intermediate filaments attach to dense bodies throughout the sarcoplasm.

Some smooth muscle fibers in the stomach and small intestine are *pacemaker cells*: Once excited, they act as "drummers" to set the pace of contraction for the entire muscle sheet. These pacemakers have fluctuating membrane potentials and are self-excitatory, that is, they depolarize spontaneously in the absence of external stimuli. However, neural and chemical stimuli can modify both the rate and the intensity of smooth muscle contraction.

Contraction in smooth muscle is like contraction in skeletal muscle in the following ways:

- Actin and myosin interact by the sliding filament mechanism.
- The final trigger for contraction is a rise in the intracellular calcium ion level.
- ATP energizes the sliding process.

During excitation-contraction coupling, the tubules of the SR release Ca^{2+}, but, as mentioned above, Ca^{2+} also moves into the cell from the extracellular space via membrane channels. In all striated muscle types, calcium ions activate myosin by binding to troponin. In smooth muscle, calcium activates myosin by interacting with a regulatory molecule called **calmodulin**, a cytoplasmic calcium-binding protein. Calmodulin, in turn, interacts with a kinase enzyme called **myosin kinase** or **myosin light chain kinase** which phosphorylates the myosin, activating it **(Figure 9.28)**.

As in skeletal muscle, smooth muscle relaxes when intracellular Ca^{2+} levels drop—but getting smooth muscle to stop contracting is more complex. Events known to be involved include calcium detachment from calmodulin, active transport of Ca^{2+} into the SR and extracellular fluid, and dephosphorylation of myosin by a phosphorylase enzyme, which reduces the activity of the myosin ATPases.

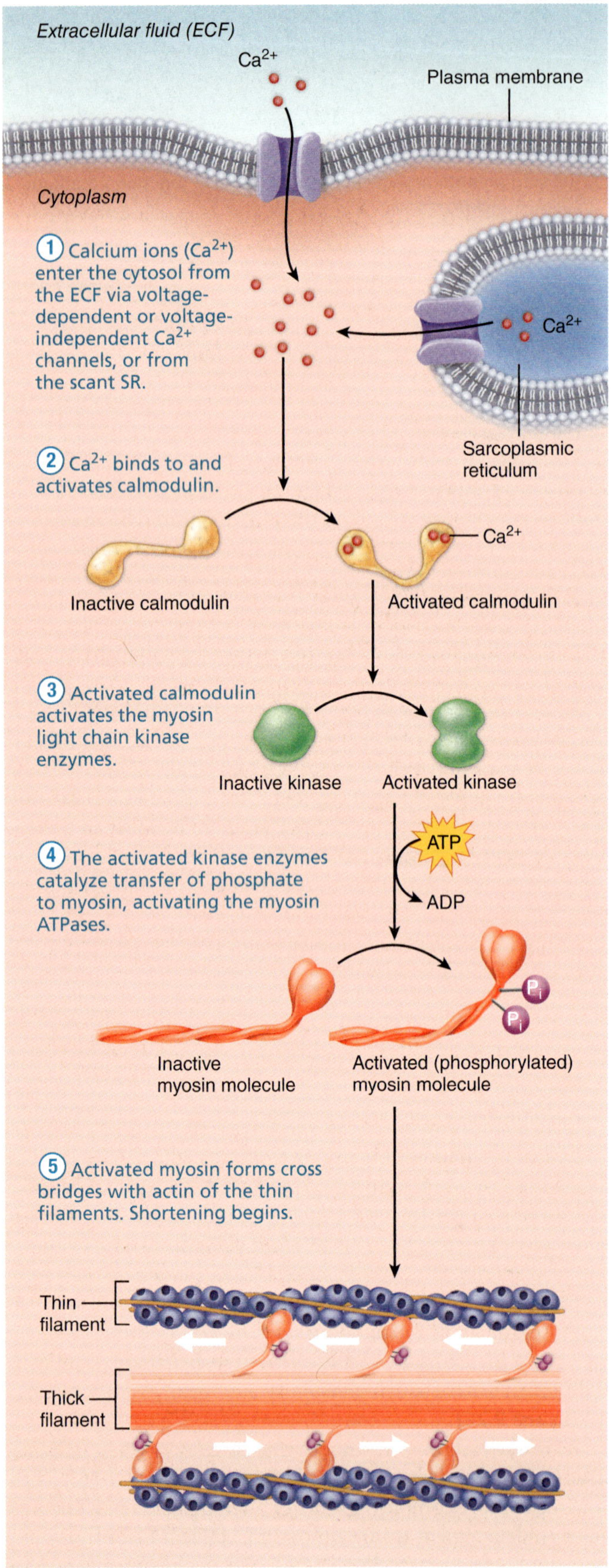

Figure 9.28 **Sequence of events in excitation-contraction coupling of smooth muscle.**

Energy Efficiency of Smooth Muscle Contraction

Smooth muscle takes 30 times longer to contract and relax than does skeletal muscle, but it can maintain the same contractile tension for prolonged periods at less than 1% of the energy cost. If skeletal muscle is like a speedy windup car that quickly runs down, then smooth muscle is like a steady, heavy-duty engine that lumbers along tirelessly.

Part of the striking energy economy of smooth muscle is the sluggishness of its ATPases compared to those in skeletal muscle. Moreover, smooth muscle myofilaments may latch together during prolonged contractions, saving energy in that way as well. Smooth muscle cells may maintain that *latch state* even after myosin is dephosphorylated.

The smooth muscle in small arterioles and other visceral organs routinely maintains a moderate degree of contraction, called *smooth muscle tone*, day in and day out without fatiguing. Smooth muscle has low energy requirements, and as a rule, it makes enough ATP via aerobic pathways to keep up with the demand.

Regulation of Contraction

The contraction of smooth muscle can be regulated by nerves, hormones, or local chemical changes. Let's briefly consider each of these methods.

Neural Regulation In some cases, the activation of smooth muscle by a neural stimulus is identical to that in skeletal muscle: Neurotransmitter binding generates an action potential, which is coupled to a rise in calcium ions in the cytosol. However, some types of smooth muscle respond to neural stimulation with graded potentials (local electrical signals) only.

Recall that all somatic nerve endings, that is, nerve endings that excite skeletal muscle, release the neurotransmitter acetylcholine. However, different autonomic nerves serving the smooth muscle of visceral organs release different neurotransmitters, each of which may excite or inhibit a particular group of smooth muscle cells.

The effect of a specific neurotransmitter on a smooth muscle cell depends on the type of receptor molecules on the cell's sarcolemma. For example, when acetylcholine binds to ACh receptors on smooth muscle in the bronchioles (small air passageways of the lungs), the response is strong contraction that narrows the bronchioles. When norepinephrine, released by a different type of autonomic nerve fiber, binds to norepinephrine receptors on the *same* smooth muscle cells, the effect is inhibitory—the muscle relaxes, which dilates the bronchioles. However, when norepinephrine binds to smooth muscle in the walls of most blood vessels, it stimulates the smooth muscle cells to contract and constrict the vessel.

Hormones and Local Chemical Factors Some smooth muscle layers have no nerve supply at all. Instead, they depolarize spontaneously or in response to chemical stimuli that bind to G protein–linked receptors. Other smooth muscle cells respond to both neural and chemical stimuli.

Several chemical factors cause smooth muscle to contract or relax without an action potential by enhancing or inhibiting

Ca^{2+} entry into the sarcoplasm. They include certain hormones, histamine, excess carbon dioxide, low pH, and lack of oxygen. The direct response to these chemical stimuli alters smooth muscle activity according to local tissue needs and probably is most responsible for smooth muscle tone. For example, the hormone gastrin stimulates stomach smooth muscle to contract so it can churn foodstuffs more efficiently. We will consider activation of smooth muscle in specific organs as we discuss each organ in subsequent chapters.

Special Features of Smooth Muscle Contraction

Smooth muscle is intimately involved in the functioning of most hollow organs and has a number of unique characteristics. We have already considered some of these—smooth muscle tone, slow prolonged contractions, and low energy requirements. But smooth muscle also responds differently to stretch and can lengthen and shorten more than other muscle types. Let's take a look.

Response to Stretch Up to a point, when skeletal muscle is stretched, it responds with more vigorous contractions. Stretching of smooth muscle also provokes contraction, which automatically moves substances along an internal tract. However, the increased tension persists only briefly, and soon the muscle adapts to its new length and relaxes, while still retaining the ability to contract on demand.

This **stress-relaxation response** allows a hollow organ to fill or expand slowly to accommodate a greater volume without causing strong contractions that would expel its contents. This is an important attribute, because organs such as the stomach and intestines must store their contents long enough to digest and absorb the nutrients. Likewise, your urinary bladder must be able to store the continuously made urine until it is convenient to empty your bladder, or you would spend all your time in the bathroom.

Length and Tension Changes Smooth muscle stretches much more and generates more tension than skeletal muscles stretched to a comparable extent. As we saw in Figure 9.22, precise, highly organized sarcomeres limit how far a skeletal muscle can stretch before it is unable to generate force.

In contrast, the irregular, overlapping arrangement of smooth muscle filaments and the lack of sarcomeres allow them to generate considerable force, even when they are substantially stretched. The total length change that skeletal muscles can undergo and still function efficiently is about 60% (from 30% shorter to 30% longer than resting length), but smooth muscle can contract when it is anywhere from half to twice its resting length—a total range of 150%. This capability allows hollow organs to tolerate tremendous changes in volume without becoming flabby when they empty.

Hyperplasia All muscle cells can hypertrophy (increase in cell size), but certain smooth muscle fibers can also undergo *hyperplasia*, that is, they divide to increase their numbers. Consider the response of the uterus to the hormone estrogen. At puberty, girls' blood estrogen levels rise. As estrogen binds to uterine smooth muscle receptors, it stimulates the synthesis of more uterine smooth muscle, causing the uterus to grow to adult size. During pregnancy, high blood levels of estrogen stimulate uterine hyperplasia to accommodate the growing fetus.

Types of Smooth Muscle

The smooth muscle in different body organs varies substantially in its (1) fiber arrangement and organization, (2) innervation, and (3) responsiveness to various stimuli. For simplicity, however, smooth muscle is usually categorized into two major types: *unitary* and *multi unit.*

Unitary Smooth Muscle

Unitary smooth muscle, commonly called **visceral muscle** because it is in the walls of all hollow organs except the heart, is far more common. All the smooth muscle characteristics described so far pertain to unitary smooth muscle.

For example, the cells of unitary smooth muscle

- Are arranged in opposing (longitudinal and circular) sheets
- Are innervated by varicosities of autonomic nerve fibers and often exhibit rhythmic spontaneous action potentials
- Are electrically coupled by gap junctions and so contract as a unit (for this reason recruitment is not an option in unitary smooth muscle)
- Respond to various chemical stimuli

Multi Unit Smooth Muscle

The smooth muscles in the large airways to the lungs and in large arteries, the arrector pili muscles attached to hair follicles, and the internal eye muscles that adjust pupil size and allow the eye to focus visually are all examples of **multi unit smooth muscle**.

In contrast to unitary muscle, gap junctions and spontaneous depolarizations are rare. Like skeletal muscle, multi unit smooth muscle

- Consists of muscle fibers that are structurally independent of one another
- Is richly supplied with nerve endings, each of which forms a motor unit with a number of muscle fibers
- Responds to neural stimulation with graded contractions that involve recruitment

However, skeletal muscle is served by the somatic (voluntary) division of the nervous system. Multi unit smooth muscle, like unitary smooth muscle, is innervated by the autonomic (involuntary) division and also responds to hormones.

☑ Check Your Understanding

17. Compare the structures of skeletal and smooth muscle fibers.
18. Calcium is the trigger for contraction of all muscle types. How does its binding site differ in skeletal and smooth muscle fibers?
19. How does the stress-relaxation response suit the role of smooth muscle in hollow organs?

For answers, see Appendix H.

(Text continues on p. 312.)

Table 9.3 Comparison of Skeletal, Cardiac, and Smooth Muscle

<table>
<tr><th>CHARACTERISTIC</th><th>SKELETAL</th><th>CARDIAC</th><th>SMOOTH</th></tr>
<tr><td>Body location</td><td>Attached to bones or (some facial muscles) to skin
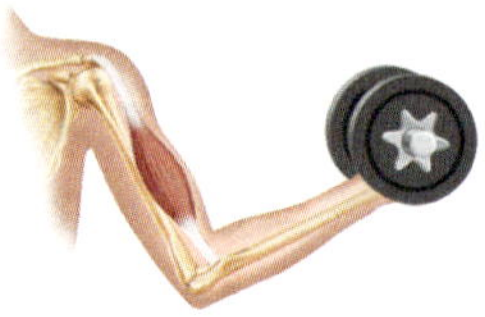</td><td>Walls of the heart
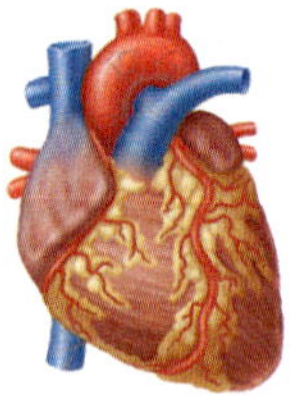</td><td>Unitary muscle in walls of hollow visceral organs (other than the heart); multi unit muscle in intrinsic eye muscles, airways, large arteries
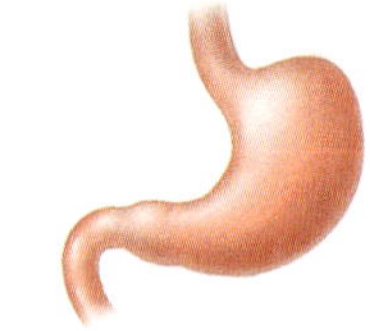</td></tr>
<tr><td>Cell shape and appearance</td><td>Single, very long, cylindrical, multinucleate cells with obvious striations
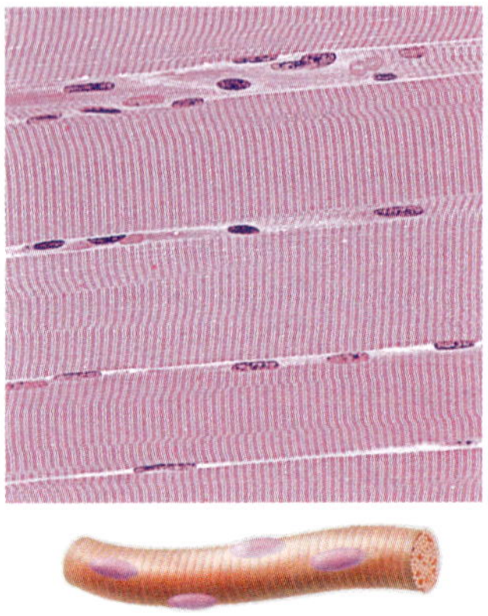</td><td>Branching chains of cells; uni- or binucleate; striations
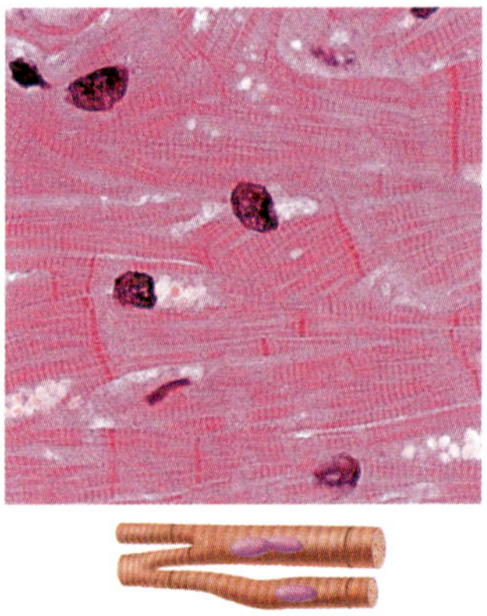</td><td>Single, fusiform, uninucleate; no striations
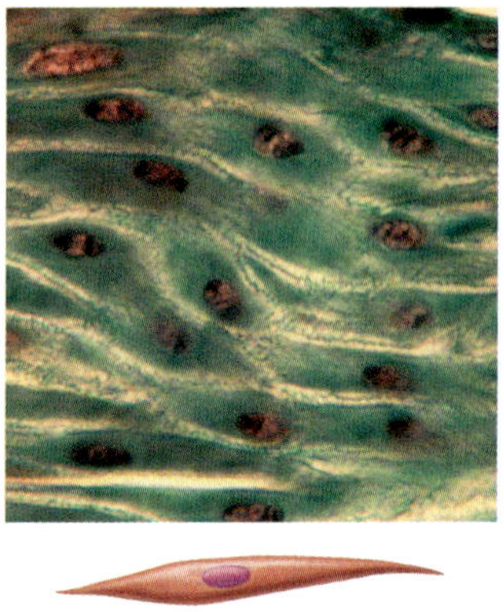</td></tr>
<tr><td>Connective tissue components</td><td>Epimysium, perimysium, and endomysium
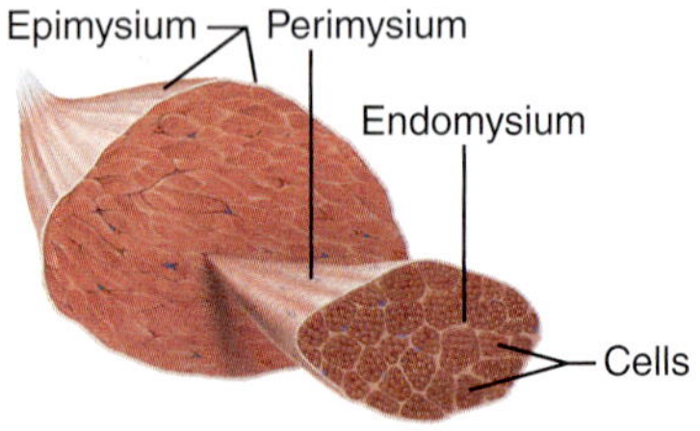</td><td>Endomysium attached to fibrous skeleton of heart
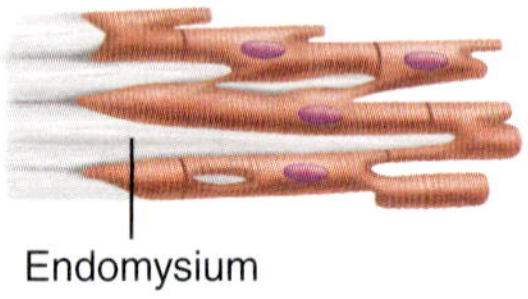</td><td>Endomysium
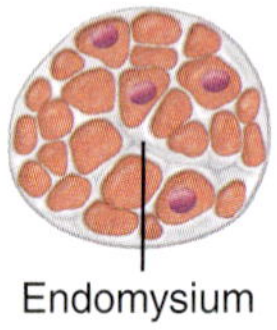</td></tr>
<tr><td>Presence of myofibrils composed of sarcomeres</td><td>Yes</td><td>Yes, but myofibrils are of irregular thickness</td><td>No, but actin and myosin filaments are present throughout; dense bodies anchor actin filaments</td></tr>
<tr><td>Presence of T tubules and site of invagination</td><td>Yes; two in each sarcomere at A-I junctions
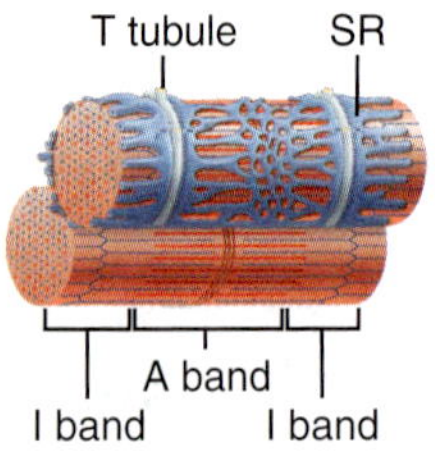</td><td>Yes; one in each sarcomere at Z disc; larger diameter than those of skeletal muscle
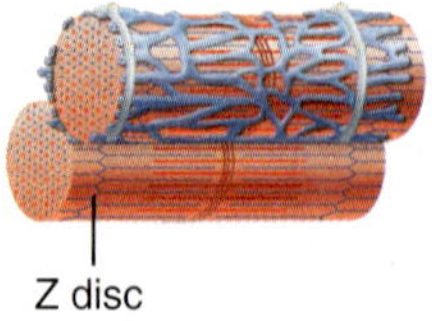</td><td>No; only caveolae</td></tr>
</table>

Table 9.3 *(continued)*

CHARACTERISTIC	SKELETAL	CARDIAC	SMOOTH
Elaborate sarcoplasmic reticulum	Yes	Less than skeletal muscle (1–8% of cell volume); scant terminal cisterns	Equivalent to cardiac muscle (1–8% of cell volume); some SR contacts the sarcolemma
Presence of gap junctions	No	Yes; at intercalated discs	Yes; in unitary muscle
Cells exhibit individual neuromuscular junctions	Yes 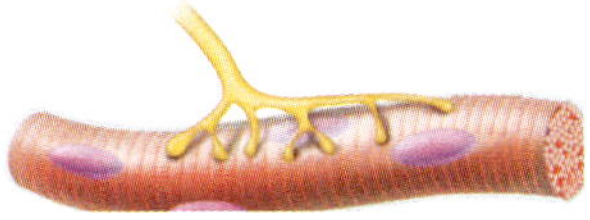	No	Not in unitary muscle; yes in multi unit muscle 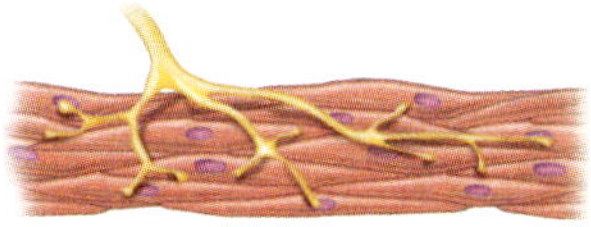
Regulation of contraction	Voluntary via axon terminals of the somatic nervous system 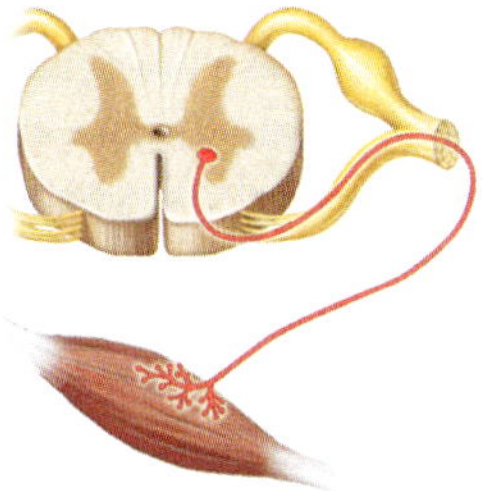	Involuntary; intrinsic system regulation; also autonomic nervous system controls; hormones; stretch 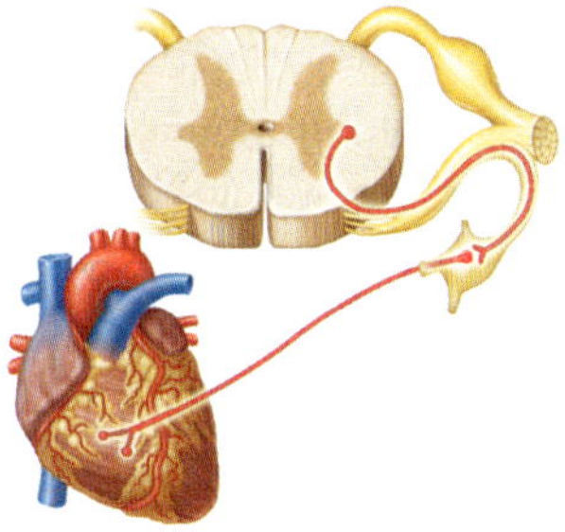	Involuntary; autonomic nerves, hormones, local chemicals; stretch 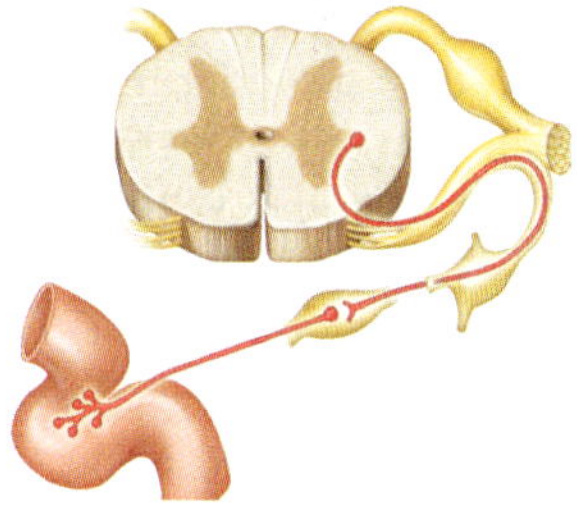
Source of Ca^{2+} for calcium pulse	Sarcoplasmic reticulum (SR)	SR and from extracellular fluid	SR and from extracellular fluid
Site of calcium regulation	Troponin on actin-containing thin filaments 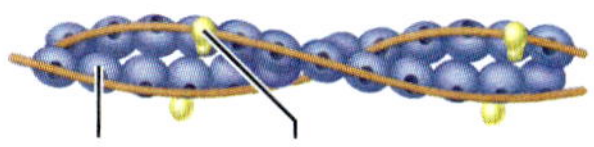	Troponin on actin-containing thin filaments 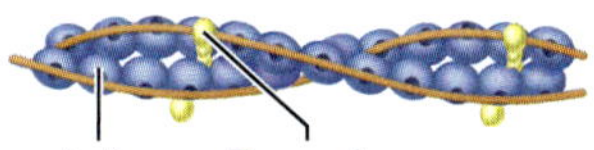	Calmodulin in the cytosol 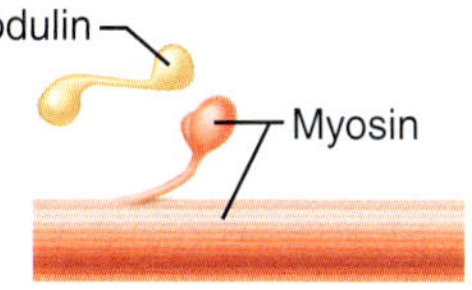
Presence of pacemaker(s)	No	Yes	Yes (in unitary muscle only)
Effect of nervous system stimulation	Excitation	Excitation or inhibition	Excitation or inhibition
Speed of contraction	Slow to fast 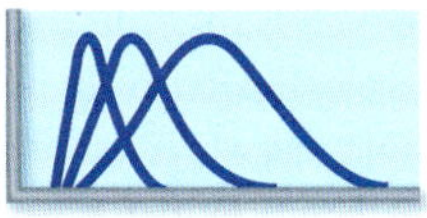	Slow 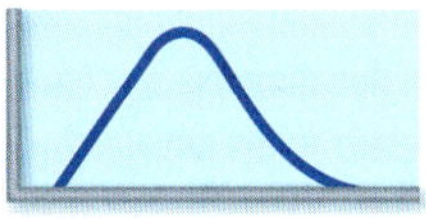	Very slow 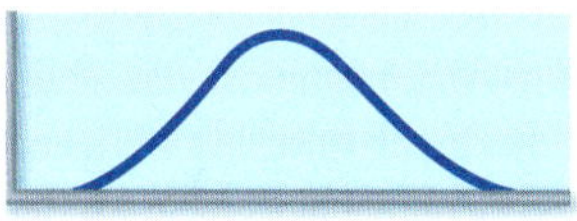
Rhythmic contraction	No	Yes	Yes in unitary muscle
Response to stretch	Contractile strength increases with degree of stretch (to a point)	Contractile strength increases with degree of stretch	Stress-relaxation response
Respiration	Aerobic and anaerobic	Aerobic	Mainly aerobic

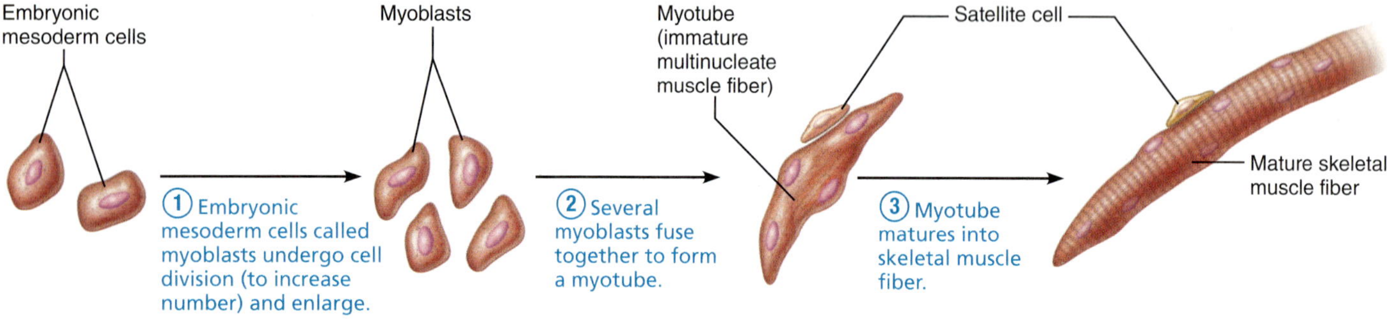

Figure 9.29 **Myoblasts fuse to form a multinucleate skeletal muscle fiber.**

Developmental Aspects of Muscles

✓ Describe embryonic development of muscle tissues and the changes that occur in skeletal muscles with age.

With rare exceptions, all three types of muscle tissue develop from embryonic mesoderm cells called **myoblasts**. In forming skeletal muscle tissue, several myoblasts fuse to form multinuclear *myotubes* **(Figure 9.29)**. Integrins (cell adhesion proteins) in the myoblast membranes guide this process and soon functional sarcomeres appear. Skeletal muscle fibers are contracting by week 7 when the embryo is only about 2.5 cm (1 inch) long.

Initially, ACh receptors "sprout" over the entire surface of the developing myoblasts. As spinal nerves invade the muscle masses, the nerve endings target individual myoblasts and release the growth factor *agrin*. This chemical activates a muscle kinase (MuSK), which stimulates clustering and maintenance of ACh receptors at the newly forming neuromuscular junction in each muscle fiber. Then, the nerve endings release a different chemical that eliminates the receptor sites not innervated or stabilized by agrin.

Electrical activity in the neurons serving the muscle fibers also plays a critical role in muscle fiber maturation. As the somatic nervous system assumes control of muscle fibers, the number of fast and slow contractile fiber types is determined.

Myoblasts producing cardiac and smooth muscle cells do not fuse but develop gap junctions at a very early embryonic stage. Cardiac muscle is pumping blood just 3 weeks after fertilization. Specialized skeletal and cardiac muscle cells stop dividing early on but retain the ability to lengthen and thicken in a growing child and to hypertrophy in adults.

- *Satellite cells,* myoblast-like cells associated with skeletal muscle, help repair injured fibers and allow limited regeneration of dead skeletal muscle, a capability that declines with age.
- Cardiac muscle was thought to have no regenerative capability whatsoever, but recent studies suggest that cardiac cells do divide at a modest rate. Nonetheless, injured heart muscle is repaired mostly by scar tissue.
- Smooth muscles have a good regenerative capacity and smooth muscle cells of blood vessels divide regularly throughout life.

At birth, a baby's movements are uncoordinated and largely reflexive. Muscular development reflects the level of neuromuscular coordination, which develops in a head-to-toe and proximal-to-distal direction. In other words, a baby can lift its head before it can walk, and gross movements precede fine ones.

All through childhood, our control of our skeletal muscles becomes more and more sophisticated. By midadolescence, we reach the peak of our natural neural control of muscles, but can improve it by athletic or other types of training.

A frequently asked question is whether the strength difference between women and men has a biological basis. It does. Individuals vary, but on average, women's skeletal muscles make up approximately 36% of body mass, whereas men's account for about 42%. Men's greater muscular development is due primarily to the effects of testosterone on skeletal muscle, not to the effects of exercise. Body strength per unit muscle mass, however, is the same in both sexes. Strenuous muscle exercise causes more muscle enlargement in males than in females, again because of the influence of testosterone. Some athletes take large doses of synthetic male sex hormones ("steroids") to increase their muscle mass. *A Closer Look* discusses this illegal and physiologically dangerous practice.

Because of its rich blood supply, skeletal muscle is amazingly resistant to infection. Given good nutrition and moderate exercise, relatively few problems afflict skeletal muscles. However, muscular dystrophy, the world's most common genetic disorder, is a serious condition that deserves more than a passing mention.

Homeostatic Imbalance 9.4

The term **muscular dystrophy** refers to a group of inherited muscle-destroying diseases that generally appear during childhood. The affected muscles initially enlarge due to deposits of fat and connective tissue, but the muscle fibers atrophy and degenerate.

The most common and serious form is **Duchenne muscular dystrophy (DMD)**, which is inherited as a sex-linked recessive disease. It is expressed almost exclusively in males (one in every 3600 male births). This tragic disease is usually diagnosed when the boy is between 2 and 7 years old. Active, normal-appearing children become clumsy and fall frequently as their skeletal muscles weaken. The disease progresses relentlessly from the extremities upward, finally affecting the head and chest muscles and cardiac muscle. Victims rarely live beyond their early 20s, dying of respiratory failure.

DMD is caused by a defective gene for *dystrophin*, a cytoplasmic protein that links the cytoskeleton to the extracellular matrix and, like a girder, helps stabilize the sarcolemma. The fragile sarcolemma of DMD patients tears during contraction, allowing entry of excess Ca^{2+}. The deranged calcium homeostasis damages

A CLOSER LOOK

Athletes Looking Good and Doing Better with Anabolic Steroids?

Society loves a winner and top **athletes** reap large social and monetary rewards. It is not surprising that some will grasp at anything that might increase their **performance**—including "juice," or anabolic **steroids**.

These drugs are variants of the male sex hormone **testosterone** engineered by pharmaceutical companies. They were introduced in the 1950s to treat anemia and certain muscle-wasting diseases and to prevent muscle atrophy in patients immobilized after surgery. Testosterone is responsible for the increase in muscle and bone mass and other physical changes that occur during puberty and converts boys into men.

Convinced that megadoses of steroids could produce enhanced masculinizing effects in grown men, many athletes and bodybuilders were using them by the early 1960s, a practice that is still going on. Investigations have stunned sports fans with revelations of steroid use by many elite athletes including Barry Bonds, formerly of the San Francisco Giants; Mark McGwire, formerly with the St. Louis Cardinals; and Marion Jones, one of the most celebrated women athletes of all time.

However, steroid use is not confined to professional athletes. It is estimated that nearly one in every 10 young men has tried them, and their use is also spreading among young women.

It is difficult to determine the extent of anabolic steroid use because most international competitions ban the use of drugs. Users (and prescribing physicians or drug dealers) are naturally reluctant to talk about it, and users stop doping before the event, aware that evidence of drug use is hard to find a week after they stop. Additionally, "underground" suppliers of performance-enhancing drugs keep producing new versions of designer steroids that evade standard antidoping tests. The Olympic Analytical Laboratory in Los Angeles rocked the sports world when it revealed that a number of elite athletes tested positive for tetrahydrogestrinone (THG), a designer steroid not previously known or tested for.

There is little question that many professional bodybuilders and athletes competing in events that require muscle strength (e.g., shot put, discus throwing, and weight lifting) are heavy users. Football players have also admitted using steroids as an adjunct to training, diet, and psychological preparation for games. These athletes claim that anabolic steroids enhance muscle mass and strength, and raise oxygen-carrying capability owing to greater volume of red blood cells.

Typically, bodybuilders who use steroids combine high doses (up to 200 mg/day) via injection or transdermal skin patches with heavy resistance training. Intermittent use begins several months before an event, and commonly entails taking many anabolic steroid supplements (a method called stacking). They increase doses gradually as the competition nears.

Do the drugs do all that is claimed? Research studies report increased isometric strength and body weight in steroid users. While these are results weight lifters dream about, for runners and others requiring fine muscle coordination and endurance these changes may not translate into better performance. The "jury is still out" on this question.

Do the alleged advantages of steroids outweigh their risks? Absolutely not. Anabolic steroids cause: bloated faces (Cushingoid sign of steroid excess), acne and hair loss, shriveled testes and infertility, liver damage that promotes liver cancer, and changes in blood cholesterol levels that may predispose users to heart disease.

In addition, females can develop masculine characteristics such as smaller breasts, enlarged clitoris, excess body hair, and thinning scalp hair. The psychiatric

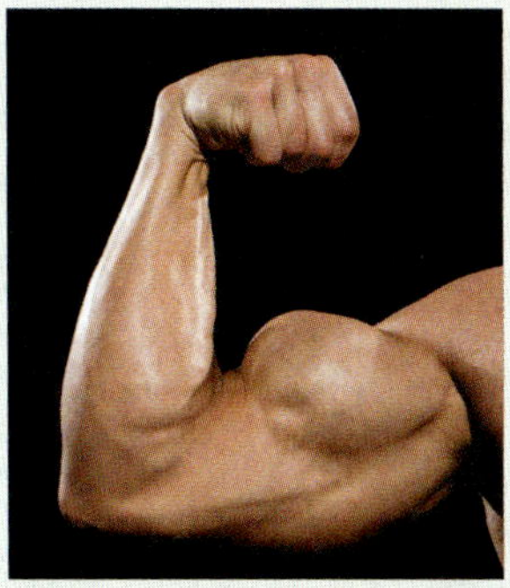

hazards of anabolic steroid use may be equally threatening: Recent studies indicate that one-third of users suffer serious mental problems. Depression, delusions, and manic behavior—in which users undergo Jekyll-and-Hyde personality swings and become extremely violent (termed *'roid rage*)—are all common.

Another recent arrival on the scene, sold over the counter as a "nutritional performance-enhancer," is androstenedione, which is converted to testosterone in the body. Though it is taken orally (and the liver destroys much of it soon after ingestion), the few milligrams that survive temporarily boost testosterone levels. Reports of athletic wannabes from the fifth grade up sweeping the supplement off the drugstore shelves are troubling, particularly since it is not regulated by the U.S. Food and Drug Administration (FDA) and its long-term effects are unknown.

A study at Massachusetts General Hospital found that males who took androstenedione developed higher levels of the female hormone estrogen as well as testosterone, raising their risk of feminizing effects such as enlarged breasts. Youths with elevated levels of estrogen or testosterone may enter puberty early, stunting bone growth and leading to shorter-than-normal adult height.

Some people seem willing to try almost anything to win, short of killing themselves. Are they unwittingly doing this as well?

9

the contractile fibers, and inflammatory cells (macrophages and lymphocytes) accumulate in the surrounding connective tissue. As the regenerative capacity of the muscle is lost, and damaged cells undergo apoptosis, muscle mass drops.

There is still no cure for DMD. Current treatments are aimed at preventing or reducing spine and joint deformities and helping those with DMD remain mobile as long as possible. Thus far the only medication that has improved muscle strength and function is the steroid prednisone, but other immunosuppressant drugs may delay muscle deterioration.

One initially promising technique, *myoblast transfer therapy* (injecting healthy myoblast cells that fuse with diseased myoblasts) has been disappointing. Newer experimental therapies have reversed disease symptoms in dystrophic animal models. One of these involves injection of adeno-associated viruses carrying pared-down microdystrophin genes. A different approach

Homeostatic Interrelationships Between the Muscular System and Other Body Systems

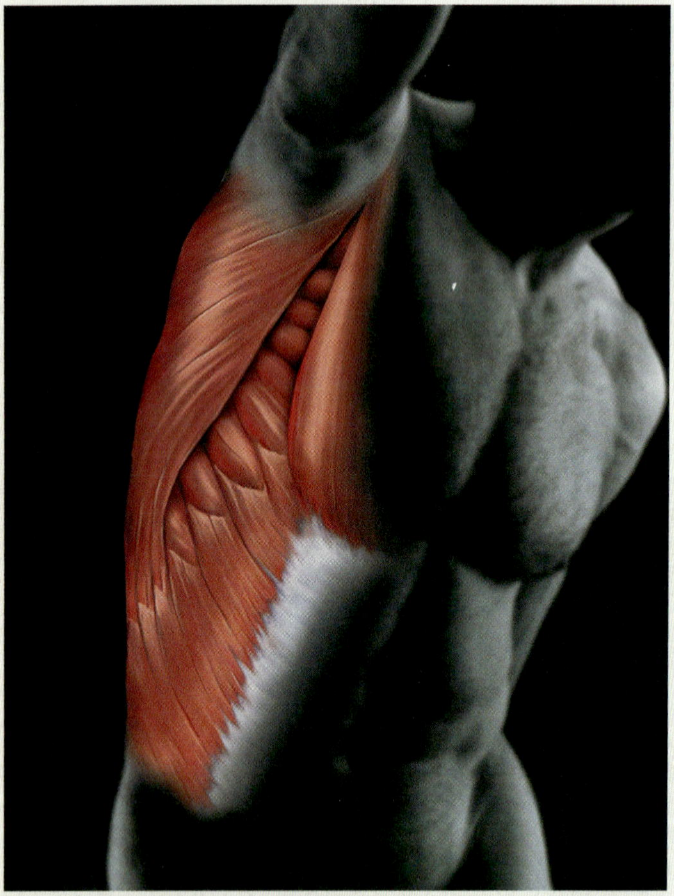

Integumentary System Chapter 5

- Muscular exercise enhances circulation to skin and improves skin health
- Skin protects the muscles by external enclosure; helps dissipate heat generated by the muscles

Skeletal System Chapters 6–8

- Skeletal muscle activity maintains bone health and strength
- Bones provide levers for muscle activity

Nervous System Chapters 11–15

- Facial muscle activity allows emotions to be expressed
- Nervous system stimulates and regulates muscle activity
- Nervous system activity maintains muscle mass

Endocrine System Chapter 16

- Growth hormone and androgens influence skeletal muscle strength and mass; other hormones help regulate cardiac and smooth muscle activity

Cardiovascular System Chapters 17–19

- Skeletal muscle activity increases efficiency of cardiovascular functioning; helps prevent atherosclerosis and causes cardiac hypertrophy
- Cardiovascular system delivers needed oxygen and nutrients to muscles

Lymphatic System/Immunity Chapters 20–21

- Physical exercise may enhance or depress immunity depending on its intensity
- Lymphatic vessels drain leaked tissue fluids; immune system protects muscles from disease

Respiratory System Chapter 22

- Muscular exercise increases respiratory capacity and efficiency of gas exchange
- Respiratory system provides oxygen and disposes of carbon dioxide

Digestive System Chapter 23

- Physical activity increases gastrointestinal motility and elimination when at rest
- Digestive system provides nutrients needed for muscle health; liver metabolizes lactic acid

Urinary System Chapters 25–26

- Physical activity promotes normal voiding behavior; skeletal muscle forms the voluntary sphincter of the urethra
- Urinary system disposes of nitrogenous wastes

Reproductive System Chapter 27

- Skeletal muscle helps support pelvic organs (e.g., uterus); assists erection of penis and clitoris
- Testicular androgen promotes increased skeletal muscle

being tested is coaxing dystrophic muscles to produce more *utrophin*, a similar protein present in low amounts in adults but at much higher levels in fetal muscles. In mice at least, utrophin can compensate for dystrophin deficiency. ✚

As we age, the amount of connective tissue in our skeletal muscles increases, the number of muscle fibers decreases, and the muscles become stringier, or more sinewy. By age 30, even in healthy people, a gradual loss of muscle mass, called *sarcopenia* (sar-co-pe′ne-ah), begins. Apparently the same regulatory molecules (transcription factors, enzymes, hormones, and others) that promote muscle growth also oversee this type of muscle atrophy. Because skeletal muscles form so much of the body mass, body weight and muscle strength decline in tandem. By age 80, muscle strength usually decreases by about 50%. This "flesh wasting" condition has serious health implications for the elderly, particularly because falling becomes a common event.

Muscles can also suffer indirectly. Aging of the cardiovascular system affects nearly every organ in the body, and muscles are no exception. As atherosclerosis takes its toll and begins to block distal arteries, a circulatory condition called *intermittent claudication* (klaw″dĭ-ka′shun; "limping") occurs in some individuals. This condition restricts blood delivery to the legs, leading to excruciating pains in the leg muscles during walking, which forces the person to stop and rest.

But we don't have to slow up during old age. Regular exercise helps reverse sarcopenia, and frail elders who begin to "pump iron" (lift leg and hand weights) can rebuild muscle mass and dramatically increase their strength. Performing those lifting exercises rapidly can improve our ability to carry out the "explosive" movements needed to rise from a chair. Even moderate activity, like taking a walk daily, improves neuromuscular function and enhances independent living.

Smooth muscle is remarkably trouble free. Most problems that impair gastrointestinal function, for instance, stem from irritants such as excess alcohol, spicy foods, or bacterial infection. Under such conditions, smooth muscle motility increases in an attempt to rid the body of irritating agents, and diarrhea or vomiting occur.

☑ Check Your Understanding

20. How is the multinucleate condition achieved during development of skeletal muscle fibers?
21. What does it mean when we say "muscles get stringier with age"?
22. How can we defer (or reverse) some of the effects of age on skeletal muscles?

For answers, see Appendix H.

The capacity for movement is a property of all cells but, with the exception of muscle, these movements are largely restricted to intracellular events. Skeletal muscles, the major focus of this chapter, permit us to interact with our external environment in an amazing number of ways, and they also contribute to our internal homeostasis as summarized in *System Connections*.

In this chapter we have covered muscle anatomy from gross to molecular levels and have considered muscle physiology in some detail. Chapter 10 continues from this point to explain how skeletal muscles interact with bones and with each other, and then describes the individual skeletal muscles that make up the muscular system of the body.

Chapter Summary

MAP™ For more chapter study tools, go to the Study Area of MasteringA&P at **www.masteringaandp.com**.
There you will find:

- Interactive Physiology iP
- A&PFlix A&PFlix
- Practice Anatomy Lab PAL
- PhysioEx PEx
- Videos, Practice Quizzes and Tests, MP3 Tutor Sessions, Case Studies, and much more!

Overview of Muscle Tissues (pp. 276–278)

Types of Muscle Tissue (p. 277)

1. Skeletal muscle is attached to the skeleton, is striated, and can be controlled voluntarily.
2. Cardiac muscle forms the heart, is striated, and is controlled involuntarily.
3. Smooth muscle, located chiefly in the walls of hollow organs, is controlled involuntarily. Its fibers are not striated.

Special Characteristics of Muscle Tissue (p. 277)

4. Special functional characteristics of muscle include excitability, contractility, extensibility, and elasticity.

Muscle Functions (pp. 277–278)

5. Muscles move internal and external body parts, maintain posture, stabilize joints, generate heat, and protect some visceral organs.

Skeletal Muscle (pp. 278–305)

Gross Anatomy of a Skeletal Muscle (pp. 278–279)

1. Connective tissue coverings protect and strengthen skeletal muscle fibers (cells). Superficial to deep, these are epimysium, perimysium, and endomysium.
2. Skeletal muscle attachments (origins/insertions) may be direct or indirect via tendons or aponeuroses. Indirect attachments withstand friction better.

Microscopic Anatomy of a Skeletal Muscle Fiber (pp. 279–285)

3. Skeletal muscle fibers are long, striated, and multinucleate.
4. Myofibrils are contractile elements that occupy most of the cell volume. Their banded appearance results from a regular alternation of dark (A) and light (I) bands. Myofibrils are chains of sarcomeres; each sarcomere contains thick (myosin) and thin (actin) myofilaments arranged in a regular array. The heads of myosin molecules form cross bridges that interact with the thin filaments.
5. The sarcoplasmic reticulum (SR) is a system of membranous tubules surrounding each myofibril. Its function is to release and then sequester calcium ions.

6. T tubules are invaginations of the sarcolemma that run between the terminal cisterns of the SR. They allow an electrical stimulus to be delivered quickly deep into the cell.

Sliding Filament Model of Contraction (p. 285)

7. According to the sliding filament model, cross bridge (myosin head) activity of the thick filaments pulls the thin filaments toward the sarcomere centers.

Physiology of Skeletal Muscle Fibers (pp. 285–293)

8. Regulation of skeletal muscle cell contraction involves (a) generating and transmitting an action potential along the sarcolemma and (b) excitation-contraction coupling.
9. An end plate potential is set up when acetylcholine released by a nerve ending binds to ACh receptors on the sarcolemma, causing local changes in membrane permeability which allow ion flows that depolarize the membrane at that site.
10. The flow of current from the locally depolarized area spreads to the adjacent area of the sarcolemma, opening voltage-gated Na^+ channels, which allows Na^+ influx. These events generate the action potential. Once initiated, the action potential is self-propagating and unstoppable.
11. Then as the action potential travels away from a region, Na^+ channels close and voltage-gated K^+ channels open, repolarizing the membrane.
12. In excitation-contraction coupling the action potential is propagated down the T tubules, causing calcium to be released from the SR into the cytosol.
13. Sliding of the filaments is triggered by a rise in intracellular calcium ion levels. Troponin binding of calcium moves tropomyosin away from myosin-binding sites on actin, allowing cross bridge binding. Myosin ATPases split ATP, which energizes the power strokes. ATP binding to the myosin head is necessary for cross bridge detachment. Cross bridge activity ends when calcium is pumped back into the SR.

iP Muscular System; Topic: Sliding Filament Theory, pp. 18–29.

Contraction of a Skeletal Muscle (pp. 293–298)

14. A motor unit is one motor neuron and all the muscle cells it innervates. The neuron's axon has several branches, each of which forms a neuromuscular junction with one muscle cell.
15. A motor unit's response to a single brief threshold stimulus is a twitch. A twitch has three phases: latent (preparatory events occurring), contraction (the muscle tenses and may shorten), and relaxation (muscle tension declines and the muscle returns to its resting length).
16. Graded responses of muscles to rapid stimuli are wave summation and unfused and fused tetanus. A graded response to increasingly strong stimuli is multiple motor unit summation, or recruitment. The type and order of motor unit recruitment follows the size principle.
17. Isotonic contractions occur when the muscle shortens (concentric contraction) or lengthens (eccentric contraction) as the load is moved. Isometric contractions occur when muscle tension produces neither shortening nor lengthening.

iP Muscular System; Topic: Contraction of Motor Units, pp. 1–11.

Muscle Metabolism (pp. 298–301)

18. The energy source for muscle contraction is ATP, obtained from a coupled reaction of creatine phosphate with ADP and from aerobic and anaerobic metabolism of glucose.
19. When ATP is produced by anaerobic pathways, lactic acid accumulates and ionic imbalances disturb the membrane potential. To return the muscles to their resting state, ATP must be produced aerobically and used to regenerate creatine phosphate, glycogen reserves must be restored, and accumulated lactic acid must be metabolized. Oxygen used to accomplish this repayment is called excess postexercise oxygen consumption (EPOC).
20. Only about 40% of energy released during ATP hydrolysis powers contractile activity. The rest is liberated as heat.

iP Muscular System; Topic: Muscle Metabolism, pp. 1–7.

Force of Muscle Contraction (pp. 301–302)

21. The force of muscle contraction is affected by the number and size of contracting muscle cells (the more and the larger the cells, the greater the force), the frequency of stimulation, and the degree of muscle stretch.
22. In twitch contractions, the external tension exerted on the load is always less than the internal tension. When a muscle is tetanized, the external tension equals the internal tension.
23. When the thick and thin filaments are optimally overlapping, the muscle can generate maximum force. With excessive increase or decrease in muscle length, force declines.

Velocity and Duration of Contraction (pp. 302–304)

24. Factors determining the velocity and duration of muscle contraction include the load (the greater the load, the slower the contraction) and muscle fiber types.
25. The three types of muscle fibers are: (1) fast glycolytic (fatigable) fibers, (2) slow oxidative (fatigue-resistant) fibers, and (3) fast oxidative (fatigue-resistant) fibers. Most muscles contain a mixture of fiber types. The fast muscle fiber types can interconvert with certain exercise regimens.

Adaptations to Exercise (pp. 304–305)

26. Regular aerobic exercise gives skeletal muscles increased efficiency, endurance, strength, and resistance to fatigue.
27. In skeletal muscle, resistance exercises cause hypertrophy and large gains in strength.
28. Immobilizing muscles leads to muscle weakness and severe atrophy.
29. Improper training and excessive exercise result in overuse injuries, which may be disabling.

Smooth Muscle (pp. 305–311)

Microscopic Structure of Smooth Muscle Fibers (pp. 305–307)

1. A smooth muscle fiber is spindle shaped and uninucleate, and has no striations.
2. Smooth muscle cells are most often arranged in sheets. They lack elaborate connective tissue coverings.
3. The SR is poorly developed and T tubules are absent. Actin and myosin filaments are present, but sarcomeres are not. Intermediate filaments and dense bodies form an intracellular network that harnesses the pull generated during cross bridge activity and transfers it to the extracellular matrix.

Contraction of Smooth Muscle (pp. 307–309)

4. Smooth muscle fibers may be electrically coupled by gap junctions.
5. ATP energizes smooth muscle contraction, which is activated by a calcium pulse. However, calcium binds to calmodulin rather than to troponin (which is not present in smooth muscle fibers), and myosin must be phosphorylated to become active in contraction.
6. Smooth muscle contracts for extended periods at low energy cost and without fatigue.
7. Neurotransmitters of the autonomic nervous system may inhibit or stimulate smooth muscle fibers. Smooth muscle contraction may also be initiated by pacemaker cells, hormones, or local chemical factors that influence intracellular calcium levels, and by mechanical stretch.

8. Special features of smooth muscle contraction include the stress-relaxation response, the ability to generate large amounts of force when extensively stretched, and hyperplasia under certain conditions.

Types of Smooth Muscle (p. 309)

9. Unitary smooth muscle has electrically coupled fibers that contract synchronously and often spontaneously.
10. Multi unit smooth muscle has independent, well-innervated fibers that lack gap junctions and pacemaker cells. Stimulation occurs via autonomic nerves (or hormones). Multi unit muscle contractions are rarely synchronous.

Developmental Aspects of Muscles (pp. 312–313, 315)

1. Muscle tissue develops from embryonic mesoderm cells called myoblasts. Several myoblasts fuse to form a skeletal muscle fiber. Smooth and cardiac cells develop from single myoblasts and display gap junctions.
2. For the most part, specialized skeletal and cardiac muscle cells lose their ability to divide but retain the ability to hypertrophy. Smooth muscle regenerates well and undergoes hyperplasia.
3. Skeletal muscle development reflects maturation of the nervous system and occurs in head-to-toe and proximal-to-distal directions. Natural neuromuscular control reaches its peak in midadolescence.
4. Women's muscles account for about 36% of their total body weight and men's for about 42%, a difference due chiefly to the effects of male hormones on skeletal muscle growth.
5. Skeletal muscle is richly vascularized and quite resistant to infection, but in old age, skeletal muscles become fibrous, decline in strength, and atrophy. Regular exercise can offset some of these changes.

Review Questions

Multiple Choice/Matching

(Some questions have more than one correct answer. Select the best answer or answers from the choices given.)

1. The connective tissue covering that encloses the sarcolemma of an individual muscle fiber is called the **(a)** epimysium, **(b)** perimysium, **(c)** endomysium, **(d)** periosteum.
2. A fascicle is a **(a)** muscle, **(b)** bundle of muscle fibers enclosed by a connective tissue sheath, **(c)** bundle of myofibrils, **(d)** group of myofilaments.
3. Thick and thin myofilaments have different compositions. For each descriptive phrase, indicate whether the filament is **(a)** thick or **(b)** thin.

    ____ **(1)** contains actin
    ____ **(2)** contains ATPases
    ____ **(3)** attaches to the Z disc
    ____ **(4)** contains myosin
    ____ **(5)** contains troponin
    ____ **(6)** does not lie in the I band

4. The function of the T tubules in muscle contraction is to **(a)** make and store glycogen, **(b)** release Ca^{2+} into the cell interior and then pick it up again, **(c)** transmit the action potential deep into the muscle cells, **(d)** form proteins.
5. The sites where the motor nerve impulse is transmitted from the nerve endings to the skeletal muscle cell membranes are the **(a)** neuromuscular junctions, **(b)** sarcomeres, **(c)** myofilaments, **(d)** Z discs.
6. Contraction elicited by a single brief stimulus is called **(a)** a twitch, **(b)** wave summation, **(c)** multiple motor unit summation, **(d)** fused tetanus.
7. A smooth, sustained contraction resulting from very rapid stimulation of the muscle, in which no evidence of relaxation is seen, is called **(a)** a twitch, **(b)** wave summation, **(c)** multiple motor unit summation, **(d)** fused tetanus.
8. Characteristics of isometric contractions include all but **(a)** shortening, **(b)** increased muscle tension throughout the contraction phase, **(c)** absence of shortening, **(d)** used in resistance training.
9. During muscle contraction, ATP is provided by **(a)** a coupled reaction of creatine phosphate with ADP, **(b)** aerobic respiration of glucose, and **(c)** anaerobic glycolysis.

    ____ **(1)** Which provides ATP fastest?
    ____ **(2)** Which does (do) not require that oxygen be available?
    ____ **(3)** Which provides the highest yield of ATP per glucose molecule?
    ____ **(4)** Which results in the formation of lactic acid?
    ____ **(5)** Which has carbon dioxide and water products?
    ____ **(6)** Which is most important in endurance sports?

10. The neurotransmitter released by somatic motor neurons is **(a)** acetylcholine, **(b)** acetylcholinesterase, **(c)** norepinephrine.
11. The ions that enter the skeletal muscle cell during the generation of an action potential are **(a)** calcium ions, **(b)** chloride ions, **(c)** sodium ions, **(d)** potassium ions.
12. Myoglobin has a special function in muscle tissue. It **(a)** breaks down glycogen, **(b)** is a contractile protein, **(c)** holds a reserve supply of oxygen in the muscle.
13. Aerobic exercise results in all of the following except **(a)** increased cardiovascular system efficiency, **(b)** more mitochondria in the muscle cells, **(c)** increased size and strength of existing muscle cells, **(d)** increased neuromuscular system coordination.
14. The smooth muscle type found in the walls of digestive and urinary system organs and that exhibits gap junctions and pacemaker cells is **(a)** multi unit, **(b)** unitary.

Short Answer Essay Questions

15. Name and describe the four special functional abilities of muscle that are the basis for muscle response.
16. Distinguish between (a) direct and indirect muscle attachments and (b) a tendon and an aponeurosis.
17. (a) Describe the structure of a sarcomere and indicate the relationship of the sarcomere to myofilaments. (b) Explain the sliding filament model of contraction using appropriately labeled diagrams of a relaxed and a contracted sarcomere.
18. What is the importance of acetylcholinesterase in muscle cell contraction?
19. Explain how a slight (but smooth) contraction differs from a vigorous contraction of the same muscle. Use the concepts of multiple motor unit summation.
20. Explain what is meant by the term excitation-contraction coupling.
21. Define and draw a motor unit.
22. Describe the three distinct types of skeletal muscle fibers.
23. True or false: Most muscles contain a predominance of one skeletal muscle fiber type. Explain the reasoning behind your choice.
24. Describe some cause(s) of muscle fatigue and define this term clearly.

25. Define EPOC.
26. Smooth muscle has some unique properties, such as low energy usage, and the ability to maintain contraction over long periods. Tie these properties to the function of smooth muscle in the body.

Critical Thinking and Clinical Application Questions

1. Jim Fitch decided that his physique left much to be desired, so he joined a local health club and began to "pump iron" three times weekly. After three months of training, during which he lifted increasingly heavier weights, he noticed that his arm and chest muscles were substantially larger. Explain the structural and functional basis of these changes.
2. When a suicide victim was found, the coroner was unable to remove the drug vial clutched in his hand. Explain the reasons for this. If the victim had been discovered three days later, would the coroner have had the same difficulty? Explain.
3. Muscle-relaxing drugs are administered to a patient during major surgery. Which of the two chemicals described next would be a good skeletal muscle relaxant and why?
   - Chemical A binds to and blocks ACh receptors of muscle cells.
   - Chemical B floods the muscle cells' cytoplasm with Ca^{2+}.
4. Michael is answering a series of questions dealing with skeletal muscle cell excitation and contraction. In response to "What protein changes shape when Ca^{2+} binds to it?" he writes "tropomyosin." What should he have responded and what is the result of that calcium ion binding?

AT THE CLINIC

Related Clinical Terms

Fibromyositis (*fibro* = fiber; *itis* = inflammation) Also known as **fibromyalgia**; a group of conditions involving chronic inflammation of a muscle, its connective tissue coverings and tendons, and capsules of nearby joints. Symptoms are nonspecific and involve varying degrees of tenderness associated with specific trigger points, as well as fatigue and frequent awakening from sleep.

Hernia Protrusion of an organ through its body cavity wall. May be congenital (owing to failure of muscle fusion during development), but most often is caused by heavy lifting or obesity and subsequent muscle weakening.

Myalgia (mi-al′je-ah; *algia* = pain) Muscle pain resulting from any muscle disorder.

Myofascial pain syndrome Pain caused by a tightened band of muscle fibers, which twitch when the skin over them is touched. Mostly associated with overused or strained postural muscles.

Myopathy (mi-op′ah-the; *path* = disease, suffering) Any disease of muscle.

Myotonic dystrophy A form of muscular dystrophy that is less common than DMD; in the U.S. it affects about 14 of 100,000 people. Symptoms include a gradual reduction in muscle mass and control of the skeletal muscles, abnormal heart rhythm, and diabetes mellitus. May appear at any time; not sex-linked. Underlying genetic defect is multiple repeats of a particular gene on chromosome 19. Because the number of repeats tends to increase from generation to generation, subsequent generations develop more severe symptoms. No effective treatment.

RICE Acronym for rest, ice, compression, and elevation. The standard treatment for a pulled muscle, or excessively stretched tendons or ligaments.

Spasm A sudden, involuntary twitch in smooth or skeletal muscle ranging from merely irritating to very painful; may be due to chemical imbalances. In spasms of the eyelid or facial muscles, called tics, psychological factors may be involved. Stretching and massaging the affected area may help end the spasm. A cramp is a prolonged spasm; usually occurs at night or after exercise.

Strain Commonly called a "pulled muscle," a strain is excessive stretching and possible tearing of a muscle due to muscle overuse or abuse. The injured muscle becomes painfully inflamed (myositis), and adjacent joints are usually immobilized.

Tetanus (1) A state of sustained contraction of a muscle that is a normal aspect of skeletal muscle functioning. (2) An acute infectious disease caused by the anaerobic bacterium *Clostridium tetani* and resulting in persistent painful spasms of some skeletal muscles. Progresses to fixed rigidity of the jaws (lockjaw) and spasms of trunk and limb muscles. Usually fatal due to respiratory failure.

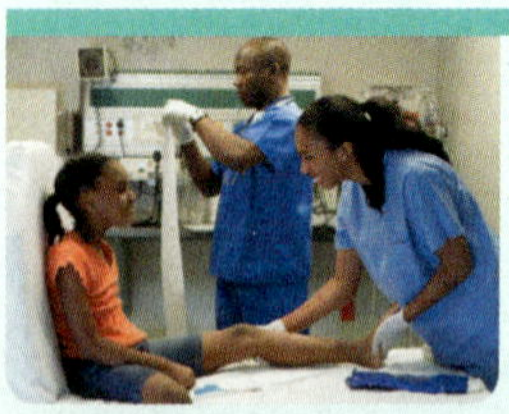

Case Study Muscular System

Let's continue our tale of Mrs. DeStephano's medical problems, this time looking at the notes made detailing observations of her skeletal musculature.

- Severe lacerations of the muscles of the right leg and knee
- Damage to the blood vessels serving the right leg and knee
- Transection of the sciatic nerve (the large nerve serving most of the lower limb), just above the right knee

Her physician orders daily passive range-of-motion (ROM) exercise and electrical stimulation for her right leg and a diet high in protein, carbohydrates, and vitamin C.

1. Describe the step-by-step process of wound healing that will occur in her fleshy (muscle) wounds, and note the consequences of the specific restorative process that occurs.
2. What complications in healing can be anticipated owing to vascular (blood vessel) damage in the right leg?
3. What complications in muscle structure and function result from transection of the sciatic nerve? Why are passive ROM and electrical stimulation of her right leg muscles ordered?
4. Explain the reasoning behind the dietary recommendations.

(Answers in Appendix H)

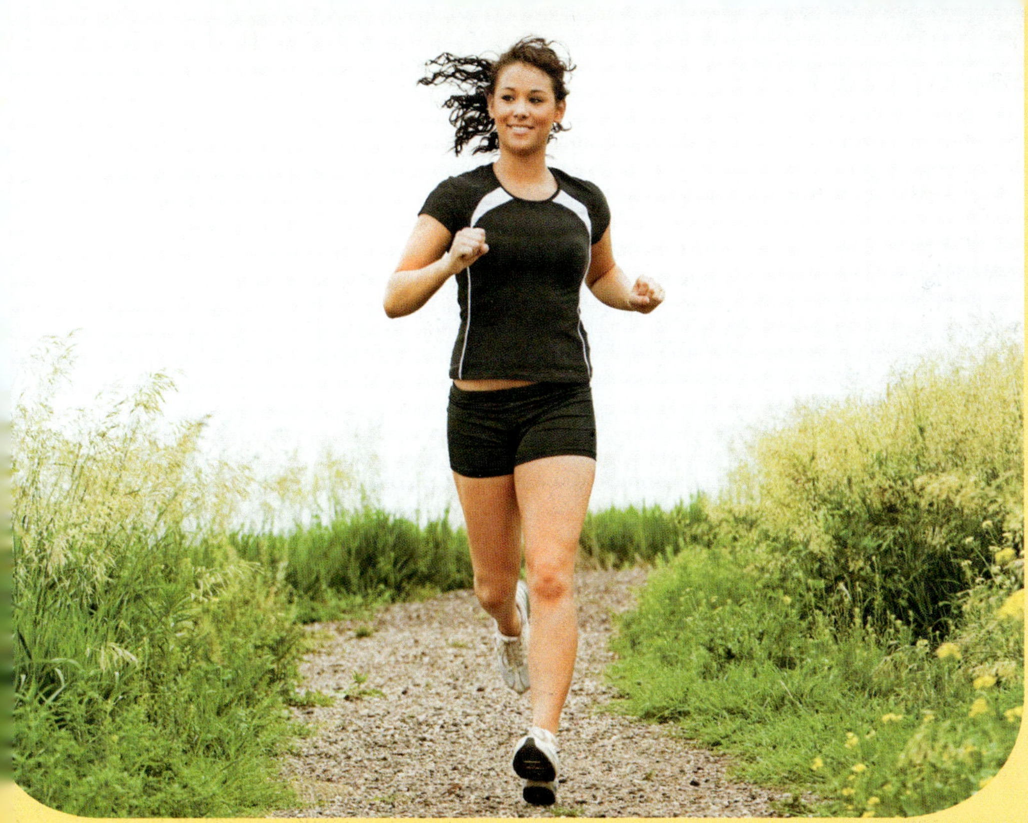

10 The Muscular System

The human body enjoys an incredibly wide range of movements. The gentle blinking of your eye, standing on tiptoe, and wielding a sledgehammer are just a sample of the actions made possible by your muscular system.

Muscle tissue includes all contractile tissues (skeletal, cardiac, and smooth muscle), but when we study the muscular system, **skeletal muscles** take center stage. This chapter focuses on these muscular "machines" that enable us to perform so many different activities. However, before describing the individual muscles in detail, we will consider

- The manner in which muscles "play" with or against each other to bring about movement
- The criteria used for naming muscles
- The principles of leverage

Actions and Interactions of Skeletal Muscles

✓ Describe the functions of prime movers, antagonists, synergists, and fixators.

✓ Explain how a muscle's position relative to a joint affects its action.

The arrangement of body muscles permits them to work either together or in opposition to produce a wide variety of movements. As you eat, for example, you alternately raise your fork to your lips and lower it to your plate, and both sets of actions are accomplished by your arm and hand muscles. But muscles can only *pull*; they never *push*. Generally as a muscle shortens, its *insertion* (attachment on the movable bone) moves toward its *origin* (its fixed or immovable point of attachment). Whatever one muscle or muscle group can do, another muscle or group of muscles can "undo."

Muscles can be classified into four *functional* groups: prime movers, antagonists, synergists, and fixators. A muscle that has the major responsibility for producing a specific movement is a **prime mover**, or **agonist** (ag′o-nist; "leader"), of that movement. The pectoralis major muscle, which fleshes out the anterior chest (and inserts on the humerus), is a prime mover of arm flexion.

Muscles that oppose, or reverse, a particular movement are **antagonists** (an-tag′o-nists; "against the leaders"). When a prime mover is active, the antagonist muscles may stretch or remain relaxed. Usually, however, antagonists help to regulate the action of a prime mover by contracting slightly to provide some resistance, thus helping to prevent overshooting the mark or to slow or stop the movement. As you might expect, a prime mover and its antagonist are located on opposite sides of the joint across which they act, as shown in *Focus on Muscle Action* **(Figure 10.1)**.

Antagonists can also be prime movers in their own right. For example, flexion of the arm by the pectoralis major muscle is antagonized by the latissimus dorsi, the prime mover for extending the arm.

In addition to agonists and antagonists, most movements involve the action of one or more **synergists** (sin′er-jists; *syn* = together, *erg* = work). Synergists help prime movers in one of these ways:

- Adding a little extra force to the same movement
- Reducing undesirable or unnecessary movements that might occur as the prime mover contracts

Let's look at the second function more closely. When a muscle crosses two or more joints, its contraction causes movement at all of the spanned joints unless other muscles act as joint stabilizers. For example, the finger flexor muscles cross both the wrist and the interphalangeal joints, but you can make a fist without bending your wrist because synergistic muscles stabilize the wrist. Additionally, as some flexors act, they may cause several other (undesirable) movements at the same joint. Synergists can prevent this, allowing all of the prime mover's force to be exerted in the desired direction.

When synergists immobilize a bone, or a muscle's origin so that the prime mover has a stable base on which to act, they are called **fixators** (fik′sa-terz). Recall from Chapter 7 that the scapula is held to the axial skeleton only by muscles and is quite freely movable. The fixator muscles that run from the axial skeleton to the scapula can immobilize the scapula so that only the desired movements occur at the mobile shoulder joint. Additionally, muscles that help maintain upright posture are fixators.

In summary, although prime movers seem to get all the credit for causing certain movements, antagonistic and synergistic muscles are also important in producing smooth, coordinated, and precise movements. Furthermore, a muscle may act as a prime mover in one movement, an antagonist for another movement, a synergist for a third movement, and so on.

Naming Skeletal Muscles

✓ List the criteria used in naming muscles. Provide an example to illustrate the use of each criterion.

Skeletal muscles are named according to a number of criteria. To simplify the task of learning muscle names and actions, pay attention to the following cues.

- **Muscle location.** Some muscle names indicate the bone or body region with which the muscle is associated.
  Examples: The temporalis (tem″por-ă′lis) muscle overlies the temporal bone, and intercostal (*costal* = rib) muscles run between the ribs.
- **Muscle shape.** Some muscles are named for their distinctive shapes.
  Examples: The deltoid (del′toid) muscle is roughly triangular (*deltoid* = triangle), and together the right and left trapezius (trah-pe′ze-us) muscles form a trapezoid.
- **Muscle size.** Terms such as *maximus* (largest), *minimus* (smallest), *longus* (long), and *brevis* (short) are often used in muscle names.
  Examples: The gluteus maximus and gluteus minimus are the large and small gluteus muscles, respectively.
- **Direction of muscle fibers.** The names of some muscles reveal the direction in which their fibers (and fascicles) run in reference to some imaginary line, usually the midline of the body or the longitudinal axis of a limb bone. In muscles with the term *rectus* (straight) in their names, the fibers run parallel to that imaginary line (axis). *Transversus* indicates that the muscle fibers run at right angles to that line, and *oblique* indicates that the fibers run obliquely to it.
  Examples: The rectus femoris (straight muscle of the thigh, or femur) and transversus abdominis (transverse muscle of the abdomen).
- **Number of origins.** When *biceps*, *triceps*, or *quadriceps* forms part of a muscle's name, you can assume that the muscle has two, three, or four origins, respectively.
  Example: The biceps brachii (bra′ke-i) muscle of the arm has two origins, or *heads*.
- **Location of the attachments.** Some muscles are named according to their points of origin and insertion. The origin is always named first.
  Example: The sternocleidomastoid (ster″no-kli″do-mas′toid) muscle of the neck has a dual origin on the sternum (*sterno*) and clavicle (*cleido*), and it inserts on the mastoid process of the temporal bone.
- **Muscle action.** When muscles are named for the movement they produce, action words such as *flexor*, *extensor*, or *adductor* appear in the muscle's name.
  Example: The adductor longus, located on the medial thigh, brings about thigh adduction. (To review the terminology for various actions, see Chapter 8, Figures 8.5, 8.6, pp. 256–259.)

Often, several criteria are combined in naming a muscle. For instance, the name *extensor carpi radialis longus* tells us the muscle's action (extensor), what joint it acts on (*carpi* = wrist), and that it lies close to the radius of the forearm (radialis). It also hints at the size (longus) relative to other wrist extensor muscles. Unfortunately, not all muscle names are this descriptive.

Figure 10.1 The action of a muscle can be inferred by the position of the muscle relative to the joint it crosses. (Examples given relate to the shoulder joint.) A&P Flix Available at www.masteringaandp.com

(a) A muscle that crosses on the anterior side of a joint produces flexion*

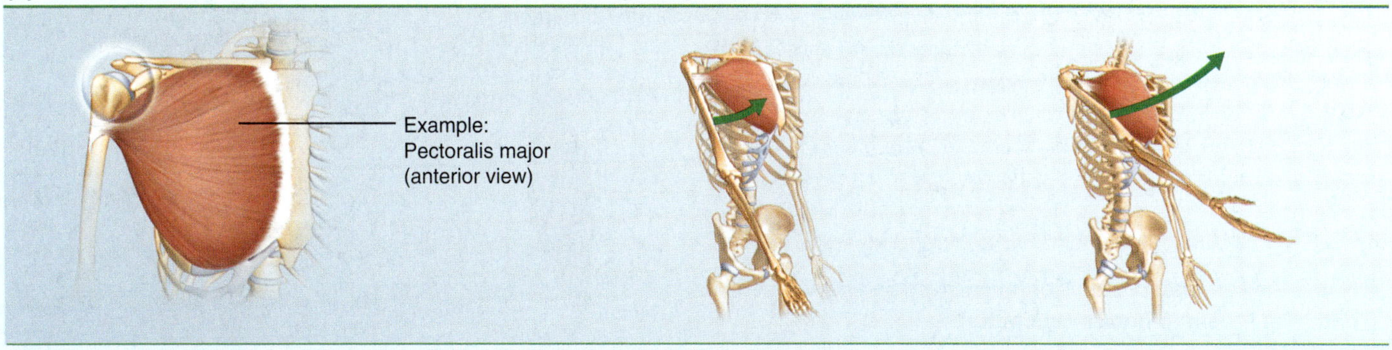

(b) A muscle that crosses on the posterior side of a joint produces extension*

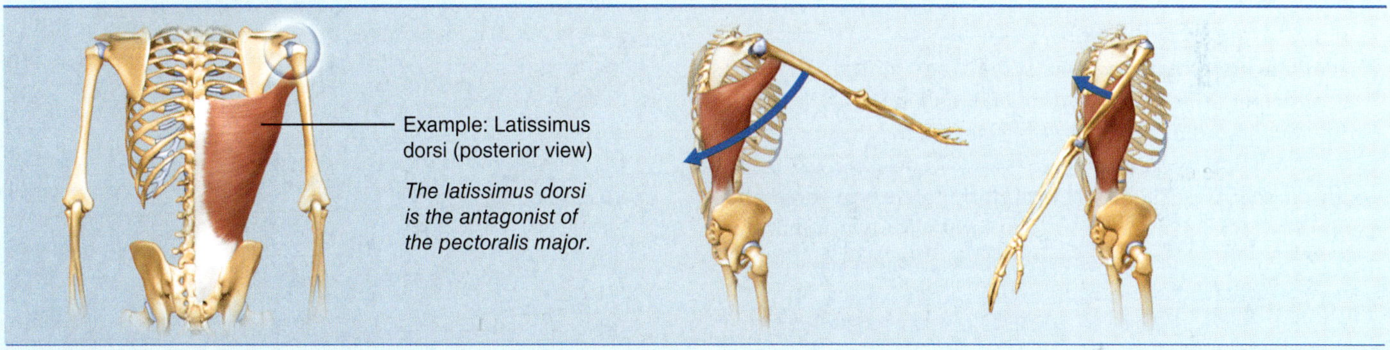

(c) A muscle that crosses on the lateral side of a joint produces abduction

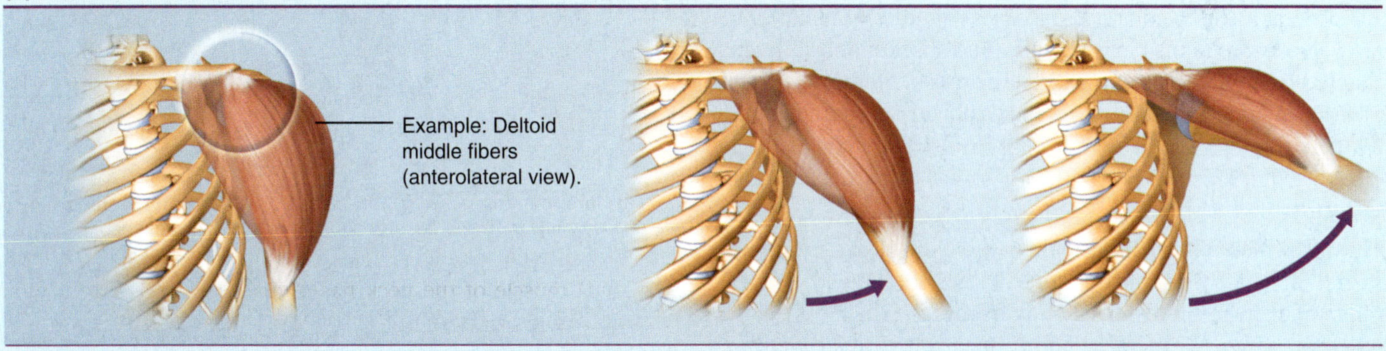

(d) A muscle that crosses on the medial side of a joint produces adduction

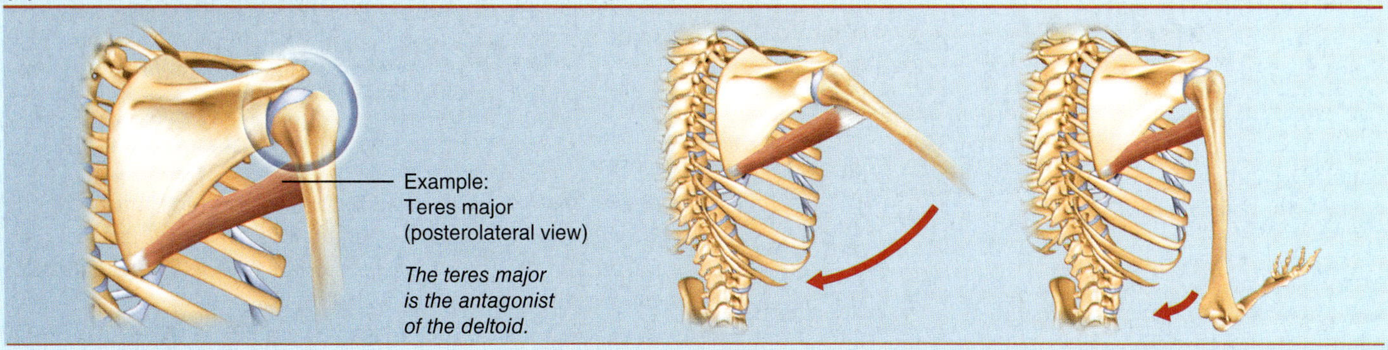

*These generalities do not apply to the knee and ankle because the lower limb is rotated during development. The muscles that cross these joints posteriorly produce flexion, and those that cross anteriorly produce extension.

☑ Check Your Understanding

1. The term "prime mover" is used in the business world to indicate people that get things done—the movers and shakers. What is its physiological meaning?
2. What criteria are used in naming each of the following muscles? Iliacus, adductor brevis, quadriceps femoris.

For answers, see Appendix H.

Muscle Mechanics: Importance of Fascicle Arrangement and Leverage

✓ Name the common patterns of muscle fascicle arrangement and relate them to power generation.

✓ Define lever, and explain how a lever operating at a mechanical advantage differs from one operating at a mechanical disadvantage.

✓ Name the three types of lever systems and indicate the arrangement of effort, fulcrum, and load in each. Also note the advantages of each type of lever system.

We discussed most factors contributing to muscle force and speed (load, fiber type, etc.) in Chapter 9 with two important exceptions—fascicle arrangement and lever systems. We attend to these factors next.

Arrangement of Fascicles

All skeletal muscles consist of fascicles (bundles of fibers), but fascicle arrangements vary, resulting in muscles with different shapes and functional capabilities. The most common patterns of fascicle arrangement are circular, convergent, parallel, and pennate **(Figure 10.2)**.

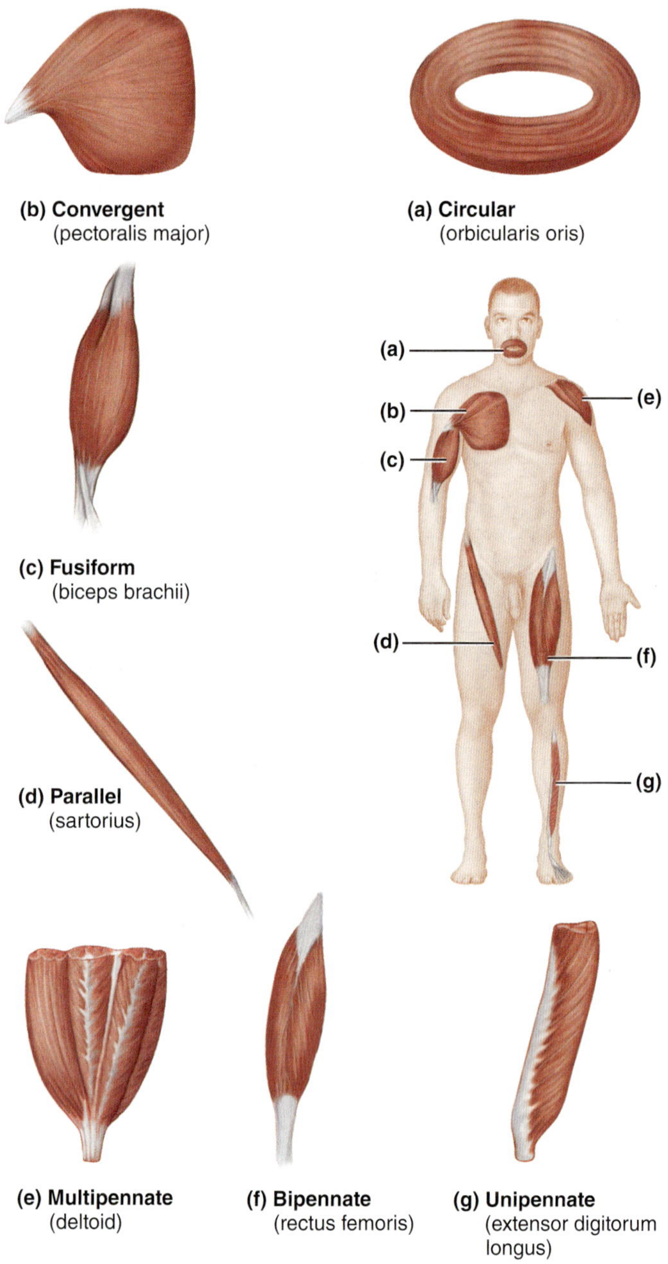

Figure 10.2 **Patterns of fascicle arrangement in muscles.**

Circular

The fascicular pattern is **circular** when the fascicles are arranged in concentric rings (Figure 10.2a). Muscles with this arrangement surround external body openings, which they close by contracting. A general term for such muscles is *sphincters* ("squeezers"). Examples are the orbicularis muscles surrounding the eyes and the mouth.

Convergent

A **convergent** muscle has a broad origin, and its fascicles *converge* toward a single tendon of insertion. Such a muscle is triangular or fan shaped like the pectoralis major muscle of the anterior thorax (Figure 10.2b).

Parallel

In a **parallel** arrangement, the length of the fascicles runs parallel to the long axis of the muscle. Such muscles are either *straplike* like the sartorius muscle of the thigh (Figure 10.2d), or *spindle shaped* with an expanded belly (midsection), like the biceps brachii muscle of the arm (Figure 10.2c). However, some authorities classify spindle-shaped muscles into a separate class as **fusiform muscles**. This is the approach we use here in Figure 10.2.

Pennate

In a **pennate** (pen′āt) pattern, the fascicles (and muscle fibers) are short and they attach obliquely (*penna* = feather) to a central tendon that runs the length of the muscle. Pennate muscles come in three forms:

- *Unipennate*, in which the fascicles insert into only one side of the tendon, as in the extensor digitorum longus muscle of the leg (Figure 10.2g).

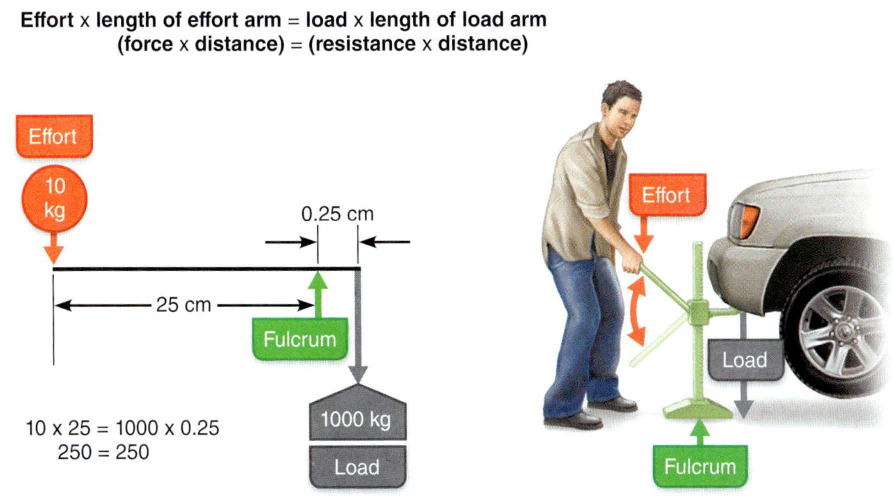

(a) Mechanical advantage with a power lever

Figure 10.3 Lever systems operating at a mechanical advantage and a mechanical disadvantage. The equation at the top expresses the relationships among the forces and relative distances in any lever system. **(a)** Mechanical advantage with a power lever. When using a jack, the load lifted is greater than the applied muscular effort. Only 10 kg of force (the effort) is needed to lift a 1000-kg car (the load).

(Figure continues on p. 324.)

10

- *Bipennate*, in which the fascicles insert into the tendon from opposite sides so the muscle's "grain" resembles a feather (Figure 10.2f). The rectus femoris of the thigh is bipennate.
- *Multipennate*, which looks like many feathers side by side, with all their quills inserted into one large tendon. The deltoid muscle, which forms the roundness of the shoulder, is multipennate (Figure 10.2e).

The arrangement of a muscle's fascicles determines its range of motion (the amount of movement produced when a muscle shortens) and its power. Because skeletal muscle fibers may shorten to about 70% of their resting length when they contract, the longer and the more nearly parallel the muscle fibers are to a muscle's long axis, the more the muscle can shorten. Muscles with parallel fascicle arrangements shorten the most, but are not usually very powerful. Muscle power depends more on the total number of muscle fibers in the muscle: The greater the number of muscle fibers, the greater the power. The stocky bipennate and multipennate muscles, which "pack in" the most fibers, shorten very little but are very powerful.

☑ Check Your Understanding

3. Of the muscles illustrated in Figure 10.2, which could shorten most? Which two would likely be most powerful? Why?

For answers, see Appendix H.

Lever Systems: Bone-Muscle Relationships

The operation of most skeletal muscles involves leverage—using a lever to move some object. A **lever** is a rigid bar that moves on a fixed point called the **fulcrum**, when a force is applied to it. The applied force, or **effort**, is used to move a resistance, or **load**. In your body, your joints are the fulcrums, and your bones act as levers. Muscle contraction provides the effort that is applied at the muscle's insertion point on a bone. The load is the bone itself, along with overlying tissues and anything else you are trying to move with that lever.

Levers: Power Versus Speed

A lever allows a given effort to move a heavier load, or to move a load farther or faster, than it otherwise could. If the load is close to the fulcrum and the effort is applied far from the fulcrum, a small effort exerted over a relatively large distance can move a large load over a small distance (**Figure 10.3a**). Such lever is said to operate at a **mechanical advantage** and is commonly called a *power lever*. For example, as shown to the right in Figure 10.3a, a person can lift a car with a power lever, in this case, a jack. The car moves up only a small distance with each downward "push" of the jack handle, but relatively little muscle effort is needed.

If, on the other hand, the load is far from the fulcrum and the effort is applied near the fulcrum, the force exerted by the muscle must be greater than the load to be moved or supported (Figure 10.3b on p. 324). This lever system is a *speed lever* and operates at a **mechanical disadvantage**. Speed levers are useful because they allow a load to be moved rapidly over a large distance with a wide range of motion. Wielding a shovel is an example. As you can see, small differences in the site of a muscle's insertion (relative to the fulcrum or joint) can translate into large differences in the amount of force a muscle must generate to move a given load or resistance.

Regardless of type, all levers follow the same basic principle:

Effort farther than load from fulcrum	=	lever operates at a mechanical advantage
Effort nearer than load to fulcrum	=	lever operates at a mechanical disadvantage

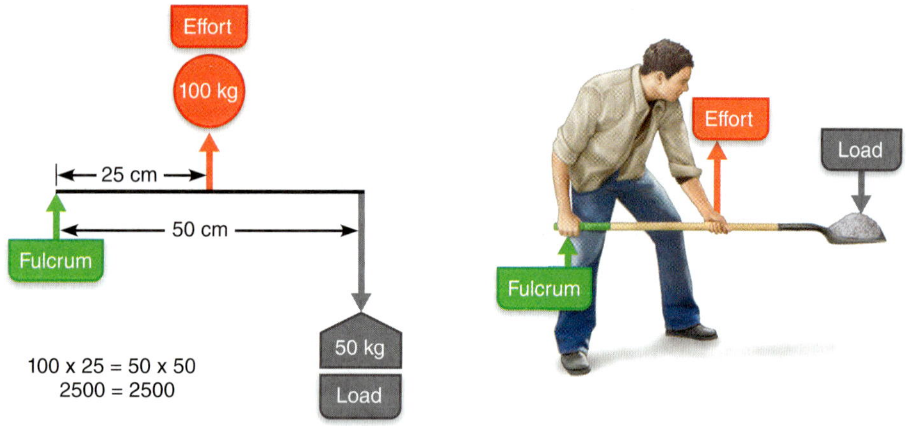

(b) Mechanical disadvantage with a speed lever

Figure 10.3 *(continued)* **Lever systems operating at a mechanical advantage and a mechanical disadvantage.** **(b)** Mechanical disadvantage with a speed lever. When using a shovel to lift dirt, the muscular force is greater than the load lifted. A muscular force (effort) of 100 kg is used to lift 50 kg of dirt (the load). Levers operating at a mechanical disadvantage are common in the body.

10

Classes of Levers

Depending on the relative position of the three elements—effort, fulcrum, and load—a lever belongs to one of three classes.

In a **first-class lever**, the effort is applied at one end of the lever and the load is at the other, with the fulcrum somewhere between. Seesaws and scissors are first-class levers. First-class leverage also occurs when you lift your head off your chest (**Figure 10.4a**). Some first-class levers in the body operate at a mechanical advantage (for strength), but others, such as the action of the triceps muscle in extending the forearm against resistance, operate at a mechanical disadvantage (for speed and distance).

In a **second-class lever**, the effort is applied at one end of the lever and the fulcrum is located at the other, with the load between them. A wheelbarrow demonstrates this type of lever system. Second-class levers are uncommon in the body, but the best example is the act of standing on your toes (Figure 10.4b). All second-class levers in the body work at a mechanical advantage because the muscle insertion is always farther from the fulcrum than is the load. Second-class levers are levers of strength, but speed and range of motion are sacrificed for that strength.

In a **third-class lever**, the effort is applied between the load and the fulcrum. These levers are speedy and always operate at a mechanical disadvantage—think of tweezers and forceps. Most skeletal muscles of the body act in third-class lever systems. An example is the activity of the biceps muscle of the arm, lifting the distal forearm and anything carried in the hand (Figure 10.4c). Third-class lever systems permit a muscle to be inserted very close to the joint across which movement occurs, which allows rapid, extensive movements (as in throwing) with relatively little shortening of the muscle. Muscles involved in third-class levers tend to be thicker and more powerful.

In conclusion, differences in the positioning of the three elements modify muscle activity with respect to speed of contraction, range of movement, and the weight of the load that can be lifted.

In lever systems that operate at a mechanical disadvantage (speed levers), force is lost but speed and range of movement are gained. Systems that operate at a mechanical advantage (power levers) are slower, more stable, and used where strength is a priority.

☑ Check Your Understanding

4. Which of the three lever systems involved in muscle mechanics would be the fastest lever—first-, second-, or third-class?
5. What benefit is provided by a lever that operates at a mechanical advantage?

For answers, see Appendix H.

Major Skeletal Muscles of the Body

✓ Name and identify the muscles described in Tables 10.1 to 10.17. State the origin, insertion, and action of each.

The grand plan of the muscular system is all the more impressive because of the sheer number of skeletal muscles in the body—more than 600 of them (many more than in **Figures 10.5** and **10.6** combined)! Remembering all the names, locations, and actions of these muscles is a monumental task. Take heart; here we consider only the principal muscles (approximately 125 pairs of them). Although this number is far fewer than 600, the job of learning about all these muscles will still require a concerted effort on your part.

Memorization will be easier if you apply what you learn in a practical, or clinical, way; that is, with a *functional anatomy focus*. Once you are satisfied that you have learned the name of a muscle and can identify it on a cadaver, model, or diagram, flesh out your learning by asking yourself, "What does it do?" [It might be a good idea to review body movements (pp. 256–259) before you get to this point.]

(Text continues on p. 328.)

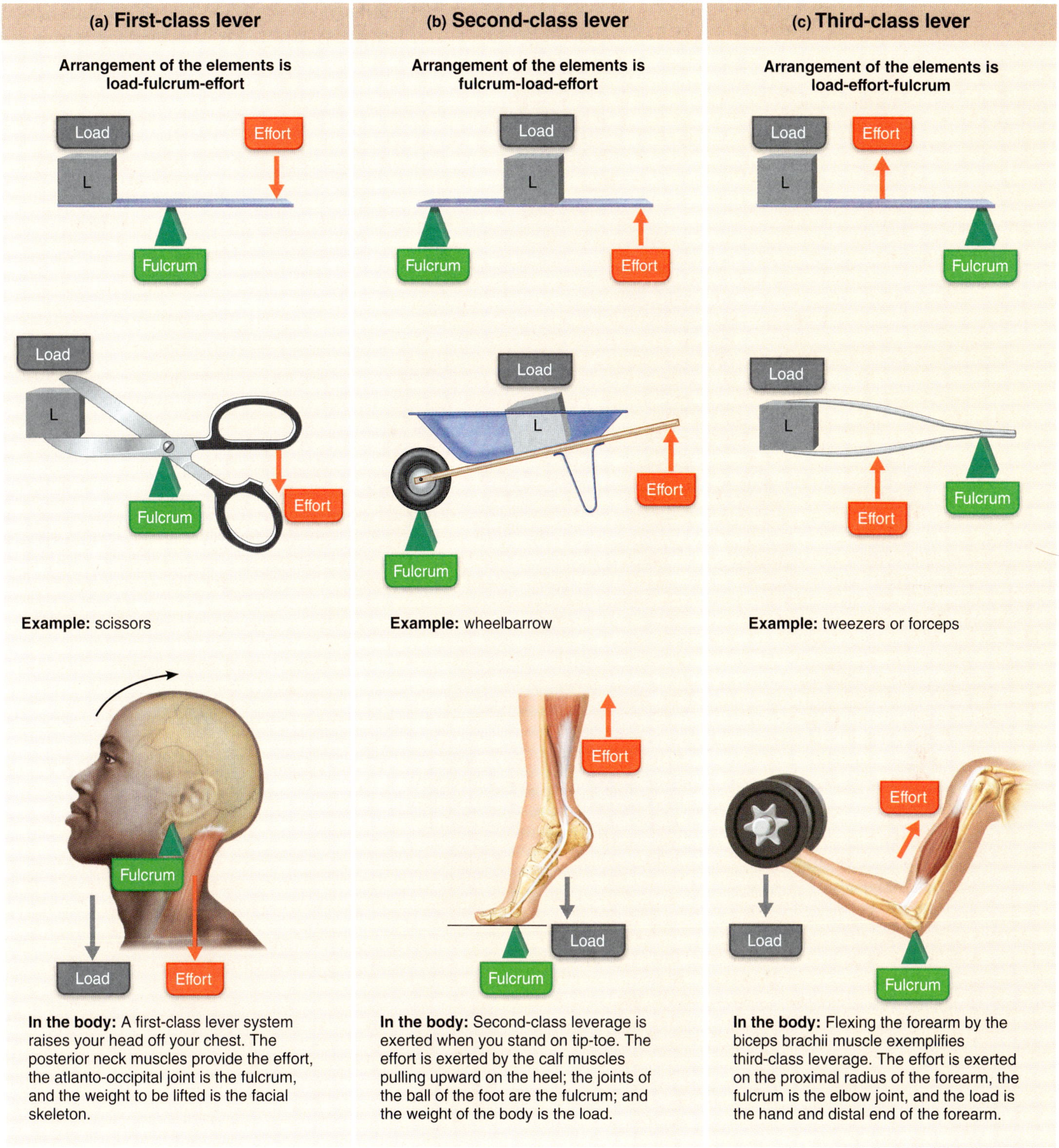

Figure 10.4 Lever systems.

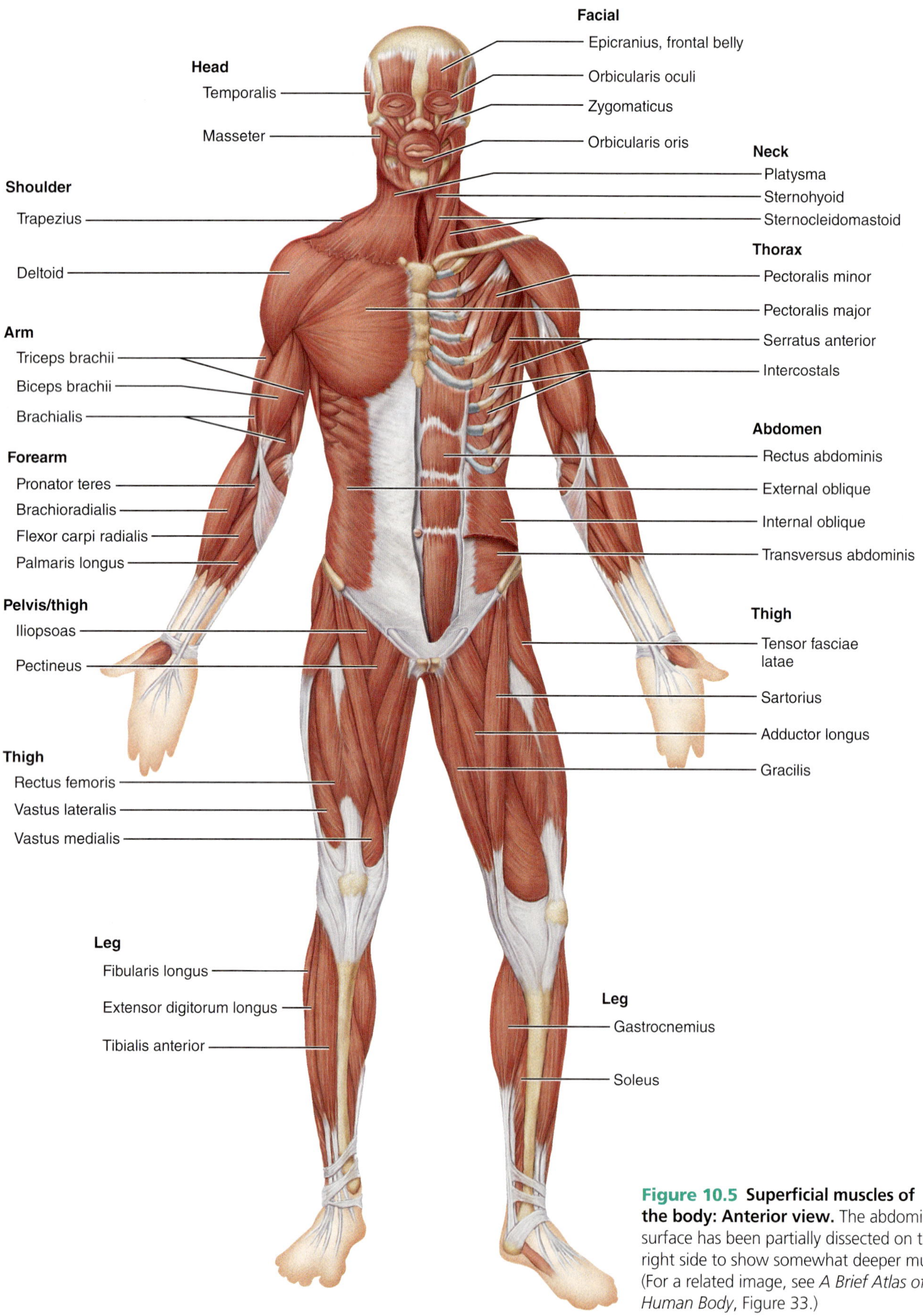

Figure 10.5 Superficial muscles of the body: Anterior view. The abdominal surface has been partially dissected on the right side to show somewhat deeper muscles. (For a related image, see *A Brief Atlas of the Human Body*, Figure 33.)

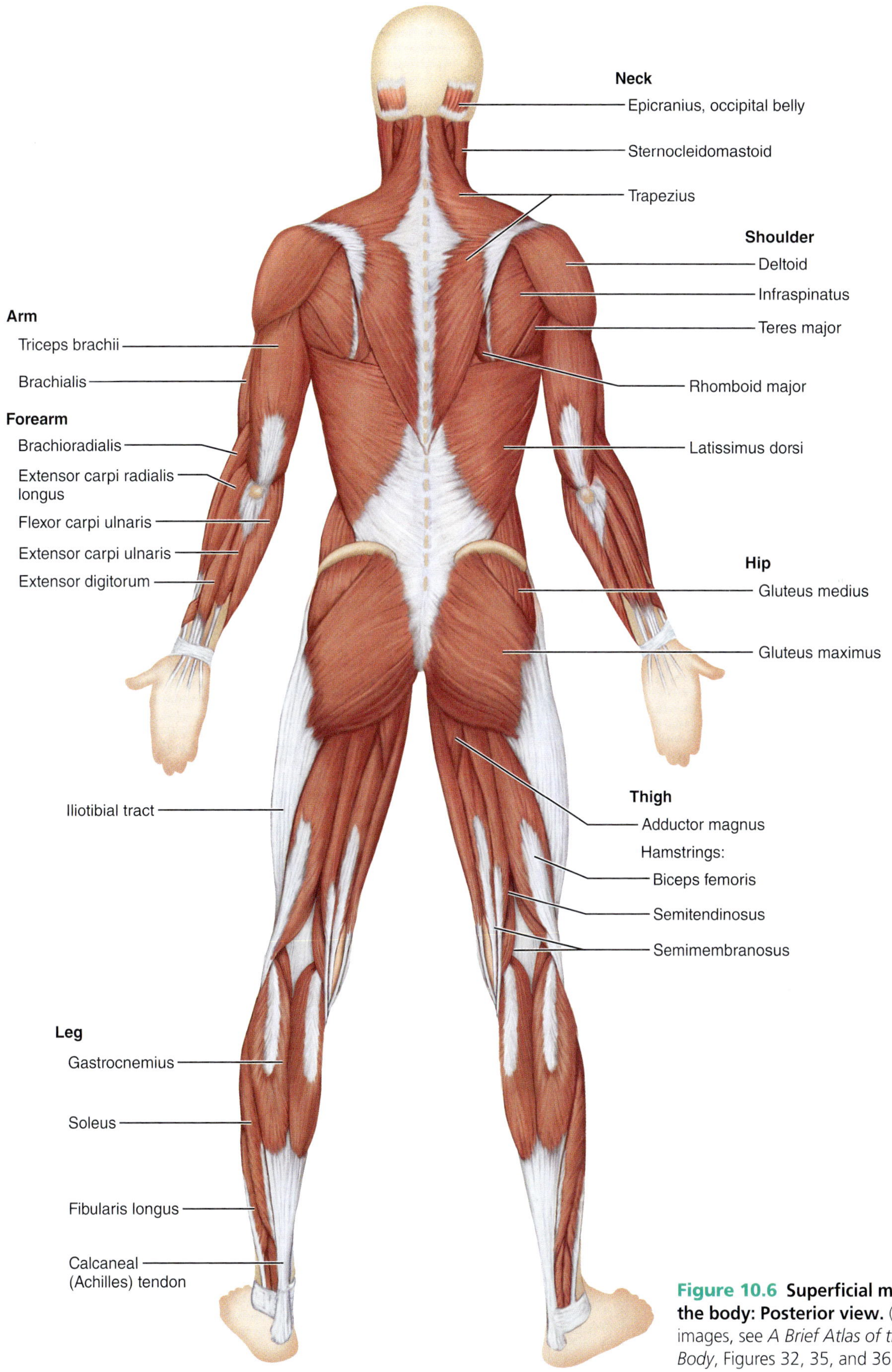

Figure 10.6 Superficial muscles of the body: Posterior view. (For related images, see *A Brief Atlas of the Human Body*, Figures 32, 35, and 36.)

The tables that follow group the muscles of the body by function and by location, roughly from head to foot. Each table is keyed to a particular figure or group of figures illustrating the muscles it describes. The legend at the beginning of each table summarizes the types of movements produced by the muscles listed and gives pointers on the way those muscles interact with one another. The table itself describes each muscle's shape, location relative to other muscles, origin and insertion, primary actions, and innervation. (Some instructors want students to defer learning the muscle innervations until they study the nervous system, so check on what is expected of you in this regard.)

As you consider each muscle, we recommend the following plan of action:

1. Be alert to the information provided by the muscle's name.
2. Read its entire description and identify the muscle on the corresponding figure. If it's a superficial muscle, also identify it on Figure 10.5 or Figure 10.6. Doing so will help you to link the description in the table to a visual image of the muscle's location in the body.
3. Relate the muscle's attachments and location to its actions. This will focus your attention on functional details that often escape student awareness. For example, both the elbow and knee joints are hinge joints that allow flexion and extension. However, the knee flexes to the dorsum of the body (the calf moves toward the posterior thigh), whereas elbow flexion carries the forearm toward the anterior aspect of the arm. Therefore, leg flexors are located on the posterior thigh, while forearm flexors are found on the anterior aspect of the humerus. A visual example of this relationship is shown in Figure 10.1a and b with the action of the muscles acting at the shoulder. Because many muscles have several actions, we indicate the primary action of each muscle in blue type in the tables.
4. Finally, keep in mind the *best* way to learn muscle actions: Act out their movements yourself while feeling for the muscles contracting (bulging) beneath your skin.

Now you are ready to tackle these tables:

(Text continues on p. 382.)

MUSCLE GALLERY

Table 10.1 Muscles of the Head, Part I: Facial Expression (Figure 10.7)

The muscles that promote facial expression lie in the scalp and face just deep to the skin. They are thin and variable in shape and strength, and adjacent muscles tend to be fused. They are unusual muscles in that they insert into skin (or other muscles), not bones.

In the scalp, the main muscle is the **epicranius**, which has distinct anterior and posterior parts. The lateral scalp muscles are vestigial in humans. Muscles clothing the facial bones lift the eyebrows, flare the nostrils, open and close the eyes and mouth, and provide one of the best tools for influencing others—the smile. The tremendous importance of facial muscles in nonverbal communication becomes especially clear when they are paralyzed, as in some stroke victims and in the expressionless "mask" of patients with Parkinson's disease.

Cranial nerve VII, the *facial nerve*, innervates all muscles listed in this table (see Table 13.2).

Chapter 15 describes the external muscles of the eyes, which direct the eyeballs, and the levator palpebrae superioris muscles that raise the eyelids.

MUSCLE	DESCRIPTION	ORIGIN (O) AND INSERTION (I)	ACTION	NERVE SUPPLY
MUSCLES OF THE SCALP				
Epicranius (occipitofrontalis) (ep″ĭ-kra′ne-us; ok-sip″ĭ-to-fron-ta′lis) (*epi* = over; *cran* = skull)	Bipartite muscle consisting of the frontal and occipital bellies connected by the epicranial aponeurosis. The alternate actions of these two muscles pull scalp forward and backward.			
▪ **Frontal belly** (fron′tal) (*front* = forehead)	Covers forehead and dome of skull; no bony attachments	O—epicranial aponeurosis I—skin of eyebrows and root of nose	With aponeurosis fixed, raises the eyebrows (as in surprise). Wrinkles forehead skin horizontally	Facial nerve (cranial VII)
▪ **Occipital belly** (ok-sip′ĭ-tal′) (*occipito* = base of skull)	Overlies posterior occiput; by pulling on the epicranial aponeurosis, fixes origin of frontal belly	O—occipital and temporal bones I—epicranial aponeurosis	Fixes aponeurosis and pulls scalp posteriorly	Facial nerve
MUSCLES OF THE FACE				
Corrugator supercilii (kor′ah-ga-ter soo″per-sĭ′le-i) (*corrugo* = wrinkle; *supercilium* = eyebrow)	Small muscle; activity associated with that of orbicularis oculi	O—arch of frontal bone above nasal bone I—skin of eyebrow	Draws eyebrows together and inferiorly; wrinkles skin of forehead vertically (as in frowning)	Facial nerve

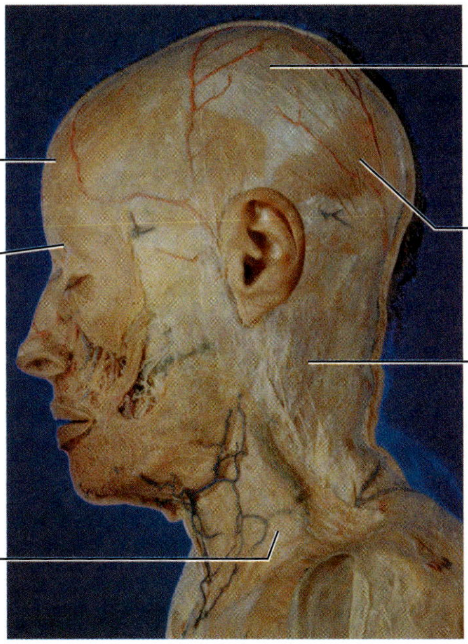

Figure 10.7 Lateral view of muscles of the scalp, face, and neck. (a) Photograph.

MUSCLE GALLERY

Table 10.1 Muscles of the Head, Part I: Facial Expression (Figure 10.7) *(continued)*

MUSCLE	DESCRIPTION	ORIGIN (O) AND INSERTION (I)	ACTION	NERVE SUPPLY
Orbicularis oculi (or-bik′u-lar-is ok′u-li) (*orb* = circular; *ocul* = eye)	Thin, flat sphincter muscle of eyelid; surrounds rim of the orbit	O—frontal and maxillary bones and ligaments around orbit I—tissue of eyelid	Closes eye; various parts can be activated individually; produces blinking and squinting; draws eyebrows inferiorly	Facial nerve (cranial VII)
Zygomaticus—major and minor (zi-go-mat′ĭ-kus) (*zygomatic* = cheekbone)	Muscle pair extending diagonally from cheekbone to corner of mouth	O—zygomatic bone I—skin and muscle at corner of mouth	Raises lateral corners of mouth upward (smiling muscle)	Facial nerve
Risorius (ri-zor′e-us) (*risor* = laughter)	Slender muscle inferior and lateral to zygomaticus	O—lateral fascia associated with masseter muscle I—skin at angle of mouth	Draws corner of lip laterally; tenses lips; synergist of zygomaticus	Facial nerve
Levator labii superioris (lĕva′tor la′be-i soo-per″e-or′is) (*leva* = raise; *labi* = lip; *superior* = above, over)	Thin muscle between orbicularis oris and inferior eye margin	O—zygomatic bone and infraorbital margin of maxilla I—skin and muscle of upper lip	Opens lips; raises and furrows upper lip	Facial nerve
Depressor labii inferioris (de-pres′or la′be-i in-fer″e-or′is) (*depressor* = depresses; *infer* = below)	Small muscle running from mandible to lower lip	O—body of mandible lateral to its midline I—skin and muscle of lower lip	Draws lower lip inferiorly (as in a pout)	Facial nerve
Depressor anguli oris (ang′gu-li or-is) (*angul* = angle, corner; *or* = mouth)	Small muscle lateral to depressor labii inferioris	O—body of mandible below incisors I—skin and muscle at angle of mouth below insertion of zygomaticus	Draws corners of mouth down and laterally (a "tragedy mask" grimace); zygomaticus antagonist	Facial nerve
Orbicularis oris	Complicated, multilayered muscle of the lips with fibers that run in many different directions; most run circularly	O—arises indirectly from maxilla and mandible; fibers blend with fibers of other facial muscles associated with the lips I—encircles mouth; inserts into muscle and skin at angles of mouth	Closes lips; purses and protrudes lips; kissing and whistling muscle	Facial nerve
Mentalis (men-ta′lis) (*ment* = chin)	One of the muscle pair forming a V-shaped muscle mass on chin	O—mandible below incisors I—skin of chin	Wrinkles chin; protrudes lower lip	Facial nerve
Buccinator (bu′sĭ-na″ter) (*bucc* = cheek or "trumpeter")	Thin, horizontal cheek muscle; principal muscle of cheek; deep to masseter (see also Figure 10.8)	O—molar region of maxilla and mandible I—orbicularis oris	Compresses cheek (as in whistling and sucking); trampoline-like action holds food between teeth during chewing; draws corner of mouth laterally; well developed in nursing infants	Facial nerve
Platysma (plah-tiz′mah) (*platy* = broad, flat)	Unpaired, thin, sheetlike superficial neck muscle; not strictly a head muscle, but plays a role in facial expression	O—fascia of chest (over pectoral muscles and deltoid) I—lower margin of mandible, and skin and muscle at corner of mouth	Tenses skin of neck (as during shaving); helps depress mandible; pulls lower lip back and down, producing downward sag of mouth	Facial nerve

MUSCLE GALLERY

Table 10.1 *(continued)*

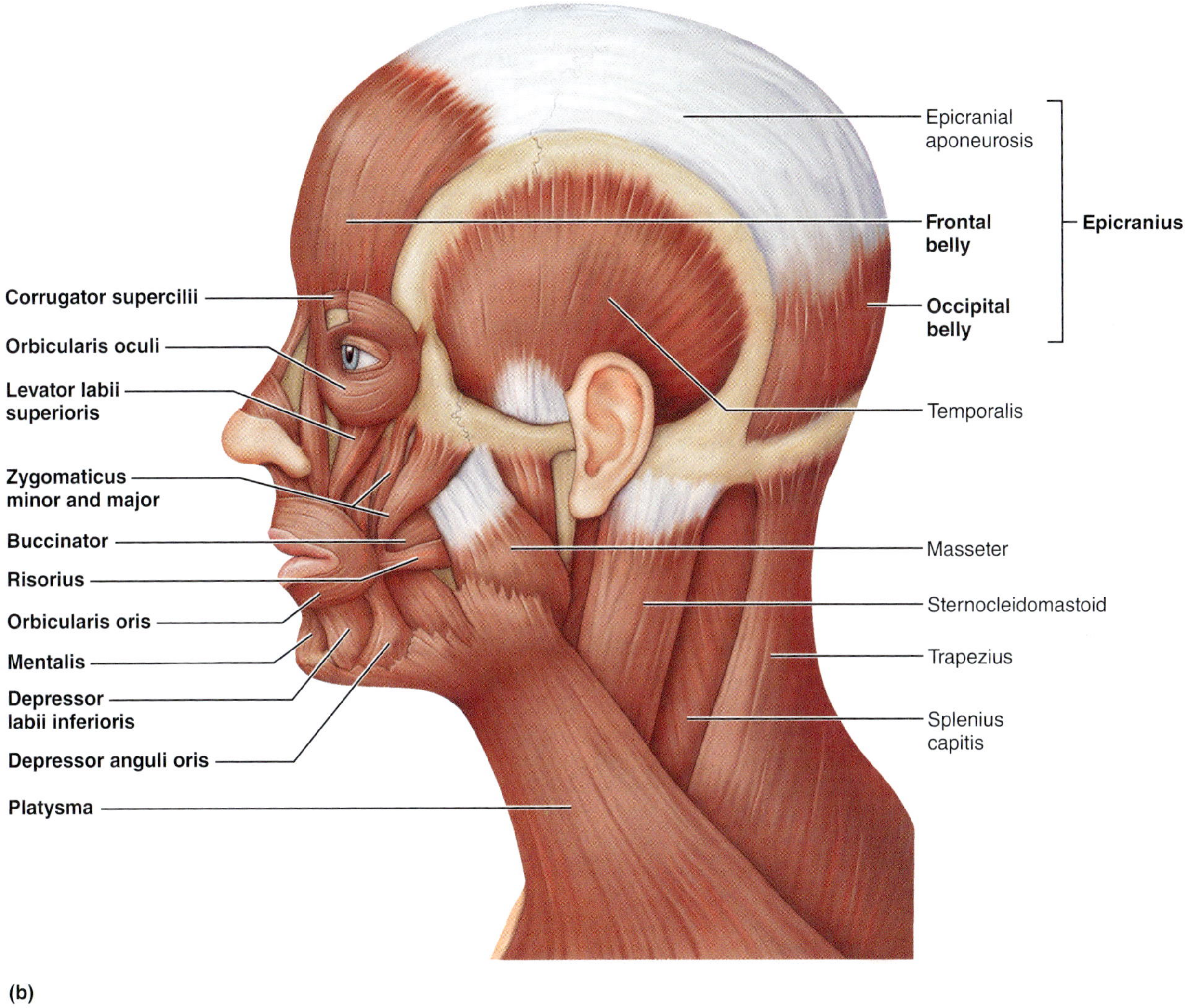

Figure 10.7 *(continued)* **Lateral view of muscles of the scalp, face, and neck. (b)** Superficial muscles.

10

MUSCLE GALLERY

Table 10.2 Muscles of the Head, Part II: Mastication and Tongue Movement (Figure 10.8)

Four pairs of muscles are involved in mastication (chewing). All are innervated by the *mandibular branch* of *cranial nerve V*.

The prime movers of jaw closure (and biting) are the powerful **masseter** and **temporalis** muscles, which are easily palpated when the teeth are clenched (Figure 10.8a). The **pterygoid** muscles produce side-to-side grinding (Figure 10.8b). The **buccinator** muscles (see Table 10.1) also play a role in chewing. Normally, gravity is sufficient to depress the mandible, but if there is resistance to jaw opening, neck muscles such as the digastric and mylohyoid muscles (see Table 10.3) are activated.

The tongue is composed of muscle fibers that curl, squeeze, and fold the tongue during speaking and chewing. These **intrinsic tongue muscles** change the shape of the tongue and contribute to its exceptional nimbleness, but they do not really move the tongue. We discuss them in Chapter 23 with the digestive system.

In this table, we consider only the **extrinsic tongue muscles**, which anchor and move the tongue (Figure 10.8c). *Cranial nerve XII*, the *hypoglossal nerve*, innervates all extrinsic tongue muscles (see Table 13.2).

MUSCLE	DESCRIPTION	ORIGIN (O) AND INSERTION (I)	ACTION	NERVE SUPPLY
MUSCLES OF MASTICATION				
Masseter (mah-se′ter) (*maseter* = chewer)	Powerful muscle that covers lateral aspect of mandibular ramus	O—zygomatic arch and zygomatic bone I—angle and ramus of mandible	Prime mover of jaw closure; elevates mandible	Trigeminal nerve (cranial V)
Temporalis (tem″por-ă′lis) (*tempora* = time; pertaining to the temporal bone)	Fan-shaped muscle that covers parts of the temporal, frontal, and parietal bones	O—temporal fossa I—coronoid process of mandible via a tendon that passes deep to zygomatic arch	Closes jaw; elevates and retracts mandible; maintains position of the mandible at rest; deep anterior part may help protract mandible	Trigeminal nerve
Medial pterygoid (me′de-ul ter′ĭ-goid) (*medial* = toward median plane; *pterygoid* = winglike)	Deep two-headed muscle that runs along internal surface of mandible and is largely concealed by that bone	O—medial surface of lateral pterygoid plate of sphenoid bone, maxilla, and palatine bone I—medial surface of mandible near its angle	Acts with the lateral pterygoid muscle to protrude (pull anteriorly) the mandible and promote side-to-side (grinding) movements; synergist of temporalis and masseter muscles in elevation of the mandible	Trigeminal nerve
Lateral pterygoid (*lateral* = away from median plane)	Deep two-headed muscle; lies superior to medial pterygoid muscle	O—greater wing and lateral pterygoid plate of sphenoid bone I—condylar process of mandible and capsule of temporomandibular joint	Provides forward sliding and side-to-side grinding movements of the lower teeth; protrudes mandible	Trigeminal nerve
Buccinator	See Table 10.1	See Table 10.1	Compresses the cheek; keeps food between grinding surfaces of teeth during chewing	Facial nerve (cranial VII)
MUSCLES PROMOTING TONGUE MOVEMENTS (EXTRINSIC TONGUE MUSCLES)				
Genioglossus (je″ne-o-glah′sus) (*geni* = chin; *glossus* = tongue)	Fan-shaped muscle; forms bulk of inferior part of tongue; its attachment to mandible prevents tongue from falling backward and obstructing breathing	O—internal surface of mandible near symphysis I—inferior aspect of the tongue and body of hyoid bone	Protracts tongue; can depress or act in concert with other extrinsic muscles to retract tongue	Hypoglossal nerve (cranial XII)
Hyoglossus (hi′o-glos″us) (*hyo* = pertaining to hyoid bone)	Flat, quadrilateral muscle	O—body and greater horn of hyoid bone I—inferolateral tongue	Depresses tongue and draws its sides inferiorly	Hypoglossal nerve
Styloglossus (sti-lo-glah′sus) (*stylo* = pertaining to styloid process)	Slender muscle running superiorly to and at right angles to hyoglossus	O—styloid process of temporal bone I—inferolateral tongue	Retracts and elevates tongue	Hypoglossal nerve

MUSCLE GALLERY

Table 10.2 *(continued)*

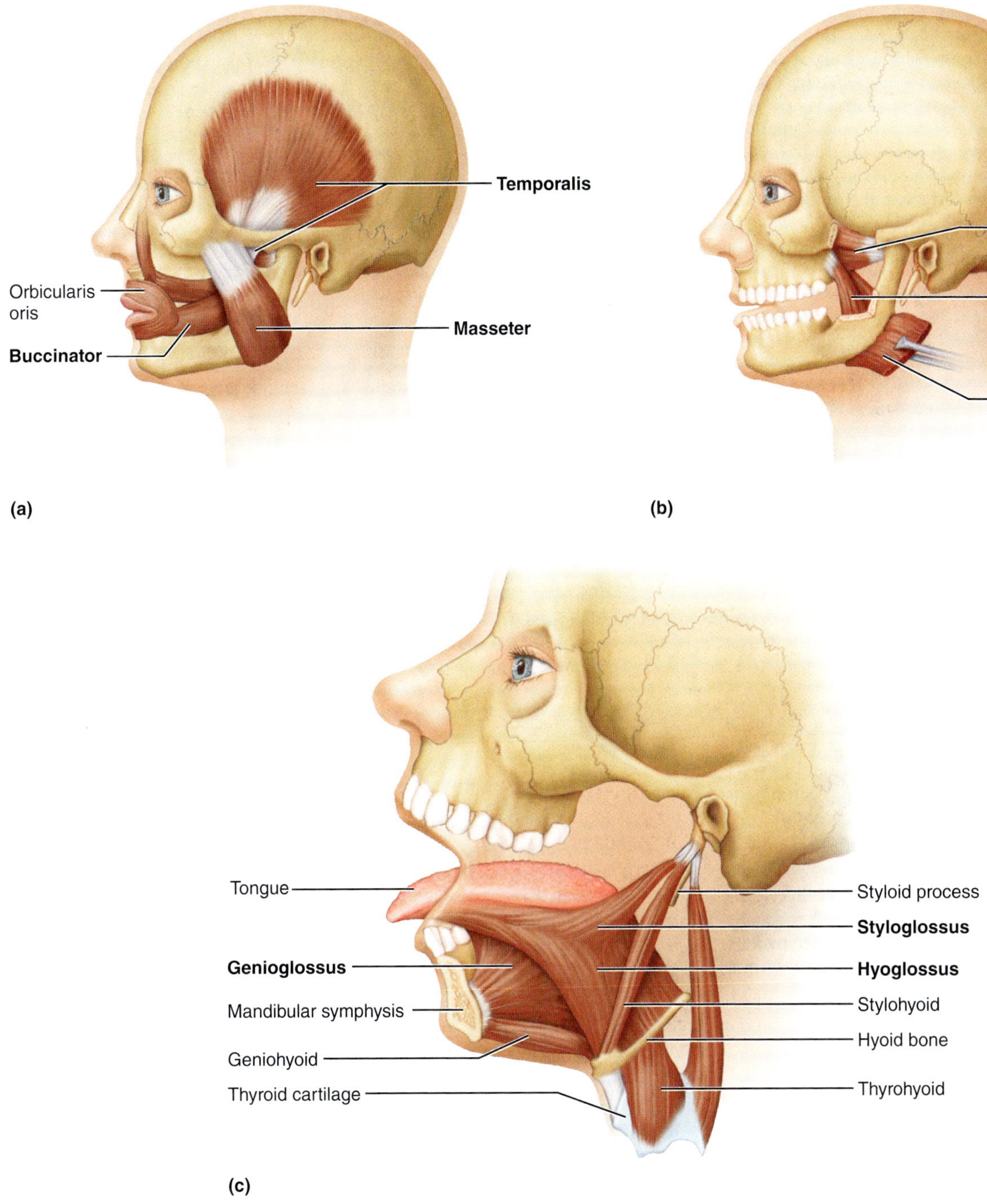

Figure 10.8 Muscles promoting mastication and tongue movements. (a) Lateral view of superficial muscles of mastication (temporalis, masseter, and buccinator muscles). **(b)** Lateral view of the deep chewing muscles. **(c)** Extrinsic muscles of the tongue and associated suprahyoid muscles of the throat.

MUSCLE GALLERY

Table 10.3 Muscles of the Anterior Neck and Throat: Swallowing (Figure 10.9)

The sternocleidomastoid muscle divides the neck into two triangles (anterior and posterior; Figure 10.9a). In this table, we consider the muscles of the *anterior* triangle, which are divided into **suprahyoid** and **infrahyoid muscles** (above and below the hyoid bone, respectively). Most of these muscles participate in swallowing.

Swallowing begins when the tongue and buccinator muscles of the cheeks squeeze the food back along the roof of the mouth toward the pharynx. A rapid series of sequential muscular movements in the posterior mouth and pharynx complete the process:

1. The *suprahyoid muscles* pull the hyoid bone superiorly and anteriorly toward the mandible, which widens the pharynx to receive the food (Figure 10.9c). The larynx is also pulled superiorly and anteriorly under the cover of the flaplike epiglottis, a maneuver that closes off the respiratory passageway (larynx) so that food is not inhaled into the lungs.
2. Small muscles that elevate the soft palate close off the nasal passages to prevent food from entering the superior nasal cavity. (These muscles, the *tensor* and *levator veli palatini*, are not described in the table but are illustrated in Figure 10.9c.)
3. The **pharyngeal constrictor muscles** in the wall of the pharynx propel food inferiorly into the esophagus.
4. The *infrahyoid muscles* pull the hyoid bone and larynx to their more inferior positions as swallowing ends.

10

MUSCLE	DESCRIPTION	ORIGIN (O) AND INSERTION (I)	ACTION	NERVE SUPPLY
SUPRAHYOID MUSCLES (soo″prah-hi′oid)	Muscles that help form floor of oral cavity, anchor tongue, elevate hyoid, and move larynx superiorly during swallowing; lie superior to hyoid bone			
Digastric (di-gas′trik) (*di* = two; *gaster* = belly)	Consists of two bellies united by an intermediate tendon, forming a V shape under the chin	O—lower margin of mandible (anterior belly) and mastoid process of temporal bone (posterior belly) I—by a connective tissue loop to hyoid bone	Open mouth and depress mandible; acting in concert, the digastric muscles elevate hyoid bone and steady it during swallowing and speech	Mandibular branch of trigeminal nerve (cranial V) for anterior belly; facial nerve (cranial VII) for posterior belly
Stylohyoid (sti″lo-hi′oid) (also see Figure 10.8)	Slender muscle below angle of jaw; parallels posterior belly of digastric muscle	O—styloid process of temporal bone I—hyoid bone	Elevates and retracts hyoid, thereby elongating floor of mouth during swallowing	Facial nerve
Mylohyoid (mi″lo-hi′oid) (*myle* = molar)	Flat, triangular muscle just deep to digastric muscle; this muscle pair make a sling that forms the floor of the anterior mouth	O—medial surface of mandible I—hyoid bone and median raphe (a median strip of connective tissue between the mylohyoid muscles)	Elevates hyoid bone and floor of mouth, enabling tongue to exert backward and upward pressure that forces food into pharynx	Mandibular branch of trigeminal nerve
Geniohyoid (je′ne-o-hi″oid) (also see Figure 10.8) (*geni* = chin)	Narrow muscle in contact with its partner medially; runs from chin to hyoid bone deep to mylohyoid	O—inner surface of mandibular symphysis I—hyoid bone	Pulls hyoid bone superiorly and anteriorly, shortening floor of mouth and widening pharynx to receive food	First cervical spinal nerve via hypoglossal nerve (cranial XII)
INFRAHYOID MUSCLES	Straplike muscles that depress the hyoid bone and larynx during swallowing and speaking (see also Figure 10.10c)			
Sternohyoid (ster″no-hi′oid) (*sterno* = sternum)	Most medial muscle of the neck: thin; superficial except inferiorly, where covered by sternocleidomastoid	O—manubrium and medial end of clavicle I—lower margin of hyoid bone	Depresses larynx and hyoid bone if mandible is fixed; may also flex skull	Cervical spinal nerves 1–3 (C_1–C_3) through ansa cervicalis (slender nerve root in cervical plexus)
Sternothyroid (ster′no-thi′roid) (*thyro* = thyroid cartilage)	Lateral and deep to sternohyoid	O—posterior surface of manubrium of sternum I—thyroid cartilage	Pulls larynx and hyoid bone inferiorly	As for sternohyoid
Omohyoid (o″mo-hi′oid) (*omo* = shoulder)	Straplike muscle with two bellies united by an intermediate tendon; lateral to sternohyoid	O—superior surface of scapula I—hyoid bone, lower border	Depresses and retracts hyoid bone	As for sternohyoid
Thyrohyoid (thi″ro-hi′oid) (also see Figure 10.8)	Appears as a superior continuation of sternothyroid muscle	O—thyroid cartilage I—hyoid bone	Depresses hyoid bone or elevates larynx if hyoid is fixed	First cervical nerve via hypoglossal nerve

MUSCLE GALLERY

Table 10.3 *(continued)*

MUSCLE	DESCRIPTION	ORIGIN (O) AND INSERTION (I)	ACTION	NERVE SUPPLY
PHARYNGEAL CONSTRICTOR MUSCLES (far-rin′je-al)				
Superior, middle, and inferior pharyngeal constrictor muscles	Three paired muscles whose fibers run circularly in pharynx wall; superior muscle is innermost and inferior one is outermost; substantial overlap	O—attached anteriorly to mandible and medial pterygoid plate (superior), hyoid bone (middle), and laryngeal cartilages (inferior) I—posterior median raphe of pharynx	Constrict pharynx during swallowing, which propels food to esophagus (via a massagelike action called peristalsis)	Pharyngeal plexus [branches of vagus nerve (X)]

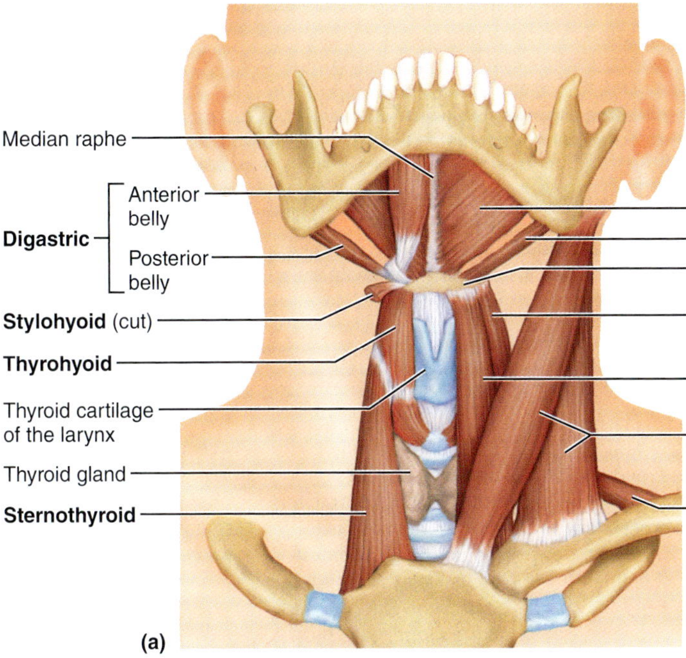

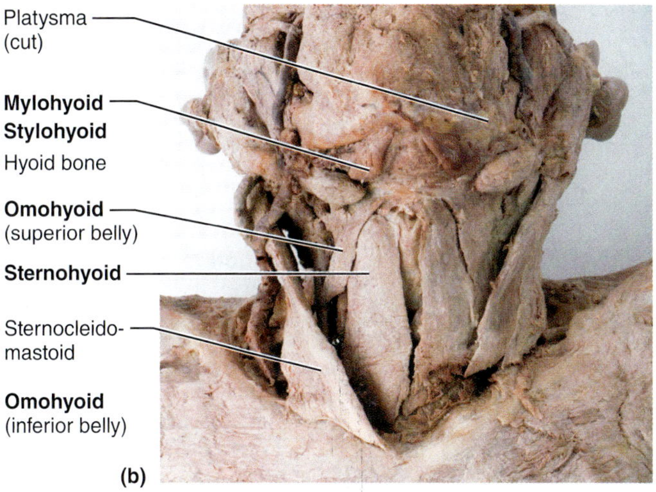

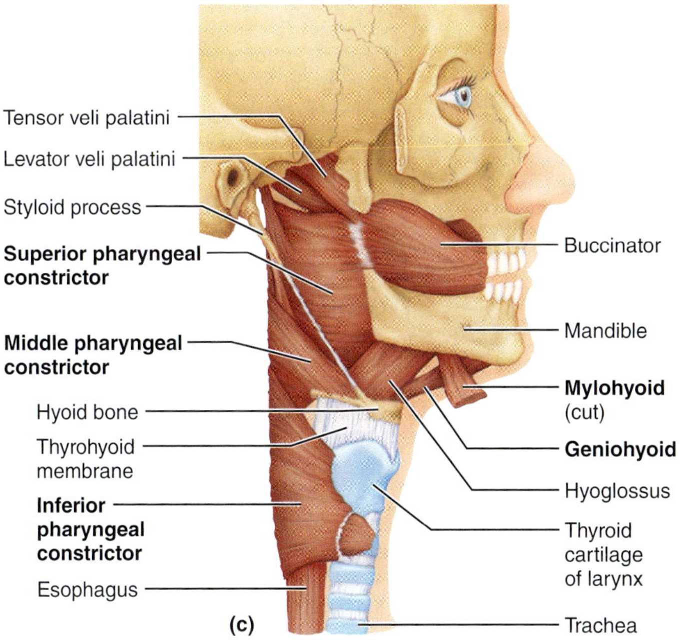

Figure 10.9 Muscles of the anterior neck and throat used in swallowing. (a) Anterior view of the suprahyoid and infrahyoid muscles. The sternocleidomastoid muscle (not involved in swallowing) is shown on the right side of the illustration to provide an anatomical landmark. Deeper neck muscles are illustrated on the left side. Note that a raphe is a seam of fibrous tissue. **(b)** Cadaver photo of suprahyoid and infrahyoid muscles. (For related images, see *A Brief Atlas of the Human Body*, Figures 44 and 45.) **(c)** Lateral view of the constrictor muscles of the pharynx shown in their proper anatomical relationship to the buccinator (a chewing muscle) and the hyoglossus muscle (which moves the tongue).

MUSCLE GALLERY

Table 10.4 Muscles of the Neck and Vertebral Column: Head Movements and Trunk Extension (Figure 10.10)

Head movements

Muscles originating from the axial skeleton move the head. The major head flexors are the **sternocleidomastoid muscles** (Figure 10.10a, c), with help from the suprahyoid and infrahyoid muscles described in Table 10.3. Lateral head movements (rotating or tilting the head) result when the muscles on only one side of the neck contract. These actions are produced by the sternocleidomastoids and a number of deeper neck muscles, considered in this table. Head extension is aided by the trapezius muscles of the back, but the main extensors of the head are the **splenius** muscles deep to the trapezius muscles (Figure 10.10b).

Trunk extension

Trunk extension is brought about by the *deep* or *intrinsic back muscles* associated with the bony vertebral column. These muscles also maintain the normal curvatures of the spine, acting as postural muscles. As you consider these back muscles, keep in mind that they are deep. The superficial back muscles that cover them are concerned primarily with moving the shoulder girdle and upper limbs (see Tables 10.8 and 10.9).

The deep muscles of the back form a broad, thick column extending from the sacrum to the skull. Many muscles of varying length contribute to this mass. Think of each muscle as a string that when pulled causes one or several vertebrae to extend or to rotate on the vertebrae below. The largest deep back muscle group is the **erector spinae** group (Figure 10.10d). Because the origins and insertions of the different muscle groups overlap extensively, and many of these muscles are long, large regions of the vertebral column can be moved simultaneously and smoothly. Acting together, the deep back muscles extend (or hyperextend) the spine, but muscle contraction on only one side causes the spine to bend laterally (flex). Lateral flexion is automatically accompanied by some degree of rotation of the vertebral column. During vertebral movements, the articular facets of the vertebrae glide on each other.

In addition to the long back muscles, there are a number of short muscles that extend from one vertebra to the next. These small muscles act primarily as synergists in extending and rotating the spine and as spine stabilizers. They are not described in the table but you can deduce their actions by examining their origins and insertions in Figure 10.10e.

The trunk *muscles* that we consider in this table are extensors. The more superficial muscles, which have other functions, are considered in subsequent tables. For example, the anterior muscles of the abdominal wall that cause trunk *flexion* are described in Table 10.6.

MUSCLE	DESCRIPTION	ORIGIN (O) AND INSERTION (I)	ACTION	NERVE SUPPLY
ANTEROLATERAL NECK MUSCLES (Figure 10.10a and c)				
Sternocleidomastoid (ster″no-kli″do-mas′toid) (*sterno* = breastbone; *cleido* = clavicle; *mastoid* = mastoid process)	Two-headed muscle located deep to platysma on anterolateral surface of neck; fleshy parts on either side of neck delineate limits of anterior and posterior triangles; key muscular landmark in neck; spasms of one of these muscles may cause torticollis (wryneck)	O—manubrium of sternum and medial portion of clavicle I—mastoid process of temporal bone and superior nuchal line of occipital bone	Flexes and laterally rotates the head; simultaneous contraction of both muscles flexes neck, generally against resistance as when raising head when lying on back; acting alone, each muscle rotates head toward shoulder on opposite side and tilts or laterally flexes head to its own side	Accessory nerve (cranial nerve XI) and branches of cervical spinal nerves C_2 and C_3 (ventral rami)
Scalenes (ska′lēnz)—anterior, middle, and posterior (*scalene* = uneven)	Located more laterally than anteriorly on neck; deep to platysma and sternocleidomastoid	O—transverse processes of cervical vertebrae I—anterolaterally on first two ribs	Elevate first two ribs (aid in inspiration); flex and rotate neck	Cervical spinal nerves
INTRINSIC MUSCLES OF THE BACK (Figure 10.10b, d, e)				
Splenius (sple′ne-us)—capitis and cervicis portions (kă′pĭ-tis; ser-vis′us) (*splenion* = bandage; *caput* = head; *cervi* = neck) (Figures 10.10b and 10.7)	Broad bipartite superficial muscle (capitis and cervicis parts) extending from upper thoracic vertebrae to skull; capitis portion known as "bandage muscle" because it covers and holds down deeper neck muscles	O—ligamentum nuchae,* spinous processes of vertebrae C_7–T_6 I—mastoid process of temporal bone and occipital bone (capitis); transverse processes of C_2–C_4 vertebrae (cervicis)	Extend or hyperextend head; when splenius muscles on one side are activated, head rotates and bends laterally toward same side	Cervical spinal nerves (dorsal rami)

*The ligamentum nuchae (lig″ah-men′tum noo′ke) is a strong, elastic ligament extending from the occipital bone of the skull along the tips of the spinous processes of the cervical vertebrae. It binds the cervical vertebrae together and inhibits excessive head and neck flexion, thus preventing damage to the spinal cord in the vertebral canal.

MUSCLE GALLERY

Table 10.4 *(continued)*

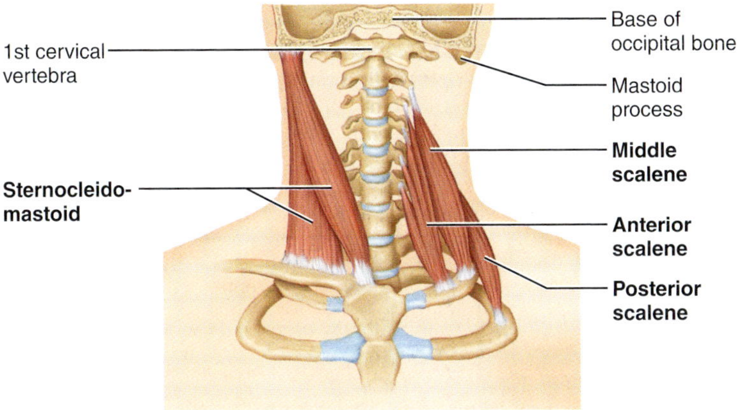

(a) Anterior

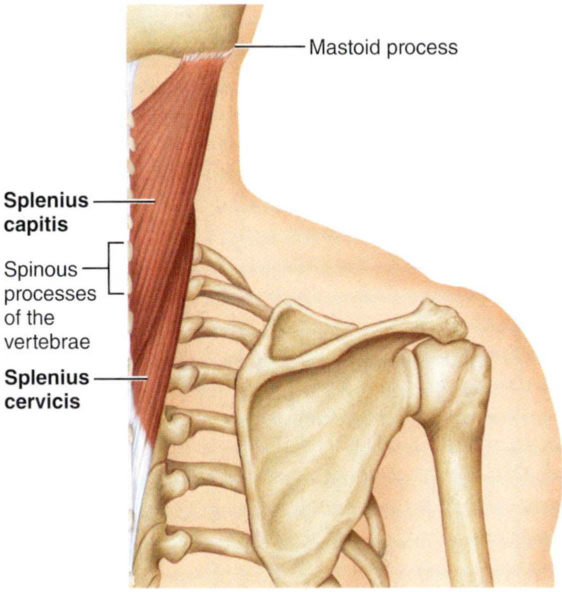

(b) Posterior

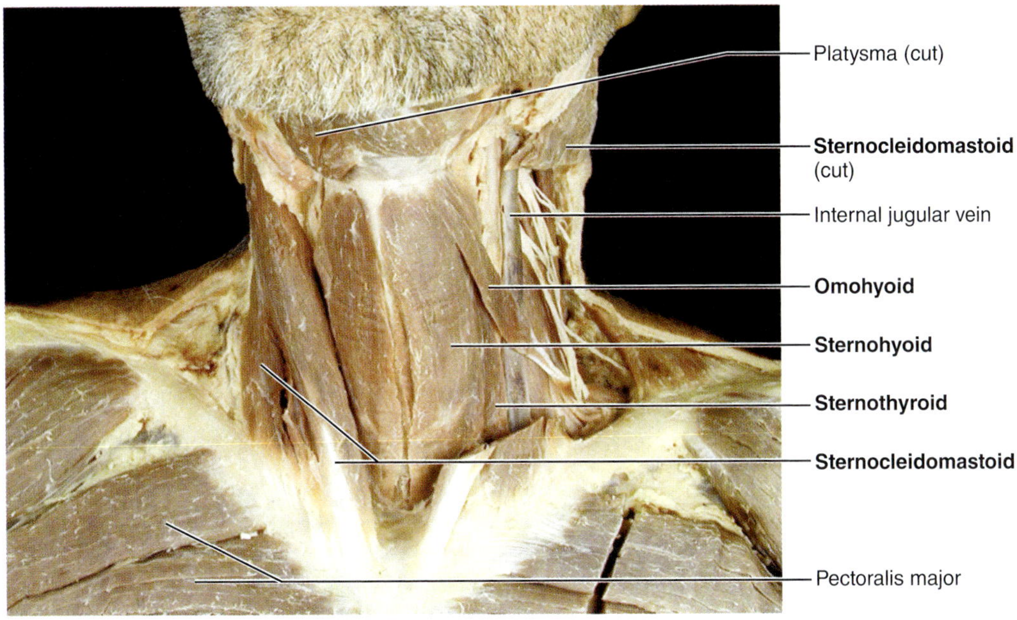

(c)

Figure 10.10 Muscles of the neck and vertebral column that move the head and trunk. (For a related image, see *A Brief Atlas of the Human Body*, Plate 44.) **(a)** Muscles of the anterolateral neck; superficial platysma muscle and the deeper neck muscles removed. **(b)** Deep muscles of the posterior neck; superficial muscles removed. **(c)** Photograph of the anterior and lateral regions of the neck.

MUSCLE GALLERY

Table 10.4 Muscles of the Neck and Vertebral Column: Head Movements and Trunk Extension (Figure 10.10) *(continued)*

MUSCLE	DESCRIPTION	ORIGIN (O) AND INSERTION (I)	ACTION	NERVE SUPPLY
Erector spinae (e-rek′tor spi′ne) Also called **sacrospinalis** (Figure 10.10d, left side)	Prime mover of back extension. Each side consists of three columns—the iliocostalis, longissimus, and spinalis muscles—forming intermediate layer of intrinsic back muscles. Erector spinae provide resistance that helps control action of bending forward at the waist and act as powerful extensors to promote return to erect position. During full flexion (i.e., when touching fingertips to floor), erector spinae are relaxed and strain is borne entirely by ligaments of back. On reversing the movement, these muscles are initially inactive, and extension is initiated by hamstring muscles of thighs and gluteus maximus muscles of buttocks. As a result of this peculiarity, lifting a load or moving suddenly from a bent-over position can injure muscles and ligaments of back and intervertebral discs. Erector spinae muscles readily go into painful spasms following injury to back structures.			
▪ **Iliocostalis** (il″e-o-kos-tă′lis)—lumborum, thoracis, and cervicis portions (lum′bor-um; tho-ra′sis) (*ilio* = ilium; *cost* = rib; *thorac* = thorax)	Most lateral muscle group of erector spinae muscles; extend from pelvis to neck	O—iliac crests (lumborum); inferior 6 ribs (thoracis); ribs 3 to 6 (cervicis) I—angles of ribs (lumborum and thoracis); transverse processes of cervical vertebrae C_6–C_4 (cervicis)	Extend and laterally flex the vertebral column; maintain erect posture; acting on one side, bend vertebral column to same side	Spinal nerves (dorsal rami)
▪ **Longissimus** (lon-jis′ĭ-mus)—thoracis, cervicis, and capitis parts (*longissimus* = longest)	Intermediate tripartite muscle group of erector spinae; extend by many muscle slips from lumbar region to skull; mainly pass between transverse processes of vertebrae	O—transverse processes of lumbar through cervical vertebrae I—transverse processes of thoracic or cervical vertebrae and to ribs superior to origin as indicated by name; capitis inserts into mastoid process of temporal bone	Thoracis and cervicis act together to extend and laterally flex vertebral column; capitis extends head and turns the face toward same side	Spinal nerves (dorsal rami)
▪ **Spinalis** (spi-nă′lis)—thoracis and cervicis parts (*spin* = vertebral column, spine)	Most medial muscle column of erector spinae; cervicis usually rudimentary and poorly defined	O—spinous process of upper lumbar and lower thoracic vertebrae I—spinous process of upper thoracic and cervical vertebrae	Extends vertebral column	Spinal nerves (dorsal rami)
Semispinalis (sem′e-spĭ-nă′lis)—thoracis, cervicis, and capitis regions (*semi* = half) (Figure 10.10d, right side)	Composite muscle forming part of deep layer of intrinsic back muscles; extends from thoracic region to head	O—transverse processes of C_7–T_{12} I—occipital bone (capitis) and spinous processes of cervical (cervicis) and thoracic vertebrae T_1–T_4 (thoracis)	Extends vertebral column and head and rotates them to opposite side; acts synergistically with sternocleidomastoid muscles of opposite side	Spinal nerves (dorsal rami)
Quadratus lumborum (kwod-ra′tus lum-bor′um) (*quad* = four-sided; *lumb* = lumbar region) (See also Figure 10.20a)	Fleshy muscle forming part of posterior abdominal wall	O—iliac crest and lumbar fascia I—transverse processes of lumbar vertebrae L_1–L_4 and lower margin of 12th rib	Flexes vertebral column laterally when acting separately; when pair acts jointly, lumbar spine is extended and 12th rib is fixed; maintains upright posture; assists in forced inspiration	T_{12} and upper lumbar spinal nerves (ventral rami)

MUSCLE GALLERY

Table 10.4 *(continued)*

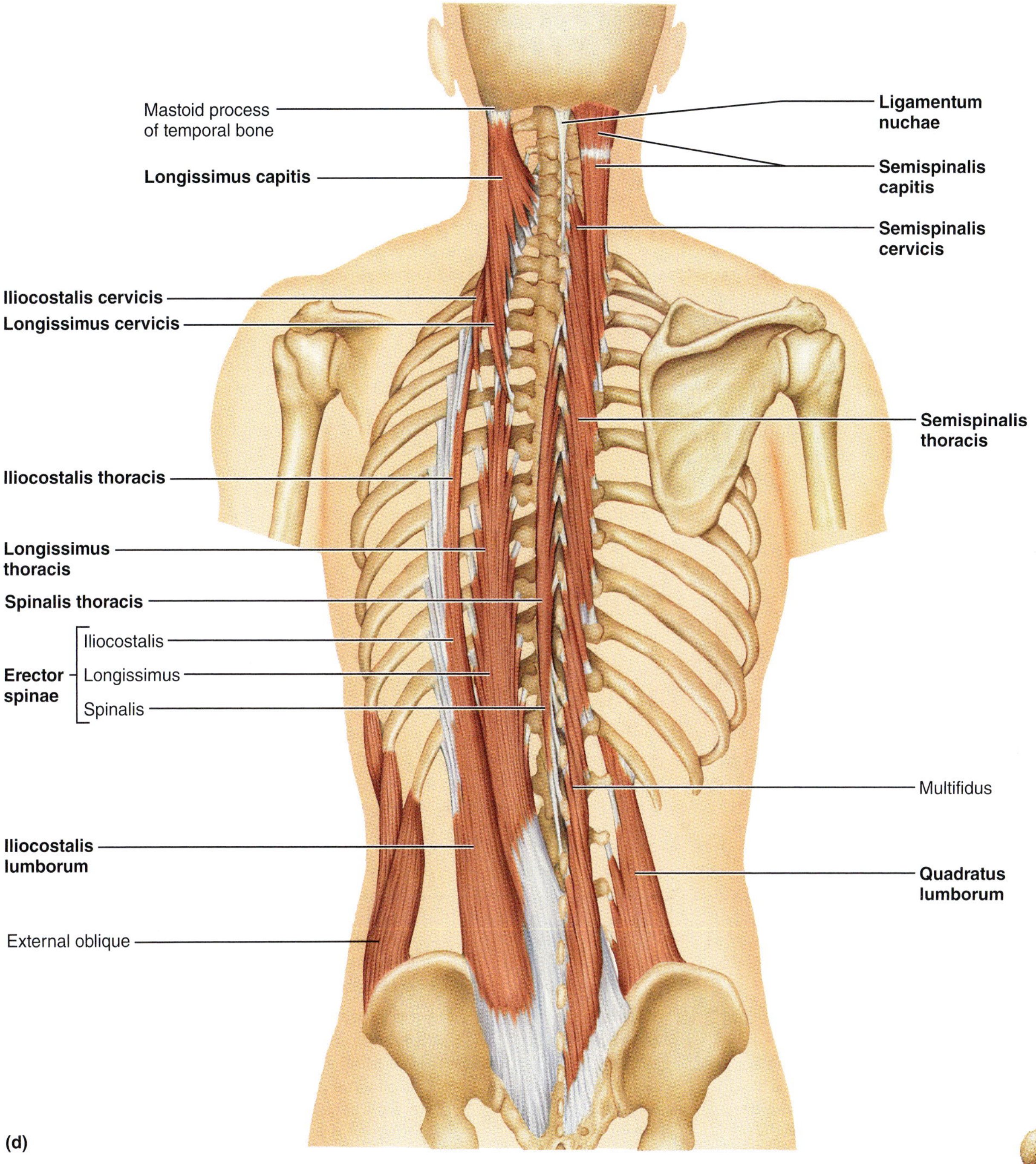

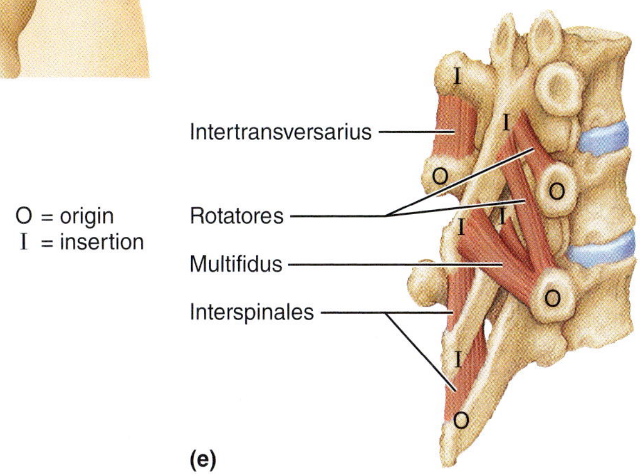

Figure 10.10 *(continued)* **Muscles of the neck and vertebral column that move the head and trunk. (d)** Deep muscles of the back; superficial, intermediate, and splenius muscles removed. The erector spinae muscles are shown on the left; deeper semispinalis muscles are shown on the right. **(e)** The deepest muscles of the back associated with the vertebral column.

MUSCLE GALLERY

Table 10.5 Deep Muscles of the Thorax: Breathing (Figure 10.11)

The deep muscles of the thorax promote movements necessary for breathing. Breathing consists of two phases—inspiration (inhaling) and expiration (exhaling)—caused by cyclic changes in the volume of the thoracic cavity.

Two main layers of muscles help form the anterolateral wall of the thorax.* The thoracic muscles are very short, most extending only from one rib to the next. On contraction, they draw the somewhat flexible ribs closer together. The **external intercostal muscles**, considered inspiratory muscles, form the more superficial layer (Figure 10.11a). They lift the rib cage, which increases the anterior to posterior and side-to-side dimensions of the thorax. The **internal intercostal muscles** form the deeper layer and may aid active (forced) expiration by depressing the rib cage. (However, quiet expiration is largely passive, resulting from relaxation of the external intercostals and diaphragm and elastic recoil of the lungs.)

The **diaphragm**, the most important muscle of inspiration, forms a muscular partition between the thoracic and abdominopelvic cavities (Figure 10.11b, c). In the relaxed state, the diaphragm is dome shaped. When it contracts it moves inferiorly and flattens, increasing the volume of the thoracic cavity, which draws air into the respiratory passageways. The alternating rhythmic contraction and relaxation of the diaphragm also causes pressure changes in the abdominopelvic cavity below that facilitate the return of blood to the heart.

In addition you can contract the diaphragm voluntarily to push down on the abdominal viscera and increase the pressure in the abdominopelvic cavity to help evacuate pelvic organ contents (urine, feces, or a baby) or lift weights. When you take a deep breath to fix the diaphragm, the abdomen becomes a firm pillar that will not buckle under the weight being lifted. Needless to say, it is important to have good control of the urinary bladder and anal sphincters during such maneuvers.

With the exception of the diaphragm, which is served by the *phrenic nerves*, the muscles listed in this table are served by the *intercostal nerves*, which run between the ribs.

Forced breathing (as during exercise) calls into play a number of other muscles that insert into the ribs. For example, during forced inspiration the scalene and sternocleidomastoid muscles of the neck help lift the ribs. Forced expiration is aided by muscles that pull the ribs inferiorly and those that push the diaphragm superiorly by compressing the abdominal contents (abdominal wall muscles).

MUSCLE	DESCRIPTION	ORIGIN (O) AND INSERTION (I)	ACTION	NERVE SUPPLY
External intercostals (in″ter-kos′talz) (*external* = toward the outside; *inter* = between; *cost* = rib)	11 pairs lie between ribs; fibers run obliquely (down and forward) from each rib to rib below; in lower intercostal spaces, fibers are continuous with external oblique muscle, forming part of abdominal wall	O—inferior border of rib above I—superior border of rib below	With first ribs fixed by scalene muscles, pull ribs toward one another to elevate rib cage; aid in inspiration; synergists of diaphragm	Intercostal nerves
Internal intercostals (*internal* = toward the inside, deep)	11 pairs lie between ribs; fibers run deep to and at right angles to those of external intercostals (i.e., run downward and posteriorly); lower internal intercostal muscles are continuous with fibers of internal oblique muscle of abdominal wall	O—superior border of rib below I—inferior border (costal groove) of rib above	With 12th ribs fixed by quadratus lumborum, muscles of posterior abdominal wall, and oblique muscles of the abdominal wall, they draw ribs together and depress rib cage; aid forced expiration; antagonistic to external intercostals	Intercostal nerves
Diaphragm (di′ah-fram) (*dia* = across; *phragm* = partition)	Broad muscle pierced by the aorta, inferior vena cava, and esophagus, forms floor of thoracic cavity; dome shaped in relaxed state; fibers converge from margins of thoracic cage toward a boomerang-shaped central tendon	O—inferior, internal surface of rib cage and sternum, costal cartilages of last six ribs and lumbar vertebrae I—central tendon	Prime mover of inspiration; flattens on contraction, increasing vertical dimensions of thorax; when strongly contracted, dramatically increases intra-abdominal pressure	Phrenic nerves

*Although there is a third (deepest) muscle layer of the thoracic wall, the muscles are small and discontinuous. Additionally, their function is unclear, so they are not included in this table.

MUSCLE GALLERY

Table 10.5 *(continued)*

Figure 10.11 Muscles of respiration. (a) Deep muscles of the thorax. The external intercostals (inspiratory muscles) are shown on the left and the internal intercostals (expiratory muscles) are shown on the right. These two muscle layers run obliquely and at right angles to each other. **(b)** Inferior view of the diaphragm, the prime mover of inspiration. Notice that its muscle fibers converge toward a central tendon, an arrangement that causes the diaphragm to flatten and move inferiorly as it contracts. **(c)** Photograph of the diaphragm, superior view.

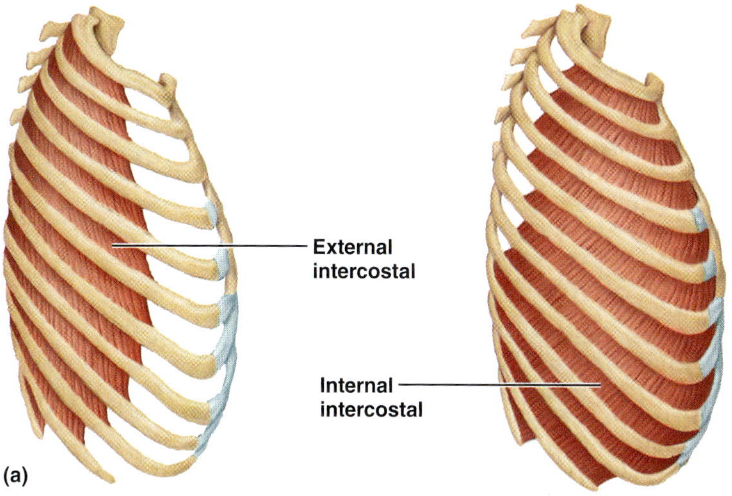

(a)

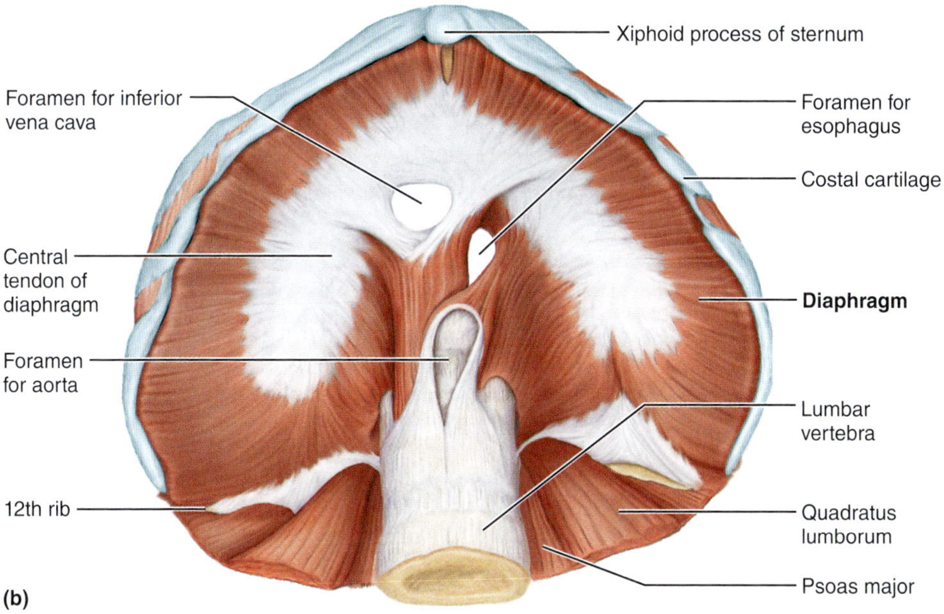

(b)

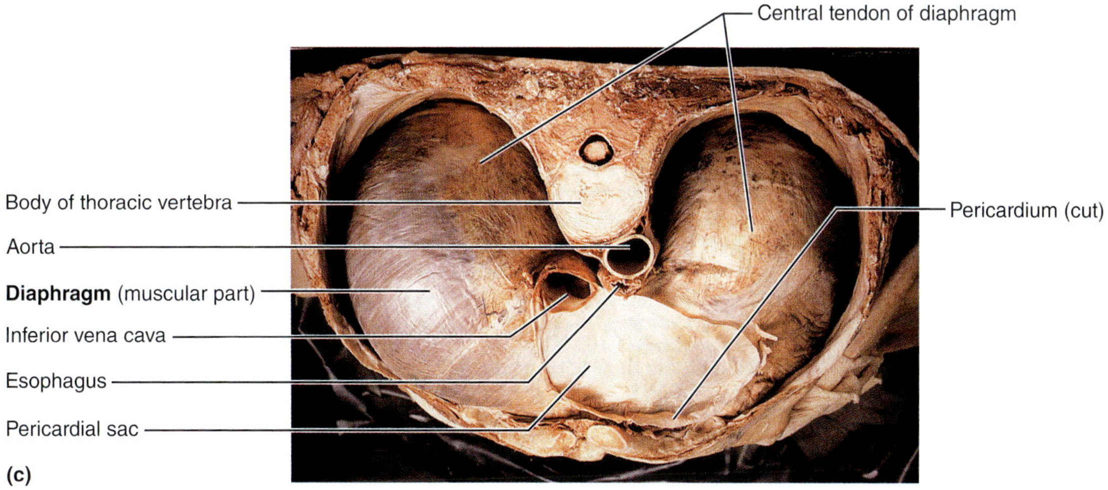

(c)

10

MUSCLE GALLERY

Table 10.6 Muscles of the Abdominal Wall: Trunk Movements and Compression of Abdominal Viscera (Figure 10.12)

Unlike the thorax, the anterior and lateral abdominal wall has no bony reinforcements (ribs). Instead, it is a composite of four paired muscles, their investing fasciae, and aponeuroses.

Three broad flat muscle pairs, layered one atop the next, form the lateral abdominal walls: The fibers of the **external oblique muscle** run inferomedially and at right angles to those of the **internal oblique**, which immediately underlies it (Figure 10.12a, b). The fibers of the deep **transversus abdominis muscle** run horizontally across the abdomen at an angle to both. This alternation of fascicle directions is similar to the construction of plywood (which is made of sheets with different grains) and provides great strength.

These three muscles blend into broad insertion aponeuroses anteriorly. The aponeuroses, in turn, enclose a fourth muscle pair medially, the straplike **rectus abdominis muscles**, and then fuse, forming the **linea alba** ("white line"), a tendinous raphe (seam) that runs from the sternum to the pubic symphysis (Figure 10.12a, c). The snug enclosure of the rectus abdominis muscles within the aponeuroses, the so-called *rectus sheath*, prevents them from "bowstringing" (protruding anteriorly) when they contract. Table 10.4 describes the quadratus lumborum muscles of the *posterior* abdominal wall.

The abdominal muscles protect and support the viscera most effectively when they are well toned. When weak or severely stretched (as during pregnancy), they allow the abdomen to become pendulous (i.e., to form a potbelly). Additional functions include lateral flexion and rotation of the trunk and flexion of the trunk against resistance (as in sit-ups).

During inspiration, the abdominal muscles relax, allowing the descending diaphragm to push the abdominal viscera inferiorly. When these abdominal muscles contract, several different activities may occur. For example, when they contract simultaneously, they pull the ribs inferiorly and compress the abdominal contents. This forces the visceral organs upward on the diaphragm, aiding forced expiration. When the abdominal muscles contract with the diaphragm and the glottis is closed (the Valsalva maneuver), the increased intra-abdominal pressure promotes urination, defecation, childbirth, vomiting, coughing, screaming, sneezing, burping, and nose blowing. (Next time you perform one of these activities, feel your abdominal muscles contract under your skin.)

These muscles also contract during heavy lifting— sometimes so forcefully that hernias result. Contracting the abdominal muscles as the deep back muscles contract helps prevent hyperextension of the spine and splints the entire body trunk.

10

MUSCLE	DESCRIPTION	ORIGIN (O) AND INSERTION (I)	ACTION	NERVE SUPPLY
MUSCLES OF THE ANTERIOR AND LATERAL ABDOMINAL WALL	Four paired flat muscles; important in supporting and protecting abdominal viscera; promote lateral flexion and flexion of vertebral column			
Rectus abdominis (rek′tus ab-dom′ĭ-nis) (*rectus* = straight; *abdom* = abdomen)	Medial superficial muscle pair; extend from pubis to rib cage; ensheathed by aponeuroses of lateral muscles; segmented by three tendinous intersections	O—pubic crest and symphysis I—xiphoid process and costal cartilages of ribs 5–7	Flex and rotate lumbar region of vertebral column; fix and depress ribs, stabilize pelvis during walking, increase intra-abdominal pressure; used in sit-ups, curls	Intercostal nerves (T_6 or T_7–T_{12})
External oblique (o-blēk′) (*external* = toward outside; *oblique* = running at an angle)	Largest and most superficial of the three lateral muscles; fibers run downward and medially (same direction outstretched fingers take when hands are in pants pockets); aponeurosis turns under inferiorly, forming inguinal ligament	O—by fleshy strips from outer surfaces of lower eight ribs I—most fibers insert into linea alba via a broad aponeurosis; some insert into pubic crest and tubercle and iliac crest	When pair contract simultaneously, flex vertebral column and compress abdominal wall and increase intra-abdominal pressure; acting individually, aid muscles of back in rotating trunk and flexing laterally; used in oblique curls	Intercostal nerves (T_7–T_{12})
Internal oblique (*internal* = toward the inside; deep)	Most fibers run upward and medially; however, the muscle fans so its inferior fibers run downward and medially	O—lumbar fascia, iliac crest, and inguinal ligament I—linea alba, pubic crest, last three or four ribs, and costal margin	As for external oblique	Intercostal nerves (T_7–T_{12}) and L_1
Transversus abdominis (trans-ver′sus) (*transverse* = running straight across)	Deepest (innermost) muscle of abdominal wall; fibers run horizontally	O—inguinal ligament, lumbar fascia, cartilages of last six ribs; iliac crest I—linea alba, pubic crest	Compresses abdominal contents	Intercostal nerves (T_7–T_{12}) and L_1

MUSCLE GALLERY

Table 10.6 *(continued)*

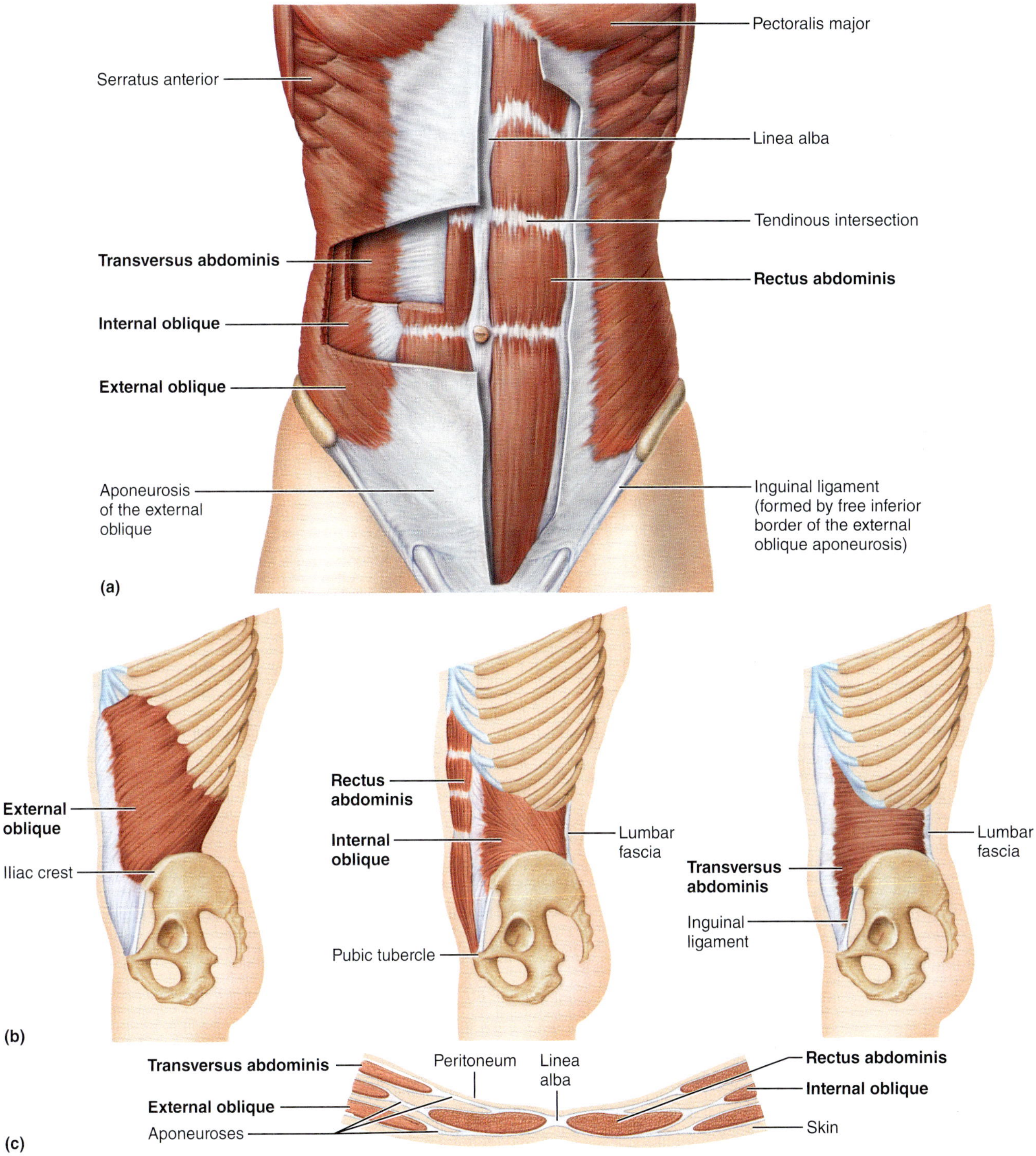

Figure 10.12 Muscles of the abdominal wall. (a) Anterior view of the muscles forming the anterolateral abdominal wall; superficial muscles partially cut away to reveal the deeper muscles. **(b)** Lateral view of the trunk, illustrating the fiber direction and attachments of the abdominal muscles. Although shown in the same view, the rectus abdominis is deep to the fascia of the internal oblique muscle. **(c)** Transverse section through the anterolateral abdominal wall (midregion), showing how the aponeuroses of the lateral abdominal muscles contribute to the rectus abdominis sheath.

MUSCLE GALLERY

Table 10.7 Muscles of the Pelvic Floor and Perineum: Support of Abdominopelvic Organs (Figure 10.13)

Two paired muscles, the **levator ani** and **coccygeus**, form the funnel-shaped pelvic floor, or **pelvic diaphragm** (Figure 10.13a). This diaphragm (1) seals the inferior opening of the bony pelvis, (2) supports the pelvic organs, (3) lifts the pelvic floor superiorly to release feces, and (4) resists increased intra-abdominal pressure (which would expel contents of the urinary bladder, rectum, and uterus). The pelvic diaphragm is pierced by the rectum and urethra (urinary tube), and by the vagina in females.

The body region inferior to the pelvic diaphragm is the *perineum*. The **urogenital diaphragm** sits inferior to the muscles of the pelvic floor, and stretches between the two sides of the pubic arch in the anterior half of the perineum (Figure 10.13b). This thin triangular sheet of muscle contains the **external urethral sphincter**, a sphincter muscle that surrounds the urethra and allows voluntary control of urination. Superficial to the urogenital diaphragm, and covered by the skin of the perineum, is the *superficial perineal space*, which contains muscles (**ischiocavernosus** and **bulbospongiosus**) that help maintain erection of the penis and clitoris (Figure 10.13c). In the posterior half of the perineum encircling the anus is the **external anal sphincter**, which allows voluntary control of defecation. Just anterior to this sphincter is the **central tendon of the perineum**, a strong tendon into which many of the perineal muscles insert.

10

MUSCLE	DESCRIPTION	ORIGIN (O) AND INSERTION (I)	ACTION	NERVE SUPPLY
MUSCLES OF THE PELVIC DIAPHRAGM (Figure 10.13a)				
Levator ani (lĕ-va′tor a′ne) (*levator* = raises; *ani* = anus)	Broad, thin, tripartite muscle (pubococcygeus, puborectalis, and iliococcygeus); its fibers extend inferomedially, forming a muscular "sling" around male prostate (or female vagina), urethra, and anorectal junction before meeting in the median plane	O—extensive linear origin inside pelvis from pubis to ischial spine I—inner surface of coccyx, levator ani of opposite side, and (in part) into the structures that penetrate it	Supports and maintains position of pelvic viscera; resists downward thrusts that accompany rises in intrapelvic pressure during coughing, vomiting, and expulsive efforts of abdominal muscles; forms sphincters at anorectal junction and vagina; lifts anal canal during defecation	S_3, S_4, and inferior rectal nerve (branch of pudendal nerve)
Coccygeus (kok-sij′e-us) (*coccy* = coccyx)	Small triangular muscle lying posterior to levator ani; forms posterior part of pelvic diaphragm	O—spine of ischium I—sacrum and coccyx	Supports pelvic viscera; supports coccyx and pulls it forward after it has been reflected posteriorly by defecation and childbirth	S_4 and S_5
MUSCLES OF THE UROGENITAL DIAPHRAGM (Figure 10.13b)				
Deep transverse perineal muscle (per″ĭ-ne′al) (*deep* = far from surface; *transverse* = across; *perine* = near anus)	Together the pair spans distance between ischial rami; in females, lies posterior to vagina	O—ischial rami I—midline central tendon of perineum; some fibers into vaginal wall in females	Supports pelvic organs; steadies central tendon	Pudendal nerve
External urethral sphincter (*sphin* = squeeze)	Muscle encircling urethra and vagina (female)	O—ischiopubic rami I—midline raphe	Constricts urethra; allows voluntary inhibition of urination; helps support pelvic organs	Pudendal nerve
MUSCLES OF THE SUPERFICIAL PERINEAL SPACE (Figure 10.13c)				
Ischiocavernosus (is″ke-o-kav″ern-o′sus) (*ischi* = hip; *caverna* = hollow chamber)	Runs from pelvis to base of penis or clitoris	O—ischial tuberosities I—crus of corpora cavernosa of male penis or female clitoris	Retards venous drainage and maintains erection of penis or clitoris	Pudendal nerve
Bulbospongiosus (bul″bo-spun″je-o′sus) (*bulbon* = bulb; *spongio* = sponge)	Encloses base of penis (bulb) in males and lies deep to labia in females	O—central tendon of perineum and midline raphe of penis I—anteriorly into corpora cavernosa of penis or clitoris	Empties male urethra; assists in erection of penis and of clitoris	Pudendal nerve
Superficial transverse perineal muscles (*superficial* = closer to surface)	Paired muscle bands posterior to urethral (and in females, vaginal) opening; variable; sometimes absent	O—ischial tuberosity I—central tendon of perineum	Stabilizes and strengthens central tendon of perineum	Pudendal nerve

MUSCLE GALLERY

Table 10.7 *(continued)*

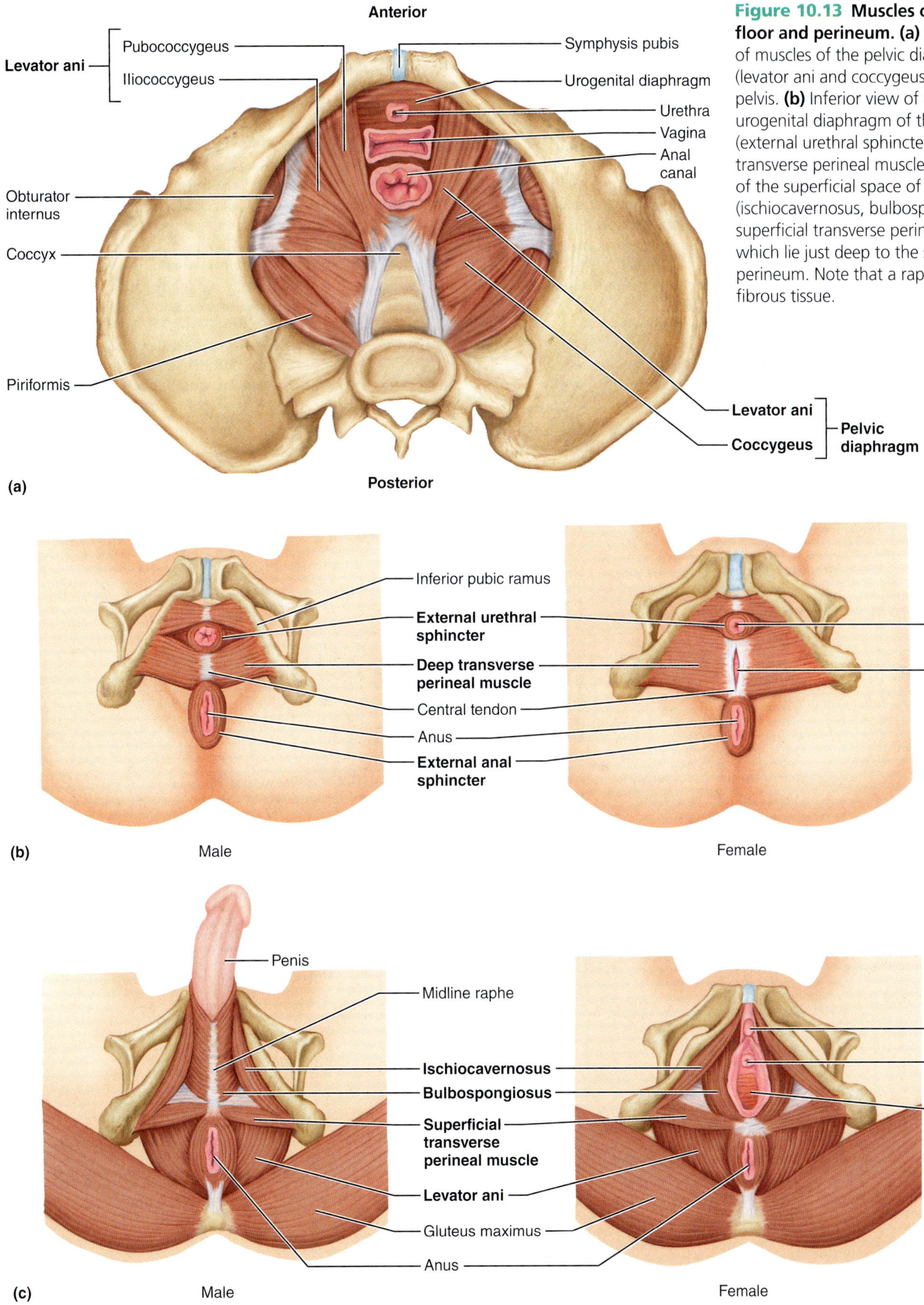

Figure 10.13 Muscles of the pelvic floor and perineum. (a) Superior view of muscles of the pelvic diaphragm (levator ani and coccygeus) in a female pelvis. **(b)** Inferior view of muscles of the urogenital diaphragm of the perineum (external urethral sphincter and deep transverse perineal muscles). **(c)** Muscles of the superficial space of the perineum (ischiocavernosus, bulbospongiosus, and superficial transverse perineal muscle), which lie just deep to the skin of the perineum. Note that a raphe is a seam of fibrous tissue.

10

10

MUSCLE GALLERY

Table 10.8 Superficial Muscles of the Anterior and Posterior Thorax: Movements of the Scapula and Arm (Figure 10.14)

Most superficial thorax muscles are *extrinsic shoulder muscles*, which run from the ribs and vertebral column to the shoulder girdle. They both fix the scapula in place and move it to increase the range of arm movements.

The anterior muscles of this group include the **pectoralis major**, **pectoralis minor**, **serratus anterior**, and **subclavius** (Figure 10.14a). Except for the pectoralis major, which inserts into the humerus, all muscles of the anterior group insert into the pectoral girdle.

The posterior muscles include the **latissimus dorsi** and **trapezius muscles** superficially and the underlying **levator scapulae** and **rhomboids** (Figure 10.14c). The latissimus dorsi, like the pectoralis major muscles anteriorly, insert into the humerus and are more concerned with moving the arm than the scapula, so we defer their consideration to Table 10.9 (arm-moving muscles).

The important movements of the pectoral girdle involve displacing the scapula, i.e., its elevation and depression, rotation, lateral (forward) movements, and medial (backward) movements. The clavicles rotate around their own axes to provide stability and precision to scapular movements.

Except for the serratus anterior, the anterior muscles stabilize and depress the shoulder girdle. Thus, most scapular movements are promoted by the serratus anterior muscles anteriorly and by posterior thoracic muscles. The arrangement of muscle attachments to the scapula is such that one muscle cannot bring about a simple (linear) movement on its own. To effect scapular movements, several muscles must act in combination.

The prime movers of shoulder (scapular) elevation are the superior trapezius fibers and the levator scapulae. When acting together to shrug the shoulder, their opposite rotational effects counterbalance each other. The scapula is depressed largely by gravity (weight of the arm), but when it is depressed against resistance, the inferior part of the trapezius, the pectoralis minor, and the serratus anterior (along with the latissimus dorsi, Table 10.9) are active. Anterolateral movements (abduction) of the scapula on the thorax wall, as in pushing or punching, mainly reflect serratus anterior activity. Posteromedial movement (adduction) of the scapula is effected mainly by the trapezius (midpart) and the rhomboids. Although the serratus anterior and trapezius muscles are antagonists in forward/backward movements of the scapulae, they act together to coordinate *rotational* scapular movements.

MUSCLE	DESCRIPTION	ORIGIN (O) AND INSERTION (I)	ACTION	NERVE SUPPLY
MUSCLES OF THE ANTERIOR THORAX (Figure 10.14a)				
Pectoralis minor (pek″to-ra′lis mi′nor) (*pectus* = chest, breast; *minor* = lesser)	Flat, thin muscle directly beneath and obscured by pectoralis major	O—anterior surfaces of ribs 3–5 (or 2–4) I—coracoid process of scapula	With ribs fixed, draws scapula forward and downward; with scapula fixed, draws rib cage superiorly	Medial and lateral pectoral nerves (C_6–C_8)
Serratus anterior (ser-a′tus) (*serratus* = saw)	Fan-shaped muscle; lies deep to scapula, deep and inferior to pectoral muscles on lateral rib cage; forms medial wall of axilla; origins have serrated (sawtooth) appearance; paralysis results in "winging" of vertebral border of scapula away from chest wall, making arm elevation impossible	O—by a series of muscle slips from ribs 1–8 (or 9) I—entire anterior surface of vertebral border of scapula	Rotates scapula so its inferior angle moves laterally and upward; prime mover to protract and hold scapula against chest wall; raises point of shoulder; important role in abducting and raising arm and in horizontal arm movements (pushing, punching); called "boxer's muscle"	Long thoracic nerve (C_5–C_7)
Subclavius (sub-kla′ve-us) (*sub* = under, beneath; *clav* = clavicle)	Small cylindrical muscle extending from rib 1 to clavicle	O—costal cartilage of rib 1 I—groove on inferior surface of clavicle	Helps stabilize and depress pectoral girdle	Nerve to subclavius (C_5 and C_6)

MUSCLE GALLERY

Table 10.8 *(continued)*

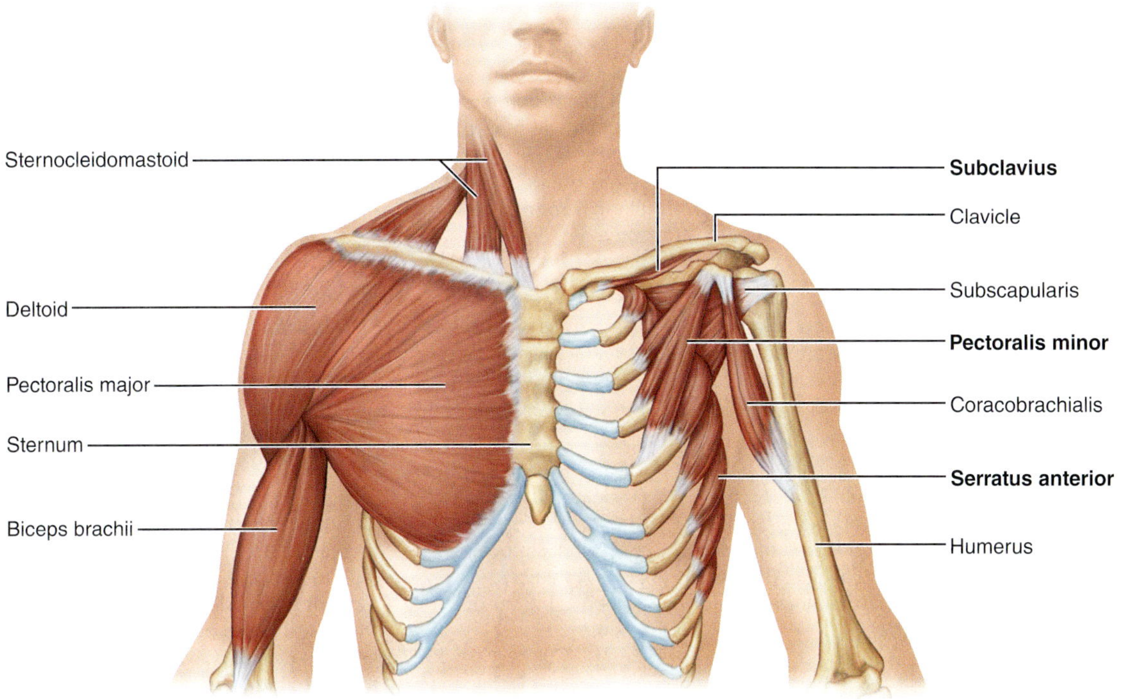

(a)

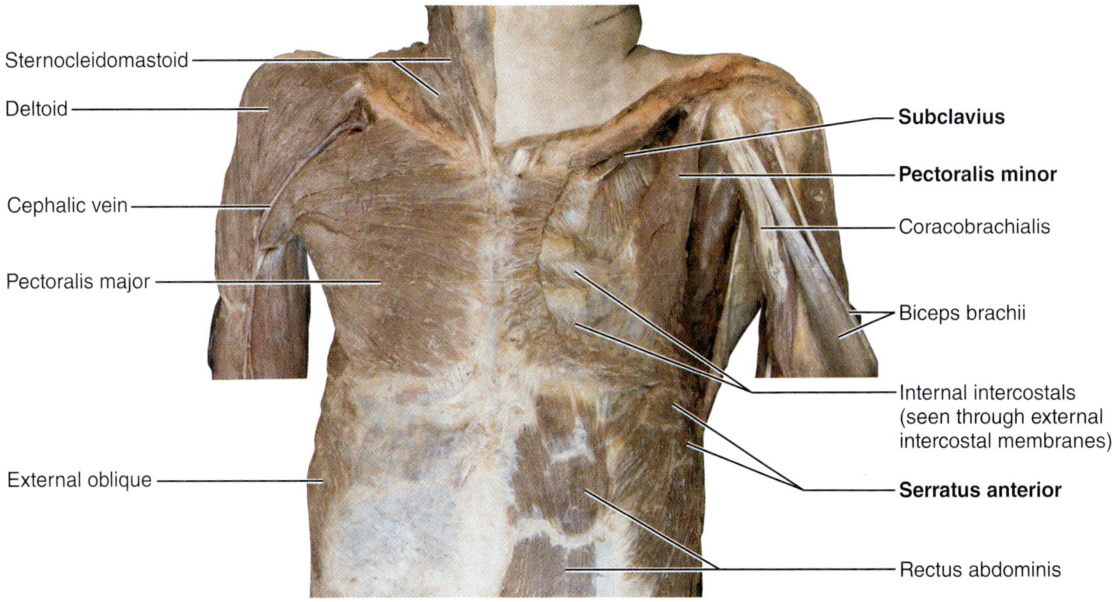

(b)

Figure 10.14 Superficial muscles of the thorax and shoulder acting on the scapula and arm. (a) Anterior view. The superficial muscles, which effect arm movements, are shown on the left side of the illustration. These muscles are removed on the right to show the muscles that stabilize or move the pectoral girdle. **(b)** Cadaver dissection, anterior view of superficial muscles of anterior thorax.

Table 10.8 Superficial Muscles of the Anterior and Posterior Thorax: Movements of the Scapula and Arm (Figure 10.14) *(continued)*

MUSCLE	DESCRIPTION	ORIGIN (O) AND INSERTION (I)	ACTION	NERVE SUPPLY
MUSCLES OF THE POSTERIOR THORAX (Figure 10.14c–e)				
Trapezius (trah-pe′ze-us) (*trapezion* = irregular four-sided figure)	Most superficial muscle of posterior thorax; flat and triangular in shape; upper fibers run inferiorly to scapula; middle fibers run horizontally to scapula; lower fibers run superiorly to scapula	O—occipital bone, ligamentum nuchae, and spinous processes of C_7 and all thoracic vertebrae I—a continuous insertion along acromion and spine of scapula and lateral third of clavicle	Stabilizes, raises, retracts, and rotates scapula; middle fibers retract (adduct) scapula; superior fibers elevate scapula (as in shrugging the shoulders) or help extend head with scapula fixed; inferior fibers depress scapula (and shoulder)	Accessory nerve (cranial nerve XI); C_3 and C_4
Levator scapulae (skap′u-le) (*levator* = raises)	Located at back and side of neck, deep to trapezius; thick straplike muscle	O—transverse processes of C_1–C_4 I—medial border of scapula, superior to spine	Elevates/adducts scapula in concert with superior fibers of trapezius; tilts glenoid cavity downward when scapula is fixed, flexes neck to same side	Cervical spinal nerves and dorsal scapular nerve (C_3–C_5)
Rhomboids (rom′boidz)—major and minor (*rhomboid* = diamond shaped)	Two roughly diamond-shaped muscles lying deep to trapezius and inferior to levator scapulae; rhomboid minor is the more superior muscle	O—spinous processes of C_7 and T_1 (minor) and spinous processes of T_2–T_5 (major) I—medial border of scapula	Stabilize scapula; act together (and with middle trapezius fibers) to retract (adduct) scapula, thus "squaring shoulders"; rotate scapula so that glenoid cavity is downward (as when lowering arm against resistance; e.g., paddling a canoe)	Dorsal scapular nerve (C_4 and C_5)

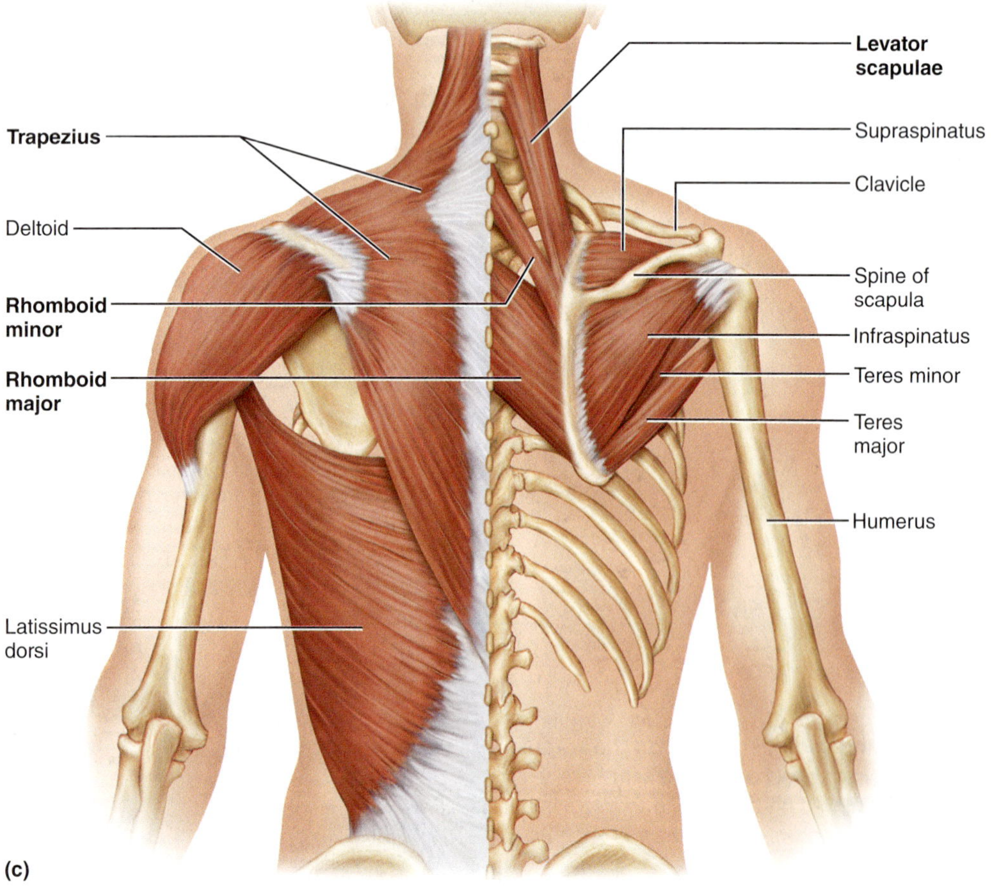

Figure 10.14 *(continued)* **Superficial muscles of the thorax and shoulder acting on the scapula and arm.** **(c)** Posterior view. The superficial muscles are shown on the left side of the illustration. Superficial muscles are removed on the right side to reveal the deeper muscles acting on the scapula, and the rotator cuff muscles that help stabilize the shoulder joint.

MUSCLE GALLERY

Table 10.8 *(continued)*

Figure 10.14 *(continued)* **Superficial muscles of the thorax and shoulder acting on the scapula and arm. (d)** and **(e)** Cadaver dissections showing views similar to (c).

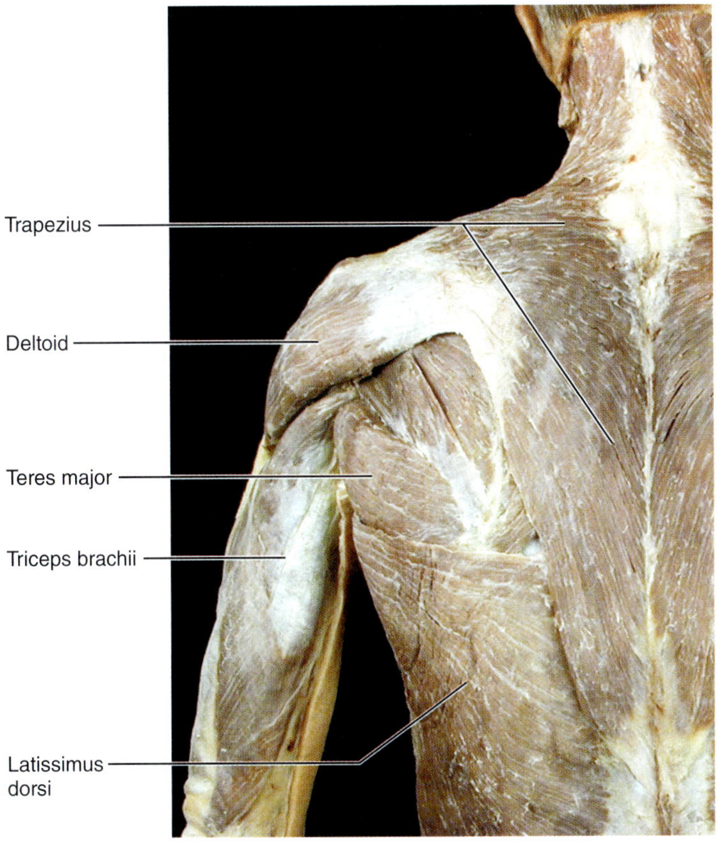

(d)

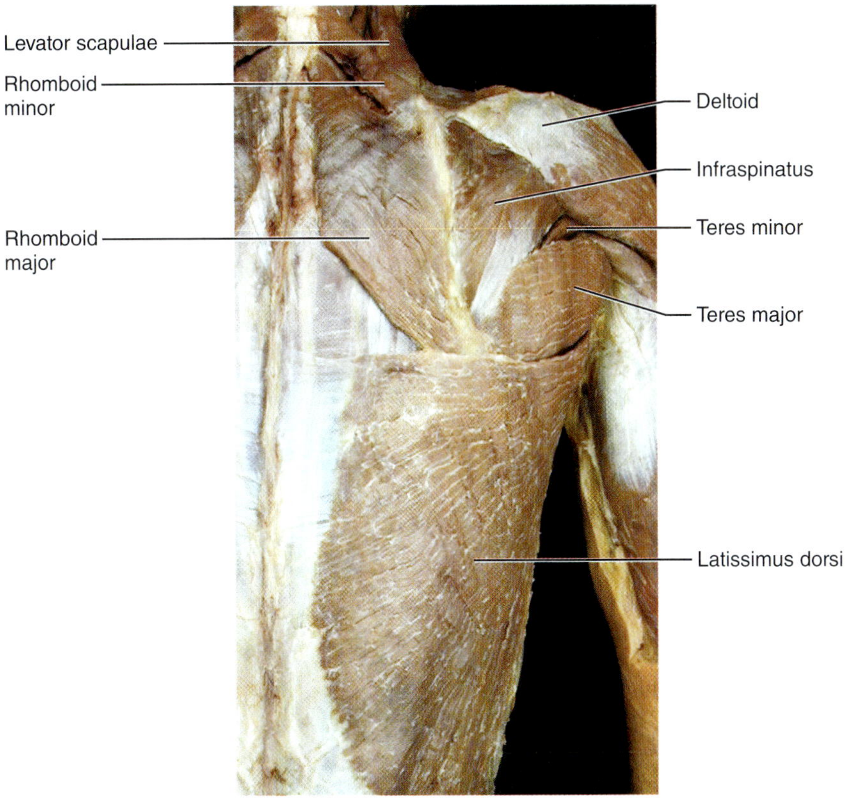

(e)

MUSCLE GALLERY

Table 10.9 Muscles Crossing the Shoulder Joint: Movements of the Arm (Humerus) (Figure 10.15)

Recall that the ball-and-socket shoulder joint is the most flexible joint in the body, but pays the price of instability. Several muscles cross each shoulder joint to insert on the humerus. All muscles acting on the humerus originate from the pectoral girdle. However, two of these—the latissimus dorsi and pectoralis major—primarily originate on the axial skeleton.

Of the nine muscles covered here, only the **pectoralis major**, **latissimus dorsi**, and **deltoid muscles** are prime movers of arm movements (Figure 10.15a, b). The remaining six are synergists and fixators. Four of these, the **supraspinatus**, **infraspinatus**, **teres minor**, and **subscapularis** (marked with an asterisk* in Figure 10.15b, d), are *rotator cuff muscles.* They originate on the scapula, and their tendons blend with the fibrous capsule of the shoulder joint en route to the humerus. Although the rotator cuff muscles act as synergists in angular and rotational movements of the arm, their main function is to reinforce the capsule of the shoulder joint to prevent dislocation of the humerus. The remaining two muscles, the small **teres major** and **coracobrachialis**, cross the shoulder joint but do not reinforce it.

Generally speaking, muscles that originate *anterior* to the shoulder joint (pectoralis major, coracobrachialis, and anterior fibers of the deltoid) *flex* the arm, i.e., lift it anteriorly. The prime mover of arm flexion is the pectoralis major. The biceps brachii of the arm assists in this action (Figure 10.15a, c; see Table 10.10).

Muscles originating *posterior* to the shoulder joint extend the arm. These include the latissimus dorsi and posterior fibers of the deltoid muscles (both prime movers of arm extension) and the teres major. Note that the pectoralis and latissimus dorsi muscles are *antagonists* of one another in flexing and extending the arm.

The middle region of the fleshy deltoid muscle of the shoulder, which extends over the superolateral side of the humerus, is the prime mover of arm abduction. The main arm adductors are the pectoralis major anteriorly and latissimus dorsi posteriorly. The small muscles acting on the humerus promote lateral and medial rotation of the arm. The interactions among these nine muscles are complex and each contributes to several movements. Table 10.12 (Part I) summarizes their actions.

10

MUSCLE	DESCRIPTION	ORIGIN (O) AND INSERTION (I)	ACTION	NERVE SUPPLY
Pectoralis major (pek″to-ra′lis ma′jer) (*pectus* = breast, chest; *major* = larger)	Large, fan-shaped muscle covering superior portion of chest; forms anterior axillary fold; divided into clavicular and sternal parts	O—sternal end of clavicle, sternum, cartilage of ribs 1–6 (or 7), and aponeurosis of external oblique muscle I—fibers converge to insert by a short tendon into intertubercular sulcus and greater tubercle of humerus	Prime mover of arm flexion; rotates arm medially; adducts arm against resistance; with scapula (and arm) fixed, pulls rib cage upward, thus can help in climbing, throwing, pushing, and forced inspiration	Lateral and medial pectoral nerves (C_5–C_8 and T_1)
Deltoid (del′toid) (*delta* = triangular)	Thick, multipennate muscle forming rounded shoulder muscle mass; a common site for intramuscular injection, particularly in males, where it tends to be quite fleshy	O—embraces insertion of the trapezius; lateral third of clavicle; acromion and spine of scapula I—deltoid tuberosity of humerus	Prime mover of arm abduction when all its fibers contract simultaneously; antagonist of pectoralis major and latissimus dorsi, which adduct the arm; if only anterior fibers are active, can act powerfully in flexing and rotating humerus medially, therefore synergist of pectoralis major; if only posterior fibers are active, causes extension and lateral rotation of arm; active during rhythmic arm-swinging movements while walking	Axillary nerve (C_5 and C_6)

MUSCLE GALLERY

Table 10.9 *(continued)*

MUSCLE	DESCRIPTION	ORIGIN (O) AND INSERTION (I)	ACTION	NERVE SUPPLY
Latissimus dorsi (lah-tis′ĭ-mus dor′si) (*latissimus* = widest; *dorsi* = back)	Broad, flat, triangular muscle of lower back (lumbar region); extensive superficial origins; covered by trapezius superiorly; contributes to the posterior wall of axilla	O—indirect attachment via lumbodorsal fascia into spines of lower six thoracic vertebrae, lumbar vertebrae, lower 3 to 4 ribs, and iliac crest; also from scapula's inferior angle I—spirals around teres major to insert in floor of intertubercular sulcus of humerus	Prime mover of arm extension; powerful arm adductor; medially rotates arm at shoulder; depresses scapula; plays important role in lowering arm in a power stroke, as in striking a blow, hammering, swimming, and rowing; with arms fixed overhead, it pulls the rest of the body upward and forward	Thoracodorsal nerve (C_6–C_8)

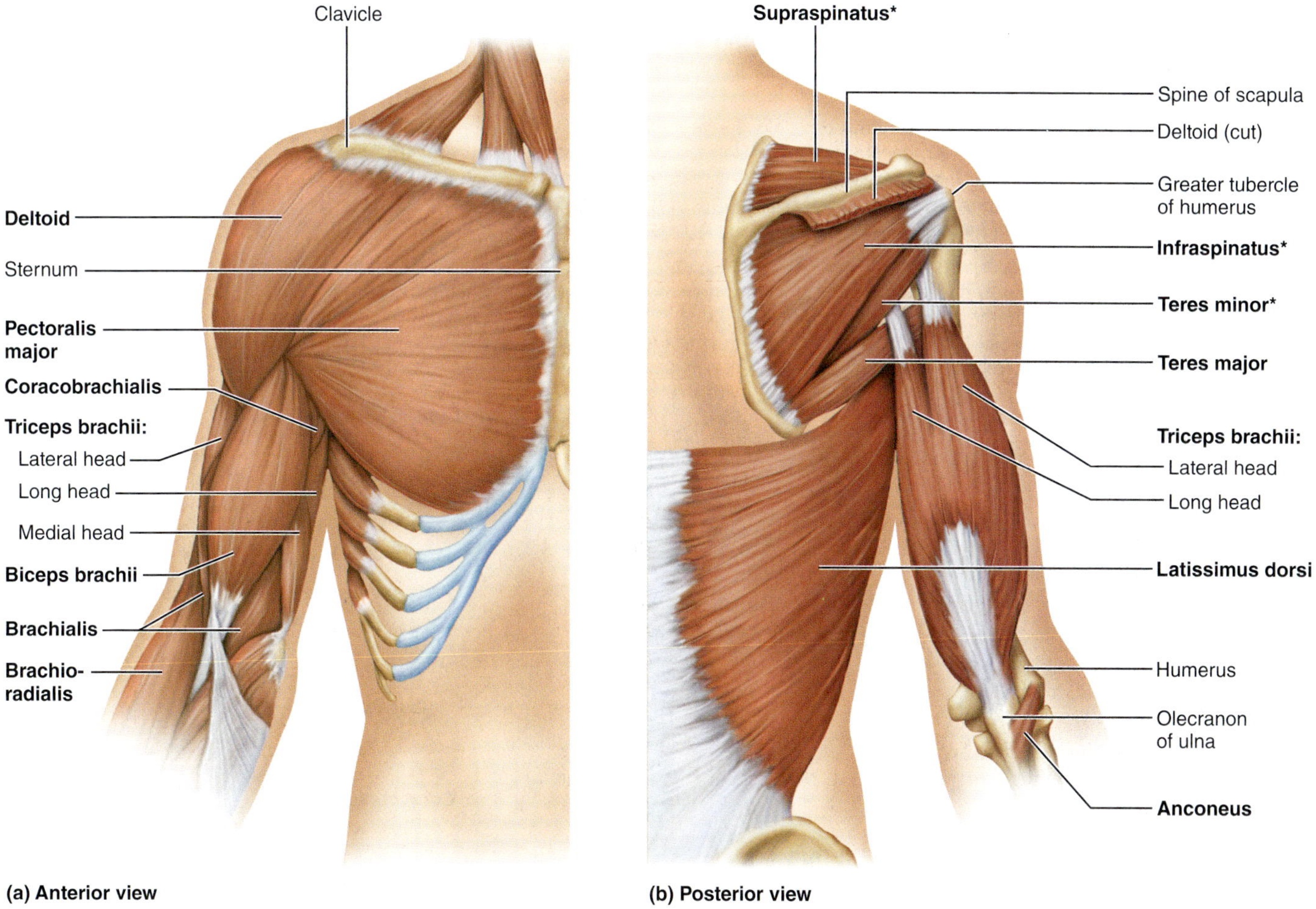

Figure 10.15 Muscles crossing the shoulder and elbow joints, causing movements of the arm and forearm, respectively. (For related images, see *A Brief Atlas of the Human Body*, Figures 35 and 36.) **(a)** Superficial muscles of the anterior thorax, shoulder, and arm, anterior view. **(b)** Muscles of the posterior thorax and arm. The triceps brachii muscle of the posterior arm is shown in relation to the deep scapular muscles. The deltoid muscle of the shoulder and the trapezius muscle have been removed.

*Rotator cuff muscles

MUSCLE GALLERY

Table 10.9 Muscles Crossing the Shoulder Joint: Movements of the Arm (Humerus) (Figure 10.15) *(continued)*

MUSCLE	DESCRIPTION	ORIGIN (O) AND INSERTION (I)	ACTION	NERVE SUPPLY
Subscapularis (sub-scap″u-lar′is) (*sub* = under; *scapular* = scapula)	Forms part of posterior wall of axilla; tendon of insertion passes in front of shoulder joint; a rotator cuff muscle	O—subscapular fossa of scapula I—lesser tubercle of humerus	Chief medial rotator of humerus; assisted by pectoralis major; helps hold head of humerus in glenoid cavity, stabilizing shoulder joint	Subscapular nerves (C_5–C_7)
Supraspinatus (soo″prah-spi-nah′tus) (*supra* = above, over; *spin* = spine)	Named for its location on posterior aspect of scapula; deep to trapezius; a rotator cuff muscle	O—supraspinous fossa of scapula I—superior part of greater tubercle of humerus	Initiates abduction; stabilizes shoulder joint; helps prevent downward dislocation of humerus, as when carrying a heavy suitcase	Suprascapular nerve
Infraspinatus (in″frah-spi-nah′tus) (*infra* = below)	Partially covered by deltoid and trapezius; named for its scapular location; a rotator cuff muscle	O—infraspinous fossa of scapula I—greater tubercle of humerus posterior to insertion of supraspinatus	Rotates humerus laterally; helps hold head of humerus in glenoid cavity, stabilizing the shoulder joint	Suprascapular nerve
Teres minor (te′rēz) (*teres* = round; *minor* = lesser)	Small, elongated muscle; lies inferior to infraspinatus and may be inseparable from that muscle; a rotator cuff muscle	O—lateral border of dorsal scapular surface I—greater tubercle of humerus inferior to infraspinatus insertion	Same action(s) as infraspinatus muscle	Axillary nerve
Teres major	Thick, rounded muscle; located inferior to teres minor; helps form posterior wall of axilla (along with latissimus dorsi and subscapularis)	O—posterior surface of scapula at inferior angle I—crest of lesser tubercle on anterior humerus; insertion tendon fused with that of latissimus dorsi	Extends, medially rotates, and adducts humerus; synergist of latissimus dorsi	Lower subscapular nerve (C_6 and C_7)
Coracobrachialis (kor″ah-ko-bra″ke-al′is) (*coraco* = coracoid; *brachi* = arm)	Small, cylindrical muscle	O—coracoid process of scapula I — medial surface of humerus shaft	Flexes and adducts humerus; synergist of pectoralis major	Musculocutaneous nerve (C_5–C_7)

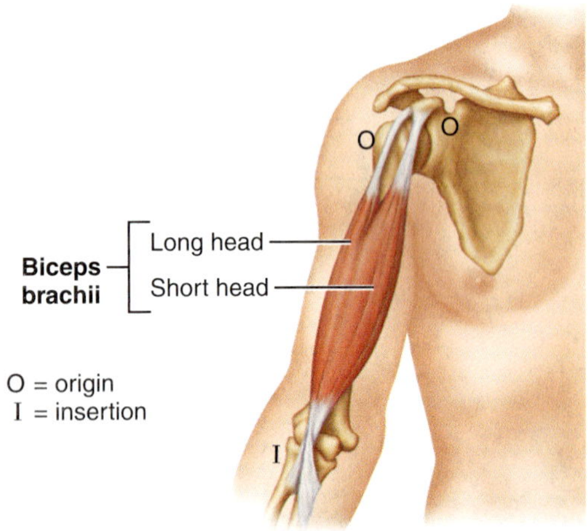

(c)

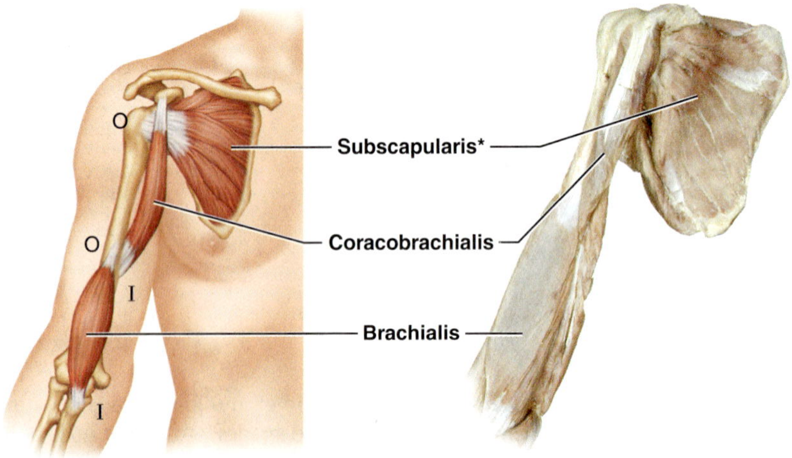

(d)

Figure 10.15 *(continued)* **Muscles crossing the shoulder and elbow joints, causing movements of the arm and forearm, respectively. (c)** The isolated biceps brachii muscle of the anterior arm. **(d)** The brachialis muscle and the coracobrachialis and subscapularis muscles shown in isolation in the diagram on the left, and in a dissection on the right.

*Rotator cuff muscles

MUSCLE GALLERY

Table 10.10 Muscles Crossing the Elbow Joint: Flexion and Extension of the Forearm (Figure 10.15)

Muscles fleshing out the arm cross the elbow joint to insert on the forearm bones. Since the elbow is a hinge joint, movements promoted by these arm muscles are limited almost entirely to flexing and extending the forearm. Walls of fascia divide the arm into two muscle compartments—the *posterior extensors* and *anterior flexors*. The main forearm extensor is the bulky **triceps brachii** muscle, which forms nearly the entire musculature of the posterior compartment (Figure 10.15a, b).

All anterior arm muscles flex the forearm (elbow). In order of decreasing strength, these are the **brachialis, biceps brachii**, and **brachioradialis** (Figure 10.15a, c, d). The brachialis and biceps insert (respectively) into the ulna and radius and contract simultaneously during flexion; they are the chief forearm flexors. The biceps brachii, a muscle that bulges when the forearm is flexed, is familiar to almost everyone. The brachialis, which lies deep to the biceps, is less known but is equally important in flexing the elbow. Because the brachioradialis arises from the distal humerus and inserts on the distal forearm, it resides mainly in the forearm. Its force is exerted far from the fulcrum, so the brachioradialis is a weak forearm flexor. The biceps muscle also supinates the forearm and is ineffective in flexing the elbow when the forearm *must* stay pronated. (This is why doing chin-ups with palms facing anteriorly is harder than with palms facing posteriorly.)

Table 10.12 (Part II) summarizes the actions of the muscles described here.

MUSCLE	DESCRIPTION	ORIGIN (O) AND INSERTION (I)	ACTION	NERVE SUPPLY
POSTERIOR MUSCLES				
Triceps brachii (tri′seps bra′ke-i) (*triceps* = three heads; *brachi* = arm)	Large fleshy muscle; the only muscle of posterior compartment of arm; three-headed origin; long and lateral heads lie superficial to medial head	O—long head: infraglenoid tubercle of scapula; lateral head: posterior shaft of humerus; medial head: posterior humeral shaft distal to radial groove I—by common tendon into olecranon of ulna	Powerful forearm extensor (prime mover, particularly medial head); antagonist of forearm flexors; long and lateral heads mainly active in extending the forearm against resistance; long head tendon may help stabilize shoulder joint and assist in arm adduction	Radial nerve (C_6–C_8)
Anconeus (an-ko′ne-us) (*ancon* = elbow) (see Figure 10.17)	Short triangular muscle; partially blended with distal end of triceps on posterior humerus	O—lateral epicondyle of humerus I—lateral aspect of olecranon of ulna	May control ulnar abduction during forearm pronation; synergist of triceps brachii in elbow extension	Radial nerve
ANTERIOR MUSCLES				
Biceps brachii (bi′seps) (*biceps* = two heads)	Two-headed fusiform muscle; bellies unite as insertion point is approached; tendon of long head helps stabilize shoulder joint	O—short head: coracoid process; long head: supraglenoid tubercle and lip of glenoid cavity; tendon of long head runs within capsule and into intertubercular sulcus of humerus I—by common tendon into radial tuberosity	Flexes elbow joint and supinates forearm; these actions usually occur at same time (e.g., when you open a bottle of wine, it turns the corkscrew and pulls the cork); weak flexor of arm at shoulder	Musculocutaneous nerve (C_5 and C_6)
Brachialis (bra′ke-al-is)	Strong muscle that is immediately deep to biceps brachii on distal humerus	O—front of distal humerus; embraces insertion of deltoid muscle I—coronoid process of ulna and capsule of elbow joint	A major forearm flexor (lifts ulna as biceps lifts the radius)	Musculocutaneous nerve
Brachioradialis (bra″ke-o-ra″de-al′is) (*radi* = radius, ray) (also see Figure 10.16)	Superficial muscle of lateral forearm; forms lateral boundary of cubital fossa; extends from distal humerus to distal forearm	O—lateral supracondylar ridge at distal end of humerus I—base of radial styloid process	Synergist in flexing forearm; acts to best advantage when forearm is partially flexed and semipronated; stabilizes elbow during rapid flexion *and* extension	Radial nerve (an important exception: the radial nerve typically serves extensor muscles)

MUSCLE GALLERY

Table 10.11 Muscles of the Forearm: Movements of the Wrist, Hand, and Fingers (Figures 10.16 and 10.17)

The many muscles in the forearm perform several basic functions. Some cause wrist movements, some move the fingers and thumb, and a few help pronate and supinate the forearms. In most cases, their fleshy portions contribute to the roundness of the proximal forearm and then they taper to long tendons distally to insert into the hand.

At the wrist, these tendons are securely anchored by bandlike thickenings of deep fascia called **flexor** and **extensor retinacula** ("retainers") (Figure 10.16a). These "wrist bands" keep the tendons from jumping outward when tensed. Crowded together in the wrist and palm, the muscle tendons are surrounded by slippery tendon sheaths that minimize friction as they slide against one another.

Although many forearm muscles arise from the humerus (and thus cross both the elbow and wrist joints), their actions on the elbow are slight. Flexion and extension are the movements typically effected at both the wrist and finger joints. In addition, the forearm muscles can abduct and adduct the wrist.

Fascia subdivides the forearm muscles into two main compartments: the *anterior flexors* and *posterior extensors*. Each has superficial and deep muscle layers. Most flexors in the anterior compartment arise from a common tendon on the humerus and are innervated largely by the median nerve. Two anterior compartment muscles are not flexors but pronators, the **pronator teres** and **pronator quadratus** (Figure 10.16a–c). Pronation is one of the most important forearm movements.

Muscles of the posterior compartment extend the wrist and fingers. One exception is the **supinator** muscle, which assists the biceps brachii muscle of the arm in supinating the forearm (Figures 10.16b, c and 10.17b). (Also residing in the posterior compartment is the brachioradialis muscle, the weak elbow flexor considered in Table 10.10.) Most muscles of the posterior compartment arise from a common tendon on the humerus. The radial nerve supplies all posterior forearm muscles.

As described above, most muscles that move the hand are located in the forearm and "operate" the fingers via their long tendons, like operating a puppet by strings. This design makes the hand less bulky and enables it to perform finer movements. The hand movements promoted by the forearm muscles are assisted by the small *intrinsic* muscles of the hand, which control the most delicate and precise finger movements (see Table 10.13). Table 10.12 (Parts II and III) summarizes the actions of the forearm muscles.

10

MUSCLE	DESCRIPTION	ORIGIN (O) AND INSERTION (I)	ACTION	NERVE SUPPLY
PART I: ANTERIOR MUSCLES (Figure 10.16)	These eight muscles of the anterior fascial compartment are listed from the lateral to the medial aspect. Most arise from a common flexor tendon attached to the medial epicondyle of the humerus and have additional origins as well. Most of their tendons of insertion are held in place at the wrist by a thickening of deep fascia called the *flexor retinaculum*.			
Superficial Muscles				
Pronator teres (pro-na′tor te′rēz) (*pronation* = turning palm posteriorly, or down; *teres* = round)	Two-headed muscle; seen in superficial view between proximal margins of brachioradialis and flexor carpi radialis; forms medial boundary of cubital fossa	O—medial epicondyle of humerus; coronoid process of ulna I—by common tendon into lateral radius, midshaft	Pronates forearm; weak flexor of elbow	Median nerve
Flexor carpi radialis (flek′sor kar′pe ra″de-al′is) (*flex* = decrease angle between two bones; *carpi* = wrist; *radi* = radius)	Runs diagonally across forearm; midway, its fleshy belly is replaced by a flat tendon that becomes cordlike at wrist	O—medial epicondyle of humerus I—base of second and third metacarpals; insertion tendon easily seen and provides guide to position of radial artery at wrist (used for taking pulse)	Powerful flexor of wrist; abducts hand; weak synergist of elbow flexion	Median nerve
Palmaris longus (pahl-ma′ris lon′gus) (*palma* = palm; *longus* = long)	Small fleshy muscle with a long insertion tendon; often absent; may be used as guide to find median nerve that lies lateral to it at wrist	O—medial epicondyle of humerus I—palmar aponeurosis; (fascia of palm)	Tenses skin and fascia of palm during hand movements; weak wrist flexor; weak synergist for elbow flexion	Median nerve
Flexor carpi ulnaris (ul-na′ris) (*ulnar* = ulna)	Most medial muscle of this group; two-headed; ulnar nerve lies lateral to its tendon	O—medial epicondyle of humerus; olecranon and posterior surface of ulna I—pisiform and hamate bones and base of fifth metacarpal	Powerful flexor of wrist; also adducts hand in concert with extensor carpi ulnaris (posterior muscle); stabilizes wrist during finger extension	Ulnar nerve (C_7 and C_8)

MUSCLE GALLERY

Table 10.11 *(continued)*

MUSCLE	DESCRIPTION	ORIGIN (O) AND INSERTION (I)	ACTION	NERVE SUPPLY
Flexor digitorum superficialis (dĭ″jĭ-tor′um soo″per-fish″e-al′is) (*digit* = finger, toe; *superficial* = close to surface)	Two-headed muscle; more deeply placed (therefore, actually forms an intermediate layer); overlain by muscles above but visible at distal end of forearm	O—medial epicondyle of humerus, coronoid process of ulna; shaft of radius I—by four tendons into middle phalanges of fingers 2–5	Flexes wrist and middle phalanges of fingers 2–5; the important finger flexor for speed and flexion against resistance	Median nerve (C_7, C_8, and T_1)
Deep Muscles				
Flexor pollicis longus (pah′lĭ-kis) (*pollix* = thumb)	Partly covered by flexor digitorum superficialis; parallels flexor digitorum profundus laterally	O—anterior surface of radius and interosseous membrane I—distal phalanx of thumb	Flexes distal phalanx of thumb	Branch of median nerve (C_8,T_1)
Flexor digitorum profundus (pro-fun′dus) (*profund* = deep)	Extensive origin; overlain entirely by flexor digitorum superficialis	O—coronoid process, anteromedial surface of ulna, and interosseous membrane I—by four tendons into distal phalanges of fingers 2–5	Flexes distal interphalangeal joints; slow-acting flexor of any or all fingers; helps flex wrist	Medial half by ulnar nerve; lateral half by median nerve

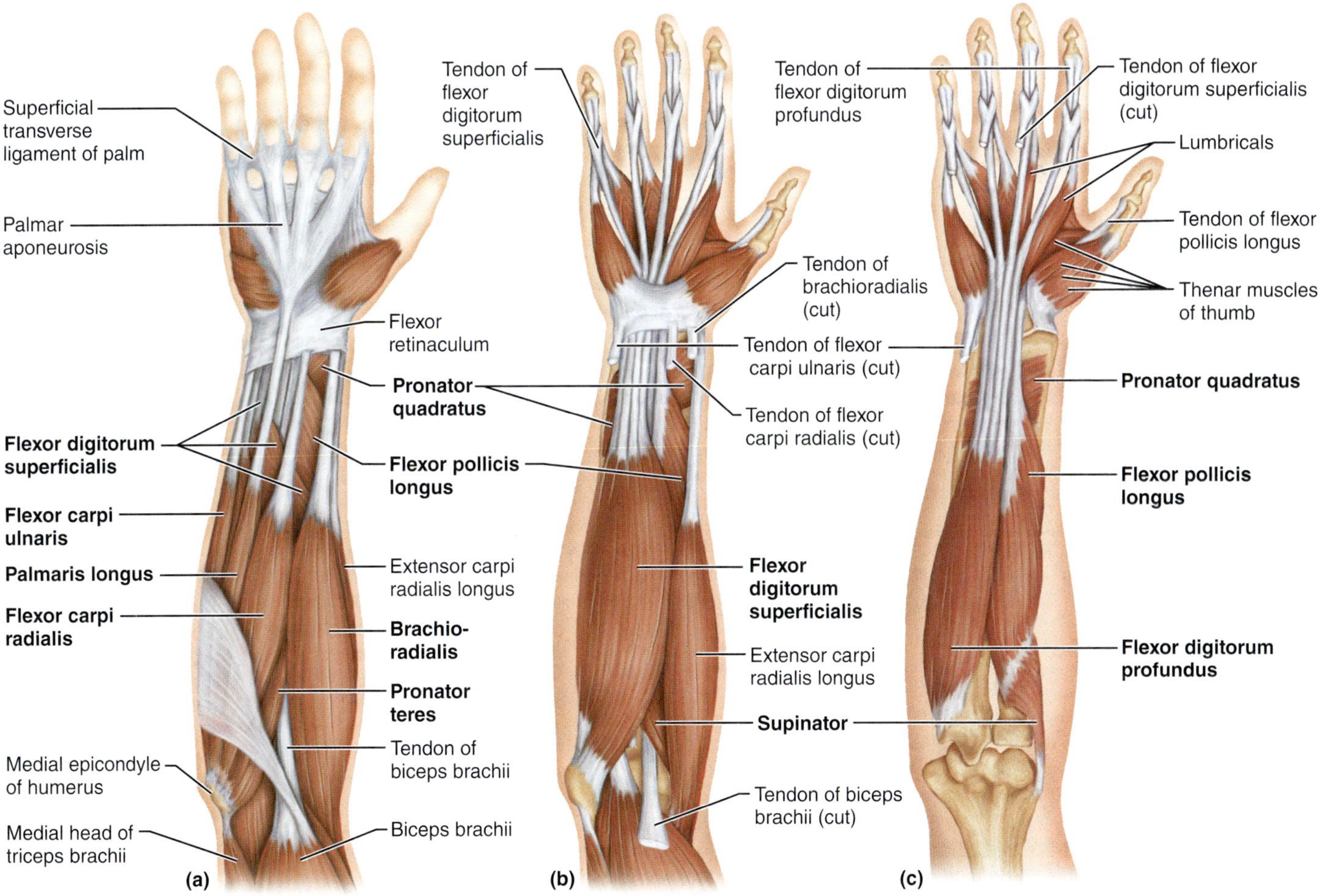

Figure 10.16 Muscles of the anterior fascial compartment of the forearm acting on the right wrist and fingers. **(a)** Superficial view. **(b)** The brachioradialis, flexors carpi radialis and ulnaris, and palmaris longus muscles have been removed to reveal the flexor digitorum superficialis. **(c)** Deep muscles of the anterior compartment. The lumbricals and thenar muscles (intrinsic hand muscles) are also illustrated. (For a related image, see *A Brief Atlas of the Human Body*, Figure 37.)

MUSCLE GALLERY

Table 10.11 Muscles of the Forearm: Movements of the Wrist, Hand, and Fingers (Figures 10.16 and 10.17) *(continued)*

MUSCLE	DESCRIPTION	ORIGIN (O) AND INSERTION (I)	ACTION	NERVE SUPPLY
Pronator quadratus (kwod-ra′tus) (*quad* = square, four-sided)	Deepest muscle of distal forearm; passes downward and laterally; only muscle that arises solely from ulna and inserts solely into radius	O—distal portion of anterior ulnar shaft I—distal surface of anterior radius	Prime mover of forearm pronation; acts with pronator teres; also helps hold ulna and radius together	Median nerve (C_8 and T_1)
PART II: POSTERIOR MUSCLES (Figure 10.17)	These muscles of the posterior fascial compartment are listed from the lateral to the medial aspect. They are all innervated by the radial nerve or its branches. More than half of the posterior compartment muscles arise from a common extensor origin tendon attached to the posterior surface of the lateral epicondyle of the humerus and adjacent fascia. The extensor tendons are held in place at the posterior aspect of the wrist by the *extensor retinaculum,* which prevents "bowstringing" of these tendons when the wrist is hyperextended. The *extensor* muscles of the fingers end in a broad hood over the dorsal side of the digits, the extensor expansion.			
Superficial Muscles				
Brachioradialis (see Table 10.10)	See Table 10.10	See Table 10.10	See Table 10.10	See Table 10.10
Extensor carpi radialis longus (ek-sten′sor) (*extend* = increase angle between two bones)	Parallels brachioradialis on lateral forearm, and may blend with it	O—lateral supracondylar ridge of humerus I—base of second metacarpal	Extends wrist in conjunction with extensor carpi ulnaris and abducts wrist in conjunction with flexor carpi radialis	Radial nerve (C_6 and C_7)
Extensor carpi radialis brevis (brĕ′vis) (*brevis* = short)	Shorter than extensor carpi radialis longus and lies deep to it	O—lateral epicondyle of humerus I—base of third metacarpal	Extends and abducts wrist; acts synergistically with extensor carpi radialis longus to steady wrist during finger flexion	Deep branch of radial nerve
Extensor digitorum	Lies medial to extensor carpi radialis brevis; a detached portion of this muscle, called *extensor digiti minimi,* extends little finger	O—lateral epicondyle of humerus I—by four tendons into extensor expansions and distal phalanges of fingers 2–5	Prime mover of finger extension; extends wrist; can abduct (flare) fingers	Posterior interosseous nerve, a branch of radial nerve (C_5 and C_6)
Extensor carpi ulnaris	Most medial of superficial posterior muscles; long, slender muscle	O—lateral epicondyle of humerus and posterior border of ulna I—base of fifth metacarpal	Extends wrist in conjunction with extensor carpi radialis and adducts wrist in conjunction with flexor carpi ulnaris	Posterior interosseous nerve
Deep Muscles				
Supinator (soo″pĭ-na′tor) (*supination* = turning palm anteriorly or upward)	Deep muscle at posterior aspect of elbow; largely concealed by superficial muscles	O—lateral epicondyle of humerus; proximal ulna I—proximal end of radius	Assists biceps brachii to forcibly supinate forearm; works alone in slow supination; antagonist of pronator muscles	Posterior interosseous nerve
Abductor pollicis longus (ab-duk′tor) (*abduct* = movement away from median plane)	Lateral and parallel to extensor pollicis longus; just distal to supinator	O—posterior surface of radius and ulna; interosseous membrane I—base of first metacarpal and trapezium	Abducts and extends thumb	Posterior interosseous nerve
Extensor pollicis brevis and longus	Deep muscle pair with a common origin and action; overlain by extensor carpi ulnaris	O—dorsal shaft of radius and ulna; interosseous membrane I—base of proximal (brevis) and distal (longus) phalanx of thumb	Extends thumb	Posterior interosseous nerve

10

MUSCLE GALLERY

Table 10.11 *(continued)*

MUSCLE	DESCRIPTION	ORIGIN (O) AND INSERTION (I)	ACTION	NERVE SUPPLY
Extensor indicis (in′dĭ-kis) (*indicis* = index finger)	Tiny muscle arising close to wrist	O—posterior surface of distal ulna; interosseous membrane I—extensor expansion of index finger; joins tendon of extensor digitorum	Extends index finger and assists in extending wrist	Posterior interosseous nerve

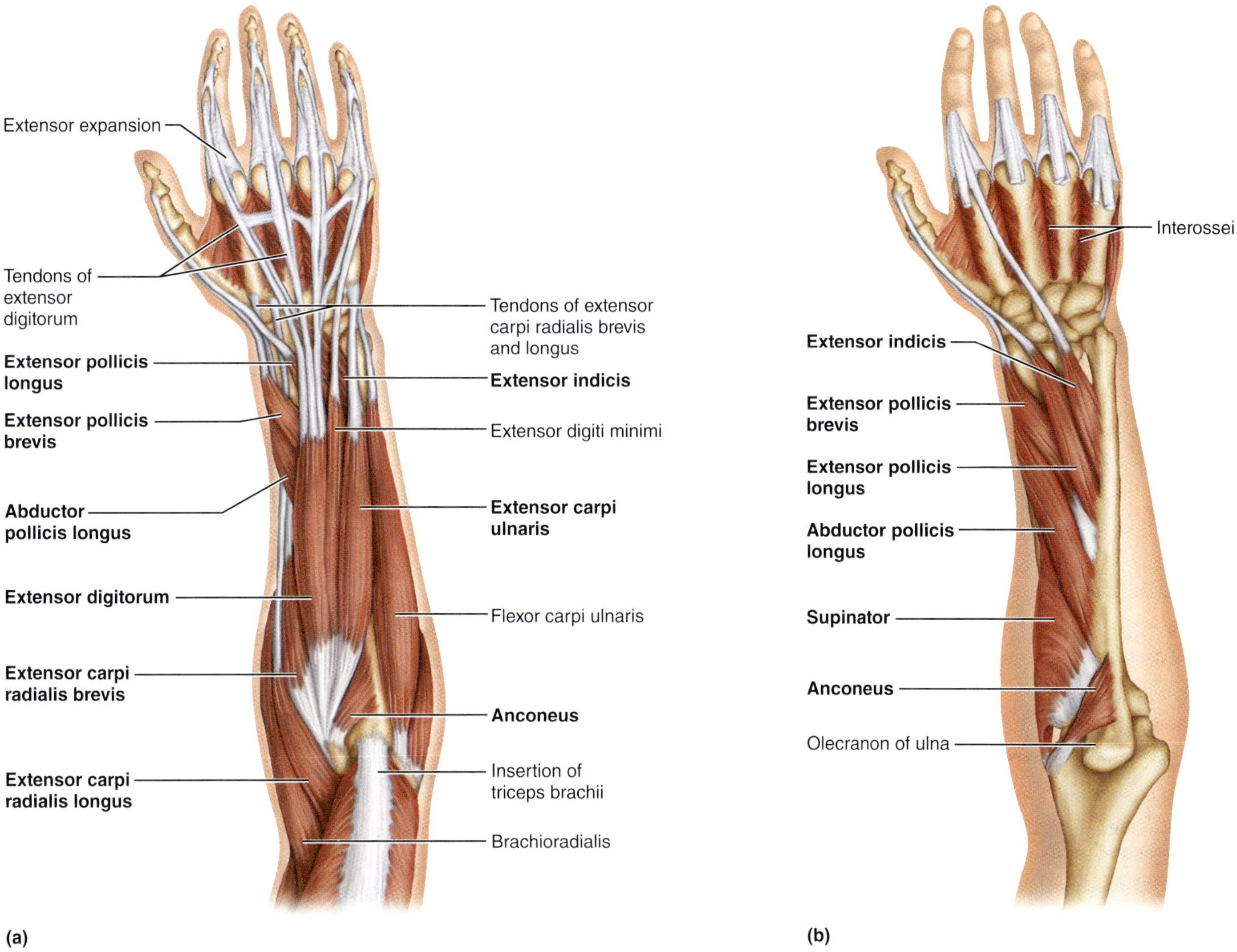

Figure 10.17 Muscles of the posterior fascial compartment of the right forearm acting on the wrist and fingers. (a) Superficial muscles, posterior view. (For a related image, see *A Brief Atlas of the Human Body*, Figure 37b.) **(b)** Deep posterior muscles, superficial muscles removed. The interossei, the deepest layer of intrinsic hand muscles, are also illustrated.

MUSCLE GALLERY

Table 10.12 Summary: Actions of Muscles Acting on the Arm, Forearm, and Hand (Figure 10.18)

PART I: Muscles Acting on the Arm (Humerus) (PM = Prime Mover)	Actions at the Shoulder					
	Flexion	Extension	Abduction	Adduction	Medial Rotation	Lateral Rotation
Pectoralis major	× (PM)			× (PM)	×	
Latissimus dorsi		× (PM)		× (PM)	×	
Teres major		×		×	×	
Deltoid	× (PM) (anterior fibers)	× (PM) (posterior fibers)	× (PM)		× (anterior fibers)	× (posterior fibers)
Subscapularis					× (PM)	
Supraspinatus			×			
Infraspinatus						× (PM)
Teres minor				× (weak)		× (PM)
Coracobrachialis	×			×		
Biceps brachii	× (weak)					
Triceps brachii				×		

PART II: Muscles Acting on the Forearm	Actions on the Forearm			
	Elbow Flexion	Elbow Extension	Pronation	Supination
Biceps brachii	× (PM)			×
Brachialis	× (PM)			
Triceps brachii		× (PM)		
Anconeus		×		
Pronator teres	× (weak)		×	
Pronator quadratus			× (PM)	
Supinator				×
Brachioradialis	×			

PART III: Muscles Acting on the Wrist and Fingers	Actions on the Wrist				Actions on the Fingers	
	Flexion	Extension	Abduction	Adduction	Flexion	Extension
Anterior Compartment						
Flexor carpi radialis	× (PM)		×			
Palmaris longus	× (weak)					
Flexor carpi ulnaris	× (PM)			×		
Flexor digitorum superficialis	× (PM)				×	
Flexor pollicis longus					× (thumb)	
Flexor digitorum profundus	×				×	
Posterior Compartment						
Extensor carpi radialis longus and brevis		×	×			
Extensor digitorum		× (PM)				× (and abducts)
Extensor carpi ulnaris		×		×		
Abductor pollicis longus			×		(abducts thumb)	
Extensor pollicis longus and brevis						× (thumb)
Extensor indicis		× (weak)				× (index finger)

MUSCLE GALLERY

Table 10.12 *(continued)*

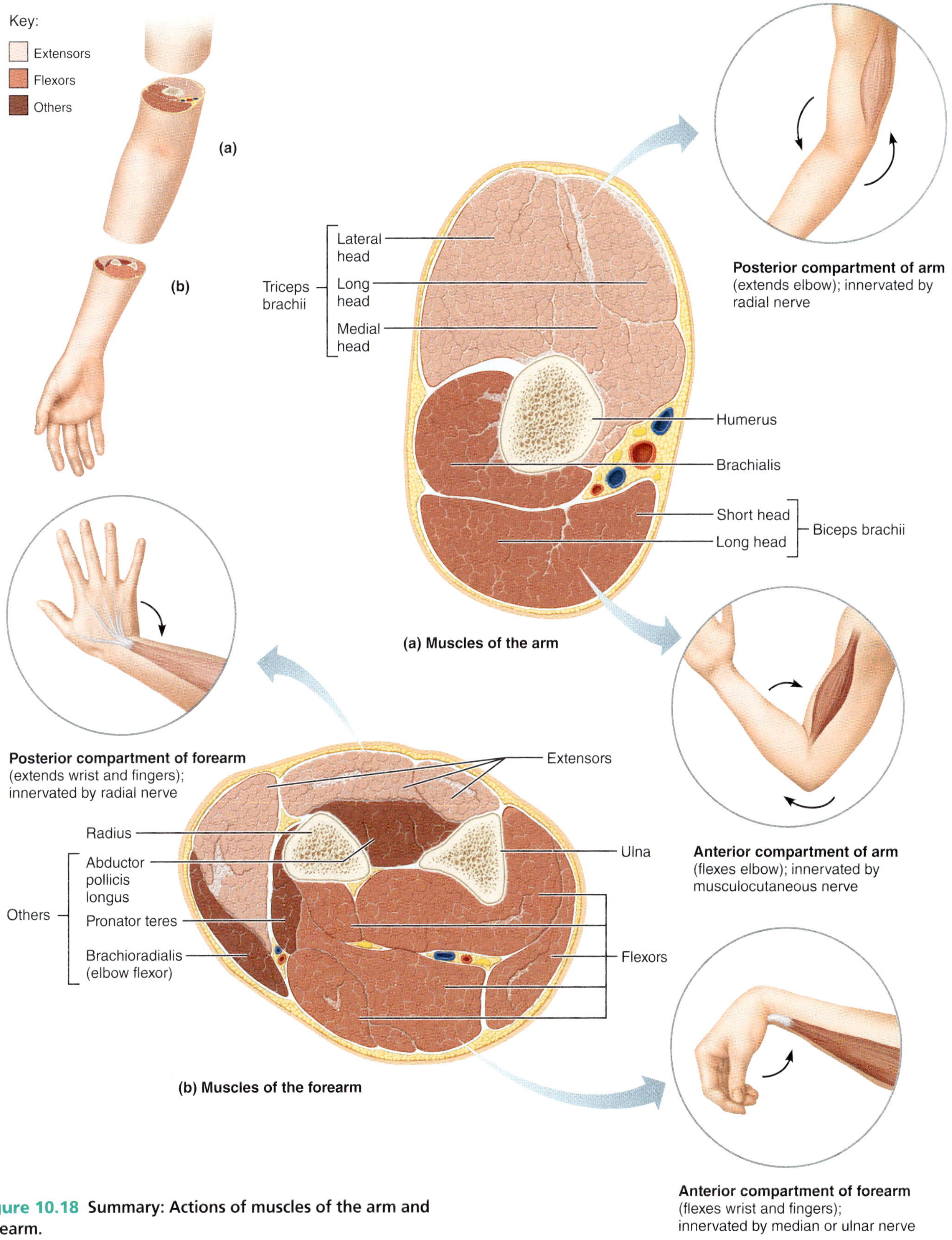

Figure 10.18 Summary: Actions of muscles of the arm and forearm.

MUSCLE GALLERY

Table 10.13 Intrinsic Muscles of the Hand: Fine Movements of the Fingers (Figure 10.19)

In this table we consider the small muscles that lie entirely in the hand. All are in the palm, none on the hand's dorsal side. All move the metacarpals and fingers. Small, weak muscles, they mostly control precise movements (such as threading a needle), leaving the powerful movements of the fingers ("power grip") to the forearm muscles.

The intrinsic muscles include the main abductors and adductors of the fingers, as well as muscles that produce the movement of opposition—moving the thumb toward the little finger—that enables you to grip objects. Many palm muscles are specialized to move the thumb, and surprisingly many move the little finger.

Thumb movements are defined differently from movements of other fingers because the thumb lies at a right angle to the rest of the hand. The thumb flexes by bending medially along the palm, not by bending anteriorly, as do the other fingers. (To demonstrate this difference, start with your hand in the anatomical position or this will not be clear!) The thumb extends by pointing laterally (as in hitchhiking), not posteriorly, as do the other fingers. To abduct the fingers is to splay them laterally, but to abduct the thumb is to point it anteriorly. Adduction of the thumb brings it back posteriorly.

The intrinsic muscles of the palm are divided into three groups, those in

1. The *thenar eminence* (ball of the thumb)
2. The *hypothenar eminence* (ball of the little finger)
3. The midpalm

Thenar and hypothenar muscles are almost mirror images of each other, each containing a small flexor, an abductor, and an opponens muscle. The midpalmar muscles, called **lumbricals** and **interossei**, extend our fingers at the interphalangeal joints. The interossei are also the main finger abductors and adductors.

10

MUSCLE	DESCRIPTION	ORIGIN (O) AND INSERTION (I)	ACTION	NERVE SUPPLY
THENAR MUSCLES IN BALL OF THUMB (the′nar) (*thenar* = palm)				
Abductor pollicis brevis (*pollex* = thumb)	Lateral muscle of thenar group; superficial	O—flexor retinaculum and nearby carpals I—lateral base of thumb's proximal phalanx	Abducts thumb (at carpometacarpal joint)	Median nerve (C_8, T_1)
Flexor pollicis brevis	Medial and deep muscle of thenar group	O—flexor retinaculum and nearby carpals I—lateral side of base of proximal phalanx of thumb	Flexes thumb (at carpometacarpal and metacarpophalangeal joints)	Median (or occasionally ulnar) nerve (C_8, T_1)
Opponens pollicis (o-pōn′enz) (*opponens* = opposition)	Deep to abductor pollicis brevis, on metacarpal I	O—flexor retinaculum and trapezium I—whole anterior side of metacarpal I	Opposition: moves thumb to touch tip of little finger	Median (or occasionally ulnar) nerve
Adductor pollicis	Fan-shaped with horizontal fibers; distal to other thenar muscles; oblique and transverse heads	O—capitate bone and bases of metacarpals II–IV; front of metacarpal III I—medial side of base of proximal phalanx of thumb	Adducts and helps to oppose thumb	Ulnar nerve (C_8, T_1)
HYPOTHENAR MUSCLES IN BALL OF LITTLE FINGER				
Abductor digiti minimi (dĭ′jĭ-ti min′ĭ-mi) (*digiti minimi* = little finger)	Medial muscle of hypothenar group; superficial	O—pisiform bone I—medial side of proximal phalanx of little finger	Abducts little finger at metacarpophalangeal joint	Ulnar nerve
Flexor digiti minimi brevis	Lateral deep muscle of hypothenar group	O—hamate bone and flexor retinaculum I—same as abductor digiti minimi	Flexes little finger at metacarpophalangeal joint	Ulnar nerve
Opponens digiti minimi	Deep to abductor digiti minimi	O—same as flexor digiti minimi brevis I—most of length of medial side of metacarpal V	Helps in opposition: brings metacarpal V toward thumb to cup the hand	Ulnar nerve

MUSCLE GALLERY

Table 10.13 *(continued)*

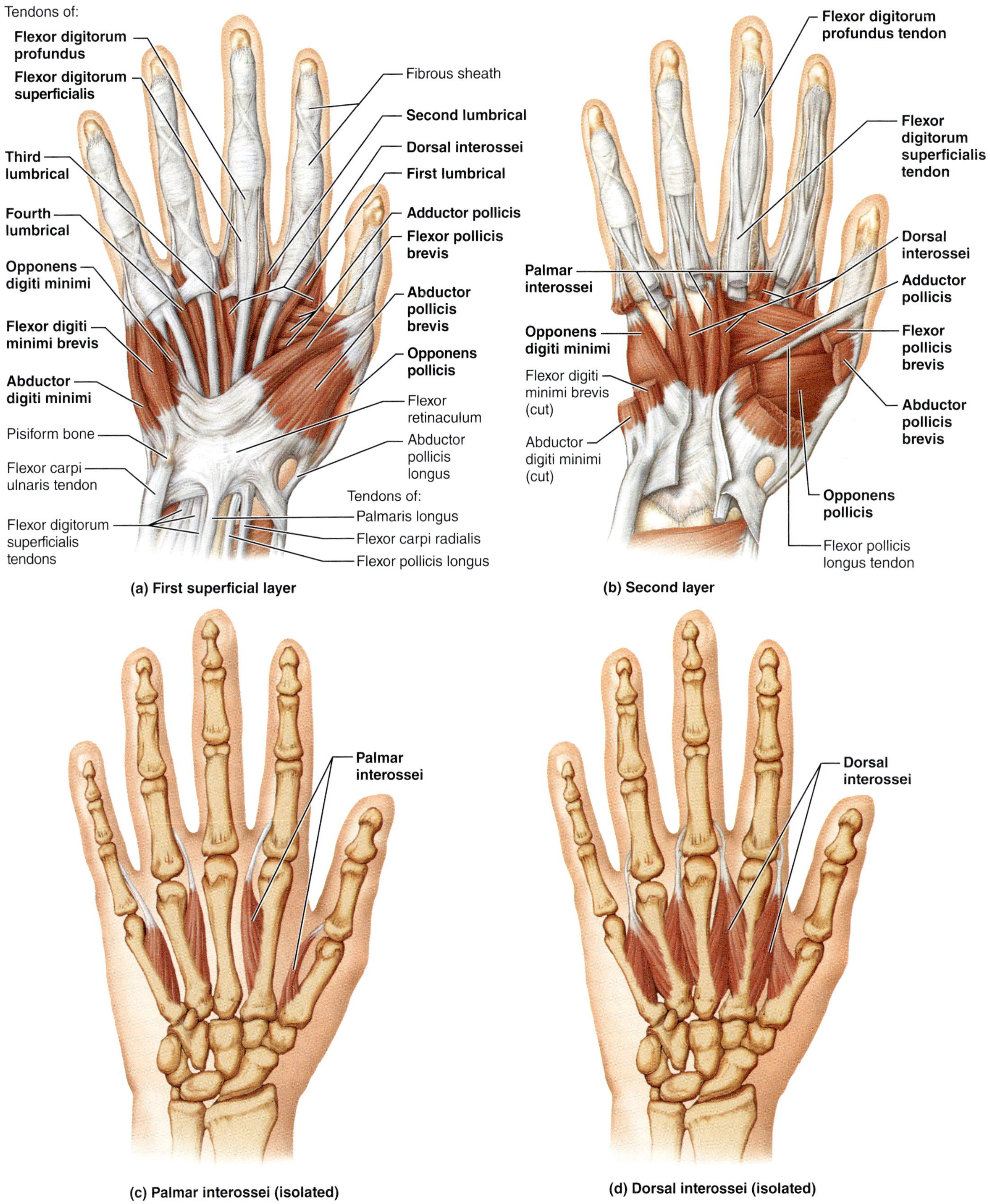

Figure 10.19 Hand muscles, ventral views of right hand.

MUSCLE GALLERY

Table 10.13 Intrinsic Muscles of the Hand: Fine Movements of the Fingers (Figure 10.19) *(continued)*

MUSCLE	DESCRIPTION	ORIGIN (O) AND INSERTION (I)	ACTION	NERVE SUPPLY
MIDPALMAR MUSCLES				
Lumbricals (lum′brĭ-klz) (*lumbric* = earthworm)	Four worm-shaped muscles in palm, one to each finger (except thumb); unusual because they originate from the tendons of another muscle	O—lateral side of each tendon of flexor digitorum profundus in palm I—lateral edge of extensor expansion on proximal phalanx of fingers 2–5	Flex fingers at metacarpophalangeal joints but extend fingers at interphalangeal joints	Median nerve (lateral two) and ulnar nerve (medial two)
Palmar interossei (in″ter-os′e-i) (*interossei* = between bones)	Four long, cone-shaped muscles in the spaces between the metacarpals; lie ventral to the dorsal interossei	O—the side of each metacarpal that faces the midaxis of the hand (metacarpal III) but absent from metacarpal III I—extensor expansion on first phalanx of each finger (except finger 3), on side facing midaxis of hand	Adduct fingers: pull fingers in toward third digit; act with lumbricals to extend fingers at interphalangeal joints and flex them at metacarpophalangeal joints	Ulnar nerve
Dorsal interossei	Four bipennate muscles filling spaces between the metacarpals; deepest palm muscles, also visible on dorsal side of hand (Figure 10.17b)	O—sides of metacarpals I—extensor expansion over proximal phalanx of fingers 2–4 on side opposite midaxis of hand (finger 3), but on *both* sides of finger 3	Abduct (diverge) fingers; extend fingers at interphalangeal joints and flex them at metacarpophalangeal joints	Ulnar nerve

MUSCLE GALLERY

Table 10.14 Muscles Crossing the Hip and Knee Joints: Movements of the Thigh and Leg (Figures 10.20 and 10.21)

The muscles fleshing out the thigh are difficult to segregate into groups on the basis of action. Some thigh muscles act only at the hip joint, others only at the knee, while still others act at both joints. However, *most anterior* muscles of the hip and thigh flex the femur at the hip and extend the leg at the knee, producing the foreswing phase of walking. The *posterior* muscles of the hip and thigh, by contrast, mostly extend the thigh and flex the leg—the backswing phase of walking. A third group of muscles in this region, the *medial*, or *adductor*, muscles, all adduct the thigh; they have no effect on the leg.

In the thigh, the anterior, posterior, and adductor muscles are separated by walls of fascia into *anterior*, *posterior*, and *medial compartments* (see Figure 10.26a). The deep fascia of the thigh, the *fascia lata*, surrounds and encloses all three groups of muscles like a support stocking.

Movements of the thigh (occurring at the hip joint) are accomplished largely by muscles anchored to the pelvic girdle. Like the shoulder joint, the hip joint is a ball-and-socket joint permitting flexion, extension, abduction, adduction, circumduction, and rotation. Muscles effecting these movements are among the most powerful muscles of the body.

For the most part, the thigh *flexors* pass in front of the hip joint. The most important thigh flexors are the **iliopsoas** (the prime mover), **tensor fasciae latae**, and **rectus femoris** (Figure 10.20a). They are assisted in this action by the **adductor muscles** of the medial thigh and the straplike **sartorius**.

Thigh *extension* is effected primarily by the massive **hamstring muscles** of the posterior thigh (Figure 10.21a). During forceful extension, the **gluteus maximus** of the buttocks is called into play. Buttock muscles that lie lateral to the hip joint (**gluteus medius** and **minimus**) *abduct* the thigh (Figure 10.21c).

Thigh adduction is the role of the adductor muscles of the medial thigh. Abduction and adduction of the thighs are extremely important during walking to shift the trunk from side to side and balance the body's weight over the limb that is on the ground. Many different muscles bring about medial and lateral rotation of the thigh.

At the knee joint, flexion and extension are the main movements. The sole knee *extensor* is the **quadriceps femoris** muscle of the anterior thigh, the most powerful muscle in the body (Figure 10.20a). The quadriceps is antagonized by the hamstrings of the posterior compartment, which are the prime movers of knee flexion.

Table 10.17 (Part I) summarizes the actions of these muscles.

10

MUSCLE	DESCRIPTION	ORIGIN (O) AND INSERTION (I)	ACTION	NERVE SUPPLY
PART I: ANTERIOR AND MEDIAL MUSCLES (Figure 10.20)				
Origin on the Pelvis or Spine				
Iliopsoas (il″e-o-so′us)	Iliopsoas is a composite of two closely related muscles (iliacus and psoas major) whose fibers pass under the inguinal ligament (see Figure 10.12) to insert via a common tendon on the femur.			
▪ **Iliacus** (il-e-ak′us) (*iliac* = ilium)	Large, fan-shaped, more lateral muscle	O—iliac fossa and crest, ala of sacrum I—lesser trochanter of femur via iliopsoas tendon	Iliopsoas is the prime mover for flexing thigh, or for flexing trunk on thigh as during a bow	Femoral nerve (L_2 and L_3)
▪ **Psoas major** (so′us) (*psoa* = loin muscle; *major* = larger)	Longer, thicker, more medial muscle of the pair (butchers refer to this muscle as the tenderloin)	O—by fleshy slips from transverse processes, bodies, and discs of lumbar vertebrae and T_{12} I—lesser trochanter of femur via iliopsoas tendon	As above; also flexes vertebral column laterally; important postural muscle	Ventral rami (L_1–L_3)
Sartorius (sar-tor′e-us) (*sartor* = tailor)	Straplike superficial muscle running obliquely across anterior surface of thigh to knee; longest muscle in body; crosses both hip and knee joints	O—anterior superior iliac spine I—winds around medial aspect of knee and inserts into medial aspect of proximal tibia	Flexes, abducts, and laterally rotates thigh; flexes knee (weak) as in a soccer kick; helps produce the cross-legged position	Femoral nerve

➤

Table 10.14 Muscles Crossing the Hip and Knee Joints: Movements of the Thigh and Leg (Figures 10.20 and 10.21) *(continued)*

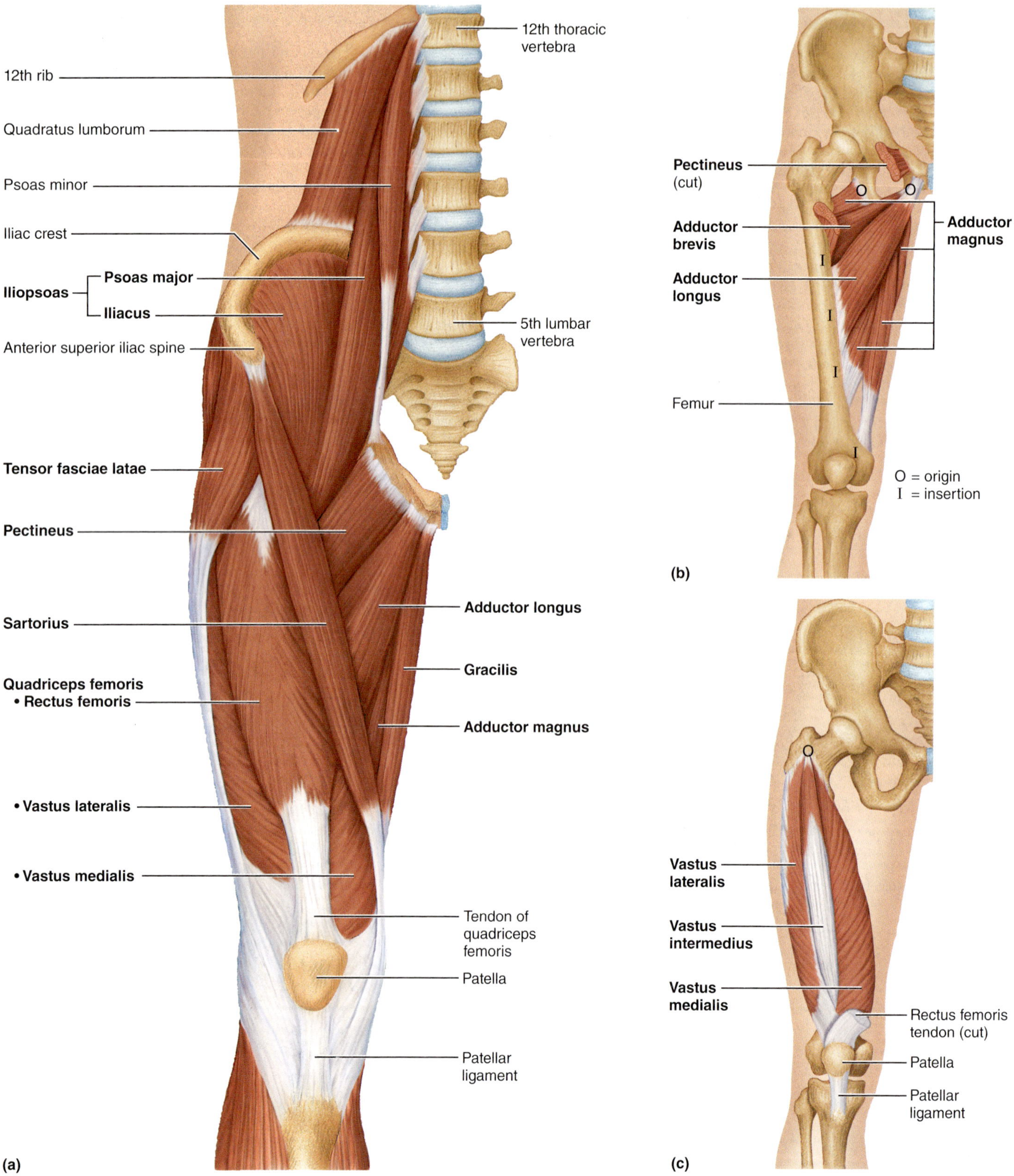

Figure 10.20 Anterior and medial muscles promoting movements of the thigh and leg. (For a related image, see *A Brief Atlas of the Human Body*, Figure 40.) **(a)** Anterior view of the deep muscles of the pelvis and superficial muscles of the right thigh. **(b)** Adductor muscles of the medial compartment of the thigh, isolated. **(c)** Vastus muscles of the quadriceps group, isolated.

MUSCLE GALLERY

Table 10.14 *(continued)*

Muscles of the Medial Compartment of the Thigh				
Adductors (ah-duk′torz)	Large muscle mass consisting of three muscles (magnus, longus, and brevis) forming medial aspect of thigh; arise from inferior part of pelvis and insert at various levels on femur. All are used in movements that press thighs together, as when astride a horse; important in pelvic tilting movements that occur during walking and in fixing the hip when the knee is flexed and the foot is off the ground. Obturator nerve innervates entire group. Strain or stretching of this muscle group is called a "pulled groin."			
▪ **Adductor magnus** (mag′nus) (*adduct* = move toward midline; *magnus* = large)	Triangular muscle with a broad insertion; a composite muscle that is part adductor and part hamstring in action	O—ischial and pubic rami and ischial tuberosity I—linea aspera and adductor tubercle of femur	Anterior part adducts and medially rotates and flexes thigh; posterior part is a synergist of hamstrings to extend thigh	Obturator nerve and sciatic nerve (L_2–L_4)
▪ **Adductor longus** (*longus* = long)	Overlies middle aspect of adductor magnus; most anterior of adductor muscles	O—pubis near pubic symphysis I—linea aspera	Adducts, flexes, and medially rotates thigh	Obturator nerve (L_2–L_4)
▪ **Adductor brevis** (*brevis* = short)	In contact with obturator externus muscle; largely concealed by adductor longus and pectineus	O—body and inferior pubic ramus I—linea aspera above adductor longus	Adducts, flexes, and medially rotates thigh	Obturator nerve
Pectineus (pek-tin′e-us) (*pecten* = comb)	Short, flat muscle; overlies adductor brevis on proximal thigh; abuts adductor longus medially	O—pubis (and superior ramus) I—from lesser trochanter inferior to the linea aspera on posterior aspect of femur	Adducts, flexes, and medially rotates thigh	Femoral and sometimes obturator nerve
Gracilis (grah-sĭ′lis) (*gracilis* = slender)	Long, thin, superficial muscle of medial thigh	O—inferior ramus and body of pubis and adjacent ischial ramus I—medial surface of tibia just inferior to its medial condyle	Adducts thigh, flexes and medially rotates leg, especially during walking	Obturator nerve
Muscles of the Anterior Compartment of the Thigh				
Quadriceps femoris (kwod′rĭ-seps fem′o-ris)	Arises from four separate heads (*quadriceps* = four heads) that form the flesh of front and sides of thigh. These heads (rectus femoris, and lateral, medial, and intermediate vasti muscles) have a common insertion tendon, the *quadriceps tendon*, which inserts into the patella and then via the *patellar ligament* into tibial tuberosity. The quadriceps is a powerful knee extensor used in climbing, jumping, running, and rising from seated position. The tone of quadriceps plays important role in strengthening the knee joint. Femoral nerve innervates the group.			
▪ **Rectus femoris** (rek′tus) (*rectus* = straight; *femoris* = femur)	Superficial muscle of anterior thigh; runs straight down thigh; longest head and only muscle of group to cross hip joint	O—anterior inferior iliac spine and superior margin of acetabulum I—patella and tibial tuberosity via patellar ligament	Extends knee and flexes thigh at hip	Femoral nerve (L_2–L_4)
▪ **Vastus lateralis** (vas′tus lat″er-a′lis) (*vastus* = large; *lateralis* = lateral)	Largest head of the group, forms lateral aspect of thigh; a common intramuscular injection site, particularly in infants (who have poorly developed buttock and arm muscles)	O—greater trochanter, intertrochanteric line, linea aspera I—as for rectus femoris	Extends and stabilizes knee	Femoral nerve
▪ **Vastus medialis** (me″de-a′lis) (*medialis* = medial)	Forms inferomedial aspect of thigh	O—linea aspera, intertrochanteric and medial supracondylar lines I—as for rectus femoris	Extends knee	Femoral nerve

MUSCLE GALLERY

Table 10.14 Muscles Crossing the Hip and Knee Joints: Movements of the Thigh and Leg (Figures 10.20 and 10.21) *(continued)*

MUSCLE	DESCRIPTION	ORIGIN (O) AND INSERTION (I)	ACTION	NERVE SUPPLY
▪ **Vastus intermedius** (in″ter-me′de-us) (*intermedius* = intermediate)	Obscured by rectus femoris; lies between vastus lateralis and vastus medialis on anterior thigh	O—anterior and lateral surfaces of proximal femur shaft I—as for rectus femoris	Extends knee	Femoral nerve
Tensor fasciae latae (ten′sor fă′she-e la′te) (*tensor* = to make tense; *fascia* = band; *lata* = wide)	Enclosed between fascia layers of anterolateral aspect of thigh; functionally associated with medial rotators and flexors of thigh	O—anterior aspect of iliac crest and anterior superior iliac spine I—iliotibial tract*	Steadies the knee and trunk on thigh by making iliotibial tract taut; flexes and abducts thigh; rotates thigh medially	Superior gluteal nerve (L_4 and L_5)
PART II: POSTERIOR MUSCLES (Figure 10.21)				
Gluteal Muscles—Origin on Pelvis				
Gluteus maximus (gloo′te-us mak′sĭ-mus) (*glutos* = buttock; *maximus* = largest)	Largest and most superficial gluteus muscle; forms bulk of buttock mass; fibers are thick and coarse; important site of intramuscular injection (dorsal gluteal site); overlies large sciatic nerve; covers ischial tuberosity only when standing; when sitting, moves superiorly, leaving ischial tuberosity exposed in the subcutaneous position	O—dorsal ilium, sacrum, and coccyx I—gluteal tuberosity of femur; iliotibial tract	Major extensor of thigh; complex, powerful, and most effective when thigh is flexed and force is necessary, as in rising from a forward flexed position and in thrusting the thigh posteriorly in climbing stairs and running; generally inactive during standing and walking; laterally rotates and abducts thigh	Inferior gluteal nerve (L_5, S_1, and S_2)
Gluteus medius (me′de-us) (*medius* = middle)	Thick muscle largely covered by gluteus maximus; important site for intramuscular injections (ventral gluteal site); considered safer than dorsal gluteal site because less chance of injuring sciatic nerve	O—between anterior and posterior gluteal lines on lateral surface of ilium I—by short tendon into lateral aspect of greater trochanter of femur	Abducts and medially rotates thigh; steadies pelvis; its action is extremely important in walking; e.g., muscle of limb planted on ground tilts or holds pelvis in abduction so that pelvis on side of swinging limb does not sag and foot of swinging limb can clear the ground	Superior gluteal nerve (L_5, S_1)
Gluteus minimus (mĭ′nĭ-mus) (minimus = smallest)	Smallest and deepest gluteal muscle	O—between anterior and inferior gluteal lines on external surface of ilium I—anterior border of greater trochanter of femur	As for gluteus medius	Superior gluteal nerve (L_5, S_1)
Lateral Rotators				
Piriformis (pir′ĭ-form-is) (*piri* = pear; *forma* = shape)	Pyramidal muscle located on posterior aspect of hip joint; inferior to gluteus minimus; issues from pelvis via greater sciatic notch	O—anterolateral surface of sacrum (opposite greater sciatic notch) I—superior border of greater trochanter of femur	Rotates extended thigh laterally; because inserted above head of femur, can also help abduct thigh when hip is flexed; stabilizes hip joint	S_1 and S_2, L_5

*The iliotibial tract is a thickened lateral portion of the *fascia lata* (the fascia that ensheathes all the muscles of the thigh). It extends as a tendinous band from the iliac crest to the knee (see Figure 10.21a).

MUSCLE GALLERY

Table 10.14 *(continued)*

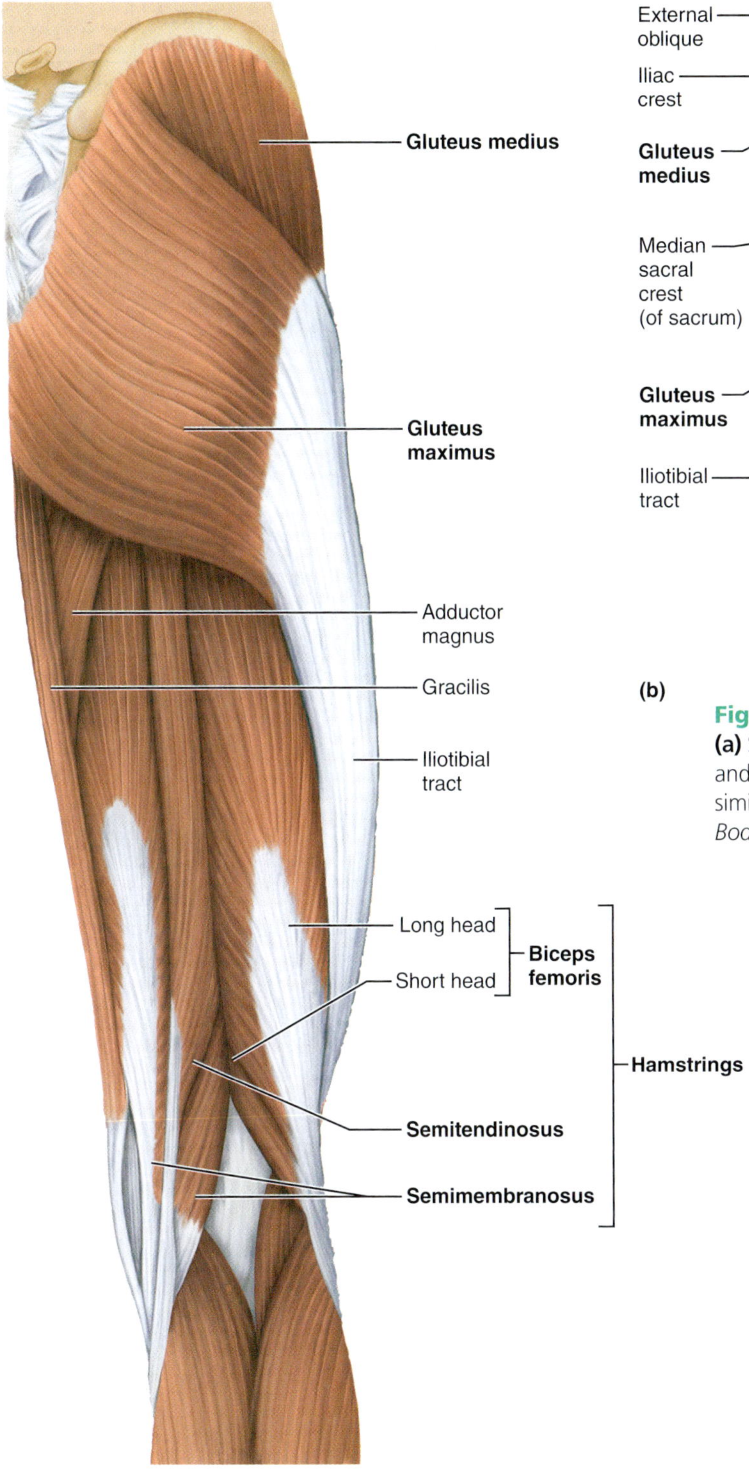

(a)

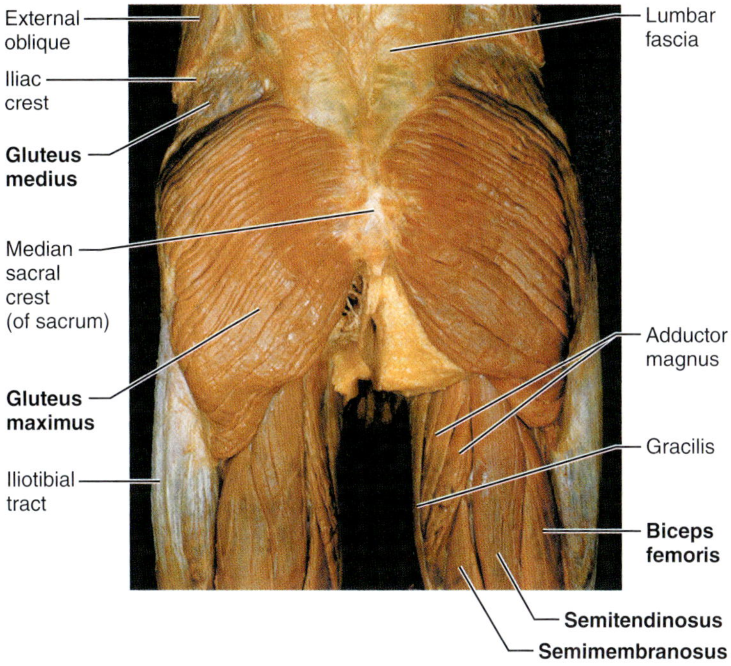

(b)

Figure 10.21 Posterior muscles of the right hip and thigh. **(a)** Superficial view showing the gluteus muscles of the buttock and hamstring muscles of the thigh. **(b)** Cadaver dissection of view similar to (a). (For a related image, see *A Brief Atlas of the Human Body*, Figure 41.)

MUSCLE GALLERY

Table 10.14 Muscles Crossing the Hip and Knee Joints: Movements of the Thigh and Leg (Figures 10.20 and 10.21) *(continued)*

MUSCLE	DESCRIPTION	ORIGIN (O) AND INSERTION (I)	ACTION	NERVE SUPPLY
Obturator externus (ob″tu-ra′tor ek-ster′nus) (*obturator* = obturator foramen; *externus* = outside)	Flat, triangular muscle deep in superomedial aspect of thigh	O—outer surfaces of obturator membrane, pubis, and ischium, margins of obturator foramen I—by a tendon into trochanteric fossa of posterior femur	As for piriformis	Obturator nerve
Obturator internus (in-ter′nus) (*internus* = inside)	Surrounds obturator foramen within pelvis; leaves pelvis via lesser sciatic notch and turns acutely forward to insert on femur	O—inner surface of obturator membrane, greater sciatic notch, and margins of obturator foramen I—greater trochanter in front of piriformis	As for piriformis	L_5 and S_1
Gemellus (jĕ-mĕ′lis)—superior and inferior (*gemin* = twin, double; *superior* = above; *inferior* = below)	Two small muscles with common insertions and actions; considered extrapelvic portions of obturator internus	O—ischial spine (superior); ischial tuberosity (inferior) I—greater trochanter of femur	As for piriformis	L_5 and S_1
Quadratus femoris (*quad* = four-sided square)	Short, thick muscle; most inferior lateral rotator muscle; extends laterally from pelvis	O—ischial tuberosity I—intertrochanteric crest of femur	Rotates thigh laterally and stabilizes hip joint	L_5 and S_1

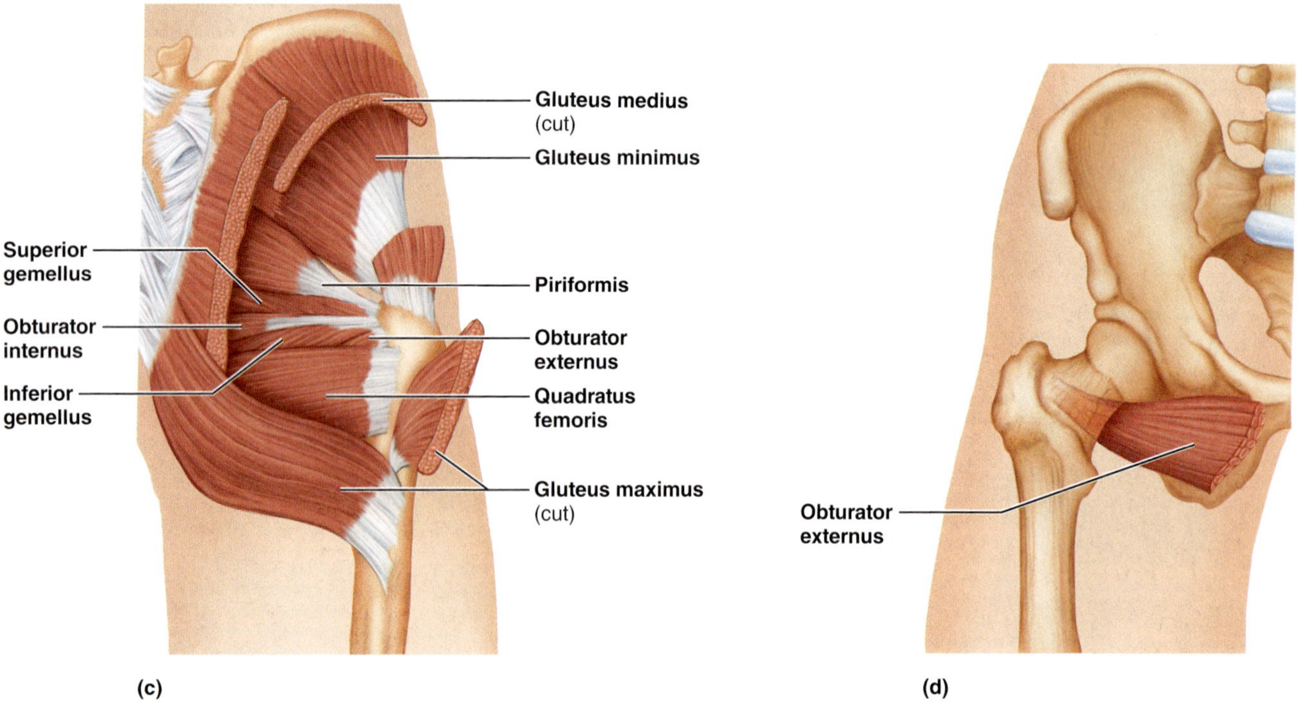

Figure 10.21 *(continued)* **Posterior muscles of the right hip and thigh. (c)** Deep muscles of the gluteal region, which act primarily to rotate the thigh laterally. The superficial gluteus maximus and medius have been removed. **(d)** Anterior view of the isolated obturator externus muscle.

MUSCLE GALLERY

Table 10.14 *(continued)*

MUSCLE	DESCRIPTION	ORIGIN (O) AND INSERTION (I)	ACTION	NERVE SUPPLY
Muscles of the Posterior Compartment of the Thigh				
Hamstrings	The hamstrings are fleshy muscles of the posterior thigh (biceps femoris, semitendinosus, and semimembranosus). They cross both the hip and knee joints and are prime movers of thigh extension and knee flexion. The group has a common origin site and is innervated by sciatic nerve (actually two nerves, the tibial and common fibular nerves wrapped in a common sheath). Ability of hamstrings to act on one of the two joints spanned depends on which joint is fixed—if knee is fixed (extended), they extend hip; if hip is extended, they flex knee. However, when hamstrings are stretched, they tend to restrict full accomplishment of antagonistic movement; e.g., if knees are fully extended, it is difficult to flex the hip fully (and touch your toes), and when the thigh is fully flexed as in kicking a football, it is almost impossible to extend the knee fully at the same time (without considerable practice). Name of this muscle group comes from old butchers' practice of using their tendons to hang hams for smoking. "Pulled hamstrings" are common sports injuries in those who run very hard, e.g., football halfbacks.			
▪ **Biceps femoris** (*biceps* = two heads)	Most lateral muscle of the group; arises from two heads	O—ischial tuberosity (long head); linea aspera, lateral supracondylar line, and distal femur (short head) I—common tendon passes downward and laterally (forming lateral border of popliteal fossa) to insert into head of fibula and lateral condyle of tibia	Extends thigh and flexes knee; laterally rotates leg, especially when knee is flexed	Sciatic nerve—tibial nerve to long head, common fibular nerve to short head (L_5–S_2)
▪ **Semitendinosus** (sem″e-ten″dĭ-no′sus) (*semi* = half; *tendinosus* = tendon)	Lies medial to biceps femoris; although its name suggests that this muscle is largely tendinous, it is quite fleshy; its long slender tendon begins about two-thirds of the way down thigh	O—ischial tuberosity in common with long head of biceps femoris I—medial aspect of upper tibial shaft	Extends thigh and flexes knee; with semimembranosus, medially rotates leg	Sciatic nerve—tibial nerve portion (L_5–S_2)
▪ **Semimembranosus** (sem″e-mem″-brah-no′sus) (*membranosus* = membrane)	Deep to semitendinosus	O—ischial tuberosity I—medial condyle of tibia; via oblique popliteal ligament to lateral condyle of femur	Extends thigh and flexes knee; medially rotates leg	Sciatic nerve—tibial nerve portion (L_5–S_2)

10

MUSCLE GALLERY

Table 10.15 Muscles of the Leg: Movements of the Ankle and Toes (Figures 10.22 to 10.24)

The deep fascia of the leg is continuous with the fascia lata that ensheathes the thigh. Like a snug "knee sock" beneath the skin, the leg fascia binds the leg muscles tightly, preventing excessive muscle swelling during exercise and aiding venous return. Its inward extensions segregate the leg muscles into *anterior*, *lateral*, and *posterior compartments* (see Figure 10.26b), each with its own nerve and blood supply. Distally the leg fascia thickens to form the **flexor**, **extensor**, and **fibular** (or peroneal) **retinacula**, "ankle brackets" that hold the tendons in place where they run to the foot (Figures 10.22a, 10.23a).

The various muscles of the leg promote movements at the ankle joint (dorsiflex and plantar flex), at the intertarsal joints (invert and evert the foot), and/or at the toes (flex and extend). Muscles in the *anterior extensor compartment of the leg* are primarily toe extensors and ankle dorsiflexors. Although dorsiflexion is not a powerful movement, it is important in preventing the toes from dragging during walking. Lateral compartment muscles are the **fibular**, formerly *peroneal* (*peron* = fibula), **muscles** that plantar flex and evert the foot. Muscles of the *posterior flexor compartment* primarily plantar flex the foot and flex the toes (Figure 10.24b–d). Plantar flexion is the most powerful movement of the ankle (and foot) because it lifts the entire weight of our body. It is essential for standing on tiptoe and provides the forward thrust when walking and running. The **popliteus muscle**, which crosses the knee, has a unique function. It "unlocks" the extended knee in preparation for flexion (Figure 10.24b, f).

We consider the tiny intrinsic muscles of the sole of the foot (lumbricals, interossei, and others) in Table 10.16.

Table 10.17 (Part II) summarizes the actions of the muscles in this table.

MUSCLE	DESCRIPTION	ORIGIN (O) AND INSERTION (I)	ACTION	NERVE SUPPLY
PART I: MUSCLES OF THE ANTERIOR COMPARTMENT (Figures 10.22 and 10.23)	All muscles of the anterior compartment dorsiflex the ankle and have a common innervation, the deep fibular nerve. Paralysis of the anterior muscle group causes *foot drop*, which requires that the leg be lifted unusually high during walking to prevent tripping over one's toes. One cause of "shin splints," also called anterior compartment syndrome, is painful inflammation of the anterior compartment muscles.			
Tibialis anterior (tib″e-a′lis) (*tibial* = tibia; *anterior* = toward the front)	Superficial muscle of anterior leg; laterally parallels sharp anterior margin of tibia	O—lateral condyle and upper 2/3 of tibial shaft; interosseous membrane I—by tendon into inferior surface of medial cuneiform and first metatarsal bone	Prime mover of dorsiflexion; inverts foot; helps support medial longitudinal arch of foot	Deep fibular nerve (L_4 and L_5)
Extensor digitorum longus (*extensor* = increases angle at a joint; *digit* = finger or toe; *longus* = long)	Unipennate muscle on anterolateral surface of leg; lateral to tibialis anterior muscle	O—lateral condyle of tibia; proximal 3/4 of fibula; interosseous membrane I—middle and distal phalanges of toes 2–5 via extensor expansion	Prime mover of toe extension (acts mainly at metatarsophalangeal joints); dorsiflexes foot	Deep fibular nerve (L_5 and S_1)
Fibularis (peroneus) tertius (fib-u-lar′ris ter′shus) (*fibular* = fibula; *tertius* = third)	Small muscle; usually continuous and fused with distal part of extensor digitorum longus; not always present	O—distal anterior surface of fibula and interosseous membrane I—tendon inserts on dorsum of fifth metatarsal	Dorsiflexes and everts foot	Deep fibular nerve (L_5 and S_1)
Extensor hallucis longus (hal′yu-kis) (*hallux* = great toe)	Deep to extensor digitorum longus and tibialis anterior; narrow origin	O—anteromedial fibula shaft and interosseous membrane I—tendon inserts on distal phalanx of great toe	Extends great toe; dorsiflexes foot	Deep fibular nerve (L_5 and S_1)

MUSCLE GALLERY

Table 10.15 *(continued)*

Figure 10.22 Muscles of the anterior compartment of the right leg. (a) Superficial view of anterior leg muscles. (For a related image, see *A Brief Atlas of the Human Body*, Figure 40.) **(b–d)** Some of the same muscles shown in isolation to visualize their origins and insertions.

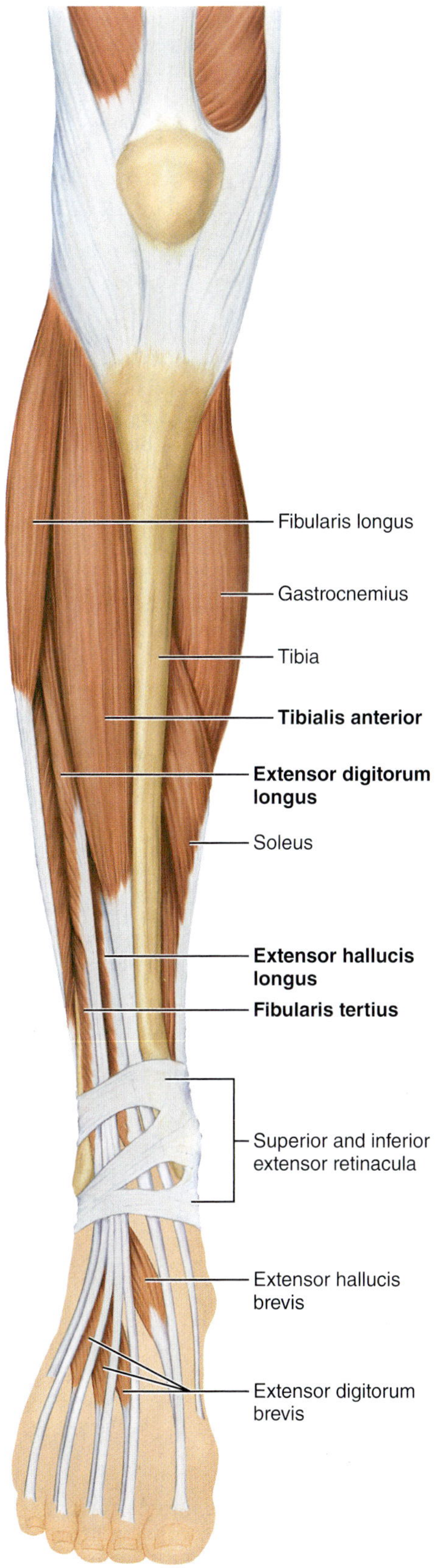

(a)

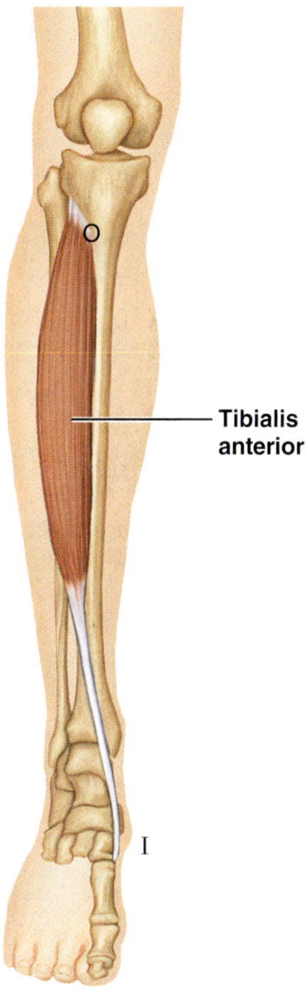

(b)

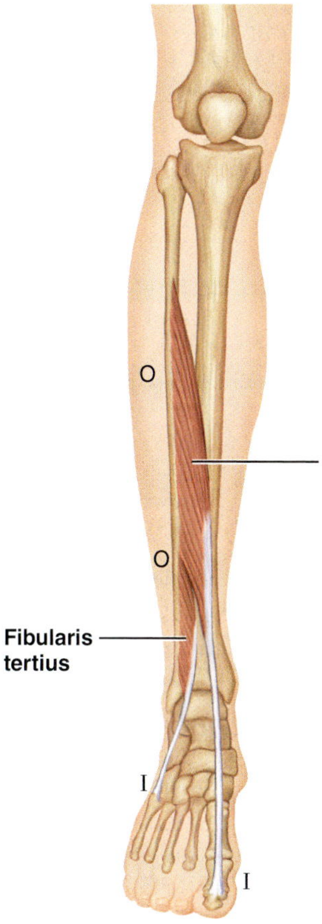

(c)

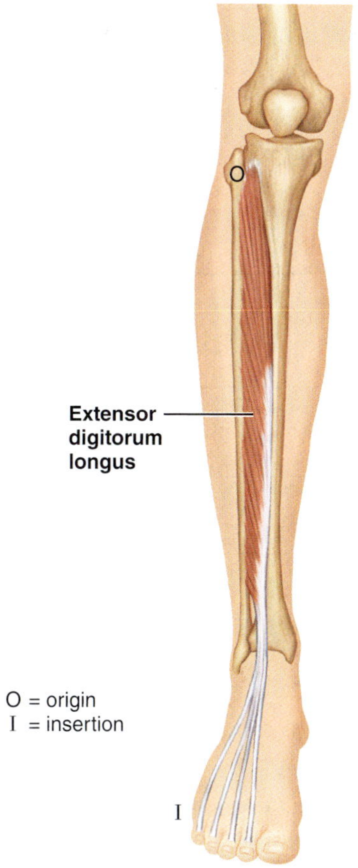

(d)

MUSCLE GALLERY

Table 10.15 Muscles of the Leg: Movements of the Ankle and Toes (Figures 10.22 to 10.24) *(continued)*

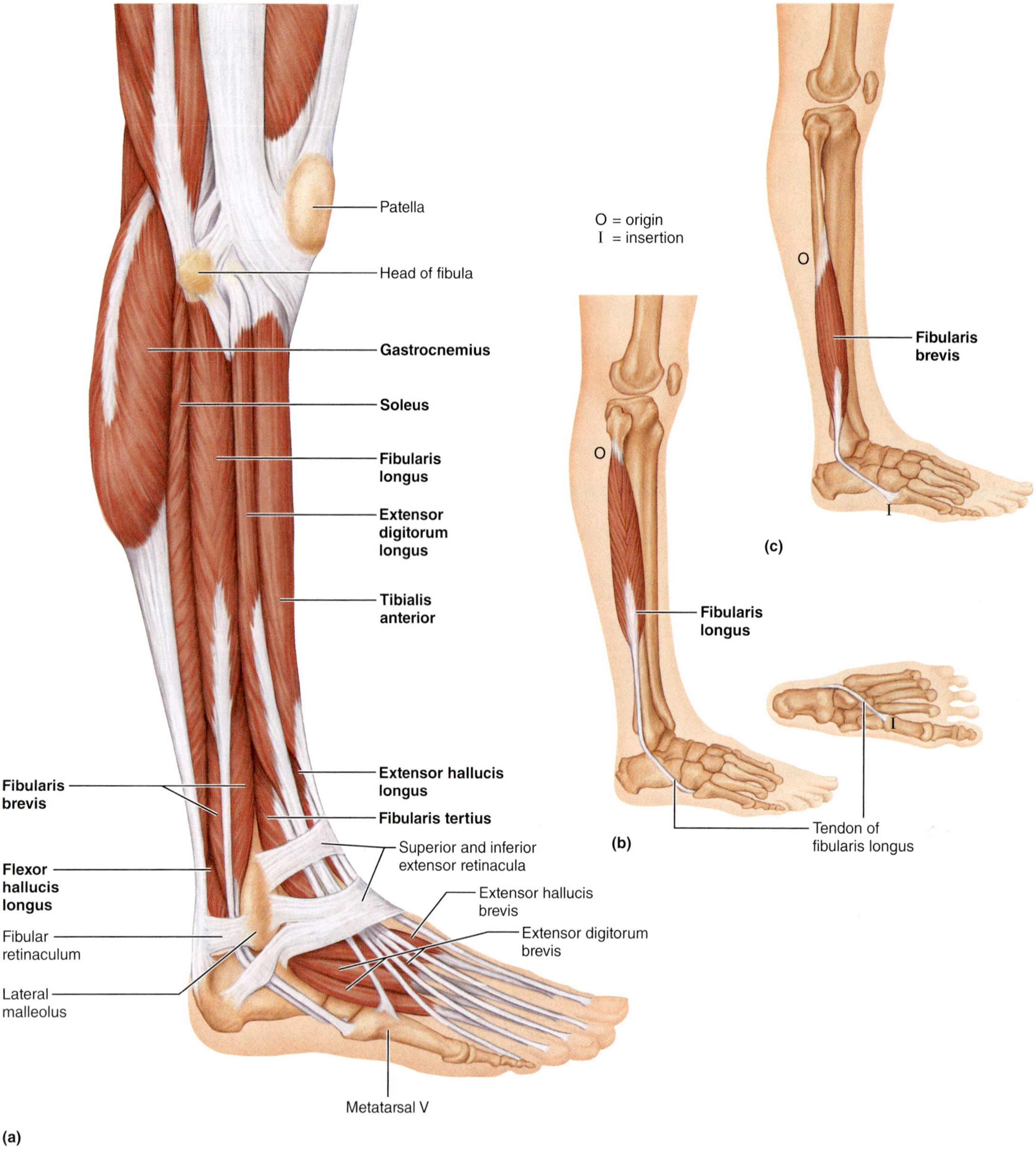

Figure 10.23 Muscles of the lateral compartment of the right leg. **(a)** Superficial view of lateral aspect of the leg, illustrating positions of lateral compartment muscles (fibularis longus and brevis) relative to anterior and posterior leg muscles. **(b)** Isolated view of fibularis longus; inset illustrates the insertion of the fibularis longus on the plantar surface of the foot. **(c)** Isolated view of fibularis brevis. (For a related image, see *A Brief Atlas of the Human Body*, Figure 42.)

MUSCLE GALLERY

Table 10.15 *(continued)*

MUSCLE	DESCRIPTION	ORIGIN (O) AND INSERTION (I)	ACTION	NERVE SUPPLY
PART II: MUSCLES OF THE LATERAL COMPARTMENT (Figures 10.23 and 10.24) These muscles have a common innervation, the superficial fibular nerve. Besides plantar flexion and foot eversion, these muscles stabilize the lateral ankle and lateral longitudinal arch of the foot.				
Fibularis (peroneus) longus (See also Figure 10.22)	Superficial lateral muscle; overlies fibula	O—head and upper portion of lateral fibula I—by long tendon that curves under foot to first metatarsal and medial cuneiform	Plantar flexes and everts foot; may help keep foot flat on ground	Superficial fibular nerve (L_5–S_2)
Fibularis (peroneus) brevis (*brevis* = short)	Smaller muscle; deep to fibularis longus; enclosed in a common sheath	O—distal fibula shaft I—by tendon running behind lateral malleolus to insert on proximal end of fifth metatarsal	Plantar flexes and everts foot	Superficial fibular nerve
PART III: MUSCLES OF THE POSTERIOR COMPARTMENT (Figure 10.24) The muscles of the posterior compartment have a common innervation, the tibial nerve. They act in concert to plantar flex the ankle.				
Superficial Muscles				
Triceps surae (tri″seps sur′e) (See also Figure 10.23)	Refers to muscle pair (gastrocnemius and soleus) that shapes the posterior calf and inserts via a common tendon into the calcaneus of the heel; this *calcaneal* or *Achilles tendon* is the largest tendon in the body. Prime movers of ankle plantar flexion.			
▪ **Gastrocnemius** (gas″truk-ne′me-us) (*gaster* = belly; *kneme* = leg)	Superficial muscle of pair; two prominent bellies that form proximal curve of calf	O—by two heads from medial and lateral condyles of femur I—posterior calcaneus via calcaneal tendon	Plantar flexes foot when knee is extended; because it also crosses knee joint, it can flex knee when foot is dorsiflexed	Tibial nerve (S_1, S_2)
▪ **Soleus** (so′le-us) (*soleus* = fish)	Broad, flat muscle, deep to gastrocnemius on posterior surface of calf	O—extensive origin from superior tibia, fibula, and interosseous membrane I—as for gastrocnemius	Plantar flexes foot; important locomotor and postural muscle during walking, running, and dancing	Tibial nerve
Plantaris (plan-tar′is) (*planta* = sole of foot)	Generally a small, feeble muscle, but varies in size and extent; may be absent	O—posterior femur above lateral condyle I—via a long, thin tendon into calcaneus or its tendon	Helps to flex knee and plantar flex foot	Tibial nerve
Deep Muscles (Figure 10.24c–f)				
Popliteus (pop-lit′e-us) (*poplit* = back of knee)	Thin, triangular muscle at posterior knee; passes inferomedially to tibial surface	O—lateral condyle of femur and lateral meniscus of knee I—proximal tibia	Flexes and rotates leg medially to unlock extended knee when flexion begins; with tibia fixed, rotates thigh laterally	Tibial nerve (L_4–S_1)
Flexor digitorum longus (*flexor* = decreases angle at a joint)	Long, narrow muscle; runs medial to and partially overlies tibialis posterior	O—extensive origin on the posterior tibia I—tendon runs behind medial malleolus and inserts into distal phalanges of toes 2–5	Plantar flexes and inverts foot; flexes toes; helps foot "grip" ground	Tibial nerve (L_5–S_2)
Flexor hallucis longus (See also Figure 10.23)	Bipennate muscle; lies lateral to inferior aspect of tibialis posterior	O—midshaft of fibula; interosseous membrane I—tendon runs under foot to distal phalanx of great toe	Plantar flexes and inverts foot; flexes great toe at all joints; "push off" muscle during walking	Tibial nerve (L_5–S_2)
Tibialis posterior (*posterior* = toward the back)	Thick, flat muscle deep to soleus; placed between posterior flexors	O—superior tibia and fibula and interosseous membrane I—tendon passes behind medial malleolus and under arch of foot; inserts into several tarsals and metatarsals II–IV	Prime mover of foot inversion; plantar flexes foot; stabilizes medial longitudinal arch of foot (as during ice skating)	Tibial nerve (L_4 and L_5)

10

MUSCLE GALLERY

Table 10.15 Muscles of the Leg: Movements of the Ankle and Toes (Figures 10.22 to 10.24) *(continued)*

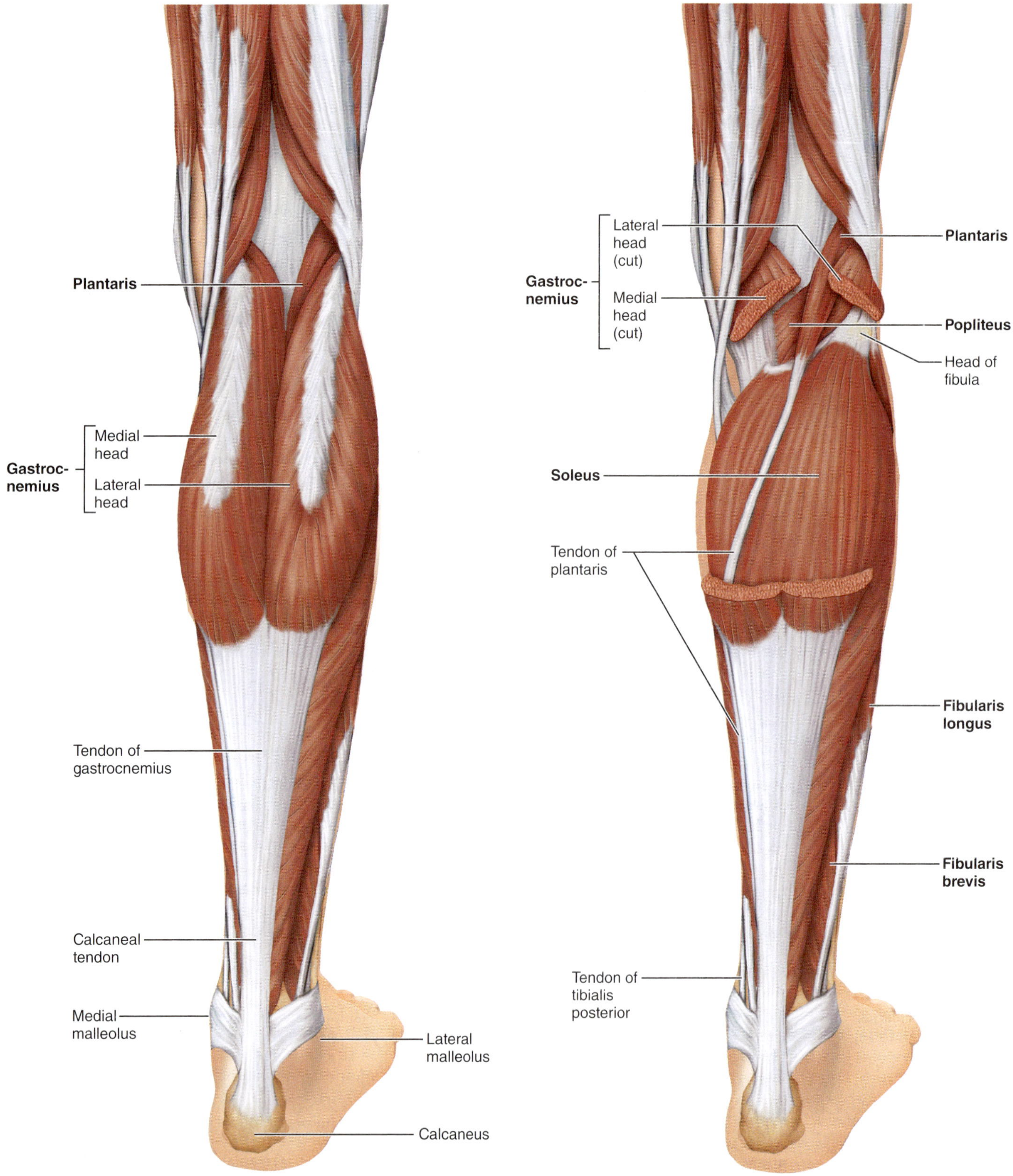

(a) Superficial view of the posterior leg.

(b) The gastrocnemius has been removed to show the soleus immediately deep to it.

Figure 10.24 Muscles of the posterior compartment of the right leg.

MUSCLE GALLERY

Table 10.15 *(continued)*

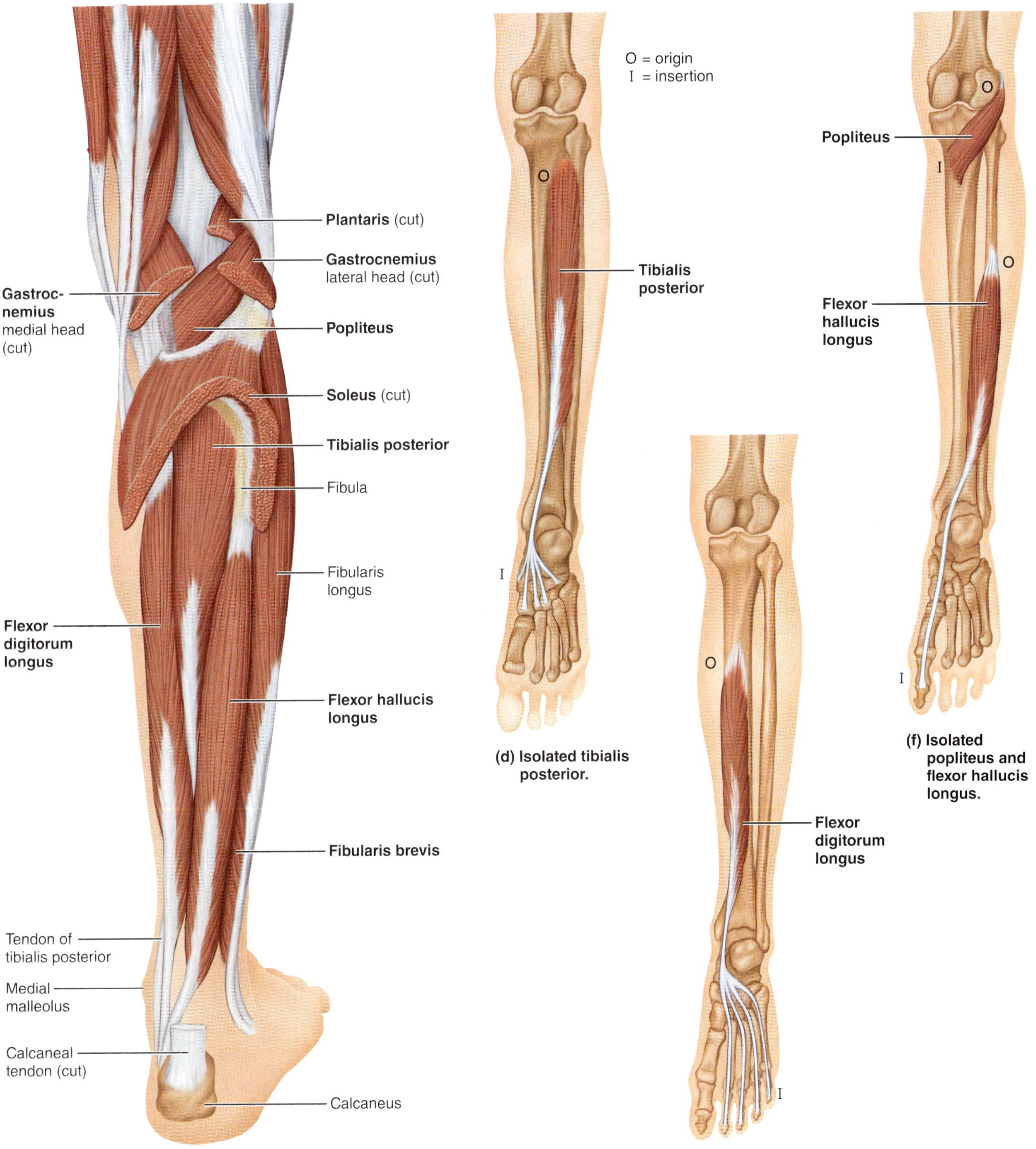

(c) The triceps surae has been removed to show the deep muscles of the posterior compartment.

(d) Isolated tibialis posterior.

(e) Isolated flexor digitorum longus.

(f) Isolated popliteus and flexor hallucis longus.

Figure 10.24 *(continued)*

MUSCLE GALLERY

Table 10.16 Intrinsic Muscles of the Foot: Toe Movement and Arch Support (Figure 10.25)

The intrinsic muscles of the foot help to flex, extend, abduct, and adduct the toes. Collectively, along with the tendons of some leg muscles that enter the sole, the foot muscles help support the arches of the foot. There is a single muscle on the foot's dorsum (superior aspect), and several muscles on the plantar aspect (the sole). The plantar muscles occur in four layers, from superficial to deep. Overall, the foot muscles are remarkably similar to those in the palm of the hand.

MUSCLE	DESCRIPTION	ORIGIN (O) AND INSERTION (I)	ACTION	NERVE SUPPLY
MUSCLES ON DORSUM OF FOOT				
Extensor digitorum brevis (Figures 10.22a and 10.23a)	Small, four-part muscle on dorsum of foot; deep to the tendons of extensor digitorum longus; corresponds to the extensor indicis and extensor pollicis muscles of forearm	O—anterior part of calcaneus bone; extensor retinaculum I—base of proximal phalanx of great toe; extensor expansions on toes 2 to 4 or 5	Helps extend toes at metatarsophalangeal joints	Deep fibular nerve (L_5 and S_1)
MUSCLES ON SOLE OF FOOT—FIRST LAYER (MOST SUPERFICIAL) (Figure 10.25)				
Flexor digitorum brevis	Bandlike muscle in middle of sole; corresponds to flexor digitorum superficialis of forearm and inserts into digits in the same way	O—calcaneal tuberosity I—middle phalanx of toes 2–4	Helps flex toes	Medial plantar nerve (a branch of tibial nerve, S_1 and S_2)
Abductor hallucis (hal′yu-kis) (*hallux* = great toe)	Lies medial to flexor digitorum brevis (recall the similar thumb muscle, abductor pollicis brevis)	O—calcaneal tuberosity and flexor retinaculum I—proximal phalanx of great toe, medial side, in the tendon of flexor hallucis brevis)	Abducts great toe	Medial plantar nerve
Abductor digiti minimi	Most lateral of the three superficial sole muscles (recall similar abductor muscle in palm)	O—calcaneal tuberosity I—lateral side of base of little toe's proximal phalanx	Abducts and flexes little toe	Lateral plantar nerve (a branch of tibial nerve, S_1, S_2, and S_3)
MUSCLES ON SOLE OF FOOT—SECOND LAYER				
Flexor accessorius (quadratus plantae)	Rectangular muscle just deep to flexor digitorum brevis in posterior half of sole; two heads (see also Figure 10.25c)	O—medial and lateral sides of calcaneus I—tendon of flexor digitorum longus in midsole	Straightens out the oblique pull of flexor digitorum longus	Lateral plantar nerve
Lumbricals	Four little "worms" (like lumbricals in hand)	O—from each tendon of flexor digitorum longus I—extensor expansion on proximal phalanx of toes 2–5, medial side	By pulling on extensor expansion, flex toes at metatarsophalangeal joints and extend toes at interphalangeal joints	Medial plantar nerve (first lumbrical) and lateral plantar nerve (second to fourth lumbrical)

MUSCLE GALLERY

Table 10.16 *(continued)*

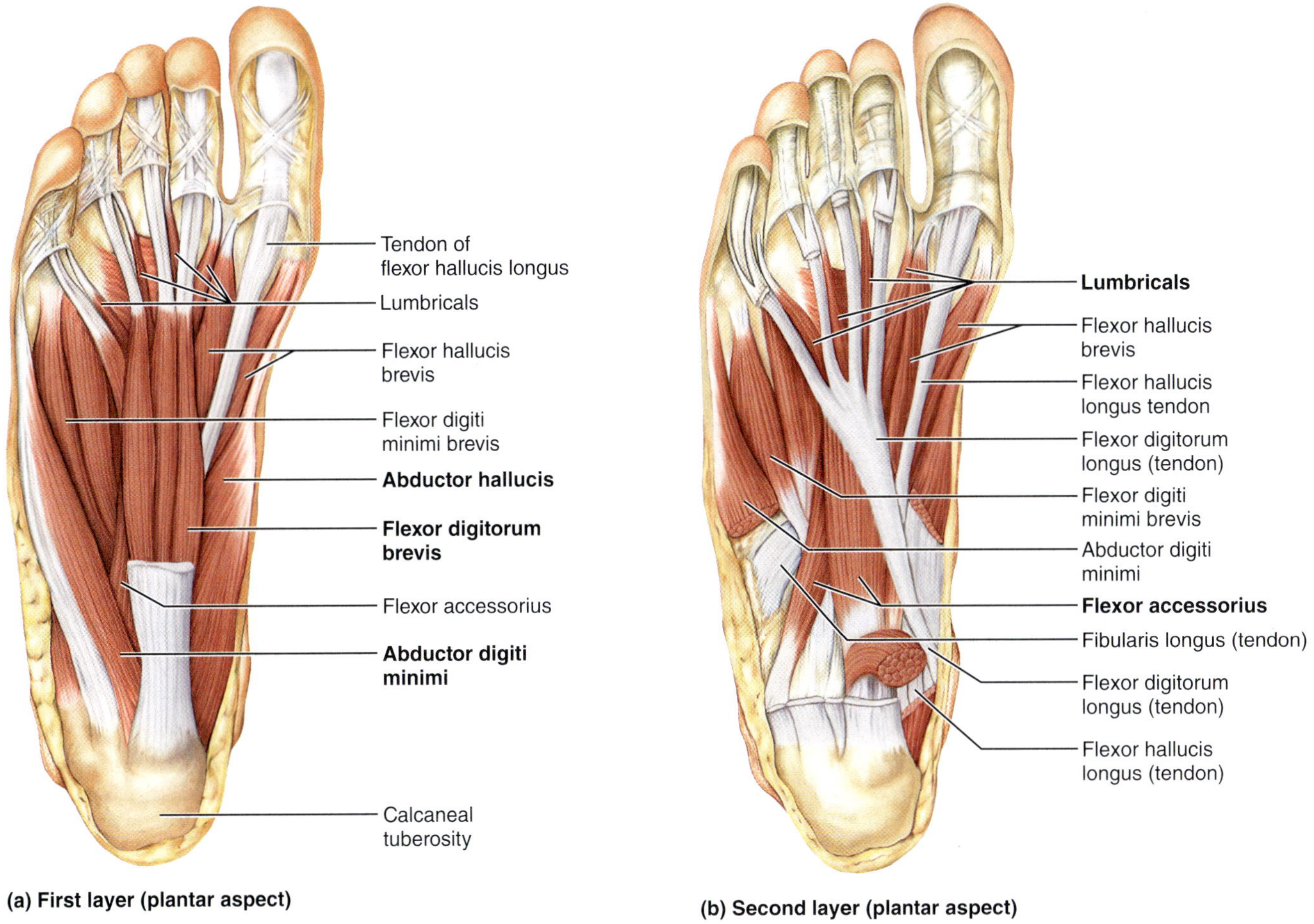

Figure 10.25 Muscles of the right foot, plantar aspect. (For a related image, see *A Brief Atlas of the Human Body*, Figure 43.)

MUSCLE GALLERY

Table 10.16 Intrinsic Muscles of the Foot: Toe Movement and Arch Support (Figure 10.25) *(continued)*

MUSCLE	DESCRIPTION	ORIGIN (O) AND INSERTION (I)	ACTION	NERVE SUPPLY
MUSCLES ON SOLE OF FOOT—THIRD LAYER				
Flexor hallucis brevis	Covers metatarsal I; splits into two bellies—recall flexor pollicis brevis of thumb	O—lateral cuneiform and cuboid bones I—via two tendons onto base of the proximal phalanx of great toe; each insertion tendon contains a sesamoid bone	Flexes great toe's metatarsophalangeal joint	Medial plantar nerve
Adductor hallucis	Oblique and transverse heads; deep to lumbricals (recall adductor pollicis in thumb)	O—from bases of metatarsals II–IV and from fibularis longus tendon sheath (oblique head); from a ligament across metatarsophalangeal joints (transverse head) I—base of proximal phalanx of great toe, lateral side	Helps maintain the transverse arch of foot; weak adductor of great toe	Lateral plantar nerve (S_2 and S_3)
Flexor digiti minimi brevis	Covers metatarsal V (recall same muscle in hand)	O—base of metatarsal V and tendon sheath of fibularis longus I—base of proximal phalanx of toe 5	Flexes little toe at metatarsophalangeal joint	Lateral plantar nerve
MUSCLES ON SOLE OF FOOT—FOURTH LAYER (DEEPEST)				
Plantar (3) and dorsal interossei (4)	Similar to palmar and dorsal interossei of hand in locations, attachments, and actions; however, these muscles orient around the second digit, not the third	See palmar and dorsal interossei (Table 10.13)	See palmar and dorsal interossei (Table 10.13)	Lateral plantar nerve

10

MUSCLE GALLERY

Table 10.16 *(continued)*

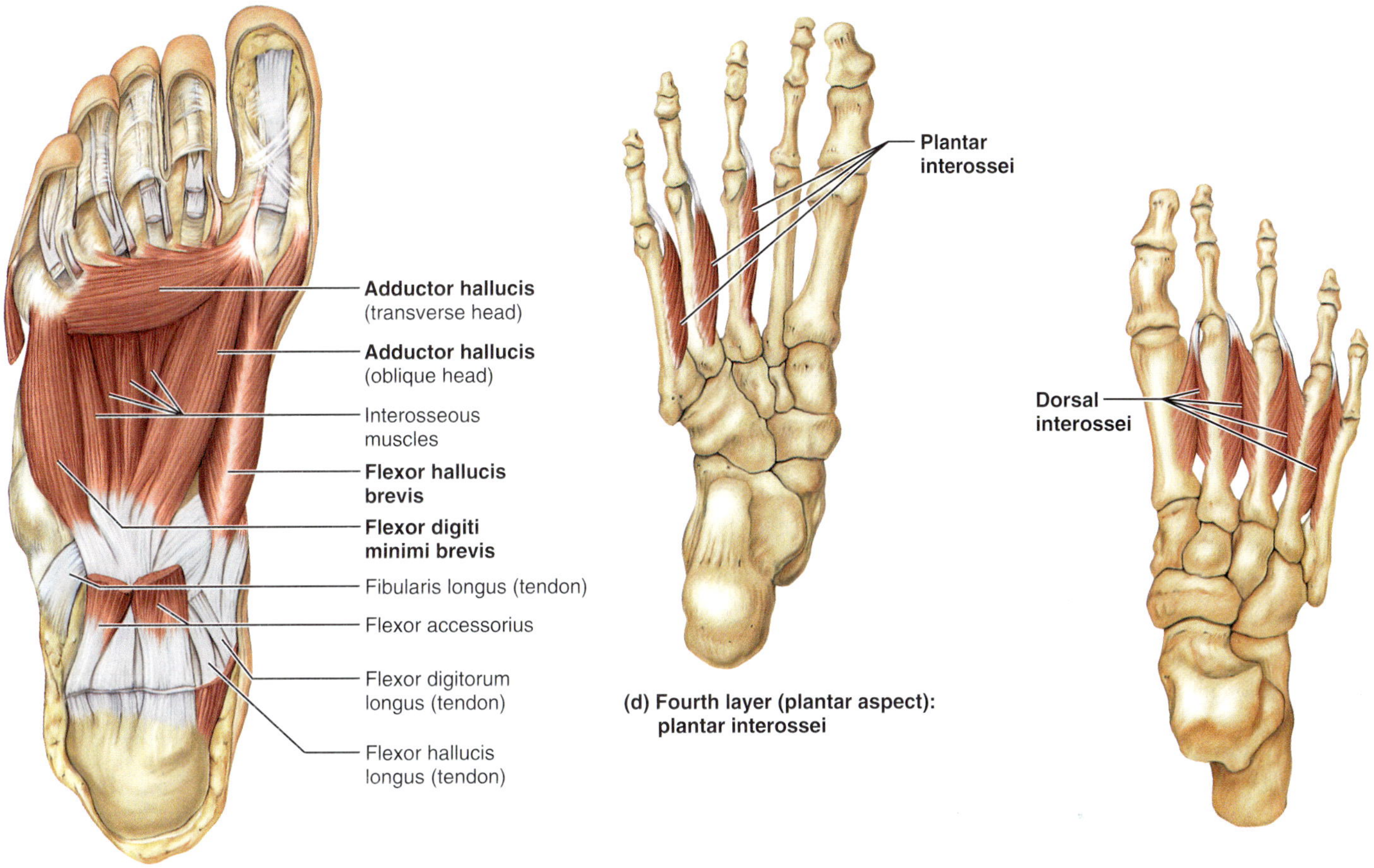

(c) Third layer (plantar aspect)

(d) Fourth layer (plantar aspect): plantar interossei

(e) Fourth layer (dorsal aspect): dorsal interossei

Figure 10.25 *(continued)* **Muscles of the right foot, plantar aspect.**

MUSCLE GALLERY

Table 10.17 Summary: Actions of Muscles Acting on the Thigh, Leg, and Foot (Figure 10.26)

PART I: Muscles Acting on the Thigh and Leg (PM = Prime Mover)	Actions at the Hip Joint						Actions at the Knee	
	Flexion	Extension	Abduction	Adduction	Medial Rotation	Lateral Rotation	Flexion	Extension
Anterior and Medial Muscles								
Iliopsoas	× (PM)							
Sartorius	×		×			×	×	
Tensor fasciae latae	×		×		×			
Rectus femoris	×							× (PM)
Vastus muscles								× (PM)
Adductor magnus	×	×		×	×			
Adductor longus	×			×	×			
Adductor brevis	×			×	×			
Pectineus	×			×	×			
Gracilis				×	×		×	
Posterior Muscles								
Gluteus maximus		× (PM)	×			×		
Gluteus medius			× (PM)		×			
Gluteus minimus			×		×			
Piriformis			×			×		
Obturator internus			× (flexed) × (thigh)			×		
Obturator externus						×		
Gemelli						×		
Quadratus femoris						×		
Biceps femoris		× (PM)					× (PM)	
Semitendinosus		×					× (PM)	
Semimembranosus		×					× (PM)	
Gastrocnemius							×	
Plantaris							×	
Popliteus							× (and rotates leg medially)	

PART II: Muscles Acting on the Ankle and Toes	Actions at the Ankle Joint				Actions at the Toes	
	Plantar Flexion	Dorsiflexion	Inversion	Eversion	Flexion	Extension
Anterior Compartment						
Tibialis anterior		× (PM)	×			
Extensor digitorum longus		×				× (PM)
Fibularis tertius		×		×		
Extensor hallucis longus		×	× (weak)			× (great toe)
Lateral Compartment						
Fibularis longus and brevis	×			×		
Posterior Compartment						
Gastrocnemius	× (PM)					
Soleus	× (PM)					
Plantaris	×					
Flexor digitorum longus	×		×		× (PM)	
Flexor hallucis longus	×		×		× (great toe)	
Tibialis posterior	×		× (PM)			

MUSCLE GALLERY

Table 10.17 *(continued)*

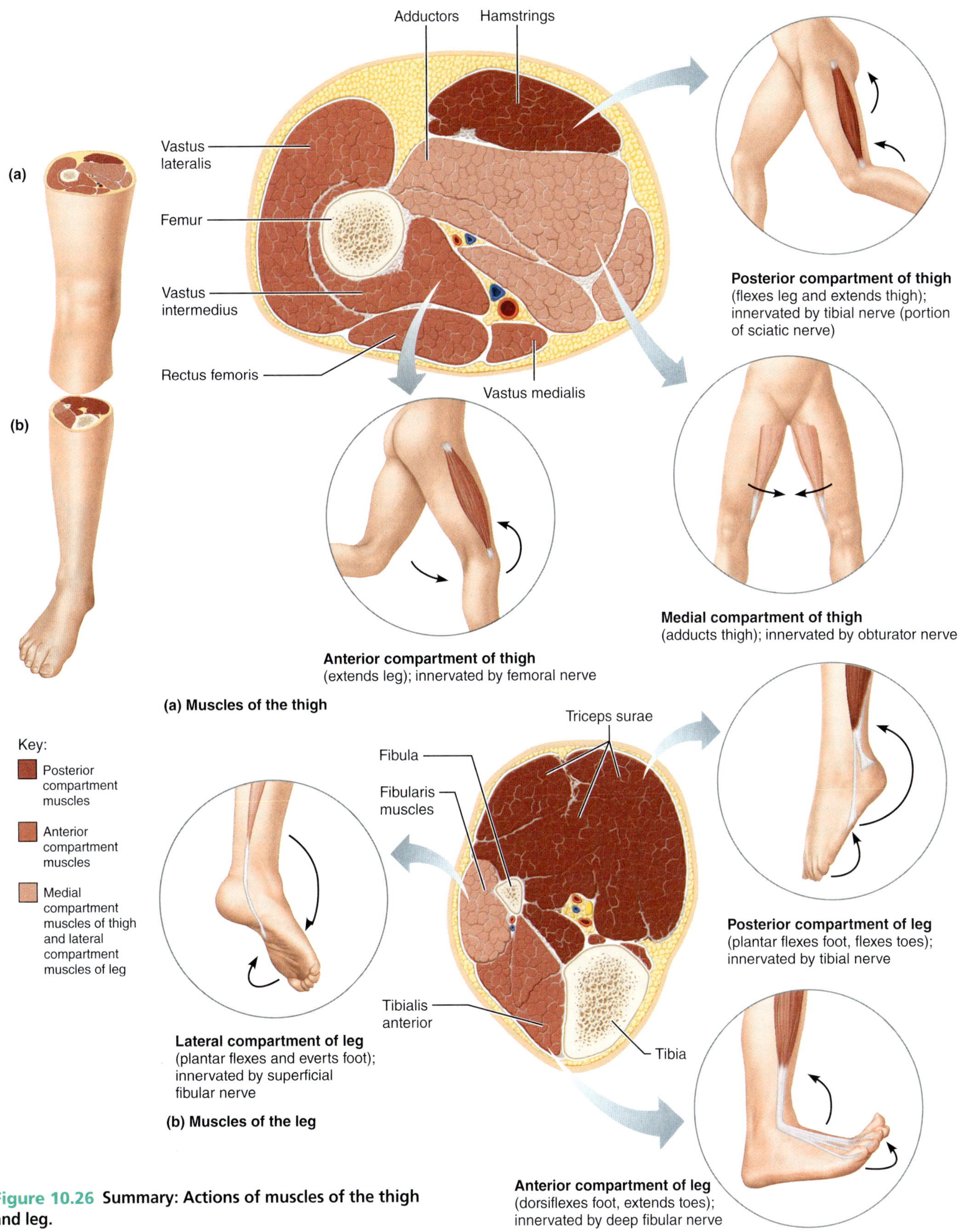

Figure 10.26 Summary: Actions of muscles of the thigh and leg.

10

Check Your Understanding

6. As John listened to Roger's account of how he flirted with his neighbor, he raised his eyebrows and then winked at Sarah. What facial muscles was he using?
7. What muscles would you contract to make a "sad clown's face"?
8. How can the deltoid muscles both extend and flex the arm? Aren't these antagonistic movements?
9. Which of the thenar muscles does not have an insertion on bones of the thumb?

For answers, see Appendix H.

Chapter Summary

MAP™ For more chapter study tools, go to the Study Area of MasteringA&P at **www.masteringaandp.com**.
There you will find:

- Interactive Physiology iP
- A&PFlix A&PFlix
- Practice Anatomy Lab PAL
- PhysioEx PEx
- Videos, Practice Quizzes and Tests, MP3 Tutor Sessions, Case Studies, and much more!

Actions and Interactions of Skeletal Muscles (pp. 319–320)

1. Skeletal muscles are arranged in opposing groups across body joints so that one group can reverse or modify the action of the other.
2. Muscles are classified as prime movers (agonists), antagonists, synergists, and fixators.

Naming Skeletal Muscles (pp. 320–322)

1. Criteria used to name muscles include a muscle's location, shape, relative size, fiber (fascicle) direction, number of origins, attachment sites (origin/insertion), and action. Several criteria are combined to name some muscles.

Muscle Mechanics: Importance of Fascicle Arrangement and Leverage (pp. 322–324)

1. Common patterns of fascicle arrangement are circular, convergent, parallel, fusiform, and pennate. Muscles with fibers that run parallel to the long axis of the muscle shorten most; stocky pennate muscles shorten little but are the most powerful muscles.
2. A lever is a bar that moves on a fulcrum. When an effort is applied to the lever, a load is moved. In the body, bones are the levers, joints are the fulcrums, and skeletal muscles exert the effort at their insertions.
3. When the effort is farther from the fulcrum than is the load, the lever operates at a mechanical advantage (it's slow and strong). When the effort is exerted closer to the fulcrum than is the load, the lever operates at a mechanical disadvantage (it's fast and promotes a large degree of movement).
4. First-class levers (effort-fulcrum-load) may operate at a mechanical advantage or disadvantage. Second-class levers (fulcrum-load-effort) all operate at a mechanical advantage. Third-class levers (fulcrum-effort-load) always operate at a mechanical disadvantage. Most skeletal muscles of the body act in third-class lever systems.

Major Skeletal Muscles of the Body (pp. 324–382)

1. Muscles of the head that produce facial expression tend to be small and to insert into soft tissue (skin and other muscles) rather than into bone. These muscles open and close the eyes and mouth, compress the cheeks, allow smiling and other types of facial language (see Table 10.1*).
2. Muscles of the head involved in mastication include the masseter and temporalis that elevate the mandible and two deep muscle pairs that promote grinding and sliding jaw movements (see Table 10.2*). Extrinsic muscles of the tongue anchor the tongue and control its movements.
3. Deep muscles of the anterior neck promote swallowing movements, including elevation/depression of the hyoid bone, closing off the respiratory passages, and peristalsis of the pharynx (see Table 10.3*).
4. Neck muscles and deep muscles of the vertebral column promote head and trunk movements (see Table 10.4*). The deep muscles of the posterior trunk can extend large regions of the vertebral column (and head) simultaneously. The anteriorly located sternocleidomastoid and scalene muscles effect head flexion and rotation.
5. The diaphragm and external intercostal muscles of the thorax promote movements of quiet breathing (see Table 10.5*). Downward movement of the diaphragm increases intra-abdominal pressure.
6. The four muscle pairs forming the abdominal wall are layered like plywood to form a natural muscular girdle that protects, supports, and compresses abdominal contents. These muscles also flex and laterally rotate the trunk (see Table 10.6*).
7. Muscles of the pelvic floor and perineum (see Table 10.7*) support the pelvic viscera, resist increases in intra-abdominal pressure, inhibit urination and defecation, and aid erection.
8. Except for the pectoralis major and the latissimus dorsi, the superficial muscles of the thorax fix or promote movements of the scapula (see Table 10.8*). Scapular movements are effected primarily by posterior thoracic muscles.
9. Nine muscles cross the shoulder joint to move the humerus (see Table 10.9*). Of these, seven originate on the scapula and two arise from the axial skeleton. Four muscles contribute to the "rotator cuff" helping to stabilize the multiaxial shoulder joint. Generally speaking, muscles located anteriorly flex, rotate, and adduct the arm. Those located posteriorly extend, rotate, and adduct the arm. The deltoid muscle of the shoulder is the prime mover of shoulder abduction.
10. Muscles that move the forearm form the flesh of the arm (see Table 10.10*). Anterior arm muscles are forearm flexors; posterior muscles are forearm extensors.
11. Muscles originating on the forearm mainly move the wrist, hand, and fingers (see Table 10.11*). Except for the two pronator muscles, the anterior forearm muscles are wrist and/or finger flexors; those of the posterior compartment are wrist and finger extensors.
12. The intrinsic muscles of the hand aid in precise movements of the fingers (Table 10.13*) and in opposition, which helps us grip things. These small muscles are divided into thenar, hypothenar, and midpalmar groups.

13. Muscles crossing the hip and knee joints move the thigh and leg (see Table 10.14*). Anteromedial muscles flex and/or adduct the thigh and flex the knee. Muscles of the posterior gluteal region extend and rotate the thigh. Posterior thigh muscles extend the hip and flex the knee.
14. Muscles in the leg act on the ankle and toes (see Table 10.15*). Anterior compartment muscles are largely ankle dorsiflexors. Lateral compartment muscles are plantar flexors and foot everters. Those of the posterior leg are plantar flexors.
15. The intrinsic muscles of the foot (Table 10.16*) support the foot arches and help move the toes. Most occur in the sole, arranged in four layers. They resemble the small muscles in the palm of the hand.

*See specific table cited for detailed description of each muscle in the group.

Review Questions

Multiple Choice/Matching

(Some questions have more than one correct answer. Select the best answer or answers from the choices given.)

1. A muscle that assists an agonist by causing a like movement or by stabilizing a joint over which an agonist acts is a(n) **(a)** antagonist, **(b)** prime mover, **(c)** synergist, **(d)** agonist.
2. The arrangement of muscle fibers in which the fibers are arranged at an angle to a central longitudinal tendon is **(a)** circular, **(b)** longitudinal, **(c)** pennate, **(d)** parallel.
3. Match the muscle names in column B to the facial muscles described in column A.

Column A	Column B
____ (1) squints the eyes	(a) corrugator supercilii
____ (2) raises the eyebrows	(b) depressor anguli oris
____ (3) smiling muscle	(c) frontal belly of epicranius
____ (4) puckers the lips	
____ (5) pulls the scalp posteriorly	(d) occipital belly of epicranius
	(e) orbicularis oculi
	(f) orbicularis oris
	(g) zygomaticus

4. The prime mover of inspiration is the **(a)** diaphragm, **(b)** internal intercostals, **(c)** external intercostals, **(d)** abdominal wall muscles.
5. The arm muscle that both flexes the elbow and supinates the forearm is the **(a)** brachialis, **(b)** brachioradialis, **(c)** biceps brachii, **(d)** triceps brachii.
6. The chewing muscles that protrude the mandible and produce side-to-side grinding movements are the **(a)** buccinators, **(b)** masseters, **(c)** temporalis, **(d)** pterygoids.
7. Muscles that depress the hyoid bone and larynx include all but the **(a)** sternohyoid, **(b)** omohyoid, **(c)** geniohyoid, **(d)** sternothyroid.
8. Intrinsic muscles of the back that promote extension of the spine (or head) include all but **(a)** splenius muscles, **(b)** semispinalis muscles, **(c)** scalene muscles, **(d)** erector spinae.
9. Several muscles act to move and/or stabilize the scapula. Which of the following are small rectangular muscles that square the shoulders as they act together to retract the scapula? **(a)** levator scapulae, **(b)** rhomboids, **(c)** serratus anterior, **(d)** trapezius.
10. The quadriceps include all but **(a)** vastus lateralis, **(b)** vastus intermedius, **(c)** vastus medialis, **(d)** biceps femoris, **(e)** rectus femoris.
11. A prime mover of hip flexion is the **(a)** rectus femoris, **(b)** iliopsoas, **(c)** vastus muscles, **(d)** gluteus maximus.
12. The prime mover of hip extension *against* resistance is the **(a)** gluteus maximus, **(b)** gluteus medius, **(c)** biceps femoris, **(d)** semimembranosus.
13. Muscles that cause plantar flexion include all but the **(a)** gastrocnemius, **(b)** soleus, **(c)** tibialis anterior, **(d)** tibialis posterior, **(e)** fibularis muscles.
14. In walking, which two lower limb muscles keep the forward-swinging foot from dragging on the ground? **(a)** pronator teres and popliteus, **(b)** flexor digitorum longus and popliteus, **(c)** adductor longus and abductor digiti minimi in foot, **(d)** gluteus medius and tibialis anterior.
15. Which criterion (or criteria) is/are used in naming the gluteus medius? **(a)** relative size, **(b)** muscle location, **(c)** muscle shape, **(d)** action, **(e)** number of origins.
16. Which of the following is a large, deep muscle that protracts the scapula during punching? **(a)** serratus anterior, **(b)** rhomboids, **(c)** levator scapulae, **(d)** subscapularis.

10

Short Answer Essay Questions

17. Name four criteria used in naming muscles, and provide an example (other than those used in the text) that illustrates each criterion.
18. Differentiate between the arrangement of elements (load, fulcrum, and effort) in first-, second-, and third-class levers.
19. What does it mean when we say that a lever operates at a mechanical disadvantage, and what benefits does such a lever system provide?
20. Which muscles act to propel food down the length of the pharynx to the esophagus?
21. Name and describe the action of muscles used to shake your head no; to nod yes.
22. (a) Name the four muscle pairs that act in unison to compress the abdominal contents. (b) How does their arrangement (fiber direction) contribute to the strength of the abdominal wall? (c) Which of these muscles can effect lateral rotation of the spine? (d) Which can act alone to flex the spine?
23. List all six possible movements that can occur at the shoulder joint and name the prime mover(s) of each movement. Then name their antagonists.
24. (a) Name two forearm muscles that are powerful extensors and abductors of the wrist. (b) Name the sole forearm muscle that can flex the distal interphalangeal joints.
25. Name the muscles usually grouped together as the lateral rotators of the hip.
26. Name three thigh muscles that help you keep your seat astride a horse.
27. (a) Name three muscles or muscle groups used as sites for intramuscular injections. (b) Which of these is used most often in infants, and why?
28. Name two muscles in each of the following compartments or regions: (a) thenar eminence (ball of thumb), (b) posterior compartment of forearm, (c) anterior compartment of forearm—deep muscle group, (d) anterior muscle group in the arm,

(e) muscles of mastication, (f) third muscle layer of the foot, (g) posterior compartment of leg, (h) medial compartment of thigh, (i) posterior compartment of thigh.

Critical Thinking and Clinical Application Questions

1. Assume you have a 10-lb weight in your right hand. Explain why it is easier to flex the right elbow when your forearm is supinated than when it is pronated.
2. When Mrs. O'Brien returned to her doctor for a follow-up visit after childbirth, she complained that she was having problems controlling her urine flow (incontinent) when she sneezed. The physician asked his nurse to give Mrs. O'Brien instructions on how to perform exercises to strengthen the muscles of the pelvic floor. To which muscles was he referring?
3. Mr. Ahmadi, an out-of-shape 45-year-old man, was advised by his physician to lose weight and to exercise on a regular basis. He followed his diet faithfully and began to jog daily. One day, while on his morning jog, he heard a snapping sound that was immediately followed by a severe pain in his right lower calf. When his leg was examined, a gap was seen between his swollen upper calf region and his heel, and he was unable to plantar flex that ankle. What do you think happened? Why was the upper part of his calf swollen?
4. As Peter watched Sue walk down the runway at the fashion show, he contracted his right orbicularis oculi muscle, raised his arm, and contracted his opponens pollicis. Was he pleased or displeased with her performance? How do you know?
5. What type of lever system do the following activities describe? (a) The soleus muscle plantar flexes the foot. (b) The deltoid abducts the arm. (c) The triceps brachii is strained while doing pushups.

AT THE CLINIC

Related Clinical Terms

Charley horse A muscle contusion, i.e., tearing of muscle followed by bleeding into the tissues (hematoma) and severe, prolonged pain. A common contact sports injury; football players frequently suffer a charley horse of the quadriceps muscle of the thigh.

Electromyography Recording and interpretation of graphic records of the electrical activity of contracting muscles. Electrodes inserted into the muscles record the impulses that pass over muscle-cell membranes to stimulate contraction. The best and most important technique for determining the functions of muscles and muscle groups.

Hernia An abnormal protrusion of abdominal contents (typically coils of the small intestine) through a weak point in the muscles of the abdominal wall. Most often caused by increased intra-abdominal pressure during lifting or straining. The hernia penetrates the muscle wall but not the skin and so appears as a visible bulge in the body surface. Common abdominal hernias include the inguinal and umbilical hernias.

Quadriceps and hamstring strains Also called quad and hamstring pulls, these conditions involve tearing these muscles or their tendons; happen mainly in athletes who do not warm up properly and then fully extend their hip (quad pull) or knee (hamstring pull) quickly or forcefully (e.g., sprinters, tennis players). Not painful at first, but pain intensifies within three to six hours (30 minutes if the tearing is severe). After a week of rest, stretching is the best therapy.

Ruptured calcaneal tendon Although the calcaneal (Achilles) tendon is the largest, strongest tendon in the body, its rupture is surprisingly common, particularly in older people as a result of stumbling and in young sprinters when the tendon is traumatized during takeoff. The rupture is followed by abrupt pain; a gap is seen just above the heel, and the calf bulges as the triceps surae are released from their insertion. Plantar flexion is weak or impossible, but dorsiflexion is exaggerated. Usually repaired surgically.

Shin splints Common term for pain in the anterior compartment of the leg caused by irritation of the tibialis anterior muscle as might follow extreme or unusual exercise without adequate prior conditioning. Because it is tightly wrapped by fascia, the inflamed tibialis anterior cuts off its own circulation as it swells and presses painfully on its own nerves.

Tennis elbow Tenderness due to trauma or overuse of the tendon of origin of the forearm extensor muscles at the lateral epicondyle of the humerus. Caused and aggravated when these muscles contract forcefully to extend the hand at the wrist—as in executing a tennis backhand or lifting a loaded snow shovel. Despite its name, tennis elbow does not involve the elbow joint; most cases caused by work activities.

Torticollis (tor″tĭ-kol′is; *tort* = twisted) A twisting of the neck in which there is a chronic rotation and tilting of the head to one side, due to injury of the sternocleidomastoid muscle on one side; also called wryneck. Sometimes present at birth when the muscle fibers are torn during difficult delivery. Exercise that stretches the affected muscle is the usual treatment.

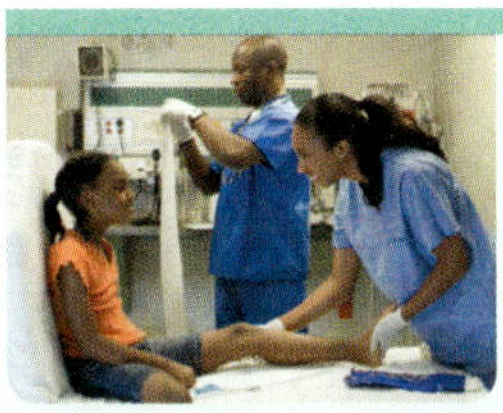

Case Study Muscular System

In Chapters 7 and 8, you were introduced to Kayla Tanner, a 45-year-old mother of four who had suffered a dislocated right hip in the bus accident on Route 91. Six weeks after the injury, Mrs. Tanner reported that she was still unable to walk or run without hip pain, and had weakness in her hip, knee, and ankle. Mrs. Tanner walked with a limp that her doctors attributed to weaknesses in flexion at the knee, inversion of the foot, and plantar flexion.

Electromyography (which measures muscle electrical activity) and nerve conduction studies (which measure the speed of nerve impulses) revealed that Mrs. Tanner's sciatic nerve had been damaged as a result of her injuries—most likely as a result of the nerve being compressed when the hip was dislocated. This large nerve innervates a large number of lower limb muscles. Since her surgery, Mrs. Tanner has been undergoing intense physical therapy and has shown significant improvement.

1. During her initial visit with the physical therapist, Mrs. Tanner presented with significant "foot drop" (the inability to dorsiflex the foot when taking a step). Mrs. Tanner was asked to perform a variety of movements with her right lower extremity. The therapist focused her attention on the *prime movers* and *synergists* of the hip, knee, and ankle. What are "prime movers" and "synergists"?
2. In order to assess the function and strength of a specific muscle, a physical therapist will often apply resistance (push against the moving limb) to mimic the action of an *antagonist muscle*. What is an antagonist muscle, and why would the therapist mimic its action?
3. Mrs. Tanner's physical therapist performed a variety of assessments in order to establish a baseline from which her recovery could be measured. For each of the descriptions below, name the muscle (or muscles) that the therapist was assessing.
   - **a.** With Mrs. Tanner in the seated position, the therapist positioned Mrs. Tanner's legs shoulder-width apart, then asked Mrs. Tanner to bring her feet together while the therapist applied resistance to the right leg.
   - **b.** The therapist applied resistance to the top of Mrs. Tanner's foot and asked her to pull her forefoot up toward her shin.
   - **c.** With Mrs. Tanner in the prone position (on her stomach), the therapist applied resistance to the leg while Mrs. Tanner was instructed to bring her heel up toward her buttocks (flex her knee).
4. Using descriptions similar to those listed in the question above, explain how you would assess the function of the following muscles.
   - **a.** Extensor hallucis longus
   - **b.** Fibularis (peroneus) longus
   - **c.** Gastrocnemius

(Answers in Appendix H)

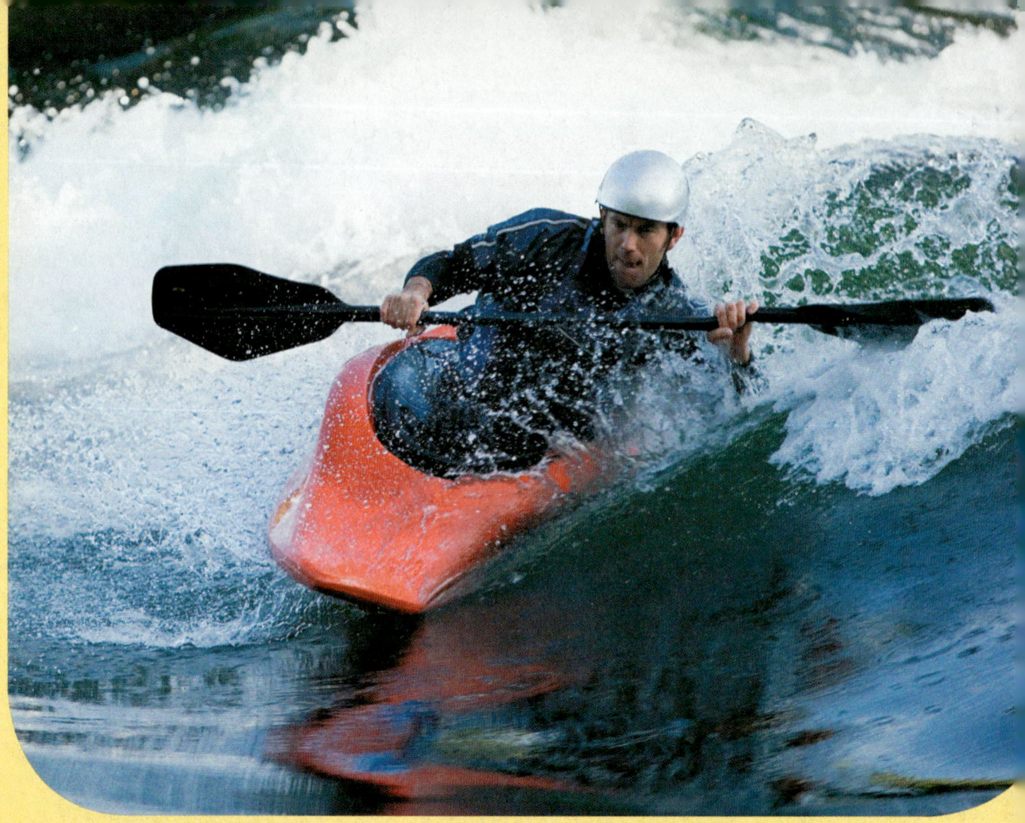

11

Fundamentals of the Nervous System and Nervous Tissue

You are driving down the freeway, and a horn blares to your right. You immediately swerve to your left. Charlie leaves a note on the kitchen table: "See you later. Have the stuff ready at 6." You know the "stuff" is chili with taco chips. You are dozing but you awaken instantly when your infant son cries softly.

What do these three events have in common? They are all everyday examples of the functioning of your nervous system, which has your body cells humming with activity nearly all the time.

The **nervous system** is the master controlling and communicating system of the body. Every thought, action, and emotion reflects its activity. Its cells communicate by electrical and chemical signals, which are rapid and specific, and usually cause almost immediate responses.

We begin this chapter with a brief overview of the functions and organization of the nervous system. Then we focus on the functional anatomy of nervous tissue, especially the nerve cells, or *neurons*, which are the key to neural communication.

Functions and Divisions of the Nervous System

✓ List the basic functions of the nervous system.

✓ Explain the structural and functional divisions of the nervous system.

The nervous system has three overlapping functions, illustrated by the example of a thirsty person seeing and then lifting a glass of water **(Figure 11.1)**:

1. **Sensory input.** The nervous system uses its millions of sensory receptors to monitor changes occurring both inside and outside the body. The gathered information is called **sensory input**.
2. **Integration.** The nervous system processes and interprets sensory input and decides what should be done at each moment—a process called **integration**.
3. **Motor output.** The nervous system activates *effector organs*—the muscles and glands—to cause a *response*, called **motor output.**

Here's another example: You are driving and see a red light ahead (sensory input). Your nervous system integrates this information (red light means "stop"), and your foot goes for the brake (motor output).

We have only one highly integrated nervous system. For convenience, it is divided into two principal parts, *central* and *peripheral.*

The **central nervous system (CNS)** consists of the *brain* and *spinal cord*, which occupy the dorsal body cavity. The CNS is the integrating and control center of the nervous system. It interprets sensory input and dictates motor output based on reflexes, current conditions, and past experience **(Figure 11.2)**.

The **peripheral nervous system (PNS)** is the part of the nervous system *outside* the CNS. The PNS consists mainly of the nerves (bundles of axons) that extend from the brain and spinal cord. *Spinal nerves* carry impulses to and from the spinal cord, and *cranial nerves* carry impulses to and from the brain. These peripheral nerves serve as communication lines that link all parts of the body to the CNS.

The PNS has two functional subdivisions, as Figure 11.2 shows. The **sensory**, or **afferent**, **division** (af′er-ent; "carrying toward") consists of nerve fibers (axons) that convey impulses *to* the central nervous system from sensory receptors located throughout the body (see the blue fibers in Figure 11.2).

- *Somatic sensory fibers* convey impulses from the skin, skeletal muscles, and joints (*soma* = body)
- *Visceral sensory fibers* transmit impulses from the visceral organs (organs within the ventral body cavity)

The sensory division keeps the CNS constantly informed of events going on both inside and outside the body.

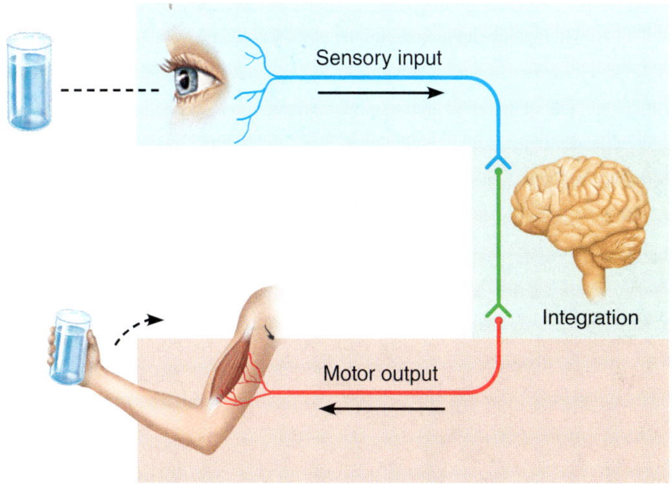

Figure 11.1 The nervous system's functions.

The **motor**, or **efferent**, **division** (ef′er-ent; "carrying away") of the PNS transmits impulses *from* the CNS to effector organs, which are the muscles and glands (see the red fibers in Figure 11.2). These impulses activate muscles to contract and glands to secrete. In other words, they *effect* (bring about) a motor response.

The motor division also has two main parts:

- The **somatic nervous system** is composed of somatic motor nerve fibers that conduct impulses from the CNS to skeletal muscles. It is often referred to as the **voluntary nervous system** because it allows us to consciously control our skeletal muscles.
- The **autonomic nervous system (ANS)** consists of visceral motor nerve fibers that regulate the activity of smooth muscles, cardiac muscles, and glands. *Autonomic* means "a law unto itself," and because we generally cannot control such activities as the pumping of our heart or the movement of food through our digestive tract, the ANS is also called the **involuntary nervous system**.

As we will describe in Chapter 14, the ANS has two functional subdivisions, the **sympathetic division** and the **parasympathetic division**. Typically these divisions work in opposition to each other—whatever one stimulates, the other inhibits.

☑ Check Your Understanding

1. What is meant by "integration," and does it primarily occur in the CNS or the PNS?
2. Which subdivision of the PNS is involved in (a) relaying the feeling of a "full stomach" after a meal, (b) contracting the muscles to lift your arm, and (c) increasing your heart rate?

For answers, see Appendix H.

Histology of Nervous Tissue

The nervous system consists mostly of nervous tissue, which is highly cellular. For example, less than 20% of the CNS is extracellular space, which means that the cells are densely packed

11

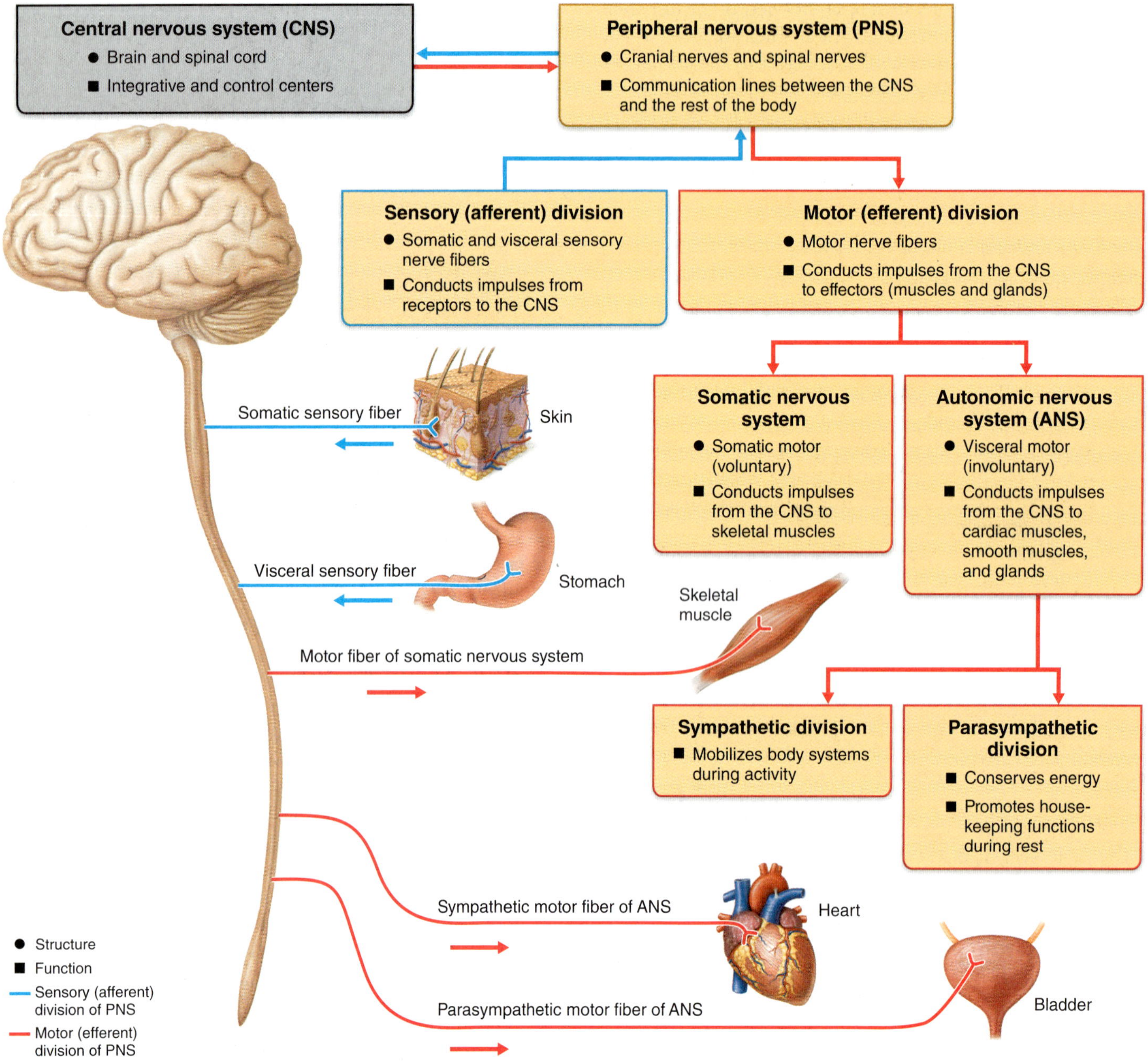

Figure 11.2 Levels of organization in the nervous system. The human nervous system is organized into two major divisions, the central nervous system (CNS) and peripheral nervous system (PNS). Visceral organs (primarily located in the ventral body cavity) are served by visceral sensory fibers and by motor fibers of the autonomic nervous system. The somata (limbs and body wall) are served by motor fibers of the somatic nervous system and by somatic sensory fibers. Arrows indicate the direction of nerve impulses. (Connections to spinal cord are not anatomically accurate.)

and tightly intertwined. Although it is very complex, nervous tissue is made up of just two principal types of cells:

- Supporting cells called *neuroglia*, small cells that surround and wrap the more delicate neurons
- *Neurons*, nerve cells that are excitable (responsive to stimuli) and transmit electrical signals

See Figure 4.10 on p. 140 to refresh your memory.

Neuroglia

✓ List the types of neuroglia and cite their functions.

Neurons associate closely with much smaller cells called **neuroglia** (nu-rog′le-ah; "nerve glue") or **glial cells** (gle′al). There are six types of neuroglia—four in the CNS and two in the PNS **(Figure 11.3)**. Once considered merely the "glue" or scaffolding that supports the neurons, neuroglia are now known to have many other important and unique functions.

Neuroglia in the CNS

Neuroglia in the CNS include *astrocytes*, *microglial cells*, *ependymal cells*, and *oligodendrocytes* (Figure 11.3a–d). Like neurons, most neuroglia have branching processes (extensions) and a central cell body. They can be distinguished, however, by their much smaller size and their darker-staining nuclei. They outnumber neurons in the CNS by about 10 to 1, and make up about half the mass of the brain.

Astrocytes Shaped like delicate branching sea anemones, **astrocytes** (as′tro-sītz; "star cells") are the most abundant and versatile glial cells. Their numerous radiating processes cling to neurons and their synaptic endings, and cover nearby capillaries. They support and brace the neurons and anchor them to their nutrient supply lines (Figure 11.3a).

Astrocytes play a role in making exchanges between capillaries and neurons, helping determine capillary permeability. They guide the migration of young neurons, and formation of synapses (junctions) between neurons. Astrocytes also control the chemical environment around neurons, where their most important job is "mopping up" leaked potassium ions and recapturing and recycling released neurotransmitters. Furthermore, astrocytes have been shown to respond to nearby nerve impulses and released neurotransmitters.

Connected by gap junctions, astrocytes signal each other both by taking in calcium, creating slow-paced intracellular calcium pulses (calcium waves), and by releasing extracellular chemical messengers. Recent research shows they also influence neuronal functioning and therefore participate in information processing in the brain.

Microglial Cells **Microglial cells** (mi-kro′gle-al) are small and ovoid with relatively long "thorny" processes (Figure 11.3b). Their processes touch nearby neurons, monitoring their health, and when they sense that certain neurons are injured or in other trouble, the microglial cells migrate toward them. Where invading microorganisms or dead neurons are present, the microglial cells transform into a special type of macrophage that phagocytizes the microorganisms or neuronal debris. This protective role of the microglial cells is important because cells of the immune system have limited access to the CNS.

Ependymal Cells **Ependymal cells** (ĕ-pen′dĭ-mul; "wrapping garment") range in shape from squamous to columnar, and many are ciliated (Figure 11.3c). They line the central cavities of the brain and the spinal cord, where they form a fairly permeable barrier between the cerebrospinal fluid that fills those cavities and the tissue fluid bathing the cells of the CNS. The beating of their cilia helps to circulate the cerebrospinal fluid that cushions the brain and spinal cord.

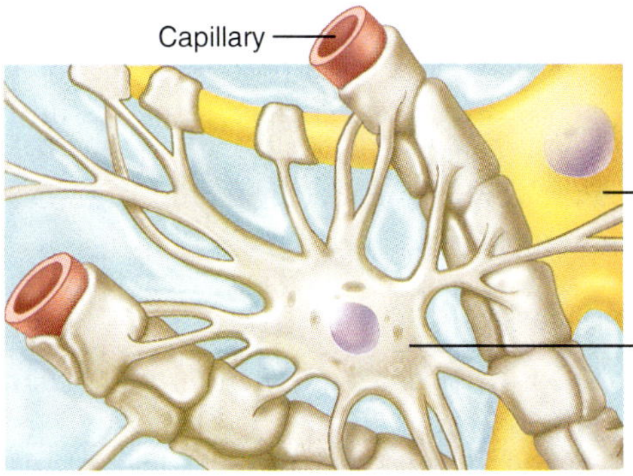

(a) Astrocytes are the most abundant CNS neuroglia.

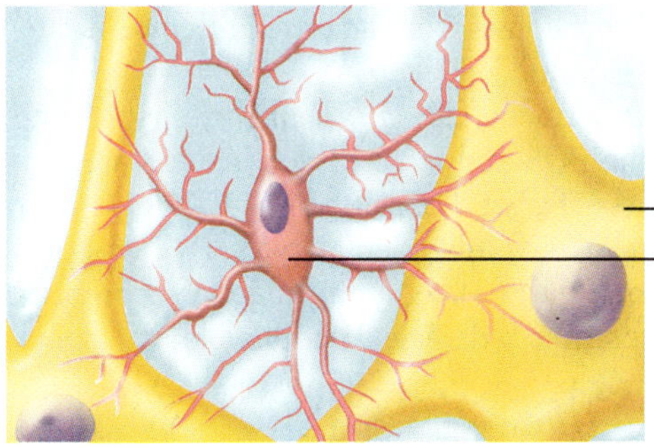

(b) Microglial cells are defensive cells in the CNS.

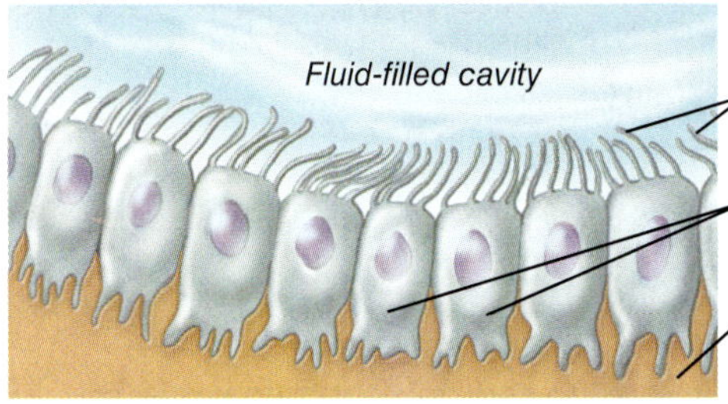

(c) Ependymal cells line cerebrospinal fluid–filled cavities.

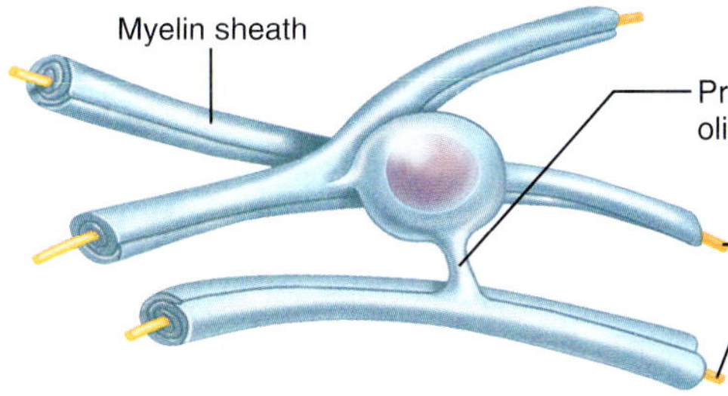

(d) Oligodendrocytes have processes that form myelin sheaths around CNS nerve fibers.

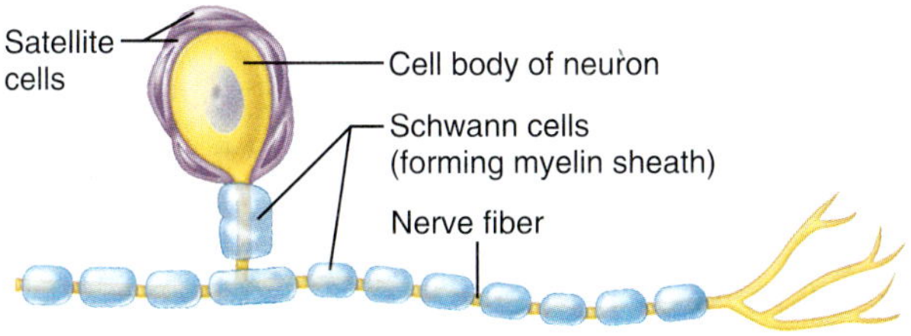

(e) Satellite cells and Schwann cells (which form myelin) surround neurons in the PNS.

Figure 11.3 Neuroglia. (a–d) The four types of neuroglia of the CNS. **(e)** Neuroglia of the PNS.

Oligodendrocytes Though they also branch, the **oligodendrocytes** (ol″ĭ-go-den′dro-sīts) have fewer processes (*oligo* = few; *dendr* = branch) than astrocytes. Oligodendrocytes line up along the thicker nerve fibers in the CNS and wrap their processes tightly around the fibers, producing an insulating covering called a *myelin sheath* (Figure 11.3d).

Neuroglia in the PNS

The two kinds of PNS neuroglia—*satellite cells* and *Schwann cells*—differ mainly in location.

Satellite cells surround neuron cell bodies located in the peripheral nervous system (Figure 11.3e), and are thought to have many of the same functions in the PNS as astrocytes do in the CNS. Their name comes from a fancied resemblance to the moons (satellites) around a planet.

Schwann cells (also called *neurolemmocytes*) surround all nerve fibers in the PNS and form myelin sheaths around the thicker nerve fibers (Figure 11.3e and 11.4a). In this way, they are functionally similar to oligodendrocytes. (We describe the formation of myelin sheaths later in this chapter.) Schwann cells are vital to regeneration of damaged peripheral nerve fibers.

☑ Check Your Understanding

3. Which type of neuroglia controls the extracellular fluid environment around neuron cell bodies in the CNS? In the PNS?
4. Which two types of neuroglia form insulating coverings called myelin sheaths?

For answers, see Appendix H.

11

Neurons

✓ Define neuron, describe its important structural components, and relate each to a functional role.

✓ Differentiate between (1) a nerve and a tract, and (2) a nucleus and a ganglion.

✓ Explain the importance of the myelin sheath and describe how it is formed in the central and peripheral nervous systems.

The billions of **neurons**, also called *nerve cells*, are the structural units of the nervous system. They are typically large, highly specialized cells that conduct messages in the form of nerve impulses from one part of the body to another. Besides their ability to conduct nerve impulses, they have three other special characteristics:

- Neurons have *extreme longevity*. Given good nutrition, they can function optimally for a lifetime (over 100 years).
- Neurons are *amitotic*. As neurons assume their roles as communicating links of the nervous system, they lose their ability to divide. We pay a high price for this feature because neurons cannot be replaced if destroyed. There *are* exceptions to this rule. For example, olfactory epithelium and some hippocampal regions contain stem cells that can produce new neurons throughout life. (The hippocampus is a brain region involved in memory.)
- Neurons have an exceptionally *high metabolic rate* and require continuous and abundant supplies of oxygen and glucose. They cannot survive for more than a few minutes without oxygen.

Although neurons vary in structure, they all have a *cell body* and one or more slender *processes* (**Figure 11.4**).

Neuron Cell Body

The **neuron cell body** consists of a spherical nucleus with a conspicuous nucleolus surrounded by cytoplasm. Also called the **perikaryon** (*peri* = around, *kary* = nucleus) or **soma**, the cell body ranges in diameter from 5 to 140 μm. The cell body is the major *biosynthetic center* of a neuron and so it contains the usual organelles needed to synthesize proteins and other chemicals.

The neuron cell body's protein- and membrane-making machinery, consisting of clustered free ribosomes and rough endoplasmic reticulum (ER), is probably the most active and best developed in the body. This rough ER, also called the **chromatophilic substance** (*chromatophilic* = color loving) or *Nissl bodies* (nis′l), stains darkly with basic dyes. The Golgi apparatus is also well developed and forms an arc or a complete circle around the nucleus.

Mitochondria are scattered among the other organelles. Microtubules and **neurofibrils**, which are bundles of intermediate filaments (*neurofilaments*), are important in maintaining cell shape and integrity. They form a network throughout the cell body.

The cell body of some neurons also contains pigment inclusions. For example, some contain a black melanin, a red iron-containing pigment, or a golden-brown pigment called *lipofuscin* (lip″o-fu′sin). Lipofuscin, a harmless by-product of lysosomal activity, is sometimes called the "aging pigment" because it accumulates in neurons of elderly individuals.

The cell body is the focal point for the outgrowth of neuron processes during embryonic development. In most neurons, the plasma membrane of the cell body also acts as *part of the receptive region* that receives information from other neurons.

Most neuron cell bodies are located in the CNS, where they are protected by the bones of the skull and vertebral column. Clusters of cell bodies in the CNS are called **nuclei**, whereas those that lie along the nerves in the PNS are called **ganglia** (gang′gle-ah; *ganglion* = "knot on a string," "swelling").

Neuron Processes

Armlike **processes** extend from the cell body of all neurons. The brain and spinal cord (CNS) contain both neuron cell bodies and their processes. The PNS consists chiefly of neuron processes. Bundles of neuron processes are called **tracts** in the CNS and **nerves** in the PNS.

The two types of neuron processes, *dendrites* and *axons* (ak′sonz), differ in the structure and function of their plasma membranes. The convention is to describe these processes using a motor neuron as an example. We shall follow this practice, but keep in mind that many sensory neurons and some tiny CNS neurons differ from the "typical" pattern we present here.

Dendrites **Dendrites** of motor neurons are short, tapering, diffusely branching extensions. Typically, motor neurons have hundreds of twiglike dendrites clustering close to the cell body. Virtually all organelles present in the cell body also occur in dendrites.

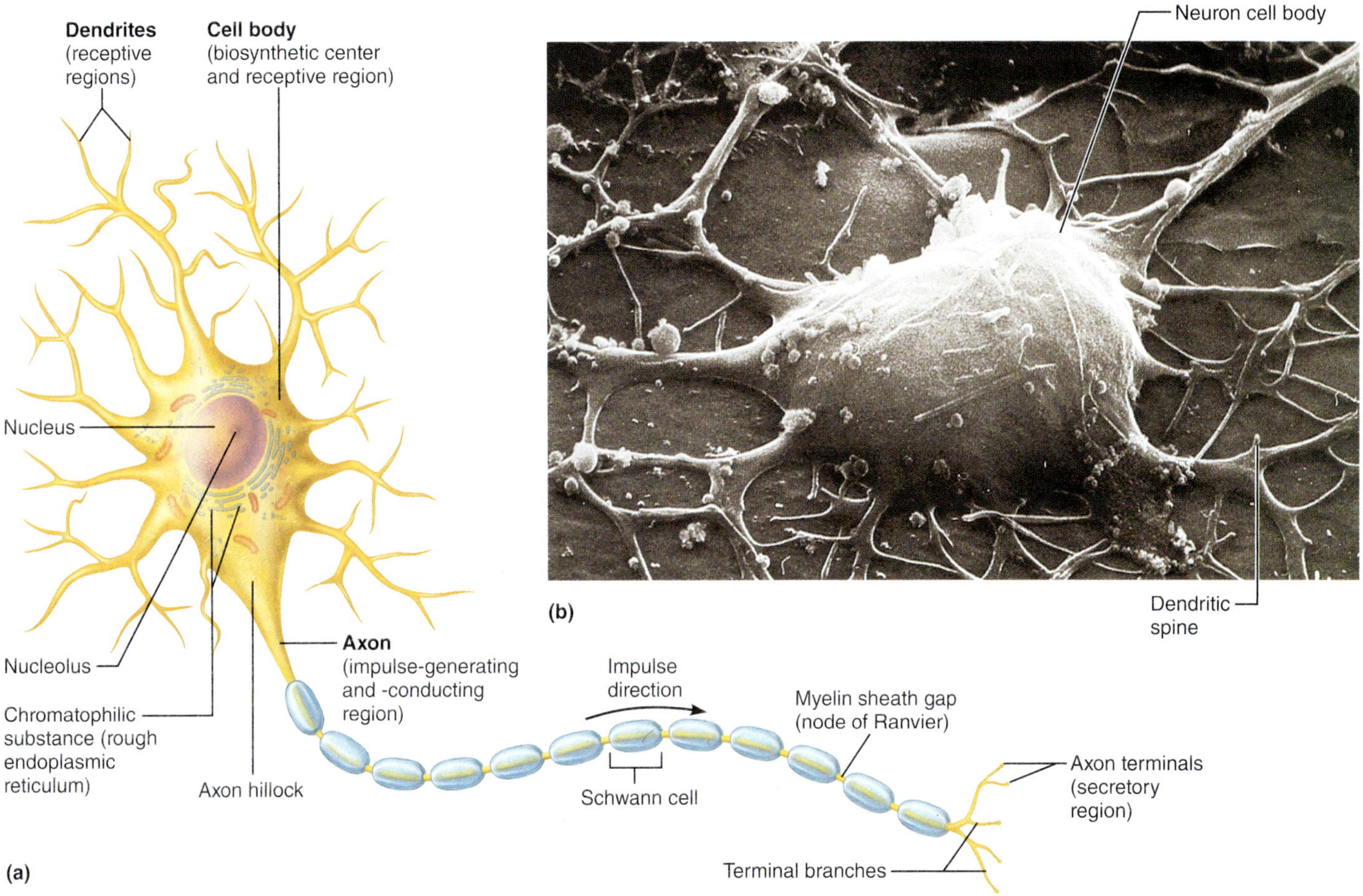

Figure 11.4 Structure of a motor neuron. (a) Diagrammatic view. **(b)** Scanning electron micrograph showing the cell body and dendrites with obvious dendritic spines (2000×).

Dendrites, the main **receptive** or **input regions**, provide an enormous surface area for receiving signals from other neurons. In many brain areas, the finer dendrites are highly specialized for collecting information. They bristle with *dendritic spines*—thorny appendages having bulbous or spiky ends—which represent points of close contact (synapses) with other neurons (Figure 11.4b).

Dendrites convey incoming messages *toward* the cell body. These electrical signals are usually *not* action potentials (nerve impulses) but are short-distance signals called *graded potentials*, as we will describe shortly.

The Axon: Structure Each neuron has a single **axon** (*axo* = axis, axle). The initial region of the axon arises from a cone-shaped area of the cell body called the **axon hillock** ("little hill") and then narrows to form a slender process that is uniform in diameter for the rest of its length (Figure 11.4a). In some neurons, the axon is very short or absent, but in others it accounts for nearly the entire length of the neuron. For example, axons of the motor neurons controlling the skeletal muscles of your great toe extend a meter or more (3–4 feet) from the lumbar region of your spine to your foot, making them among the longest cells in the body. Any long axon is called a **nerve fiber**.

Each neuron has only one axon, but axons may have occasional branches along their length. These branches, called **axon collaterals**, extend from the axon at more or less right angles. Whether an axon is undivided or has collaterals, it usually branches profusely at its end (terminus): 10,000 or more **terminal branches** (also called *terminal arborizations*) per neuron is not unusual. The knoblike distal endings of the terminal branches are called **axon terminals** or **terminal boutons** (boo-tonz′; "buttons"). Take your pick!

The Axon: Functional Characteristics Functionally, the axon is the **conducting region** of the neuron (Figure 11.4). It *generates nerve impulses* and *transmits them*, typically away from the cell body, along the plasma membrane, or **axolemma** (ak″so-lem′ah). In motor neurons, the nerve impulse is generated at the junction of the axon hillock and axon (which for this reason is called the *trigger zone*) and conducted along the axon to the axon terminals, which are the **secretory region** of the neuron.

When the impulse reaches the axon terminals, it causes *neurotransmitters*—signaling chemicals usually stored in vesicles—to be released into the extracellular space. The neurotransmitters either excite or inhibit neurons (or effector cells) with which the axon is in close contact. Because each neuron both receives signals from and sends signals to scores of other neurons, it carries on "conversations" with many different neurons at the same time.

An axon contains the same organelles found in the dendrites and cell body with two important exceptions—it lacks rough

11

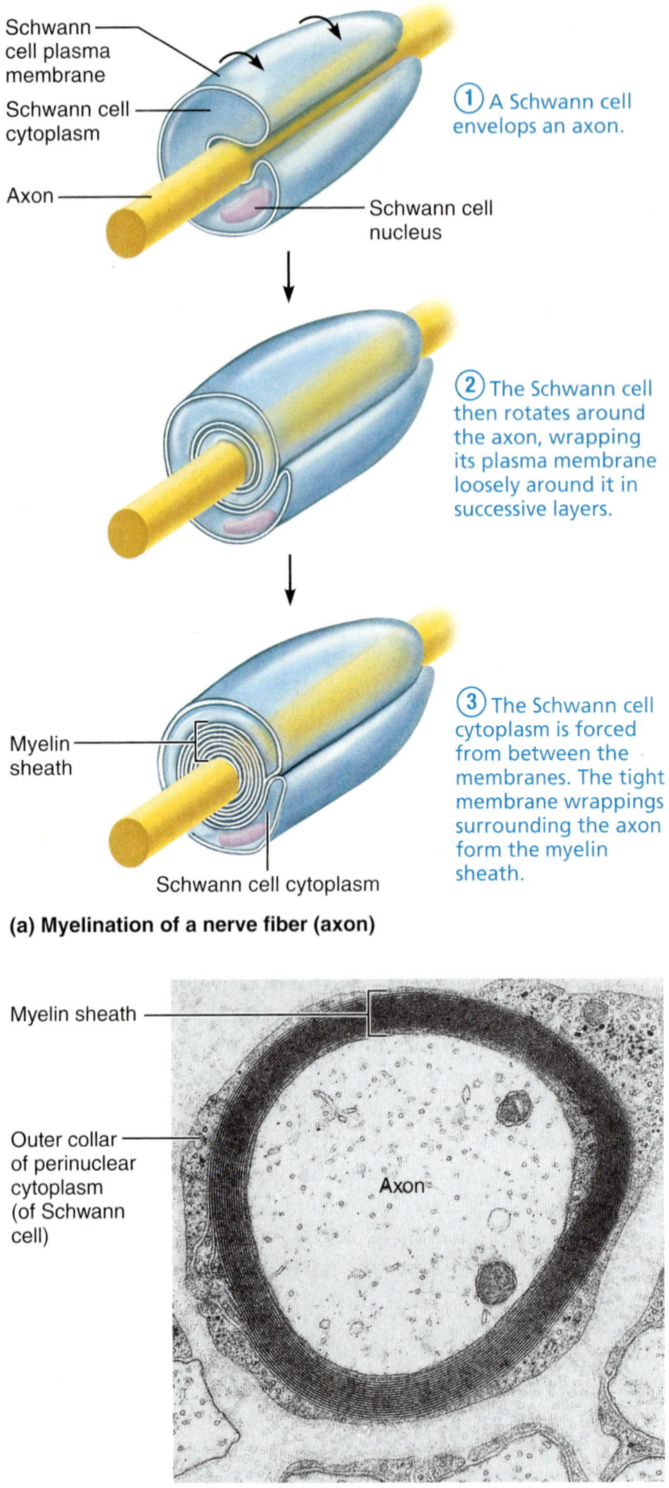

(a) Myelination of a nerve fiber (axon)

(b) Cross-sectional view of a myelinated axon (electron micrograph 24,000×)

Figure 11.5 Nerve fiber myelination by Schwann cells in the PNS.

endoplasmic reticulum and a Golgi apparatus, the structures involved with protein synthesis and packaging. Consequently, an axon depends (1) on its cell body to renew the necessary proteins and membrane components, and (2) on efficient transport mechanisms to distribute them. Axons quickly decay if cut or severely damaged.

Transport Along the Axon Because axons are often very long, the task of moving molecules along their length might appear difficult. However, through the cooperative efforts of motor proteins and cytoskeletal elements (microtubules and actin filaments), substances travel continuously along the axon both away from and toward the cell body. Movement away from the cell body is *anterograde movement*, and that in the opposite direction is *retrograde movement*.

Substances moved in the anterograde direction include mitochondria, cytoskeletal elements, membrane components used to renew the axon plasma membrane, and enzymes needed to synthesize certain neurotransmitters. (Some neurotransmitters are synthesized in the cell body and then transported to the axon terminals.)

Substances transported through the axon in the retrograde direction are mostly organelles returning to the cell body to be degraded or recycled. Retrograde transport is also an important means of intracellular communication to "advise" the cell body of conditions at the axon terminals, and deliver to the cell body vesicles containing signal molecules (like nerve growth factor, which activates certain nuclear genes promoting growth).

One basic bidirectional transport mechanism appears to be responsible for axonal transport. It uses ATP-dependent "motor" proteins (kinesin and dynein), depending on the direction of transport. These proteins propel cellular components along the microtubules like trains along tracks at speeds up to 40 cm (15 inches) per day.

Homeostatic Imbalance 11.1

Certain viruses and bacterial toxins that damage neural tissues use retrograde axonal transport to reach the cell body. This transport mechanism has been demonstrated for polio, rabies, and herpes simplex viruses and for tetanus toxin. Researchers are investigating using retrograde transport to treat genetic diseases by introducing viruses containing "corrected" genes or microRNA to suppress defective genes. +

Myelin Sheath Many nerve fibers, particularly those that are long or large in diameter, are covered with a whitish, fatty (protein-lipoid), segmented **myelin sheath** (mi′ĕ-lin). Myelin protects and electrically insulates fibers, and it increases the transmission speed of nerve impulses. **Myelinated fibers** (axons bearing a myelin sheath) conduct nerve impulses rapidly, whereas **nonmyelinated fibers** conduct impulses more slowly. Note that myelin sheaths are associated only with axons. Dendrites are *always* nonmyelinated.

Myelination in the PNS Myelin sheaths in the PNS are formed by Schwann cells, which indent to receive an axon and then wrap themselves around it in a jelly roll fashion (Figure 11.5). Initially the wrapping is loose, but the Schwann cell cytoplasm is gradually squeezed from between the membrane layers.

When the wrapping process is complete, many concentric layers of Schwann cell plasma membrane enclose the axon, much like gauze wrapped around an injured finger. This tight coil of wrapped membranes is the myelin sheath, and its thickness depends on the number of spirals. The nucleus and most of the cytoplasm of the Schwann cell end up as a bulge just external to the myelin sheath. This portion of the Schwann cell, next to the exposed part of its plasma membrane, is called the *outer collar of perinuclear cytoplasm* (formerly known as the *neurilemma*) (Figure 11.5b).

Plasma membranes of myelinating cells contain much less protein than the plasma membranes of most body cells. Channel and carrier proteins are notably absent, a characteristic that makes myelin sheaths exceptionally good electrical insulators. Another unique characteristic of these membranes is the presence of specific protein molecules that interlock to form a sort of molecular Velcro between adjacent myelin membranes.

Adjacent Schwann cells along an axon do not touch one another, so there are gaps in the sheath. These **myelin sheath gaps**, or **nodes of Ranvier** (ran′vē-ā″), occur at regular intervals (about 1 mm apart) along a myelinated axon. Axon collaterals can emerge from the axon at these gaps.

Sometimes Schwann cells surround peripheral nerve fibers but the coiling process does not occur. In such instances, a single Schwann cell can partially enclose 15 or more axons, each of which occupies a separate recess in the Schwann cell surface. Nerve fibers associated with Schwann cells in this manner are said to be *nonmyelinated* and are typically thin fibers.

Myelination in the CNS The central nervous system contains both myelinated and nonmyelinated axons. However, in the CNS, it is the oligodendrocytes that form myelin sheaths (Figure 11.3d).

Unlike a Schwann cell, which forms only one segment of a myelin sheath, an oligodendrocyte has multiple flat processes that can coil around as many as 60 axons at the same time. As in the PNS, myelin sheath gaps separate adjacent sections of an axon's myelin sheath. However, CNS myelin sheaths lack an outer collar of perinuclear cytoplasm because cell extensions do the coiling and the squeezed-out cytoplasm is forced back toward the centrally located nucleus instead of peripherally.

As in the PNS, the smallest-diameter axons are nonmyelinated. These nonmyelinated axons are covered by the long extensions of adjacent glial cells.

Regions of the brain and spinal cord containing dense collections of myelinated fibers are referred to as **white matter** and are primarily fiber tracts. **Gray matter** contains mostly nerve cell bodies and nonmyelinated fibers.

☑ Check Your Understanding

5. Which part of the neuron is its fiber? How do nerve fibers differ from the fibers of connective tissue (see Chapter 4) and the fibers in muscle (see Chapter 9)?
6. How does a nucleus within the brain differ from a nucleus within a neuron?
7. How is a myelin sheath formed in the CNS, and what is its function?

For answers, see Appendix H.

Classification of Neurons

✓ Classify neurons by structure and by function.

Neurons are classified both structurally and functionally. We describe both classifications here but use the functional classification in most discussions.

Structural Classification Neurons are grouped structurally according to the number of processes extending from their cell body. Three major neuron groups make up this classification: multipolar (*polar* = end, pole), bipolar, and unipolar neurons. (Table 11.1 is organized according to these three neuron types, and the top row shows their structures.)

Multipolar neurons have three or more processes—one axon and the rest dendrites. They are the most common neuron type in humans, with more than 99% of neurons belonging to this class. Multipolar neurons are the major neuron type in the CNS.

Bipolar neurons have two processes—an axon and a dendrite—that extend from opposite sides of the cell body. These rare neurons are found in some of the special sense organs. Examples include some neurons in the retina of the eye and in the olfactory mucosa.

Unipolar neurons have a single short process that emerges from the cell body and divides T-like into proximal and distal branches. The more distal process, the **peripheral process**, is often associated with a sensory receptor. The **central process** enters the CNS (Table 11.1). Unipolar neurons are more accurately called **pseudounipolar neurons** (*pseudo* = false) because they originate as bipolar neurons. Then, during early embryonic development, the two processes converge and partially fuse to form the short single process that issues from the cell body. Unipolar neurons are found chiefly in ganglia in the PNS, where they function as sensory neurons.

The fact that the fused peripheral and central processes of unipolar neurons are continuous and function as a single fiber might make you wonder whether they are axons or dendrites. The central process is definitely an axon because it conducts impulses away from the cell body (one definition of axon). However, the peripheral process is perplexing. Three facts favor classifying it as an axon: (1) It generates and conducts an impulse (functional definition of axon); (2) when large, it is heavily myelinated; and (3) it has a uniform diameter and is indistinguishable microscopically from an axon. However, the older definition of a dendrite as a process that transmits impulses *toward* the cell body interferes with that conclusion.

So which is it? In this book, we have chosen to emphasize the newer definition of an axon as generating and transmitting an impulse. For *unipolar neurons*, we will refer to the combined length of the peripheral and central process as an axon. In place of "dendrites," unipolar neurons have *receptive endings* (sensory terminals) at the end of the peripheral process.

Functional Classification This scheme groups neurons according to the direction in which the nerve impulse travels relative to the central nervous system. Based on this criterion, there are sensory neurons, motor neurons, and interneurons (Table 11.1, last row).

Table 11.1 Comparison of Structural Classes of Neurons

NEURON TYPE		
MULTIPOLAR	**BIPOLAR**	**UNIPOLAR (PSEUDOUNIPOLAR)**
Structural Class: Neuron Type According to the Number of Processes Extending from the Cell Body		
Many processes extend from the cell body. All are dendrites except for a single axon.	Two processes extend from the cell body. One is a fused dendrite, the other is an axon.	One process extends from the cell body and forms central and peripheral processes, which together comprise an axon.
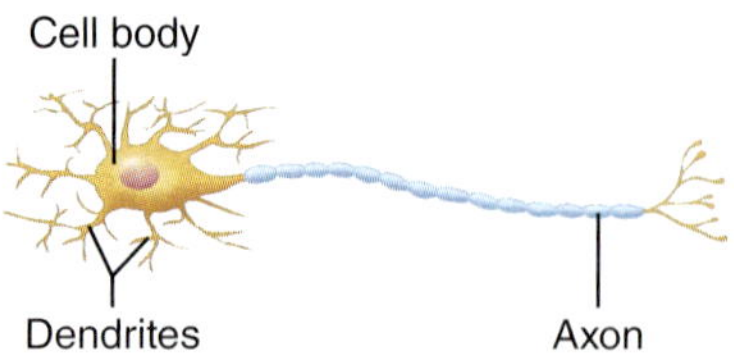	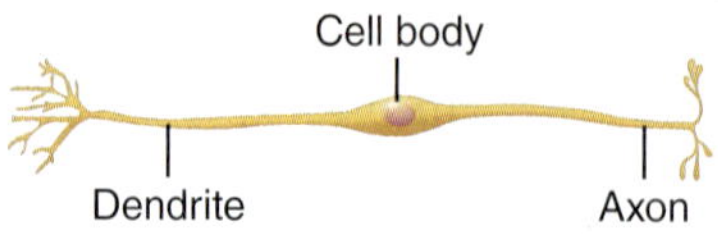	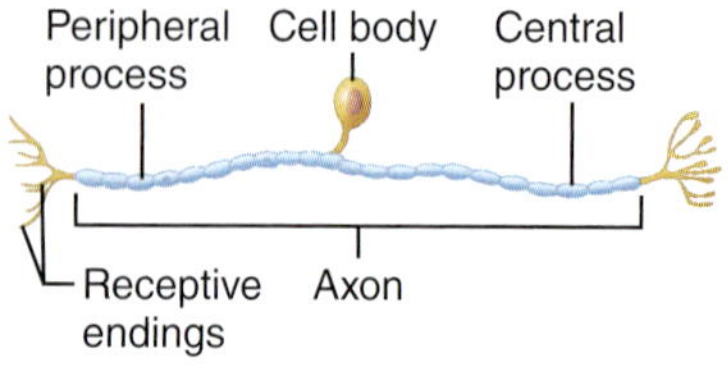
Relationship of Anatomy to the Three Functional Regions		
Receptive region (receives stimulus). Conducting region (generates/transmits action potential). Secretory region (axon terminals release neurotransmitters). 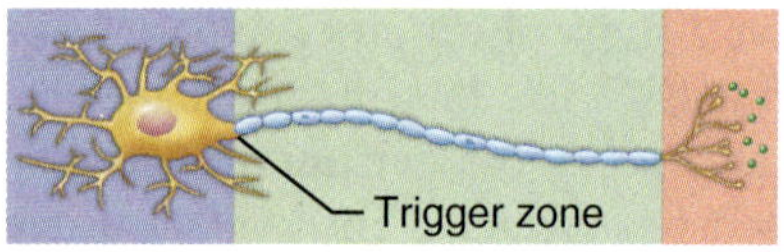	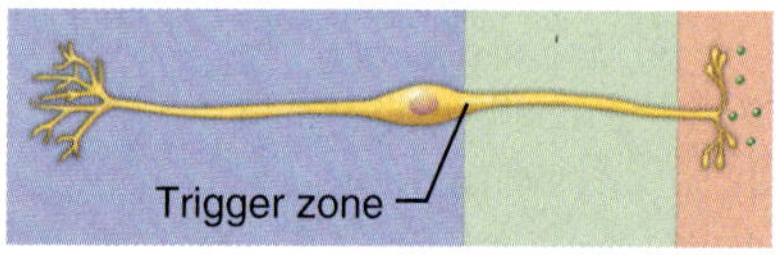 (Many bipolar neurons do not generate action potentials. In those that do, the location of the trigger zone is not universal.)	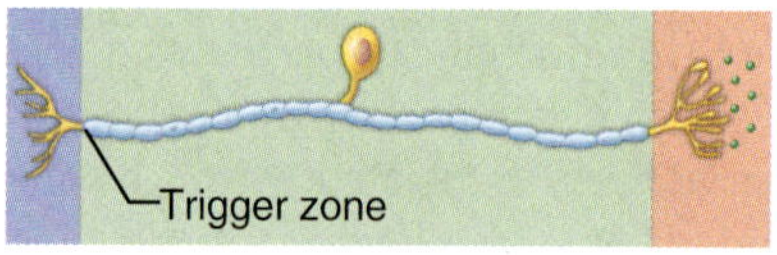
Relative Abundance and Location in Human Body		
Most abundant in body. Major neuron type in the CNS.	Rare. Found in some special sensory organs (olfactory mucosa, eye, ear).	Found mainly in the PNS. Common only in dorsal root ganglia of the spinal cord and sensory ganglia of cranial nerves.
Structural Variations		
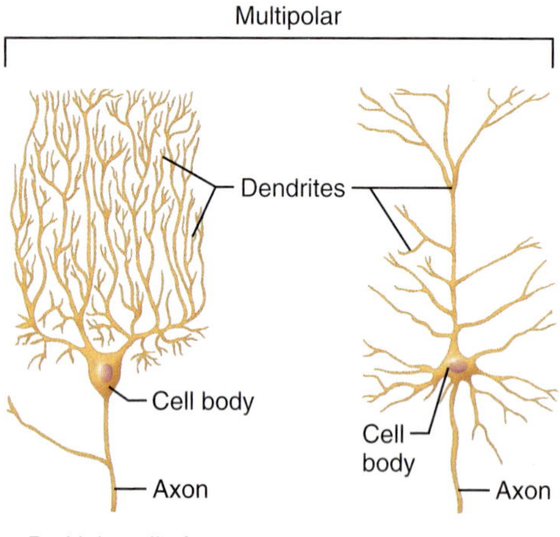 Purkinje cell of cerebellum Pyramidal cell	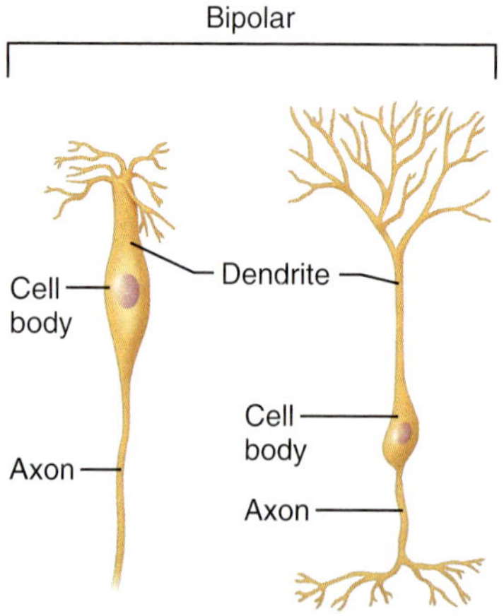 Olfactory cell Retinal cell	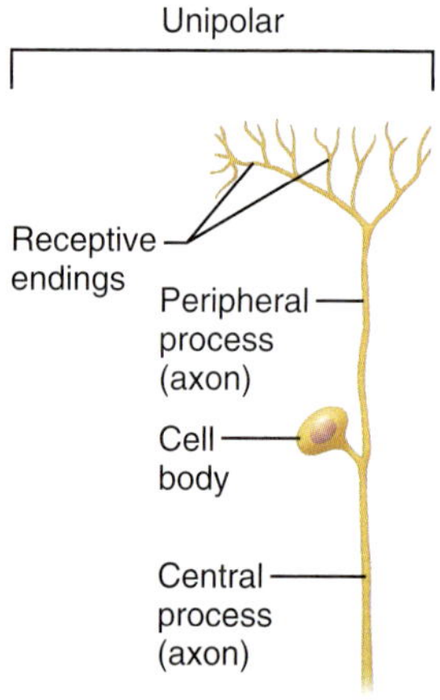 Dorsal root ganglion cell

Table 11.1 *(continued)*

	NEURON TYPE	
MULTIPOLAR	**BIPOLAR**	**UNIPOLAR (PSEUDOUNIPOLAR)**
Functional Class: Neuron Type According to Direction of Impulse Conduction		
1. Most multipolar neurons are **interneurons** that conduct impulses within the CNS, integrating sensory input or motor output. May be one of a chain of CNS neurons, or a single neuron connecting sensory and motor neurons. 2. Some multipolar neurons are **motor neurons** that conduct impulses along the efferent pathways from the CNS to an effector (muscle/gland).	Essentially all bipolar neurons are **sensory neurons** that are located in some special sense organs. For example, bipolar cells of the retina are involved with transmitting visual inputs from the eye to the brain (via an intermediate chain of neurons).	Most unipolar neurons are **sensory neurons** that conduct impulses along afferent pathways to the CNS for interpretation. (These sensory neurons are called primary or first-order sensory neurons.)

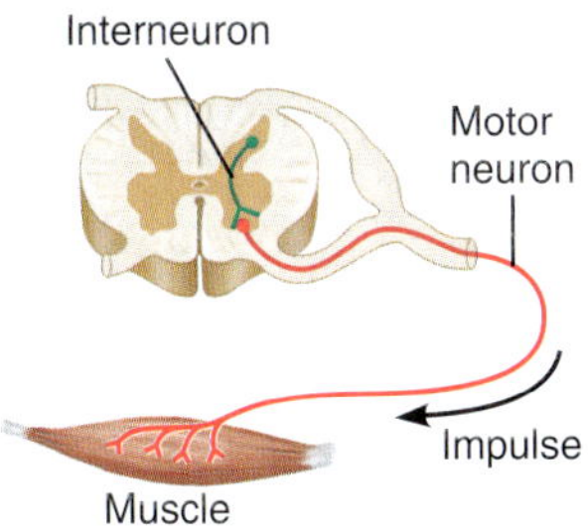

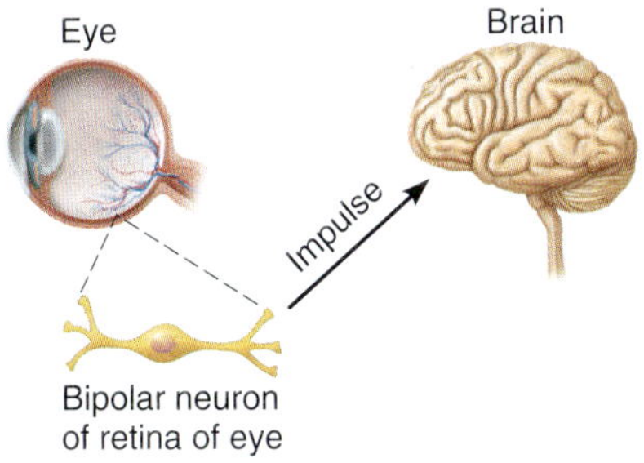

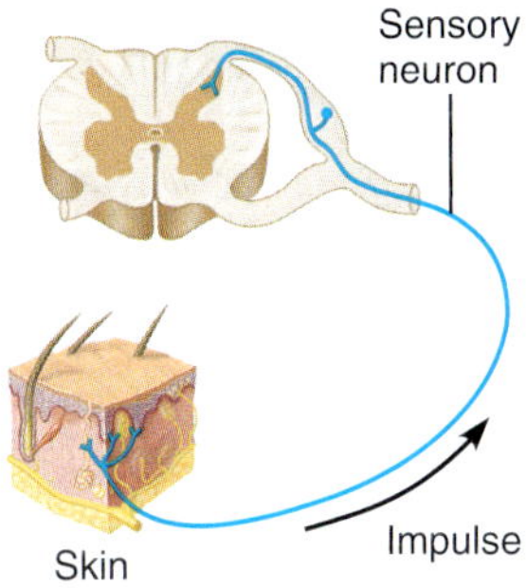

Sensory, or **afferent**, **neurons** transmit impulses from sensory receptors in the skin or internal organs *toward* or *into* the central nervous system. Except for certain neurons found in some special sense organs, virtually all sensory neurons are unipolar, and their cell bodies are located in sensory ganglia *outside* the CNS. Only the most distal parts of these unipolar neurons act as impulse receptor sites, and the peripheral processes are often very long. For example, fibers carrying sensory impulses from the skin of your great toe travel for more than a meter before they reach their cell bodies in a ganglion close to the spinal cord.

The receptive endings of some sensory neurons are naked, in which case those terminals themselves function as sensory receptors, but many sensory neuron endings bear receptors that include other cell types. We describe the various types of general sensory receptor end organs, such as those of the skin, in Chapter 13. The special sensory receptors (of the ear, eye, etc.) are the topic of Chapter 15.

Motor, or **efferent**, **neurons** carry impulses *away from* the CNS to the effector organs (muscles and glands) of the body periphery. Motor neurons are multipolar. Except for some neurons of the autonomic nervous system, their cell bodies are located in the CNS.

Interneurons, or *association neurons*, lie between motor and sensory neurons in neural pathways and shuttle signals through CNS pathways where integration occurs. Most interneurons are confined within the CNS. They make up over 99% of the neurons of the body, including most of those in the CNS.

Almost all interneurons are multipolar, but there is considerable diversity in both size and fiber-branching patterns. The Purkinje and pyramidal cells illustrated as structural variations in Table 11.1 are just two examples of their variety.

☑ Check Your Understanding

8. Which structural and functional type of neuron is activated first when you burn your finger? Which type is activated last to move your finger away from the source of heat?

For answers, see Appendix H.

Membrane Potentials

When a neuron is adequately stimulated, an electrical impulse is generated and conducted along the length of its axon. This response, called the *action potential* or *nerve impulse*, is always the same regardless of the source or type of stimulus, and it underlies virtually all functional activities of the nervous system.

In this section, we will consider how neurons are excited or inhibited and how they communicate with other cells. First, however, we need to explore some basic principles of electricity and revisit the resting membrane potential.

Basic Principles of Electricity

The human body is electrically neutral—it has the same number of positive and negative charges. However, there are regions where one type of charge predominates, making those regions positively or negatively charged. Because opposite charges attract each other, energy must be used (work must be done) to separate them. On the other hand, the coming together of opposite charges liberates energy that can be used to do work. For this reason, situations in which there are separated electrical charges of opposite sign have potential energy.

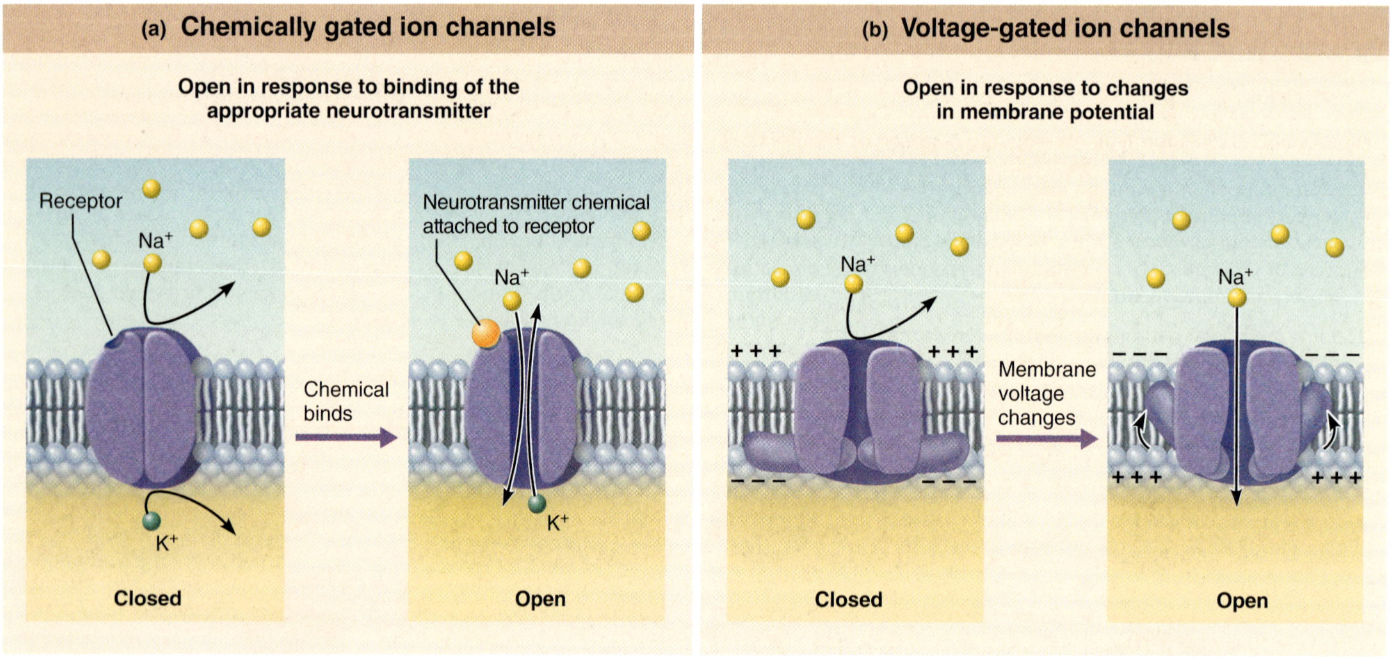

Figure 11.6 Operation of gated channels. (a) A chemically gated channel permeable to both Na^+ and K^+, and **(b)** a voltage-gated Na^+ channel.

11

Some Definitions: Voltage, Resistance, Current

Voltage, the measure of potential energy generated by separated charge, is measured in either *volts* (V) or *millivolts* (1 mV = 0.001 V). Voltage is always measured between two points and is called the **potential difference** or simply the **potential** between the points. The greater the difference in charge between two points, the higher the voltage.

The flow of electrical charge from one point to another is a **current**, and it can be used to do work—for example, to power a flashlight. The amount of charge that moves between the two points depends on two factors: voltage and resistance. **Resistance** is the hindrance to charge flow provided by substances through which the current must pass. Substances with high electrical resistance are *insulators*, and those with low resistance are *conductors*.

Ohm's law gives the relationship between voltage, current, and resistance:

$$\text{Current } (I) = \frac{\text{voltage } (V)}{\text{resistance } (R)}$$

Ohm's law tells us three things:

- Current (I) is directly proportional to voltage. The greater the voltage (potential difference), the greater the current.
- There is no net current flow between points that have the same potential, as you can see by inserting a value of 0 V into the equation.
- Current is inversely related to resistance: The greater the resistance, the smaller the current.

In the body, electrical currents reflect the flow of ions (rather than free electrons) across cellular membranes. (Unlike the electrons flowing along your house wiring, there are no free electrons "running around" in a living system.) As we described in Chapter 3, there is a slight difference in the numbers of positive and negative ions on the two sides of cellular plasma membranes (there is a charge separation), so there is a potential across those membranes. The plasma membranes provide the resistance to current flow.

Role of Membrane Ion Channels

Recall that plasma membranes are peppered with a variety of membrane proteins that act as *ion channels*. Each of these channels is selective as to the type of ion (or ions) it allows to pass. For example, a potassium ion channel allows only potassium ions to pass.

Membrane channels are large proteins, often with several subunits, whose amino acid chains snake back and forth across the membrane. Some channels, **leakage** or **nongated channels**, are always open. Other channels are *gated*: Part of the protein forms a molecular "gate" that changes shape to open and close the channel in response to specific signals. There are three main types of gated channels:

- **Chemically gated**, or **ligand-gated**, **channels** open when the appropriate chemical (in this case a neurotransmitter) binds **(Figure 11.6a)**.
- **Voltage-gated channels** open and close in response to changes in the membrane potential (Figure 11.6b).
- **Mechanically gated channels** open in response to physical deformation of the receptor (as in sensory receptors for touch and pressure).

When gated ion channels open, ions diffuse quickly across the membrane following their electrochemical gradients, creating electrical currents and voltage changes across the membrane according to the rearranged Ohm's law equation:

$$\text{Voltage } (V) = \text{current } (I) \times \text{resistance } (R)$$

Ions move along chemical *concentration gradients* when they diffuse passively from an area of their higher concentration to an area of lower concentration. They move along *electrical gradients* when they move toward an area of opposite electrical charge. Together, electrical and concentration gradients constitute the **electrochemical gradient**. Ions flowing along electrochemical gradients underlie all electrical events in neurons.

The Resting Membrane Potential

✓ Define resting membrane potential and describe its electrochemical basis.

A voltmeter is used to measure the potential difference between two points. When one microelectrode of the voltmeter is inserted into a neuron and the other is in the extracellular fluid, it records a voltage across the membrane of approximately −70 mV **(Figure 11.7)**. The minus sign indicates that the cytoplasmic side (inside) of the membrane is negatively charged relative to the outside. This potential difference in a resting neuron (V_r) is called the **resting membrane potential**, and the membrane is said to be **polarized**. The value of the resting membrane potential varies (from −40 mV to −90 mV) in different types of neurons.

The resting potential exists only across the membrane. In other words, the bulk solutions inside and outside the cell are electrically neutral. Two factors generate the resting membrane potential: differences in the ionic composition of the intracellular and extracellular fluids, and differences in the permeability of the plasma membrane to those ions.

Differences in Ionic Composition

First, let's compare the ionic makeup of the intracellular and extracellular fluids, as shown in *Focus on Resting Membrane Potential* **(Figure 11.8)**. The cell cytosol contains a lower concentration of Na^+ and a higher concentration of K^+ than the extracellular fluid. Negatively charged (anionic) proteins (not shown) help to balance the positive charges of intracellular cations (primarily K^+). In the extracellular fluid, the positive charges of Na^+ and other cations are balanced chiefly by chloride ions (Cl^-). Although there are many other solutes (glucose, urea, and other ions) in both fluids, potassium (K^+) plays the most important role in generating the membrane potential.

Differences in Plasma Membrane Permeability

Next, let's consider the differential permeability of the membrane to various ions (Figure 11.8, bottom). At rest the membrane is impermeable to the large anionic cytoplasmic proteins, very slightly permeable to sodium, approximately 25 times more permeable to potassium than to sodium, and quite permeable to chloride ions. These resting permeabilities reflect the properties of the leakage ion channels in the membrane. Potassium ions diffuse out of the cell along their *concentration gradient* much

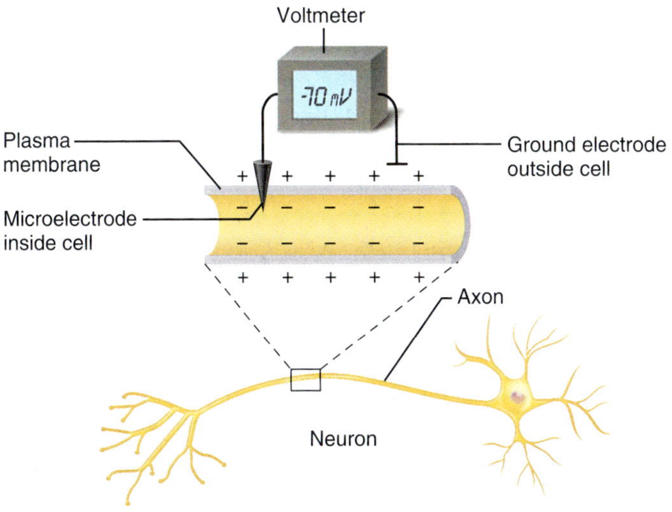

Figure 11.7 Measuring membrane potential in neurons. The potential difference between an electrode inside a neuron and the ground electrode in the extracellular fluid is approximately −70 mV (inside negative).

more easily than sodium ions can enter the cell along theirs. K^+ flowing out of the cell causes the cell to become more negative inside. Na^+ trickling into the cell makes the cell just slightly more positive than it would be if only K^+ flowed. Therefore, at resting membrane potential, the negative interior of the cell is due to a much greater ability for K^+ to diffuse out of the cell than for Na^+ to diffuse into the cell.

Because some K^+ is always leaking out of the cell and some Na^+ is always leaking in, you might think that the concentration gradients would eventually "run down," resulting in equal concentrations of Na^+ and K^+ inside and outside the cell. This does not happen because the ATP-driven sodium-potassium pump first ejects three Na^+ from the cell and then transports two K^+ back into the cell. In other words, the **sodium-potassium pump (Na^+-K^+ ATPase)** stabilizes the resting membrane potential by maintaining the concentration gradients for sodium and potassium.

Check Your Understanding

9. For an open channel, what factors determine in which direction ions will move through that channel?
10. For which cation is there the greatest amount of leakage (through leakage channels) across the plasma membrane?

For answers, see Appendix H.

Membrane Potentials That Act as Signals

✓ Compare and contrast graded potentials and action potentials.

✓ Explain how action potentials are generated and propagated along neurons.

✓ Define absolute and relative refractory periods.

✓ Define saltatory conduction and contrast it to continuous conduction.

11

Figure 11.8 Generating a resting membrane potential depends on (1) differences in K^+ and Na^+ concentrations inside and outside cells, and (2) differences in permeability of the plasma membrane to these ions. A&PFlix *Available at www.masteringaandp.com*

The concentrations of Na^+ and K^+ on each side of the membrane are different.

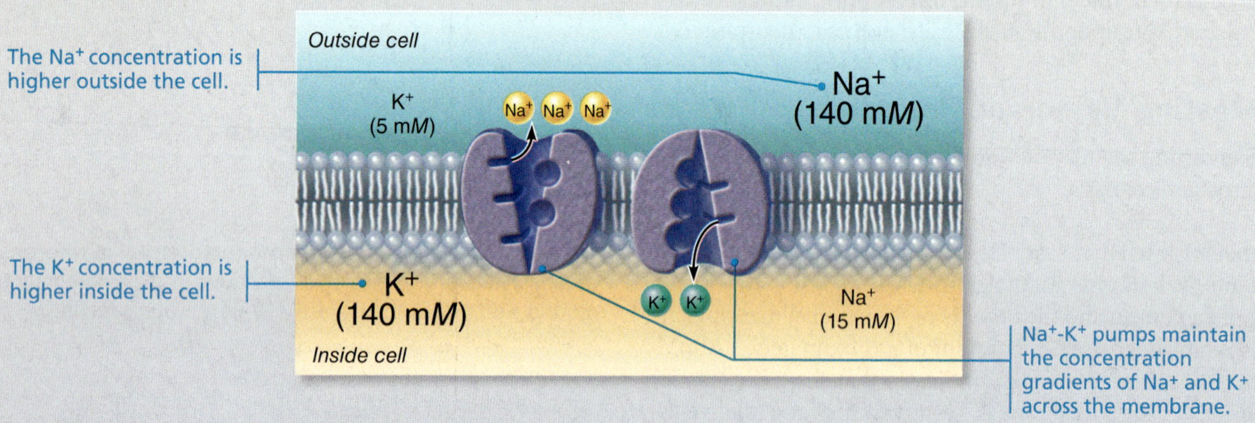

The permeabilities of Na^+ and K^+ across the membrane are different. In the next three panels, we will build the resting membrane potential step by step.

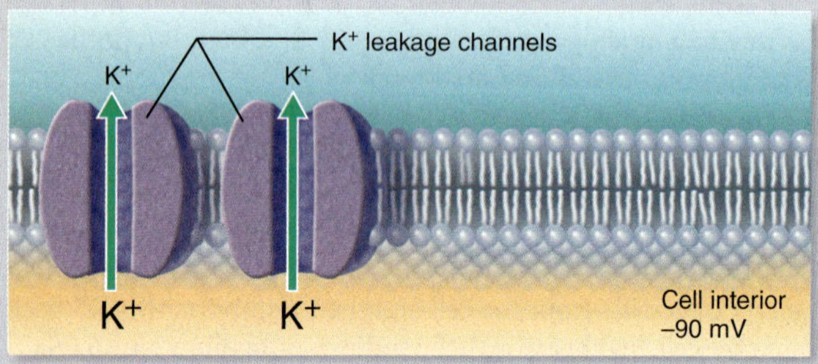

Suppose a cell has only K^+ channels...

K^+ loss through abundant leakage channels establishes a negative membrane potential. K^+ flows down its large concentration gradient because the membrane is highly permeable to K^+. As the positive K^+ ions leak out, the negative voltage that develops on the membrane interior counteracts the concentration gradient, pulling K^+ back into the cell. At -90 mV, the concentration and electrical gradients for K^+ are balanced.

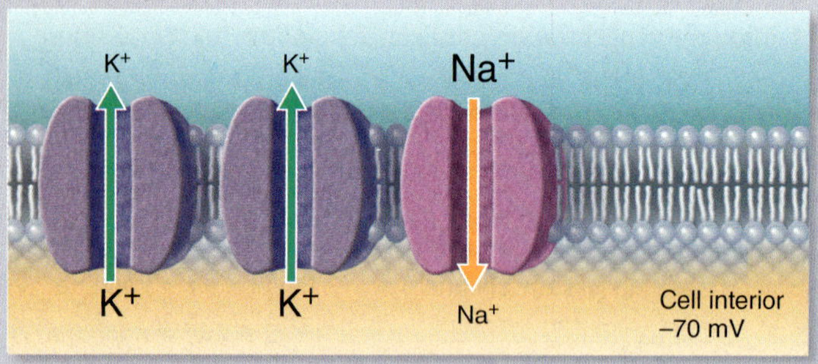

Now, let's add some Na^+ channels to our cell...

Na^+ entry through leakage channels reduces the negative membrane potential slightly. Na^+ flows down its large concentration gradient, but the membrane is only slightly permeable to Na^+. As a result, Na^+ entering the cell makes the membrane potential slightly less negative than if there were only K^+ channels.

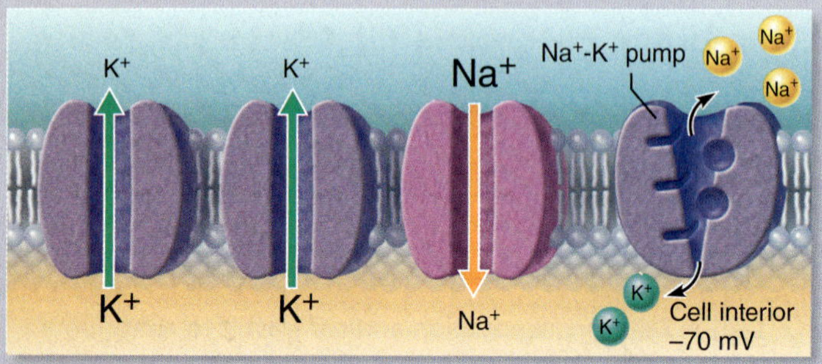

Finally, let's add a pump to compensate for leaking ions.

Na^+-K^+ pumps maintain the concentration gradients, resulting in the resting membrane potential. A cell at rest is like a leaky boat that is constantly leaking K^+ out and Na^+ in through open channels. The "bailing pump" for this boat is the **Na^+-K^+ pump**, which counteracts the leaks by transporting Na^+ out and K^+ in.

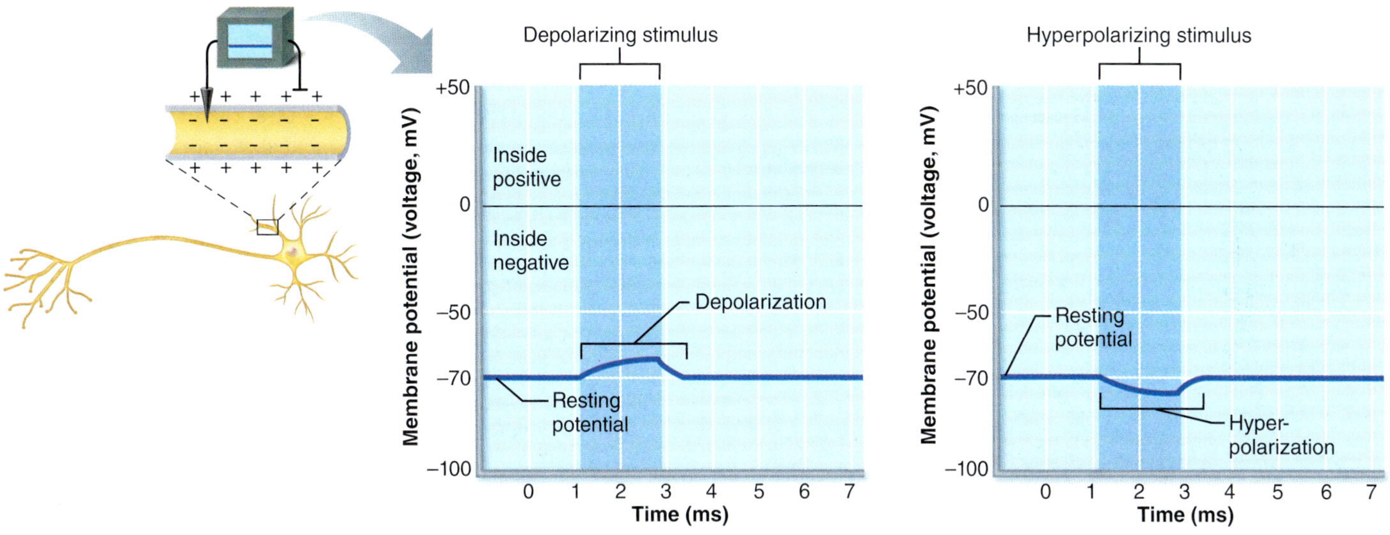

(a) Depolarization: The membrane potential moves toward 0 mV, the inside becoming less negative (more positive).

(b) Hyperpolarization: The membrane potential increases, the inside becoming more negative.

Figure 11.9 Depolarization and hyperpolarization of the membrane. The resting membrane potential is approximately −70 mV (inside negative) in neurons.

Neurons use changes in their membrane potential as communication signals to receive, integrate, and send information. A change in membrane potential can be produced by (1) anything that alters ion concentrations on the two sides of the membrane, or (2) anything that changes membrane permeability to any ion. However, only permeability changes (changes in the number of open channels) are important for transferring information.

Changes in membrane potential can produce two types of signals:

- *Graded potentials*, which are usually incoming signals operating over short distances
- *Action potentials*, which are long-distance signals of axons

The terms *depolarization* and *hyperpolarization* describe changes in membrane potential *relative to resting membrane potential*. It is important to clearly understand these terms.

Depolarization is a decrease in membrane potential: The inside of the membrane becomes *less negative* (moves closer to zero) than the resting potential. For instance, a change in resting potential from −70 mV to −65 mV is a depolarization **(Figure 11.9a)**. By convention, depolarization also includes events in which the membrane potential reverses and moves above zero to become positive.

Hyperpolarization is an increase in membrane potential: The inside of the membrane becomes *more negative* (moves further from zero) than the resting potential. For example, a change from −70 mV to −75 mV is hyperpolarization (Figure 11.9b). As we will describe shortly, depolarization increases the probability of producing nerve impulses, whereas hyperpolarization reduces this probability.

Graded Potentials

Graded potentials are short-lived, localized changes in membrane potential that can be either depolarizations or hyperpolarizations. These changes cause current flows that decrease in magnitude with distance. Graded potentials are called "graded" because their magnitude varies directly with stimulus strength. The stronger the stimulus, the more the voltage changes and the farther the current flows.

Graded potentials are triggered by some change (a stimulus) in the neuron's environment that opens gated ion channels. Graded potentials are given different names, depending on where they occur and the functions they perform.

- When the receptor of a sensory neuron is excited by some form of energy (heat, light, or other), the resulting graded potential is called a *receptor potential* or *generator potential*. We will consider these types of graded potentials in Chapter 13.
- When the stimulus is a neurotransmitter released by another neuron, the graded potential is called a *postsynaptic potential*, because the neurotransmitter is released into a fluid-filled gap called a synapse and influences the neuron beyond (post) the synapse.

Fluids inside and outside cells are fairly good conductors, and current, carried by ions, flows through these fluids whenever voltage changes. Suppose a stimulus depolarizes a small area of a neuron's plasma membrane **(Figure 11.10a)**. Current (ions) flows on both sides of the membrane between the depolarized (active) membrane area and the adjacent polarized (resting) areas. Positive ions migrate toward more negative areas (the direction of cation movement is the direction of current flow),

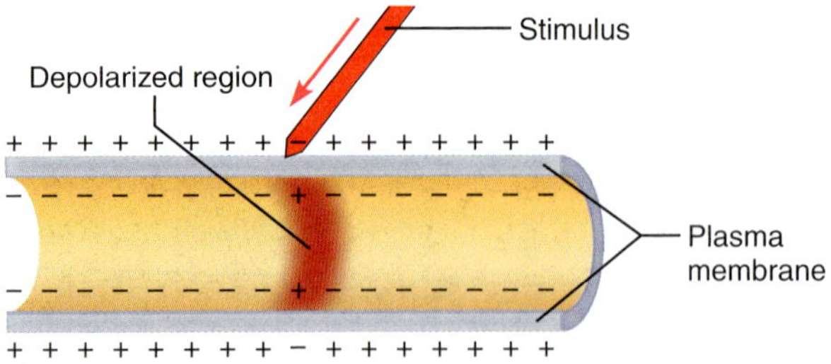

(a) Depolarization: A small patch of the membrane (red area) depolarizes.

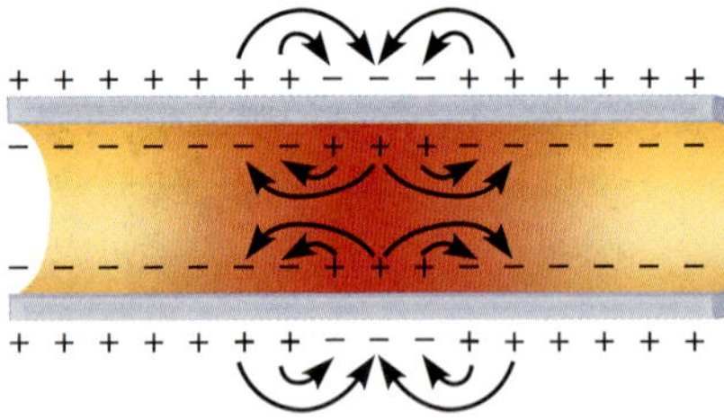

(b) Depolarization spreads: Opposite charges attract each other. This creates local currents (black arrows) that depolarize adjacent membrane areas, spreading the wave of depolarization.

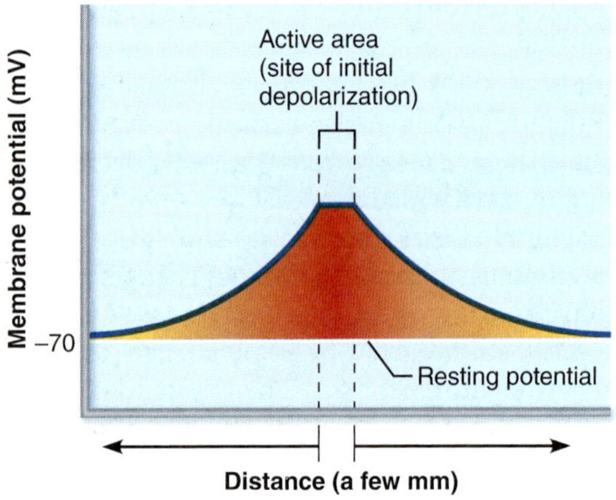

(c) Membrane potential decays with distance: Because current is lost through the "leaky" plasma membrane, the voltage declines with distance from the stimulus (the voltage is *decremental*). Consequently, graded potentials are short-distance signals.

Figure 11.10 The spread and decay of a graded potential.

and negative ions simultaneously move toward more positive areas (Figure 11.10b).

For our patch of plasma membrane, positive ions (mostly K^+) inside the cell move away from the depolarized area and accumulate on the neighboring membrane areas, where they neutralize negative ions. Meanwhile, positive ions on the outer membrane face move toward the region of reversed membrane polarity (the depolarized region), which is momentarily less positive. As these positive ions move, their "places" on the membrane become occupied by negative ions (such as Cl^- and HCO_3^-), sort of like ionic musical chairs. In this way, at regions abutting the depolarized region, the inside becomes less negative and the outside becomes less positive. In other words, the depolarization spreads as the neighboring membrane "patch" is, in turn, depolarized.

As just explained, the flow of current to adjacent membrane areas changes the membrane potential there as well. However, the plasma membrane is permeable like a leaky water hose, and most of the charge is quickly lost through leakage channels. Consequently, the current dies out within a few millimeters of its origin and is said to be *decremental* (Figure 11.10c).

Because the current dissipates quickly and decays (declines) with increasing distance from the site of initial depolarization, graded potentials can act as signals only over very short distances. Nonetheless, they are essential in initiating action potentials, the long-distance signals.

Action Potentials (AP)

The principal way neurons send signals over long distances is by generating and propagating (transmitting) action potentials. Only cells with *excitable membranes*—neurons and muscle cells—can generate action potentials.

An **action potential (AP)** is a brief reversal of membrane potential with a total amplitude (change in voltage) of about 100 mV (from −70 mV to +30 mV). Depolarization is followed by repolarization and often a short period of hyperpolarization. The whole event is over in a few milliseconds. Unlike graded potentials, action potentials do not decay with distance.

The events of action potential generation and transmission are identical in skeletal muscle cells and neurons. As we have noted, in a neuron, an AP is also called a **nerve impulse**, and is typically generated *only in axons.* A neuron generates a nerve impulse only when adequately stimulated. The stimulus changes the permeability of the neuron's membrane by opening specific voltage-gated channels on the axon.

These channels open and close in response to changes in the membrane potential. They are activated by local currents (graded potentials) that spread toward the axon along the dendritic and cell body membranes.

In many neurons, the transition from local graded potential to long-distance action potential takes place at the axon hillock. In sensory neurons, the action potential is generated by the peripheral (axonal) process just proximal to the receptor region. However, for simplicity, we will just use the term axon in our discussion. We'll look first at the generation of an action potential and then at its propagation.

Generation of an Action Potential *Focus on an Action Potential* **(Figure 11.11)** on pp. 402–403 describes how an action potential is generated. Let's start with a neuron in the resting (polarized) state.

(1) **Resting state: All gated Na^+ and K^+ channels are closed.** Only the leakage channels are open, maintaining resting membrane potential. Each Na^+ channel has two gates: a voltage-sensitive *activation gate* that is closed at rest and responds to depolarization by opening, and an *inactivation gate* that blocks the channel once it is open. Thus, *depolarization opens and then inactivates sodium channels.*

Both gates must be open in order for Na^+ to enter, but the closing of *either* gate effectively closes the channel. By contrast, each active potassium channel has a single voltage-sensitive gate that is closed in the resting state and opens slowly in response to depolarization.

(2) **Depolarization: Na^+ channels open.** As local currents depolarize the axon membrane, the voltage-gated sodium channels open and Na^+ rushes into the cell. This influx of positive charge depolarizes that local patch of membrane further, opening more Na^+ channels so the cell interior becomes progressively less negative.

When depolarization at the stimulation site reaches a certain critical level called **threshold** (often between −55 and −50 mV), depolarization becomes self-generating, urged on by positive feedback. That is, after being initiated by the stimulus, depolarization is driven by the ionic currents created by Na^+ influx. As more Na^+ enters, the membrane depolarizes further and opens still more channels until all Na^+ channels are open. At this point, Na^+ permeability is about 1000 times greater than in a resting neuron. As a result, the membrane potential becomes less and less negative and then overshoots to about +30 mV as Na^+ rushes in along its electrochemical gradient. This rapid depolarization and polarity reversal produces the sharp upward *spike* of the action potential (Figure 11.11).

Earlier, we stated that membrane potential depends on membrane permeability, but here we say that membrane permeability depends on membrane potential. Can both statements be true? Yes, because these two relationships establish a *positive feedback cycle*: Increasing Na^+ permeability due to increased channel openings leads to greater depolarization, which increases Na^+ permeability, and so on. This explosive positive feedback cycle is responsible for the rising (depolarizing) phase of an action potential—it puts the "action" in the action potential.

(3) **Repolarization: Na^+ channels are inactivating, and K^+ channels open.** The explosively rising phase of the action potential persists for only about 1 ms. It is self-limiting because the slow inactivation gates of the Na^+ channels begin to close at this point. As a result, the membrane permeability to Na^+ declines to resting levels, and the net influx of Na^+ stops completely. Consequently, the AP spike stops rising.

As Na^+ entry declines, the slow voltage-gated K^+ channels open and K^+ rushes out of the cell, following its electrochemical gradient. This restores the internal negativity of the resting neuron, an event called **repolarization**. Both the abrupt decline in Na^+ permeability and the increased permeability to K^+ contribute to repolarization.

(4) **Hyperpolarization: Some K^+ channels remain open, and Na^+ channels reset.** The period of increased K^+ permeability typically lasts longer than needed to restore the resting state. As a result of the excessive K^+ efflux before the potassium channels close, a hyperpolarization is seen on the AP curve as a slight dip following the spike. Also at this point, the Na^+ channels begin to reset to their original position by changing shape to reopen their inactivation gates and close their activation gates.

Repolarization restores resting electrical conditions, but it does *not* restore resting ionic conditions. After repolarization, the *sodium-potassium pump* redistributes the ions. While it might appear that tremendous numbers of Na^+ and K^+ ions change places during an action potential, this is not the case. Only small amounts of sodium and potassium cross the membrane. (The Na^+ influx required to reach threshold produces only a 0.012% change in intracellular Na^+ concentration.) These small ionic changes are quickly corrected because an axon membrane has thousands of Na^+-K^+ pumps.

Threshold and the All-or-None Phenomenon Not all local depolarization events produce APs. The depolarization must reach threshold values if an axon is to "fire." What determines the *threshold point*?

One explanation is that threshold is the membrane potential at which the outward current created by K^+ movement is exactly equal to the inward current created by Na^+ movement. Threshold is typically reached when the membrane has been depolarized by 15 to 20 mV from the resting value. This depolarization status represents an unstable equilibrium state. If one more Na^+ enters, further depolarization occurs, opening more Na^+ channels and allowing more Na^+ to enter. If, on the other hand, one more K^+ leaves, the membrane potential is driven away from threshold, Na^+ channels close, and K^+ continues to diffuse outward until the potential returns to its resting value.

Recall that local depolarizations are graded potentials and their magnitude increases when stimuli become more intense. Brief weak stimuli (*subthreshold stimuli*) produce subthreshold depolarizations that are not translated into nerve impulses. On the other hand, stronger *threshold stimuli* produce depolarizing currents that push the membrane potential toward and beyond the threshold voltage. As a result, Na^+ permeability rises to such an extent that entering sodium ions "swamp" (exceed) the outward movement of K^+, establishing the positive feedback cycle and generating an AP.

The critical factor here is the total amount of current that flows through the membrane during a stimulus (electrical charge × time). Strong stimuli depolarize the membrane to threshold quickly. Weaker stimuli must be applied for longer periods to provide the crucial amount of current flow. Very weak stimuli do not trigger an AP because the local current flows they produce are so slight that they dissipate long before threshold is reached.

An AP is an **all-or-none phenomenon**: It either happens completely or doesn't happen at all. We can compare the generation of an AP to lighting a match under a small dry twig. The changes occurring where the twig is heated are analogous to the change in membrane permeability that initially allows more Na^+ to enter the cell. When that part of the twig becomes hot enough (when enough Na^+ enters the cell), it reaches the flash point (threshold) and the flame consumes the entire twig, even if you blow out the match. Similarly, the AP is generated and propagated whether or not the stimulus continues. But if you blow out the match before the twig reaches the threshold temperature, ignition will not take

(Text continues on p. 404.)

11

Figure 11.11 The action potential (AP) is a brief change in membrane potential in a "patch" of membrane that is depolarized by local currents.

A&P Flix Available at www.masteringaandp.com

The big picture

This graph shows how voltage changes over time at a given point inside an axon during the course of an action potential.

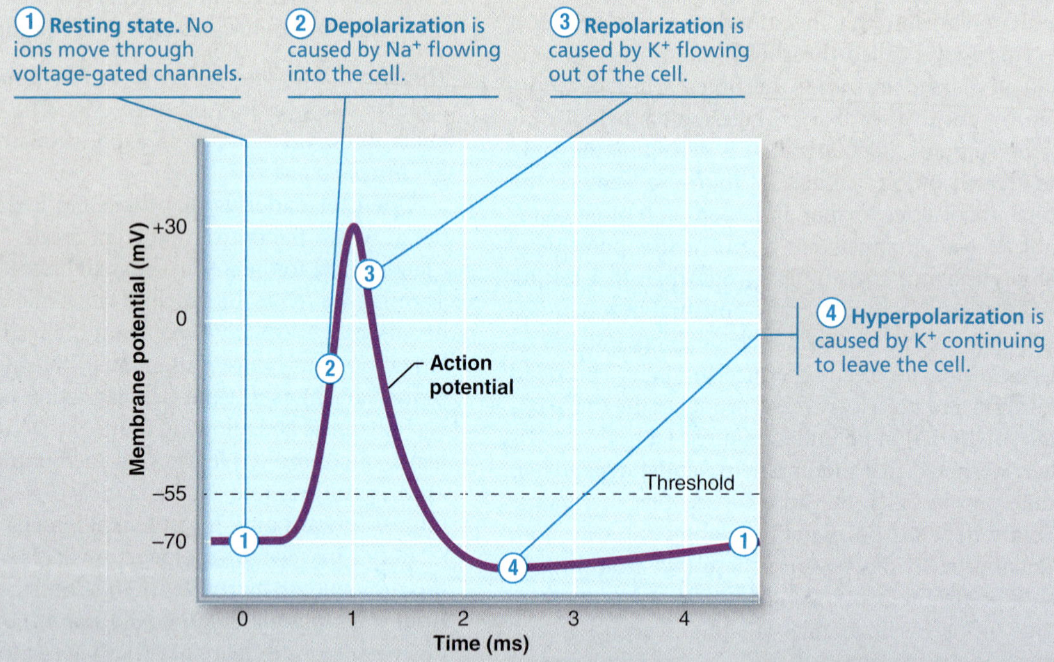

The AP is caused by permeability changes in the plasma membrane:

Relative membrane permeability tells you the relative number of ion channels that are open for each ion. Remember that open ion channels make the plasma membrane permeable to those ions.

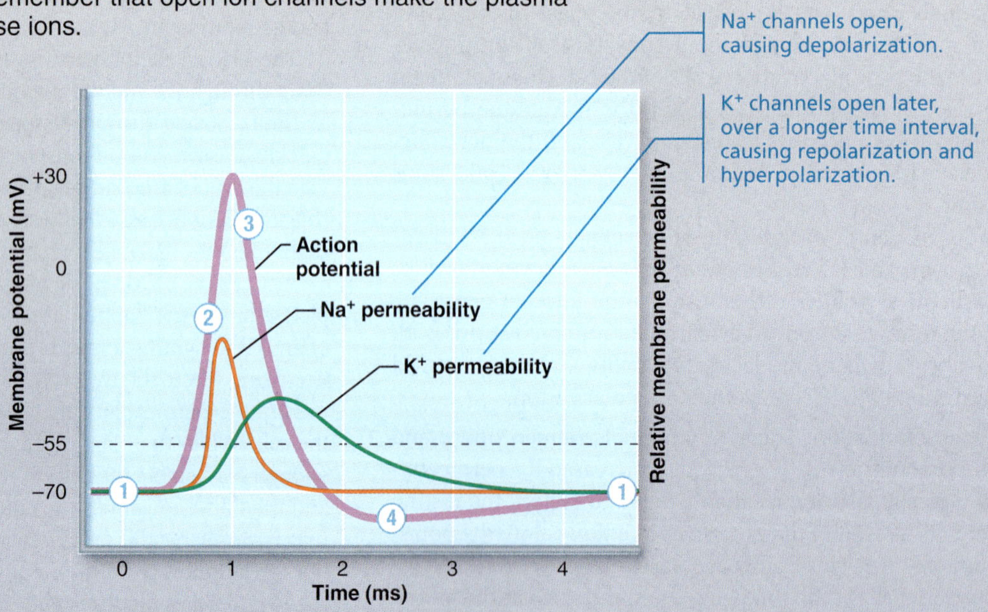

The key players

Voltage-gated Na^+ channels have two gates and alternate between three different states.

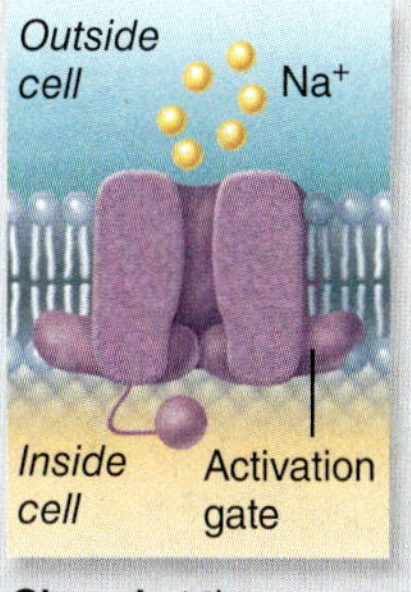

Closed at the resting state, so no Na^+ enters the cell through them

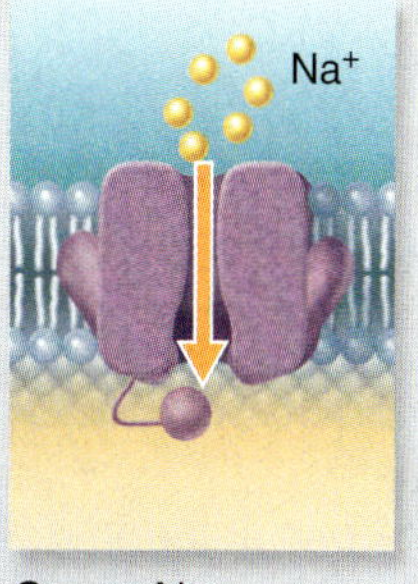

Opened by depolarization, allowing Na^+ to enter the cell

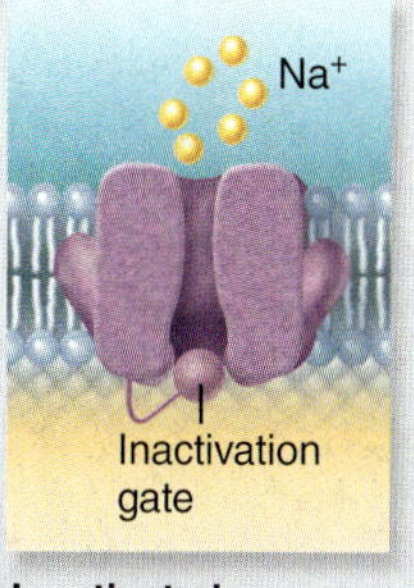

Inactivated—channels automatically blocked by inactivation gates soon after they open

Voltage-gated K^+ channels have one gate and two states.

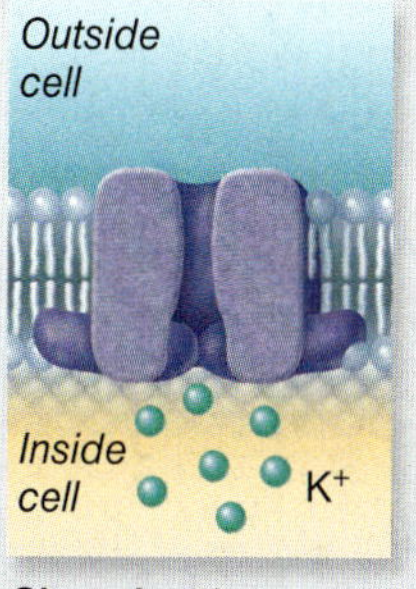

Closed at the resting state, so no K^+ exits the cell through them

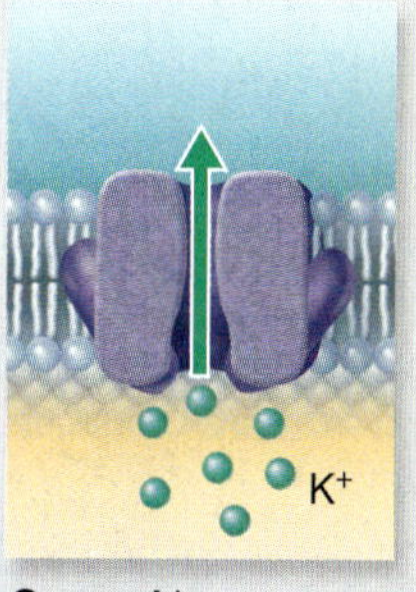

Opened by depolarization, after a delay, allowing K^+ to exit the cell

The events

Each step corresponds to one part of the AP graph.

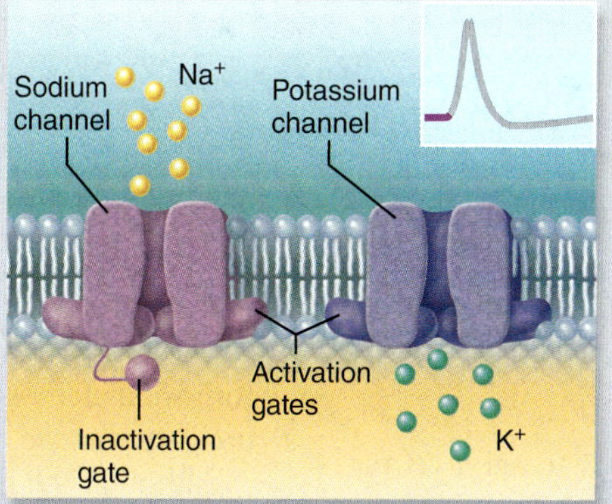

(1) **Resting state:** All gated Na^+ and K^+ channels are closed.

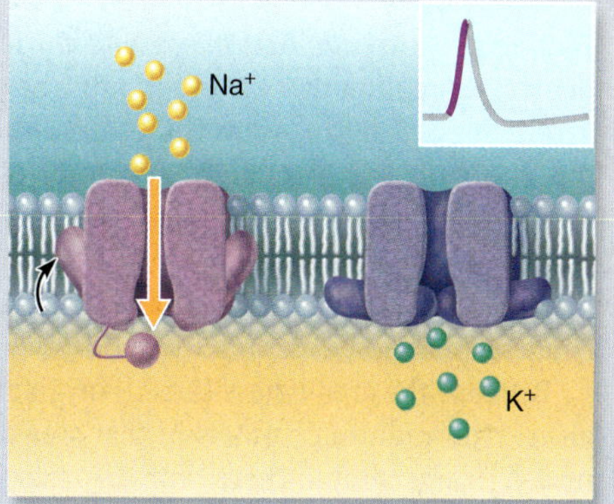

(2) **Depolarization:** Na^+ channels open.

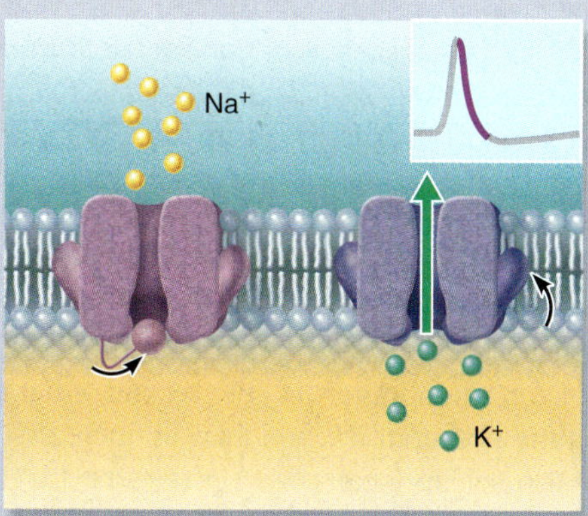

(3) **Repolarization:** Na^+ channels are inactivating, and K^+ channels open.

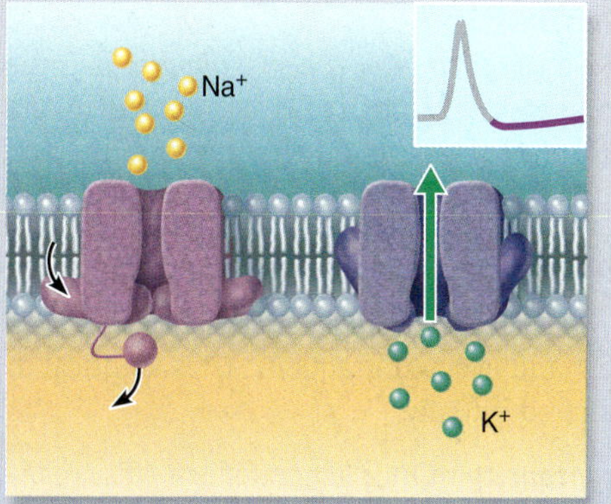

(4) **Hyperpolarization:** Some K^+ channels remain open, and Na^+ channels reset.

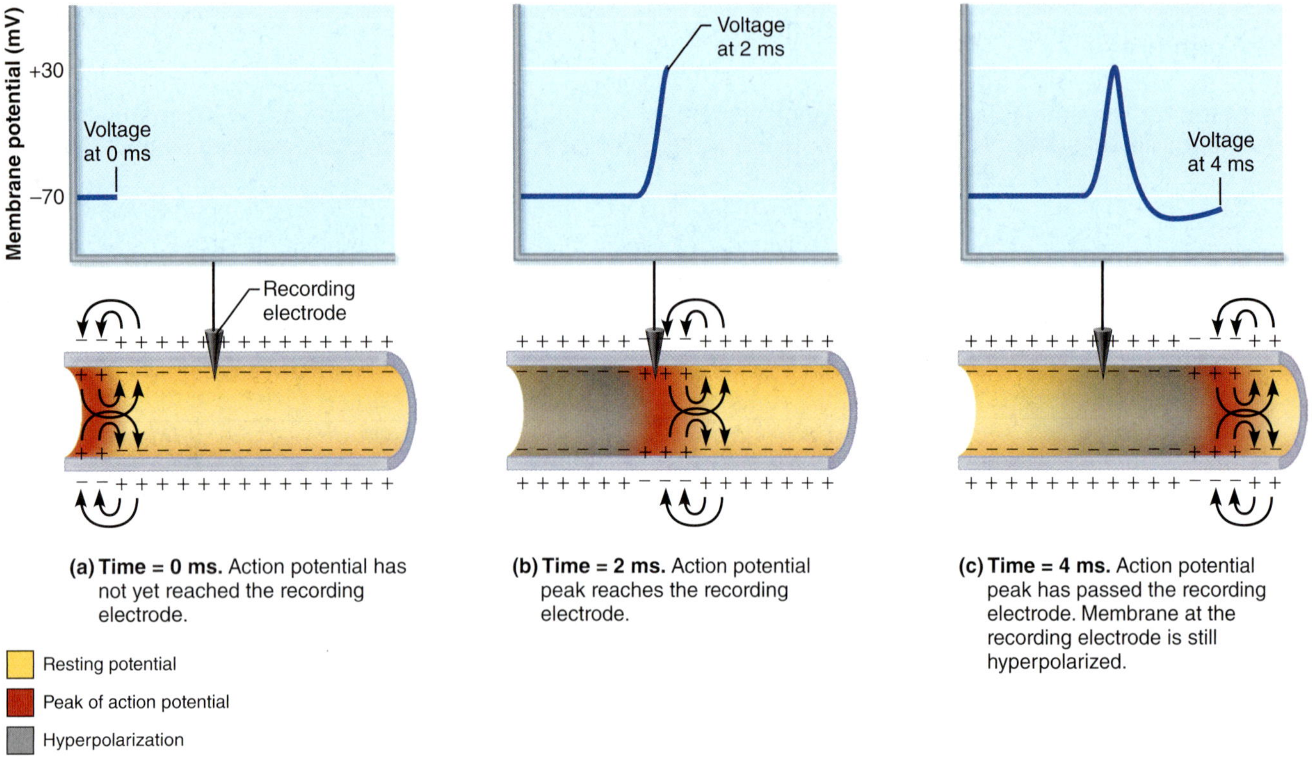

Figure 11.12 Propagation of an action potential (AP). Recordings at three successive times as an AP propagates along an axon (from left to right). The arrows show the direction of local current flow generated by the movement of positive ions. This current brings the resting membrane at the leading edge of the AP to threshold, propagating the AP forward.

place. Likewise, if the number of Na^+ ions entering the cell is too low to achieve threshold, no AP will occur.

Propagation of an Action Potential If it is to serve as the neuron's signaling device, an AP must be **propagated** along the axon's entire length. As we have seen, the AP is generated by the influx of Na^+ through a given area of the membrane. This influx establishes local currents that depolarize adjacent membrane areas in the forward direction (away from the origin of the nerve impulse), which opens voltage-gated channels and triggers an action potential there **(Figure 11.12)**.

Because the area where the AP originated has just generated an AP, the sodium channels in that area are inactivated and no new AP is generated there. For this reason, the AP propagates away from its point of origin. (If an *isolated* axon is stimulated by an electrode, the nerve impulse will move away from the point of stimulus in all directions along the membrane.) In the body, APs are initiated at one end of the axon and conducted away from that point toward the axon's terminals. Once initiated, an AP is *self-propagating* and continues along the axon at a constant velocity—something like a domino effect.

Following depolarization, each segment of axon membrane repolarizes, which restores the resting membrane potential in that region. Because these electrical changes also set up local currents, the repolarization wave chases the depolarization wave down the length of the axon.

The propagation process we have just described occurs on nonmyelinated axons. On p. 405, we will describe propagation along myelinated axons.

Although the phrase *conduction of a nerve impulse* is commonly used, nerve impulses are not really conducted in the same way that an insulated wire conducts current. In fact, neurons are fairly poor conductors, and as noted earlier, local current flows decline with distance because the charges leak through the membrane. The expression *propagation of a nerve impulse* is more accurate, because the AP is *regenerated anew* at each membrane patch, and every subsequent AP is identical to the one that was generated initially.

Coding for Stimulus Intensity Once generated, all APs are independent of stimulus strength, and all APs are alike. So how can the CNS determine whether a particular stimulus is intense or weak—information it needs to initiate an appropriate response?

The answer is really quite simple: Strong stimuli generate nerve impulses more *often* in a given time interval than do weak stimuli. Stimulus intensity is coded for by the number of impulses per second—that is, by the *frequency of action potentials*—rather than by increases in the strength (amplitude) of the individual APs **(Figure 11.13)**.

Refractory Periods When a patch of neuron membrane is generating an AP and its voltage-gated sodium channels are open, the neuron cannot respond to another stimulus, no matter how

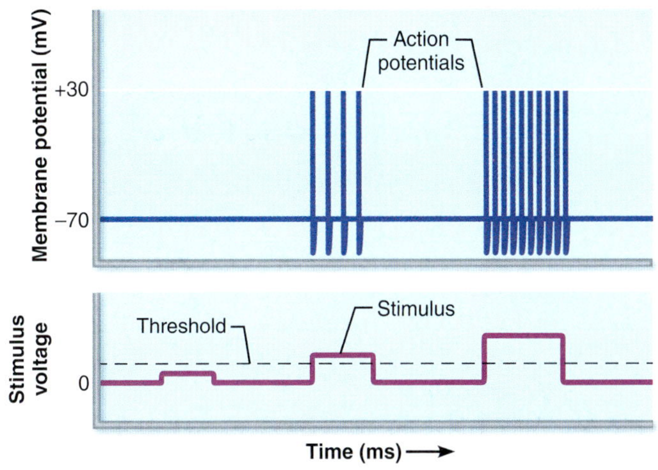

Figure 11.13 Relationship between stimulus strength and action potential frequency. APs are shown as vertical lines in the upper trace. The lower trace shows the intensity of the applied stimulus. A subthreshold stimulus does not generate an AP, but once threshold voltage is reached, the stronger the stimulus, the more frequently APs are generated.

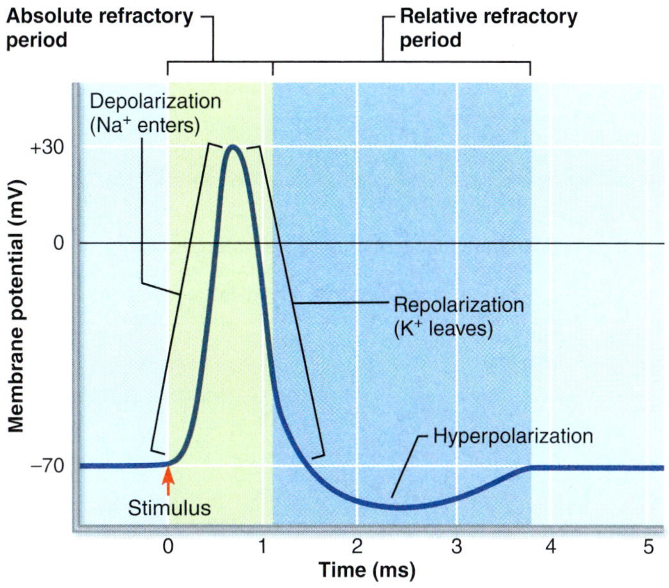

Figure 11.14 Absolute and relative refractory periods in an AP.

strong. This period, from the opening of the Na^+ channels until the Na^+ channels begin to reset to their original resting state, is called the **absolute refractory period (Figure 11.14)**. It ensures that each AP is a separate, *all-or-none event* and enforces one-way transmission of the AP.

The **relative refractory period** is the interval following the absolute refractory period. During the relative refractory period, most Na^+ channels have returned to their resting state, some K^+ channels are still open, and repolarization is occurring. During this time, the axon's threshold for AP generation is substantially elevated. A stimulus that would normally generate an AP is no longer sufficient, but an exceptionally strong stimulus can reopen the Na^+ channels that have already returned to their resting state and generate another AP. Strong stimuli trigger more frequent APs by intruding into the relative refractory period.

Conduction Velocity How fast do APs travel? Conduction velocities of neurons vary widely. Nerve fibers that transmit impulses most rapidly (100 m/s or more) are found in neural pathways where speed is essential, such as those that mediate postural reflexes. Axons that conduct impulses more slowly typically serve internal organs (the gut, glands, blood vessels), where slower responses are not a handicap. The rate of impulse propagation depends largely on two factors:

- **Axon diameter.** As a rule, the larger the axon's diameter, the faster it conducts impulses. Larger axons conduct more rapidly because they offer less resistance to the flow of local currents, bringing adjacent areas of the membrane to threshold more quickly.
- **Degree of myelination.** Action potentials propagate because they are regenerated by voltage-gated channels in the membrane **(Figure 11.15a, b)**. In **continuous conduction**, AP propagation involving nonmyelinated axons, these channels are immediately adjacent to each other. Continuous conduction is relatively slow.

The presence of a myelin sheath dramatically increases the rate of AP propagation. By acting as an insulator, myelin prevents almost all charge from leaking from the axon and allows the membrane voltage to change more rapidly. Current can pass through the membrane of a myelinated axon *only* at the myelin sheath gaps, where there is no myelin sheath and the axon is bare. Nearly all the voltage-gated Na^+ channels are concentrated in these gaps.

When an AP is generated in a myelinated fiber, the local depolarizing current does not dissipate through the adjacent membrane regions, which are nonexcitable. Instead, the current is maintained and moves rapidly to the next myelin sheath gap, a distance of approximately 1 mm, where it triggers another AP. Consequently, APs are triggered only at the gaps, a type of conduction called **saltatory conduction** (*saltare* = to leap) because the electrical signal appears to jump from gap to gap along the axon (Figure 11.15c). Saltatory conduction is about 30 times faster than continuous conduction.

Homeostatic Imbalance 11.2

The importance of myelin to nerve transmission is painfully clear to people with demyelinating diseases such as **multiple sclerosis (MS)**. This autoimmune disease affects mostly young adults.

Multiple sclerosis gradually destroys myelin sheaths in the CNS, reducing them to nonfunctional hardened lesions called *scleroses*. The loss of myelin (a result of the immune system's attack on myelin proteins) shunts and short-circuits the current so that successive gaps are excited more and more slowly, and eventually impulse conduction ceases. However, the axons themselves are not damaged and growing numbers of Na^+ channels appear spontaneously in the demyelinated fibers. This

11

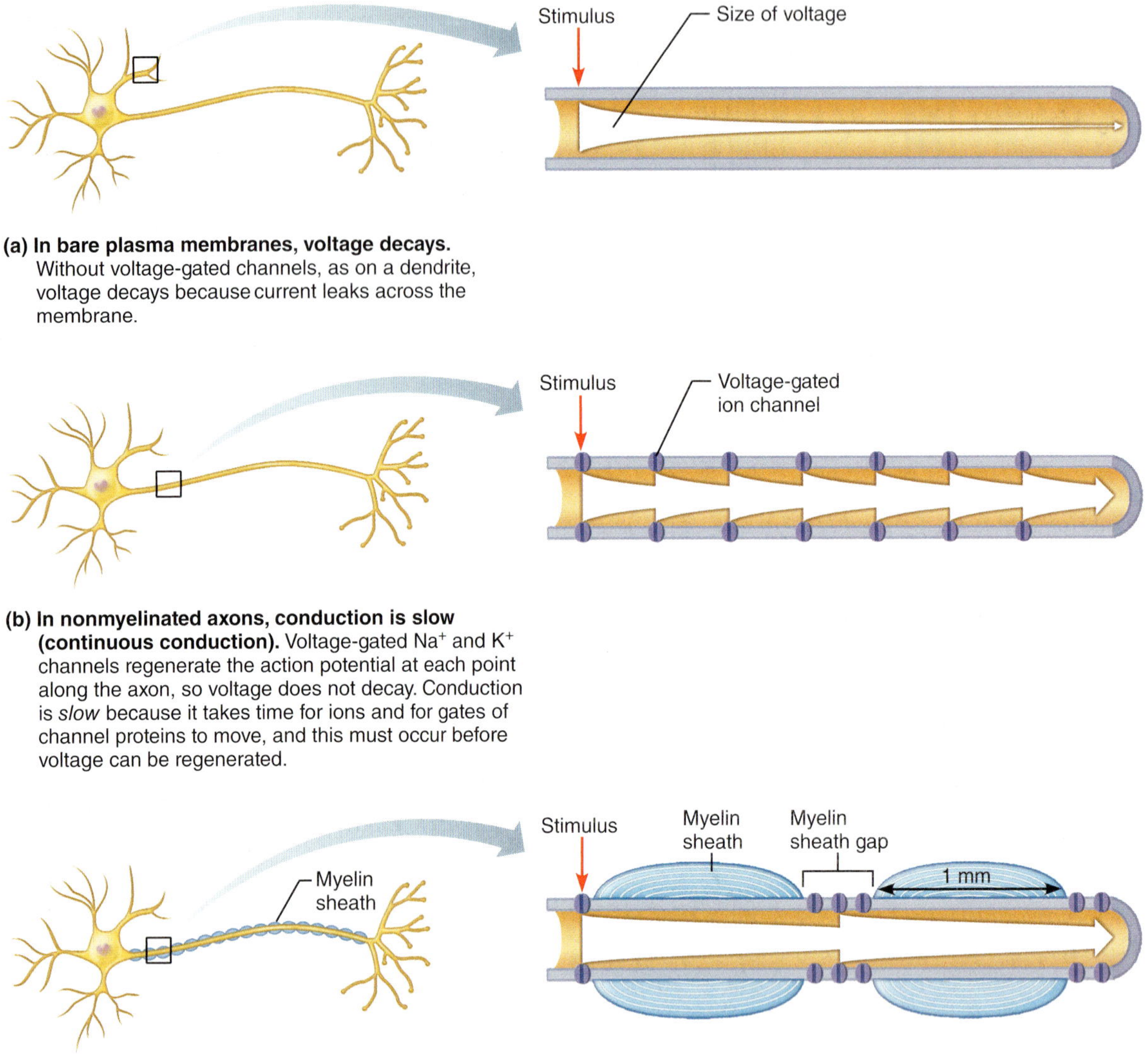

(a) In bare plasma membranes, voltage decays. Without voltage-gated channels, as on a dendrite, voltage decays because current leaks across the membrane.

(b) In nonmyelinated axons, conduction is slow (continuous conduction). Voltage-gated Na^+ and K^+ channels regenerate the action potential at each point along the axon, so voltage does not decay. Conduction is *slow* because it takes time for ions and for gates of channel proteins to move, and this must occur before voltage can be regenerated.

(c) In myelinated axons, conduction is fast (saltatory conduction). Myelin keeps current in axons (voltage doesn't decay much). APs are generated *only* in the myelin sheath gaps and appear to jump *rapidly* from gap to gap.

Figure 11.15 Action potential propagation in nonmyelinated and myelinated axons.

may account for the remarkably variable cycles of remission (symptom-free periods) and relapse (disability) typical of this disease. Common symptoms are visual disturbances (including blindness), problems controlling muscles (weakness, clumsiness, and ultimately paralysis), speech disturbances, and urinary incontinence.

The advent of drugs that modify the immune system's activity (such as interferons, glatiramer, and fingolimod) will continue to improve the lives of people with MS. These drugs seem to hold symptoms at bay, reducing complications and disability. Recent studies show that high blood levels of vitamin D reduce the risk of developing MS in the first place. +

Nerve fibers may be classified according to diameter, degree of myelination, and conduction speed.

- **Group A fibers** are mostly somatic sensory and motor fibers serving the skin, skeletal muscles, and joints. They have the largest diameter and thick myelin sheaths, and conduct impulses at speeds ranging up to 150 m/s (over 300 miles per hour).
- **Group B fibers**, lightly myelinated fibers of intermediate diameter, transmit impulses at an average rate of 15 m/s (about 30 mi/h).
- **Group C fibers** have the smallest diameter and are nonmyelinated. Consequently, they are incapable of saltatory conduction and conduct impulses at a leisurely pace—1 m/s (2 mi/h) or less.

The B and C fiber groups include autonomic nervous system motor fibers serving the visceral organs; visceral sensory fibers; and the smaller somatic sensory fibers transmitting sensory impulses from the skin (such as pain and small touch fibers).

What happens when an action potential arrives at the end of a neuron's axon? That is the subject of the next section.

Homeostatic Imbalance 11.3

A number of chemical and physical factors impair impulse propagation. Local anesthetics like those used by your dentist act by blocking voltage-gated Na^+ channels. As we have seen, no Na^+ entry—no AP.

Cold and continuous pressure interrupt blood circulation, hindering the delivery of oxygen and nutrients to neuron processes and impairing their ability to conduct impulses. For example, your fingers get numb when you hold an ice cube for more than a few seconds, and your foot "goes to sleep" when you sit on it. When you remove the cold object or pressure, impulses are transmitted again, leading to an unpleasant prickly feeling. ✚

Check Your Understanding

11. Which is bigger, a graded potential or an action potential? Which travels farthest? Which initiates the other?
12. An action potential does not get smaller as it propagates along an axon. Why not?
13. Why does a myelinated axon conduct action potentials faster than a nonmyelinated axon?
14. If an axon receives two stimuli close together in time, only one AP occurs. Why?

For answers, see Appendix H.

The Synapse

✓ Define synapse. Distinguish between electrical and chemical synapses by structure and by the way they transmit information.

The operation of the nervous system depends on the flow of information through chains of neurons functionally connected by synapses. A **synapse** (sin′aps), from the Greek *syn*, "to clasp or join," is a junction that mediates information transfer from one neuron to the next or from a neuron to an effector cell—it's where the action is.

Synapses between the axon endings of one neuron and the dendrites of other neurons are **axodendritic synapses**. Those between axon endings of one neuron and cell bodies (soma) of other neurons are **axosomatic synapses** (**Figure 11.16**). Less common (and far less understood) are synapses between axons (*axoaxonal*), between dendrites (*dendrodendritic*), or between cell bodies and dendrites (*somatodendritic*).

The neuron conducting impulses toward the synapse is the **presynaptic neuron**, and the neuron transmitting the electrical signal away from the synapse is the **postsynaptic neuron.** At a given synapse, the presynaptic neuron sends the information, and the postsynaptic neuron receives the information. As you might anticipate, most neurons function as both presynaptic and postsynaptic neurons. Neurons have anywhere from 1000 to 10,000 axon terminals making synapses and are stimulated by an equal number of other neurons. Outside the central nervous system, the postsynaptic cell may be either another neuron or an effector cell (a muscle cell or gland cell).

Now let's look at the two varieties of synapses: *electrical* and *chemical.*

Electrical Synapses

Electrical synapses, the less common variety, consist of gap junctions like those found between certain other body cells. They contain protein channels, called connexons, that intimately connect the cytoplasm of adjacent neurons and allow ions and small molecules to flow directly from one neuron to the next. These neurons are *electrically coupled*, and transmission across these synapses is very rapid. Depending on the nature of the synapse, communication may be unidirectional or bidirectional.

A key feature of electrical synapses between neurons is that they provide a simple means of synchronizing the activity of all interconnected neurons. In adults, electrical synapses are found in regions of the brain responsible for certain stereotyped movements, such as the normal jerky movements of the eyes. They also occur in axoaxonal synapses in the hippocampus, a brain region intimately involved in emotions and memory.

Electrical synapses are far more abundant in embryonic nervous tissue, where they permit exchange of guiding cues during early neuronal development so that neurons can connect properly with one another. As the nervous system develops, chemical synapses replace some electrical synapses. Gap junctions also exist between glial cells of the CNS.

Chemical Synapses

In contrast to electrical synapses, which are specialized to allow the flow of ions between neurons, **chemical synapses** are specialized to allow the release and reception of chemical neurotransmitters. A typical chemical synapse is made up of two parts:

- A knoblike *axon terminal* of the presynaptic neuron, which contains many tiny, membrane-bounded sacs called **synaptic vesicles**, each containing thousands of neurotransmitter molecules
- A neurotransmitter *receptor region* on the postsynaptic neuron's membrane, usually located on a dendrite or the cell body

Although close to each other, presynaptic and postsynaptic membranes are always separated by the **synaptic cleft**, a fluid-filled space approximately 30 to 50 nm (about one-millionth of an inch) wide. (If an electrical synapse with its gap junctions is like the threshold of a doorway between neurons, a synaptic cleft is like a good-size lake between them.)

Because the current from the presynaptic membrane dissipates in the fluid-filled cleft, chemical synapses effectively prevent a nerve impulse from being *directly* transmitted from one neuron to another. Instead, an impulse is transmitted via a *chemical event* that depends on the release, diffusion, and receptor binding of neurotransmitter molecules and results in *unidirectional communication* between neurons.

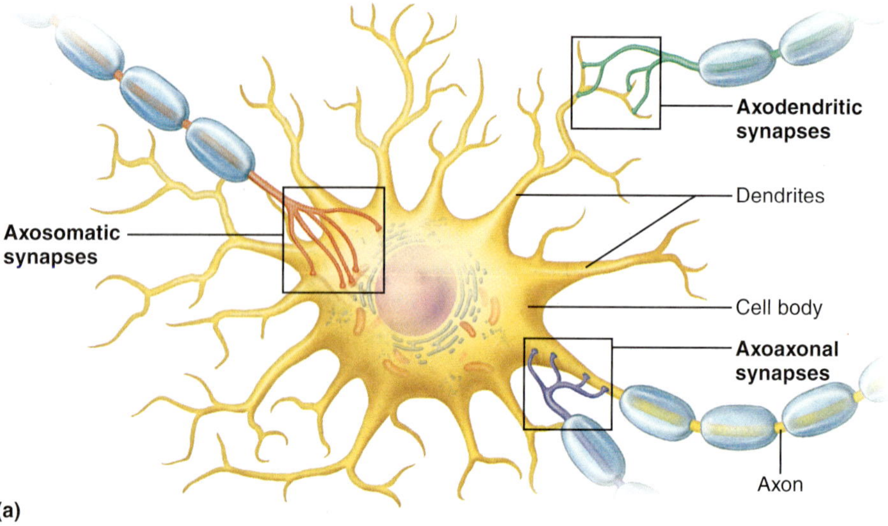

(a)

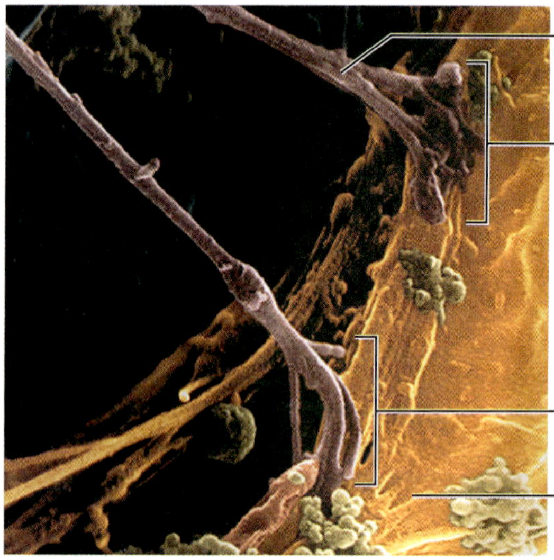

(b)

Figure 11.16 Synapses. (a) Axodendritic, axosomatic, and axoaxonal synapses. **(b)** Scanning electron micrograph of incoming fibers at axosomatic synapses (5300×).

In short, transmission of nerve impulses along an axon and across electrical synapses is a purely electrical event. However, chemical synapses convert the electrical signals to chemical signals (neurotransmitters) that travel across the synapse to the postsynaptic cells, where they are converted back into electrical signals.

Information Transfer Across Chemical Synapses

In Chapter 9 we introduced a specialized chemical synapse called a neuromuscular junction (p. 286). The chain of events that occurs at the neuromuscular junction is simply one example of the general process that we will discuss next and show in *Focus on a Chemical Synapse* **(Figure 11.17)**:

① **Action potential arrives at axon terminal.** Neurotransmission at a chemical synapse begins with the arrival of an action potential at the presynaptic axon terminal.

② **Voltage-gated Ca^{2+} channels open and Ca^{2+} enters the axon terminal.** Depolarization of the membrane by the action potential opens not only Na^+ channels but voltage-gated Ca^{2+} channels as well. During the brief time the Ca^{2+} channels are open, Ca^{2+} floods down its electrochemical gradient from the extracellular fluid into the terminal.

③ **Ca^{2+} entry causes synaptic vesicles to release neurotransmitter by exocytosis.** The surge of Ca^{2+} into the axon terminal acts as an intracellular messenger. A Ca^{2+}-sensing protein (*synaptotagmin*) binds Ca^{2+} and interacts with the SNARE proteins that control membrane fusion (see Figure 3.14). As a result, synaptic vesicles fuse with the axon membrane and empty their contents by exocytosis into the synaptic cleft. Ca^{2+} is then quickly removed from the terminal—either taken up into the mitochondria or ejected from the neuron by an active Ca^{2+} pump.

Figure 11.17 Chemical synapses transmit signals from one neuron to another using neurotransmitters.

A&P Flix Available at www.masteringaandp.com

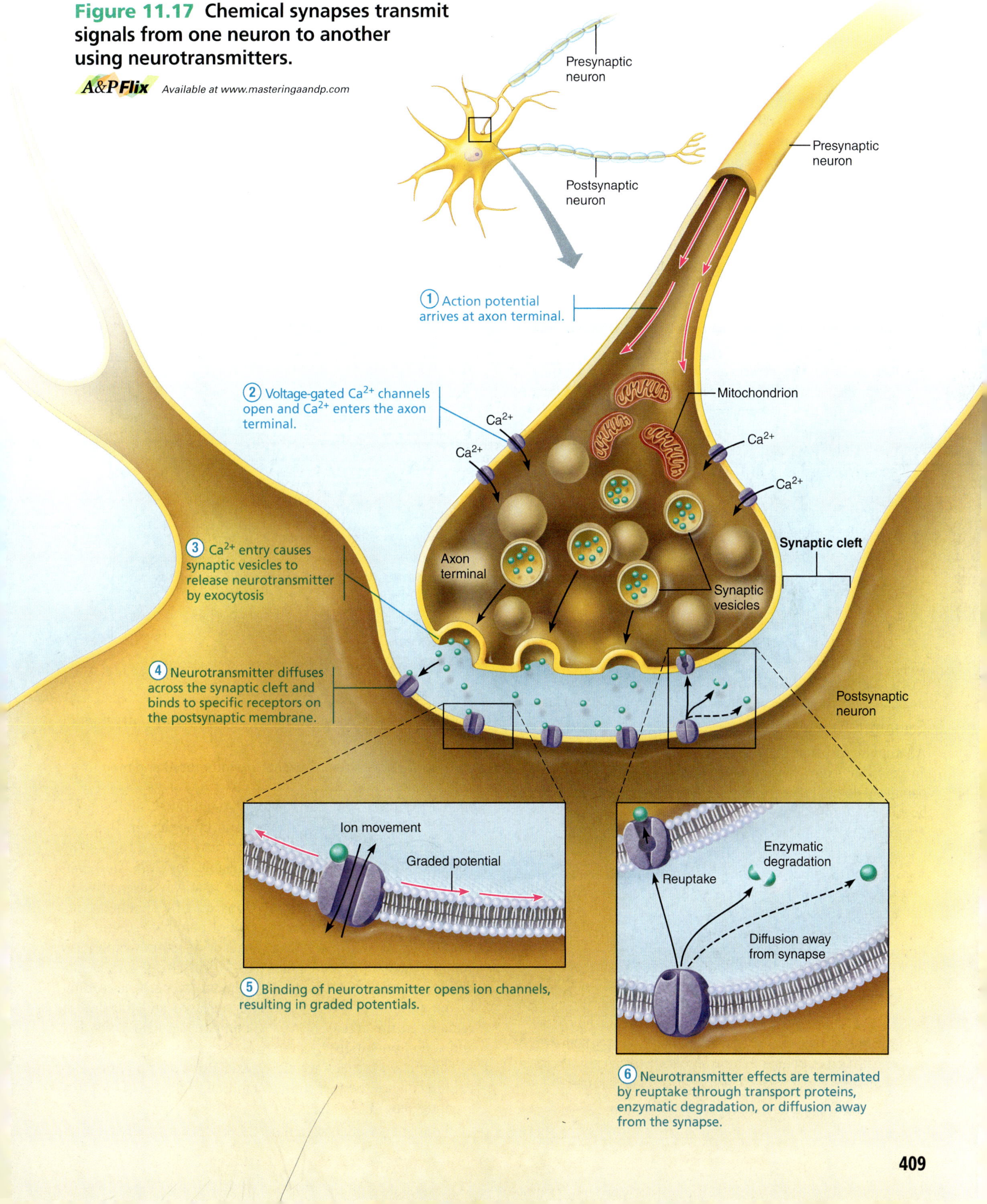

5 Binding of neurotransmitter opens ion channels, resulting in graded potentials.

6 Neurotransmitter effects are terminated by reuptake through transport proteins, enzymatic degradation, or diffusion away from the synapse.

For each nerve impulse reaching the presynaptic terminal, many vesicles (perhaps 300) empty into the synaptic cleft. The higher the impulse frequency (that is, the more intense the stimulus), the greater the number of synaptic vesicles that fuse and spill their contents, and the greater the effect on the postsynaptic cell.

4. **Neurotransmitter diffuses across the synaptic cleft and binds to specific receptors on the postsynaptic membrane.**

5. **Binding of neurotransmitter opens ion channels, creating graded potentials.** When neurotransmitter binds to the receptor protein, this receptor changes its three-dimensional shape. This change in turn opens ion channels and creates graded potentials. Postsynaptic membranes often contain receptor proteins and ion channels packaged together as chemically gated ion channels. Depending on the receptor protein to which the neurotransmitter binds and the type of channel the receptor controls, the postsynaptic neuron may be either excited or inhibited.

6. **Neurotransmitter effects are terminated.** The binding of a neurotransmitter to its receptor is reversible. As long as it is bound to a postsynaptic receptor, a neurotransmitter continues to affect membrane permeability and block reception of additional signals from presynaptic neurons. For this reason, some means of "wiping the postsynaptic slate clean" is necessary. The effects of neurotransmitters generally last a few milliseconds before being terminated in one of three ways, depending on the particular neurotransmitter:
   - *Reuptake* by astrocytes or the presynaptic terminal, where the neurotransmitter is stored or destroyed by enzymes, as with norepinephrine
   - *Degradation* by enzymes associated with the postsynaptic membrane or present in the synapse, as with acetylcholine
   - *Diffusion* away from the synapse

Synaptic Delay

An impulse may travel at speeds of up to 150 m/s (300 mi/h) down an axon, but neural transmission across a chemical synapse is comparatively slow. It reflects the time required for neurotransmitter to be released, diffuse across the synaptic cleft, and bind to receptors. Typically, this **synaptic delay** lasts 0.3–5.0 ms, making transmission across the chemical synapse the *rate-limiting* (slowest) step of neural transmission. Synaptic delay helps explain why transmission along neural pathways involving only two or three neurons occurs rapidly, but transmission along multisynaptic pathways typical of higher mental functioning occurs much more slowly. However, in practical terms these differences are not noticeable.

Check Your Understanding

15. What structure joins two neurons at an electrical synapse?

16. Events at a chemical synapse usually involve opening both voltage-gated ion channels and chemically gated ion channels. Where are these ion channels located and what causes each to open?

For answers, see Appendix H.

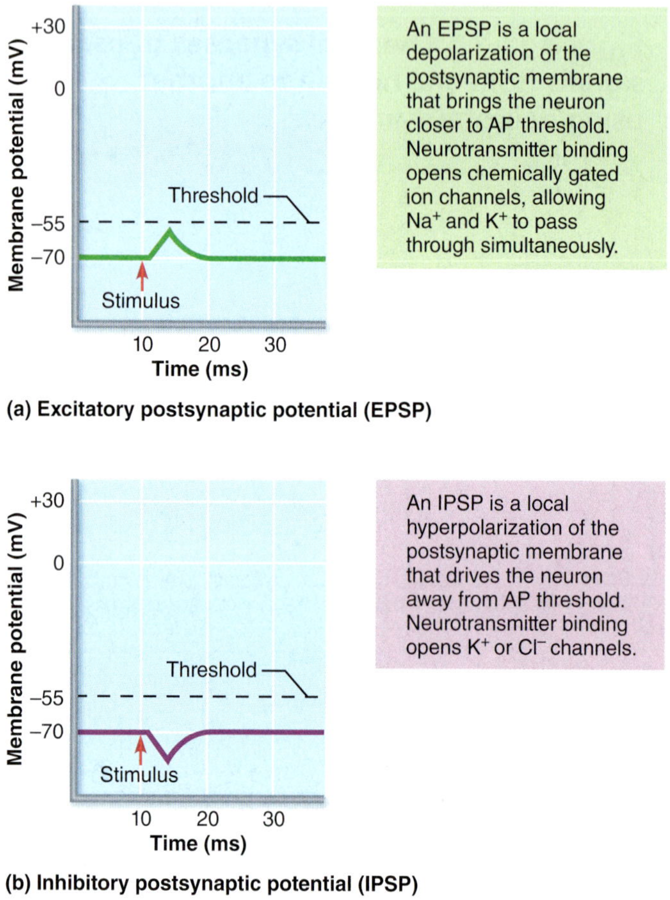

Figure 11.18 Postsynaptic potentials can be excitatory or inhibitory.

Postsynaptic Potentials and Synaptic Integration

✓ Distinguish between excitatory and inhibitory postsynaptic potentials.

✓ Describe how synaptic events are integrated and modified.

Many receptors on postsynaptic membranes at chemical synapses are specialized to open ion channels, in this way converting chemical signals to electrical signals. Unlike the voltage-gated ion channels responsible for APs, however, these chemically gated channels are relatively insensitive to changes in membrane potential. Consequently, channel opening at postsynaptic membranes cannot possibly become self-amplifying or self-generating. Instead, neurotransmitter receptors mediate graded potentials—local changes in membrane potential that are *graded* (vary in strength) according to the amount of neurotransmitter released and the time it remains in the area. **Table 11.2** compares graded potentials and action potentials.

Chemical synapses are either excitatory or inhibitory, depending on how they affect the membrane potential of the postsynaptic neuron.

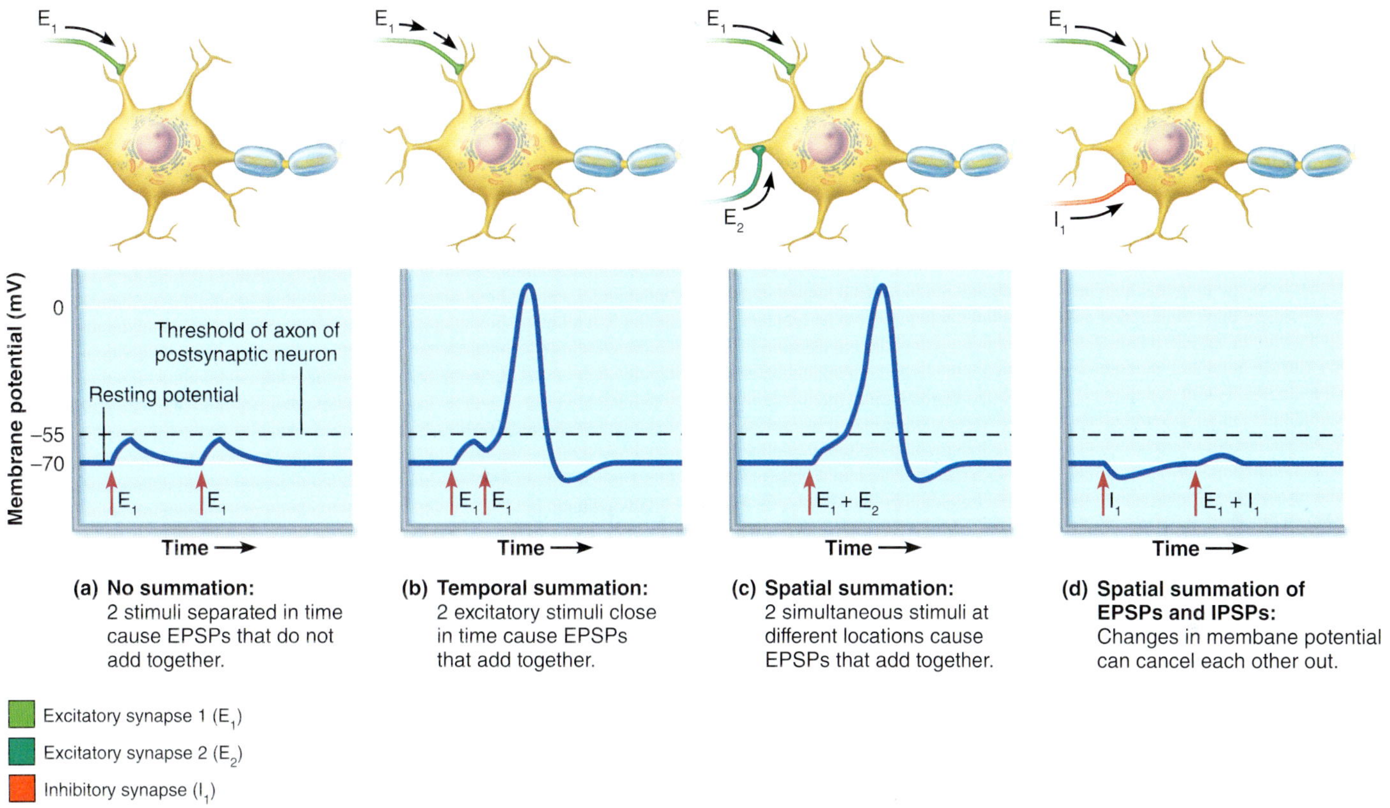

Figure 11.19 Neural integration of EPSPs and IPSPs.

Excitatory Synapses and EPSPs

At excitatory synapses, neurotransmitter binding depolarizes the postsynaptic membrane. However, in contrast to what happens on axon membranes, *chemically gated* ion channels open on postsynaptic membranes (those of dendrites and neuronal cell bodies). Each channel allows Na^+ and K^+ to diffuse *simultaneously* through the membrane but in opposite directions.

Although this two-way cation flow may appear to be self-defeating when depolarization is the goal, remember that the electrochemical gradient for sodium is much steeper than that for potassium. As a result, Na^+ influx is greater than K^+ efflux, and *net* depolarization occurs.

If enough neurotransmitter binds, depolarization of the postsynaptic membrane can reach 0 mV, which is well above an axon's threshold (about −50 mV) for "firing off" an AP. However, unlike axons which have voltage-gated channels that make an AP possible, *postsynaptic membranes generally do not generate APs*. The dramatic polarity reversal seen in axons never occurs in membranes containing *only* chemically gated channels because the opposite movements of K^+ and Na^+ prevent excessive positive charge from accumulating inside the cell. For this reason, instead of APs, local graded depolarization events called **excitatory postsynaptic potentials (EPSPs)** occur at excitatory postsynaptic membranes **(Figure 11.18a)**.

Each EPSP lasts a few milliseconds and then the membrane returns to its resting potential. The only function of EPSPs is to help trigger an AP distally at the axon hillock of the postsynaptic neuron. Although currents created by individual EPSPs decline with distance, they can and often do spread all the way to the axon hillock. If currents reaching the hillock are strong enough to depolarize the axon to threshold, axonal voltage-gated channels open and an AP is generated.

Inhibitory Synapses and IPSPs

Binding of neurotransmitters at inhibitory synapses *reduces* a postsynaptic neuron's ability to generate an AP. Most inhibitory neurotransmitters hyperpolarize the postsynaptic membrane by making the membrane more permeable to K^+ or Cl^-. Sodium ion permeability is not affected.

If K^+ channels open, K^+ moves out of the cell. If Cl^- channels open, Cl^- moves in. In either case, the charge on the inner face of the membrane becomes more negative. As the membrane potential increases and is driven farther from the axon's threshold, the postsynaptic neuron becomes *less and less likely* to "fire," and larger depolarizing currents are required to induce an AP. Hyperpolarizing changes in potential are called **inhibitory postsynaptic potentials (IPSPs)** (Figure 11.18b).

Integration and Modification of Synaptic Events

Summation by the Postsynaptic Neuron A single EPSP cannot induce an AP in the postsynaptic neuron **(Figure 11.19a)**. But if thousands of excitatory axon terminals fire on the same postsynaptic membrane, or if a small number of terminals deliver impulses rapidly, the probability of reaching threshold soars. EPSPs can add together, or **summate**, to influence the

Table 11.2 Comparison of Graded Potentials and Action Potentials

	GRADED POTENTIAL (GP)	ACTION POTENTIAL (AP)
Location of event	Cell body and dendrites, typically	Axon hillock and axon
	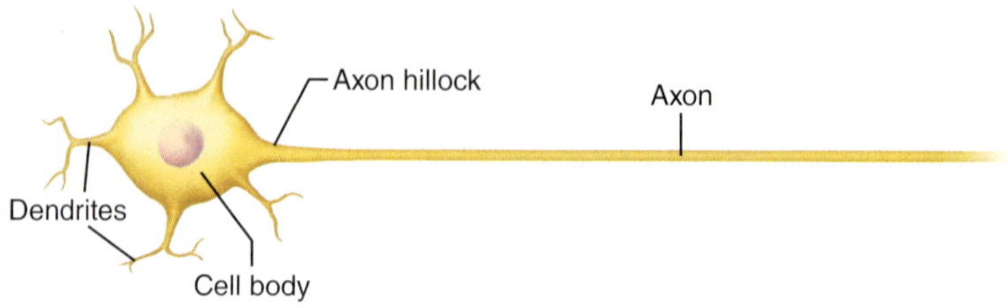	
Distance traveled	Short distance—typically within cell body to axon hillock (0.1–1.0 mm)	Long distance—from trigger zone at axon hillock through entire length of axon (a few mm to over a meter)
	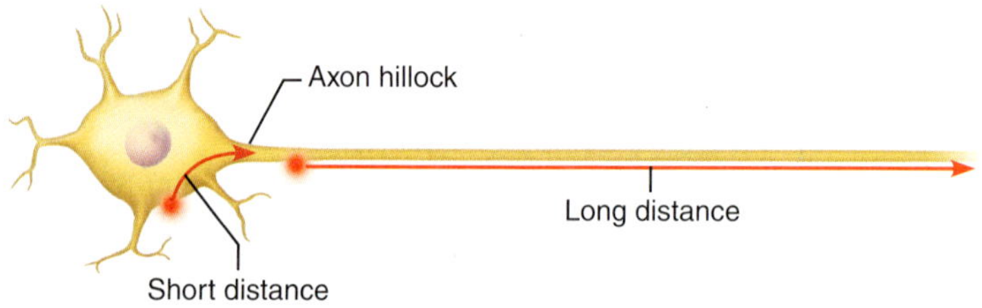	
Amplitude (size)	Various sizes (graded); decays with distance	Always the same size (all-or-none); does not decay with distance
Stimulus for opening ion channels	Chemical (neurotransmitter) or sensory stimulus (e.g., light, pressure, temperature)	Voltage (depolarization, triggered by GP reaching threshold)
Positive feedback cycle	Absent	Present
Repolarization	Voltage independent; occurs when stimulus is no longer present	Voltage regulated; occurs when Na^+ channels inactivate and K^+ channels open
Summation	Stimulus responses can summate to increase amplitude of graded potential	Does not occur; an all-or-none phenomenon
	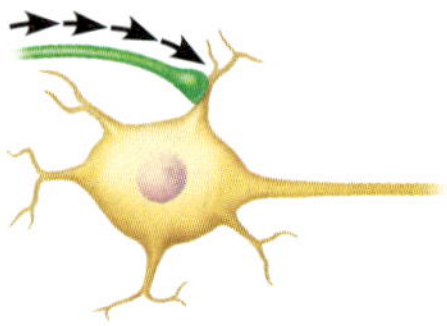 Temporal: increased frequency of stimuli 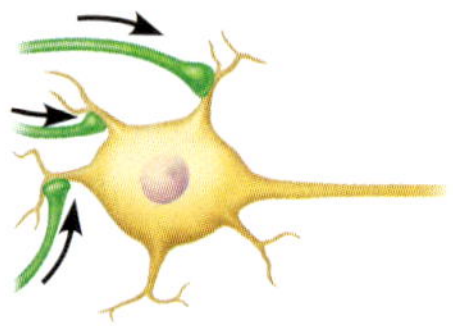 Spatial: stimuli from multiple sources	

activity of a postsynaptic neuron. Otherwise, nerve impulses would never result.

Two types of summation occur: temporal and spatial.

- **Temporal summation** (*temporal* = time) occurs when one or more presynaptic neurons transmit impulses in rapid-fire order and bursts of neurotransmitter are released in quick succession. The first impulse produces a small EPSP, and before it dissipates, successive impulses trigger more EPSPs. These summate, causing the postsynaptic membrane to depolarize much more than it would from a single EPSP (Figure 11.19b).
- **Spatial summation** occurs when the postsynaptic neuron is stimulated simultaneously by a large number of terminals from one or, more commonly, many presynaptic neurons. Huge numbers of its receptors bind neurotransmitter and simultaneously initiate EPSPs, which summate and dramatically enhance depolarization (Figure 11.19c).

Although we have focused on EPSPs here, IPSPs also summate, both temporally and spatially. In this case, the postsynaptic neuron is inhibited to a greater degree.

Most neurons receive both excitatory and inhibitory inputs from thousands of other neurons. Additionally, the same axon may form different types of synapses (in terms

Table 11.2 *(continued)*

	GRADED POTENTIAL (GP)		ACTION POTENTIAL (AP)
	POSTSYNAPTIC POTENTIAL (A TYPE OF GP)		
	EXCITATORY (EPSP)	**INHIBITORY (IPSP)**	
Function	Short-distance signaling; depolarization that spreads to axon hillock; moves membrane potential *toward* threshold for generating an AP	Short-distance signaling; hyperpolarization that spreads to axon hillock; moves membrane potential *away* from threshold for generating an AP	Long-distance signaling; constitutes the nerve impulse
Initial effect of stimulus	Opens chemically gated channels that allow simultaneous Na^+ and K^+ fluxes 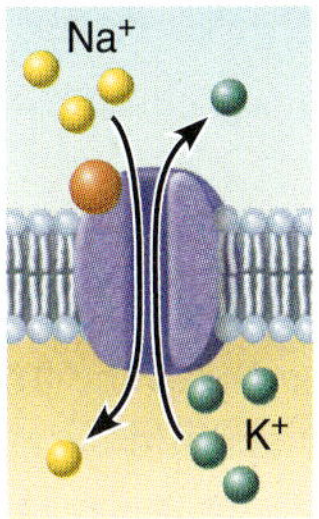	Opens chemically gated K^+ or Cl^- channels 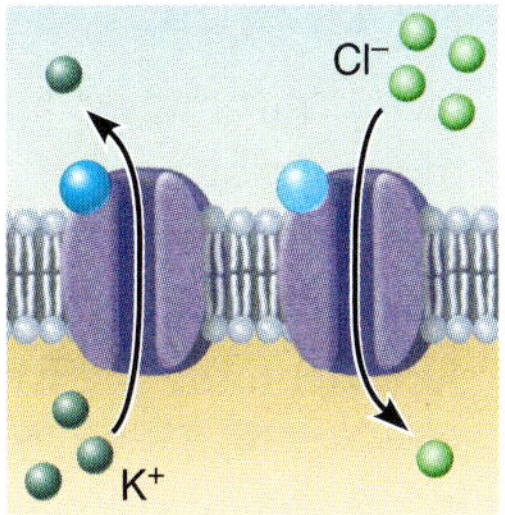	Opens voltage-gated channels; first opens Na^+ channels, then K^+ channels 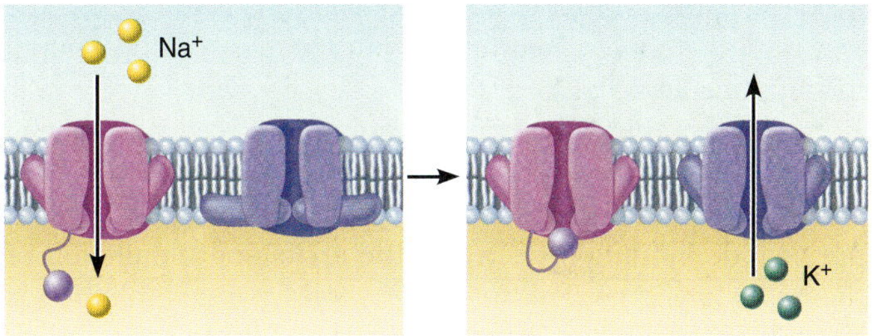
Peak membrane potential	Depolarizes; moves toward 0 mV 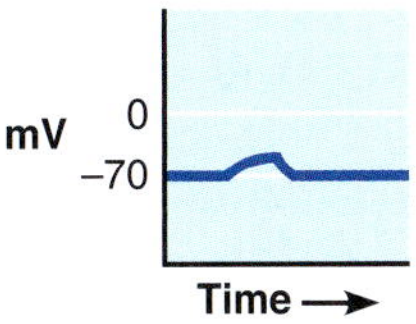	Hyperpolarizes; moves toward −90 mV 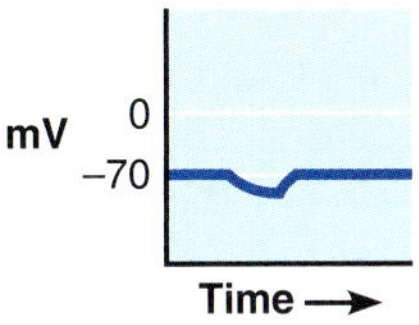	+30 to +50 mV 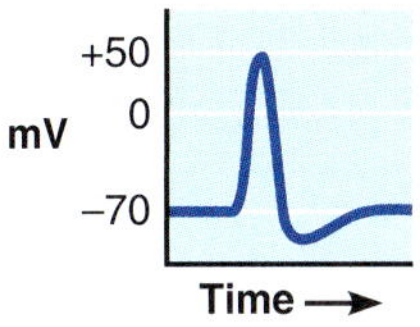

of biochemical and electrical characteristics) with different types of target neurons. How is all this conflicting information sorted out?

Each neuron's axon hillock keeps a running account of all the signals it receives. Not only do EPSPs summate and IPSPs summate, but also EPSPs summate with IPSPs. If the stimulatory effects of EPSPs dominate the membrane potential enough to reach threshold, the neuron will fire. If summation yields only subthreshold depolarization or hyperpolarization, the neuron fails to generate an AP (Figure 11.19d).

However, partially depolarized neurons are **facilitated**—that is, more easily excited by successive depolarization events—because they are already near threshold. Thus, axon hillock membranes function as *neural integrators*, and their potential at any time reflects the sum of all incoming neural information.

Because EPSPs and IPSPs are graded potentials that decay the farther they spread, the most effective synapses are those closest to the axon hillock. Specifically, inhibitory synapses are most effective when located between the site of excitatory inputs and the site of action potential generation (the axon hillock). Accordingly, inhibitory synapses occur most often on the cell body and excitatory synapses occur most often on the dendrites (Figure 11.19d).

Synaptic Potentiation Repeated or continuous use of a synapse (even for short periods) enhances the presynaptic neuron's ability to excite the postsynaptic neuron, producing larger-than-expected EPSPs. This phenomenon is called **synaptic potentiation**. The presynaptic terminals at such synapses contain relatively high Ca^{2+} concentrations, a condition that triggers the release of more neurotransmitter, which in turn produces larger EPSPs.

Synaptic potentiation also brings about Ca^{2+} influx via dendritic spines into the postsynaptic neuron. Brief high-frequency stimulation partially depolarizes the postsynaptic membrane. This partial depolarization causes certain chemically gated channels called *NMDA (N-methyl-D-aspartate) receptors* to allow Ca^{2+} to enter, something that only happens when the membrane is depolarized. As Ca^{2+} floods into the cell, it activates certain kinase enzymes that promote changes resulting in more effective responses to subsequent stimuli.

In some neurons, APs generated at the axon hillock propagate back up into the dendrites. This current flow may alter the effectiveness of synapses by opening voltage-gated Ca^{2+} channels, again allowing Ca^{2+} into the dendrites and promoting synaptic potentiation.

Synaptic potentiation can be viewed as a learning process that increases the efficiency of neurotransmission along a particular pathway. Indeed, the hippocampus of the brain, which plays a special role in memory and learning, exhibits an important type of synaptic plasticity called *long-term potentiation* (LTP).

Presynaptic Inhibition Events at the presynaptic membrane can also influence postsynaptic activity. **Presynaptic inhibition** occurs when the release of excitatory neurotransmitter by one neuron is inhibited by the activity of another neuron via an axoaxonal synapse. More than one mechanism is involved, but the end result is that less neurotransmitter is released and bound, forming smaller EPSPs.

Notice that this is the opposite of what we see with synaptic potentiation. In contrast to postsynaptic inhibition by IPSPs, which decreases the excitability of the postsynaptic neuron, presynaptic inhibition decreases the excitatory stimulation of the postsynaptic neuron. In this way, presynaptic inhibition is like a functional synaptic "pruning."

11

☑ Check Your Understanding

17. Which ions flow through chemically gated channels to produce IPSPs? EPSPs?
18. What is the difference between temporal summation and spatial summation?

For answers, see Appendix H.

Neurotransmitters and Their Receptors

✓ Define neurotransmitter and name several classes of neurotransmitters.

Neurotransmitters, along with electrical signals, are the "language" of the nervous system—the means by which each neuron communicates with others to process and send messages to the rest of the body. Sleep, thought, rage, hunger, memory, movement, and even your smile reflect the "doings" of these versatile molecules. Most factors that affect synaptic transmission do so by enhancing or inhibiting neurotransmitter release or destruction, or by blocking their binding to receptors. Just as speech defects may hinder interpersonal communication, anything that interferes with neurotransmitter activity may short-circuit the brain's "conversations" or internal talk (see *A Closer Look* on pp. 418–419).

At present, more than 50 neurotransmitters or neurotransmitter candidates have been identified. Although some neurons produce and release only one kind of neurotransmitter, most make two or more and may release any one or all of them at a given time. It appears that in most cases, different neurotransmitters are released at different stimulation frequencies, a restriction that avoids producing a jumble of nonsense messages. However, co-release of two neurotransmitters from the same vesicles has been documented. The coexistence of more than one neurotransmitter in a single neuron makes it possible for that cell to exert several influences rather than one discrete effect.

Neurotransmitters are classified chemically and functionally. **Table 11.3** provides a detailed overview of neurotransmitters, and we describe some of them here. No one expects you to memorize this table at this point, but it will be a handy reference for you to look back at when you read about neurotransmitters in subsequent chapters.

Classification of Neurotransmitters by Chemical Structure

Neurotransmitters fall into several chemical classes based on molecular structure.

Acetylcholine

Acetylcholine (ACh) (as″ĕ-til-ko′lēn), the first neurotransmitter identified, is still the best understood because it is released at neuromuscular junctions, which are much easier to study than synapses buried in the CNS.

ACh is synthesized from acetic acid (as acetyl CoA) and choline by the enzyme *choline acetyltransferase*, then transported into synaptic vesicles for later release. Once released by the presynaptic terminal, ACh binds briefly to the postsynaptic receptors. Then it is released and degraded to acetic acid and choline by the enzyme **acetylcholinesterase (AChE)**, located in the synaptic cleft and on postsynaptic membranes. Presynaptic terminals recapture the released choline and reuse it to synthesize more ACh.

ACh is released by all neurons that stimulate skeletal muscles and by some neurons of the autonomic nervous system. ACh-releasing neurons are also found in the CNS.

Biogenic Amines

The **biogenic amines** (bi″o-jen′ik) include the **catecholamines** (kat″ĕ-kol′ah-mēnz), such as dopamine, norepinephrine (NE), and epinephrine, and the **indolamines**, which include serotonin and histamine. *Dopamine* and *NE* are synthesized from the amino acid tyrosine in a common pathway consisting of several steps. The epinephrine-releasing cells of the brain and adrenal medulla use the same pathway. *Serotonin* is synthesized from the amino acid tryptophan. *Histamine* is synthesized from the amino acid histidine.

Biogenic amine neurotransmitters are broadly distributed in the brain, where they play a role in emotional behavior and help regulate the biological clock. Additionally, some motor neurons of the autonomic nervous system release catecholamines, particularly NE. Imbalances of these neurotransmitters are associated with mental illness. For example, overactive dopamine signaling occurs in schizophrenia. Additionally, certain psychoactive

Table 11.3 Neurotransmitters and Neuromodulators

NEUROTRANSMITTER	FUNCTIONAL CLASSES	SITES WHERE SECRETED	COMMENTS
Acetylcholine (ACh)			
▪ At *nicotinic ACh receptors* (on skeletal muscles, autonomic ganglia, and in the CNS) ▪ At *muscarinic ACh receptors* (on visceral effectors and in the CNS)	Excitatory Direct action Excitatory or inhibitory depending on subtype of muscarinic receptor Indirect action via second messengers	CNS: widespread throughout cerebral cortex, hippocampus, and brain stem PNS: all neuromuscular junctions with skeletal muscle; some autonomic motor endings (all preganglionic and parasympathetic postganglionic fibers)	Effects prolonged when AChE blocked by nerve gas or organophosphate insecticides (malathion), leading to tetanic muscle spasms. Release inhibited by botulinum toxin; binding to nicotinic ACh receptors inhibited by curare (a muscle paralytic agent) and to muscarinic ACh receptors by atropine. ACh levels decrease in certain brain areas in Alzheimer's disease; nicotinic ACh receptors destroyed in myasthenia gravis. Binding of nicotine to nicotinic receptors in the brain enhances dopamine release, which may account for the behavioral effects of nicotine in smokers.
Biogenic Amines			
Norepinephrine (NE)	Excitatory or inhibitory depending on receptor type bound Indirect action via second messengers	CNS: brain stem, particularly in the locus coeruleus of the midbrain; limbic system; some areas of cerebral cortex PNS: main neurotransmitter of postganglionic neurons in the sympathetic nervous system	A "feel good" neurotransmitter. Release enhanced by amphetamines; removal from synapse blocked by tricyclic antidepressants [amitriptyline (Elavil) and others] and cocaine. Brain levels reduced by reserpine (an antihypertensive drug), leading to depression.
Dopamine	Excitatory or inhibitory depending on the receptor type bound Indirect action via second messengers	CNS: substantia nigra of midbrain; hypothalamus; the principal neurotransmitter of indirect motor pathways PNS: some sympathetic ganglia	A "feel good" neurotransmitter. Release enhanced by L-dopa and amphetamines; reuptake blocked by cocaine. Deficient in Parkinson's disease; dopamine neurotransmission increases in schizophrenia.
Serotonin (5-HT)	Mainly inhibitory Indirect action via second messengers; direct action at 5-HT_3 receptors	CNS: brain stem, especially midbrain; hypothalamus; limbic system; cerebellum; pineal gland; spinal cord	Plays a role in sleep, appetite, nausea, migraine headaches, and regulating mood. Drugs that block its uptake [fluoxetine (Prozac)] relieve anxiety and depression. Activity blocked by LSD and enhanced by ecstasy (MDMA).
Histamine	Excitatory or inhibitory depending on receptor type bound Indirect action via second messengers	CNS: hypothalamus	Involved in wakefulness, appetite control, and learning and memory. Also a paracrine (local signal) released from stomach (causes acid secretion) and connective tissue mast cells (mediates inflammation and vasodilation).
Amino Acids			
GABA (γ-aminobutyric acid)	Generally inhibitory Direct and indirect actions via second messengers	CNS: cerebral cortex, hypothalamus, Purkinje cells of cerebellum, spinal cord, granule cells of olfactory bulb, retina	Principal inhibitory neurotransmitter in the brain; important in presynaptic inhibition at axoaxonal synapses. Inhibitory effects augmented by alcohol, antianxiety drugs of the benzodiazepine class (e.g., Valium), and barbiturates, impairing motor coordination. Substances that block its synthesis, release, or action induce convulsions.

➤

Table 11.3 Neurotransmitters and Neuromodulators *(continued)*

NEUROTRANSMITTER	FUNCTIONAL CLASSES	SITES WHERE SECRETED	COMMENTS
Amino Acids, continued			
Glutamate	Generally excitatory Direct action	CNS: spinal cord; widespread in brain where it represents the major excitatory neurotransmitter	Important in learning and memory. The "stroke neurotransmitter": excessive release produces excitotoxicity—neurons literally stimulated to death; most commonly caused by ischemia (oxygen deprivation, usually due to a blocked blood vessel).
Glycine	Generally inhibitory Direct action	CNS: spinal cord and brain stem, retina	Principal inhibitory neurotransmitter of the spinal cord. Strychnine blocks glycine receptors, resulting in uncontrolled convulsions and respiratory arrest.
Peptides			
Endorphins, e.g., beta endorphin, dynorphin, enkephalins	Generally inhibitory Indirect action via second messengers	CNS: widely distributed in brain; hypothalamus; limbic system; pituitary; spinal cord	Natural opiates; inhibit pain by inhibiting substance P. Effects mimicked by morphine, heroin, and methadone.
Tachykinins: substance P, neurokinin A (NKA)	Excitatory Indirect action via second messengers	CNS: basal nuclei, midbrain, hypothalamus, cerebral cortex PNS: certain sensory neurons of dorsal root ganglia (pain afferents), enteric neurons	Substance P mediates pain transmission in the PNS. In the CNS, tachykinins are involved in respiratory and cardiovascular controls and in mood.
Somatostatin	Generally inhibitory Indirect action via second messengers	CNS: hypothalamus, septum, basal nuclei, hippocampus, cerebral cortex Pancreas	Often released with GABA. A gut-brain peptide. Inhibits growth hormone release.
Cholecystokinin (CCK)	Generally excitatory Indirect action via second messengers	Throughout CNS Small intestine	Involved in anxiety, pain, memory. A gut-brain peptide hormone. Inhibits appetite.
Purines			
ATP	Excitatory or inhibitory depending on receptor type bound Direct and indirect actions via second messengers	CNS: basal nuclei, induces Ca^{2+} wave propagation in astrocytes PNS: dorsal root ganglion neurons	ATP released by sensory neurons (as well as that released by injured cells) provokes pain sensation.
Adenosine	Generally inhibitory Indirect action via second messengers	Throughout CNS and PNS	Caffeine (coffee), theophylline (tea), and theobromine (chocolate) stimulate by blocking brain adenosine receptors. May be involved in sleep-wake cycle and terminating seizures. Dilates arterioles, increasing blood flow to heart and other tissues as needed.
Gases and Lipids			
Nitric oxide (NO)	Excitatory or inhibitory Indirect action via second messengers	CNS: brain, spinal cord PNS: adrenal gland; nerves to penis	Its release potentiates stroke damage. Some types of male impotence treated by enhancing NO action [e.g., with sildenafil (Viagra)].
Carbon monoxide (CO)	Excitatory or inhibitory Indirect action via second messengers	Brain and some neuromuscular and neuroglandular synapses	
Endocannabinoids, e.g., 2-arachidonoylglycerol, anandamide	Inhibitory Indirect action via second messengers	Throughout CNS	Involved in memory (as a retrograde messenger), appetite control, nausea and vomiting, neuronal development. Receptors activated by THC, the principal active ingredient of cannabis. Receptors also found on immune cells.

drugs (LSD and mescaline) can bind to biogenic amine receptors and induce hallucinations.

Amino Acids

It is difficult to prove a neurotransmitter role when the suspect is an amino acid, because amino acids occur in all cells of the body and are important in many biochemical reactions. The amino acids for which a neurotransmitter role is certain include **glutamate**, **aspartate**, **glycine**, and **gamma (γ)-aminobutyric acid (GABA)**, but there may be others.

Peptides

The **neuropeptides**, essentially strings of amino acids, include a broad spectrum of molecules with diverse effects. For example, a neuropeptide called **substance P** is an important mediator of pain signals. By contrast, **endorphins**, which include **beta endorphin**, **dynorphin**, and **enkephalins** (en-kef′ah-linz), act as natural opiates, reducing our perception of pain under stressful conditions. Enkephalin activity increases dramatically in pregnant women in labor. Endorphin release is enhanced when an athlete gets a so-called second wind and is probably responsible for the "runner's high." Additionally, some researchers claim that the placebo effect is due to endorphin release. These painkilling neurotransmitters remained undiscovered until investigators began to ask why morphine and other opiates reduce anxiety and pain, and found that these drugs attach to the same receptors that bind natural opiates, producing similar but stronger effects.

Some neuropeptides, known as **gut-brain peptides**, are also produced by nonneural body tissues and are widespread in the gastrointestinal tract. Examples include somatostatin and cholecystokinin (CCK).

Purines

Purines are nitrogen-containing chemicals (such as guanine and adenine) that are breakdown products of nucleic acids. **Adenosine triphosphate (ATP)**, the cell's universal form of energy, is now recognized as a major neurotransmitter (perhaps the most primitive one) in both the CNS and PNS. Like the receptors for glutamate and acetylcholine, certain receptors produce fast excitatory responses when ATP binds, while other ATP receptors trigger slow, second-messenger responses. Upon binding to receptors on astrocytes, ATP mediates Ca^{2+} influx.

In addition to the neurotransmitter action of extracellular ATP, **adenosine**, a part of ATP, also acts outside of cells on adenosine receptors. Adenosine is a potent inhibitor in the brain. Caffeine's well-known stimulatory effects result from blocking these adenosine receptors.

Gases and Lipids

Not so long ago, it would have been scientific suicide to suggest that small, short-lived, toxic gas molecules might be neurotransmitters. Nonetheless, the discovery of these unlikely messengers has opened up a new chapter in the story of neurotransmission.

Gasotransmitters These gases—the so-called "gasotransmitters" nitric oxide, carbon monoxide, and hydrogen sulfide—defy all the classical descriptions of neurotransmitters. Rather than being stored in vesicles and released by exocytosis, they are synthesized on demand and diffuse out of the cells that make them. Instead of attaching to surface receptors, they zoom through the plasma membrane of nearby cells to bind with particular intracellular receptors.

Both **nitric oxide (NO)** and **carbon monoxide (CO)** activate *guanylyl cyclase*, the enzyme that makes the second messenger *cyclic GMP*. NO and CO are found in different brain regions and appear to act in different pathways, but their mode of action is similar. NO participates in a variety of processes in the brain, including the formation of new memories by increasing the strength of certain synapses. In this process, neurotransmitter binding to the postsynaptic receptors indirectly activates *nitric oxide synthase* (*NOS*), the enzyme that makes NO. The newly synthesized NO diffuses out of the postsynaptic cell back to the presynaptic terminal, where it activates guanylyl cyclase. In this way NO is thought to act as a retrograde messenger that sends a signal to increase synaptic strength.

Excessive release of NO contributes to much of the brain damage seen in stroke patients (see p. 463). In the myenteric plexus of the intestine, NO causes intestinal smooth muscle to relax.

Less is known about **hydrogen sulfide (H_2S)**, the most recently discovered gasotransmitter. Unlike NO and CO, it appears to act directly on ion channels and other proteins to alter their function.

11

Endocannabinoids Just as there are natural opiate neurotransmitters in the brain, our brains make natural neurotransmitters, the **endocannabinoids** (en″do-kă-nă′bĭ-noids), that act at the same receptors as tetrahydrocannabinol (THC), the active ingredient in marijuana. Their receptors, the *cannabinoid receptors*, are the most common G protein–linked receptors in the brain.

Like the gasotransmitters, the endocannabinoids are lipid soluble and are synthesized on demand, rather than stored and released from vesicles. Endocannabinoids are formed by clipping the cell's own plasma membrane lipids. The newly synthesized endocannabinoids diffuse freely from the postsynaptic neuron to their receptors on presynaptic terminals where they act as a retrograde messenger to decrease neurotransmitter release. Like NO, they are thought to be involved in learning and memory. We are only beginning to understand the many other processes these neurotransmitters may be involved in, which include neuronal development, controlling appetite, and suppressing nausea.

Classification of Neurotransmitters by Function

In this text we can only sample the incredible diversity of functions that neurotransmitters mediate. We limit our discussion here to two broad ways of classifying neurotransmitters according to function, adding more details in subsequent chapters.

A CLOSER LOOK

Pleasure Me, Pleasure Me!

Sex! Drugs! Rock 'n' roll! Eat, drink, and be merry! Why do we find these activities so compelling? Our brains are wired to **reward** us with **pleasure** when we engage in behavior that is necessary for our own and our species' **survival**. This reward system consists of dopamine-releasing neurons in areas of the brain called the *ventral tegmental area* (VTA), the *nucleus accumbens*, and the *amygdala*.

Our ability to "feel good" involves brain neurotransmitters in this reward system. For example, the ecstasy of romantic love may be just a brain bath of glutamate and norepinephrine, which act on the reward system to release dopamine.

Unfortunately, drugs of abuse can subvert this powerful system. The 1930s songwriter Cole Porter knew what he was talking about when he wrote "I get a kick out of you," because these neurotransmitters are chemical cousins of the amphetamines. People who use "crystal meth" (methamphetamine) artificially stimulate their brains to provide their highly addictive pleasure flush. However, their pleasure is short-lived, because when the brain is flooded with neurotransmitter-like chemicals from the outside, it makes less of its own (why bother?).

Cocaine, another reward system titillater, has been around since ancient times. Once a toy of the rich, its granular form is inhaled, or "snorted." The laws of supply and demand have now brought cheaper cocaine to the masses, notably "crack"—a cheaper, more potent, smokable form of cocaine. For $50 or so, a novice user can experience a rush of intense pleasure. But crack is treacherous and intensely addictive. It produces not only a higher high than the inhaled form of cocaine, but also a deeper crash that leaves the user desperate for more.

How does cocaine produce its effects? Basically, the drug stimulates the reward system and then "squeezes it dry." Cocaine produces its rush by hooking up to the dopamine reuptake transporter protein, blocking the reabsorption of dopamine. The neurotransmitter remains in the synapse and stimulates the postsynaptic receptor cells again and again, allowing the body to feel its effects over a prolonged period. This sensation is accompanied by increases in heart rate, blood pressure, and sexual appetite.

As repeated doses of cocaine continue to block dopamine uptake, the body releases less and less dopamine and the reward system effectively goes dry. The cocaine user becomes anxious and, in a very real sense, unable to experience pleasure without the drug. The postsynaptic cells

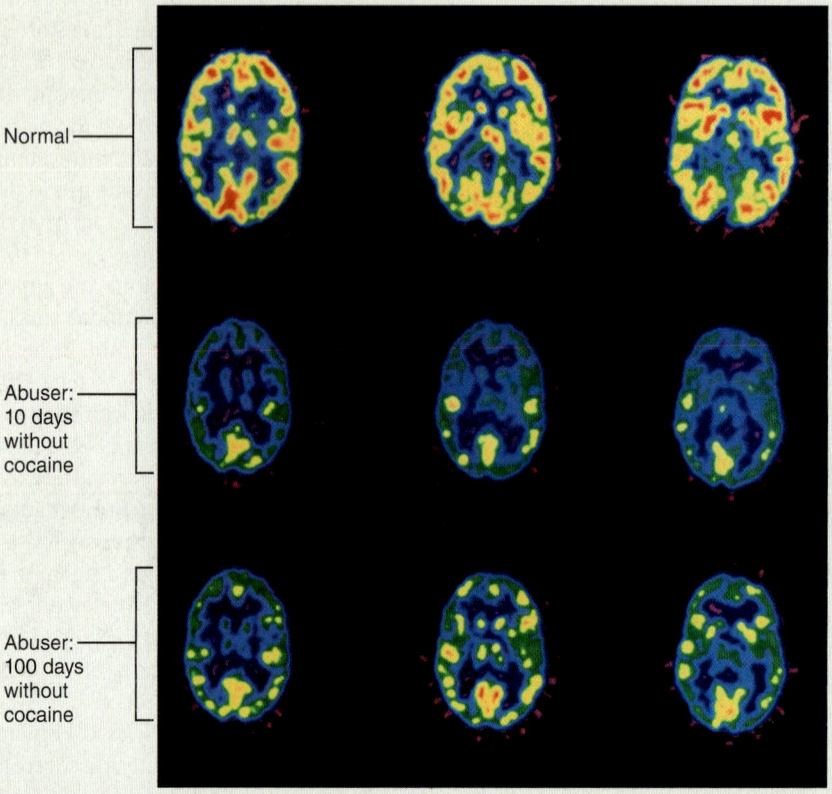

PET scans show that normal levels of brain activity (yellow and red) are depressed in cocaine users long after they stop using the drug.

The important idea to keep in mind is this: The function of a neurotransmitter is determined by the receptor to which it binds.

Effects: Excitatory Versus Inhibitory

Some neurotransmitters are excitatory (cause depolarization). Some are inhibitory (cause hyperpolarization). Others exert both effects, depending on the specific receptor types with which they interact.

For example, the amino acids GABA and glycine are usually inhibitory, whereas glutamate is typically excitatory (Table 11.3). On the other hand, ACh and NE each bind to at least two receptor types that cause opposite effects. For example, acetylcholine is excitatory at neuromuscular junctions in skeletal muscle and inhibitory in cardiac muscle.

Actions: Direct Versus Indirect

Neurotransmitters that act *directly* are those that bind to and open ion channels. These neurotransmitters provoke rapid responses in postsynaptic cells by altering membrane potential. ACh and the amino acid neurotransmitters are typically direct-acting neurotransmitters.

become hypersensitive and sprout new receptors in a desperate effort to pick up dopamine signals. A vicious cycle of addiction begins: Cocaine is needed to experience pleasure, but using it suppresses dopamine release even more.

The dopamine effect alone is not enough to establish addiction. Another neurotransmitter, glutamate, which plays an important role in learning, is required to maintain addiction. Glutamate signaling seems to cause more permanent changes in the brain (synaptic potentiation) that lead to compulsive drug-seeking behaviors elicited by external cues. Take, for example, mice genetically engineered to lack a particular glutamate receptor (GluR5). These mice are perfectly willing to try cocaine but never become addicted. (Of course, no GluR5 means they're none too bright, either.)

Current thinking, then, is that the rush of pleasure on taking cocaine is due to dopamine. Glutamate, on the other hand, is thought to be responsible for the learning that makes true the perception "once an addict, always an addict." So strong is the combined dopamine and glutamate system that, even years later, certain settings can trigger intense cravings for the drug.

These out-of-control, desperate cravings are notoriously difficult to manage. Drug abusers call it "jonesing." Traditional antiaddiction drugs take so long to reduce the cravings that users commonly drop out of treatment programs.

How can we break this cycle of addiction? One way is to prevent cocaine from ever reaching the brain. Promising results have been obtained from a vaccine that prompts the immune system to bind cocaine molecules, preventing them from entering the brain. In a clinical trial, this vaccine dampened addicts' pleasurable responses to cocaine and reduced their use of the drug.

Another approach to breaking the addiction cycle is to even out the highs and lows experienced by the drug user by leveling out brain dopamine levels and keep the user from "crashing" so badly. Possibilities include using a much longer-acting inhibitor of dopamine reuptake or taking a drug that binds but only partially activates dopamine receptors.

A final approach to breaking the addiction cycle is to interrupt the learned reinforcement that brings on cravings. An effective ancient African folk remedy called ibogaine may do exactly this. However, ibogaine itself is too toxic for clinical use, as some unfortunate "underground" users have discovered. A close synthetic cousin, 18-methoxycoronaridine (18-MC) is much less toxic and promises to be effective against not only cocaine but also a number of other abused drugs. Future studies will show if it truly works.

The craving for drugs has made some addicts very creative home pharmacologists, willing to experiment with practically anything, no matter how toxic or dangerous, to get the "buzz" they need. A cheap mixture of cold medications, match heads, and iodine in acetone yields crystal meth—the highly addictive and once-again popular drug that wrecks people's lives and often explodes their home laboratories. Another creative mixture, with the street name of "ill face" or "illy," involves dipping marijuana in formaldehyde, drying and then smoking it. Other remarkable combinations are the "H-bomb" (ecstasy mixed with heroin), "A-bomb" (marijuana with heroin or opium), "sextasy" [ecstasy mixed with sildenafil (Viagra)], "octane" (PCP laced with gasoline), and "ozone" (marijuana, PCP, and crack in a cigarette). Formaldehyde is known to cause cancer and gasoline damages the liver, but the real damage comes from the drugs themselves.

Take, for example, ecstasy, a drug that many of its users believe to be innocuous. In reality, ecstasy (MDMA) targets serotonin-releasing neurons. The "rush" of pleasure and energy that users feel is due to release of serotonin and other neurotransmitters. However, it damages and may destroy these neurons, causing the loss of verbal and spatial memory. Depression, sleeplessness, and memory problems may be permanent consequences—a steep price for a few moments of pleasure!

People who want pure, effective, and "safe" drugs of abuse don't get them on the street. They get them from doctors or "pill ladies" [female senior citizens who sell oxycodone (OxyContin), a powerful prescription opioid with effects similar to heroin]. Even people who would never dream of taking illicit drugs can be caught in the addictive cycle of prescription drugs. Prescribed legitimately to relieve severe pain, oxycodone is meant to be swallowed whole. Abusers crush the tablets and snort the powder or dissolve it in water and inject the solution. Abuse of oxycodone and its chemical cousin hydrocodone is spreading rapidly, doubling over the past four years. Medical examiners across North America report soaring rates of oxycodone-related emergency room visits and deaths. Indeed, emergency room visits caused by abuse of prescription or over-the-counter drugs now equal those for illicit drugs.

The brain, with its complex biochemistry, always circumvents attempts to keep it in a euphoric haze. Perhaps this means that pleasure must be transient by nature, experienced only against a background of its absence.

Neurotransmitters that act *indirectly* promote broader, longer-lasting effects by acting through intracellular *second-messenger* molecules, typically via G protein pathways (see Figure 3.16). In this way their action is similar to that of many hormones. The biogenic amines, neuropeptides, and dissolved gases are indirect neurotransmitters.

Neuromodulator is a term used to describe a chemical messenger released by a neuron that does not directly cause EPSPs or IPSPs but instead affects the strength of synaptic transmission. A neuromodulator may act presynaptically to influence the synthesis, release, degradation, or reuptake of neurotransmitter. Alternatively, a neuromodulator may act postsynaptically by altering the sensitivity of the postsynaptic membrane to neurotransmitter.

Receptors for neuromodulators are not necessarily found at a synapse. Instead, a neuromodulator may be released from one cell to act at many cells in its vicinity, similar to paracrines (chemical messengers that act locally and are quickly destroyed). The distinction between neurotransmitters and neuromodulators is fuzzy, but chemical messengers such as NO, adenosine, and a number of neuropeptides are often referred to as neuromodulators.

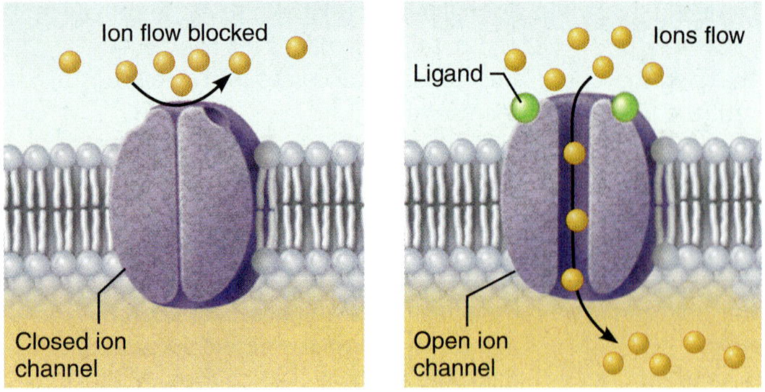

Figure 11.20 Direct neurotransmitter receptor mechanism: Channel-linked receptors. These chemically gated ion channels promote rapid synaptic transmission. In this case, ligand binding directly opens the channel.

Neurotransmitter Receptors

In Chapter 3, we introduced the various receptors involved in cell signaling. Now we are ready to pick up that thread again as we examine the action of receptors that bind neurotransmitters. For the most part, neurotransmitter receptors are either channel-linked receptors, which mediate fast synaptic transmission, or G protein–linked receptors, which oversee slow synaptic responses.

Channel-Linked Receptors: Mechanism of Action

Channel-linked receptors (*ionotropic receptors*) are ligand-gated ion channels that mediate direct neurotransmitter action. They are composed of several protein subunits in a "rosette" around a central pore. As the ligand binds to one (or more) receptor subunits, the proteins change shape. This event opens the central channel and allows ions to pass **(Figure 11.20)**. As a result, the membrane potential of the target cell changes.

Channel-linked receptors are always located precisely opposite sites of neurotransmitter release, and their ion channels open instantly upon ligand binding and remain open 1 ms or less while the ligand is bound. At excitatory receptor sites (nicotinic ACh channels and receptors for glutamate, aspartate, and ATP), the channel-linked receptors are cation channels that allow small cations (Na^+, K^+, Ca^{2+}) to pass, but Na^+ entry contributes most to membrane depolarization. Channel-linked receptors that respond to GABA and glycine, and allow Cl^- to pass, mediate fast inhibition (hyperpolarization).

G Protein–Linked Receptors: Mechanism of Action

Unlike responses to neurotransmitter binding at channel-linked receptors, which are immediate, simple, and brief, the activity mediated by **G protein–linked receptors** is indirect, complex, slow (hundreds of milliseconds or more), and often prolonged—ideal as a basis for some types of learning. Receptors in this class

11

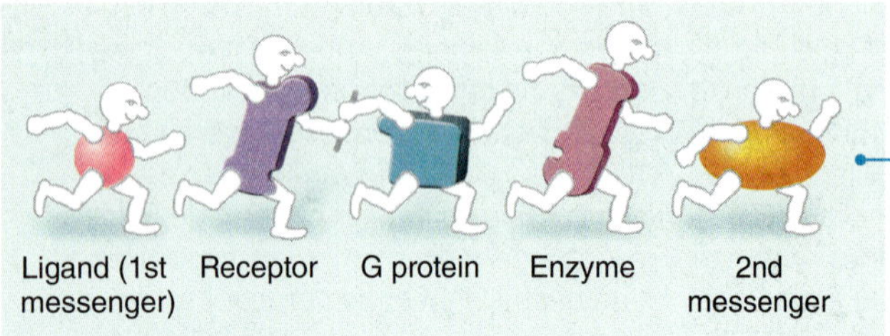

Recall from Chapter 3 that G protein signaling mechanisms are like a molecular relay race.

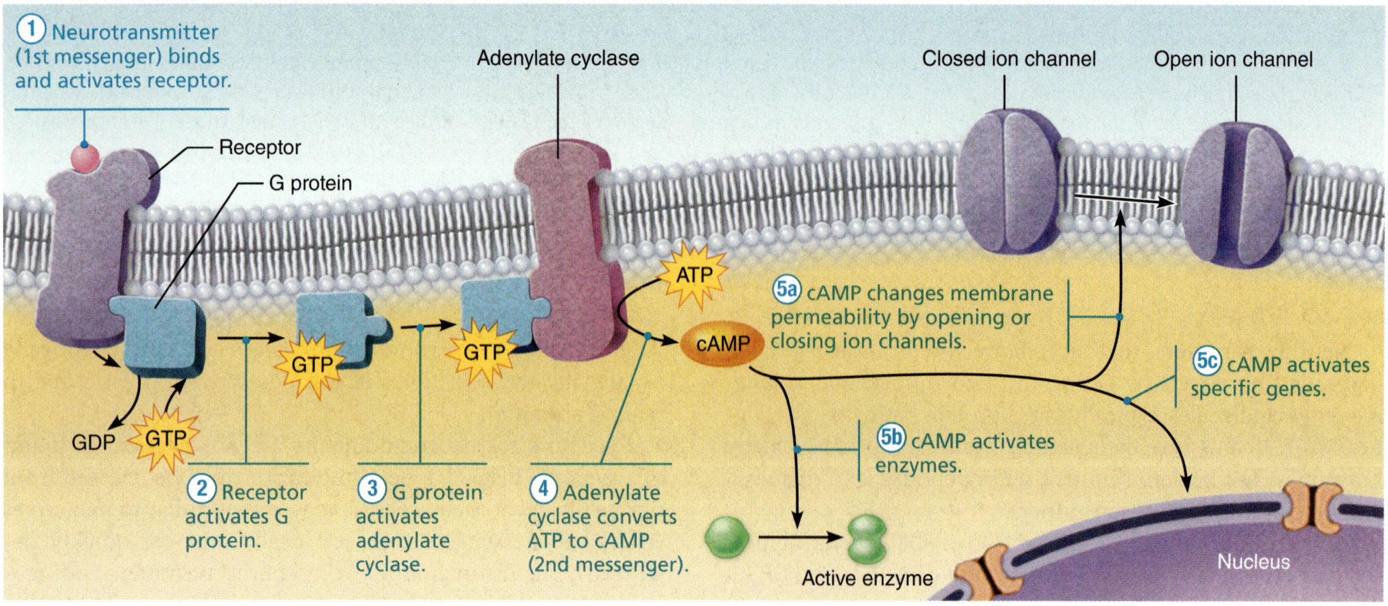

Figure 11.21 Indirect neurotransmitter receptor mechanism: G protein–linked receptors. These receptors cause the formation of intracellular second messengers—cyclic AMP (cAMP) in this example—that indirectly bring about the cell's response.

are transmembrane protein complexes. They include muscarinic ACh receptors and those that bind the biogenic amines and neuropeptides. Because their effects tend to bring about widespread metabolic changes, G protein–linked receptors are commonly called *metabotropic receptors*.

When a neurotransmitter binds to a G protein–linked receptor, the G protein is activated **(Figure 11.21)**. (To orient yourself, refer back to the simpler G protein explanation in Figure 3.16 on p. 82.) Activated G proteins typically work by controlling the production of second messengers such as **cyclic AMP**, **cyclic GMP**, **diacylglycerol**, or **Ca^{2+}**.

These second messengers, in turn, act as go-betweens to regulate (open or close) ion channels or activate kinase enzymes that initiate a cascade of enzymatic reactions in the target cells. Some second messengers modify (activate or inactivate) other proteins, including channel proteins, by attaching phosphate groups to them. Others interact with nuclear proteins that activate genes and induce synthesis of new proteins in the target cell.

Check Your Understanding

19. ACh excites skeletal muscle and yet it inhibits heart muscle. How can this be?
20. Why is cyclic AMP called a second messenger?

For answers, see Appendix H.

Basic Concepts of Neural Integration

Until now, we have concentrated on the activities of individual neurons. However, neurons function in groups, and each group contributes to still broader neural functions. In this way, the organization of the nervous system is hierarchical.

Any time you have a large number of *anything*—people included—there must be *integration*. In other words, the parts must be fused into a smoothly operating whole.

In this section, we move to the first level of **neural integration**: *neuronal pools* and their patterns of communicating with other parts of the nervous system. In Chapter 12 we discuss the highest levels of neural integration—how we think and remember. With this understanding of the basics and of the larger picture, in Chapter 13 we examine how sensory inputs interface with motor activity.

Organization of Neurons: Neuronal Pools

✓ Describe common patterns of neuronal organization and processing.

The billions of neurons in the CNS are organized into **neuronal pools**. These functional groups of neurons integrate incoming information received from receptors or different neuronal pools and then forward the processed information to other destinations.

In a simple type of neuronal pool **(Figure 11.22)**, one incoming presynaptic fiber branches profusely as it enters the pool and then synapses with several different neurons in the pool. When the incoming fiber is excited, it will excite some postsynaptic neurons and facilitate others. Neurons most likely to generate impulses are those closely associated with the incoming fiber, because they receive the bulk of the synaptic contacts. Those neurons are in the *discharge zone* of the pool.

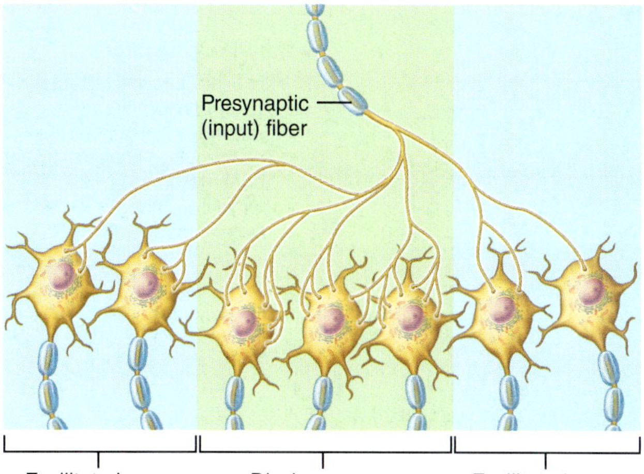

Figure 11.22 Simple neuronal pool. Postsynaptic neurons in the discharge zone receive more synapses and are more likely to discharge (generate APs). Postsynaptic neurons in the facilitated zone receive fewer synapses and are facilitated (brought closer to threshold).

Neurons farther from the center are not usually excited to threshold, but they are facilitated and can easily be brought to threshold by stimuli from another source. For this reason, the periphery of the pool is the *facilitated zone*. Keep in mind, however, that our figure is a gross oversimplification. Most neuronal pools consist of thousands of neurons and include inhibitory as well as excitatory neurons.

11

Types of Circuits

Individual neurons in a neuronal pool both send and receive information, and synaptic contacts may cause either excitation or inhibition. The patterns of synaptic connections in neuronal pools, called **circuits**, determine the pool's functional capabilities. **Figure 11.23** describes four basic circuit patterns and their properties: diverging, converging, reverberating, and parallel after-discharge circuits.

Patterns of Neural Processing

✓ Distinguish between serial and parallel processing.

Input processing is both *serial* and *parallel*. In serial processing, the input travels along one pathway to a specific destination. In parallel processing, the input travels along several different pathways to be integrated in different CNS regions. Each mode has unique advantages, but as an information processor, the brain derives its power from its ability to process in parallel.

Serial Processing

In **serial processing**, the whole system works in a predictable all-or-nothing manner. One neuron stimulates the next, which stimulates the next, and so on, eventually causing a specific, anticipated response. The most clear-cut examples of serial processing are spinal reflexes, but straight-through sensory

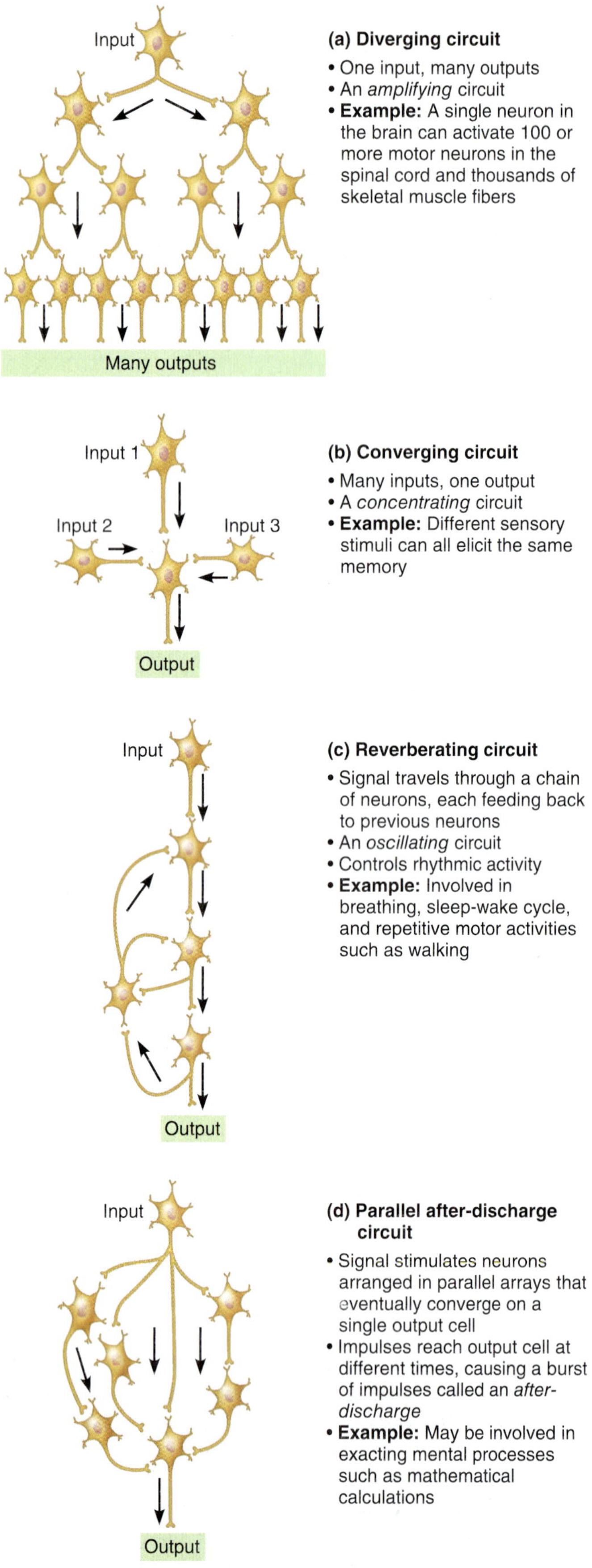

Figure 11.23 **Types of circuits in neuronal pools.**

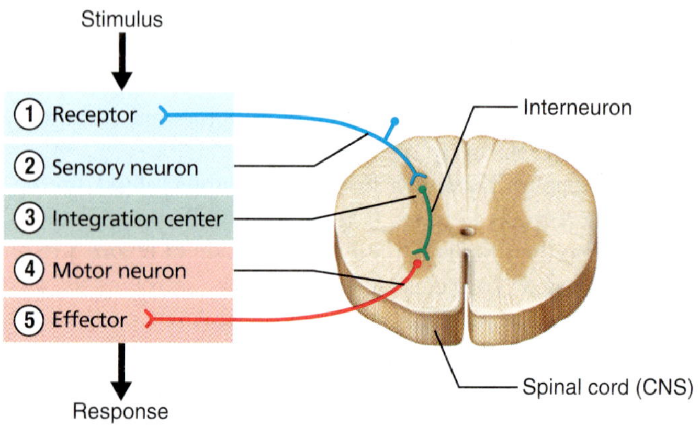

Figure 11.24 **A simple reflex arc.** Receptors detect a change in the internal or external environment that elicits a rapid stereotyped response. Effectors are muscles or glands.

pathways from receptors to the brain are also examples. Because reflexes are the functional units of the nervous system, it is important that you understand them early on.

Reflexes are rapid, automatic responses to stimuli, in which a particular stimulus always causes the same response. Reflex activity, which produces the simplest behaviors, is stereotyped and dependable. For example, if you touch a hot object you jerk your hand away, and an object approaching your eye triggers a blink. Reflexes occur over neural pathways called **reflex arcs** that have five essential components—receptor, sensory neuron, CNS integration center, motor neuron, and effector **(Figure 11.24)**.

Parallel Processing

In **parallel processing**, inputs are segregated into many pathways, and different parts of the neural circuitry deal simultaneously with the information delivered by each pathway. For example, smelling a pickle (the input) may cause you to remember picking cucumbers on a farm; or it may remind you that you don't like pickles or that you must buy some at the market; or perhaps it will call to mind *all* these thoughts. For each person, parallel processing triggers unique pathways. The same stimulus—pickle smell, in our example—promotes many responses beyond simple awareness of the smell. Parallel processing is not repetitious because the circuits do different things with the information, and each pathway or "channel" is decoded in relation to all the others to produce a total picture.

Think, for example, about what happens when you step on something sharp while walking barefoot. The serially processed withdrawal reflex causes you to remove your foot immediately from the sharp object (painful stimulus). At the same time, pain and pressure impulses are speeding up to your brain along parallel pathways that allow you to decide whether to simply rub the hurt spot to soothe it or seek first aid.

Parallel processing is extremely important for higher-level mental functioning—for putting the parts together to understand the whole. For example, you can recognize a dollar bill in a split second. This task takes a serial-based computer a fairly long time, but your recognition is rapid because you use parallel processing. A single neuron sends information along several pathways instead of just one, so you process a large amount of information much more quickly.

Check Your Understanding

21. Which types of neural circuits would give a prolonged output after a single input?
22. What pattern of neural processing occurs when your finger accidentally touches a hot grill? What is this response called?
23. What pattern of neural processing occurs when we smell freshly baked apple pie and remember Thanksgiving at our grandparents' house, the odor of freshly cooked turkey, sitting by the fire, and other such memories?

For answers, see Appendix H.

Developmental Aspects of Neurons

✓ Describe how neurons develop and form synapses.

We cover the nervous system in several chapters, so we limit our attention here to the development of neurons. Let's begin with two questions, How do neurons originate? and How do they mature?

The nervous system originates from a dorsal *neural tube* and the *neural crest*, formed from surface ectoderm (see Figure 12.33 ②, ③, p. 475). The neural tube, whose walls begin as a layer of *neuroepithelial* cells, becomes the CNS. The neuroepithelial cells then begin a three-phase process of differentiation, which occurs largely in the second month of development:

1. They *proliferate* to produce the appropriate number of cells needed for nervous system development.
2. The potential neurons, **neuroblasts**, become amitotic and *migrate* externally into their characteristic positions.
3. The neuroblasts sprout axons to *connect with* their functional targets and in so doing become neurons.

How does a neuroblast's growing axon "know" where to go—and once it gets there, where to make the proper connection? The growth of an axon toward an appropriate target requires multiple steps and is guided by multiple signals.

The growing tip of an axon, called a **growth cone**, is a prickly, fanlike structure that gives the axon the ability to interact with its environment **(Figure 11.25)**. Extracellular and cell surface adhesion proteins such as laminin, integrin, and *nerve cell adhesion molecule* (*N-CAM*) provide anchor points for the growth cone, saying, "It's okay to grow here." *Neurotropins* are chemicals that signal to the growth cone "come this way" (netrin) or "go away" (ephrin, slit) or "stop here" (semaphorin). Throughout this growth and development, neurotrophic factors such as *nerve growth factor* (*NGF*) must be present to keep the neuroblast alive.

Failure of any of these guiding signals results in catastrophic developmental problems. For example, lack of N-CAM action causes developing neural tissue to fall into a tangled, spaghetti-like mass and hopelessly impairs neural function.

The growth cone gropes along like an amoeba, with oozing processes called *filopodia* which detect the guiding signals in the surrounding environment. Receptors for these signals generate various second messengers that cause the filopodia to move by rearranging their actin protein cores.

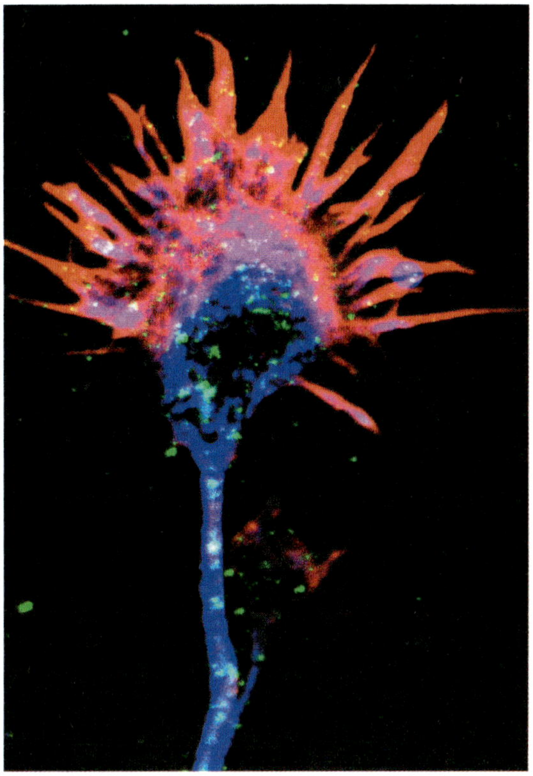

Figure 11.25 A neuronal growth cone. Fluorescent stains show the locations of cannabinoid receptors (green), tubulin (blue), and actin (pink) in this photomicrograph (1400×).

Once the axon reaches its target area, it must select the right site on the target cell to form a synapse. Special cell adhesion molecules couple the presynaptic and postsynaptic membranes together and generate intracellular signals that recruit vesicles containing preformed synaptic components. This results in the rapid formation of a synapse. In the brain and spinal cord, astrocytes provide both physical support and the cholesterol essential for constructing synapses. Both dendrites and astrocytes are active partners in the process of synapse formation. In the presence of thrombospondin released by astrocytes, dendrites actually reach out and grasp migrating axons, and synapses begin sprouting.

If neurons fail to make appropriate or functional synaptic contacts, they die. Besides cell death resulting from unsuccessful synapse formation, *apoptosis* (programmed cell death) is also a normal part of the developmental process. Of the neurons formed during the embryonic period, perhaps two-thirds die before we are born or shortly thereafter. Those that remain constitute most of our neural endowment for life.

The generally amitotic nature of neurons is important because their activity depends on the synapses they've formed, and if neurons were to divide, their connections might be hopelessly disrupted. This aside, there *do* appear to be some special neuronal populations where stem cells are found and new neurons can be formed—notably olfactory neurons and some cells of the hippocampus, a brain region involved in learning and memory.

Check Your Understanding

24. What is the name of the growing tip of an axon that "sniffs out" where to go during development? What is the general name for the chemicals that tell it where to go?

For answers, see Appendix H.

In this chapter, we have examined how the amazingly complex neurons, via electrical and chemical signals, serve the body in a variety of ways. Some serve as "lookouts," others process information for immediate use or for future reference, and still others stimulate the body's muscles and glands into activity. With this background, we are ready to study the most sophisticated mass of neural tissue in the entire body—the brain (and its continuation, the spinal cord), the focus of Chapter 12.

Chapter Summary

MAP™ For more chapter study tools, go to the Study Area of MasteringA&P at **www.masteringaandp.com**. There you will find:

- Interactive Physiology iP
- A&PFlix A&PFlix
- Practice Anatomy Lab PAL
- PhysioEx PEx
- Videos, Practice Quizzes and Tests, MP3 Tutor Sessions, Case Studies, and much more!

11

Functions and Divisions of the Nervous System (p. 387)

1. The nervous system bears a major responsibility for maintaining body homeostasis. It monitors, integrates, and responds to information in the environment.
2. The nervous system is divided anatomically into the central nervous system (brain and spinal cord) and the peripheral nervous system (mainly cranial and spinal nerves).
3. The major functional divisions of the PNS are the sensory (afferent) division, which conveys impulses to the CNS, and the motor (efferent) division, which conveys impulses from the CNS.
4. The efferent division includes the somatic (voluntary) system, which serves skeletal muscles, and the autonomic (involuntary) system, which innervates smooth and cardiac muscle and glands.

Histology of Nervous Tissue (pp. 387–395)

Neuroglia (pp. 388–390)

1. Neuroglia (supporting cells) segregate and insulate neurons and assist neurons in various other ways.
2. CNS neuroglia include astrocytes, microglial cells, ependymal cells, and oligodendrocytes. PNS neuroglia include Schwann cells and satellite cells.

Neurons (pp. 390–395)

3. Neurons have a cell body and cytoplasmic processes called axons and dendrites.
4. A bundle of nerve fibers is called a tract in the CNS and a nerve in the PNS. A collection of cell bodies is called a nucleus in the CNS and a ganglion in the PNS.
5. The cell body is the biosynthetic (and receptive) center of the neuron. Except for those found in ganglia, cell bodies are found in the CNS.
6. Most neurons have many dendrites, receptive processes that conduct signals from other neurons toward the nerve cell body. With few exceptions, all neurons have one axon, which generates and conducts nerve impulses away from the nerve cell body. Axon terminals release neurotransmitter.
7. Bidirectional transport along axons uses ATP-dependent motor proteins "walking" along microtubule tracks. It moves vesicles, mitochondria, and cytosolic proteins toward the axon terminals and conducts substances destined for degradation back to the cell body.
8. Large nerve fibers (axons) are myelinated. The myelin sheath is formed in the PNS by Schwann cells and in the CNS by oligodendrocytes. The myelin sheath gaps are also called nodes of Ranvier. Nonmyelinated fibers are surrounded by supporting cells, but the membrane-wrapping process does not occur.
9. Anatomically, neurons are classified according to the number of processes issuing from the cell body as multipolar, bipolar, or unipolar.
10. Functionally, neurons are classified according to the direction of nerve impulse conduction. Sensory neurons conduct impulses toward the CNS, motor neurons conduct away from the CNS, and interneurons (association neurons) lie between sensory and motor neurons in the neural pathways.

iP Nervous System I; Topic: Anatomy Review, pp. 1–12.

Membrane Potentials (pp. 395–407)

Basic Principles of Electricity (pp. 395–397)

1. The measure of the potential energy of separated electrical charges is called voltage (V) or potential. Current (I) is the flow of electrical charge from one point to another. Resistance (R) is hindrance to current flow. Ohm's law gives the relationship among these: $I = V/R$.
2. In the body, ions provide the electrical charges; cellular plasma membranes provide resistance to ion flow. The membranes contain leakage channels (nongated, always open) and gated channels.

iP Nervous System I; Topic: Ion Channels, pp. 1–10.

The Resting Membrane Potential (p. 397)

3. A resting neuron exhibits a resting membrane potential, which is -70 mV (inside negative). It is due both to differences in sodium and potassium ion concentrations inside and outside the cell and to differences in permeability of the membrane to these ions.
4. The ionic concentration differences result from the operation of the sodium-potassium pump, which ejects 3 Na^+ from the cell for each 2 K^+ transported in.

iP Nervous System I; Topic: The Membrane Potential, pp. 1–16.

Membrane Potentials That Act as Signals (pp. 397–407)

5. Depolarization is a reduction in membrane potential (inside becomes less negative); hyperpolarization is an increase in membrane potential (inside becomes more negative).
6. Graded potentials are small, brief, local changes in membrane potential that act as short-distance signals. The current produced dissipates with distance.

7. An action potential (AP), or nerve impulse, is a large, but brief, depolarization signal (and polarity reversal) that underlies long-distance neural communication. It is an all-or-none phenomenon.
8. In the AP graph, an AP begins and ends at resting membrane potential. Depolarization to approximately +30 mV (inside positive) is caused by Na^+ influx. Depolarization ends when Na^+ channels inactivate. Repolarization and hyperpolarization are caused by K^+ efflux.
9. If threshold is reached, an AP is generated. If not, depolarization remains local.
10. In nerve impulse propagation, each AP provides the depolarizing stimulus for triggering an AP in the next membrane patch. Regions that have just generated APs are refractory; for this reason, the nerve impulse propagates in one direction only.
11. APs are independent of stimulus strength: Strong stimuli cause APs to be generated more frequently but not with greater amplitude.
12. During the absolute refractory period, a neuron cannot respond to another stimulus because it is already generating an AP. During the relative refractory period, the neuron's threshold is elevated because repolarization is ongoing.
13. In nonmyelinated fibers, APs are produced in a wave all along the axon, that is, by continuous conduction. In myelinated fibers, APs are generated only at myelin sheath gaps and are propagated more rapidly by saltatory conduction.

iP Nervous System I; Topic: The Action Potential, pp. 1–18.

The Synapse (pp. 407–414)

1. A synapse is a functional junction between neurons. The information-transmitting neuron is the presynaptic neuron; the information-receiving neuron is the postsynaptic neuron.

Electrical Synapses (p. 407)

2. Electrical synapses allow ions to flow directly from one neuron to another; the cells are electrically coupled.

Chemical Synapses (pp. 407–410)

3. Chemical synapses are sites of neurotransmitter release and binding. When the impulse reaches the presynaptic axon terminals, voltage-gated Ca^{2+} channels open, and Ca^{2+} enters the cell and mediates neurotransmitter release. Neurotransmitters diffuse across the synaptic cleft and attach to postsynaptic membrane receptors, opening ion channels. After binding, the neurotransmitters are removed from the synapse by diffusion, enzymatic breakdown, or reuptake into the presynaptic terminal or astrocytes.

iP Nervous System II; Topics: Anatomy Review, pp. 1–9, Ion Channels, pp. 1–8, Synaptic Transmission, pp. 1–7.

Postsynaptic Potentials and Synaptic Integration (pp. 410–414)

4. Binding of neurotransmitter at excitatory chemical synapses results in local graded potentials called EPSPs, caused by the opening of channels that allow simultaneous passage of Na^+ and K^+.
5. Neurotransmitter binding at inhibitory chemical synapses results in hyperpolarizations called IPSPs, caused by the opening of K^+ or Cl^- channels. IPSPs drive the membrane potential farther from threshold.
6. EPSPs and IPSPs summate temporally and spatially. The membrane of the axon hillock acts as a neuronal integrator.
7. Synaptic potentiation, which enhances the postsynaptic neuron's response, is produced by intense repeated stimulation. Ionic calcium appears to mediate such effects, which may be the basis of learning.
8. Presynaptic inhibition is mediated by axoaxonal synapses that reduce the amount of neurotransmitter released by the inhibited neuron.

iP Nervous System II; Topic: Synaptic Potentials and Cellular Integration, pp. 1-10.

Neurotransmitters and Their Receptors (pp. 414–421)

Classification of Neurotransmitters by Chemical Structure (pp. 414–417)

1. The major classes of neurotransmitters based on chemical structure are acetylcholine, biogenic amines, amino acids, peptides, purines, dissolved gases, and lipids.

Classification of Neurotransmitters by Function (pp. 417–419)

2. Functionally, neurotransmitters are classified as (1) inhibitory or excitatory (or both) and (2) direct or indirect action. Direct-acting neurotransmitters bind to and open ion channels. Indirect-acting neurotransmitters act through second messengers. Neuromodulators also act indirectly presynaptically or postsynaptically to change synaptic strength.

Neurotransmitter Receptors (pp. 420–421)

3. Neurotransmitter receptors are either channel-linked receptors that open ion channels, leading to fast changes in membrane potential, or G protein–linked receptors that oversee slow synaptic responses mediated by G proteins and intracellular second messengers. Second messengers most often activate kinases, which in turn act on ion channels or activate other proteins.

iP Nervous System II; Topic: Synaptic Transmission, pp. 6–15.

11

Basic Concepts of Neural Integration (pp. 421–423)

Organization of Neurons: Neuronal Pools (p. 421)

1. CNS neurons are organized into several types of neuronal pools, each with distinguishing patterns of synaptic connections called circuits.

Types of Circuits (p. 421)

2. The four basic circuit types are diverging, converging, reverberating, and parallel after-discharge.

Patterns of Neural Processing (pp. 421–423)

3. In serial processing, one neuron stimulates the next in sequence, producing specific, predictable responses, as in spinal reflexes. A reflex is a rapid, involuntary motor response to a stimulus.
4. Reflexes are mediated over neural pathways called reflex arcs. The minimum number of elements in a reflex arc is five: receptor, sensory neuron, integration center, motor neuron, and effector.
5. In parallel processing, which underlies complex mental functions, impulses travel along several pathways to different integration centers.

Developmental Aspects of Neurons (pp. 423–424)

1. Neuron development involves proliferation, migration, and the formation of interconnections. The formation of interconnections involves axons finding their targets and forming synapses, and the synthesis of specific neurotransmitters.
2. Axon outgrowth and synapse formation are guided by other neurons, glial cells, and chemicals (such as N-CAM and nerve growth factor). Neurons that do not make appropriate synapses die, and approximately two-thirds of neurons formed in the embryo undergo programmed cell death.

Review Questions

Multiple Choice/Matching

(Some questions have more than one correct answer. Select the best answer or answers from the choices given.)

1. Which of the following structures is not part of the central nervous system? **(a)** the brain, **(b)** a nerve, **(c)** the spinal cord, **(d)** a tract.
2. Match the names of the supporting cells found in column B with the appropriate descriptions in column A.

Column A	Column B
____ **(1)** myelinates nerve fibers in the CNS	**(a)** astrocyte
____ **(2)** lines brain cavities	**(b)** ependymal cell
____ **(3)** myelinates nerve fibers in the PNS	**(c)** microglial cell
____ **(4)** CNS phagocyte	**(d)** oligodendrocyte
____ **(5)** helps regulate the ionic composition of CNS extracellular fluid	**(e)** satellite cell
	(f) Schwann cell

3. What type of current flows through the axolemma during the steep phase of repolarization? **(a)** chiefly a sodium current, **(b)** chiefly a potassium current, **(c)** sodium and potassium currents of approximately the same magnitude.
4. Assume that an EPSP is being generated on the dendritic membrane. Which will occur? **(a)** specific Na^+ channels will open, **(b)** specific K^+ channels will open, **(c)** a single type of channel will open, permitting simultaneous flow of Na^+ and K^+, **(d)** Na^+ channels will open first and then close as K^+ channels open.
5. The velocity of nerve impulse conduction is greatest in **(a)** heavily myelinated, large-diameter fibers, **(b)** myelinated, small-diameter fibers, **(c)** nonmyelinated, small-diameter fibers, **(d)** nonmyelinated, large-diameter fibers.
6. Chemical synapses are characterized by all of the following except **(a)** the release of neurotransmitter by the presynaptic membranes, **(b)** postsynaptic membranes bearing receptors that bind neurotransmitter, **(c)** ions flowing through protein channels from the presynaptic to the postsynaptic neuron, **(d)** a fluid-filled gap separating the neurons.
7. Biogenic amine neurotransmitters include all but **(a)** norepinephrine, **(b)** acetylcholine, **(c)** dopamine, **(d)** serotonin.
8. The neuropeptides that act as natural opiates are **(a)** substance P, **(b)** somatostatin and cholecystokinin, **(c)** tachykinins, **(d)** enkephalins.
9. Inhibition of acetylcholinesterase by poisoning blocks neurotransmission at the neuromuscular junction because **(a)** ACh is no longer released by the presynaptic terminal, **(b)** ACh synthesis in the presynaptic terminal is blocked, **(c)** ACh is not degraded, hence prolonged depolarization is enforced on the postsynaptic cell, **(d)** ACh is blocked from attaching to the postsynaptic ACh receptors.
10. The anatomical region of a multipolar neuron that has the lowest threshold for generating an AP is the **(a)** soma, **(b)** dendrites, **(c)** axon hillock, **(d)** distal axon.
11. An IPSP is inhibitory because **(a)** it hyperpolarizes the postsynaptic membrane, **(b)** it reduces the amount of neurotransmitter released by the presynaptic terminal, **(c)** it prevents calcium ion entry into the presynaptic terminal, **(d)** it changes the threshold of the neuron.
12. Identify the neuronal circuits described by choosing the correct response from the key.

Key: **(a)** converging **(b)** diverging **(c)** parallel after-discharge **(d)** reverberating

____ **(1)** Impulses continue around and around the circuit until one neuron stops firing.
____ **(2)** One or a few inputs ultimately influence large numbers of neurons.
____ **(3)** Many neurons influence a few neurons.
____ **(4)** May be involved in exacting types of mental activity.

Short Answer Essay Questions

13. Explain both the anatomical and functional divisions of the nervous system. Include the subdivisions of each.
14. (a) Describe the composition and function of the cell body. (b) How are axons and dendrites alike? In what ways (structurally and functionally) do they differ?
15. (a) What is myelin? (b) How does the myelination process differ in the CNS and PNS?
16. (a) Contrast unipolar, bipolar, and multipolar neurons structurally. (b) Indicate where each is most likely to be found.
17. What is the polarized membrane state? How is it maintained? (Note the relative roles of both passive and active mechanisms.)
18. Describe the events that must occur to generate an AP. Relate the sequence of changes in permeability to changes in the ion channels, and explain why the AP is an all-or-none phenomenon.
19. Since all APs generated by a given nerve fiber have the same magnitude, how does the CNS "know" whether a stimulus is strong or weak?
20. (a) Explain the difference between an EPSP and an IPSP. (b) What specifically determines whether an EPSP or IPSP will be generated at the postsynaptic membrane?
21. Since at any moment a neuron is likely to have thousands of neurons releasing neurotransmitters at its surface, how is neuronal activity (to fire or not to fire) determined?
22. The effects of neurotransmitter binding are very brief. Explain.
23. During a neurobiology lecture, a professor repeatedly refers to group A and group B fibers, absolute refractory period, and myelin sheath gaps. Define these terms.
24. Distinguish between serial and parallel processing.
25. Briefly describe the three stages of neuron development.
26. What factors appear to guide the outgrowth of an axon and its ability to make the "correct" synaptic contacts?

Critical Thinking and Clinical Application Questions

1. Mr. Miller is hospitalized for cardiac problems. Somehow, medical orders are mixed up and Mr. Miller is infused with a K^+-enhanced intravenous solution meant for another patient who is taking potassium-wasting diuretics (i.e., drugs that cause excessive loss of potassium from the body in urine). Mr. Miller's potassium levels are normal before the IV is administered. What do you think will happen to Mr. Miller's resting membrane potentials? To his neurons' ability to generate APs?
2. Local anesthetics block voltage-gated Na^+ channels. General anesthetics are thought to activate chemically gated Cl^- channels,

thereby rendering the nervous system quiescent while surgery is performed. What specific process do anesthetics impair, and how does this interfere with nerve impulse transmission?

3. When admitted to the emergency room, John was holding his right hand, which had a deep puncture hole in its palm. He explained that he had fallen on a nail while exploring a barn. John was given an antitetanus shot to prevent neural complications. Tetanus bacteria fester in deep, dark wounds, but how do their toxins travel in neural tissue?
4. Rochelle developed multiple sclerosis when she was 27. After eight years she had lost a good portion of her ability to control her skeletal muscles. How did this happen?
5. In the Netherlands a young man named Jan was admitted to the emergency room. He and his friends had been to a rave. His friends say he started twitching and having muscle spasms which progressed until he was "stiff as a board." On examination, staff found a marked increase in muscle tone and hyperreflexia involving facial and limb muscles. In his pocket, he had unmarked dark yellow tablets with dark flecks. Analysis of the tablets showed them to contain a mixture of ecstasy and strychnine. Ecstasy would not cause this clinical picture, but strychnine, which blocks glycine receptors, could. Explain how.

AT THE CLINIC

Related Clinical Terms

Neuroblastoma (nu″ro-blas-to′mah; *oma* = tumor) A malignant tumor in children; arises from cells that retain a neuroblast-like structure. These tumors sometimes arise in the brain, but most occur in the peripheral nervous system.

Neurologist (nu-rol′o-jist) A medical specialist in the study of the nervous system and its functions and disorders.

Neuropathy (nu-rop′ah-the) Any disease of nervous tissue, but particularly degenerative diseases of nerves.

Neuropharmacology (nu″ro-far″mah-kol′o-je) Scientific study of the effects of drugs on the nervous system.

Neurotoxin Substance that is poisonous or destructive to nervous tissue, e.g., botulinum and tetanus toxins.

Rabies (*rabies* = madness) A viral infection of the nervous system transmitted by the bite of an infected mammal (such as a dog, bat, or skunk). After entry, the virus travels via axonal transport in peripheral nerve axons to the CNS, where it causes brain inflammation, delirium, and death. A vaccine- and antibody-based treatment is effective if given before symptoms appear. Rabies in humans is very rare in the United States.

Shingles (herpes zoster) Inflammation of virally infected sensory neurons serving the skin. Caused by the varicella-zoster virus, which causes chicken pox (generally during childhood); during the initial infection the virus is transported from the skin lesions to the sensory cell bodies in the sensory ganglia. Typically, the immune system holds the virus in check. It remains dormant until the immune system is weakened, often by stress. Then viral particles multiply, causing nerve pain (neuralgia), and travel back to the skin, producing characteristic scaly blisters. This rash is usually confined to one side of the body trunk. Attacks last several weeks, alternating between periods of healing and relapse. Seen mostly in those over 50 years old. Vaccination can prevent occurrence and minimize pain.

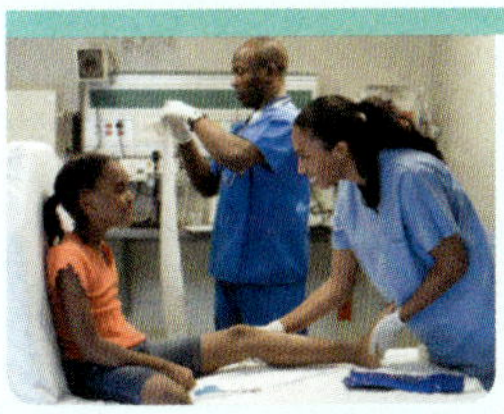

Case Study Nervous System

Elaine Sawyer, 35, was on her way to the local elementary school with her three children when the accident on Route 91 occurred. As Mrs. Sawyer swerved to avoid the bus, the right rear corner of her minivan struck the side of the bus, causing the minivan to tip over and slide on its side. Her children were shaken but unhurt. Mrs. Sawyer, however, suffered a severe head injury that caused post-traumatic seizures.

The drugs initially prescribed for her treatment were insufficient to control these seizures. Her doctor additionally prescribed Valium (diazepam), but suggested that she use it only for a month because Valium induces tolerance (loses its effectiveness). After a month of Valium treatment, Mrs. Sawyer no longer had seizures and gradually reduced and eliminated her use of Valium. After being seizure-free for another year, restrictions on her driver's license were lifted.

1. Seizures reflect uncontrolled electrical activity of groups of neurons in the brain. Valium is described as a drug that can "quiet the nerves," which means that it inhibits the ability of neurons to generate electrical signals. What are these electrical signals called, and what is happening at the level of the cell when they are generated?
2. Valium enhances inhibitory postsynaptic potentials (IPSPs). What is an IPSP? How does it affect action potential generation?
3. Valium enhances the natural effects of the neurotransmitter GABA [gamma (γ)-aminobutyric acid]. What chemical class of neurotransmitters does GABA belong to? What are some of the other neurotransmitters that fall into this same class?
4. Theoretically, there are a number of possible ways that a drug such as Valium could act to enhance the action of GABA. What are three such possibilities?
5. Valium actually works postsynaptically to promote binding of GABA to its receptor, thereby enhancing the influx of Cl^- ions into the postsynaptic cell (the natural effect produced by GABA). Why would this effect reduce the likelihood that this cell would be able to produce an electrical signal?

(Answers in Appendix H)

12

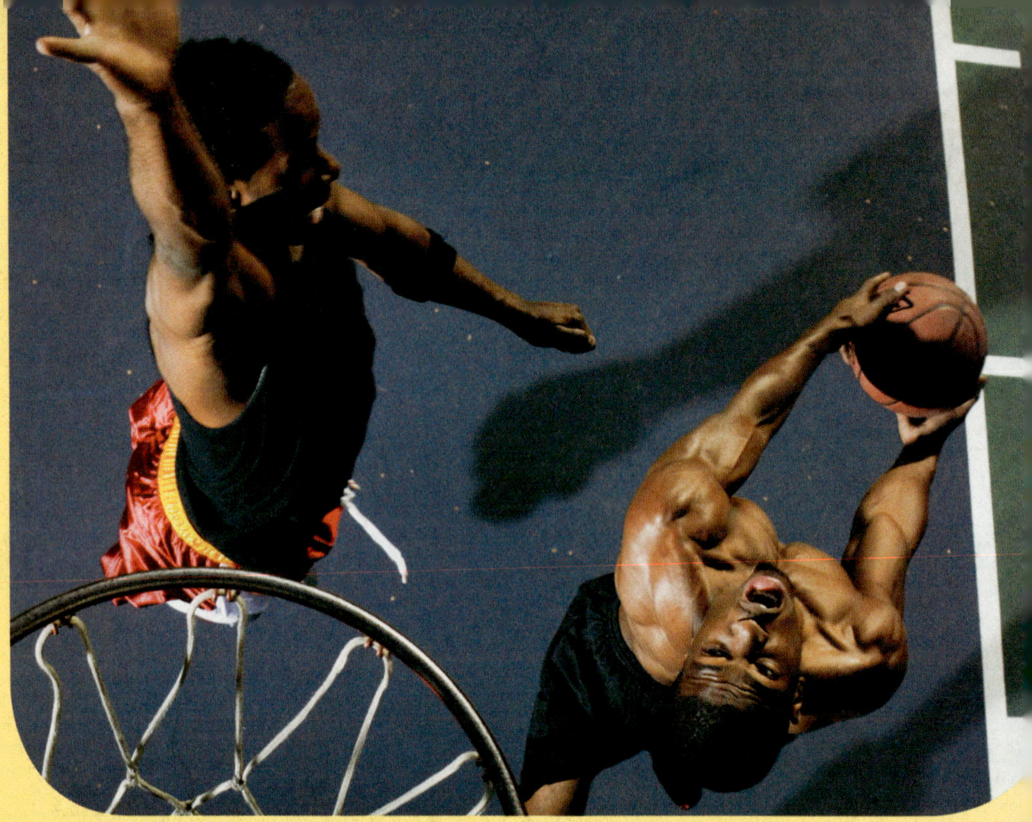

The Central Nervous System

Interconnecting and directing a dizzying number of incoming and outgoing calls, the central switchboard of a telephone system historically seemed an apt comparison for the **central nervous system (CNS)**—brain and spinal cord. Nowadays, many people compare the CNS to a "cloud" of networked computers. These analogies may explain some workings of the spinal cord, but neither does justice to the fantastic complexity of the human brain. Whether we view the brain as an evolved biological organ, an impressive network of computers, or simply a miracle, it is one of the most amazing things known.

During the course of animal evolution, **cephalization** (sĕ″fah-lĭ-za′shun) has occurred. That is, there has been an elaboration of the *rostral* ("toward the snout"), or anterior, portion of the CNS, along with an increase in the number of neurons in the head. This phenomenon reaches its highest level in the human brain.

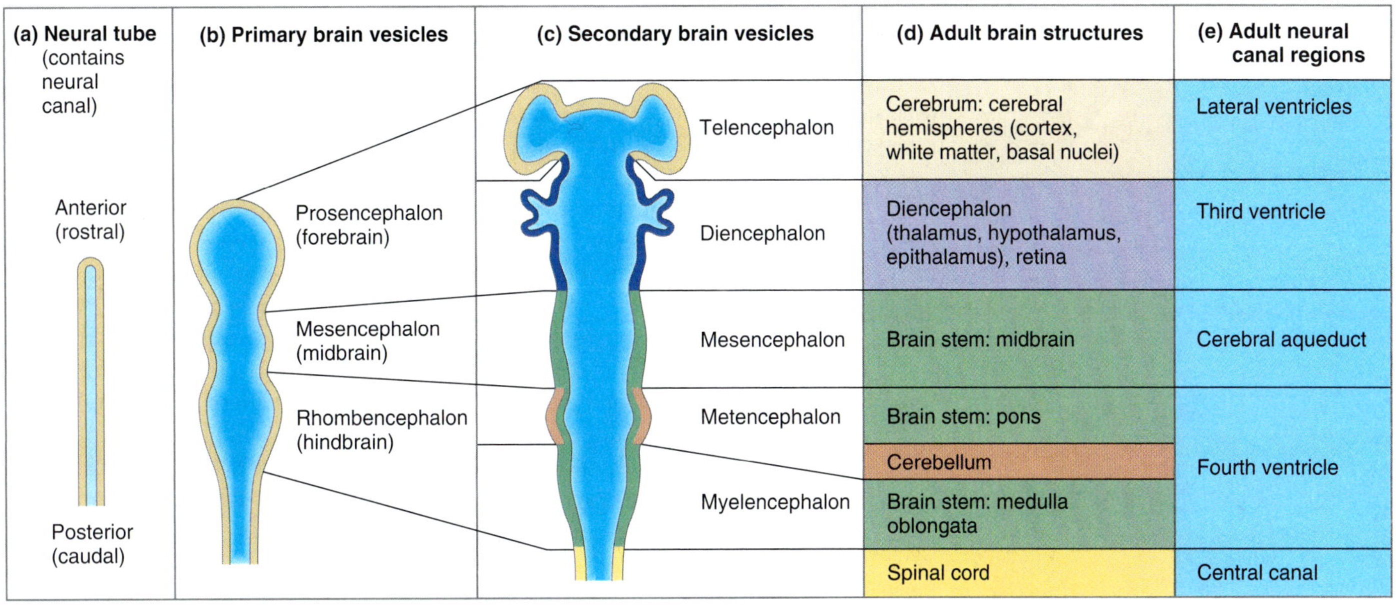

Figure 12.1 Embryonic development of the human brain. (a) Formed by week 4, the neural tube quickly subdivides into **(b)** the primary brain vesicles, which subsequently form **(c)** the secondary brain vesicles by week 5. These five vesicles differentiate into **(d)** the adult brain structures. **(e)** The adult structures derived from the neural canal.

In this chapter, we examine the structure of the CNS and the functions associated with its various regions. We also touch on complex integrative functions, such as sleep-wake cycles and memory.

The Brain

The unimpressive appearance of the human **brain** gives few hints of its remarkable abilities. It is about two good fistfuls of quivering pinkish gray tissue, wrinkled like a walnut, with a consistency somewhat like cold oatmeal. The average adult human brain has a mass of about 1500 g (3.3 lb).

Embryonic Development

✓ Describe how space constraints affect brain development.

✓ Name the major regions of the adult brain.

✓ Name and locate the ventricles of the brain.

We begin with an introduction to brain embryology, as the terminology used for the structural divisions of the adult brain is easier to follow when you understand brain development.

The brain and spinal cord begin as an embryonic structure called the **neural tube** (Figure 12.1a). As soon as the neural tube forms, its anterior (rostral) end begins to expand and constrictions appear that mark off the three **primary brain vesicles** (Figure 12.1b):

- **Prosencephalon** (pros″en-sef′ah-lon), or **forebrain**
- **Mesencephalon** (mes″en-sef′ah-lon), or **midbrain**
- **Rhombencephalon** (romb″en-sef′ah-lon), or **hindbrain**

(Note that *encephalo* means "brain.") The remaining *caudal* ("toward the tail"), or posterior, portion of the neural tube becomes the spinal cord, which we will discuss later in the chapter.

The primary vesicles give rise to the **secondary brain vesicles** (Figure 12.1c). The forebrain divides into the **telencephalon** ("endbrain") and **diencephalon** ("interbrain"), and the hindbrain constricts, forming the **metencephalon** ("afterbrain") and **myelencephalon** ("spinal brain"). The midbrain remains undivided.

Each of the five secondary vesicles then develops rapidly to produce the major structures of the adult brain (Figure 12.1d). The greatest change occurs in the telencephalon, which sprouts two lateral swellings that look like Mickey Mouse's ears. These become the two *cerebral hemispheres*, referred to collectively as the **cerebrum** (ser′ĕ-brum). The diencephalon specializes to form the *hypothalamus* (hi″po-thal′ah-mus), *thalamus*, *epithalamus*, and *retina* of the eye. Less dramatic changes occur in the mesencephalon, metencephalon, and myelencephalon as these regions transform into the *midbrain*, the *pons* and *cerebellum*, and the *medulla oblongata*, respectively. All these midbrain and hindbrain structures, except the cerebellum, form the **brain stem**.

The central cavity of the neural tube remains continuous and enlarges in four areas to form the fluid-filled *ventricles* (*ventr* = little belly) of the brain (Figure 12.1e). We will describe the ventricles shortly.

Because the brain grows more rapidly than the membranous skull that contains it, it folds up to occupy the available space. The *midbrain* and *cervical flexures* move the forebrain toward the brain stem (Figure 12.2a). The cerebral hemispheres are forced to take a horseshoe-shaped course and grow posteriorly and laterally (indicated by black arrows in Figure 12.2b). As a result, they grow back over and almost completely envelop the diencephalon and midbrain. By week 26, the continued growth

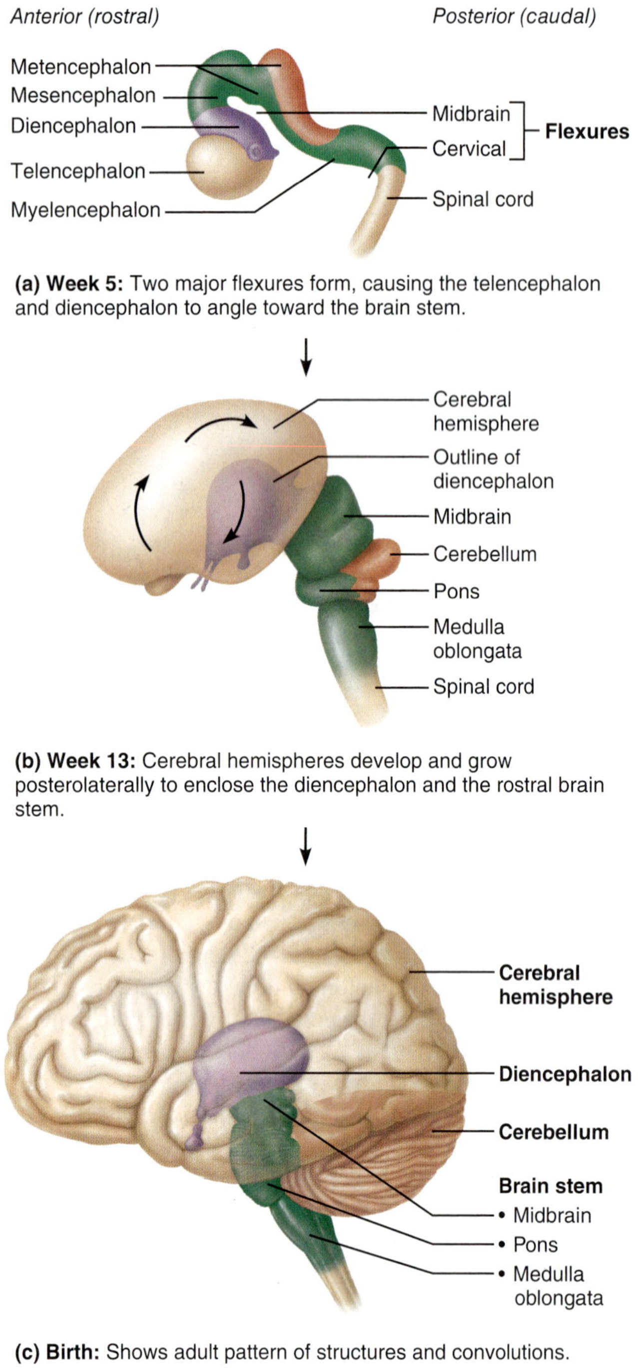

Figure 12.2 Brain development. Initially, the cerebral surface is smooth. Folding begins in month 6, and convolutions become more obvious as development continues. See-through view in (b) and (c).

of the cerebral hemispheres causes their surfaces to crease and fold into *convolutions* (Figure 12.2c), which increases their surface area and allows more neurons to occupy the limited space.

Regions and Organization

Some textbooks discuss brain anatomy in terms of the *embryonic scheme* (see Figure 12.1c), but in this text, we will consider the brain in terms of the medical scheme and the four adult brain regions shown in Figure 12.2c: (1) cerebral hemispheres, (2) diencephalon, (3) brain stem (midbrain, pons, and medulla oblongata), and (4) cerebellum.

The basic pattern of the CNS is a central cavity surrounded by gray matter (mostly neuron cell bodies), external to which is white matter (myelinated fiber tracts). The spinal cord exhibits this basic pattern, but the brain has additional regions of gray matter not present in the spinal cord. Both the cerebral hemispheres and the cerebellum have an outer layer or "bark" of gray matter called a cortex. This pattern changes with descent through the brain stem—the cortex disappears, but scattered gray matter nuclei are seen within the white matter. At the caudal end of the brain stem, the basic pattern is evident. Knowledge of the basic pattern of the CNS will help you explore the brain, moving from the most rostral region (cerebrum) to the most caudal (brain stem). But first, let's explore the central hollow cavities that lie deep within the brain—the ventricles.

Ventricles

The brain **ventricles** are continuous with one another and with the central canal of the spinal cord **(Figure 12.3)**. The hollow ventricular chambers are filled with cerebrospinal fluid and lined by *ependymal cells*, a type of neuroglia (see Figure 11.3c on p. 389).

The paired **lateral ventricles**, one deep within each cerebral hemisphere, are large C-shaped chambers that reflect the pattern of cerebral growth. Anteriorly, the lateral ventricles lie close together, separated only by a thin median membrane called the **septum pellucidum** (pĕ-lu′sid-um; "transparent wall"). (See Figure 12.10, p. 440.)

Each lateral ventricle communicates with the narrow **third ventricle** in the diencephalon via a channel called an **interventricular foramen**.

The third ventricle is continuous with the **fourth ventricle** via the canal-like **cerebral aqueduct** that runs through the midbrain. The fourth ventricle lies in the hindbrain dorsal to the pons and superior medulla. It is continuous with the central canal of the spinal cord inferiorly. Three openings mark the walls of the fourth ventricle: the paired **lateral apertures** in its side walls and the **median aperture** in its roof. These apertures connect the ventricles to the *subarachnoid space* (sub″ah-rak′noid), a fluid-filled space surrounding the brain.

Check Your Understanding

1. Which ventricle is surrounded by the diencephalon?
2. Which two areas of the adult brain have an outside layer of gray matter in addition to central gray matter and surrounding white matter?
3. What is the function of convolutions of the brain?

For answers, see Appendix H.

Cerebral Hemispheres

✓ List the major lobes, fissures, and functional areas of the cerebral cortex.

✓ Explain lateralization of hemisphere function.

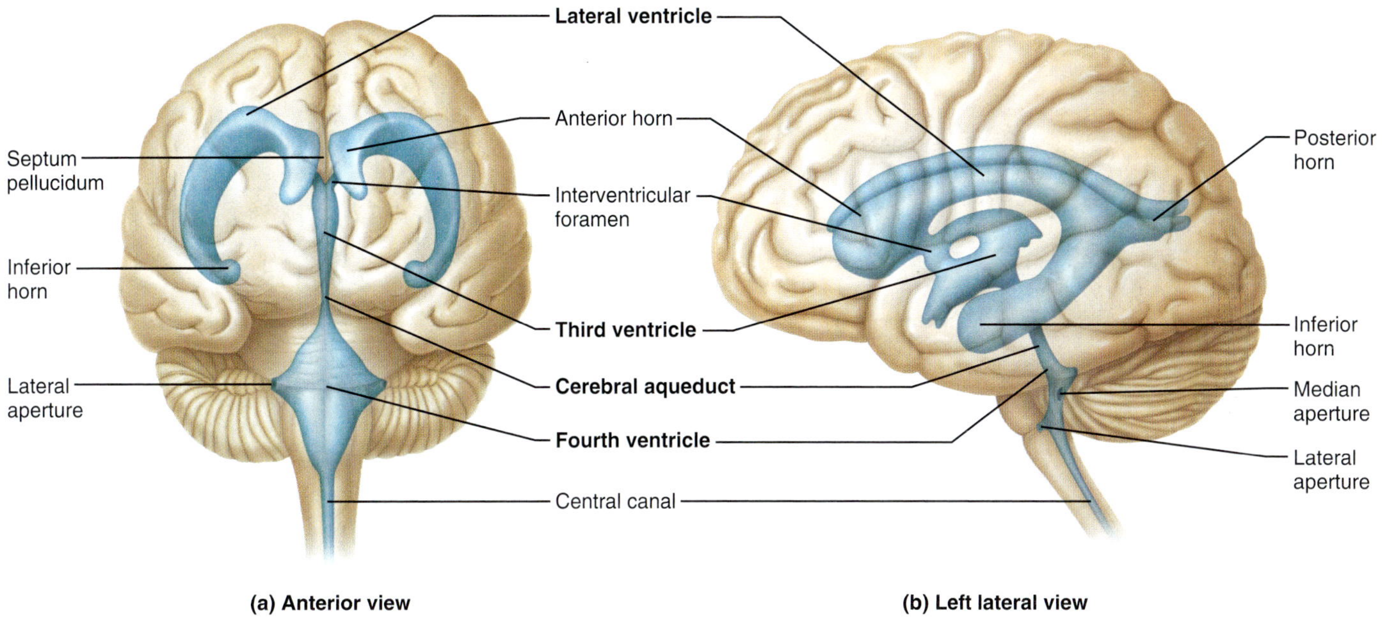

Figure 12.3 Ventricles of the brain. Different regions of the large lateral ventricles are labeled anterior horn, posterior horn, and inferior horn.

✓ Differentiate between commissures, association fibers, and projection fibers.

✓ Describe the general function of the basal nuclei (basal ganglia).

The **cerebral hemispheres** form the superior part of the brain **(Figure 12.4)**. The most conspicuous parts of an intact brain, together they account for about 83% of total brain mass. Picture how a mushroom cap covers the top of its stalk, and you have a good idea of how the paired cerebral hemispheres cover and obscure the diencephalon and the top of the brain stem (see Figure 12.2c).

Elevated ridges of tissue called **gyri** (ji′ri; singular: *gyrus;* "twisters")—separated by shallow grooves called **sulci** (sul′ki; singular: *sulcus;* "furrows")—mark nearly the entire surface of the cerebral hemispheres. Deeper grooves, called **fissures**, separate large regions of the brain (Figure 12.4c).

The more prominent gyri and sulci are important anatomical landmarks that are similar in all humans. The median **longitudinal fissure** separates the cerebral hemispheres (Figure 12.4a). Another large fissure, the **transverse cerebral fissure**, separates the cerebral hemispheres from the cerebellum below (Figure 12.4b, c).

Several sulci divide each hemisphere into five lobes—frontal, parietal, temporal, occipital, and insula (Figure 12.4c, d). All but the last are named for the cranial bones that overlie them (see Figure 7.5, pp. 204–205). The **central sulcus**, which lies in the frontal plane, separates the **frontal lobe** from the **parietal lobe**. Bordering the central sulcus are the **precentral gyrus** anteriorly and the **postcentral gyrus** posteriorly. The **parieto-occipital sulcus** (pah-ri″ĕ-to-ok-sip′ĭ-tal), located more posteriorly on the medial surface of the hemisphere, separates the **occipital lobe** from the parietal lobe.

The deep **lateral sulcus** outlines the flaplike **temporal lobe** and separates it from the parietal and frontal lobes. A fifth lobe of the cerebral hemisphere, the **insula** (in′su-lah; "island"), is buried deep within the lateral sulcus and forms part of its floor (Figure 12.4d). The insula is covered by portions of the temporal, parietal, and frontal lobes.

The cerebral hemispheres fit snugly in the skull. The frontal lobes lie in the anterior cranial fossa, and the anterior parts of the temporal lobes fill the middle cranial fossa (see Figure 7.2b, c, p. 201). The posterior cranial fossa, however, houses the brain stem and cerebellum. The occipital lobes are located well superior to that cranial fossa.

Each cerebral hemisphere has three basic regions:

- A superficial *cerebral cortex* of gray matter, which looks gray in fresh brain tissue
- Internal *white matter*
- *Basal nuclei*, islands of gray matter situated deep within the white matter

We consider these regions next.

12

Cerebral Cortex

The **cerebral cortex** is the "executive suite" of the nervous system, where our *conscious mind* is found. It enables us to be aware of ourselves and our sensations, to communicate, remember, understand, and initiate voluntary movements.

The cerebral cortex is composed of gray matter: neuron cell bodies, dendrites, associated glia and blood vessels, but no fiber tracts. It contains billions of neurons arranged in six layers. Although only 2–4 mm (about 1/8 inch) thick, it accounts for roughly 40% of total brain mass. Its many convolutions effectively triple its surface area.

Modern imaging techniques allow us to see the brain in action—PET scans show maximal metabolic activity in the brain,

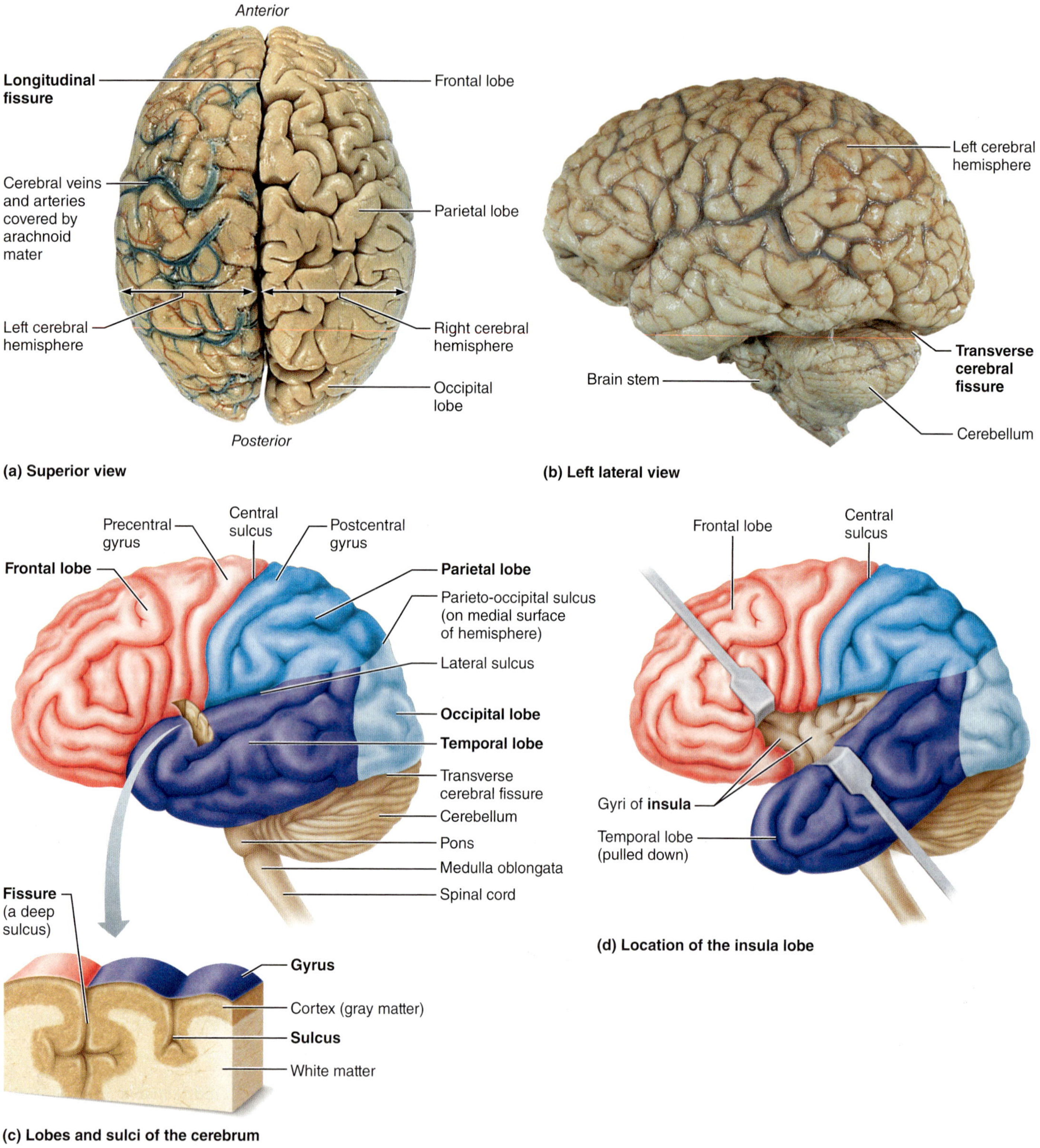

Figure 12.4 Lobes, sulci, and fissures of the cerebral hemispheres.

and functional MRI scans reveal blood flow **(Figure 12.5)**. They show that specific motor and sensory functions are localized in discrete cortical areas called *domains*. However, many higher mental functions, such as memory and language, appear to be spread over large areas of the cortex in overlapping domains.

Before we examine the functional regions of the cerebral cortex, let's consider four generalizations:

- The cerebral cortex contains three kinds of functional areas: *motor areas*, *sensory areas*, and *association areas*. As you read about these areas, do not confuse the sensory and motor areas of the cortex with sensory and motor neurons. All neurons in the cortex are interneurons.

- Each hemisphere is chiefly concerned with the sensory and motor functions of the **contralateral** (literally, "opposite") side of the body.
- Although largely symmetrical in structure, the two hemispheres are not entirely equal in function. Instead, there is lateralization (specialization) of cortical functions.
- And finally, keep in mind that our approach is a gross oversimplification. No functional area of the cortex acts alone, and conscious behavior involves the entire cortex in one way or another.

Motor Areas The following **motor areas** of the cortex, which control voluntary movement, lie in the posterior part of the frontal lobes: primary motor cortex, premotor cortex, Broca's area, and the frontal eye field (**Figure 12.6a**, dark and light red areas).

1. **Primary motor cortex.** The **primary (somatic) motor cortex** is located in the precentral gyrus of the frontal lobe of each hemisphere (Figure 12.6, dark red area). Large neurons, called **pyramidal cells,** in these gyri allow us to consciously control the precise or skilled voluntary movements of our skeletal muscles. Their long axons, which project to the spinal cord, form the massive voluntary motor tracts called *pyramidal tracts* or *corticospinal tracts* (kor″tĭ-ko-spi′nal). All other descending motor tracts issue from brain stem nuclei and consist of chains of two or more neurons.

   The entire body is represented spatially in the primary motor cortex of each hemisphere. For example, the pyramidal cells that control foot movements are in one place and those that control hand movements are in another. Such mapping of the body in CNS structures is called **somatotopy** (so″mah-to-to′pe).

   As illustrated in **Figure 12.7** (p. 435), in somatotopy the body is represented upside down—with the head at the inferolateral part of the precentral gyrus, and the toes at the superomedial end. Most of the neurons in these gyri control muscles in body areas having the most precise motor control—that is, the face, tongue, and hands. Consequently, these regions are disproportionately large in the caricature-like **motor homunculus** (ho-mung′ku-lus; "little man") drawn in Figure 12.7. The motor innervation of the body is contralateral: In other words, the left primary motor gyrus controls muscles on the right side of the body, and vice versa.

   The motor homunculus view of the primary motor cortex, shown at the left in Figure 12.7, implies a one-to-one correspondence between cortical neurons and the muscles they control, but this is somewhat misleading. In fact, a given muscle is controlled by multiple spots on the cortex, and individual cortical neurons actually send impulses to more than one muscle. In other words, individual pyramidal motor neurons control muscles that work together in a synergistic way to perform a given movement.

   For example, reaching forward with one arm involves some muscles acting at the shoulder and some acting at the elbow. Instead of the discrete map offered by the motor homunculus, the primary motor cortex map is an orderly but fuzzy map with neurons arranged in useful ways to control and coordinate sets of muscles. Neurons controlling the arm, for instance, intermingle and overlap with those controlling the hand and shoulder. However, neurons controlling unrelated movements, such as those controlling the arm and those controlling body trunk muscles, do not cooperate in motor activity.

   Thus, the motor homunculus is useful to show that broad areas of the primary cortex are devoted to the leg, arm, torso, and head, but neuron organization within those broad areas is much more diffuse than initially imagined.

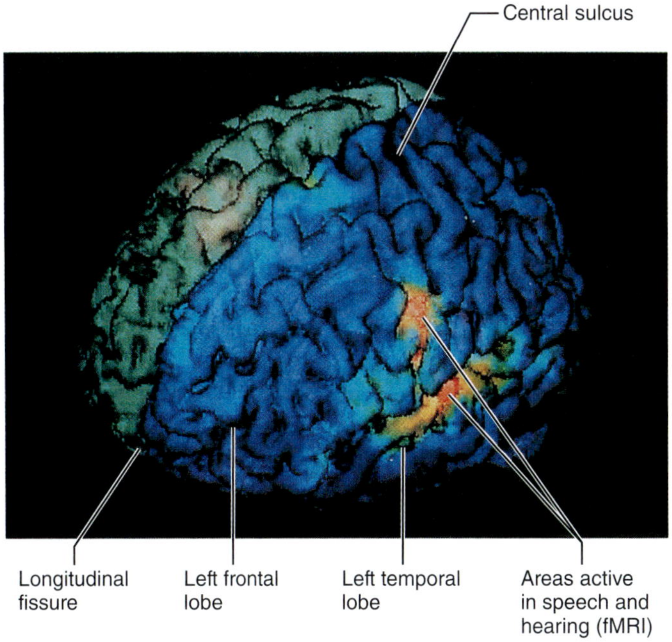

Figure 12.5 Functional neuroimaging (fMRI) of the cerebral cortex. Speaking and hearing increase activity (blood flow, shown by yellow and orange areas) in the posterior frontal and superior temporal lobes, respectively.

2. **Premotor cortex.** Just anterior to the precentral gyrus in the frontal lobe is the **premotor cortex** (see Figure 12.6, light red area). The premotor cortex helps plan movements. This region selects and sequences basic motor movements into more complex tasks, such as playing a musical instrument or typing. Using highly processed sensory information received from other cortical areas, it can control voluntary actions that depend on sensory feedback, such as moving an arm through a maze to grasp a hidden object.

   The premotor cortex coordinates the movement of several muscle groups either simultaneously or sequentially, mainly by sending activating impulses to the primary motor cortex. However, the premotor cortex also influences motor activity more directly by supplying about 15% of pyramidal tract fibers. Think of this region as the staging area for skilled motor activities.
3. **Broca's area. Broca's area** (bro′kahz) lies anterior to the inferior region of the premotor area. It has long been

12

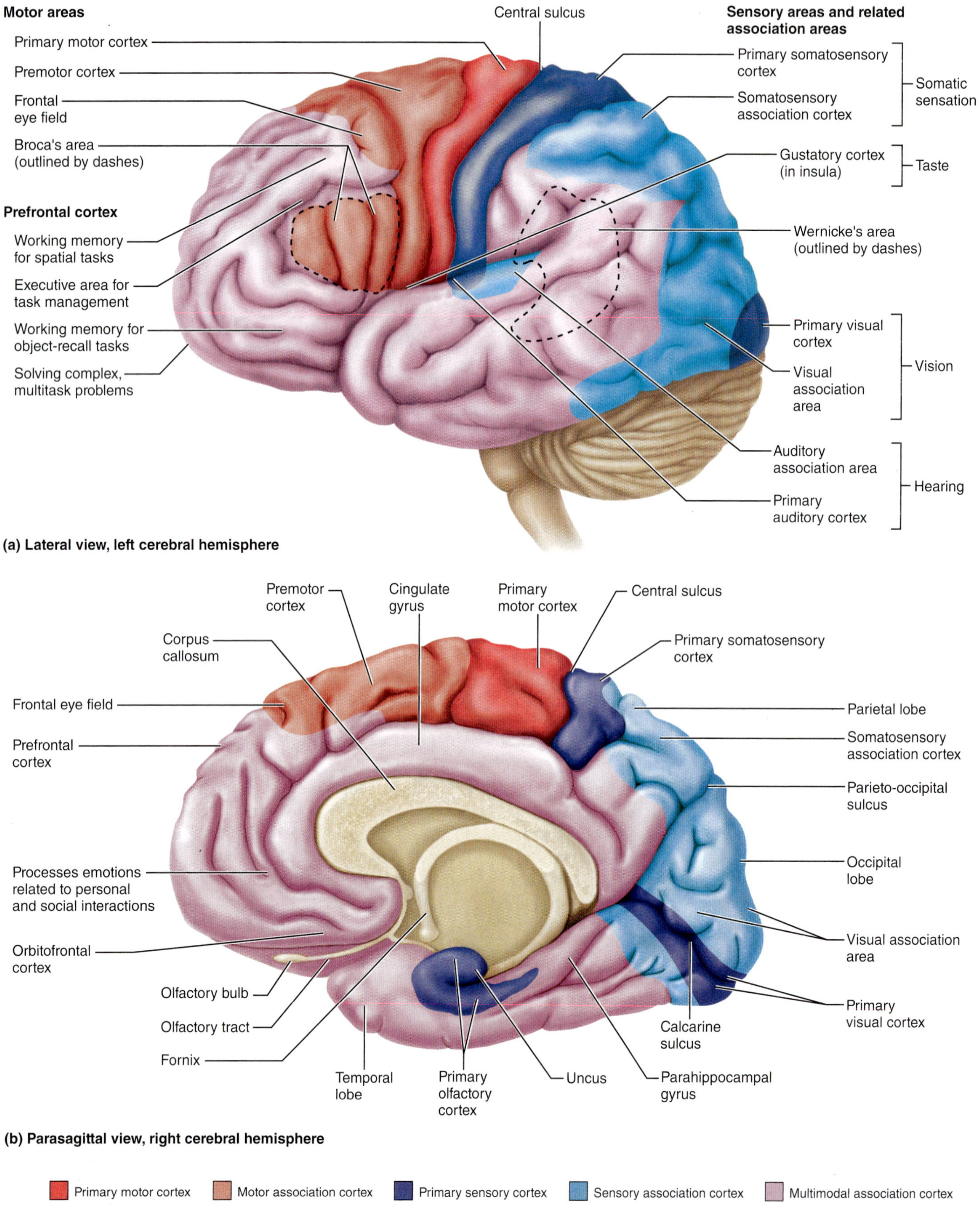

Figure 12.6 Functional and structural areas of the cerebral cortex.

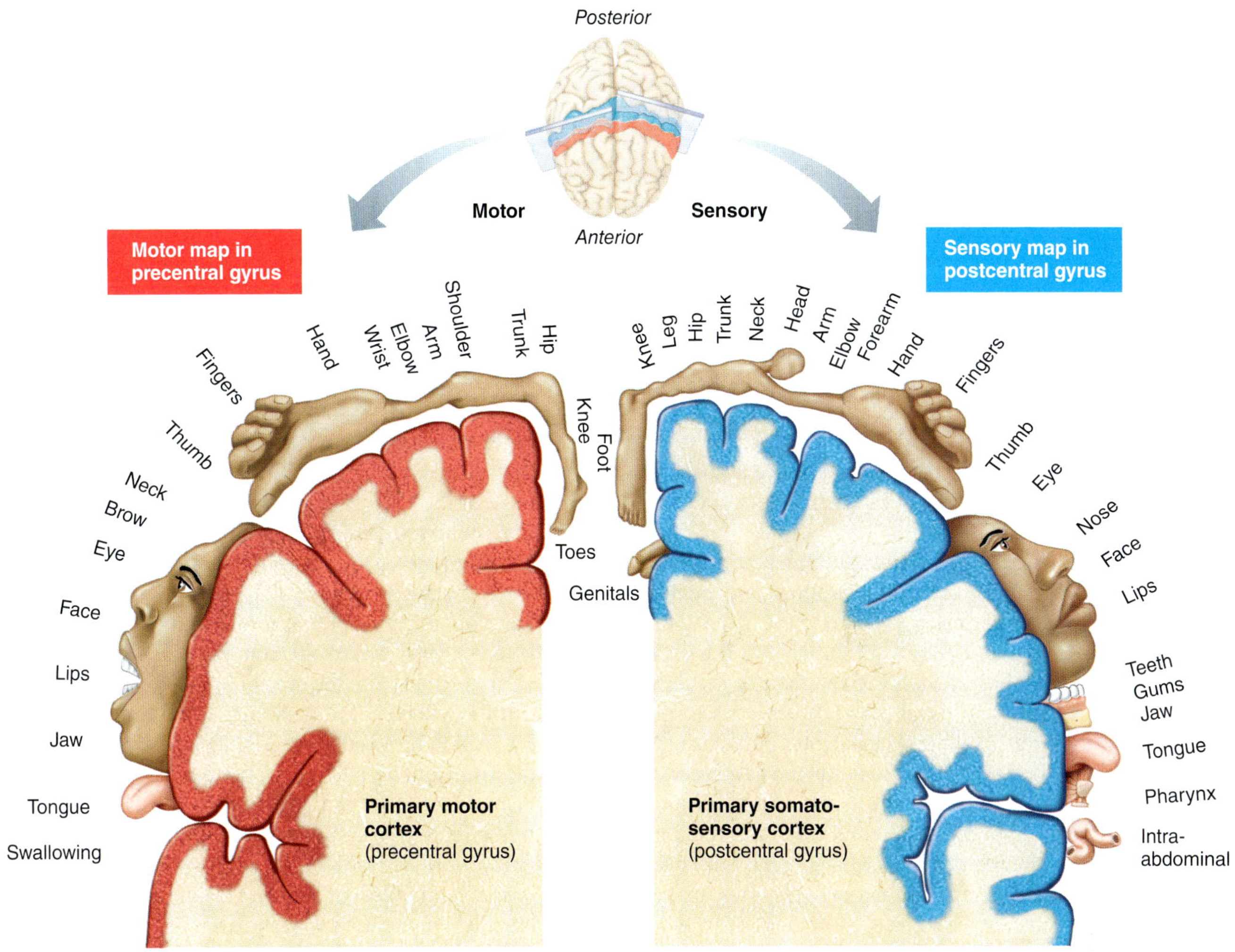

Figure 12.7 Body maps in the primary motor cortex and somatosensory cortex of the cerebrum. The relative amount and location of cortical tissue devoted to each function is proportional to the distorted body diagrams (homunculi).

considered to be (1) present in one hemisphere only (usually the left) and (2) a special *motor speech area* that directs the muscles involved in speech production. However, imaging studies indicate that Broca's area also becomes active as we prepare to speak and even as we think about (plan) many voluntary motor activities other than speech.

4. **Frontal eye field.** The **frontal eye field** is located partially in and anterior to the premotor cortex and superior to Broca's area. This cortical region controls voluntary movement of the eyes.

Homeostatic Imbalance 12.1

Damage to localized areas of the *primary motor cortex* (as from a stroke) paralyzes the body muscles controlled by those areas. If the lesion is in the right hemisphere, the left side of the body will be paralyzed. Only *voluntary* control is lost, however, as the muscles can still contract reflexively.

Destruction of the *premotor cortex*, or part of it, results in loss of the motor skill(s) programmed by that region, but does not impair muscle strength and the ability to perform the discrete individual movements. For example, if the premotor area controlling the flight of your fingers over a computer keyboard were damaged, you couldn't type with your usual speed, but you could still make the same movements with your fingers. Reprogramming the skill into another set of premotor neurons would require practice, just as the initial learning process did. ✚

Sensory Areas Areas concerned with conscious awareness of sensation, the sensory areas of the cortex, occur in the parietal, insular, temporal, and occipital lobes (see Figure 12.6, dark and light blue areas).

1. **Primary somatosensory cortex.** The **primary somatosensory cortex** resides in the postcentral gyrus of the parietal lobe, just posterior to the primary motor cortex. Neurons in this gyrus receive information from the general (somatic) sensory receptors in the skin and from proprioceptors (position sense receptors) in skeletal muscles, joints, and tendons. The neurons then identify the body region being stimulated, an ability called **spatial discrimination**.

As with the primary motor cortex, the body is represented spatially and upside down according to the site of stimulus input, and the right hemisphere receives input from the left side of the body. The amount of sensory cortex devoted to a particular body region is related to that region's sensitivity (that is, to how many receptors it has), not its size. In humans, the face (especially the lips) and fingertips are the most sensitive body areas, so these regions are the largest parts of the **somatosensory homunculus** (shown in the right half of Figure 12.7).

2. **Somatosensory association cortex.** The **somatosensory association cortex** lies just posterior to the primary somatosensory cortex and has many connections with it. The major function of this area is to integrate sensory inputs (temperature, pressure, and so forth) relayed to it via the primary somatosensory cortex to produce an understanding of an object being felt: its size, texture, and the relationship of its parts.

   For example, when you reach into your pocket, your somatosensory association cortex draws upon stored memories of past sensory experiences to perceive the objects you feel as coins or keys. Someone with damage to this area could not recognize these objects without looking at them.

3. **Visual areas.** The **primary visual (striate) cortex** is seen on the extreme posterior tip of the occipital lobe, but most of it is buried deep in the *calcarine sulcus* in the medial aspect of the occipital lobe (Figure 12.6b). The largest cortical sensory area, the primary visual cortex receives visual information that originates on the retina of the eye. There is a contralateral map of visual space on the primary visual cortex, analogous to the body map on the somatosensory cortex.

   The **visual association area** surrounds the primary visual cortex and covers much of the occipital lobe. Communicating with the primary visual cortex, the visual association area uses past visual experiences to interpret visual stimuli (color, form, and movement), enabling us to recognize a flower or a person's face and to appreciate what we are seeing. We do our "seeing" with these cortical neurons. However, complex visual processing involves the entire posterior half of the cerebral hemispheres. Particularly important are two visual "streams"—one running along the top of the brain and handling spatial relationships and object location, the other taking the lower road and focusing on recognizing faces, words, and objects.

4. **Auditory areas.** Each **primary auditory cortex** is located in the superior margin of the temporal lobe abutting the lateral sulcus. Sound energy exciting the hearing receptors of the inner ear causes impulses to be transmitted to the primary auditory cortex, where they are interpreted as pitch, loudness, and location.

   The more posterior **auditory association area** then permits the perception of the sound stimulus, which we "hear" as speech, a scream, music, thunder, noise, and so on. Memories of sounds heard in the past appear to be stored here for reference. Wernicke's area, which we describe later, includes parts of the auditory cortex.

5. **Vestibular (equilibrium) cortex.** Imaging studies show that the part of the cortex responsible for conscious awareness of balance (the position of the head in space) is located in the posterior part of the insula and adjacent parietal cortex.

6. **Olfactory cortex.** The **primary olfactory (smell) cortex** lies on the medial aspect of the temporal lobe in a small region called the *piriform lobe* which is dominated by the hooklike *uncus* (Figure 12.6b). Afferent fibers from smell receptors in the superior nasal cavities send impulses along the olfactory tracts that are ultimately relayed to the olfactory cortices. The outcome is conscious awareness of different odors.

   The olfactory cortex is part of the primitive **rhinencephalon** (ri″nen-sef′ah-lon; "nose brain"), which includes all parts of the cerebrum that receive olfactory signals—the orbitofrontal cortex, uncus, and associated regions located on or in the medial aspects of the temporal lobes, and the protruding olfactory tracts and bulbs that extend to the nose. During the course of evolution, most of the "old" rhinencephalon has taken on new functions concerned chiefly with emotions and memory. It has become part of the "newer" emotional brain, called the *limbic system*, which we will consider later in this chapter. The only portions of the human rhinencephalon still devoted to smell are the olfactory bulbs and tracts (described in Chapter 13) and the greatly reduced olfactory cortices.

7. **Gustatory cortex.** The **gustatory (taste) cortex** (gus′tah-tor-e), a region involved in perceiving taste stimuli, is located in the insula just deep to the temporal lobe (Figure 12.6a).

8. **Visceral sensory area.** The cortex of the insula just posterior to the gustatory cortex is involved in conscious perception of visceral sensations. These include upset stomach, full bladder, and the feeling that your lungs will burst when you hold your breath too long.

Homeostatic Imbalance 12.2

Damage to the *primary visual cortex* (Figure 12.6) results in functional blindness. By contrast, individuals with a damaged visual association area can see, but they do not comprehend what they are looking at. +

Multimodal Association Areas The association areas that we have considered so far (colored light red or light blue in Figure 12.6) have all been tightly tied to one kind of primary motor or sensory cortex (colored dark red or dark blue). Most of the cortex, though, consists of complexly connected **multimodal association areas** (colored light violet in Figure 12.6) that receive inputs from multiple senses and send outputs to multiple areas.

In general, information flows from sensory receptors to the appropriate primary sensory cortex, then to a sensory association cortex and then on to the multimodal association cortex. Multimodal association cortex allows us to give meaning to the information that we receive, store it in memory, tie it to previous experience and knowledge, and decide what action to take. Those decisions are relayed to the premotor cortex, which in turn communicates with the motor cortex. The multimodal association cortex seems to be where sensations, thoughts, and emotions become conscious. It is what makes us who we are.

Suppose, for example, you drop a bottle of acid in the chem lab and it splashes on you. You see the bottle shatter, hear the crash, feel your skin burning, and smell the acid fumes. These individual perceptions come together in the multimodal association areas. Along with feelings of panic, these perceptions are woven into a seamless whole, which (hopefully) recalls instructions about what to do in this situation. As a result your premotor and primary motor cortices direct your legs to propel you to the safety shower.

The multimodal association areas can be broadly divided into three parts: the anterior association, posterior association, and limbic association areas.

1. **Anterior association area.** The **anterior association area** in the frontal lobe, also called the **prefrontal cortex**, is the most complicated cortical region of all (Figure 12.6). It is involved with intellect, complex learning abilities (called cognition), recall, and personality. It contains working memory, which is necessary for abstract ideas, judgment, reasoning, persistence, and planning. These abilities develop slowly in children, which implies that the prefrontal cortex matures slowly and depends heavily on positive and negative feedback from our social environment.
2. **Posterior association area.** The **posterior association area** is a large region encompassing parts of the temporal, parietal, and occipital lobes. This area plays a role in recognizing patterns and faces, localizing us and our surroundings in space, and binding different sensory inputs into a coherent whole. In the spilled acid example above, your awareness of the entire scene originates from this area. Attention to an area of space or an area of one's own body is also a function of this part of the brain. Many parts of the posterior association area (including Wernicke's area, Figure 12.6a) are also involved in understanding written and spoken language.
3. **Limbic association area.** The **limbic association area** includes the cingulate gyrus, parahippocampal gyrus, and hippocampus (see Figures 12.6b and 12.16). Part of the limbic system (which we describe later), the limbic association area provides the emotional impact that makes a scene important to us. In our example above, it provides the sense of "danger" when the acid splashes on our legs. The hippocampus establishes memories that allow us to remember this incident. More on this later.

Homeostatic Imbalance 12.3

Tumors or other lesions of the *anterior association area* may cause mental and personality disorders including loss of judgment, attentiveness, and inhibitions. The affected individual may be oblivious to social restraints, perhaps becoming careless about personal appearance, or rashly attacking a 7-foot opponent rather than running.

Different problems arise for individuals with lesions in the part of the *posterior association area* that provides awareness of self in space. They may refuse to wash or dress the side of their body opposite to the lesion because "that doesn't belong to me." +

Lateralization of Cortical Functioning We use both cerebral hemispheres for almost every activity, and the hemispheres appear nearly identical. Nonetheless, there is a division of labor, and each hemisphere has abilities not completely shared by its partner. This phenomenon is called **lateralization**.

Although one cerebral hemisphere or the other "dominates" each task, the term **cerebral dominance** designates the hemisphere that is *dominant for language*. In most people (about 90%), the left hemisphere has greater control over language abilities, math, and logic. This so-called dominant hemisphere is working when we compose a sentence, balance a checkbook, and memorize a list. The other hemisphere (usually the right) is more free-spirited, more involved in visual-spatial skills, intuition, emotion, and artistic and musical skills. It is the poetic, creative, and the "Ah-ha!" (insightful) side of our nature, and in males it is better at recognizing faces.

Most individuals with left cerebral dominance are right-handed. In the remaining 10% of people, the roles of the hemispheres are reversed or the hemispheres share their functions equally. Typically, right-cerebral-dominant people are left-handed and male. Some "lefties" who have a cerebral cortex that functions bilaterally are ambidextrous.

The two cerebral hemispheres have almost instantaneous communication with each other via connecting fiber tracts, as well as complete functional integration. Furthermore, although lateralization means that each hemisphere is better than the other at certain functions, neither hemisphere is better at everything.

Cerebral White Matter

The second of the three basic regions of each cerebral hemisphere is the internal **cerebral white matter**. From what we have already described, you know that communication within the brain is extensive. The white matter deep to the cortical gray matter is responsible for communication between cerebral areas and between the cerebral cortex and lower CNS centers.

White matter consists largely of myelinated fibers bundled into large tracts. These fibers and tracts are classified according to the direction in which they run as *association*, *commissural*, or *projection* **(Figure 12.8)**.

- **Association fibers** connect different parts of the same hemisphere. Short association fibers connect adjacent gyri. Long association fibers are bundled into tracts and connect different cortical lobes.
- **Commissural fibers** connect corresponding gray areas of the two hemispheres. These **commissures** (kom′ĭ-shūrz) allow the two hemispheres to function as a coordinated whole. The largest commissure is the **corpus callosum** (kah-lo′sum; "thickened body"), which lies superior to the lateral ventricles, deep within the longitudinal fissure. Less prominent examples are the **anterior** and **posterior commissures** (see Figure 12.10, p. 440).
- **Projection fibers** either enter the cerebral cortex from lower brain or cord centers or descend from the cortex to lower areas. Sensory information reaches the cerebral cortex and motor output leaves it through these projection fibers. They tie the cortex to the rest of the nervous system and to the body's receptors and effectors. In contrast to commissural and association fibers, which run horizontally, projection fibers run vertically (Figure 12.8a).

  At the top of the brain stem, the projection fibers on each side form a compact band, the **internal capsule**, that passes between the thalamus and some of the basal nuclei. Beyond that point, the fibers radiate fanlike through the cerebral white matter to the cortex. This distinctive arrangement is called the **corona radiata** ("radiating crown").

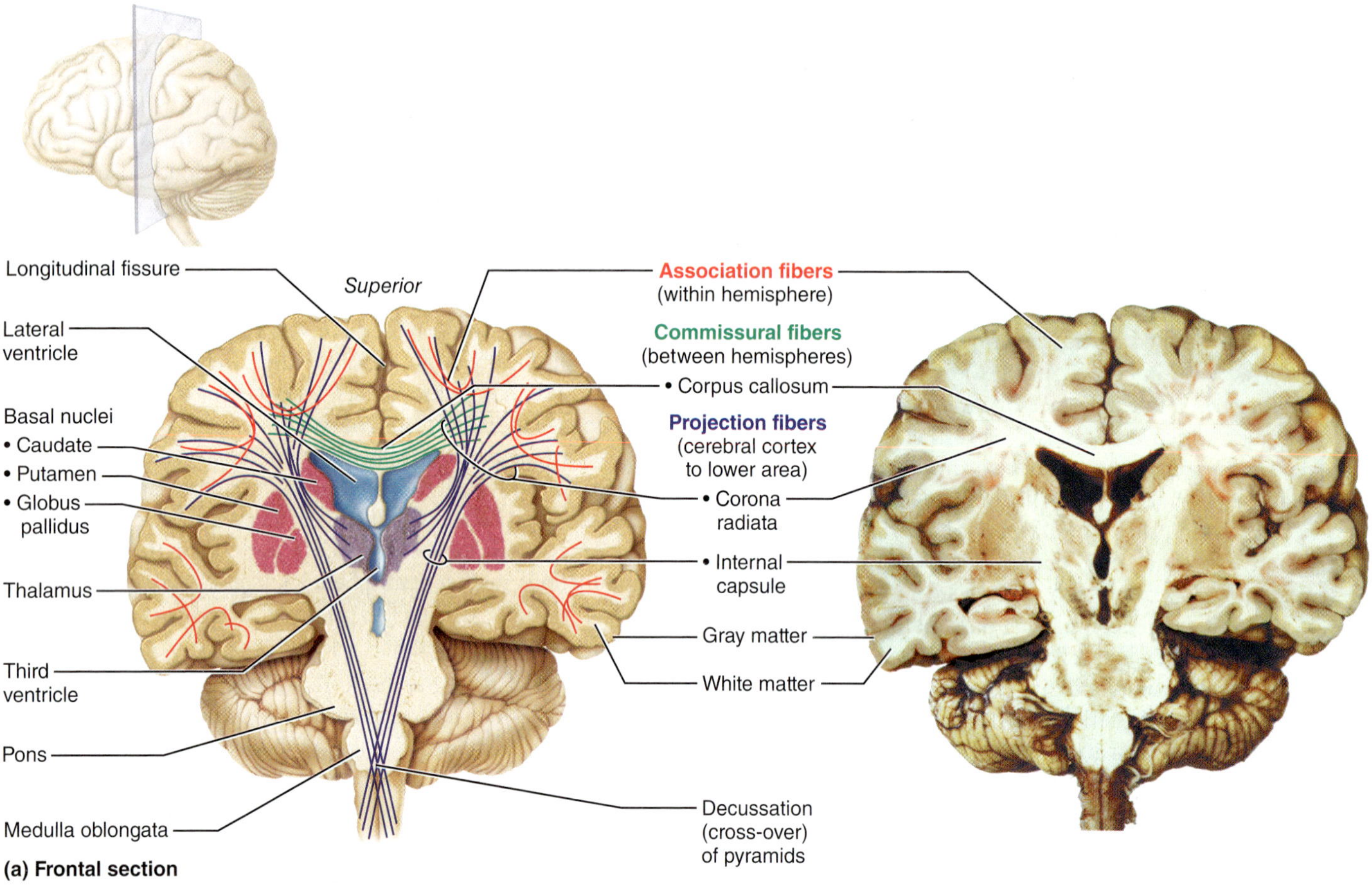

(a) Frontal section

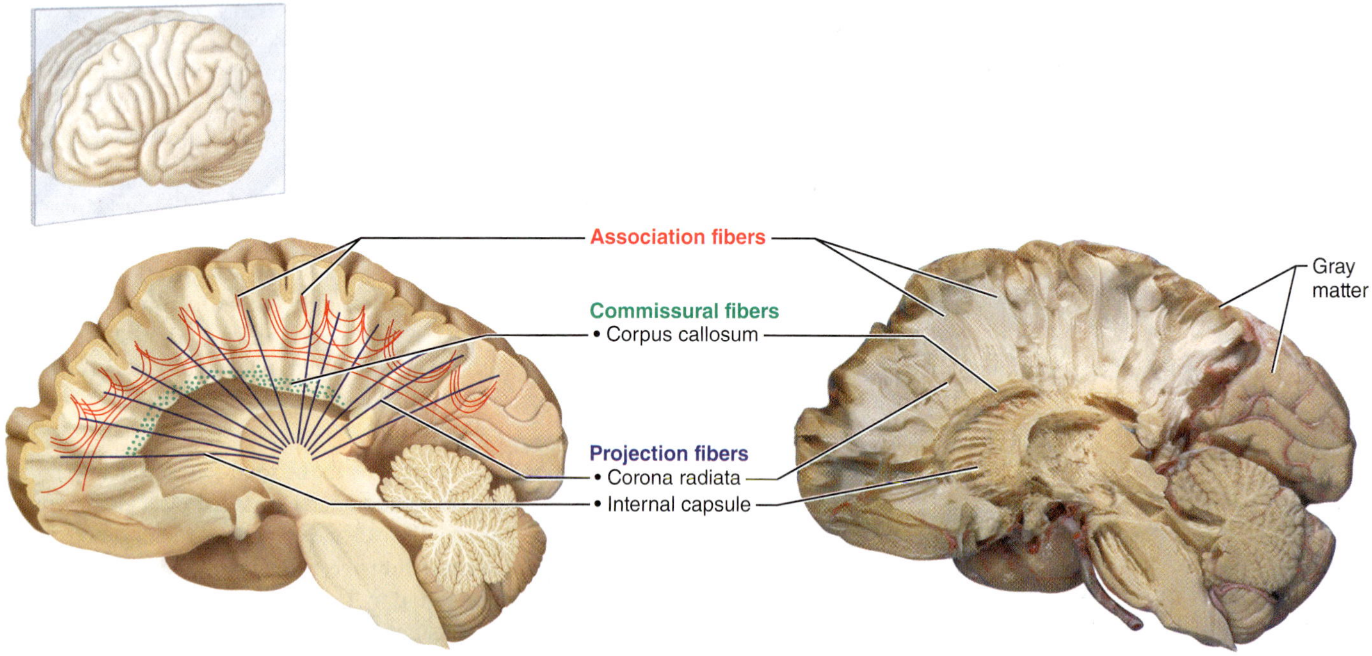

(b) Parasagittal section and dissection

Figure 12.8 White fiber tracts of the cerebral hemispheres. Commissural, association, and projection fibers run within the cerebrum, and between the cerebrum and lower CNS centers. In all views, notice the tight band of projection fibers, called the internal capsule, that passes between the thalamus and the basal nuclei, and then fans out as the corona radiata.

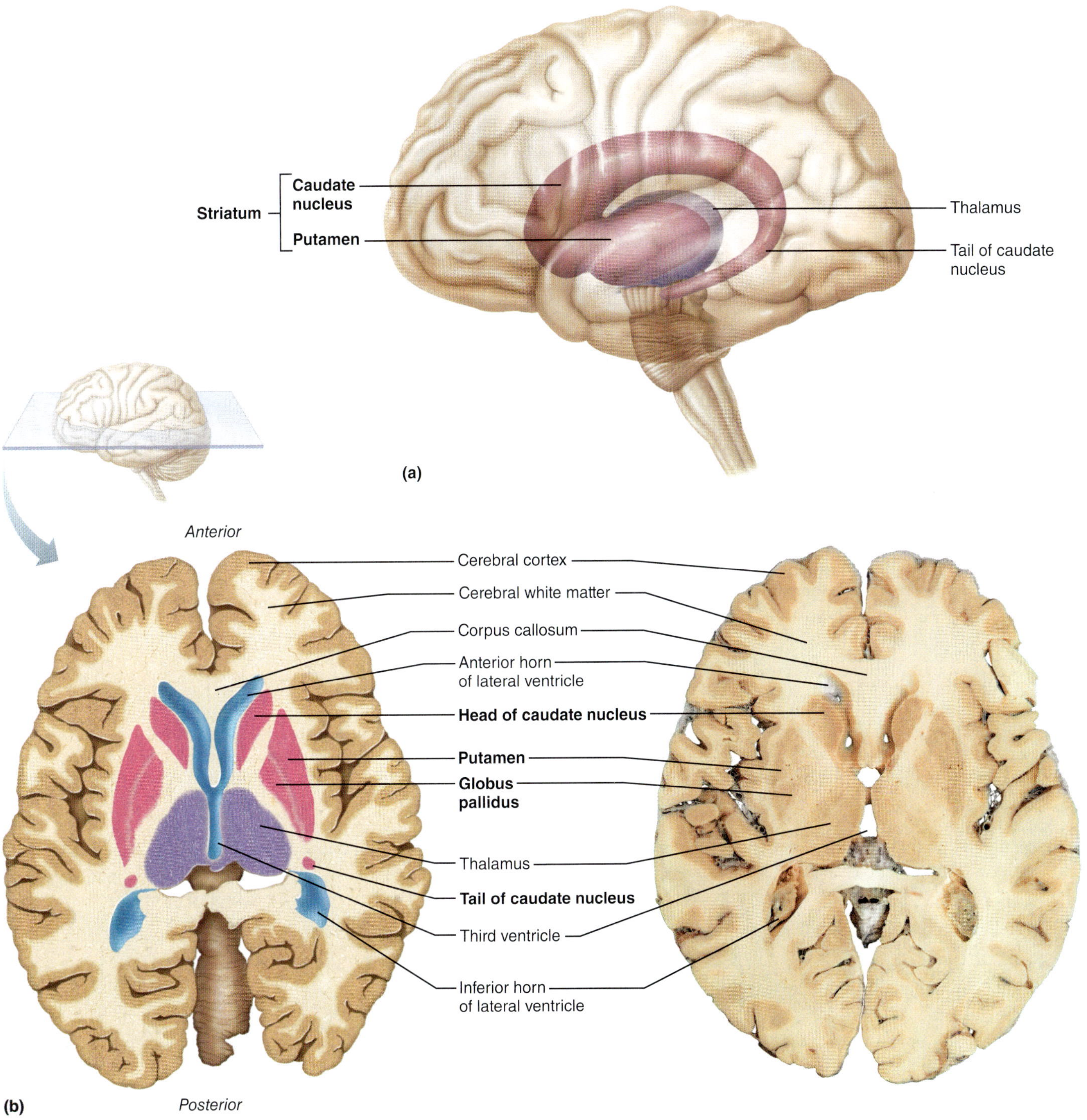

Figure 12.9 Basal nuclei. (a) Three-dimensional view of the basal nuclei (basal ganglia), showing their position in the cerebrum. **(b)** Transverse section of cerebrum and diencephalon showing the relationship of the basal nuclei to the thalamus and the lateral and third ventricles.

Basal Nuclei

Deep within the cerebral white matter is the third basic region of each hemisphere, a group of subcortical nuclei called the **basal nuclei** or **basal ganglia**.* Although the definition of the precise structures forming the basal nuclei is controversial, most anatomists agree each hemisphere's basal nuclei include the **caudate nucleus** (kaw′dāt), **putamen** (pu-ta′men), and **globus pallidus** (glo′bis pal′ĭ-dus) **(Figure 12.9)**.

The comma-shaped caudate nucleus arches superiorly over the diencephalon. Together with the putamen, it forms the **striatum** (stri-a′tum), so called because the fibers of the internal capsule passing through them create a striped appearance. Although

*Because a nucleus is a collection of nerve cell bodies within the CNS, the term *basal nuclei* is technically correct. The more frequently used but misleading historical term *basal ganglia* is a misnomer and should be abandoned, because ganglia are PNS structures.

12

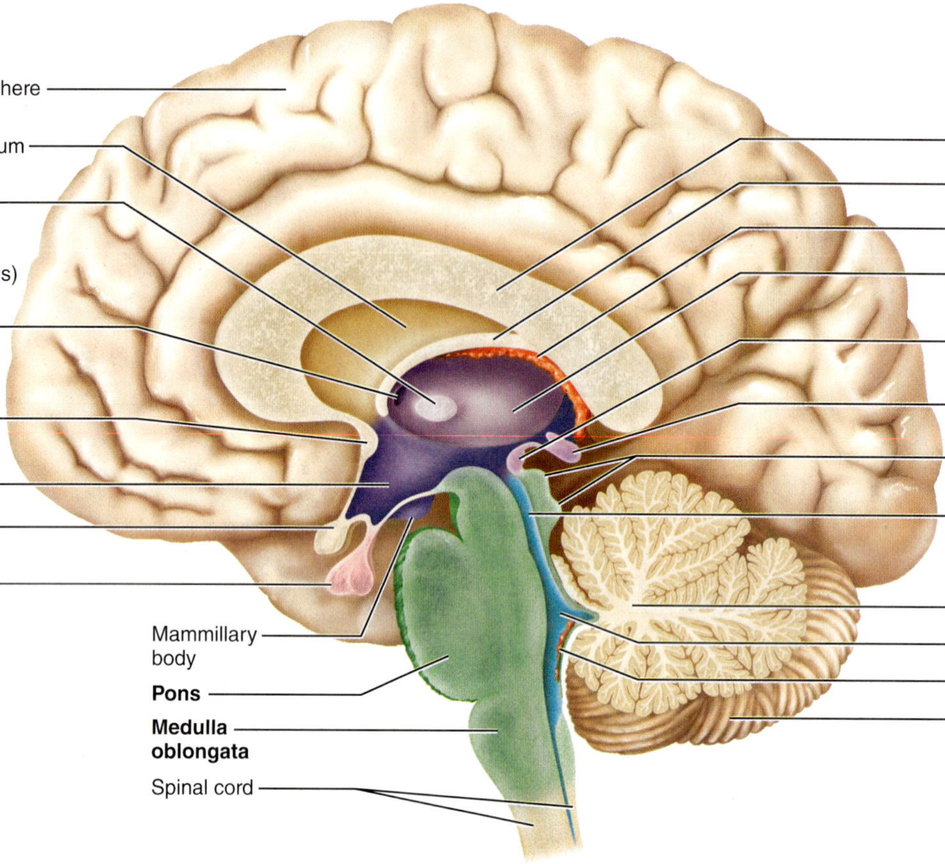

(a)

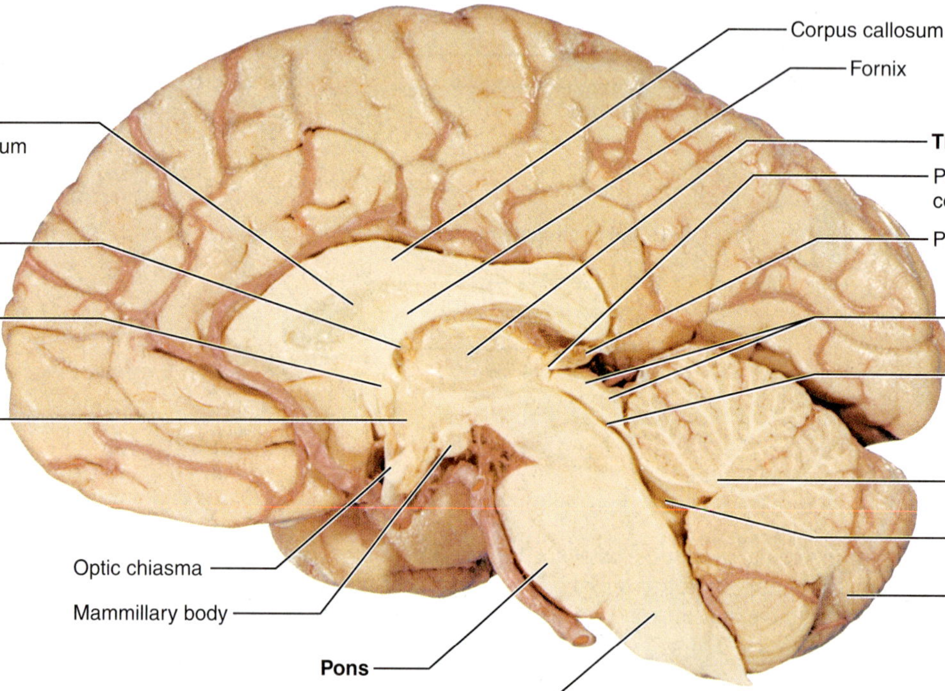

(b)

Figure 12.10 Midsagittal section of the brain. (a) Illustration highlighting the diencephalon (purple) and brain stem (green). **(b)** Photo of same view.

the putamen ("pod") and globus pallidus ("pale globe") together form a lens-shaped mass, sometimes called the *lentiform nucleus*, these two nuclei are functionally separate.

The basal nuclei are functionally associated with the *subthalamic nuclei* (located in the lateral "floor" of the diencephalon) and the *substantia nigra* of the midbrain (see Figure 12.14a).

The basal nuclei receive input from the entire cerebral cortex, as well as from other subcortical nuclei and each other. Via relays through the thalamus, the output nucleus of the basal nuclei (globus pallidus) and the substantia nigra project to the premotor and prefrontal cortices and so influence muscle movements directed by the primary motor cortex. The basal nuclei have no direct access to motor pathways.

The precise role of the basal nuclei has been elusive because of their inaccessible location and because their motor functions overlap with those of the cerebellum. In addition to their motor functions, the basal nuclei play a role in cognition and emotion. In all of these cases, the basal nuclei seem to filter out incorrect or inappropriate responses, passing only the best response on to the cortex.

For example, in motor activity, the basal nuclei are particularly important in starting, stopping, and monitoring the intensity of movements executed by the cortex, especially those that are relatively slow or stereotyped, such as arm-swinging during walking. Additionally, they inhibit antagonistic or unnecessary movements. Disorders of the basal nuclei result in either too much movement (as in Huntington's disease) or too little movement (Parkinson's disease); see p. 464.

☑ Check Your Understanding

4. What anatomical landmark of the cerebral cortex separates primary motor areas from somatosensory areas?
5. Mike, who is left-handed, decided to wear his favorite T-shirt to his anatomy class. On his T-shirt were the words "Only left-handed people are in their right minds." What does this statement mean?
6. Which type of fiber allows the two cerebral hemispheres to "talk to each other"?
7. Name the components of the basal nuclei.

For answers, see Appendix H.

Diencephalon

✓ Describe the location of the diencephalon, and name its subdivisions and functions.

Forming the central core of the forebrain and surrounded by the cerebral hemispheres, the **diencephalon** consists largely of three paired structures—the thalamus, hypothalamus, and epithalamus. These gray matter areas collectively enclose the third ventricle **(Figure 12.10)**.

Thalamus

The **thalamus** consists of bilateral egg-shaped nuclei, which form the superolateral walls of the third ventricle (Figures 12.8 and 12.10). In most people, an **interthalamic adhesion** (**intermediate mass**) connects the nuclei. *Thalamus* is a Greek word meaning "inner room," which well describes this deep, well-hidden brain region that makes up 80% of the diencephalon.

The thalamus is *the* relay station for information coming into the cerebral cortex. Within the thalamus are a large number of nuclei, most named according to their location **(Figure 12.11a)**. Each nucleus has a functional specialty, and each projects fibers to and receives fibers from a specific region of the cerebral cortex.

Afferent impulses from all senses and all parts of the body converge on the thalamus and synapse with at least one of its nuclei. For example, the ventral posterolateral nuclei receive impulses from the general somatic sensory receptors (touch, pressure, pain, etc.), and the *lateral* and *medial geniculate bodies* (jĕ-nik′u-lāt; "knee shaped") are important visual and auditory relay centers, respectively.

Within the thalamus, information is sorted out and "edited." Impulses having to do with similar functions are relayed as a group via the internal capsule to the appropriate area of the sensory cortex as well as to specific cortical association areas. As the afferent impulses reach the thalamus, we have a crude recognition of the sensation as pleasant or unpleasant. However, specific stimulus localization and discrimination occur in the cerebral cortex.

In addition to sensory inputs, virtually *all* other inputs ascending to the cerebral cortex funnel through thalamic nuclei. These include:

- Inputs that help regulate emotion and visceral function from the hypothalamus (via the anterior nuclei)
- Instructions that help direct the activity of the motor cortices from the cerebellum and basal nuclei (via the ventral lateral and ventral anterior nuclei, respectively)
- Inputs for memory or sensory integration that are projected to specific association cortices (via pulvinar, lateral dorsal, and lateral posterior nuclei)

In summary, the thalamus plays a key role in mediating sensation, motor activities, cortical arousal, learning, and memory. It is truly the gateway to the cerebral cortex.

Hypothalamus

Named for its position below (*hypo*) the thalamus, the **hypothalamus** caps the brain stem and forms the inferolateral walls of the third ventricle (Figure 12.10). Merging into the midbrain inferiorly, the hypothalamus extends from the optic chiasma (crossover point of the optic nerves) to the posterior margin of the mammillary bodies.

The **mammillary bodies** (mam′mil-er-e; "little breast"), paired pealike nuclei that bulge anteriorly from the hypothalamus, are relay stations in the olfactory pathways. Between the optic chiasma and mammillary bodies is the **infundibulum** (in″fun-dib′u-lum), a stalk of hypothalamic tissue that connects the **pituitary gland** to the base of the hypothalamus. Like the thalamus, the hypothalamus contains many functionally important nuclei (Figure 12.11b).

Despite its small size, the hypothalamus is the main visceral control center of the body and is vitally important to overall

12

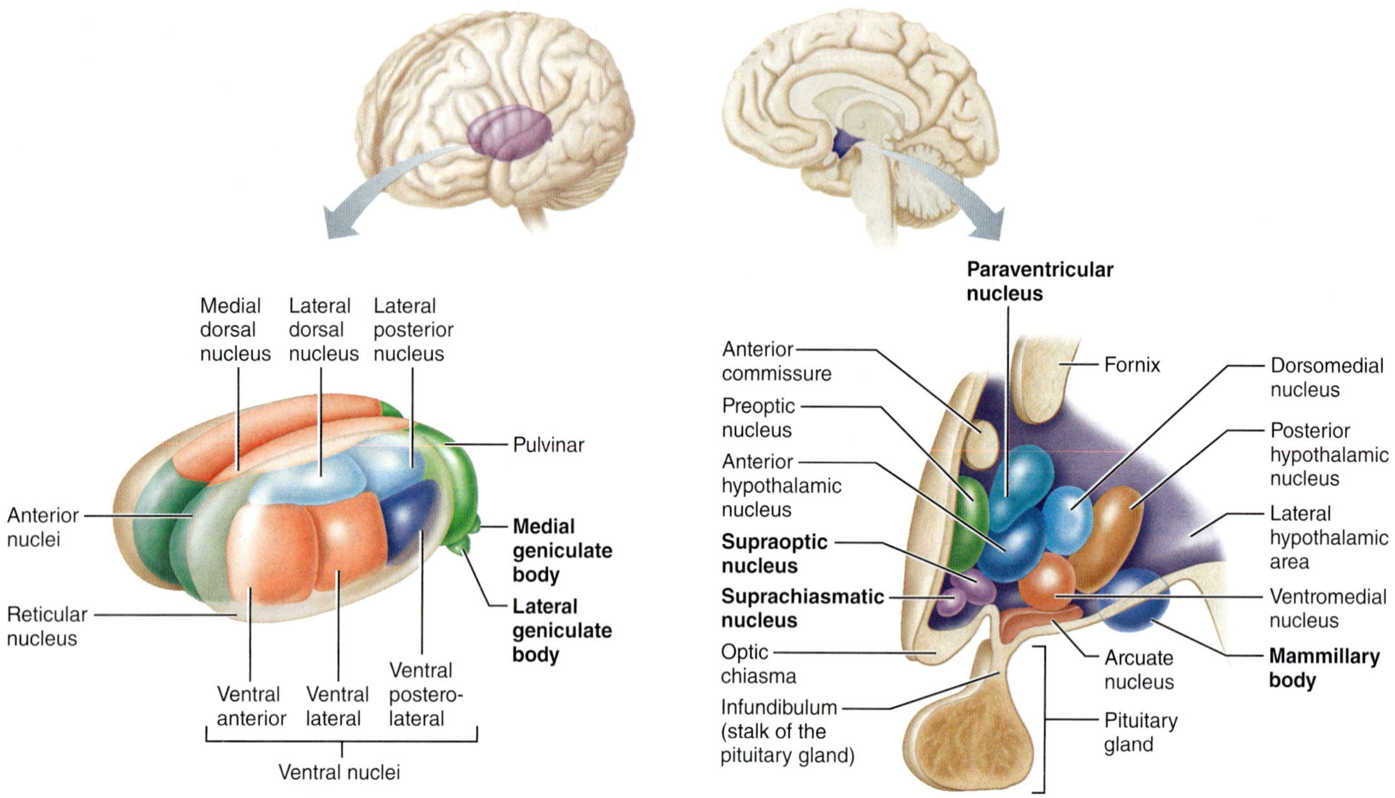

(a) The main thalamic nuclei. (The reticular nuclei that "cap" the thalamus laterally are depicted as curving translucent structures.)

(b) The main hypothalamic nuclei.

12

Figure 12.11 Selected structures of the diencephalon.

body homeostasis. Few tissues in the body escape its influence. Its chief homeostatic roles are to:

- **Control the autonomic nervous system.** Recall that the autonomic nervous system (ANS) is a system of peripheral nerves that regulates cardiac and smooth muscle and secretion by the glands. The hypothalamus regulates ANS activity by controlling the activity of centers in the brain stem and spinal cord. In this role, the hypothalamus influences blood pressure, rate and force of heartbeat, digestive tract motility, eye pupil size, and many other visceral activities.
- **Initiate physical responses to emotions.** The hypothalamus lies at the "heart" of the limbic system (the emotional part of the brain). It contains nuclei involved in perceiving pleasure, fear, and rage, as well as those involved in biological rhythms and drives (such as the sex drive).

  The hypothalamus acts through ANS pathways to initiate most physical expressions of emotion. For example, a fearful person has a pounding heart, high blood pressure, pallor, sweating, and a dry mouth.
- **Regulate body temperature.** The body's thermostat is in the hypothalamus. Hypothalamic neurons monitor blood temperature and receive input from other thermoreceptors in the brain and body periphery. Accordingly, the hypothalamus initiates cooling (sweating) or heat-generating actions (shivering) as needed to maintain a relatively constant body temperature (see Figure 24.26, p. 946).
- **Regulate food intake.** In response to changing blood levels of certain nutrients (glucose and amino acids) or hormones (cholecystokinin, ghrelin, and others), the hypothalamus regulates feelings of hunger and satiety.
- **Regulate water balance and thirst.** When body fluids become too concentrated, hypothalamic neurons called *osmoreceptors* are activated. Osmoreceptors excite hypothalamic nuclei that trigger the release of antidiuretic hormone (ADH) from the posterior pituitary. ADH causes the kidneys to retain water. The same conditions also stimulate hypothalamic neurons in the *thirst center*, causing us to feel thirsty and drink more fluids.
- **Regulate sleep-wake cycles.** Acting with other brain regions, the hypothalamus helps regulate sleep. Its *suprachiasmatic nucleus* (our biological clock) sets the timing of the sleep cycle in response to daylight-darkness cues received from the visual pathways.
- **Control endocrine system function.** The hypothalamus acts as the helmsman of the endocrine system in two important ways. First, its *releasing* and *inhibiting hormones* control the secretion of hormones by the anterior pituitary gland. Second, its *supraoptic* and *paraventricular nuclei* produce the hormones ADH and oxytocin.

Homeostatic Imbalance 12.4

Hypothalamic disturbances cause a number of disorders including severe body wasting, obesity, sleep disturbances, dehydration, and emotional imbalances. For example, the hypothalamus is implicated in *failure to thrive*, a condition characterized by delay in growth or development that occurs when a child is deprived of a warm, nurturing relationship. +

Epithalamus

The most dorsal portion of the diencephalon, the **epithalamus** forms the roof of the third ventricle. Extending from its posterior border and visible externally is the **pineal gland** or **body** (pin′e-al; "pine cone shaped") (see Figures 12.10 and 12.13c). The pineal gland secretes the hormone *melatonin* (a sleep-inducing signal and antioxidant; see Chapter 16) and, along with hypothalamic nuclei, helps regulate the sleep-wake cycle. The *posterior commissure* forms the caudal border of the epithalamus.

☑ Check Your Understanding

8. Why is the thalamus called the "gateway to the cerebral cortex"?
9. The hypothalamus oversees a branch of the peripheral nervous system. Which branch?

For answers, see Appendix H.

Brain Stem

✓ Identify the three major regions of the brain stem, and note the functions of each area.

From superior to inferior, the brain stem regions are midbrain, pons, and medulla oblongata (Figures 12.10, 12.12, and 12.13). Each roughly an inch long, collectively they account for only 2.5% of total brain mass. Histologically, the organization of the brain stem is similar (but not identical) to that of the spinal cord—deep gray matter surrounded by white matter fiber tracts. However, the brain stem has nuclei of gray matter embedded in the white matter, a feature not found in the spinal cord.

Brain stem centers produce the rigidly programmed, automatic behaviors necessary for survival. Positioned between the cerebrum and the spinal cord, the brain stem also provides a pathway for fiber tracts running between higher and lower neural centers. Additionally, brain stem nuclei are associated with 10 of the 12 pairs of cranial nerves (which we will describe in Chapter 13), so it is heavily involved with innervating the head.

Midbrain

The **midbrain** is located between the diencephalon and pons (**Figure 12.12** and **Figure 12.13**). On its ventral aspect two bulging **cerebral peduncles** (pĕ-dung′klz) form vertical pillars that seem to hold up the cerebrum, hence their name meaning "little feet of the cerebrum" (Figure 12.13a, b, and **Figure 12.14a**). The *crus cerebri* ("leg of the cerebrum") of each peduncle contains a large pyramidal (corticospinal) motor tract descending toward the spinal cord. The *superior*

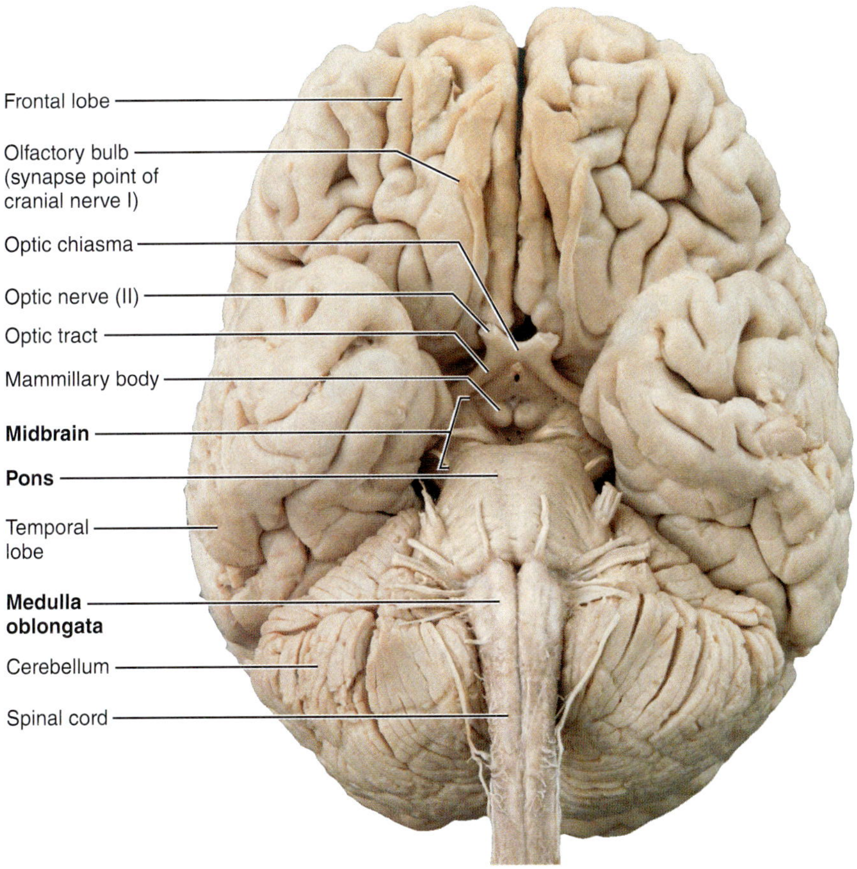

Figure 12.12 Inferior view of the brain, showing the three parts of the brain stem: midbrain, pons, and medulla oblongata. Only a small portion of the midbrain is visible in this view. (For a related image, see *A Brief Atlas of the Human Body*, Figure 49.)

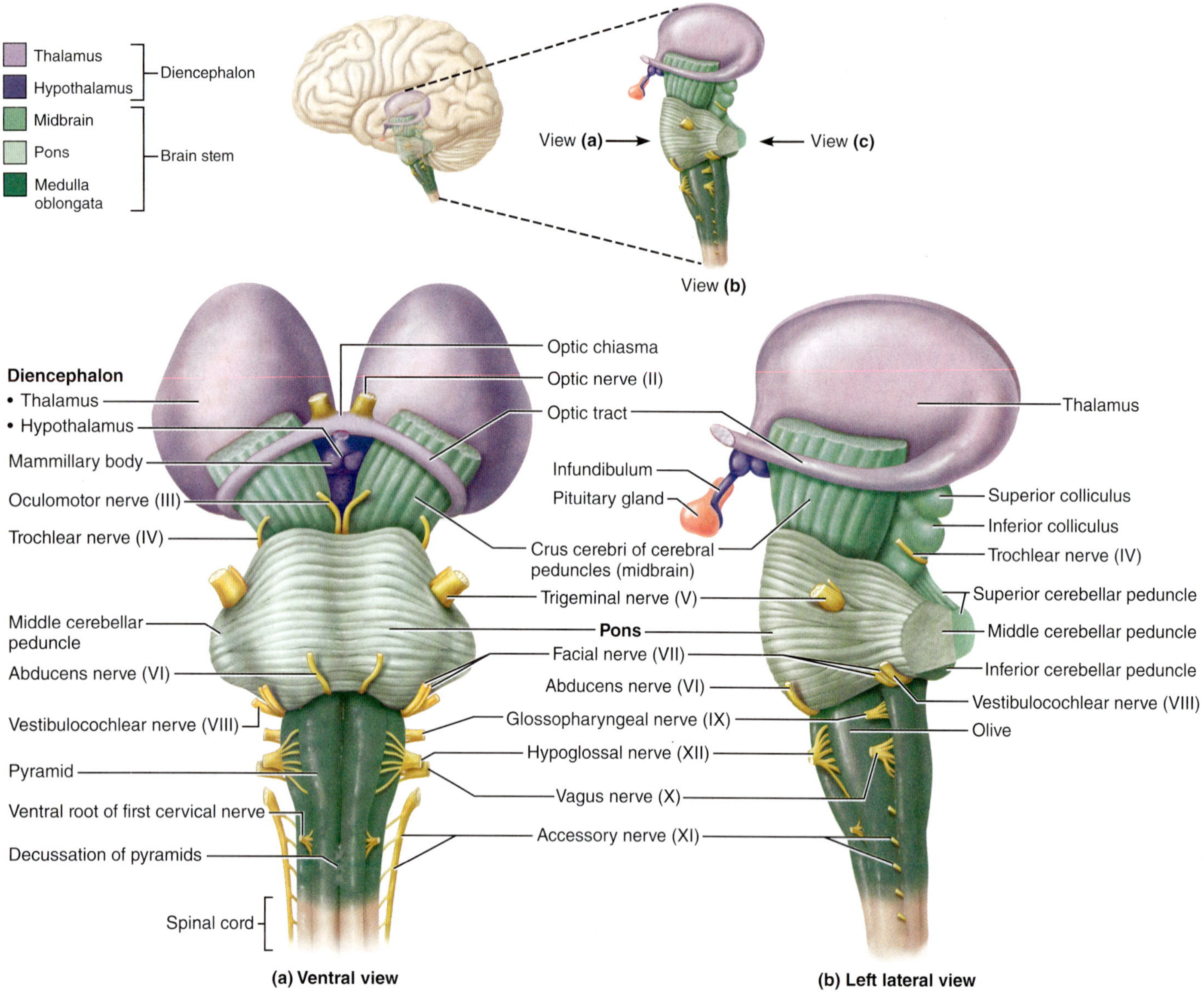

Figure 12.13 **Three views of the brain stem (green) and the diencephalon (purple).**

cerebellar peduncles, also fiber tracts, connect the midbrain to the cerebellum dorsally (Figure 12.13b, c).

Running through the midbrain is the hollow *cerebral aqueduct*, which connects the third and fourth ventricles (Figures 12.10 and 12.14a). It delineates the cerebral peduncles ventrally from the *tectum*, the midbrain's roof. Surrounding the aqueduct is the *periaqueductal gray matter*, which is involved in pain suppression and links the fear-perceiving amygdaloid body and ANS pathways that control the "fight-or-flight" response. The periaqueductal gray matter also includes nuclei that control two cranial nerves, the *oculomotor* and the *trochlear nuclei* (trok′le-ar).

Nuclei are also scattered in the surrounding white matter of the midbrain. The **corpora quadrigemina** (kor′por-ah kwod″rĭ-jem′ĭ-nah; "quadruplets"), the largest midbrain nuclei, raise four domelike protrusions on the dorsal midbrain surface (Figures 12.10 and 12.13c). The superior pair, the **superior colliculi** (kŏ-lik′ū-li), are visual reflex centers that coordinate head and eye movements when we visually follow a moving object, even if we are not consciously looking at it. The **inferior colliculi** are part of the auditory relay from the hearing receptors of the ear to the sensory cortex. They also act in reflexive responses to sound, such as the *startle reflex* which causes you to turn your head toward an unexpected noise.

Also embedded in each side of the midbrain white matter are two pigmented nuclei, the substantia nigra and red nucleus. The bandlike **substantia nigra** (sub-stan′she-ah ni′grah) is located deep to the cerebral peduncle (Figure 12.14a). Its dark (*nigr* = black) color reflects a high content of melanin pigment, a precursor of the neurotransmitter (dopamine) released by these neurons. The substantia nigra is functionally linked to the basal nuclei (its axons project to the putamen), and many authorities consider it part of the basal nuclear complex. Degeneration of the dopamine-releasing neurons of the substantia nigra is the ultimate cause of Parkinson's disease.

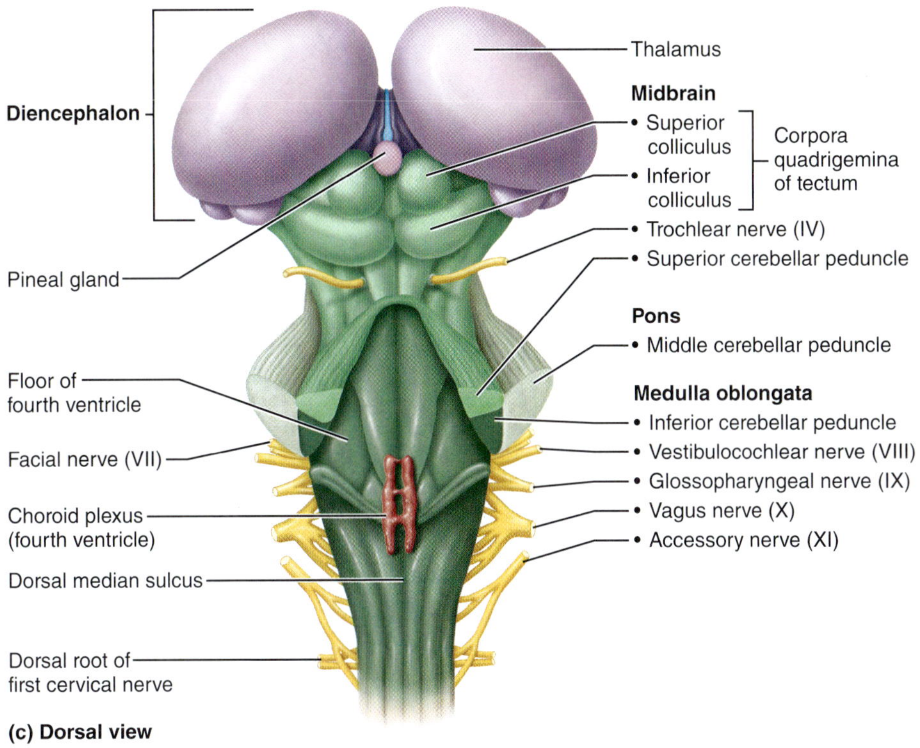

Figure 12.13 *(continued)*

12

The oval **red nucleus** lies deep to the substantia nigra (Figure 12.14a). Its reddish hue is due to its rich blood supply and to the presence of iron pigment in its neurons. The red nuclei are relay nuclei in some descending motor pathways that effect limb flexion, and they are embedded in the *reticular formation*, a system of small nuclei scattered through the core of the brain stem (see pp. 450–451).

Pons

The **pons** is the bulging brain stem region wedged between the midbrain and the medulla oblongata (see Figures 12.10, 12.12, and 12.13). Dorsally, the fourth ventricle separates it from the cerebellum.

As its name suggests (*pons* = bridge), the pons is chiefly composed of conduction tracts. They are oriented in two different directions:

- The deep projection fibers run longitudinally as part of the pathway between higher brain centers and the spinal cord.
- The more superficial ventral fibers are oriented transversely and dorsally. They form the *middle cerebellar peduncles* and connect the pons bilaterally with the two sides of the cerebellum dorsally (Figure 12.13). These fibers issue from numerous *pontine nuclei*, which relay "conversations" between the motor cortex and cerebellum.

Several cranial nerve pairs issue from pontine nuclei. They include the *trigeminal* (tri-jem′ĭ-nal), *abducens* (ab-du′senz), and *facial nerves* (Figures 12.13a, b and 12.14b). We discuss the cranial nerves and their functions in Chapter 13.

Other important pontine nuclei are part of the reticular formation and some help the medulla oblongata maintain the normal rhythm of breathing.

Medulla Oblongata

The conical **medulla oblongata** (mĕ-dul′ah ob″long-gah′tah), or simply **medulla**, is the most inferior part of the brain stem. It blends imperceptibly into the spinal cord at the level of the foramen magnum of the skull (Figures 12.10 and 12.12; see Figure 7.6, p. 206).

The central canal of the spinal cord continues upward into the medulla, where it broadens out to form the cavity of the fourth ventricle. Together, the medulla and the pons form the ventral wall of the fourth ventricle. [The dorsal ventricular wall is formed by a thin capillary-rich membrane called a choroid plexus which abuts the cerebellum dorsally (Figure 12.10).]

Structures of the Medulla Oblongata Flanking the midline on the medulla's ventral aspect are two longitudinal ridges called **pyramids**, formed by the large pyramidal (corticospinal) tracts descending from the motor cortex (Figure 12.14c). Just above the medulla–spinal cord junction, most of these fibers cross over to the opposite side before continuing into the spinal cord. This crossover point is called the **decussation of the pyramids** (de″kus-sa′shun; "a crossing"). As a result of this crossover, each cerebral hemisphere chiefly controls the voluntary movements of muscles on the opposite side of the body.

Several other structures are visible externally. The *inferior cerebellar peduncles* are fiber tracts that connect the medulla to the cerebellum dorsally. Situated lateral to the pyramids,

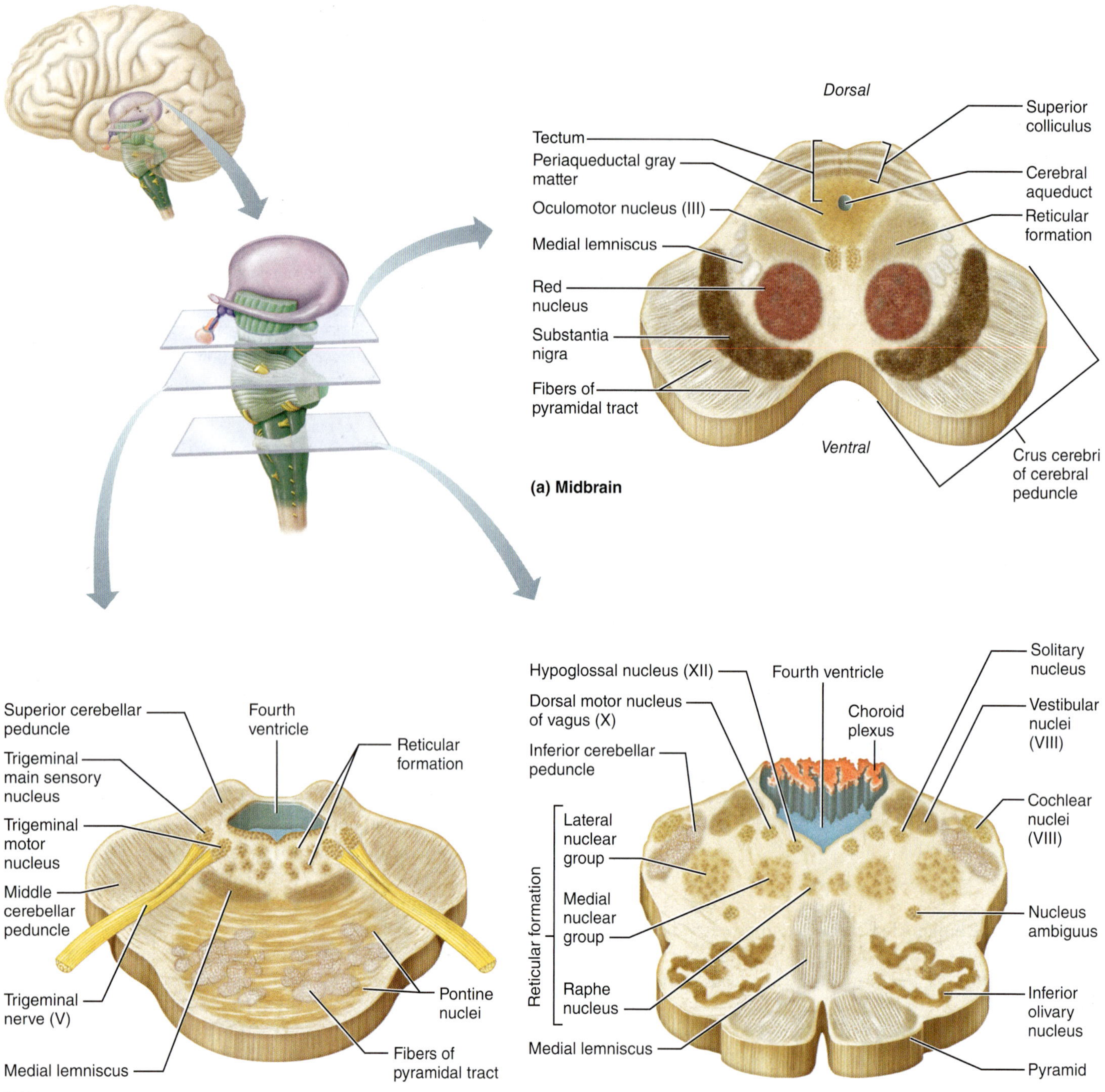

Figure 12.14 **Cross sections through different regions of the brain stem.**

the **olives** are oval swellings (which *do* resemble olives) (Figure 12.13b). These swellings are caused mainly by the wavy folds of gray matter of the underlying **inferior olivary nuclei** (Figure 12.14c). These nuclei relay sensory information on the degree of stretch in muscles and joints to the cerebellum. The rootlets of the *hypoglossal nerves* emerge from the groove between the pyramid and olive on each side of the brain stem. Other cranial nerves associated with the medulla are the *glossopharyngeal nerves* and *vagus nerves*. Additionally, the fibers of the *vestibulocochlear nerves* (ves-tib″u-lo-kok′le-ar) synapse with the **cochlear nuclei** (auditory relays), and with numerous **vestibular nuclei** in both the pons and medulla. The vestibular nuclei mediate responses that maintain equilibrium.

Also housed in the medulla are several nuclei associated with ascending sensory tracts. The most prominent are the dorsally located **nucleus gracilis** (grah-sĭ′lis) and **nucleus cuneatus** (ku′ne-āt-us), associated with a tract called the *medial lemniscus* (Figure 12.14). These serve as relay nuclei in a pathway by which general somatic sensory information ascends from the spinal cord to the somatosensory cortex.

Functions of the Medulla Oblongata The small size of the medulla belies its crucial role as an autonomic reflex center involved in maintaining body homeostasis. The medulla contains these important functional groups of visceral motor nuclei:

- **Cardiovascular center.** This includes the *cardiac center*, which adjusts the force and rate of heart contraction to meet the body's needs, and the *vasomotor center*, which changes blood vessel diameter to regulate blood pressure.
- **Respiratory centers.** These generate the respiratory rhythm and (in concert with pontine centers) control the rate and depth of breathing.
- **Various other centers.** Additional centers regulate such activities as vomiting, hiccuping, swallowing, coughing, and sneezing.

Notice that many functions listed above are also attributed to the hypothalamus (pp. 441–442). The overlap is easily explained. The hypothalamus controls many visceral functions by relaying its instructions through medullary reticular centers, which carry them out.

Check Your Understanding

10. What are the pyramids of the medulla? What is the result of decussation of the pyramids?
11. Which region of the brain stem is associated with the cerebral peduncles and the superior and inferior colliculi?

For answers, see Appendix H.

Cerebellum

✓ Describe the structure and function of the cerebellum.

The cauliflower-like **cerebellum** (ser″ĕ-bel′um; "small brain"), exceeded in size only by the cerebrum, accounts for about 11% of total brain mass. The cerebellum is located dorsal to the pons and medulla (and to the intervening fourth ventricle). It protrudes under the occipital lobes of the cerebral hemispheres, from which it is separated by the transverse cerebral fissure (see Figure 12.4b).

By processing inputs received from the cerebral motor cortex, various brain stem nuclei, and sensory receptors, the cerebellum provides the precise timing and appropriate patterns of skeletal muscle contraction for smooth, coordinated movements and agility needed for our daily living—driving, typing, and for some of us, playing the tuba. Cerebellar activity occurs subconsciously—we have no awareness of it.

Cerebellar Anatomy

The cerebellum is bilaterally symmetrical. The wormlike **vermis** connects its two apple-sized **cerebellar hemispheres** medially **(Figure 12.15)**. Its surface is heavily convoluted, with fine, transversely oriented pleatlike gyri known as **folia** ("leaves"). Deep fissures subdivide each hemisphere into **anterior**, **posterior**, and **flocculonodular lobes** (flok″u-lo-nod′u-lar). The small propeller-shaped flocculonodular lobes, situated deep to the vermis and posterior lobe, cannot be seen in a surface view.

Like the cerebrum, the cerebellum has a thin outer cortex of gray matter, internal white matter, and small, deeply situated, paired masses of gray matter, the most familiar of which are the *dentate nuclei*. Several types of neurons populate the cerebellar cortex, including **Purkinje cells** (see Table 11.1 on p. 394). These large cells, with their extensively branched dendrites, are the only cortical neurons that send axons through the white matter to synapse with the central nuclei of the cerebellum. The distinctive pattern of white matter in the cerebellum resembles a branching tree, a pattern fancifully called the **arbor vitae** (ar′bor vi′te; "tree of life") (Figure 12.15a, b).

The anterior and posterior lobes of the cerebellum, which coordinate body movements, have three sensory maps of the entire body as indicated by the homunculi in Figure 12.15d. The part of the cerebellar cortex that receives sensory input from a body region influences motor output to that region. The medial portions influence the motor activities of the trunk and girdle muscles. The intermediate parts of each hemisphere influence the distal parts of the limbs and skilled movements. The lateral-most parts of each hemisphere integrate information from the association areas of the cerebral cortex and appear to play a role in planning movements rather than executing them. The flocculonodular lobes receive inputs from the equilibrium apparatus of the inner ears, and adjust posture to maintain balance.

Cerebellar Peduncles

As noted earlier, three paired fiber tracts—the cerebellar peduncles—connect the cerebellum to the brain stem (see Figures 12.13 and 12.15b). Unlike the contralateral fiber distribution to and from the cerebral cortex, virtually all fibers entering and leaving the cerebellum are **ipsilateral** (*ipsi* = same)—from and to the same side of the body.

- The **superior cerebellar peduncles** connecting cerebellum and midbrain carry instructions from neurons in the deep cerebellar nuclei to the cerebral motor cortex via thalamic relays. Like the basal nuclei, the cerebellum has no *direct* connections to the cerebral cortex.
- The **middle cerebellar peduncles** carry one-way communications from the pons to the cerebellum, advising the cerebellum of voluntary motor activities initiated by the motor cortex (via relays in the pontine nuclei).
- The **inferior cerebellar peduncles** connect medulla and cerebellum. These peduncles convey sensory information to the cerebellum from (1) muscle proprioceptors throughout the body, and (2) the vestibular nuclei of the brain stem, which are concerned with equilibrium and balance.

Cerebellar Processing

Cerebellar processing fine-tunes motor activity as follows:

1. The motor areas of the cerebral cortex, via relay nuclei in the brain stem, notify the cerebellum of their intent to initiate voluntary muscle contractions.

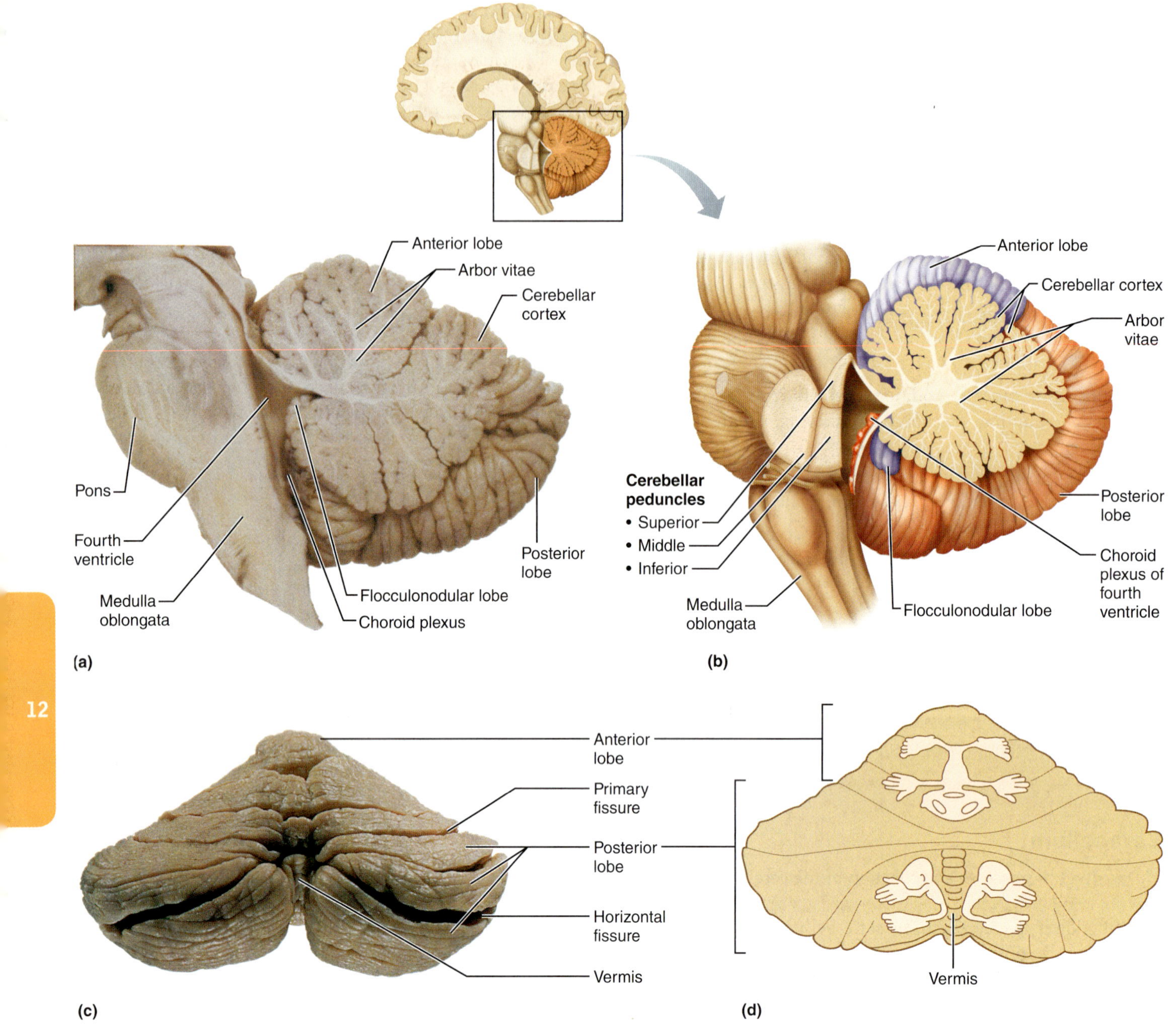

Figure 12.15 Cerebellum. (a) Photo of midsagittal section. **(b)** Drawing of parasagittal section. **(c)** Photograph of the posterior aspect of the cerebellum. **(d)** Three body maps of the cerebellar cortex (in the form of homunculi).

2. At the same time, the cerebellum receives information from proprioceptors throughout the body (regarding tension in the muscles and tendons, and joint position) and from visual and equilibrium pathways. This information enables the cerebellum to evaluate body position and momentum—where the body is and where it is going.
3. The cerebellar cortex calculates the best way to coordinate the force, direction, and extent of muscle contraction to prevent overshoot, maintain posture, and ensure smooth, coordinated movements.
4. Then, via the superior peduncles, the cerebellum dispatches to the cerebral motor cortex its "blueprint" for coordinating movement. Cerebellar fibers also send information to brain stem nuclei, which in turn influence motor neurons of the spinal cord.

Just as an automatic pilot compares a plane's instrument readings with the planned course, the cerebellum continually compares the body's performance with the higher brain's intention and sends out messages to initiate appropriate corrective measures. Cerebellar injury results in loss of muscle tone and clumsy, unsure movements.

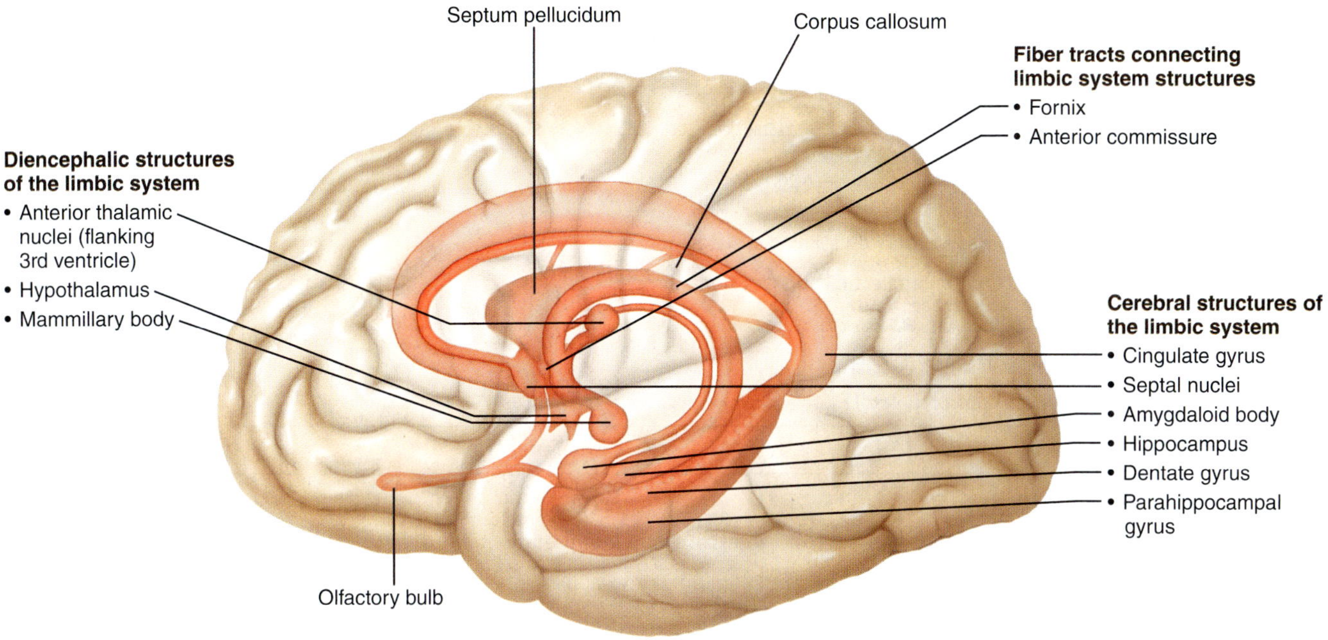

Figure 12.16 The limbic system. Lateral view of the brain, showing some of the structures of the limbic system, the emotional-visceral brain. The brain stem is not illustrated.

Cognitive Functions of the Cerebellum

Neuroanatomy, imaging studies, and observations of patients with cerebellar injuries suggest that the cerebellum also plays a role in thinking, language, and emotion. As in the motor system, the cerebellum may compare the actual output of these systems with the expected output and adjust accordingly. Much still remains to be discovered about the precise role of the cerebellum in nonmotor functions.

Check Your Understanding

12. In what ways are the cerebellum and the cerebrum similar? In what ways are they different?

For answers, see Appendix H.

Functional Brain Systems

✓ Locate the limbic system and the reticular formation, and explain the role of each functional system.

Functional brain systems are networks of neurons that work together but span relatively large distances in the brain, so they cannot be localized to specific regions. The *limbic system* and the *reticular formation* are excellent examples. Table 12.1 summarizes their functions, as well as those of the cerebral hemispheres, diencephalon, brain stem, and cerebellum.

The Limbic System

The **limbic system** is a group of structures located on the medial aspect of each cerebral hemisphere and diencephalon. Its cerebral structures encircle (*limbus* = ring) the upper part of the brain stem (Figure 12.16). The limbic system includes the **amygdaloid body** (ah-mig′dah-loid), an almond-shaped nucleus that sits on the tail of the caudate nucleus, and other parts of the rhinencephalon (*cingulate gyrus*, *septal nuclei*, the C-shaped *hippocampus*, *dentate gyrus*, and *parahippocampal gyrus*). In the diencephalon, the main limbic structures are the *hypothalamus* and the *anterior thalamic nuclei*. The **fornix** ("arch") and other fiber tracts link these limbic system regions together.

The limbic system is our *emotional*, or *affective* (feelings), *brain*. The amygdaloid body and the anterior part of the **cingulate gyrus** seem especially important in emotions. The amygdaloid body is critical for responding to perceived threats (such as angry or fearful facial expressions) with fear or aggression. The cingulate gyrus plays a role in expressing our emotions through gestures and in resolving mental conflicts when we are frustrated.

Odors often trigger emotional reactions and memories. These responses reflect the origin of much of the limbic system in the primitive "smell brain" (rhinencephalon). Our reactions to odors are rarely neutral (a skunk smells *bad* and repulses us), and odors often recall memories of emotion-laden events.

Extensive connections between the limbic system and lower and higher brain regions allow the system to integrate and respond to a variety of environmental stimuli. Most limbic system output is relayed through the hypothalamus. Because the hypothalamus is the neural clearinghouse for both autonomic (visceral) function and emotional response, it is not surprising that some people under acute or unrelenting emotional stress fall prey to visceral illnesses, such as high blood pressure and heartburn. Such emotion-induced illnesses are called **psychosomatic illnesses**.

Because the limbic system interacts with the prefrontal lobes, there is an intimate relationship between our feelings (mediated

12

Table 12.1 Functions of Major Brain Regions

REGION	FUNCTION
Cerebral Hemispheres (pp. 430–441)	
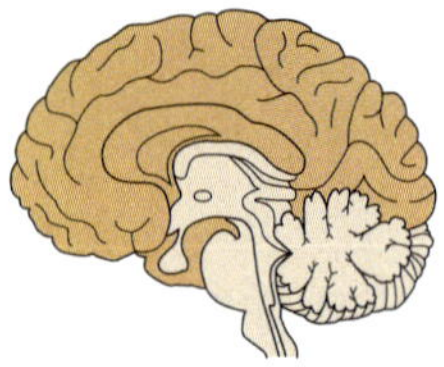	**Cortical gray matter:** ▪ Localizes and interprets sensory inputs ▪ Controls voluntary and skilled skeletal muscle activity ▪ Functions in intellectual and emotional processing **Basal nuclei (ganglia):** ▪ Subcortical motor centers ▪ Help control skeletal muscle movements
Diencephalon (pp. 441–443)	
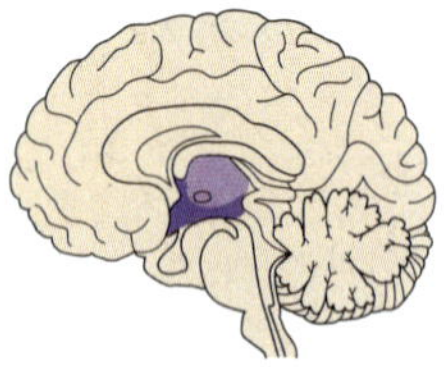	**Thalamus:** ▪ Relays sensory impulses to cerebral cortex for interpretation ▪ Relays impulses between cerebral motor cortex and lower (subcortical) motor centers, including cerebellum ▪ Involved in memory processing **Hypothalamus:** ▪ Chief integration center of autonomic (involuntary) nervous system ▪ Regulates body temperature, food intake, water balance, thirst, and biological rhythms and drives ▪ Regulates hormonal output of anterior pituitary gland ▪ Acts as an endocrine organ, producing posterior pituitary hormones ADH and oxytocin
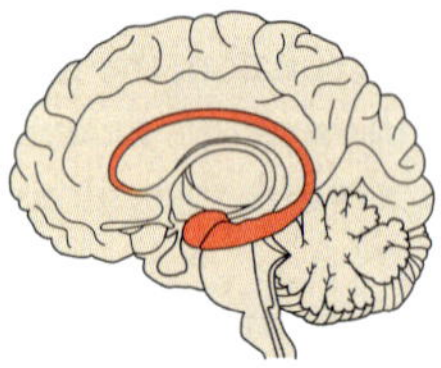	**Limbic System** (pp. 449–450)—A functional system: ▪ Includes cerebral and diencephalon structures (e.g., hypothalamus and anterior thalamic nuclei) ▪ Mediates emotional response ▪ Involved in memory processing

by the emotional brain) and our thoughts (mediated by the cognitive brain). As a result, we (1) react emotionally to things we consciously understand to be happening, and (2) are consciously aware of the emotional richness of our lives. Communication between the cerebral cortex and limbic system explains why emotions sometimes override logic and, conversely, why reason can stop us from expressing our emotions in inappropriate situations. Particular limbic system structures—the **hippocampus** and amygdaloid body—also play a role in memory.

The Reticular Formation

The **reticular formation** extends through the central core of the medulla oblongata, pons, and midbrain **(Figure 12.17)**. It is composed of loosely clustered neurons in what is otherwise white matter. These neurons form three broad columns along the length of the brain stem (Figure 12.14c): (1) the midline **raphe nuclei** (ra′fe; *raphe* = seam or crease), which are flanked laterally by (2) the **medial (large cell) group of nuclei** and (3) the **lateral (small cell) group of nuclei**.

The outstanding feature of the reticular neurons is their far-flung axonal connections. Individual reticular neurons project to the hypothalamus, thalamus, cerebral cortex, cerebellum, and spinal cord, making reticular neurons ideal for governing the arousal of the brain as a whole.

For example, unless inhibited by other brain areas, the neurons of the part of the reticular formation known as the **reticular activating system (RAS)** send a continuous stream of impulses to the cerebral cortex, keeping the cortex alert and conscious and enhancing its excitability. Impulses from all the great ascending sensory tracts synapse with RAS neurons, keeping them active and enhancing their arousing effect on the cerebrum. (This may explain why many students, stimulated by a bustling environment, like to study in a crowded cafeteria.)

The RAS also filters this flood of sensory inputs. Repetitive, familiar, or weak signals are filtered out, but unusual, significant, or strong impulses do reach consciousness. For example, you are probably unaware of your watch encircling your wrist, but would immediately notice it if the clasp broke. Between them, the RAS and the cerebral cortex disregard perhaps 99% of all sensory stimuli as unimportant. If this filtering did not occur, the sensory overload would drive us crazy. The drug LSD interferes with these sensory dampers, promoting an often overwhelming sensory overload.

Table 12.1 *(continued)*

REGION	FUNCTION
Brain Stem (pp. 443–447)	
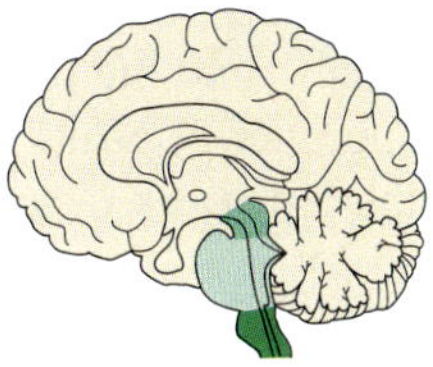	**Midbrain:** ▪ Contains visual (superior colliculi) and auditory (inferior colliculi) reflex centers ▪ Contains subcortical motor centers (substantia nigra and red nuclei) ▪ Contains nuclei for cranial nerves III and IV ▪ Contains projection fibers (e.g., fibers of the pyramidal tracts) **Pons:** ▪ Relays information from the cerebrum to the cerebellum ▪ Cooperates with the medullary respiratory centers to control respiratory rate and depth ▪ Contains nuclei of cranial nerves V–VII ▪ Contains projection fibers **Medulla oblongata:** ▪ Relays ascending sensory pathway impulses from skin and proprioceptors through nuclei cuneatus and gracilis ▪ Contains visceral nuclei controlling heart rate, blood vessel diameter, respiratory rate, vomiting, coughing, etc. ▪ Relays sensory information to the cerebellum through inferior olivary nuclei ▪ Contains nuclei of cranial nerves VIII–XII ▪ Contains projection fibers ▪ Site of decussation of pyramids
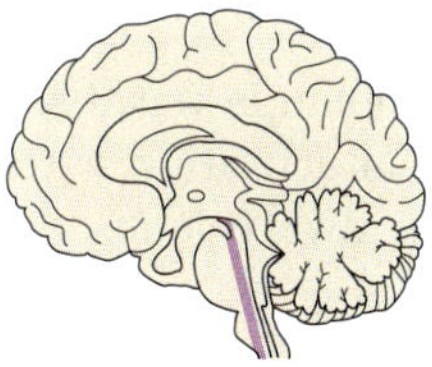	**Reticular formation** (pp. 450–451)—A functional system: ▪ Maintains cerebral cortical alertness (reticular activating system) ▪ Filters out repetitive stimuli ▪ Helps regulate skeletal and visceral muscle activity
Cerebellum (pp. 447–449)	
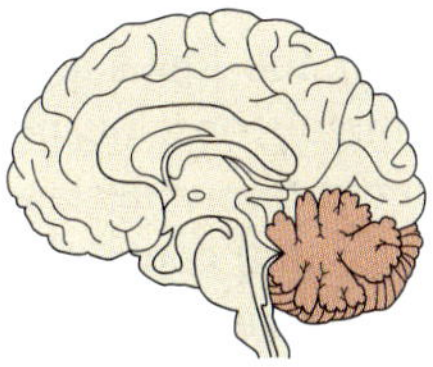	**Cerebellum:** ▪ Processes information from cerebral motor cortex, proprioceptors, and visual and equilibrium pathways ▪ Provides "instructions" to cerebral motor cortex and subcortical motor centers, resulting in smooth, coordinated skeletal muscle movements ▪ Responsible for proper balance and posture

- Take a moment to become aware of all the stimuli in your environment. Notice all the colors, shapes, odors, sounds, and so on. How many of these sensory stimuli are you usually aware of?

The RAS is inhibited by sleep centers located in the hypothalamus and other neural regions, and is depressed by alcohol, sleep-inducing drugs, and tranquilizers. Severe injury to this system, as might follow a knockout punch that twists the brain stem, results in permanent unconsciousness (irreversible *coma*). Although the RAS is central to wakefulness, some of its nuclei are also involved in sleep, which we will discuss later in this chapter.

The reticular formation also has a *motor* arm. Some of its motor nuclei project to motor neurons in the spinal cord via the *reticulospinal tracts*, and help control skeletal muscles during coarse limb movements. Other reticular motor nuclei, such as the vasomotor, cardiac, and respiratory centers of the medulla, are autonomic centers that regulate visceral motor functions.

☑ Check Your Understanding

13. The limbic system is sometimes called the emotional-visceral brain. Which part of the limbic system is responsible for the visceral connection?
14. When Taylor begins to feel drowsy while driving, she opens her window, turns up the volume of the car stereo, and sips ice-cold water. How do these actions keep her awake?

For answers, see Appendix H.

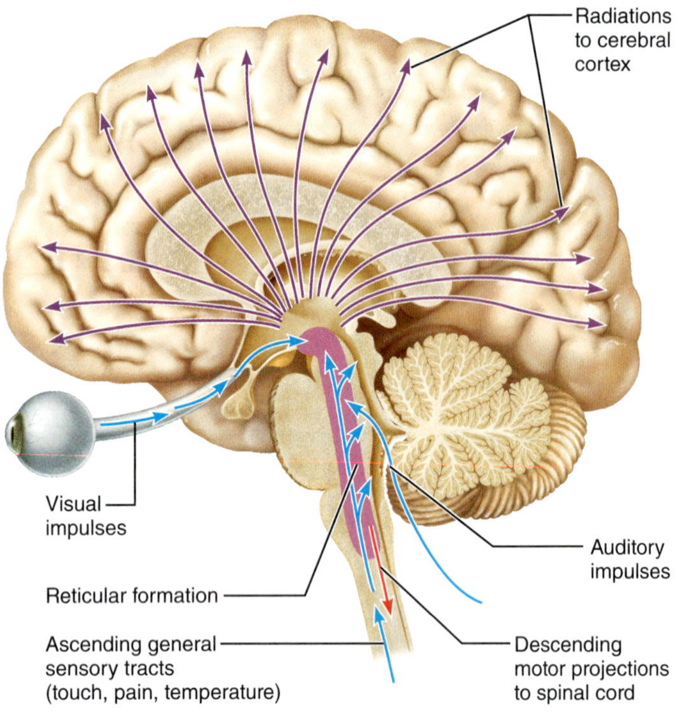

Figure 12.17 The reticular formation. This functional brain system extends the length of the brain stem. Part of this formation, the reticular activating system (RAS), maintains alert wakefulness of the cerebral cortex. Ascending blue arrows indicate sensory input to the RAS. Purple arrows indicate reticular output (some via thalamic relays) to the cerebral cortex. Descending red arrow represents motor output involved in regulating muscle tone.

12

Higher Mental Functions

During the last four decades, an exciting exploration of our "inner space," or what we commonly call the *mind*, has been going on. But researchers in the field of cognition are still struggling to understand how the mind's qualities spring from living tissue and electrical impulses. Souls and synapses are hard to reconcile!

Because brain waves reflect the electrical activity on which higher mental functions are based, we will consider them first, along with the related topics of consciousness and sleep. We will then examine language and memory, an area of ongoing research that is of particular interest to our aging population.

Brain Wave Patterns and the EEG

✓ Define EEG and distinguish between alpha, beta, theta, and delta brain waves.

Normal brain function involves continuous electrical activity of neurons. An **electroencephalogram** (e-lek"tro-en-sef'ah-lo-gram), or **EEG**, records some aspects of this activity. An EEG is made by placing electrodes on the scalp and connecting the electrodes to an apparatus that measures voltage differences between various cortical areas **(Figure 12.18a)**. The patterns of neuronal electrical activity recorded, called **brain waves**, are generated by synaptic activity at the surface of the cortex, rather than by action potentials in the white matter.

Each of us has a brain wave pattern that is as unique as our fingerprints. For simplicity, however, we can group brain waves into the four frequency classes shown in Figure 12.18b. Each wave is a continuous train of peaks and troughs, and the wave frequency, expressed in hertz (Hz), is the number of peaks in one second. A frequency of 1 Hz means that one peak occurs each second.

The amplitude or intensity of any wave is represented by how high the wave peaks rise and how low the troughs dip. The amplitude of brain waves reflects the synchronous activity of many neurons and not the degree of electrical activity of individual neurons. Usually, brain waves are complex and low amplitude. During some stages of sleep, neurons tend to fire synchronously, producing similar, high-amplitude brain waves.

- **Alpha waves** (8–13 Hz) are relatively regular and rhythmic, low-amplitude, synchronous waves. In most cases, they indicate a brain that is "idling"—a calm, relaxed state of wakefulness.
- **Beta waves** (14–30 Hz) are also rhythmic, but less regular than alpha waves and with a higher frequency. Beta waves occur when we are mentally alert, as when concentrating on some problem or visual stimulus.
- **Theta waves** (4–7 Hz) are still more irregular. Though common in children, theta waves are uncommon in awake adults but may appear when concentrating.
- **Delta waves** (4 Hz or less) are high-amplitude waves seen during deep sleep and when the reticular activating system is damped, such as during anesthesia. In awake adults, they indicate brain damage.

Brain waves change with age, sensory stimuli, brain disease, and the chemical state of the body. EEGs are used for diagnosing epilepsy and sleep disorders, and in research on brain function. Brain waves whose frequency is too high or too low suggest problems with cerebral cortical functions, and unconsciousness occurs at both extremes. Because spontaneous brain waves are always present, even during unconsciousness and coma, their absence—a "flat EEG"—is clinical evidence of brain death.

Homeostatic Imbalance 12.5

Almost without warning, a person with epilepsy may lose consciousness and fall stiffly to the ground, wracked by uncontrollable jerking. These **epileptic seizures** reflect a torrent of electrical discharges by groups of brain neurons, and during their uncontrolled activity no other messages can get through.

Epilepsy, manifested by one out of 100 of us, is not associated with, nor does it cause, intellectual impairment. Genetic factors induce some cases, but epilepsy can also result from brain injuries caused by blows to the head, stroke, infections, or tumors.

Epileptic seizures vary tremendously in their expression and severity.

- *Absence seizures*, formerly known as *petit mal*, are mild forms in which the expression goes blank for a few seconds as

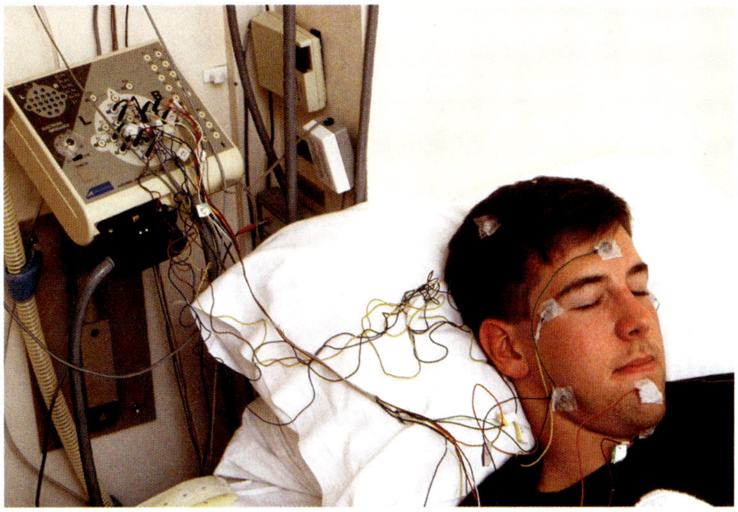

(a) Scalp electrodes are used to record brain wave activity.

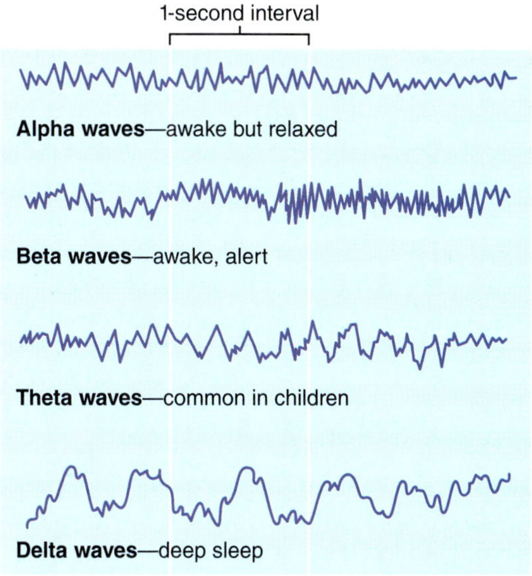

(b) Brain waves shown in EEGs fall into four general classes.

Figure 12.18 Electroencephalography (EEG) and brain waves.

consciousness disappears. These are typically seen in young children and usually disappear by age 10.

- *Tonic-clonic seizures*, formerly called *grand mal*, are the most severe, convulsive form of epileptic seizures. The person loses consciousness, often breaking bones during the intense convulsions, showing the incredible strength of these muscle contractions. Loss of bowel and bladder control and severe biting of the tongue are common. The seizure lasts for a few minutes, then the muscles relax and the person awakens but remains disoriented for several minutes.

Many seizure sufferers experience a sensory hallucination, such as a taste, smell, or flashes of light, just before the seizure begins. This phenomenon, called an **aura**, is helpful because it gives the person time to lie down and avoid falling to the floor.

Epilepsy can usually be controlled by anticonvulsive drugs. If drugs fail to control the seizures, a *vagus nerve stimulator* or *deep brain stimulator* can be implanted. These devices deliver pulses to the vagus nerve or directly to the brain at predetermined intervals to stabilize the brain's electrical activity. A current line of research seeks to implant electrodes in the brain to detect and prevent oncoming seizures. +

Consciousness

✓ Describe consciousness clinically.

Consciousness encompasses conscious perception of sensations, voluntary initiation and control of movement, and capabilities associated with higher mental processing (memory, logic, judgment, perseverance, and so on). Clinically, consciousness is defined on a continuum that grades behavior in response to stimuli as (1) *alertness*, (2) *drowsiness* or *lethargy* (which proceeds to sleep), (3) *stupor*, and (4) *coma*. Alertness is the highest state of consciousness and cortical activity, and coma the most depressed.

Consciousness is difficult to define. And to be frank, reducing our response to a Key West sunset to a series of interactions between dendrites, axons, and neurotransmitters does not capture what makes that event so special. A sleeping person obviously lacks something that he or she has when awake, and we call this "something" consciousness.

Current suppositions about consciousness are as follows:

- **Consciousness involves simultaneous activity of large areas of the cerebral cortex.**
- **It is superimposed on other types of neural activity.** At any time, specific neurons and neuronal pools are involved both in localized activities (such as motor control) and in cognition.
- **It is holistic and totally interconnected.** Information for "thought" can be claimed from many locations in the cerebrum simultaneously. For example, retrieval of a specific memory can be triggered by several routes—a smell, a place, a particular person, and so on.

Homeostatic Imbalance 12.6

Except during sleep, unconsciousness is always a signal that brain function is impaired. A brief loss of consciousness is called **fainting** or **syncope** (sing′ko-pe; "cut short"). Most often, syncope indicates inadequate cerebral blood flow due to low blood pressure, as might follow hemorrhage or sudden emotional stress.

Significant unresponsiveness to sensory stimuli for an extended period is called **coma**. Coma is *not* deep sleep. During sleep, the brain remains active and oxygen consumption resembles that of the waking state. In coma patients, oxygen use is always below normal resting levels.

Factors that can induce coma include: (1) blows to the head that cause widespread cerebral or brain stem trauma, (2) tumors or infections that invade the brain stem, (3) metabolic disturbances such as hypoglycemia (abnormally low blood sugar levels), (4) drug overdose, (5) liver or kidney failure. Strokes rarely cause coma unless they are massive and accompanied by extreme swelling of the brain, or are located in the brain stem.

When the brain has suffered irreparable damage, irreversible coma occurs, even though life-support measures may restore vitality to other body organs. The result is **brain death**, a dead brain in an otherwise living body. Because life support can be removed only after death, physicians must determine whether a patient in an irreversible coma is legally alive or dead. ✚

Sleep and Sleep-Wake Cycles

✓ Compare and contrast the events and importance of slow-wave and REM sleep, and indicate how their patterns change through life.

Sleep is defined as a state of partial unconsciousness from which a person can be aroused by stimulation. This distinguishes sleep from coma, a state of unconsciousness from which a person *cannot* be aroused by even the most vigorous stimuli.

For the most part, cortical activity is depressed during sleep, but brain stem functions continue, such as control of respiration, heart rate, and blood pressure. Even environmental monitoring continues to some extent, as illustrated by the fact that strong stimuli ("things that go bump in the night") immediately arouse us. In fact, people who sleepwalk can avoid objects and navigate stairs while truly asleep.

12

Types of Sleep

The two major types of sleep, which alternate through most of the sleep cycle, are **non–rapid eye movement (NREM) sleep** and **rapid eye movement (REM) sleep**, defined in terms of their EEG patterns **(Figure 12.19)**. During the first 30 to 45 minutes of the sleep cycle, we pass through the first two stages of NREM sleep and into NREM stages 3 and 4, also called **slow-wave sleep**. As we pass through these stages and slip into deeper and deeper sleep, the frequency of the EEG waves declines, but their amplitude increases. Blood pressure and heart rate also decrease.

About 90 minutes after sleep begins, after reaching NREM stage 4, the EEG pattern changes abruptly. It becomes very irregular and appears to backtrack quickly through the stages until alpha waves (more typical of the awake state) reappear, indicating the onset of REM sleep. This brain wave change is coupled with increases in heart rate, respiratory rate, and blood pressure and a decrease in gastrointestinal motility. Oxygen use by the brain is tremendous during REM—greater than during the awake state.

Although the eyes move rapidly under the lids during REM, most of the body's skeletal muscles are actively inhibited and go limp. This temporary paralysis prevents us from acting out our dreams. Most dreaming occurs during REM sleep, and some suggest that the flitting eye movements are following the visual imagery of our dreams. (Note, however, that most nightmares and night terrors occur during NREM stages 3 and 4.) In adolescents and adults, REM episodes are frequently associated with erection of the penis or engorgement of the clitoris.

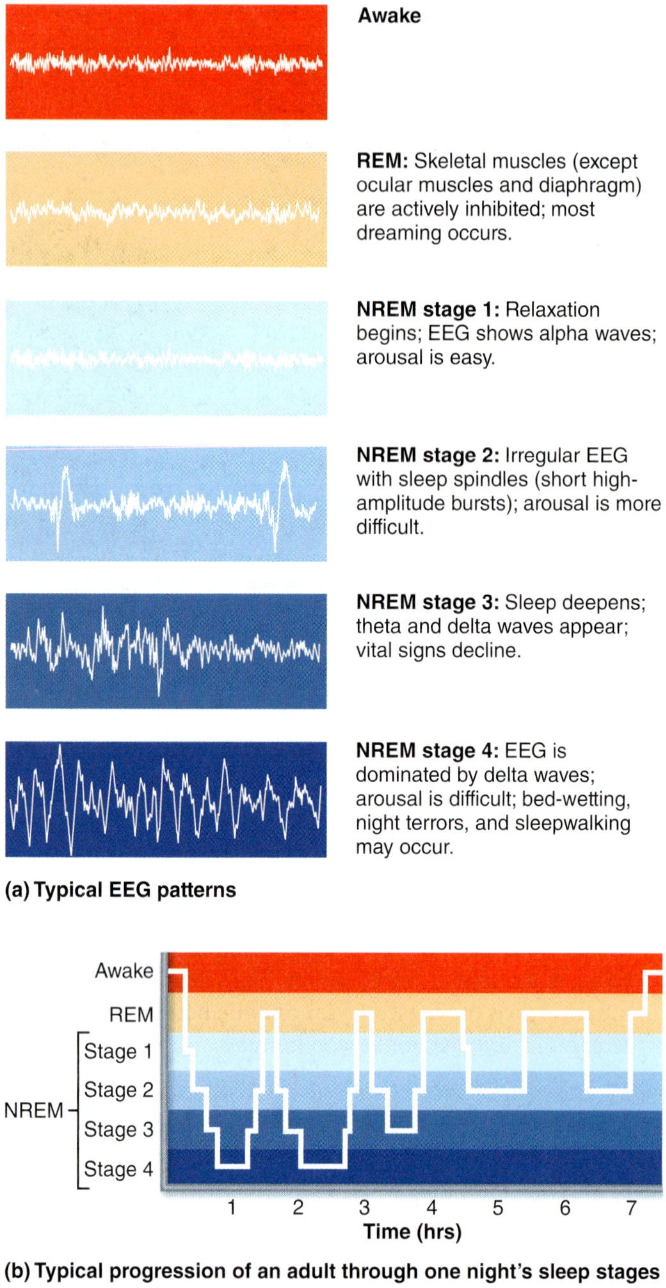

Figure 12.19 Types and stages of sleep. The four stages of non–rapid eye movement (NREM) sleep and rapid eye movement (REM) sleep are shown.

Sleep Patterns

The alternating cycles of sleep and wakefulness reflect a natural *circadian*, or 24-hour, *rhythm*. The hypothalamus is responsible for the timing of the sleep cycle. Its *suprachiasmatic nucleus* (a biological clock) regulates its *preoptic nucleus* (a sleep-inducing center). By inhibiting the brain stem's reticular activating system (RAS; see Figure 12.17), the preoptic nucleus puts the cerebral cortex to sleep. However, sleep is much more than simply turning off the arousal system. RAS centers not only help maintain the awake state but also mediate some sleep stages, especially dreaming sleep.

In young and middle-aged adults, a typical night's sleep starts with the four stages of NREM sleep and then alternates between REM and NREM sleep with occasional partial arousals. Following each REM episode, the sleeper descends toward stage 4 again. REM recurs about every 90 minutes, with each REM period getting longer. The first REM of the night lasts 5–10 minutes and the final one 20 to 50 minutes (Figure 12.19b). Consequently, our longest dreams occur at the end of the sleep period. Just before we wake, hypothalamic neurons release peptides called *orexins*, which in this situation act as "wake-up" chemicals. As a result, certain neurons of the brain stem reticular formation fire at maximal rates, arousing the sleepy cortex.

The slow theta and delta waves of deep sleep are the result of synchronized firing of thalamic neurons that is normally inhibited during wakefulness by the RAS of the pons. Some pontine neurons of the reticular formation control the transition from NREM sleep to REM sleep, and others suppress motor activity, inducing paralysis. A large number of chemical substances in the body cause sleepiness, but the relative importance of these various sleep-inducing substances is not known.

Importance of Sleep

Why do we sleep? Slow-wave (NREM stages 3 and 4) and REM sleep seem to be important in different ways. Slow-wave sleep is presumed to be restorative—the time when most neural activity can wind down to basal levels. When deprived of sleep, we spend more time than usual in slow-wave sleep during the next sleep episode.

A person persistently deprived of REM sleep becomes moody and depressed, and exhibits various personality disorders. REM sleep may give the brain an opportunity to analyze the day's events and work through emotional problems in dream imagery.

Another idea is that REM sleep is reverse learning. According to this hypothesis, accidental, repetitious, and meaningless communications continually occur. Dreaming eliminates them from our neural networks so the cortex remains a well-behaved and efficient thinking system. In other words, we dream to forget.

Alcohol and some sleep medications (barbiturates and others) suppress REM sleep but not slow-wave sleep. On the other hand, certain tranquilizers, such as diazepam (Valium) reduce slow-wave sleep much more than REM sleep.

Whatever its importance, a person's daily sleep requirement declines steadily from 16 hours or so in infants to approximately 7½ to 8½ hours in early adulthood. It then levels off before declining again in old age. Sleep patterns also change throughout life. REM sleep occupies about half the total sleeping time in infants and then declines until age 10, when it stabilizes at about 25%. In contrast, stage 4 sleep declines steadily from birth and often disappears completely in those over 60.

Homeostatic Imbalance 12.7

People with **narcolepsy** lapse abruptly into REM sleep from the awake state. These sleep episodes last about 15 minutes, can occur without warning, and are often triggered by a pleasurable event—a good joke, a game of poker.

In most patients with narcolepsy, an emotionally intense experience can also trigger *cataplexy*, a sudden loss of voluntary muscle control similar to that seen during REM sleep. During cataplectic attacks, lasting seconds to minutes, the patient remains fully conscious but unable to move. Obviously this can be extremely hazardous if the person is driving a car or swimming!

Cells in the hypothalamus that secrete peptides called orexins (the peptides mentioned above as a wake-up chemical; also called hypocretins) are selectively destroyed in patients with narcolepsy, probably by the patient's own immune system. Replacing the orexins may be a key to future treatments.

Conversely, drugs that block the actions of orexin and promote sleep may treat **insomnia**, a chronic inability to obtain the *amount* or *quality* of sleep needed to function adequately during the day. Sleep requirements vary from four to nine hours a day in healthy people, so there is no way to determine the "right" amount. Insomniacs tend to overestimate the extent of their sleeplessness, and some come to rely on hypnotics (sleep medications), which can exacerbate the problem.

True insomnia often reflects normal age-related changes, but perhaps the most common cause is psychological disturbance. We have difficulty falling asleep when we are anxious or upset, and depression is often accompanied by early awakening.

Sleep apnea, a temporary cessation of breathing during sleep, is scary. The victim awakes abruptly due to hypoxia (lack of oxygen)—a condition that may occur several hundred times per night.

Obstructive sleep apnea, the most common form, occurs when the loss of muscle tone during sleep allows excess fatty tissue or other structural abnormalities to block the upper airway. It is associated with obesity and made worse by alcohol and other depressants. Aside from weight loss, effective treatments are either a mask that blows air in through the nose, keeping the airway open, or surgery to correct the problem. ✚

12

☑ Check Your Understanding

15. When would you see delta waves in an EEG?
16. Which two states of consciousness are between alertness and coma?
17. During which sleep stage are most skeletal muscles actively inhibited?

For answers, see Appendix H.

Language

Language is such an important function of the brain that it involves practically all of the association cortex on the left side in one way or another. Pioneering studies of patients with *aphasias* (the loss of language abilities due to damage to specific areas of the brain) pointed to two critically important regions, Broca's area and Wernicke's area (see areas outlined by dashes in Figure 12.6a).

Patients with lesions involving **Broca's area** can understand language but have difficulty speaking (and sometimes cannot write or type or use sign language). On the other hand, patients with lesions involving **Wernicke's area** are able to speak but

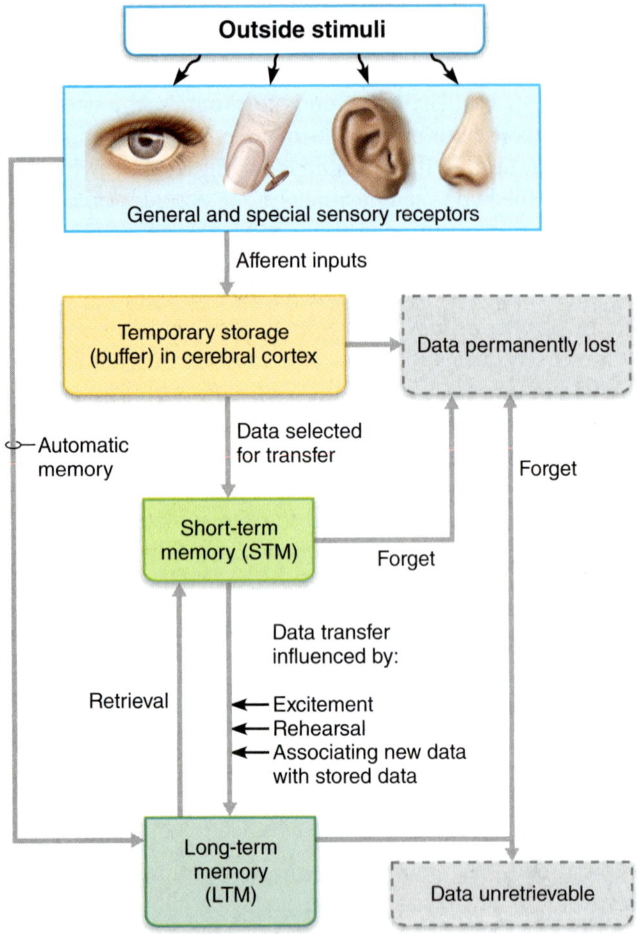

Figure 12.20 **Memory processing.**

produce a type of nonsense often referred to as "word salad." They also have great difficulty understanding language.

Recent imaging studies of the brain indicate that this picture is clinically useful, but oversimplified. In fact, Broca's and Wernicke's areas together with the basal nuclei form a single language implementation system that analyzes incoming and produces outgoing word sounds and grammatical structures. A surrounding set of cortical areas forms a bridge between this system and the regions of cortex that hold concepts and ideas, which are distributed throughout the remainder of the association cortices.

The corresponding areas in the right or non-language-dominant hemisphere are involved in "body language"—the nonverbal emotional (affective) components of language. These areas allow the lilt or tone of our voice and our gestures to express our emotions when we speak, and permit us to comprehend the emotional content of what we hear. For example, a soft, melodious response to your question conveys quite a different meaning than a sharp reply.

Memory

✓ Compare and contrast the stages and categories of memory.

✓ Describe the roles of the major brain structures believed to be involved in declarative and procedural memories.

Memory is the storage and retrieval of information. Memories are essential for learning and incorporating our experiences into behavior and are part and parcel of our consciousness. Stored somewhere in your 3 pounds of wrinkled brain are zip codes, the face of your grandfather, and the taste of yesterday's pizza. Your memories reflect your lifetime.

Stages of Memory

Memory storage involves two distinct stages: short-term memory and long-term memory **(Figure 12.20)**.

Short-term memory (STM), also called *working memory*, is the preliminary step, as well as the power that lets you look up a telephone number, dial it, and then never think of it again. STM is limited to seven or eight chunks of information, such as the digits of a telephone number or the sequence of words in an elaborate sentence.

In contrast, **long-term memory (LTM)** seems to have a limitless capacity. Although our STM cannot recall numbers much longer than a telephone number, we can remember scores of telephone numbers by committing them to LTM. However, long-term memories can be forgotten, and so our memory bank continually changes with time. Furthermore, our ability to store and retrieve information declines with aging.

We do not remember or even consciously notice much of what is going on around us. As sensory inputs flood into our cerebral cortex, they are processed (yellow box in Figure 12.20). Some 5% of this information is selected for transfer to STM (light green box in Figure 12.20). STM serves as a temporary holding bin for data that we may or may not want to retain.

Information is then transferred from STM to LTM (dark green box in Figure 12.20). Many factors can influence this transfer, including:

- **Emotional state.** We learn best when we are alert, motivated, surprised, and aroused. For example, when we witness shocking events, transferral is almost immediate. Norepinephrine, a neurotransmitter involved in memory processing of emotionally charged events, is released when we are excited or "stressed out," which helps to explain this phenomenon.
- **Rehearsal.** Rehearsing or repeating the material enhances memory.
- **Association.** Tying "new" information to "old" information already stored in LTM appears to be important in remembering facts.
- **Automatic memory.** Not all impressions that become part of LTM are consciously formed. A student concentrating on a lecturer's speech may record an automatic memory of the pattern of the lecturer's tie.

Memories transferred to LTM take time to become permanent. The process of **memory consolidation** apparently involves fitting new facts into the categories of knowledge already stored in the cerebral cortex.

Categories of Memory

The brain distinguishes between factual knowledge and skills, and we process and store these two kinds of information in different ways.

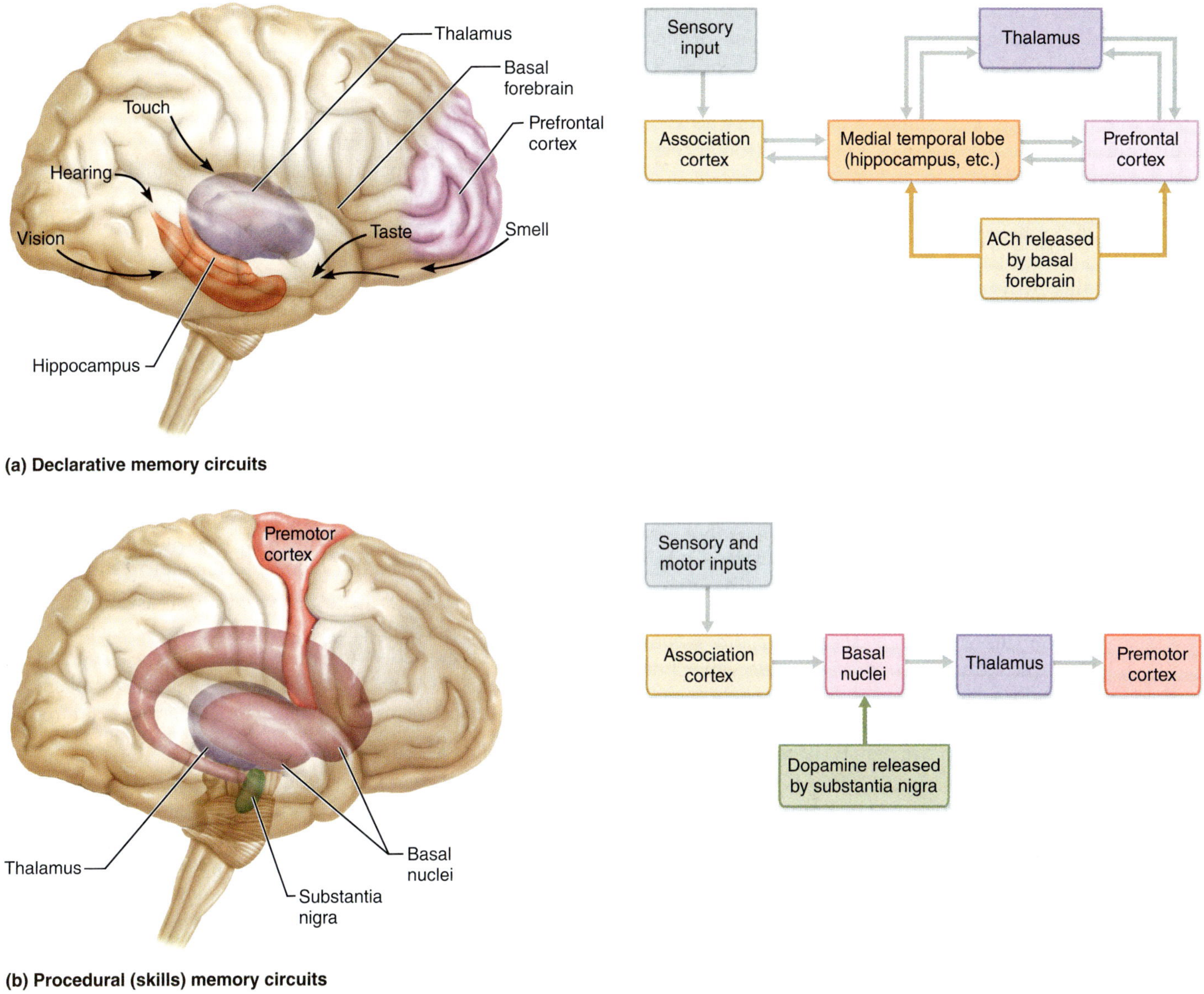

Figure 12.21 Proposed memory circuits. **(a)** Information from association cortices flows to the medial temporal lobe (including the hippocampus), which communicates with the thalamus and prefrontal cortex. The association cortices receive feedback from these structures. Acetylcholine from the basal forebrain is necessary for this circuit to function. **(b)** Sensory and motor inputs flow through the association cortices and are relayed to the premotor cortex. Dopamine from the substantia nigra is necessary for this circuit to function.

Declarative (fact) memory entails learning explicit information, such as names, faces, words, and dates. It is related to our conscious thoughts and our ability to manipulate symbols and language. When fact memories are committed to LTM, they are usually filed with the context in which they were learned. For instance, when you think of your new acquaintance Joe, you probably picture him at the basketball game where you met him.

Nondeclarative memory is less conscious or even unconscious learning. Categories of nondeclarative memory are **procedural (skills) memory** (piano playing), **motor memory** (riding a bike), and **emotional memory** (your pounding heart when you hear a rattlesnake nearby). We acquire nondeclarative memories through experience and usually repetition. They do not preserve the circumstances of learning, and in fact, they are best remembered in the doing. You do not have to think through how to tie your shoes. Once learned, nondeclarative memories are hard to unlearn.

Brain Structures Involved in Memory

Specific pieces of each memory are thought to be stored near regions of the brain that need them so new inputs can be quickly associated with the old. Accordingly, visual memories are stored in the occipital cortex, memories of music in the temporal cortex, and so on.

But how do we create new memories? It seems that different types of memory are created in different parts of the brain. **Figure 12.21a** shows a proposed scheme of information flow for declarative memory.

When sensory input is processed in the association cortices, the cortical neurons dispatch impulses to the medial temporal lobe, which includes the hippocampus and surrounding temporal cortical areas. These temporal lobe areas play a major role in memory consolidation and memory access by communicating with the thalamus and the prefrontal cortex. The prefrontal cortex and medial temporal lobe receive input from acetylcholine-releasing neurons in the basal forebrain. The sprinkling of acetylcholine (ACh) onto these structures is thought to prime them to allow the formation of memories. The loss of this ACh input, for example in Alzheimer's disease, seems to disrupt both the formation of new memories and the retrieval of old ones. Memories are retrieved when the same sets of neurons that were initially involved in forming the memories are stimulated.

Homeostatic Imbalance 12.8

Damage to the hippocampus and surrounding medial temporal lobe structures on either side results in only slight memory loss, but bilateral destruction causes widespread amnesia. Consolidated memories are not lost, but new sensory inputs cannot be associated with old, and the person lives in the here and now from that point on. This condition is called *anterograde amnesia* (an′ter-o-grād″), in contrast to *retrograde amnesia*, which is the loss of memories formed in the distant past. You could carry on an animated conversation with a person with anterograde amnesia, excuse yourself, return five minutes later, and that person would not remember you. +

Individuals suffering from anterograde amnesia can still learn skills such as drawing, so procedural memory must involve a different learning circuit. As Figure 12.21b shows, the basal nuclei (pink) are key players for procedural memory. Sensory and motor inputs pass through the association cortex to the basal nuclei. These inputs are then relayed via the thalamus to the premotor cortex. Note that the basal nuclei receive input from dopamine-releasing neurons in the substantia nigra of the midbrain. Just as acetylcholine is necessary for declarative memory, dopamine appears to be necessary for this procedural memory circuit to function. The loss of this dopamine input, as in Parkinson's disease, interferes with procedural memory.

The two other kinds of nondeclarative memory involve yet other brain regions. The cerebellum is involved in motor memory, while the amygdaloid body is crucial for emotional memory (see Figure 12.16). We will not describe these pathways here.

Molecular Basis of Memory

What happens at the molecular level when we form memories? Human memory is notoriously difficult to study. Animal experimental studies reveal that during learning:

- Neuronal RNA content is altered and newly synthesized mRNAs are delivered to axons and dendrites.
- Dendritic spines change shape.
- Unique extracellular proteins are deposited at synapses involved in long-term memory.
- The number and size of presynaptic terminals may increase.
- Presynaptic neurons release more neurotransmitter.

Each of these changes is an aspect of **long-term potentiation (LTP)**, a persistent increase in synaptic strength that has been shown to be crucial for memory formation. LTP was first identified in hippocampal neurons that use the amino acid glutamate as a neurotransmitter. One kind of glutamate receptor, the *NMDA receptor*, can act as a calcium channel and initiate the cellular changes that bring about LTP.

Normally, NMDA receptors are blocked, preventing calcium entry. When glutamate binds to different receptors and depolarizes the postsynaptic terminal, as would happen upon the rapid arrival of action potentials at the synapse, this NMDA block is removed and calcium flows into the postsynaptic cell.

Calcium influx activates enzymes that carry out two main tasks:

- The enzymes modify the proteins in the postsynaptic terminal, and also in the presynaptic terminal via retrograde messengers such as nitric oxide and endocannabinoids. These changes strengthen the response to subsequent stimuli.
- They activate genes in the postsynaptic neuron's nucleus, which leads to synthesis of synaptic proteins. The molecular messenger that alerts the nucleus that more protein is needed is a molecule called CREB (cAMP response-element binding protein). A neurotrophic factor called BDNF (brain-derived neurotrophic factor) is required for the protein synthesis phase of LTP.

Together, these changes create long-lasting increases in synaptic strength that are believed to underlie memory.

The events underlying memory at a cellular level suggest several approaches to enhancing memory formation. Currently several drugs to improve memory are undergoing clinical trials. Among these are drugs that enhance CREB production—the more CREB, the more protein synthesis and the stronger the synapse becomes.

Check Your Understanding

18. Name three factors that can enhance transfer of information from STM to LTM.
19. Which functional areas of the cerebrum are involved in the formation of procedural (skills) memory, but not involved in declarative memory?

For answers, see Appendix H.

Protection of the Brain

✓ Describe how meninges, cerebrospinal fluid, and the blood brain barrier protect the CNS.

✓ Explain how cerebrospinal fluid is formed and describe its circulatory pathway.

Nervous tissue is soft and delicate, and even slight pressure can injure neurons. However, the brain is protected by bone (the skull), membranes (the meninges), and a watery cushion

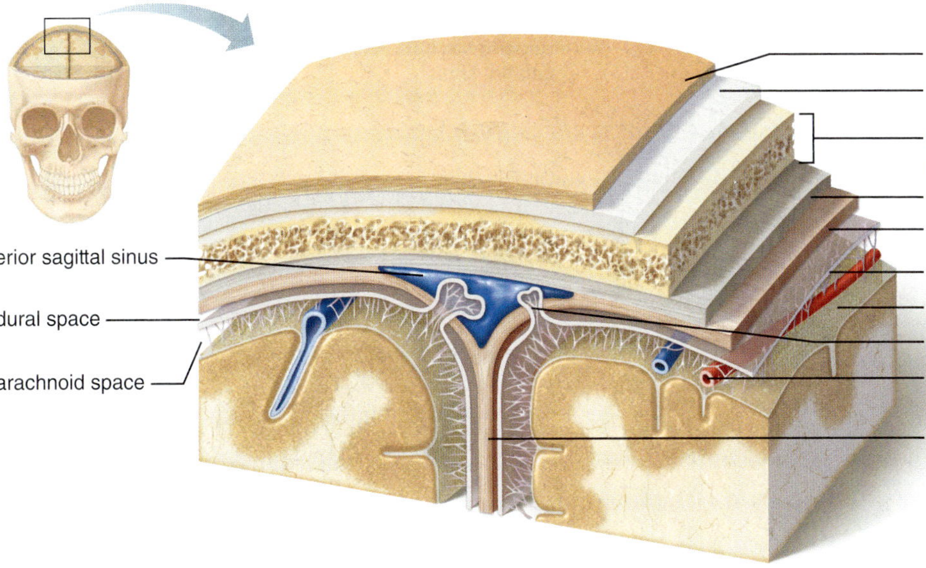

Figure 12.22 Meninges: dura mater, arachnoid mater, and pia mater. The meningeal dura forms the falx cerebri fold. A dural sinus, the superior sagittal sinus, is enclosed by the dural membranes superiorly. Arachnoid villi return cerebrospinal fluid to the dural sinus. (Frontal section.)

(cerebrospinal fluid). Furthermore, the blood brain barrier protects the brain from harmful substances in the blood. We described the cranium, the brain's bony encasement, in Chapter 7. Here we will consider the other protective elements.

Meninges

The **meninges** (mĕ-nin′jēz; *mening* = membrane) are three connective tissue membranes that lie just external to the CNS organs. The meninges:

- Cover and protect the CNS
- Protect blood vessels and enclose venous sinuses
- Contain cerebrospinal fluid
- Form partitions in the skull

From external to internal, the meninges (singular: **meninx**) are the dura mater, arachnoid mater, and pia mater **(Figure 12.22)**.

Dura Mater

The leathery **dura mater** (du′rah ma′ter), meaning "tough mother," is the strongest meninx. Where it surrounds the brain, it is a two-layered sheet of fibrous connective tissue. The more superficial *periosteal layer* attaches to the inner surface of the skull (the periosteum). (There is no dural periosteal layer surrounding the spinal cord.) The deeper *meningeal layer* forms the true external covering of the brain and continues caudally in the vertebral canal as the spinal dura mater. The brain's two dural layers are fused together except in certain areas, where they separate to enclose **dural venous sinuses** that collect venous blood from the brain and direct it into the internal jugular veins of the neck **(Figure 12.23)**.

In several places, the meningeal dura mater extends inward to form flat partitions that subdivide the cranial cavity. These **dural septa**, which limit excessive movement of the brain within the cranium, include the following (Figure 12.23a):

- **Falx cerebri** (falks ser′ĕ-bri). A large sickle-shaped (*falx* = sickle) fold that dips into the longitudinal fissure between the cerebral hemispheres. Anteriorly, it attaches to the crista galli of the ethmoid bone.
- **Falx cerebelli** (ser″ĕ-bel′i). Continuing inferiorly from the posterior falx cerebri, this small midline partition runs along the vermis of the cerebellum.
- **Tentorium cerebelli** (ten-to′re-um; "tent"). Resembling a tent over the cerebellum, this nearly horizontal dural fold extends into the transverse fissure between the cerebral hemispheres (which it helps to support) and the cerebellum.

Arachnoid Mater

The middle meninx, the **arachnoid mater** (ah-rak′noid), forms a loose brain covering, never dipping into the sulci at the cerebral surface. It is separated from the dura mater by a narrow serous cavity, the **subdural space**, which contains a film of fluid. Beneath the arachnoid membrane is the wide **subarachnoid space**. Spider-web-like extensions span this space and secure the arachnoid mater to the underlying pia mater (*arachnida* means "spider"). The subarachnoid space is filled with cerebrospinal fluid and also contains the largest blood vessels serving the brain. Because the arachnoid mater is fine and elastic, these blood vessels are poorly protected.

Knoblike projections of the arachnoid mater called **arachnoid villi** (vil′i) protrude superiorly through the dura mater and into the superior sagittal sinus (see Figure 12.22). These villi absorb cerebrospinal fluid into the venous blood of the sinus.

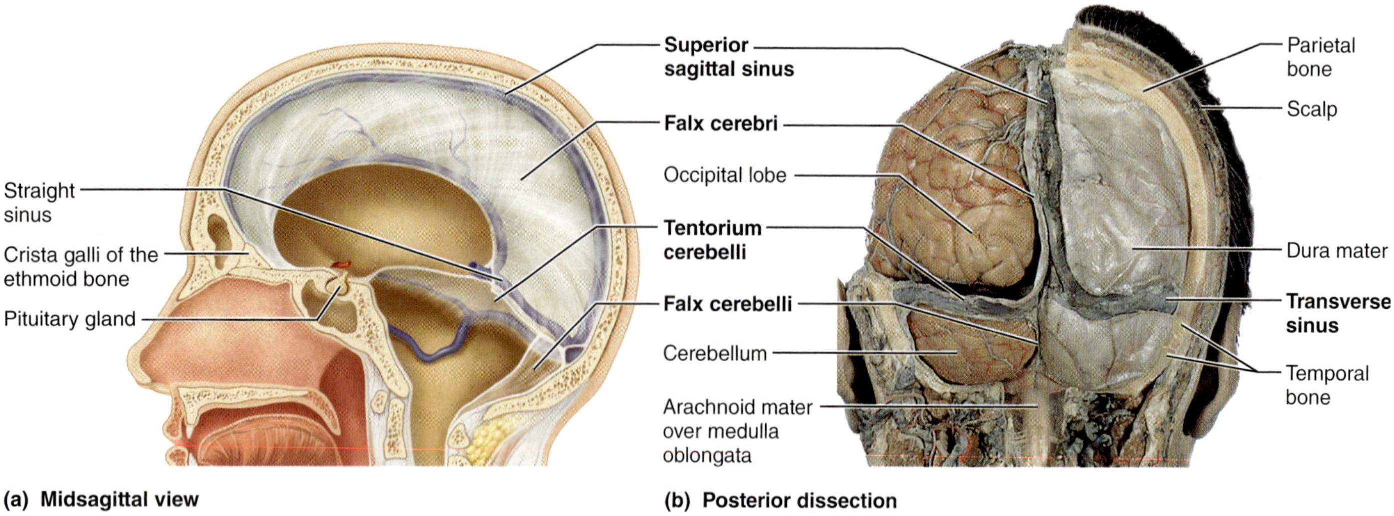

Figure 12.23 Dural septa and dural venous sinuses. (a) Dural septa are partitioning folds of dura mater in the cranial cavity. **(b)** Dural venous sinuses (injected with blue latex) are spaces between the periosteal and meningeal dura containing venous blood.

Pia Mater

The **pia mater** (pi′ah), meaning "gentle mother," is composed of delicate connective tissue and richly invested with tiny blood vessels. It is the only meninx that clings tightly to the brain like cellophane wrap, following its every convolution. Small arteries entering the brain tissue carry ragged sheaths of pia mater inward with them for short distances.

12

Homeostatic Imbalance 12.9

Meningitis, inflammation of the meninges, is a serious threat to the brain because a bacterial or viral meningitis may spread to the CNS. Brain inflammation is called *encephalitis* (en-sef″ah-li′tis). Meningitis is usually diagnosed by obtaining a sample of cerebrospinal fluid via a lumbar tap (see Figure 12.27, p. 466) and examining it for microbes. ✚

Cerebrospinal Fluid (CSF)

Cerebrospinal fluid, found in and around the brain and spinal cord, forms a liquid cushion that gives buoyancy to CNS structures. By floating the jellylike brain, the CSF effectively reduces brain weight by 97% and prevents the delicate brain from crushing under its own weight. CSF also protects the brain and spinal cord from blows and other trauma. Additionally, although the brain has a rich blood supply, CSF helps nourish the brain, and there is some evidence that it carries chemical signals (such as hormones and sleep- and appetite-inducing molecules) from one part of the brain to another.

CSF is a watery "broth" similar in composition to blood plasma, from which it is formed. However, it contains less protein than plasma and its ion concentrations are different. For example, CSF contains more Na^+, Cl^-, and H^+ than does blood plasma, and less Ca^{2+} and K^+.

The **choroid plexuses** that hang from the roof of each ventricle form CSF. These plexuses are frond-shaped clusters of broad, thin-walled capillaries (*plex* = interwoven) enclosed first by pia mater and then by a layer of ependymal cells lining the ventricles (Figure 12.24b). These capillaries are fairly permeable, and tissue fluid filters continuously from the bloodstream. However, the choroid plexus ependymal cells are joined by tight junctions, and they have ion pumps that allow them to modify this filtrate by actively transporting only certain ions across their membranes into the CSF pool. This careful regulation of CSF composition is important because CSF mixes with the extracellular fluid bathing neurons and influences the composition of this fluid. Ion pumping also sets up ionic gradients that cause water to diffuse into the ventricles.

In adults, the total CSF volume of about 150 ml (about half a cup) is replaced every 8 hours or so. About 500 ml of CSF is formed daily. The choroid plexuses also help cleanse the CSF by removing waste products and unnecessary solutes.

Once produced, CSF moves freely through the ventricles. CSF enters the subarachnoid space via the lateral and median apertures in the walls of the fourth ventricle (Figure 12.24a). The long cilia of the ependymal cells lining the ventricles help keep the CSF in constant motion. In the subarachnoid space, CSF bathes the outer surfaces of the brain and spinal cord and then returns to the blood in the dural sinuses via the arachnoid villi.

Homeostatic Imbalance 12.10

Ordinarily, CSF is produced and drained at a constant rate. However, if something (such as a tumor) obstructs its circulation or drainage, CSF accumulates and exerts pressure on the brain. This condition is called *hydrocephalus* ("water on the brain").

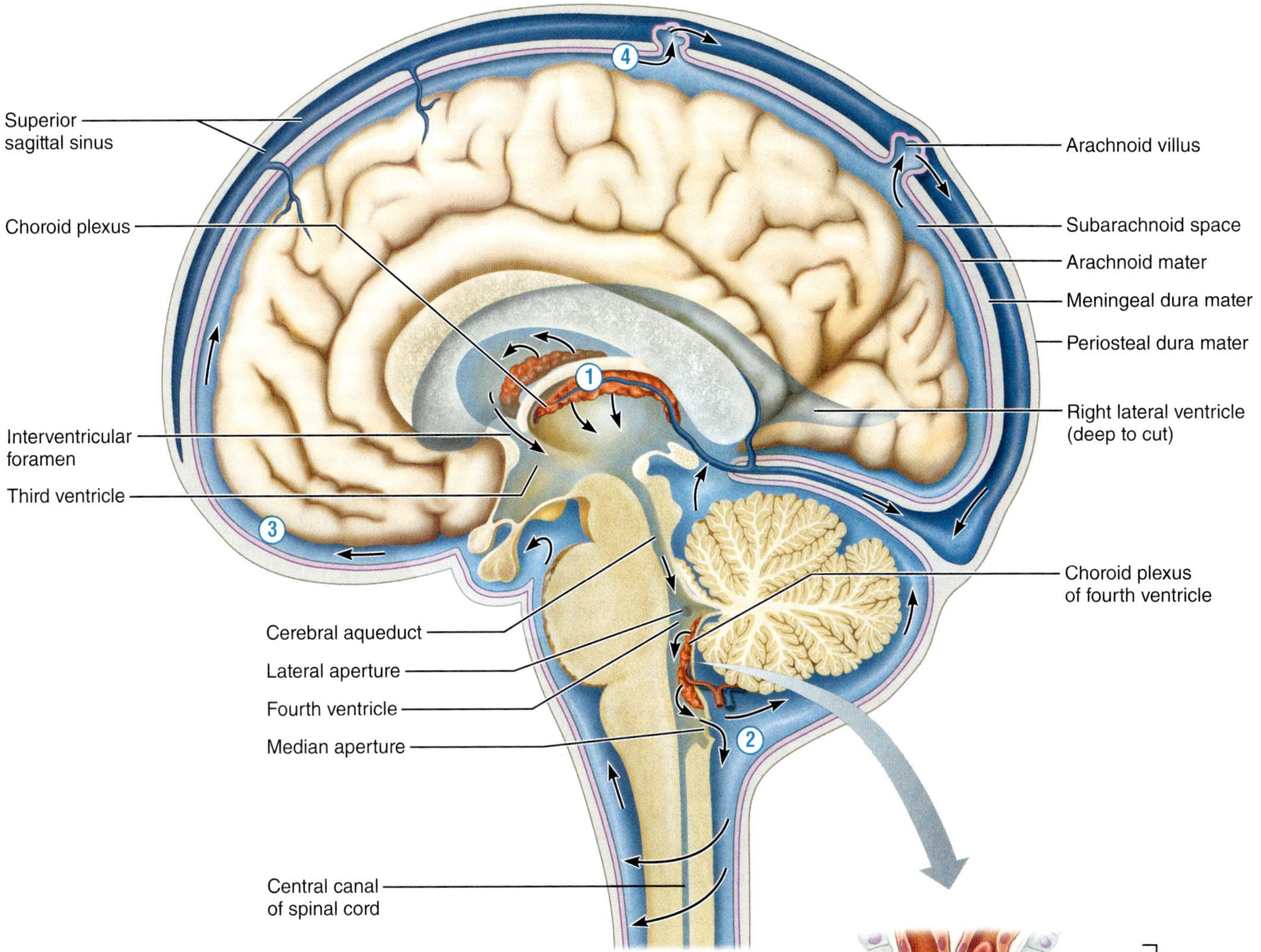

(a) CSF circulation

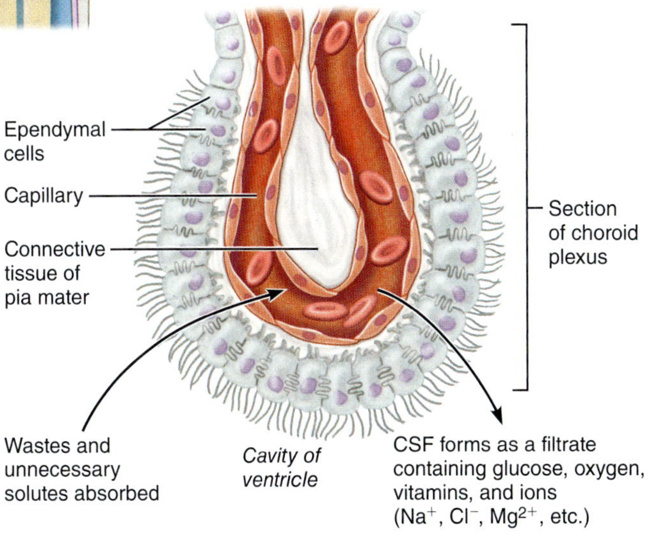

(b) CSF formation by choroid plexuses

Figure 12.24 Formation, location, and circulation of CSF. (a) Location and circulatory pattern of cerebrospinal fluid (CSF). Arrows indicate the direction of flow. **(b)** Each choroid plexus consists of a knot of porous capillaries surrounded by a single layer of ependymal cells joined by tight junctions and bearing long cilia. Fluid leaking from porous capillaries is processed by the ependymal cells to form the CSF in the ventricles.

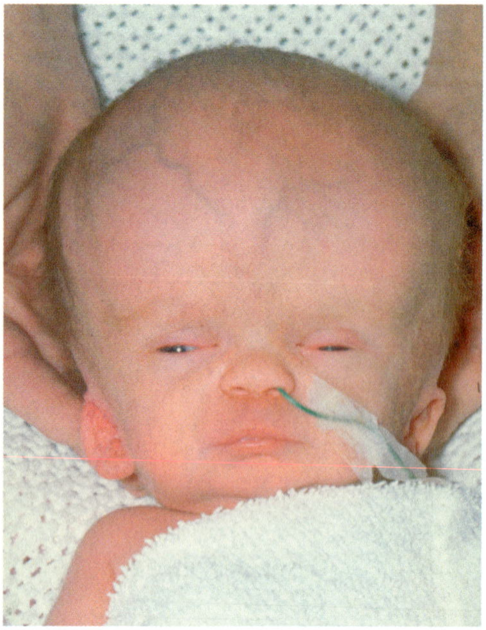

Figure 12.25 Hydrocephalus in a newborn.

Hydrocephalus enlarges the head of a newborn baby because the skull bones have not yet fused **(Figure 12.25)**. In adults, however, the skull is rigid and hard, and hydrocephalus is likely to damage the brain because accumulating fluid compresses blood vessels and crushes the soft nervous tissue. Hydrocephalus is treated by inserting a shunt into the ventricles to drain excess fluid into the abdominal cavity. +

12

Blood Brain Barrier

The **blood brain barrier** is a protective mechanism that helps maintain a stable environment for the brain. No other body tissue is so absolutely dependent on a constant internal environment as is the brain. In other body regions, the extracellular concentrations of hormones, amino acids, and ions are in constant flux, particularly after eating or exercise. If the brain were exposed to such chemical variations, its neurons would fire uncontrollably, because some hormones and amino acids serve as neurotransmitters and certain ions (particularly K^+) modify the threshold for neuronal firing.

Bloodborne substances in the brain's capillaries must pass through three layers before they reach the neurons: (1) the endothelium of the capillary wall, (2) a relatively thick basal lamina surrounding the external face of each capillary, and (3) the bulbous "feet" of the astrocytes clinging to the capillaries.

Which of these layers constitutes the blood brain barrier? As you might expect, the astrocyte "feet" play a role but they are not themselves the barrier. Instead, they supply required signals to the endothelial cells, causing them to make *tight junctions*. These tight junctions seamlessly join together the endothelial cells, forming the blood brain barrier and making these the least permeable capillaries in the body.

The blood brain barrier is selective, not absolute. Nutrients such as glucose, essential amino acids, and some electrolytes move passively by facilitated diffusion through the endothelial cell membranes. Bloodborne metabolic wastes, proteins, certain toxins, and most drugs are denied entry. Small nonessential amino acids and potassium ions not only are prevented from entering the brain, but also are actively pumped from the brain across the capillary endothelium.

The barrier is ineffective against fats, fatty acids, oxygen, carbon dioxide, and other fat-soluble molecules that diffuse easily through all plasma membranes. This explains why bloodborne alcohol, nicotine, and anesthetics can affect the brain.

The structure of the blood brain barrier is not completely uniform. In some brain areas surrounding the third and fourth ventricles, the barrier is entirely absent and the capillary endothelium is quite permeable, allowing bloodborne molecules easy access to the neural tissue. One such region is the vomiting center of the brain stem, which monitors the blood for poisonous substances. Another is in the hypothalamus, which regulates water balance, body temperature, and many other metabolic activities. Lack of a blood brain barrier here is essential to allow the hypothalamus to sample the chemical composition of the blood. The barrier is incomplete in newborn and premature infants, and potentially toxic substances can enter the CNS and cause problems not seen in adults.

Injury to the brain, whatever the cause, may result in a localized breakdown of the blood brain barrier. Most likely, this breakdown reflects some change in the capillary endothelial cells or their tight junctions.

Homeostatic Imbalances of the Brain

✓ Describe the cause (if known) and major signs and symptoms of cerebrovascular accidents, Alzheimer's disease, Parkinson's disease, and Huntington's disease.

Brain dysfunctions are unbelievably varied and extensive. We have mentioned some of them already, but here we will focus on traumatic brain injuries, cerebrovascular accidents, and degenerative brain disorders.

Traumatic Brain Injuries

Head injuries are a leading cause of accidental death in North America. Consider, for example, what happens if you forget to fasten your seat belt and then rear-end another car. Your head is moving and then stops suddenly as it hits the windshield. Brain damage is caused not only by localized injury at the site of the blow (the *coup* injury), but also by the ricocheting effect as the brain hits the opposite end of the skull (the *contrecoup* injury).

A **concussion** is an alteration in brain function, usually temporary, following a blow to the head. The victim may be dizzy or lose consciousness. Although typically mild and short-lived, even a seemingly mild concussion can be damaging, and multiple concussions over time produce cumulative damage.

More serious concussions can bruise the brain and cause permanent neurological damage, a condition called a **contusion**. In cortical contusions, the individual may remain conscious. Severe brain stem contusions always cause coma, lasting from hours to a lifetime because of injury to the reticular activating system.

Following a head blow, death may result from **subdural** or **subarachnoid hemorrhage** (bleeding from ruptured vessels into those spaces). Individuals who are initially lucid and then begin to deteriorate neurologically are, in all probability, hemorrhaging intracranially. Blood accumulating in the skull increases intracranial pressure and compresses brain tissue. If the pressure forces the brain stem inferiorly through the foramen magnum, control of blood pressure, heart rate, and respiration is lost. Intracranial hemorrhages are treated by surgically removing the hematoma (localized blood mass) and repairing the ruptured vessels.

Another consequence of traumatic head injury is **cerebral edema**, swelling of the brain. At best, cerebral edema aggravates the injury. At worst, it can be fatal in and of itself.

Cerebrovascular Accidents (CVAs)

The single most common nervous system disorder and the third leading cause of death in North America are **cerebrovascular accidents (CVAs)** (ser″ĕ-bro-vas′ku-lar), also called *strokes* or "brain attacks." CVAs occur when blood circulation to a brain area is blocked and brain tissue dies. [**Ischemia** (is-ke′me-ah; "to hold back blood"), deprivation of blood supply to any tissue, impairs the delivery of oxygen and nutrients to cells.]

The most common cause of CVA is a blood clot that blocks a cerebral artery. A clot can originate outside the brain (from the heart, for example) or form on the roughened interior wall of a brain artery narrowed by atherosclerosis. Less frequently, strokes are caused by bleeding, which compresses brain tissue.

Those who survive a CVA are typically paralyzed on one side of the body (*hemiplegia*). Many exhibit sensory deficits or have difficulty understanding or vocalizing speech. Even so, the picture is not hopeless. Some patients recover at least part of their lost faculties, because undamaged neurons sprout new branches that spread into the injured area and take over some lost functions. Physical therapy should start as soon as possible to prevent muscle contractures (abnormally shortened muscles due to differences in strength between opposing muscle groups).

Not all strokes are "completed." Temporary episodes of reversible cerebral ischemia, called **transient ischemic attacks (TIAs)**, are common. TIAs last from 5 to 50 minutes and are characterized by temporary numbness, paralysis, or impaired speech. These deficits are not permanent, but TIAs do constitute "red flags" that warn of impending, more serious CVAs.

A CVA is like an undersea earthquake. It's not the initial temblor that does most of the damage, it's the tsunami that floods the coast later. Similarly, the initial vascular blockage during a stroke is not usually disastrous because there are many blood vessels in the brain that can pick up the slack. Rather, it's the neuron-killing events outside the initial ischemic zone that wreak the most havoc.

Experimental evidence indicates that the main culprit is *glutamate*, an excitatory neurotransmitter also involved in learning and memory. Normally, glutamate binding to NMDA receptors opens NMDA channels that allow Ca^{2+} to enter the stimulated neuron. After brain injury, neurons totally deprived of oxygen begin to disintegrate, unleashing the cellular equivalent of "buckets" of glutamate. Under these conditions, glutamate acts as an *excitotoxin*, literally exciting surrounding cells to death.

The initial events in excitotoxicity are identical to those in LTP: Ca^{2+} flows in through NMDA receptor channels (see p. 458). In excitotoxicity, however, the amount of Ca^{2+} swamps the cell's ability to cope and Ca^{2+} homeostasis breaks down. High levels of Ca^{2+} kill cells in two ways:

- Ca^{2+} damages mitochondria, causing them to produce the free radical superoxide, which damages cells directly and can also cause programmed cell death (apoptosis).
- Ca^{2+} turns on the synthesis of certain proteins. Some of these promote apoptosis while others are enzymes that produce the free radical NO and other powerful inflammatory agents.

Although the NMDA receptor and the enzyme that makes NO are attractive targets for drug therapies to decrease damage around the stroke epicenter, clinical trials so far have all failed. At present, the most successful treatment for stroke is tissue plasminogen activator (tPA), which dissolves blood clots in the brain. Alternatively, a mechanical device can drill into a blood clot and pull it from a blood vessel like a cork from a bottle.

Other approaches currently under study focus on recovering function after a stroke. One method implants immature neurons into stroke-damaged brain regions in the hope that they will take on properties of nearby mature neurons. Another tries to coax adult brain stem cells to replace damaged neurons. Mice with strokes can generate new tissue and recover motor function when treated with a combination of growth factors during a critical time following injury. Hopefully, this will be true for humans, too.

Degenerative Brain Disorders

Alzheimer's Disease

Alzheimer's disease (AD) (altz′hi-merz), a progressive degenerative disease of the brain, ultimately results in **dementia** (mental deterioration). Alzheimer's patients represent nearly half of the people living in nursing homes. Between 5 and 15% of people over 65 develop this condition, and for up to half of those over 85 it is a major contributing cause in their deaths.

Its victims exhibit memory loss (particularly for recent events), shortened attention span, disorientation, and eventual language loss. Over a period of several years, formerly good-natured people may become irritable, moody, and confused. Hallucinations may ultimately occur.

Examinations of brain tissue reveal senile plaques littering the brain like shrapnel between the neurons. The plaques consist of extracellular aggregations of *beta-amyloid peptide*, which is cut from a normal membrane precursor protein (APP) by enzymes. One form of Alzheimer's disease is caused by an inherited mutation in the gene for APP, which suggests that too much beta-amyloid may be toxic. New evidence suggests that the beta-amyloid peptide may exert its toxic effect through the prion protein, the same protein that (in an altered form) causes mad cow disease. Current clinical trials focus on using the immune system to clear away beta-amyloid peptide.

Another hallmark of Alzheimer's disease is the presence of *neurofibrillary tangles* inside neurons. These tangles involve a protein called tau, which functions like railroad ties to bind microtubule "tracks" together. In the brains of AD victims, tau abandons its microtubule-stabilizing role and grabs onto other tau molecules, forming spaghetti-like neurofibrillary tangles, which kill the neurons by disrupting their transport mechanisms.

As the brain cells die, the brain shrinks. Particularly vulnerable brain areas include the hippocampus and the basal forebrain, regions involved in thinking and memory (see Figure 12.21). Loss of neurons in the basal forebrain is associated with a shortage of the neurotransmitter acetylcholine, and drugs that inhibit breakdown of acetylcholine slightly enhance cognitive function in AD patients. Interestingly, a drug that blocks NMDA receptors, memantine, also slightly improves thinking in more advanced stages of AD, suggesting that glutamate excitotoxicity is also involved in this disease.

Parkinson's Disease

Typically striking people in their 50s and 60s, **Parkinson's disease** results from a degeneration of the dopamine-releasing neurons of the substantia nigra. As those neurons deteriorate, the dopamine-deprived basal nuclei they target become overactive. Afflicted individuals have a persistent tremor at rest (exhibited by "pill-rolling" movements of the fingers and wrist), a forward-bent walking posture and shuffling gait, and a stiff facial expression. They are slow initiating and executing movement.

12

The cause of Parkinson's disease is still unknown, but multiple factors may interact to destroy dopamine-releasing neurons. Recent evidence points to abnormalities in certain mitochondrial proteins and protein degradation pathways. The drug *L-dopa* helps to alleviate some symptoms. It passes through the blood brain barrier and is then converted into dopamine.

However, as more and more neurons die off, L-dopa becomes ineffective. Mixing L-dopa with drugs that inhibit the breakdown of dopamine (for example, deprenyl) can prolong its effectiveness. In addition, deprenyl by itself, early in the disease, slows the neurological deterioration to some extent and delays the need to administer L-dopa for up to 18 months.

Deep brain stimulation via implanted electrodes shuts down abnormal brain activity and can alleviate tremors. This treatment (for patients who no longer respond to drug therapy) is expensive and risky, but it works. Another possibility is to use gene therapy to insert genes into adult brain cells, causing them to secrete the inhibitory neurotransmitter GABA. GABA then inhibits the abnormal brain activity just as the electrical stimulation does. Replacing dead or damaged cells by implanting stem cells is promising, but results to date are no better than more conventional treatments.

Huntington's Disease

Huntington's disease, a fatal hereditary disorder, strikes during middle age. Mutant *huntingtin* protein accumulates in brain cells and the tissue dies, leading to massive degeneration of the basal nuclei and later of the cerebral cortex. Its initial symptoms in many are wild, jerky, almost continuous "flapping" movements called *chorea* (Greek for "dance"). Although the movements appear to be voluntary, they are not. Late in the disease, marked mental deterioration occurs. Huntington's disease is progressive and usually fatal within 15 years of onset of symptoms.

The hyperkinetic manifestations of Huntington's disease are essentially the opposite of those of Parkinson's disease (overstimulation rather than inhibition of the motor drive). Huntington's is usually treated with drugs that block, rather than enhance, dopamine's effects. As with Parkinson's disease, stem cell implants may be a promising treatment in the future.

Check Your Understanding

20. What is CSF? Where is it produced? What are its functions?
21. What is a transient ischemic attack (TIA) and how is it different from a stroke?
22. Mrs. Lee, a neurology patient, seldom smiles, has a shuffling, stooped gait, and often spills her coffee. What degenerative brain disorder might she have?

For answers, see Appendix H.

The Spinal Cord

✓ Describe the gross and microscopic structure of the spinal cord.

✓ List the major spinal cord tracts, and classify each as a motor or sensory tract.

Gross Anatomy and Protection

The spinal cord, enclosed in the vertebral column, extends from the foramen magnum of the skull to the first or second lumbar vertebra, just inferior to the ribs **(Figure 12.26)**. About 42 cm (17 inches) long and 1.8 cm (3/4 of an inch) thick, the glistening-white **spinal cord** provides a two-way conduction pathway to and from the brain. It is a major reflex center: Spinal reflexes are initiated and completed at the spinal cord level. We discuss reflex functions and motor activity of the cord in subsequent chapters. In this section we focus on the anatomy of the spinal cord and its ascending and descending tracts.

Like the brain, the spinal cord is protected by bone, meninges, and cerebrospinal fluid. The single-layered **spinal dura mater** (Figure 12.26c) is not attached to the bony walls of the vertebral column. Between the bony vertebrae and the spinal dura mater is an **epidural space** filled with a soft padding of fat and a network of veins (see Figure 12.28a). Cerebrospinal fluid fills the subarachnoid space between the *arachnoid* and *pia mater* meninges.

Inferiorly, the dural and arachnoid membranes extend to the level of S_2, well beyond the end of the spinal cord. The spinal cord typically ends between L_1 and L_2 (Figure 12.26a). For this reason, the subarachnoid space within the meningeal sac inferior to that point provides a nearly ideal spot for removing cerebrospinal fluid for testing, a procedure called a **lumbar**

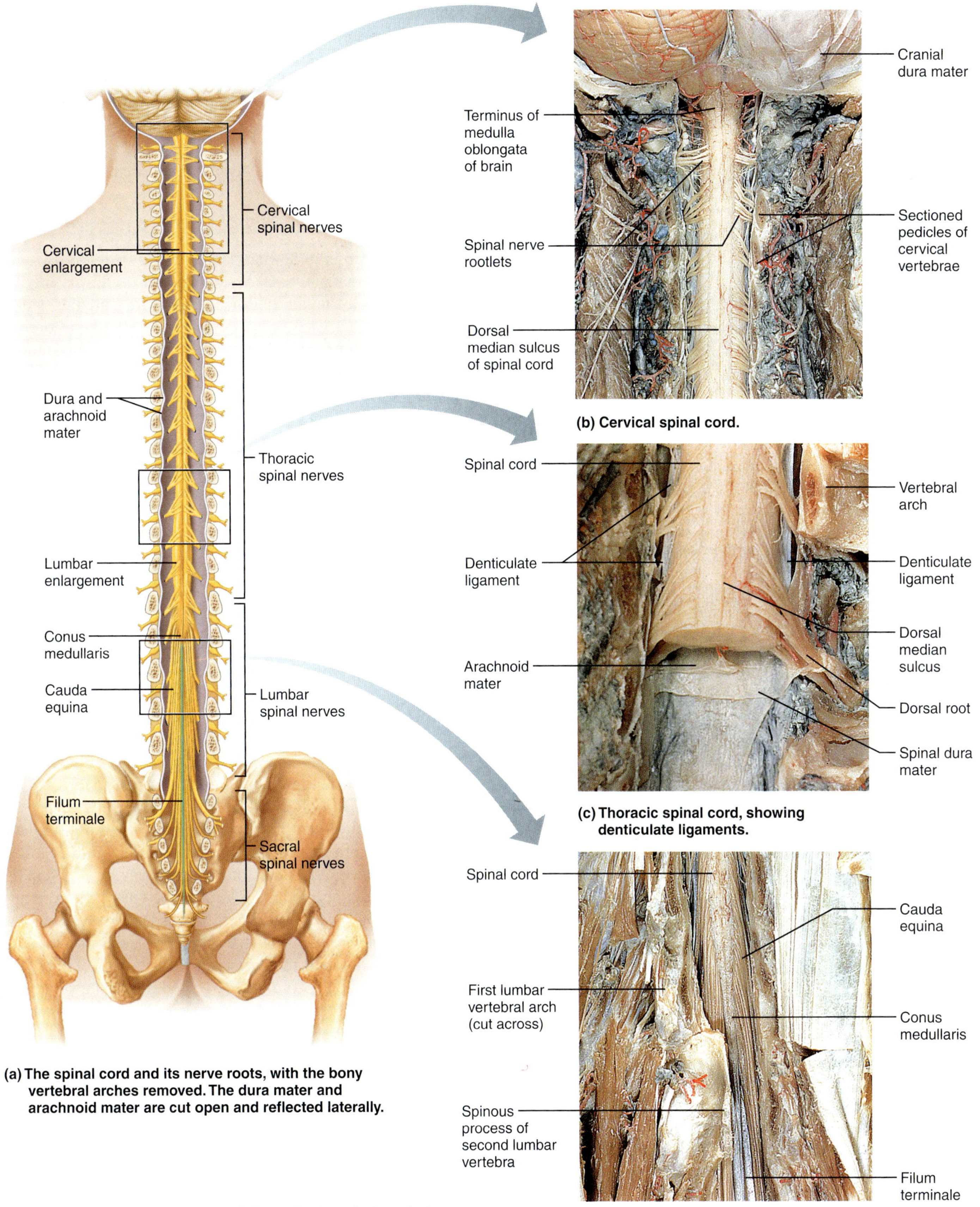

(a) The spinal cord and its nerve roots, with the bony vertebral arches removed. The dura mater and arachnoid mater are cut open and reflected laterally.

(b) Cervical spinal cord.

(c) Thoracic spinal cord, showing denticulate ligaments.

(d) Inferior end of spinal cord, showing conus medullaris, cauda equina, and filum terminale.

Figure 12.26 Gross structure of the spinal cord, dorsal view. (For related images, see *A Brief Atlas of the Human Body*, Figures 52, 53, and 55.)

12

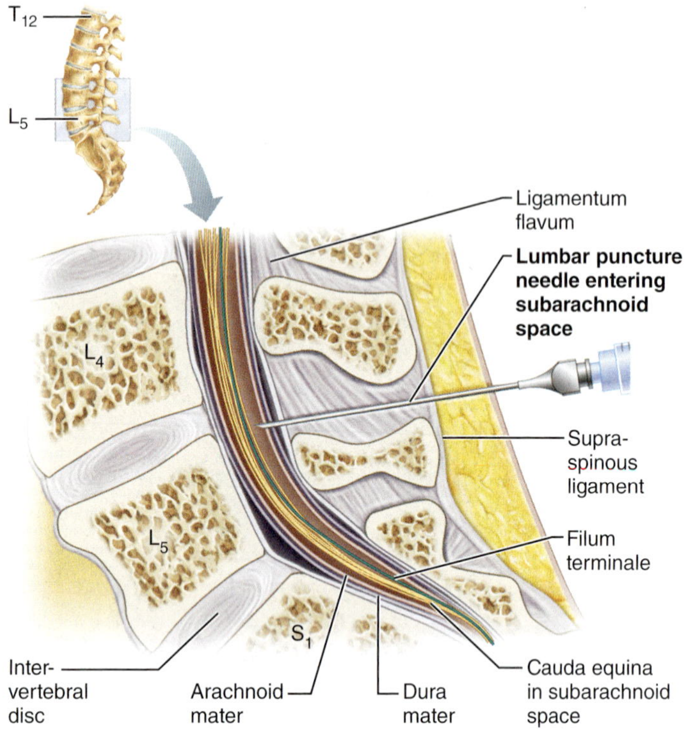

Figure 12.27 Diagram of a lumbar tap. This procedure removes CSF for testing.

12

puncture or **tap (Figure 12.27)**. Because the spinal cord is absent there and the delicate nerve roots drift away from the point of needle insertion, there is little or no danger of damaging the cord (or spinal roots) beyond L_3.

Inferiorly, the spinal cord terminates in a tapering cone-shaped structure called the **conus medullaris** (ko′nus mĕ″dul-ar′is). The **filum terminale** (fi′lum ter″mĭ-nah′le; "terminal filament"), a fibrous extension of the conus covered by pia mater, extends inferiorly from the conus medullaris to the coccyx, where it anchors the spinal cord so it is not jostled by body movements (Figure 12.26a, d). Furthermore, saw-toothed shelves of pia mater called **denticulate ligaments** (den-tik′u-lāt; "toothed") secure the spinal cord to the tough dura mater meninx throughout its length (Figure 12.26c).

In humans, 31 pairs of *spinal nerves*—part of the peripheral nervous system—attach to the cord by paired roots. Each nerve exits from the vertebral column by passing superior to its corresponding vertebra via the intervertebral foramen, and travels to the body region it serves. While each nerve pair defines a segment of the cord, the spinal cord is, in fact, continuous throughout its length and its internal structure changes gradually.

The spinal cord is about the width of a thumb for most of its length, but it has obvious enlargements in the cervical and lumbosacral regions, where the nerves serving the upper and lower limbs arise. These enlargements are the **cervical** and **lumbar enlargements**, respectively (Figure 12.26a).

Because the cord does not reach the end of the vertebral column, the lumbar and sacral spinal nerve roots angle sharply downward and travel inferiorly through the vertebral canal for some distance before reaching their intervertebral foramina. The collection of nerve roots at the inferior end of the vertebral canal is named the **cauda equina** (kaw′da e-kwi′nuh) because it resembles a horse's tail (Figure 12.26a, d). This strange arrangement reflects the fact that during fetal development, the vertebral column grows faster than the spinal cord, forcing the lower spinal nerve roots to "chase" their exit points inferiorly through the vertebral canal.

We will discuss the spinal nerves in more detail in Chapter 13.

Spinal Cord Cross-Sectional Anatomy

The spinal cord is somewhat flattened from front to back and two grooves mark its surface: the **ventral (anterior) median fissure** and the shallower **dorsal (posterior) median sulcus (Figure 12.28b)**. These grooves run the length of the cord and partially divide it into right and left halves. The gray matter of the cord is located in its core, the white matter outside.

Gray Matter and Spinal Roots

In cross section the gray matter of the cord looks like the letter H or like a butterfly (Figure 12.28b). It consists of mirror-image lateral gray masses connected by a crossbar of gray matter, the **gray commissure**, that encloses the central canal. The two dorsal projections of the gray matter are the **dorsal (posterior) horns**, and the ventral pair are the **ventral (anterior) horns**. In 3-D, these horns form columns of gray matter that run the entire length of the spinal cord. The thoracic and superior lumbar segments of the cord have an additional pair of gray matter columns, the small **lateral horns**.

All neurons whose cell bodies are in the spinal cord gray matter are multipolar. The dorsal horns consist entirely of interneurons. The ventral horns have some interneurons but mainly house cell bodies of somatic motor neurons. These motor neurons send their axons out to the skeletal muscles (their effector organs) via the *ventral rootlets* that fuse together to become the **ventral roots** of the spinal cord (Figure 12.28b).

The amount of ventral gray matter present at a given level of the spinal cord reflects the amount of skeletal muscle innervated at that level. As a result, the ventral horns are largest in the limb-innervating cervical and lumbar regions of the cord and are responsible for the cord enlargements seen in those regions.

The lateral horns consist mostly of the cell bodies of autonomic (sympathetic division) motor neurons that serve visceral organs. Their axons leave the cord via the ventral root along with those of the somatic motor neurons. Because the ventral roots contain both somatic and autonomic efferent fibers, they serve both motor divisions of the peripheral nervous system **(Figure 12.29)**.

Afferent fibers carrying impulses from peripheral sensory receptors form the **dorsal roots** of the spinal cord that fan out as the *dorsal rootlets* before they enter the spinal cord (Figure 12.28). The cell bodies of the associated sensory neurons are found in an enlarged region of the dorsal root called the **dorsal root ganglion** or **spinal ganglion**. After entering the cord, the axons of these neurons may take a number of routes. Some enter the dorsal white matter of the cord directly and travel to synapse at higher cord or brain levels. Others synapse with interneurons in the dorsal horns of the spinal cord gray matter at their entry level. The

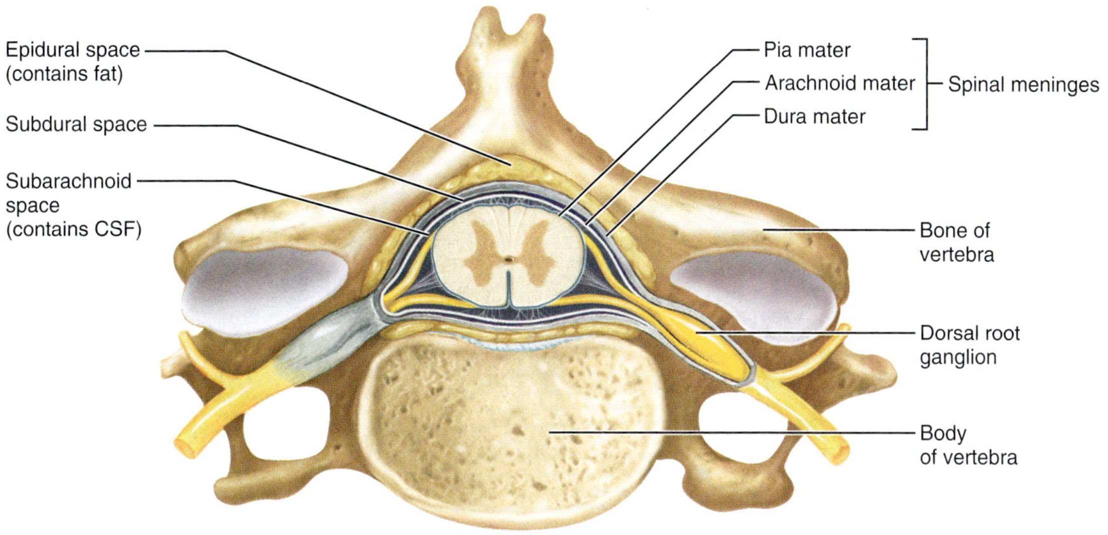

(a) Cross section of spinal cord and vertebra

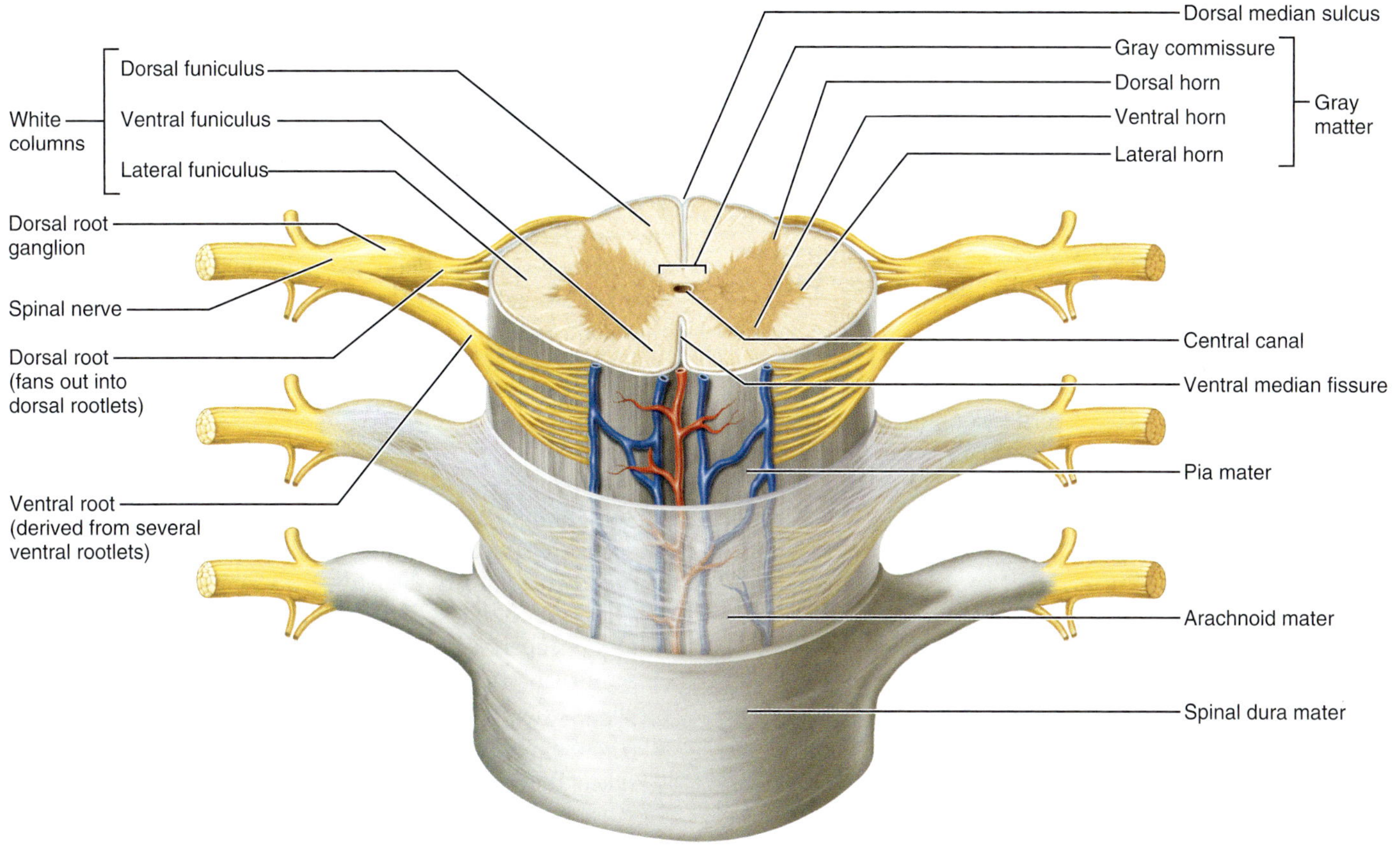

(b) The spinal cord and its meningeal coverings

Figure 12.28 Anatomy of the spinal cord. (a) Cross section through the spinal cord illustrating its relationship to the surrounding vertebral column. **(b)** Anterior view of the spinal cord and its meningeal coverings.

12

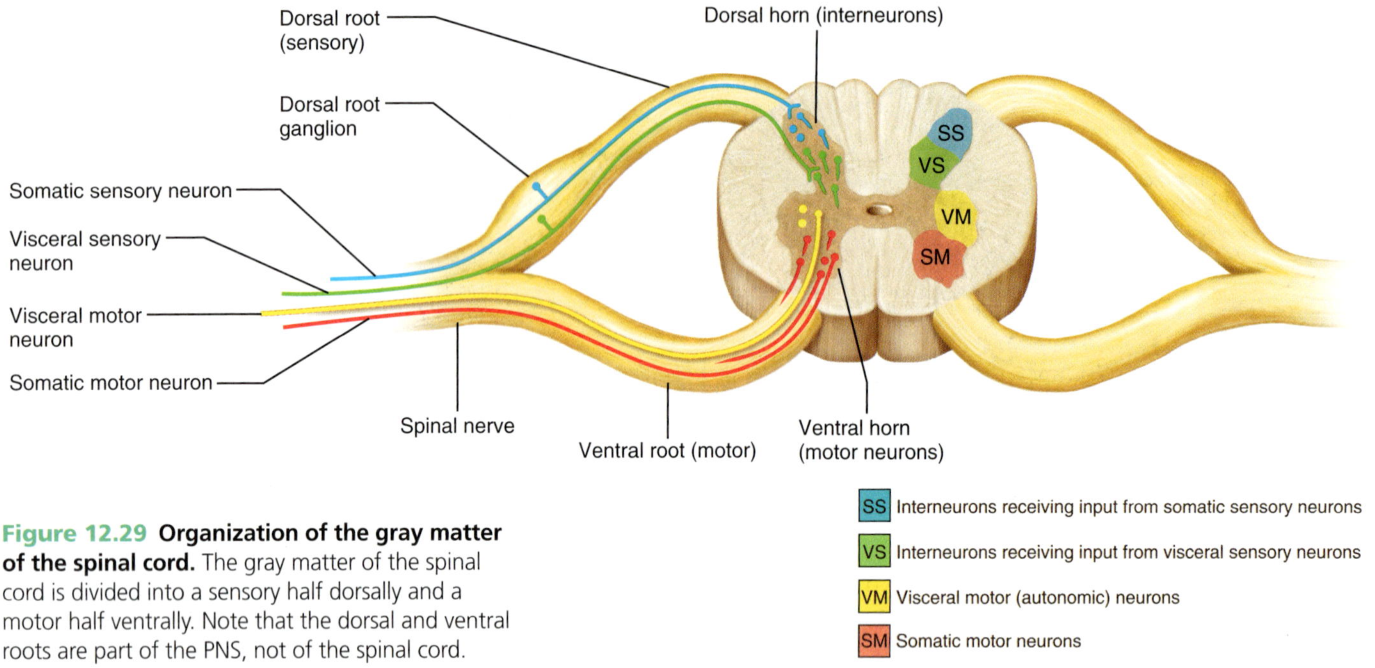

Figure 12.29 Organization of the gray matter of the spinal cord. The gray matter of the spinal cord is divided into a sensory half dorsally and a motor half ventrally. Note that the dorsal and ventral roots are part of the PNS, not of the spinal cord.

dorsal and ventral roots are very short and fuse laterally to form the **spinal nerves** (see Chapter 13).

The spinal gray matter can be divided further according to its neurons' relative involvement in innervating the somatic and visceral regions of the body. Spinal gray matter has the following four zones (Figure 12.29): **somatic sensory (SS)**, **visceral sensory (VS)**, **visceral (autonomic) motor (VM)**, **somatic motor (SM)**.

12

White Matter

The white matter of the spinal cord is composed of myelinated and nonmyelinated nerve fibers that allow communication between different parts of the spinal cord and between the cord and brain. These fibers run in three directions:

- *Ascending*—up to higher centers (sensory inputs)
- *Descending*—down to the cord from the brain or within the cord to lower levels (motor outputs)
- *Transverse*—across from one side of the cord to the other (commissural fibers)

Ascending and descending tracts make up most of the white matter.

The white matter on each side of the cord is divided into three **white columns**, or **funiculi** (fu-nik′u-li; "long ropes"), named according to their position as **dorsal (posterior)**, **lateral**, and **ventral (anterior) funiculi** (Figure 12.28b). Each funiculus contains several fiber tracts, and each tract is made up of axons with similar destinations and functions. With a few exceptions, the names of the spinal tracts reveal both their origin and destination. **Figure 12.30** schematically illustrates the principal ascending and descending tracts of the spinal cord in cross-sectional view.

Neuronal Pathways

All major spinal tracts are part of *multineuron pathways* that connect the brain to the body periphery. These great ascending and descending pathways contain not only spinal cord neurons but also parts of peripheral neurons and neurons in the brain. Before we get specific about the individual tracts, we will note four key generalizations about them and the pathways to which they contribute:

- **Decussation.** Most pathways cross from one side of the CNS to the other (decussate) at some point along their journey.
- **Relay.** Most pathways consist of a chain of two or three neurons (a relay) that contribute to successive tracts of the pathway.
- **Somatotopy.** Most pathways exhibit *somatotopy*, a precise spatial relationship among the tract fibers that reflects the orderly mapping of the body. For example, in an ascending sensory tract, fibers transmitting inputs from sensory receptors in superior body regions lie lateral to those conveying sensory information from inferior body regions.
- **Symmetry.** All pathways and tracts are paired symmetrically (right and left), with a member of the pair present on each side of the spinal cord or brain.

Ascending Pathways to the Brain

The ascending pathways conduct sensory impulses upward, typically through chains of three successive neurons (first-, second-, and third-order neurons) to various areas of the brain. Note that both second- and third-order neurons are interneurons.

- **First-order neurons**, whose cell bodies reside in a ganglion (dorsal root or cranial), conduct impulses from the cutaneous receptors of the skin and from proprioceptors to the spinal cord or brain stem, where they synapse with second-order neurons. Impulses from the facial area are transmitted by cranial nerves,

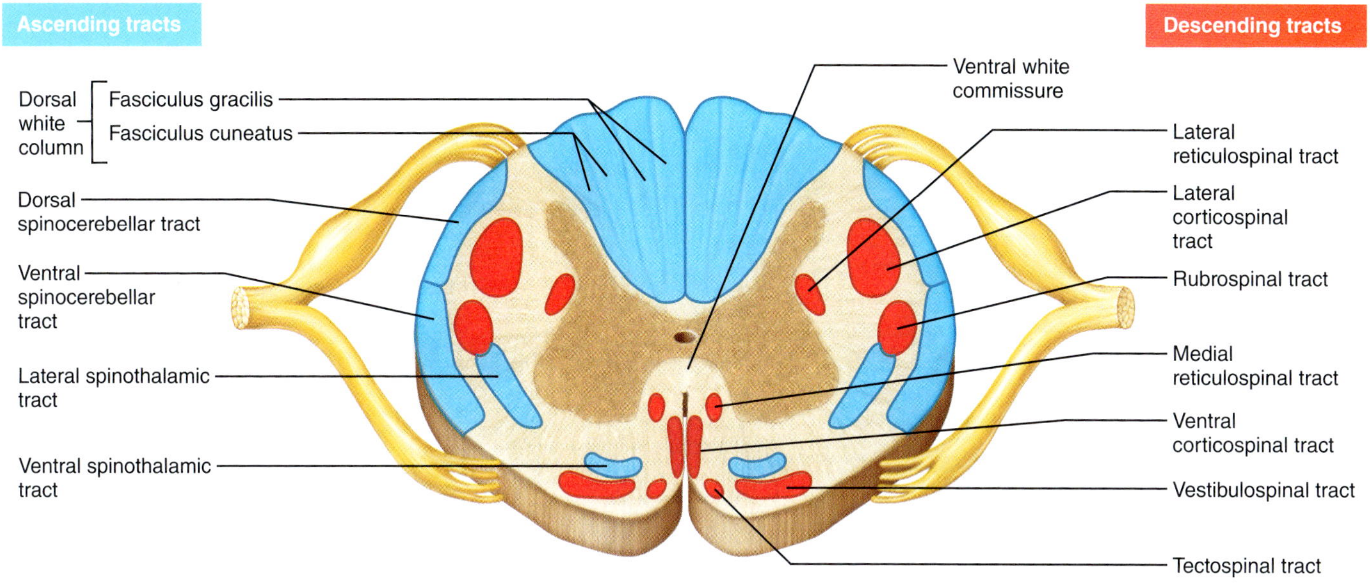

Figure 12.30 Major ascending (sensory) and descending (motor) tracts of the spinal cord, cross-sectional view.

and spinal nerves conduct somatic sensory impulses from the rest of the body to the CNS. First-order neurons entering the spinal cord are shown at the bottom of **Figure 12.31**.

- The cell bodies of **second-order neurons** (Figure 12.31, middle) reside in the dorsal horn of the spinal cord or in medullary nuclei. They transmit impulses to the thalamus or to the cerebellum where they synapse.
- **Third-order neurons** have cell bodies in the thalamus (Figure 12.31, top). They relay impulses to the somatosensory cortex of the cerebrum. (There are no third-order neurons in the cerebellum.)

In general, somatosensory information travels along three main pathways on each side of the spinal cord. Two of these pathways (the *dorsal column–medial lemniscal* and *spinothalamic pathways*) transmit impulses via the thalamus to the sensory cortex for conscious interpretation. Collectively the inputs of these sister tracts provide *discriminative touch* and *conscious proprioception*. Both pathways decussate—the first in the medulla and the second in the spinal cord.

The third pathway, the *spinocerebellar pathway*, terminates in the cerebellum, and does not contribute to sensory perception. Let's examine these pathways more closely.

1. **Dorsal column–medial lemniscal pathways.** The **dorsal column–medial lemniscal pathways** (lem-nis′kul; "ribbon") mediate precise, straight-through transmission of inputs from a single type (or a few related types) of sensory receptor that can be localized precisely on the body surface, such as discriminative touch and vibrations. These pathways are formed by the paired tracts of the **dorsal white column** of the spinal cord—**fasciculus cuneatus** and **fasciculus gracilis**—and the **medial lemniscus**.

   The medial lemniscus arises in the medulla and terminates in the thalamus (Figure 12.31a and **Table 12.2**). From the thalamus, impulses are forwarded to specific areas of the somatosensory cortex.
2. **Spinothalamic pathways.** The **spinothalamic pathways** receive input from many different types of sensory receptors and make multiple synapses in the brain stem. These pathways consist of the **lateral** and **ventral (anterior) spinothalamic tracts** (see Figure 12.31b and Table 12.2). Their fibers cross over in the spinal cord.

   The fibers in these pathways primarily transmit impulses for pain and temperature, but also for coarse touch and pressure. All are sensations that we are aware of but have difficulty localizing precisely on the body surface.
3. **Spinocerebellar pathways.** The third ascending pathway consists of the **ventral** and **dorsal spinocerebellar tracts**. They convey information about muscle or tendon stretch to the cerebellum, which uses this information to coordinate skeletal muscle activity (see Figure 12.31a and Table 12.2). As noted earlier, these pathways do not contribute to conscious sensation. The fibers of the spinocerebellar pathways either do not decussate or else cross over twice (thus "undoing" the decussation).

Descending Pathways and Tracts

The descending pathways that deliver efferent impulses from the brain to the spinal cord are divided into two groups: (1) the *direct pathways*, equivalent to the pyramidal tracts, and (2) the *indirect pathways*, essentially all others. Motor pathways involve two neurons, referred to as the upper and lower motor neurons:

- *Upper motor neurons* are the pyramidal cells of the motor cortex (see p. 433) and the neurons of subcortical motor nuclei.
- *Lower motor neurons* are the ventral horn motor neurons. These directly innervate the skeletal muscles (their effectors).

We give a brief overview of these pathways on p. 471. See **Table 12.3** on p. 473 for more information.

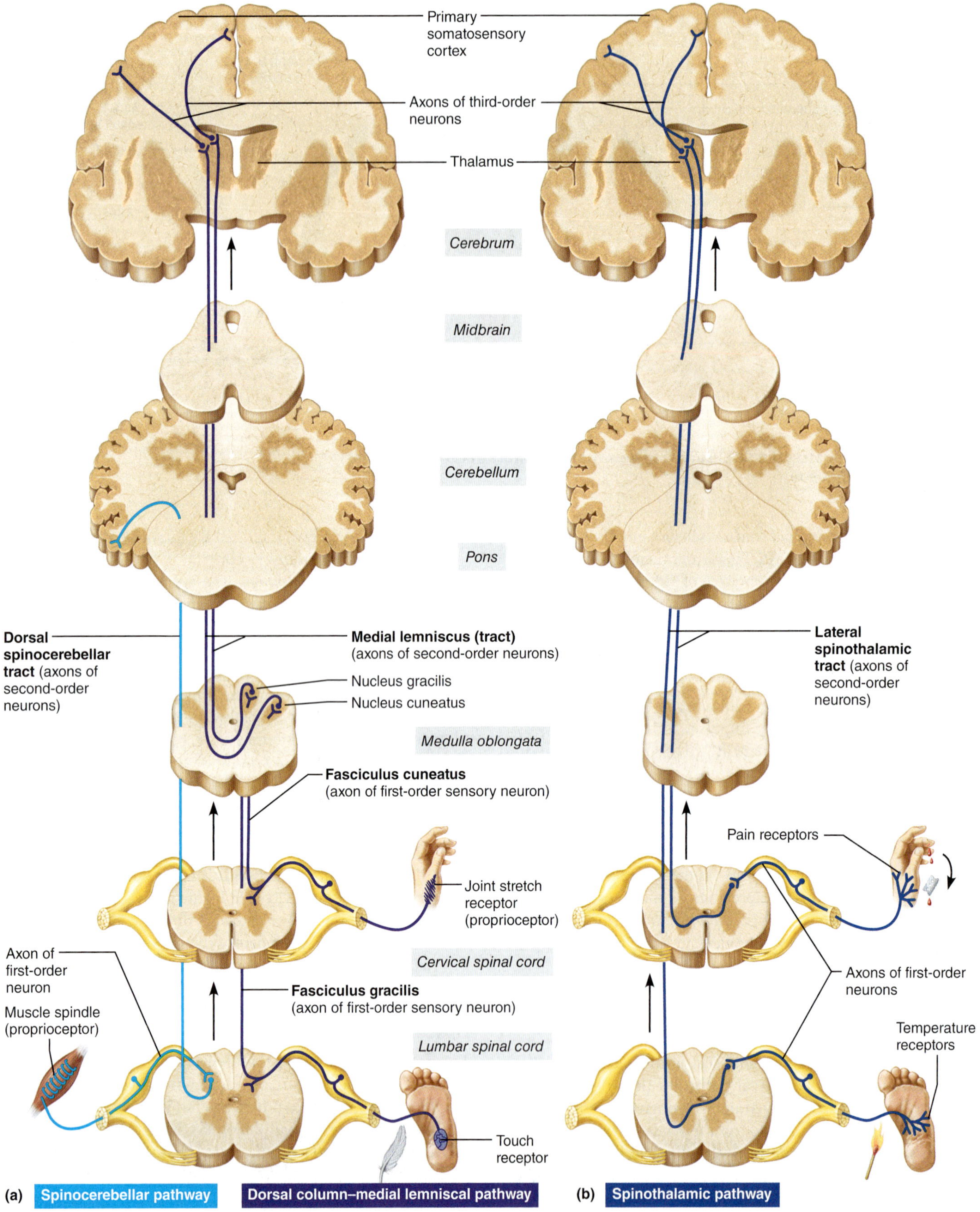

Figure 12.31 Pathways of selected ascending spinal cord tracts. Cross sections up to the cerebrum, which is shown in frontal section. **(a)** The spinocerebellar pathway (left) transmits proprioceptive information only to the cerebellum, and so is subconscious. The dorsal column–medial lemniscal pathway transmits discriminative touch and conscious proprioception signals to the cerebral cortex. **(b)** The lateral spinothalamic pathway transmits pain and temperature.

Table 12.2 Major Ascending (Sensory) Pathways and Spinal Cord Tracts

SPINAL CORD TRACT	LOCATION (FUNICULUS)	ORIGIN	TERMINATION	FUNCTION
Dorsal Column–Medial Lemniscal Pathways				
Fasciculus cuneatus and fasciculus gracilis (dorsal white column)	Dorsal	Central axons of sensory (first-order) neurons enter dorsal root of the spinal cord and branch. Branches enter dorsal white column on same side without synapsing.	By synapse with second-order neurons in nucleus cuneatus and nucleus gracilis in medulla. Fibers of medullary neurons cross over and ascend in medial lemniscus to thalamus, where they synapse with third-order neurons. Thalamic neurons then transmit impulses to somatosensory cortex.	Both tracts transmit sensory impulses from general sensory receptors of skin and proprioceptors, which are interpreted as discriminative touch, pressure, and "body sense" (limb and joint position) in opposite somatosensory cortex. Cuneatus transmits afferent impulses from upper limbs, upper trunk, and neck. Gracilis carries impulses from lower limbs and inferior body trunk.
Spinothalamic Pathways				
Lateral spinothalamic	Lateral	Interneurons (second-order neurons) in dorsal horns. Fibers cross to opposite side before ascending.	By synapse with third-order neurons in thalamus. Thalamic neurons then convey impulses to somatosensory cortex.	Transmits impulses concerned with pain and temperature to opposite side of brain for interpretation by somatosensory cortex.
Ventral spinothalamic	Ventral	Interneurons (second-order neurons) in dorsal horns. Fibers cross to opposite side before ascending.	By synapse with third-order neurons in thalamus. Thalamic neurons eventually convey impulses to somatosensory cortex.	Transmits impulses concerned with crude touch and pressure to opposite side of brain for interpretation by somatosensory cortex.
Spinocerebellar Pathways				
Dorsal spinocerebellar*	Lateral (dorsal part)	Interneurons (second-order neurons) in dorsal horn on same side of cord. Fibers ascend without crossing.	By synapse in cerebellum	Transmits impulses from trunk and lower limb proprioceptors on one side of body to same side of cerebellum for subconscious proprioception.
Ventral spinocerebellar*	Lateral (ventral part)	Interneurons (second-order neurons) of dorsal horn. Contains crossed fibers that cross back to the opposite side in the pons.	By synapse in cerebellum	Transmits impulses from the trunk and lower limb on the same side of body to cerebellum for subconscious proprioception.

*These spinocerebellar tracts carry information from the lower limbs and trunk only. The corresponding tracts for the upper limb and neck (rostral spinocerebellar and others) are beyond the scope of this book.

Direct (Pyramidal) Pathways The direct pathways originate mainly with the pyramidal neurons located in the precentral gyri. These neurons send impulses through the brain stem via the large **pyramidal (corticospinal) tracts** (Figure 12.32a). The direct pathways are so called because their axons descend without synapsing from the pyramidal neurons to the spinal cord. There they synapse either with interneurons or with ventral horn motor neurons.

Stimulation of the ventral horn neurons activates the skeletal muscles with which they are associated. The direct pathway primarily regulates fast and fine (or skilled) movements such as doing needlework and writing.

Indirect Pathways The indirect pathways include brain stem motor nuclei and *all motor pathways except* the pyramidal pathways. These pathways were formerly lumped together as

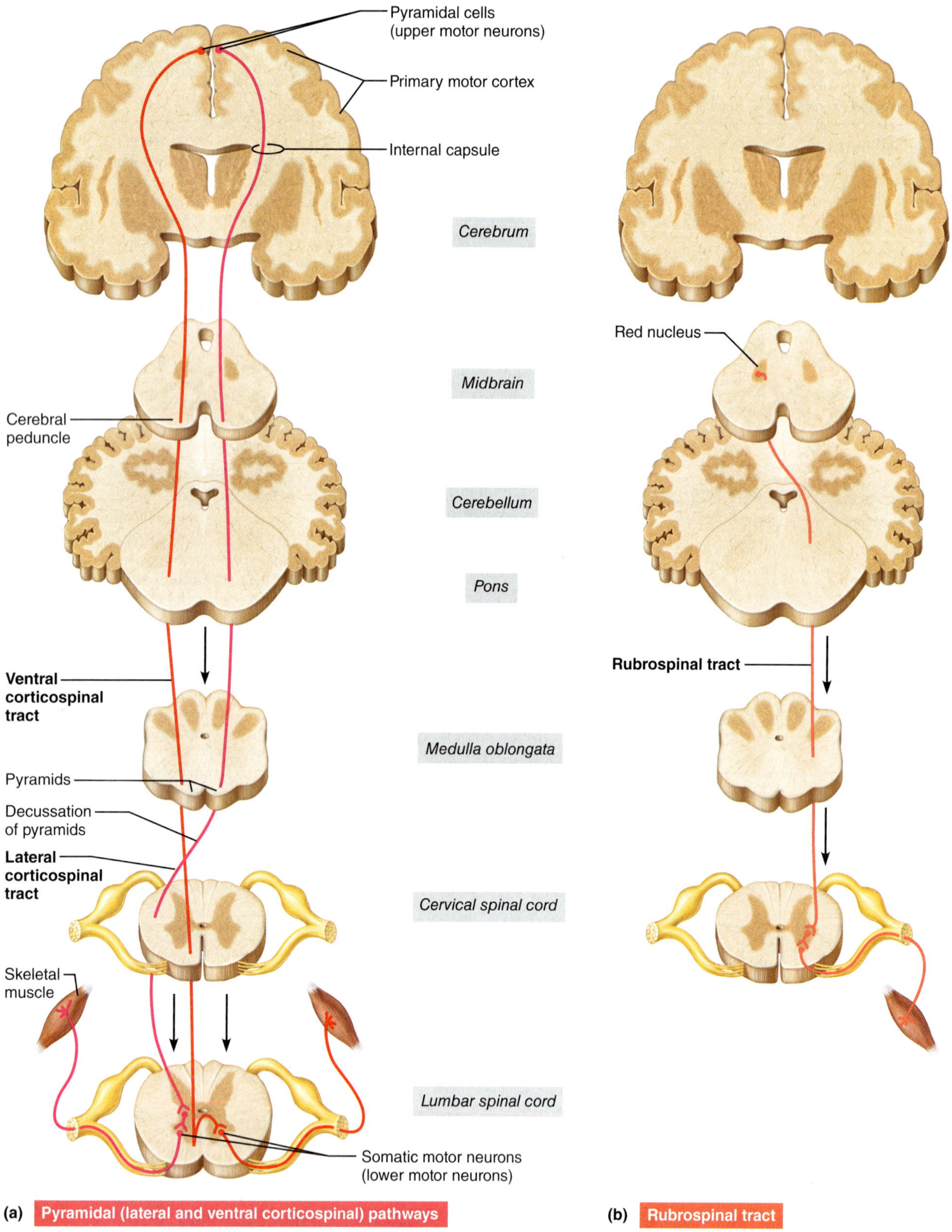

Figure 12.32 Three descending pathways by which the brain influences movement. Cross sections up to the cerebrum, which is shown in frontal section. **(a)** Pyramidal (lateral and ventral corticospinal pathways) are direct pathways that control skilled voluntary movements. **(b)** The rubrospinal tract, one of the indirect pathways, helps regulate muscle tone.

Table 12.3 Major Descending (Motor) Pathways and Spinal Cord Tracts

SPINAL CORD TRACT	LOCATION (FUNICULUS)	ORIGIN	TERMINATION	FUNCTION
Direct (Pyramidal) Pathways				
Lateral corticospinal	Lateral	Pyramidal neurons of motor cortex of the cerebrum. Cross over in pyramids of medulla.	By synapse with ventral horn interneurons that influence motor neurons and occasionally with ventral horn motor neurons directly.	Transmits motor impulses from cerebrum to spinal cord motor neurons (which activate skeletal muscles on opposite side of body). A voluntary motor tract.
Ventral corticospinal	Ventral	Pyramidal neurons of motor cortex. Fibers cross over at the spinal cord level.	Ventral horn (as above).	Same as lateral corticospinal tract.
Indirect Pathways				
Tectospinal	Ventral	Superior colliculus of midbrain of brain stem (fibers cross to opposite side of cord).	Ventral horn (as above).	Turns neck so eyes can follow a moving object.
Vestibulospinal	Ventral	Vestibular nuclei in medulla of brain stem (fibers descend without crossing).	Ventral horn (as above).	Transmits motor impulses that maintain muscle tone and activate ipsilateral limb and trunk extensor muscles and muscles that move head. Helps maintain balance during standing and moving.
Rubrospinal	Lateral	Red nucleus of midbrain of brain stem (fibers cross to opposite side just inferior to the red nucleus).	Ventral horn (as above).	In experimental animals, transmits motor impulses concerned with muscle tone of distal limb muscles (mostly flexors) on opposite side of body. In humans, functions are largely assumed by corticospinal tracts.
Reticulospinal (ventral, medial, and lateral)	Ventral and lateral	Reticular formation of brain stem (medial nuclear group of pons and medulla). Both crossed and uncrossed fibers.	Ventral horn (as above).	Transmits impulses concerned with muscle tone and many visceral motor functions. May control most unskilled movements.

the *extrapyramidal system* because their nuclei of origin were presumed to be independent of ("extra to") the pyramidal tracts. This term is still widely used clinically. However, pyramidal tract neurons are now known to project to and influence the activity of most "extrapyramidal" nuclei, so modern anatomists prefer the term **indirect**, or **multineuronal**, **pathways**, or even just the names of the individual motor pathways.

Indirect motor pathways are complex and multisynaptic. They are most involved in regulating:

- Axial muscles that maintain balance and posture
- Muscles controlling coarse limb movements
- Head, neck, and eye movements that follow objects in the visual field

Many of the activities controlled by subcortical motor nuclei depend heavily on reflex activity. Figure 12.32b illustrates one of these tracts, the rubrospinal tract.

Overall, the **reticulospinal** and **vestibulospinal tracts** maintain balance by varying the tone of postural muscles (Table 12.3). The **rubrospinal tracts** control flexor muscles, whereas the **tectospinal tracts** and the *superior colliculi* mediate head movements in response to visual stimuli.

Check Your Understanding

23. What is the explanation for the cervical and lumbar enlargements of the spinal cord?
24. Where are the cell bodies of the first-, second-, and third-order sensory neurons in the spinothalamic pathway located?

For answers, see Appendix H.

12

Spinal Cord Trauma and Disorders

✓ Distinguish between flaccid and spastic paralysis, and between paralysis and paresthesia.

Spinal Cord Trauma

The spinal cord is elastic, stretching with every turn of the head or bend of the trunk, but it is exquisitely sensitive to direct pressure. Any localized damage to the spinal cord or its roots leads to some functional loss, either **paralysis** (loss of motor function) or **paresthesias** (par″es-the′ze-ahz) (abnormal sensations).

Severe damage to ventral root or ventral horn cells results in **flaccid paralysis** (flak′sid) of the skeletal muscles served. Nerve impulses do not reach these muscles, which consequently cannot move either voluntarily or involuntarily. Without stimulation, the muscles atrophy.

When only the upper motor neurons of the primary motor cortex are damaged, **spastic paralysis** occurs. In this case, the spinal motor neurons remain intact and spinal reflex activity continues to stimulate the muscles irregularly. As a result, the muscles remain healthy longer, but their movements are no longer subject to voluntary control. In many cases, the muscles shorten permanently.

Transection (cross sectioning) of the spinal cord at any level results in total motor and sensory loss in body regions inferior to the site of damage.

- If the transection occurs between T_1 and L_1, both lower limbs are affected, resulting in **paraplegia** (par″ah-ple′je-ah; *para* = beside, *plegia* = a blow).
- If the injury occurs in the cervical region, all four limbs are affected and the result is **quadriplegia**.

12

Hemiplegia, paralysis of one side of the body, usually reflects brain injury rather than spinal cord injury.

Anyone with a spinal cord transection must be watched for symptoms of **spinal shock**, a transient period of functional loss that follows the injury. Spinal shock immediately depresses all reflex activity caudal to the lesion site. Bowel and bladder reflexes stop, blood pressure falls, and all muscles (somatic and visceral alike) below the injury are paralyzed and insensitive. Neural function usually returns within a few hours following injury. If function does not resume within 48 hours, paralysis is permanent in most cases.

Poliomyelitis

Poliomyelitis (po″le-o-mi″ĕ-li′tis; *polio* = gray matter; *myelitis* = inflammation of the spinal cord) results from the poliovirus, which typically enters the body in feces-contaminated water and destroys ventral horn motor neurons. Early symptoms include fever, headache, muscle pain and weakness, and loss of certain somatic reflexes. Later, paralysis develops and the muscles served atrophy. The victim may die from paralyzed respiratory muscles or from cardiac arrest. Fortunately, vaccines have nearly eliminated this disease and a global effort is ongoing to eradicate it completely.

However, many survivors of the great polio epidemic of the late 1940s and 1950s have begun to experience extreme lethargy, sharp burning pains in their muscles, and progressive muscle weakness and atrophy. These disturbing symptoms are referred to as **postpolio syndrome**. The cause of postpolio syndrome is not known, but a likely explanation is that its victims, like the rest of us, continue to lose neurons throughout life. While a healthy nervous system can recruit nearby neurons to compensate, polio survivors have already drawn on that "pool" and have few neurons left to take over. Ironically, those who worked hardest to overcome their disease are its newest victims.

Amyotrophic Lateral Sclerosis (ALS)

Amyotrophic lateral sclerosis (*ALS*) (ah-mi″o-trof′ik), also called Lou Gehrig's disease, is a devastating neuromuscular condition that progressively destroys ventral horn motor neurons and fibers of the pyramidal tracts. As the disease progresses, the sufferer loses the ability to speak, swallow, and breathe. Death typically occurs within five years.

Environmental and genetic factors interact to cause ALS. In 10% of cases mutations are inherited; spontaneous mutations are probably involved in the rest. Recently, the mutations have been localized to genes that are involved in RNA processing. While the exact mechanism is not clear, the presence of excess extracellular glutamate suggests that excitotoxic cell death is involved. Riluzole, a drug that interferes with glutamate signaling, is the only available life-prolonging treatment.

Diagnostic Procedures for Assessing CNS Dysfunction

✓ List and explain several techniques used to diagnose brain disorders.

If you have had a routine physical examination, you are familiar with the reflex tests done to assess neural function. A tap with a reflex hammer stretches your quadriceps tendon and your anterior thigh muscles contract. This produces the knee-jerk response, which shows that your spinal cord and upper brain centers are functioning normally.

Abnormal responses to a reflex test may indicate such serious disorders as intracranial hemorrhage, multiple sclerosis, or hydrocephalus. They indicate that more sophisticated neurological tests are needed to identify the problem.

New imaging techniques have revolutionized the diagnosis of brain lesions (see *A Closer Look*, pp. 18–19). Together, various *CT* and *MRI scanning techniques* allow quick identification of most tumors, intracranial lesions, multiple sclerosis plaques, and areas of dead brain tissue (infarcts). PET scans can localize brain lesions that generate seizures (epileptic tissue), and new radiotracer dyes that bind to beta-amyloid promise earlier, more reliable diagnosis of Alzheimer's disease.

Take, for example, a patient arriving in the emergency room with a stroke. A race against time begins to save the affected area of the patient's brain. The first step is to determine if the stroke is due to a clot or a bleed by imaging the brain, most often with CT. If the stroke is due to a clot, the clot-busting drug tPA can be used, but only within the first hours. tPA is usually given intravenously, but a longer time window is possible if tPA is applied directly to the clot using a catheter guided into position.

To visualize the location of the clot and the catheter, dye is injected to make arteries stand out in an X ray, a procedure called *cerebral angiography*. Cerebral angiography can also help patients who have had a warning stroke, or TIA.

Another test to assess risk of a CVA uses ultrasound. The carotid arteries of the neck, which feed most of the cerebral vessels, often narrow with age, which can lead to strokes. Cheaper and less invasive than angiography, ultrasound can be used to quickly examine the carotid arteries and even measure blood flow through them.

☑ Check Your Understanding

25. Roy was tackled while playing football. After hitting the ground, he was unable to move his lower limbs. What is a loss of motor function called? What level of his spinal cord do you think was injured (cervical, thoracic, lumbar, or sacral)? Is this a permanent injury? What diagnostic procedures might be helpful?

For answers, see Appendix H.

Developmental Aspects of the Central Nervous System

- ✓ Describe the development of the brain and spinal cord.
- ✓ Indicate several maternal factors that can impair development of the nervous system in an embryo.
- ✓ Explain the effects of aging on the brain.

Figure 12.33 shows the earliest phase of CNS development. Starting in the three-week-old embryo:

① The ectoderm (cell layer at the dorsal surface) thickens along the dorsal midline axis of the embryo to form the **neural plate**. The neural plate invaginates, forming a **neural groove** flanked by **neural folds**.

② Small groups of neural fold cells migrate laterally from between the surface ectoderm and the neural groove, forming the **neural crest**. Neural crest cells give rise (among other things) to some neurons destined to reside in ganglia.

③ As the neural groove deepens, the superior edges of the neural folds fuse, forming the **neural tube**, which soon detaches from the surface ectoderm and sinks to a deeper position.

The neural tube, formed by the fourth week of pregnancy, differentiates rapidly into the CNS. The brain forms rostrally, as we described on p. 429, and the spinal cord develops from the caudal portion of the neural tube.

By the sixth week, each side of the developing spinal cord has two recognizable clusters of neuroblasts that have migrated outward from the original neural tube: a dorsal **alar plate** (a′lar) and a ventral **basal plate** **(Figure 12.34)**. Alar plate neuroblasts become interneurons. Basal plate neuroblasts develop into motor neurons and sprout axons that grow out to the effector organs. Axons that emerge from alar plate cells (and some basal plate cells) form the white matter of the cord. As development progresses, these plates

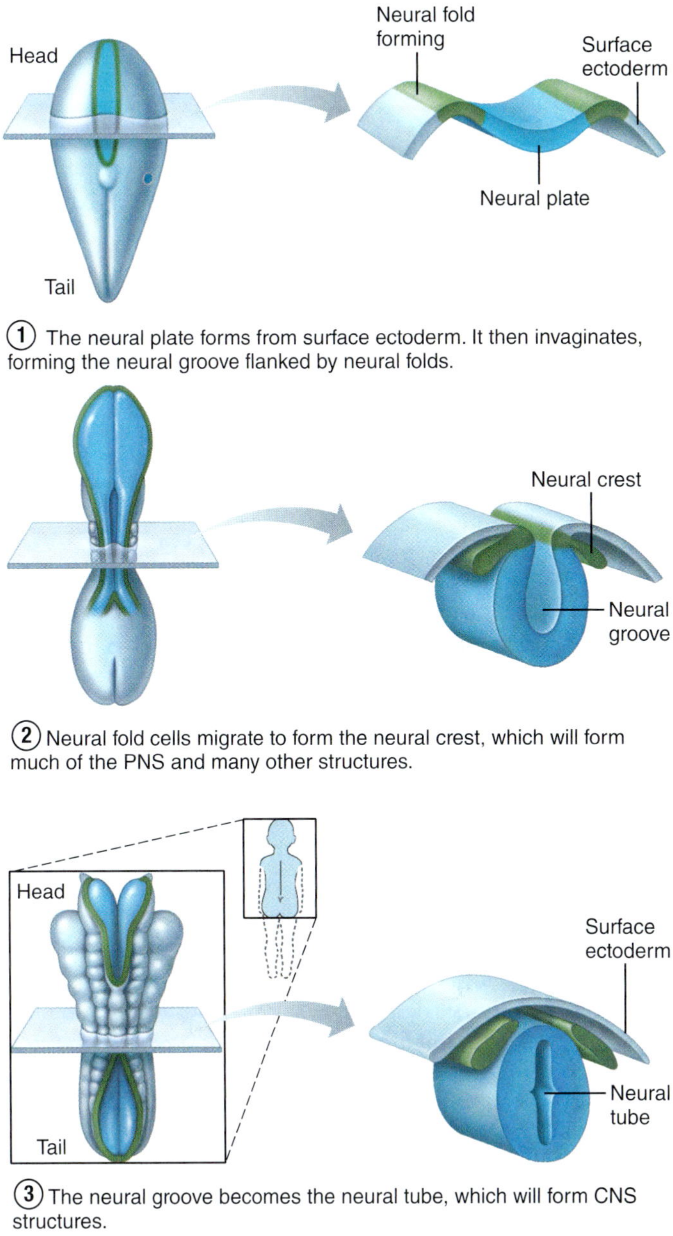

Figure 12.33 Development of the neural tube from embryonic ectoderm. Left: Dorsal surface views of the embryo. Right: Transverse sections at days 17, 20, and 22.

expand dorsally and ventrally to produce the H-shaped central mass of gray matter in the adult spinal cord.

Neural crest cells that come to lie alongside the cord form the *dorsal root ganglia* containing sensory neuron cell bodies. These sensory neurons send their axons into the dorsal aspect of the cord.

As the brain and spinal cord grow and mature throughout the prenatal period, gender-specific areas appear. For example, certain hypothalamic nuclei concerned with regulating typical male sexual behavior and clusters of neurons in the spinal cord that serve the external genitals are much larger in males. Females have a larger corpus callosum, and gender differences are seen in the language and auditory areas of the cerebral cortex. The key to CNS gender-specific development is whether or not the fetus is secreting testosterone. If it is, the male pattern develops.

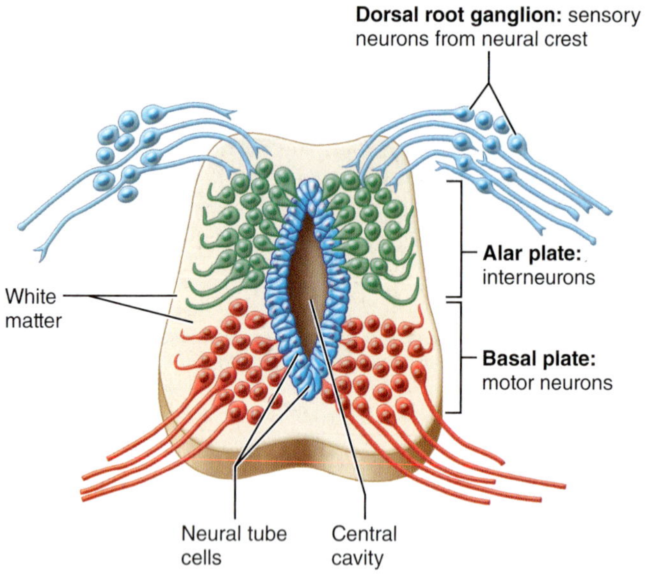

Figure 12.34 Structure of the embryonic spinal cord. At six weeks of development, aggregations of gray matter called the alar plates (future interneurons) and basal plates (future motor neurons) have formed. Dorsal root ganglia (future sensory neurons) have arisen from neural crest cells.

12

Maternal exposure to radiation, various drugs (alcohol, opiates, and others), and infections can harm a developing infant's nervous system, particularly during the initial formative stages. For example, rubella (German measles) often leads to deafness and other types of CNS damage in the newborn. Smoking decreases the amount of oxygen in the blood, and lack of oxygen for even a few minutes destroys neurons. A mother who smokes may sentence her infant to some degree of brain damage.

Homeostatic Imbalance 12.11

Cerebral palsy is a neuromuscular disability in which the voluntary muscles are poorly controlled or paralyzed as a result of brain damage. It may be caused by temporary lack of oxygen during a difficult delivery, or by any of the factors listed above.

In addition to spasticity, speech difficulties, and other motor impairments, about half of cerebral palsy victims have seizures, half are mentally retarded, and about a third have some degree of deafness. Visual impairments are also common. Cerebral palsy does not get worse over time, but its deficits are irreversible. It is the largest single cause of physical disability in children, affecting three out of every 1000 births.

The CNS is plagued by a number of other congenital malformations triggered by genetic or environmental factors during early development. The most serious are congenital hydrocephalus (discussed previously), anencephaly, and spina bifida.

In **anencephaly** (an″en-sef′ah-le; "without brain"), the cerebrum and part of the brain stem never develop because the neural folds fail to fuse rostrally. The child is totally vegetative, unable to see, hear, or process sensory inputs. Muscles are flaccid, and no voluntary movement is possible. Mental life as we know it does not exist. Mercifully, death occurs soon after birth.

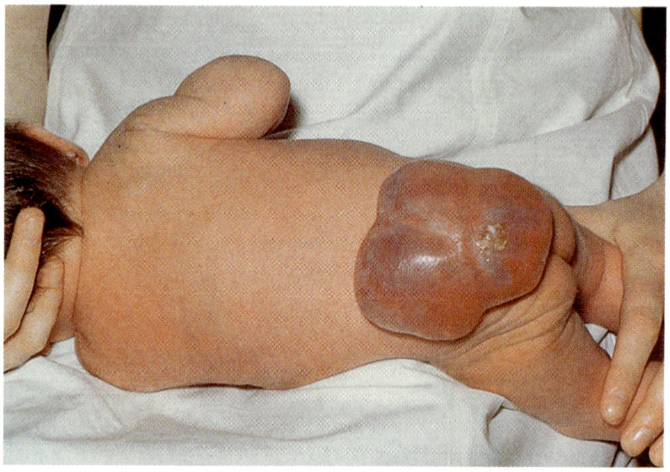

Figure 12.35 Newborn with a lumbar myelomeningocele.

Spina bifida (spi′nah bif′ĭ-dah; "forked spine") results from incomplete formation of the vertebral arches and typically involves the lumbosacral region. The technical definition is that laminae and spinous processes are missing on at least one vertebra. If the condition is severe, neural deficits occur as well.

Spina bifida occulta, the least serious type, involves one or only a few vertebrae and causes no neural problems. Other than a small dimple or tuft of hair over the site of nonfusion, it has no external manifestations.

In *spina bifida cystica*, the more common and severe form, a saclike cyst protrudes dorsally from the child's spine. The cyst may contain meninges and cerebrospinal fluid [a *meningocele* (mě-ning′go-sēl)], or even portions of the spinal cord and spinal nerve roots (a *myelomeningocele*, "spinal cord in a meningeal sac," Figure 12.35). The larger the cyst and the more neural structures it contains, the greater the neurological impairment. In the worst case, where the inferior spinal cord is functionless, the infant experiences bowel incontinence, bladder muscle paralysis (which promotes urinary tract infection and kidney failure), and lower limb paralysis. Infections occur continually because the cyst wall is thin and porous and tends to rupture or leak. Hydrocephalus accompanies spina bifida cystica in 90% of cases.

In the past, up to 70% of cases of spina bifida were caused by inadequate amounts of the B vitamin folic acid in the maternal diet. The incidence of spina bifida has dropped significantly in countries (such as the U.S.) that have introduced mandatory supplementation of folic acid in bread, flour, and pasta products. ✚

One of the last CNS areas to mature is the hypothalamus. Since the hypothalamus contains body temperature regulatory centers, premature babies have problems controlling their loss of body heat and must be kept in temperature-controlled environments. PET scans reveal that the thalamus and somatosensory cortex are active in a 5-day-old baby, but the visual cortex is not. This explains why infants of this age respond to touch but have poor vision. By 11 weeks, more of the cortex is active, and the baby can reach for a rattle. By 8 months, the cortex is very active and the child can think about what he or she sees.

Growth and maturation of the nervous system continue throughout childhood and largely reflect progressive myelination. As described in Chapter 9, neuromuscular coordination progresses in a superior-to-inferior direction and in a proximal-to-distal direction, and we know that myelination also occurs in this sequence.

The brain reaches its maximum weight in the young adult. Over the next 60 years or so, neurons are damaged and die, and brain weight and volume steadily decline. However, the number of neurons lost over the decades is normally only a small percentage of the total, and the remaining neurons can change their synaptic connections, providing for continued learning throughout life.

Although age brings some cognitive declines in spatial ability, speed of perception, decision making, reaction time, and working memory, these losses are not significant in the healthy individual until after the seventh decade. Then the brain becomes increasingly fragile, presumably due to less efficient calcium clearance in aging neurons (as we have seen, elevated Ca^{2+} levels are neurotoxic). A fairly rapid decline occurs in some, but not all, of these abilities.

However, mathematical skills, verbal fluency, and the ability to build on experience do not decline with age, and many people continue to enjoy intellectual lives and work at mentally demanding tasks their entire life. Fewer people over 65 than you might think demonstrate true dementia. Sadly, many cases of "reversible dementia" are caused by prescription drug side effects, low blood pressure, poor nutrition, hormone imbalances, depression, and/or dehydration that go undiagnosed. The best way to maintain your mental abilities in old age may be to seek regular medical checkups throughout life.

Although eventual shrinking of the brain is normal and accelerates in old age, alcoholics and professional boxers hasten the process. Whether a boxer wins the match or not, the likelihood of brain damage and atrophy increases with every blow. And everyone recognizes that alcohol profoundly affects both the mind and the body. CT scans of alcoholics reveal reduced brain size and density starting at a fairly early age. Both boxers and alcoholics exhibit signs of mental deterioration unrelated to the aging process.

☑ Check Your Understanding

26. What functional type of neuron is derived from the alar plate? From the basal plate?
27. Premature babies have problems controlling their body temperature. Why?
28. List several causes of reversible dementia in the elderly.

For answers, see Appendix H.

The human cerebral hemispheres—our "thinking caps"—are awesome in their complexity. But no less amazing are the brain regions that oversee our subconscious, autonomic body functions—the diencephalon and brain stem—particularly when you consider their relatively insignificant size. The spinal cord, which acts as a reflex center and a communication link between the brain and body periphery, is equally important to body homeostasis.

We have introduced a good deal of new terminology in this chapter, and much of it will come up again in the remaining nervous system chapters. Chapter 13, your next challenge, considers the structures of the peripheral nervous system that work hand in hand with the CNS to keep it informed and deliver its orders to the effectors of the body.

Chapter Summary

For more chapter study tools, go to the Study Area of Mastering A&P at **www.masteringaandp.com**.
There you will find:

- Interactive Physiology iP
- A&PFlix A&PFlix
- Practice Anatomy Lab PAL
- PhysioEx PEx
- Videos, Practice Quizzes and Tests, MP3 Tutor Sessions, Case Studies, and much more!

The Brain (pp. 429–452)

1. The brain provides for voluntary movements, interpretation and integration of sensation, consciousness, and cognitive function.

Embryonic Development (pp. 429–430)

2. Early brain development yields the three primary brain vesicles: the prosencephalon (cerebral hemispheres and diencephalon), mesencephalon (midbrain), and rhombencephalon (pons, medulla oblongata, and cerebellum).
3. As a result of cephalization, the diencephalon and superior brain stem are enveloped by the cerebral hemispheres.

Regions and Organization (p. 430)

4. In a widely used system, the adult brain is divided into the cerebral hemispheres, diencephalon, brain stem, and cerebellum.
5. The cerebral hemispheres and cerebellum have gray matter nuclei surrounded by white matter and an outer cortex of gray matter. The diencephalon and brain stem lack a cortex.

Ventricles (p. 430)

6. The brain contains four ventricles filled with cerebrospinal fluid. The lateral ventricles are in the cerebral hemispheres; the third ventricle is in the diencephalon; the fourth ventricle is between the brain stem and the cerebellum and connects with the central canal of the spinal cord.

Cerebral Hemispheres (pp. 430–441)

7. The two cerebral hemispheres exhibit gyri, sulci, and fissures. The longitudinal fissure partially separates the hemispheres; other fissures or sulci subdivide each hemisphere into lobes.
8. Each cerebral hemisphere consists of the cerebral cortex, the cerebral white matter, and basal nuclei (ganglia).

9. Each cerebral hemisphere receives sensory impulses from, and dispatches motor impulses to, the opposite side of the body. The body is represented in an upside-down fashion in the sensory and motor cortices.
10. Functional areas of the cerebral cortex include (1) motor areas: primary motor and premotor cortices of the frontal lobe, the frontal eye field, and Broca's area in the frontal lobe of one hemisphere (usually the left); (2) sensory areas: primary somatosensory cortex and somatosensory association cortex in the parietal lobe; visual areas in the occipital lobe; olfactory and auditory areas in the temporal lobe; gustatory, visceral, and vestibular areas in the insula; (3) association areas: anterior association area in the frontal lobe, and posterior and limbic association areas spanning several lobes.
11. The cerebral hemispheres show lateralization of cortical function. In most people, the left hemisphere is dominant (i.e., specialized for language and mathematical skills); the right hemisphere is more concerned with visual-spatial skills and creative endeavors.
12. Fiber tracts of the cerebral white matter include commissures, association fibers, and projection fibers.
13. The paired basal nuclei (also called basal ganglia) include the globus pallidus, putamen, and caudate nucleus. The basal nuclei are subcortical nuclei that help control movements. Functionally they are closely associated with the substantia nigra of the midbrain.

Diencephalon (pp. 441–443)

14. The diencephalon includes the thalamus, hypothalamus, and epithalamus and encloses the third ventricle.
15. The thalamus is the major relay station for (1) sensory impulses ascending to the sensory cortex, (2) inputs from subcortical motor nuclei and the cerebellum traveling to the cerebral motor cortex, and (3) impulses traveling to association cortices from lower centers.
16. The hypothalamus is an important control center of the autonomic nervous system and a pivotal part of the limbic system. It maintains water balance and regulates thirst, eating behavior, gastrointestinal activity, body temperature, and the activity of the anterior pituitary gland.
17. The epithalamus includes the pineal gland, which secretes the hormone melatonin.

12

Brain Stem (pp. 443–447)

18. The brain stem includes the midbrain, pons, and medulla oblongata.
19. The midbrain contains the corpora quadrigemina (visual and auditory reflex centers), the red nucleus (subcortical motor centers), and the substantia nigra. The periaqueductal gray matter is involved in pain suppression and contains the motor nuclei of cranial nerves III and IV. The cerebral peduncles on its ventral face house the pyramidal fiber tracts. The midbrain surrounds the cerebral aqueduct.
20. The pons is mainly a conduction area. Its nuclei contribute to regulating respiration and cranial nerves V–VII.
21. The pyramids (descending corticospinal tracts) form the ventral face of the medulla oblongata. These fibers cross over (decussation of the pyramids) before entering the spinal cord. Important nuclei in the medulla regulate respiratory rhythm, heart rate, and blood pressure and serve cranial nerves VIII–XII. The olivary nuclei and cough, sneezing, swallowing, and vomiting centers are also in the medulla.

Cerebellum (pp. 447–449)

22. The cerebellum consists of two hemispheres, marked by convolutions and separated by the vermis. It is connected to the brain stem by superior, middle, and inferior peduncles.
23. The cerebellum processes and interprets impulses from the motor cortex and sensory pathways and coordinates motor activity so that smooth, well-timed movements occur. It also plays a poorly understood role in cognition.

Functional Brain Systems (pp. 449–452)

24. The limbic system consists of numerous structures that encircle the brain stem. It is the "emotional-visceral brain." It also plays a role in memory.
25. The reticular formation is a diffuse network of neurons and nuclei spanning the length of the brain stem. It maintains the alert state of the cerebral cortex (RAS), and its motor nuclei serve both somatic and visceral motor activities.

Higher Mental Functions (pp. 452–458)

Brain Wave Patterns and the EEG (pp. 452–453)

1. Patterns of electrical activity of the brain are called brain waves; a record of this activity is an electroencephalogram (EEG). Brain wave patterns, identified by their frequencies, include alpha, beta, theta, and delta waves.
2. Epilepsy results from abnormal electrical activity of brain neurons. Involuntary muscle contractions and sensory auras are typical during some epileptic seizures.

Consciousness (pp. 453–454)

3. Consciousness is described clinically on a continuum from alertness to drowsiness to stupor and finally to coma.
4. Human consciousness is thought to involve holistic information processing, which is (1) not localizable, (2) superimposed on other types of neural activity, and (3) totally interconnected.
5. Fainting (syncope) is a temporary loss of consciousness that usually reflects inadequate blood delivery to the brain. Coma is loss of consciousness in which the victim is unresponsive to stimuli.

Sleep and Sleep-Wake Cycles (pp. 454–455)

6. Sleep is a state of partial consciousness from which a person can be aroused by stimulation. The two major types of sleep are non-rapid eye movement (NREM) sleep and rapid eye movement (REM) sleep.
7. During stages 1–4 of NREM sleep, brain wave frequency decreases and amplitude increases until delta wave sleep (stage 4) is achieved. REM sleep is indicated by a return to alpha waves on the EEG. During REM, the eyes move rapidly under the lids. NREM and REM sleep alternate throughout the night.
8. Slow-wave sleep (stages 3 and 4 of NREM) appears to be restorative. REM sleep is important for emotional stability.
9. REM occupies half of an infant's sleep time and then declines to about 25% of sleep time by age 10. Time spent in slow-wave sleep declines steadily throughout life.
10. Narcolepsy is involuntary lapses into REM sleep that occur without warning during waking periods. Insomnia is a chronic inability to obtain the amount or quality of sleep needed to function adequately. A person with sleep apnea stops breathing temporarily during sleep, causing hypoxia.

Language (pp. 455–456)

11. In most people the left hemisphere controls language. The language implementation system, which includes Broca's and Wernicke's areas and the basal nuclei, analyzes incoming and produces outgoing language. The opposite hemisphere deals with the emotional content of language.

Memory (pp. 456–458)

12. Memory is the storage and retrieval of information. It is essential for learning and is part of consciousness.
13. Memory storage has two stages: short-term memory (STM) and long-term memory (LTM). Transfer of information from STM to LTM takes minutes to hours, but more time is required for LTM consolidation.
14. Declarative memory is the ability to learn and consciously remember information. Procedural memory is the learning of motor skills, which are then performed without conscious thought.
15. Declarative memory appears to involve the medial temporal lobe (hippocampus and surrounding temporal cortical areas), thalamus, basal forebrain, and prefrontal cortex. Procedural memory (a type of nondeclarative memory) relies on the basal nuclei.
16. The nature of memory formation at the molecular level is not fully known, but NMDA receptors (essentially calcium channels), activated by depolarization and glutamate binding, play a major role in long-term potentiation (LTP). The calcium influx that follows NMDA receptor activation mobilizes enzymes that mediate events necessary for memory formation.

Protection of the Brain (pp. 458–462)

1. The delicate brain is protected by bone, meninges, cerebrospinal fluid, and the blood brain barrier.

Meninges (pp. 459–460)

2. The meninges from superficial to deep are the dura mater, arachnoid mater, and pia mater. They enclose the brain and spinal cord and their blood vessels. Inward folds of the inner layer of the dura mater secure the brain to the skull.

Cerebrospinal Fluid (pp. 460–462)

3. Cerebrospinal fluid (CSF), formed by the choroid plexuses from blood plasma, circulates through the ventricles and into the subarachnoid space. It returns to the dural venous sinuses via the arachnoid villi. CSF supports and cushions the brain and cord and helps to nourish them.

Blood Brain Barrier (p. 462)

4. The blood brain barrier reflects the relative impermeability of the epithelium of capillaries of the brain. It allows water, respiratory gases, essential nutrients, and fat-soluble molecules to enter the neural tissue, but blocks other, water-soluble, potentially harmful substances.

Homeostatic Imbalances of the Brain (pp. 462–464)

Traumatic Brain Injuries (pp. 462–463)

1. Head trauma may cause brain injuries called concussions or, in severe cases, contusions (bruising). When the brain stem is affected, unconsciousness (temporary or permanent) occurs. Trauma-induced brain injuries may be aggravated by intracranial hemorrhage or cerebral edema, both of which compress brain tissue.

Cerebrovascular Accidents (CVAs) (p. 463)

2. Cerebrovascular accidents (strokes) result when blood circulation to brain neurons is impaired and brain tissue dies. The result may be hemiplegia, sensory deficits, or speech impairment.

Degenerative Brain Disorders (pp. 463–464)

3. Alzheimer's disease is a degenerative brain disease in which beta-amyloid peptide deposits and neurofibrillary tangles appear. Marked by a deficit of ACh, it results in slow, progressive loss of memory and motor control and increasing dementia.
4. Parkinson's disease and Huntington's disease are neurodegenerative disorders of the basal nuclei. Both involve abnormalities of the neurotransmitter dopamine (too little or too much secreted) and are characterized by abnormal movements.

The Spinal Cord (pp. 464–474)

Gross Anatomy and Protection (pp. 464–466)

1. The spinal cord, a two-way impulse conduction pathway and a reflex center, resides within the vertebral column and is protected by meninges and cerebrospinal fluid. It extends from the foramen magnum to the end of the first lumbar vertebra.
2. Thirty-one pairs of spinal nerves issue from the cord. The cord is enlarged in the cervical and lumbar regions, where spinal nerves serving the limbs arise.

Spinal Cord Cross-Sectional Anatomy (pp. 466–468)

3. The central gray matter of the cord is H shaped. Ventral horns mainly contain somatic motor neurons. Lateral horns contain visceral (autonomic) motor neurons. Dorsal horns contain interneurons.
4. Axons of neurons of the lateral and ventral horns emerge in common from the cord via the ventral roots. Axons of sensory neurons (with cell bodies located in the dorsal root ganglion) form the dorsal roots and enter the dorsal aspect of the cord. The ventral and dorsal roots combine to form the spinal nerves.
5. Each side of the white matter of the cord has dorsal, lateral, and ventral columns (funiculi), and each funiculus contains a number of ascending and descending tracts. All tracts are paired and most decussate.

Neuronal Pathways (pp. 468–473)

6. Ascending (sensory) tracts include the fasciculi gracilis and cuneatus, spinothalamic tracts, and spinocerebellar tracts.
7. The dorsal column–medial lemniscal pathway consists of the dorsal white column (fasciculus cuneatus, fasciculus gracilis) and the medial lemniscus, which are concerned with straight-through, precise transmission of one or a few related types of sensory input. The spinothalamic pathways transmit pain, temperature, and coarse touch, and permit brain stem processing of ascending impulses. The spinocerebellar tracts, which terminate in the cerebellum, serve muscle sense, not conscious sensory perception.
8. Descending tracts include the pyramidal tracts (ventral and lateral corticospinal tracts) and a number of motor tracts originating from subcortical motor nuclei. These descending fibers issue from the brain stem motor areas [indirect system] and cortical motor areas [direct (pyramidal) system].

Spinal Cord Trauma and Disorders (p. 474)

9. Injury to the ventral horn neurons or the ventral roots results in flaccid paralysis. (Injury to the upper motor neurons in the brain results in spastic paralysis.) If the dorsal roots or sensory tracts are damaged, paresthesias occur.

10. Poliomyelitis results from inflammation and destruction of the ventral horn neurons by the poliovirus. Paralysis and muscle atrophy ensue.
11. Amyotrophic lateral sclerosis (ALS) results from destruction of the ventral horn neurons and the pyramidal tracts. The victim eventually loses the ability to swallow, speak, and breathe. Death generally occurs within five years.

Diagnostic Procedures for Assessing CNS Dysfunction (pp. 474–475)

1. Diagnostic procedures used to assess neurological condition and function range from routine reflex testing to sophisticated techniques such as cerebral angiography, CT scans, MRI scans, and PET scans.

Developmental Aspects of the Central Nervous System (pp. 475–477)

1. The CNS develops from the embryonic neural tube—the brain from the rostral part and the spinal cord from the caudal part.
2. The gray matter of the spinal cord forms from the alar and basal plates. Fiber tracts form the outer white matter. The neural crest forms the sensory (dorsal root) ganglia.
3. Maternal and environmental factors may impair embryonic brain development, and oxygen deprivation destroys brain cells. Severe congenital brain disorders include cerebral palsy, anencephaly, hydrocephalus, and spina bifida.
4. Premature babies have trouble regulating body temperature because the hypothalamus is one of the last brain areas to mature prenatally.
5. Development of motor control indicates progressive myelination and maturation of a child's nervous system.
6. Brain growth ends in young adulthood. Neurons die throughout life and most are not replaced; brain weight and volume decline with age.
7. Healthy elders maintain nearly optimal intellectual function. Disease—particularly cardiovascular disease—is the major cause of declining mental function with age.

Review Questions

12

Multiple Choice/Matching

(Some questions have more than one correct answer. Select the best answer or answers from the choices given.)

1. The primary motor cortex, Broca's area, and the premotor cortex are located in which lobe? **(a)** frontal, **(b)** parietal, **(c)** temporal, **(d)** occipital.
2. The innermost layer of the meninges, delicate and closely apposed to the brain tissue, is the **(a)** dura mater, **(b)** corpus callosum, **(c)** arachnoid mater, **(d)** pia mater.
3. Cerebrospinal fluid is formed by **(a)** arachnoid villi, **(b)** dura mater, **(c)** choroid plexuses, **(d)** all of these.
4. A patient has suffered a cerebral hemorrhage that has caused dysfunction of the precentral gyrus of his right cerebral cortex. As a result, **(a)** he cannot voluntarily move his left arm or leg, **(b)** he feels no sensation on the left side of his body, **(c)** he feels no sensation on his right side.
5. Choose the correct term from the key to respond to the statements describing various brain areas.

Key:

(a) cerebellum	**(d)** striatum	**(g)** midbrain
(b) corpora quadrigemina	**(e)** hypothalamus	**(h)** pons
(c) corpus callosum	**(f)** medulla	**(i)** thalamus

____ (1) basal nuclei involved in fine control of motor activities
____ (2) region where there is a gross crossover of fibers of descending pyramidal tracts
____ (3) control of temperature, autonomic nervous system reflexes, hunger, and water balance
____ (4) houses the substantia nigra and cerebral aqueduct
____ (5) relay stations for visual and auditory stimuli input; found in midbrain
____ (6) houses vital centers for control of the heart, respiration, and blood pressure
____ (7) brain area through which all the sensory input is relayed to get to the cerebral cortex
____ (8) brain area most concerned with equilibrium, body posture, and coordination of motor activity

6. Which of the following tracts convey vibration and other specific sensations that can be precisely localized? **(a)** pyramidal tract, **(b)** medial lemniscus, **(c)** lateral spinothalamic tract, **(d)** reticulospinal tract.
7. Destruction of the ventral horn cells of the spinal cord results in loss of **(a)** integrating impulses, **(b)** sensory impulses, **(c)** voluntary motor impulses, **(d)** all of these.
8. Fiber tracts that allow neurons within the same cerebral hemisphere to communicate are **(a)** association fibers, **(b)** commissures, **(c)** projection fibers.
9. A number of brain structures are listed below. If an area is primarily gray matter, write **a** in the answer blank; if mostly white matter, respond with **b**.

____ (1) cerebral cortex
____ (2) corpus callosum and corona radiata
____ (3) red nucleus
____ (4) medial and lateral nuclear groups
____ (5) medial lemniscus
____ (6) cranial nerve nuclei
____ (7) spinothalamic tract
____ (8) fornix
____ (9) cingulate and precentral gyri

10. A professor unexpectedly blew a loud horn in his anatomy and physiology class. The students looked up, startled. The reflexive movements of their eyes were mediated by the **(a)** cerebral cortex, **(b)** inferior olives, **(c)** raphe nuclei, **(d)** superior colliculi, **(e)** nucleus gracilis.
11. Identify the stage of sleep described by using choices from the key. (Note that responses a–d refer to NREM sleep.)

Key: **(a)** stage 1 **(b)** stage 2 **(c)** stage 3 **(d)** stage 4 **(e)** REM

____ (1) the stage when blood pressure and heart rate reach their lowest levels
____ (2) indicated by movement of the eyes under the lids; dreaming occurs
____ (3) when nightmares are likely to occur
____ (4) when the sleeper is very easily awakened; EEG shows alpha waves

12. All of the following descriptions refer to dorsal column–medial lemniscal ascending pathways except one: **(a)** they include the fasciculus gracilis and fasciculus cuneatus; **(b)** they include a chain of three neurons; **(c)** their connections are diffuse and poorly localized; **(d)** they are concerned with precise transmission of one or a few related types of sensory input.

Short Answer Essay Questions

13. Make a diagram showing the three primary (embryonic) brain vesicles. Name each and then use clinical terminology to name the resulting adult brain regions.
14. (a) What is the advantage of having a cerebrum that is highly convoluted? (b) What term is used to indicate its grooves? Its outward folds? (c) Which groove divides the cerebrum into two hemispheres? (d) What divides the parietal from the frontal lobe? The parietal from the temporal lobe?
15. (a) Make a rough drawing of the lateral aspect of the left cerebral hemisphere. (b) You may be thinking, "But I just can't draw!" So, name the hemisphere involved with most people's ability to draw. (c) On your drawing, locate the following areas and provide the major function of each: primary motor cortex, premotor cortex, somatosensory association cortex, primary somatosensory cortex, visual and auditory areas, prefrontal cortex, Wernicke's and Broca's areas.
16. (a) What does lateralization of cortical functioning mean? (b) Why is the term cerebral dominance a misnomer?
17. (a) What is the function of the basal nuclei? (b) Which basal nuclei form the striatum? (c) Which arches over the diencephalon?
18. Explain how the cerebellum is physically connected to the brain stem.
19. Describe the role of the cerebellum in maintaining smooth, coordinated skeletal muscle activity.
20. (a) Where is the limbic system located? (b) Which structures make up this system? (c) How is the limbic system important in behavior?
21. (a) Localize the reticular formation in the brain. (b) What does RAS mean, and what is its function?
22. What is an aura?
23. How do sleep patterns, extent of sleeping time, and amount of time spent in REM and NREM sleep change through life?
24. Compare and contrast short-term memory (STM) and long-term memory (LTM) relative to storage capacity and duration of the memory.
25. Define memory consolidation.
26. Compare and contrast declarative and procedural memory relative to the types of things remembered and the importance of conscious retrieval.
27. List four ways in which the CNS is protected.
28. (a) How is cerebrospinal fluid formed and drained? Describe its pathway within and around the brain. (b) What happens if CSF does not drain properly? Why is this consequence more harmful in adults?
29. What constitutes the blood brain barrier?
30. A brain surgeon is about to make an incision. Name all the tissue layers that she cuts through from the skin to the brain.
31. (a) Define concussion and contusion. (b) Why does severe brain stem injury result in unconsciousness?
32. Describe the spinal cord, depicting its extent, its composition of gray and white matter, and its spinal roots.
33. How do the types of motor activity controlled by the direct (pyramidal) and indirect systems differ?
34. Describe the functional problems that would be experienced by a person in which these fiber tracts have been cut: (a) lateral spinothalamic, (b) ventral and dorsal spinocerebellar, (c) tectospinal.
35. Differentiate between spastic and flaccid paralysis.
36. How do the conditions paraplegia, hemiplegia, and quadriplegia differ?
37. (a) Define cerebrovascular accident or CVA. (b) Describe its possible causes and consequences.
38. (a) What factors account for brain growth after birth? (b) List some structural brain changes observed with aging.

Critical Thinking and Clinical Application Questions

1. A 10-month-old infant has an enlarging head circumference and delayed overall development. She has a bulging anterior fontanelle and her CSF pressure is elevated. Based on these findings, answer the following questions: (a) What are the possible cause(s) of an enlarged head? (b) Which tests might be helpful in obtaining information about this infant's problem? (c) Assuming the tests conducted showed the cerebral aqueduct to be constricted, which ventricles or CSF-containing areas would you expect to be enlarged? Which would likely not be visible? Respond to the same questions based on a finding of obstructed arachnoid villi.
2. Mrs. Jones has had a progressive decline in her mental capabilities in the last five or six years. At first her family attributed her occasional memory lapses, confusion, and agitation to grief over her husband's death six years earlier. When examined, Mrs. Jones was aware of her cognitive problems and was shown to have an IQ score approximately 30 points less than would be predicted by her work history. A CT scan showed diffuse cerebral atrophy. The physician prescribed an acetylcholinesterase inhibitor and Mrs. Jones showed slight improvement. What is Mrs. Jones's problem? Why did the acetylcholinesterase inhibitor help?
3. Robert, a brilliant computer analyst, suffered a blow to his anterior skull from a falling rock while mountain climbing. Shortly thereafter, it was obvious to his coworkers that his behavior had undergone a dramatic change. Although previously a smart dresser, he was now unkempt. One morning, he was observed defecating into the wastebasket. His supervisor ordered Robert to report to the company's doctor immediately. Which region of Robert's brain was affected by the cranial blow?
4. Mrs. Adams is ready to deliver her first baby. Unfortunately, the baby appears to have a myelomeningocele. Would a vaginal or surgical (C-section) delivery be more appropriate and why?
5. The medical chart of a 68-year-old man includes the following notes: "Slight tremor of right hand at rest; stony facial expression; difficulty in initiating movements." (a) Based on your present knowledge, what is the diagnosis? (b) What brain areas are most likely involved in this man's disorder, and what is the deficiency? (c) How is this condition currently treated?
6. Cynthia, a 16-year-old girl, was rushed to the hospital after taking a bad spill off the parallel bars. After she had a complete neurological workup, her family was told that she would be permanently paralyzed from the waist down. The neurologist then outlined for Cynthia's parents the importance of preventing complications in such cases. Common complications include urinary infection, bed sores, and muscular spasms. Using your knowledge of neuroanatomy, explain the underlying reasons for these complications.

7. Five-year-old Amy wakes her parents up at 3 AM crying and complaining of a sore neck, severe headache, and feeling sick to her stomach. She has a temperature of 40°C (104°F) and hides her eyes, saying that the lights are too bright. The emergency physician suspects meningitis and performs a lumbar tap. Using your knowledge of neuroanatomy, explain into which space and at what level of the vertebral column the needle will be inserted to perform this test. Which fluid is being obtained and why?

AT THE CLINIC

Related Clinical Terms

Autism A complex developmental neurological disorder, typically appearing in the first three years of life, characterized by difficulty in communicating, forming relationships with others, and responding appropriately to the environment. A wide variety of mutations in functionally related genes can give rise to autism and its related disorders. Occurs in about two per 1000 people, and early behavioral intervention is beneficial.

Cordotomy (kor-dot′o-me) A procedure in which a tract in the spinal cord is severed surgically; usually done to relieve unremitting pain.

Dyslexia A learning disability in 5 to 15% of the population that specifically affects the ability of otherwise intelligent people to read. This deficit in visual symbol and language processing is thought to result from errors arising in one hemisphere. Several genes that predispose children to dyslexia have been identified, but dyslexia can also be acquired by brain injury or degeneration.

Encephalopathy (en-sef″ah-lop′ah-the; *enceph* = brain; *path* = disease) Any disease or disorder of the brain.

12

Hypersomnia (*hyper* = excess; *somnus* = sleep) A condition in which affected individuals sleep as much as 15 hours daily.

Microcephaly (mi″kro-sef′ah-le; *micro* = small) Congenital condition involving the formation of a small brain, as evidenced by reduced skull size; most microcephalic children are mentally retarded.

Myelitis (mi″ĕ-li′tis; *myel* = spinal cord; *itis* = inflammation) Inflammation of the spinal cord.

Myelogram (*gram* = recording) X ray of the spinal cord after injection of a contrast medium.

Myoclonus (mi″o-klo′nus; *myo* = muscle; *clon* = violent motion, tumult) Sudden contraction of a muscle or muscle part, usually involving muscles of the limbs. Myoclonal jerks can occur in normal individuals as they are falling asleep; others may be due to diseases of the reticular formation or cerebellum.

Neuroses (nu-ro′sēs) A less debilitating class of mental illness; examples include severe anxiety (panic attacks), phobias (irrational fears), and obsessive-compulsive behaviors (e.g., washing one's hands every few minutes). However, the affected individual retains contact with reality.

Psychoses (si-ko′sēs) A class of severe mental illness in which affected individuals lose touch with reality and exhibit bizarre behaviors; the legal word for psychotic behavior is insanity. Psychoses include schizophrenia (skit-so-fre′ne-ah), bipolar disorder, and some forms of depression.

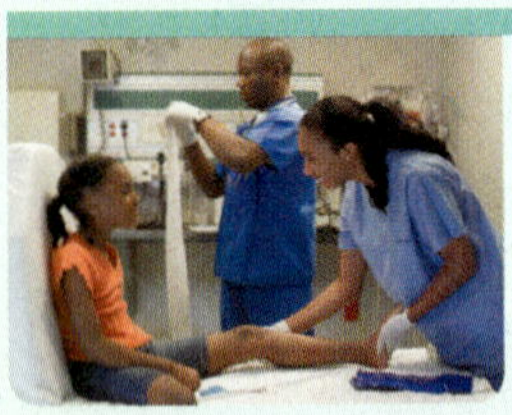

Case Study Central Nervous System

Margaret Bryans, a 39-year-old female, was a passenger on the bus that crashed on Route 91. When paramedics arrived on the scene, she was unconscious, with cuts on her arms, face, and scalp. She regained consciousness en route to the hospital and appeared agitated and combative. Paramedics observed that she had a right hemiparesis (muscle weakness), with a near complete paresis of her right upper extremity and a partial paresis of the right lower extremity. A head CT scan revealed an acute subdural hematoma and an extensive subarachnoid hemorrhage. Doctors noted that she was able to follow commands from medical personnel. With difficulty, she could speak haltingly, using only simple words.

Surgery to remove large clots from the subarachnoid space was performed immediately. Two weeks after the surgery, she showed significant improvement in her speech and motor function.

1. The adult brain can be broken down into four functional regions (see Table 12.1). Based on the observed signs in this case, which of these four brain regions is involved? What evidence did you use to determine this?
2. Which side of the brain is involved in Mrs. Bryans's injury? What evidence did you use to determine this?
3. What specific parts of the region of the brain you identified in question 1 are being affected by the injury to cause the muscle weakness and language problems?
4. What are the three membranes that make up the meninges? Describe their positions relative to the brain.
5. Relative to the meninges, describe the location of the bleeding revealed on the CT scan.

(Answers in Appendix H)

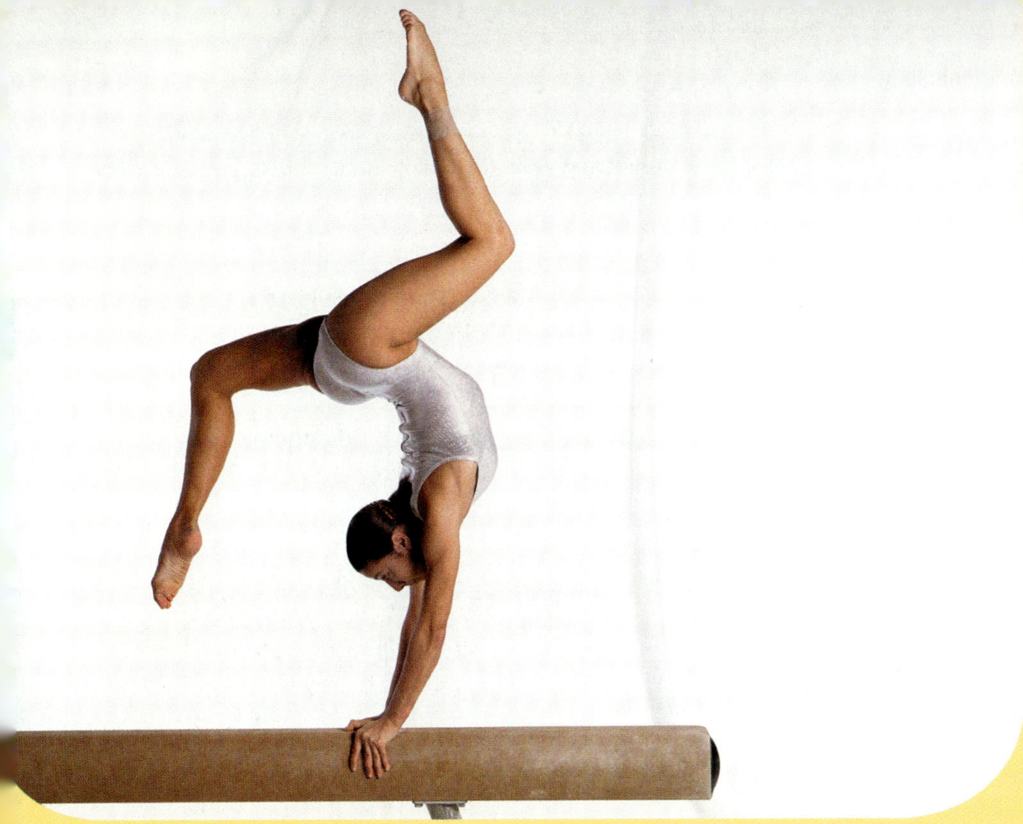

13

The Peripheral Nervous System and Reflex Activity

✓ Define peripheral nervous system and list its components.

The human brain, for all its sophistication, would be useless without its links to the outside world. Consider one experiment that illustrates this point. Volunteers who were deprived of sensory input by being blindfolded and suspended in warm water in a sensory deprivation tank hallucinated. One saw charging pink and purple elephants. Another heard a chorus, still others had taste hallucinations. Our very sanity depends on a continuous flow of information from the outside.

Equally important to our well-being are the orders sent from the CNS to voluntary muscles and other effectors of the body, which allow us to move and take care of our own

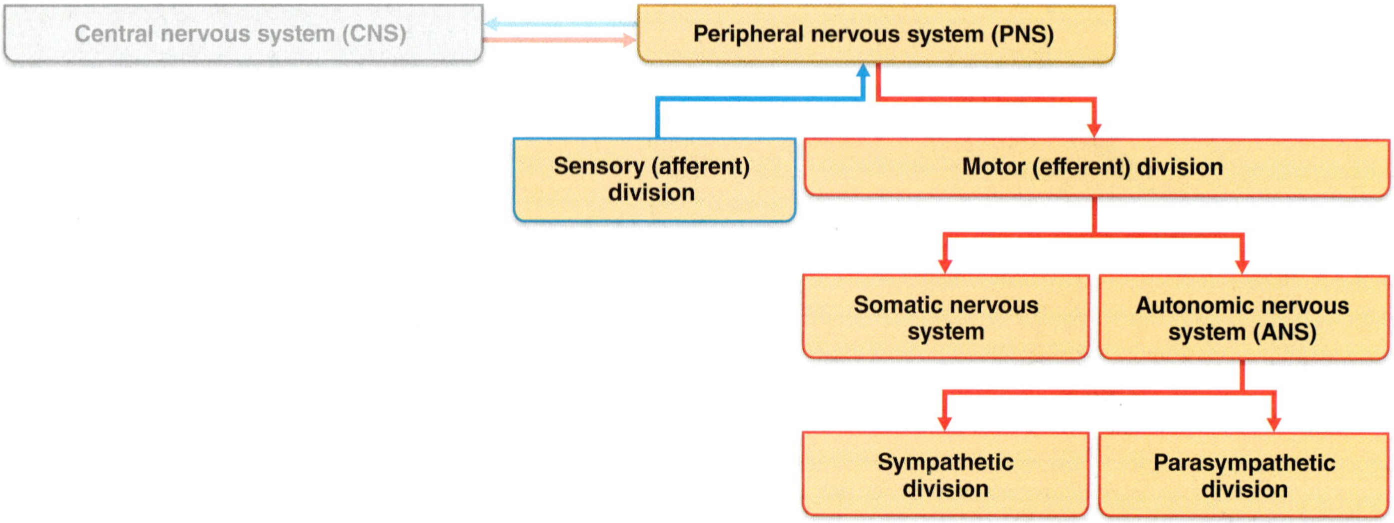

Figure 13.1 Place of the PNS in the structural organization of the nervous system.

needs. The **peripheral nervous system (PNS)** provides these links from and to the world outside our bodies. Ghostly white nerves thread through virtually every part of the body, enabling the CNS to receive information and carry out its decisions.

The PNS includes all neural structures outside the brain and spinal cord, that is, the *sensory receptors*, peripheral *nerves* and their associated *ganglia*, and efferent *motor endings*. **Figure 13.1** diagrams its basic components.

13

In the first portion of this chapter we deal with the functional anatomy of each PNS element. Then we consider the components of reflex arcs and some important somatic reflexes, played out almost entirely in PNS structures, that help maintain homeostasis.

PART 1
Sensory Receptors and Sensation

Sensory Receptors

✓ Classify general sensory receptors by structure, stimulus detected, and body location.

Sensory receptors are specialized to respond to changes in their environment, which are called **stimuli**. Typically, activation of a sensory receptor by an adequate stimulus results in graded potentials that in turn trigger nerve impulses along the afferent PNS fibers coursing to the CNS. *Sensation* (awareness of the stimulus) and *perception* (interpretation of the meaning of the stimulus) occur in the brain. But we are getting ahead of ourselves here.

For now, let's just examine how sensory receptors are classified. Basically, there are three ways to classify sensory receptors: (1) by the type of stimulus they detect; (2) by their body location; and (3) by their structural complexity.

Classification by Stimulus Type

These categories are easy to remember because the name usually indicates the stimulus that activates the receptor.

- **Mechanoreceptors** respond to mechanical force such as touch, pressure (including blood pressure), vibration, and stretch.
- **Thermoreceptors** respond to temperature changes.
- **Photoreceptors**, such as those of the retina of the eye, respond to light.
- **Chemoreceptors** respond to chemicals in solution (molecules smelled or tasted, or changes in blood or interstitial fluid chemistry).
- **Nociceptors** (no″se-sep′torz; *noci* = harm) respond to potentially damaging stimuli that result in pain. For example, searing heat, extreme cold, excessive pressure, and inflammatory chemicals are all interpreted as painful. These signals stimulate subtypes of thermoreceptors, mechanoreceptors, and chemoreceptors.

Classification by Location

Receptors can be grouped into three receptor classes according to either their location or the location of the activating stimulus: exteroceptors, interoceptors, and proprioceptors.

- **Exteroceptors** (ek″ster-o-sep′torz) are sensitive to stimuli arising outside the body (*extero* = outside), so most exteroceptors are near or at the body surface. They include touch, pressure, pain, and temperature receptors in the skin and most receptors of the special senses (vision, hearing, equilibrium, taste, smell).
- **Interoceptors** (in″ter-o-sep′torz), also called *visceroceptors*, respond to stimuli within the body (*intero* = inside), such as from the internal viscera and blood vessels. Interoceptors monitor a variety of stimuli, including chemical changes,

Table 13.1 General Sensory Receptors Classified by Structure and Function

STRUCTURAL CLASS	ILLUSTRATION	FUNCTIONAL CLASSES ACCORDING TO LOCATION (L) AND STIMULUS TYPE (S)	BODY LOCATION
Nonencapsulated			
Free nerve endings of sensory neurons	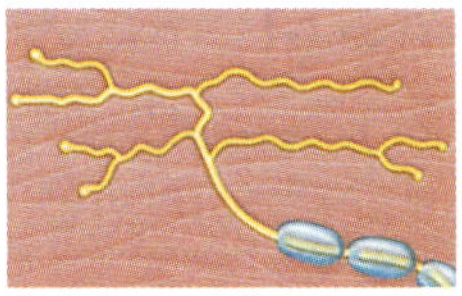	L: Exteroceptors, interoceptors, and proprioceptors S: Thermoreceptors (warm and cool), chemoreceptors (itch, pH, etc.), mechanoreceptors (pressure), nociceptors (pain, hot, cold, pinch, and chemicals)	Most body tissues; most dense in connective tissues (ligaments, tendons, dermis, joint capsules, periostea) and epithelia (epidermis, cornea, mucosae, and glands)
Modified free nerve endings: Tactile (Merkel) discs	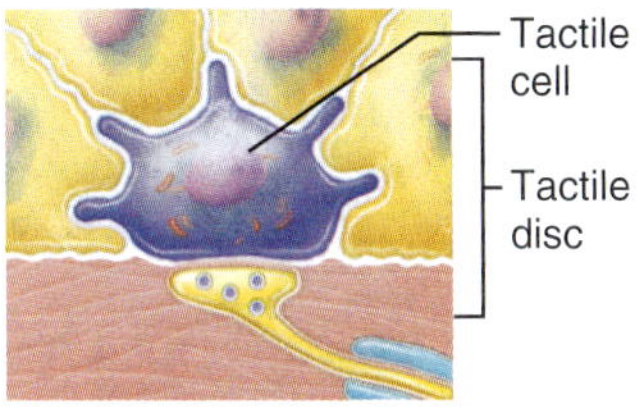	L: Exteroceptors S: Mechanoreceptors (light pressure); slowly adapting	Basal layer of epidermis
Hair follicle receptors	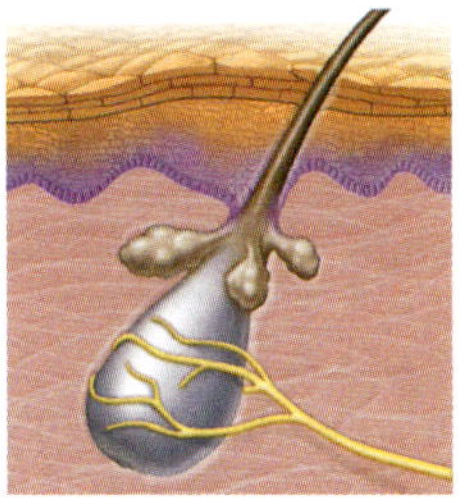	L: Exteroceptors S: Mechanoreceptors (hair deflection); rapidly adapting	In and surrounding hair follicles

➤

tissue stretch, and temperature. Sometimes their activity causes us to feel pain, discomfort, hunger, or thirst. However, we are usually unaware of their workings.

- **Proprioceptors** (pro″pre-o-sep′torz), like interoceptors, respond to internal stimuli. However, their location is much more restricted. Proprioceptors occur in skeletal muscles, tendons, joints, and ligaments and in connective tissue coverings of bones and muscles. (Some authorities include the equilibrium receptors of the inner ear in this class.) Proprioceptors constantly advise the brain of our body movements (*propria* = one's own) by monitoring how much the organs containing these receptors are stretched.

Classification by Receptor Structure

The overwhelming majority of sensory receptors belong to the **general senses** and are simply the modified dendritic endings of sensory neurons. They are found throughout the body and monitor most types of general sensory information.

Receptors for the **special senses** (vision, hearing, equilibrium, smell, and taste) are housed in complex **sense organs**. For example, the sense organ we know as the eye is composed not only of sensory neurons but also of nonneural cells that form its supporting wall, lens, and other associated structures.

Though the special senses are most familiar to us, the simple sensory receptors associated with the general senses are no less important, and we will concentrate on their structure and function in this chapter. The special senses are the topic of Chapter 15.

Simple Receptors of the General Senses

The widely distributed general sensory receptors are involved in tactile sensation (a mix of touch, pressure, stretch, and vibration), temperature monitoring, and pain, as well as the "muscle sense" provided by proprioceptors. As you read about these receptors, notice that there is no perfect "one-receptor–one-function" relationship. Instead, one type of receptor can respond to several different kinds of stimuli. Likewise, different types of receptors can respond to similar stimuli. Anatomically, general sensory receptors are nerve endings that are either *nonencapsulated* (*free*) or *encapsulated*. Table 13.1 illustrates the general sensory receptors. You may find it helpful to refer to this table throughout the discussion that follows.

Nonencapsulated (Free) Nerve Endings Present nearly everywhere in the body, **nonencapsulated (free) nerve endings** of sensory neurons are particularly abundant in epithelia and connective tissues. Most of these sensory fibers are nonmyelinated, small-diameter group C fibers, and their distal endings (the sensory terminals) usually have small knoblike swellings.

Free nerve endings respond chiefly to temperature and painful stimuli, but some respond to tissue movements caused by pressure as well. Nerve endings that respond to

Table 13.1 General Sensory Receptors Classified by Structure and Function *(continued)*

STRUCTURAL CLASS	ILLUSTRATION	FUNCTIONAL CLASSES ACCORDING TO LOCATION (L) AND STIMULUS TYPE (S)	BODY LOCATION
Encapsulated			
Tactile (Meissner's) corpuscles	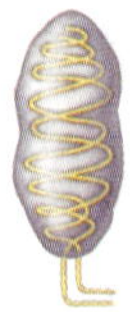	L: Exteroceptors S: Mechanoreceptors (light pressure, discriminative touch, vibration of low frequency); rapidly adapting	Dermal papillae of hairless skin, particularly nipples, external genitalia, fingertips, soles of feet, eyelids
Lamellar (Pacinian) corpuscles	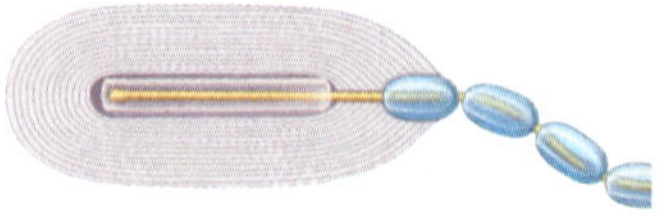	L: Exteroceptors, interoceptors, and some proprioceptors S: Mechanoreceptors (deep pressure, stretch, vibration of high frequency); rapidly adapting	Dermis and hypodermis; periostea, mesentery, tendons, ligaments, joint capsules; most abundant on fingers, soles of feet, external genitalia, nipples
Bulbous corpuscles (Ruffini endings)	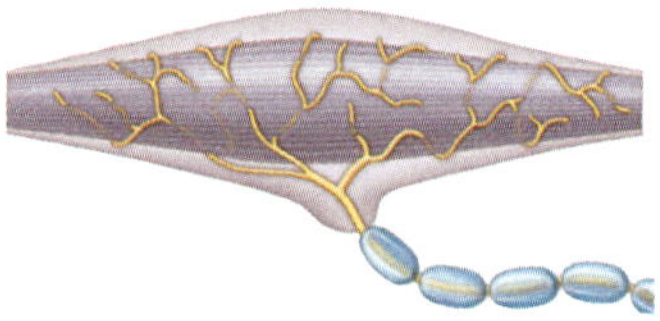	L: Exteroceptors and proprioceptors S: Mechanoreceptors (deep pressure and stretch); slowly or nonadapting	Deep in dermis, hypodermis, and joint capsules
Muscle spindles	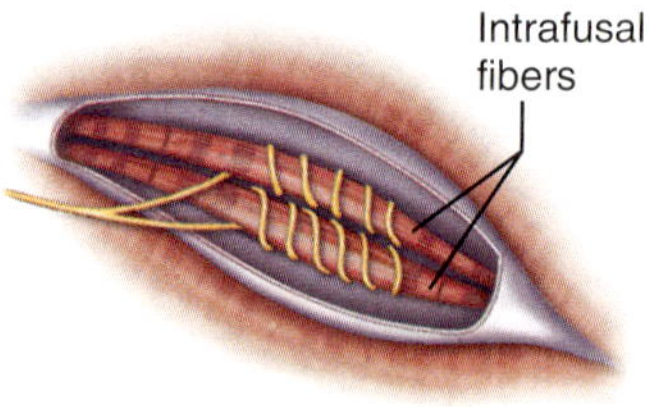	L: Proprioceptors S: Mechanoreceptors (muscle stretch, length)	Skeletal muscles, particularly in the extremities
Tendon organs	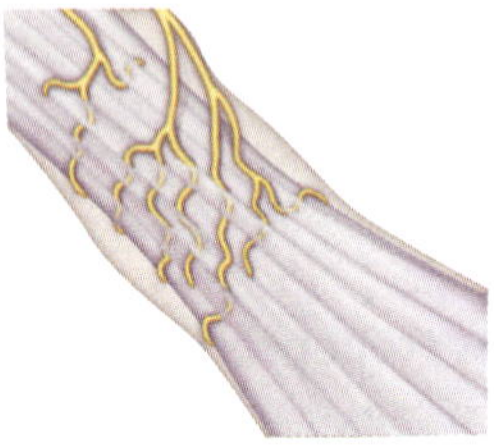	L: Proprioceptors S: Mechanoreceptors (tendon stretch, tension)	Tendons
Joint kinesthetic receptors		L: Proprioceptors S: Mechanoreceptors and nociceptors	Joint capsules of synovial joints

cold (10–40°C, or 50–104°F) are located in the superficial dermis. Those responding to heat (32–48°C, or 90–120°F) are deeper in the dermis.

Heat or cold outside the range of thermoreceptors activates nociceptors and is perceived as painful. Nociceptors also respond to pinch and chemicals released from damaged tissue. A key player in detecting painful stimuli is a plasma membrane protein called the *vanilloid receptor*. This protein is an ion channel that is opened by heat, low pH, and various chemicals including capsaicin, the substance found in red peppers.

Another sensation mediated by free nerve endings is itch. Located in the dermis, the *itch receptor* escaped detection for years because of its thin diameter. A number of chemicals—notably histamine—present at inflamed sites activate these nerve endings.

Other nonencapsulated nerve endings include:

- **Tactile (Merkel) discs**, which lie in the deepest layer of the epidermis, function as light touch receptors. Certain free nerve endings associate with enlarged, disc-shaped epidermal cells (*tactile* or *Merkel cells*) to form tactile discs.
- **Hair follicle receptors**, free nerve endings that wrap basketlike around hair follicles, are light touch receptors that detect bending of hairs. The tickle of a mosquito landing on your skin is mediated by hair follicle receptors.

Encapsulated Nerve Endings All **encapsulated nerve endings** consist of one or more fiber terminals of sensory neurons enclosed in a connective tissue capsule. Virtually all encapsulated receptors are mechanoreceptors, but they vary greatly in shape, size, and distribution in the body. They include tactile corpuscles, lamellar corpuscles, bulbous corpuscles, muscle spindles, tendon organs, and joint kinesthetic receptors.

- **Tactile corpuscles** or *Meissner's corpuscles* are small receptors in which a few spiraling sensory terminals are surrounded by Schwann cells and then by a thin egg-shaped connective tissue capsule. Tactile corpuscles are found just beneath the epidermis in the dermal papillae and are especially numerous in sensitive and hairless skin areas such as the nipples, fingertips, and soles of the feet. They are receptors for discriminative touch, and apparently play the same role in sensing light touch in hairless skin that hair follicle receptors do in hairy skin.
- **Lamellar corpuscles**, also called *Pacinian corpuscles*, are scattered deep in the dermis, and in subcutaneous tissue underlying the skin. Although they are mechanoreceptors stimulated by deep pressure, they respond only when the pressure is first applied, and thus are best suited to monitoring vibration (an "on/off" pressure stimulus). They are the largest corpuscular receptors. Some are over 3 mm long and half as wide and are visible to the naked eye as white, egg-shaped bodies. In section, a lamellar corpuscle resembles a cut onion. Its single dendrite is surrounded by a capsule containing up to 60 layers of collagen fibers and flattened supporting cells.
- **Bulbous corpuscles** or *Ruffini endings*, which lie in the dermis, subcutaneous tissue, and joint capsules, contain a spray of receptor endings enclosed by a flattened capsule. They bear a striking resemblance to tendon organs (which monitor tendon stretch) and probably play a similar role in other dense connective tissues where they respond to deep and *continuous* pressure.
- **Muscle spindles** are fusiform (spindle-shaped) proprioceptors found throughout the perimysium of a skeletal muscle. Each muscle spindle consists of a bundle of modified skeletal muscle fibers, called *intrafusal fibers* (in″trah-fu′zal), enclosed in a connective tissue capsule (Table 13.1). Muscle spindles detect muscle stretch and initiate a reflex that resists the stretch. We will consider the details of their innervation later when we describe the stretch reflex (see p. 515).
- **Tendon organs** are proprioceptors located in tendons, close to the skeletal muscle insertion. They consist of small bundles of tendon (collagen) fibers enclosed in a layered capsule, with sensory terminals coiling between and around the fibers. When muscle contraction stretches the tendon fibers, the resulting compression of the nerve fibers activates the tendon organs. This initiates a reflex that causes the contracting muscle to relax.
- **Joint kinesthetic receptors** (kin″es-thet′ik) are proprioceptors that monitor stretch in the articular capsules that enclose synovial joints. This receptor category contains at least four receptor types: lamellar corpuscles, bulbous corpuscles, free nerve endings, and receptors resembling tendon organs. Together these receptors provide information on joint position and motion (*kines* = movement), a sensation of which we are highly conscious. Close your eyes and flex and extend your fingers—you can feel exactly which joints are moving.

Check Your Understanding

1. Your PNS mostly consists of nerves. What else belongs to your PNS?
2. You've cut your finger on a broken beaker in your A&P lab. Using stimulus type, location, and receptor structure, classify the sensory receptors that allow you to feel the pain.

For answers, see Appendix H.

Sensory Integration: From Sensation to Perception

✓ Outline the events that lead to sensation and perception.

✓ Describe receptor and generator potentials and sensory adaptation.

✓ Describe the main aspects of sensory perception.

Our survival depends not only on **sensation** (awareness of changes in the internal and external environments) but also on **perception** (conscious interpretation of those stimuli). For example, a pebble in your shoe causes the *sensation* of localized deep pressure, but your *perception* of it is an awareness of discomfort. Perception in turn determines how we will respond: In this case, you take off your shoe to get rid of the pesky pebble.

General Organization of the Somatosensory System

The **somatosensory system**—the part of the sensory system serving the body wall and limbs—receives inputs from exteroceptors, proprioceptors, and interoceptors. Consequently, it transmits information about several different sensory modalities, or types of sensation.

Three main levels of neural integration operate in the somatosensory (or any sensory) system **(Figure 13.2)**:

① **Receptor level:** sensory receptors

② **Circuit level:** processing in ascending pathways

③ **Perceptual level:** processing in cortical sensory areas

Sensory input is generally relayed toward the head, but note that it is also processed along the way.

Let's examine the events that must occur at each level along the pathway.

Processing at the Receptor Level

For sensation to occur, a stimulus must excite a receptor and action potentials must reach the CNS (Figure 13.2, ①). For this to happen:

- The stimulus energy must match the *specificity* of the receptor. For example, a touch receptor may be sensitive to mechanical pressure, stretch, and vibration, but not to light

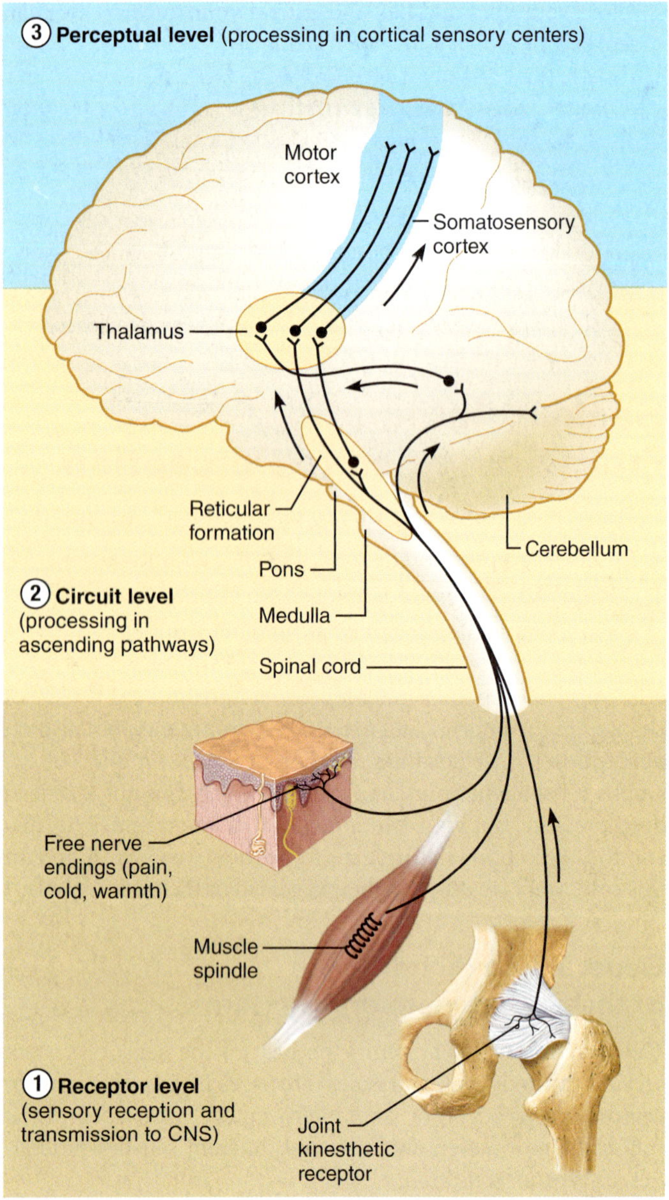

Figure 13.2 Three basic levels of neural integration in sensory systems.

energy (which is the province of receptors in the eye). The more complex the sensory receptor, the more specific it is.

- The stimulus must be applied within a sensory receptor's *receptive field*—the area the receptor monitors. Typically, the smaller the receptive field, the greater the ability of the brain to accurately localize the stimulus site.
- The stimulus energy must be converted into the energy of a *graded potential*, a process called **transduction**. This graded potential may be depolarizing or hyperpolarizing, similar to the EPSPs or IPSPs generated at postsynaptic membranes in response to neurotransmitter binding (see Chapter 11, p. 411).

  Receptors can produce one of two types of graded potentials. When the receptor region is part of a sensory neuron (as with free dendrites or the encapsulated receptors of most general sense receptors), the graded potential is called a **generator potential** because it generates action potentials in a sensory neuron.

  When the receptor is a separate cell (as in most special senses), the graded potential is called a **receptor potential** because it occurs in a separate receptor cell. The receptor potential changes the amount of neurotransmitter released by the receptor cell onto the sensory neuron. The neurotransmitters then generate graded potentials in the sensory neuron.
- Graded potentials in the first-order sensory neuron must reach *threshold* so that voltage-gated sodium channels on the axon are opened and nerve impulses are generated and propagated to the CNS.

Adaptation Information about a stimulus—its strength, duration, and pattern—is encoded in the frequency of nerve impulses: the greater the frequency, the stronger the stimulus. Many but not all sensory receptors exhibit **adaptation**, a change in sensitivity (and nerve impulse generation) in the presence of a constant stimulus. For example, when you step into bright sunlight from a darkened room, your eyes are initially dazzled, but your photoreceptors rapidly adapt, allowing you to see both bright areas and dark areas in the scene.

Phasic receptors are *fast adapting*, often giving bursts of impulses at the beginning and the end of the stimulus. Phasic receptors report changes in the internal or external environment. Examples are lamellar and tactile corpuscles.

Tonic receptors provide a sustained response with little or no adaptation. Nociceptors and most proprioceptors are tonic receptors because of the protective importance of their information.

Processing at the Circuit Level

At the second level of integration, the circuit level, the task is to deliver impulses to the appropriate region of the cerebral cortex for localization and perception of the stimulus (Figure 13.2, ②).

Recall from Chapter 12 that ascending sensory pathways typically consist of a chain of three neurons called first-, second-, and third-order sensory neurons. The axons of first-order sensory neurons, whose cell bodies are in the dorsal root or cranial ganglia, link the receptor and circuit levels of processing. Central processes of first-order neurons branch diffusely when they enter the spinal cord. Some branches take part in local spinal cord reflexes. Others synapse with second-order sensory neurons, which then synapse with the third-order sensory neurons that take the message to the cortex of the cerebrum.

As we saw in Chapter 12, the different ascending pathways (spinothalamic, dorsal column–medial lemniscal, and spinocerebellar) carry various types of information to different destinations in the brain. You may wish to review this information on p. 469.

Processing at the Perceptual Level

Sensory input is interpreted in the cerebral cortex (Figure 13.2, ③). The ability to identify and appreciate sensations depends on the location of the target neurons in the sensory cortex, not on the nature of the message (which is, after all, just an action potential). Each sensory fiber is analogous to a "labeled line" that tells the brain "who" is calling—a taste bud or a pressure receptor—and from "where." The brain always interprets the activity of a specific sensory receptor ("who") as a specific sensation, no matter how it is activated.

For example, pressing on your eyeball activates photoreceptors, but what you "see" is light. The exact point in the cortex that is activated always refers to the same "where," regardless of how it is activated, a phenomenon called **projection**. Electrically stimulating a particular spot in the visual cortex causes you to "see" light in a particular place.

Let's examine the major features of sensory perception.

- **Perceptual detection** is the ability to detect that a stimulus has occurred. This is the simplest level of perception. As a general rule, inputs from several receptors must be summed for perceptual detection to occur.
- **Magnitude estimation** is the ability to detect how *intense* the stimulus is. Perceived intensity increases as stimulus intensity increases because of frequency coding (see Figure 11.13).
- **Spatial discrimination** allows us to identify the site or pattern of stimulation. A common tool for studying this quality in the laboratory is the **two-point discrimination** test. The test determines how close together two points on the skin can be and still be perceived as two points rather than as one. This test provides a crude map of the density of tactile receptors in the various regions of the skin. The distance between perceived points varies from less than 5 mm on highly sensitive body areas (tip of the tongue) to more than 50 mm on less sensitive areas (the back).
- **Feature abstraction** is the mechanism by which a neuron or circuit is tuned to one feature, or property, of a stimulus in preference to others. Sensation usually involves an interplay of several stimulus features.

  For example, one touch tells us that velvet is warm, compressible, and smooth but not completely continuous, each a feature that contributes to our perception of "velvet." Feature abstraction enables us to identify more complex aspects of a sensation.
- **Quality discrimination** is the ability to differentiate the submodalities of a particular sensation. Each sensory modality has several **qualities**, or submodalities. For example, taste is a sensory modality and its submodalities include sweet and bitter.
- **Pattern recognition** is the ability to take in the scene around us and recognize a familiar pattern, an unfamiliar one, or one that has special significance for us. For example, we can look at an image made of dots and recognize it as the portrait of a familiar face. We can listen to music and hear a melody, not just a string of notes.

Perception of Pain

Everyone has suffered pain—the cruel persistence of a headache, the smart of a bee sting or a cut finger. Although we may not appreciate it at the time, pain is invaluable because it warns us of actual or impending tissue damage and strongly motivates us to take protective action. Managing a patient's pain can be difficult because pain is an intensely personal experience that cannot be measured objectively.

Pain receptors are activated by extremes of pressure and temperature as well as a veritable soup of chemicals released from injured tissue. Histamine, K^+, ATP, acids, and bradykinin are among the most potent pain-producing chemicals. All of these chemicals act on small-diameter fibers.

When you cut your finger, you may have noticed that you first felt a sharp pain followed some time later by burning or aching. Sharp pain is carried by the smallest of the myelinated sensory fibers, the A delta fibers, while burning pain is carried more slowly by small nonmyelinated C fibers. Both types of fibers release the neurotransmitters *glutamate* and *substance P*, which activate second-order sensory neurons. Axons from these second-order neurons ascend to the brain via the spinothalamic tract and other pathways.

If you cut your finger while fighting off an attacker, you might not notice the cut at all. How can that be? The brain has its own pain-suppressing analgesic systems in which the endogenous opioids such as *endorphins* and *enkephalins* (p. 417) play a key role. Various nuclei in the brain stem, including the periaqueductal gray matter of the midbrain, relay descending cortical and hypothalamic pain-suppressing signals. Descending fibers activate interneurons in the spinal cord, which release enkephalins. Enkephalins are inhibitory neurotransmitters that quash the pain signals generated by nociceptors.

Pain Tolerance

We all have the same *pain threshold*—that is, we begin to perceive pain at roughly the same stimulus intensity. However, our tolerance to pain varies widely. When we say that someone is "sensitive" to pain, we mean that the person has a low *pain tolerance* rather than a low pain threshold.

A number of genes help determine a person's pain tolerance and response to pain medications. The genetics of pain is currently an area of intense research, aimed at allowing an individual's genes to determine the best pain treatment.

Homeostatic Imbalance 13.1

Normally the body maintains a steady state that correlates injury and pain. Long-lasting or very intense pain inputs, such as limb amputation, can disrupt this system, leading to **hyperalgesia** (pain amplification), chronic pain, and **phantom limb pain**. Intense or long-lasting pain activates *NMDA receptors*, the same receptors that strengthen neural connections during certain kinds of learning. Essentially, the spinal cord *learns* hyperalgesia. In light of this, it is crucial that health professionals effectively manage pain early to prevent chronic pain from becoming established.

Phantom limb pain (pain perceived in tissue that is no longer present) is a curious example of hyperalgesia. Until recently, surgical limb amputations were conducted under general anesthesia only and the spinal cord still experienced the pain of amputation. Epidural anesthetics block neurotransmission in the spinal cord, and using them during surgery greatly reduces the incidence of phantom limb pain. ✚

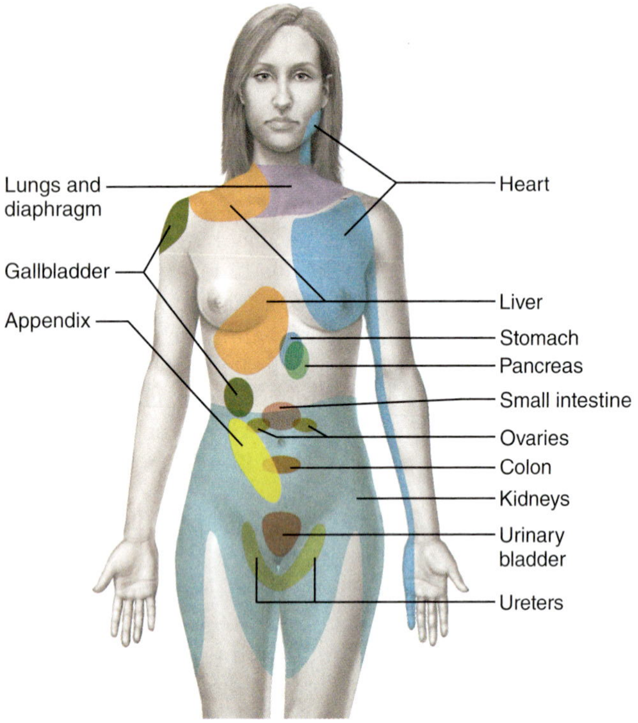

Figure 13.3 Map of referred pain. This map shows the anterior skin areas to which pain is referred from certain visceral organs.

13

Visceral and Referred Pain

Visceral pain results from noxious stimulation of receptors in the organs of the thorax and abdominal cavity. Like deep somatic pain, it is usually a vague sensation of dull aching, gnawing, or burning. Important stimuli for visceral pain are extreme stretching of tissue, ischemia (low blood flow), irritating chemicals, and muscle spasms.

The fact that visceral pain afferents travel along the same pathways as somatic pain fibers helps explain the phenomenon of **referred pain**, in which pain stimuli arising in one part of the body are perceived as coming from another part. For example, a person experiencing a heart attack may feel pain that radiates along the medial aspect of the left arm. Because the same spinal segments (T_1–T_5) innervate both the heart and arm, the brain interprets these inputs as coming from the more common somatic pathway. **Figure 13.3** shows cutaneous areas to which visceral pain is commonly referred.

☑ Check Your Understanding

3. What are the three levels of sensory integration?
4. What is the key difference between tonic and phasic receptors? Why are pain receptors tonic?
5. Your cortex decodes incoming action potentials from sensory pathways. How does it tell the difference between hot and cold? Between cool and cold? Between ice on your finger and ice on your foot?

For answers, see Appendix H.

PART 2
Transmission Lines: Nerves and Their Structure and Repair

Nerves and Associated Ganglia

✓ Define ganglion and indicate the general body location of ganglia.

✓ Describe the general structure of a nerve.

✓ Follow the process of nerve regeneration.

Structure and Classification

A **nerve** is a cordlike organ that is part of the peripheral nervous system. Nerves vary in size, but every nerve consists of parallel bundles of peripheral axons (some myelinated and some not) enclosed by successive wrappings of connective tissue **(Figure 13.4)**:

- Each axon is surrounded by **endoneurium** (en″do-nu′re-um), a delicate layer of loose connective tissue that also encloses the fiber's associated Schwann cells.
- A coarser connective tissue wrapping, the **perineurium,** binds groups of fibers into bundles called **fascicles**.
- A tough fibrous sheath, the **epineurium**, encloses all the fascicles to form the nerve.

Axons constitute only a small fraction of a nerve's bulk. The balance consists chiefly of myelin, the protective connective tissue wrappings, blood vessels, and lymphatic vessels.

Recall that the PNS is divided into *sensory* (afferent) and *motor* (efferent) divisions. Nerves are also classified according to the direction in which they transmit impulses:

- **Mixed nerves** contain both sensory and motor fibers and transmit impulses both to and from the central nervous system.
- **Sensory (afferent) nerves** carry impulses only toward the CNS.
- **Motor (efferent) nerves** carry impulses only away from the CNS.

Most nerves are mixed. Pure sensory or motor nerves are rare.

Because mixed nerves often carry both somatic and autonomic (visceral) nervous system fibers, the fibers in them may be classified according to the region they innervate as *somatic afferent*, *somatic efferent*, *visceral afferent*, and *visceral efferent*.

For convenience, the peripheral nerves are classified as *cranial* or *spinal* depending on whether they arise from the brain or spinal cord. Although we mention autonomic efferents of cranial nerves, in this chapter we will focus on somatic functions. We will defer the discussion of the autonomic nervous system and its visceral functions to Chapter 14.

Recall from Chapter 11 that **ganglia** are collections of neuron cell bodies associated with nerves in the PNS, whereas *nuclei* are collections of neuron cell bodies in the CNS. Ganglia associated with *afferent* nerve fibers contain cell bodies of sensory neurons.

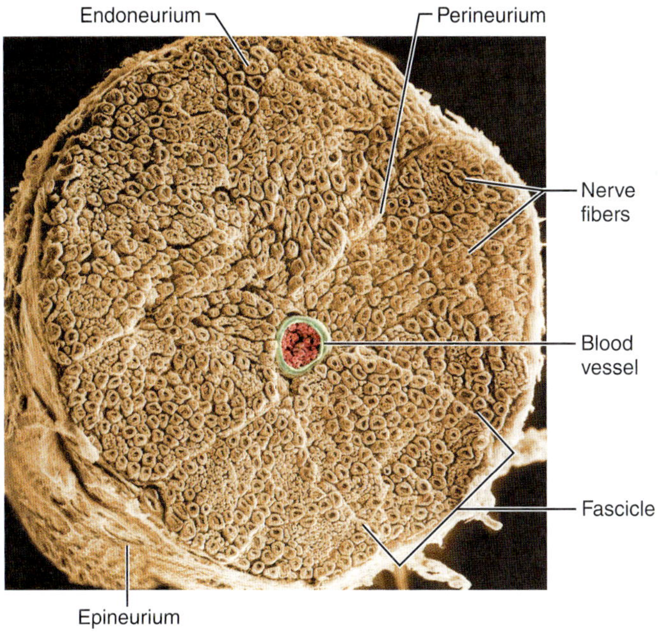

(a)

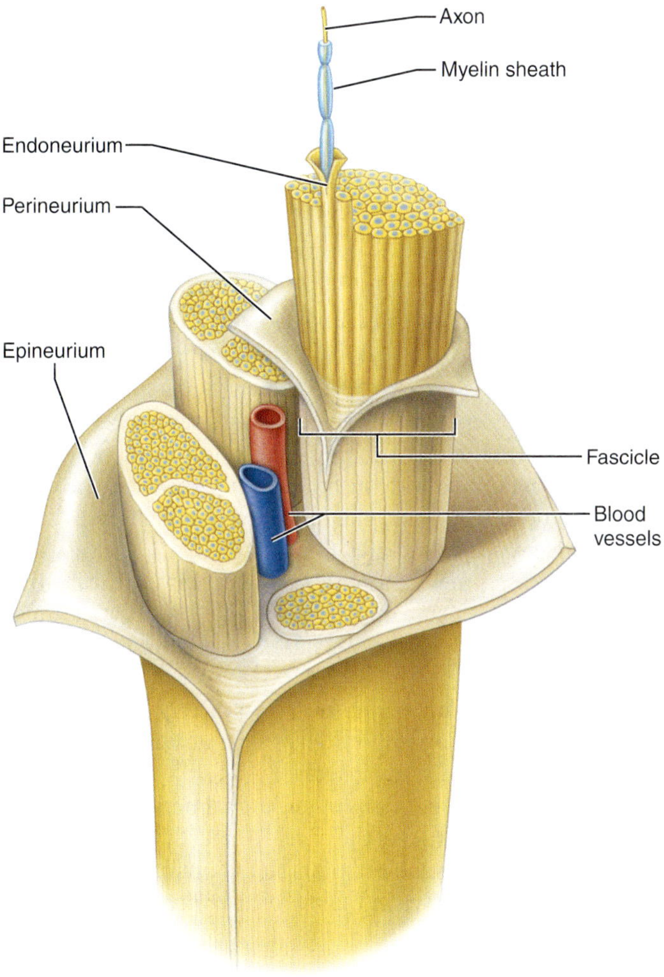

(b)

Figure 13.4 Structure of a nerve. (a) Scanning electron micrograph of a cross section of a portion of a nerve (90×). **(b)** Three-dimensional view of a portion of a nerve, showing connective tissue wrappings.

(These are the *dorsal root ganglia* described in Chapter 12.) Ganglia associated with *efferent* nerve fibers mostly contain cell bodies of autonomic motor neurons. We will describe these more complicated ganglia in Chapter 14.

Regeneration of Nerve Fibers

Damage to nervous tissue is serious because, as a rule, mature neurons do not divide. If the damage is severe or close to the cell body, the entire neuron may die, and other neurons that are normally stimulated by its axon may die as well. However, if the cell body remains intact, cut or compressed axons of peripheral nerves can regenerate successfully.

PNS Fibers

What happens if a peripheral axon is severed or crushed? As shown in **Figure 13.5**:

1. **The axon fragments.** Almost immediately, the separated ends seal themselves off and then swell as substances being transported along the axon accumulate in the sealed ends. Within a few hours, the axon and its myelin sheath distal to the injury site begin to disintegrate because they cannot receive nutrients from the cell body. This process, **Wallerian degeneration**, spreads distally from the injury site, fragmenting the distal part of the axon.
2. **Macrophages clean out the dead axon.** Within a week, macrophages generally degrade the entire axon distal to the injury, disposing of the debris. However, the myelin sheath remains intact within the endoneurium. The macrophages also release chemicals that stimulate the Schwann cells to divide.
3. **Axon filaments grow through a regeneration tube.** Surviving Schwann cells proliferate in response to the mitosis-stimulating chemicals, and migrate into the injury site. Once there, they release growth factors and begin to express cell adhesion molecules (CAMs) that encourage axonal growth. Additionally, they form a *regeneration tube*, a system of cellular cords that guide the regenerating axon "sprouts" across the gap to their original contacts.
4. **The axon regenerates and a new myelin sheath forms.** The same Schwann cells protect, support, and remyelinate the regenerating axons.

Changes also occur in the neuronal cell body after the axon has been destroyed. Within two days, its rough endoplasmic reticulum breaks apart, and then the cell body swells as protein synthesis revs up to support regeneration of its axon.

Axons regenerate at the approximate rate of 1.5 mm a day. The greater the distance between the severed ends, the less the chance of recovery because adjacent tissues block growth by protruding into the gaps, and axonal sprouts fail to find the regeneration tube. Neurosurgeons align cut nerve ends surgically to promote successful regeneration, and scaffolding devices can help guide the axons.

Whatever the measures taken, post-trauma axon regrowth never exactly matches what existed before the injury. Patients must often "retrain" the nervous system to respond appropriately so that stimulus and response are coordinated.

13

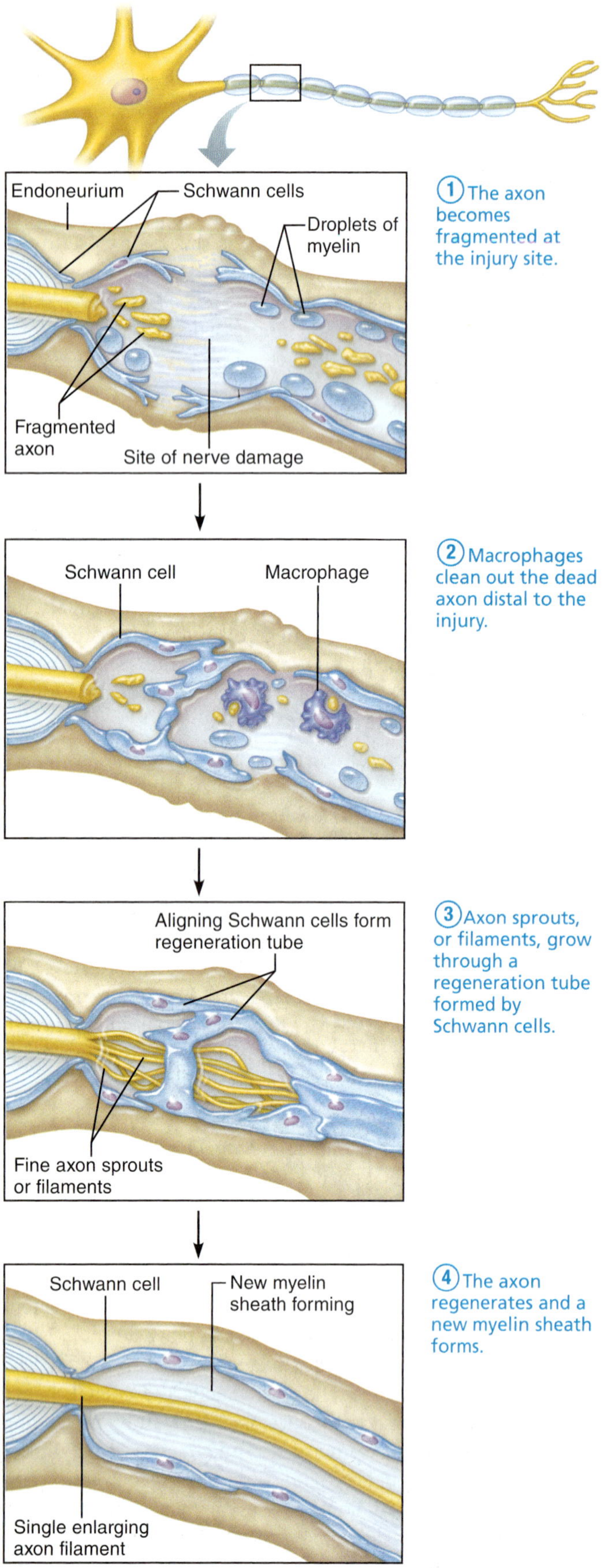

Figure 13.5 Regeneration of a nerve fiber in a peripheral nerve.

CNS Fibers

Unlike peripheral nerve fibers, most CNS fibers never regenerate. Consequently, damage to the brain or spinal cord has been viewed as irreversible. This difference in regenerative capacity seems to have less to do with the neurons themselves than with the "company they keep"—oligodendrocytes, their supporting cells.

Oligodendrocytes are studded with growth-inhibiting proteins. Consequently, the neuronal growth cone collapses and the fiber fails to regrow. Moreover, astrocytes at the site of injury form scar tissue rich in chondroitin sulfate (see p. 127) that blocks axonal regrowth.

For the clinician treating spinal cord injury, this means that multiple inhibitory processes need to be blocked simultaneously to promote axon regrowth. To date, experimentally neutralizing the myelin-bound growth inhibitors, blocking the receptors for the inhibitory proteins, or enzymatically destroying chondroitin sulfate have yielded promising results.

☑ Check Your Understanding

6. What are ganglia?
7. What is in a nerve besides axons?
8. Bill's femoral nerve was crushed while clinicians tried to control bleeding from his femoral artery. This resulted in loss of function and sensation in his leg, which gradually returned over the course of a year. Which cells were important in his recovery?

For answers, see Appendix H.

Cranial Nerves

✓ Name the 12 pairs of cranial nerves; indicate the body region and structures innervated by each.

Twelve pairs of **cranial nerves** are associated with the brain **(Figure 13.6)**. The first two pairs attach to the forebrain, and the rest are associated with the brain stem. Other than the vagus nerves, which extend into the abdomen, cranial nerves serve only head and neck structures.

In most cases, the names of the cranial nerves reveal either the structures they serve or their functions. The nerves are also numbered (using Roman numerals) from the most rostral to the most caudal.

We will begin with a brief overview of each cranial nerve and then describe the composition of all cranial nerves (p. 501). After that, you will be ready to tackle **Table 13.2** (p. 494), which provides detailed descriptions of the cranial nerves. Notice that it describes the pathways of the purely or mostly sensory nerves (I, II, and VIII) from the receptors to the brain, and the pathways of the other nerves in the oppositive direction (from the brain distally).

An Overview

I. Olfactory. These are the tiny sensory nerves (filaments) of smell, which run from the nasal mucosa to synapse with the olfactory bulbs. Note that the olfactory bulbs and tracts, shown in

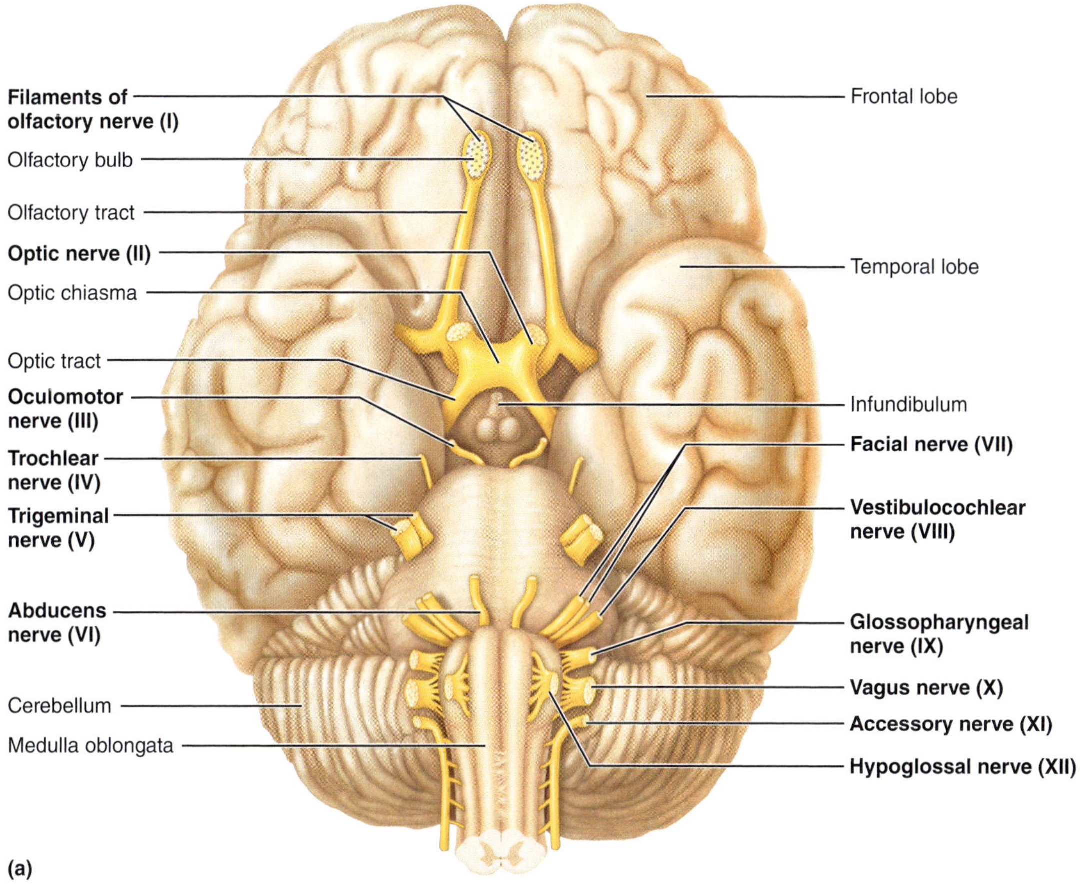

Cranial nerves I – VI	Sensory function	Motor function	PS* fibers
I Olfactory	Yes (smell)	No	No
II Optic	Yes (vision)	No	No
III Oculomotor	No	Yes	Yes
IV Trochlear	No	Yes	No
V Trigeminal	Yes (general sensation)	Yes	No
VI Abducens	No	Yes	No

Cranial nerves VII – XII	Sensory function	Motor function	PS* fibers
VII Facial	Yes (taste)	Yes	Yes
VIII Vestibulocochlear	Yes (hearing and balance)	Some	No
IX Glossopharyngeal	Yes (taste)	Yes	Yes
X Vagus	Yes (taste)	Yes	Yes
XI Accessory	No	Yes	No
XII Hypoglossal	No	Yes	No

(b) *PS = parasympathetic

Figure 13.6 Location and function of cranial nerves. (a) Ventral view of the human brain, showing the cranial nerves. **(b)** Summary of cranial nerves by function. Two cranial nerves (I and II) have sensory function only, no motor function. Four nerves (III, VII, IX, and X) carry parasympathetic fibers that serve visceral muscles and glands. All cranial nerves that innervate muscles also carry afferent fibers from proprioceptors in the muscles served. Only sensory functions other than proprioception are indicated.

Figure 13.6a, are brain structures and not part of cranial nerve I. (See Table 13.2 art for the olfactory nerve filaments.)

II. Optic. Because this sensory nerve of vision develops as an outgrowth of the brain, it is really a brain tract.

III. Oculomotor. The name *oculomotor* means "eye mover." This nerve supplies four of the six extrinsic muscles that move the eyeball in the orbit.

IV. Trochlear. The term *trochlear* means "pulley" and it innervates an extrinsic eye muscle that loops through a pulley-shaped ligament in the orbit.

V. Trigeminal. Three (*tri*) branches spring from this, the largest cranial nerve. It supplies sensory fibers to the face and motor fibers to the chewing muscles.

VI. Abducens. This nerve controls the extrinsic eye muscle that *abducts* the eyeball (turns it laterally).

VII. Facial. A large nerve that innervates muscles of *facial* expression (among other things).

VIII. Vestibulocochlear. This mostly sensory nerve for hearing and balance was formerly called the *auditory nerve*.

(Text continues on p. 500.)

Table 13.2 Cranial Nerves

I Olfactory Nerves (ol-fak′to-re)

Origin and course: Olfactory nerve fibers arise from olfactory sensory neurons located in olfactory epithelium of nasal cavity and pass through cribriform plate of ethmoid bone to synapse in olfactory bulb. Fibers of olfactory bulb neurons extend posteriorly as olfactory tract, which runs beneath frontal lobe to enter cerebral hemispheres and terminates in primary olfactory cortex. See also Figure 15.20.

Function: Purely sensory; carry afferent impulses for sense of smell.

Clinical testing: Ask subject to sniff and identify aromatic substances, such as oil of cloves and vanilla.

Homeostatic Imbalance Fracture of ethmoid bone or lesions of olfactory fibers may result in partial or total loss of smell, a condition known as *anosmia* (an-oz′me-ah). +

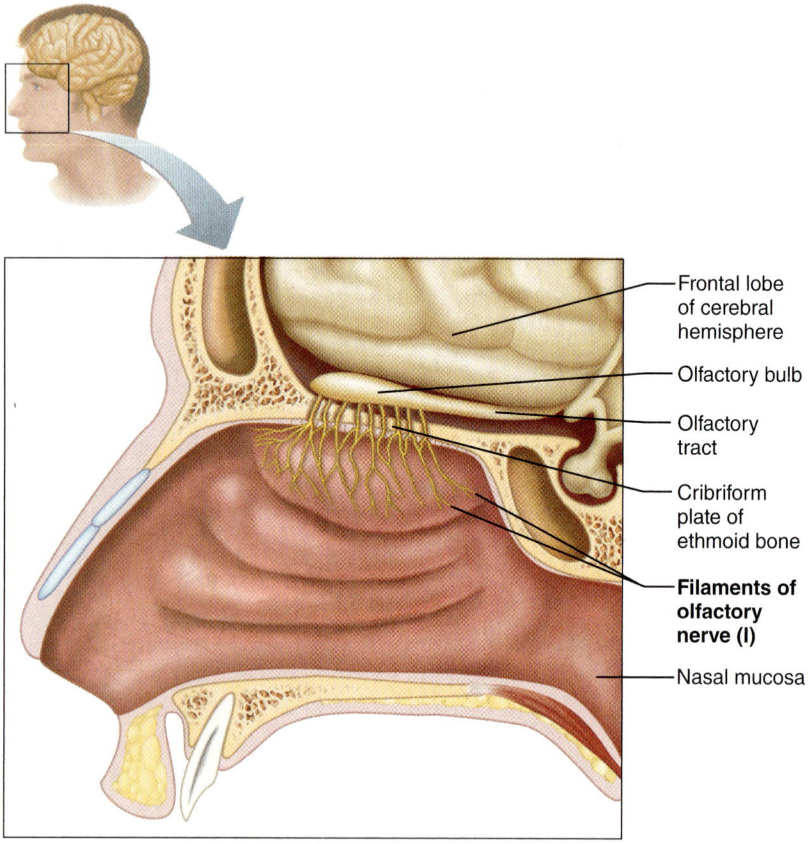

II Optic Nerves

Origin and course: Fibers arise from retina of eye to form optic nerve, which passes through optic canal of orbit. The optic nerves converge to form the optic chiasma (ki-az′mah) where fibers partially cross over, continue on as optic tracts, enter thalamus, and synapse there. Thalamic fibers run (as the optic radiation) to occipital (visual) cortex, where visual interpretation occurs. See also Figure 15.19.

Function: Purely sensory; carry afferent impulses for vision.

Clinical testing: Assess vision and visual field with eye chart and by testing the point at which the person first sees an object (finger) moving into the visual field. View fundus of eye with ophthalmoscope to detect papilledema (swelling of optic disc, the site where the optic nerve leaves the eyeball) and examine optic disc and retinal blood vessels.

Homeostatic Imbalance Damage to optic nerve results in blindness in eye served by nerve. Damage to visual pathway beyond the optic chiasma results in partial visual losses. Visual defects are called *anopsias* (ah-nop′se-ahz). +

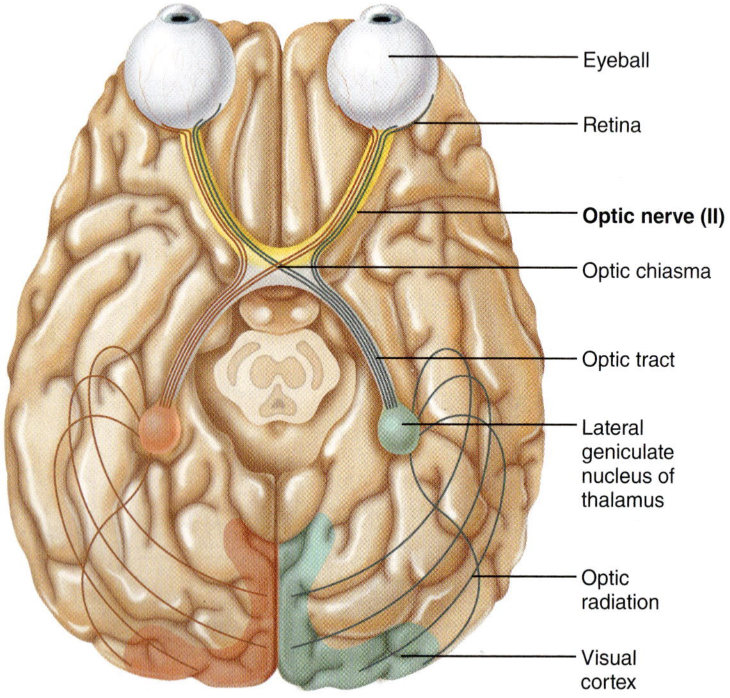

Table 13.2 *(continued)*

III Oculomotor Nerves (ok″u-lo-mo′tor)

Origin and course: Fibers extend from ventral midbrain (near its junction with pons) and pass through bony orbit, via superior orbital fissure, to eye.

Function: Chiefly motor nerves (*oculomotor* = motor to the eye); contain a few proprioceptive afferents. Each nerve includes the following:

- Somatic motor fibers to four of the six extrinsic eye muscles (inferior oblique and superior, inferior, and medial rectus muscles) that help direct eyeball, and to levator palpebrae superioris muscle, which raises upper eyelid.
- Parasympathetic (autonomic) motor fibers to sphincter pupillae (circular muscles of iris), which cause pupil to constrict, and to ciliary muscle, controlling lens shape for visual focusing. Some parasympathetic cell bodies are in the ciliary ganglia.
- Sensory (proprioceptor) afferents, which run from same four extrinsic eye muscles to midbrain.

Clinical testing: Examine pupils for size, shape, and equality. Test pupillary reflex with penlight (pupils should constrict when illuminated). Test convergence for near vision and subject's ability to follow objects with the eyes.

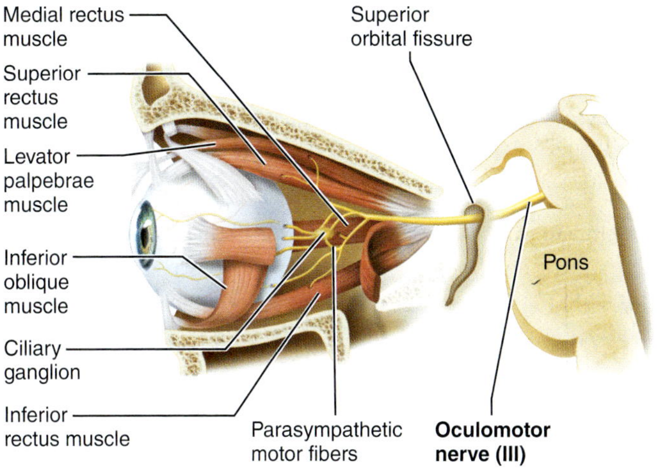

Homeostatic Imbalance In oculomotor nerve paralysis, eye cannot be moved up, down, or inward. At rest, eye rotates laterally [*external strabismus* (strah-biz′mus)] because the actions of the two extrinsic eye muscles not served by cranial nerves III are unopposed. Upper eyelid droops (*ptosis*), and the person has double vision and trouble focusing on close objects. ✚

IV Trochlear Nerves (trok′le-ar)

Origin and course: Fibers emerge from dorsal midbrain and course ventrally around midbrain to enter orbit through superior orbital fissure along with oculomotor nerves.

Function: Primarily motor nerves; supply somatic motor fibers to (and carry proprioceptor fibers from) one of the extrinsic eye muscles, the superior oblique muscle, which passes through the pulley-shaped trochlea.

Clinical testing: Test with cranial nerve III (oculomotor).

Homeostatic Imbalance Damage to a trochlear nerve results in double vision and impairs ability to rotate eye inferolaterally. ✚

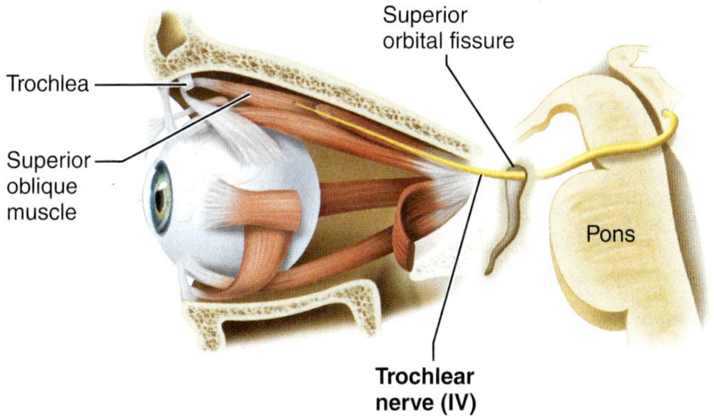

Table 13.2 Cranial Nerves *(continued)*

V Trigeminal Nerves

Largest cranial nerves; fibers extend from pons to face, and form three divisions (*trigemina* = threefold): ophthalmic, maxillary, and mandibular divisions. As main general sensory nerves of face, transmit afferent impulses from touch, temperature, and pain receptors. Cell bodies of sensory neurons of all three divisions are located in large *trigeminal ganglion*.

The mandibular division also contains motor fibers that innervate chewing muscles.

Dentists desensitize upper and lower jaws by injecting local anesthetic (such as Novocain) into alveolar branches of maxillary and mandibular divisions, respectively. Since this blocks pain-transmitting fibers of teeth, the surrounding tissues become numb.

	Ophthalmic division (V_1)	Maxillary division (V_2)	Mandibular division (V_3)
Origin and course	Fibers run from face to pons via superior orbital fissure.	Fibers run from face to pons via foramen rotundum.	Fibers pass through skull via foramen ovale.
Function	Conveys sensory impulses from skin of anterior scalp, upper eyelid, and nose, and from nasal cavity mucosa, cornea, and lacrimal gland.	Conveys sensory impulses from nasal cavity mucosa, palate, upper teeth, skin of cheek, upper lip, lower eyelid.	Conveys sensory impulses from anterior tongue (except taste buds), lower teeth, skin of chin, temporal region of scalp. Supplies motor fibers to, and carries proprioceptor fibers from, muscles of mastication.
Clinical testing	Corneal reflex test: Touching cornea with wisp of cotton should elicit blinking.	Test sensations of pain, touch, and temperature with safety pin and hot and cold objects.	Assess motor branch by asking person to clench his teeth, open mouth against resistance, and move jaw side to side.

Homeostatic Imbalance *Trigeminal neuralgia* (nu-ral′je-ah), or *tic douloureux* (tik doo″loo-roo′; *tic* = twitch, *douloureux* = painful), caused by inflammation of trigeminal nerve, is widely considered to produce most excruciating pain known. The stabbing pain lasts for a few seconds to a minute, but it can be relentless, occurring a hundred times a day. Usually provoked by some sensory stimulus, such as brushing teeth or even a passing breeze hitting the face. Thought to be caused by a loop of artery or vein that compresses the trigeminal nerve near its exit from the brain stem. Analgesics and carbamazepine (an anticonvulsant) are only partially effective. In severe cases, surgery relieves the agony—either by moving the compressing vessel or by destroying the nerve. Nerve destruction results in loss of sensation on that side of face. +

13

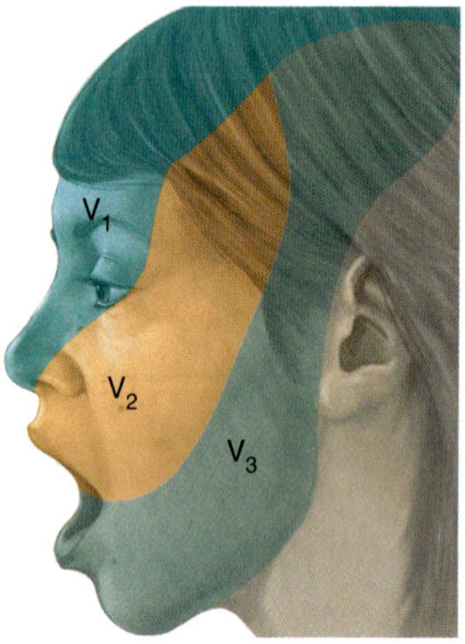

(b) Distribution of sensory fibers of each division

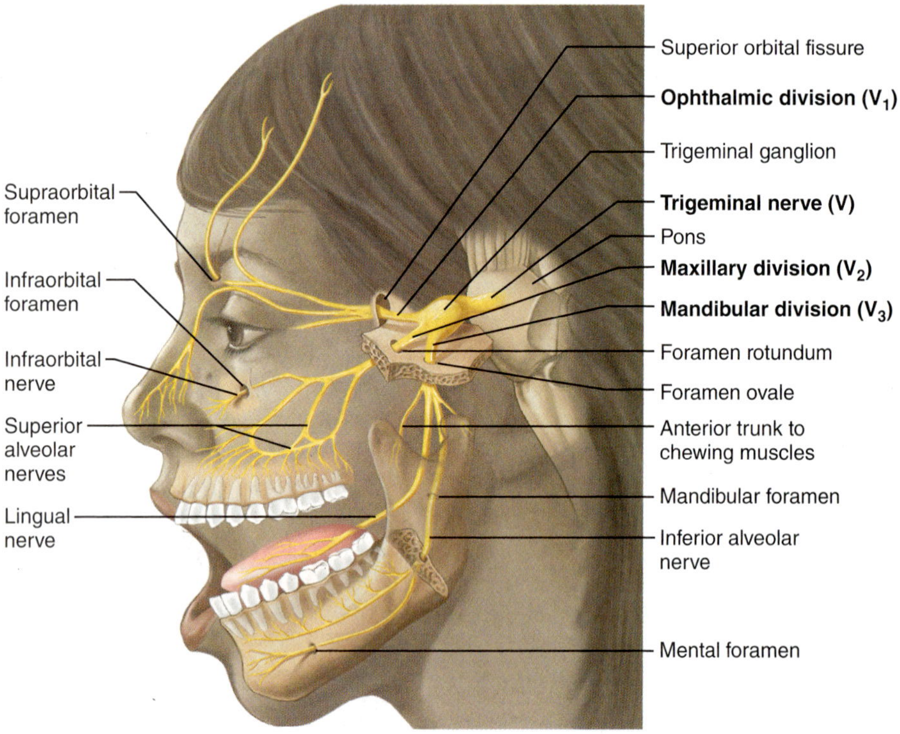

(a) Distribution of the trigeminal nerve

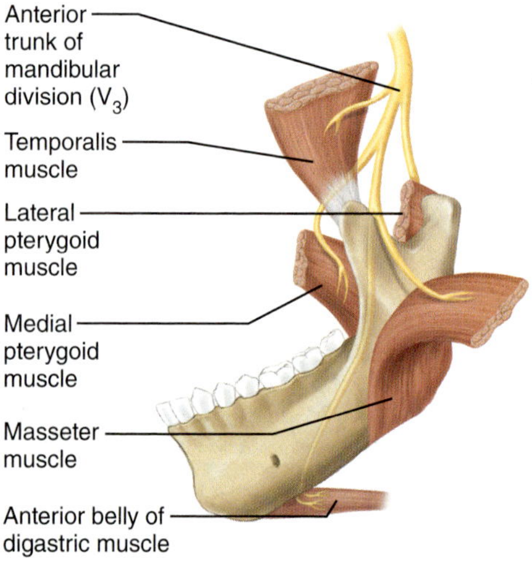

(c) Motor branches of the mandibular division (V_3)

Table 13.2 *(continued)*

VI Abducens Nerves (ab-du'senz)

Origin and course: Fibers leave inferior pons and enter orbit via superior orbital fissure to run to eye.

Function: Primarily motor; supply somatic motor fibers to lateral rectus muscle, an extrinsic muscle of the eye. Convey proprioceptor impulses from same muscle to brain.

Clinical testing: Test in common with cranial nerve III (oculomotor).

Homeostatic Imbalance In abducens nerve paralysis, eye cannot be moved laterally. At rest, eyeball rotates medially *(internal strabismus)*. ✚

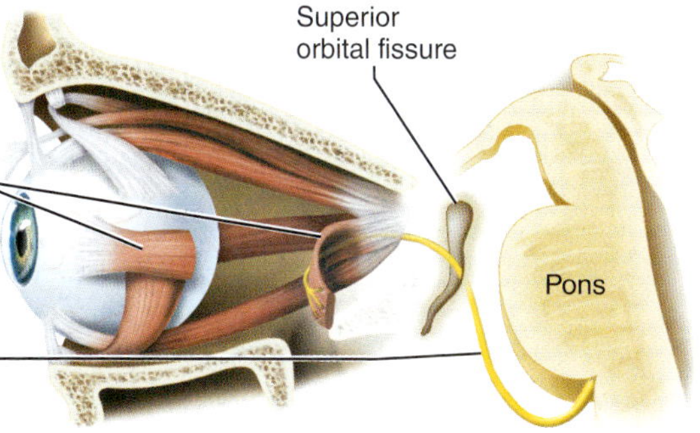

VII Facial Nerves

Origin and course: Fibers issue from pons, just lateral to abducens nerves (see Figure 13.6), enter temporal bone via *internal acoustic meatus*, and run within bone (and through inner ear cavity) before emerging through *stylomastoid foramen*. Nerve then courses to lateral aspect of face.

Function: Mixed nerves that are the chief motor nerves of face. Five major branches: temporal, zygomatic, buccal, mandibular, and cervical (see **c** on next page).

- Convey motor impulses to skeletal muscles of face (muscles of facial expression), except for chewing muscles served by trigeminal nerves, and transmit proprioceptor impulses from same muscles to pons (see **b**).
- Transmit parasympathetic (autonomic) motor impulses to lacrimal (tear) glands, nasal and palatine glands, and submandibular and sublingual salivary glands. Some of the cell bodies of these parasympathetic motor neurons are in *pterygopalatine* (ter″eh-go-pal'ah-tīn) and *submandibular ganglia* on the trigeminal nerve (see **a**).
- Convey sensory impulses from taste buds of anterior two-thirds of tongue; cell bodies of these sensory neurons are in *geniculate ganglion* (see **a**).

Clinical testing: Test anterior two-thirds of tongue for ability to taste sweet (sugar), salty, sour (vinegar), and bitter (quinine) substances. Check symmetry of face. Ask subject to close eyes, smile, whistle, and so on. Assess tearing with ammonia fumes.

Homeostatic Imbalance *Bell's palsy* is characterized by paralysis of facial muscles on affected side and partial loss of taste sensation. May develop rapidly (often overnight). Caused by inflamed and swollen facial nerve, possibly due to herpes simplex 1 viral infection. Lower eyelid droops, corner of mouth sags (making it difficult to eat or speak normally), tears drip continuously from eye and eye cannot be completely closed (conversely, dry-eye syndrome may occur). Treated with corticosteroids. Recovery is complete in 70% of cases. ✚

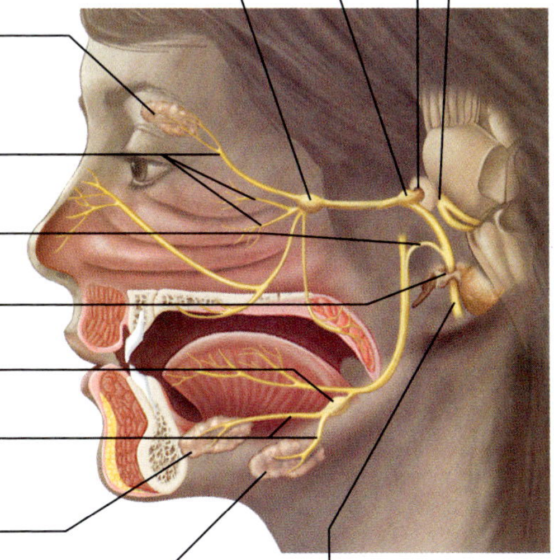

(a) Parasympathetic efferents and sensory afferents

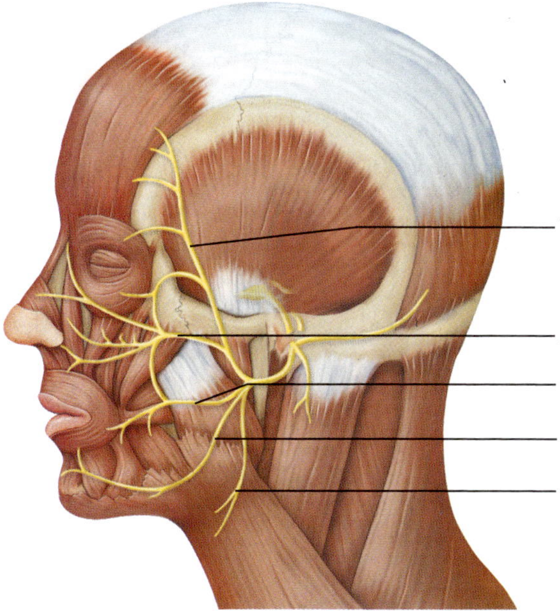

(b) Motor branches to muscles of facial expression and scalp muscles (see pp. 329–331)

➤

13

Table 13.2 Cranial Nerves *(continued)*

VII Facial Nerves *(continued)*

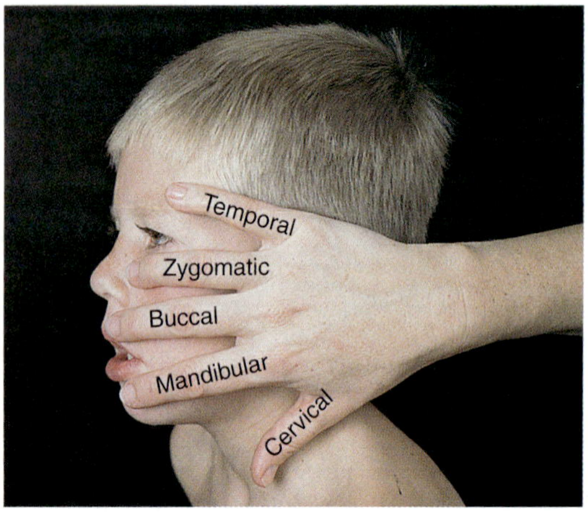

(c) A simple way to remember the courses of the five major branches of the facial nerve

VIII Vestibulocochlear Nerves (ves-tib″u-lo-kok′le-ar)

Origin and course: Fibers arise from hearing and equilibrium apparatus located within inner ear of temporal bone and pass through internal acoustic meatus to enter brain stem at pons-medulla border. Afferent fibers from hearing receptors in cochlea form the *cochlear division*; those from equilibrium receptors in semicircular canals and vestibule form the *vestibular division* (vestibular nerve). The two divisions merge to form vestibulocochlear nerve. See also Figure 15.26.

Function: Mostly sensory. Vestibular branch transmits afferent impulses for sense of equilibrium, and sensory nerve cell bodies are located in *vestibular ganglia*. Cochlear branch transmits afferent impulses for sense of hearing, and sensory nerve cell bodies are located in *spiral ganglion* within cochlea. Small motor component adjusts the sensitivity of sensory receptors. See also Figure 15.27.

Clinical testing: Check hearing by air and bone conduction using tuning fork.

Homeostatic Imbalance Lesions of cochlear nerve or cochlear receptors result in *central*, or *nerve*, *deafness*. Damage to vestibular division produces dizziness, rapid involuntary eye movements, loss of balance, nausea, and vomiting. +

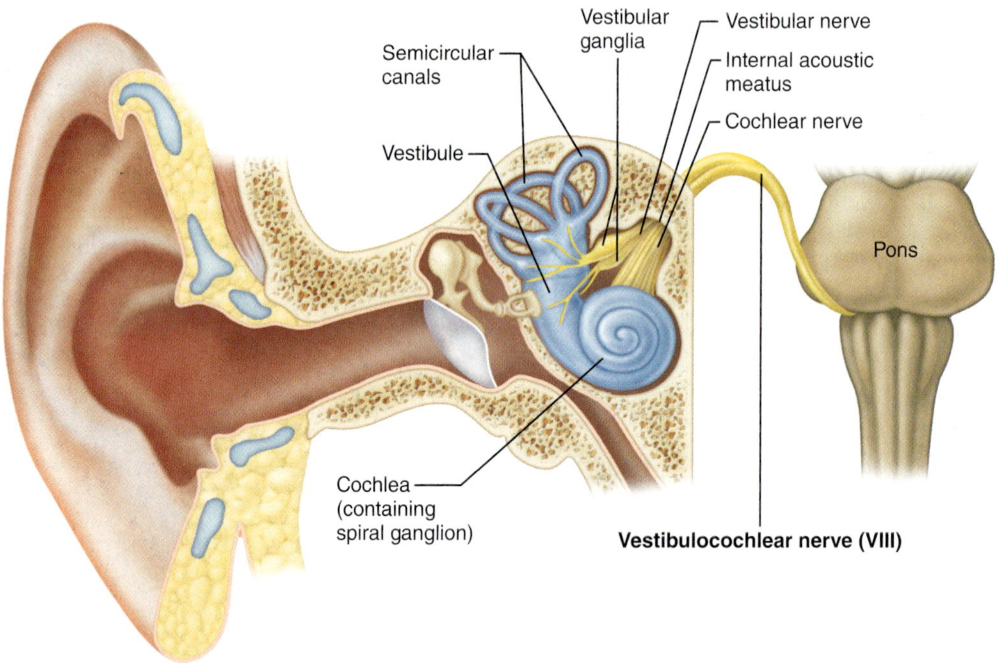

13

IX Glossopharyngeal Nerves (glos″o-fah-rin′je-al)

Origin and course: Fibers emerge from medulla and leave skull via *jugular foramen* to run to throat.

Function: Mixed nerves that innervate part of tongue and pharynx. Provide somatic motor fibers to, and carry proprioceptor fibers from, a superior pharyngeal muscle called the *stylopharyngeus*, which elevates the pharynx in swallowing. Provide parasympathetic motor fibers to parotid salivary glands (some of the nerve cell bodies of these parasympathetic motor neurons are located in *otic ganglion*).

Sensory fibers conduct taste and general sensory (touch, pressure, pain) impulses from pharynx and posterior tongue, from chemoreceptors in the carotid body (which monitor O_2 and CO_2 levels in the blood and help regulate respiratory rate and depth), and from baroreceptors of carotid sinus (which monitor blood pressure). Sensory neuron cell bodies are located in *superior* and *inferior ganglia*.

Clinical testing: Check position of uvula; check gag and swallowing reflexes. Ask subject to speak and cough. Test posterior third of tongue for taste.

Homeostatic Imbalance Injured or inflamed glossopharyngeal nerves impair swallowing and taste. +

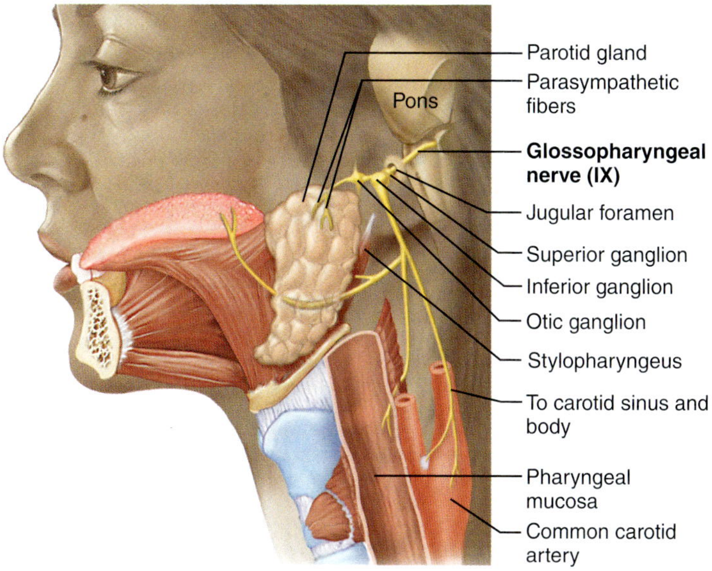

X Vagus Nerves (va′gus)

Origin and course: The only cranial nerves to extend beyond head and neck region. Fibers emerge from medulla, pass through skull via jugular foramen, and descend through neck region into thorax and abdomen. See also Figure 14.4.

Function: Mixed nerves. Nearly all motor fibers are parasympathetic efferents, except those serving skeletal muscles of pharynx and larynx (involved in swallowing). Parasympathetic motor fibers supply heart, lungs, and abdominal viscera and are involved in regulating heart rate, breathing, and digestive system activity. Transmit sensory impulses from thoracic and abdominal viscera, from the aortic arch baroreceptors (for blood pressure) and the carotid and aortic bodies (chemoreceptors for respiration), and taste buds on the epiglottis. Carry proprioceptor fibers from muscles of larynx and pharynx.

Clinical testing: As for cranial nerve IX (glossopharyngeal; IX and X are tested in common, since they both innervate muscles of throat and mouth).

Homeostatic Imbalance Since laryngeal branches of the vagus innervate nearly all muscles of the larynx ("voice box"), vagal nerve paralysis can lead to hoarseness or loss of voice. Other symptoms are difficulty swallowing and impaired digestive system motility. These parasympathetic nerves are important for maintaining the normal state of visceral organ activity. Without their influence, the sympathetic nerves, which mobilize and accelerate vital body processes (and shut down digestion), would dominate. +

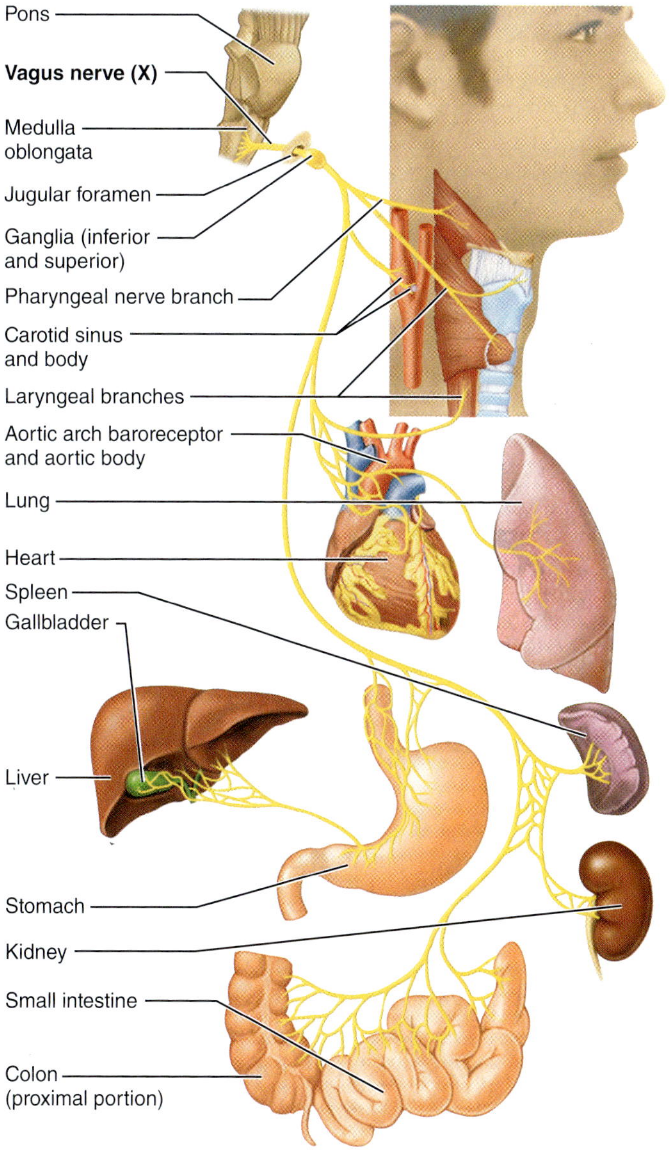

Table 13.2 Cranial Nerves *(continued)*

XI Accessory Nerves

Origin and course: Unique in that they form from rootlets that emerge from the spinal cord, not the brain stem. These rootlets arise laterally from superior region (C_1–C_5) of spinal cord, pass upward along spinal cord, and enter the skull as the accessory nerves via foramen magnum. The accessory nerves exit from skull through *jugular foramen* together with the vagus nerves, and supply two large neck muscles.

Until recently, was considered to have both a cranial and spinal portion, but the cranial rootlets are actually part of the vagus nerves. This raises an interesting question: Should the accessory nerves still be considered cranial nerves? Some anatomists say "no" because they don't arise from the brain. Others say "yes" because their origin is different from a typical spinal nerve and they pass through the skull. Stay tuned!

Function: Mixed nerves, but primarily motor in function. Supply motor fibers to trapezius and sternocleidomastoid muscles, which together move head and neck, and convey proprioceptor impulses from same muscles.

Clinical testing: Check strength of sternocleidomastoid and trapezius muscles by asking person to rotate head and shrug shoulders against resistance.

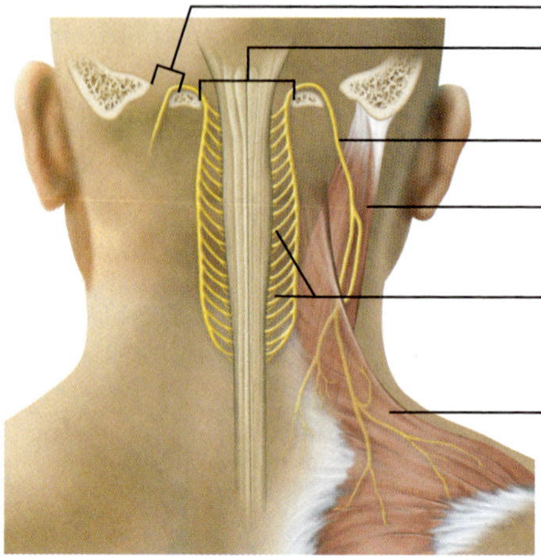

Homeostatic Imbalance Injury to one accessory nerve causes head to turn toward injury side as result of sternocleidomastoid muscle paralysis. Shrugging that shoulder (role of trapezius muscle) becomes difficult. ✚

XII Hypoglossal Nerves (hi″po-glos′al)

Origin and course: As their name implies (*hypo* = below; *glossal* = tongue), hypoglossal nerves mainly serve the tongue. Fibers arise by a series of roots from medulla and exit from skull via *hypoglossal canal* to travel to tongue. See also Figure 13.6.

Function: Mixed nerves, but primarily motor in function. Carry somatic motor fibers to intrinsic and extrinsic muscles of tongue, and proprioceptor fibers from same muscles to brain stem. Hypoglossal nerve control allows tongue movements that mix and manipulate food during chewing, and contribute to swallowing and speech.

Clinical testing: Ask subject to protrude and retract tongue. Note any deviations in position.

Homeostatic Imbalance Damage to hypoglossal nerves causes difficulties in speech and swallowing. If both nerves are impaired, the person cannot protrude tongue. If only one side is affected, tongue deviates (points) toward affected side; eventually paralyzed side begins to atrophy. ✚

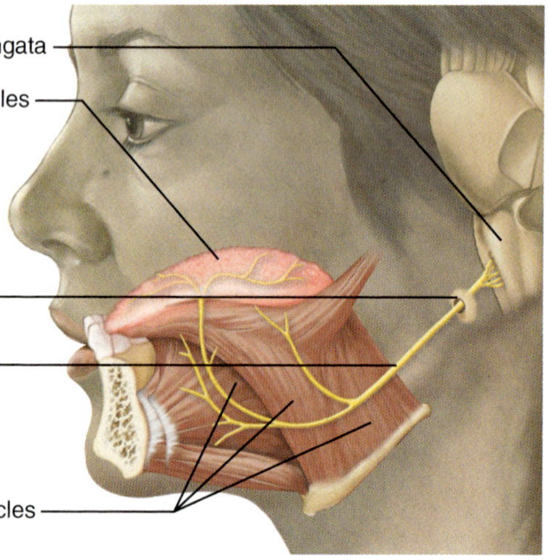

IX. Glossopharyngeal. The name *glossopharyngeal* means "tongue and pharynx," the structures that this nerve helps to innervate.

X. Vagus. This nerve's name means "wanderer" or "vagabond," and it is the only cranial nerve to extend beyond the head and neck to the thorax and abdomen.

XI. Accessory. Considered an *accessory* part of the vagus nerve, this nerve was formerly called the *spinal accessory nerve*.

XII. Hypoglossal. The name *hypoglossal* means under the tongue. This nerve runs inferior to the tongue and innervates the tongue muscles.

You might make up your own saying to remember the first letters of the cranial nerves in order, or use the following memory jog sent by a student: "**O**n **o**ccasion, **o**ur **t**rusty **t**ruck **a**cts **f**unny—**v**ery **g**ood **v**ehicle **a**ny**h**ow."

Composition of Cranial Nerves

In the last chapter, we described how ventral (motor) and dorsal (sensory) roots fuse to form spinal nerves. Cranial nerves, on the other hand, vary markedly in their composition.

Most cranial nerves are mixed nerves, as shown in Figure 13.6b. However, two nerve pairs (the olfactory and optic) associated with special sense organs are generally considered purely sensory. The cell bodies of the sensory neurons in the olfactory and optic nerves are located *within* their respective special sense organs. In other sensory neurons contributing to cranial nerves (V, VII, IX, and X), the cell bodies are located in **cranial sensory ganglia** just outside the brain. Some cranial nerves have a single sensory ganglion, others have several, and still others have none.

Several of the mixed cranial nerves contain both somatic and autonomic motor fibers and hence serve both skeletal muscles and visceral organs. Except for some autonomic motor neurons located in ganglia, the cell bodies of motor neurons contributing to the cranial nerves are located in the ventral gray matter regions (nuclei) of the brain stem.

Remembering the primary functions of the cranial nerves (as **s**ensory, **m**otor, or **b**oth) can be a challenge. This sentence might help: "**S**ome say **m**arry **m**oney, **b**ut **m**y **b**rother **b**elieves (it's) **b**ad **b**usiness (to) **m**arry **m**oney."

Check Your Understanding

9. Name the cranial nerve(s) most involved in each of the following: moving your eyeball; sticking out your tongue; controlling your heart rate and digestive activity; shrugging your shoulders.

For answers, see Appendix H.

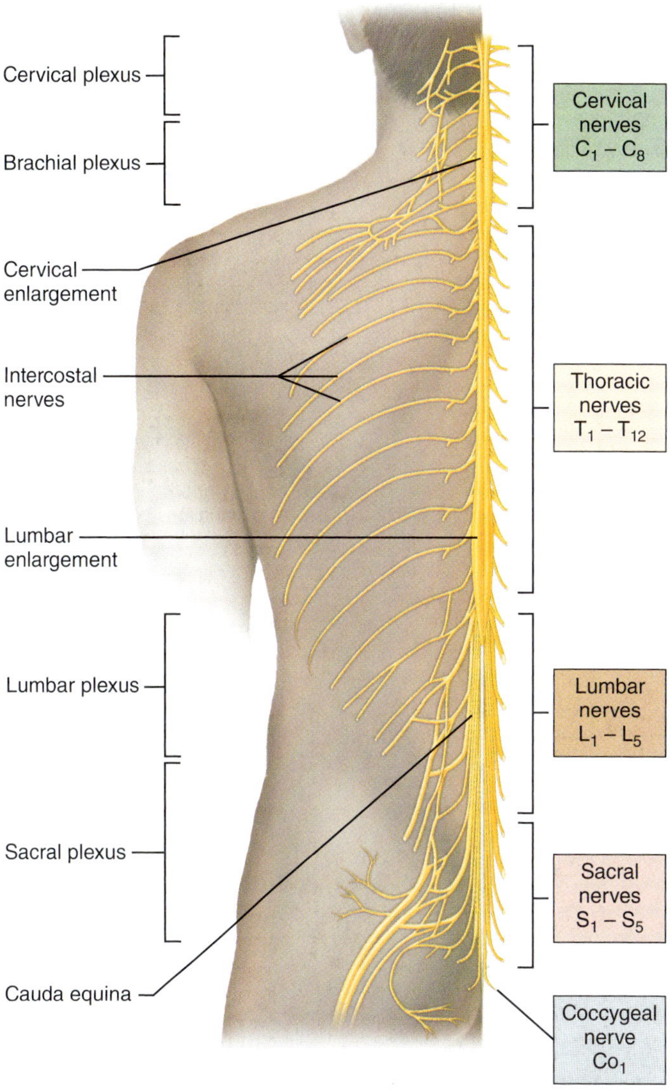

Figure 13.7 Spinal nerves. (Posterior view.) The spinal nerves are shown at right; their ventral rami are shown at left. Most ventral rami form nerve plexuses (cervical, brachial, lumbar, and sacral).

Spinal Nerves

- ✓ Describe the general structure of a spinal nerve and the general distribution of its rami.
- ✓ Define plexus. Name the major plexuses and describe the distribution and function of the peripheral nerves arising from each plexus.

Thirty-one pairs of **spinal nerves**, each containing thousands of nerve fibers, arise from the spinal cord and supply all parts of the body except the head and some areas of the neck. All are mixed nerves.

Spinal nerves are named according to where they issue from the spinal cord **(Figure 13.7)**. The spinal nerves include:

- 8 pairs of cervical spinal nerves (C_1–C_8)
- 12 pairs of thoracic nerves (T_1–T_{12})
- 5 pairs of lumbar nerves (L_1–L_5)
- 5 pairs of sacral nerves (S_1–S_5)
- 1 pair of tiny coccygeal nerves (Co_1)

Notice that there are eight pairs of cervical nerves but only seven cervical vertebrae. This "discrepancy" is easily explained. The first seven pairs exit the vertebral canal *superior* to the vertebrae for which they are named, but C_8 emerges *inferior* to the seventh cervical vertebra (between C_7 and T_1). Below the cervical level, each spinal nerve leaves the vertebral column *inferior* to the same-numbered vertebra.

As we mentioned in Chapter 12, each spinal nerve connects to the spinal cord by a dorsal root and a ventral root **(Figure 13.8)**. Each root forms from a series of **rootlets** that attach along the length of the corresponding spinal cord segment (Figure 13.8a).

- **Ventral roots** contain *motor* (efferent) fibers that arise from ventral horn motor neurons and extend to and innervate the skeletal muscles. (In Chapter 14, we describe autonomic nervous system efferents that are also contained in the ventral roots.)
- **Dorsal roots** contain *sensory* (afferent) fibers that arise from sensory neurons in the dorsal root ganglia and conduct impulses from peripheral receptors to the spinal cord.

The spinal roots pass laterally from the cord and unite just distal to the dorsal root ganglion to form a spinal nerve before emerging from the vertebral column via their respective

13

Figure 13.8 Formation of spinal nerves and rami distribution. Notice the dorsal and ventral roots and rami. In the thorax, each ventral ramus continues as an intercostal nerve. (The small meningeal branch is not illustrated.)

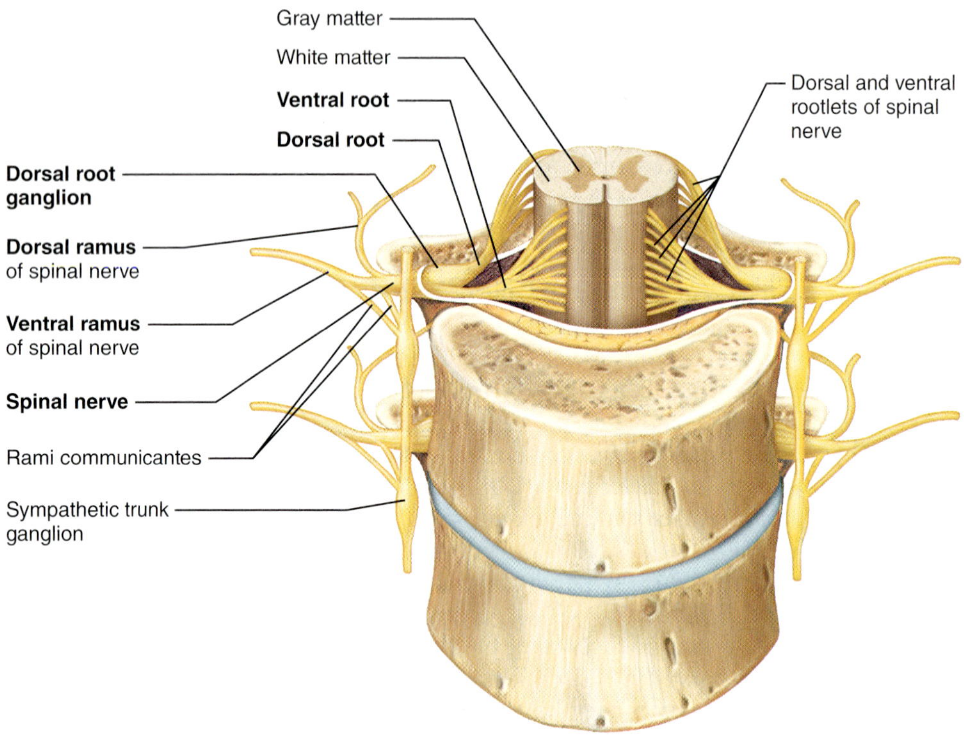

(a) Anterior view showing spinal cord, associated nerves, and vertebrae. The dorsal and ventral roots arise medially as rootlets and join laterally to form the spinal nerve.

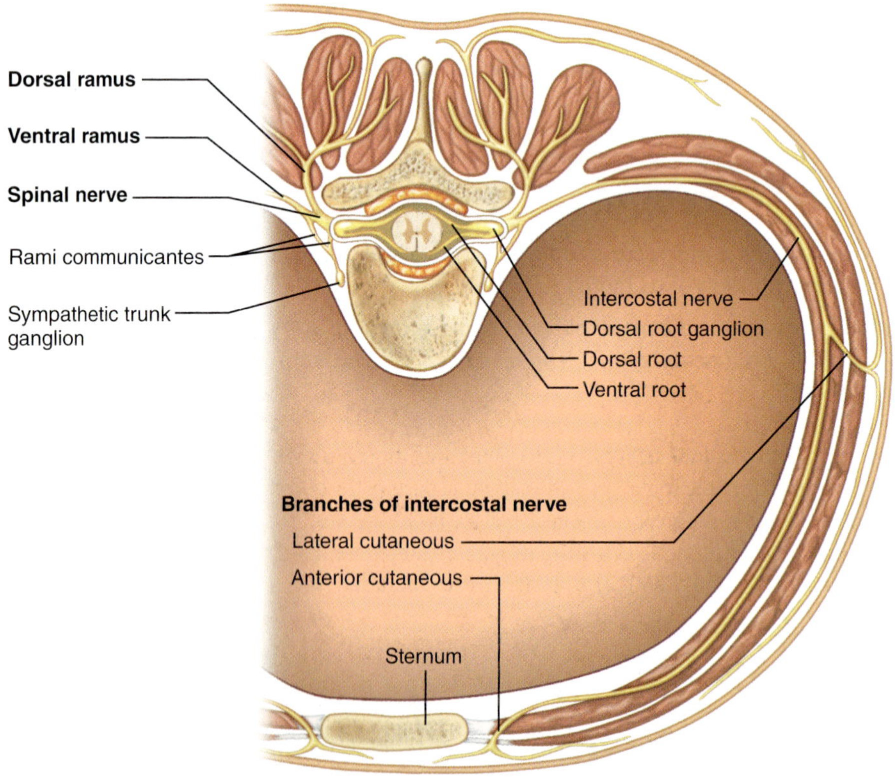

(b) Cross section of thorax showing the main roots and branches of a spinal nerve.

intervertebral foramina. Because motor and sensory fibers mingle in a spinal nerve, it contains both efferent and afferent fibers.

The spinal roots become progressively longer from the superior to the inferior aspect of the cord. In the cervical region, the roots are short and run horizontally, but the roots of the lumbar and sacral nerves extend inferiorly for some distance through the lower vertebral canal as the *cauda equina* before exiting the vertebral column (Figure 13.7).

A spinal nerve is quite short (only 1–2 cm). Almost immediately after emerging from its foramen, it divides into a small **dorsal ramus** (ra′mus; "branch"), a larger **ventral ramus**, and a tiny **meningeal branch** (mĕ-nin′je-al) that reenters the vertebral canal to innervate the meninges and blood vessels within. Each ramus, like the spinal nerve itself, is mixed.

Special rami called **rami communicantes**, which contain autonomic (visceral) nerve fibers, attach to the base of the ventral rami of the thoracic spinal nerves (Figure 13.8).

Innervation of Specific Body Regions

The spinal nerve rami and their main branches supply the entire somatic region of the body (skeletal muscles and skin) from the neck down. The dorsal rami supply the posterior body trunk. The thicker ventral rami supply the rest of the trunk and the limbs.

To be clear, let's review the difference between roots and rami:

- Roots lie medial to and form the spinal nerves. Each root is strictly sensory or motor.
- Rami lie distal to and are lateral branches of the spinal nerves. Like spinal nerves, rami carry both sensory and motor fibers.

Before we get into the specifics of how the body is innervated, it is important for you to understand some points about the ventral rami of the spinal nerves. Except for T_2–T_{12}, all ventral rami branch and join one another lateral to the vertebral column, forming complicated interlacing nerve networks called **nerve plexuses** (Figure 13.7). Nerve plexuses occur in the cervical, brachial, lumbar, and sacral regions and primarily serve the limbs. Notice that *only ventral rami form plexuses.*

Within a plexus, fibers from the various ventral rami crisscross one another and become redistributed so that (1) each resulting branch of the plexus contains fibers from several spinal nerves and (2) fibers from each ventral ramus travel to the body periphery via several routes. As a result, each muscle in a limb receives its nerve supply from more than one spinal nerve. An advantage of this fiber regrouping is that damage to one spinal segment or root cannot completely paralyze any limb muscle.

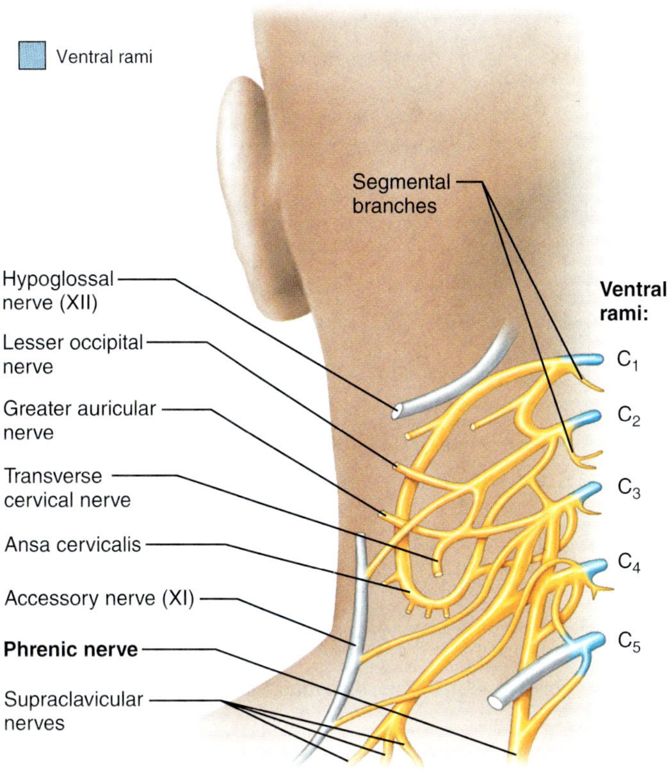

Figure 13.9 The cervical plexus. The nerves colored gray connect to the plexus but do not belong to it. See Table 13.3 for structures served. (Posterior view.)

In the rest of this section, we summarize the major groups of skeletal muscles served. For more specific information on muscle innervations, see Tables 10.1–10.17.

Cervical Plexus and the Neck

Buried deep in the neck under the sternocleidomastoid muscle, the ventral rami of the first four cervical nerves form the looping **cervical plexus** (Figure 13.9). Most of its branches are **cutaneous nerves** that supply only the skin (Table 13.3).

Table 13.3 Branches of the Cervical Plexus (See Figure 13.9)

NERVES	VENTRAL RAMI	STRUCTURES SERVED
Cutaneous Branches (Superficial)		
Lesser occipital	C_2 (C_3)	Skin on posterolateral aspect of head and neck
Greater auricular	C_2, C_3	Skin of ear, skin over parotid gland
Transverse cervical	C_2, C_3	Skin on anterior and lateral aspect of neck
Supraclavicular (medial, intermediate, and lateral)	C_3, C_4	Skin of shoulder and clavicular region
Motor Branches (Deep)		
Ansa cervicalis (superior and inferior roots)	C_1–C_3	Infrahyoid muscles of neck (omohyoid, sternohyoid, and sternothyroid)
Segmental and other muscular branches	C_1–C_5	Deep muscles of neck (geniohyoid and thyrohyoid) and portions of scalenes, levator scapulae, trapezius, and sternocleidomastoid muscles
Phrenic	C_3–C_5	Diaphragm (sole motor nerve supply)

13

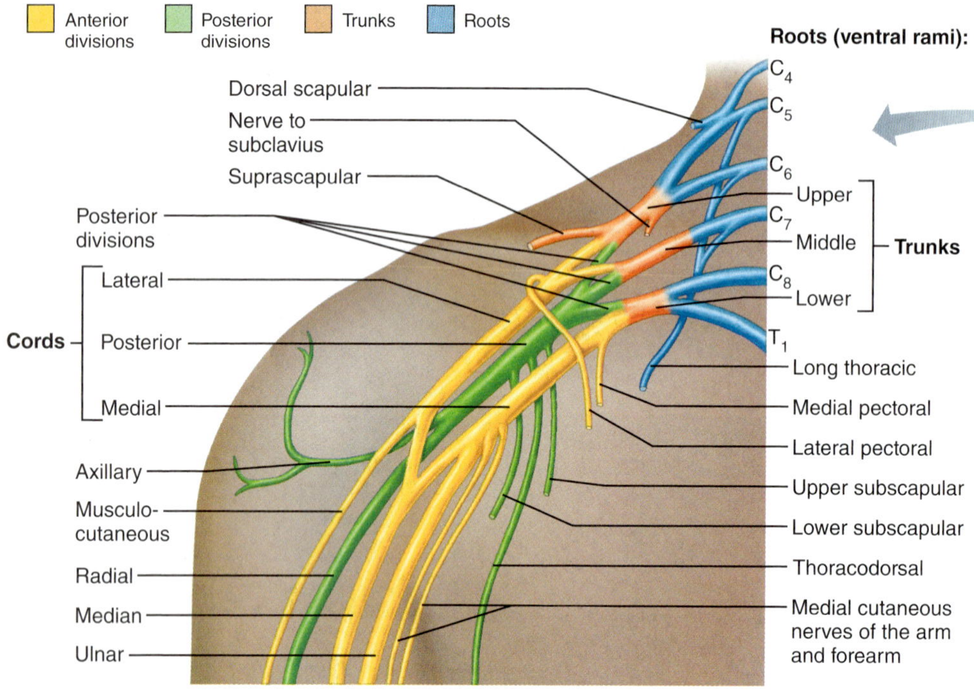

(a) Roots (rami C_5–T_1), trunks, divisions, and cords

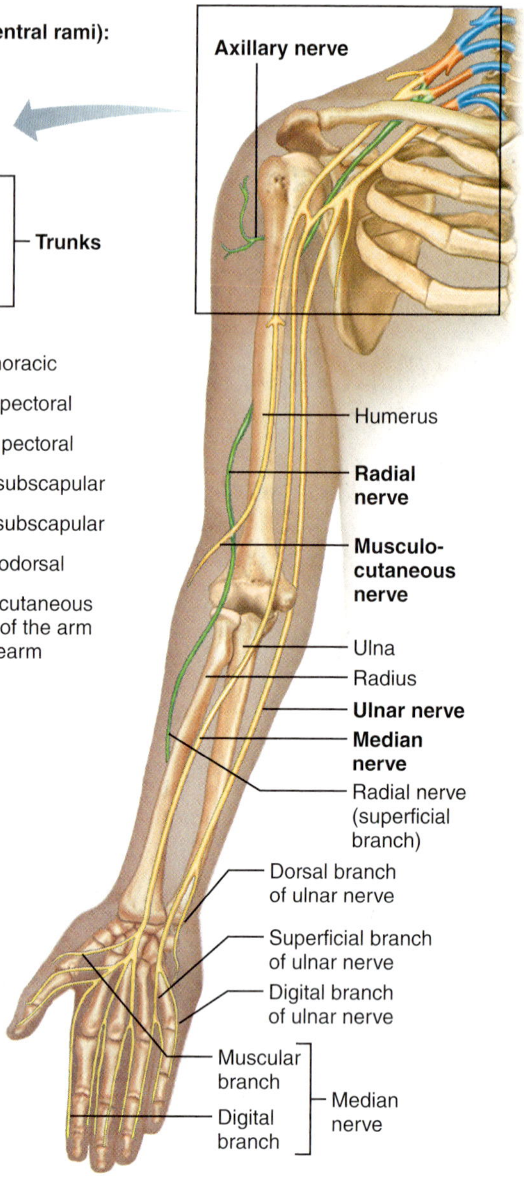

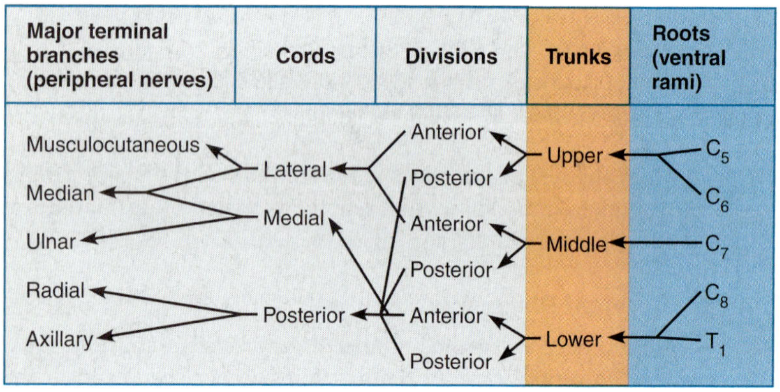

(b) Flowchart summarizing relationships within the brachial plexus

(c) The major nerves of the upper limb

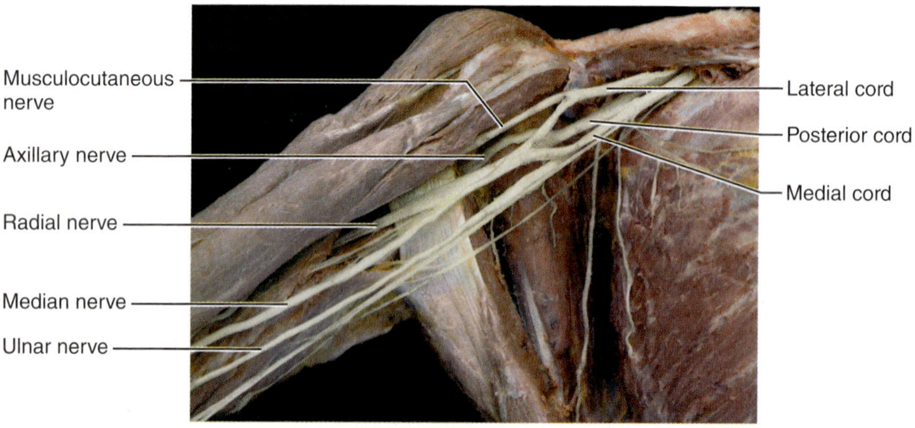

(d) Cadaver photo

Figure 13.10 The brachial plexus. (Anterior view.)

Table 13.4 Branches of the Brachial Plexus (See Figure 13.10 and Appendix G)

NERVES	CORD AND VENTRAL RAMI	STRUCTURES SERVED
Musculocutaneous	Lateral cord (C_5–C_7)	Muscular branches: flexor muscles in anterior arm (biceps brachii, brachialis, coracobrachialis) Cutaneous branches: skin on lateral forearm (extremely variable)
Median	By two branches, one from medial cord (C_8, T_1) and one from the lateral cord (C_5–C_7)	Muscular branches to flexor group of anterior forearm (palmaris longus, flexor carpi radialis, flexor digitorum superficialis, flexor pollicis longus, lateral half of flexor digitorum profundus, and pronator muscles); intrinsic muscles of lateral palm and digital branches to the fingers Cutaneous branches: skin of lateral two-thirds of hand on ventral side and dorsum of fingers 2 and 3
Ulnar	Medial cord (C_8, T_1)	Muscular branches: flexor muscles in anterior forearm (flexor carpi ulnaris and medial half of flexor digitorum profundus); most intrinsic muscles of hand Cutaneous branches: skin of medial third of hand, both anterior and posterior aspects
Radial	Posterior cord (C_5–C_8, T_1)	Muscular branches: posterior muscles of arm and forearm (triceps brachii, anconeus, supinator, brachioradialis, extensors carpi radialis longus and brevis, extensor carpi ulnaris, and several muscles that extend the fingers) Cutaneous branches: skin of posterolateral surface of entire limb (except dorsum of fingers 2 and 3)
Axillary	Posterior cord (C_5, C_6)	Muscular branches: deltoid and teres minor muscles Cutaneous branches: some skin of shoulder region
Dorsal scapular	Branches of C_5 rami	Rhomboid muscles and levator scapulae
Long thoracic	Branches of C_5–C_7 rami	Serratus anterior muscle
Subscapular	Posterior cord; branches of C_5 and C_6 rami	Teres major and subscapularis muscles
Suprascapular	Upper trunk (C_5, C_6)	Shoulder joint; supraspinatus and infraspinatus muscles
Pectoral (lateral and medial)	Branches of lateral and medial cords (C_5–T_1)	Pectoralis major and minor muscles

They transmit sensory impulses from the skin of the neck, the ear area, the back of the head, and the shoulder. Other branches innervate muscles of the anterior neck.

The single most important nerve from this plexus is the **phrenic nerve** (fren′ik), which receives fibers from C_3, C_4, and C_5. The phrenic nerve runs inferiorly through the thorax and supplies both motor and sensory fibers to the diaphragm (*phren* = diaphragm), which is the chief muscle causing breathing movements.

Homeostatic Imbalance 13.2

Irritation of the phrenic nerve causes spasms of the diaphragm, or hiccups. If both phrenic nerves are severed, or if the C_3–C_5 region of the spinal cord is crushed or destroyed, the diaphragm is paralyzed and respiratory arrest occurs. Mechanical respirators keep victims alive by forcing air into their lungs—literally breathing for them. +

Brachial Plexus and Upper Limb

The large, important **brachial plexus**, situated partly in the neck and partly in the axilla, gives rise to virtually all the nerves that innervate the upper limb (Table 13.4). It can be palpated (felt) in a living person just superior to the clavicle at the lateral border of the sternocleidomastoid muscle. Ventral rami of C_5–C_8 and most of the T_1 ramus intermix to form the brachial plexus. Additionally, it often receives fibers from C_4 or T_2 or both.

The brachial plexus is very complex (some consider it the anatomy student's nightmare). Perhaps the simplest approach is to master the terms used for its four major groups of branches (**Figure 13.10a, b**). From medial to lateral, these are (1) the ventral rami, misleadingly called *roots*, which form (2) *trunks*, which form (3) *divisions*, which form (4) *cords*. You might want to use the saying "**R**eally **t**ired? **D**rink **c**offee" to help you remember this branching sequence.

The five **roots** (ventral rami C_5–T_1) of the brachial plexus lie deep to the sternocleidomastoid muscle. At the lateral border of that muscle, these roots unite to form **upper**, **middle**, and **lower trunks**, each of which divides almost immediately into an **anterior division** and a **posterior division**.

The anterior and posterior divisions, which generally indicate which fibers serve the front or back of the limb, pass deep to the clavicle and enter the axilla. There they give rise to three large fiber bundles called the **lateral**, **medial**, and **posterior cords**. (The cords are named for their relationship to the axillary artery, which runs through the axilla; see Figure 19.23.) All along the plexus, small nerves branch off. These supply the muscles and skin of the shoulder and superior thorax.

Homeostatic Imbalance 13.3

Injuries to the brachial plexus are common. When severe, they weaken or paralyze the entire upper limb. Such injuries may occur when the upper limb is pulled hard, stretching the plexus (as when a football tackler yanks the arm of the running back), or by blows to the top of the shoulder that force the humerus inferiorly (as when a cyclist pitches headfirst off a motorcycle and his shoulder grinds into the pavement). +

The brachial plexus ends in the axilla, where its three cords wind along the axillary artery and give rise to the main nerves of the upper limb (Figure 13.10c, d). Five of these nerves are especially important: the axillary, musculocutaneous, median, ulnar, and radial nerves. We describe their distribution and targets briefly here. For more detail, see Table 13.4 and Appendix G.

Axillary Nerve The **axillary nerve** branches off the posterior cord and runs posterior to the surgical neck of the humerus. It innervates the deltoid and teres minor muscles and the skin and joint capsule of the shoulder.

Musculocutaneous Nerve The **musculocutaneous nerve**, the major end branch of the lateral cord, courses inferiorly in the anterior arm, supplying motor fibers to the biceps brachii, brachialis, and coracobrachialis muscles. Distal to the elbow, it provides cutaneous sensation in the lateral forearm.

Median Nerve The **median nerve** descends through the arm to the anterior forearm, where it gives off branches to the skin and to most flexor muscles. On reaching the hand, it innervates five intrinsic muscles of the lateral palm. The median nerve activates muscles that pronate the forearm, flex the wrist and fingers, and oppose the thumb.

13

Homeostatic Imbalance 13.4

Median nerve injury makes it difficult to use the pincer grasp (opposed thumb and index finger) to pick up small objects. Because this nerve runs down the midline of the forearm and wrist, it is a frequent casualty of wrist-slashing suicide attempts. In carpal tunnel syndrome (see p. 234), the median nerve is compressed. +

Ulnar Nerve The **ulnar nerve** branches off the medial cord of the plexus. It descends along the medial aspect of the arm toward the elbow, swings behind the medial epicondyle, and then follows the ulna along the medial forearm. There it supplies the flexor carpi ulnaris and the medial part of the flexor digitorum profundus (the flexors not supplied by the median nerve).

The ulnar nerve continues into the hand, where it innervates most intrinsic hand muscles and the skin of the medial aspect of the hand. It causes the wrist and fingers to flex, and (with the median nerve) adducts and abducts the medial fingers.

Homeostatic Imbalance 13.5

Where it takes a superficial course, the ulnar nerve is very vulnerable to injury. Striking the "funny bone"—the spot where this nerve rests against the medial epicondyle—makes the little finger tingle. Severe or chronic damage can lead to sensory loss, paralysis, and muscle atrophy. Affected individuals have trouble making a fist and gripping objects. As the little and ring fingers become hyperextended at the knuckles and flexed at the distal interphalangeal joints, the hand contorts into a *clawhand*. +

Radial Nerve The **radial nerve**, the largest branch of the brachial plexus, is a continuation of the posterior cord. This nerve wraps around the humerus (in the radial groove), and then runs anteriorly around the lateral epicondyle at the elbow. There it divides into a superficial branch that follows the lateral edge of the radius to the hand and a deep branch (not illustrated) that runs posteriorly. It supplies the posterior skin of the limb along its entire course. Its motor branches innervate essentially all the extensor muscles of the upper limb. Muscles controlled by the radial nerve extend the elbow, supinate the forearm, extend the wrist and fingers, and abduct the thumb.

Homeostatic Imbalance 13.6

Trauma to the radial nerve results in *wrist drop*, inability to extend the hand at the wrist. Improper use of a crutch or "Saturday night paralysis," in which an intoxicated person falls asleep with an arm draped over the back of a chair or sofa edge, can compress the radial nerve and impair its blood supply. +

Lumbosacral Plexus and Lower Limb

The sacral and lumbar plexuses overlap substantially. Because many fibers of the lumbar plexus contribute to the sacral plexus via the **lumbosacral trunk**, the two plexuses are often referred to as the **lumbosacral plexus**. Although the lumbosacral plexus serves mainly the lower limb, it also sends some branches to the abdomen, pelvis, and buttock.

Lumbar Plexus The **lumbar plexus** arises from spinal nerves L_1–L_4 and lies within the psoas major muscle **(Figure 13.11)**. Its proximal branches innervate parts of the abdominal wall muscles and the psoas muscle, but its major branches descend to innervate the anterior and medial thigh. Appendix G shows the distribution and targets of the major lumbosacral nerves.

The **femoral nerve**, the largest terminal nerve of this plexus, runs deep to the inguinal ligament to enter the thigh and then divides into several large branches. The motor branches innervate anterior thigh muscles (quadriceps), which are the principal thigh flexors and knee extensors. The cutaneous branches serve the skin of the anterior thigh and the medial surface of the leg from knee to foot.

The **obturator nerve** (ob″tu-ra′tor) enters the medial thigh via the obturator foramen and innervates the adductor muscles. **Table 13.5** summarizes the branches of the lumbar plexus.

Homeostatic Imbalance 13.7

When the spinal roots of the lumbar plexus are compressed, as by a herniated disc, gait problems occur because the femoral nerve serves the prime movers that flex the hip and extend the knee. Other symptoms are pain or numbness of the anterior thigh and (if the obturator nerve is impaired) of the medial thigh. +

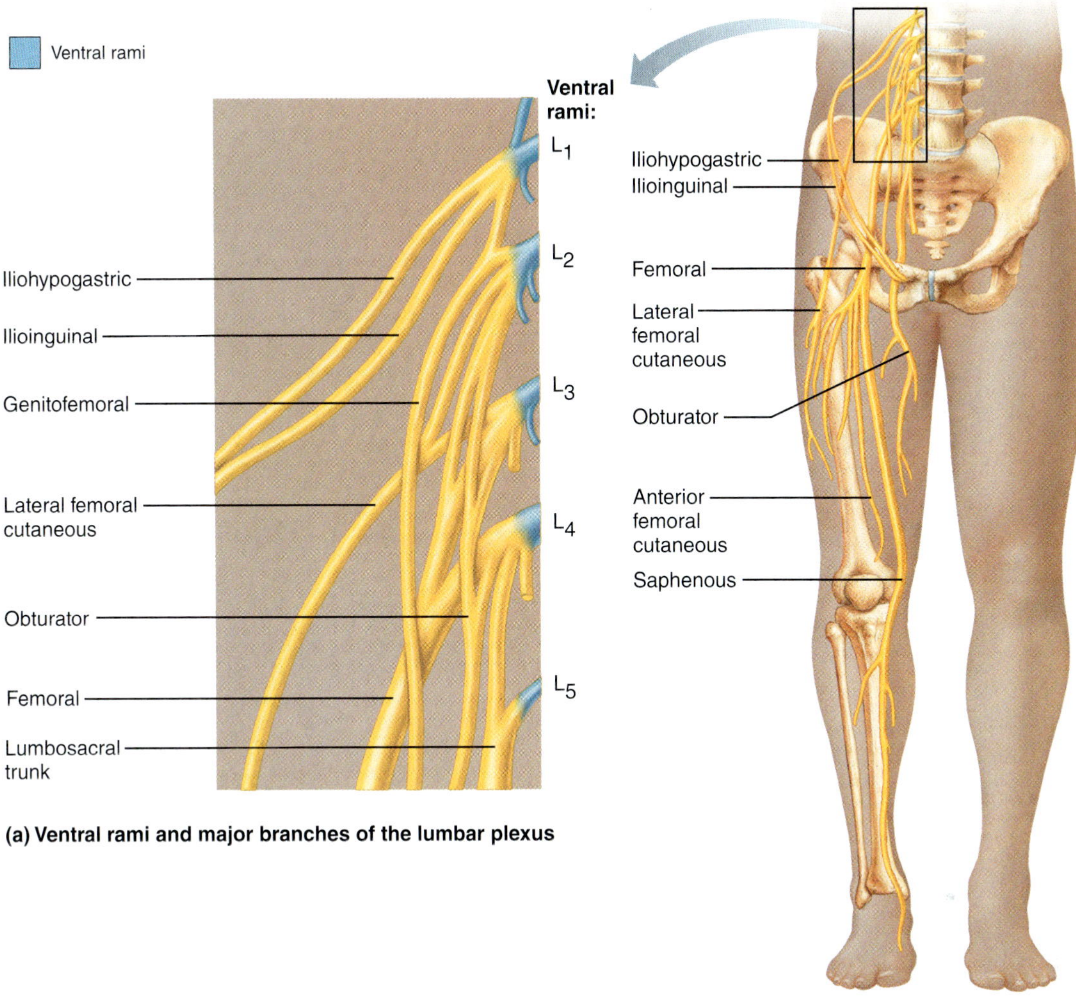

(a) Ventral rami and major branches of the lumbar plexus

(b) Distribution of the major nerves from the lumbar plexus to the lower limb

Figure 13.11 The lumbar plexus. (Anterior view.)

Table 13.5 Branches of the Lumbar Plexus (See Figure 13.11 and Appendix G)

NERVES	VENTRAL RAMI	STRUCTURES SERVED
Femoral	L_2–L_4	Skin of anterior and medial thigh via *anterior femoral cutaneous* branch; skin of medial leg and foot, hip and knee joints via *saphenous* branch; motor to anterior muscles (quadriceps and sartorius) of thigh and to pectineus, iliacus
Obturator	L_2–L_4	Motor to adductor magnus (part), longus, and brevis muscles, gracilis muscle of medial thigh, obturator externus; sensory for skin of medial thigh and for hip and knee joints
Lateral femoral cutaneous	L_2, L_3	Skin of lateral thigh; some sensory branches to peritoneum
Iliohypogastric	L_1	Skin of lower abdomen and hip; muscles of anterolateral abdominal wall (internal obliques and transversus abdominis)
Ilioinguinal	L_1	Skin of external genitalia and proximal medial aspect of the thigh; inferior abdominal muscles
Genitofemoral	L_1, L_2	Skin of scrotum in males, of labia majora in females, and of anterior thigh inferior to middle portion of inguinal region; cremaster muscle in males

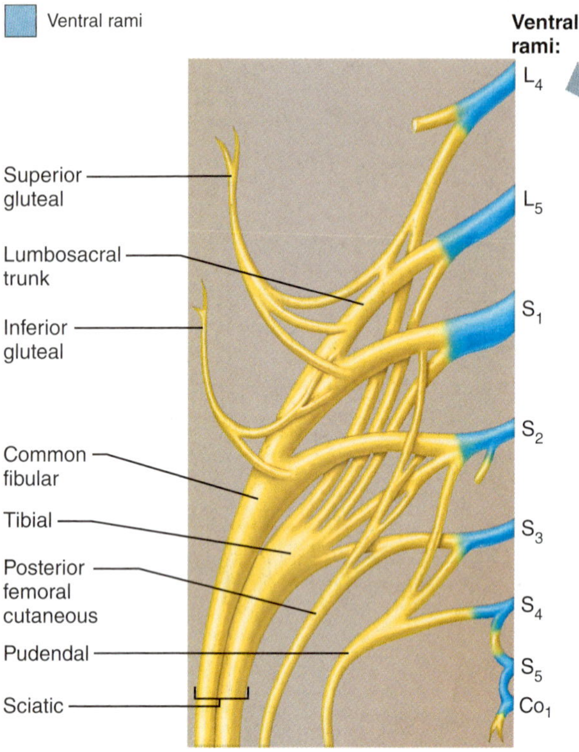

(a) Ventral rami and major branches of the sacral plexus

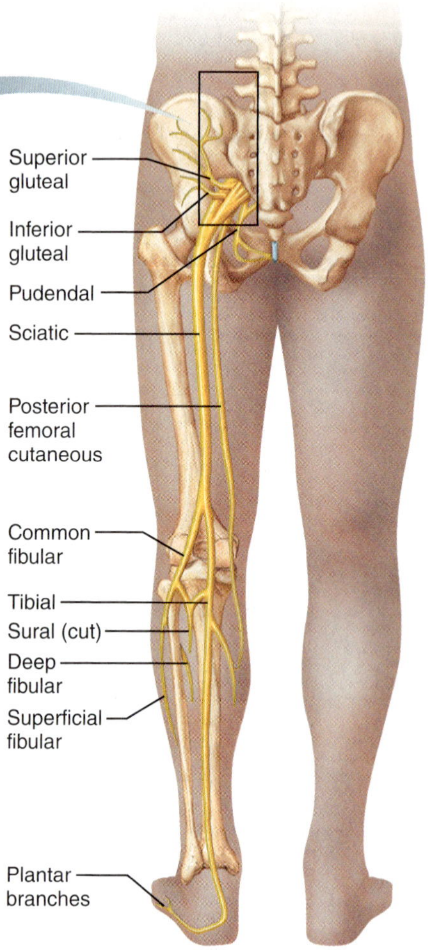

(b) Distribution of the major nerves from the sacral plexus to the lower limb

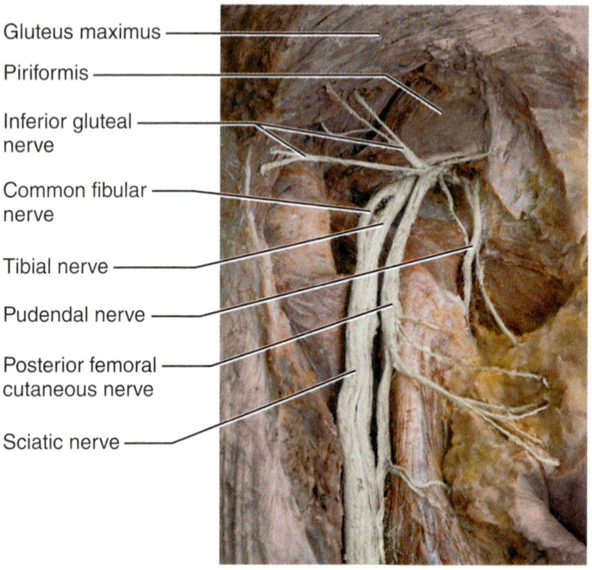

(c) Cadaver photo

Figure 13.12 The sacral plexus. (Posterior view.)

Sacral Plexus The **sacral plexus** arises from spinal nerves L_4–S_4 and lies immediately caudal to the lumbar plexus **(Figure 13.12)**. Some fibers of the lumbar plexus contribute to the sacral plexus via the *lumbosacral trunk*, as mentioned earlier.

The sacral plexus has about a dozen named branches. About half of these serve the buttock and lower limb; the others innervate pelvic structures and the perineum. Here we describe the most important branches. **Table 13.6** summarizes all but the smallest ones.

The largest branch of the sacral plexus is the **sciatic nerve** (si-at′ik), the thickest and longest nerve in the body. It supplies the entire lower limb, except the anteromedial thigh.

The sciatic nerve is actually two nerves—the *tibial* and *common fibular*—wrapped in a common sheath. The sciatic nerve leaves the pelvis via the greater sciatic notch. It courses deep to the gluteus maximus muscle and enters the posterior thigh just medial to the hip joint (*sciatic* = of the hip). There it gives off motor branches to the hamstring muscles

Table 13.6 Branches of the Sacral Plexus (See Figure 13.12 and Appendix G)

NERVES	VENTRAL RAMI	STRUCTURES SERVED
Sciatic nerve	L_4, L_5, S_1–S_3	Composed of two nerves (tibial and common fibular) in a common sheath; they diverge just proximal to the knee
▪ Tibial (including sural, medial and lateral plantar, and medial calcaneal branches)	L_4–S_3	Cutaneous branches: to skin of posterior surface of leg and sole of foot Motor branches: to muscles of back of thigh, leg, and foot [hamstrings (except short head of biceps femoris), posterior part of adductor magnus, triceps surae, tibialis posterior, popliteus, flexor digitorum longus, flexor hallucis longus, and intrinsic muscles of foot]
▪ Common fibular (superficial and deep branches)	L_4–S_2	Cutaneous branches: to skin of anterior and lateral surface of leg and dorsum of foot Motor branches: to short head of biceps femoris of thigh, fibular muscles of lateral compartment of leg, tibialis anterior, and extensor muscles of toes (extensor hallucis longus, extensors digitorum longus and brevis)
Superior gluteal	L_4, L_5, S_1	Motor branches: to gluteus medius and minimus and tensor fasciae latae
Inferior gluteal	L_5–S_2	Motor branches: to gluteus maximus
Posterior femoral cutaneous	S_1–S_3	Skin of buttock, posterior thigh, and popliteal region; length varies; may also innervate part of skin of calf and heel
Pudendal	S_2–S_4	Supplies most of skin and muscles of perineum (region encompassing external genitalia and anus and including clitoris, labia, and vaginal mucosa in females, and scrotum and penis in males); external anal sphincter

(all thigh extensors and knee flexors) and to the adductor magnus. Immediately above the knee, the two divisions of the sciatic nerve diverge.

The **tibial nerve** continues through the popliteal fossa (the region just posterior to the knee joint) and supplies the posterior compartment muscles of the leg and the skin of the posterior calf and sole of the foot.

- In the vicinity of the knee, the tibial nerve gives off the **sural nerve**, which serves the skin of the posterolateral leg.
- At the ankle the tibial nerve divides into the **medial** and **lateral plantar nerves**, which serve most of the foot.

The **common fibular nerve**, or *common peroneal nerve* (*perone* = fibula), descends from its point of origin, wraps around the neck of the fibula, and then divides into superficial and deep branches. These branches innervate the knee joint, skin of the anterior and lateral leg and dorsum of the foot, and muscles of the anterolateral leg (the extensors that dorsiflex the foot).

The next largest sacral plexus branches are the **superior** and **inferior gluteal nerves**. Together, they innervate the buttock (gluteal) and tensor fasciae latae muscles. The **pudendal nerve** (pu-den′dal; "shameful") innervates the muscles and skin of the perineum, and helps stimulate erection and control urination (see Table 10.7). Other branches of the sacral plexus supply the thigh rotators and muscles of the pelvic floor.

Homeostatic Imbalance 13.8

Injury to the proximal part of the sciatic nerve—as might follow a fall, disc herniation, or badly placed injection into the buttock—can impair the lower limbs in a variety of ways depending on the nerve roots injured.

Sciatica (si-at′ĭ-kah), characterized by stabbing pain radiating over the course of the sciatic nerve, is common. When the nerve is transected, the leg is nearly useless. The leg cannot be flexed (because the hamstrings are paralyzed), and the foot and ankle cannot move at all. The foot drops into plantar flexion (it dangles), a condition called *footdrop*. Recovery from sciatic nerve injury is usually slow and incomplete.

If the lesion occurs below the knee, thigh muscles are spared. When the tibial nerve is injured, the paralyzed calf muscles cannot plantar flex the foot and a shuffling gait develops. The common fibular nerve is susceptible to injury largely because of its superficial location at the head and neck of the fibula. Even a tight leg cast, or lying too long on your side on a firm mattress, can compress this nerve and cause footdrop. ✚

Anterolateral Thorax and Abdominal Wall

Only in the thorax are the ventral rami arranged in a simple segmental pattern corresponding to that of the dorsal rami. The ventral rami of T_1–T_{12} mostly course anteriorly, deep to each rib, as the **intercostal nerves**. These nerves supply the intercostal muscles, the muscle and skin of the anterolateral thorax, and most of the abdominal wall. Along their course, these nerves give off *cutaneous branches* to the skin (Figure 13.8b).

Two thoracic nerves are unusual: the tiny T_1 (most fibers enter the brachial plexus) and T_{12}, which lies inferior to the twelfth rib, making it a **subcostal nerve**.

Back

The dorsal rami innervate the posterior body trunk in a neat, segmented pattern. Via its several branches, each dorsal ramus innervates the narrow strip of muscle (and skin) in line with where it emerges from the spinal column (Figure 13.8b).

Innervation of Skin: Dermatomes

A **dermatome** (der′mah-tōm; "skin segment") is an area of skin innervated by the cutaneous branches of a single spinal nerve. Every spinal nerve except C_1 innervates dermatomes. In patients

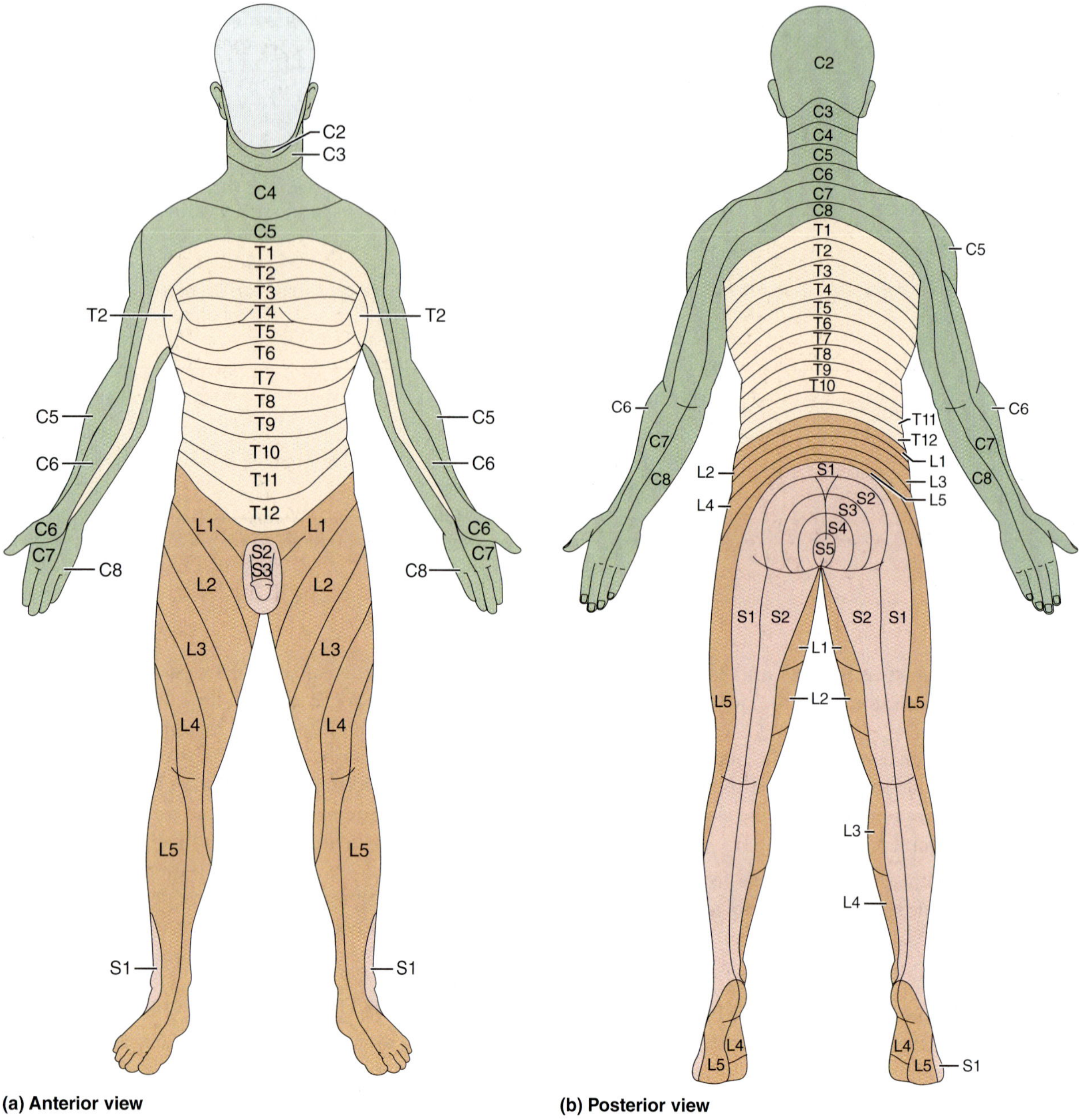

Figure 13.13 Map of dermatomes. Each dermatome is the skin segment innervated by the cutaneous sensory branches of a single spinal nerve. All spinal nerves except C_1 participate in the innervation of the dermatomes.

with spinal cord injuries, you can pinpoint the damaged nerves and the injured region of the spinal cord by determining which dermatomes are affected.

Adjacent dermatomes on the body trunk are fairly uniform in width, almost horizontal, and in direct line with their spinal nerves **(Figure 13.13)**. The dermatome arrangement in the limbs is less obvious. (It is also more variable—different clinicians have mapped a variety of areas for the same dermatomes.) The skin of the upper limbs is supplied by ventral rami of C_5–T_1 (or T_2). The lumbar nerves supply most of the anterior surfaces of the thighs and legs, and the sacral nerves serve most of the posterior surfaces of the lower limbs. (This distribution basically reflects the areas supplied by the lumbar and sacral plexuses, respectively.)

Adjacent dermatomes are not as cleanly separated as a typical dermatome map indicates. On the trunk, neighboring dermatomes overlap considerably (about 50%). As a result, destruction of a single spinal nerve will not cause complete numbness anywhere. In the limbs, the overlap is less complete and some skin regions are innervated by just one spinal nerve.

Innervation of Joints

The easiest way to remember which nerves serve which synovial joint is to use **Hilton's law**: *Any nerve serving a muscle that produces movement at a joint also innervates the joint and the skin over* *the joint.* Hence, once you learn which nerves serve the various major muscles and muscle groups, no new learning is necessary.

For example, the quadriceps, gracilis, and hamstring muscles all cross the knee. The nerves to these muscles are the femoral nerve anteriorly and branches of the sciatic and obturator nerves posteriorly. Consequently, these nerves innervate the knee joint as well.

Check Your Understanding

10. Spinal nerves have both *dorsal roots* and *dorsal rami*. How are these different from each other in location and composition?
11. After his horse-riding accident, the actor Christopher Reeve was unable to breathe on his own. Which spinal nerve roots, spinal nerve, and spinal nerve plexus were involved?

For answers, see Appendix H.

PART 3 Motor Endings and Motor Activity

Peripheral Motor Endings

✓ Compare and contrast the motor endings of somatic and autonomic nerve fibers.

So far we have covered the sensory receptors that detect stimuli and the nerves containing the afferent and efferent fibers that deliver impulses to and from the CNS. We now turn to **motor endings**, the PNS elements that activate effectors by releasing neurotransmitters. Because we discussed that topic in Chapter 9 with the innervation of body muscles, all we need to do here is recap. We will follow the recap with a brief overview of motor integration.

Innervation of Skeletal Muscle

Recall that the terminals of somatic motor fibers that innervate voluntary muscles form elaborate **neuromuscular junctions** with their effector cells (Figure 9.8, p. 287). As each axon branch reaches its target, a single muscle fiber, the ending splits into a cluster of *axon terminals* that branch treelike over the junctional folds of the sarcolemma of the muscle fiber. The axon terminals contain mitochondria and synaptic vesicles filled with the neurotransmitter acetylcholine (ACh).

When a nerve impulse reaches an axon terminal, ACh is released by exocytosis, diffuses across the fluid-filled synaptic cleft (about 50 nm wide), and attaches to ACh receptors on the sarcolemma at the junction. ACh binding opens ligand-gated channels that allow both Na^+ and K^+ to pass. Because more Na^+ enters the cell than K^+ leaves, the muscle cell interior at that point depolarizes. The resulting graded potential is called an *end plate potential.*

The end plate potential spreads to adjacent areas of the membrane where it triggers the opening of voltage-gated sodium channels. This event causes an action potential to propagate along the sarcolemma, which stimulates the muscle fiber to contract. The synaptic cleft at somatic neuromuscular junctions is filled with a glycoprotein-rich basal lamina, a structure not seen at other synapses. The basal lamina contains *acetylcholinesterase*, the enzyme that breaks down ACh.

Innervation of Visceral Muscle and Glands

The junctions between autonomic motor endings and their effectors (smooth and cardiac muscle and glands) are much simpler than the junctions formed between somatic fibers and skeletal muscle cells. The autonomic motor axons branch repeatedly, each branch forming *synapses en passant* ("synapses in passing") with its effector cells. Instead of a cluster of bulblike terminals, an axon ending serving smooth muscle or a gland (but not cardiac muscle) has a series of **varicosities**, knoblike swellings containing mitochondria and synaptic vesicles, that make it look like a string of beads (see Figure 9.26, p. 306).

The autonomic synaptic vesicles typically contain either acetylcholine or norepinephrine, both of which act indirectly on their targets via second messengers. Consequently, visceral motor responses tend to be slower than those induced by somatic motor fibers, which directly open ion channels.

Motor Integration: From Intention to Effect

✓ Outline the three levels of the motor hierarchy.

✓ Compare the roles of the cerebellum and basal nuclei in controlling motor activity.

13

How does integration in the motor system compare with integration in sensory systems? In the motor system, we have motor endings serving effectors (muscle fibers) instead of sensory receptors, descending efferent circuits instead of ascending afferent circuits, and motor behavior instead of perception. However, as in sensory systems, the basic mechanisms of motor systems operate at three levels.

Levels of Motor Control

The cerebral cortex is at the highest level of our conscious motor pathways, but it is *not* the ultimate planner and coordinator of complex motor activities. The cerebellum and basal nuclei (ganglia) play this role and are therefore at the top of the motor control hierarchy. Motor control exerted by lower levels is mediated by *reflex arcs* in some cases, but complex motor behavior, such as walking and swimming, depends on more complex patterns. Currently, we define three levels of motor control: the *segmental level*, *projection level*, and *precommand level* **(Figure 13.14)**.

The Segmental Level

The lowest level of the motor hierarchy, the **segmental level**, consists of reflexes and spinal cord circuits that control automatic movements. A segmental circuit activates a network of ventral horn neurons in a group of cord segments, causing them to stimulate specific groups of muscles.

Circuits that control locomotion and other specific and oft-repeated motor activities are called **central pattern generators**

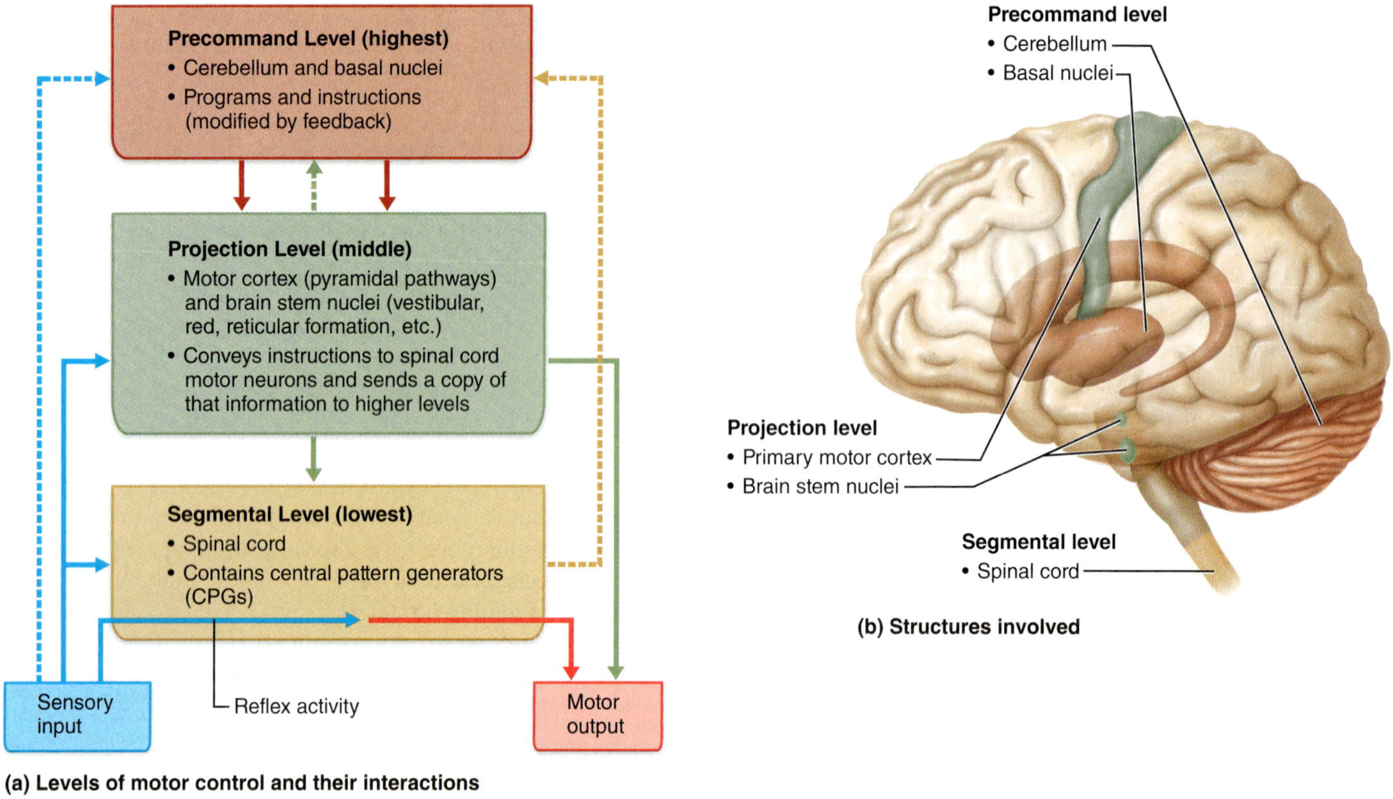

Figure 13.14 Hierarchy of motor control. Dashed lines in (a) indicate feedback.

13

(CPGs). CPGs consist of networks of oscillating inhibitory and excitatory neurons, which set crude rhythms and alternating patterns of movement.

The Projection Level

The spinal cord is under the direct control of the **projection level** of motor control. The projection level consists of neurons acting through the direct and indirect motor pathways (see Table 12.3 and pp. 469–473):

- *Upper motor neurons* of the motor cortex initiate the *direct (pyramidal) pathways*. Axons of direct pathway neurons produce discrete voluntary movements of the skeletal muscles.
- Brain stem motor nuclei oversee the *indirect pathways*. Axons of these pathways help control reflex and CPG-controlled motor actions, modifying and controlling the activity of the segmental apparatus.

Projection motor pathways convey information to lower motor neurons, and send a copy of that information as *internal feedback* to higher command levels, continually informing them of what is supposed to happen. The direct (pyramidal) and indirect pathways provide separate and parallel pathways for controlling the spinal cord, but these systems are interrelated at all levels.

The Precommand Level

Two other systems of brain neurons, located in the cerebellum and basal nuclei, regulate motor activity. They precisely start or stop movements, coordinate movements with posture, block unwanted movements, and monitor muscle tone. Collectively called **precommand areas**, these systems *control the outputs* of the cortex and brain stem motor centers and stand at the highest level of the motor hierarchy.

The key center for "online" sensorimotor integration and control is the **cerebellum**. Remember the cerebellum is a target of ascending proprioceptor, tactile, equilibrium, and visual inputs—feedback that it needs to rapidly correct "errors" in motor activity. It also receives information via branches from descending pyramidal tracts, and from various brain stem nuclei.

The cerebellum lacks direct connections to the spinal cord. It acts on motor pathways through the projection areas of the brain stem and on the motor cortex via the thalamus to fine-tune motor activity.

The **basal nuclei** receive inputs from *all* cortical areas and send their output back mainly to premotor and prefrontal cortical areas via the thalamus. Compared to the cerebellum, the basal nuclei appear to be involved in more complex aspects of motor control. Under resting conditions, the basal nuclei inhibit various motor centers of the brain. When the motor centers are released from inhibition, coordinated motions can begin.

Cells in both the basal nuclei and the cerebellum are involved in this unconscious planning and discharge *in advance* of willed movements. When you actually move your fingers, both the precommand areas and the primary motor cortex are active. At the risk of oversimplifying, it appears that the cortex says, "I want to do this," and then lets the precommand areas take over to provide the proper timing and patterns to execute the desired movements. The precommand areas control the motor cortex and provide its readiness to initiate a voluntary act. The conscious cortex then chooses to act or not act, but the groundwork has already been laid.

Check Your Understanding

12. What are varicosities and where would you find them?
13. Which parts of the nervous system ultimately plan and coordinate complex motor activities?

For answers, see Appendix H.

PART 4
Reflex Activity

The Reflex Arc

✓ Name the components of a reflex arc and distinguish between autonomic and somatic reflexes.

Many of the body's control systems are reflexes, which can be either inborn or learned.

An *inborn* (*intrinsic*) *reflex* is a rapid, predictable motor response to a stimulus. It is unlearned, unpremeditated, and involuntary, and is built into our neural anatomy. Reflexes prevent us from having to *think* about all the little details of staying upright, intact, and alive—helping us maintain posture, avoid pain, and control visceral activities.

For instance, what happens when you splash a pot of boiling water on your arm? You are likely to drop the pot instantly and involuntarily even before you feel any pain. Your response is triggered by an inborn spinal reflex without any help from the brain. In many cases we are aware of the final response of a basic reflex (you know you've dropped the pot of boiling water). In other cases, reflex activities go on without any awareness on our part. This is typical of many visceral reflexes, which are regulated by the subconscious lower regions of the CNS, specifically the brain stem and spinal cord.

The second type of reflex, a *learned* (*acquired*) *reflex,* results from practice or repetition. Take, for instance, the complex sequence of reactions that occurs when an experienced driver drives a car. The process is largely automatic, but only because substantial time and effort were expended to acquire driving skills.

In reality, the distinction between inborn and learned reflexes is not clear-cut and most inborn reflex actions can be modified by learning and conscious effort. For instance, if a 3-year-old child was standing by your side when you scalded your arm, you most likely would set the pot down (rather than just letting go) because you consciously recognized the danger to the child.

Recall the discussion in Chapter 11 about serial and parallel processing of sensory input. What happens when you scald your arm is a good example of how these two processing modes work together. You drop the pot before feeling any pain, but the pain signals picked up by the interneurons of the spinal cord are quickly transmitted to the brain, so that within the next few seconds you do become aware of pain, and you also know what happened to cause it. The withdrawal reflex is serial processing mediated by the spinal cord, and pain awareness reflects simultaneous parallel processing of the sensory input.

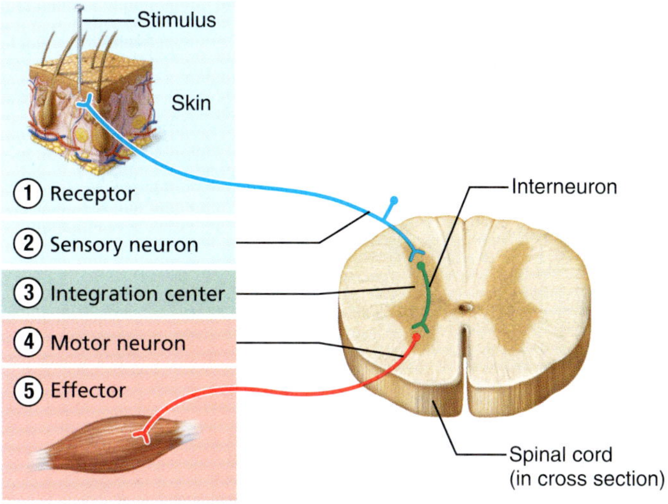

Figure 13.15 The five basic components of all reflex arcs. The reflex arc illustrated is polysynaptic.

Components of a Reflex Arc

As you learned in Chapter 11, reflexes occur over highly specific neural paths called reflex arcs. All reflex arcs have five essential components (**Figure 13.15**):

1. **Receptor:** Site of the stimulus action.
2. **Sensory neuron:** Transmits afferent impulses to the CNS.
3. **Integration center:** In simple reflex arcs, the integration center may be a single synapse between a sensory neuron and a motor neuron (**monosynaptic reflex**). More complex reflex arcs involve multiple synapses with chains of interneurons (**polysynaptic reflex**). The integration center for the reflexes we will describe in this chapter is within the CNS.
4. **Motor neuron:** Conducts efferent impulses from the integration center to an effector organ.
5. **Effector:** Muscle fiber or gland cell that responds to the efferent impulses (by contracting or secreting).

Reflexes are classified functionally as **somatic reflexes** if they activate skeletal muscle, or as **autonomic (visceral) reflexes** if they activate visceral effectors (smooth or cardiac muscle or glands). Here we describe some common somatic reflexes mediated by the spinal cord. We will consider autonomic reflexes in later chapters along with the visceral processes they help to regulate.

Spinal Reflexes

✓ Compare and contrast stretch, flexor, crossed-extensor, and tendon reflexes.

Spinal reflexes are somatic reflexes that are mediated by the spinal cord. Many spinal reflexes occur without the direct involvement of higher brain centers. Generally, these reflexes are even present in animals whose brains have been destroyed as long as the spinal cord is still functional.

13

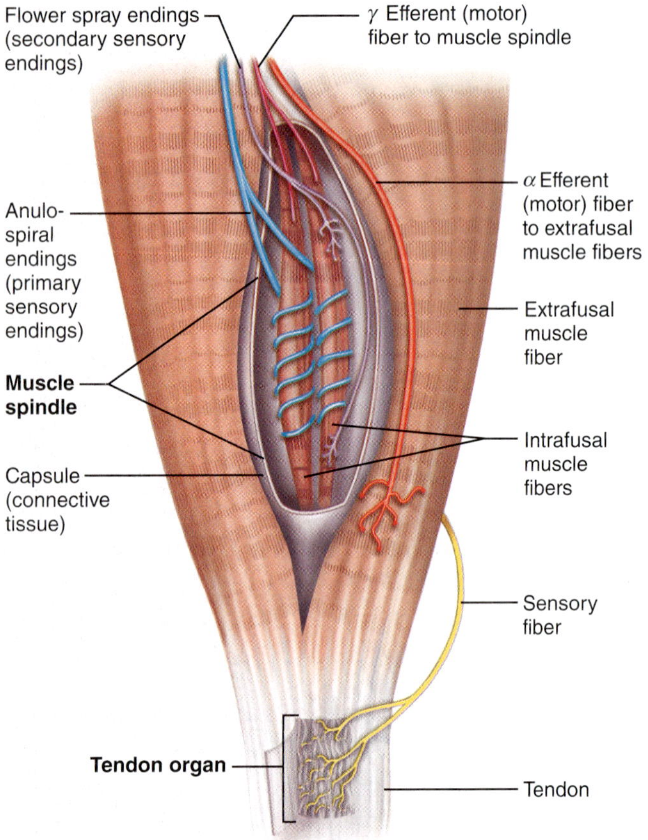

Figure 13.16 Anatomy of the muscle spindle and tendon organ. Notice the afferent fibers from and efferent fibers to the muscle spindle. Myelin has been omitted from all nerve fibers for clarity.

13

However, the brain is "advised" of most spinal reflex activity and can facilitate, inhibit, or adapt it, depending on the circumstances (as we described in the example of the hot water–filled pot). Moreover, continuous facilitating signals from the brain are required for normal spinal reflex activity. As we saw in Chapter 12, *spinal shock* occurs when the spinal cord is transected, immediately depressing all functions controlled by the cord.

Tests of somatic reflexes are important clinically to assess the condition of the nervous system. Exaggerated, distorted, or absent reflexes indicate degeneration or pathology of specific nervous system regions, often before other signs appear.

Stretch and Tendon Reflexes

What information does your nervous system need to smoothly coordinate the activity of your skeletal muscles? Two types of information about the current state of a muscle are key. First, the nervous system needs to know the length of the muscle. This information comes from the *muscle spindles*, found in skeletal muscles. Second, it needs to know the amount of tension in the muscle and its associated tendons. *Tendon organs* provide this information.

These two types of proprioceptors play an important role in spinal reflexes and also provide essential feedback to the cerebral cortex and cerebellum. Just remember, muscle spindles measure **l**ength and tendon organs measure **t**ension. Let's take a closer look at the functional anatomy of these proprioceptors and their roles in certain spinal reflexes.

Functional Anatomy of Muscle Spindles

Each muscle spindle consists of three to ten modified skeletal muscle fibers called **intrafusal muscle fibers** (*intra* = within; *fusal* = the spindle) enclosed in a connective tissue capsule **(Figure 13.16)**. These fibers are less than one-quarter the size of the effector fibers of the muscle, called **extrafusal muscle fibers**.

The central regions of the intrafusal fibers lack myofilaments and are noncontractile. These regions are the receptive surfaces of the spindle. Two types of afferent endings send sensory inputs to the CNS:

- **Anulospiral endings** (also called *primary sensory endings*) are the endings of large axons that wrap around the spindle center. They are stimulated by both the rate and degree of stretch.
- **Flower spray endings** (also called *secondary sensory endings*) are formed by smaller axons that supply the spindle ends. They are stimulated only by degree of stretch.

The intrafusal muscle fibers have contractile regions at their ends, which are the only areas containing actin and myosin myofilaments. These regions are innervated by **gamma (γ) efferent fibers** that arise from small motor neurons in the ventral horn of the spinal cord. These γ motor fibers, which maintain spindle sensitivity (as described shortly), are distinct from the **alpha (α) efferent fibers** of the large **alpha (α) motor neurons** that stimulate the extrafusal muscle fibers to contract.

The muscle spindle is stretched (and excited) in one of two ways:

- By applying an external force that lengthens the entire muscle, such as when we carry a heavy weight or when antagonistic muscles contract (external stretch)
- By activating the γ motor neurons that stimulate the distal ends of the intrafusal fibers to contract, thereby stretching the middle of the spindle (internal stretch).

Whenever the muscle spindle is stretched, its associated sensory neurons transmit impulses at higher frequency to the spinal cord **(Figure 13.17a)**.

During voluntary skeletal muscle contraction, the muscle shortens. If the intrafusal muscle fibers didn't contract along with the extrafusal fibers, the muscle spindle would go slack and cease generating action potentials (Figure 13.17b). At this point it would be unable to signal further changes in muscle length, so it would be useless.

Fortunately, **α-γ coactivation** prevents this from happening. Descending fibers of motor pathways synapse with both α and γ motor neurons, and motor impulses are simultaneously sent to the large extrafusal fibers and to muscle spindle intrafusal fibers. Stimulating the intrafusal fibers maintains the spindle's tension (and sensitivity) during muscle contraction, so that the brain continues to be notified of changes in the muscle length (Figure 13.17b). Without such a system, information on changes in muscle length would cease to flow from contracting muscles.

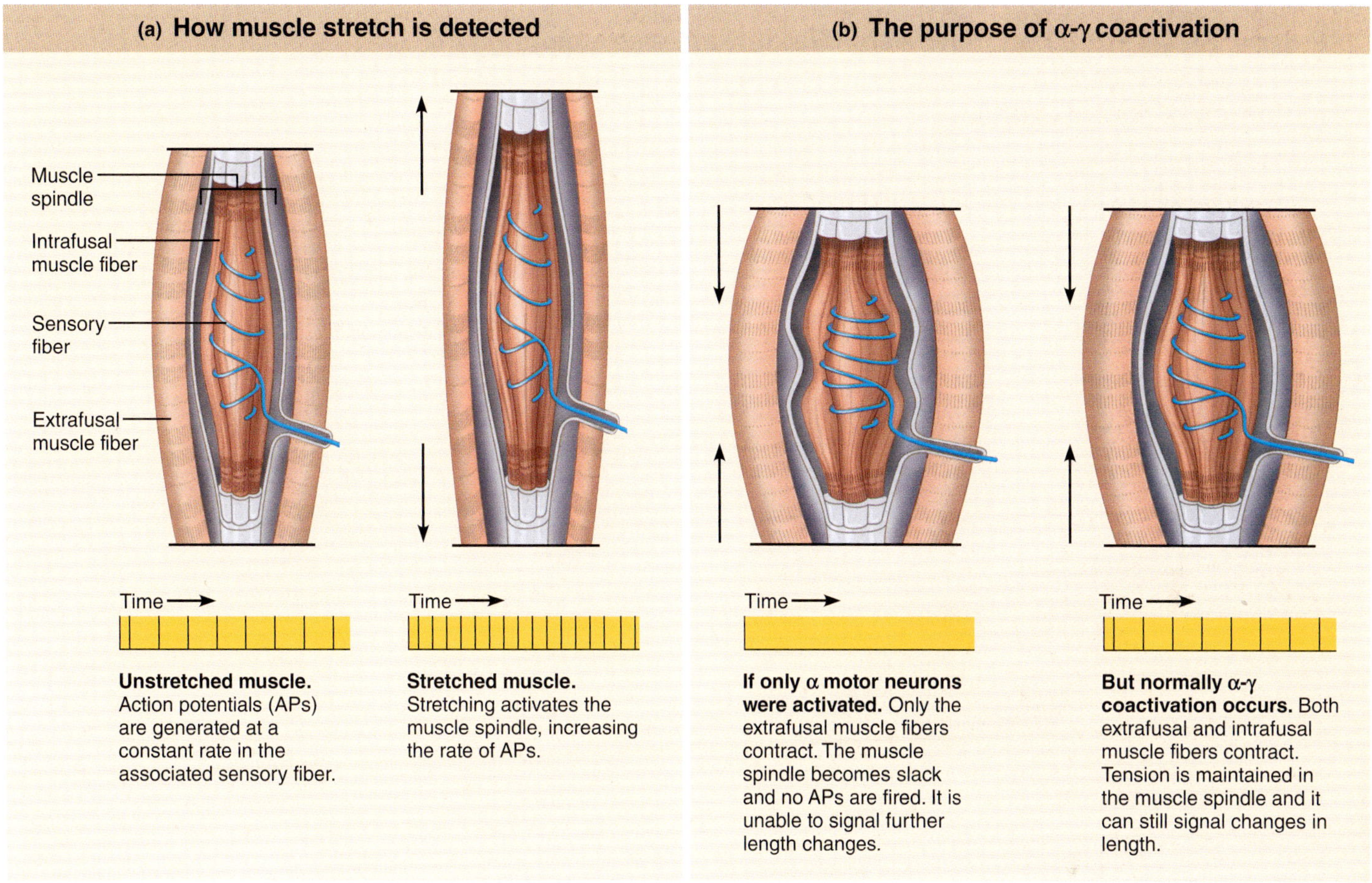

Figure 13.17 Operation of the muscle spindle. The action potentials generated in the sensory fibers are shown for each case as black lines in yellow bars.

The Stretch Reflex

By sending commands to the motor neurons, the brain essentially sets a muscle's length. The **stretch reflex** makes sure that the muscle stays at that length. For example, the **patellar** (pah-tel′ar) or **knee-jerk reflex** is a stretch reflex that helps keep your knees from buckling when you are standing upright. As your knees begin to buckle and the quadriceps lengthens, the stretch reflex causes the quadriceps to contract without your having to think about it. *Focus on the Stretch Reflex* **(Figure 13.18)** shows the stretch reflex and a specific example—the knee-jerk reflex.

The stretch reflex is important for maintaining muscle tone and adjusting it reflexively. It is most important in the large extensor muscles that sustain upright posture and in postural muscles of the trunk. For example, stretch reflexes initiated first on one side of the spine and then on the other regulate contractions of the postural muscles of the spine almost continuously.

Let's look at how the stretch reflex works. As we've just seen in Figure 13.17, when stretch activates sensory neurons of muscle spindles, they transmit impulses at a higher frequency to the spinal cord. There the sensory neurons synapse directly with α motor neurons, which rapidly excite the extrafusal muscle fibers of the stretched muscle (Figure 13.18). The reflexive muscle contraction that follows (an example of serial processing) resists further muscle stretching.

Branches of the afferent fibers also synapse with interneurons that inhibit motor neurons controlling antagonistic muscles (parallel processing), and the resulting inhibition is called **reciprocal inhibition**. Consequently, the stretch stimulus causes the antagonists to relax so that they cannot resist the shortening of the "stretched" muscle caused by the main reflex arc. While this spinal reflex is occurring, information on muscle length and the speed of muscle shortening is being relayed (mainly via the dorsal white columns) to higher brain centers (more parallel processing).

The most familiar clinical example of a stretch reflex is the knee-jerk reflex we have just described. Stretch reflexes can be elicited in any skeletal muscle by a sudden jolt to the tendon or the muscle itself. All stretch reflexes are **monosynaptic** and **ipsilateral**. In other words, they involve a single synapse and motor activity on the same side of the body. Stretch reflexes are the only monosynaptic reflexes in the body. However, even in these reflexes, the part of the reflex arc that inhibits the motor neurons serving the antagonistic muscles is polysynaptic.

A positive knee jerk (or a positive result for any other stretch reflex test) provides two important pieces of information. First, it proves that the sensory and motor connections between that muscle and the spinal cord are intact. Second, the vigor of the response indicates the degree of excitability of the spinal cord. When the spinal motor neurons are highly facilitated by impulses

FOCUS Stretch Reflex

Figure 13.18 Stretched muscle spindles initiate a stretch reflex, causing contraction of the stretched muscle and inhibition of its antagonist.

The events by which muscle stretch is damped

① When stretch activates muscle spindles, the associated sensory neurons (blue) transmit afferent impulses at higher frequency to the spinal cord.

② The sensory neurons synapse directly with alpha motor neurons (red), which excite extrafusal fibers of the stretched muscle. Sensory fibers also synapse with interneurons (green) that inhibit motor neurons (purple) controlling antagonistic muscles.

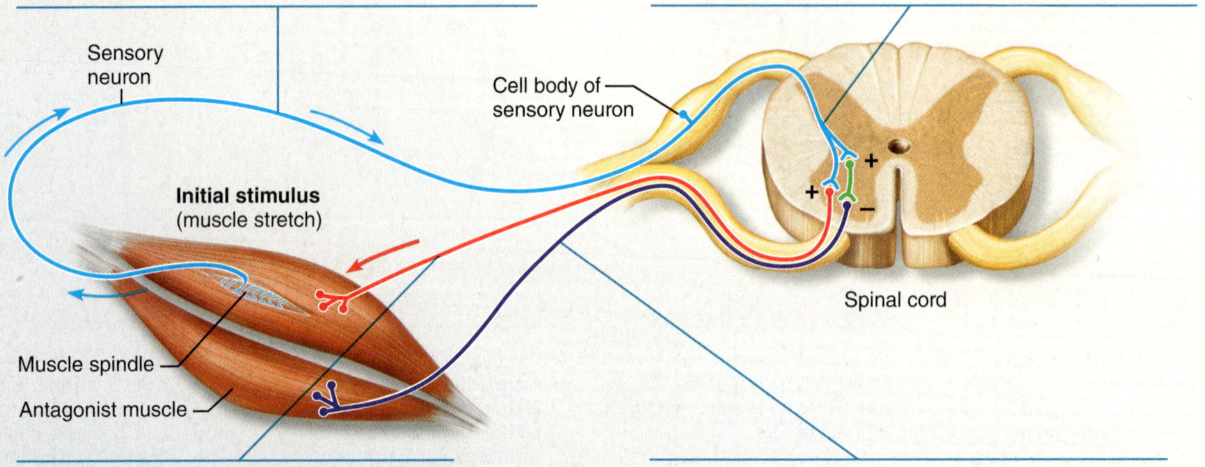

③a Efferent impulses of alpha motor neurons cause the stretched muscle to contract, which resists or reverses the stretch.

③b Efferent impulses of alpha motor neurons to antagonist muscles are reduced (reciprocal inhibition).

The patellar (knee-jerk) reflex—an example of a stretch reflex

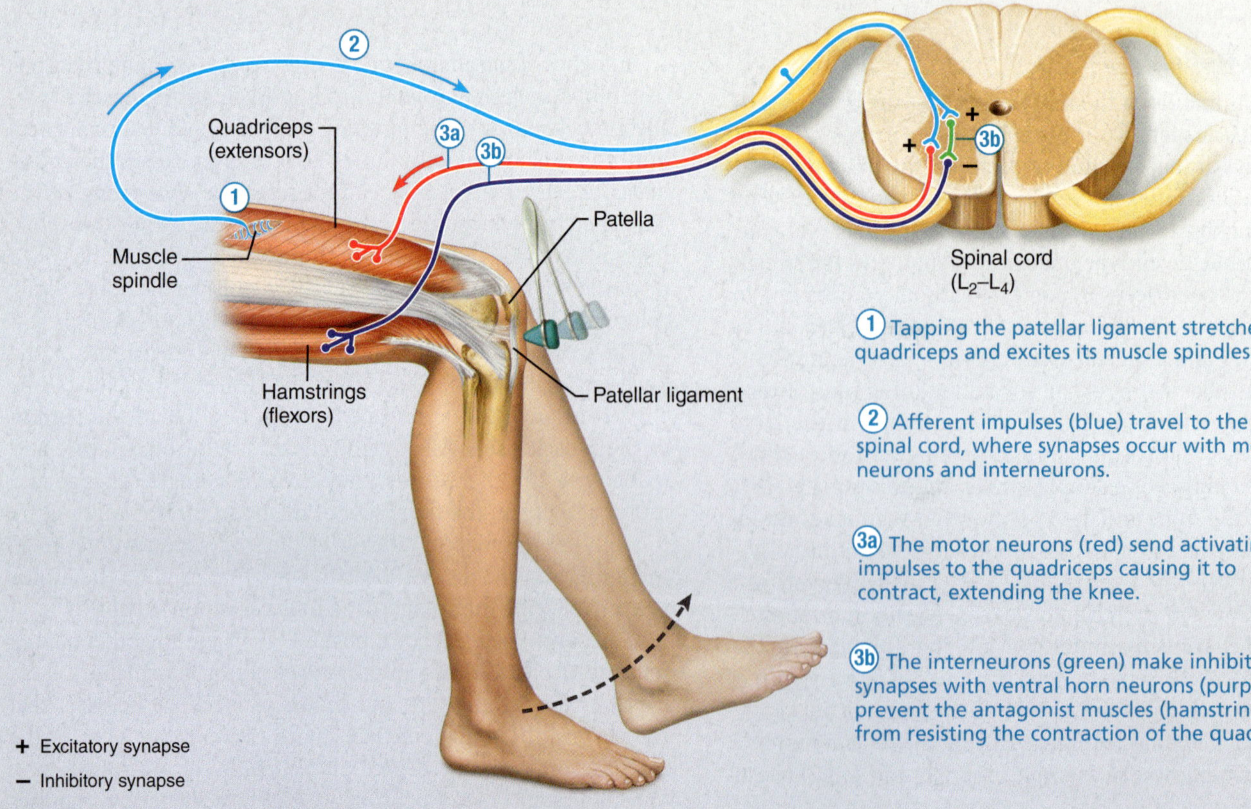

① Tapping the patellar ligament stretches the quadriceps and excites its muscle spindles.

② Afferent impulses (blue) travel to the spinal cord, where synapses occur with motor neurons and interneurons.

③a The motor neurons (red) send activating impulses to the quadriceps causing it to contract, extending the knee.

③b The interneurons (green) make inhibitory synapses with ventral horn neurons (purple) that prevent the antagonist muscles (hamstrings) from resisting the contraction of the quadriceps.

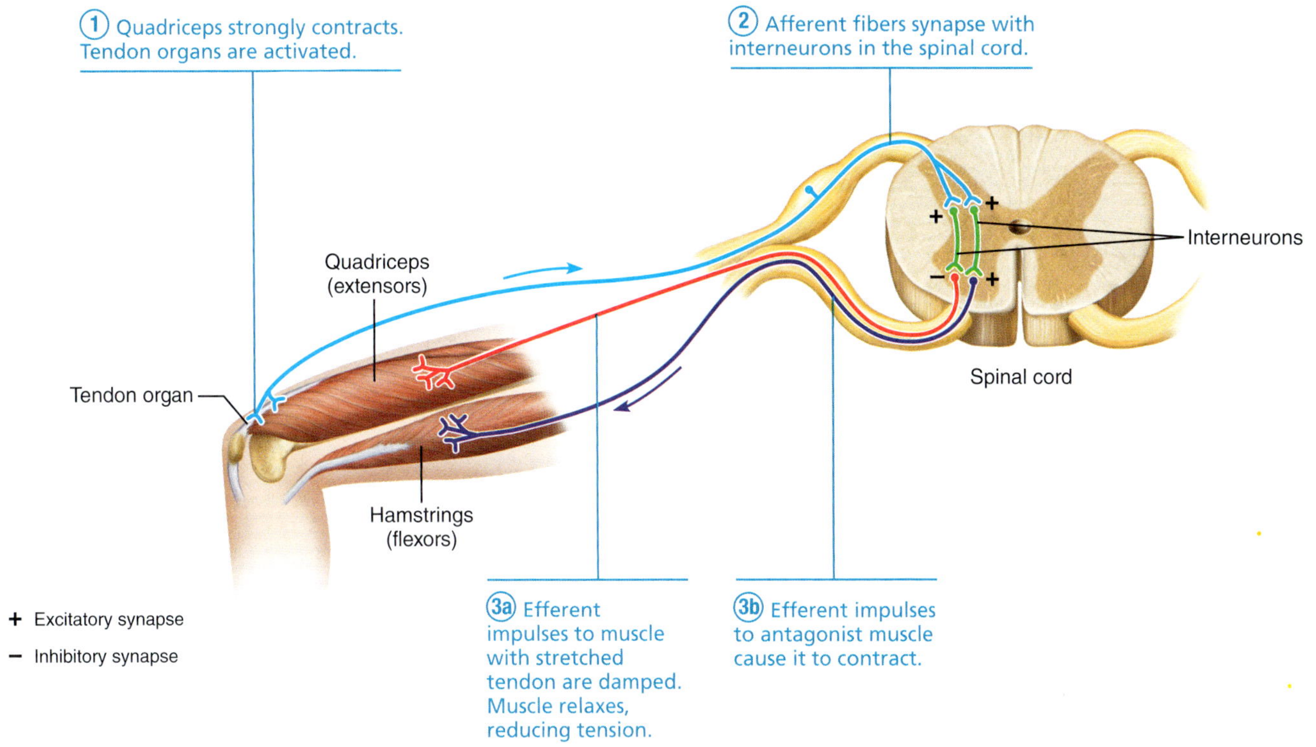

Figure 13.19 **The tendon reflex.**

descending from higher centers, just touching the muscle tendon produces a vigorous reflex response. On the other hand, when inhibitory signals bombard the lower motor neurons, even pounding on the tendon may fail to trigger the reflex response.

Homeostatic Imbalance 13.9

Stretch reflexes tend to be hypoactive or absent in cases of peripheral nerve damage or ventral horn injury involving the tested area. These reflexes are absent in those with chronic diabetes mellitus or neurosyphilis and during coma. However, they are hyperactive when lesions of the corticospinal tract reduce the inhibitory effect of the brain on the spinal cord (as in stroke patients). ✚

Adjusting Muscle Spindle Sensitivity

The motor supply to the muscle spindle allows the brain to voluntarily modify the stretch reflex response and the firing rate of α motor neurons. When the γ neurons are vigorously stimulated by impulses from the brain, the spindle is stretched and highly sensitive, and muscle contraction force is maintained or increased. When the γ motor neurons are inhibited, the spindle resembles a loose rubber band and is nonresponsive, and the extrafusal muscles relax.

The ability to modify the stretch reflex is important in many situations. As the speed and difficulty of a movement increase, the brain increases γ motor output to make the muscle spindles more sensitive. This sensitivity is highest when balance reflexes must be razor sharp, as for a gymnast on a balance beam. On the other hand, if you want to wind up to pitch a baseball, it is essential to suppress the stretch reflex so that your muscles can produce a large degree of motion (i.e., circumduct your pitching arm). Other athletes who require movements of maximum force learn to stretch muscles as much and as quickly as possible just before the movement. This advantage is demonstrated by the crouch that athletes assume just before jumping or running.

As we have seen, muscle tone and smooth coordination of movement depend upon intact stretch reflex pathways. Both afferent and efferent fibers to the muscle spindle are vitally important. If either afferent or efferent fibers are cut, the muscle immediately loses its tone and becomes flaccid.

The Tendon Reflex

Stretch reflexes cause muscle contraction in response to increased muscle length (stretch). The polysynaptic **tendon reflexes**, on the other hand, produce exactly the opposite effect: Muscles relax and lengthen in response to tension.

When muscle tension increases substantially during contraction or passive stretching, high-threshold *tendon organs* may be activated. Afferent impulses are transmitted to the spinal cord, and then to the cerebellum, where the information is used to adjust muscle tension. Simultaneously, motor neurons in spinal cord circuits supplying the contracting muscle are inhibited and antagonist muscles are activated, a phenomenon called **reciprocal activation**. As a result, the contracting muscle relaxes as its antagonist is activated **(Figure 13.19)**.

Tendon organs help to prevent muscles and tendons from tearing when they are subjected to possibly damaging stretching force. Tendon organs also function at normal muscle tensions. In the normal range, tendon organs help to ensure smooth onset and termination of muscle contraction.

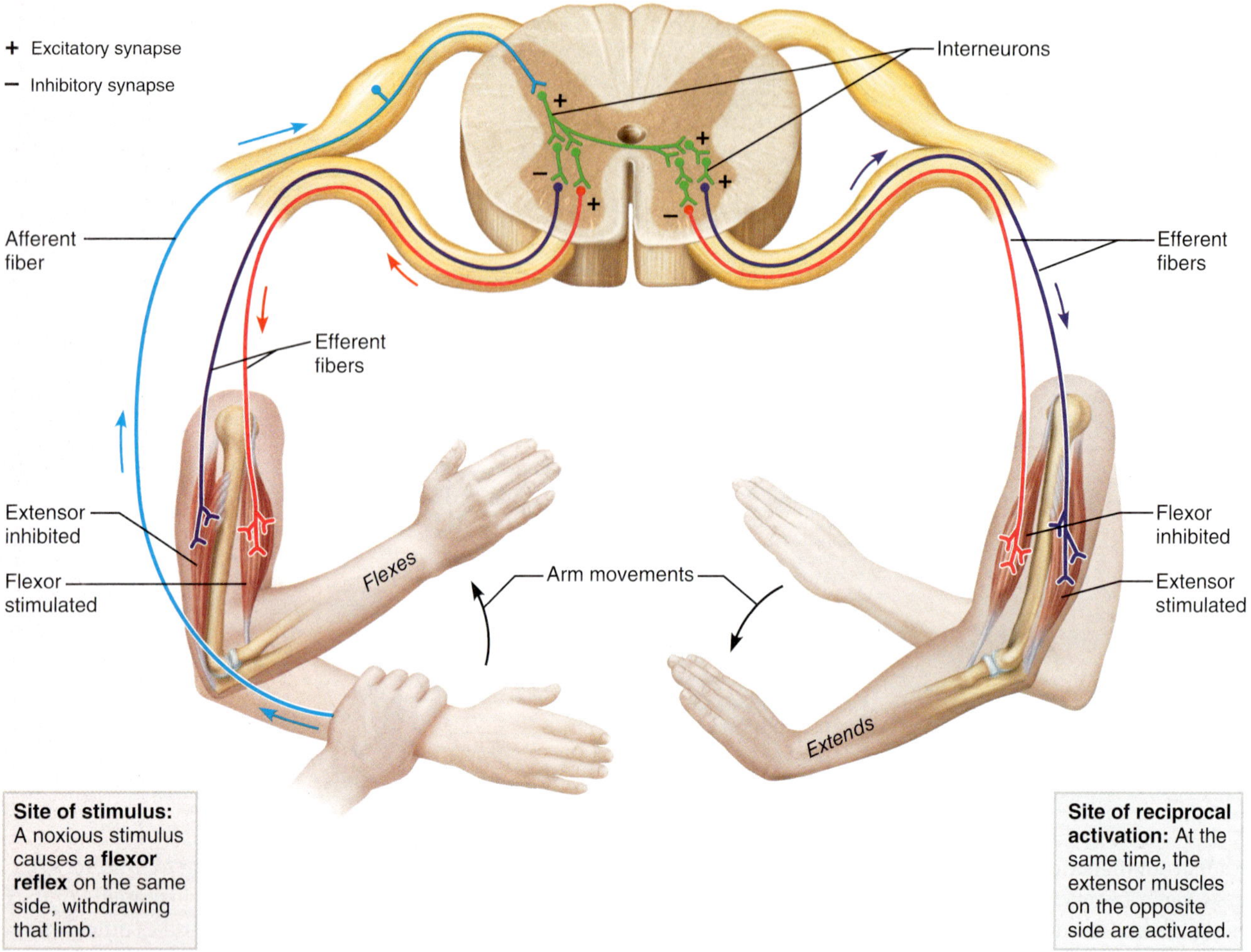

13

Figure 13.20 The crossed-extensor reflex. In this example, a stranger suddenly grasps the right arm, which is withdrawn reflexively while the opposite (left) arm reflexively extends and pushes the stranger away.

The Flexor and Crossed-Extensor Reflexes

A painful stimulus initiates the **flexor**, or **withdrawal**, **reflex**, which causes automatic withdrawal of the threatened body part from the stimulus (**Figure 13.20**, left). Think of the response that occurs when you prick your finger. Flexor reflexes are ipsilateral and polysynaptic, the latter a necessity when several muscles must be recruited to withdraw the injured body part.

Because flexor reflexes are protective and important to our survival, they override the spinal pathways and prevent any other reflexes from using them at the same time. However, like other spinal reflexes, descending signals from the brain can override flexor reflexes. This happens when you are expecting a painful stimulus, for example a skin prick as a lab technician prepares to draw blood from a vein.

The **crossed-extensor reflex** often accompanies the flexor reflex in weight-bearing limbs and is particularly important in maintaining balance. It is a complex spinal reflex consisting of an ipsilateral withdrawal reflex and a contralateral extensor reflex. Incoming afferent fibers synapse with interneurons that control the flexor withdrawal response on the same side of the body and with other interneurons that control the extensor muscles on the opposite side.

The crossed-extensor reflex is obvious when you step barefoot on broken glass. The ipsilateral response causes you to quickly lift your cut foot, while the contralateral response activates the extensor muscles of your opposite leg to support the weight suddenly shifted to it. The crossed-extensor reflex also occurs when someone unexpectedly grabs your arm. The grasped arm is withdrawn as the opposite arm pushes you away from the attacker (Figure 13.20).

Superficial Reflexes

Superficial reflexes are elicited by gentle cutaneous stimulation, such as that produced by stroking the skin with a tongue depressor. These clinically important reflexes depend both on functional upper motor pathways and on cord-level reflex arcs. The best known are the plantar and abdominal reflexes.

Plantar Reflex

The **plantar reflex** tests the integrity of the spinal cord from L_4 to S_2 and indirectly determines if the corticospinal tracts are functioning properly. To elicit the plantar reflex, draw a blunt object downward along the lateral aspect of the plantar surface (sole) of the foot. The normal response is for the toes to flex downward (curl). However, if the primary motor cortex or corticospinal tract is damaged, the plantar reflex is replaced by an abnormal reflex called **Babinski's sign**, in which the great toe dorsiflexes and the smaller toes fan laterally.

Infants exhibit Babinski's sign until they are about a year old because their nervous systems are incompletely myelinated. Despite its clinical significance, the physiological mechanism of Babinski's sign is not understood.

Abdominal Reflexes

Stroking the skin of the lateral abdomen above, to the side, or below the umbilicus induces a reflex contraction of the abdominal muscles in which the umbilicus moves toward the stimulated site. These reflexes, called **abdominal reflexes**, check the integrity of the spinal cord and ventral rami from T_8 to T_{12}.

Abdominal reflexes vary in intensity from one person to another. However, their absence indicates lesions in the corticospinal tract.

☑ Check Your Understanding

14. Name the five components of a reflex arc.
15. What is the role of the stretch reflex? The flexor reflex?
16. Juan injured his back in a fall. When his ER physician stroked the bottom of Juan's foot, she noted that his big toe pointed up and his other toes fanned out. What is this response called and what does it indicate?

For answers, see Appendix H.

Developmental Aspects of the Peripheral Nervous System

✓ Describe the developmental relationship between the segmented arrangement of peripheral nerves, skeletal muscles, and skin dermatomes.

✓ List changes that occur in the peripheral nervous system with aging.

Most skeletal muscles derive from paired blocks of mesoderm (somites) distributed segmentally down the posteromedial aspect of the embryo. The spinal nerves branch from the developing spinal cord and adjacent neural crest and exit between the forming vertebrae, and each nerve becomes associated with the adjacent muscle mass. The spinal nerves supply both sensory and motor fibers to the developing muscles and help direct their maturation. Cranial nerves innervate muscles of the head in a comparable manner.

The distribution of cutaneous nerves to the skin follows a similar pattern. The trigeminal nerves innervate most of the scalp and facial skin. Spinal nerves supply cutaneous branches to specific (adjacent) dermatomes that eventually become dermal segments. As a result, the distribution and growth of the spinal nerves correlate with the segmented body plan, which is established by the fourth week of embryonic development.

Growth of the limbs and unequal growth of other body areas result in an adult pattern of dermatomes with unequal sizes and shapes and varying degrees of overlap. Because embryonic muscle cells migrate extensively, much of the early segmental pattern is lost.

It's crucial that physicians understand the general pattern of sensory nerve distribution. For example, in areas where several dermatomes overlap, two or three spinal nerves must be blocked (anesthetized) to perform local surgery.

Sensory receptors atrophy to some degree with age, and muscle tone decreases in the face and neck. Reflexes occur a bit more slowly during old age. This deterioration seems to reflect a general loss of neurons, fewer synapses per neuron, and a slowdown in central processing rather than any major changes in the peripheral nerve fibers. In fact, peripheral nerves remain viable and normally functional throughout life unless subjected to traumatic injury or ischemia. The most common symptoms of ischemia are sensations of tingling or numbness in the affected region.

13

☑ Check Your Understanding

17. Segmentation in the embryo gives rise to segmentation in the adult. Name two examples of segmentation in the adult body.

For answers, see Appendix H.

The PNS is an essential part of any functional nervous system. Without it, the CNS would lack its rich bank of information about events of the external and internal environments. Now that we have connected the CNS to both of these environments, we are ready to consider the autonomic nervous system, the topic of Chapter 14.

Chapter Summary

MAP™ For more chapter study tools, go to the Study Area of MasteringA&P at **www.masteringaandp.com**.
There you will find:

- Interactive Physiology iP
- A&PFlix *A&PFlix*
- Practice Anatomy Lab PAL
- PhysioEx PEx
- Videos, Practice Quizzes and Tests, MP3 Tutor Sessions, Case Studies, and much more!

1. The peripheral nervous system consists of sensory receptors, nerves conducting impulses to and from the CNS, their associated ganglia, and motor endings.

PART 1 Sensory Receptors and Sensation

Sensory Receptors (pp. 484–487)

1. Sensory receptors are specialized to respond to environmental changes (stimuli).
2. Sensory receptors include the receptors for the general senses—pain, touch, pressure, and temperature receptors in the skin—as

well as receptors in skeletal muscles and tendons and in the visceral organs. Sense organs contain sensory receptors and other cells that serve the special senses (vision, hearing, equilibrium, smell, and taste).
3. Receptors are classified according to stimulus detected as mechanoreceptors, thermoreceptors, photoreceptors, chemoreceptors, and nociceptors, and according to location as exteroceptors, interoceptors, and proprioceptors.
4. The general sensory receptors are classified structurally as free or encapsulated nerve endings of sensory neurons. The free endings are mainly receptors for temperature and pain, although two are for light touch (tactile discs and hair follicle receptors). The encapsulated endings, which are mechanoreceptors, include tactile corpuscles, lamellar corpuscles, bulbous corpuscles, muscle spindles, tendon organs, and joint kinesthetic receptors.

Sensory Integration: From Sensation to Perception (pp. 487–490)

1. Sensation is awareness of internal and external stimuli. Perception is conscious interpretation of those stimuli.
2. The three levels of sensory integration are the receptor, circuit, and perceptual levels. These levels are functions of the sensory receptors, the ascending pathways, and the cerebral cortex, respectively.
3. Sensory receptors transduce (convert) stimulus energy via receptor or generator potentials into action potentials. Stimulus strength is frequency coded. Adaptation (decreased response to a continuous or unchanging stimulus) occurs in all general receptors except pain and proprioceptors.
4. The circuit level consists of the ascending pathways—the axons of the first-, second-, and third-order sensory neurons. These were discussed in Chapter 12.
5. Perception—the internal, conscious image of the stimulus that serves as the basis for response—is the result of cortical processing.
6. The main features of sensory perception are perceptual detection, magnitude estimation, spatial discrimination, feature abstraction, quality discrimination, and pattern recognition.

13

PART 2 Transmission Lines: Nerves and Their Structure and Repair

Nerves and Associated Ganglia (pp. 490–492)

1. A nerve is a bundle of axons in the PNS. Each fiber is enclosed by an endoneurium, fascicles of fibers are wrapped by a perineurium, and the whole nerve is bundled by the epineurium.
2. Nerves are classified according to the direction of impulse conduction as sensory, motor, or mixed; most nerves are mixed. Efferent fibers may be somatic or autonomic.
3. Ganglia are collections of neuron cell bodies associated with nerves in the PNS. Examples are the dorsal root (sensory) ganglia and autonomic (motor) ganglia.
4. Injured PNS fibers may regenerate if macrophages enter the area, phagocytize the debris, and promote the proliferation of Schwann cells. Schwann cells then form a channel and secrete chemicals to guide axon sprouts to their original contacts. Fibers in the CNS do not normally regenerate because the oligodendrocytes inhibit axonal sprouting and regrowth.

Cranial Nerves (pp. 492–501)

1. Twelve pairs of cranial nerves issue through the skull to innervate the head and neck. Only the vagus nerves extend into the thoracic and abdominal cavities. All but the accessory nerve originate from the brain.
2. Cranial nerves are (generally) numbered from rostral to caudal in order of emergence from the brain. Their names reflect structures served or function or both. The cranial nerves and their numbers are
   - I. Olfactory nerves: purely sensory. Concerned with the sense of smell.
   - II. Optic nerves: purely sensory. Transmit visual impulses from the retina to the thalamus.
   - III. Oculomotor nerves: primarily motor. Emerge from the midbrain and serve four extrinsic eye muscles, the levator palpebrae superioris of the eyelid, and the intrinsic ciliary muscle of the eye and constrictor fibers of the iris. Also carry proprioceptive impulses from the skeletal muscles served.
   - IV. Trochlear nerves: primarily motor. Issue from the dorsal midbrain and carry motor and proprioceptor impulses to and from superior oblique muscles of the eyeballs.
   - V. Trigeminal nerves: mixed nerves. Emerge from the lateral pons as the main general sensory nerves of the face. Each has three sensory divisions: ophthalmic, maxillary, and mandibular. The mandibular branch also contains motor fibers that innervate the chewing muscles.
   - VI. Abducens nerves: primarily motor. Emerge from the pons and serve the motor and proprioceptive functions of the lateral rectus muscles of the eyeballs.
   - VII. Facial nerves: mixed nerves. Emerge from the pons as the major motor nerves of the face. Also carry sensory impulses from the taste buds of anterior two-thirds of the tongue.
   - VIII. Vestibulocochlear nerves: mostly sensory. Transmit impulses from the hearing and equilibrium receptors of the inner ears.
   - IX. Glossopharyngeal nerves: mixed nerves. Issue from the medulla. Transmit sensory impulses from the taste buds of the posterior tongue, the pharynx, and chemo- and baroreceptors of the carotid bodies and sinuses. Innervate some pharyngeal muscles and parotid glands.
   - X. Vagus nerves: mixed nerves. Arise from the medulla. Almost all motor fibers are autonomic parasympathetic fibers; motor efferents to, and sensory fibers from, the pharynx, larynx, and visceral organs of the thoracic and abdominal cavities.
   - XI. Accessory nerves: primarily motor. Arise as spinal rootlets from the cervical spinal cord and enter the foramen magnum. Supply somatic efferents to the trapezius and sternocleidomastoid muscles of the neck and carry proprioceptor afferents from the same muscles.
   - XII. Hypoglossal nerves: primarily motor. Issue from the medulla and carry somatic motor efferents to, and proprioceptive fibers from, the tongue muscles.

Spinal Nerves (pp. 501–511)

1. The 31 pairs of spinal nerves (all mixed nerves) are numbered successively according to the region of the spinal cord from which they issue.
2. Dorsal and ventral roots of the spinal cord fuse to form spinal nerves. Spinal nerves are short, confined to the intervertebral foramina.
3. Branches of each spinal nerve include dorsal and ventral rami, a meningeal branch, and in the thoracic region, rami communicantes (ANS branches).
4. Ventral rami, except T_2–T_{12}, form plexuses that serve the limbs.

5. The cervical plexus (C_1–C_4) innervates the muscles and skin of the neck and shoulder. Its phrenic nerve serves the diaphragm.
6. The brachial plexus serves the shoulder, some thorax muscles, and the upper limb. It arises primarily from C_5–T_1. Proximal to distal, the brachial plexus has roots, trunks, divisions, and cords. The main nerves arising from the cords are the axillary, musculocutaneous, median, radial, and ulnar nerves.
7. The lumbar plexus (L_1–L_4) provides the motor supply to the anterior and medial thigh muscles and the cutaneous supply to the anterior thigh and part of the leg. Its chief nerves are the femoral and obturator.
8. The sacral plexus (L_4–S_4) supplies the posterior muscles and skin of the lower limb. Its principal nerve is the large sciatic nerve composed of the tibial and common fibular nerves.
9. Dorsal rami serve the muscles and skin of the posterior body trunk. T_1–T_{12} ventral rami give rise to intercostal nerves that serve the thorax wall and abdominal surface.
10. Joints are innervated by the same nerves that serve the muscles acting at the joint. All spinal nerves except C_1 innervate specific segments of the skin called dermatomes.

PART 3 Motor Endings and Motor Activity

Peripheral Motor Endings (p. 511)

1. Motor endings of somatic nerve fibers (axon terminals) form neuromuscular junctions with skeletal muscle cells. Axon terminals contain synaptic vesicles filled with acetylcholine, which (when released) signals the muscle cell to contract. An elaborate basal lamina fills the synaptic cleft.
2. Autonomic motor endings, called varicosities, are functionally similar, but structurally simpler, beaded terminals that innervate smooth muscle and glands. They do not form specialized neuromuscular junctions and the motor responses elicited are generally slower.

Motor Integration: From Intention to Effect (pp. 511–513)

1. Motor mechanisms operate at the level of the effectors (muscle fibers), descending circuits, and control levels of motor behavior.
2. The motor control hierarchy consists of the segmental level, the projection level, and the precommand level.
3. The segmental level is the spinal cord circuitry that activates ventral horn motor neurons to stimulate the muscles. It consists of reflexes and central pattern generators (CPGs), segmental circuits controlling locomotion.
4. The projection level consists of descending fibers that project to and control the segmental level. These fibers issue from the brain stem motor areas (indirect system) and cortical motor areas [direct (pyramidal) system]. Neurons in the brain stem appear to turn CPGs on and off, or to modulate them.
5. The cerebellum and basal nuclei constitute the precommand areas that subconsciously integrate mechanisms mediated by the projection level.

PART 4 Reflex Activity

The Reflex Arc (p. 513)

1. A reflex is a rapid, involuntary motor response to a stimulus. The reflex arc has five elements: receptor, sensory neuron, integration center, motor neuron, and effector.

Spinal Reflexes (pp. 513–519)

1. Testing of somatic spinal reflexes provides information on the integrity of the reflex pathway and the degree of excitability of the spinal cord.
2. Somatic spinal reflexes include stretch, tendon, flexor, crossed-extensor, and superficial reflexes.
3. A stretch reflex, initiated by stretching of muscle spindles, causes contraction of the stimulated muscle and inhibits its antagonist. It is monosynaptic and ipsilateral. Stretch reflexes maintain muscle tone and body posture.
4. Tendon reflexes, initiated by stimulation of tendon organs by excessive muscle tension, are polysynaptic reflexes. They cause relaxation of the stimulated muscle and contraction of its antagonist to prevent muscle and tendon damage.
5. Flexor reflexes are initiated by painful stimuli. They are polysynaptic, ipsilateral reflexes that are protective in nature.
6. Crossed-extensor reflexes consist of an ipsilateral flexor reflex and a contralateral extensor reflex.
7. Superficial reflexes (plantar and abdominal reflexes) are elicited by cutaneous stimulation. They require functional cord reflex arcs and corticospinal pathways.

Developmental Aspects of the Peripheral Nervous System (p. 519)

1. Each spinal nerve provides the sensory and motor supply of an adjacent muscle mass (destined to become skeletal muscles) and the cutaneous supply of a dermatome (skin segment).
2. Reflexes slow down with age; this probably reflects neuronal loss or sluggish CNS integration circuits.

Review Questions

Multiple Choice/Matching

(Some questions have more than one correct answer. Select the best answer or answers from the choices given.)

1. The large onion-shaped receptors that are found deep in the dermis and in subcutaneous tissue and that respond to deep pressure are **(a)** tactile discs, **(b)** lamellar corpuscles, **(c)** free nerve endings, **(d)** muscle spindles.
2. Proprioceptors include all of the following except **(a)** muscle spindles, **(b)** tendon organs, **(c)** tactile discs, **(d)** joint kinesthetic receptors.
3. The aspect of sensory perception by which the cerebral cortex identifies the site or pattern of stimulation is **(a)** perceptual detection, **(b)** feature abstraction, **(c)** pattern recognition, **(d)** spatial discrimination.
4. The neural machinery of the spinal cord is at the **(a)** precommand level, **(b)** projection level, **(c)** segmental level.
5. Dorsal root ganglia contain **(a)** cell bodies of somatic motor neurons, **(b)** axon terminals of somatic motor neurons, **(c)** cell bodies of autonomic motor neurons, **(d)** axon terminals of sensory neurons, **(e)** cell bodies of sensory neurons.
6. The connective tissue sheath that surrounds a fascicle of nerve fibers is the **(a)** epineurium, **(b)** endoneurium, **(c)** perineurium, **(d)** epimysium.

7. Match the receptor type in column B to the correct description in column A.

Column A	Column B
_____ (1) pain, itch, and temperature receptors	(a) bulbous corpuscles
_____ (2) contains intrafusal fibers and anulospiral and flower spray endings	(b) tendon organ
_____ (3) discriminative touch receptor in hairless skin (fingertips)	(c) muscle spindle
_____ (4) contains receptor endings wrapped around thick collagen bundles	(d) free nerve endings
_____ (5) rapidly adapting deep-pressure receptor	(e) lamellar corpuscle
_____ (6) slowly adapting deep-pressure receptor	(f) tactile corpuscle

8. Match the names of the cranial nerves in column B to the appropriate description in column A.

Column A	Column B
_____ (1) causes pupillary constriction	(a) abducens
_____ (2) the major sensory nerve of the face	(b) accessory
_____ (3) serves the sternocleidomastoid and trapezius muscles	(c) facial
_____ (4) purely sensory (two nerves)	(d) glossopharyngeal
_____ (5) serves the tongue muscles	(e) hypoglossal
_____ (6) allows you to chew your food	(f) oculomotor
_____ (7) impaired in Bell's palsy	(g) olfactory
_____ (8) helps regulate heart activity	(h) optic
_____ (9) helps you hear and maintain your balance	(i) trigeminal
_____, _____, _____, _____, (10) contain parasympathetic motor fibers (four nerves)	(j) trochlear
	(k) vagus
	(l) vestibulocochlear

9. For each of the following muscles or body regions, identify the plexus and the peripheral nerve(s) (or branch of one) involved. Use choices from keys A and B.

_____; _____ (1) the diaphragm
_____; _____ (2) muscles of the posterior leg
_____; _____ (3) anterior thigh muscles
_____; _____ (4) medial thigh muscles
_____; _____ (5) anterior arm muscles that flex the forearm
_____; _____ (6) muscles that flex the wrist and digits (two nerves)
_____; _____ (7) muscles that extend the wrist and digits
_____; _____ (8) skin and extensor muscles of the posterior arm
_____; _____ (9) fibularis muscles, tibialis anterior, and toe extensors
_____; _____, _____, _____, (10) elbow joint

Key A: Plexuses
(a) brachial
(b) cervical
(c) lumbar
(d) sacral

Key B: Nerves
(1) common fibular
(2) femoral
(3) median
(4) musculocutaneous
(5) obturator
(6) phrenic
(7) radial
(8) tibial
(9) ulnar

10. Characterize each receptor activity described below by choosing the appropriate letter and number(s) from keys A and B.

_____, _____ (1) You are enjoying an ice cream cone.
_____, _____ (2) You have just scalded yourself with hot coffee.
_____, _____ (3) The retinas of your eyes are stimulated.
_____, _____ (4) You bump (lightly) into someone.
_____, _____ (5) You are in a completely dark room and reaching toward the light switch.
_____, _____ (6) You feel uncomfortable after a large meal.

Key A:
(a) exteroceptor
(b) interoceptor
(c) proprioceptor

Key B:
(1) chemoreceptor
(2) mechanoreceptor
(3) nociceptor
(4) photoreceptor
(5) thermoreceptor

11. A reflex that causes reciprocal activation of the antagonist muscle is the **(a)** crossed-extensor, **(b)** flexor, **(c)** tendon, **(d)** muscle stretch.

Short Answer Essay Questions

12. What is the functional relationship of the peripheral nervous system to the central nervous system?
13. List the structural components of the peripheral nervous system, and describe the function of each component.
14. Differentiate clearly between sensation and perception.
15. Central pattern generators (CPGs) are found at the segmental level of motor control. (a) What is the job of the CPGs? (b) What controls them, and where is this control localized?
16. Make a diagram of the hierarchy of motor control. Position the CPGs, motor cortex, brain stem nuclei, cerebellum, and basal nuclei in this scheme.
17. Why are the cerebellum and basal nuclei called precommand areas?
18. Explain why damage to peripheral nerve fibers is often reversible, whereas damage to CNS fibers rarely is.
19. (a) Describe the formation and composition of a spinal nerve. (b) Name the branches of a spinal nerve (other than the rami communicantes), and indicate their distribution.
20. (a) Define plexus. (b) Indicate the spinal roots of origin of the four major nerve plexuses, and name the general body regions served by each.
21. Differentiate between ipsilateral and contralateral reflexes.
22. What is the homeostatic value of flexor reflexes?
23. Compare and contrast flexor and crossed-extensor reflexes.
24. Explain how a crossed-extensor reflex exemplifies both serial and parallel processing.
25. What clinical information can be gained by conducting somatic reflex tests?
26. What is the structural and functional relationship between spinal nerves, skeletal muscles, and dermatomes?

Critical Thinking and Clinical Application Questions

1. In 1962 a boy playing in a train yard fell under a train. The train wheel cleanly cut off his right arm. Surgeons reattached the arm, sewing nerves and vessels back together. The boy was told he should eventually regain the use of his arm but that it would never be strong enough to pitch a baseball. Explain why full recovery of strength was unlikely.
2. Jefferson, a football quarterback, suffered torn menisci in his right knee joint when tackled from the side. The same injury crushed his common fibular nerve against the head of the fibula. What locomotor problems did Jefferson have after this?
3. As Harry fell off a ladder, he grabbed a tree branch with his right hand, but unfortunately lost his grip and fell heavily to the

ground. Days later, Harry complained that his upper limb was numb. What was damaged in his fall?

4. Mr. Frank, a former stroke victim who had made a remarkable recovery, suddenly began to have problems reading. He complained of seeing double and also had problems navigating steps. He was unable to move his left eye downward and laterally. Which cranial nerve was the site of lesion? (Right or left?)
5. One of a group of rabbit hunters was accidentally sprayed with buckshot in both of his gluteal prominences. When his companions saw that he would survive, they laughed and joked about where he had been shot. They were horrified and ashamed a week later when they learned their friend would be permanently paralyzed and without sensation in both legs from the knee down, as well as on the back of his thighs. What had happened?
6. You are at a party at Mary's house. After you are blindfolded, an object (a key or a rabbit's foot) is placed in your hand. Which spinal tracts carry the signals to the cortex that will allow you to differentiate between these objects, and what aspects of sensory perception are operating?
7. Mr. Jake was admitted to the hospital with excruciating pain in his left shoulder and arm. He was found to have suffered a heart attack. Explain the phenomenon of referred pain as exhibited by Mr. Jake.

AT THE CLINIC

Related Clinical Terms

Analgesia (an″al-je′zeah; *an* = without; *algos* = pain) Reduced ability to feel pain, but without losing consciousness. An analgesic is a pain-relieving drug.

Dysarthria (dis-ar′thre-ah) Difficulty in articulating speech due to motor pathway disorders that result in weakness, uncoordinated motion, or altered respiration or rhythm. For example, lesions of cranial nerves IX, X, and XII result in nasal, breathy speech, and lesions in upper motor pathways produce a hoarse, strained voice. Not to be confused with *dysphasia* or *aphasia*, which are disorders of language processing.

Dystonia (dis-to′ne-ah) Impaired muscle tone.

Nerve conduction studies Diagnostic tests that assess nerve integrity as indicated by their conduction velocities. The nerve is stimulated at one point, activity is recorded at a second point a known distance away, and the time required for the response to reach the recording electrode is measured. Used to assess suspected *peripheral neuropathies* (see entry in this list).

Neuralgia (nu-ral′je-ah; *neuro* = nerve) Sharp spasmlike pain along the course of one or more nerves. May be caused by inflammation or injury to the nerve(s) (for example, trigeminal neuralgia).

Paresthesia (par″es-the′ze-ah) An abnormal sensation (burning, numbness, tingling) in the absence of stimuli. Caused by a sensory nerve disorder.

Peripheral neuropathy (nu-rop′ah-the) Disease of the peripheral nerves characterized by muscle weakness and atrophy, pain, and numbness. Diabetes is a common cause. Other causes are genetic, other metabolic disorders, infections or inflammation, and toxins.

Tabes dorsalis (ta′bēz dor-sa′lis) A slowly progressive condition caused by deteriorating dorsal tracts (gracilis and cuneatus) and associated dorsal roots. A late sign of the neurological damage caused by the syphilis bacterium. Because joint proprioceptor tracts are destroyed, affected individuals have poor muscle coordination and an unstable gait. Bacterial invasion of the sensory (dorsal) roots results in pain, which ends when dorsal roots have been completely destroyed.

13

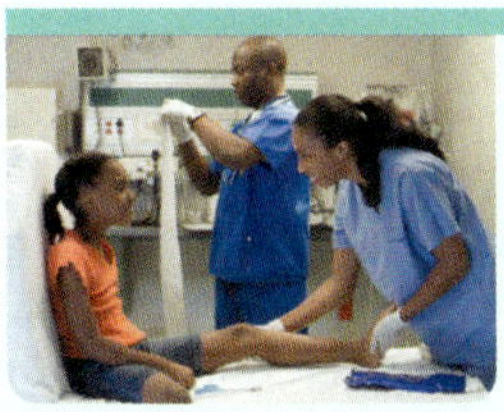

Case Study Peripheral Nervous System

William Hancock, a 44-year-old male, was a passenger on the bus involved in the accident on Route 91. When emergency personnel arrived on the scene, they found Mr. Hancock unconscious, but with stable vital signs. As paramedics placed him on a backboard to stabilize his head, neck, and back, they noted watery blood leaking from his right ear. In the hospital, Mr. Hancock regained consciousness and was treated for deep lacerations on his scalp and face. Head CT scans revealed both longitudinal and transverse fractures of the right petrous temporal and sphenoid bones that extended through the foramen rotundum and foramen ovale.

The following observations were recorded on Mr. Hancock's chart on admission:

- Complete loss of hearing in the right ear.
- Paresthesia (sensation of "pins and needles") at the right corner of the mouth, extending to the lower lip and chin.
- Numbness of the right upper lip, lower eyelid, and cheek.
- Right eye turned slightly inward when looking straight ahead. Diplopia (double vision), particularly when looking to the right.

Mr. Hancock was given a course of antibiotics, the head of his bed was elevated by 30°, and he was placed under close observation. After 24 hours, doctors noted that the right side of Mr. Hancock's face showed signs of drooping, with incomplete eye closure and asymmetric facial expressions. Mr. Hancock's right eye showed minimal tear production. The weakness and asymmetry on the right side of his face began to subside after a few days, and the leak of fluid from his ear stopped, but he continued to complain of paresthesia, diplopia, and an inability to hear with his right ear.

1. In addition to blood, which fluid was leaking from Mr. Hancock's right ear? Which structures must have been damaged to allow this to happen? Why would this lead Mr. Hancock's doctors to give him antibiotics? Why was the head of his bed elevated?
2. Each of the four observations on Mr. Hancock's chart indicates damage to a cranial nerve. Identify each cranial nerve involved. If applicable, identify which specific branch of that nerve is involved.
3. The observations after 24 hours suggest that yet another cranial nerve has been damaged. Which one? How can you explain the lack of tear production in the right eye?

(Answers in Appendix H)

14

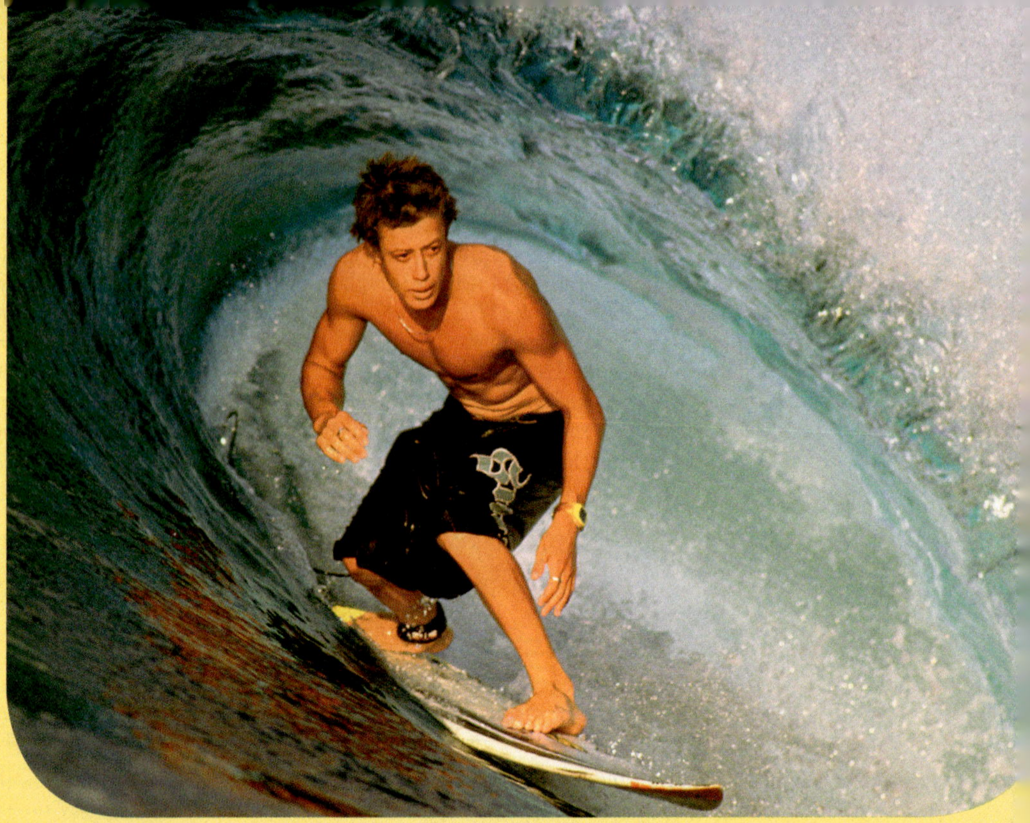

The Autonomic Nervous System

The human body is exquisitely sensitive to changes in its internal environment, and engages in a lifelong struggle to balance competing demands for resources under ever-changing conditions. Although all body systems contribute, the stability of our internal environment depends largely on the **autonomic nervous system (ANS)**, the system of motor neurons that innervates smooth and cardiac muscle and glands **(Figure 14.1)**.

At every moment, signals stream from visceral organs into the CNS, and autonomic nerves make adjustments as necessary to ensure optimal support for body activities. In response to changing conditions, the ANS shunts blood to "needy" areas, speeds or slows heart rate, adjusts blood pressure and body temperature, and increases or decreases stomach secretions.

Most of this fine-tuning occurs without our awareness or attention. Can you tell when your arteries are constricting or your pupils are dilating? Probably not—but if you've ever been stuck in a checkout line, and your full bladder was contracting as if it had a mind of its own, you've been very aware of visceral activity. The ANS controls all these functions, both those we're aware of and those we're not. Indeed, as the term *autonomic* (*auto* = self; *nom* = govern) implies, this motor subdivision of the peripheral nervous system has a certain amount of functional independence. The ANS is also called the **involuntary nervous system**, which reflects its subconscious control, or the **general visceral motor system**, which indicates the location of most of its effectors.

Overview

✓ Define autonomic nervous system and explain its relationship to the peripheral nervous system.

✓ Compare the somatic and autonomic nervous systems relative to effectors, efferent pathways, and neurotransmitters released.

✓ Compare and contrast the functions of the parasympathetic and sympathetic divisions.

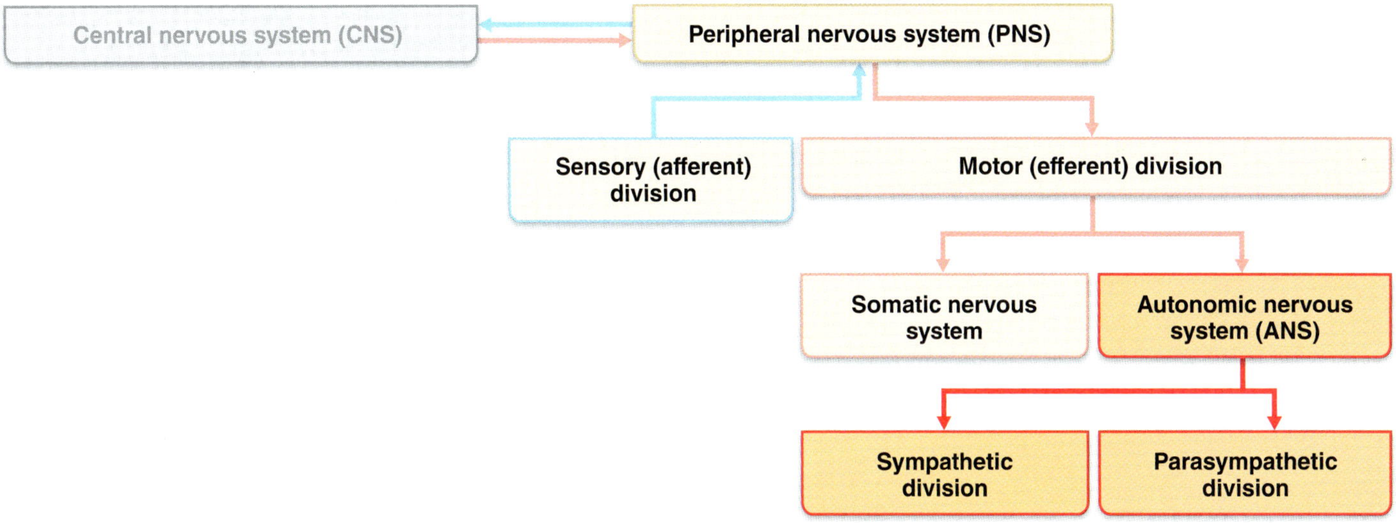

Figure 14.1 Place of the ANS in the structural organization of the nervous system.

Comparison of the Somatic and Autonomic Nervous Systems

In our previous discussions of motor nerves, we have focused largely on the somatic nervous system. So, before describing autonomic nervous system anatomy, let's point out key differences between the somatic and autonomic systems as well as areas of functional overlap.

Both systems have motor fibers, but the somatic and autonomic nervous systems differ in: (1) their effectors, (2) their efferent pathways and ganglia, and (3) target organ responses to their neurotransmitters. Consult **Figure 14.2** for a summary of the differences as we discuss them next.

Effectors

The somatic nervous system stimulates skeletal muscles, whereas the ANS innervates cardiac and smooth muscle and glands. Differences in the physiology of the effector organs account for most of the remaining differences between somatic and autonomic effects on their target organs.

Efferent Pathways and Ganglia

In the somatic nervous system, the motor neuron cell bodies are in the CNS, and their axons extend in spinal or cranial nerves all the way to the skeletal muscles they activate. Somatic motor fibers are typically thick, heavily myelinated group A fibers that conduct nerve impulses rapidly.

In contrast, the ANS uses a *two-neuron chain* to reach its effectors:

1. The cell body of the first neuron, the **preganglionic neuron**, resides in the brain or spinal cord. Its axon, the **preganglionic axon**, synapses with the second motor neuron.
2. The **postganglionic neuron** (sometimes called the *ganglionic neuron*), is the second motor neuron. Its cell body is in an **autonomic ganglion** outside the CNS. Its axon, the **postganglionic axon,** extends to the effector organ.

If you think about the meanings of all these terms while referring to Figure 14.2, understanding the rest of the chapter will be much easier.

Preganglionic axons are thin, lightly myelinated fibers, and postganglionic axons are even thinner and nonmyelinated. Consequently, conduction through the autonomic efferent chain is slower than conduction in the somatic motor system. For most of their course, many pre- and postganglionic fibers are incorporated into spinal or cranial nerves.

Keep in mind that autonomic ganglia are *motor* ganglia, containing the cell bodies of motor neurons. Technically, they are sites of synapse and information transmission from preganglionic to postganglionic neurons. Also, remember that the somatic motor division *lacks* ganglia entirely. The dorsal root ganglia are part of the sensory, not the motor, division of the PNS.

Neurotransmitter Effects

All somatic motor neurons release **acetylcholine (ACh)** at their synapses with skeletal muscle fibers. The effect is always *excitatory*, and if stimulation reaches threshold, the muscle fibers contract.

Autonomic postganglionic fibers release two neurotransmitters: **norepinephrine (NE)** secreted by most sympathetic fibers, and ACh secreted by parasympathetic fibers. Depending on the type of receptors on the target organ, the effect may be excitatory or inhibitory (Figure 14.2; see Table 14.2 on p. 534).

Overlap of Somatic and Autonomic Function

Higher brain centers regulate and coordinate both somatic and autonomic motor activities, and most spinal nerves (and many cranial nerves) contain both somatic and autonomic fibers. Moreover, most of the body's adaptations to changing internal and external conditions involve both skeletal muscles and visceral organs. For example, when skeletal muscles are working hard, they need more oxygen and glucose, so autonomic

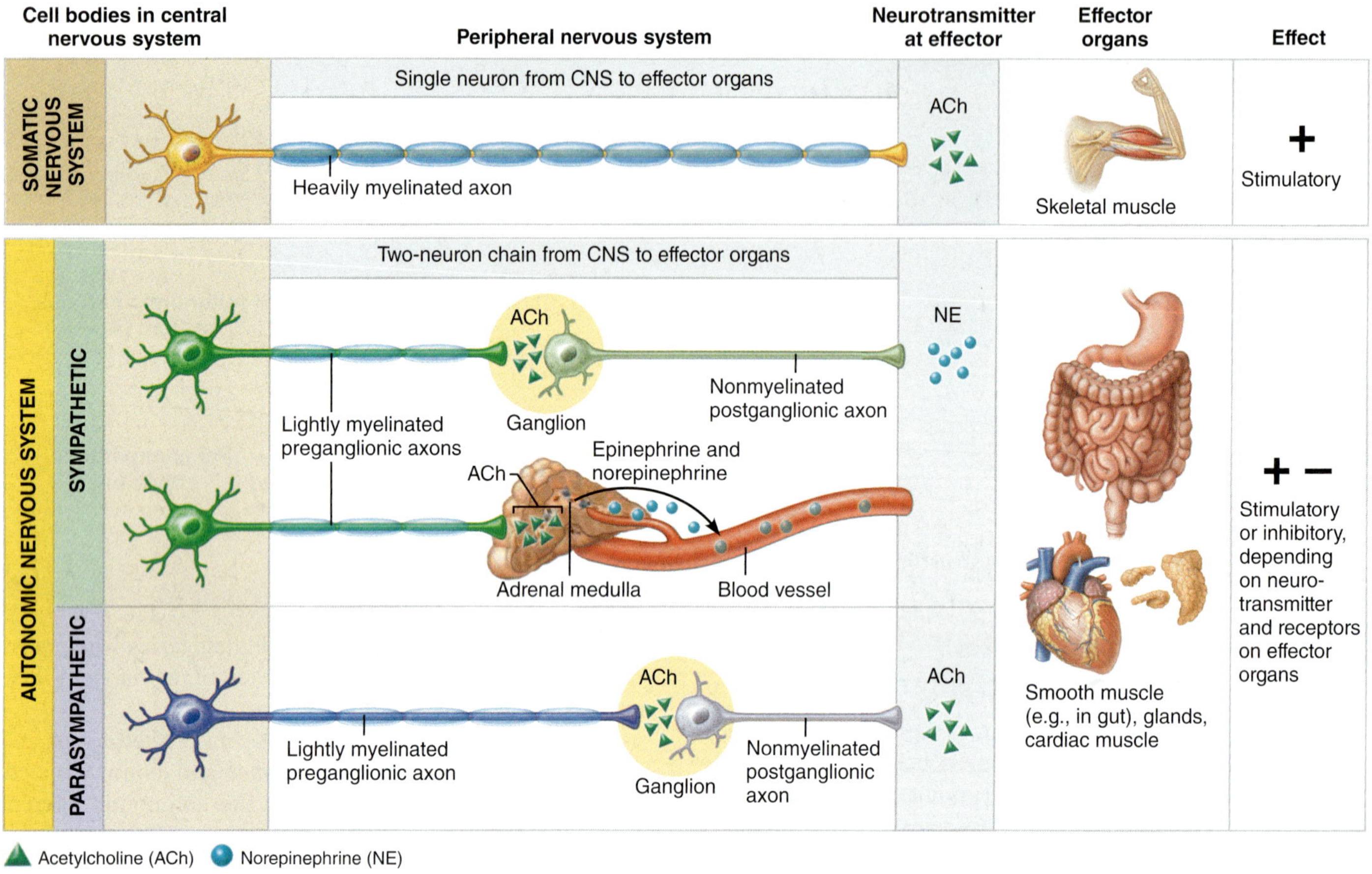

Figure 14.2 Comparison of motor neurons in the somatic and autonomic nervous systems.

control mechanisms speed up heart rate and dilate airways to meet these needs and maintain homeostasis.

Next, we will describe the role of the ANS. But as you read, remember that the ANS does not act in isolation—it is only one part of our highly integrated nervous system.

ANS Divisions

The ANS has two arms, parasympathetic and sympathetic. The *parasympathetic division* promotes maintenance functions and conserves body energy, whereas the *sympathetic division* mobilizes the body during activity.

Both divisions generally serve the same visceral organs but cause opposite effects: While one division stimulates certain smooth muscles to contract or a gland to secrete, the other division inhibits that action. Through this **dual innervation**, the two divisions counterbalance each other to keep body systems running smoothly. Let's elaborate on these functional differences by focusing briefly on extreme situations in which each division exerts primary control.

Role of the Parasympathetic Division

The **parasympathetic division**, sometimes called the "rest and digest" system, keeps body energy use as low as possible, even as it directs vital "housekeeping" activities like digesting food and eliminating feces and urine. (This explains why it is a good idea to relax after a heavy meal: so sympathetic activity does not interfere with digestion.)

Parasympathetic activity is best illustrated in a person who relaxes after a meal and reads a magazine. Blood pressure and heart rate are regulated at low normal levels, and the gastrointestinal tract is actively digesting food. In the eyes, the pupils are constricted and the lenses are accommodated for close vision to improve the clarity of the close-up image (such as your magazine).

Role of the Sympathetic Division

The activity of the **sympathetic division** (often called the "fight-or-flight" system) is evident when we are excited or find ourselves in emergency or threatening situations, such as being frightened by street toughs late at night. A rapidly pounding heart; deep breathing; dry mouth; cold, sweaty skin; and dilated eye pupils are sure signs of sympathetic nervous system mobilization.

During any type of vigorous physical activity, the sympathetic division also promotes a number of other adjustments. It:

- Constricts visceral (and sometimes cutaneous) blood vessels, shunting blood to active skeletal muscles and the vigorously working heart

- Dilates the bronchioles in the lungs, increasing ventilation (and thus increasing oxygen delivery to body cells)
- Causes the liver to release more glucose into the blood to accommodate the increased energy needs of body cells

At the same time, the sympathetic division temporarily damps nonessential activities, such as gastrointestinal tract motility. If you are running from a mugger, digesting lunch can wait! It is far more important to give your muscles everything they need to get you out of danger. In such active situations, the sympathetic division generates a head of steam that enables the body to cope with situations that threaten homeostasis. It provides the optimal conditions for an appropriate response to some threat, whether that response is to run, see distant objects better, or think more clearly.

We have just looked at two extreme situations in which one or the other branch of the ANS dominates. Think of the parasympathetic division as the **D** division [digestion, defecation, and diuresis (urination)], and the sympathetic division as the **E** division (exercise, excitement, emergency, embarrassment). Table 14.4 (p. 536) presents a more detailed summary of how each division affects various organs.

Remember, however, that the two ANS divisions rarely work in an all-or-none fashion as described above. A dynamic antagonism exists between the divisions, and both make continuous fine adjustments to maintain homeostasis.

Check Your Understanding

1. Name the three types of effectors of the autonomic nervous system.
2. Which relays instructions from the CNS to muscles more quickly, the somatic nervous system or the ANS? Explain why.
3. Which branch of the ANS would predominate if you were lying on the beach enjoying the sun and the sound of the waves? Which branch would predominate if you were on a surfboard and a shark appeared within a few feet of you?

For answers, see Appendix H.

ANS Anatomy

✓ For the parasympathetic and sympathetic divisions, describe the site of CNS origin, locations of ganglia, and general fiber pathways.

Anatomically, the sympathetic and parasympathetic divisions differ in

- **Sites of origin.** Parasympathetic fibers are craniosacral—they originate in the brain (cranium) and sacral spinal cord. Sympathetic fibers are thoracolumbar—they originate in the thoracic and lumbar regions of the spinal cord.
- **Relative lengths of their fibers.** The parasympathetic division has long preganglionic and short postganglionic fibers. The sympathetic division has the opposite condition—the preganglionic fibers are short and the postganglionic fibers are long.

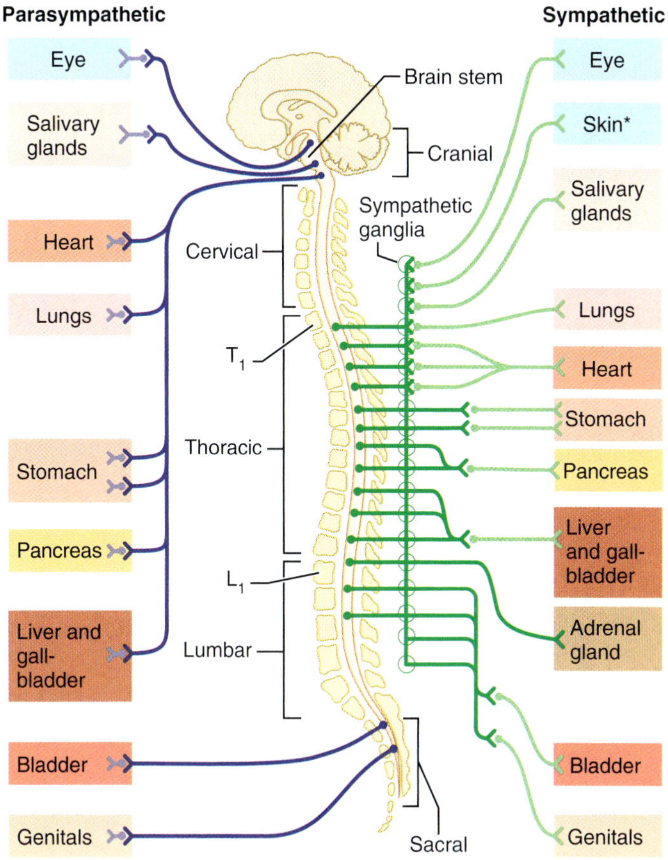

Figure 14.3 The subdivisions of the ANS. The parasympathetic and sympathetic divisions differ anatomically in the (1) sites where their nerves originate, (2) relative lengths of their preganglionic and postganglionic fibers, and (3) locations of their ganglia (indicated here by synapse sites).

*Although sympathetic innervation to the skin is mapped to the cervical region here, all nerves to the periphery carry postganglionic sympathetic fibers.

- **Location of their ganglia.** Most parasympathetic ganglia are located in the visceral effector organs. Sympathetic ganglia lie close to the spinal cord.

Figure 14.3 illustrates these and other key differences, which are summarized in **Table 14.1**.

We begin our detailed exploration of the ANS with the anatomically simpler parasympathetic division.

Parasympathetic (Craniosacral) Division

The parasympathetic division is also called the **craniosacral division** because its preganglionic fibers spring from opposite ends of the CNS—the brain stem and the sacral region of the spinal cord **(Figure 14.4)**. The preganglionic axons extend from the CNS nearly all the way to the structures they innervate. There the axons synapse with postganglionic neurons located in **terminal ganglia** that lie close to or within the target organs. Very short postganglionic axons issue from the terminal ganglia and synapse with effector cells in their immediate area.

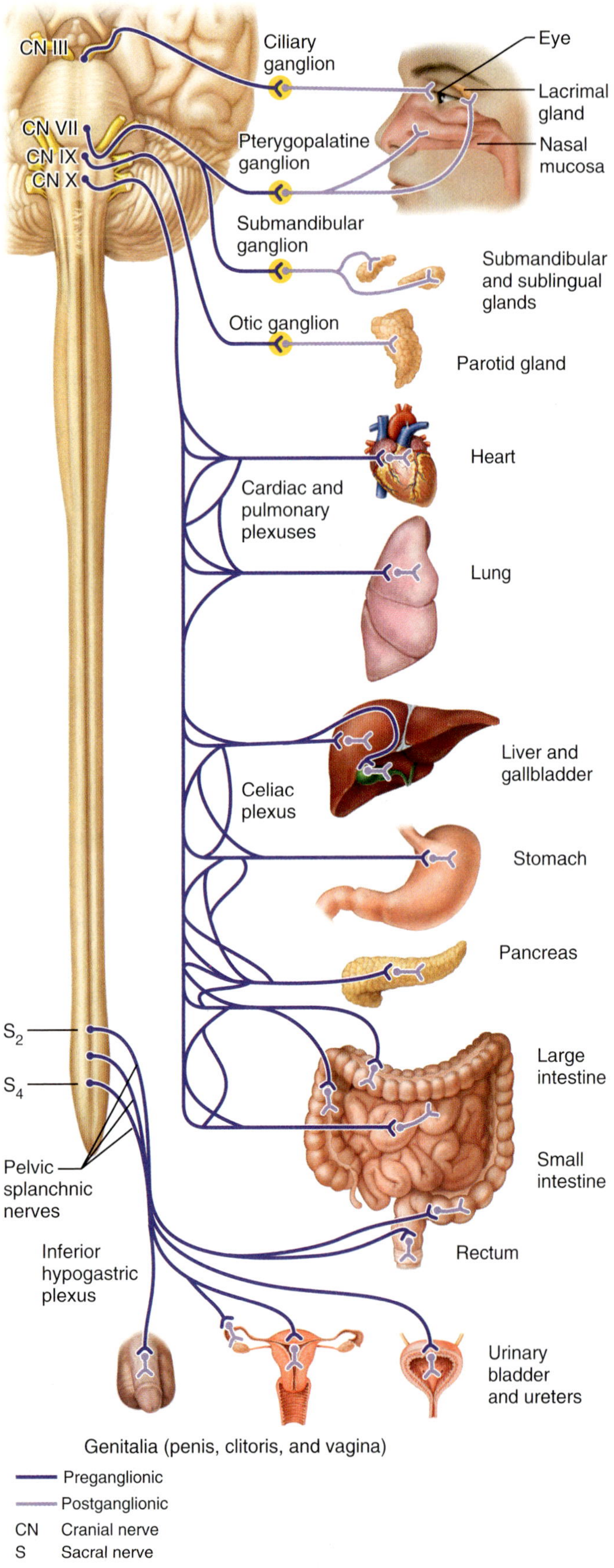

Figure 14.4 **Parasympathetic division of the ANS.**

Cranial Part

Preganglionic fibers run in the oculomotor, facial, glossopharyngeal, and vagus cranial nerves. Their cell bodies lie in associated motor cranial-nerve nuclei in the brain stem (see Figures 12.13 and 12.14). Next, let's look at where the neurons of the cranial parasympathetics are located.

Oculomotor Nerves The parasympathetic fibers of the **oculomotor nerves (III)** innervate smooth muscles in the eyes that cause the pupils to constrict and the lenses to bulge—actions needed to focus on close objects. The preganglionic axons found in the oculomotor nerves issue from the *accessory oculomotor (Edinger-Westphal) nuclei* in the midbrain. The cell bodies of the postganglionic neurons are in the **ciliary ganglia** within the eye orbits (see Table 13.2, p. 495).

Facial Nerves The parasympathetic fibers of the **facial nerves (VII)** stimulate many large glands in the head.

Fibers that activate the nasal glands and the lacrimal glands of the eyes originate in the *lacrimal nuclei* of the pons. The preganglionic fibers synapse with postganglionic neurons in the **pterygopalatine ganglia** (ter″eh-go-pal′ah-tīn) just posterior to the maxillae.

The preganglionic neurons that stimulate the submandibular and sublingual salivary glands originate in the *superior salivatory nuclei* of the pons. They synapse with postganglionic neurons in the **submandibular ganglia**, deep to the mandibular angles (see Table 13.2, p. 497).

Glossopharyngeal Nerves The parasympathetics in the **glossopharyngeal nerves (IX)** originate in the *inferior salivatory nuclei* of the medulla and synapse in the **otic ganglia**, located just inferior to the foramen ovale of the skull. The postganglionic fibers course to and activate the parotid salivary glands anterior to the ears (see Table 13.2, p. 499).

Cranial nerves III, VII, and IX supply the entire parasympathetic innervation of the head. Note that only the *preganglionic* fibers lie within these three pairs of cranial nerves—*postganglionic* fibers do not. Many of the postganglionic fibers "hitch a ride" with branches of the *trigeminal nerve* (*V*), taking advantage of its wide distribution.

Vagus Nerves Between them, the two **vagus nerves (X)** account for about 90% of all preganglionic parasympathetic fibers in the body. They provide fibers to the neck and to nerve plexuses (interweaving networks of nerves) that serve virtually every organ in the thoracic and abdominal cavities.

The vagal nerve fibers (preganglionic axons) arise mostly from the *dorsal motor nuclei* of the medulla and synapse in terminal ganglia usually located in the walls of the target organ. Rather than having individual names, most of the terminal ganglia are collectively called *intramural ganglia*, literally, "ganglia within the walls."

As the vagus nerves pass into the thorax, they send branches to the **cardiac plexuses** supplying fibers to the heart that slow heart rate, the **pulmonary plexuses** serving the lungs and bronchi, and the **esophageal plexuses** (ĕ-sof″ah-je′al) supplying the esophagus.

Table 14.1 Anatomical and Physiological Differences Between the Parasympathetic and Sympathetic Divisions

CHARACTERISTIC	PARASYMPATHETIC	SYMPATHETIC
Origin	Craniosacral part: brain stem nuclei of cranial nerves III, VII, IX, and X; spinal cord segments S_2–S_4.	Thoracolumbar part: lateral horns of gray matter of spinal cord segments T_1–L_2.
Location of ganglia	Ganglia (terminal ganglia) are within the visceral organ (intramural) or close to the organ served.	Ganglia are within a few centimeters of CNS: alongside vertebral column (sympathetic trunk ganglia) and anterior to vertebral column (collateral, or prevertebral, ganglia).
Relative length of pre- and postganglionic fibers	Long preganglionic; short postganglionic.	Short preganglionic; long postganglionic.
Rami communicantes	None.	Gray and white rami communicantes. White rami contain myelinated preganglionic fibers. Gray contain nonmyelinated postganglionic fibers.
Degree of branching of preganglionic fibers	Minimal.	Extensive.
Functional role	Maintenance functions; conserves and stores energy; "rest and digest."	Prepares body for activity; "fight or flight."
Neurotransmitters	All preganglionic and postganglionic fibers release ACh (cholinergic fibers).	All preganglionic fibers release ACh. Most postganglionic fibers release norepinephrine (adrenergic fibers). Postganglionic fibers serving sweat glands release ACh. Neurotransmitter activity is augmented by release of adrenal medullary hormones (norepinephrine and epinephrine).

When the main trunks of the vagus nerves reach the esophagus, their fibers intermingle, forming the **anterior** and **posterior vagal trunks**, each containing fibers from both vagus nerves. These vagal trunks then "ride" the esophagus down to the abdominal cavity. There they send fibers *through* the large **abdominal aortic plexus** [formed by a number of smaller plexuses (e.g., *celiac, superior mesenteric*, and *hypogastric*) that run along the aorta] before giving off branches to the abdominal viscera. The vagus nerves innervate the liver, gallbladder, stomach, small intestine, kidneys, pancreas, and the proximal half of the large intestine.

Sacral Part

The sacral part of the parasympathetic division serves the pelvic organs and the distal half of the large intestine. The sacral part arises from neurons located in the lateral gray matter of spinal cord segments S_2–S_4. Axons of these neurons run in the ventral roots of the spinal nerves to the ventral rami and then branch off to form the **pelvic splanchnic nerves** (splank′nik; *splanchni* = viscera), which pass through the **inferior hypogastric (pelvic) plexus** in the pelvic floor (Figure 14.4). Some preganglionic fibers synapse with ganglia in this plexus, but most synapse in intramural ganglia in the walls of the following organs: distal half of the large intestine, urinary bladder, ureters, and reproductive organs.

Sympathetic (Thoracolumbar) Division

The sympathetic division is anatomically more complex than the parasympathetic division, partly because it innervates more organs. It supplies not only the visceral organs in the internal body cavities but also all visceral structures in the superficial (somatic) part of the body. This sounds impossible, but there is an explanation—some glands and smooth muscle structures in the soma (sweat glands and the hair-raising arrector pili muscles of the skin) require autonomic innervation and are served only by sympathetic fibers. In addition, sympathetic fibers innervate smooth muscle in the walls of all arteries and veins, both deep and superficial. But we will explain these matters later—let's get on with the anatomy of the sympathetic division.

All preganglionic fibers of the sympathetic division arise from cell bodies of preganglionic neurons in spinal cord segments T_1 through L_2 (Figure 14.3). For this reason, the sympathetic division is also referred to as the **thoracolumbar division** (tho-rah″ko-lum′bar).

The numerous preganglionic sympathetic neurons in the gray matter of the spinal cord form the **lateral horns** (see Figures 12.28b, p. 467, and 12.29, p. 468). The lateral horns are just posterolateral to the ventral horns that house somatic motor neurons. (Parasympathetic preganglionic neurons in the sacral cord are far less abundant than the comparable sympathetic neurons in the thoracolumbar regions, so there are no lateral horns in the sacral region of the spinal cord. This is a major anatomical difference between the two divisions.)

After leaving the cord via the ventral root, preganglionic sympathetic fibers pass through a **white ramus communicans** [plural: **rami communicantes** (kom-mu″nĭ-kan′tēz)] to enter an adjoining **sympathetic trunk ganglion** forming part of the **sympathetic trunk** (or *sympathetic chain*, **Figure 14.5**). Looking like strands of glistening white beads, the sympathetic trunks flank each side of the vertebral column. They consist of the sympathetic ganglia and fibers running from one ganglion to another. The sympathetic trunk ganglia are also called *chain ganglia* or *paravertebral* ("near the vertebrae") *ganglia.*

Although the sympathetic *trunks* extend from neck to pelvis, sympathetic *fibers* arise only from the thoracic and lumbar

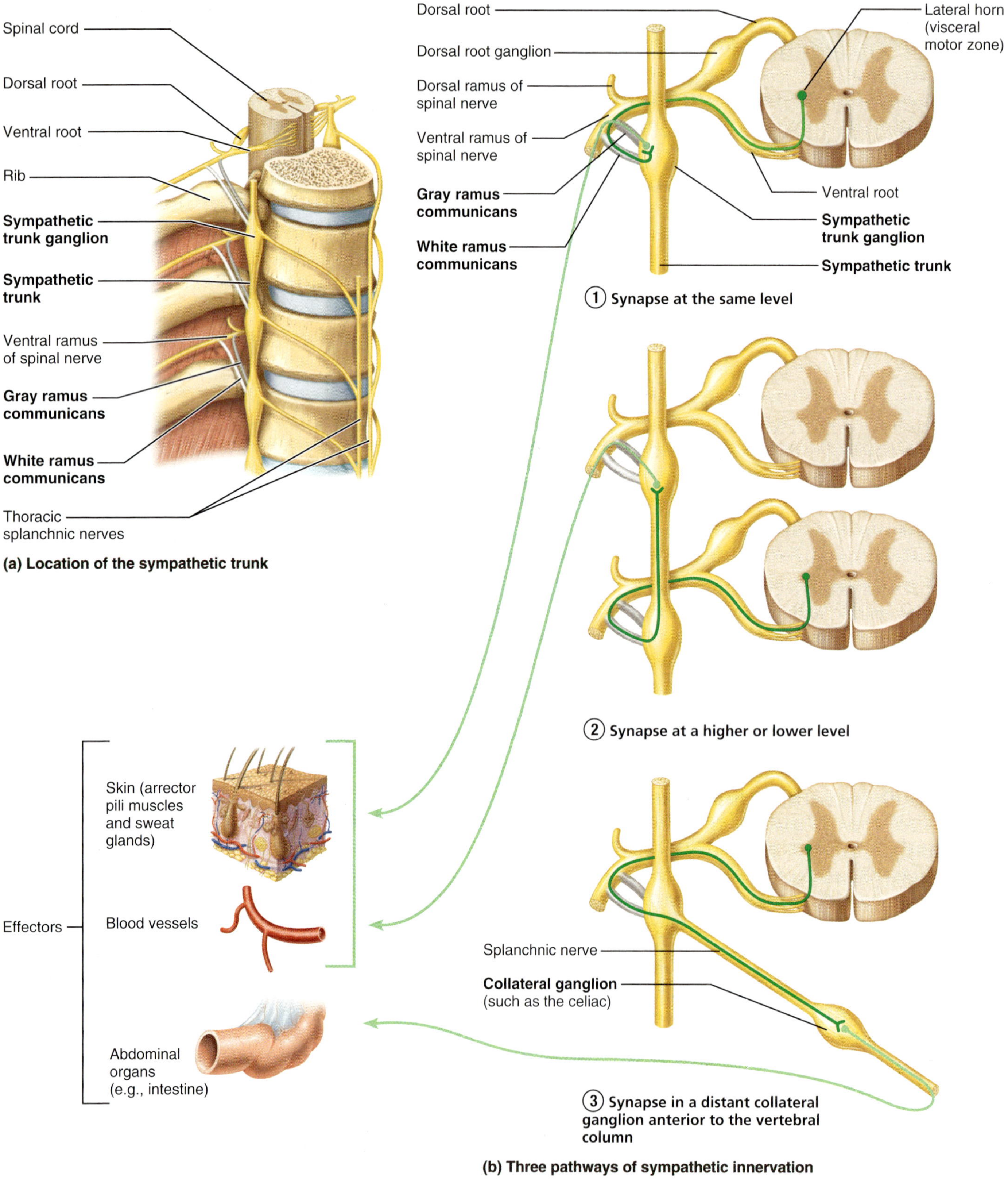

Figure 14.5 Sympathetic trunks and pathways. (a) Diagram of the right sympathetic trunk in the posterior thorax. **(b)** Synapses between preganglionic and postganglionic sympathetic neurons can occur at three different locations—in a sympathetic trunk ganglion at the same level, in a sympathetic trunk ganglion at a different level, or in a collateral ganglion.

cord segments, as shown in Figure 14.3. The ganglia vary in size, position, and number, but typically there are 23 in each sympathetic trunk—3 cervical, 11 thoracic, 4 lumbar, 4 sacral, and 1 coccygeal.

Once a preganglionic axon reaches a trunk ganglion, one of three things can happen to the axon (see the three pathways in Figure 14.5b). The preganglionic and postganglionic neurons can:

① **Synapse at the same level.** In this case, the synapse is in the same trunk ganglion.

② **Synapse at a higher or lower level.** The preganglionic axon ascends or descends the sympathetic trunk to another trunk ganglion.

③ **Synapse in a distant collateral ganglion.** The preganglionic axon passes through the trunk ganglion and emerges from the sympathetic trunk without synapsing. These preganglionic fibers help form several *splanchnic nerves* and synapse in **collateral**, or *prevertebral*, **ganglia** located anterior to the vertebral column. Unlike sympathetic trunk ganglia, the collateral ganglia are neither paired nor segmentally arranged. They occur only in the abdomen and pelvis.

Regardless of where the synapse occurs, all sympathetic ganglia are close to the spinal cord, and their postganglionic fibers are typically much longer than their preganglionic fibers. Recall that the opposite condition exists in the parasympathetic division, an important anatomical distinction.

Pathways with Synapses in Trunk Ganglia

When synapses are made in sympathetic trunk ganglia, the postganglionic axons enter the ventral (or dorsal) ramus of the adjoining spinal nerves by way of communicating branches called **gray rami communicantes** (Figure 14.5). From there they travel via branches of the rami to their effectors, including sweat glands and arrector pili muscles of the skin. Anywhere along their path, the postganglionic axons may transfer over to nearby blood vessels and innervate the vascular smooth muscle all the way to the final branches of the blood vessels.

Notice that the names of the rami communicantes—*white* or *gray*—reflect their appearance, revealing whether or not their fibers are myelinated. Preganglionic fibers composing the white rami are myelinated. Postganglionic axons forming the gray rami are not. (This has no relationship to the white and gray matter of the CNS.)

The white rami, which carry preganglionic axons to the sympathetic trunks, are found only in the T_1–L_2 cord segments, regions of sympathetic outflow. However, gray rami carrying postganglionic fibers headed for the periphery issue from every trunk ganglion from the cervical to the sacral region, allowing sympathetic output to reach all parts of the body.

Note that *rami communicantes are associated only with the sympathetic division*. They never carry parasympathetic fibers.

Pathways to the Head Sympathetic preganglionic fibers serving the head emerge from spinal cord segments T_1–T_4 and ascend the sympathetic trunk to synapse with postganglionic neurons in the **superior cervical ganglion** (Figure 14.6). This ganglion contributes sympathetic fibers that run in several cranial nerves and in the upper three or four cervical spinal nerves.

Besides serving the skin and blood vessels of the head, fibers from the superior cervical ganglion stimulate the dilator muscles of the irises of the eyes, inhibit the nasal and salivary glands (the reason your mouth goes dry when you are scared), and innervate the smooth (tarsal) muscle that lifts the upper eyelid. The superior cervical ganglion also sends direct branches to the heart.

Pathways to the Thorax Sympathetic preganglionic fibers innervating the thoracic organs originate at T_1–T_6. From there the preganglionic fibers run to synapse in the cervical trunk ganglia. Postganglionic fibers emerging from the **middle** and **inferior cervical ganglia** enter cervical nerves C_4–C_8 (Figure 14.6). Some of these fibers innervate the heart via the cardiac plexus, and some innervate the thyroid gland, but most serve the skin. Additionally, some T_1–T_6 preganglionic fibers synapse in the nearest trunk ganglion, and the postganglionic fibers pass directly to the organ served. Fibers to the heart, aorta, lungs, and esophagus take this direct route. Along the way, they run through the plexuses associated with those organs.

Pathways with Synapses in Collateral Ganglia

Most of the preganglionic fibers from T_5 down synapse in collateral ganglia, and so most of these fibers enter and leave the sympathetic trunks without synapsing. They form several nerves called **splanchnic nerves**, including the thoracic splanchnic nerves (greater, lesser, and least) and the **lumbar** and **sacral splanchnic nerves**.

14

The splanchnic nerves contribute to a number of interweaving nerve plexuses known collectively as the *abdominal aortic plexus*, which clings to the surface of the abdominal aorta. This complex plexus contains several ganglia that together serve the abdominopelvic viscera. From superior to inferior, the most important of these ganglia (and related subplexuses) are the **celiac**, **superior mesenteric**, and **inferior mesenteric**, named for the arteries with which they most closely associate (Figure 14.6). Postganglionic fibers issuing from these ganglia generally travel to their target organs in the company of the arteries serving these organs.

Pathways to the Abdomen Sympathetic preganglionic fibers from T_5 to L_2 innervate the abdomen. They travel in the thoracic splanchnic nerves to synapse mainly at the celiac and superior mesenteric ganglia. Postganglionic fibers issuing from these ganglia serve the stomach, intestines (except the distal half of the large intestine), liver, spleen, and kidneys.

Pathways to the Pelvis Preganglionic fibers innervating the pelvis originate from T_{10} to L_2 and then descend in the sympathetic trunk to the lumbar and sacral trunk ganglia. Some fibers synapse there and the postganglionic fibers run in lumbar and sacral splanchnic nerves to plexuses on the lower aorta and in the pelvis. Other preganglionic fibers pass directly to these autonomic plexuses and synapse in collateral ganglia, such as the inferior mesenteric ganglion.

Postganglionic fibers proceed from these plexuses to the pelvic organs (the urinary bladder and reproductive organs) and

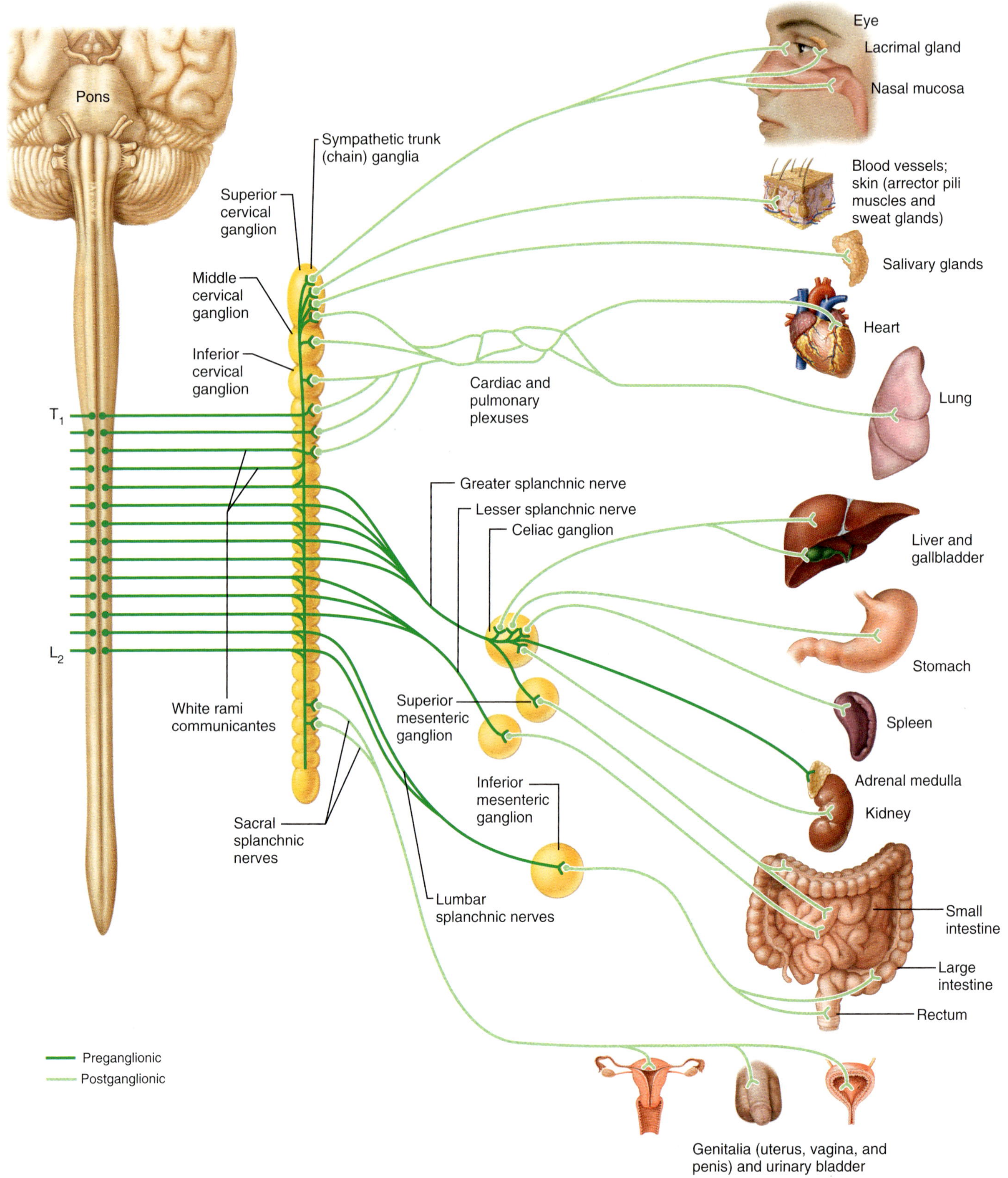

Figure 14.6 Sympathetic division of the ANS. Sympathetic innervation to peripheral structures (blood vessels, glands, and arrector pili muscles) occurs in all areas but is shown only in the cervical area.

14

also the distal half of the large intestine. For the most part, sympathetic fibers *inhibit* the activity of muscles and glands in the abdominopelvic visceral organs.

Pathways with Synapses in the Adrenal Medulla

Some fibers traveling in the thoracic splanchnic nerves pass through the celiac ganglion without synapsing and terminate by synapsing with the hormone-producing medullary cells of the adrenal gland. When stimulated by preganglionic fibers, the medullary cells secrete *norepinephrine* and *epinephrine* (also called *noradrenaline* and *adrenaline*, respectively) into the blood, producing the excitatory effects we have all felt as a "surge of adrenaline."

Embryologically, sympathetic ganglia and the adrenal medulla arise from the same tissue. For this reason, the adrenal medulla is sometimes viewed as a "misplaced" sympathetic ganglion, and its hormone-releasing cells, although lacking nerve processes, are considered equivalent to postganglionic sympathetic neurons.

Visceral Reflexes

Because most anatomists consider the ANS to be a visceral motor system, the presence of sensory fibers (mostly visceral pain afferents) is often overlooked. However, **visceral sensory neurons**, which send information concerning chemical changes, stretch, and irritation of the viscera, are the first link in autonomic reflexes.

Visceral reflex arcs have essentially the same components as somatic reflex arcs—receptor, sensory neuron, integration center, motor neuron, and effector. However, a key difference is that a visceral reflex arc has *two* neurons in its motor component (**Figure 14.7**; compare with Figure 13.15). Two examples of visceral reflexes are the reflexes that empty the rectum and bladder, which we discuss in Chapters 23 and 25.

Nearly all the sympathetic and parasympathetic fibers we have described so far are accompanied by afferent fibers conducting sensory impulses from glands or muscles. This means that peripheral processes of visceral sensory neurons are found in cranial nerves VII, IX, and X, splanchnic nerves, and the sympathetic trunk, as well as in spinal nerves.

Like sensory neurons serving somatic structures (skeletal muscles and skin), the cell bodies of visceral sensory neurons are located either in sensory ganglia of cranial nerves or in dorsal root ganglia of the spinal cord. Visceral sensory neurons are also found in sympathetic ganglia where preganglionic neurons synapse.

Furthermore, complete three-neuron reflex arcs (with sensory neurons, interneurons, and motor neurons) exist entirely within the walls of the gastrointestinal tract. Neurons composing these reflex arcs make up the *enteric nervous system*, which plays an important role in controlling gastrointestinal tract activity. We will discuss the enteric nervous system in more detail in Chapter 23.

Visceral sensory neurons are also involved in the phenomenon of referred pain that we described in Chapter 13 (p. 490).

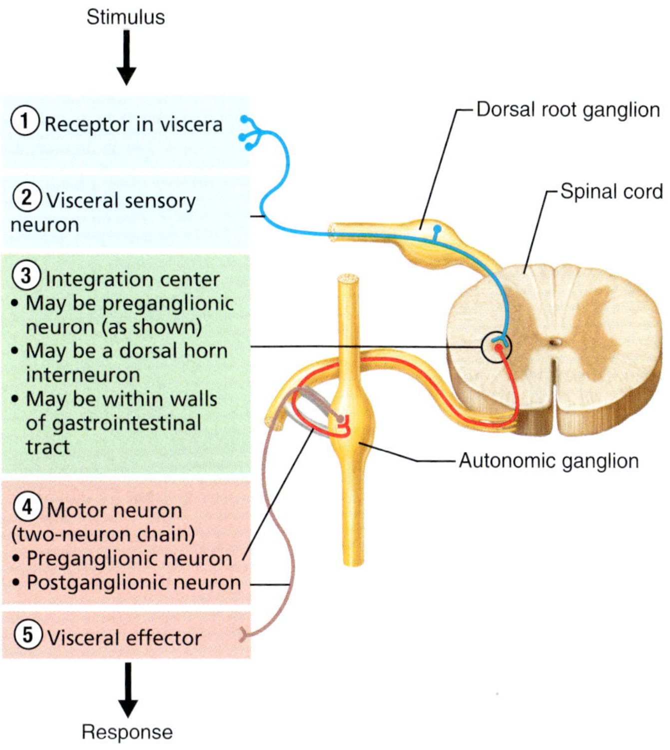

Figure 14.7 Visceral reflexes. Visceral reflex arcs have the same five elements as somatic reflex arcs. The visceral afferent (sensory) fibers are found both in spinal nerves (as depicted here) and in autonomic nerves.

☑ Check Your Understanding

4. State whether each of the following is a characteristic of the sympathetic or parasympathetic nervous system: short preganglionic fibers; origin from thoracolumbar region of spinal cord; terminal ganglia; collateral ganglia; innervates adrenal medulla.
5. How does a visceral reflex differ from a somatic reflex?

For answers, see Appendix H.

14

ANS Physiology

- ✓ Define cholinergic and adrenergic fibers, and list the different types of their receptors.
- ✓ Describe the clinical importance of drugs that mimic or inhibit adrenergic or cholinergic effects.
- ✓ State the effects of the parasympathetic and sympathetic divisions on the following organs: heart, blood vessels, gastrointestinal tract, lungs, adrenal medulla, and external genitalia.
- ✓ Describe autonomic nervous system controls.

Neurotransmitters and Receptors

The major neurotransmitters released by ANS neurons are *acetylcholine* (*ACh*) and *norepinephrine* (*NE*). ACh, the same neurotransmitter secreted by somatic motor neurons, is released by (1) all ANS preganglionic axons and (2) all parasympathetic postganglionic axons at synapses with their effectors. Fibers that release ACh are called **cholinergic fibers** (ko″lin-er′jik).

Table 14.2 Cholinergic and Adrenergic Receptors

NEUROTRANSMITTER	RECEPTOR TYPE	MAJOR LOCATIONS*	EFFECT OF BINDING
Acetylcholine (ACh)	**Cholinergic**		
	Nicotinic	All postganglionic neurons; adrenal medullary cells (also neuromuscular junctions of skeletal muscle)	Excitation
	Muscarinic	All parasympathetic target organs	Excitation in most cases; inhibition of cardiac muscle
		Limited sympathetic targets (e.g., eccrine sweat glands†)	Activation
Norepinephrine (NE) (and epinephrine released by adrenal medulla)	**Adrenergic**		
	β_1	Heart predominantly, but also kidneys and adipose tissue	Increases heart rate and force of contraction; stimulates kidneys to release renin
	β_2	Lungs and most other sympathetic target organs; abundant on blood vessels serving the heart, liver, and skeletal muscle	Effects mostly inhibitory; dilates blood vessels and bronchioles; relaxes smooth muscle walls of digestive and urinary visceral organs; relaxes uterus
	β_3	Adipose tissue	Stimulates lipolysis by fat cells
	α_1	Most importantly blood vessels serving the skin, mucosae, abdominal viscera, kidneys, and salivary glands; also, virtually all sympathetic target organs except heart	Constricts blood vessels and visceral organ sphincters; dilates pupils of the eyes
	α_2	Membrane of adrenergic axon terminals; pancreas; blood platelets	Inhibits NE release from adrenergic terminals; inhibits insulin secretion by pancreas; promotes blood clotting

* Note that all of these receptor subtypes are also found in the CNS.

† Sympathetic cholinergic vasodilator fibers are found in other animals, but do not appear to be present in humans.

14

In contrast, most sympathetic postganglionic axons release NE and are called **adrenergic fibers** (ad″ren-er′jik). An exception is sympathetic postganglionic fibers that secrete ACh onto sweat glands.

Unfortunately for memorization purposes, the effects of ACh and NE on their effectors are not consistently excitatory or inhibitory. Why not? Because the action of any neurotransmitter depends on the receptor to which it binds. Each autonomic neurotransmitter binds with two or more kinds of receptors, allowing it to exert different effects (activation or inhibition) at different body targets. **Table 14.2** summarizes the receptor types that we introduce next.

Cholinergic Receptors

The two types of cholinergic (ACh-binding) receptors are named for drugs that bind to them and mimic acetylcholine's effects. **Nicotinic receptors** (nik″o-tin′ik) respond to nicotine. **Muscarinic receptors**, the other set of ACh receptors, can be activated by the mushroom poison *muscarine* (mus′kah-rin). All ACh receptors are either nicotinic or muscarinic.

Nicotinic Receptors Nicotinic receptors are found on:

- The sarcolemma of skeletal muscle cells at neuromuscular junctions (which, as you will recall, are somatic and not autonomic targets)
- *All* postganglionic neurons, both sympathetic and parasympathetic
- The hormone-producing cells of the adrenal medulla

When ACh binds to nicotinic receptors anywhere, the effect is *always* stimulatory. Just as at the sarcolemma of skeletal muscle (examined in Chapter 9), ACh binding to any nicotinic receptor directly opens ion channels, depolarizing the postsynaptic cell.

Muscarinic Receptors Muscarinic receptors occur on all effector cells stimulated by postganglionic cholinergic fibers—that is, all parasympathetic target organs and a few sympathetic targets, such as eccrine sweat glands. When ACh binds to muscarinic receptors, the effect can be either inhibitory or stimulatory, depending on the subclass of muscarinic receptor on the target organ. For example, ACh binding to cardiac muscle receptors slows heart activity, whereas ACh binding to receptors on smooth muscle of the gastrointestinal tract increases its motility.

Adrenergic Receptors

There are also two major classes of adrenergic (NE-binding) receptors: **alpha (α)** and **beta (β)**. These receptors are further divided into subclasses (α_1 and α_2; β_1, β_2, and β_3). Organs that

Table 14.3 Selected Drug Classes That Influence the Autonomic Nervous System

DRUG CLASS	RECEPTOR BOUND	EFFECTS	EXAMPLE	CLINICAL APPLICATION
Nicotinic agents (little therapeutic value, but important for public health because tobacco contains nicotine)	Nicotinic ACh receptors on all postganglionic neurons and in CNS	Typically stimulates sympathetic effects; blood pressure rises	Nicotine	Smoking cessation products
Parasympathomimetic agents (muscarinic agents)	Muscarinic ACh receptors	Enhance parasympathetic activity by mimicking effects of ACh	Pilocarpine	Glaucoma (opens aqueous humor drainage pores)
			Bethanechol	Difficulty urinating (increases bladder contraction)
Acetylcholinesterase inhibitors	None; bind to the enzyme (AChE) that degrades ACh	Indirect effect at all ACh receptors; prolong the effect of ACh	Neostigmine	Myasthenia gravis (increases availability of ACh)
			Sarin	Used as chemical warfare agent (similar to widely used insecticides)
Sympathomimetic agents	Adrenergic receptors	Enhance sympathetic activity by binding to adrenergic receptors or increasing NE release	Albuterol (Ventolin)	Asthma (dilates bronchioles by binding to β_2 receptors)
			Phenylephrine	Colds (nasal decongestant, binds to α_1 receptors)
Sympatholytic agents	Adrenergic receptors	Decrease sympathetic activity by blocking adrenergic receptors or inhibiting NE release	Propranolol	Hypertension (member of a class of drugs called *beta-blockers* that block β receptors, decreasing blood pressure)

respond to NE (or to epinephrine) have one or more of these receptor subtypes.

NE or epinephrine can be either excitatory or inhibitory depending on which subclass of receptor predominates in the target organ. For example, NE binding to the β_1 receptors of cardiac muscle prods the heart into more vigorous activity, whereas epinephrine binding to β_2 receptors in bronchiole smooth muscle causes it to relax, dilating the bronchiole.

The Effects of Drugs

Knowing the locations of the cholinergic and adrenergic receptor subtypes allows clinicians to prescribe specific drugs to stimulate or inhibit selected target organs.

For example, *atropine* is an anticholinergic drug that blocks muscarinic ACh receptors. It is routinely administered before surgery to prevent salivation and dry up respiratory system secretions. Ophthalmologists also administer atropine to dilate the pupils for eye examination.

The anticholinesterase drug *neostigmine* inhibits the enzyme acetylcholinesterase that breaks down ACh. This allows ACh to accumulate in synapses. Neostigmine is used to treat myasthenia gravis, a condition in which inadequate ACh stimulation impairs skeletal muscle activity.

As we described in Chapter 11, NE is one of our "feel good" neurotransmitters, and drugs that prolong the activity of NE on postsynaptic membranes in the brain help to relieve depression. Hundreds of over-the-counter drugs used to treat colds, coughs, allergies, and nasal congestion contain *sympathomimetics*—sympathetic-mimicking drugs such as phenylephrine that stimulate α-adrenergic receptors. This constricts the blood vessels in the nasal mucosa, inhibiting secretions.

Much pharmaceutical research is directed toward finding medications that affect only one subclass of receptor without upsetting the whole adrenergic or cholinergic system. An important breakthrough was finding drugs that mainly activate β_2 receptors. People with asthma use such β_2 activators to dilate their lung bronchioles without activating β_1 receptors, which would increase their heart rate. **Table 14.3** summarizes selected drug classes that influence ANS activity.

Interactions of the Autonomic Divisions

As we mentioned earlier, most visceral organs receive *dual innervation* from both the parasympathetic and sympathetic divisions. Normally, both ANS divisions are partially active. Action potentials continually fire down both sympathetic and parasympathetic axons, producing a dynamic antagonism that precisely controls visceral activity. However, one division or the other usually predominates in given circumstances, and in a few cases, the two divisions actually cooperate with each other. **Table 14.4** contains an organ-by-organ summary of how their effects differ.

Table 14.4 Effects of the Parasympathetic and Sympathetic Divisions on Various Organs

TARGET ORGAN OR SYSTEM	PARASYMPATHETIC EFFECTS	SYMPATHETIC EFFECTS
Eye (iris)	Stimulates sphincter pupillae muscles; constricts pupils	Stimulates dilator pupillae muscles; dilates pupils
Eye (ciliary muscle)	Stimulates muscle, which makes lens bulge for close vision	Weakly inhibits muscle, which flattens lens for far vision
Glands (nasal, lacrimal, gastric, pancreas)	Stimulates secretory activity	Inhibits secretory activity; constricts blood vessels supplying the glands
Salivary glands	Stimulates secretion of watery saliva	Stimulates secretion of thick, viscous saliva
Sweat glands	No effect (no innervation)	Stimulates copious sweating (cholinergic fibers)
Adrenal medulla	No effect (no innervation)	Stimulates medulla cells to secrete epinephrine and norepinephrine
Arrector pili muscles attached to hair follicles	No effect (no innervation)	Stimulates contraction (erects hairs and produces "goosebumps")
Heart (muscle)	Decreases rate; slows heart	Increases rate and force of heartbeat
Heart (coronary blood vessels)	No effect (no innervation)	Dilates blood vessels (vasodilation)*
Urinary bladder/urethra	Contracts smooth muscle of bladder wall; relaxes urethral sphincter; promotes voiding	Relaxes smooth muscle of bladder wall; constricts urethral sphincter; inhibits voiding
Lungs	Constricts bronchioles	Dilates bronchioles*
Digestive tract organs	Increases motility (peristalsis) and amount of secretion by digestive organs; relaxes sphincters to allow foodstuffs to move through tract	Decreases activity of glands and muscles of digestive system; constricts sphincters (e.g., anal sphincter)
Liver	Increases glucose uptake from blood	Stimulates release of glucose to blood*
Gallbladder	Excites (gallbladder contracts to expel bile)	Inhibits (gallbladder is relaxed)
Kidney	No effect (no innervation)	Promotes renin release; causes vasoconstriction; decreases urine output
Penis	Causes erection (vasodilation)	Causes ejaculation
Vagina/clitoris	Causes erection (vasodilation) of clitoris; increases vaginal lubrication	Causes vagina to contract
Blood vessels	Little or no effect	Constricts most vessels and increases blood pressure; constricts vessels of abdominal viscera and skin to divert blood to muscles, brain, and heart when necessary; epinephrine weakly dilates vessels of skeletal muscles during exercise*
Blood coagulation	No effect (no innervation)	Increases coagulation*
Cellular metabolism	No effect (no innervation)	Increases metabolic rate*
Adipose tissue	No effect (no innervation)	Stimulates lipolysis (fat breakdown)

*Effects are mediated by epinephrine release into the bloodstream from the adrenal medulla.

Antagonistic Interactions

Antagonistic effects, described earlier, are most clearly seen on the activity of the heart, respiratory system, and gastrointestinal organs. In a fight-or-flight situation, the sympathetic division increases heart rate, dilates airways, and inhibits digestion and elimination. When the emergency is over, the parasympathetic division restores heart rate and airway diameter to resting levels and then attends to processes that refuel your body cells and discard wastes.

Sympathetic and Parasympathetic Tone

We have described the parasympathetic division as the "rest and digest" division, but the sympathetic division is the major actor in controlling blood pressure, even at rest. With few exceptions, the vascular system is entirely innervated by sympathetic fibers that keep the blood vessels in a continual state of partial constriction called **sympathetic**, or **vasomotor**, **tone**.

When blood pressure is too low to maintain blood flow, the sympathetic fibers fire more rapidly, causing blood vessels to constrict and raising blood pressure. When blood pressure becomes too high, sympathetic fibers fire less rapidly and the vessels dilate. *Alpha-blockers*, drugs that block the responses in these **vasomotor fibers**, are sometimes used to treat hypertension (high blood pressure).

During circulatory shock (inadequate blood flow to body tissues), or when more blood is needed to meet the soaring needs of working skeletal muscles, blood vessels serving the skin and abdominal viscera strongly constrict. This blood "shunting" helps maintain circulation to vital organs and skeletal muscles.

In contrast to the sympathetic division's dominance of blood vessels, parasympathetic effects normally dominate the heart and the smooth muscle of digestive and urinary tract organs. These organs exhibit **parasympathetic tone**. The parasympathetic division slows the heart and dictates the normal activity levels of the digestive and urinary tracts. However, the sympathetic division can override these parasympathetic effects during times of stress. Drugs that block parasympathetic responses increase heart rate and cause fecal and urinary retention. Parasympathetic fibers activate most glands, except for the adrenal glands and sweat glands of the skin.

Cooperative Effects

The best example of cooperative ANS effects occurs in the external genitalia. Parasympathetic stimulation dilates blood vessels in the external genitalia, producing the erection of the male penis or female clitoris during sexual excitement. (This may explain why anxiety can impair sexual performance—the sympathetic division is in charge.) Sympathetic stimulation then causes ejaculation of semen by the penis or reflex contractions of the vagina.

Homeostatic Imbalance 14.1

Autonomic neuropathy (damage to autonomic nerves) is a common complication of diabetes mellitus. One of the earliest and most troubling symptoms is sexual dysfunction. Up to 75% of male diabetics experience erectile dysfunction, and female diabetics often experience reduced vaginal lubrication. Other frequent manifestations of autonomic neuropathy include dizziness after standing suddenly (poor blood pressure control), urinary incontinence, sluggish eye pupil reactions, and impaired sweating. Maintaining tight control of blood glucose levels is the best way to prevent diabetic neuropathy. ✚

Unique Roles of the Sympathetic Division

The adrenal medulla, sweat glands and arrector pili muscles of the skin, the kidneys, and most blood vessels receive only sympathetic fibers. It is easy to remember that the sympathetic system innervates these structures because most of us sweat under stress, our scalp "prickles" during fear, and our blood pressure skyrockets (from widespread constriction of blood vessels) when we get excited.

We have already described how sympathetic control of blood vessels regulates blood pressure and shunting of blood in the vascular system. We will now consider several other uniquely sympathetic functions.

Thermoregulatory Responses to Heat The sympathetic division mediates reflexes that regulate body temperature. For example, applying heat to the skin causes blood vessels in that area to dilate reflexively. When systemic body temperature rises, sympathetic nerves (1) dilate the skin's blood vessels, allowing heat to escape from skin flushed with warm blood, and (2) activate the sweat glands to help cool the body. When body temperature falls, skin blood vessels constrict, preventing heat loss from the skin.

Release of Renin from the Kidneys Sympathetic impulses stimulate the kidneys to release *renin*, an enzyme that causes the formation of blood pressure–increasing hormones. We describe this renin-triggered mechanism in Chapter 25.

Metabolic Effects Through both direct neural stimulation and release of adrenal medullary hormones, the sympathetic division promotes a number of metabolic effects not reversed by parasympathetic activity. It (1) increases the metabolic rate of body cells; (2) raises blood glucose levels; and (3) mobilizes fats for use as fuels.

The medullary hormones also cause skeletal muscle to contract more strongly and quickly. As a side effect, this stimulates muscle spindles more often and, consequently, nerve impulses traveling to the muscles occur more synchronously. These neural bursts, which put muscle contractions on a "hair trigger," are great if you have to make a quick jump or run, but they can be embarrassing or even disabling to the nervous musician or surgeon.

Localized Versus Diffuse Effects

In the parasympathetic division, one preganglionic neuron synapses with one (or at most a few) postganglionic neurons. Additionally, all parasympathetic fibers release ACh, which is quickly destroyed (hydrolyzed) by acetylcholinesterase. Consequently, the parasympathetic division exerts short-lived, highly localized control over its effectors.

In contrast, in the sympathetic division, preganglionic axons branch profusely as they enter the sympathetic trunk, and they synapse with postganglionic neurons at several levels. As a result, when the sympathetic division is activated, it responds in a diffuse and highly interconnected way. Indeed, the literal translation of sympathetic (*sym* = together; *pathos* = feeling) relates to the bodywide mobilization this division provokes. Nevertheless, parts of the sympathetic nervous system can be activated individually. For example, just because your eye pupils dilate in dim light doesn't necessarily mean that your heart rate also speeds up.

Sympathetic activation produces much longer-lasting effects than parasympathetic activation. The sympathetic system's neurotransmitter, NE, is inactivated more slowly than the parasympathetic system's ACh, because NE must be taken back up into the presynaptic ending before being hydrolyzed or stored. More importantly, adrenal medullary cells secrete NE and epinephrine into the blood when the sympathetic division is mobilized. These hormones reinforce and prolong the effects of the sympathetic nervous system. Although epinephrine is more potent at increasing heart rate and raising blood glucose levels and metabolic rate, these hormones have essentially the same effects as NE released by sympathetic neurons. In fact, circulating adrenal medullary hormones produce 25–50% of all the sympathetic effects acting on the body at a given time. These effects continue for several minutes until the liver destroys the hormones.

In short, sympathetic nerve impulses act only briefly, but the hormonal effects they provoke linger. The widespread and prolonged effect of sympathetic activation explains why we need time to "come down" after an extremely stressful experience.

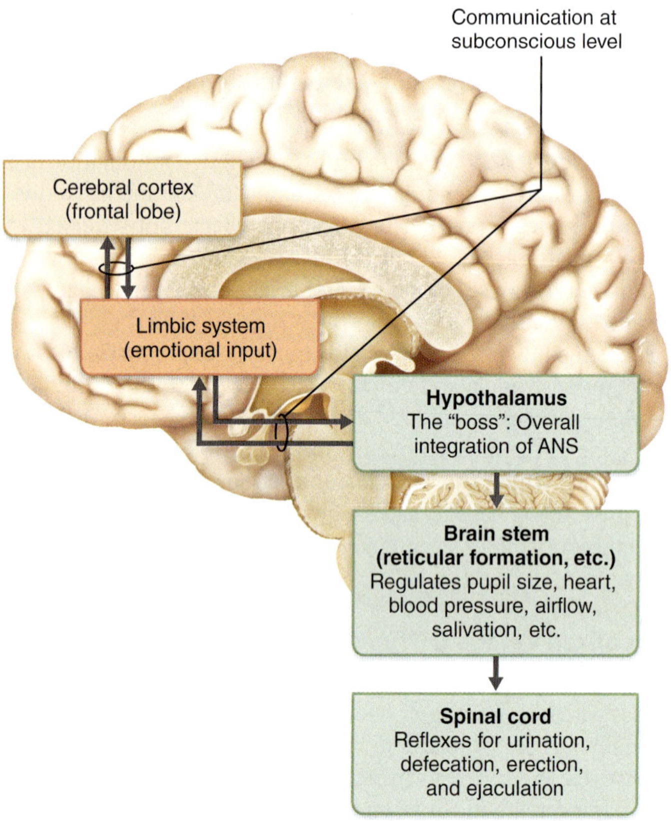

Figure 14.8 Levels of ANS control. The hypothalamus stands at the top of the control hierarchy as the integrator of ANS activity, but it is influenced by subconscious cerebral inputs via limbic system connections.

14

Control of Autonomic Function

Although the ANS is not usually considered to be under voluntary control, its activity is regulated by CNS controls in the spinal cord, brain stem, hypothalamus, and cerebral cortex **(Figure 14.8)**. In general, the hypothalamus is the integrative center at the top of the ANS control hierarchy. From there, orders flow to lower and lower CNS centers for execution. Although the cerebral cortex may modify the workings of the ANS, it does so at the subconscious level and by acting through limbic system structures on hypothalamic centers.

Brain Stem and Spinal Cord Controls

The hypothalamus is the "boss," but the brain stem reticular formation appears to exert the most *direct* influence over autonomic functions (see Figure 12.14 on p. 446). For example, certain motor centers in the ventrolateral medulla (*cardiac* and *vasomotor centers*) reflexively regulate heart rate and blood vessel diameter. Other medullary regions oversee gastrointestinal activities. Most sensory impulses involved in these autonomic reflexes reach the brain stem via vagus nerve afferents. Midbrain centers (*oculomotor nuclei*) control the muscles concerned with pupil diameter and lens focus.

Defecation and micturition (urination) reflexes that empty the rectum and urinary bladder are integrated at the spinal cord level but are subject to conscious inhibition. We will describe all of these autonomic reflexes in later chapters in relation to the organ systems they serve.

Hypothalamic Controls

As we noted, the hypothalamus is the main integration center of the autonomic nervous system. In general, anterior hypothalamic regions direct parasympathetic functions, and posterior areas direct sympathetic functions. Hypothalamic centers exert their effects both directly and via relays through the *reticular formation*, which in turn influences the preganglionic motor neurons in the brain stem and spinal cord (Figure 14.8). The hypothalamus, acting through the ANS, coordinates heart activity, blood pressure, body temperature, water balance, and endocrine activity.

The hypothalamus also mediates our reactions to fear via its associations with the amygdala and the periaqueductal gray matter. Emotional responses of the limbic system of the cerebrum to danger and stress signal the hypothalamus to activate the sympathetic system to fight-or-flight status. In this way, the hypothalamus serves as the keystone of the emotional and visceral brain. Through its centers, emotions influence ANS function and behavior.

Cortical Controls

Originally, scientists believed the ANS was not subject to voluntary controls. However, we have all had occasions when just remembering a frightening event made our heart race (sympathetic response) or the thought of a favorite food, pecan pie for example, made our mouth water (parasympathetic response). These inputs converge on the hypothalamus through its connections to the limbic lobe.

Additionally, studies have shown that voluntary cortical control of visceral activities is possible—a capability untapped by most people.

Influence of Biofeedback on Autonomic Function **Biofeedback** is a way of becoming aware of physiological conditions (such as heart rate and blood pressure), with the goal of being able to influence them consciously. During **biofeedback training**, subjects are connected to monitoring devices that detect and amplify changes in these physiological processes. The feedback comes in the form of flashing lights or audible tones.

Subjects try to alter or control some "involuntary" function by concentrating on calming, pleasant thoughts. The monitor allows them to identify changes in the desired direction, so they can recognize the feelings associated with these changes and learn to produce the changes at will.

Biofeedback techniques have been successful in helping individuals plagued by migraine headaches. Some cardiac patients also use them to manage stress and reduce their risk of heart attack. However, biofeedback training is time-consuming and often frustrating, and the training equipment is expensive and difficult to use.

☑ Check Your Understanding

6. Name the division of the ANS that does each of the following: increases digestive activity; increases blood pressure; dilates bronchioles; decreases heart rate; stimulates the adrenal medulla to release its hormones; causes ejaculation.
7. Would you find nicotinic receptors on skeletal muscle? Smooth muscle? Eccrine sweat glands? The adrenal medulla? CNS neurons?

8. Which part of the brain is the main integration center of the ANS? Which part exerts the most direct influence over autonomic functions?

For answers, see Appendix H.

Homeostatic Imbalances of the ANS

✓ Explain the relationship of some types of hypertension, Raynaud's disease, and autonomic dysreflexia to disorders of autonomic function.

The ANS is involved in nearly every important process that goes on in the body, so it is not surprising that abnormalities of autonomic function can have far-reaching effects. Most autonomic disorders reflect exaggerated or deficient controls of smooth muscle activity. The most devastating involve blood vessels and include conditions such as hypertension, Raynaud's disease, and autonomic dysreflexia.

- *Hypertension*, or high blood pressure, may result from an overactive sympathetic vasoconstrictor response promoted by continuous high levels of stress. Hypertension is always serious because it forces the heart to work harder, which may precipitate heart disease, and increases the wear and tear on artery walls. Hypertension is sometimes treated with adrenergic receptor–blocking drugs that counteract the effects of the sympathetic nervous system on the cardiovascular system. We will discuss hypertension in more detail in Chapter 19.
- *Raynaud's disease* is characterized by intermittent attacks causing the skin of the fingers and toes to become pale, then cyanotic (bluish) and painful. Commonly provoked by exposure to cold or emotional stress, it is an exaggerated vasoconstriction response. The severity of Raynaud's disease ranges from merely uncomfortable to severe blood vessel constriction that causes ischemia and gangrene (tissue death).

  Vasodilators (for example, adrenergic blockers) usually suffice. To treat very severe cases, preganglionic sympathetic fibers serving the affected regions are severed (a procedure called *sympathectomy*). The involved vessels then dilate, reestablishing adequate blood flow to the region.
- *Autonomic dysreflexia* is a life-threatening condition involving uncontrolled activation of autonomic neurons. It occurs in a majority of individuals with quadriplegia and in others with spinal cord injuries above the T_6 level, usually in the first year after injury. The usual trigger is a painful stimulus to the skin or an overfilled visceral organ, such as the urinary bladder. Arterial blood pressure skyrockets to life-threatening levels, which may rupture a blood vessel in the brain, precipitating stroke. Symptoms include headache, flushed face, sweating above the level of the injury, and cold, clammy skin below. The precise mechanism of autonomic dysreflexia is not yet clear.

☑ Check Your Understanding

9. Jackson works long, stress-filled shifts as an air traffic controller at a busy airport. His doctor has prescribed a beta-blocker. Why might his doctor have done this? What does a beta-blocker do?

For answers, see Appendix H.

Developmental Aspects of the ANS

✓ Describe several effects of aging on the autonomic nervous system.

ANS preganglionic neurons derive from the embryonic *neural tube*, as do somatic motor neurons. ANS structures in the PNS—postganglionic neurons, the adrenal medulla, and all autonomic ganglia—derive from the **neural crest** (along with all sensory neurons) (see Figure 12.33, ②).

Neural crest cells reach their ultimate destinations by migrating along growing axons. Forming ganglia receive axons from preganglionic neurons in the spinal cord or brain and send their axons to synapse with their effector cells in the body periphery. This process depends on the presence of **nerve growth factor**, and is guided by a number of signaling chemicals similar to those acting in the CNS.

During youth, impairments of ANS function are usually due to injuries to the spinal cord or autonomic nerves. In old age, the efficiency of the ANS declines. At least part of the problem is due to structural changes in some preganglionic axon terminals, which become congested with neurofilaments.

Many elderly people complain of constipation (a result of reduced gastrointestinal tract motility), and of dry eyes and frequent eye infections (both a result of a diminished ability to form tears). Additionally, when they stand up they may have fainting episodes due to **orthostatic hypotension** (*ortho* = straight; *stat* = standing), low blood pressure following changes in position. Orthostatic hypotension occurs because aging pressure receptors become less responsive to changes in blood pressure, and aging cardiovascular centers fail to maintain healthy blood pressure.

These problems are distressing, but not usually life threatening, and most can be managed by lifestyle changes or artificial aids. For example, changing position slowly gives the sympathetic nervous system time to adjust blood pressure, and eye drops (artificial tears) can alleviate the dry-eye problem.

☑ Check Your Understanding

10. Which embryonic structure gives rise to both the autonomic ganglia and the adrenal medulla?

For answers, see Appendix H.

In this chapter, we have described the structure and function of the ANS, one arm of the motor division of the peripheral nervous system. Because virtually every organ system still to be considered depends on autonomic controls, you will be hearing more about the ANS in chapters that follow. Now that we have explored most of the nervous system, this is a good time to examine how it interacts with the rest of the body as summarized in *System Connections*, p. 540.

Homeostatic Interrelationships Between the Nervous System and Other Body Systems

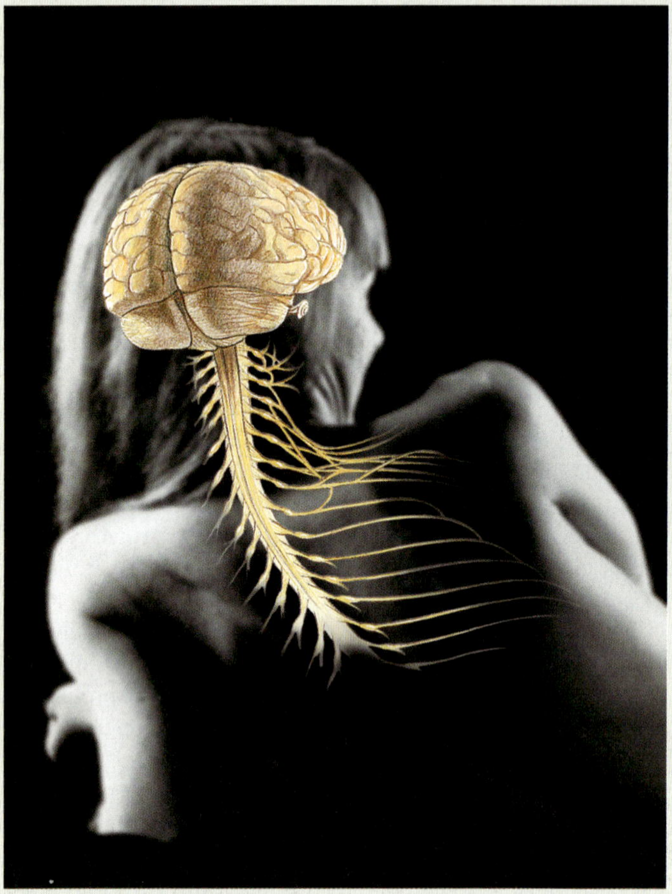

Integumentary System Chapter 5

- Sympathetic division of the ANS regulates sweat glands and blood vessels of skin (therefore heat loss/retention)
- Skin serves as heat loss surface

Skeletal System Chapters 6–8

- Nerves innervate bones and joints, providing for pain and joint sense
- Bones serve as depot for calcium needed for neural function; skeletal system protects CNS structures

Muscular System Chapters 9–10

- Somatic division of nervous system activates skeletal muscles; maintains muscle health
- Skeletal muscles are the effectors of the somatic division

Endocrine System Chapter 16

- Sympathetic division of the ANS activates the adrenal medulla; hypothalamus helps regulate the activity of the anterior pituitary gland and produces the two posterior pituitary hormones
- Hormones influence neuronal metabolism

Cardiovascular System Chapters 17–19

- ANS helps regulate heart rate and blood pressure
- Cardiovascular system provides blood containing oxygen and nutrients to the nervous system and carries away wastes

Lymphatic System/Immunity Chapters 20–21

- Nerves innervate lymphoid organs; the brain plays a role in regulating immune function
- Lymphatic vessels carry away leaked tissue fluids from tissues surrounding nervous system structures; immune elements protect all body organs from pathogens (CNS has additional mechanisms as well)

Respiratory System Chapter 22

- Nervous system initiates and regulates respiratory rhythm and depth
- Respiratory system provides life-sustaining oxygen; disposes of carbon dioxide

Digestive System Chapter 23

- ANS (particularly the parasympathetic division) regulates digestive motility and glandular activity
- Digestive system provides nutrients needed for neuronal health

Urinary System Chapters 25–26

- ANS regulates bladder emptying and renal blood pressure
- Kidneys help dispose of metabolic wastes and maintain proper electrolyte composition and pH of blood for neural functioning

Reproductive System Chapter 27

- ANS regulates sexual erection and ejaculation in males; erection of the clitoris in females
- Testosterone causes masculinization of the brain and underlies sex drive and aggressive behavior

Chapter Summary

For more chapter study tools, go to the Study Area of MasteringA&P at **www.masteringaandp.com**.
There you will find:

- Interactive Physiology iP
- A&PFlix A&PFlix
- Practice Anatomy Lab PAL
- PhysioEx PEx
- Videos, Practice Quizzes and Tests, MP3 Tutor Sessions, Case Studies, and much more!

1. The autonomic nervous system (ANS) is the motor division of the PNS that controls visceral activities, with the goal of maintaining internal homeostasis.

Overview (pp. 524–527)

Comparison of the Somatic and Autonomic Nervous Systems (pp. 525–526)

1. The somatic (voluntary) nervous system provides motor fibers to skeletal muscles. The autonomic (involuntary or visceral motor) nervous system provides motor fibers to smooth and cardiac muscles and glands.
2. In the somatic division, a single motor neuron forms the efferent pathway from the CNS to the effectors. The efferent pathway of the autonomic division consists of a two-neuron chain: the preganglionic neuron in the CNS and the postganglionic neuron in a ganglion.
3. Acetylcholine, the neurotransmitter of somatic motor neurons, is stimulatory to skeletal muscle fibers. Neurotransmitters released by autonomic motor neurons (acetylcholine and norepinephrine) may excite or inhibit target cells.

iP Nervous System II; Topic: Synaptic Transmission, pp. 8–11.

ANS Divisions (pp. 526–527)

4. The ANS consists of two divisions, parasympathetic and sympathetic, which normally exert antagonistic effects on many of the same target organs.
5. The parasympathetic division (the rest-digest system) conserves body energy and maintains body activities at basal levels.
6. Parasympathetic effects include constricted pupils, glandular secretion, increased digestive tract motility, and smooth muscle activity leading to elimination of feces and urine.
7. The sympathetic division prepares the body for activity (the fight-or-flight system).
8. Sympathetic responses include dilated pupils, increased heart rate, increased blood pressure, dilated bronchioles of the lungs, increased blood glucose levels, and sweating. During exercise, sympathetic vasoconstriction shunts blood from the skin and digestive viscera to the heart, brain, and skeletal muscles.

ANS Anatomy (pp. 527–533)

Parasympathetic (Craniosacral) Division (pp. 527–529)

1. Parasympathetic preganglionic neurons arise from the brain stem and from the sacral (S_2–S_4) region of the spinal cord.
2. Preganglionic fibers synapse with postganglionic neurons in terminal ganglia located in (intramural ganglia) or close to their effector organs. Preganglionic fibers are long; postganglionic fibers are short.
3. Cranial fibers arise in the brain stem nuclei of cranial nerves III, VII, IX, and X and synapse in ganglia of the head, thorax, and abdomen. The vagus nerves serve virtually all organs of the thoracic and abdominal cavities.
4. Sacral fibers (S_2–S_4) issue from the lateral region of the cord and form pelvic splanchnic nerves that innervate the pelvic viscera. The preganglionic axons do not travel within rami communicantes.

Sympathetic (Thoracolumbar) Division (pp. 529–533)

5. Preganglionic sympathetic neurons arise from the lateral horns of the spinal cord from the level of T_1 through L_2.
6. Preganglionic axons leave the cord via white rami communicantes and enter the sympathetic trunk ganglia in the sympathetic trunk. An axon may synapse in a trunk ganglion at the same or at a different level, or it may issue from the sympathetic trunk without synapsing. Preganglionic fibers are short; postganglionic fibers are long.
7. When the synapse occurs in a trunk ganglion, the postganglionic fiber may enter the spinal nerve ramus via the gray ramus communicans to travel to the body periphery. Postganglionic fibers issuing from the cervical ganglia also serve visceral organs and blood vessels of the head, neck, and thorax.
8. When synapses do not occur in the trunk ganglia, the preganglionic fibers form splanchnic nerves (thoracic, lumbar, and sacral). Most splanchnic nerve fibers synapse in collateral ganglia, and the postganglionic fibers serve the abdominal viscera. Exceptions are that (1) some splanchnic nerve fibers synapse with cells of the adrenal medulla, and (2) some lumbar and sacral splanchnic nerve fibers *do* synapse in trunk ganglia.

Visceral Reflexes (p. 533)

9. Visceral reflex arcs have the same components as somatic reflexes: receptor, sensory neuron, integration center, motor neurons, effector.
10. Cell bodies of visceral sensory neurons are located in dorsal root ganglia, sensory ganglia of cranial nerves, or autonomic ganglia. Visceral afferents are located in spinal nerves and in virtually all autonomic nerves.

ANS Physiology (pp. 533–539)

Neurotransmitters and Receptors (pp. 533–535)

1. Autonomic motor neurons release two major neurotransmitters, acetylcholine (ACh) and norepinephrine (NE). Based on the neurotransmitter they release, fibers are classified as cholinergic (ACh) or adrenergic (NE).
2. ACh is released by all preganglionic fibers and all parasympathetic postganglionic fibers. NE is released by all sympathetic postganglionic fibers except those serving the sweat glands of the skin.
3. Neurotransmitter effects depend on the receptors to which the neurotransmitter binds. Cholinergic (ACh) receptors are classified as nicotinic or muscarinic. Adrenergic (NE) receptors are classified as α_1 or α_2, or β_1, β_2, or β_3.

iP Nervous System II; Topic: Synaptic Transmission, pp. 8–11, 14.

14

The Effects of Drugs (p. 535)

4. Drugs that mimic, enhance, or inhibit the action of ANS neurotransmitters are used to treat conditions caused by excessive, inadequate, or inappropriate ANS function. Some drugs bind with only one receptor subtype, blocking or enhancing specific ANS-mediated activities.

Interactions of the Autonomic Divisions (pp. 535–537)

5. Most visceral organs are innervated by both parasympathetic and sympathetic divisions. The divisions interact in various ways but usually exert a dynamic antagonism. Antagonistic interactions mainly involve the heart, respiratory system, and gastrointestinal organs. Sympathetic activity increases heart activity, dilates bronchioles, and depresses gastrointestinal activity. Parasympathetic activity reverses these effects.
6. Most blood vessels are innervated only by sympathetic fibers and exhibit vasomotor tone. Parasympathetic activity dominates the heart and muscles of the gastrointestinal tract (which normally exhibit parasympathetic tone) and glands.
7. The two ANS divisions exert cooperative effects on the external genitalia.
8. Roles unique to the sympathetic division are regulating blood pressure, shunting blood in the vascular system, regulating body temperature, stimulating the kidneys to release renin, and metabolic effects.
9. Activation of the sympathetic division can cause widespread, long-lasting mobilization of the fight-or-flight response. Parasympathetic effects are highly localized and short-lived.

Control of Autonomic Function (pp. 538–539)

10. Autonomic function is controlled at several levels: (1) The spinal cord and brain stem (particularly medullary) centers mediate reflex activity. (2) Hypothalamic integration centers interact with both higher and lower centers to orchestrate autonomic, somatic, and endocrine responses. (3) Cortical centers influence autonomic function via connections with the limbic system. Conscious control of autonomic function is rare but possible, as illustrated by biofeedback training.

Homeostatic Imbalances of the ANS (p. 539)

1. Most autonomic disorders reflect problems with smooth muscle control. Abnormalities in vascular control, such as hypertension, Raynaud's disease, and autonomic dysreflexia, are most devastating.

Developmental Aspects of the ANS (p. 539)

1. Preganglionic neurons develop from the neural tube; postganglionic neurons develop from the embryonic neural crest.
2. The efficiency of the autonomic nervous system declines in old age, as reflected by decreased gland secretion, reduced gastrointestinal motility, and slower sympathetic vasomotor responses to changes in position.

14

Review Questions

Multiple Choice/Matching

(Some questions have more than one correct answer. Select the best answer or answers from the choices given.)

1. All of the following characterize the ANS except **(a)** a two-neuron efferent chain, **(b)** presence of nerve cell bodies in the CNS, **(c)** presence of nerve cell bodies in the ganglia, **(d)** innervation of skeletal muscles.
2. Relate each of the following terms or phrases to either the sympathetic **(S)** or parasympathetic **(P)** division of the autonomic nervous system:

    ____ **(1)** short preganglionic, long postganglionic fibers
    ____ **(2)** intramural ganglia
    ____ **(3)** craniosacral part
    ____ **(4)** adrenergic fibers
    ____ **(5)** cervical ganglia
    ____ **(6)** otic and ciliary ganglia
    ____ **(7)** generally short-duration action
    ____ **(8)** increases heart rate and blood pressure
    ____ **(9)** increases gastric motility and secretion of lacrimal, salivary, and digestive juices
    ____ **(10)** innervates blood vessels
    ____ **(11)** most active when you are relaxing in a hammock
    ____ **(12)** active when you are running in the Boston Marathon

3. Preganglionic neurons develop from **(a)** neural crest cells, **(b)** neural tube cells, **(c)** alar plate cells, **(d)** endoderm.
4. The white rami communicantes contain what kind of fibers? **(a)** preganglionic parasympathetic, **(b)** postganglionic parasympathetic, **(c)** preganglionic sympathetic, **(d)** postganglionic sympathetic.
5. Collateral sympathetic ganglia are involved with innervating **(a)** abdominal organs, **(b)** thoracic organs, **(c)** head, **(d)** arrector pili, **(e)** all of these.

Short Answer Essay Questions

6. Briefly explain why the following terms are sometimes used to refer to the autonomic nervous system: involuntary nervous system and emotional-visceral system.
7. Describe the anatomical relationship of the white and gray rami communicantes to the spinal nerve, and indicate the kind of fibers found in each ramus type.
8. Indicate the results of sympathetic activation of the following structures: sweat glands, eye pupils, adrenal medullae, heart, bronchioles of the lungs, liver, blood vessels of vigorously working skeletal muscles, blood vessels of digestive viscera, salivary glands.
9. Which of the effects listed in response to question 8 would be reversed by parasympathetic activity?
10. Which ANS fibers release acetylcholine? Which release norepinephrine?
11. Describe the meaning and importance of sympathetic tone and parasympathetic tone.
12. List the receptor subtypes for ACh and NE, and indicate the major sites where each type is found.
13. Which area of the brain is most directly involved in mediating autonomic reflexes?
14. Describe the importance of the hypothalamus in controlling the autonomic nervous system.
15. Describe the basis and uses of biofeedback training.

16. What manifestations of decreased autonomic nervous system efficiency are seen in elderly individuals?
17. Postganglionic neurons are also called ganglionic neurons. Why is the latter term more accurate?

Critical Thinking and Clinical Application Questions

1. Mr. Johnson suffers from urinary retention and a hypoactive urinary bladder. Bethanechol, a drug that mimics acetylcholine's autonomic effects, is prescribed to manage his problem. First explain the rationale for prescribing bethanechol, and then predict which of the following adverse effects Mr. Johnson might experience while taking this drug (select all that apply): dizziness, low blood pressure, deficient tear formation, wheezing, increased mucus production in bronchi, deficient salivation, diarrhea, cramping, excessive sweating, undesirable erection of penis.
2. A 32-year-old woman complains of intermittent aching pains in the medial two fingers of both hands. During such episodes, the fingers become blanched and then blue. Her history is taken, and it is noted that she is a heavy smoker. The physician advises her that she must stop smoking and states that she will not prescribe any medication until the patient has discontinued smoking for a month. What is this patient's condition, and why was she told to stop smoking?
3. Tiffany, a 21-year-old college student, is having trouble sleeping, crying frequently, and having recurrent thoughts of suicide. An antidepressant is prescribed. Like many such drugs, this antidepressant has anticholinergic side effects. What side effects might Tiffany experience in the first week of treatment?
4. As the aroma of freshly brewed coffee drifted by dozing Henry's nose, his mouth started to water and his stomach began to rumble. Explain his reactions in terms of ANS activity.

AT THE CLINIC

Related Clinical Terms

Atonic bladder (ah-ton′ik; *a* = without; *ton* = tone, tension) A condition in which the urinary bladder becomes flaccid and overfills, allowing urine to dribble through the sphincters. Results from temporary loss of the micturition reflex following spinal cord injury.

Horner's syndrome A condition due to damage to the superior sympathetic trunk on one side of the body. On the affected side, the upper eyelid droops (ptosis) and the pupil constricts, and the person does not sweat on that side of the head.

Vagotomy (va-got′o-me) Cutting or severing the vagus nerve to decrease secretion of gastric juice. Treatment for peptic ulcers that do not respond to medication.

Vasovagal syncope Vasovagal syncope, also called *neurocardiogenic syncope*, is the most common cause of fainting. Although it may be provoked by emotional stress, pain, or dehydration, it typically occurs during prolonged standing. Fainting is due to a drop in blood pressure, which decreases blood flow to the brain.

Case Study Autonomic Nervous System

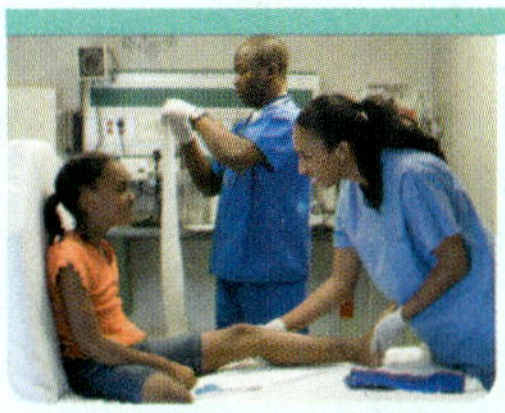

On arrival at Holyoke Hospital, Jimmy Chin, a 10-year-old boy, is immobilized on a rigid stretcher so that he is unable to move his head or trunk. The paramedics report that when they found him some 50 feet from the bus, he was awake and alert, but crying and complaining that he couldn't "get up to find his mom" and he had a "wicked headache." He has severe bruises on his upper back and head, and lacerations of his back and scalp. His blood pressure is low, body temperature is below normal, lower limbs are paralyzed, and he is insensitive to painful stimuli below the nipples. Although still alert on arrival, Jimmy soon begins to drift in and out of unconsciousness.

Jimmy is immediately scheduled for a CT scan, and an operating room is reserved.

Relative to Jimmy's condition:

1. Why were his head and torso immobilized for transport to the hospital?
2. What do his worsening neurological signs (drowsiness, incoherence, etc.) probably indicate? Relate this to the type of surgery that will be performed.
3. Assuming that Jimmy's sensory and motor deficits are due to a spinal cord injury, at what level do you expect to find a spinal cord lesion?
4. Two days after his surgery, Jimmy is alert and his MRI scan shows no residual brain injury, but pronounced swelling and damage to the spinal cord at T_4. On physical examination, Jimmy shows no reflex activity below the level of the spinal cord injury. His blood pressure is still low. Why are there no reflexes in his lower limbs and abdomen?
5. Over the next few days, his reflexes return in his lower limbs and become exaggerated. He is incontinent. Why is Jimmy hyperreflexive and incontinent?

On one occasion, Jimmy complains of a massive headache and his blood pressure is way above normal. On examination, he is sweating intensely above the nipples but has cold, clammy skin below the nipples and his heart rate is very slow.

6. What is this condition called and what precipitates it?
7. How does Jimmy's excessively high blood pressure put him at risk?

(Answers in Appendix H)

15

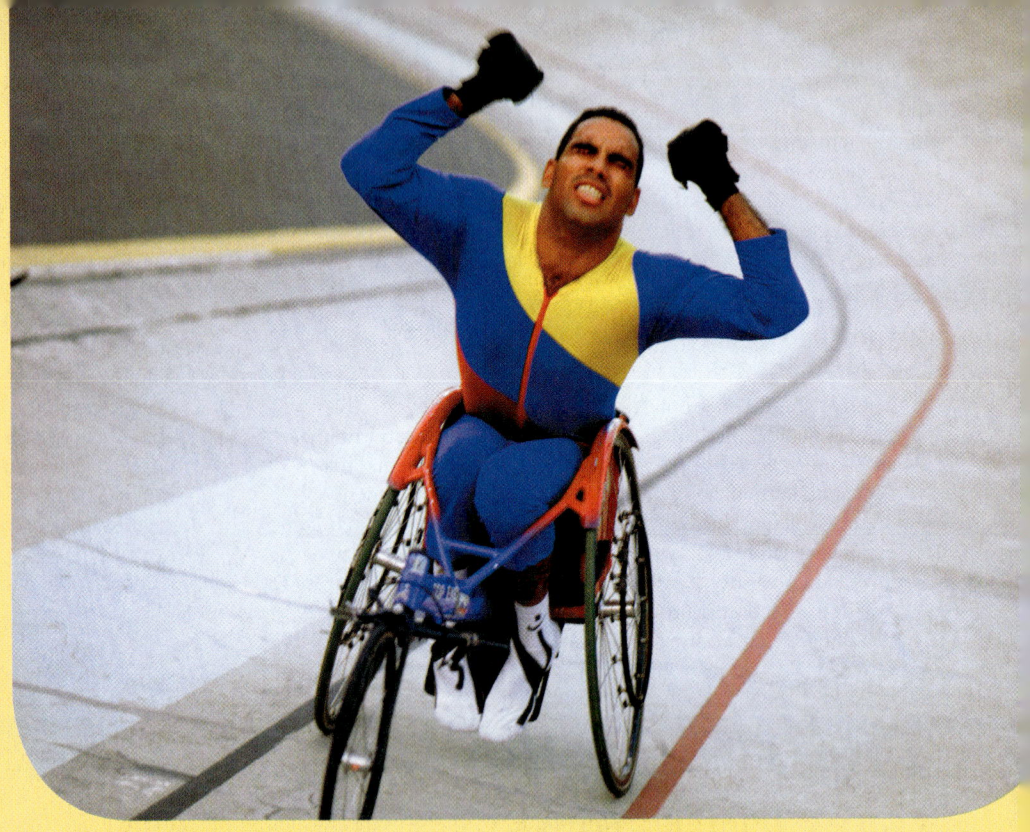

The Special Senses

People are responsive creatures. The aroma of freshly baked bread makes our mouths water. A sudden clap of thunder makes us jump. These stimuli and many others continually greet us and are interpreted by our nervous systems.

When people are asked to list the senses, they usually come up with five: vision, taste, smell, hearing, and touch. Actually, touch reflects the combined activity of the general senses that we considered in Chapter 13. The remaining senses—*vision, taste, smell, hearing,* and *equilibrium*—are called **special senses.** Most of us tend to forget the sense of equilibrium, whose receptors are housed in the ear along with the organ of hearing.

In contrast to the widely distributed general receptors (most of which are modified nerve endings of sensory neurons), the **special sensory receptors** are distinct *receptor cells.* These receptor cells are confined to the head region and are highly localized, either housed within complex sensory organs (eyes and ears) or in distinct epithelial structures (taste buds and olfactory epithelium).

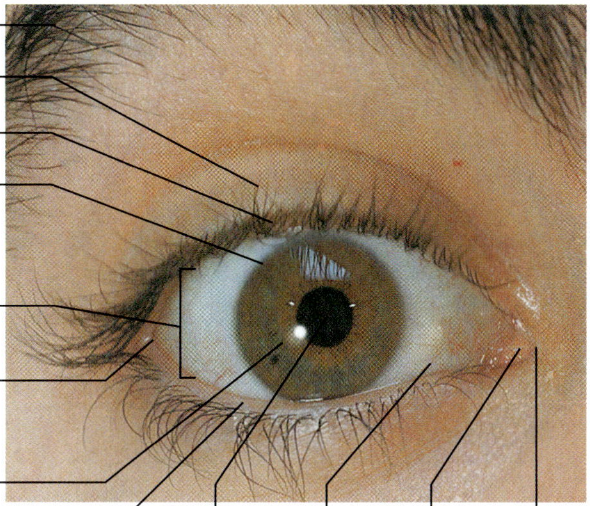

(a) Surface anatomy of the right eye

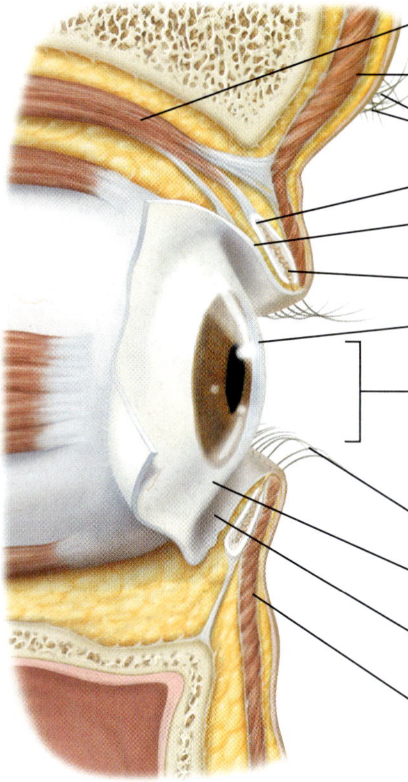

(b) Lateral view; some structures shown in sagittal section

Figure 15.1 **The eye and accessory structures.**

In this chapter we consider each of the five special senses in turn. But keep in mind that our perceptions of sensory inputs overlap. What we finally experience—our "feel" of the world—is a blending of stimulus effects.

The Eye and Vision

✓ Describe the structure and function of accessory eye structures, eye layers, the lens, and humors of the eye.

✓ Outline the causes and consequences of cataracts and glaucoma.

Vision is our dominant sense: Some 70% of all the sensory receptors in the body are in the eyes, and nearly half of the cerebral cortex is involved in some aspect of visual processing.

The adult **eye** is a sphere with a diameter of about 2.5 cm (1 inch). Only the anterior one-sixth of the eye's surface is visible **(Figure 15.1a)**. The rest is enclosed and protected by a cushion of fat and the walls of the bony orbit. The fat pad occupies nearly all of the orbit not occupied by the eye itself. The eye is a complex structure and only a small portion of its tissues are actually involved in photoreception. Before turning our attention to the eye itself, let us consider the accessory structures that protect it or aid its function.

Accessory Structures of the Eye

The **accessory structures** of the eye include the eyebrows, eyelids, conjunctiva, lacrimal apparatus, and extrinsic eye muscles.

Eyebrows

The **eyebrows** are short, coarse hairs that overlie the supraorbital margins of the skull (Figure 15.1). They help shade the eyes from sunlight and prevent perspiration trickling down the forehead from reaching the eyes.

Eyelids

Anteriorly, the eyes are protected by the mobile **eyelids** or **palpebrae** (pal′pĕ-bre). The eyelids are separated by the **palpebral fissure** ("eyelid slit") and meet at the medial and lateral angles of the eye—the **medial** and **lateral commissures** (*canthi*), respectively (Figure 15.1a).

The medial commissure sports a fleshy elevation called the **lacrimal caruncle** (kar′ung-kl; "a bit of flesh"). The caruncle contains sebaceous and sweat glands and produces the whitish, oily secretion (fancifully called the Sandman's eye-sand) that sometimes collects at the medial commissure, especially during sleep. In most Asian peoples, a vertical fold of skin called the *epicanthic fold* commonly appears on both sides of the nose and sometimes covers the medial commissure.

The eyelids are thin, skin-covered folds supported internally by connective tissue sheets called **tarsal plates** (Figure 15.1b). The tarsal plates also anchor the **orbicularis oculi** and **levator palpebrae superioris** muscles that run within the eyelid. The orbicularis muscle encircles the eye, and the eye closes when it contracts. Of the two eyelids, the larger, upper one is much more mobile, mainly because of the levator palpebrae superioris muscle, which raises that eyelid to open the eye.

15

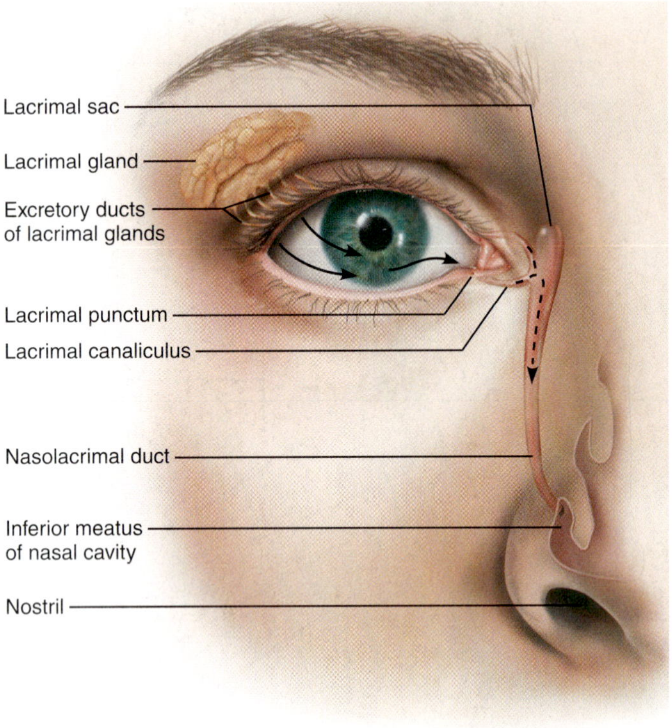

Figure 15.2 The lacrimal apparatus. Arrows indicate the flow of lacrimal fluid (tears) from the lacrimal gland to the nasal cavity.

15

The eyelid muscles are activated reflexively to cause blinking every 3–7 seconds and to protect the eye when it is threatened by foreign objects. Each time we blink, accessory structure secretions (oil, mucus, and saline solution) spread across the eyeball surface, keeping the eyes moist.

Projecting from the free margin of each eyelid are the **eyelashes**. The follicles of the eyelash hairs are richly innervated by nerve endings (hair follicle receptors), and anything that touches the eyelashes (even a puff of air) triggers reflex blinking.

Several types of glands are associated with the eyelids. The **tarsal glands** are embedded in the tarsal plates (Figure 15.1b), and their ducts open at the eyelid edge just posterior to the eyelashes. These modified sebaceous glands produce an oily secretion that lubricates the eyelid and the eye and prevents the eyelids from sticking together. Associated with the eyelash follicles are a number of smaller, more typical sebaceous glands, and modified sweat glands called ciliary glands lie between the hair follicles (*cilium* = eyelash).

Homeostatic Imbalance 15.1

An infected tarsal gland results in an unsightly cyst called a *chalazion* (kah-la′ze-on; "swelling"). Inflammation of any of the smaller glands is called a sty. ✚

Conjunctiva

The **conjunctiva** (kon″junk-ti′vah; "joined together") is a transparent mucous membrane. It lines the eyelids as the **palpebral conjunctiva** and reflects (folds back) over the anterior surface of the eyeball as the **bulbar conjunctiva** (Figure 15.1b). The bulbar conjunctiva covers only the white of the eye, not the cornea (the clear "window" over the iris and pupil). The bulbar conjunctiva is very thin, and blood vessels are clearly visible beneath it. (They are even more visible in irritated "bloodshot" eyes.)

When the eye is closed, a slitlike space occurs between the conjunctiva-covered eyeball and eyelids. This so-called **conjunctival sac** is where a contact lens lies, and eye medications are often administered into its inferior recess. The major function of the conjunctiva is to produce a lubricating mucus that prevents the eyes from drying out.

Homeostatic Imbalance 15.2

Inflammation of the conjunctiva, called *conjunctivitis*, results in reddened, irritated eyes. *Pinkeye*, a conjunctival infection caused by bacteria or viruses, is highly contagious. ✚

Lacrimal Apparatus

The **lacrimal apparatus** (lak′rĭ-mal; "tear") consists of the lacrimal gland and the ducts that drain lacrimal secretions into the nasal cavity **(Figure 15.2)**. The **lacrimal gland** lies in the orbit above the lateral end of the eye and is visible through the conjunctiva when the lid is everted. It continually releases a dilute saline solution called **lacrimal secretion**—or, more commonly, **tears**—into the superior part of the conjunctival sac through several small excretory ducts.

Blinking spreads the tears downward and across the eyeball to the medial commissure, where they enter the paired **lacrimal canaliculi** via two tiny openings called **lacrimal puncta** (literally, "prick points"), visible as tiny red dots on the medial margin of each eyelid. From the lacrimal canaliculi, the tears drain into the **lacrimal sac** and then into the **nasolacrimal duct**, which empties into the nasal cavity at the inferior nasal meatus.

Lacrimal fluid contains mucus, antibodies, and **lysozyme**, an enzyme that destroys bacteria. Thus, it cleanses and protects the eye surface as it moistens and lubricates it. When lacrimal secretion increases substantially, tears spill over the eyelids and fill the nasal cavities, causing congestion and the "sniffles." This spillover (tearing) happens when the eyes are irritated or when we are emotionally upset. In the case of eye irritation, enhanced tearing washes away or dilutes the irritating substance. The importance of emotionally induced tears is poorly understood.

Homeostatic Imbalance 15.3

Because the nasal cavity mucosa is continuous with that of the lacrimal duct system, a cold or nasal inflammation often causes the lacrimal mucosa to swell. This swelling constricts the ducts and prevents tears from draining, causing "watery" eyes. ✚

Extrinsic Eye Muscles

How do our eyes move? Six straplike **extrinsic eye muscles** control the movement of each eyeball. These muscles originate from the walls of the orbit and insert into the outer surface of

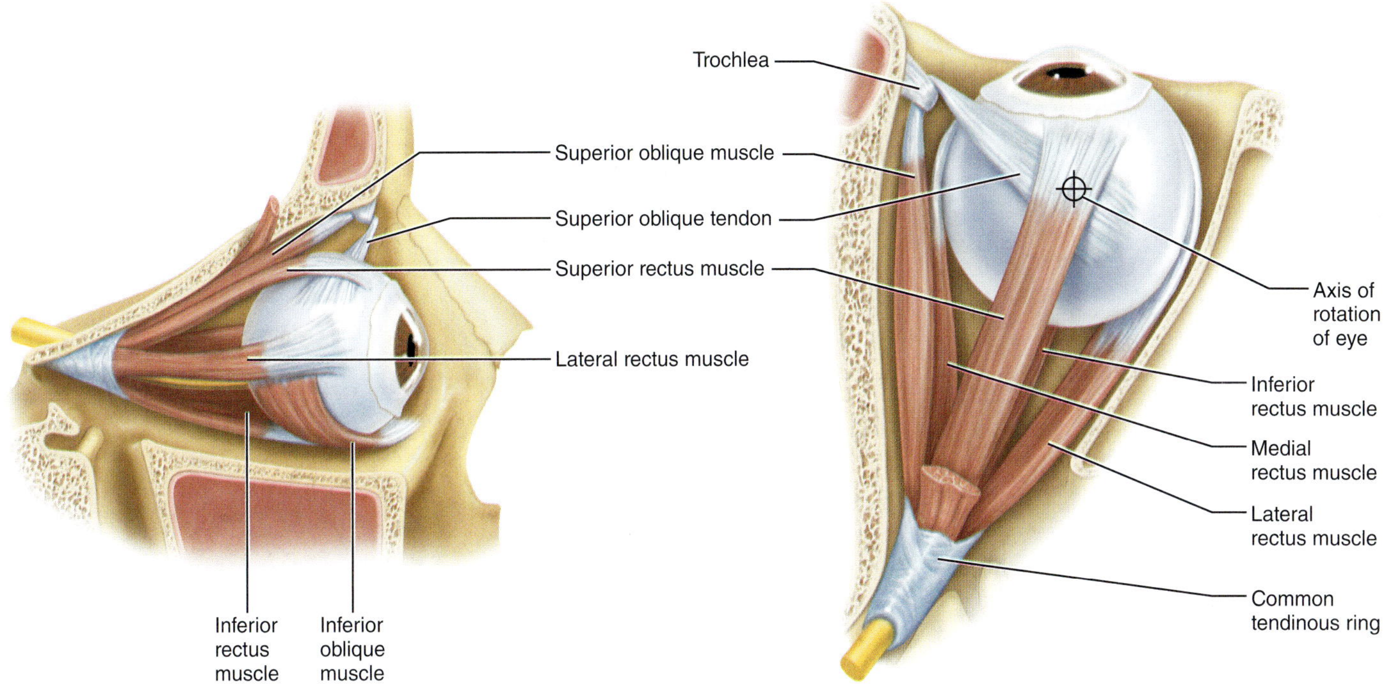

(a) Lateral view of the right eye

(b) Superior view of the right eye

Muscle	Action	Controlling cranial nerve
Lateral rectus	Moves eye laterally	VI (abducens)
Medial rectus	Moves eye medially	III (oculomotor)
Superior rectus	Elevates eye and turns it medially	III (oculomotor)
Inferior rectus	Depresses eye and turns it medially	III (oculomotor)
Inferior oblique	Elevates eye and turns it laterally	III (oculomotor)
Superior oblique	Depresses eye and turns it laterally	IV (trochlear)

(c) Summary of muscle actions and innervating cranial nerves

Figure 15.3 Extrinsic eye muscles.

the eyeball **(Figure 15.3)**. They allow the eyes to follow a moving object, and provide external "guy-wires" that help maintain the shape of the eyeball and hold it in the orbit.

The four *rectus muscles* originate from the **common tendinous ring** (or annular ring) at the back of the orbit and run straight to their insertion on the eyeball. Their locations and the movements that they promote are clearly indicated by their names: **superior, inferior, lateral**, and **medial rectus muscles**.

The actions of the two *oblique muscles* are less easy to deduce because they take rather strange paths through the orbit. They move the eye in the vertical plane when the eyeball is already turned medially by the rectus muscles. The **superior oblique muscle** originates in common with the rectus muscles, runs along the medial wall of the orbit, and then makes a right-angle turn and passes through a fibrocartilaginous loop called the **trochlea** (trok′le-ah; "pulley") suspended from the frontal bone before inserting on the superolateral aspect of the eyeball. It rotates the eye downward and somewhat laterally.

The **inferior oblique muscle** originates from the medial orbit surface and runs laterally and obliquely to insert on the inferolateral eye surface. It rotates the eye up and laterally.

The four rectus muscles would seem to provide all the eye movements we require—medial, lateral, superior, and inferior—so why the two oblique muscles? The simplest way to answer this question is to point out that the superior and inferior recti cannot elevate or depress the eye *without also turning it medially* because they approach the eye from a posteromedial direction. For an eye to be *directly* elevated or depressed, the lateral pull of the oblique muscles is necessary to cancel the medial pull of the superior and inferior recti.

Except for the lateral rectus and superior oblique muscles, which are innervated respectively by the *abducens* and *trochlear nerves*, the *oculomotor nerves* serve all extrinsic eye muscles. Figure 15.3c summarizes the actions and nerve supply of these muscles. Table 13.2 (pp. 495–497) illustrates the courses of the associated cranial nerves.

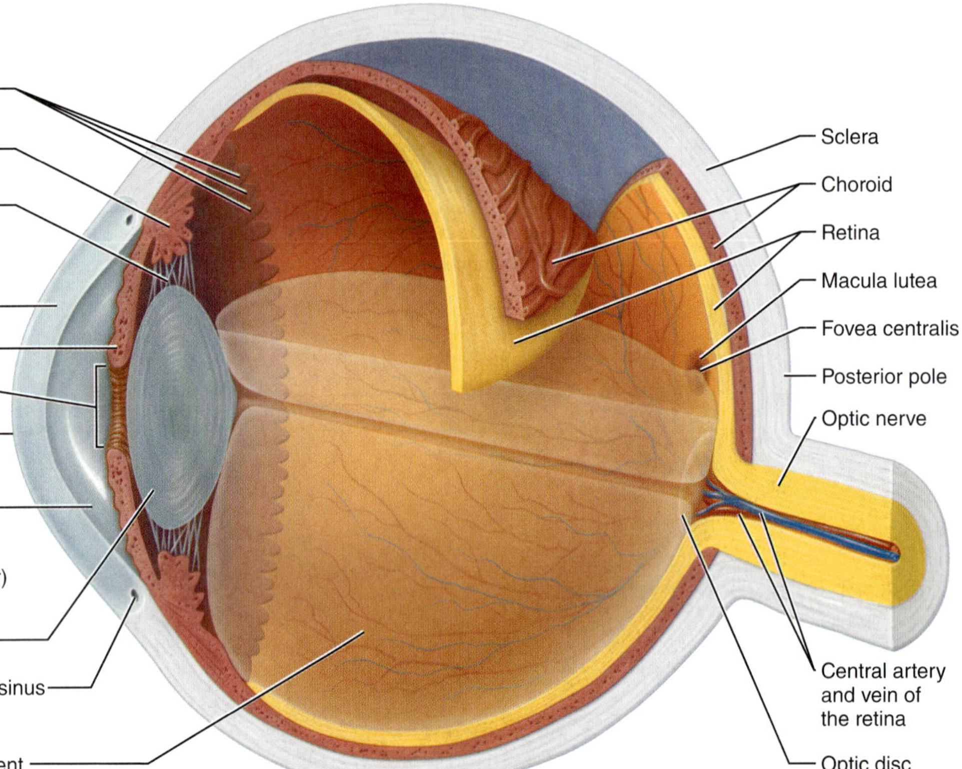

(a) Diagrammatic view. The vitreous humor is illustrated only in the bottom part of the eyeball.

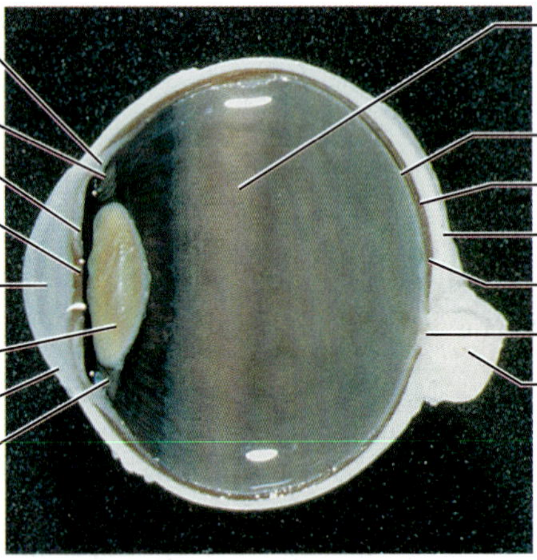

(b) Photograph of the human eye.

Figure 15.4 Internal structure of the eye (sagittal section).

The extrinsic eye muscles are among the most precisely and rapidly controlled skeletal muscles in the entire body. This precision reflects their high axon-to-muscle-fiber ratio: The motor units of these muscles contain only 8 to 12 muscle cells and in some cases as few as two or three.

Homeostatic Imbalance 15.4

When movements of the external muscles of the two eyes are not perfectly coordinated, a person cannot properly focus the images of the same area of the visual field from each eye and so sees two images instead of one. This condition is called **diplopia** (dĭ-plo′pe-ah), or *double vision*. It can result from paralysis or weakness of certain extrinsic muscles, neurological disorders, or it may be a temporary consequence of acute alcohol intoxication.

Congenital weakness of the external eye muscles may cause **strabismus** (strah-biz′mus; "cross-eyed"), in which the affected eye rotates medially or laterally. To compensate, the eyes may alternate in focusing on objects. In other cases, only the controllable eye is used, and the brain begins to disregard inputs from the deviant eye, which then becomes functionally blind. Strabismus is treated either with eye exercises to strengthen the weak muscles or by temporarily placing a patch on the stronger eye, which forces the child to use the weaker eye. Surgery is needed for unyielding conditions.+

Structure of the Eyeball

The eye itself, commonly called the **eyeball**, is a slightly irregular hollow sphere **(Figure 15.4)**. Because the eyeball is shaped roughly like the globe of the earth, it is said to have poles. Its most anterior point is the **anterior pole**, and its most posterior point is the **posterior pole**. Its wall is composed of three layers: the fibrous, vascular, and inner layers. Its internal cavity is filled with fluids called *humors* that help to maintain its shape. The lens, the adjustable focusing apparatus of the eye, is supported vertically within the eyeball, dividing it into *anterior* and *posterior segments*.

Fibrous Layer

The outermost coat of the eyeball, the **fibrous layer**, is composed of dense avascular connective tissue. It has two obviously different regions: the sclera and the cornea.

Sclera The **sclera** (skle′rah), forming the posterior portion and the bulk of the fibrous layer, is glistening white and opaque. Seen anteriorly as the "white of the eye," the tough, tendonlike sclera (*sclera* = hard) protects and shapes the eyeball and provides a sturdy anchoring site for the extrinsic eye muscles. Posteriorly, where the sclera is pierced by the optic nerve, it is continuous with the dura mater of the brain.

Cornea The anterior sixth of the fibrous layer is modified to form the transparent **cornea**, which bulges anteriorly from its junction with the sclera. The crystal-clear cornea forms a window that lets light enter the eye, and is a major part of the light-bending apparatus of the eye.

Epithelial sheets cover both faces of the cornea. The external sheet, a stratified squamous epithelium that protects the cornea from abrasion, merges with the bulbar conjunctiva at the corneoscleral junction. Epithelial cells that continually renew the cornea are located here. The deep *corneal endothelium*, composed of simple squamous epithelium, lines the inner face of the cornea. Its cells have active sodium pumps that maintain the clarity of the cornea by keeping its water content low.

The cornea is well supplied with nerve endings, most of which are pain receptors. (For this reason, some people can never adjust to wearing contact lenses.) When the cornea is touched, blinking and increased tearing occur reflexively. Even so, the cornea is the most exposed part of the eye and is vulnerable to damage from dust, slivers, and the like. Luckily, its capacity for regeneration and repair is extraordinary.

The cornea has no blood vessels and so it is beyond the reach of the immune system. As a result, the cornea is the only tissue in the body that can be transplanted from one person to another with little risk of rejection.

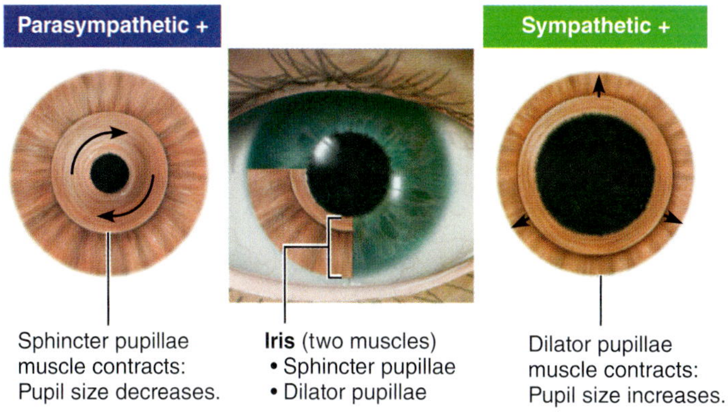

Figure 15.5 Pupil constriction and dilation, anterior view. (+ means activation.)

Vascular Layer

The **vascular layer** forms the middle coat of the eyeball. Also called the *uvea* (u′ve-ah; "grape"), this pigmented layer has three regions: choroid, ciliary body, and iris (Figure 15.4).

Choroid The **choroid** is a blood vessel–rich, dark brown membrane (*choroid* = membrane) that forms the posterior five-sixths of the vascular layer. Its blood vessels nourish all eye layers. Its brown pigment, produced by melanocytes, helps absorb light, preventing it from scattering and reflecting within the eye (which would cause visual confusion). The choroid is incomplete posteriorly where the optic nerve leaves the eye.

Ciliary Body Anteriorly, the choroid becomes the **ciliary body**, a thickened ring of tissue that encircles the lens. The ciliary body consists chiefly of interlacing smooth muscle bundles called **ciliary muscles**, which act to control lens shape. Near the lens, its posterior surface is thrown into radiating folds called **ciliary processes**, which secrete the fluid that fills the cavity of the anterior segment of the eyeball. The **ciliary zonule** (*suspensory ligament*) extends from the ciliary processes to the lens. This halo of fine fibers encircles and helps hold the lens in its upright position.

Iris The **iris**, the visible colored part of the eye, is the most anterior portion of the vascular layer. Shaped like a flattened doughnut, it lies between the cornea and the lens and is continuous with the ciliary body posteriorly. Its round central opening, the **pupil**, allows light to enter the eye. The iris is made up of two smooth muscle layers with bunches of sticky elastic fibers that congeal into a random pattern before birth. Its muscle fibers allow it to act as a reflexively activated diaphragm to vary pupil size **(Figure 15.5)**. In close vision and bright light, the *sphincter pupillae* (circular muscles) contract and the pupil constricts. In distant vision and dim light, the *dilator pupillae* (radial muscles) contract and the pupil dilates, allowing more light to enter. Sympathetic fibers control pupillary dilation and parasympathetic fibers control constriction.

Changes in pupil size may also reflect our interests and emotional reactions. Our pupils often dilate when the subject matter

15

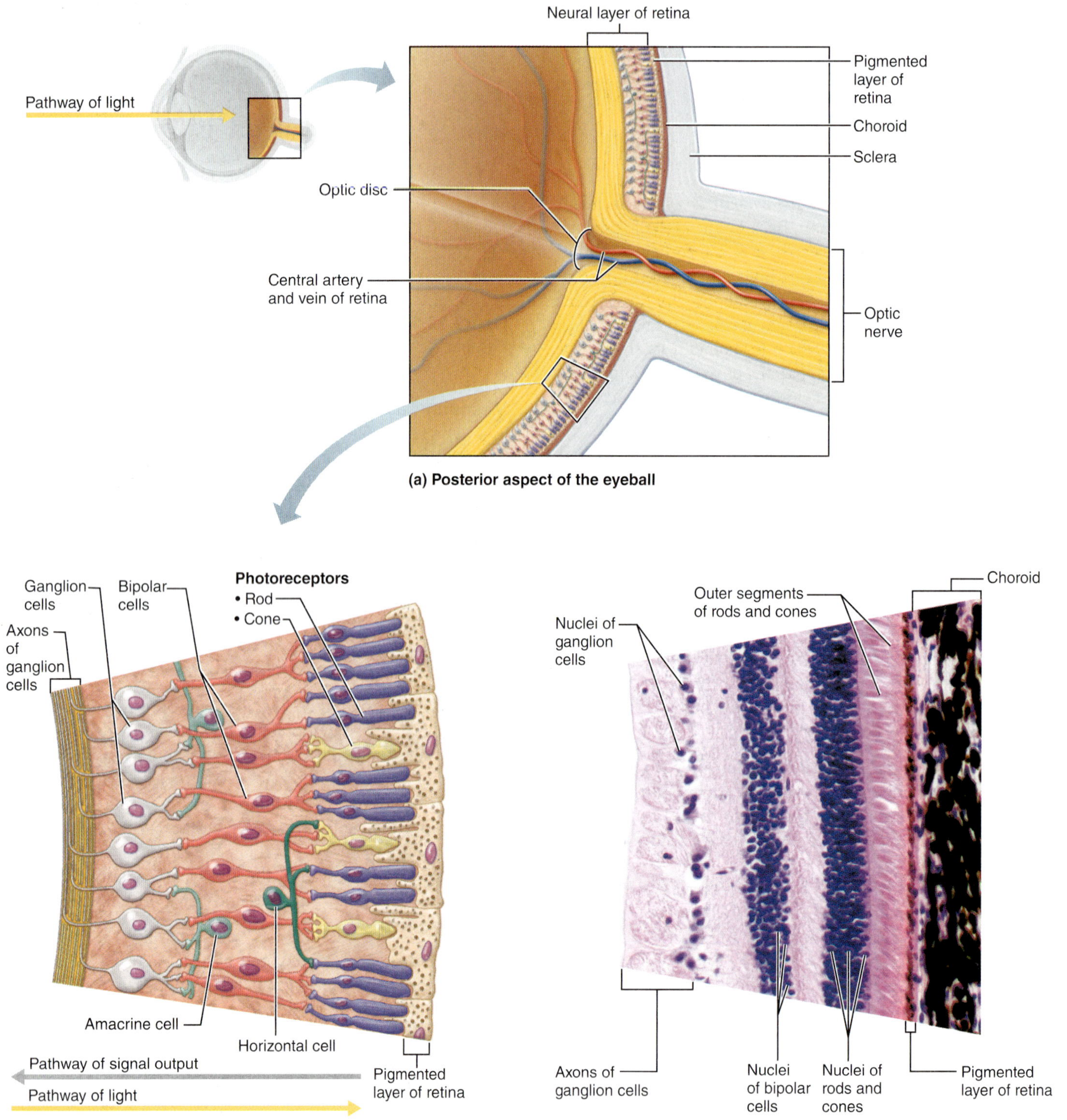

(a) Posterior aspect of the eyeball

(b) Cells of the neural layer of the retina

(c) Photomicrograph of retina

Figure 15.6 Microscopic anatomy of the retina. (a) The axons of the ganglion cells form the optic nerve, which leaves the back of the eyeball at the optic disc. **(b)** Light (indicated by the yellow arrow) passes through the retina to excite the photoreceptor cells (rods and cones). Information (output signals; gray arrow) flows in the opposite direction via bipolar and ganglion cells. **(c)** Photomicrograph (145×).

is appealing, in response to fear, and during problem solving. (Computing your taxes should make your pupils get bigger and bigger.) On the other hand, boredom or repulsive subject matter causes pupils to constrict.

Although irises come in different colors (*iris* = rainbow), they contain only brown pigment. When they have a lot of pigment, the eyes appear brown or black. If the amount of pigment is small and restricted to the posterior surface of the iris, the unpigmented parts simply scatter the shorter wavelengths of light and the eyes appear blue, green, or gray. Most newborn babies' eyes are slate gray or blue because their iris pigment is not yet developed.

Inner Layer (Retina)

The innermost layer of the eyeball is the delicate **retina** (ret′ĭ-nah), which originates as an outpocketing of the brain. It contains millions of photoreceptors that transduce (convert) light energy, other neurons involved in processing light responses, and glia. The retina consists of two layers: an outer *pigmented layer* and an inner *neural layer* **(Figure 15.6)**. Although the pigmented and neural layers are very close together, they are not fused. Only the neural layer of the retina plays a direct role in vision.

Pigmented Layer of the Retina The outer **pigmented layer**, a single-cell-thick lining, abuts the choroid, and extends anteriorly to cover the ciliary body and the posterior face of the iris. These pigment cells, like those of the choroid, absorb light and prevent it from scattering in the eye. They also act as phagocytes participating in photoreceptor cell renewal (described on p. 559), and store vitamin A needed by the photoreceptor cells.

Neural Layer of the Retina The transparent inner **neural layer** extends anteriorly to the posterior margin of the ciliary body. This junction is called the **ora serrata**, literally, the saw-toothed margin (see Figure 15.4).

From posterior to anterior, the neural layer is composed of three main types of neurons: **photoreceptors**, **bipolar cells**, and **ganglion cells** (Figure 15.6). Signals are produced in response to light and spread from the photoreceptors (abutting the pigmented layer) to the bipolar cells and then to the innermost ganglion cells, where action potentials are generated. The ganglion cell axons make a right-angle turn at the inner face of the retina, then leave the posterior aspect of the eye as the thick optic nerve. The retina also contains other types of neurons—horizontal cells and amacrine cells—which play a role in visual processing.

The **optic disc**, where the optic nerve exits the eye, is a weak spot in the **fundus** (posterior wall) of the eye because it is not reinforced by the sclera. The optic disc is also called the **blind spot** because it lacks photoreceptors, so light focused on it cannot be seen. Nonetheless, we do not usually notice these gaps in our vision because the brain uses a sophisticated process called *filling in* to deal with absence of input.

The quarter-billion photoreceptors found in the neural layer are of two types: rods and cones.

- **Rods** are our dim-light and peripheral vision receptors. They are more numerous and far more sensitive to light than cones are, but they do not provide sharp images or color vision. This is why colors disappear and the edges of objects appear fuzzy in dim light and at the edges of our visual field.
- **Cones**, by contrast, are our vision receptors for bright light and provide high-resolution color vision.

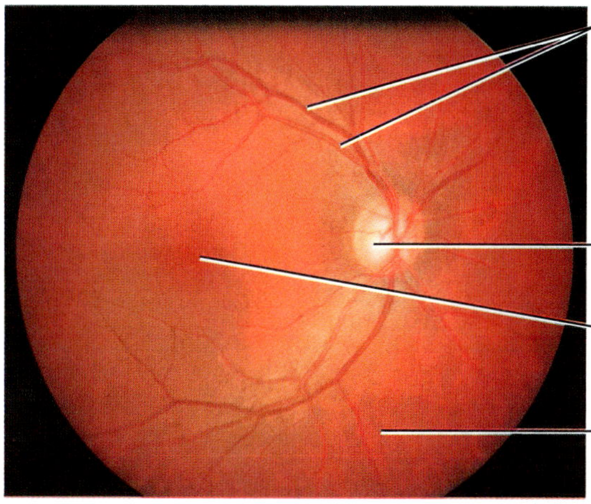

Figure 15.7 Part of the posterior wall (fundus) of the right eye as seen with an ophthalmoscope.

Lateral to the blind spot of each eye, and located precisely at the eye's posterior pole, is an oval region called the **macula lutea** (mak′u-lah lu′te-ah; "yellow spot") with a minute (0.4 mm) pit in its center called the **fovea centralis** (see Figure 15.4). In this region, the retinal structures abutting the vitreous humor are displaced to the sides. This allows light to pass almost directly to the photoreceptors rather than through several retinal layers, greatly enhancing visual acuity (the ability to resolve detail). The fovea contains only cones, the macula contains mostly cones, and from the edge of the macula toward the retina periphery, cone density declines gradually. The retina periphery contains mostly rods, which continuously decrease in density from there to the macula.

Only the foveae (plural of fovea) have a sufficient cone density to provide detailed color vision, so anything we wish to view critically is focused on the foveae. Because each fovea is only about the size of the head of a pin, only a thousandth of the entire visual field is in *hard focus* (foveal focus) at a given moment. Consequently, for us to visually comprehend a scene that is rapidly changing (as when we drive in traffic), our eyes must flick rapidly back and forth to provide the foveae with images of different parts of the visual field.

The neural layer of the retina receives its blood supply from two sources. Vessels in the choroid supply the outer third (containing photoreceptors). The inner two-thirds is served by the **central artery** and **central vein of the retina**, which enter and leave the eye through the center of the optic nerve (see Figure 15.4a). Radiating outward from the optic disc, these vessels give rise to a rich vascular network. This is the only place where small blood vessels are visible in a living person **(Figure 15.7)**. Physicians may observe these tiny vessels with an ophthalmoscope for signs of hypertension, diabetes, and other vascular diseases.

15

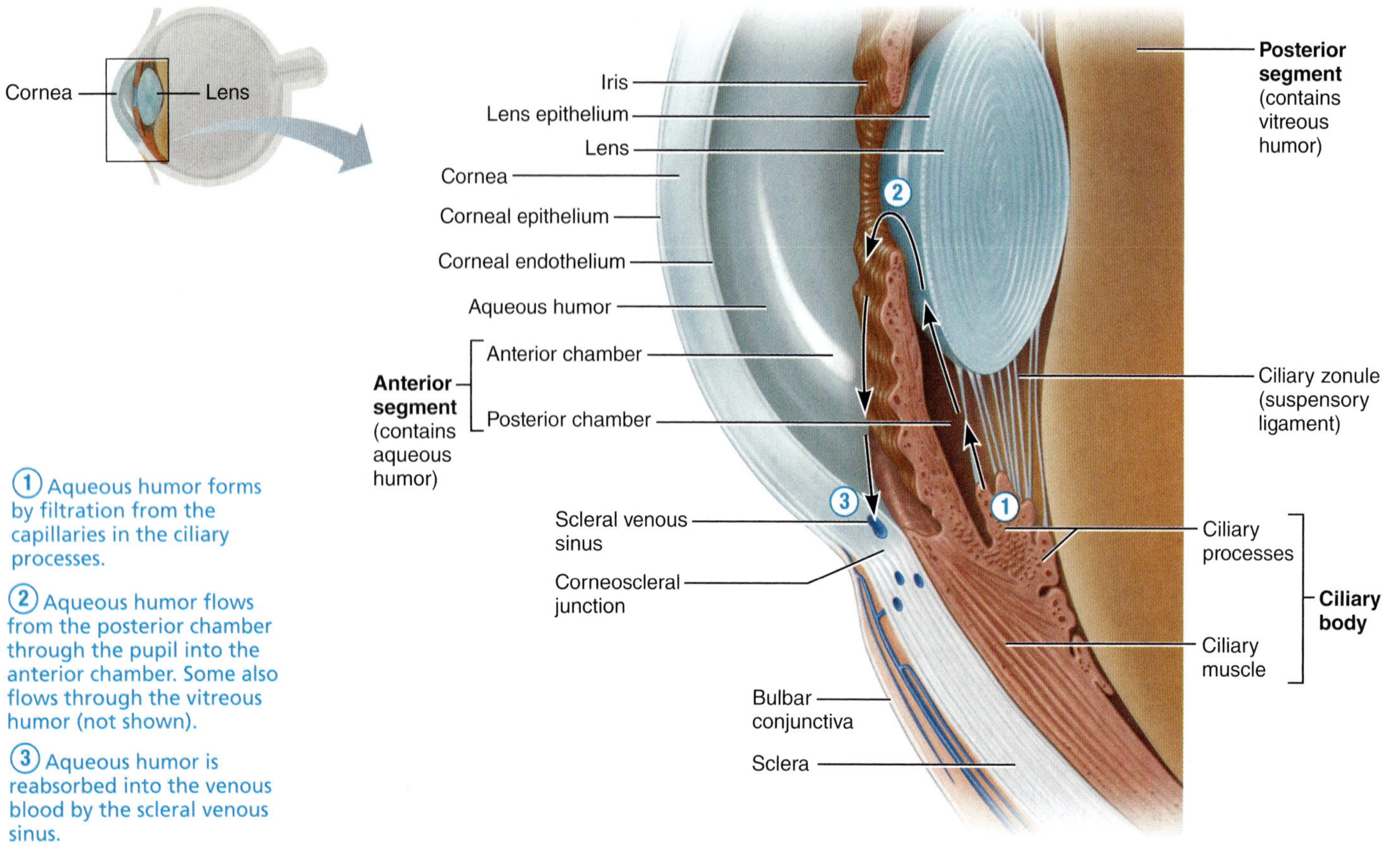

Figure 15.8 Circulation of aqueous humor. The arrows indicate the circulation pathway.

15

Homeostatic Imbalance 15.5

The pattern of vascularization of the retina makes it susceptible to *retinal detachment*. This condition, in which the pigmented and neural layers separate (detach) and allow the jellylike vitreous humor to seep between them, can cause permanent blindness because it deprives the photoreceptors of nutrients.

Retinal detachment usually happens when the retina is torn during a traumatic blow to the head or when the head stops moving suddenly and then jerks in the opposite direction (as in bungee jumping). The symptom that victims most often describe is "a curtain being drawn across the eye," but some people see sootlike spots or light flashes. If diagnosed early, it is often possible to reattach the retina with a laser before photoreceptors are permanently damaged. +

Internal Chambers and Fluids

As we noted earlier, the lens and its halolike ciliary zonule divide the eye into two segments, the anterior segment in front of the lens and the larger posterior segment behind it (see Figure 15.4a). The **posterior segment** is filled with a clear gel called **vitreous humor** (*vitre* = glassy) that binds tremendous amounts of water. Vitreous humor

- Transmits light
- Supports the posterior surface of the lens and holds the neural layer of the retina firmly against the pigmented layer
- Contributes to intraocular pressure, helping to counteract the pulling force of the extrinsic eye muscles

Vitreous humor forms in the embryo and lasts for a lifetime.

The iris divides the **anterior segment** into the **anterior chamber** (between the cornea and the iris) and the **posterior chamber** (between the iris and the lens) (**Figure 15.8**). The *entire* anterior segment is filled with **aqueous humor**, a clear fluid similar in composition to blood plasma. Unlike the vitreous humor, aqueous humor forms and drains continually and is in constant motion.

1. The capillaries of the ciliary processes form the aqueous humor by filtering plasma into the posterior chamber.
2. A portion of the fluid freely diffuses through the vitreous humor in the posterior segment while the remainder flows into the anterior chamber.
3. After flowing through the pupil into the anterior chamber, aqueous humor drains into the venous blood via the **scleral venous sinus**, an unusual venous channel that encircles the eye in the angle at the corneoscleral junction.

Normally, aqueous humor forms and drains at the same rate, maintaining a constant intraocular pressure of about 16 mm Hg, which helps to support the eyeball internally. Aqueous humor supplies nutrients and oxygen to the lens and cornea and to some cells of the retina, and it carries away their metabolic wastes.

Homeostatic Imbalance 15.6

If the drainage of aqueous humor is blocked, fluid backs up as in a clogged sink. Pressure within the eye may increase to dangerous levels and compress the retina and optic nerve—a condition called **glaucoma** (glaw-ko′mah). The eventual result is blindness (*glaucoma* = vision growing gray) unless the condition is detected early. Unfortunately, many forms of glaucoma steal sight so slowly and painlessly that people do not realize they have a problem until the damage is done. Late signs include seeing halos around lights and blurred vision.

The glaucoma examination is simple. The intraocular pressure is determined by directing a puff of air at the cornea and measuring the amount of corneal deformation it causes. This exam should be done yearly after age 40. The most common treatment is eye drops that increase the rate of aqueous humor drainage or decrease its production. Laser therapy or surgery can also help. ✚

Lens

The **lens** is a biconvex, transparent, flexible structure that can change shape to precisely focus light on the retina. It is enclosed in a thin, elastic capsule and held in place just posterior to the iris by the ciliary zonule (Figure 15.8). Like the cornea, the lens is avascular; blood vessels interfere with transparency.

The lens has two regions: the **lens epithelium** and the lens fibers. The lens epithelium, confined to the anterior lens surface, consists of cuboidal cells that eventually differentiate into the **lens fibers** that form the bulk of the lens. The lens fibers, which are packed tightly together like the layers in an onion, contain no nuclei and few organelles. They do, however, contain transparent, precisely folded proteins called **crystallins** that form the body of the lens. Since new lens fibers are continually added, the lens enlarges throughout life, becoming denser, more convex, and less elastic, all of which gradually impair its ability to focus light properly.

Homeostatic Imbalance 15.7

A **cataract** ("waterfall") is a clouding of the lens that causes the world to appear distorted, as if seen through frosted glass **(Figure 15.9)**. Some cataracts are congenital, but most result from age-related hardening and thickening of the lens or are a secondary consequence of diabetes mellitus. Heavy smoking and frequent exposure to intense sunlight increase the risk for cataracts.

Oxidative stress and metabolic changes in the deeper lens fibers promote clumping of the crystallin proteins. A recent study unexpectedly showed that supplementation with the antioxidant vitamin C actually increases cataract formation. Fortunately, the offending lens can be surgically removed and an artificial lens implanted to save the patient's sight. ✚

Check Your Understanding

1. What are tears and what structure secretes them?
2. What is the blind spot and why is it blind?

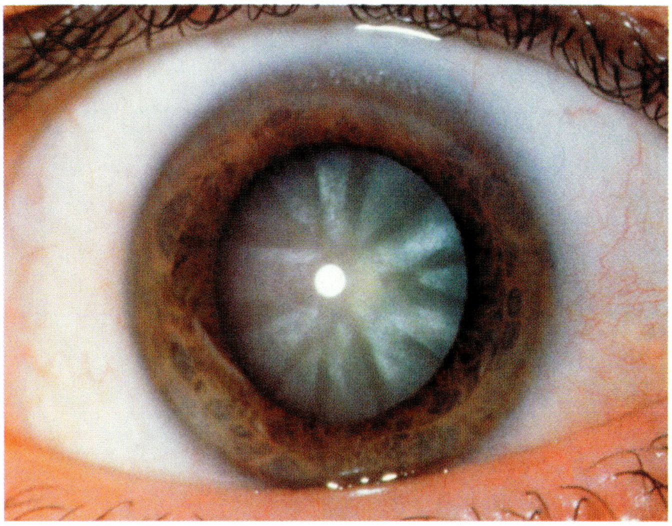

Figure 15.9 Photograph of a cataract. The lens, not the cornea, is milky and opaque.

3. Sam's optometrist tells him that his intraocular pressure is high. What is this condition called and which fluid does it involve?

For answers, see Appendix H.

15

Optics and the Eye

✓ Trace the pathway of light through the eye to the retina, and explain how light is focused for distant and close vision.

✓ Outline the causes and consequences of astigmatism, myopia, hyperopia, and presbyopia.

Overview: Light and Optics

To comprehend the function of the eye as a photoreceptor organ, we need to understand the properties of light.

Wavelength and Color **Electromagnetic radiation** includes all energy waves, from long radio waves (with wavelengths measured in meters) to very short gamma (γ) waves and X rays with wavelengths of 1 nm and less. Our eyes respond to the part of the spectrum called **visible light**, which has a wavelength range of approximately 400–700 nm **(Figure 15.10a)**. (1 nm = 10^{-9} m, or one-billionth of a meter.)

Visible light travels in the form of waves, and its wavelengths can be measured very accurately. However, light can also be envisioned as small particles or packets of energy called **photons** or **quanta**. Attempts to reconcile these two findings have led to the present concept of light as packets of energy (photons) traveling in a wavelike fashion at very high speeds (300,000 km/s or about 186,000 mi/s). We can think of light as a vibration of pure energy ("a bright wiggle") rather than a material substance.

When visible light passes through a prism, each of its component waves bends to a different degree, dispersing the beam of

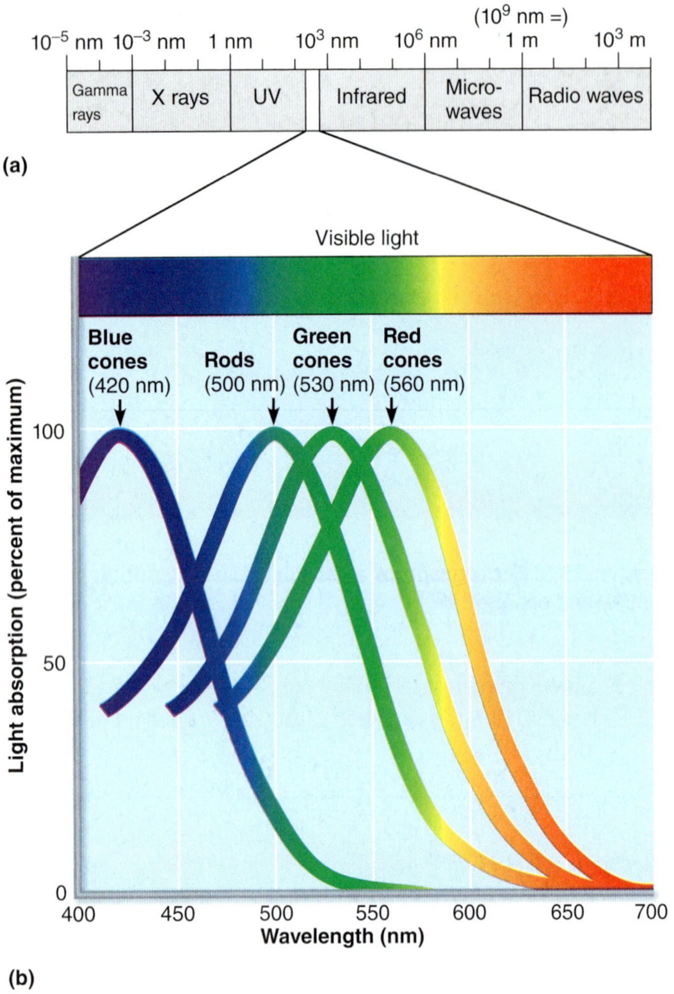

Figure 15.10 The electromagnetic spectrum and photoreceptor sensitivities. (a) The electromagnetic spectrum, of which visible light constitutes only a small portion. (nm = nanometers.) **(b)** Sensitivities of rods and the three cone types to the different wavelengths of the visible spectrum.

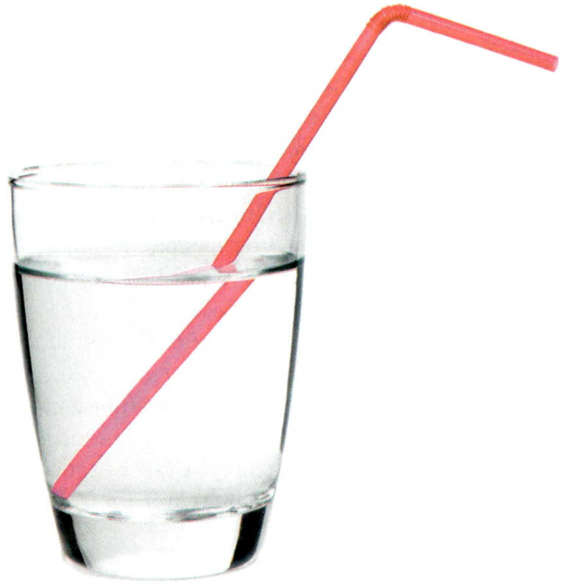

Figure 15.11 Refraction. A straw standing in a glass of water appears to be broken at the water-air interface. This occurs because light bends toward the perpendicular when it travels from a less dense medium (such as air) to a more dense medium (such as water).

light into a **visible spectrum**, or band of colors (Figure 15.10b). (A rainbow that appears during a summer shower represents the collective prismatic effects of all the tiny water droplets suspended in air.) Red wavelengths are the longest and have the lowest energy, while violet wavelengths are the shortest and most energetic.

Like sound, light can reflect, or bounce, off a surface. This *reflection* of light by objects in our environment accounts for most of the light reaching our eyes. Objects have color because they absorb some wavelengths and reflect others. A red apple reflects mostly red light, while grass reflects more of the green. Things that look white reflect all wavelengths of light, whereas black objects absorb them all.

Refraction and Lenses Light travels in straight lines (rays) and is blocked by any nontransparent object. When light travels in a given medium, its speed is constant. But when it passes from one transparent medium into another with a different density, its speed changes. Light speeds up as it passes into a less dense medium and slows as it passes into a denser medium. Because of these changes in speed, bending or **refraction** of a light ray occurs when it meets the surface of a different medium at an oblique angle rather than at a right angle (perpendicular). The greater this angle, the greater the amount of bending. **Figure 15.11** shows refraction: A straw in a glass of water appears to break at the air-water interface.

A lens is a transparent object curved on one or both surfaces. Since light hits the curve at an angle, it is refracted. If the lens surface is convex, that is, thickest in the center like a camera lens, the light rays bend so that they converge or intersect at a single point called the **focal point (Figure 15.12a)**. In general, the thicker (more convex) the lens, the more the light bends and the shorter the focal distance (distance between the lens and focal point). The image formed by a convex lens, called a **real image**, is inverted—upside down and reversed from left to right (Figure 15.12b).

Concave lenses, which are thicker at the edges than at the center, diverge the light (bend it outward) so that the light rays move away from each other. Consequently, concave lenses prevent light from focusing and extend the focal distance.

Focusing Light on the Retina

As light passes from air into the eye, it moves sequentially through the cornea, aqueous humor, lens, and vitreous humor, and then passes *through the entire neural layer of the retina* to excite the photoreceptors that abut the pigmented layer (see

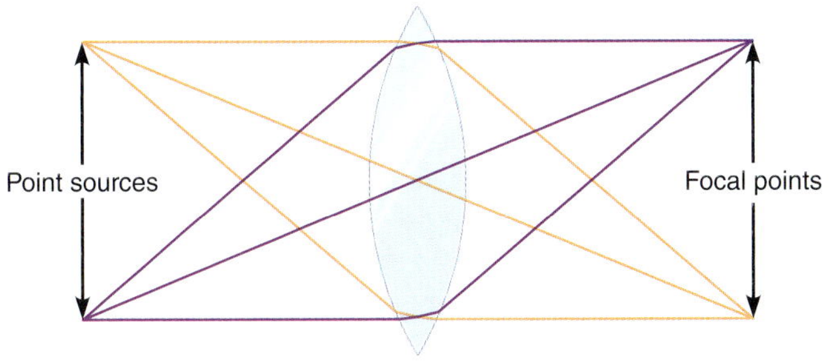

(a) Focusing of two points of light.

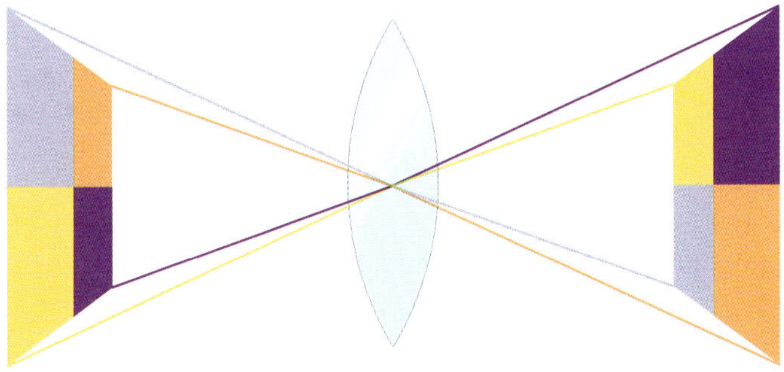

(b) The image is inverted—upside down and reversed.

Figure 15.12 Light is focused by a convex lens. The lens bends, or refracts, light rays so they converge on a focal point.

Figures 15.4 and 15.6). During its passage, light is bent three times: (1) entering the cornea, (2) entering the lens, and (3) leaving the lens.

The cornea accounts for the majority of the refractory power of the eye. However, the refractory power of the cornea is constant. On the other hand, the lens is highly elastic, and its curvature and light-bending power can actively change to allow fine focusing.

Focusing for Distant Vision Our eyes are best adapted ("preset to focus") for distant vision. To look at distant objects, we need only aim our eyeballs so that they are both fixated on the same spot. The **far point of vision** is that distance beyond which no change in lens shape (accommodation) is needed for focusing. For the normal or **emmetropic** (em″ĕ-tro′pik) eye, the far point is 6 m (20 feet).

Any object being viewed can be said to consist of many small points, with light radiating outward in all directions from each point. However, because distant objects appear smaller, light from an object at or beyond the far point of vision approaches the eyes as nearly parallel rays. The cornea and the at-rest lens focus the light from these distant objects precisely on the retina **(Figure 15.13a)**.

During distant vision, the sphincterlike ciliary muscles are completely relaxed, and tension in the ciliary zonule stretches the lens flat. Consequently, the lens is as thin as it gets and is at its lowest refractory power when at rest. The ciliary muscles relax when sympathetic input to them increases and parasympathetic input decreases.

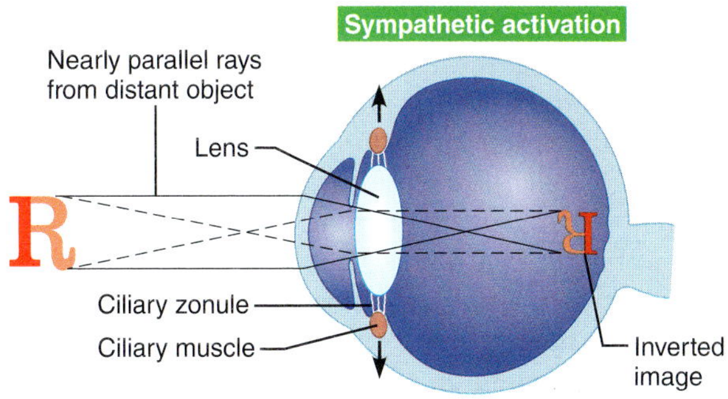

(a) Lens flattens for distant vision. Sympathetic input relaxes the ciliary muscle, tightening the ciliary zonule, and flattening the lens.

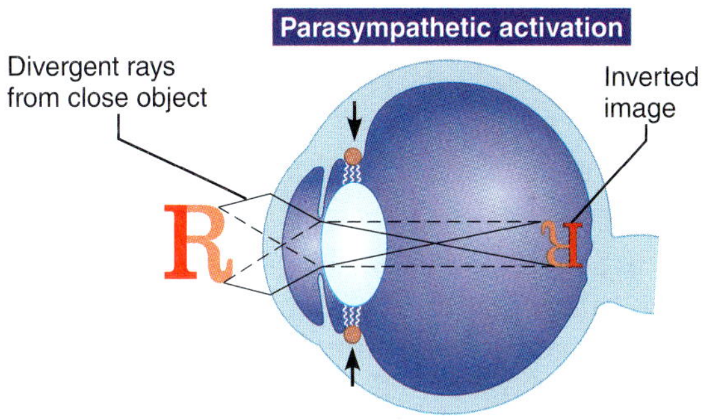

(b) Lens bulges for close vision. Parasympathetic input contracts the ciliary muscle, loosening the ciliary zonule, allowing the lens to bulge.

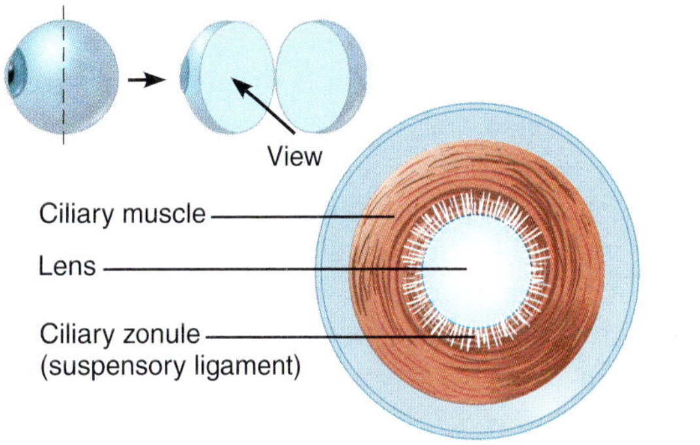

(c) The ciliary muscle and ciliary zonule are arranged sphincterlike around the lens. As a result, contraction loosens the ciliary zonule fibers and relaxation tightens them.

Figure 15.13 Focusing for distant and close vision.

Focusing for Close Vision Light from close objects (less than 6 m away) diverges as it approaches the eyes and comes to a focal point farther from the lens. For this reason, close vision demands that the eye make active adjustments. To restore focus, three processes must occur simultaneously: accommodation of the lenses, constriction of the pupils, and convergence of the eyeballs. The signal that induces this trio of reflex responses is blurring of the retinal image.

- **Accommodation of the lenses. Accommodation** is the process that increases the refractory power of the lens. The ciliary muscles contract, pulling the ciliary body anteriorly toward the pupil and inward, releasing tension in the ciliary zonule. No longer stretched, the elastic lens recoils and bulges, providing the shorter focal length needed to focus the image of a close object on the retina (Figure 15.13b). Parasympathetic fibers of the oculomotor nerves control the contraction of the ciliary muscles.

  The closest point on which we can focus clearly is called the **near point of vision**, and it represents the maximum bulge the lens can achieve. In young adults with emmetropic vision, the near point is 10 cm (4 inches) from the eye. However, it is closer in children and gradually recedes with age, explaining why children can hold their books very close to their faces while many elderly people must hold the newspaper at arm's length. The gradual loss of accommodation with age reflects the lens's decreasing elasticity. In many people over age 50, the lens is nonaccommodating, a condition known as **presbyopia** (pres″be-o′pe-ah), literally "old person's vision."
- **Constriction of the pupils.** The sphincter pupillae muscles of the iris enhance the effect of accommodation by reducing the size of the pupil toward 2 mm (see Figure 15.5). This **accommodation pupillary reflex**, mediated by parasympathetic fibers of the oculomotor nerves, prevents the most divergent light rays from entering the eye. Such rays would pass through the extreme edge of the lens and would not focus properly, causing blurred vision.
- **Convergence of the eyeballs.** The visual goal is always to keep the object being viewed focused on the retinal foveae. When we look at distant objects, both eyes are directed either straight ahead or to one side to the same degree, but when we fixate on a close object, our eyes converge. **Convergence**, controlled by somatic motor fibers of the oculomotor nerves, is medial rotation of the eyeballs by the medial rectus muscles so that each is directed toward the object being viewed. The closer that object, the greater the degree of convergence required. For example, when you focus on the tip of your nose, you "go cross-eyed."

Reading or other close work requires almost continuous accommodation, pupillary constriction, and convergence. This is why prolonged periods of reading tire the eye muscles and can result in eyestrain. When you read for an extended time, it helps to look up and stare into the distance occasionally to relax your intrinsic eye muscles.

Homeostatic Imbalance 15.8

Theoretically, visual problems related to refraction could result from a hyperrefractive (overconverging) or hyporefractive (underconverging) lens or from structural abnormalities of the eyeball. In practice, 99% of refractive problems are related to eyeball shape—either too long or too short.

Myopia (mi-o′pe-ah; "short vision") occurs when distant objects focus in front of the retina, rather than on it (**Figure 15.14**, left). Myopic people see close objects without problems because they can focus them on the retina, but distant objects are blurred. The common name for myopia is *nearsightedness*. (Notice that this terminology names the aspect of vision that is *unimpaired*.) Myopia typically results from an eyeball that is too long.

Correction has traditionally involved using concave lenses that diverge the light before it enters the eye. Laser procedures to flatten the cornea slightly offer other treatment options.

Hyperopia (hy′per-o″pe-ah; "far vision"), or *farsightedness*, occurs when the parallel light rays from distant objects focus *behind* the retina (Figure 15.14, right). Hyperopic individuals can see distant objects perfectly well because their ciliary muscles contract almost continuously to increase the light-bending power of the lens, which moves the focal point forward onto the retina. However, diverging light rays from *nearby* objects focus so far behind the retina that the lens cannot bring the focal point onto the retina even at its full refractory power. As a result, close objects appear blurry, and convex corrective lenses are needed to converge the light more strongly for close vision. Hyperopia usually results from an eyeball that is too short.

Unequal curvatures in different parts of the cornea or lens also lead to blurry images. This refractory problem is **astigmatism** (*astigma* = not a point). Special cylindrically ground lenses or laser procedures are used to correct this problem. +

Check Your Understanding

4. Arrange the following in the order that light passes through them to reach the photoreceptors (rods and cones) in the retina: lens, bipolar cells, vitreous humor, cornea, aqueous humor, ganglion cells. (Hint: See Figure 15.6 if you need a reminder of where ganglion cells and bipolar cells are.)
5. You have been reading this book for a while now and your eyes are beginning to tire. Which intrinsic eye muscles are relaxing as you stare thoughtfully into the distance?
6. Why does your near point of vision move farther away as you age?

For answers, see Appendix H.

Photoreceptors and Phototransduction

- ✓ Describe the events that convert light into a neural signal.
- ✓ Compare and contrast the roles of rods and cones in vision.
- ✓ Compare and contrast light and dark adaptation.

Once light is focused on the retina, the photoreceptors come into play. First, we will describe the functional anatomy of the rod and cone photoreceptor cells, then the chemistry and response of their visual pigments to light, and finally, photoreceptor activation, phototransduction, and information processing in the retina. **Phototransduction** is the process by which light energy is converted into a graded receptor potential.

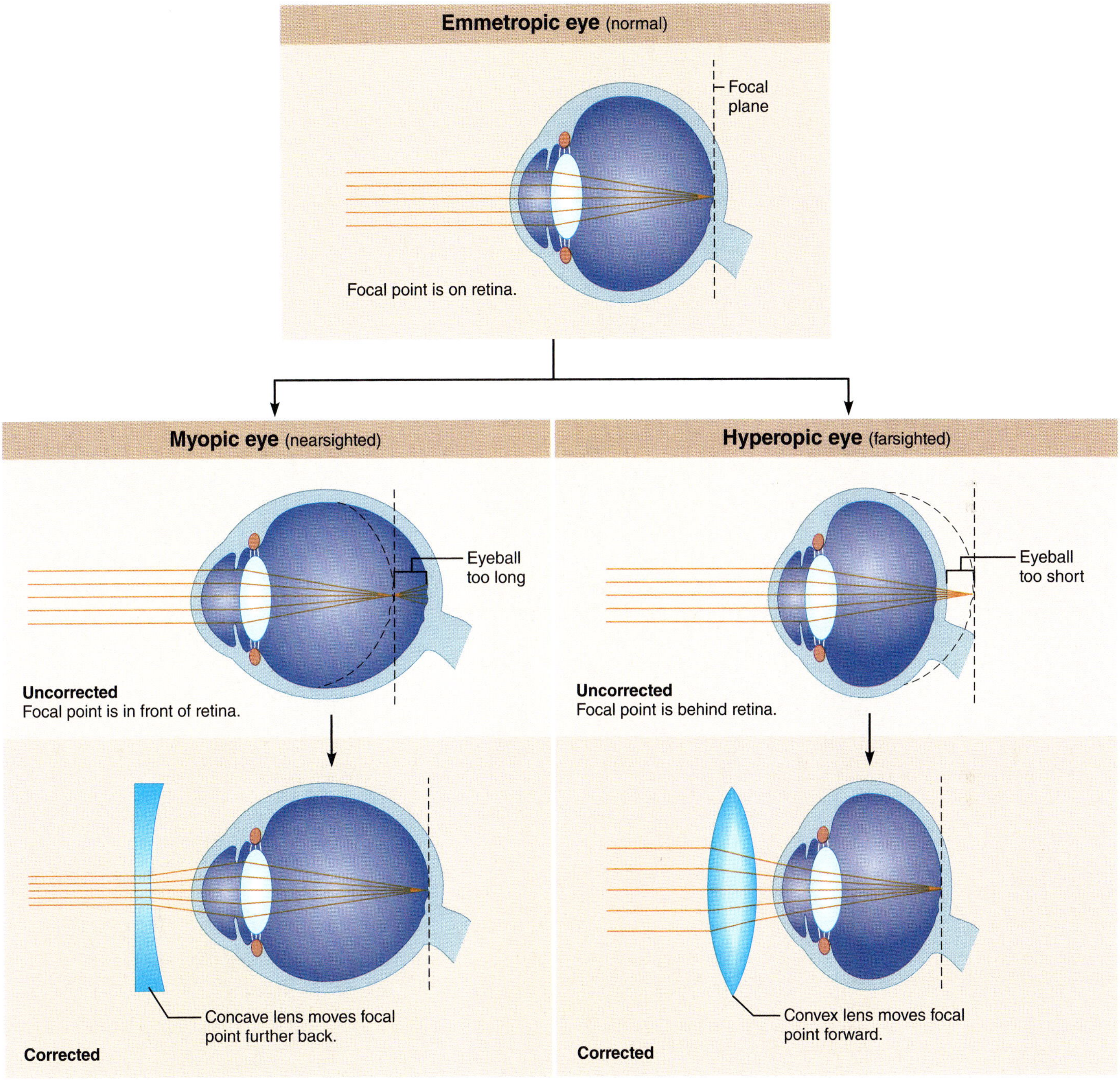

Figure 15.14 Problems of refraction. The refractive power of the cornea, which normally supplies about two-thirds of the light-bending power of the eye, is ignored here.

Functional Anatomy of the Photoreceptors

Photoreceptors are modified neurons, but structurally they resemble tall epithelial cells turned upside down with their "tips" immersed in the pigmented layer of the retina (**Figure 15.15a**). These "tips" are the receptive regions of rods and cones and are called the **outer segments**. Moving from the pigmented layer into the neural layer, a connecting cilium joins the outer segment of a rod or cone to the **inner segment**. The inner segment then connects to the *cell body*, which is continuous with an *inner fiber* bearing *synaptic terminals*.

In rods, the outer segment is slender and rod shaped (hence their name) and the inner segment connects to the cell body by the *outer fiber*. By contrast, the cones have a short conical outer segment and the inner segment directly joins the cell body.

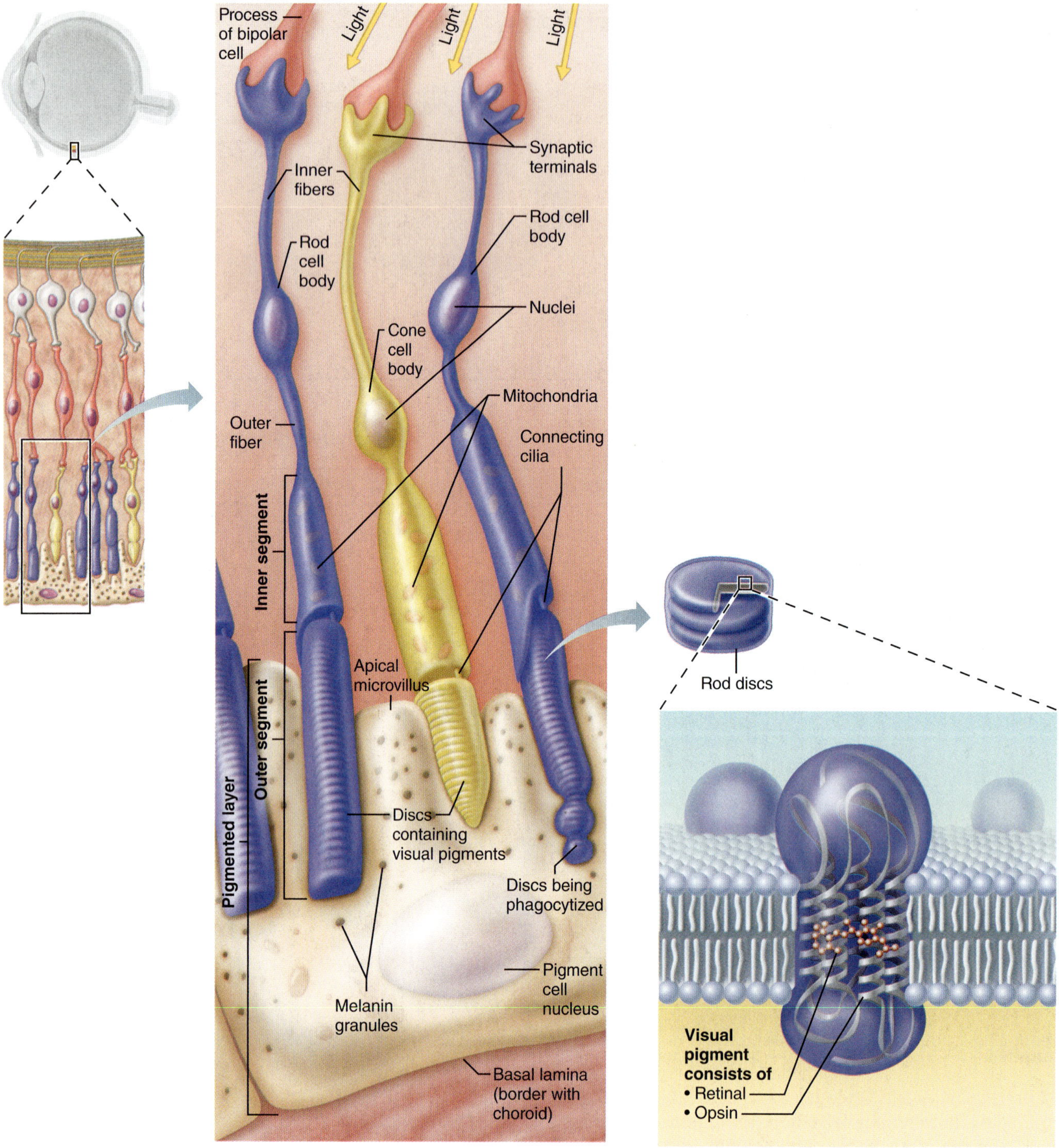

(a) **The outer segments of rods and cones are embedded in the pigmented layer of the retina.**

(b) **Rhodopsin, the visual pigment in rods, is embedded in the membrane that forms discs in the outer segment.**

Figure 15.15 Photoreceptors of the retina.

The outer segments contain an elaborate array of **visual pigments (photopigments)** that change shape as they absorb light. These pigments are embedded in areas of the plasma membrane that form discs (Figure 15.15b). Folding the plasma membrane into discs increases the surface area available for trapping light. In rods, the discs are discontinuous—stacked inside a cylinder of plasma membrane like pennies in a coin wrapper. In cones, the disc membranes are continuous with the plasma membrane, so the interiors of the cone discs are continuous with the extracellular space.

Photoreceptor cells are highly vulnerable to damage and immediately begin to degenerate if the retina becomes detached. They are also destroyed by intense light, the very energy they detect. How is it, then, that we do not all gradually go blind? The answer lies in the photoreceptors' unique system for renewing their light-trapping outer segment. Every 24 hours, new components are synthesized in the cell body and added to the base of the outer segment. As new discs are made, the discs at the tip of the outer segment continually fragment off and pigment cells phagocytize them.

Comparing Rod and Cone Vision

Rods and cones have different thresholds for activation. Rods, for example, are very sensitive (they respond to very dim light—a single photon), making them best suited for night vision and peripheral vision. Cones, on the other hand, need bright light for activation (have low sensitivity), but react more rapidly. Cones have one of three different pigments that furnish a vividly colored view of the world, but rods contain a single kind of visual pigment so their inputs are perceived only in gray tones.

Rods and cones are also "wired" differently to other retinal neurons. Rods participate in converging pathways, and as many as 100 rods may ultimately feed into each ganglion cell. As a result, rod effects are summated and considered collectively, resulting in vision that is fuzzy and indistinct. (The visual cortex has no way of knowing exactly *which* rods of the large number influencing a particular ganglion cell are actually activated.)

In contrast, each cone in the fovea (or at most a few) has a straight-through pathway via its "own personal bipolar cell" to a ganglion cell (see Figure 15.6b). Essentially, each foveal cone has its own "labeled line" to the higher visual centers—permitting detailed, high-acuity (high-resolution) views of very small areas of the visual field.

Because rods are absent from the foveae and cones do not respond to low-intensity light, we see dimly lit objects best when we do not look at them directly, and we recognize them best when they move. If you doubt this, go out into your backyard on a moonlit evening and see how much you can actually discriminate.

Table 15.1 summarizes the differences between rods and cones.

Table 15.1 Comparison of Rods and Cones

RODS	CONES
Noncolor vision (one visual pigment)	Color vision (three visual pigments)
High sensitivity; function in dim light	Low sensitivity; function in bright light
Low acuity (many rods converge onto one ganglion cell)	High acuity (one cone per ganglion cell in fovea)
More numerous (20 rods for every cone)	Less numerous
Mostly in peripheral retina	Mostly in central retina

The Chemistry of Visual Pigments

How do photoreceptors translate incoming light into electrical signals? The key is a light-absorbing molecule called **retinal** that combines with proteins called **opsins** to form four types of visual pigments. Depending on the type of opsin to which it is bound, retinal absorbs different wavelengths of the visible spectrum.

The cone opsins differ both from the opsin of the rods and from one another. The naming of cones reflects the colors (that is, wavelengths) of light that each cone variety absorbs best. Blue cones respond maximally to wavelengths around 420 nm, green cones to wavelengths of 530 nm, and red cones to wavelengths at or close to 560 nm (see Figure 15.10b).

How do we see other colors besides blue, green, and red? Cones' absorption spectra overlap, and our perception of intermediate hues, such as yellow, orange, and purple, results from differential activation of more than one type of cone at the same time. For example, yellow light stimulates both red and green cone receptors, but if the red cones are stimulated more than the green cones, we see orange instead of yellow. When all cones are stimulated equally, we see white.

Homeostatic Imbalance 15.9

Color blindness is due to a congenital lack of one or more cone pigments. Inherited as an X-linked condition, it is far more common in males than in females. As many as 8–10% of males have some form of color blindness.

The most common type is red-green color blindness, resulting from a deficit or absolute absence of either red or green cone pigments. Red and green are seen as the same color—either red or green, depending on the cone pigment present. Many color-blind people are unaware of their condition because they have learned to rely on other cues—such as different intensities of the same color—to distinguish something green from something red, such as traffic signals. +

Retinal is chemically related to vitamin A and is made from it. The cells of the pigmented layer of the retina absorb vitamin A from the blood and serve as the local vitamin A depot for rods and cones.

Retinal can assume a variety of distinct three-dimensional forms, each form called an isomer. When bound to opsin, retinal has a bent, or kinked, shape called **11-*cis*-retinal**, as shown at the top of Figure 15.16. However, when the pigment is struck by light and absorbs a photon, retinal twists and snaps into a new configuration, **all-*trans*-retinal**, shown at the bottom of Figure 15.16. This change, in turn, causes opsin to change shape and assume its activated form.

The capture of light by visual pigments is the *only* light-dependent stage, and this simple photochemical event initiates a whole chain of chemical and electrical reactions in rods and cones that ultimately causes electrical impulses to be transmitted

15

Figure 15.16 The formation and breakdown of rhodopsin. 11-*cis*-retinal can either be regenerated from all-*trans*-retinal or made from vitamin A.

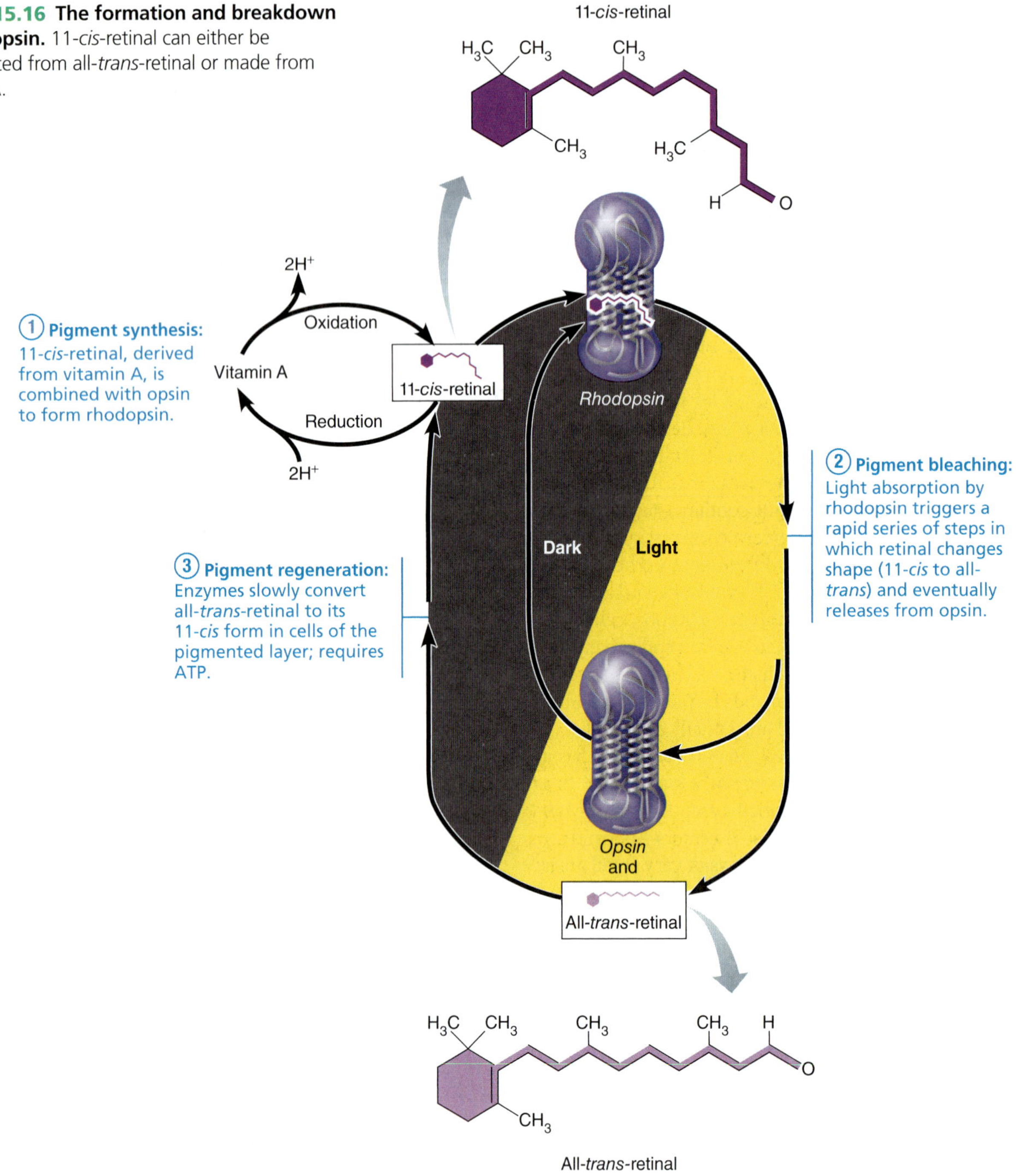

along the optic nerve. Let's look more closely at these events in rods and in cones.

Phototransduction

Phototransduction begins when a visual pigment captures a photon of light.

Capturing Light The visual pigment of rods is a deep purple pigment called **rhodopsin** (ro-dop′sin; *rhodo* = rose, *opsis* = vision). (Do you suppose the person who coined the expression "looking at the world through rose-colored glasses" knew the meaning of "rhodopsin"?) Rhodopsin molecules are arranged in a single layer in the membranes of each of the thousands of discs in the rods' outer segments. The formation and breakdown of rhodopsin is shown in Figure 15.16.

① **Pigment synthesis:** Rhodopsin forms and accumulates in the dark. Vitamin A is oxidized (and isomerized) to the 11-*cis*-retinal form and then combined with opsin to form rhodopsin.

② **Pigment bleaching:** When rhodopsin absorbs light, retinal changes shape to its all-*trans* isomer, allowing the surrounding protein to quickly relax like an uncoiling spring into its light-activated form. Eventually, the retinal-opsin

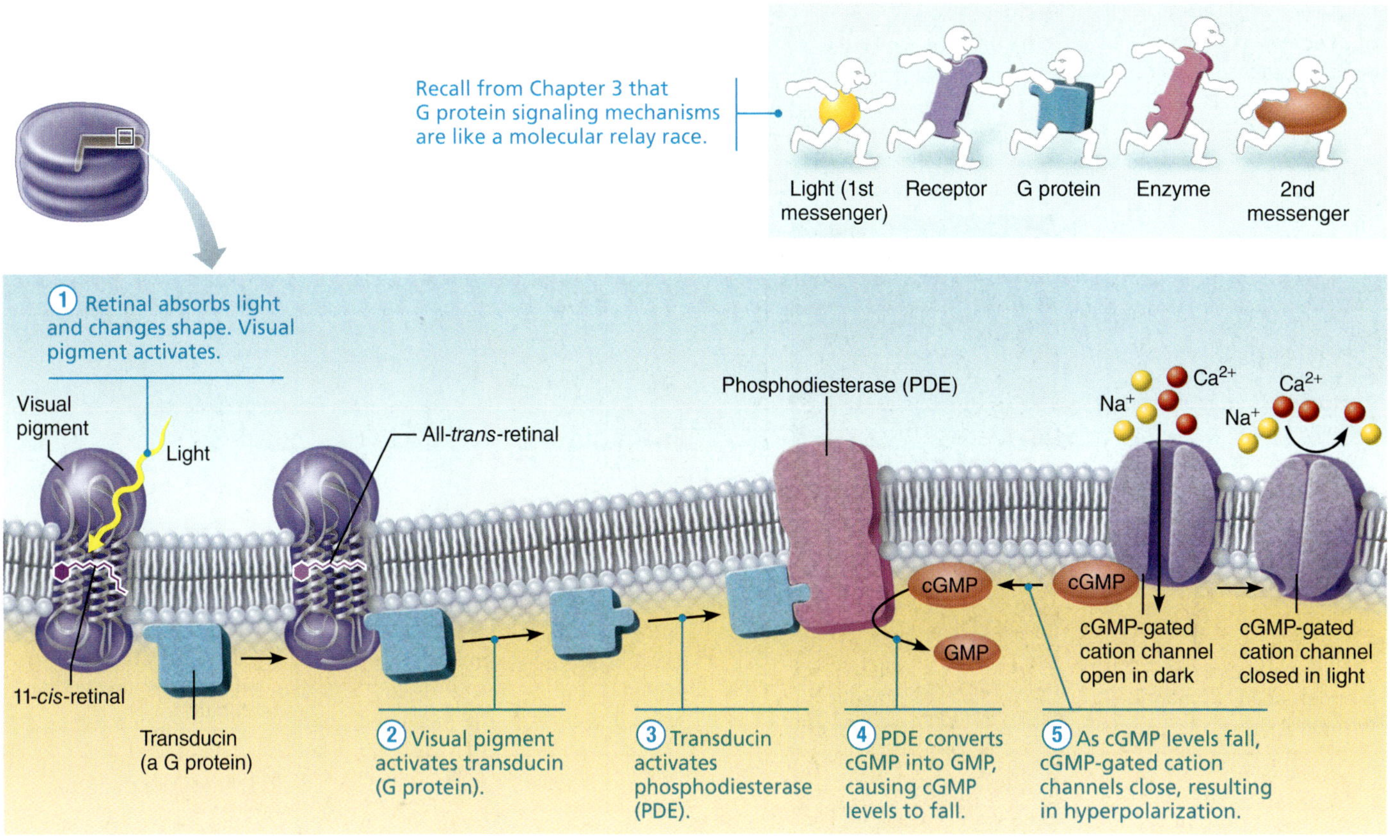

Figure 15.17 Events of phototransduction. A portion of photoreceptor disc membrane is shown. The G protein conversion of GTP to GDP has been omitted for clarity. For simplicity, the channels gated by cyclic GMP (cGMP) are shown on the same membrane as the visual pigment instead of in the plasma membrane.

combination breaks down, allowing retinal and opsin to separate. The breakdown of rhodopsin to retinal and opsin is known as the **bleaching of the pigment**.

3. **Pigment regeneration:** Once the light-struck all-*trans*-retinal detaches from opsin, enzymes within the pigmented epithelium reconvert it to its 11-*cis* isomer. Then, retinal heads "homeward" again to the photoreceptor cells' outer segments. Rhodopsin is regenerated when 11-*cis*-retinal is rejoined to opsin.

The breakdown and regeneration of visual pigments in cones is essentially the same as for rhodopsin. However, cones are about a hundred times less sensitive than rods, which means that it takes higher-intensity (brighter) light to activate cones.

Light Transduction Reactions What happens when light changes opsin's shape? An enzymatic cascade occurs that ultimately results in closing cation channels that are normally kept open in the dark. **Figure 15.17** illustrates this process in more detail, but in short, light-activated rhodopsin activates a G protein called **transducin**. Transducin, in turn, activates *PDE (phosphodiesterase)*, the enzyme that breaks down **cyclic GMP (cGMP)**. In the dark, cGMP binds to cation channels in the outer segments of photoreceptor cells, holding them open. This allows Na^+ and Ca^{2+} to enter, depolarizing the cell to its *dark potential* of about −40 mV. In the light, cGMP breaks down, the cation channels close, Na^+ and Ca^{2+} stop entering the cell, and the cell hyperpolarizes to about −70 mV.

This arrangement can seem bewildering, to say the least. Here we have receptors built to detect light that depolarize in the dark and hyperpolarize when exposed to light! However, all that is required is a signal and hyperpolarization is just as good a signal as depolarization.

Information Processing in the Retina

How is the hyperpolarization of the photoreceptors transmitted through the retina and on to the brain? **Figure 15.18** illustrates this process. As you study this sequence, notice that the photoreceptors do not generate action potentials (APs), and neither do the bipolar cells that lie between them and the ganglion cells. Photoreceptors and bipolar cells only generate graded potentials—excitatory postsynaptic potentials (EPSPs) and inhibitory postsynaptic potentials (IPSPs).

This is not surprising if you remember that the primary function of APs is to carry information rapidly over long distances. Retinal cells are small cells that are very close together. Graded potentials can serve quite adequately as signals that directly

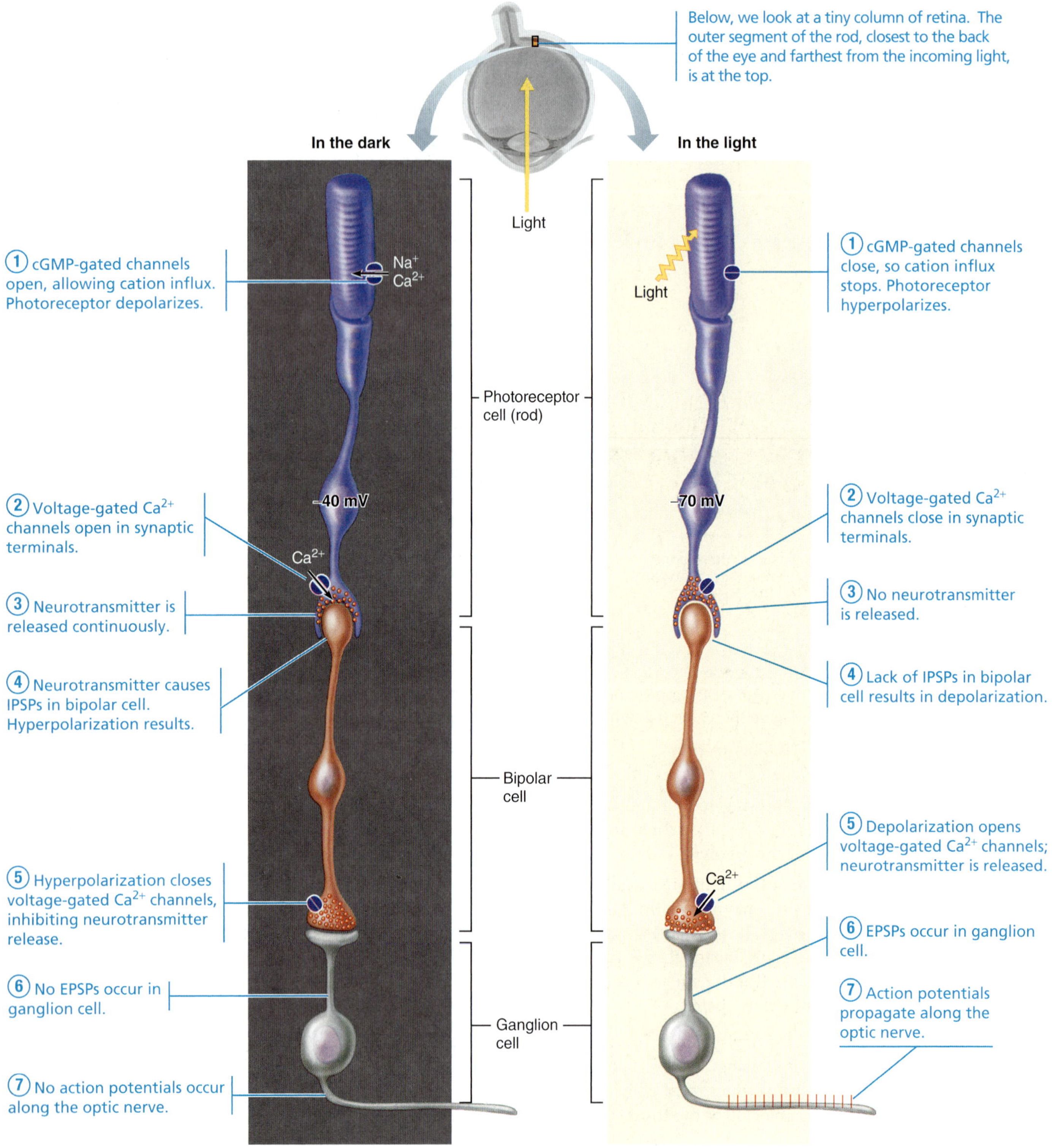

Figure 15.18 Signal transmission in the retina. EPSP = excitatory postsynaptic potential; IPSP = inhibitory postsynaptic potential.

regulate neurotransmitter release at the synapse by opening or closing voltage-gated Ca^{2+} channels.

As shown in the right panel of Figure 15.18, for example, light hyperpolarizes photoreceptors, which then stop releasing their inhibitory neurotransmitter (glutamate). No longer inhibited, bipolar cells depolarize and release neurotransmitter onto ganglion cells. Once the signal reaches the ganglion cells, it is converted into an AP. This AP is transmitted to the brain along the ganglion cell axons that make up the optic nerve.

Light and Dark Adaptation

Rhodopsin is amazingly sensitive. Even starlight bleaches some of its molecules. As long as the light is low intensity, relatively little rhodopsin bleaches and the retina continues to respond to light stimuli. However, in high-intensity light, there is wholesale bleaching of the pigment, and rhodopsin bleaches as fast as it is re-formed. At this point, the rods are nonfunctional, but cones still respond. Hence, retinal sensitivity automatically adjusts to the amount of light present.

Light Adaptation **Light adaptation** occurs when we move from darkness into bright light, as when leaving a movie matinee. We are momentarily dazzled—all we see is white light—because the sensitivity of the retina is still "set" for dim light. Both rods and cones are strongly stimulated, and large amounts of the visual pigments break down almost instantaneously, producing a flood of signals that accounts for the glare.

Under such conditions, compensations occur. The rod system turns off—all of the transducins "pack up and move" to the inner segment, uncoupling rhodopsin from the rest of the transduction cascade. Without transducin in the outer segment, light hitting rhodopsin cannot produce a signal. At the same time, the less sensitive cone system and other retinal neurons rapidly adapt, and retinal sensitivity decreases dramatically. Within about 60 seconds, the cones, initially overexcited by the bright light, are sufficiently desensitized to take over. Visual acuity and color vision continue to improve over the next 5–10 minutes. Thus, during light adaptation, we lose retinal sensitivity (rod function) but gain visual acuity.

Dark Adaptation **Dark adaptation**, essentially the reverse of light adaptation, occurs when we go from a well-lit area into a dark one. Initially, we see nothing but velvety blackness because (1) our cones stop functioning in low-intensity light, and (2) the bright light bleached our rod pigments, and the rods are still turned off.

But once we are in the dark, rhodopsin accumulates, transducin returns to the outer segment, and retinal sensitivity increases. Dark adaptation is much slower than light adaptation and can go on for hours. However, there is usually enough rhodopsin within 20–30 minutes to allow adequate dim-light vision.

During both light and dark adaptation, reflexive changes occur in pupil size. Bright light shining in one or both eyes constricts both pupils (elicits the *pupillary* and *consensual light reflexes*). These pupillary reflexes are mediated by the pretectal nucleus of the midbrain and by parasympathetic fibers. In dim light, the pupils dilate, allowing more light to enter the eye.

Homeostatic Imbalance 15.10

Night blindness, or *nyctalopia* (nic″tă-lo′pe-uh), is a condition in which rod function is seriously hampered, impairing one's ability to drive safely at night. In countries where malnutrition is common, the most common cause of night blindness is prolonged vitamin A deficiency, which leads to rod degeneration. Vitamin A supplements restore function if they are administered early.

In countries where nutrition isn't a problem, *retinitis pigmentosa*—a group of degenerative retinal diseases that destroy rods—are the most common causes of night blindness. Retinitis pigmentosa results from pigment epithelial cells that are unable to recycle the tips of the rods as they get sloughed off. +

Check Your Understanding

7. For each of the following, indicate whether it applies to rods or cones: vision in bright light; only one type of visual pigment; most abundant in the periphery of the retina; many feed into one ganglion cell; color vision; higher sensitivity; higher acuity.
8. What does bleaching of the pigment mean and when does it happen?

For answers, see Appendix H.

Visual Pathways and Processing

✓ Trace the visual pathway to the visual cortex, and briefly describe the steps in visual processing.

The Visual Pathway to the Brain

As we described earlier, the axons of the retinal ganglion cells exit the eye in the **optic nerves** (**Figure 15.19**). At the X-shaped **optic chiasma** (*chiasm* = cross), fibers from the medial aspect of each eye cross over to the opposite side and then continue on via the **optic tracts**. As a result, each optic tract

- Contains fibers from the lateral (temporal) aspect of the eye on the same side and fibers from the medial (nasal) aspect of the opposite eye
- Carries all the information from the same half of the visual field

Notice that, because the lens system of each eye reverses all images, the medial half of each retina receives light rays from the *temporal* (lateralmost) part of the visual field (that is, from the far left or far right rather than from straight ahead), and the lateral half of each retina receives an image of the nasal (central) part of the visual field. Consequently, the left optic tract carries (and sends on) a complete representation of the right half of the visual field, and the opposite is true for the right optic tract.

The paired optic tracts sweep posteriorly around the hypothalamus and send most of their axons to synapse with neurons in the **lateral geniculate nuclei** (contained within the lateral geniculate bodies) of the thalamus. The lateral geniculate nuclei maintain the fiber separation established at the chiasma, but they balance and combine the retinal input for delivery to the visual cortex. Axons of these thalamic neurons project through the internal capsule to form the **optic radiation** of fibers in the cerebral white matter (Figure 15.19). These fibers project to the **primary visual cortex** in the occipital lobes, where conscious perception of visual images (seeing) occurs.

Some nerve fibers in the optic tracts send branches to the midbrain. One set of these fibers ends in the **superior colliculi**,

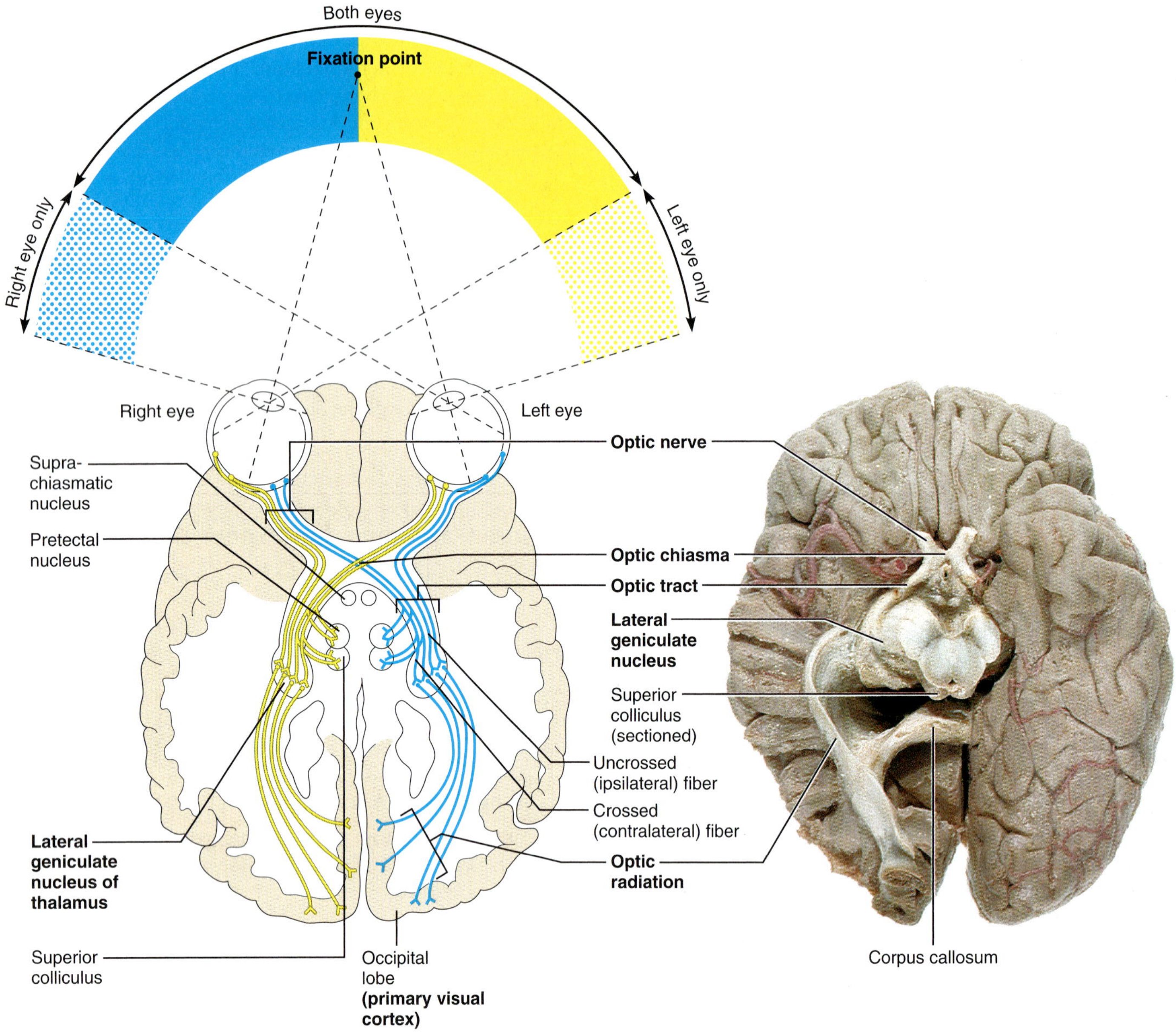

(a) The visual fields of the two eyes overlap considerably. Note that fibers from the lateral portion of each retinal field do not cross at the optic chiasma.

(b) Photograph of human brain, with the right side dissected to reveal internal structures.

Figure 15.19 Visual pathway to the brain and visual fields, inferior view.

15

visual reflex centers controlling the extrinsic muscles of the eyes. Another set comes from a small subset of ganglion cells in the retina that contain the visual pigment *melanopsin,* dubbed the circadian pigment. These ganglion cells respond directly to light stimuli and their fibers project to the **pretectal nuclei**, which mediate pupillary light reflexes, and to the **suprachiasmatic nucleus** of the hypothalamus, which functions as the "timer" to set our daily biorhythms.

Depth Perception

Notice that both eyes are set anteriorly and look in approximately the same direction. Their visual fields, each about 170 degrees, overlap to a considerable extent, and each eye sees a slightly different view (Figure 15.19a). The visual cortex fuses the slightly different images delivered by the two eyes, providing us with **depth perception** (or **three-dimensional vision**), an accurate means of locating objects in space.

In contrast, many animals (pigeons, rabbits, and others) have *panoramic vision.* Their eyes are placed more laterally on the head, so that the visual fields overlap very little, and crossover of the optic nerve fibers is almost complete. Consequently, each visual cortex receives input principally from a single eye and a totally different visual field.

Depth perception depends on the two eyes working together. If only one eye is used, depth perception is lost, and the person must learn to judge an object's position based on learned cues (for example, nearer objects appear larger, and parallel lines converge with distance).

Homeostatic Imbalance 15.11

The visual system's pathways explain patterns of blindness that follow damage to different visual structures. Loss of an eye or destruction of one optic nerve eliminates true depth perception entirely, and peripheral vision on the damaged side. For example, if the "left eye" in Figure 15.19 was lost in a hunting accident, nothing would be seen in the visual field area that is stippled yellow in that figure.

If neural destruction occurs beyond the optic chiasma—in an optic tract, the thalamus, or visual cortex—then part or all of the opposite half of the visual field is lost. For example, a stroke affecting the left visual cortex leads to blindness in the right half of the visual field. However, since the right (undamaged) visual cortex still receives inputs from both eyes, depth perception in the remaining half of the visual field is retained.+

Visual Processing

How does information received by rods and cones become vision? Visual processing begins in the retina.

Retinal cells simplify and condense the information from rods and cones, splitting it into a number of different "channels," each with its own type of ganglion cell. These "channels" include information about color and brightness, but also about more complex aspects of what we see—the angle, direction and speed of movement of *edges* (sudden changes in brightness or color). Extracting information about edges depends on a type of processing called *lateral inhibition*, a kind of contrast enhancement, which is the job of the amacrine and horizontal cells mentioned on p. 551.

The ganglion cells pass the processed information to the lateral geniculate nuclei of the thalamus. There, the retinal axons from each visual field of the two eyes are combined in preparation for depth perception, input from cones is emphasized, and contrast is further sharpened.

The *primary visual cortex*, also called the **striate cortex**, receives the thick bundle of fibers coming in from the lateral geniculate nucleus. This area contains an accurate topographical map of the retina, with the left visual cortex receiving input from the right visual field and vice versa. Visual processing here occurs at a relatively basic level, with the processing neurons responding to dark and bright edges (contrast information) and object orientation.

The striate cortex also provides form, color, and motion inputs to *visual association areas* collectively called the **prestriate cortices**. The more anterior prestriate cortices are occipital lobe centers that continue processing visual information concerned with form, color, and movement.

Functional neuroimaging of humans has revealed that complex visual processing extends well forward into the temporal, parietal, and frontal lobes via two parallel streams:

- The "what" processing stream extends through the ventral part of the temporal lobe and specializes in identifying objects in the visual field.
- The "where" processing stream takes a dorsal path through the parietal cortex all the way to the postcentral gyrus and uses information from the primary visual cortex to assess the location of objects in space.

Output from both these regions then passes to the frontal cortex, which uses that information to direct activities that, among other things, can guide movements such as reaching for a juicy peach.

Check Your Understanding

9. Which part of the visual field would be affected by a tumor in the right visual cortex? By a tumor compressing the right optic nerve?

For answers, see Appendix H.

The Chemical Senses: Smell and Taste

✓ Describe the location, structure, and afferent pathways of smell and taste receptors, and explain how these receptors are activated.

Smell and taste are gritty, primitive senses that alert us to whether that "stuff" nearby (or in our mouth) is to be savored or avoided. The receptors for smell (olfaction) and taste (gustation) are **chemoreceptors** (they respond to chemicals in an aqueous solution). They complement each other and respond to different classes of chemicals. Smell receptors are excited by airborne chemicals that dissolve in fluids coating nasal membranes, and taste receptors are excited by food chemicals dissolved in saliva.

Olfactory Epithelium and the Sense of Smell

Although our olfactory sense (*olfact* = to smell) is far less acute than that of many other animals, the human nose is still no slouch in picking up small differences in odors. Some people capitalize on this ability by becoming wine tasters.

Location and Structure of Olfactory Receptors

Olfaction detects chemicals (*odorants*) in solution. The organ of smell is a yellow-tinged patch (about 5 cm^2) of pseudostratified epithelium, called the **olfactory epithelium**, located in the roof of the nasal cavity (Figure 15.20a). Air entering the nasal cavity must make a hairpin turn to stimulate olfactory receptors before entering the respiratory passageway below, so the human olfactory epithelium is in a poor position for doing its job. (This is why sniffing, which draws more air superiorly across the olfactory epithelium, intensifies the sense of smell.)

The olfactory epithelium covers the superior nasal concha on each side of the nasal septum, and contains millions of bowling pin–shaped receptor cells—the **olfactory sensory neurons**. These are surrounded and cushioned by columnar **supporting cells**, which make up the bulk of the penny-thin epithelial

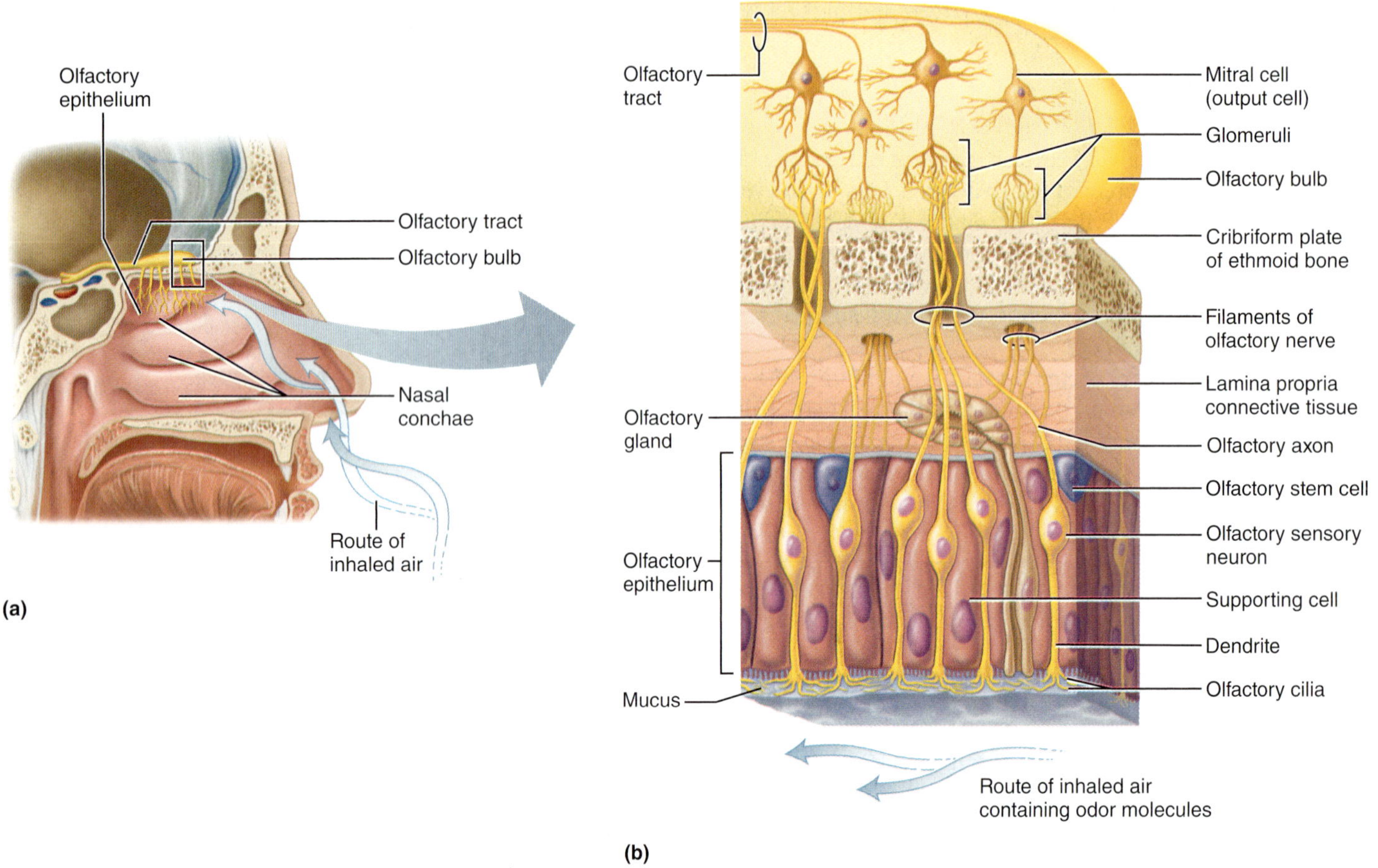

15

Figure 15.20 Olfactory receptors. (a) Site of olfactory epithelium in the superior nasal cavity. **(b)** An enlarged view of the olfactory epithelium showing the course of the fibers [filaments of the olfactory nerve (I)] through the ethmoid bone. These synapse in the glomeruli of the overlying olfactory bulb. The mitral cells are the output cells of the olfactory bulb.

membrane (Figure 15.20b). The supporting cells contain a yellow-brown pigment similar to lipofuscin, which gives the olfactory epithelium its yellow hue. At the base of the epithelium lie the short **olfactory stem cells**.

The olfactory sensory neurons are unusual bipolar neurons. Each has a thin apical dendrite that terminates in a knob from which several long cilia radiate. These **olfactory cilia**, which substantially increase the receptive surface area, typically lie flat on the nasal epithelium and are covered by a coat of thin mucus produced by the supporting cells and by olfactory glands in the underlying connective tissue. This mucus is a solvent that "captures" and dissolves airborne odorants. Unlike other cilia in the body, which beat rapidly in a coordinated manner, olfactory cilia are largely nonmotile.

The slender, nonmyelinated axons of the olfactory sensory neurons are gathered into small fascicles that collectively form the **filaments of the olfactory nerve** (cranial nerve I). They project superiorly through the openings in the cribriform plate of the ethmoid bone, where they synapse in the overlying olfactory bulbs.

Olfactory sensory neurons are also unusual because they are one of the few types of *neurons* that undergo noticeable turnover throughout adult life. Their superficial location puts them at risk for damage, and their typical life span is 30–60 days. Olfactory stem cells in the olfactory epithelium differentiate to replace them.

Specificity of Olfactory Receptors

Smell is difficult to research because any given odor (say, tobacco smoke) may be made up of hundreds of different chemicals. Taste has been neatly packaged into five taste qualities as you will see, but science has yet to discover any similar means for classifying smell. Humans can distinguish 10,000 or so odors, but research suggests that our olfactory sensory neurons are stimulated by different combinations of a more limited number of olfactory qualities.

There are about 400 "smell genes" in humans that are active only in the nose. Each gene encodes a unique receptor protein. It appears that each protein responds to one or more odors and each odor binds to several different receptor types. However, each receptor cell has only one type of receptor protein.

Olfactory neurons are exquisitely sensitive—in some cases, just a few molecules activate them. Some of what we call smell is really pain. The nasal cavities contain pain and temperature receptors that respond to irritants such as the sharpness of

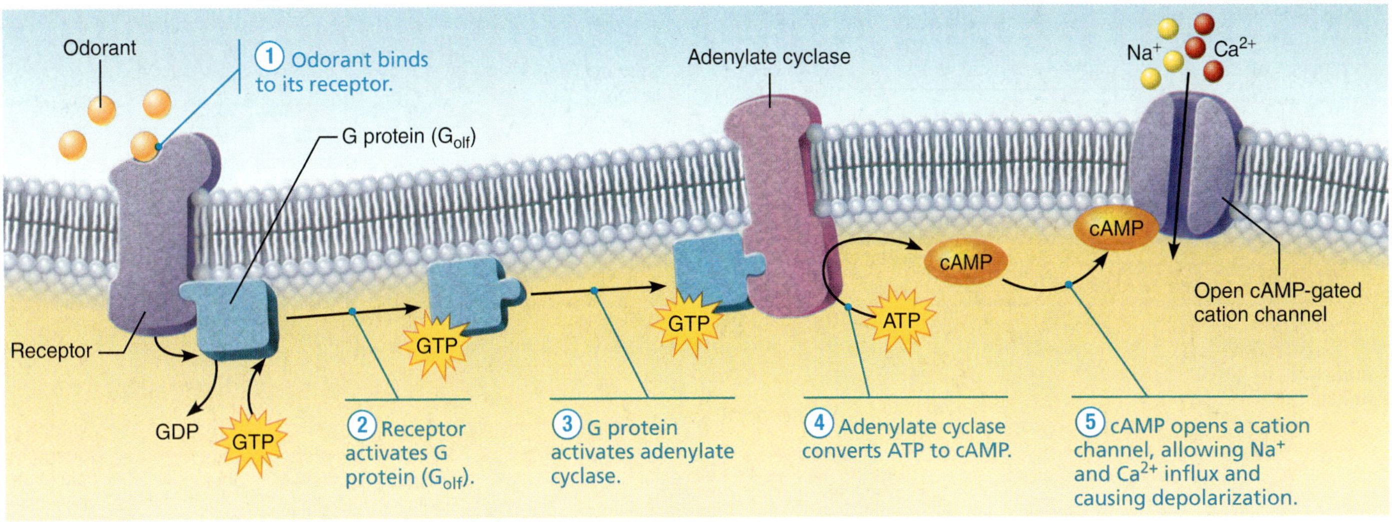

Figure 15.21 Olfactory transduction process. A portion of olfactory cilium membrane is shown.

ammonia, the hotness of chili peppers, and the "chill" of menthol. Impulses from these receptors reach the central nervous system via afferent fibers of the trigeminal nerves.

Physiology of Smell

For us to smell a particular odorant, it must be *volatile*—that is, it must be in the gaseous state as it enters the nasal cavity. Additionally, it must dissolve in the fluid coating the olfactory epithelium.

Activation of Olfactory Sensory Neurons Dissolved odorants stimulate olfactory sensory neurons by binding to receptor proteins in the olfactory cilium membranes, opening cation channels and generating a receptor potential. Ultimately (assuming threshold stimulation) an action potential is conducted to the first relay station in the olfactory bulb.

Smell Transduction Transduction of odorants uses a receptor linked to a G protein. The events that follow odorant binding will be easy for you to remember if you compare them to what you already know: general mechanisms of receptors and G proteins (see Figure 11.21) and phototransduction (see Figure 15.17).

As **Figure 15.21** shows, olfactory transduction begins when an odorant binds to a receptor. This event activates G proteins (G_{olf}), which activate enzymes (adenylate cyclases) that synthesize cyclic AMP as a second messenger. Cyclic AMP then acts directly on a plasma membrane cation channel, causing it to open, allowing Na^+ and Ca^{2+} to enter.

Na^+ influx leads to depolarization and impulse transmission. Ca^{2+} influx causes the transduction process to adapt, decreasing its response to a sustained stimulus. This *olfactory adaptation* helps explain how a person working in a paper mill or sewage treatment plant can still enjoy lunch!

The Olfactory Pathway

As we have already noted, axons of the olfactory sensory neurons form the olfactory nerves that synapse in the overlying **olfactory bulbs**, the distal ends of the olfactory tracts (see Table 13.2 on p. 494). There, the filaments of the olfactory nerves synapse with **mitral cells** (mi′tral), which are second-order sensory neurons, in complex structures called **glomeruli** (glo-mer′u-li; "little balls") (see Figure 15.20).

Axons from neurons bearing the same kind of receptor converge on a given type of glomerulus. That is, each glomerulus represents a single aspect of an odor (like one note in a chord) but each odor activates a unique set of glomeruli (the chord itself). Different odors activate different subsets of glomeruli (making different chords which may have some of the same notes). The mitral cells refine the signal, amplify it, and then relay it. The olfactory bulbs also house *amacrine granule cells*, GABA-releasing cells that inhibit mitral cells, so that only highly excitatory olfactory impulses are transmitted.

When the mitral cells are activated, impulses flow from the olfactory bulbs via the **olfactory tracts** (composed mainly of mitral cell axons) to the piriform lobe of the olfactory cortex. From there, two major pathways take information to various parts of the brain. One pathway brings information to part of the frontal lobe just above the orbit, where smells are consciously interpreted and identified. Only some of this information passes through the thalamus.

The other pathway flows to the hypothalamus, amygdala, and other regions of the limbic system. There, emotional responses to odors are elicited. Smells associated with danger—smoke, cooking gas, or skunk scent—trigger the sympathetic fight-or-flight response. Appetizing odors stimulate salivation and the digestive tract, and unpleasant odors can trigger protective reflexes such as sneezing and choking.

15

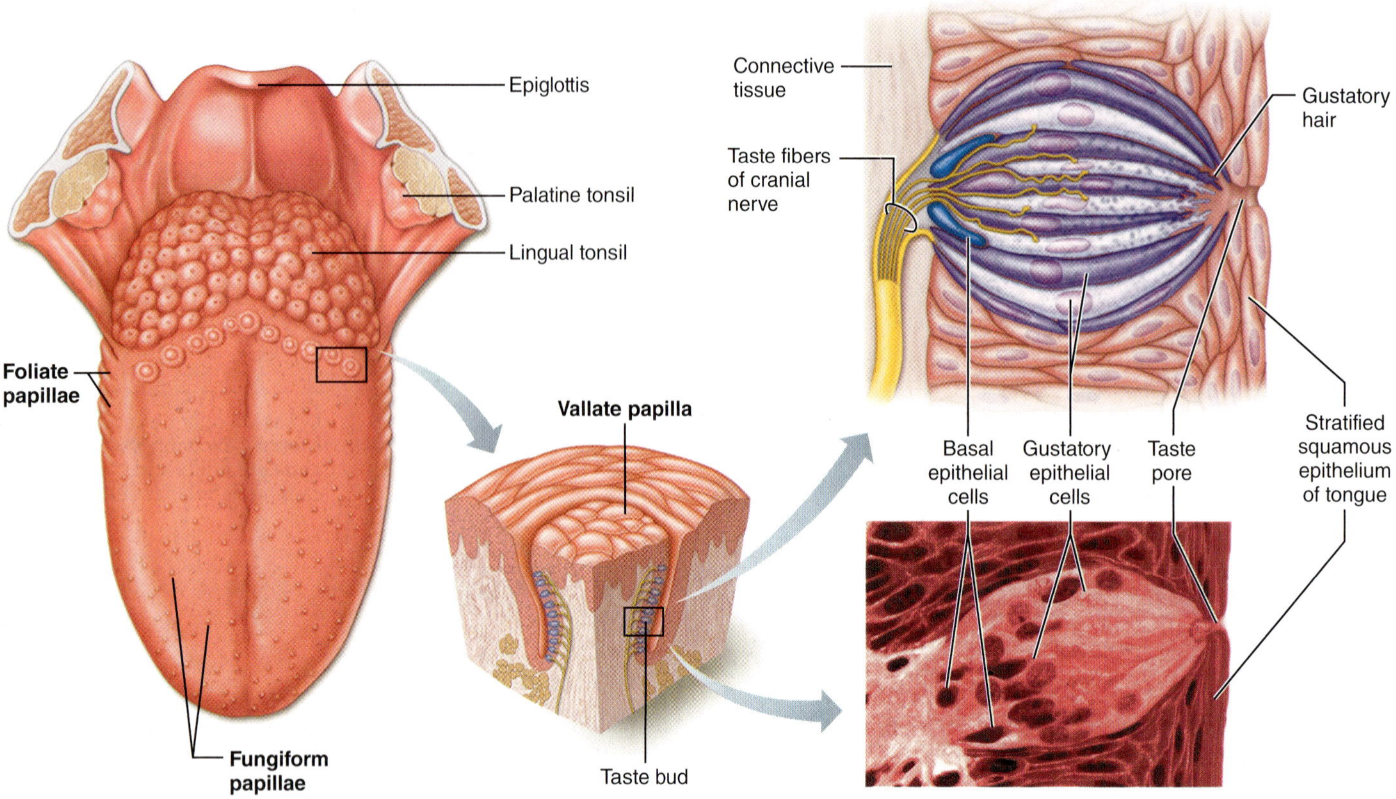

(a) **Taste buds are associated with fungiform, foliate, and vallate papillae.**

(b) **Enlarged section of a vallate papilla.**

(c) **Enlarged view of a taste bud (210×).**

Figure 15.22 **Location and structure of taste buds on the tongue.** (For a related image, see *A Brief Atlas of the Human Body*, Figure 62.)

Taste Buds and the Sense of Taste

The word *taste* comes from the Latin *taxare*, meaning "to touch, estimate, or judge." When we taste things, we are in fact intimately testing or judging our environment, and the sense of taste is considered by many to be the most pleasurable of the special senses.

Location and Structure of Taste Buds

Most of our 10,000 or so **taste buds**—the sensory organs for taste—are located on the tongue. A few taste buds are scattered on the soft palate, inner surface of the cheeks, pharynx, and epiglottis of the larynx, but most are found in **papillae** (pah-pil′e), peglike projections of the tongue mucosa that make the tongue surface slightly abrasive. Taste buds are located mainly on the tops of the mushroom-shaped **fungiform papillae** (fun′jĭ-form) (which are scattered over the entire tongue surface) and in the epithelium of the side walls of the **foliate papillae** and of the large round **vallate papillae** (val′āt). The vallate papillae are the largest and least numerous papillae, and 7 to 12 of them form an inverted V at the back of the tongue **(Figure 15.22a, b)**.

Each flask-shaped taste bud consists of 50 to 100 *epithelial cells* of two major types: *gustatory epithelial cells* and *basal epithelial cells* (Figure 15.22c).

Gustatory Epithelial Cells The **gustatory epithelial cells** are the receptor cells for taste—the *taste cells*. Long microvilli called **gustatory hairs** project from the tips of all gustatory epithelial cells and extend through a **taste pore** to the surface of the epithelium, where they are bathed by saliva. The gustatory hairs are the sensitive portions (*receptor membranes*) of the gustatory epithelial cells. Coiling intimately around the gustatory epithelial cells are sensory dendrites that represent the initial part of the gustatory pathway to the brain. Each afferent fiber receives signals from several gustatory epithelial cells within the taste bud.

There are at least three kinds of gustatory epithelial cells. One kind forms traditional synapses with the sensory dendrites and releases the neurotransmitter serotonin. The other two kinds lack synaptic vesicles, but at least one releases ATP that acts as a neurotransmitter.

Basal Epithelial Cells Because of their location, taste bud cells are subjected to friction and are routinely burned by hot foods. Luckily, they are among the most dynamic cells in the body, and they are replaced every seven to ten days. **Basal epithelial cells** act as stem cells, dividing and differentiating into new gustatory epithelial cells.

Basic Taste Sensations

Normally, our taste sensations are complicated mixtures of qualities. However, when taste is tested with pure chemical compounds, all taste sensations can be grouped into one of five basic modalities: sweet, sour, salty, bitter, and umami.

- *Sweet* taste is elicited by many organic substances including sugars, saccharin, alcohols, some amino acids, and some lead salts (such as those found in lead paint).
- *Sour* taste is produced by acids, specifically their hydrogen ions (H^+) in solution.
- *Salty* taste is produced by metal ions (inorganic salts); table salt (sodium chloride) tastes the "saltiest."
- *Bitter* taste is elicited by alkaloids (such as quinine, nicotine, caffeine, morphine, and strychnine) as well as a number of nonalkaloid substances, such as aspirin.
- *Umami* (u-mam′e; "delicious"), a subtle taste discovered by the Japanese, is elicited by the amino acids glutamate and aspartate, which appear to be responsible for the "beef taste" of steak, the characteristic tang of aging cheese, and the flavor of the food additive monosodium glutamate.

In addition, there is growing evidence for our ability to taste long-chain fatty acids from lipids. This possible sixth modality may help explain our liking for fatty foods.

Keep in mind that many substances produce a mixture of these basic taste sensations, and taste buds generally respond to all five. However, it appears that a single taste cell has receptors for only one taste modality.

Although taste maps that assign specific tastes to various areas of the tongue are common, researchers have known for years that these maps are dubious. All areas that contain taste buds can detect all modalities of taste.

Taste likes and dislikes have homeostatic value. Umami guides the intake of proteins, and a liking for sugar and salt helps satisfy the body's need for carbohydrates and minerals (as well as some amino acids). Many sour, naturally acidic foods (such as oranges, lemons, and tomatoes) are rich sources of vitamin C, an essential vitamin. On the other hand, intensely sour tastes warn us of spoilage. Likewise, many natural poisons and spoiled foods are bitter. Consequently, our dislike for sourness and bitterness is protective.

Physiology of Taste

For a chemical to be tasted it must dissolve in saliva, diffuse into a taste pore, and contact the gustatory hairs.

Activation of Taste Receptors Gustatory epithelial cells contain neurotransmitters. When a food chemical, or *tastant*, binds to receptors in the gustatory epithelial cell membrane, it induces a graded depolarizing potential that causes neurotransmitter release. Binding of the neurotransmitter to the associated sensory dendrites triggers generator potentials that elicit action potentials in these fibers.

The different gustatory epithelial cells have different thresholds for activation. In line with their protective nature, the bitter receptors detect substances present in minute amounts. The other receptors are less sensitive. Taste receptors adapt rapidly, with partial adaptation in 3–5 seconds and complete adaptation in 1–5 minutes.

Taste Transduction The mechanisms of taste transduction are only now beginning to become clear. Three different mechanisms underlie how we taste.

- Salty taste is due to Na^+ influx through Na^+ channels, which directly depolarizes gustatory epithelial cells.
- Sour is mediated by H^+, which acts intracellularly to open channels that allow other cations to enter.
- Bitter, sweet, and umami responses share a common mechanism, but each occurs in a different cell. Each taste's unique set of receptors is coupled to a common G protein called *gustducin*. Activation leads to the release of Ca^{2+} from intracellular stores, which causes cation channels in the plasma membrane to open, thereby depolarizing the cell and releasing the neurotransmitter ATP.

The Gustatory Pathway

Afferent fibers carrying taste information from the tongue are found primarily in two cranial nerve pairs. A branch of the **facial nerve** (VII), the *chorda tympani*, transmits impulses from taste receptors in the anterior two-thirds of the tongue **(Figure 15.23)**. The lingual branch of the **glossopharyngeal nerve** (IX) services the posterior third and the pharynx just behind. Taste impulses from the few taste buds in the epiglottis and the lower pharynx are conducted primarily by the **vagus nerve** (X). 15

These afferent fibers synapse in the **solitary nucleus** of the medulla, and from there impulses stream to the thalamus and ultimately to the *gustatory cortex* in the insula. Fibers also project to the hypothalamus and limbic system structures, regions that determine our appreciation of what we are tasting.

An important role of taste is to trigger reflexes involved in digestion. As taste impulses pass through the solitary nucleus, they initiate reflexes (via synapses with parasympathetic nuclei) that increase secretion of saliva into the mouth and of gastric juice into the stomach. Saliva contains mucus that moistens food and digestive enzymes that begin digesting starch. Acidic foods are particularly strong stimulants of the salivary reflex. On the other hand, when we eat revolting or foul-tasting substances, the taste may initiate protective reactions such as gagging or reflexive vomiting.

Influence of Other Sensations on Taste

Taste is 80% smell. When nasal congestion (or just pinching your nostrils) blocks access to your olfactory receptors, food tastes bland. Without smell, our morning coffee would lack its richness and simply taste bitter.

The mouth also contains thermoreceptors, mechanoreceptors, and nociceptors, and the temperature and texture of foods can enhance or detract from their taste. "Hot" foods such as chili peppers actually bring about their pleasurable effects by exciting pain receptors in the mouth.

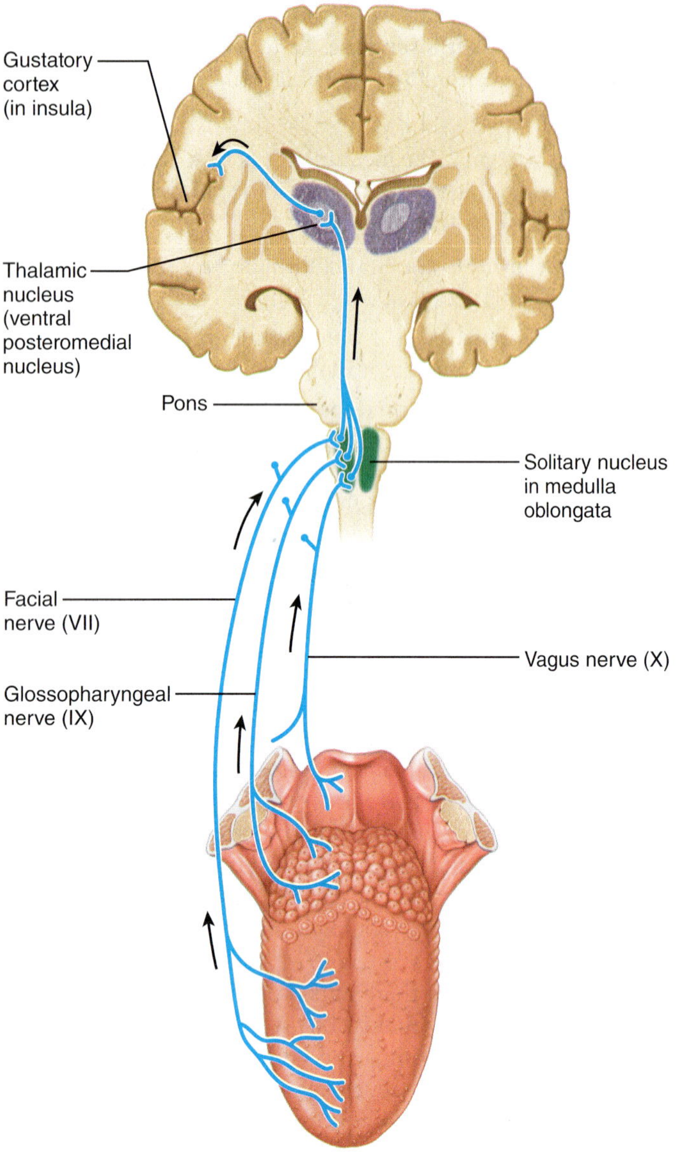

Figure 15.23 The gustatory pathway. Taste signals are relayed from the taste buds to the gustatory area of the cerebral cortex.

Homeostatic Imbalances of the Chemical Senses

Most olfactory disorders, or *anosmias* (an-oz′me-ahz; "without smells"), result from head injuries that tear the olfactory nerves, the aftereffects of nasal cavity inflammation, and neurological disorders such as Parkinson's disease. Some people have *uncinate fits* (un′sih-nāt), olfactory hallucinations during which they experience a particular (usually unpleasant) odor, such as rotting meat. *Olfactory auras* experienced by some epileptics just before they have a seizure are transient uncinate fits. These hallucinations can result from irritation of the olfactory pathway by brain surgery or head trauma.

Taste disorders are less common than disorders of smell, in part because the taste receptors are served by three different nerves and thus are less likely to be "put out of business" completely. Causes of taste disorders include upper respiratory tract infections, head injuries, chemicals or medications, or head and neck radiation for cancer treatment. Zinc supplements may help some cases of radiation-induced taste disorders.

☑ Check Your Understanding

10. Name the five taste modalities. Name the three types of papillae that have taste buds.
11. Olfactory sensory neurons have cilia and gustatory epithelial cells have hairs. How do these structures help the cells perform their functions?

For answers, see Appendix H.

The Ear: Hearing and Balance

✓ Describe the structure and general function of the outer, middle, and internal ears.

✓ Describe the sound conduction pathway to the fluids of the internal ear, and follow the auditory pathway from the spiral organ to the temporal cortex.

✓ Explain how we are able to differentiate pitch and loudness, and localize the source of sounds.

✓ List possible causes and symptoms of otitis media, deafness, and Ménière's syndrome.

At first glance, the machinery for hearing and balance appears very crude—fluids must be stirred to stimulate the mechanoreceptors of the internal ear. Nevertheless, our hearing apparatus allows us to hear an extraordinary range of sound, and our equilibrium (balance) receptors continually inform the nervous system of head movements and position. Although the organs serving these two senses are structurally interconnected within the ear, their receptors respond to different stimuli and are activated independently of one another.

Structure of the Ear

The ear is divided into three major areas: external ear, middle ear, and internal ear **(Figure 15.24a)**. The external and middle ear structures are involved with hearing only and are rather simply engineered. The internal ear functions in both equilibrium and hearing and is extremely complex.

External Ear

The **external (outer) ear** consists of the auricle and the external acoustic meatus. The **auricle**, or **pinna**, is what most people call the ear—the shell-shaped projection surrounding the opening of the external acoustic meatus. The auricle is composed of elastic cartilage covered with thin skin and an occasional hair. Its rim, the **helix**, is somewhat thicker, and its fleshy, dangling **lobule** ("earlobe") lacks supporting cartilage. The function of the auricle is to funnel sound waves into the external acoustic meatus.

The **external acoustic meatus** (auditory canal) is a short, curved tube (about 2.5 cm long by 0.6 cm wide) that extends from the auricle to the eardrum. Near the auricle, its framework is elastic cartilage; the remainder of the canal is carved into the

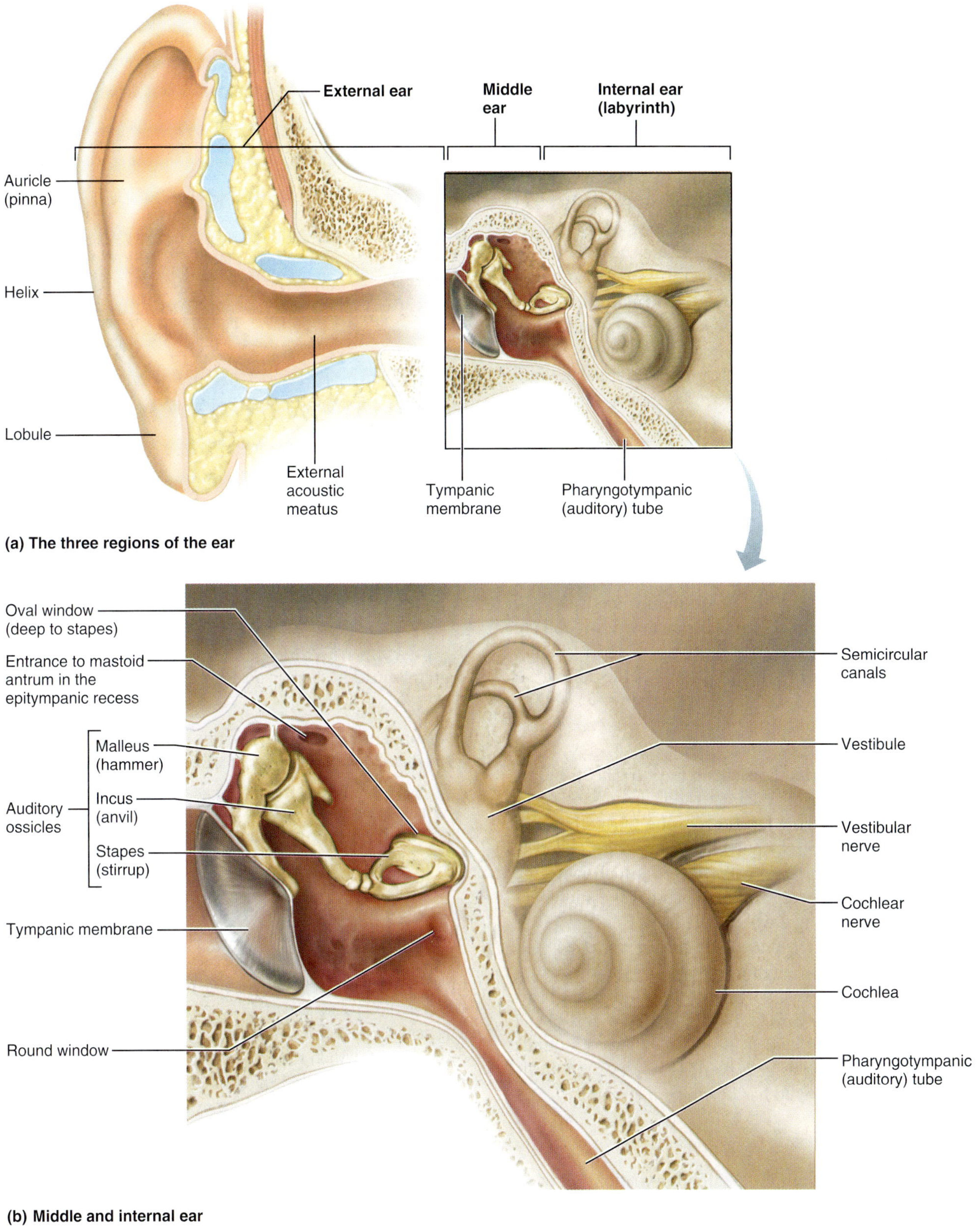

Figure 15.24 Structure of the ear. The inner ear structures in (b) appear as though they are veiled because they are cavities within the temporal bone.

temporal bone. The entire canal is lined with skin bearing hairs, sebaceous glands, and modified apocrine sweat glands called **ceruminous glands** (sĕ-roo′mĭ-nus). These glands secrete yellow-brown waxy **cerumen**, or earwax (*cere* = wax), which provides a sticky trap for foreign bodies and repels insects.

In many people, the ear is naturally cleansed as the cerumen dries and then falls out of the external acoustic meatus. Jaw movements as a person eats, talks, and so on, create an unnoticeable conveyor-belt effect that moves the wax out. In other people, cerumen builds up and becomes compacted.

Sound waves entering the external acoustic meatus eventually hit the **tympanic membrane**, or *eardrum* (*tympanum* = drum), the boundary between the outer and middle ears. The eardrum is a thin, translucent, connective tissue membrane, covered by skin on its external face and by mucosa internally. Shaped like a flattened cone, its apex protrudes medially into the middle ear.

Sound waves make the eardrum vibrate. The eardrum, in turn, transfers the sound energy to the tiny bones of the middle ear and sets them vibrating.

Middle Ear

The **middle ear**, or **tympanic cavity**, is a small, air-filled, mucosa-lined cavity in the petrous portion of the temporal bone. It is flanked laterally by the eardrum and medially by a bony wall with two openings, the superior **oval window** and the inferior **round window**. Superiorly the tympanic cavity arches upward as the **epitympanic recess**, the "roof" of the middle ear cavity. The **mastoid antrum**, a canal in the posterior wall of the tympanic cavity, allows it to communicate with *mastoid air cells* housed in the mastoid process.

15

The anterior wall of the middle ear abuts the internal carotid artery (the main artery supplying the brain) and contains the opening of the **pharyngotympanic (auditory) tube** (formerly called the eustachian tube). The pharyngotympanic tube runs obliquely downward to link the middle ear cavity with the nasopharynx (the superiormost part of the throat), and the mucosa of the middle ear is continuous with that lining the pharynx (throat).

Normally, the pharyngotympanic tube is flattened and closed, but swallowing or yawning opens it briefly to equalize pressure in the middle ear cavity with external air pressure. This is important because the eardrum vibrates freely only if the pressure on both of its surfaces is the same; otherwise sounds are distorted. The ear-popping sensation of the pressures equalizing is familiar to anyone who has flown in an airplane.

Homeostatic Imbalance 15.12

Otitis media (me′de-ah), or middle ear inflammation, is a fairly common result of a sore throat, especially in children, whose pharyngotympanic tubes are shorter and run more horizontally. Otitis media is the most frequent cause of hearing loss in children. In acute infectious forms, the eardrum bulges and becomes inflamed and red. Most cases of otitis media are treated with antibiotics. When large amounts of fluid or pus accumulate in the cavity, an emergency *myringotomy* (lancing of the eardrum) may be required to relieve the pressure, and a tiny tube implanted in the eardrum permits pus to drain into the external ear. The tube falls out by itself within a year. ✚

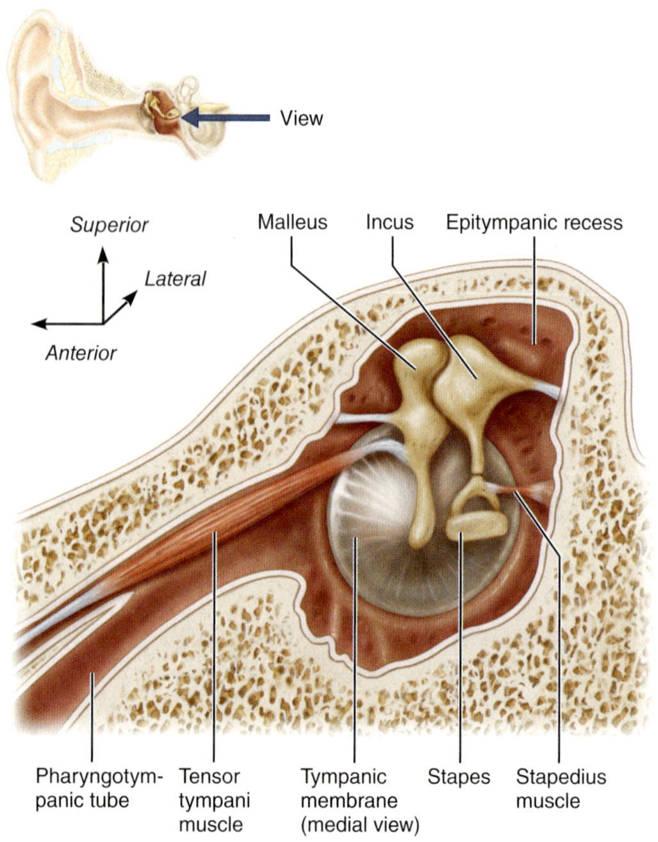

Figure 15.25 The three auditory ossicles and associated skeletal muscles. Right middle ear, medial view.

The tympanic cavity is spanned by the three smallest bones in the body: the **auditory ossicles** (Figure 15.24 and **Figure 15.25**). These bones, named for their shape, are the **malleus** (mal′e-us; "hammer"); the **incus** (ing′kus; "anvil"); and the **stapes** (sta′pēz; "stirrup"). The "handle" of the malleus is secured to the eardrum, and the base of the stapes fits into the oval window.

Tiny ligaments suspend the ossicles, and mini synovial joints link them into a chain that spans the middle ear cavity. The incus articulates with the malleus laterally and the stapes medially. The ossicles transmit the vibratory motion of the eardrum to the oval window, which in turn sets the fluids of the internal ear into motion, eventually exciting the hearing receptors.

Two tiny skeletal muscles are associated with the ossicles (Figure 15.25). The **tensor tympani** (ten′sor tim′pah-ni) arises from the wall of the pharyngotympanic tube and inserts on the malleus. The **stapedius** (stah-pe′de-us) runs from the posterior wall of the middle ear to the stapes. When loud sounds assault the ears, these muscles contract reflexively to limit the ossicles' vibration and minimize damage to the hearing receptors.

Internal Ear

The **internal ear** is also called the **labyrinth** ("maze") because of its complicated shape (see Figure 15.24). It lies deep in the temporal bone behind the eye socket and provides a secure site for all of the delicate receptor machinery.

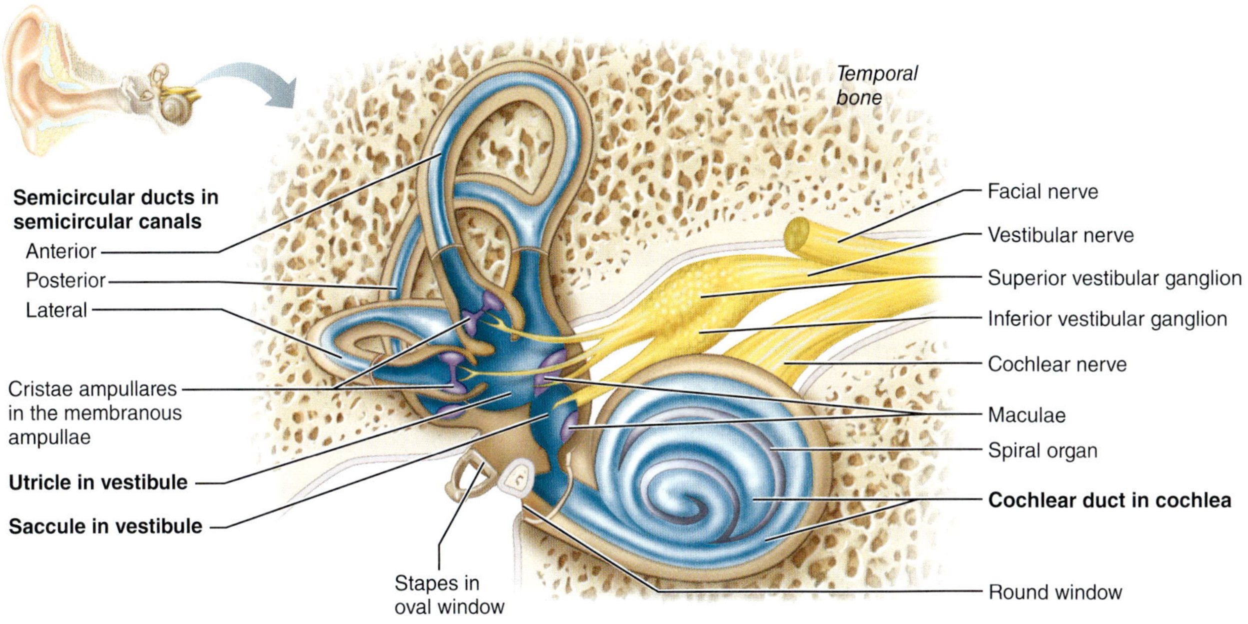

Figure 15.26 Membranous labyrinth of the internal ear. The membranous labyrinth (blue) lies within the chambers of the bony labyrinth (tan). The locations of the sensory organs for hearing (spiral organ) and equilibrium (maculae and cristae ampullares) are shown in purple.

The internal ear has two major divisions: the bony labyrinth and the membranous labyrinth.

- The **bony labyrinth** is a system of tortuous channels worming through the bone. The views of the bony labyrinth typically seen in textbooks, including this one, are somewhat misleading because we are talking about a *cavity* here. The representation in Figure 15.24 can be compared to a plaster of paris cast of the cavity or hollow space inside the bony labyrinth.
- The **membranous labyrinth** is a continuous series of membranous sacs and ducts contained within the bony labyrinth and (more or less) following its contours **(Figure 15.26)**.

The bony labyrinth is filled with **perilymph**, a fluid similar to cerebrospinal fluid and continuous with it. The membranous labyrinth is suspended in the surrounding perilymph, and its interior contains **endolymph**, which is chemically similar to K^+-rich intracellular fluid. These two fluids conduct the sound vibrations involved in hearing and respond to the mechanical forces occurring during changes in body position and acceleration.

The bony labyrinth has three regions: the *vestibule*, the *semicircular canals*, and the *cochlea*.

Vestibule The **vestibule** is the central egg-shaped cavity of the bony labyrinth. It lies posterior to the cochlea, anterior to the semicircular canals, and flanks the middle ear medially. In its lateral wall is the oval window.

Suspended in the vestibular perilymph and united by a small duct are two membranous labyrinth sacs, the **saccule** and **utricle** (u′trĭ-kl) (Figure 15.26). The smaller saccule is continuous with the membranous labyrinth extending anteriorly into the cochlea (the *cochlear duct*), whereas the utricle is continuous with the semicircular ducts extending into the semicircular canals posteriorly. The saccule and utricle house equilibrium receptor regions called *maculae* that respond to the pull of gravity and report on changes of head position.

Semicircular Canals The **semicircular canals** lie posterior and lateral to the vestibule, and each of these canals defines about two-thirds of a circle. The cavities of the bony semicircular canals project from the posterior aspect of the vestibule, each oriented in one of the three planes of space. Accordingly, there is an *anterior*, a *posterior*, and a *lateral* semicircular canal in each internal ear. The anterior and posterior canals are oriented at right angles to each other in the vertical plane, whereas the lateral canal lies horizontally (Figure 15.26).

Snaking through each semicircular canal is a corresponding membranous **semicircular duct**, which communicates with the utricle anteriorly. Each of these ducts has an enlarged swelling at one end called an **ampulla**, which houses an equilibrium receptor region called a *crista ampullaris* (literally, crest of the ampulla). These receptors respond to angular (rotational) movements of the head.

Cochlea The **cochlea** (kok′le-ah), from the Latin "snail," is a spiral, conical, bony chamber about the size of a split pea. It extends from the anterior part of the vestibule and coils for about 2½ turns around a bony pillar called the **modiolus** (mo-di′o-lus) **(Figure 15.27a)**. Running through its center like a wedge-shaped worm is the membranous **cochlear duct**, which ends blindly at the cochlear apex. The cochlear duct houses the receptor organ of hearing, called the **spiral organ** or the *organ of Corti* (Figures 15.26 and 15.27b).

The cochlear duct and the **osseous spiral lamina**, a thin shelflike extension of bone that spirals up the modiolus like the thread on a screw, together divide the cavity of the bony cochlea into three separate chambers or **scalae** (*scala* = ladder).

15

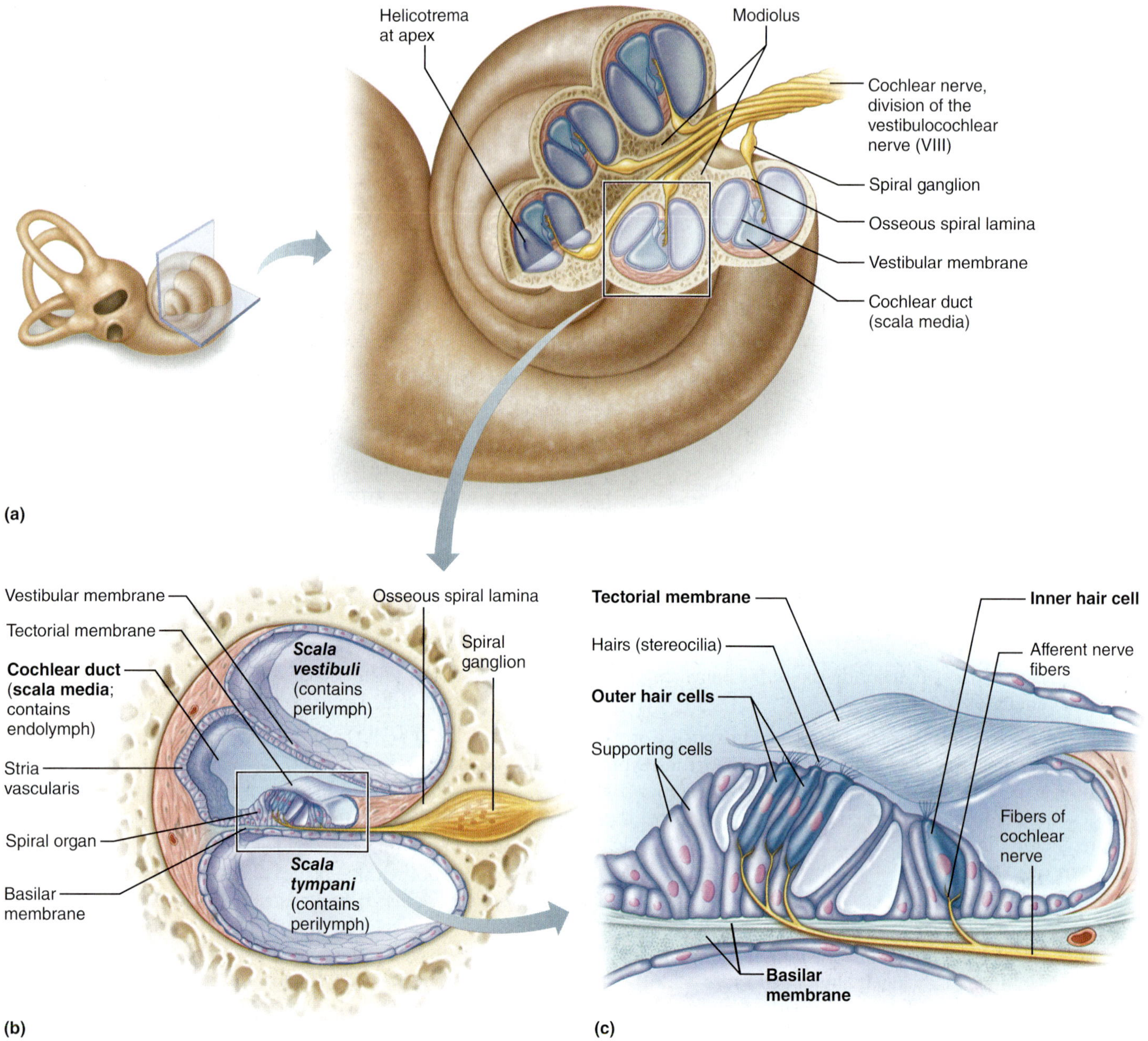

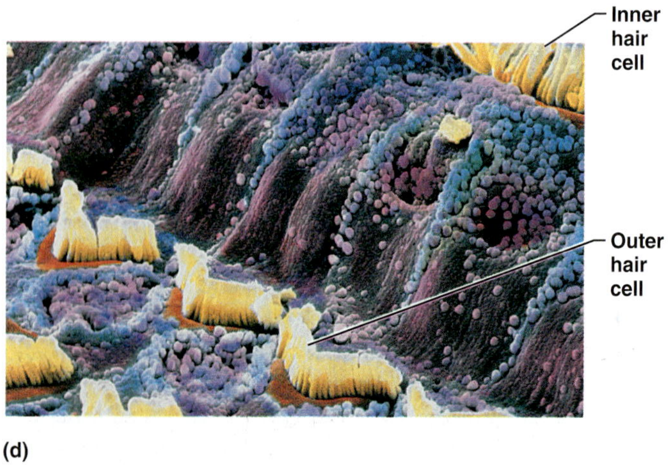

Figure 15.27 Anatomy of the cochlea. (a) Lateral view of part of the internal ear with a wedge-shaped section removed from the cochlea. **(b)** Magnified cross section of one turn of the cochlea, showing the relationship of the three scalae. This cross section has been rotated from its position in (a). **(c)** Detailed structure of the spiral organ. **(d)** Electron micrograph of cochlear hair cells (550×).

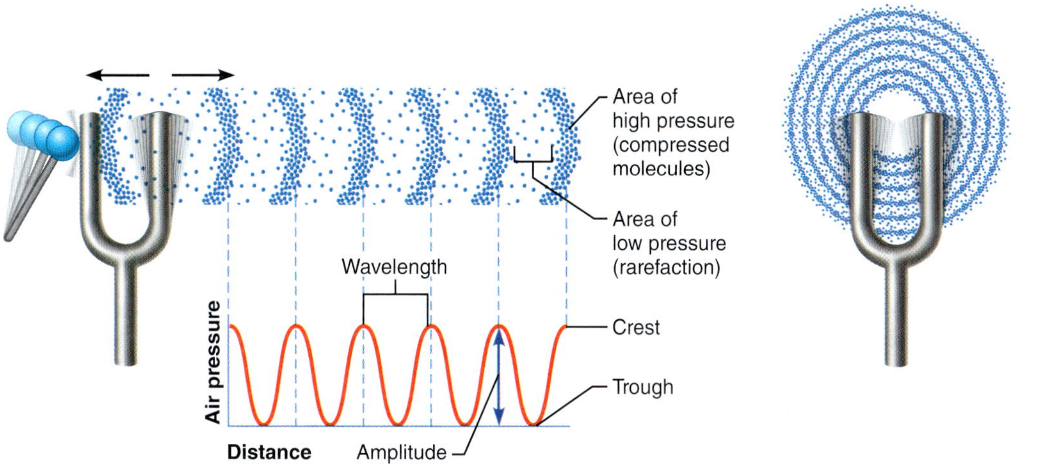

(a) A struck tuning fork alternately compresses and rarefies the air molecules around it, creating alternate zones of high and low pressure.

(b) Sound waves radiate outward in all directions.

Figure 15.28 Sound: Source and propagation. The graph in (a) shows that plotting the oscillating air pressures yields a sine wave. The height (amplitude) of the crests is proportional to the energy, or intensity, of the sound wave. The distance between two corresponding points on the wave (crests or troughs) is the wavelength.

The **scala vestibuli** (ska′lah vĕs-tĭ′bu-li), which lies superior to the cochlear duct, is continuous with the vestibule and abuts the oval window. The middle **scala media** is the cochlear duct itself. The **scala tympani**, which terminates at the membrane-covered round window, is inferior to the cochlear duct.

Since the scala media is part of the membranous labyrinth, it is filled with endolymph. The scala vestibuli and the scala tympani, both part of the bony labyrinth, contain perilymph. The perilymph-containing chambers are continuous with each other at the cochlear apex, a region called the **helicotrema** (hel″ĭ-ko-tre′mah; "the hole in the spiral").

The "roof" of the cochlear duct, separating the scala media from the scala vestibuli, is the **vestibular membrane** (Figure 15.27b). The duct's external wall, the **stria vascularis**, is composed of an unusual richly vascularized mucosa that secretes endolymph. The "floor" of the cochlear duct is composed of the osseous spiral lamina and the flexible, fibrous basilar membrane, which supports the spiral organ. (We will describe the spiral organ when we discuss hearing.) The **basilar membrane**, which plays a critical role in sound reception, is narrow and thick near the oval window and gradually widens and thins as it approaches the cochlear apex. The *cochlear nerve*, a division of the *vestibulocochlear nerve* (VIII), runs from the spiral organ through the modiolus on its way to the brain.

Table 15.2 summarizes the structures of the internal ear and their functions.

Physiology of Hearing

We can summarize human hearing in a single sprawling sentence: Sounds set up vibrations in air that beat against the eardrum that pushes a chain of tiny bones that press fluid in the internal ear against membranes that set up shearing forces that pull on the tiny hair cells that stimulate nearby neurons that give rise to impulses that travel to the brain, which interprets them—and you hear. Before we unravel this intriguing sequence, let us describe sound, the stimulus for hearing.

Overview: Properties of Sound

Light can be transmitted through a vacuum (for instance, outer space), but sound depends on an *elastic* medium for its transmission. Sound also travels much more slowly than light. Its speed in dry air is only about 331 m/s (0.2 mi/s), as opposed to about 300,000 km/s (186,000 mi/s) for light. A lightning flash is almost instantly visible, but the sound it creates (thunder) reaches our ears much more slowly. (For each second between the lightning bolt and the roll of thunder, the storm is 1/5 mile farther away.) The speed of sound is fastest in solids and slowest in gases, but it is constant in a given medium.

Sound is a pressure disturbance—alternating areas of high and low pressure—produced by a vibrating object and propagated by the molecules of the medium. Consider a vibrating tuning fork (Figure 15.28a). If the tuning fork is struck on the left, its prongs will move first to the right, creating an area of high pressure by compressing the air molecules there. Then, as the prongs rebound to the left, the air on the left will be compressed, and the region on the right will be a *rarefied*, or low-pressure, area (since most of its air molecules have been pushed farther to the right).

As the fork vibrates alternately from right to left, it produces a series of compressions and rarefactions, collectively called a *sound wave*, which moves outward in all directions (Figure 15.28b). However, the individual air molecules just vibrate back and forth for short distances as they bump other molecules and rebound. Because the outward-moving molecules give up kinetic energy

Table 15.2 Summary of the Internal Ear

BONY LABYRINTH	MEMBRANOUS LABYRINTH	FUNCTION	RECEPTOR REGION
Semicircular canals	Semicircular ducts	Equilibrium: rotational (angular) acceleration	Crista ampullaris
Vestibule	Utricle and saccule	Equilibrium: head position relative to gravity, linear acceleration	Macula
Cochlea	Cochlear duct (scala media)	Hearing	Spiral organ

to the molecules they bump, energy is always transferred in the direction the sound wave is traveling. For this reason, the energy of the wave declines with time and distance, and the sound dies a natural death.

We can illustrate a sound wave as an S-shaped curve, or *sine wave*, in which the compressed areas are crests and the rarefied areas are troughs (Figure 15.28a). Sound can be described in terms of two physical properties that you can see in this sine wave graph: frequency and amplitude.

Frequency **Frequency** is defined as the number of waves that pass a given point in a given time. The sine wave of a pure tone has crests and troughs that repeat at definite distances. The distance between two consecutive crests (or troughs) is the **wavelength** of the sound and is constant for a particular tone. The shorter the wavelength, the higher the frequency of the sound **(Figure 15.29a)**.

The frequency range of human hearing is from 20 to 20,000 waves per second, or *hertz* (*Hz*). Our ears are most sensitive to frequencies between 1500 and 4000 Hz and, in that range, we can distinguish frequencies differing by only 2–3 Hz. We perceive different sound frequencies as differences in **pitch**: the higher the frequency, the higher the pitch.

A tuning fork produces a *tone*—a pure (but bland) sound with a single frequency—but most sounds are mixtures of several frequencies. This characteristic of sound, called **quality**, enables us to distinguish between the same musical note—say, high C—sung by a soprano or played on a piano or clarinet. Sound quality also provides the richness and complexity of sounds (and music) that we hear.

Amplitude The **amplitude**, or height, of the sine wave crests reveals a sound's intensity, which is related to its energy, or the pressure differences between its compressed and rarefied areas (Figure 15.29b).

Loudness refers to our subjective interpretation of sound intensity. Because we can hear such an enormous range of intensities, from the proverbial pin drop to a jet engine 10 million times more intense, sound intensity (and loudness) is measured in logarithmic units called **decibels (dB)** (des′ĭ-belz).

On a clinical audiometer, the decibel scale is arbitrarily set to begin at 0 dB, which is the threshold of hearing (barely audible sound) for normal ears. Each 10-dB increase represents a tenfold increase in sound intensity. A sound of 10 dB has 10 times more energy than one of 0 dB, and a 20-dB sound has 100 times (10 × 10) more energy. However, the same 10-dB increase represents only a twofold increase in loudness. In other words, most people would report that a 20-dB sound seems about twice as loud as a 10-dB sound. The normal range of hearing (from barely audible to the loudest sound we can process without excruciating pain) extends over a range of 120 dB. (The threshold of pain is 120 dB.)

Severe hearing loss occurs with frequent or prolonged exposure to sounds with intensities greater than 90 dB, and in the U.S., employees exposed to occupational noise over that range must wear ear (hearing) protection. That number becomes more meaningful when you realize that a normal conversation is in the 50-dB range, a noisy restaurant has 70-dB levels, and amplified rock music is 120 dB or more, far above the 90-dB danger zone.

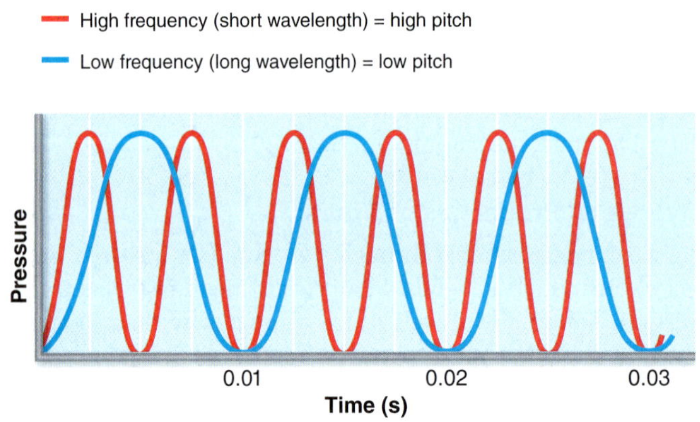

(a) Frequency is perceived as pitch.

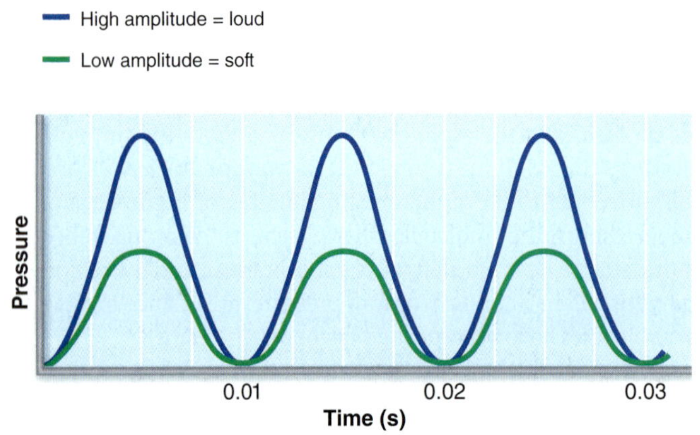

(b) Amplitude (size or intensity) is perceived as loudness.

Figure 15.29 Frequency and amplitude of sound waves.

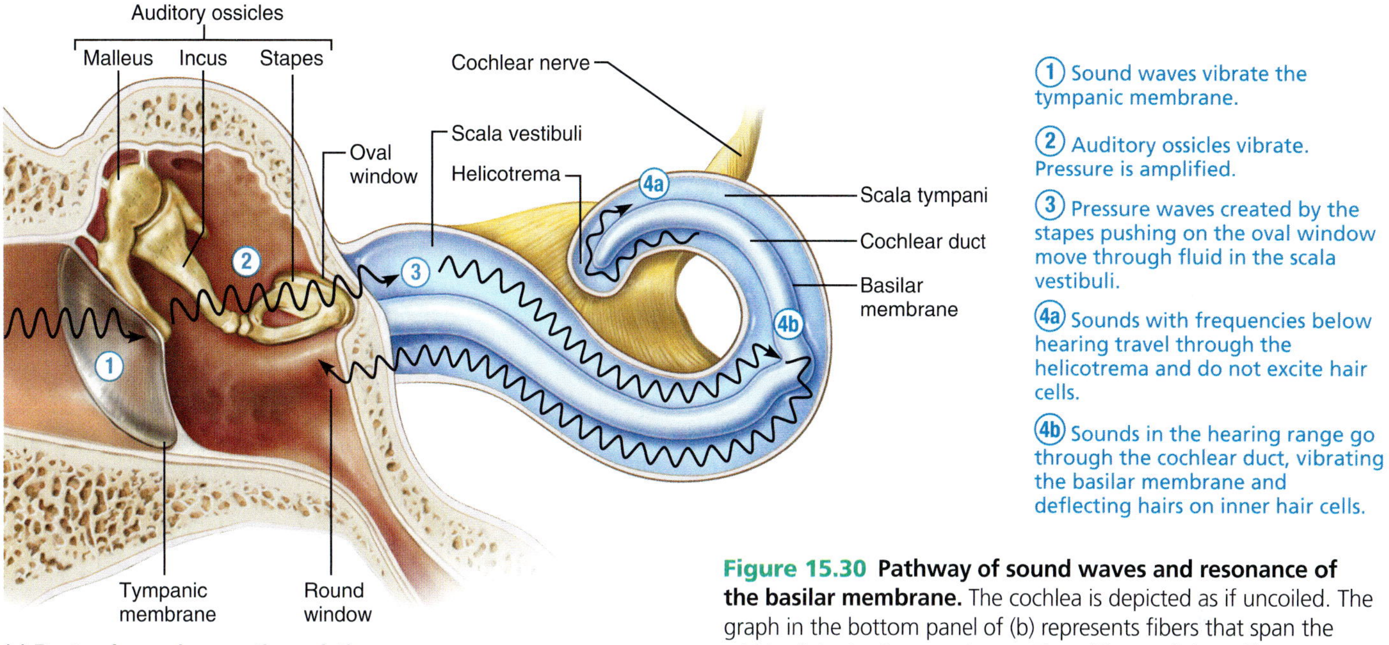

(a) Route of sound waves through the ear

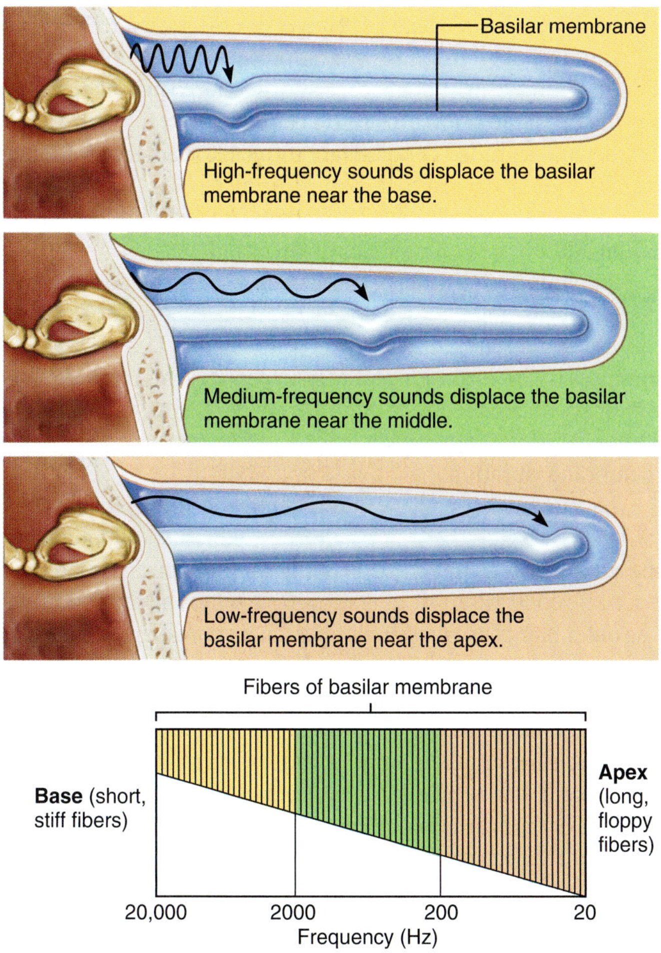

(b) Different sound frequencies cross the basilar membrane at different locations.

Figure 15.30 Pathway of sound waves and resonance of the basilar membrane. The cochlea is depicted as if uncoiled. The graph in the bottom panel of (b) represents fibers that span the width of the basilar membrane. The stiffness of these fibers "tunes" specific regions of the basilar membrane to vibrate at specific frequencies.

Transmission of Sound to the Internal Ear

Hearing occurs when the auditory area of the temporal lobe cortex is stimulated. However, before this can happen, sound waves must be propagated through air, membranes, bones, and fluids to stimulate receptor cells in the spiral organ **(Figure 15.30a)**.

Airborne sound entering the external acoustic meatus strikes the tympanic membrane and sets it vibrating at the same frequency. The greater the intensity, the farther the membrane is displaced in its vibratory motion. The motion of the tympanic membrane is amplified and transferred to the oval window by the ossicle lever system, which acts much like a hydraulic press or piston to transfer the same total force hitting the eardrum to the oval window.

Because the tympanic membrane is 17–20 times larger than the oval window, the pressure (force per unit area) actually exerted on the oval window is about 20 times that on the tympanic membrane. This increased pressure overcomes the stiffness and inertia of cochlear fluid and sets it into wave motion. This situation can be roughly compared to the difference in pressure relayed to the floor by the broad rubber heels of a man's shoes versus a woman's tiny spike heels. The man's weight—say, 70 kg (about 150 pounds)—is spread over several square inches, and his heels will not make dents in a pliable vinyl floor. But spike heels concentrate the same 70-kg force in an area of about 2.5 cm^2 (1 square inch) and *will* dent the floor.

15

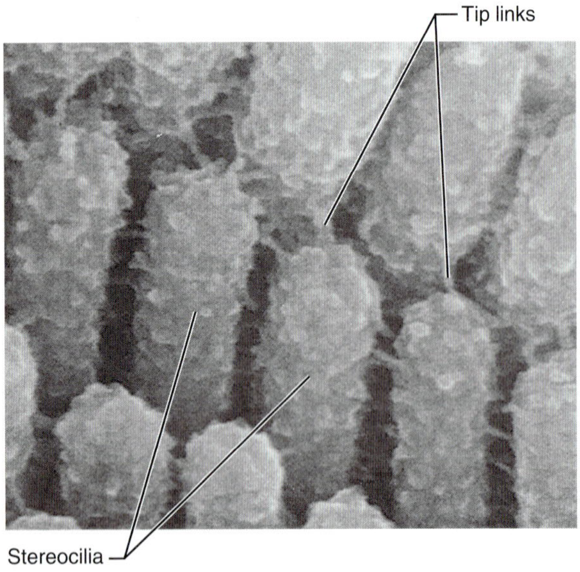

Figure 15.31 Photo of stereocilia on a hair cell. Note the precise order of the stereocilia.

Resonance of the Basilar Membrane

As the stapes rocks back and forth against the oval window, it sets the perilymph in the scala vestibuli into a similar back-and-forth motion. A pressure wave travels through the perilymph from the basal end toward the helicotrema, much as a piece of rope held horizontally can be set into wave motion by movements initiated at one end.

Fluids cannot be compressed. Think of what happens when you sit on a water bed—you sit "here" and it bulges over "there." In a similar way, each time the stapes forces the fluid adjacent to the oval window medially, the membrane of the round window bulges laterally into the middle ear cavity and acts as a pressure valve.

Sounds of very low frequency (below 20 Hz) create pressure waves that take the complete route through the cochlea—up the scala vestibuli, around the helicotrema, and back toward the round window through the scala tympani (Figure 15.30a). These low-frequency sounds do not activate the spiral organ and so are below the range of hearing.

In contrast, sounds with frequencies high enough to hear create pressure waves that take a "shortcut" and are transmitted through the cochlear duct into the perilymph of the scala tympani. As a pressure wave descends through the flexible cochlear duct, it vibrates the entire basilar membrane.

Maximal displacement of the membrane occurs where the fibers of the basilar membranes are "tuned" to a particular sound frequency (Figure 15.30b). This characteristic of maximum movement at a particular frequency is called *resonance*. The fibers of the basilar membrane span its width like the strings of a harp. The fibers near the oval window (cochlear base) are short and stiff, and they resonate in response to high-frequency pressure waves (Figure 15.30b). The longer, more floppy basilar membrane fibers near the cochlear apex resonate in time with lower-frequency pressure waves. As a result, the resonance of the basilar membrane mechanically processes sound signals before the signals ever reach the receptors.

Excitation of Hair Cells in the Spiral Organ

The spiral organ, which rests atop the basilar membrane, is composed of supporting cells and hearing receptor cells called *cochlear hair cells*. The hair cells are arranged functionally—specifically, one row of **inner hair cells** and three rows of **outer hair cells**—sandwiched between the tectorial and basilar membranes (see Figure 15.27c). Afferent fibers of the **cochlear nerve** [a division of the vestibulocochlear nerve (VIII)] coil about the bases of the hair cells.

The hair cells have numerous *stereocilia* (actually long microvilli) and a single *kinocilium* (a true cilium) protruding from their apices. The "hairs" (stereocilia) of the hair cells are stiffened by actin filaments and linked together by fine fibers called *tip links* **(Figure 15.31)**. The stereocilia protrude into the K^+-rich endolymph, and the longest are enmeshed in the overlying, stiff gel-like **tectorial membrane** (see Figure 15.27c).

Transduction of sound stimuli occurs after localized movements of the basilar membrane "tweak" or deflect the trapped stereocilia of the hair cells. Bending the stereocilia toward the kinocilium puts tension on the tip links, which in turn opens cation channels in the adjacent shorter stereocilia like a rope pulling on a trap door. This results in an inward K^+ (and Ca^{2+}) current and a graded depolarization (receptor potential). Bending the cilia away from the kinocilium relaxes the tip links, closes the mechanically gated ion channels, and allows repolarization and even a graded hyperpolarization.

Depolarization increases intracellular Ca^{2+} and so increases the hair cells' release of neurotransmitter (glutamate), which causes the afferent cochlear fibers to transmit a faster stream of impulses to the brain for auditory interpretation. Hyperpolarization produces the exact opposite effect. As you might guess, activation of the hair cells occurs at points of vigorous basilar membrane vibration.

The vast majority of the sensory fibers of the spiral ganglia (90–95%) service the inner hair cells, which shoulder nearly the entire responsibility for sending auditory messages to the brain. By contrast, most fibers coiling around the more numerous outer hair cells are *efferent* fibers that convey messages from brain to ear. So what do the outer hair cells do?

The outer hair cells act on the basilar membrane itself. When outer hair cells depolarize and hyperpolarize as the basilar membrane moves, they contract and stretch in a type of cellular boogie called *fast motility*. Their strange behavior changes the stiffness of the basilar membrane.

Outer hair cell motility serves two functions:

- It increases the responsiveness of the inner hair cells by amplifying the motion of the basilar membrane—a kind of cochlear tuning.
- It may help protect the inner hair cells from damage. Loud sounds activate a negative feedback loop from the brain

stem to the outer hair cells via the efferent fibers, which release neurotransmitters that cause the outer hair cells to stiffen. This dampens the motion of the basilar membrane and spreads the sound energy over a wider area.

The Auditory Pathway to the Brain

The ascending auditory pathway transmits auditory information primarily from the cochlear receptors (the inner hair cells) to the cerebral cortex. Impulses generated in the cochlea pass through the **spiral ganglion**, where the auditory bipolar cells reside, and along the afferent fibers of the cochlear nerve to the **cochlear nuclei** of the medulla **(Figure 15.32)**.

From there, neurons project to the **superior olivary nucleus**, which lies at the junction of the medulla and pons. Beyond this, axons ascend in the **lateral lemniscus** (a fiber tract) to the **inferior colliculus** (auditory reflex center in the midbrain), which projects to the **medial geniculate nucleus** of the thalamus. Axons of the thalamic neurons then project to the **primary auditory cortex**, which provides conscious awareness of sound.

The auditory pathway is unusual because not all of the fibers from each ear cross over to the other side of the brain. For this reason, each auditory cortex receives impulses from both ears.

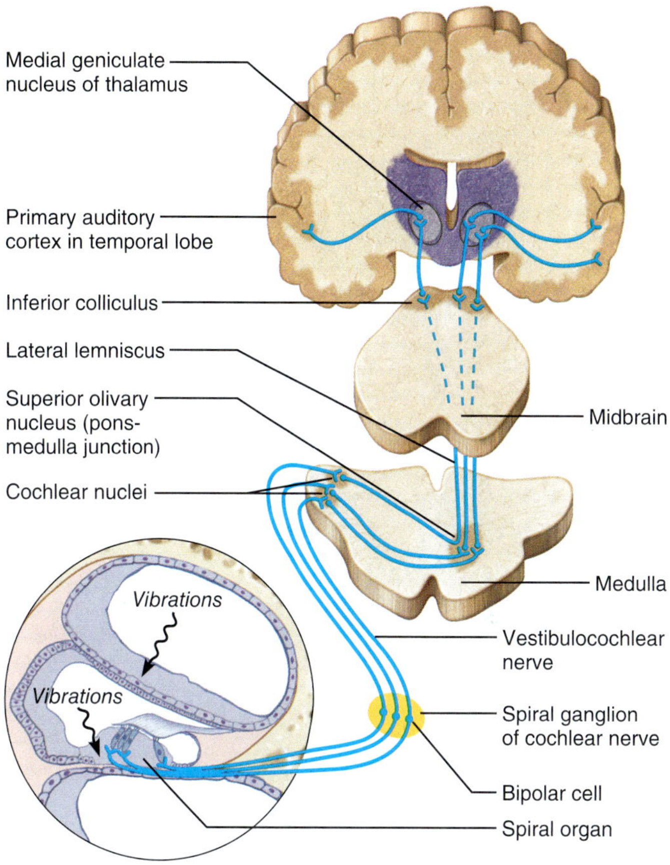

Figure 15.32 The auditory pathway. This simplified diagram shows only the pathway from the right ear.

Auditory Processing

If you are at a Broadway musical, the sound of the instruments, the actors' voices, rustling of clothing, and closing of doors are all intermingled in your awareness. Yet, your auditory cortex can distinguish the separate parts of this auditory jumble. Whenever the difference between sound wavelengths is sufficient for discrimination, you hear two separate and distinct tones. In fact, the analytic powers of the auditory cortex are so great that we are able to pick single instruments out of a whole orchestra.

Cortical processing of sound stimuli is complex. For example, certain cortical cells depolarize at the beginning of a particular tone, and others depolarize when the tone ends. Some cortical cells depolarize continuously, and others appear to have high thresholds (low sensitivity), and so on. Here we will concentrate on the more straightforward aspects of cortical perception of pitch, loudness, and sound location.

Perception of Pitch As we explained, sound waves of different frequencies activate hair cells in different positions along the length of the basilar membrane, and impulses from specific hair cells are interpreted as specific pitches. When a sound is composed of tones of many frequencies, it activates several populations of cochlear hair cells and cortical cells simultaneously, and we perceive multiple tones.

Detection of Loudness Louder sounds cause larger movements of the tympanic membrane, auditory ossicles, and oval window, and pressure waves of greater amplitude in the fluids of the cochlea. These larger waves in turn cause larger movements of the basilar membrane, larger deflections of the hairs on the hair cells, and larger graded potentials in the hair cells. As a result, they release more neurotransmitter and generate more frequent action potentials. The brain interprets more frequent action potentials as greater loudness. In addition, as more neurotransmitter is released, more of the 10 or so bipolar cells connected to a given hair cell are recruited to fire action potentials.

Localization of Sound Several brain stem nuclei (most importantly the superior olivary nuclei) help us localize a sound's source in space by means of two cues: the *relative intensity* and the *relative timing* of sound waves reaching the two ears. If the sound source is directly in front, in back, or overhead, the intensity and timing cues are the same for both ears. However, when sound comes from one side, it activates the receptors of the nearer ear slightly earlier and also more vigorously (because of the greater intensity of the sound waves entering that ear).

☑ Check Your Understanding

12. Apart from the bony boundaries, which structure separates the external from the middle ear? Which two (nonbone) structures separate the middle from the inner ear?
13. Which structure inside the spiral organ allows us to differentiate sounds of different pitch?
14. If the brain stem did not receive input from both ears, what would you not be able to do?

For answers, see Appendix H.

15

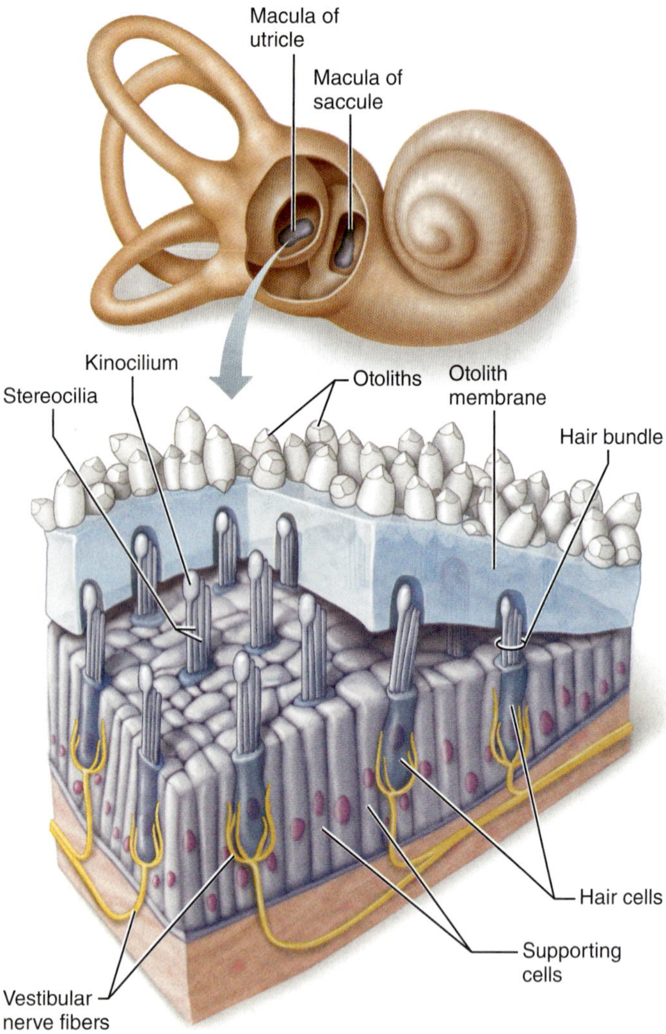

Figure 15.33 Structure of a macula. The "hairs" of the receptor cells of a macula project into the gelatinous otolith membrane. Vestibular nerve fibers surround the base of the hair cells.

15

Equilibrium and Orientation

✓ Explain how the balance organs of the semicircular canals and the vestibule help maintain equilibrium.

The equilibrium sense is not easy to describe because it does not "see," "hear," or "feel," but responds (frequently without our awareness) to various head movements. Furthermore, this sense depends not only on inputs from the internal ear but also on vision and information from stretch receptors of muscles and tendons.

The equilibrium receptors in the semicircular canals and vestibule are collectively called the **vestibular apparatus**. Under normal conditions, they send signals to the brain that initiate reflexes needed to make the simplest changes in position as well as more complex moves such as serving a tennis ball precisely to the right spot (your opponent's backhand).

The equilibrium receptors of the vestibular apparatus can be divided into two functional arms. The receptors in the vestibule monitor linear acceleration and the position of the head with respect to gravity. Because gravity is constant, this is sometimes called our sense of *static equilibrium*. The semicircular canals monitor changes in head rotation, sometimes called our sense of *dynamic equilibrium*.

The Maculae

The **maculae** (mak′u-le; "spots"), one in each saccule wall and one in each utricle wall **(Figure 15.33)**, are sensory receptor organs that monitor the position of the head in space. In so doing, they play a key role in controlling posture. They respond to *linear* acceleration, that is, changes in straight-line speed and direction, but not rotation.

Anatomy of a Macula Each macula is a flat epithelial patch containing **hair cells**. These hair cells, like all those of the internal ear, have stereocilia plus one kinocilium that project into a gel-like mass. **Supporting cells** surround the macula's scattered hair cells (Figure 15.33). The "hairs" of the hair cells are embedded in the overlying **otolith membrane** (o′to-lith), a jelly-like mass studded with tiny stones (calcium carbonate crystals) called **otoliths** ("ear stones"). The otoliths, though small, are dense and they increase the membrane's weight and its inertia (resistance to changes in motion).

In the utricle, the macula is horizontal, and the hairs are vertically oriented when the head is upright (Figure 15.33). For this reason, the utricular maculae respond best to acceleration in the horizontal plane and tilting the head to the side, because vertical (up-down) movements do not displace their horizontal otolith membrane.

In the saccule, on the other hand, the macula is nearly vertical, and the hairs protrude horizontally into the otolith membrane. The saccular maculae respond best to vertical movements, such as the sudden acceleration of an elevator.

The hair cells synapse with fibers of the **vestibular nerve**, whose endings coil around their bases. Like the cochlear nerve, the vestibular nerve is a subdivision of the vestibulocochlear nerve (VIII). The cell bodies of the sensory neurons are located in the nearby **superior** and **inferior vestibular ganglia** (see Figure 15.26).

Activating Macula Receptors What happens in the maculae that leads to sensory transduction? When your head starts or stops moving in a linear direction, inertia causes the otolith membrane to slide backward or forward like a greased plate over the hair cells, bending the hairs. For example, when you start to run, the otolith membranes of the utricle maculae lag behind, bending the hairs backward. When you suddenly stop, the otolith membrane slides abruptly forward (just as you slide forward in your car when you brake), bending the hair cells forward. Likewise, when you nod your head or fall, the otoliths roll inferiorly, bending the hairs of the maculae in the saccules.

The hair cells release neurotransmitter continuously but movement of their hairs modifies the amount they release **(Figure 15.34)**.

- When the hairs bend toward the kinocilium, the hair cells depolarize, stepping up their pace of neurotransmitter release, and more impulses travels up the vestibular nerve to the brain.

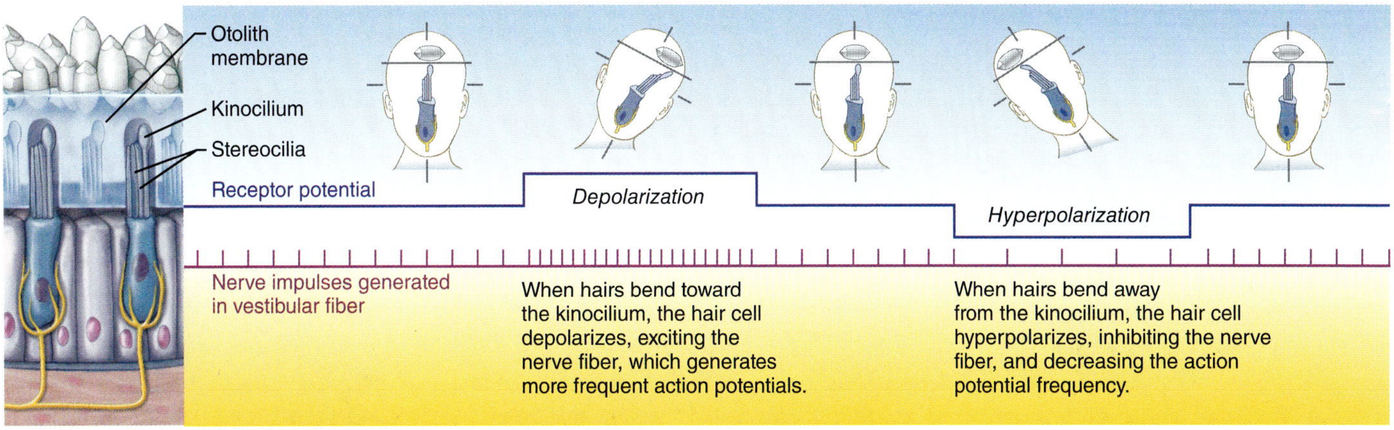

Figure 15.34 The effect of gravitational pull on a macula receptor cell in the utricle.

- When the hairs bend away from the kinocilium, the receptors hyperpolarize and release less neurotransmitter, generating fewer impulses.

In either case, the brain is informed of the changing position of the head in space.

It is important to understand that the maculae respond to *changes* in the velocity of head movement (linear acceleration or deceleration). Because most hair cells adapt quickly (resuming their basal level of neurotransmitter release), they do not report on unchanging head positions. In this way, the maculae help us to maintain normal head position with respect to gravity.

The Cristae Ampullares

The receptor for rotational acceleration, called the **crista ampullaris** or simply *crista*, is a minute elevation in the ampulla of each semicircular canal (see Figure 15.26). Like the maculae, the cristae are excited by head movement (acceleration and deceleration), but in this case the major stimuli are rotational (angular) movements. When you twirl on the dance floor or suffer through a rough boat ride, these gyroscope-like receptors are working overtime. Since the semicircular canals are located in all three planes of space, all rotational movements of the head disturb one or another *pair* of cristae (one in each ear).

Anatomy of a Crista Ampullaris Each crista is composed of supporting cells and hair cells whose structure and function are basically the same as the hair cells of the cochlea and maculae. In this case, the gelled mass is an **ampullary cupula** (ku′pu-lah), which resembles a pointed cap **(Figure 15.35)**. The cupula is a delicate, loosely organized network of gelatinous strands that radiate outward to contact the "hairs" of each hair cell. Dendrites of vestibular nerve fibers encircle the base of the hair cells.

Activating Crista Ampullaris Receptors The cristae respond to *changes* in the velocity of rotational movements of the head. Because of its inertia, the endolymph in the semicircular ducts moves briefly in the direction *opposite* the body's rotation, deforming the crista in the duct. As the hairs bend, the hair cells depolarize and impulses reach the brain at a faster rate (Figure 15.35c, middle panel). Bending the cilia in the opposite direction causes hyperpolarization and generates fewer impulses. Because the axes of the hair cells in the complementary semicircular ducts are opposite, rotation in a given direction depolarizes the receptors in one ampulla of the pair, and hyperpolarizes the receptors in the other.

If the body continues to rotate at a constant rate, the endolymph eventually comes to rest—it moves along at the same speed as the body and the hair cells are no longer stimulated. Consequently, if we are blindfolded, we cannot tell whether we are moving at a constant speed or not moving at all after the first few seconds of rotation. However, when we suddenly stop moving, the endolymph keeps on going, in effect reversing its direction within the canal. This sudden reversal in the direction of hair bending alters membrane voltage in the receptor cells and modifies the rate of impulse transmission, which tells the brain that we have slowed or stopped (Figure 15.35c, right panel).

The key point to remember when considering both types of equilibrium receptors is that the rigid bony labyrinth moves with the body, while the fluids (and gels) within the membranous labyrinth are free to move at various rates, depending on the forces (such as gravity, acceleration, and so on) acting on them.

Vestibular Nystagmus Impulses transmitted from the semicircular canals are particularly important to reflex movements of the eyes. **Vestibular nystagmus** is a complex of rather strange eye movements that occurs during and immediately after rotation.

As you rotate, your eyes slowly drift in the opposite direction, as though fixed on some object in the environment. This reaction relates to the backflow of endolymph in the semicircular canals. Then, because of CNS compensating mechanisms, the eyes jump rapidly toward the direction of rotation to establish a new fixation point. These alternating eye movements continue until the endolymph comes to rest.

When you stop rotating, at first your eyes continue to move in the direction of the previous spin, and then they jerk rapidly in the opposite direction. This sudden change is caused by the change in the direction in which the cristae bend after you stop. Nystagmus is often accompanied by vertigo.

15

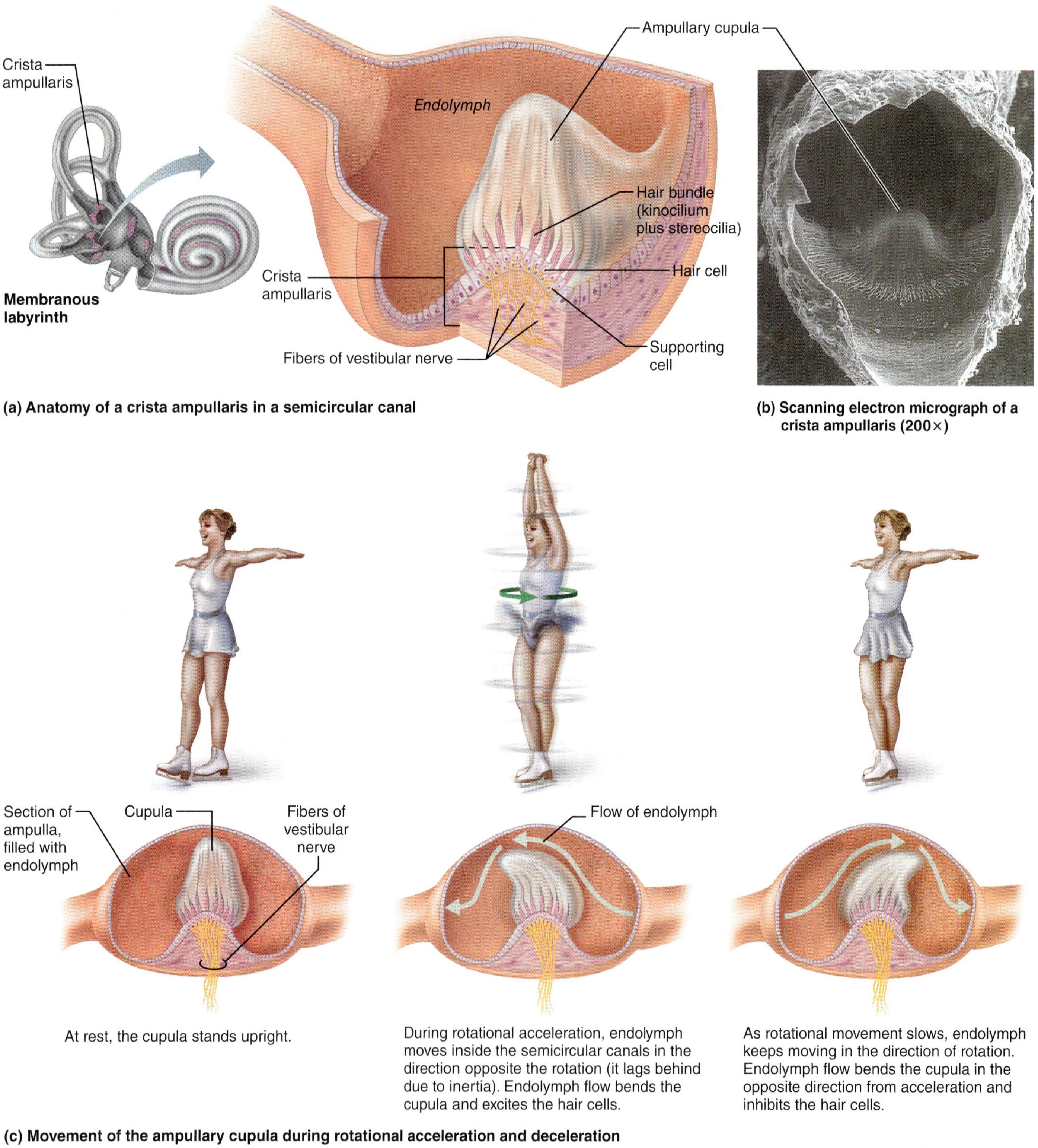

Figure 15.35 **Location, structure, and function of a crista ampullaris in the internal ear.**

The Equilibrium Pathway to the Brain

Our responses to body imbalance, such as when we stumble, must be fast and reflexive. By the time we "thought about" correcting our fall, we would already be on the ground! Accordingly, information from equilibrium receptors goes directly to reflex centers in the brain stem, rather than to the cerebral cortex as with the other special senses.

The nerve pathways connecting the vestibular apparatus with the brain are complex. The transmission sequence begins when the hair cells in the vestibular apparatus are activated. As

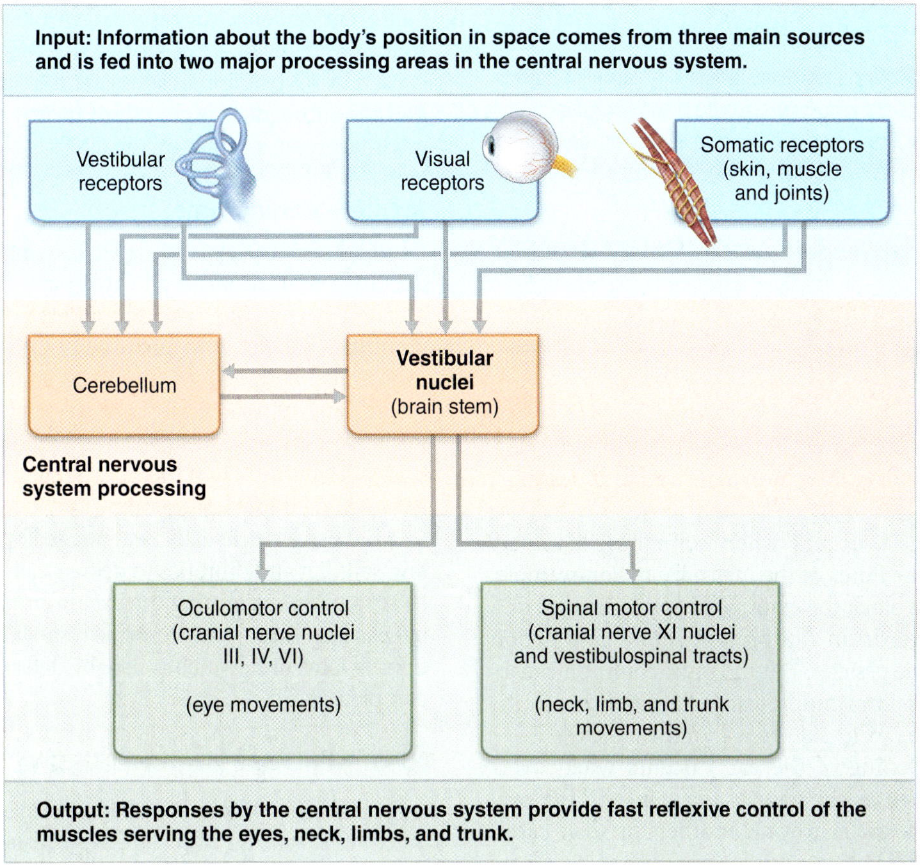

Figure 15.36 **Neural pathways of the balance and orientation system.**

depicted in **Figure 15.36**, impulses travel initially to one of two destinations: the **vestibular nuclei** in the brain stem or the **cerebellum**. The vestibular nuclei, the major integrative center for balance, also receive inputs from the visual and somatic receptors, particularly from proprioceptors in neck muscles that report on the position of the head. These nuclei integrate this information and then send commands to brain stem motor centers that control the extrinsic eye muscles (cranial nerve nuclei III, IV, and VI) and reflex movements of the neck, limb, and trunk muscles (via the vestibulospinal tracts). The ensuing reflex movements of the eyes and body allow us to remain focused on the visual field and quickly adjust our body position to maintain or regain balance.

The cerebellum also integrates inputs from the eyes and somatic receptors (as well as from the cerebrum). It coordinates skeletal muscle activity and regulates muscle tone to maintain head position, posture, and balance, often in the face of rapidly changing inputs. Its "specialty" is fine control of delicate postural movements and timing.

Notice that the vestibular apparatus *does not automatically compensate* for forces acting on the body. Its job is to send warning signals to the central nervous system, which initiates the appropriate compensations (righting) to keep your body balanced, your weight evenly distributed, and your eyes focused on what you were looking at when the disturbance occurred.

Homeostatic Imbalance 15.13

Responses to equilibrium signals are totally reflexive, and usually we are aware of vestibular apparatus activity only when its function is impaired. Equilibrium problems are usually obvious and unpleasant. Nausea, dizziness, and loss of balance are common and there may be nystagmus in the absence of rotational stimuli.

Motion sickness has been difficult to explain, but it appears to be due to sensory input mismatches. For example, if you are inside a ship during a storm, visual inputs indicate that your body is fixed with reference to a stationary environment (your cabin). But as rough seas toss the ship about, your vestibular apparatus detects movement and sends impulses that disagree with the visual information. The brain thus receives conflicting signals, and its "confusion" somehow leads to motion sickness.

Warning signals, which precede nausea and vomiting, include excessive salivation, pallor, rapid deep breathing, and profuse sweating. Removal of the stimulus usually ends the symptoms. Over-the-counter antimotion drugs, such as meclizine (Bonine), depress vestibular inputs and help alleviate the symptoms. They are most effective when taken "before the fact." Scopolamine-containing timed-release skin patches may also head off motion sickness. ✚

Check Your Understanding

15. For each of the following phrases, indicate whether it applies to a macula or a crista ampullaris: inside a semicircular canal; contains otoliths; responds to linear acceleration and deceleration; has a cupula; responds to rotational acceleration and deceleration; inside a saccule.

For answers, see Appendix H.

Homeostatic Imbalances of Hearing and Equilibrium

Deafness

Any hearing loss, no matter how slight, is **deafness** of some sort. Deafness is classified as conduction or sensorineural deafness, according to its cause.

Conduction deafness occurs when something hampers sound conduction to the fluids of the internal ear. For example, compacted earwax can block the external acoustic meatus, or a *perforated* (*ruptured*) eardrum can prevent sound conduction from the eardrum to the ossicles. But the most common causes of conduction deafness are middle ear inflammations (otitis media) and **otosclerosis** (o″to-sklě-ro′sis) of the ossicles.

Otosclerosis ("hardening of the ear") occurs when overgrowth of bony tissue fuses the base of the stapes to the oval window or welds the ossicles to one another. In such cases, vibrations of the skull bones conduct sound to the receptors of that ear, which is far less satisfactory. Otosclerosis is treated surgically.

15

Sensorineural deafness results from damage to neural structures at any point from the cochlear hair cells to and including the auditory cortical cells. This type of deafness typically results from the gradual loss of hair cells throughout life. Hair cells can also be destroyed at an earlier age by a single explosively loud noise or prolonged exposure to high-intensity sounds, such as rock bands or airport noise, which literally tear off their cilia. Other causes of sensorineural deafness are degeneration of the cochlear nerve, strokes, and tumors in the auditory cortex.

Hair cells don't normally regenerate in mammals, but researchers are seeking ways to prod supporting cells into differentiating into hair cells. For congenital defects or age- or noise-related cochlear damage, cochlear implants (devices that convert sound energy into electrical signals) can be inserted into a drilled recess in the temporal bone. The original cochlear implants made human voices sound tinny and robotlike, but modern versions are so effective that even children born deaf can hear well enough to learn to speak well.

Tinnitus

Tinnitus (tĭ-ni′tus) is a ringing or clicking sound in the ears in the absence of auditory stimuli. It is usually a symptom rather than a disease. For example, tinnitus is one of the first symptoms of cochlear nerve degeneration. It may also signal inflammation of the middle or internal ears and is a side effect of some medications, such as aspirin.

Recent evidence suggests that tinnitus is analogous to phantom limb pain. In other words, it is "phantom cochlear noise" caused by destruction of some neurons in the auditory pathway and the subsequent ingrowth of nearby neurons whose signals are interpreted as noise by the CNS.

Ménière's Syndrome

Classic **Ménière's syndrome** (men″ē-ārz′) is a labyrinth disorder that seems to affect all three parts of the internal ear. The afflicted person has repeated attacks of vertigo, nausea, and vomiting. Balance is so disturbed that standing erect is nearly impossible. A "howling" tinnitus is common, so hearing is impaired (and ultimately lost) as well. The cause is uncertain, but it may result from excessive endolymph that distorts the membranous labyrinth, or a membrane rupture that allows the perilymph and endolymph to mix.

Mild cases can usually be managed by antimotion drugs or a low-salt diet and diuretics to decrease endolymph fluid volume. In severe cases, draining the excess endolymph from the internal ear may help. A last resort is removal of the entire malfunctioning labyrinth, which is usually deferred until hearing loss is complete.

Check Your Understanding

16. Six-year-old Mohammed has a cold and says his ears feel "full" and he "can't hear well." Explain what has happened in Mohammed's ears. Which type of deafness does Mohammed have—conduction or sensorineural?

For answers, see Appendix H.

Developmental Aspects of the Special Senses

✓ List changes that occur in the special sense organs with aging.

Taste and Smell

All the special senses are functional, to a greater or lesser degree, at birth. Smell and taste are sharp, and infants relish food that adults consider bland or tasteless. Some researchers claim that smell is just as important as touch in guiding newborn infants to their mother's breast. However, very young children seem indifferent to odors and can play happily with their own feces.

There are few problems with the chemical senses during childhood and young adulthood. Women generally have a more acute sense of smell than men, and nonsmokers have a sharper sense of smell than smokers.

Beginning in the fourth decade of life, our ability to taste and smell declines due to the gradual loss of receptors, which are replaced more slowly than in younger people. More than half of people over age 65 have serious problems detecting odors, which may explain why some tend to douse themselves with large amounts of cologne, or pay little attention to formerly disagreeable odors. Additionally, their sense of taste is poor. This along with the decline in the sense of smell makes food taste bland and contributes to loss of appetite.

Vision

By the fourth week of development, the eyes begin forming as the **optic vesicles** that protrude from the diencephalon (see Figure 12.1c on p. 429). Soon these hollow vesicles indent to form double-layered **optic cups**, and their stalks form the optic nerves and provide a pathway for blood vessels to reach the eye interior.

Once an optic vesicle reaches the overlying surface ectoderm, it induces the ectoderm to thicken and then form a **lens vesicle** that pinches off into the cavity of the optic cup, where it becomes the lens. The lining (internal layer) of the optic cup becomes the neural layer of the retina, and the outer layer forms the pigmented layer. The rest of the eye tissues and the vitreous humor are formed by mesenchymal cells derived from the mesoderm that surrounds the optic cup.

In the darkness of the uterus, the fetus cannot see. Nonetheless, even before the light-sensitive portions of the photoreceptors develop, the central nervous system connections have been made and are functional. During infancy, synaptic connections are fine-tuned, and the typical cortical fields that allow binocular vision are established.

Homeostatic Imbalance 15.14

Congenital problems of the eyes are relatively uncommon, but their incidence is dramatically increased by certain maternal infections, particularly rubella (German measles) during the critical first three months of pregnancy. Common rubella sequels include blindness and cataracts. ✚

As a rule, vision is the only special sense not fully functional at birth. Because the eyeballs are foreshortened, most babies are hyperopic. The newborn infant sees only in gray tones, eye movements are uncoordinated, and often only one eye at a time is used. The lacrimal glands are not completely developed until about two weeks after birth, so babies are tearless for this period, even though they may cry lustily. By 5 months, infants can follow moving objects with their eyes, but visual acuity is still poor (20/200).

By the age of 3 years, depth perception is present and color vision is well developed. Because the eyeball has grown, visual acuity has improved to about 20/30, providing a readiness to begin reading. By first grade, emmetropia has usually replaced the initial hyperopia, and the eye reaches its adult size at 8–9 years of age. Emmetropia usually continues until presbyopia begins to set in around age 40 owing to decreasing lens elasticity.

With age, the lens loses its crystal clarity and discolors. As a result, it begins to scatter light, causing a glare that is distressing when driving at night. The dilator pupillae muscles become less efficient, so the pupils stay partly constricted. These two changes together decrease the amount of light reaching the retina, and visual acuity is dramatically lower in people over 70. In addition, the lacrimal glands are less active and the eyes tend to be dry and more susceptible to infection. Elderly persons are also at risk for certain conditions that cause blindness, such as macular degeneration, glaucoma, cataracts, atherosclerosis, and diabetes mellitus.

Hearing and Balance

The ear begins to develop in the three-week embryo. The internal ears develop first, from thickenings of the surface ectoderm called the **otic placodes** (o′tik plak′ōds), which lie lateral to the hindbrain on each side. The otic placode invaginates, forming the **otic pit** and then the **otic vesicle**, which detaches from the surface epithelium. The otic vesicle develops into the membranous labyrinth. The surrounding mesenchyme forms the bony labyrinth.

The middle ear cavity and pharyngotympanic tube of the middle ear develop from **pharyngeal pouches**, lateral outpocketings of the endoderm lining the pharynx. The auditory ossicles develop from neural crest cells.

The external acoustic meatus and external face of the tympanic membrane of the external ear differentiate from the **pharyngeal cleft** (*branchial groove*), an indentation of the surface ectoderm, and the auricle develops from swellings of the surrounding tissue.

Newborn infants can hear, but early responses to sound are mostly reflexive—for example, crying and clenching the eyelids in response to a startling noise. By the fourth month, infants will turn to the voices of family members. Critical listening begins as toddlers increase their vocabulary, and good language skills are closely tied to the ability to hear well.

Homeostatic Imbalance 15.15

Congenital abnormalities of the ears are fairly common. Examples include partly or completely missing pinnae and closed or absent external acoustic meatuses. Maternal rubella during the first trimester commonly results in sensorineural deafness. ✚

Except for ear inflammations, mostly due to infections, few problems affect the ears during childhood and adult life. By the 60s, however, deterioration of the spiral organ becomes noticeable. We are born with approximately 30,000 hair cells, but their number declines as they are damaged or destroyed by loud noises, disease, or drugs (for example, the antibiotic streptomycin). The hair cells *are* replaced, but at such a slow rate that there really is no functional regeneration. It is estimated that if we were to live 140 years, we would lose all of our hearing receptors.

The ability to hear high-pitched sounds leaves us first. This condition, called **presbycusis** (pres″bĭ-ku′sis), is a type of sensorineural deafness. Although presbycusis is considered a disability of old age, it is becoming much more common in younger people as our world grows noisier.

☑ Check Your Understanding

17. What age-related changes make it more difficult for the elderly to see at night?

For answers, see Appendix H.

Our abilities to see, hear, taste, and smell—and some of our responses to the effects of gravity—are largely the work of our brain. However, as we have discovered in this final nervous system chapter, the large and often elaborate sensory receptor organs that serve the special senses are works of art in and of themselves.

The concluding chapter of this unit describes how the body's functions are controlled by chemicals called hormones in a manner quite different from what we have described for neural control.

Chapter Summary

The Eye and Vision (pp. 545–565)

1. The eye is enclosed in the bony orbit and cushioned by fat.

Accessory Structures of the Eye (pp. 545–549)

2. Eyebrows help to shade and protect the eyes.
3. Eyelids protect and lubricate the eyes by reflex blinking. Within the eyelids are the orbicularis oculi and levator palpebrae superioris muscles, and modified sebaceous and sweat glands.
4. The conjunctiva is a mucosa that lines the eyelids and covers the anterior eyeball surface. Its mucus lubricates the eyeball surface.
5. The lacrimal apparatus consists of the lacrimal gland (which produces a saline solution containing mucus, lysozyme, and antibodies), the lacrimal canaliculi, the lacrimal sac, and the nasolacrimal duct.
6. The extrinsic eye muscles (superior, inferior, lateral, and medial rectus and superior and inferior oblique) move the eyeballs.

15

Structure of the Eyeball (pp. 549–553)

7. The wall of the eyeball is made up of three layers. The outermost fibrous layer consists of the sclera and the cornea. The sclera protects the eye and gives it shape; the cornea allows light to enter the eye.
8. The middle, pigmented vascular layer (uvea) consists of the choroid, the ciliary body, and the iris. The choroid provides nutrients to the eye and prevents light scattering within the eye. The ciliary muscles of the ciliary body control lens shape; the iris controls the size of the pupil.
9. The inner layer, or retina, consists of an outer pigmented layer and an inner neural layer. The neural layer contains photoreceptors (rods and cones), bipolar cells, and ganglion cells. Ganglion cell axons form the optic nerve, which exits via the optic disc ("blind spot").
10. The posterior segment of the eyeball, behind the lens, contains vitreous humor, which helps support the eyeball and keep the retina in place. The anterior segment, anterior to the lens, is filled with aqueous humor, formed by capillaries in the ciliary processes and drained into the scleral venous sinus. Aqueous humor is a major factor in maintaining intraocular pressure.
11. The biconvex lens is suspended within the eye by the ciliary zonule attached to the ciliary body. The lens is the only adjustable refractory structure of the eye.

Optics and the Eye (pp. 553–556)

12. Visible light is made up of those wavelengths of the electromagnetic spectrum that excite the photoreceptors.
13. Light is refracted (bent) when passing from one transparent medium to another of different density. Concave lenses disperse light; convex lenses converge light and bring its rays to a focal point. The greater the lens curvature, the more light bends.
14. As light passes through the eye, the cornea and lens bend and focus it on the retina. The cornea accounts for most of the refraction, but the lens allows active focusing for different distances.
15. Focusing for distant vision requires no special movements of the eye structures. Focusing for close-up vision requires accommodation (bulging of the lens), pupillary constriction, and convergence of the eyeballs. Cranial nerve III controls all three reflexes.
16. Refractory problems include presbyopia, myopia, hyperopia, and astigmatism.

Photoreceptors and Phototransduction (pp. 556–563)

17. The outer segments of the photoreceptors contain light-absorbing visual pigment in membrane-bounded discs.
18. The light-absorbing molecule retinal is combined with various opsins to form the visual pigments. Rod visual pigment, rhodopsin, is a combination of retinal and opsin. The three types of cones all contain retinal, but each has a different type of opsin. Each cone type responds maximally to one color of light: red, blue, or green. The chemistry of cone function is similar to that of rods.
19. Rods respond to low-intensity light and provide night and peripheral vision. Cones are bright-light, high-discrimination receptors that provide color vision. Anything that must be viewed precisely is focused on the cone-rich fovea centralis.
20. When struck by light, retinal changes shape (11-*cis* to all-*trans*) and activates opsin. Activated opsin activates transducin (a G protein) which in turn activates PDE, an enzyme that breaks down cGMP, allowing the cation channels to close. This hyperpolarizes the receptor cells and inhibits their release of neurotransmitter.
21. Photoreceptors and bipolar cells generate graded potentials only; ganglion cells generate action potentials.
22. During light adaptation, photopigments are bleached and rods are inactivated; then, as cones decrease their light sensitivity, high-acuity vision ensues. In dark adaptation, cones cease functioning, and visual acuity decreases; rod function begins when sufficient rhodopsin has accumulated.

Visual Pathways and Processing (pp. 563–565)

23. The visual pathway to the brain begins with the optic nerve fibers (ganglion cell axons) from the retina. At the optic chiasma, fibers from the medial half of each retina cross over and continue in the optic tracts to the thalamus. Thalamic neurons project to the visual cortex via the optic radiation. Fibers also project from the retina to the midbrain pretectal nuclei and the superior colliculi, and to the suprachiasmatic nucleus of the hypothalamus.

24. Each eye receives a slightly different view of the visual field. The visual cortices fuse these views to provide depth perception.
25. Retinal processing involves the selective destruction of inputs so as to emphasize bright/dark or color contrasts (edges). Thalamic processing subserves high-acuity color vision and depth perception. Cortical processing involves neurons of the striate (primary) cortex, which receive inputs from the retinal ganglion cells, and neurons of the prestriate (association) cortices, which receive inputs from striate cortical cells and mostly integrate inputs concerned with color, form, and movement. Visual processing also proceeds anteriorly in the "what" and "where" processing streams via the temporal and parietal lobes, respectively.

The Chemical Senses: Smell and Taste (pp. 565–570)

The Olfactory Epithelium and the Sense of Smell (pp. 565–567)

1. The olfactory epithelium is located in the roof of the nasal cavity. The olfactory sensory neurons are ciliated bipolar neurons. Their axons are the filaments of the olfactory nerve (cranial nerve I).
2. Individual olfactory neurons show a range of responsiveness to different chemicals. Olfactory neurons bearing the same odorant receptors synapse in the same glomerulus type.
3. Olfactory neurons are excited by volatile chemicals that bind to receptors in the olfactory cilia.
4. Action potentials of the olfactory nerve filaments are transmitted to the olfactory bulb where the filaments synapse with mitral cells. The mitral cells send impulses via the olfactory tract to the olfactory cortex. Fibers carrying impulses from the olfactory bulb also project to the limbic system.

Taste Buds and the Sense of Taste (pp. 568–570)

5. The taste buds are scattered in the oral cavity and pharynx but are most abundant on the tongue papillae.
6. Gustatory epithelial cells, the receptor cells of the taste buds, have gustatory hairs (microvilli) that serve as the receptor regions. The gustatory epithelial cells are excited by the binding of tastants (food chemicals) to receptors on their microvilli.
7. The five basic taste qualities are sweet, sour, salty, bitter, and umami.
8. The taste sense is served by cranial nerves VII, IX, and X, which send impulses to the solitary nucleus of the medulla. From there, impulses are sent to the thalamus and the gustatory cortex.

Homeostatic Imbalances of the Chemical Senses (p. 570)

9. Most chemical sense dysfunctions are olfactory disorders (anosmias). Common causes are trauma, inflammation, or neurological disorders.

The Ear: Hearing and Balance (pp. 570–584)

Structure of the Ear (pp. 570–575)

1. The auricle and external acoustic meatus compose the external ear. The tympanic membrane, the boundary between the outer and middle ears, transmits sound waves to the middle ear.
2. The middle ear is a small chamber within the temporal bone, connected by the pharyngotympanic tube to the nasopharynx. The ossicles, which help amplify sound, span the middle ear cavity and transmit sound vibrations from the tympanic membrane to the oval window.
3. The internal ear consists of the bony labyrinth, within which the membranous labyrinth is suspended. The bony labyrinth chambers contain perilymph; the membranous labyrinth ducts and sacs contain endolymph.
4. The vestibule contains the saccule and utricle. The semicircular canals extend posteriorly from the vestibule in three planes. They contain the semicircular ducts.
5. The cochlea houses the cochlear duct (scala media), containing the spiral organ, the receptor organ for hearing. Within the cochlear duct, the hair (receptor) cells rest on the basilar membrane, and their hairs project into the gelatinous tectorial membrane.

Physiology of Hearing (pp. 575–579)

6. Sound originates from a vibrating object and travels in waves consisting of alternating areas of compression and rarefaction of the medium.
7. The distance from crest to crest on a sine wave is the sound's wavelength; the shorter the wavelength, the higher the frequency (measured in hertz). Frequency is perceived as pitch.
8. The amplitude of sound is the height of the peaks of the sine wave, which reflect the sound's intensity. Sound intensity is measured in decibels. Intensity is perceived as loudness.
9. Sound passing through the external acoustic meatus sets the tympanic membrane into vibration at the same frequency. The ossicles amplify and deliver the vibrations to the oval window.
10. Pressure waves in cochlear fluids set specific locations on the basilar membrane into resonance. At points of maximal membrane vibration, the vibratory motion alternately depolarizes and hyperpolarizes the hair cells of the spiral organ. Movements of the stereocilia toward the kinocilium depolarize the hair cells and increase the rate of impulse generation in the auditory nerve fibers. Movements away from the kinocilium have the opposite effect. High-frequency sounds stimulate hair cells near the oval window; low-frequency sounds stimulate hair cells near the apex. Inner hair cells send most auditory inputs to the brain. Outer hair cells amplify the inner hair cells' responsiveness.
11. Impulses generated along the cochlear nerve travel to the cochlear nuclei of the medulla and from there through several brain stem nuclei to the medial geniculate nucleus of the thalamus and then the auditory cortex. Each auditory cortex receives impulses from both ears.
12. Auditory processing is analytic; each tone is perceived separately. Perception of pitch is related to the position of the excited hair cells along the basilar membrane. Intensity perception reflects the fact that as sound intensity increases, basilar membrane motion increases, and the frequency of impulse transmission to the cortex increases. Cues for sound localization include the intensity and timing of sound arriving at each ear.

Equilibrium and Orientation (pp. 580–584)

13. The equilibrium receptor regions of the internal ear are called the vestibular apparatus.
14. The receptors for linear acceleration and gravity are the maculae of the saccule and utricle. A macula consists of hair cells with stereocilia and a kinocilium embedded in an overlying otolith membrane. Linear movements cause the otolith membrane to move, pulling on the hair cells and changing the rate of impulse generation in the vestibular nerve fibers.
15. The receptor within each semicircular duct, the crista ampullaris, responds to angular or rotational acceleration in one plane. It consists of a tuft of hair cells whose stereocilia are embedded in the gelatinous ampullary cupula. Rotational movements cause the endolymph to flow in the opposite direction, bending the cupula and either exciting or inhibiting the hair cells.
16. Impulses from the vestibular apparatus are sent via vestibular nerve fibers mainly to the vestibular nuclei of the brain stem and

the cerebellum. These centers initiate responses that fix the eyes on objects and activate muscles to maintain balance.

Homeostatic Imbalances of Hearing and Equilibrium (p. 584)

17. Conduction deafness results from interference with conduction of sound vibrations to the fluids of the internal ear. Sensorineural deafness reflects damage to neural structures.
18. Tinnitus is an early sign of sensorineural deafness; it may also result from inflammation or certain drugs.
19. Ménière's syndrome is a disorder of the membranous labyrinth. Symptoms include tinnitus, deafness, and vertigo. Excessive endolymph accumulation is the suspected cause.

Developmental Aspects of the Special Senses (pp. 584–585)

Taste and Smell (pp. 548–585)

1. The chemical senses are sharpest at birth and gradually decline with age as receptor cells are replaced more slowly.

Vision (p. 585)

2. Congenital eye problems are uncommon, but maternal rubella can cause blindness.
3. The eye starts as an optic vesicle, an outpocketing of the diencephalon that invaginates to form the optic cup, which becomes the retina. Overlying ectoderm folds to form the lens vesicle, which gives rise to the lens. The remaining eye tissues and the accessory structures are formed by mesenchyme.
4. The eye is foreshortened at birth and reaches adult size at the age of 8–9 years. Depth perception and color vision develop before age 3.
5. With age, the lens loses its elasticity and clarity, there is a decline in the ability of the iris to dilate, and visual acuity decreases. The elderly are at risk for eye problems resulting from dry eyes and disease.

Hearing and Balance (p. 585)

6. The membranous labyrinth develops from the otic placode, an ectodermal thickening lateral to the hindbrain. Mesenchyme forms the surrounding bony structures. Pharyngeal pouch endoderm, in conjunction with mesenchyme, forms most middle ear structures; the external ear is formed largely by ectoderm.
7. Congenital ear problems are fairly common. Maternal rubella can cause deafness.
8. Response to sound in infants is reflexive. By the fourth month, an infant can locate sound. Critical listening develops in toddlers.
9. The spiral organ deteriorates throughout life as noise, disease, and drugs destroy cochlear hair cells. Age-related loss of hearing (presbycusis) occurs in the 60s and 70s.

15

Review Questions

Multiple Choice/Matching

(Some questions have more than one correct answer. Select the best answer or answers from the choices given.)

1. Accessory glands that produce an oily secretion are the **(a)** conjunctiva, **(b)** lacrimal glands, **(c)** tarsal glands.
2. The portion of the fibrous layer that is white and opaque is the **(a)** choroid, **(b)** cornea, **(c)** retina, **(d)** sclera.
3. Which sequence best describes a normal route for the flow of tears from the eyes into the nasal cavity? **(a)** lacrimal canaliculi, lacrimal sacs, nasolacrimal ducts; **(b)** lacrimal ducts, lacrimal canaliculi, nasolacrimal ducts; **(c)** nasolacrimal ducts, lacrimal canaliculi, lacrimal sacs.
4. Activation of the sympathetic nervous system causes **(a)** contraction of the sphincter pupillae muscles, **(b)** contraction of the dilator pupillae muscles, **(c)** contraction of the ciliary muscles, **(d)** a decrease in ciliary zonule tension.
5. Damage to the medial recti muscles would probably affect **(a)** accommodation, **(b)** refraction, **(c)** convergence, **(d)** pupil constriction.
6. The phenomenon of dark adaptation is best explained by the fact that **(a)** rhodopsin does not function in dim light, **(b)** rhodopsin breakdown occurs slowly, **(c)** rods exposed to intense light need time to generate rhodopsin, **(d)** cones are stimulated to function by bright light.
7. Blockage of the scleral venous sinus might result in **(a)** a sty, **(b)** glaucoma, **(c)** conjunctivitis, **(d)** a cataract.
8. Nearsightedness is more properly called **(a)** myopia, **(b)** hyperopia, **(c)** presbyopia, **(d)** emmetropia.
9. Of the neurons in the retina, the axons of which of these form the optic nerve? **(a)** bipolar cells, **(b)** ganglion cells, **(c)** cone cells, **(d)** horizontal cells.
10. Which sequence of reactions occurs when a person looks at a distant object? **(a)** pupils constrict, ciliary zonule (suspensory ligament) relaxes, lenses become less convex; **(b)** pupils dilate, ciliary zonule becomes taut, lenses become less convex; **(c)** pupils dilate, ciliary zonule becomes taut, lenses become more convex; **(d)** pupils constrict, ciliary zonule relaxes, lenses become more convex.
11. During embryonic development, the lens of the eye forms **(a)** as part of the choroid coat, **(b)** from the surface ectoderm overlying the optic cup, **(c)** as part of the sclera, **(d)** from mesodermal tissue.
12. The blind spot of the eye is **(a)** where more rods than cones are found, **(b)** where the macula lutea is located, **(c)** where only cones occur, **(d)** where the optic nerve leaves the eye.
13. Olfactory tract damage would probably affect your ability to **(a)** see, **(b)** hear, **(c)** feel pain, **(d)** smell.
14. Sensory impulses transmitted over the facial, glossopharyngeal, and vagus nerves are involved in the sensation of **(a)** taste, **(b)** touch, **(c)** equilibrium, **(d)** smell.
15. Taste buds are found on the **(a)** anterior part of the tongue, **(b)** posterior part of the tongue, **(c)** palate, **(d)** all of these.
16. Gustatory epithelial cells are stimulated by **(a)** movement of otoliths, **(b)** stretch, **(c)** substances in solution, **(d)** photons of light.
17. Cells in the olfactory bulb that act as local "integrators" of olfactory inputs are the **(a)** hair cells, **(b)** amacrine granule cells, **(c)** olfactory stem cells, **(d)** mitral cells, **(e)** supporting cells.
18. Olfactory nerve filaments are found **(a)** in the optic bulbs, **(b)** passing through the cribriform plate of the ethmoid bone, **(c)** in the optic tracts, **(d)** in the olfactory cortex.
19. Conduction of sound from the middle ear to the internal ear occurs via vibration of the **(a)** malleus against the tympanic

membrane, **(b)** stapes in the oval window, **(c)** incus in the round window, **(d)** stapes against the tympanic membrane.

20. The transmission of sound vibrations through the internal ear occurs chiefly through **(a)** nerve fibers, **(b)** air, **(c)** fluid, **(d)** bone.

21. Which of the following statements does not correctly describe the spiral organ? **(a)** Sounds of high frequency stimulate hair cells at the basal end, **(b)** the "hairs" of the receptor cells are embedded in the tectorial membrane, **(c)** the basilar membrane acts as a resonator, **(d)** the more numerous outer hair cells are largely responsible for our perception of sound.

22. Pitch is to frequency of sound as loudness is to **(a)** quality, **(b)** intensity, **(c)** overtones, **(d)** all of these.

23. The structure that allows pressure in the middle ear to be equalized with atmospheric pressure is the **(a)** pinna, **(b)** pharyngotympanic tube, **(c)** tympanic membrane, **(d)** oval window.

24. Which of the following is important in maintaining the balance of the body? **(a)** visual cues, **(b)** semicircular canals, **(c)** the saccule, **(d)** proprioceptors, **(e)** all of these.

25. Equilibrium receptors that report the position of the head in space relative to the pull of gravity are **(a)** spiral organs, **(b)** maculae, **(c)** cristae ampullares, **(d)** otoliths.

26. Which of the following is not a possible cause of conduction deafness? **(a)** impacted cerumen, **(b)** middle ear infection, **(c)** cochlear nerve degeneration, **(d)** otosclerosis.

27. Which of the following are intrinsic eye muscles? **(a)** superior rectus, **(b)** orbicularis oculi, **(c)** smooth muscles of the iris and ciliary body, **(d)** levator palpebrae superioris.

28. Which lies closest to the exact posterior pole of the eye? **(a)** optic nerve, **(b)** optic disc, **(c)** macula lutea, **(d)** point of entry of central artery into the eye.

29. Otoliths (ear stones) are **(a)** a cause of deafness, **(b)** a type of hearing aid, **(c)** important in equilibrium, **(d)** the rock-hard petrous temporal bones.

Short Answer Essay Questions

30. Why do you often have to blow your nose after crying?

31. How do rods and cones differ functionally?

32. Where is the fovea centralis, and why is it important?

33. Describe the response of rhodopsin to light stimuli. What is the outcome of this cascade of events?

34. Since there are only three types of cones, how can you explain the fact that we see many more colors?

35. Where are the olfactory sensory neurons, and why is that site poorly suited for their job?

36. Each olfactory sensory neuron responds to a single type of odorant molecule. True or false? Explain your choice.

37. Name the five primary taste qualities and the cranial nerves that serve the sense of taste.

38. Describe the effect of aging on the special sense organs.

Critical Thinking and Clinical Application Questions

1. During an ophthalmoscopic examination, Mrs. James was found to have bilateral papilledema. Further investigation indicated that this condition resulted from a rapidly growing intracranial tumor. First, define papilledema (see *Related Clinical Terms*). Then explain its presence in terms of Mrs. James's diagnosis.

2. Sally, a 9-year-old girl, told the clinic physician that her "ear lump hurt" and she kept "getting dizzy and falling down." As she told her story, she pointed to her mastoid process. An otoscopic examination of the external acoustic meatus revealed a red, swollen eardrum, and her throat was inflamed. Her condition was described as mastoiditis with secondary labyrinthitis (inflammation of the labyrinth). Describe the most likely route of infection and the infected structures in Sally's case. Also explain the cause of her dizziness and falling.

3. Mr. Gaspe appeared at the eye clinic complaining of a chip of wood in his eye. No foreign body was found, but the conjunctiva was obviously inflamed. What name is given to this inflammatory condition, and where would you look for a foreign body that has been floating around on the eye surface for a while?

4. Mrs. Orlando has been noticing flashes of light and tiny specks in her right visual field. When she begins to see a "veil" floating before her right eye, she makes an appointment to see the eye doctor. What is your diagnosis? Is the condition serious? Explain.

5. David Norris, an engineering student, has been working in a nightclub to earn money to pay for his education. After about eight months, he notices that he is having problems hearing high-pitched tones. What is the cause-and-effect relationship here?

6. Assume that a tumor in the pituitary gland or hypothalamus is protruding inferiorly and compressing the optic chiasma. What could be the visual outcome?

7. Four-year-old Gary Zammer is brought to the ophthalmologist for a routine checkup on his vision. Gary is an albino. How do you think albinism affects vision?

8. Right before Jan, a senior citizen, had a large plug of earwax cleaned from her ear, she developed a constant howling sound in her ear that would not stop. It was very annoying and stressful, and she had to go to counseling to learn how to live with this awful noise. What was her condition called?

9. During an anatomy and physiology lab exercise designed to teach the use of the ophthalmoscope, you notice that your lab partner has difficulty seeing objects in the darkened room. Upon examining her retina through the ophthalmoscope, you observe streaks and patches of dark pigmentation at the back of the eye. What might this condition be?

10. Henri, a chef in a five-star French restaurant, has been diagnosed with leukemia. He is about to undergo chemotherapy, which will kill rapidly dividing cells in his body. He needs to continue working between bouts of chemotherapy. What consequences of chemotherapy would you predict that might affect his job as a chef?

AT THE CLINIC

Related Clinical Terms

Ageusia (ah-gu′ze-ah) Loss or impairment of the taste sense.

Age-related macular degeneration (ARMD) Progressive deterioration of the macula lutea that destroys central vision; the main cause of vision loss in those over age 65. Buildup of pigments in the macula impairs functioning of the pigmented epithelium. Continued accumulation of pigment leads to the "dry" form of ARMD, in which many pigment cells and macular photoreceptors die. The dry form is largely untreatable, although a specific cocktail of vitamins and zinc slows its progression. Less common is the "wet" form in which new blood vessels from the choroid grow into the retina. Blood and fluids leak from these vessels, scarring and detaching the retina. The cause of wet ARMD is unknown, but several treatment options can slow its progression—laser treatments that destroy some of the invading vessels and drugs that prevent blood vessel growth. Clinical trials using RNA interference to inhibit vascular growth are underway.

Blepharitis (blef″ah-ri′tis; *blephar* = eyelash; *itis* = inflammation) Inflammation of the margins of the eyelids.

Enucleation (e-nu″kle-a′shun) Surgical removal of an eyeball.

Exophthalmos (ek″sof-thal′mos; *ex* = out; *ophthalmo* = the eye) Anteriorly bulging eyeballs. Seen in some cases of hyperthyroidism.

Labyrinthitis Inflammation of the labyrinth.

Ophthalmology (of″thal-mol′o-je) The science that studies the eye and eye diseases. An ophthalmologist is a medical doctor who specializes in treating eye disorders.

15

Optometrist A licensed nonphysician who measures vision and prescribes corrective lenses.

Otalgia (o-tal′je-ah; *algia* = pain) Earache.

Otitis externa Inflammation and infection of the external acoustic meatus, caused by bacteria or fungi that enter the canal from outside, especially when the canal is moist (e.g., after swimming).

Otoacoustic emissions Sounds generated by the movement of outer hair cells in the cochlea. Stimulated otoacoustic emissions are an inexpensive way to screen newborns for hearing defects.

Papilledema (pap″il-ĕ-de′mah; *papill* = nipple; *edema* = swelling) Protrusion of the optic disc into the eyeball, which can be observed by ophthalmoscopic examination; caused by conditions that increase intracranial pressure.

Scotoma (sko-to′mah; *scoto* = darkness) A blind spot other than the normal (optic disc) blind spot. Has many causes, including stroke or a brain tumor pressing on fibers of the visual pathway.

Trachoma (trah-ko′mah; *trach* = rough) A highly contagious bacterial (chlamydial) infection of the conjunctiva and cornea. Common worldwide, it blinds millions of people in poor countries of Africa and Asia. Treated with eye ointments containing antibiotic drugs.

Weber's test Hearing test during which a sounding tuning fork is held to the forehead. In those with normal hearing, the tone is heard equally in both ears. The tone will be heard best in the "good" ear if sensorineural deafness is present, and in the "bad" ear if conduction deafness is present.

Case Study Special Senses

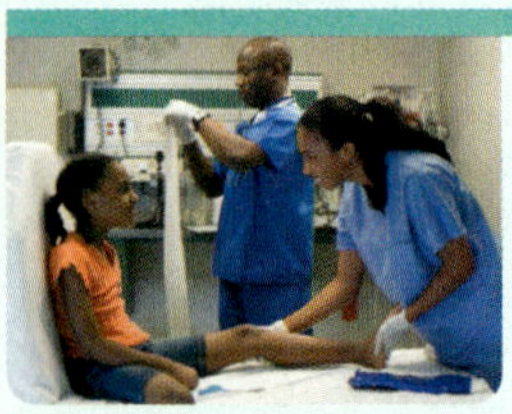

When emergency personnel arrived on the scene of the bus crash, they found Brian Rhen, 42, sitting on the side of the road holding his head in his hands. He complained of a severe headache and nausea, and was evaluated and treated for a concussion. Several days later, Mr. Rhen began to experience recurring episodes of vertigo and was referred to a neurologist. (Vertigo is a sensation of motion or movement while the person is stationary, and can be accompanied by nausea and vomiting.)

Mr. Rhen was diagnosed with *benign paroxysmal positional vertigo* (BPPV). With this condition, which can be caused by head trauma, vertigo can be provoked by specific changes in head position. Mr. Rhen reported that his vertigo usually occurred when rolling over in bed, or when turning his head from side to side while sitting up, and that these movements provoked the sensation of a spinning room, which led to nausea. The neurologist confirmed the diagnosis of BPPV by using a test called the Dix-Hallpike maneuver. During this test, the neurologist looks for nystagmus (involuntary, jerking eye movements) as he makes specific rotational changes to Mr. Rhen's head position.

1. The ear is divided into three major areas (compartments). What are these three areas, and which of these areas is involved in Mr. Rhen's BPPV?
2. What are the three main sources of sensory input that the body uses in order to control balance and equilibrium?
3. Name the two functional divisions of the vestibular apparatus. Identify the sensory receptor associated with each division, and state which aspect of equilibrium each receptor senses.
4. BPPV can be caused by otoliths that have been dislodged from the otolithic membrane of the maculae. Based on Mr. Rhen's symptoms and the head movements that provoke these symptoms, what part of the vestibular apparatus are the displaced otoliths now affecting?
5. Explain why nystagmus is associated with the Dix-Hallpike maneuver.

(Answers in Appendix H)

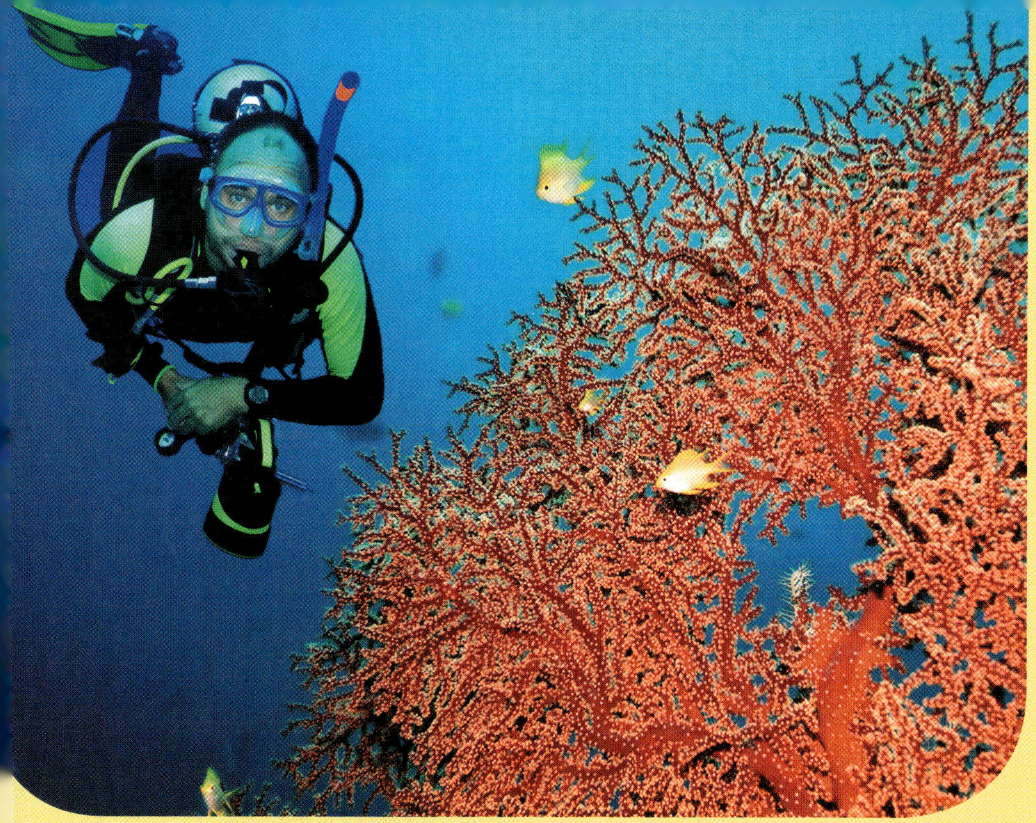

16 The Endocrine System

You don't have to watch *CSI* to experience action-packed drama. Molecules and cells inside your body have dynamic adventures on microscopic levels all the time.

For instance, when insulin molecules, carried passively along in the blood, attach to protein receptors of nearby cells, the response is dramatic: Glucose molecules disappear from the blood into the cells, and cellular activity accelerates. Such is the power of the second great control system of the body, the **endocrine system**, which interacts with the nervous system to coordinate and integrate the activity of body cells.

The Endocrine System: An Overview

✓ Indicate important differences between hormonal and neural controls of body functioning.

✓ List the major endocrine organs, and describe their body locations.

✓ Distinguish between hormones, paracrines, and autocrines.

As we have seen, the nervous system regulates the activity of muscles and glands via electrochemical impulses delivered by neurons, and those organs respond within milliseconds. The means of control and speed of the endocrine system are very different: The endocrine system influences metabolic activity by means of *hormones* (*hormone* = to excite). Hormones are chemical messengers secreted by cells into the extracellular fluids. These messengers travel through the blood and regulate the metabolic function of other cells in the body. Binding of a hormone to cellular receptors initiates responses that typically occur after a lag period of seconds or even days. But, once initiated, those responses tend to last much longer than those induced by the nervous system.

Hormones ultimately target most cells of the body, producing widespread and diverse effects. The major processes that these "mighty molecules" control and integrate include:

- Reproduction
- Growth and development
- Maintenance of electrolyte, water, and nutrient balance of the blood
- Regulation of cellular metabolism and energy balance
- Mobilization of body defenses

16

As you can see, the endocrine system orchestrates processes that go on for relatively long periods, in some instances continuously. The scientific study of hormones and the endocrine organs is called **endocrinology**.

Compared with other organs of the body, those of the endocrine system are small and unimpressive. Indeed, to collect 1 kg (2.2 lb) of hormone-producing tissue, you would need to collect all the endocrine tissue from eight or nine adults! Unlike most organ systems, the endocrine organs are not grouped together but are widely scattered about the body.

As we explained in Chapter 4, there are two kinds of glands:

- *Exocrine glands* produce nonhormonal substances, such as sweat and saliva, and have ducts that carry these substances to a membrane surface.
- **Endocrine glands**, also called *ductless glands*, produce hormones and lack ducts. They release their hormones into the surrounding tissue fluid (*endo* = within; *crine* = to secrete), and they typically have a rich vascular and lymphatic drainage that receives their hormones. Most of the hormone-producing cells in endocrine glands are arranged in cords and branching networks—a situation that maximizes contact between them and the capillaries surrounding them.

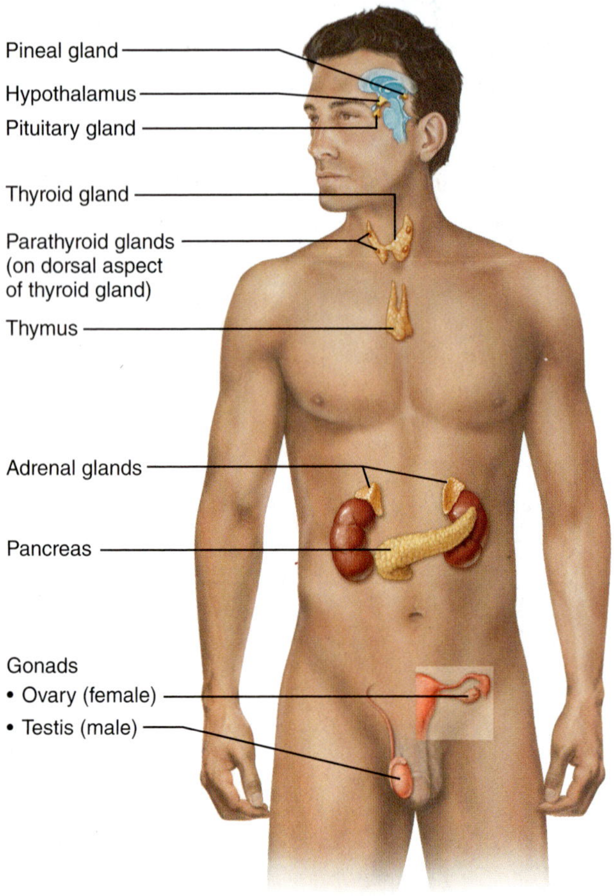

Figure 16.1 Location of selected endocrine organs of the body.

The endocrine glands include the pituitary, thyroid, parathyroid, adrenal, and pineal glands **(Figure 16.1)**. The hypothalamus, along with its neural functions, produces and releases hormones, so we can consider the hypothalamus a **neuroendocrine organ**. In addition, several organs, such as the pancreas, gonads (ovaries and testes), and placenta, contain endocrine tissue and also perform other functions.

Many other organs also contain scattered endocrine cells or small clusters of endocrine cells. For example, adipose cells release leptin, the thymus releases thymic hormones, and hormone-producing cells are found in the walls of the small intestine, stomach, kidneys, and heart—organs whose chief functions have little to do with hormone production. We describe these other hormone-producing structures on pp. 621–622.

Some physiologists include local chemical messengers—autocrines and paracrines—as part of the endocrine system, but that is not the consensus. Hormones are long-distance chemical signals that travel in blood or lymph throughout the body. Autocrines and paracrines, on the other hand, are short-distance signals. **Autocrines** are chemicals that exert their effects on the same cells that secrete them. For example, certain prostaglandins released by smooth muscle cells cause those smooth muscle cells to contract. **Paracrines** also act locally (within the same tissue) but affect cell types other than those releasing the paracrine chemicals. For example, somatostatin released by one population of pancreatic cells inhibits the release of insulin by a different population of pancreatic cells.

☑ Check Your Understanding

1. For each of the following statements, indicate whether it applies more to the endocrine system or the nervous system: rapid; discrete responses; controls growth and development; long-lasting responses.
2. Which two endocrine glands are found in the neck?
3. What is the difference between a hormone and a paracrine?

For answers, see Appendix H.

Hormones

✓ Describe how hormones are classified chemically.

✓ Describe the two major mechanisms by which hormones bring about their effects on their target tissues.

✓ Explain how hormone release is regulated.

✓ List three kinds of interaction of different hormones acting on the same target cell.

The Chemistry of Hormones

Although a large variety of hormones are produced, nearly all of them can be classified chemically as either amino acid based or steroids.

- **Amino acid based:** Most hormones are amino acid based. Molecular size varies widely in this group—from simple amino acid derivatives (which include thyroxine constructed from the amino acid tyrosine and amines), to peptides (short chains of amino acids), to proteins (long polymers of amino acids).
- **Steroids:** Steroid hormones are synthesized from cholesterol. Of the hormones produced by the major endocrine organs, only gonadal and adrenocortical hormones are steroids.

Some researchers add a third class, **eicosanoids** (i-ko′să-noyds), which include *leukotrienes* and *prostaglandins*. Nearly all cell membranes release these biologically active lipids (made from arachidonic acid). Leukotrienes are signaling chemicals that mediate inflammation and some allergic reactions. Prostaglandins have multiple targets and effects, ranging from raising blood pressure and increasing the expulsive uterine contractions of birth to enhancing blood clotting, pain, and inflammation.

Because the effects of eicosanoids are typically highly localized, affecting only nearby cells, they generally act as paracrines and autocrines and do not fit the definition of true hormones, which influence distant targets. For this reason, we will not consider this class of hormonelike chemicals here. Instead, we note their important effects in later chapters as appropriate.

Mechanisms of Hormone Action

All major hormones circulate to virtually all tissues, but a hormone influences the activity of only those tissue cells that have receptors for it. These cells are its **target cells**. Hormones bring about their characteristic effects by *altering* target cell activity. In other words, they increase or decrease the rates of normal cellular processes.

The precise response depends on the target cell type. For example, when the hormone epinephrine binds to certain smooth muscle cells in blood vessel walls, it stimulates them to contract. Epinephrine binding to cells other than muscle cells may have a totally different effect, but it does not cause those cells to contract.

A hormone typically produces one or more of the following changes:

- Alters plasma membrane permeability or membrane potential, or both, by opening or closing ion channels
- Stimulates synthesis of enzymes and other proteins within the cell
- Activates or deactivates enzymes
- Induces secretory activity
- Stimulates mitosis

How does a hormone communicate with its target cell? In other words, how is hormone receptor binding harnessed to the intracellular machinery needed for hormone action? The answer depends on the chemical nature of the hormone and the cellular location of the receptor. In general, hormones act at receptors in one of two ways.

1. *Water-soluble hormones* (all amino acid–based hormones except thyroid hormone) act on *receptors in the plasma membrane*. These receptors are usually coupled via regulatory molecules called G proteins to one or more intracellular second messengers which mediate the target cell's response.
2. *Lipid-soluble hormones* (steroid and thyroid hormones) act on *receptors inside the cell*, which directly activate genes.

This will be easy for you to remember if you think about why the hormones must bind where they do. Receptors for water-soluble hormones must be in the plasma membrane since these hormones *cannot* enter the cell, and receptors for lipid-soluble steroid and thyroid hormones are inside the cell because these hormones *can* enter the cell. Of course, things are not quite that clear-cut—steroid hormones can exert some of their more immediate effects via plasma membrane receptors, and the second messengers of some water-soluble hormones can turn genes on.

Plasma Membrane Receptors and Second-Messenger Systems

With the exception of thyroid hormone, amino acid–based hormones exert their signaling effects through intracellular **second messengers** generated when a hormone binds to a receptor in the plasma membrane. You are already familiar with

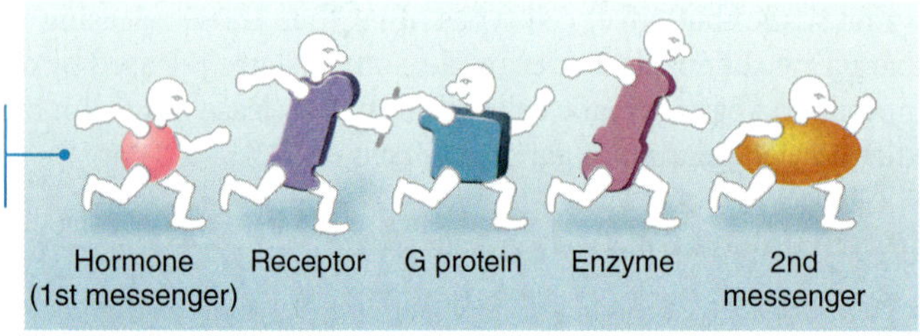

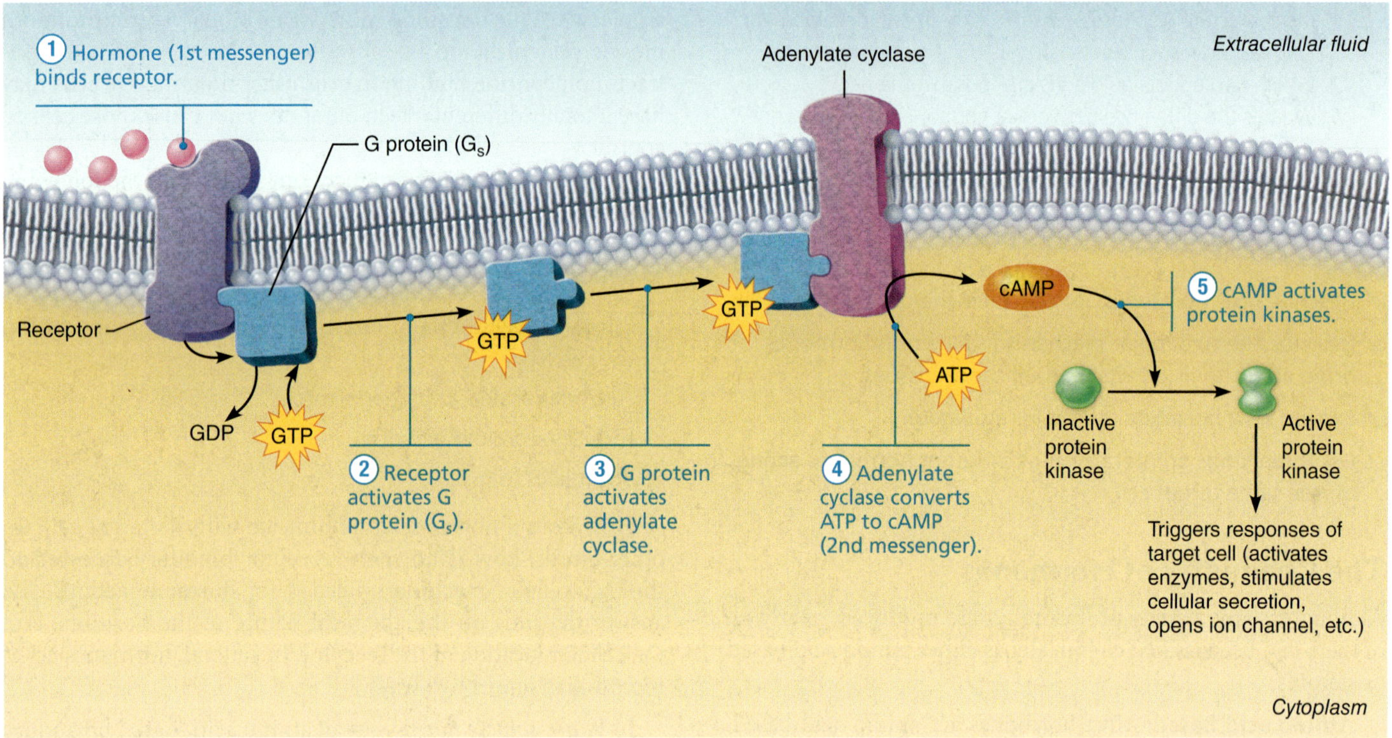

Figure 16.2 **Cyclic AMP second-messenger mechanism of water-soluble hormones.**

one of these second messengers, **cyclic AMP (cAMP)**, which is used by neurotransmitters (Chapter 11) and olfactory receptors (Chapter 15).

The Cyclic AMP Signaling Mechanism As you recall, this mechanism involves the interaction of three plasma membrane components—a hormone receptor, a G protein, and an effector enzyme (adenylate cyclase)—to determine intracellular levels of cyclic AMP. **Figure 16.2** illustrates these steps:

① **Hormone binds receptor.** The hormone, acting as the **first messenger**, binds to its receptor in the plasma membrane.

② **Receptor activates G protein.** Hormone binding causes the receptor to change shape, allowing it to bind a nearby inactive **G protein**. The G protein is activated as the guanosine diphosphate (GDP) bound to it is displaced by the high-energy compound *guanosine triphosphate* (*GTP*). The G protein behaves like a light switch: It is "off" when GDP is bound to it, and "on" when GTP is bound.

③ **G protein activates adenylate cyclase.** The activated G protein (moving along the membrane) binds to the effector enzyme **adenylate cyclase**. Some G proteins (G_s) *stimulate* adenylate cyclase (as shown in Figure 16.2), but others (G_i) *inhibit* adenylate cyclase. Eventually, the GTP bound to the G protein is hydrolyzed to GDP and the G protein becomes inactive once again. (The G protein cleaves the terminal phosphate group off GTP in much the same way that ATPase enzymes hydrolyze ATP.)

④ **Adenylate cyclase converts ATP to cyclic AMP.** For as long as activated G_s is bound to it, adenylate cyclase generates the *second messenger* cAMP from ATP.

⑤ **Cyclic AMP activates protein kinases.** cAMP, which is free to diffuse throughout the cell, triggers a cascade of chemical reactions by activating protein kinases. **Protein kinases** are enzymes that *phosphorylate* (add a phosphate group to) various proteins, many of which are other enzymes. Because phosphorylation activates some of these proteins and inhibits others, it may affect a variety of processes in the same target cell at the same time.

This type of intracellular enzymatic cascade has a huge amplification effect. Each activated adenylate cyclase generates large numbers of cAMP molecules, and a single kinase enzyme can catalyze hundreds of reactions. As the reaction cascades through one enzyme intermediate after another, the number of product molecules increases dramatically at each step. A single hormone molecule binding to a receptor can generate millions of final product molecules!

The sequence of reactions set into motion by cAMP depends on the type of target cell, the specific protein kinases it contains, and the substrates within that cell available for phosphorylation by the protein kinase. For example, in thyroid cells, binding of thyroid-stimulating hormone promotes synthesis of the thyroid hormone thyroxine; in liver cells, binding of glucagon activates enzymes that break down glycogen, releasing glucose to the blood. Since some G proteins inhibit rather than activate adenylate cyclase, thereby reducing the cytoplasmic concentration of cAMP, even slight changes in levels of antagonistic hormones can influence a target cell's activity.

The action of cAMP persists only briefly because the molecule is rapidly degraded by the intracellular enzyme **phosphodiesterase**. While at first glance this may appear to be a problem, it is quite the opposite. Because of the amplification effect, most hormones need to be present only briefly to cause results, and the quick work of phosphodiesterase means that no extracellular controls are necessary to stop the activity. It's the continued presence of hormones that maintains their continued action, if that is needed.

The PIP_2-Calcium Signaling Mechanism While cyclic AMP is the activating second messenger for many hormones, other hormones use different second messengers. For example, in the PIP_2-calcium signaling mechanism, intracellular calcium ions act as a second messenger.

Like the cAMP signaling mechanism, the PIP_2-calcium signaling mechanism involves a G protein (G_q) and a membrane-bound effector, in this case an enzyme called **phospholipase C**. Phospholipase C splits a plasma membrane phospholipid called **PIP_2** (**p**hosphatidyl **i**nositol bis**p**hosphate) into two second messengers: **diacylglycerol (DAG)** and **inositol trisphosphate (IP_3)**. DAG, like cAMP, activates a protein kinase enzyme, which triggers responses within the target cell. In addition, IP_3 releases Ca^{2+} from intracellular storage sites.

The liberated Ca^{2+} also takes on a second-messenger role, either by directly altering the activity of specific enzymes and channels or by binding to the intracellular regulatory protein **calmodulin**. Once Ca^{2+} binds to calmodulin, it activates enzymes that amplify the cellular response.

Other Signaling Mechanisms Other hormones that bind plasma membrane receptors act on their target cells through different signaling mechanisms. For example, cyclic guanosine monophosphate (cGMP) is a second messenger for selected hormones.

Still other hormones, such as insulin and certain growth factors, work without second messengers. The insulin receptor is a *tyrosine kinase* enzyme that is activated by autophosphorylation (addition of phosphate to several of its own tyrosines) when insulin binds. The activated insulin receptor provides docking sites for intracellular *relay proteins* that, in turn, initiate a series of protein phosphorylations that trigger specific cell responses.

Intracellular Receptors and Direct Gene Activation

Being lipid soluble, steroid hormones (and, strangely, thyroid hormone, a small iodinated amine) diffuse into their target cells where they bind to and activate an intracellular receptor **(Figure 16.3)**. The activated receptor-hormone complex then makes its way to the nuclear chromatin and binds to a specific region of DNA. (There are exceptions to these generalizations. For example, thyroid hormone receptors are always bound to DNA even in the absence of thyroid hormone.)

When the receptor-hormone complex binds to DNA, it "turns on" a gene; that is, it prompts transcription of DNA to produce a messenger RNA (mRNA). The mRNA is then translated on the cytoplasmic ribosomes, producing specific proteins. These proteins include enzymes that promote the metabolic activities induced by that particular hormone and, in some cases, promote synthesis of either structural proteins or proteins to be exported from the target cell.

Target Cell Specificity

In order for a target cell to respond to a hormone, the cell must have *specific* receptor proteins on its plasma membrane or in its interior to which that hormone can bind. For example, receptors for adrenocorticotropic hormone (ACTH) are normally found only on certain cells of the adrenal cortex. By contrast, thyroxine is the principal hormone stimulating cellular metabolism, and nearly all body cells have thyroxine receptors.

16

A hormone receptor responds to hormone binding by prompting the cell to perform, or turn on, some gene-determined "preprogrammed" function. As such, hormones are molecular triggers rather than informational molecules. Although binding of a hormone to a receptor is the crucial first step, target cell activation depends equally on three other factors: (1) blood levels of the hormone, (2) relative numbers of receptors for that hormone on or in the target cells, and (3) *affinity* (strength) of the binding between the hormone and the receptor.

The first two factors change rapidly in response to various stimuli and changes within the body. As a rule, for a given level of hormone in the blood, a large number of high-affinity receptors produces a pronounced hormonal effect, and a smaller number of low-affinity receptors reduces the target cell response or causes outright endocrine dysfunction.

Receptors are dynamic structures. For example, persistently low levels of a hormone can cause its target cells to form additional receptors for that hormone. This is called **up-regulation**. Likewise, prolonged exposure to high hormone concentrations can decrease the number of receptors for that hormone. This **down-regulation** desensitizes the target cells, so they respond less vigorously to hormonal stimulation, preventing them from overreacting to persistently high hormone levels. Additionally, receptors can be uncoupled from their signaling mechanism, altering the sensitivity of the response.

Hormones influence not only the number of their own receptors but also the number of receptors that respond to other hormones. For example, progesterone down-regulates estrogen receptors in the uterus, thus antagonizing estrogen's actions. On the other hand,

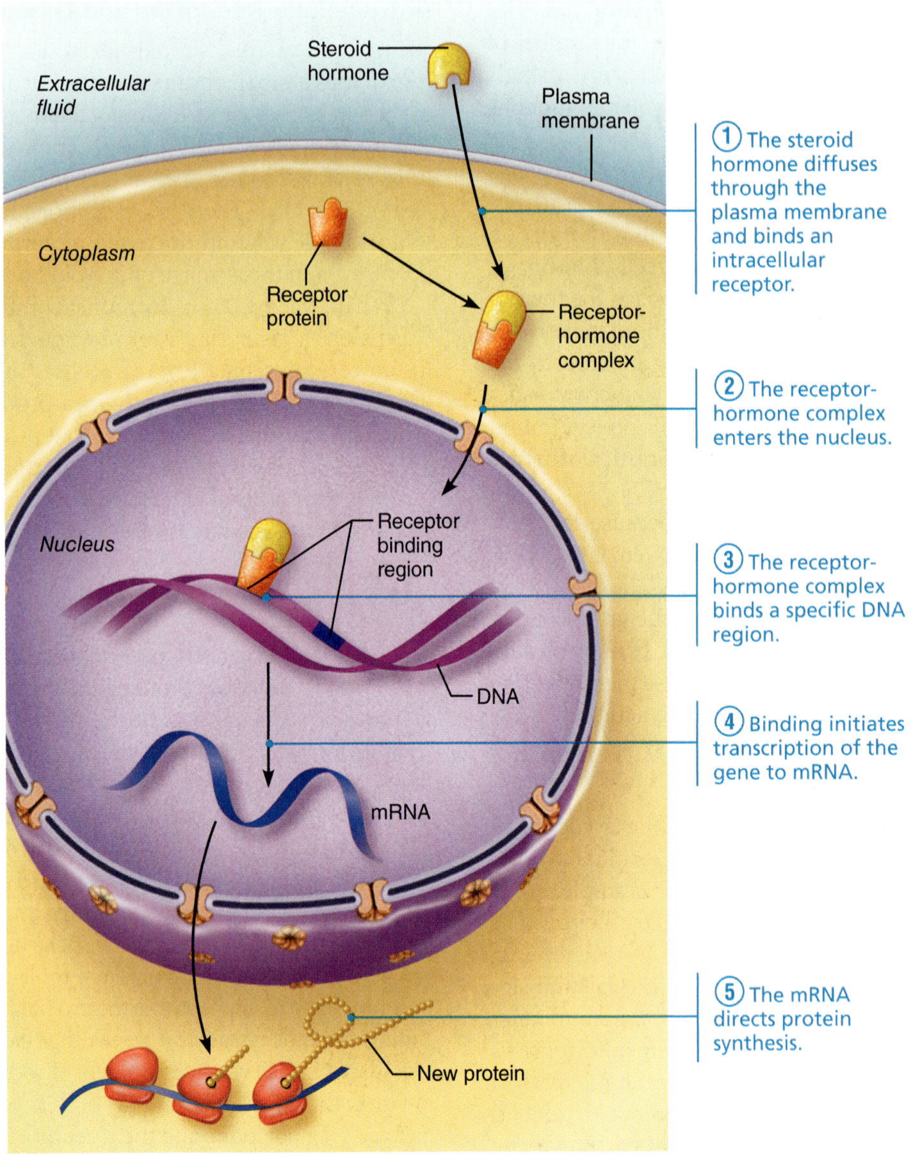

Figure 16.3 Direct gene activation mechanism of lipid-soluble hormones. Receptors may be located in the nucleus, or in the cytoplasm as shown.

estrogen causes the same cells to produce more progesterone receptors, enhancing their ability to respond to progesterone.

Control of Hormone Release

The synthesis and release of most hormones are regulated by some type of **negative feedback mechanism** (see Chapter 1). In such a mechanism, some internal or external stimulus triggers hormone secretion. As levels of a hormone rise, it causes target organ effects, which then feed back to inhibit further hormone release. As a result, blood levels of many hormones vary only within a narrow range.

Endocrine Gland Stimuli

Three types of stimuli trigger endocrine glands to manufacture and release their hormones: *humoral* (hu′mer-ul), *neural*, and *hormonal stimuli*.

Humoral Stimuli Some endocrine glands secrete their hormones in direct response to changing blood levels of certain critical ions and nutrients. These stimuli are called *humoral stimuli* to distinguish them from hormonal stimuli, which are also bloodborne chemicals. (The word *humoral* harks back to the ancient term *humor* to refer to various body fluids.)

Humoral stimuli are the simplest endocrine controls. For example, cells of the parathyroid glands monitor the body's crucial blood Ca^{2+} levels. When they detect a decline from normal values, they secrete parathyroid hormone (PTH) **(Figure 16.4a)**. Because PTH acts by several routes to reverse that decline, blood Ca^{2+} levels soon rise, ending the stimulus for PTH release. Other hormones released in response to humoral stimuli include insulin, produced by the pancreas, and aldosterone, one of the adrenal cortex hormones.

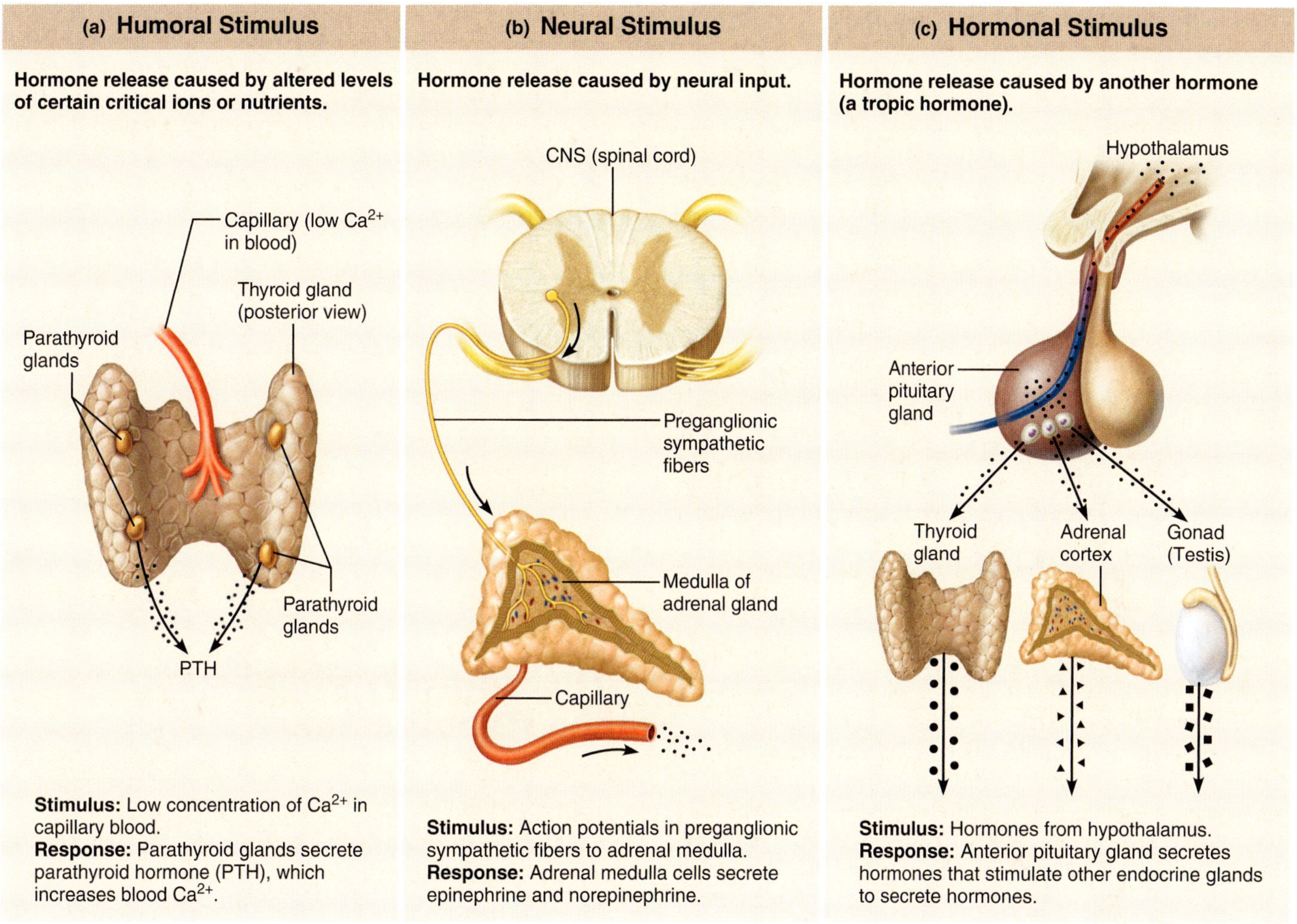

Figure 16.4 **Three types of endocrine gland stimuli.**

Neural Stimuli In a few cases, nerve fibers stimulate hormone release. The classic example of neural stimuli is the response to stress, in which the sympathetic nervous system stimulates the adrenal medulla to release norepinephrine and epinephrine (Figure 16.4b).

Hormonal Stimuli Finally, many endocrine glands release their hormones in response to hormones produced by other endocrine organs. For example, releasing and inhibiting hormones produced by the hypothalamus regulate the secretion of most anterior pituitary hormones, and many anterior pituitary hormones in turn stimulate other endocrine organs to release their hormones (Figure 16.4c). As blood levels of the hormones produced by the final target glands increase, they inhibit the release of anterior pituitary hormones and thus their own release.

This hypothalamic–pituitary–target endocrine organ feedback loop lies at the very core of endocrinology, and it will come up many times in this chapter. Hormonal stimuli promote rhythmic hormone release, with hormone blood levels rising and falling in a specific pattern.

Although these three types of stimuli are typical of most systems that control hormone release, they are by no means mutually exclusive—some endocrine organs respond to multiple stimuli.

Nervous System Modulation

The nervous system can modify both "turn-on" factors (hormonal, humoral, and neural stimuli) and "turn-off" factors (feedback inhibition and others) that affect the endocrine system. Without this added safeguard, endocrine system activity would be strictly mechanical, much like a household thermostat. A thermostat can maintain the temperature at or around its set value, but it cannot sense that your grandmother visiting from Florida feels cold at that temperature and reset itself accordingly. You must make that adjustment. In your body, it is the nervous system that makes certain adjustments to maintain homeostasis by overriding normal endocrine controls.

For example, the action of insulin and several other hormones normally keeps blood glucose levels in the range of 90–110 mg/100 ml of blood. However, when your body is under severe stress, blood glucose levels rise because the hypothalamus and sympathetic nervous system centers are strongly activated. In this way, the nervous system ensures that body cells have sufficient fuel in case vigorous activity is required.

Half-Life, Onset, and Duration of Hormone Activity

Hormones are potent chemicals, and they exert profound effects on their target organs even at very low concentrations. Hormones circulate in the blood in two forms—free or bound to a protein carrier. In general, lipid-soluble hormones (steroids and thyroid hormone) travel in the bloodstream attached to plasma proteins. Most others circulate without carriers.

The concentration of a circulating hormone in blood at any time reflects (1) its rate of release, and (2) the speed at which it is inactivated and removed from the body. Some hormones are rapidly degraded by enzymes in their target cells. However, most hormones are removed from the blood by the kidneys or liver, and the body excretes their breakdown products in urine or, to a lesser extent, in feces. As a result, the length of time for a hormone's blood level to decrease by half, referred to as its **half-life**, varies from a fraction of a minute to a week. Water-soluble hormones have the shortest half-lives.

How long does it take for a hormone to have an effect? It varies. Some hormones provoke target organ responses almost immediately, while others, particularly steroid hormones, require hours to days before their effects are seen. Additionally, some hormones are secreted in a relatively inactive form and must be activated in the target cells.

The duration of hormone action is limited, ranging from 10 seconds to several hours, depending on the hormone. Effects may disappear rapidly as blood levels drop, or they may persist for hours even at very low levels. Because of these many variations, hormonal blood levels must be precisely and individually controlled to meet the continuously changing needs of the body.

Interaction of Hormones at Target Cells

Understanding hormonal effects is a bit more complicated than you might expect because multiple hormones may act on the same target cells at the same time. In many cases the result of such an interaction is not predictable, even when you know the effects of the individual hormones. Here we will look at three types of hormone interaction—permissiveness, synergism, and antagonism.

- **Permissiveness** is the situation in which one hormone cannot exert its full effects without another hormone being present. For example, reproductive system hormones largely regulate the development of the reproductive system, as we might expect. However, thyroid hormone is also necessary (has a permissive effect) for normal *timely* development of reproductive structures. Lack of thyroid hormone delays reproductive development.
- **Synergism** occurs when more than one hormone produces the same effects at the target cell and their combined effects are amplified. For example, both glucagon (produced by the pancreas) and epinephrine cause the liver to release glucose to the blood. When they act together, the amount of glucose released is about 150% of what is released when each hormone acts alone.
- **Antagonism** occurs when one hormone opposes the action of another hormone. For example, insulin, which lowers blood glucose levels, is antagonized by glucagon, which raises blood glucose levels. How does antagonism occur? Antagonists may compete for the same receptors, act through different metabolic pathways, or even, as noted in the progesterone-estrogen interaction at the uterus, cause down-regulation of the receptors for the antagonistic hormone.

Check Your Understanding

4. Name the two major chemical classes of hormones. Which class consists entirely of lipid-soluble hormones? Name the only hormone in the other chemical class that is lipid soluble.
5. Consider the signaling mechanisms of water-soluble and lipid-soluble hormones. In each case, where are the receptors found and what is the final outcome?
6. What are the three types of stimuli that control hormone release?

For answers, see Appendix H.

The Pituitary Gland and Hypothalamus

- ✓ Describe structural and functional relationships between the hypothalamus and the pituitary gland.
- ✓ Discuss the structure of the posterior pituitary, and describe the effects of the two hormones it releases.
- ✓ List and describe the chief effects of anterior pituitary hormones.

Securely seated in the sella turcica of the sphenoid bone, the tiny **pituitary gland**, or **hypophysis** (hi-pof′ĭ-sis; "to grow under"), secretes at least eight hormones. Usually said to be the size and shape of a pea, this gland is more accurately described as a pea on a stalk. Its stalk, the funnel-shaped **infundibulum**, connects the gland to the hypothalamus superiorly as shown in *Focus on Hypothalamus and Pituitary Interactions* **(Figure 16.5)**.

In humans, the pituitary gland has two major lobes. One lobe is neural tissue and the other is glandular.

- The **posterior pituitary** (lobe) is composed largely of neural tissue such as pituicytes (glia-like supporting cells) and nerve fibers. It releases **neurohormones** (hormones secreted by neurons) received ready-made from the hypothalamus. Consequently, this lobe is a hormone-storage area and not a true endocrine gland that manufactures hormones. The posterior lobe plus the infundibulum make up the region called the **neurohypophysis** (nu″ro-hi-pof′ĭ-sis), a term commonly used (incorrectly) to indicate the posterior lobe alone.
- The **anterior pituitary** (lobe), or **adenohypophysis** (ad″ĕ-no-hi-pof′ĭ-sis), is composed of glandular tissue (*adeno* = gland). It manufactures and releases a number of hormones (**Table 16.1** on pp. 602–603).

Hypophyseal branches of the internal carotid arteries deliver arterial blood to the pituitary. The veins leaving the pituitary drain into the dural sinuses.

Pituitary-Hypothalamic Relationships

The contrasting histology of the two pituitary lobes reflects the dual origin of this tiny gland. The posterior lobe is actually part of the brain. It derives from a downgrowth of hypothalamic tissue and maintains its neural connection with the hypothalamus via a nerve bundle called the **hypothalamic-hypophyseal tract**, which runs through the infundibulum (Figure 16.5).

This tract arises from neurons in the **paraventricular** and **supraoptic nuclei** of the hypothalamus. These neurosecretory cells synthesize one of two neurohormones and transport them along their axons to the posterior pituitary. The paraventricular neurons primarily make oxytocin (ok″sĭ-to′sin), and the supraoptic neurons mainly produce antidiuretic hormone. When these hypothalamic neurons fire, they release the stored hormones into a capillary bed in the posterior pituitary for distribution throughout the body.

The glandular anterior lobe originates from epithelial tissue as a superior outpocketing of the oral mucosa. After touching the posterior lobe, the anterior lobe adheres to the neurohypophysis and loses its connection with the oral mucosa. There is no direct neural connection between the anterior lobe and hypothalamus, but there is a vascular connection. Specifically, the **primary capillary plexus** in the infundibulum communicates inferiorly via the small **hypophyseal portal veins** with a **secondary capillary plexus** in the anterior lobe. The primary and secondary capillary plexuses and the intervening hypophyseal portal veins make up the *hypophyseal portal system* (Figure 16.5). Note that a *portal system* is an unusual arrangement of blood vessels in which a capillary bed feeds into veins, which in turn feed into a second capillary bed.

Via the hypophyseal portal system, **releasing** and **inhibiting hormones** secreted by neurons in the ventral hypothalamus circulate to the anterior pituitary, where they regulate secretion of its hormones. The portal system ensures that the minute quantities of hormones released by the hypothalamus arrive rapidly at the anterior pituitary without being diluted by the systemic circulation. All these hypothalamic regulatory hormones are amino acid based, but they vary in size from a single amine to peptides to proteins.

The Posterior Pituitary and Hypothalamic Hormones

The posterior pituitary consists largely of axon terminals of hypothalamic neurons whose cell bodies are located in the supraoptic or paraventricular nuclei. These neurons synthesize one of two neurohormones in their cell bodies: Oxytocin or antidiuretic hormone (ADH). Axon terminals in the posterior pituitary release these hormones "on demand" in response to action potentials that travel down the axons of these same hypothalamic neurons.

Oxytocin and ADH, each composed of nine amino acids, are almost identical. They differ in only two amino acids, and yet they have dramatically different physiological effects, summarized in Table 16.1 and described next.

Oxytocin

A strong stimulant of uterine contraction, **oxytocin** is released in significantly higher amounts during childbirth (*oxy* = rapid; *tocia* = childbirth) and in nursing women. The number of oxytocin receptors in the uterus peaks near the end of pregnancy, and uterine smooth muscle becomes more and more sensitive to the hormone's stimulatory effects. Stretching of the uterus and cervix as birth nears dispatches afferent impulses to the hypothalamus, which responds by synthesizing oxytocin and triggering its release from the posterior pituitary. Oxytocin acts via the PIP_2-Ca^{2+} second-messenger system to mobilize Ca^{2+}, allowing stronger contractions. As blood levels of oxytocin rise, the expulsive contractions of labor gain momentum and finally end in birth.

Oxytocin also acts as the hormonal trigger for milk ejection (the "letdown" reflex) in women whose breasts are producing milk in response to prolactin. Suckling causes a reflex-initiated release of oxytocin, which targets specialized myoepithelial cells surrounding the milk-producing glands. These cells contract and force milk from the breast into the infant's mouth. Both childbirth and milk ejection result from *positive feedback mechanisms,* which Chapter 28 describes in more detail.

Both natural and synthetic oxytocic drugs are used to induce labor or to hasten labor that is progressing slowly. Less frequently, oxytocic drugs are used to stop postpartum bleeding (by compressing ruptured blood vessels at the placental site) or to stimulate the milk ejection reflex.

Oxytocin also acts as a neurotransmitter in the brain. There, it is involved in sexual and affectionate behavior (as the "cuddle hormone"), and promotes nurturing, couple bonding, and trust.

Antidiuretic Hormone (ADH)

Diuresis (di″u-re′sis) is urine production, so an *antidiuretic* is a substance that inhibits or prevents urine formation. **Antidiuretic hormone (ADH)** prevents wide swings in water balance, helping the body avoid dehydration and water overload.

Hypothalamic neurons called *osmoreceptors* continually monitor the solute concentration (and thus the water concentration) of the blood. When solutes threaten to become too concentrated (as might follow excessive perspiration or inadequate fluid intake), the osmoreceptors transmit excitatory impulses to the hypothalamic neurons, which release ADH. Liberated into the blood by the posterior pituitary, ADH targets the kidney tubules via cAMP. The tubule cells respond by reabsorbing more water from the forming urine and returning it to the bloodstream. As a result, less urine is produced and the solute concentration of the blood declines. As solute levels fall, the osmoreceptors stop depolarizing, effectively ending ADH release. Other stimuli triggering ADH release include pain, low blood pressure, and such drugs as nicotine, morphine, and barbiturates.

Figure 16.5 The hypothalamus controls release of hormones from the pituitary gland in two different ways.

Posterior Pituitary: *Action potentials* travel down the axons of hypothalamic neurons, causing hormone release from their axon terminals in the posterior pituitary.

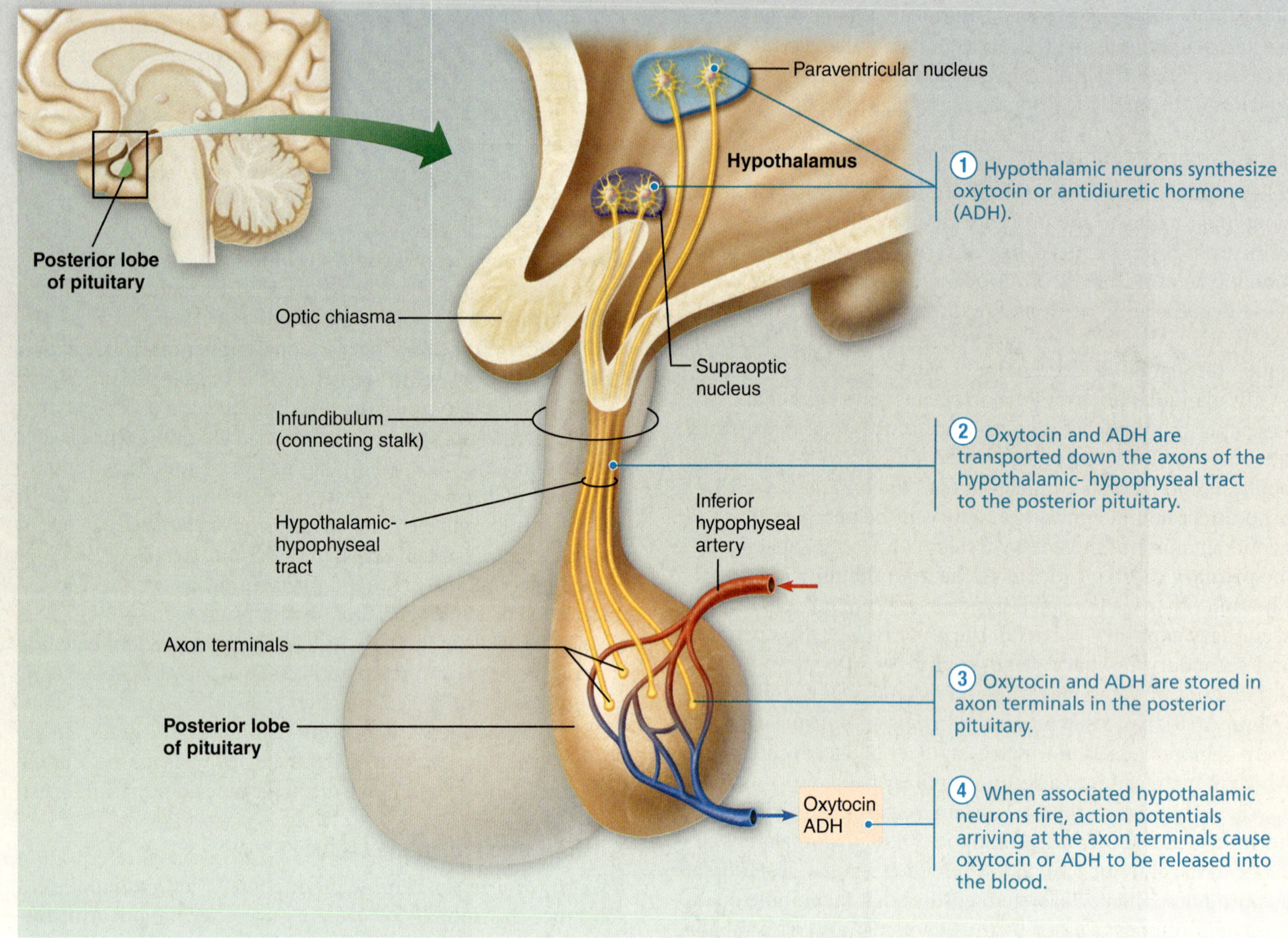

Drinking alcoholic beverages inhibits ADH secretion and causes copious urine output. The dry mouth and intense thirst of a "hangover" reflect this dehydrating effect. As you might expect, drinking lots of water also inhibits ADH release.

Diuretic drugs antagonize the effects of ADH and flush water from the body. Diuretics are used to manage some cases of hypertension and the edema (water retention in tissues) typical of congestive heart failure.

Under certain conditions, such as severe blood loss, exceptionally large amounts of ADH are released. At such high blood concentrations, ADH causes vasoconstriction, primarily of visceral blood vessels, raising blood pressure. This response targets different ADH receptors found on vascular smooth muscle. For this reason, ADH is also called **vasopressin**.

Homeostatic Imbalance 16.1

One result of ADH deficiency is **diabetes insipidus**, a syndrome marked by intense thirst and huge urine output. The name of this condition (*diabetes* = overflow; *insipidus* = tasteless) distinguishes it from diabetes mellitus (*mel* = honey), in which insulin deficiency causes large amounts of blood glucose to be lost in the urine. At one time, a clinician would taste the patient's urine to determine the type of diabetes.

Diabetes insipidus can be caused by a blow to the head that damages the hypothalamus or the posterior pituitary. Though inconvenient, the condition is not serious when the thirst center is operating properly and the person drinks enough water to prevent dehydration. However, it can be life threatening in

Anterior Pituitary: *Hypothalamic hormones* released into special blood vessels (the hypophyseal portal system) control the release of anterior pituitary hormones.

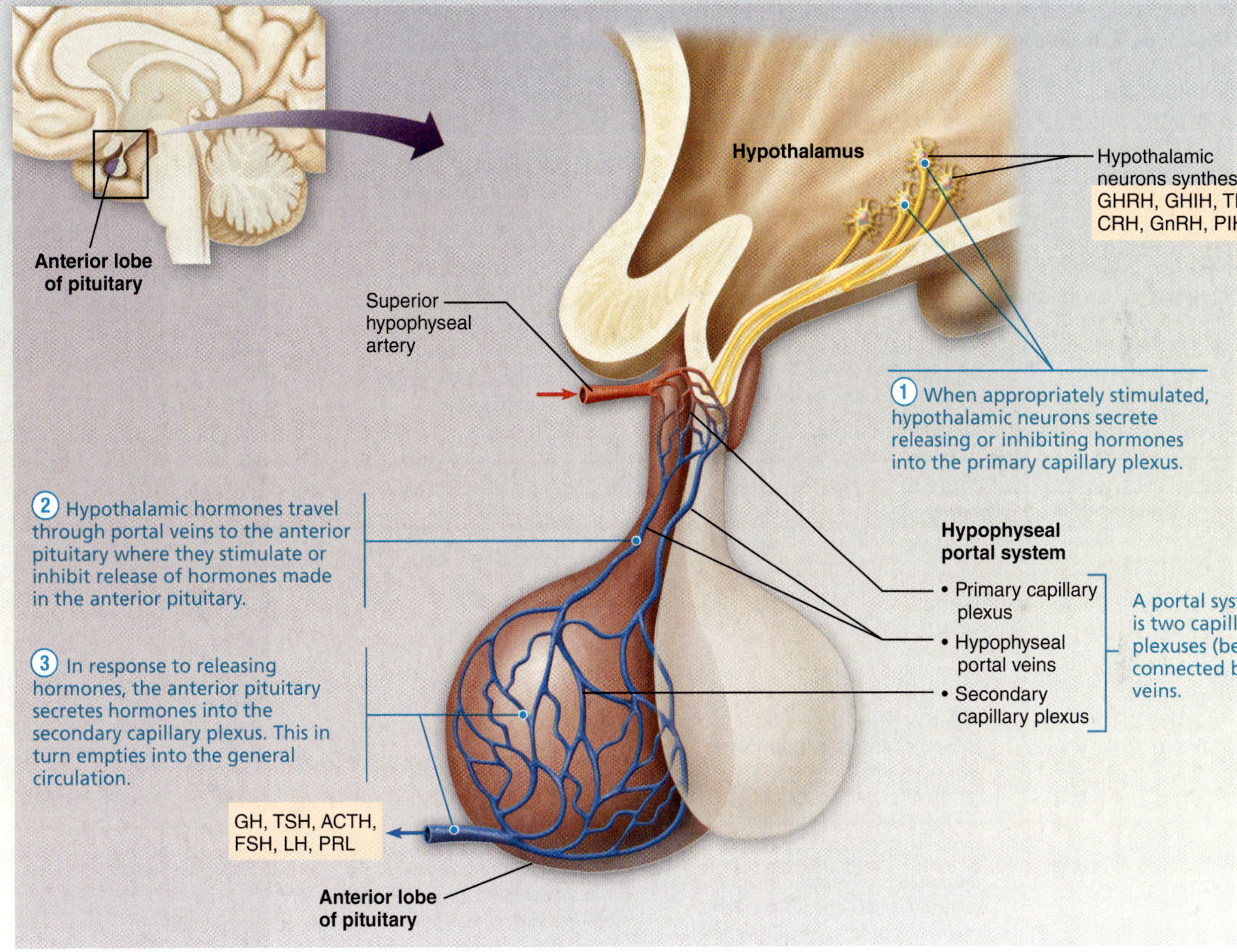

unconscious or comatose patients, so accident victims with head trauma must be carefully monitored.

The opposite problem, hypersecretion of ADH, can occur in children with meningitis, or in adults who have neurosurgery, hypothalamic injury, or cancer (particularly lung cancer) in which cancer cells are additional sources of ADH. It also may occur after general anesthesia or administration of certain drugs. The resulting condition, *syndrome of inappropriate ADH secretion* (*SIADH*), is marked by retention of fluid, headache and disorientation due to brain edema, weight gain, and decreased solute concentration in the blood. SIADH management requires restricting fluids and carefully monitoring blood sodium levels. +

Anterior Pituitary Hormones

The anterior pituitary has traditionally been called the "master endocrine gland" because many of the numerous hormones it produces regulate the activity of other endocrine glands. In recent years, however, it has been dethroned by the hypothalamus, which is now known to control the activity of the anterior pituitary.

Researchers have identified six anterior pituitary hormones, all of them proteins—growth hormone, thyroid-stimulating hormone, adrenocorticotropic hormone, follicle-stimulating hormone, luteinizing hormone, and prolactin (Table 16.1). When the anterior pituitary receives an appropriate chemical stimulus from the hypothalamus, it releases one or more of its hormones. Although many different hormones pass from the

Table 16.1 Pituitary Hormones: Summary of Regulation and Effects

HORMONE (CHEMICAL STRUCTURE AND CELL TYPE)	REGULATION OF RELEASE	TARGET ORGAN AND EFFECTS	EFFECTS OF HYPOSECRETION ↓ AND HYPERSECRETION ↑
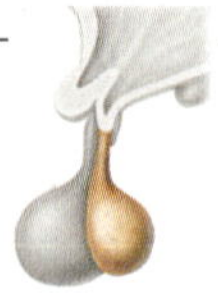 **Posterior Pituitary Hormones (Made by Hypothalamic Neurons and Stored in Posterior Pituitary**			
Oxytocin (Peptide, mostly from neurons in paraventricular nucleus of hypothalamus)	**Stimulated** by impulses from hypothalamic neurons in response to cervical/uterine stretching and suckling of infant at breast **Inhibited** by lack of appropriate neural stimuli	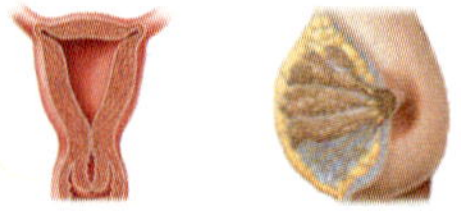 Uterus: stimulates uterine contractions; initiates labor Breast: initiates milk ejection	Unknown
Antidiuretic hormone (ADH) or vasopressin (Peptide, mostly from neurons in supraoptic nucleus of hypothalamus)	**Stimulated** by impulses from hypothalamic neurons in response to increased blood solute concentration or decreased blood volume; also stimulated by pain, some drugs, low blood pressure **Inhibited** by adequate hydration of the body and by alcohol	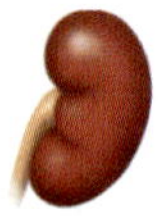 Kidneys: stimulate kidney tubule cells to reabsorb water	↓ Diabetes insipidus ↑ Syndrome of inappropriate ADH secretion (SIADH)
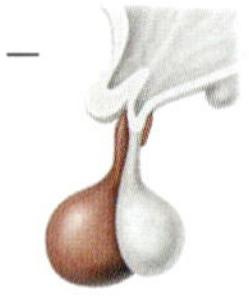 **Anterior Pituitary Hormones**			
Growth hormone (GH) (Protein, somatotropic cells)	**Stimulated** by GHRH* release, which is triggered by low blood levels of GH as well as by a number of secondary triggers including hypoglycemia, increases in blood levels of amino acids, low levels of fatty acids, exercise, and other types of stressors **Inhibited** by feedback inhibition exerted by GH and IGFs, and by hyperglycemia, hyperlipidemia, obesity, and emotional deprivation via either increased GHIH* (somatostatin) or decreased GHRH* release	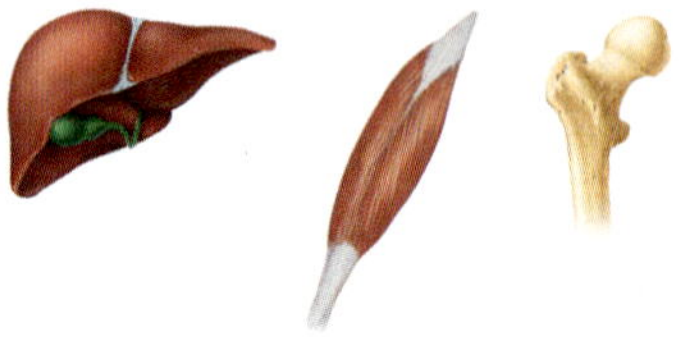 Liver, muscle, bone, cartilage, and other tissues: anabolic hormone; stimulates somatic growth; mobilizes fats; spares glucose Growth-promoting effects mediated indirectly by IGFs	↓ Pituitary dwarfism in children ↑ Gigantism in children; acromegaly in adults

hypothalamus to the anterior lobe, each target cell distinguishes the messages directed to it and responds in kind—secreting the proper hormone in response to specific releasing hormones, and shutting off hormone release in response to specific inhibiting hormones.

Four of the six anterior pituitary hormones—thyroid-stimulating hormone, adrenocorticotropic hormone, follicle-stimulating hormone, and luteinizing hormone—are **tropic hormones** or **tropins** that regulate the secretory action of other endocrine glands (*tropi* = turn on, change). All anterior pituitary hormones except growth hormone affect their target cells via a cyclic AMP second-messenger system.

Growth Hormone (GH)

Somatotropic cells of the anterior lobe produce **growth hormone** (**GH**, also called *somatotropin*). GH is essentially an anabolic (tissue building) hormone that has both metabolic and growth-promoting actions **(Figure 16.6)**.

Direct Actions on Metabolism Acting directly, GH exerts metabolic effects. It mobilizes fats from fat depots for transport to cells, increasing blood levels of fatty acids and encouraging their use for fuel. It also decreases the rate of glucose uptake and metabolism, conserving glucose. In the liver, it encourages glycogen breakdown and release of glucose to the blood.

Table 16.1 *(continued)*

HORMONE (CHEMICAL STRUCTURE AND CELL TYPE)	REGULATION OF RELEASE	TARGET ORGAN AND EFFECTS	EFFECTS OF HYPOSECRETION ↓ AND HYPERSECRETION ↑
Thyroid-stimulating hormone (TSH) (Glycoprotein, thyrotropic cells)	**Stimulated** by TRH* and in infants indirectly by cold temperature **Inhibited** by feedback inhibition exerted by thyroid hormones on anterior pituitary and hypothalamus and by GHIH*	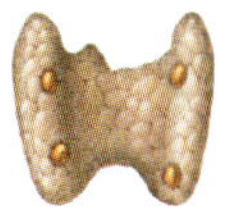 Thyroid gland: stimulates thyroid gland to release thyroid hormones	↓ Cretinism in children; myxedema in adults ↑ Hyperthyroidism; effects similar to those of Graves' disease, in which antibodies mimic TSH
Adrenocorticotropic hormone (ACTH) (Peptide, corticotropic cells)	**Stimulated** by CRH*; stimuli that increase CRH release include fever, hypoglycemia, and other stressors **Inhibited** by feedback inhibition exerted by glucocorticoids	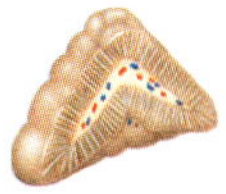 Adrenal cortex: promotes release of glucocorticoids and androgens (mineralocorticoids to a lesser extent)	↓ Rare ↑ Cushing's disease
Follicle-stimulating hormone (FSH) (Glycoprotein, gonadotropic cells)	**Stimulated** by GnRH* **Inhibited** by feedback inhibition exerted by inhibin, and estrogen in females and testosterone in males	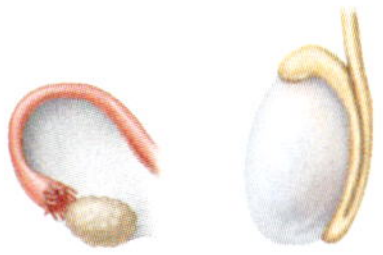 Ovaries and testes: in females, stimulates ovarian follicle maturation and estrogen production; in males, stimulates sperm production	↓ Failure of sexual maturation ↑ No important effects
Luteinizing hormone (LH) (Glycoprotein, gonadotropic cells)	**Stimulated** by GnRH* **Inhibited** by feedback inhibition exerted by estrogen and progesterone in females and testosterone in males	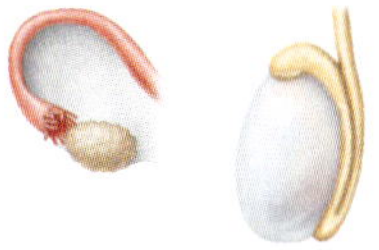 Ovaries and testes: in females, triggers ovulation and stimulates ovarian production of estrogen and progesterone; in males, promotes testosterone production	As for FSH
Prolactin (PRL) (Protein, prolactin cells)	**Stimulated** by decreased PIH*; release enhanced by estrogens, birth control pills, breast-feeding, and dopamine-blocking drugs **Inhibited** by PIH* (dopamine)	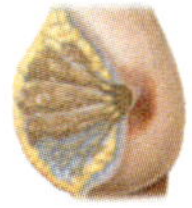 Breast secretory tissue: promotes lactation	↓ Poor milk production in nursing women ↑ Inappropriate milk production (galactorrhea); cessation of menses in females; impotence in males

*Indicates hypothalamic releasing and inhibiting hormones: GHRH = growth hormone–releasing hormone; GHIH = growth hormone–inhibiting hormone; TRH = thyrotropin-releasing hormone; CRH = corticotropin-releasing hormone; GnRH = gonadotropin-releasing hormone; PIH = prolactin-inhibiting hormone

This *glucose sparing* action, which raises blood glucose levels, is called the *anti-insulin effect* of GH because its effects oppose those of insulin. In addition, GH increases amino acid uptake into cells and their incorporation into proteins.

Indirect Actions on Growth GH mediates most of its growth-enhancing effects indirectly via a family of growth-promoting proteins called **insulin-like growth factors (IGFs)**. The liver, skeletal muscle, bone, and other tissues produce IGFs in response to GH. IGFs produced by the liver act as hormones, while IGFs made in other tissues act locally within those tissues (as paracrines).

IGFs stimulate actions required for growth: (1) uptake of nutrients from the blood and their incorporation into proteins and DNA, allowing growth by cell division; and (2) formation of collagen and deposition of bone matrix. Although GH stimulates most body cells to enlarge and divide, its major targets are bone and skeletal muscle. Stimulation of the epiphyseal plate leads to long bone growth, and stimulation of skeletal muscles increases muscle mass.

Regulation of Secretion Secretion of GH is regulated chiefly by two hypothalamic hormones with antagonistic effects. **Growth hormone–releasing hormone (GHRH)** stimulates

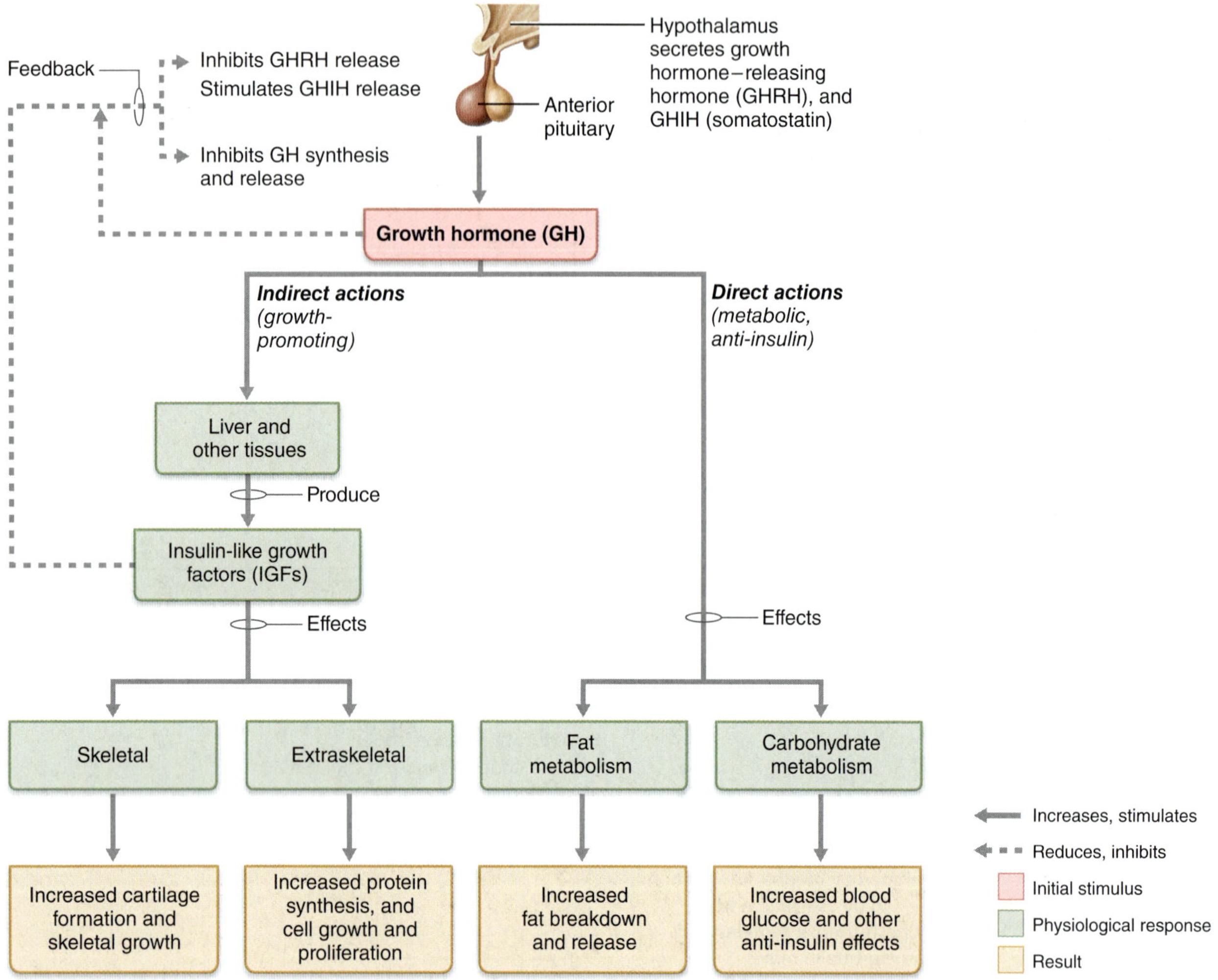

Figure 16.6 Growth-promoting and metabolic actions of growth hormone (GH).

GH release, while **growth hormone–inhibiting hormone (GHIH)**, also called **somatostatin** (so″mah-to-stat′in), inhibits it. Recent research shows that the "hunger hormone" ghrelin (produced by the stomach) also stimulates GH release.

GHIH release is triggered by the feedback of GH and IGFs. Rising levels of GH also feed back to inhibit its own release. GHIH is also produced in various locations in the gut, where it inhibits the release of virtually all gastrointestinal and pancreatic secretions—both endocrine and exocrine.

As indicated in Table 16.1, a number of secondary triggers also influence GH release. Typically, GH secretion has a daily cycle, with the highest levels occurring during evening sleep. The total amount secreted daily peaks during adolescence and then declines with age.

Homeostatic Imbalance 16.2

Both hypersecretion and hyposecretion of GH may result in structural abnormalities. Hypersecretion in children results in **gigantism** because GH targets the still-active epiphyseal (growth) plates. The person becomes abnormally tall, often reaching a height of 2.4 m (8 feet), but has relatively normal body proportions **(Figure 16.7)**.

If excessive GH is secreted after the epiphyseal plates have closed, **acromegaly** (ak″ro-meg′ah-le) results. Literally translated as "enlarged extremities," this condition is characterized by overgrowth of bony areas still responsive to GH, namely bones of the hands, feet, and face. Hypersecretion usually results from an anterior pituitary tumor that churns out excessive GH. The usual treatment is surgical removal of the tumor, but this surgery does not reverse anatomical changes that have already occurred.

Hyposecretion of GH in adults usually causes no problems, but GH deficiency in children slows long bone growth, a condition called **pituitary dwarfism** (Figure 16.7). Such individuals attain a maximum height of 1.2 m (4 feet), but usually have fairly normal body proportions. Lack of GH is often accompanied by deficiencies of other anterior pituitary hormones, and if thyroid-stimulating hormone and gonadotropins are lacking, the individual will be malproportioned and will fail to mature sexually as well. Fortunately, human GH is produced commercially by genetic engineering techniques. When pituitary dwarfism is diagnosed before puberty, growth hormone replacement therapy can promote nearly normal growth.

The availability of synthetic GH also has a downside. Athletes and the elderly have been tempted to use GH for its

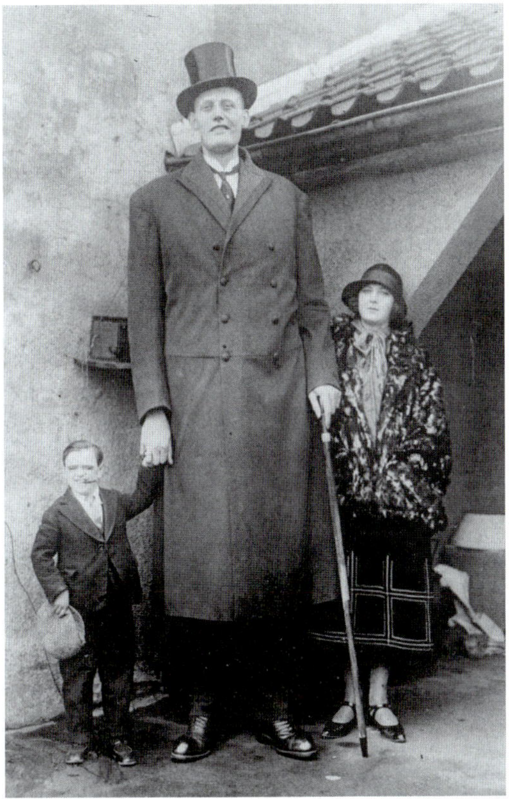

Figure 16.7 Disorders of pituitary growth hormone. An individual exhibiting gigantism (center) is flanked by a pituitary dwarf (left) and a woman of normal height (right).

bodybuilding properties, and some parents seek to give their children the hormone in an attempt to make them taller. However, while muscle mass increases, there is no objective evidence for an increase in muscle strength in either athletes or the elderly, and only minimal increases in stature occur in normal children. Moreover, taking GH can lead to fluid retention, joint and muscle pain, diabetes, and may promote cancer. ✚

Thyroid-Stimulating Hormone (TSH)

Thyroid-stimulating hormone (TSH), or **thyrotropin**, is a tropic hormone that stimulates normal development and secretory activity of the thyroid gland. Its release follows the hypothalamic–pituitary–target endocrine organ feedback loop described earlier and shown specifically for TSH in **Figure 16.8**.

The hypothalamic peptide **thyrotropin-releasing hormone (TRH)** triggers the release of TSH from **thyrotropic cells** of the anterior pituitary. Rising blood levels of thyroid hormones act on both the pituitary and the hypothalamus to inhibit TSH secretion. GHIH also inhibits TSH secretion.

Adrenocorticotropic Hormone (ACTH)

Adrenocorticotropic hormone (ACTH) (ah-dre″no-kor″tĭ-ko-trōp′ik), or **corticotropin**, is secreted by the **corticotropic cells** of the anterior pituitary. It is split from a *prohormone* (a large precursor molecule) with the tongue-twisting name **pro-opiomelanocortin**

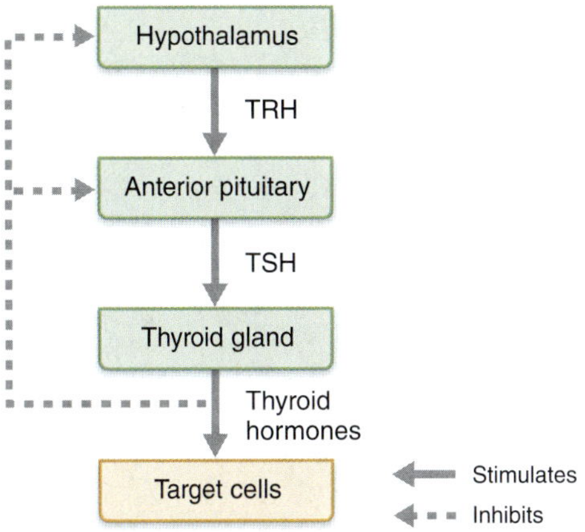

Figure 16.8 Regulation of thyroid hormone secretion. TRH = thyrotropin-releasing hormone, TSH = thyroid-stimulating hormone.

(POMC) (pro″o″pe-o-mah-lan″o-kor′tin). ACTH stimulates the adrenal cortex to release corticosteroid hormones, most importantly glucocorticoids that help the body resist stressors.

ACTH release, elicited by hypothalamic **corticotropin-releasing hormone (CRH)**, has a daily rhythm, with levels peaking in the morning, shortly before awakening. Rising levels of glucocorticoids feed back and block secretion of CRH and ACTH release. Internal and external factors that alter the normal ACTH rhythm by triggering CRH release include fever, hypoglycemia (low blood glucose levels), and stressors of all types.

16

Gonadotropins (FSH and LH)

Follicle-stimulating hormone (FSH) and **luteinizing hormone (LH)** (lu′te-in-īz″ing) are referred to collectively as **gonadotropins**. They regulate the function of the gonads (ovaries and testes). In both sexes, FSH stimulates production of gametes (sperm or eggs) and LH promotes production of gonadal hormones. In females, LH works with FSH to cause an egg-containing ovarian follicle to mature. LH then triggers ovulation and promotes synthesis and release of ovarian hormones. In males, LH stimulates the interstitial cells of the testes to produce the male hormone testosterone.

Gonadotropins are virtually absent from the blood of prepubertal boys and girls. During puberty, the **gonadotropic cells** of the anterior pituitary are activated and gonadotropin levels rise, causing the gonads to mature. In both sexes, **gonadotropin-releasing hormone (GnRH)** produced by the hypothalamus prompts gonadotropin release. Gonadal hormones, produced in response to the gonadotropins, feed back to suppress FSH and LH release.

Prolactin (PRL)

Prolactin (PRL) is a protein hormone structurally similar to GH. Produced by **prolactin cells**, PRL's only well-documented effect in humans is to stimulate milk production by the breasts (*pro* = for; *lact* = milk). The role of prolactin in males is not well understood.

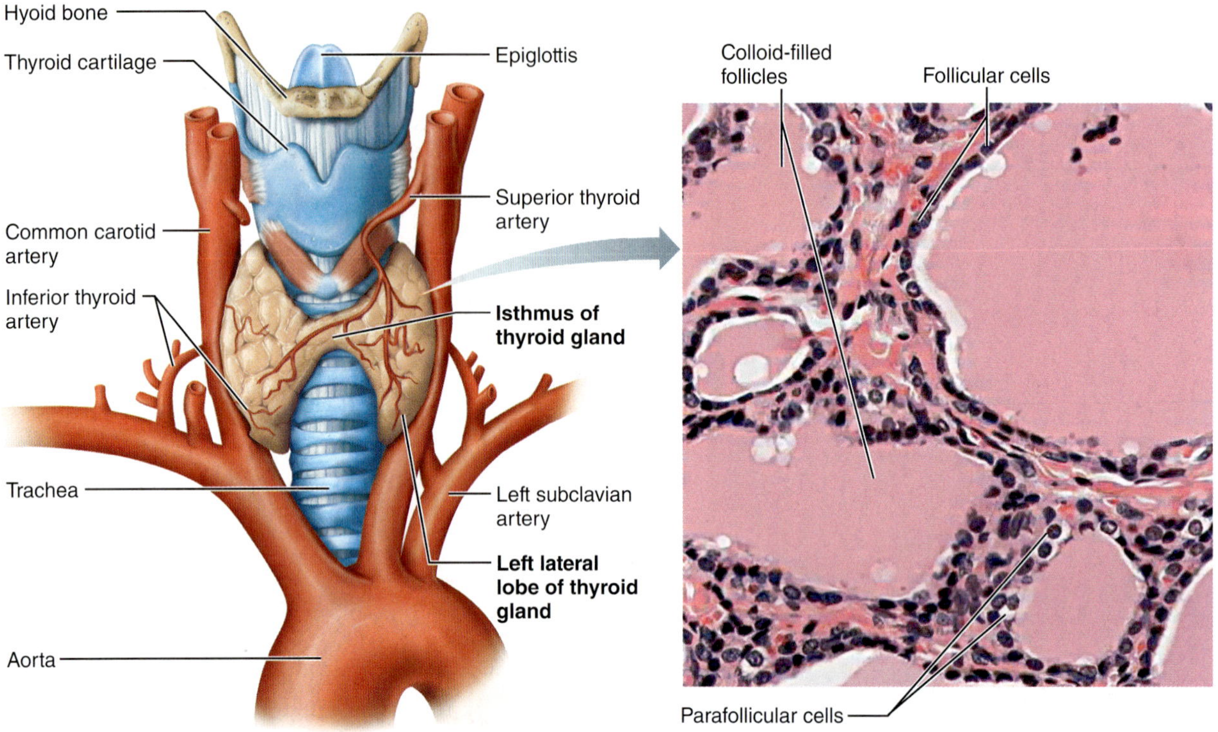

(a) Gross anatomy of the thyroid gland, anterior view

(b) Photomicrograph of thyroid gland follicles (145×)

Figure 16.9 The thyroid gland.

16

Unlike other anterior pituitary hormones, PRL release is controlled primarily by an inhibitory hormone, **prolactin-inhibiting hormone (PIH)**, now known to be **dopamine**, which prevents prolactin secretion. Decreased PIH secretion leads to a surge in PRL release. There are a number of *prolactin-releasing factors*, including TRH, but their exact roles are not well understood.

In females, prolactin levels rise and fall in rhythm with estrogen blood levels. Estrogen stimulates prolactin release, both directly and indirectly. A brief rise in prolactin levels just before the menstrual period partially accounts for the breast swelling and tenderness some women experience at that time, but because this PRL stimulation is so brief, the breasts do not produce milk. In pregnant women, PRL blood levels rise dramatically toward the end of pregnancy, and milk production becomes possible. After birth, the infant's suckling stimulates release of prolactin-releasing factors in the mother, encouraging continued milk production.

Homeostatic Imbalance 16.3

Hypersecretion of prolactin is more common than hyposecretion (which is not a problem in anyone except women who choose to nurse). In fact, hyperprolactinemia is the most frequent abnormality of anterior pituitary tumors. Clinical signs include inappropriate lactation, lack of menses, infertility in females, and impotence in males. ✚

Check Your Understanding

7. What is the key difference between the way the hypothalamus communicates with the anterior pituitary and the way it communicates with the posterior pituitary?
8. Anita drank too much alcohol one night and suffered from a headache and nausea the next morning. What caused these "hangover" effects?
9. List the four anterior pituitary hormones that are tropic hormones and name their target glands.

For answers, see Appendix H.

The Thyroid Gland

✓ Describe the effects of the two groups of hormones produced by the thyroid gland.

✓ Follow the process of thyroxine formation and release.

Location and Structure

The butterfly-shaped **thyroid gland** is located in the anterior neck, on the trachea just inferior to the larynx (Figure 16.1 and **Figure 16.9a**). A median tissue mass called the *isthmus* (is′mus) connects its two lateral *lobes*. The thyroid gland is the largest pure endocrine gland in the body. Its prodigious blood supply (from the *superior* and *inferior thyroid arteries*) makes thyroid surgery a painstaking (and bloody) endeavor.

Table 16.2 Major Effects of Thyroid Hormone (T_4 and T_3) in the Body

PROCESS OR SYSTEM AFFECTED	NORMAL PHYSIOLOGICAL EFFECTS	EFFECTS OF HYPOSECRETION	EFFECTS OF HYPERSECRETION
Basal metabolic rate (BMR)/ temperature regulation	Promotes normal oxygen use and BMR; calorigenesis; enhances effects of sympathetic nervous system	BMR below normal; decreased body temperature, cold intolerance; decreased appetite; weight gain; reduced sensitivity to catecholamines	BMR above normal; increased body temperature, heat intolerance; increased appetite; weight loss
Carbohydrate/lipid/protein metabolism	Promotes glucose catabolism; mobilizes fats; essential for protein synthesis; enhances liver's synthesis of cholesterol	Decreased glucose metabolism; elevated cholesterol/triglyceride levels in blood; decreased protein synthesis; edema	Enhanced catabolism of glucose, proteins, and fats; weight loss; loss of muscle mass
Nervous system	Promotes normal development of nervous system in fetus and infant; promotes normal adult nervous system function	In infant, slowed/deficient brain development, retardation; in adult, mental dulling, depression, paresthesias, memory impairment, hypoactive reflexes	Irritability, restlessness, insomnia, personality changes, exophthalmos (in Graves' disease)
Cardiovascular system	Promotes normal functioning of the heart	Decreased efficiency of heart's pumping action; low heart rate and blood pressure	Increased sensitivity to catecholamines leads to rapid heart rate and possible palpitations; high blood pressure; if prolonged, heart failure
Muscular system	Promotes normal muscular development and function	Sluggish muscle action; muscle cramps; myalgia	Muscle atrophy and weakness
Skeletal system	Promotes normal growth and maturation of the skeleton	In child, growth retardation, skeletal stunting and retention of child's body proportions; in adult, joint pain	In child, excessive skeletal growth initially, followed by early epiphyseal closure and short stature; in adult, demineralization of skeleton
Gastrointestinal (GI) system	Promotes normal GI motility and tone; increases secretion of digestive juices	Depressed GI motility, tone, and secretory activity; constipation	Excessive GI motility; diarrhea; loss of appetite
Reproductive system	Promotes normal female reproductive ability and lactation	Depressed ovarian function; sterility; depressed lactation	In females, depressed ovarian function; in males, impotence
Integumentary system	Promotes normal hydration and secretory activity of skin	Skin pale, thick, and dry; facial edema; hair coarse and thick	Skin flushed, thin, and moist; hair fine and soft; nails soft and thin

Internally, the gland is composed of hollow, spherical **follicles** (Figure 16.9b). The walls of each follicle are formed largely by cuboidal or squamous epithelial cells called *follicular cells*, which produce the glycoprotein **thyroglobulin** (thi″ro-glob′u-lin). The central cavity, or lumen, of the follicle stores **colloid**, an amber-colored, sticky material consisting of thyroglobulin molecules with attached iodine atoms. *Thyroid hormone* is derived from this iodinated thyroglobulin.

The *parafollicular cells*, another population of endocrine cells in the thyroid gland, produce *calcitonin*, an entirely different hormone. The parafollicular cells lie in the follicular epithelium but protrude into the soft connective tissue that separates and surrounds the thyroid follicles.

Thyroid Hormone (TH)

Often referred to as the body's major metabolic hormone, **thyroid hormone (TH)** is actually two iodine-containing amine hormones, **thyroxine** (thi-rok′sin), or **T_4**, and **triiodothyronine** (tri″i-o″do-thi′ro-nēn), or **T_3**. T_4 is the major hormone secreted by the thyroid follicles. Most T_3 is formed at the target tissues by conversion of T_4 to T_3. Both T_4 and T_3 are constructed from two linked tyrosine amino acids. The principal difference between them is that T_4 has four bound iodine atoms, and T_3 has three (thus, T_4 and T_3).

TH affects virtually every cell in the body (Table 16.2). Like steroids, TH enters a target cell, binds to intracellular receptors within the cell's nucleus, and initiates transcription of mRNA for protein synthesis. Effects of thyroid hormone include:

- Increasing basal metabolic rate and body heat production, by turning on transcription of genes concerned with glucose oxidation. This is the hormone's **calorigenic effect** (*calorigenic* = heat producing).
- Regulating tissue growth and development. TH is critical for normal skeletal and nervous system development and maturation and for reproductive capabilities.
- Maintaining blood pressure by increasing the number of adrenergic receptors in blood vessels.

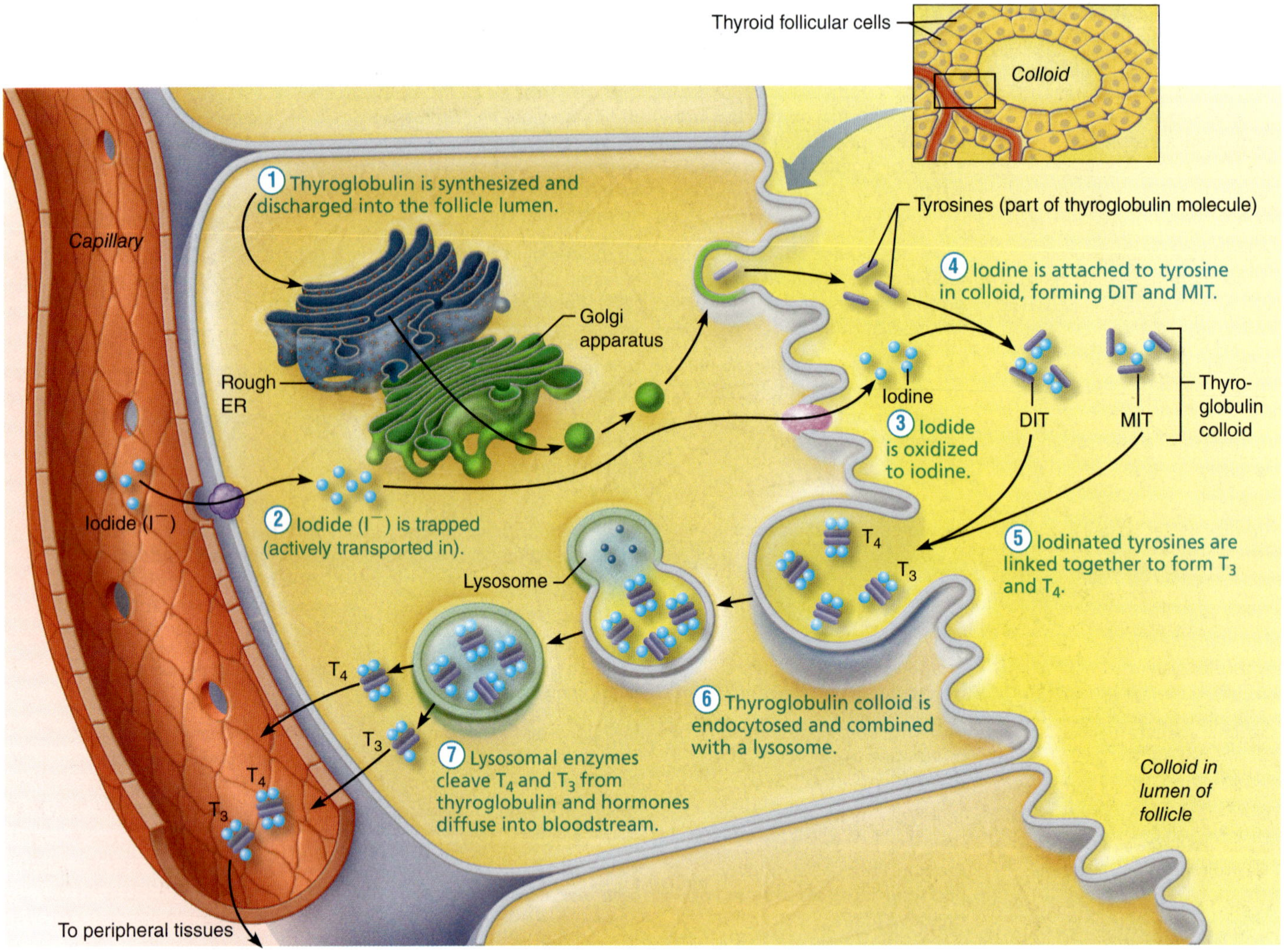

16

Figure 16.10 Synthesis of thyroid hormone. Only a few tyrosines of the thyroglobulins in the colloid are illustrated. The unstructured yellow substance in the follicle lumen is colloid. (MIT = monoiodotyrosine; DIT = diiodotyrosine.)

Synthesis

The thyroid gland is unique among the endocrine glands in its ability to store its hormone extracellularly and in large quantities. A normal thyroid gland stores enough colloid to provide normal levels of hormone for two to three months.

When TSH from the anterior pituitary binds to receptors on follicular cells, their *first* response is to secrete stored thyroid hormone. Their *second* response is to begin synthesizing more colloid to "restock" the follicle lumen. As a general rule, TSH levels are lower during the day, peak just before sleep, and remain high during the night. Consequently, thyroid hormone release and synthesis follows a similar pattern.

Let's examine how follicular cells synthesize thyroid hormone **(Figure 16.10)**:

1. **Thyroglobulin is synthesized and discharged into the follicle lumen.** After being synthesized on the ribosomes of the thyroid's follicular cells, thyroglobulin is transported to the Golgi apparatus, where sugar molecules are attached and the thyroglobulin is packed into transport vesicles. These vesicles move to the apex of the follicular cell, where they discharge their contents into the follicle lumen to become part of the stored colloid.
2. **Iodide is trapped.** To produce the functional iodinated hormones, the follicular cells must accumulate iodides (anions of iodine, I^-) from the blood. Iodide trapping depends on active transport. (The concentration of I^- is over 30 times higher inside the cell than in blood.) Once trapped inside the follicular cell, iodide then moves into the follicle lumen by facilitated diffusion.
3. **Iodide is oxidized to iodine.** At the border of the follicular cell and colloid, iodides are oxidized (by removal of electrons) and converted to iodine (I_2).
4. **Iodine is attached to tyrosine.** Once formed, iodine is attached to tyrosine amino acids that form part of the thyroglobulin colloid. This iodination reaction, mediated by peroxidase enzymes, occurs at the junction of the follicular

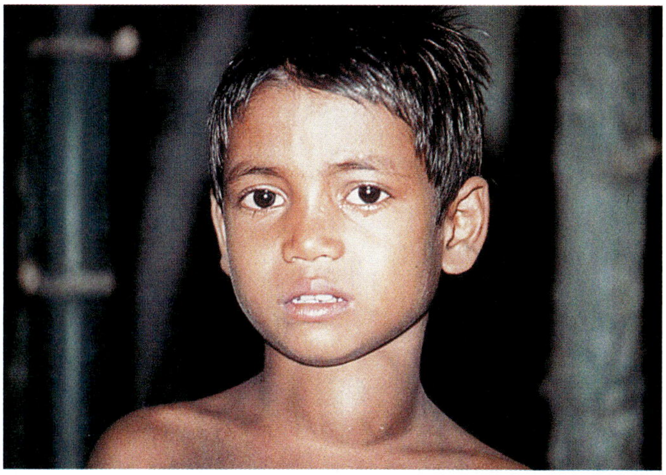

(a)

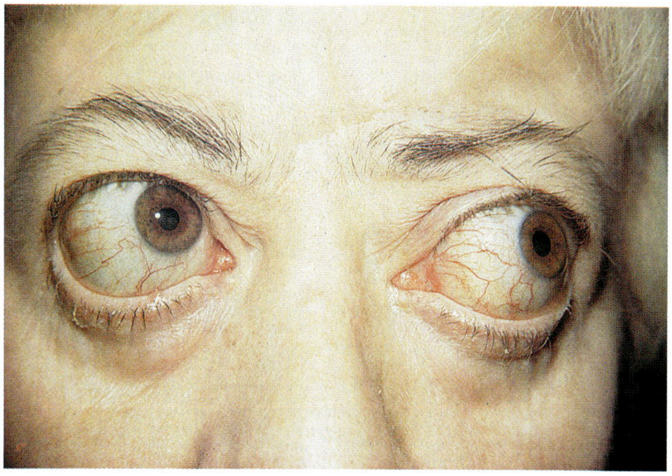

(b)

Figure 16.11 Thyroid disorders. (a) An enlarged thyroid (goiter) of a Bangladeshi boy. **(b)** Bulging eyes (exophthalmos) of Graves' disease.

cell and the colloid. Attachment of one iodine to a tyrosine produces **monoiodotyrosine** (**MIT**), and attachment of two iodines produces **diiodotyrosine** (**DIT**).

5. **Iodinated tyrosines are linked together to form T_3 and T_4.** Enzymes in the colloid link MIT and DIT together. Two linked DITs result in T_4, and coupling of MIT and DIT produces T_3. At this point, the hormones are still part of the thyroglobulin colloid.
6. **Thyroglobulin colloid is endocytosed.** To secrete the hormones, the follicular cells must reclaim iodinated thyroglobulin by endocytosis and combine the vesicles with lysosomes.
7. **Lysosomal enzymes cleave T_4 and T_3 from thyroglobulin and the hormones diffuse from the follicular cell into the bloodstream.** The main hormonal product secreted is T_4. Some T_4 is converted to T_3 before secretion, but most T_3 is generated in the peripheral tissues.

Transport and Regulation

Most released T_4 and T_3 immediately binds to *thyroxine-binding globulins* (*TBGs*) and other transport proteins produced by the liver. Both T_4 and T_3 bind to target tissue receptors, but T_3 binds more avidly and is about 10 times more active. Most peripheral tissues have the enzymes needed to convert T_4 to T_3 by removing one iodine atom.

Figure 16.8 shows the negative feedback loop that regulates blood levels of TH. Falling TH blood levels trigger release of *thyroid-stimulating hormone* (*TSH*), and ultimately of more TH. Rising TH levels feed back to inhibit the hypothalamic–anterior pituitary axis, temporarily shutting off the stimulus for TSH release.

In infants, exposure to cold stimulates the hypothalamus to secrete *thyrotropin-releasing hormone* (*TRH*), which triggers TSH release. The thyroid gland then releases larger amounts of thyroid hormones, enhancing body metabolism and heat production. Factors that inhibit TSH release include GHIH, dopamine, and rising levels of glucocorticoids. Excessively high blood iodide concentrations also inhibit TH release.

Homeostatic Imbalance 16.4

Both overactivity and underactivity of the thyroid gland can cause severe metabolic disturbances. Hypothyroid disorders may result from some thyroid gland defects or secondarily from inadequate TSH or TRH release. They also occur when the thyroid gland is removed surgically and when dietary iodine is inadequate.

16

In adults, the full-blown hypothyroid syndrome is called **myxedema** (mik″sĕ-de′mah; "mucous swelling"). Symptoms include a low metabolic rate; feeling chilled; constipation; thick, dry skin and puffy eyes; edema; lethargy; and mental sluggishness (but not mental retardation). A **goiter** (an enlarged protruding thyroid gland) occurs if myxedema results from lack of iodine **(Figure 16.11a)**. The follicular cells produce colloid but cannot iodinate it and make functional hormones. The pituitary gland secretes increasing amounts of TSH in a futile attempt to stimulate the thyroid to produce TH, but the only result is that the follicles accumulate more and more *unusable* colloid. Depending on the cause, iodine supplements or hormone replacement therapy can reverse myxedema.

Before iodized salt became available, the midwestern United States was called the "goiter belt." Goiters were common there because this area had iodine-poor soil and no access to iodine-rich seafood. In places where goiters are especially common, these goiters are called *endemic goiters*.

Like many other hormones, the important effects of TH depend on a person's age and development. Severe hypothyroidism in infants is called **cretinism** (kre′tĭ-nizm). The child is mentally retarded and has a short, disproportionately sized body and a thick tongue and neck. Cretinism may reflect a genetic deficiency of the fetal thyroid gland or maternal factors, such as lack of dietary iodine. Thyroid hormone replacement therapy can prevent cretinism if diagnosed early enough, but

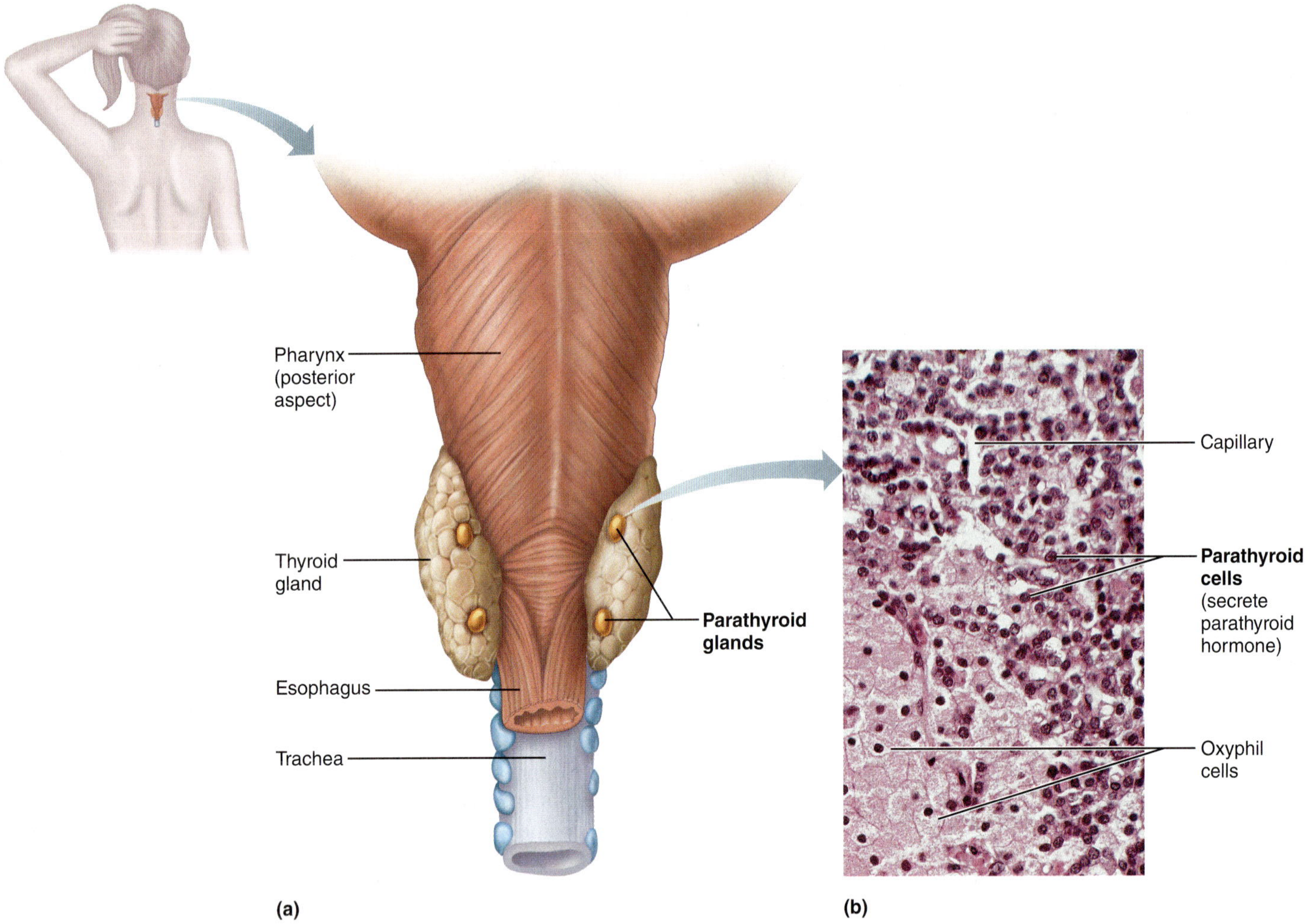

Figure 16.12 The parathyroid glands. (a) The parathyroid glands are located on the posterior aspect of the thyroid gland and may be more inconspicuous than depicted. **(b)** Photomicrograph of parathyroid gland tissue (160×).

developmental abnormalities and mental retardation are not reversible once they appear.

The most common hyperthyroid pathology is **Graves' disease**. In this autoimmune condition, a person makes abnormal antibodies directed against thyroid follicular cells. Rather than marking these cells for destruction as antibodies normally do, these antibodies paradoxically mimic TSH and continuously stimulate TH release.

Typical symptoms of Graves' disease include elevated metabolic rate; sweating; rapid, irregular heartbeat; nervousness; and weight loss despite adequate food. Eyeballs may protrude (*exophthalmos*) if the tissue behind the eyes becomes edematous and fibrous (Figure 16.11b). Treatments include surgically removing the thyroid gland or ingesting radioactive iodine (^{131}I), which destroys the most active thyroid cells. ✚

Calcitonin

Calcitonin, a polypeptide hormone released by the **parafollicular**, or **C, cells** of the thyroid gland in response to a rise in blood Ca^{2+} levels, does not have a known physiological role in humans. In fact, calcitonin does not need to be replaced in patients whose thyroid gland has been removed.

At pharmacological doses (doses higher than normally found in the body), calcitonin has a bone-sparing effect and is given therapeutically to patients to treat Paget's disease and sometimes osteoporosis (bone diseases described in Chapter 6). Calcitonin targets the skeleton, where it (1) inhibits osteoclast activity, inhibiting bone resorption and release of Ca^{2+} from the bony matrix, and (2) stimulates Ca^{2+} uptake and incorporation into bone matrix. In other animals, calcitonin rapidly (but briefly) reduces blood Ca^{2+} levels.

The Parathyroid Glands

✓ Indicate the general functions of parathyroid hormone.

The tiny, yellow-brown **parathyroid glands** are nearly hidden from view in the posterior aspect of the thyroid gland (Figure 16.12a). There are usually four of these glands, but the number varies from one individual to another—as many as eight have been reported, and some may be located in other regions of the neck or even in the thorax.

The parathyroid's glandular cells are arranged in thick, branching cords containing scattered *oxyphil cells* and large numbers of smaller **parathyroid cells** (Figure 16.12b). The parathyroid cells secrete parathyroid hormone. The function of the oxyphil cells is unclear.

The parathyroid glands were discovered by accident. Years ago, surgeons were baffled by the observation that most patients recovered uneventfully after partial (or even total) thyroid gland removal, while others suffered uncontrolled muscle spasms and severe pain, and subsequently died. Only after several such tragic deaths were the parathyroid glands discovered and their hormonal function identified.

Parathyroid hormone (PTH), or *parathormone*, the protein hormone of these glands, is the single most important hormone controlling calcium balance in the blood. Precise control of calcium levels is critical because Ca^{2+} homeostasis is essential for so many functions, including transmission of nerve impulses, muscle contraction, and blood clotting.

Falling blood Ca^{2+} levels trigger PTH release, and rising blood Ca^{2+} levels inhibit its release. PTH increases Ca^{2+} levels in blood by stimulating three target organs: the skeleton (which contains considerable amounts of calcium salts in its matrix), the kidneys, and the intestine **(Figure 16.13)**. PTH release

- Stimulates osteoclasts (bone-resorbing cells) to digest some of the bony matrix and release ionic calcium and phosphates to the blood.
- Enhances reabsorption of Ca^{2+} [and excretion of phosphate (PO_4^{3-})] by the kidneys.
- Promotes activation of vitamin D, thereby increasing absorption of Ca^{2+} by intestinal mucosal cells. Vitamin D is required for absorption of Ca^{2+} from food, but first the kidneys must convert it to its active vitamin D_3 form, *calcitriol* (1,25-dihydroxycholecalciferol). PTH stimulates this transformation.

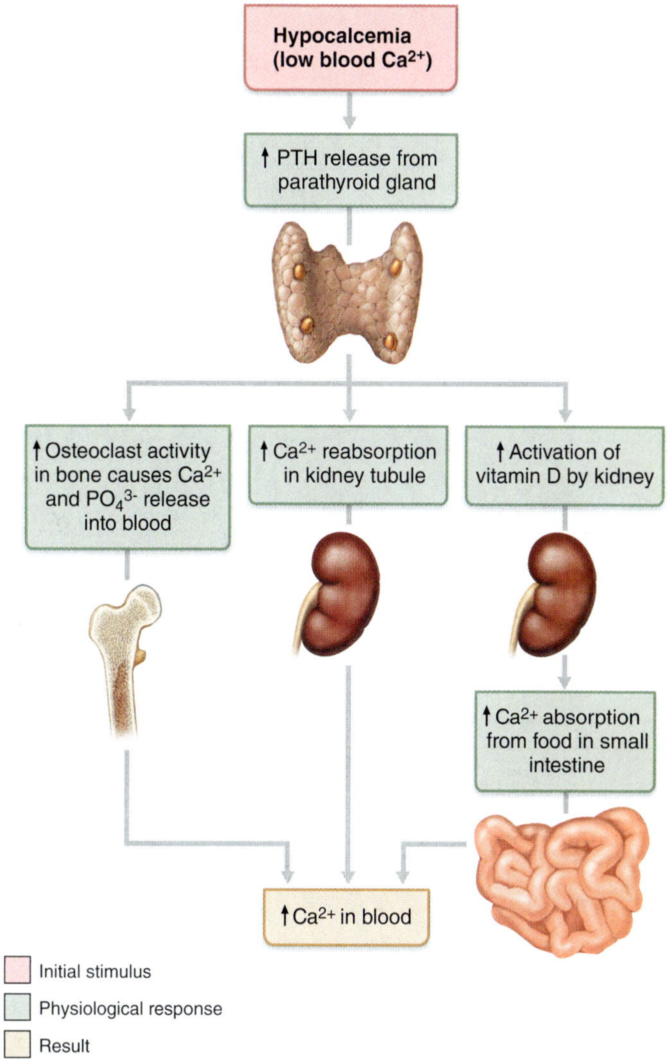

Figure 16.13 Effects of parathyroid hormone on bone, the kidneys, and the intestine.

Homeostatic Imbalance 16.5

Hyperparathyroidism (excess PTH) is rare and usually results from a parathyroid gland tumor. Calcium leaches from the bones, which soften and deform as fibrous connective tissue replaces their mineral salts. In *osteitis fibrosa cystica*, a severe form of this disorder, the bones have a moth-eaten appearance on X rays and tend to fracture spontaneously. The resulting hypercalcemia (abnormally elevated blood Ca^{2+} level) has many outcomes, but the two most notable are (1) it depresses the nervous system, which leads to abnormal reflexes and weak skeletal muscles, and (2) excess calcium salts precipitate in the kidney tubules, forming kidney stones. Calcium deposits may also form in soft tissues throughout the body and severely impair vital organ functioning, a condition called *metastatic calcification*.

Hypoparathyroidism (PTH deficiency) most often follows parathyroid gland trauma or removal during thyroid surgery. However, an extended deficiency of dietary magnesium (required for PTH secretion) can cause functional hypoparathyroidism. The resulting hypocalcemia (low blood Ca^{2+}) makes neurons more excitable and accounts for the classic symptoms of tingling sensations, *tetany* (twitching muscle), and convulsions. Untreated, the symptoms progress to respiratory paralysis and death. ✚

☑ Check Your Understanding

10. What is the major effect of thyroid hormone? Parathyroid hormone? Calcitonin?
11. Name the cells that release each of the three hormones listed above.

For answers, see Appendix H.

The Adrenal (Suprarenal) Glands

✓ List hormones produced by the adrenal gland, and cite their physiological effects.

The paired **adrenal glands** are pyramid-shaped organs perched atop the kidneys (*ad* = near; *renal* = kidney), where they are enclosed in a fibrous capsule and a cushion of fat (see Figure 16.1

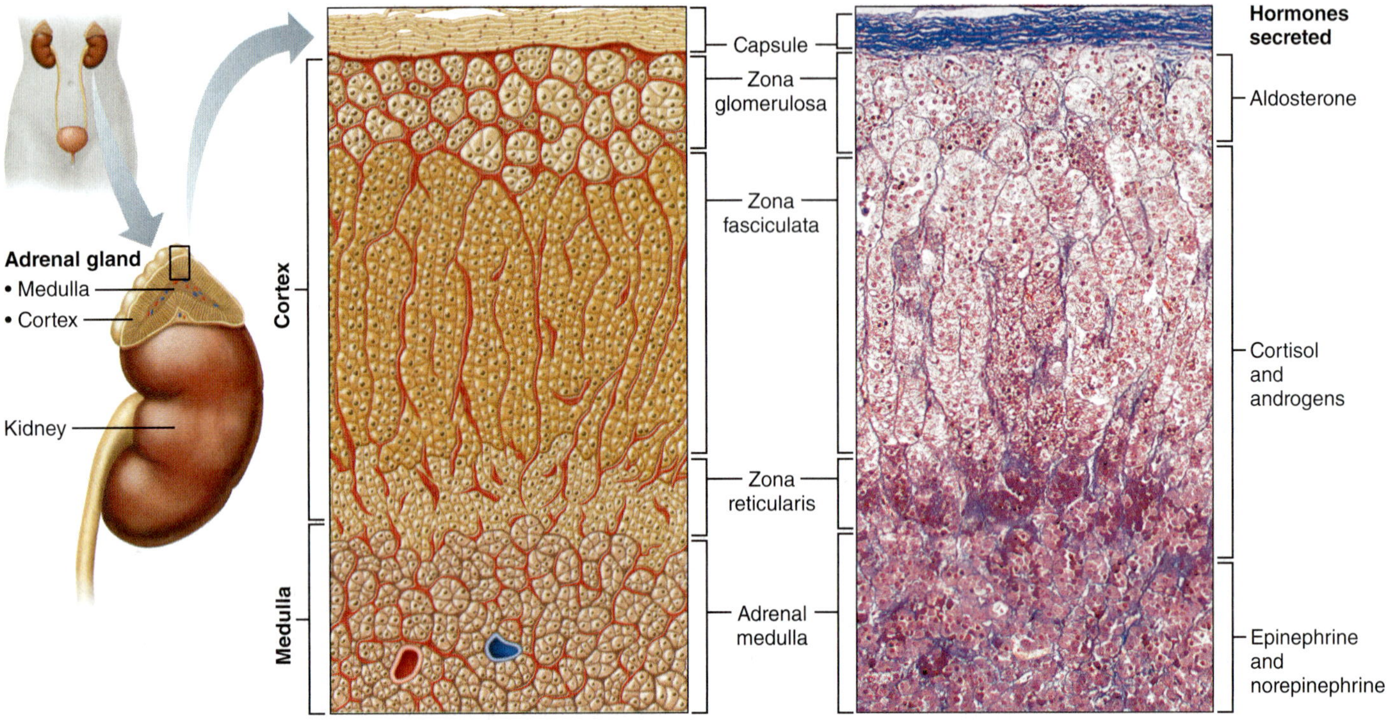

(a) Drawing of the histology of the adrenal cortex and a portion of the adrenal medulla

(b) Photomicrograph (115×)

Figure 16.14 Microscopic structure of the adrenal gland.

and **Figure 16.14**). They are also called the **suprarenal glands** (*supra* = above).

Each adrenal gland is structurally and functionally two endocrine glands. The inner **adrenal medulla**, more like a knot of nervous tissue than a gland, is part of the sympathetic nervous system. The outer **adrenal cortex**, encapsulating the medulla and forming the bulk of the gland, is glandular tissue derived from embryonic mesoderm. Each region produces its own set of hormones summarized in Table 16.3 (p. 616), but all adrenal hormones help us cope with stressful situations.

The Adrenal Cortex

The adrenal cortex synthesizes well over two dozen steroid hormones, collectively called **corticosteroids**. The multistep steroid synthesis pathway begins with cholesterol, and involves varying intermediates depending on the hormone being formed. Unlike the amino acid–based hormones, steroid hormones are not stored in cells. Consequently, their rate of release depends on their rate of synthesis.

The large, lipid-laden cortical cells are arranged in three layers or zones (Figure 16.14). From the outside in, they are:

- **Zona glomerulosa** (zo′nah glo-mer″u-lo′sah). The cell clusters forming this superficial layer produce mineralocorticoids, hormones that help control the balance of minerals and water in the blood.
- **Zona fasciculata** (fah-sik″u-la′tah). The cells of this middle layer, arranged in more or less linear cords, mainly produce the metabolic hormones called glucocorticoids.
- **Zona reticularis** (rĕ-tik″u-lar′is). The cells of this innermost layer, abutting the adrenal medulla, have a netlike arrangement. They mainly produce small amounts of adrenal sex hormones, or gonadocorticoids.

Note, however, that the two innermost layers of the adrenal cortex share production of glucocorticoids and gonadocorticoids, although each layer predominantly produces one type.

Mineralocorticoids

The essential function of **mineralocorticoids** is to regulate the electrolyte (mineral salt) concentrations in extracellular fluids, particularly of Na^+ and K^+. The single most abundant cation in extracellular fluid is Na^+, and the amount of Na^+ in the body largely determines the volume of the extracellular fluid—where Na^+ goes, water follows. Changes in Na^+ concentration lead to changes in blood volume and blood pressure. Moreover, the regulation of Na^+ is coupled to the regulation of many other ions, including K^+, H^+, HCO_3^- (bicarbonate), and Cl^- (chloride).

The extracellular concentration of K^+ is also critical—it sets the resting membrane potential of all cells and determines how easily action potentials are generated in nerve and muscle. Not surprisingly, Na^+ and K^+ regulation are crucial to overall body homeostasis. Their regulation is the primary job of **aldosterone**

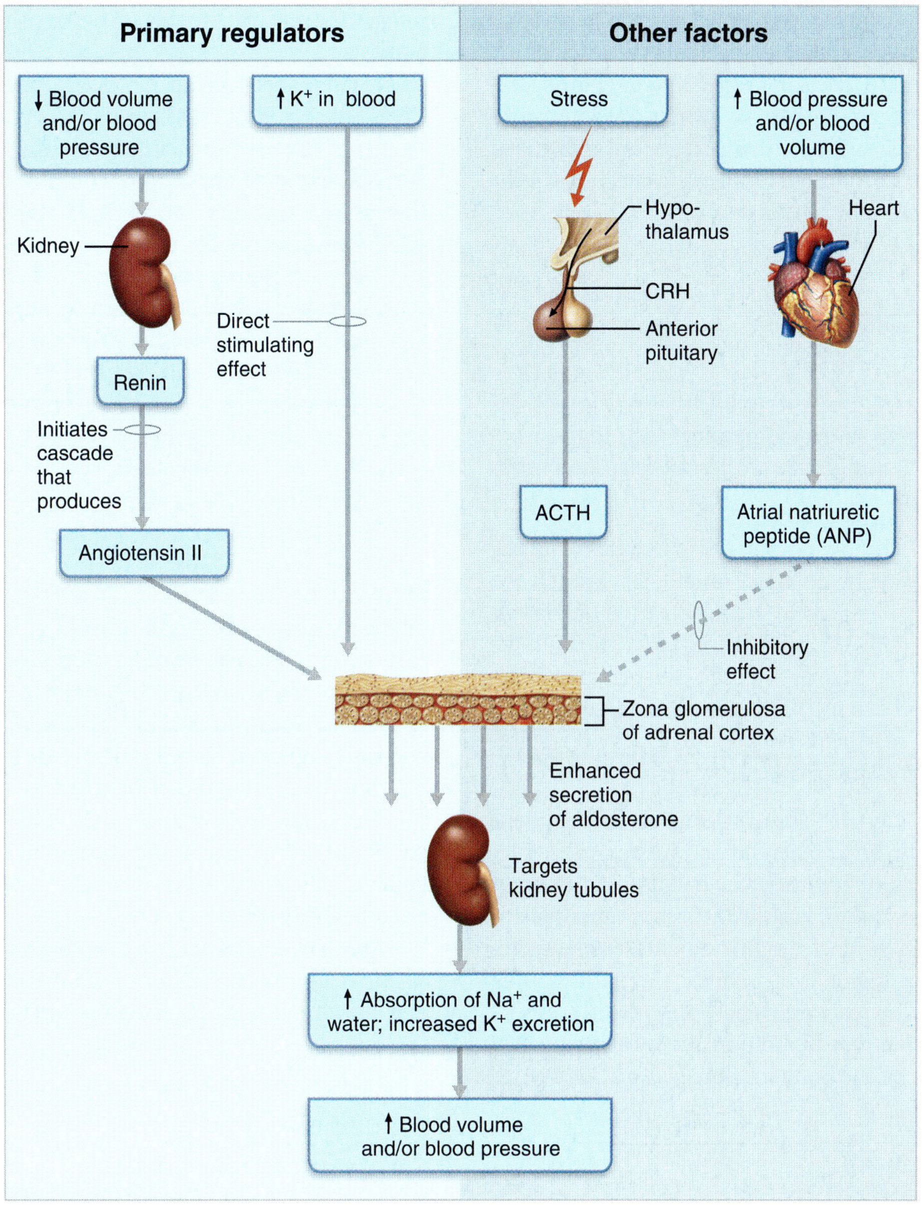

Figure 16.15 Major mechanisms controlling aldosterone release from the adrenal cortex.

(al-dos′ter-ōn), the most potent mineralocorticoid. Aldosterone accounts for more than 95% of the mineralocorticoids produced.

Aldosterone reduces excretion of Na^+ from the body. Its primary target is the distal parts of the kidney tubules, where it stimulates Na^+ reabsorption and water retention accompanied by elimination of K^+ and, in some instances, alterations in the acid-base balance of the blood (by H^+ excretion). Aldosterone also enhances Na^+ reabsorption from perspiration, saliva, and gastric juice.

Aldosterone's regulatory effects are brief (lasting approximately 20 minutes), allowing plasma electrolyte balance to be precisely controlled and continuously modified. The mechanism of aldosterone activity involves the synthesis and activation of proteins required for Na^+ transport such as Na^+-K^+ ATPase, the pump that exchanges Na^+ for K^+.

In this discussion we are focusing on the major roles of blood-borne aldosterone produced by the adrenal cortex, but aldosterone is also secreted by cardiovascular organs. There it is a paracrine and plays a completely different role in cardiac regulation.

Decreasing blood volume and blood pressure, and rising blood levels of K^+, stimulate aldosterone secretion. The reverse conditions inhibit its secretion. Four mechanisms regulate aldosterone secretion, but two of them—the renin-angiotensin-aldosterone mechanism and plasma concentrations of potassium—are by far the most important (Figure 16.15 and Table 16.3).

The Renin-Angiotensin-Aldosterone Mechanism The renin-angiotensin-aldosterone mechanism (re′nin an″je-o-ten′sin) influences both blood volume and blood pressure by regulating the release of aldosterone and therefore Na^+ and water reabsorption by the kidneys.

1. When blood pressure (or blood volume) falls, specialized cells of the *juxtaglomerular complex* in the kidneys are excited.
2. These cells respond by releasing **renin** into the blood.
3. Renin cleaves off part of the plasma protein **angiotensinogen** (an″je-o-ten′sin-o-jen), triggering an enzymatic cascade that forms **angiotensin II**, which stimulates the glomerulosa cells to release aldosterone.

However, the renin-angiotensin-aldosterone mechanism does much more than trigger aldosterone release, and all of its effects ultimately raise blood pressure. We describe these additional effects in Chapters 19 and 26.

Plasma Concentrations of Potassium Fluctuating blood levels of K^+ directly influence the zona glomerulosa cells in the adrenal cortex. Increased K^+ stimulates aldosterone release, whereas decreased K^+ inhibits it.

ACTH Under normal circumstances, ACTH released by the anterior pituitary has little or no effect on aldosterone release. However, when a person is severely stressed, the hypothalamus secretes more corticotropin-releasing hormone (CRH), and the resulting rise in ACTH blood levels steps up the rate of aldosterone secretion to a small extent. The resulting increase in blood volume and blood pressure helps deliver nutrients and respiratory gases during the stressful period.

Atrial Natriuretic Peptide (ANP) Atrial natriuretic peptide, a hormone secreted by the heart when blood pressure rises, fine-tunes blood pressure and sodium-water balance of the body. One of its major effects is to inhibit the renin-angiotensin-aldosterone mechanism. It blocks renin and aldosterone secretion and inhibits other angiotensin-induced mechanisms that enhance water and Na^+ reabsorption. Consequently, ANP's overall influence is to decrease blood pressure by allowing Na^+ (and water) to flow out of the body in urine (*natriuretic* = producing salty urine).

16

Homeostatic Imbalance 16.6

Hypersecretion of aldosterone, a condition called *aldosteronism*, typically results from adrenal tumors. Two major sets of problems result: (1) hypertension and edema due to excessive Na^+ and water retention, and (2) accelerated excretion of potassium ions. If K^+ loss is extreme, neurons become nonresponsive, leading to muscle weakness and eventually paralysis. ✚

Glucocorticoids

Essential to life, the **glucocorticoids** influence the energy metabolism of most body cells and help us resist stressors. Under normal circumstances, they help the body adapt to intermittent food intake by keeping blood glucose levels fairly constant, and maintain blood pressure by increasing the action of vasoconstrictors. However, severe stress due to hemorrhage, infection, or physical or emotional trauma evokes a dramatically higher output of glucocorticoids, which helps the body negotiate the crisis.

Glucocorticoid hormones include **cortisol (hydrocortisone)**, **cortisone**, and **corticosterone**, but only cortisol is secreted in significant amounts in humans. As with all steroid hormones, glucocorticoids act on target cells by modifying gene activity.

Negative feedback regulates glucocorticoid secretion. Cortisol release is promoted by ACTH. ACTH release is triggered in turn by the hypothalamic releasing hormone CRH. Rising cortisol levels feed back to act on both the hypothalamus and the anterior pituitary, preventing CRH release and shutting off ACTH and cortisol secretion.

Cortisol secretory bursts, driven by patterns of eating and activity, occur in a definite pattern throughout the day and night. Cortisol blood levels peak shortly before we rise in the morning. The lowest levels occur in the evening just before and shortly after we fall asleep. However, acute stress of any variety interrupts the normal cortisol rhythm as higher CNS centers override the (usually) inhibitory effects of elevated cortisol levels and trigger CRH release. The resulting increase in ACTH blood levels causes an outpouring of cortisol from the adrenal cortex.

Stress results in a dramatic rise in blood levels of glucose, fatty acids, and amino acids, all provoked by cortisol. Cortisol's prime metabolic effect is to provoke *gluconeogenesis*, that is, the formation of glucose from fats and proteins. In order to "save" glucose for the brain, cortisol mobilizes fatty acids from adipose tissue and encourages their increased use for energy. Under cortisol's influence, stored proteins are broken down to provide building blocks for repair or to make enzymes for metabolic processes. Cortisol enhances the sympathetic nervous system's vasoconstrictive effects, and the rise in blood pressure and circulatory efficiency that results helps ensure that these nutrients are quickly distributed to cells.

Note that *ideal amounts of glucocorticoids promote normal function*, but too much cortisol exerts significant anti-inflammatory and anti-immune effects. Excessive levels of glucocorticoids

- Depress cartilage and bone formation
- Inhibit inflammation by decreasing the release of inflammatory chemicals
- Depress the immune system
- Disrupt normal cardiovascular, neural, and gastrointestinal function

Glucocorticoid drugs can control symptoms of many chronic inflammatory disorders, such as rheumatoid arthritis and allergic responses. However, these potent drugs are a double-edged sword because they also cause the undesirable effects of excessive levels of these hormones.

Homeostatic Imbalance 16.7

The pathology of glucocorticoid excess, **Cushing's syndrome**, may be caused by an ACTH-releasing pituitary tumor (in which case it is called **Cushing's disease**); by an ACTH-releasing malignancy of the lungs, pancreas, or kidneys; or by a tumor of the adrenal cortex. However, it most often results from the clinical administration of glucocorticoid drugs.

The syndrome is characterized by persistent elevated blood glucose levels (*steroid diabetes*), dramatic losses in muscle and bone protein, and water and salt retention, leading to hypertension and edema. The so-called *cushingoid signs* **(Figure 16.16)**

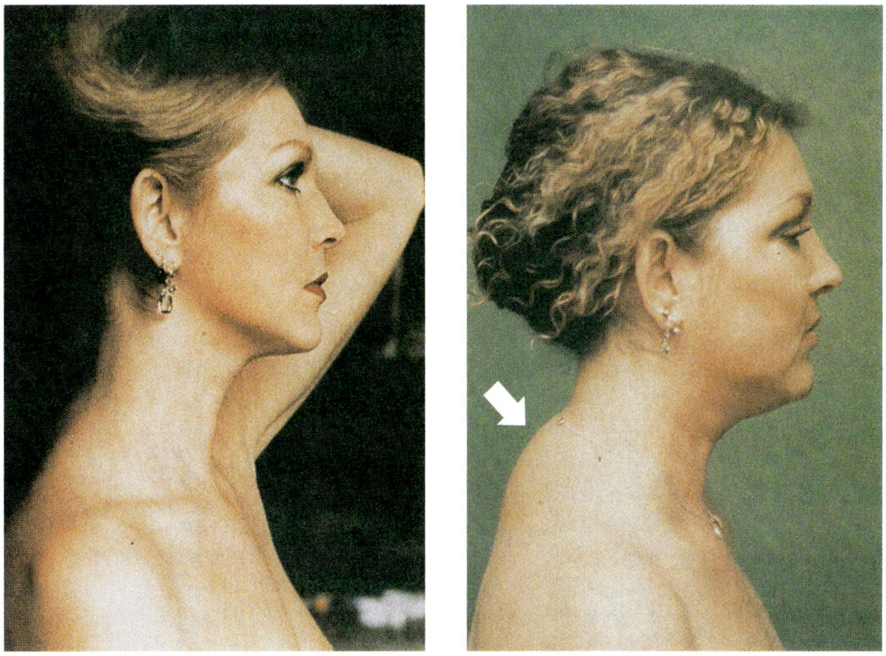

(a) Patient before onset.

(b) Same patient with Cushing's syndrome. The white arrow shows the characteristic "buffalo hump" of fat on the upper back.

Figure 16.16 The effects of excess glucocorticoid.

include a swollen "moon" face, redistribution of fat to the abdomen and the posterior neck (causing a "buffalo hump"), easy bruising, and poor wound healing. Because of enhanced anti-inflammatory effects, infections may become overwhelmingly severe before producing recognizable symptoms. Eventually, muscles weaken and spontaneous fractures force the person to become bedridden. The only treatment is to remove the cause—be it surgically removing the tumor or discontinuing the drug.

Addison's disease, the major hyposecretory disorder of the adrenal cortex, usually involves deficits in both glucocorticoids and mineralocorticoids. Its victims tend to lose weight; plasma glucose and sodium levels drop, and potassium levels rise. Severe dehydration and hypotension are common. Corticosteroid replacement therapy is the usual treatment. ✚

Gonadocorticoids (Adrenal Sex Hormones)

Most **gonadocorticoids** secreted by the adrenal cortex are weak **androgens**, or male sex hormones, such as *androstenedione* and *dehydroepiandrosterone* (*DHEA*). Most are converted in tissue cells to more potent male hormones, such as *testosterone*, and some are converted to estrogens. The amount of gonadocorticoids produced by the adrenal cortex is insignificant compared with the amounts made by the gonads during late puberty and adulthood.

The exact role of the adrenal sex hormones is still in question, but we know that they contribute to axillary and pubic hair development. In adult women adrenal androgens are thought to contribute to the sex drive, and they largely account for the estrogens produced after menopause when ovarian estrogens are no longer produced. Control of gonadocorticoid secretion is not completely understood. ACTH stimulates their release, but the gonadocorticoids do not appear to exert feedback inhibition on ACTH release.

Homeostatic Imbalance 16.8

Since androgens predominate, hypersecretion of gonadocorticoids causes *adrenogenital syndrome* (masculinization). In adult males, elevated gonadocorticoid levels may not be noticeable since testicular testosterone has already produced masculinization, but in prepubertal males and in females, the results can be dramatic. In boys, the reproductive organs mature and secondary sex characteristics appear early, and the sex drive emerges with a vengeance. Females develop a beard and a masculine distribution of body hair, and the clitoris grows to resemble a small penis. ✚

The Adrenal Medulla

We discussed the adrenal medulla in Chapter 14 as part of the autonomic nervous system, so our coverage here is brief. The spherical **medullary chromaffin cells** (kro′mah-fin), which crowd around blood-filled capillaries and sinusoids, are modified postganglionic sympathetic neurons that synthesize the *catecholamines* **epinephrine** and **norepinephrine (NE)** via a molecular sequence from tyrosine to dopamine to NE to epinephrine.

Table 16.3 Adrenal Gland Hormones: Summary of Regulation and Effects

HORMONE	REGULATION OF RELEASE	TARGET ORGAN AND EFFECTS	EFFECTS OF HYPERSECRETION ↑ AND HYPOSECRETION ↓
Adrenocortical Hormones			
Mineralocorticoids (chiefly aldosterone)	**Stimulated** by renin-angiotensin-aldosterone mechanism (activated by decreasing blood volume or blood pressure), elevated blood K^+ levels, and ACTH (minor influence) **Inhibited** by increased blood volume and pressure, and decreased blood K^+ levels	Kidneys: increase blood levels of Na^+ and decrease blood levels of K^+; since water reabsorption accompanies sodium retention, blood volume and blood pressure rise	↑ Aldosteronism ↓ Addison's disease
Glucocorticoids (chiefly cortisol)	**Stimulated** by ACTH **Inhibited** by feedback inhibition exerted by cortisol	Body cells: promote gluconeogenesis and hyperglycemia; mobilize fats for energy metabolism; stimulate protein catabolism; assist body to resist stressors; depress inflammatory and immune responses	↑ Cushing's syndrome ↓ Addison's disease
Gonadocorticoids (chiefly androgens, converted to testosterone or estrogens after release)	**Stimulated** by ACTH; mechanism of inhibition incompletely understood, but feedback inhibition not seen	Insignificant effects in males; contributes to female libido; development of pubic and axillary hair in females; source of estrogen after menopause	↑ Masculinization of females (adrenogenital syndrome) ↓ No effects known
Adrenal Medullary Hormones			
Catecholamines (epinephrine and norepinephrine)	**Stimulated** by preganglionic fibers of the sympathetic nervous system	Sympathetic nervous system target organs: effects mimic sympathetic nervous system activation; increase heart rate and metabolic rate; increase blood pressure by promoting vasoconstriction	↑ Prolonged fight-or-flight response; hypertension ↓ Unimportant

When a short-term stressor activates the body to fight-or-flight status, the sympathetic nervous system is mobilized. Blood vessels constrict and the heart beats faster (together raising the blood pressure), and blood is diverted from temporarily nonessential organs to the heart and skeletal muscles. Blood glucose levels rise, and preganglionic sympathetic nerve endings weaving through the adrenal medulla signal for release of catecholamines, which reinforce and prolong the fight-or-flight response.

Unequal amounts of the two hormones are stored and released. Approximately 80% is epinephrine and 20% norepinephrine. With a few exceptions, the two hormones exert the same effects (see Table 14.2, p. 534). Epinephrine is the more potent stimulator of metabolic activities, bronchial dilation, and increased blood flow to skeletal muscles and the heart, but norepinephrine has a greater influence on peripheral vasoconstriction and blood pressure. Epinephrine is used clinically as a heart stimulant and to dilate the bronchioles during acute asthmatic attacks.

Unlike hormones from the adrenal cortex, which promote long-lasting body responses to stressors, catecholamines cause fairly brief responses. **Figure 16.17** depicts the interrelationships of the hypothalamus, the "director" of the stress response, with adrenal hormones.

Homeostatic Imbalance 16.9

A deficiency in adrenal medulla hormones is not a problem because these hormones merely intensify activities set into motion by the sympathetic nervous system neurons. Unlike glucocorticoids and mineralocorticoids, adrenal catecholamines are not essential for life.

On the other hand, hypersecretion of catecholamines, sometimes arising from a medullary chromaffin cell tumor called a *pheochromocytoma* (fe-o-kro″mo-si-to′mah), produces symptoms of uncontrolled sympathetic nervous system activity—**hyperglycemia** (elevated blood glucose), increased metabolic rate, rapid heartbeat and palpitations, hypertension, intense nervousness, and sweating. ✚

Check Your Understanding

12. List the three classes of hormones released from the adrenal cortex and for each briefly state its major effect(s).

For answers, see Appendix H.

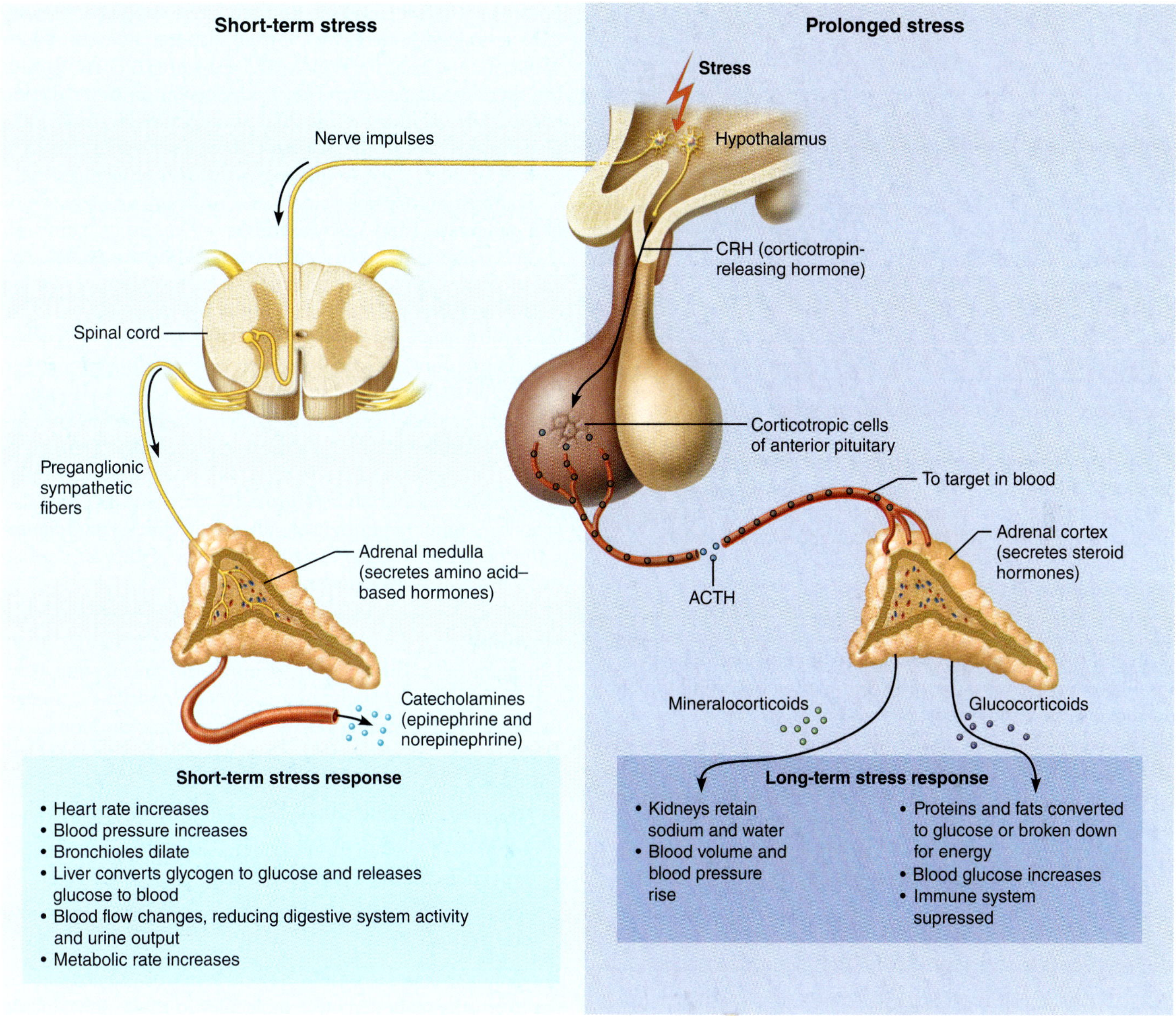

Figure 16.17 Stress and the adrenal gland. Stressful stimuli cause the hypothalamus to activate the adrenal medulla via sympathetic nerve impulses and the adrenal cortex via hormonal signals.

The Pineal Gland

✓ Briefly describe the importance of melatonin.

The tiny, pine cone–shaped **pineal gland** hangs from the roof of the third ventricle in the diencephalon (see Figure 16.1 and Figure 12.10 on p. 440). Its secretory cells, called **pinealocytes**, are arranged in compact cords and clusters. Lying between pinealocytes in adults are dense particles containing calcium salts ("brain-sand" or "pineal sand"). These salts are radiopaque, making the pineal gland a handy landmark for determining brain orientation in X rays.

The endocrine function of the pineal gland is still somewhat of a mystery. Although many peptides and amines have been isolated from this minute gland, its only major secretory product is **melatonin** (mel″ah-to′nin), an amine hormone derived from serotonin. Melatonin concentrations in the blood rise and fall in a diurnal (daily) cycle. Peak levels occur during the night and make us drowsy, and lowest levels occur around noon. Recent evidence suggests that melatonin also controls the production of protective antioxidant and detoxification molecules within cells.

The pineal gland indirectly receives input from the visual pathways (retina → suprachiasmatic nucleus of hypothalamus → superior cervical ganglion → pineal gland) concerning the intensity and duration of daylight. In some animals, mating behavior and gonadal size vary with relative lengths of light and dark periods, and melatonin mediates these effects.

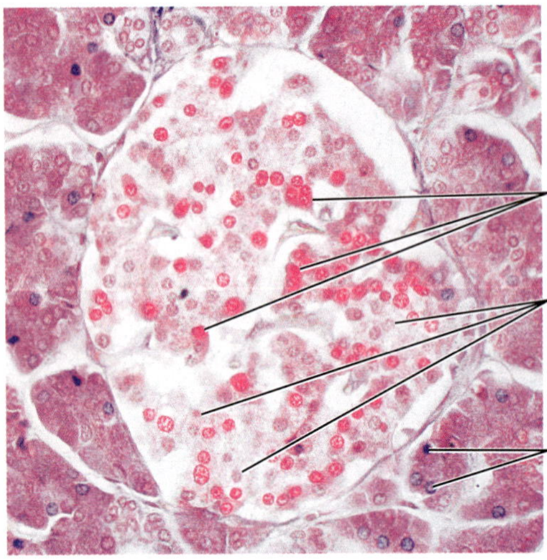

Figure 16.18 Photomicrograph of differentially stained pancreatic tissue. A pancreatic islet is surrounded by acinar cells, which produce the exocrine product (enzyme-rich pancreatic juice). The β cells of the islets that produce insulin have cytoplasm that stains pale pink, and the α cells that produce glucagon have bright pink cytoplasm (190×).

16

In children, melatonin may have an antigonadotropic effect. In other words, it may affect the timing of puberty and inhibit precocious (too early) sexual maturation.

The *suprachiasmatic nucleus* of the hypothalamus, an area referred to as our "biological clock," is richly supplied with melatonin receptors, and exposure to bright light (known to suppress melatonin secretion) can reset the clock timing. As a result, changing melatonin levels may influence rhythmic variations in physiological processes such as body temperature, sleep, and appetite.

Check Your Understanding

13. Synthetic melatonin supplements are available, although their safety and efficacy have not been proved. What do you think they might be used for?

For answers, see Appendix H.

Other Endocrine Glands and Tissues

So far, we've examined the endocrine role of the hypothalamus and of glands dedicated solely to endocrine function. We will now consider a set of organs that contain endocrine tissue but also have other major functions. These include the pancreas, gonads, and placenta.

The Pancreas

✓ Compare and contrast the effects of the two major pancreatic hormones.

Located partially behind the stomach in the abdomen, the soft, tadpole-shaped **pancreas** is a mixed gland composed of both endocrine and exocrine gland cells (see Figure 16.1). Along with the thyroid and parathyroids, it develops as an outpocketing of the epithelial lining of the gastrointestinal tract. *Acinar cells*, forming the bulk of the gland, produce an enzyme-rich juice that is carried by ducts to the small intestine during digestion.

Scattered among the acinar cells are approximately a million **pancreatic islets** (also called *islets of Langerhans*), tiny cell clusters that produce pancreatic hormones **(Figure 16.18)**. The islets contain two major populations of hormone-producing cells, the glucagon-synthesizing **alpha (α) cells** and the more numerous insulin-synthesizing **beta (β) cells.** These cells act as tiny fuel sensors, secreting glucagon and insulin appropriately during the fasting and fed states.

Insulin and glucagon are intimately but independently involved in regulating blood glucose levels. Their effects are antagonistic: Glucagon is a *hyperglycemic* hormone, whereas insulin is a *hypoglycemic* hormone **(Figure 16.19)**. Some islet cells also synthesize other peptides in small amounts, including *somatostatin, pancreatic polypeptide* (*PP*), and others. However, here we will focus on glucagon and insulin.

Glucagon

Glucagon (gloo′kah-gon), a 29-amino-acid polypeptide, is an extremely potent hyperglycemic agent: One molecule can cause the release of 100 million glucose molecules into the blood! The major target of glucagon is the liver, where it promotes the following actions:

- Breakdown of glycogen to glucose (*glycogenolysis*) (Figure 16.19)
- Synthesis of glucose from lactic acid and from noncarbohydrate molecules (*gluconeogenesis*)
- Release of glucose to the blood by liver cells, causing blood glucose levels to rise

A secondary effect is to lower blood levels of amino acids as the liver cells sequester these molecules to make new glucose molecules.

Humoral stimuli, mainly falling blood glucose levels, prompt the alpha cells to secrete glucagon. However, sympathetic nervous system stimulation and rising amino acid levels (as might follow a protein-rich meal) are also stimulatory. Glucagon release is suppressed by rising blood glucose levels, insulin, and somatostatin.

Insulin

Insulin is a small (51-amino-acid) protein consisting of two amino acid chains linked by disulfide (–S–S–) bonds. It is synthesized as part of a larger polypeptide chain called **proinsulin**. Enzymes then excise the middle portion of this chain, releasing functional insulin. This "clipping" process occurs in the secretory vesicles just before the beta cell releases insulin.

Insulin's effects are most obvious when we have just eaten. Its main effect is to lower blood glucose levels (Figure 16.19), but it also influences protein and fat metabolism. Circulating insulin lowers blood glucose levels in three ways. It

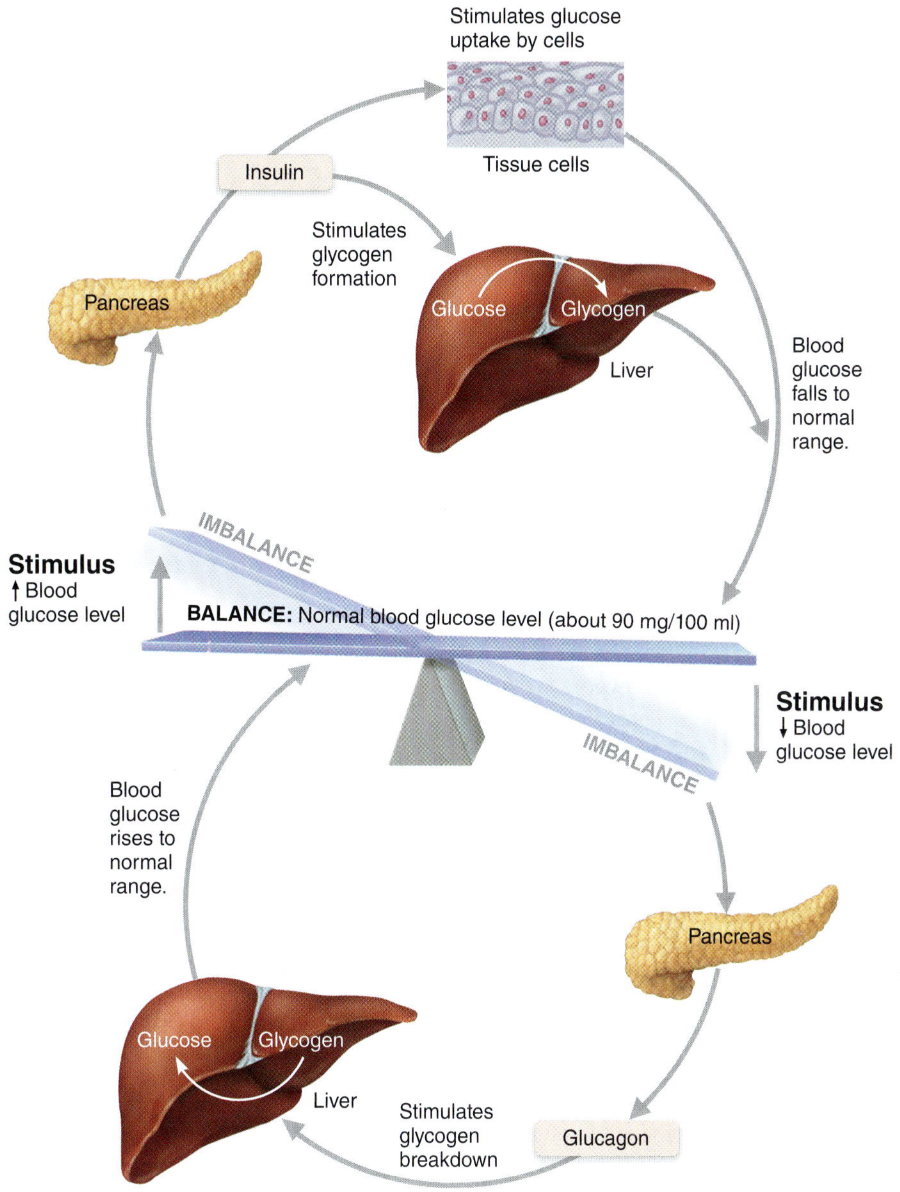

Figure 16.19 Insulin and glucagon from the pancreas regulate blood glucose levels.

- Enhances membrane transport of glucose (and other simple sugars) into most body cells, especially muscle and fat cells.
- Inhibits the breakdown of glycogen to glucose.
- Inhibits the conversion of amino acids or fats to glucose. These inhibiting effects counter any metabolic activity that would increase plasma levels of glucose.

Insulin is *not* needed for glucose entry into liver, kidney, and brain tissue, all of which have easy access to blood glucose regardless of insulin levels. However, insulin does have important roles in the brain—it participates in neuronal development, feeding behavior, and learning and memory.

Insulin activates its receptor (a tyrosine kinase enzyme), which phosphorylates specific proteins, beginning the cascade that promotes glucose uptake and insulin's other effects. After glucose enters a target cell, insulin binding triggers enzymatic activities that

1. Catalyze the oxidation of glucose for ATP production
2. Join glucose molecules together to form glycogen
3. Convert glucose to fat (particularly in adipose tissue)

As a rule, energy needs are met first, followed by glycogen formation. Finally, if excess glucose is still available, it is converted to fat. Insulin also stimulates amino acid uptake and protein synthesis in muscle tissue. In summary, insulin "sweeps" glucose out of the blood, causing it to be used for energy or converted to other forms (glycogen or fats); insulin also promotes protein synthesis and fat storage.

Factors That Influence Insulin Release Elevated blood glucose levels are the chief factor that stimulates pancreatic beta cells to secrete insulin. Other stimuli include rising blood levels of amino acids and fatty acids, and release of acetylcholine by parasympathetic nerve fibers. As body cells take up glucose and other nutrients, and blood levels of these substances drop, insulin secretion is suppressed.

Other hormones also influence insulin release. For example, any hyperglycemic hormone (such as glucagon, epinephrine, growth hormone, thyroxine, or glucocorticoids) called into action as blood glucose levels drop indirectly stimulates insulin release by promoting glucose entry into the bloodstream. Somatostatin and sympathetic nervous system activation depress insulin release.

As you can see, blood glucose levels represent a balance of humoral, neural, and hormonal influences. Insulin is the major hypoglycemic factor that counterbalances the many hyperglycemic hormones.

Homeostatic Imbalance 16.10

Diabetes mellitus (DM) results from either hyposecretion or hypoactivity of insulin. When insulin is absent, the result is *type 1 diabetes mellitus*. If insulin is present, but its effects are deficient, the result is *type 2 diabetes mellitus*. In either case, blood glucose levels remain high after a meal because glucose is unable to enter most tissue cells. Ordinarily, when blood glucose levels rise, hyperglycemic hormones are not released, but when hyperglycemia becomes excessive, the person begins to feel nauseated, which precipitates the fight-or-flight response. This response results, inappropriately, in all the reactions that normally occur in the hypoglycemic (fasting) state to make glucose available—that is, glycogenolysis, lipolysis (breakdown of fat), and gluconeogenesis. Consequently, high blood glucose levels soar even higher, and ex-

cess glucose begins to be lost from the body in urine (*glycosuria*).

When sugars cannot be used as cellular fuel, more fats are mobilized, resulting in high fatty acid levels in the blood, a condition called lipidemia. In severe cases of diabetes mellitus, blood levels of fatty acids and their metabolites (acetoacetic acid, acetone, and others) rise dramatically. The fatty acid metabolites, collectively called **ketones** (ke′tōnz) or **ketone bodies**, are organic acids. When they accumulate in the blood, the blood pH drops, resulting in **ketoacidosis**, and ketone bodies begin to spill into the urine (*ketonuria*).

Severe ketoacidosis is life threatening. The nervous system responds by initiating rapid deep breathing (hyperpnea) to blow off carbon dioxide from the blood and increase blood pH. (We will explain the physiological basis of this mechanism in Chapter 22.) If untreated, ketoacidosis disrupts heart activity and oxygen transport, and severe depression of the nervous system leads to coma and death.

The three cardinal signs of diabetes mellitus are polyuria, polydipsia, and polyphagia. Excessive glucose in the blood leads to excessive glucose in the kidney filtrate where it acts as an osmotic diuretic (that is, it inhibits water reabsorption by the kidney tubules), resulting in **polyuria**, a huge urine output that decreases blood volume and causes dehydration.

Serious electrolyte losses also occur as the body rids itself of excess ketone bodies. Ketone bodies are negatively charged and carry positive ions out with them, so sodium and potassium ions are also lost. The electrolyte imbalance leads to abdominal pain and possibly vomiting, and the stress reaction spirals even higher. Dehydration stimulates hypothalamic thirst centers, causing **polydipsia**, or excessive thirst.

The final sign, **polyphagia**, refers to excessive hunger and food consumption, a sign that the person is "starving in the land of plenty." Although plenty of glucose is available, the body cannot use it and consumes its fat and protein stores for energy metabolism instead. **Table 16.4** summarizes the consequences of insulin deficiency. DM is the focus of *A Closer Look* on pp. 624–625.

Hyperinsulinism, or excessive insulin secretion, results in low blood glucose levels, or **hypoglycemia**. This condition triggers the release of hyperglycemic hormones, which cause anxiety, nervousness, tremors, and weakness. Insufficient glucose delivery to the brain causes disorientation, progressing to convulsions, unconsciousness, and even death. In rare cases, hyperinsulinism results from an islet cell tumor. More commonly, it is caused by an overdose of insulin and is easily treated by ingesting sugar. +

Check Your Understanding

14. You've just attended a football game with your friend, Sharon, who is diabetic. While Sharon drank only one beer during the game, she is having trouble walking straight, her speech is slurred, and she is not making sense. What does it mean when we say Sharon is diabetic? What is the most likely explanation for Sharon's current behavior? How could you help her?
15. Diabetes mellitus and diabetes insipidus are both due to lack of a hormone. Which hormone causes which? What symptom do they have in common? What would you find in the urine of a patient with one but not the other?

For answers, see Appendix H.

The Gonads and Placenta

✓ Describe the functional roles of hormones of the testes, ovaries, and placenta.

The male and female **gonads** produce steroid sex hormones, identical to those produced by adrenal cortical cells (see Figure 16.1). The major distinction is the source and relative amounts produced. As described earlier, gonadotropins regulate the release of gonadal hormones.

The paired *ovaries* are small, oval organs located in the female's abdominopelvic cavity. Besides producing ova, or eggs, the ovaries produce several hormones, most importantly **estrogens** and **progesterone** (pro-jes′tĕ-rōn). Alone, the estrogens are responsible for maturation of the reproductive organs and the appearance of the secondary sex characteristics of females at puberty. Acting with progesterone, estrogens promote breast development and cyclic changes in the uterine mucosa (the menstrual cycle).

The male *testes*, located in an extra-abdominal skin pouch called the scrotum, produce sperm and male sex hormones, primarily **testosterone** (tes-tos′tĕ-rōn). During puberty, testosterone initiates the maturation of the male reproductive organs and the appearance of secondary sex characteristics and sex drive. In addition, testosterone is necessary for normal sperm production and maintains the reproductive organs in their mature functional state in adult males.

Table 16.4 Symptoms of Insulin Deficit (Diabetes Mellitus)

ORGANS/TISSUES INVOLVED	ORGAN/TISSUE RESPONSES TO INSULIN DEFICIENCY	RESULTING CONDITIONS		SIGNS AND SYMPTOMS
		IN BLOOD	IN URINE	
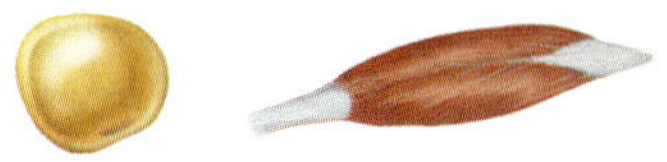 Adipose tissue; Muscle	Decreased glucose uptake and utilization	Hyperglycemia	Glycosuria Osmotic diuresis	Polyuria (and dehydration, soft eyeballs) Polydipsia (and fatigue, weight loss) Polyphagia
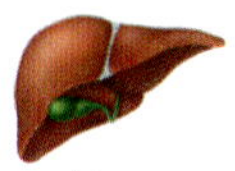 Liver	Glycogenolysis			
	Protein catabolism and gluconeogenesis			
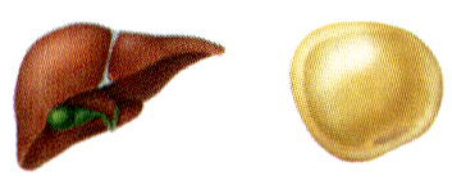	Lipolysis and ketogenesis	Lipidemia and ketoacidosis	Ketonuria Loss of Na^+, K^+; electrolyte and acid-base imbalances	Acetone breath Hyperpnea Nausea, vomiting, abdominal pain Cardiac irregularities Central nervous system depression; coma

The *placenta* is a temporary endocrine organ. Besides sustaining the fetus during pregnancy, it secretes several steroid and protein hormones that influence the course of pregnancy. Placental hormones include estrogens and progesterone (hormones more often associated with the ovary), and human chorionic gonadotropin (hCG).

We will discuss the roles of the gonadal, placental, and gonadotropic hormones in Chapters 27 and 28, where we consider the reproductive system and pregnancy.

☑ Check Your Understanding

16. Which of the two chemical classes of hormones introduced at the beginning of this chapter do the gonadal hormones belong to? Which major endocrine gland secretes hormones of this same chemical class?

For answers, see Appendix H.

Hormone Secretion by Other Organs

- ✓ Name a hormone produced by the heart.
- ✓ State the location of enteroendocrine cells.
- ✓ Briefly explain the hormonal functions of the kidney, skin, adipose tissue, bone, and thymus.

Other hormone-producing cells occur in various organs including the heart, gastrointestinal tract, kidneys, skin, adipose tissue, skeleton, and thymus (**Table 16.5**).

Adipose Tissue Adipose cells release **leptin**, which serves to tell your body how much stored energy (as fat) you have. The more fat you have, the more leptin there will be in your blood. As we describe in Chapter 24, leptin binds to CNS neurons concerned with appetite control, producing a sensation of satiety. It also appears to stimulate increased energy expenditure.

Two other hormones released by adipose cells both affect the sensitivity of cells to insulin. *Resistin* is an insulin antagonist, while *adiponectin* enhances sensitivity to insulin.

Gastrointestinal Tract *Enteroendocrine cells* are hormone-secreting cells sprinkled in the mucosa of the gastrointestinal (GI) tract. These scattered cells release several peptide hormones that help regulate a wide variety of digestive functions, some of which are summarized in Table 16.5. Enteroendocrine cells also release amines such as serotonin, which act as paracrines, diffusing to and influencing nearby target cells without first entering the bloodstream. Enteroendocrine cells have been referred to as *paraneurons* because they are similar in certain ways to neurons and many of their hormones and paracrines are chemically identical to neurotransmitters.

Heart The atria contain specialized cardiac muscle cells that secrete **atrial natriuretic peptide (ANP).** As noted on p. 614, ANP decreases the amount of sodium in the extracellular fluid, thereby reducing blood volume and blood pressure.

Kidneys Interstitial cells in the kidneys secrete **erythropoietin** (ĕ-rith″ro-poi′ĕ-tin; "red-maker"), a glycoprotein hormone that signals the bone marrow to increase production of red blood cells. The kidneys also release **renin**, which acts as an enzyme to

Table 16.5 Selected Examples of Hormones Produced by Organs Other Than the Major Endocrine Organs

SOURCE	HORMONE	CHEMICAL COMPOSITION	TRIGGER	TARGET ORGAN AND EFFECTS
Adipose tissue	Leptin	Peptide	Secretion proportional to fat stores; increased by nutrient uptake	Brain: suppresses appetite; increases energy expenditure
Adipose tissue	Resistin, adiponectin	Peptides	Secretion proportional to fat stores for resistin, inversely proportional for adiponectin	Fat, muscle, liver: resistin antagonizes insulin's action and adiponectin enhances it
Gastrointestinal (GI) tract mucosa				
▪ Stomach	Gastrin	Peptide	Secreted in response to food	Stomach: stimulates glands to release hydrochloric acid (HCl)
▪ Stomach	Ghrelin	Peptide	Secreted in response to fasting	Hypothalamus and pituitary: stimulates food intake and GH release
▪ Duodenum (of small intestine)	Secretin	Peptide	Secreted in response to food	Pancreas and liver: stimulates release of bicarbonate-rich juice Stomach: inhibits secretory activity
▪ Duodenum	Cholecystokinin (CCK)	Peptide	Secreted in response to food	Pancreas: stimulates release of enzyme-rich juice Gallbladder: stimulates expulsion of stored bile Hepatopancreatic sphincter: causes sphincter to relax, allowing bile and pancreatic juice to enter duodenum
▪ Duodenum (and other gut regions)	Incretins [glucose-dependent insulinotropic peptide (GIP) and glucagon-like peptide 1 (GLP-1)]	Peptide	Secreted in response to glucose in intestinal lumen	Pancreas: enhances glucose-dependent release of insulin and inhibition of glucagon release
Heart (atria)	Atrial natriuretic peptide (ANP)	Peptide	Secreted in response to stretching of atria (by rising blood pressure)	Kidney: inhibits sodium ion reabsorption and renin release Adrenal cortex: inhibits secretion of aldosterone; decreases blood pressure
Kidney	Erythropoietin (EPO)	Glycoprotein	Secreted in response to hypoxia	Red bone marrow: stimulates production of red blood cells
Skeleton	Osteocalcin	Peptide	Unknown; insulin promotes its activation	Increases insulin production and insulin sensitivity
Skin (epidermal cells)	Cholecalciferol (provitamin D_3)	Steroid	Activated by the kidneys to active vitamin D_3 (calcitriol) in response to parathyroid hormone	Intestine: stimulates active transport of dietary calcium across cell membranes of small intestine
Thymus	Thymulin, thymopoietins, thymosins	Peptides	Unknown	Mostly act locally as paracrines; involved in T lymphocyte development and in immune responses

16

initiate the renin-angiotensin-aldosterone mechanism of aldosterone release described earlier.

Skeleton Osteoblasts in bone secrete *osteocalcin*, a hormone that prods pancreatic beta cells to divide and secrete more insulin. It also restricts fat storage by adipocytes, and triggers the release of adiponectin. This improves glucose handling and reduces body fat.

Interestingly, insulin promotes the conversion of inactive osteocalcin to active osteocalcin in bone, forming a two-way conversation between bone and the pancreas. Osteocalcin levels are low in type 2 diabetes, and increasing its level may offer a new treatment approach.

Skin The skin produces **cholecalciferol**, an inactive form of vitamin D_3, when modified cholesterol molecules in epidermal cells are exposed to ultraviolet radiation. This compound then enters the blood via the dermal capillaries, is modified in the liver, and becomes fully activated in the kidneys. The active form of vitamin D_3, **calcitriol**, is an essential regulator of the carrier system that intestinal cells use to absorb Ca^{2+} from food. Without this vitamin, bones become soft and weak.

Thymus Located deep to the sternum in the thorax is the lobulated **thymus** (see Figure 16.1). Large and conspicuous in infants and children, the thymus shrinks throughout adulthood. By old age, it is composed largely of adipose and fibrous connective tissues.

Thymic epithelial cells secrete several different families of peptide hormones, including **thymulin, thymopoietins**, and **thymosins** (thi′mo-sinz). These hormones are thought to be involved in the normal development of *T lymphocytes* and the immune response, but their roles are not well understood. Although still called hormones, they mainly act locally as paracrines. We describe the thymus in Chapter 20 in our discussion of lymphoid organs and tissues.

☑ Check Your Understanding

17. Which hormone does the heart produce and what is its function?
18. What is the function of the hormone produced by the skin?

For answers, see Appendix H.

Developmental Aspects of the Endocrine System

✓ Describe the effects of aging on endocrine system function.

Hormone-producing glands arise from all three embryonic germ layers. Endocrine glands derived from mesoderm produce steroid hormones. All others produce amines, peptides, or protein hormones.

Effects of Environmental Pollutants

Exposure to environmental pollutants—many pesticides, industrial chemicals, arsenic, dioxin, and other soil and water pollutants—can disrupt endocrine function. So far, sex hormones, thyroid hormone, and glucocorticoids have proved vulnerable to the effects of such pollutants. Interference with glucocorticoids, which turn on many genes that may suppress cancer, may help to explain high cancer rates in certain areas of the country.

Endocrine Function Throughout Life

Barring exposure to environmental pollutants, and hypersecretory and hyposecretory disorders, most endocrine organs operate smoothly until old age. Aging may alter the rates of hormone secretion, breakdown, and excretion, or the sensitivity of target cell receptors. Endocrine function in the elderly is difficult to research, however, because it is frequently affected by the chronic illnesses common in that age group.

Structural changes in the anterior pituitary occur with age. The amount of connective tissue increases, vascularization decreases, and the number of hormone-secreting cells declines. These changes may or may not affect hormone production. In women, for example, blood levels and the release rhythm of ACTH remain constant, but levels of gonadotropins increase with age. GH levels decline in both sexes, which partially explains muscle atrophy in old age.

The adrenal glands also show structural changes with age, but normal controls of cortisol persist as long as a person is healthy and not stressed. Chronic stress, on the other hand, drives up blood levels of cortisol and appears to contribute to hippocampal (and memory) deterioration. Plasma levels of aldosterone fall by half in old age, but this change may reflect a decline in renin release by the kidneys, which become less responsive to renin-evoking stimuli. No age-related differences have been found in the release of catecholamines by the adrenal medulla.

The gonads, particularly the ovaries, undergo significant changes with age. In late middle age, the ovaries become smaller and unresponsive to gonadotropins. As female hormone production declines dramatically, the ability to bear children ends, and problems associated with estrogen deficiency appear, such as atherosclerosis and osteoporosis. Testosterone production by the testes also wanes with age, but this effect usually is not seen until very old age.

Glucose tolerance (the ability to dispose of a glucose load effectively) begins to deteriorate as early as the fourth decade of life. Blood glucose levels rise higher and return to resting levels more slowly in the elderly than in young adults. The fact that the islet cells continue to secrete near-normal amounts of insulin leads researchers to conclude that decreasing glucose tolerance with age may reflect declining receptor sensitivity to insulin (pre–type 2 diabetes).

Thyroid hormone synthesis and release diminish somewhat with age. Typically, the follicles are loaded with colloid in the elderly, and the gland becomes fibrosed. Basal metabolic rate declines with age. Mild hypothyroidism is only one cause of this decline. The increase in body fat relative to muscle is equally important, because muscle tissue is more active metabolically than fat.

The parathyroid glands change little with age, and PTH levels remain fairly normal throughout life. Estrogens protect women against the demineralizing effects of PTH, but estrogen production wanes after menopause, leaving older women vulnerable to the bone-demineralizing effects of PTH and to osteoporosis.

A CLOSER LOOK

Sweet Revenge: Taming the Diabetes Monster?

Few medical **breakthroughs** have been as electrifying as the discovery of **insulin** in 1921, an event that changed **diabetes mellitus** (DM) from a **death sentence** to a survivable disease. Nonetheless, DM is still a huge health problem: Determining blood glucose levels accurately and maintaining desirable levels sorely challenge our present biotechnology. Let's take a closer look at the characteristics and challenges of type 1 and type 2, the major forms of diabetes mellitus.

More than 1 million Americans have **type 1 diabetes mellitus**, formerly called *insulin-dependent diabetes mellitus (IDDM)*. Symptoms appear suddenly, usually before age 15, following a long asymptomatic period during which the immune system destroys the beta cells. Consequently, type 1 diabetics effectively lack insulin.

Type 1 diabetes susceptibility genes have been localized on several chromosomes, indicating that type 1 diabetes is an example of a multigene autoimmune response. However, some investigators believe that *molecular mimicry* is at least part of the problem: Some foreign substance (for example, a virus) has entered the body and is so similar to certain self (beta cell) proteins that the immune system attacks the beta cells as well as the invader. Sadly, once beta cells are destroyed, they're gone for good.

The goal of several lines of current research is to halt the destruction of beta cells. While broad-spectrum immunosuppressants have been used, these have serious side effects and a more targeted approach is necessary. Several clinical trials using various peptides and DNA vaccines are underway. A complicating factor is choosing which patients can be helped: These treatments work only if some beta cells still exist. Unfortunately in children, the main target population, beta cell destruction is rapid and virtually complete by the time of diagnosis.

Type 1 diabetes is difficult to control and patients typically develop long-term vascular and neural problems. The lipidemia and high blood cholesterol levels typical of the disease can lead to severe vascular complications including atherosclerosis, strokes, heart attacks, renal shutdown, gangrene, and blindness. Nerve damage leads to loss of sensation, impaired bladder function, and impotence. Female type 1 diabetics also tend to have lumpy breasts and to undergo premature menopause, which increases their risk for cardiac problems.

Hyperglycemia is the culprit behind these complications, and the closer to normal blood glucose levels are held, the less likely complications are. Continuous glucose monitors make this much easier than relying on finger pricks, and a new device called the e-Mosquito that uses tiny and nearly painless needles is also promising. Currently, frequent insulin injections (up to four times daily, or better yet, by a continuous infusion pump) are recommended to reduce vascular and renal complications. While some glucose sensors can talk directly to insulin pumps, problems with automatically calculating the amount of insulin to dispense mean that patients must still make these decisions. Such combined devices still fall short of being a true "artificial pancreas." A number of alternative insulin delivery methods including insulin inhalers exist.

Pancreatic islet cell transplants have become increasingly successful in helping type 1 diabetics. Still, only 33%

16

Check Your Understanding

19. In the elderly, the decline in levels of which hormone is associated with muscle atrophy? With osteoporosis in women?

For answers, see Appendix H.

In this chapter, we have covered the general mechanisms of hormone action and have provided an overview of the major endocrine organs, their chief targets, and their most important physiological effects, as summarized in *System Connections* on p. 626. However, every one of the hormones discussed here comes up in at least one other chapter, where its actions are described as part of the functional framework of a particular organ system. For example, we described the effects of PTH and calcitonin on bone mineralization in Chapter 6 along with the discussion of bone remodeling.

Chapter Summary

MAP™ For more chapter study tools, go to the Study Area of MasteringA&P at **www.masteringaandp.com**.
There you will find:

- Interactive Physiology iP
- A&PFlix *A&PFlix*
- Practice Anatomy Lab PAL
- PhysioEx PEx
- Videos, Practice Quizzes and Tests, MP3 Tutor Sessions, Case Studies, and much more!

1. The nervous and endocrine systems are the major controlling systems of the body. The nervous system exerts rapid controls via nerve impulses; the endocrine system exerts more prolonged effects via hormones.

The Endocrine System: An Overview (pp. 592–593)

1. Hormonally regulated processes include reproduction; growth and development; maintaining electrolyte, water, and nutrient balance; regulating cellular metabolism and energy balance; and mobilizing body defenses.

of patients need no injected insulin after two years. The need for long-term immunosuppression limits this treatment to only those diabetics who cannot control their blood glucose by any other means.

Over 90% of known DM cases are **type 2 diabetes mellitus**, formerly called *non-insulin-dependent diabetes mellitus* (*NIDDM*). Type 2 diabetics produce insulin, but their insulin receptors are unable to respond to it, a phenomenon called **insulin resistance**. Type 2 DM grows increasingly common with age and with the increasing size of our waistlines. About 12 million people in the U.S. have been diagnosed with type 2 diabetes, and roughly half as many are believed to be undiagnosed victims. Type 2 diabetics are at risk for the same complications as type 1 diabetics—heart disease, amputations, kidney failure, and blindness.

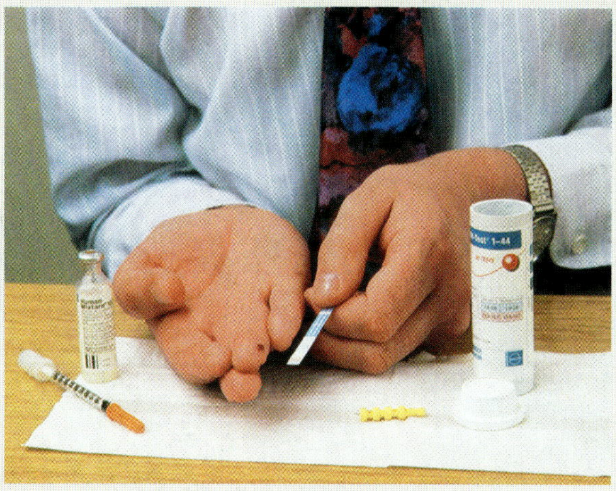

A hereditary predisposition is particularly striking in this diabetic group. Mutations in any one of several genes could lead to insulin resistance. About 25–30% of Americans carry a gene that predisposes them to type 2 diabetes, with nonwhites affected to a much greater extent. If an identical twin has type 2 diabetes mellitus, the probability that the other twin will have the disease is virtually 100%.

Lifestyle factors also play a role: Type 2 diabetics are almost always overweight and sedentary. Adipose tissue of obese people overproduces a number of signaling chemicals including *tumor necrosis factor alpha* and *resistin*, which may alter the enzymatic cascade triggered by insulin binding. The Diabetes Prevention Program, a major clinical trial, showed that weight loss and regular exercise can lower the risk of type 2 diabetes dramatically, even for people at high risk.

In many cases type 2 diabetes can be managed solely by exercise, weight loss, and a healthy diet. Some type 2 diabetics also benefit from oral medications that lower blood glucose or reduce insulin resistance. A promising new class of drugs targets the incretin hormones normally secreted by the gut, enhancing glucose-dependent insulin release from pancreatic beta cells using a normal physiological pathway. However, most type 2 diabetics must eventually inject insulin.

While we cannot yet cure diabetes, biotechnology promises to continue to improve control of blood glucose levels and thereby tame the monster that is diabetes.

2. Endocrine organs are ductless, well-vascularized glands that release hormones directly into the blood or lymph. They are small and widely separated in the body.
3. The purely endocrine organs are the pituitary, thyroid, parathyroid, adrenal, and pineal glands. The hypothalamus is a neuroendocrine organ. The pancreas, gonads, and placenta also have endocrine tissue.
4. Local chemical messengers, not generally considered part of the endocrine system, include autocrines, which act on the cells that secrete them, and paracrines, which act on a different cell type nearby.

iP Endocrine System; Topic: Endocrine System Review, p. 3.

Hormones (pp. 593–598)

The Chemistry of Hormones (p. 593)

1. Most hormones are steroids or amino acid based.

iP Endocrine System; Topic: Biochemistry, Secretion, and Transport of Hormones, p. 3.

Mechanisms of Hormone Action (pp. 593–595)

2. Hormones alter cell activity by stimulating or inhibiting characteristic cellular processes of their target cells.
3. Cell responses to hormone stimulation may involve changes in membrane permeability; enzyme synthesis, activation, or inhibition; secretory activity; and mitosis.
4. Second-messenger mechanisms employing G proteins and intracellular second messengers are a common means by which amino acid–based hormones interact with their target cells. In the cyclic AMP system, the hormone binds to a plasma membrane receptor that couples to a G protein. When the G protein is activated, it couples to adenylate cyclase, which catalyzes the synthesis of cyclic AMP from ATP. Cyclic AMP initiates reactions that activate protein kinases and other enzymes, leading to cellular responses. The PIP_2-calcium signaling mechanism, involving phosphatidyl inositol, is another important second-messenger system. Other second messengers are cyclic GMP and calcium.

iP Endocrine System; Topic: The Actions of Hormones on Target Cells, pp. 3–7.

5. Steroid hormones (and thyroid hormone) enter their target cells and effect responses by activating DNA, which initiates messenger RNA formation leading to protein synthesis.

Target Cell Specificity (pp. 595–596)

6. The ability of a target cell to respond to a hormone depends on the presence of receptors, on its plasma membrane or within the cell, to which the hormone can bind.
7. Hormone receptors are dynamic structures. High or low levels of stimulating hormones can change the number and/or sensitivity of hormone receptors.

Homeostatic Interrelationships Between the Endocrine System and Other Body Systems

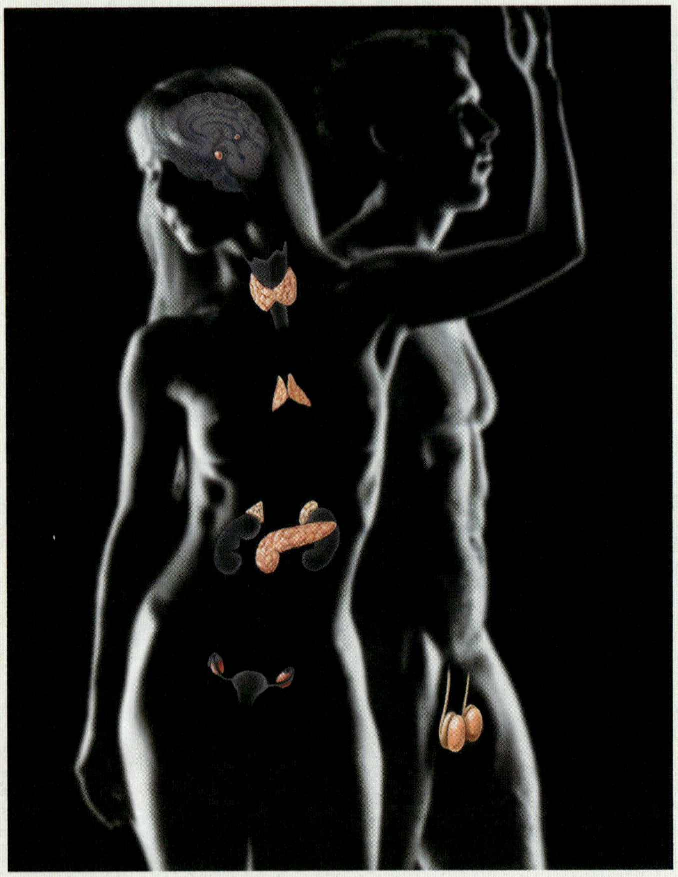

Integumentary System Chapter 5

- Androgens cause activation of sebaceous glands; estrogen increases skin hydration
- Skin produces cholecalciferol (provitamin D)

Skeletal System Chapters 6–8

- PTH regulates calcium blood levels; growth hormone, T_3, T_4, and sex hormones are necessary for normal skeletal development
- The skeleton provides some protection to endocrine organs, especially to those in the brain, chest, and pelvis

Muscular System Chapters 9–10

- Growth hormone is essential for normal muscular development; other hormones (thyroxine and catecholamines) influence muscle metabolism
- Muscular system mechanically protects some endocrine glands; muscular activity elicits catecholamine release

Nervous System Chapters 11–15

- Many hormones (growth hormone, thyroxine, sex hormones) influence normal maturation and function of the nervous system
- Hypothalamus controls anterior pituitary function and produces two hormones

Cardiovascular System Chapters 17–19

- Several hormones influence blood volume, blood pressure, and heart contractility; erythropoietin stimulates red blood cell production
- Blood is the main transport medium of hormones; heart produces atrial natriuretic peptide

Lymphatic System/Immunity Chapters 20–21

- Lymphocytes "programmed" by thymic hormones seed the lymph nodes; glucocorticoids depress the immune response and inflammation
- Chemical messengers of the immune system stimulate the release of cortisol and ACTH; lymph provides a route for transport of hormones

Respiratory System Chapter 22

- Epinephrine influences ventilation (dilates bronchioles)
- Respiratory system provides oxygen; disposes of carbon dioxide; converting enzyme in lungs converts angiotensin I to angiotensin II

Digestive System Chapter 23

- GI hormones and paracrines influence GI function; activated vitamin D necessary for absorption of calcium from diet; catecholamines influence digestive motility and secretory activity
- Digestive system provides nutrients to endocrine organs

Urinary System Chapters 25–26

- Aldosterone and ADH influence renal function; erythropoietin released by kidneys influences red blood cell formation
- Kidneys activate vitamin D (considered a hormone)

Reproductive System Chapters 27–28

- Hypothalamic, anterior pituitary, and gonadal hormones direct reproductive system development and function; oxytocin and prolactin involved in birth and breast-feeding
- Gonadal hormones feed back to influence endocrine system function

iP Endocrine System; Topic: The Actions of Hormones on Target Cells, p. 3.

Control of Hormone Release (pp. 596–597)

8. Humoral, neural, or hormonal stimuli activate endocrine organs to release their hormones. Negative feedback is important in regulating hormone levels in the blood.
9. The nervous system, acting through hypothalamic controls, can in certain cases override or modulate hormonal effects.

Half-Life, Onset, and Duration of Hormone Activity (p. 598)

10. Blood levels of hormones reflect a balance between secretion and degradation/excretion. The liver and kidneys are the major organs that degrade hormones; breakdown products are excreted in urine and feces.
11. Hormone half-life and duration of activity are limited and vary from hormone to hormone.

Interaction of Hormones at Target Cells (p. 598)

12. Permissiveness is the situation in which one hormone must be present in order for another hormone to exert its full effects.
13. Synergism occurs when two or more hormones produce the same effects in a target cell and their results together are amplified.
14. Antagonism occurs when a hormone opposes or reverses the effect of another hormone.

iP Endocrine System; Topic: The Hypothalamic–Pituitary Axis, pp. 4 and 5.

The Pituitary Gland and Hypothalamus (pp. 598–606)

Pituitary-Hypothalamic Relationships (p. 599)

1. The pituitary gland hangs from the base of the brain and is enclosed by bone. It consists of a hormone-producing glandular portion (anterior pituitary or adenohypophysis) and a neural portion (posterior pituitary or neurohypophysis), which is an extension of the hypothalamus. The neurohypophysis includes the infundibulum (stalk) and the posterior pituitary.
2. The hypothalamus (a) synthesizes two hormones that it exports to the posterior pituitary for storage and later release and (b) regulates the hormonal output of the anterior pituitary via releasing and inhibiting hormones.

The Posterior Pituitary and Hypothalamic Hormones (pp. 599–601)

3. The posterior pituitary stores and releases two hypothalamic hormones, oxytocin and antidiuretic hormone (ADH).
4. Oxytocin stimulates powerful uterine contractions, which trigger labor and delivery of an infant, and milk ejection in nursing women. Its release is mediated reflexively by the hypothalamus and represents a positive feedback mechanism.
5. Antidiuretic hormone stimulates the kidney tubules to reabsorb and conserve water, resulting in small volumes of highly concentrated urine and decreased plasma solute concentration. ADH is released in response to high solute concentrations in the blood and inhibited by low solute concentrations in the blood. Hyposecretion results in diabetes insipidus.

Anterior Pituitary Hormones (pp. 601–606)

6. Four of the six anterior pituitary hormones are tropic hormones that regulate the function of other endocrine organs. Most anterior pituitary hormones exhibit a diurnal rhythm of release, which is subject to modification by stimuli influencing the hypothalamus.
7. Growth hormone (GH) is an anabolic hormone that stimulates growth of all body tissues but especially skeletal muscle and bone. It may act directly, or indirectly, via insulin-like growth factors (IGFs). GH mobilizes fats, stimulates protein synthesis, and inhibits glucose uptake and metabolism. Its secretion is regulated by growth hormone–releasing hormone (GHRH) and growth hormone–inhibiting hormone (GHIH), or somatostatin. Hypersecretion causes gigantism in children and acromegaly in adults; hyposecretion in children causes pituitary dwarfism.
8. Thyroid-stimulating hormone (TSH) promotes normal development and activity of the thyroid gland. Thyrotropin-releasing hormone (TRH) stimulates release of TSH; negative feedback of thyroid hormone inhibits it.
9. Adrenocorticotropic hormone (ACTH) stimulates the adrenal cortex to release corticosteroids. Corticotropin-releasing hormone (CRH) triggers ACTH release; rising glucocorticoid levels inhibit it.
10. The gonadotropins—follicle-stimulating hormone (FSH) and luteinizing hormone (LH)—regulate the functions of the gonads in both sexes. FSH stimulates sex cell production; LH stimulates gonadal hormone production. Gonadotropin levels rise in response to gonadotropin-releasing hormone (GnRH). Negative feedback of gonadal hormones inhibits gonadotropin release.
11. Prolactin (PRL) promotes milk production in humans. Its secretion is inhibited by prolactin-inhibiting hormone (PIH).

The Thyroid Gland (pp. 606–610)

1. The thyroid gland is located in the anterior neck. Thyroid follicles store colloid containing thyroglobulin, a glycoprotein from which thyroid hormone is derived.
2. Thyroid hormone (TH) includes thyroxine (T_4) and triiodothyronine (T_3), which increase the rate of cellular metabolism. Consequently, oxygen use and heat production rise.
3. Secretion of thyroid hormone, prompted by TSH, requires the follicular cells to take up the stored colloid and split the hormones from the colloid for release. Rising levels of thyroid hormone feed back to inhibit the anterior pituitary and hypothalamus.
4. Most T_4 is converted to T_3 (the more active form) in the target tissues. These hormones act by turning on gene transcription and protein synthesis.
5. Graves' disease is the most common cause of hyperthyroidism. Hyposecretion causes cretinism in infants and myxedema in adults.
6. The parafollicular (C) cells of the thyroid gland produce calcitonin. It is not normally important in calcium homeostasis. At pharmacological levels, it inhibits bone matrix resorption and enhances calcium deposit in bone.

iP Endocrine System; Topic: The Hypothalamic–Pituitary Axis, p. 6.

The Parathyroid Glands (pp. 610–611)

1. The parathyroid glands, located on the dorsal aspect of the thyroid gland, secrete parathyroid hormone (PTH), which increases blood calcium levels. It targets bone, the kidneys, and the small intestine (indirectly via vitamin D activation). PTH is the key hormone for calcium homeostasis.
2. Falling blood calcium levels trigger PTH release; rising blood calcium levels inhibit its release.
3. Hyperparathyroidism results in hypercalcemia and extreme bone wasting. Hypoparathyroidism leads to hypocalcemia, evidenced by tetany and respiratory paralysis.

The Adrenal (Suprarenal) Glands (pp. 611–616)

1. The paired adrenal (suprarenal) glands sit atop the kidneys. Each adrenal gland has two functional portions, the cortex and the medulla.

The Adrenal Cortex (pp. 612–615)

2. The cortex produces three groups of steroid hormones from cholesterol.
3. Mineralocorticoids (primarily aldosterone) regulate sodium ion reabsorption and potassium ion excretion by the kidneys. Sodium ion reabsorption leads to water reabsorption, and raises blood volume and blood pressure. Release of aldosterone is stimulated by the renin-angiotensin-aldosterone mechanism, rising potassium ion levels in the blood, and ACTH. Atrial natriuretic peptide inhibits aldosterone release.
4. Glucocorticoids (primarily cortisol) are important metabolic hormones that help the body resist stressors by increasing blood glucose, fatty acid and amino acid levels, and blood pressure. High levels of glucocorticoids depress the immune system and the inflammatory response. ACTH is the major stimulus for glucocorticoid release.
5. Gonadocorticoids (mainly androgens) are produced in small amounts throughout life.
6. Hypoactivity of the adrenal cortex results in Addison's disease. Hypersecretion can result in aldosteronism, Cushing's syndrome, and adrenogenital syndrome.

The Adrenal Medulla (pp. 615–616)

16

7. The adrenal medulla produces catecholamines (epinephrine and norepinephrine) in response to sympathetic nervous system stimulation. Catecholamines enhance and prolong the fight-or-flight response to short-term stressors. Hypersecretion leads to symptoms typical of sympathetic nervous system overactivity.

iP Endocrine System; Topic: Response to Stress, pp. 5–8.

The Pineal Gland (pp. 617–618)

1. The pineal gland is located in the diencephalon. Its primary hormone is melatonin, which influences daily rhythms and may have an antigonadotropic effect in humans.

Other Endocrine Glands and Tissues (pp. 618–623)

The Pancreas (pp. 618–620)

1. The pancreas, located in the abdomen close to the stomach, is both an exocrine and an endocrine gland. The endocrine portion (pancreatic islets) releases insulin and glucagon and smaller amounts of other hormones to the blood.
2. Glucagon, released by alpha (α) cells when blood levels of glucose are low, stimulates the liver to release glucose to the blood.
3. Insulin is released by beta (β) cells when blood levels of glucose (and amino acids) are rising. It increases the rate of glucose uptake and metabolism by most body cells. Hyposecretion or hypoactivity of insulin results in diabetes mellitus; cardinal signs are polyuria, polydipsia, and polyphagia.

iP Endocrine System; Topic: The Actions of Hormones on Target Cells, pp. 5 and 8.

The Gonads and Placenta (pp. 620–621)

4. The ovaries of the female, located in the pelvic cavity, release two main hormones. The ovarian follicles begin to secrete estrogens at puberty under the influence of FSH. Estrogens stimulate maturation of the female reproductive system and development of the secondary sex characteristics. Progesterone is released in response to high blood levels of LH. It works with estrogens in establishing the menstrual cycle.
5. The testes of the male begin to produce testosterone at puberty in response to LH. Testosterone promotes maturation of the male reproductive organs, development of secondary sex characteristics, and production of sperm by the testes.
6. The placenta produces hormones of pregnancy—estrogens, progesterone, and others.

Hormone Secretion by Other Organs (pp. 621–623)

7. Many body organs not normally considered endocrine organs contain cells that secrete hormones. Examples include the heart (atrial natriuretic peptide); gastrointestinal tract organs (gastrin, secretin, and others); the kidneys (erythropoietin); skin (cholecalciferol); adipose tissue (leptin, resistin, and adiponectin); bone (osteocalcin); and thymus (thymic hormones).
8. The thymus, located in the upper thorax, declines in size and function with age. Its hormones, thymulin, thymosins, and thymopoietins, are important to the normal development of the immune response.

Developmental Aspects of the Endocrine System (pp. 623–624)

1. Endocrine glands derive from all three germ layers. Those derived from mesoderm produce steroid hormones; the others produce the amino acid–based hormones.
2. The natural decrease in function of the female's ovaries during late middle age results in menopause.
3. All endocrine glands gradually become less efficient as aging occurs. This change leads to a generalized increase in the incidence of diabetes mellitus and a lower metabolic rate.

Review Questions

Multiple Choice/Matching

(Some questions have more than one correct answer. Select the best answer or answers from the choices given.)

1. The major stimulus for release of parathyroid hormone is **(a)** hormonal, **(b)** humoral, **(c)** neural.
2. The anterior pituitary secretes all but **(a)** antidiuretic hormone, **(b)** growth hormone, **(c)** gonadotropins, **(d)** TSH.
3. A hormone not involved in glucose metabolism is **(a)** glucagon, **(b)** cortisone, **(c)** aldosterone, **(d)** insulin.
4. Parathyroid hormone **(a)** increases bone formation and lowers blood calcium levels, **(b)** increases calcium excretion from the body, **(c)** decreases calcium absorption from the gut, **(d)** demineralizes bone and raises blood calcium levels.
5. Choose from the following key to identify the hormones described.

Key:
(a) aldosterone
(b) antidiuretic hormone
(c) growth hormone
(d) luteinizing hormone
(e) oxytocin
(f) prolactin
(g) T_4 and T_3
(h) TSH

____ (1) important anabolic hormone; many of its effects mediated by IGFs
____ (2) cause the kidneys to conserve water and/or salt (two choices)
____ (3) stimulates milk production
____ (4) tropic hormone that stimulates the gonads to secrete sex hormones
____ (5) increases uterine contractions during birth
____ (6) major metabolic hormone(s) of the body
____ (7) causes reabsorption of sodium ions by the kidneys
____ (8) tropic hormone that stimulates the thyroid gland to secrete thyroid hormone
____ (9) secreted by the posterior pituitary (two choices)
____ (10) the only steroid hormone in the list

6. A hypodermic injection of epinephrine would **(a)** increase heart rate, increase blood pressure, dilate the bronchi of the lungs, and increase peristalsis, **(b)** decrease heart rate, decrease blood pressure, constrict the bronchi, and increase peristalsis, **(c)** decrease heart rate, increase blood pressure, constrict the bronchi, and decrease peristalsis, **(d)** increase heart rate, increase blood pressure, dilate the bronchi, and decrease peristalsis.
7. Testosterone is to the male as which hormone is to the female? **(a)** luteinizing hormone, **(b)** progesterone, **(c)** estrogen, **(d)** prolactin.
8. If anterior pituitary secretion is deficient in a growing child, the child will **(a)** develop acromegaly, **(b)** become a dwarf but have fairly normal body proportions, **(c)** mature sexually at an earlier than normal age, **(d)** be in constant danger of becoming dehydrated.
9. If there is adequate carbohydrate intake, secretion of insulin results in **(a)** lower blood glucose levels, **(b)** increased cell utilization of glucose, **(c)** storage of glycogen, **(d)** all of these.
10. Hormones **(a)** are produced by exocrine glands, **(b)** are carried to all parts of the body in blood, **(c)** remain at constant concentration in the blood, **(d)** affect only non-hormone-producing organs.
11. Some hormones act by **(a)** increasing the synthesis of enzymes, **(b)** converting an inactive enzyme into an active enzyme, **(c)** affecting only specific target organs, **(d)** all of these.
12. Absence of thyroid hormone would result in **(a)** increased heart rate and increased force of heart contraction, **(b)** depression of the CNS and lethargy, **(c)** exophthalmos, **(d)** high metabolic rate.
13. Medullary chromaffin cells are found in the **(a)** parathyroid gland, **(b)** anterior pituitary gland, **(c)** adrenal gland, **(d)** pineal gland.
14. Atrial natriuretic peptide secreted by the heart has exactly the opposite function of this hormone secreted by the zona glomerulosa: **(a)** antidiuretic hormone, **(b)** epinephrine, **(c)** calcitonin, **(d)** aldosterone, **(e)** androgens.

Short Answer Essay Questions

15. Define hormone.
16. Which type of hormone receptor—plasma membrane bound or intracellular—would be expected to provide the most long-lived response to hormone binding and why?
17. (a) Describe the body location of each of the following endocrine organs: anterior pituitary, pineal gland, pancreas, ovaries, testes, and adrenal glands. (b) List the hormones produced by each organ.
18. Name two endocrine glands (or regions) that are important in the stress response, and explain why they are important.
19. The anterior pituitary is often referred to as the master endocrine organ, but it, too, has a "master." What controls the release of anterior pituitary hormones?
20. The posterior pituitary is not really an endocrine gland. Why not? What is it?
21. Endemic goiter is not really the result of a malfunctioning thyroid gland. What does cause it?
22. How are the hyperglycemia and lipidemia of insulin deficiency linked?
23. Name a hormone secreted by a muscle cell and two hormones secreted by neurons.
24. List some problems that elderly people might have as a result of decreasing hormone production.

Critical Thinking and Clinical Application Questions

1. Richard Neis had symptoms of excessive secretion of PTH (high blood calcium levels), and his physicians were certain he had a parathyroid gland tumor. Yet when surgery was performed on his neck, the surgeon could not find the parathyroid glands at all. Where should the surgeon look next to find the tumorous parathyroid gland?
2. Mary Morgan has just been brought into the emergency room of City General Hospital. She is perspiring profusely and is breathing rapidly and irregularly. Her breath smells like acetone (sweet and fruity), and her blood glucose tests out at 650 mg/100 ml of blood. She is in acidosis. Which hormone drug should be administered, and why?
3. Johnny, a 5-year-old boy, has been growing by leaps and bounds; his height is 100% above normal for his age. He has been complaining of headaches and vision problems. A CT scan reveals a large pituitary tumor. (a) Which hormone is being secreted in excess? (b) What condition will Johnny exhibit if corrective measures are not taken? (c) What is the probable cause of his headaches and visual problems?
4. Sean, a 42-year-old single father, goes to his physician complaining of nausea and chronic fatigue. He reports having felt fatigued and listless for about half a year, but he had attributed this to stress. He has lost considerable weight and, strangely, his skin has a healthy tan, even though he spends long hours at work and rarely ventures outside. His doctor finds very low blood pressure and a rapid, weak pulse. Blood tests show that Sean does not have anemia, but his plasma glucose, cortisol, and Na^+ are low, and his plasma K^+ is high. His doctor orders an ACTH stimulation test, in which Sean's secretion of cortisol is measured after he is given a synthetic form of ACTH. (a) What would account for Sean's low plasma Na^+ and high plasma K^+? (b) What is the reason for doing an ACTH stimulation test? (c) Which gland is primarily affected if ACTH does not cause a normal elevation of cortisol secretion? What is this abnormality called? (d) Which gland is primarily affected if ACTH does cause an elevation of cortisol secretion?
5. Roger Proulx has severe arthritis and has been taking prednisone (a glucocorticoid) for two months. He isn't feeling well, complains of repeated "colds," and is extremely "puffy" (edematous). Explain the reason for these symptoms.

AT THE CLINIC

Related Clinical Terms

Hirsutism (her′soot-izm; *hirsut* = hairy, rough) Excessive hair growth; usually refers to this phenomenon in women and reflects excessive androgen production.

Hypophysectomy (hi-pof″ĭ-sek′to-me) Surgical removal of the pituitary gland.

Prolactinoma (pro-lak″tĭ-no′mah; *oma* = tumor) The most common type (30–40% or more) of pituitary gland tumor; evidenced by hypersecretion of prolactin and menstrual disturbances in women.

Psychosocial dwarfism Dwarfism (and failure to thrive) resulting from stress and emotional disorders that suppress hypothalamic release of growth hormone–releasing hormone and thus anterior pituitary secretion of growth hormone.

Thyroid storm (thyroid crisis) A sudden and dangerous increase in all of the manifestations of hyperthyroidism due to excessive amounts of circulating TH. Signs include fever, rapid heart rate, high blood pressure, dehydration, nervousness, and tremors. Precipitating factors include severe infection, excessive intake of TH supplements, or trauma.

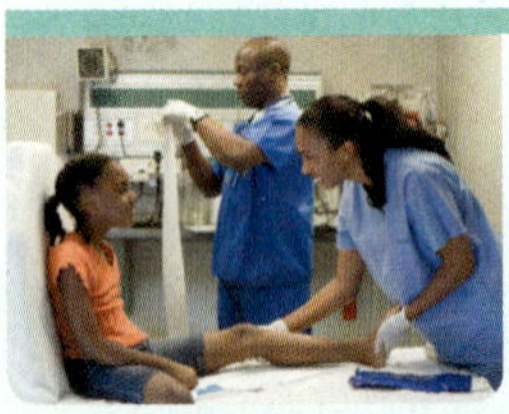

Case Study Endocrine System

We have a new patient to consider today. Mr. Gutteman, a 70-year-old male, was brought into the ER in a comatose state and has yet to come out of it. It is obvious that he suffered severe head trauma—his scalp was badly lacerated, and he has an impacted skull fracture. His initial lab tests (blood and urine) were within normal limits. His fracture was repaired and the following orders (and others) were given:

- Check qh (every hour) and record: spontaneous behavior, level of responsiveness to stimulation, movements, pupil size and reaction to light, speech, and vital signs.
- Turn patient q4h and maintain meticulous skin care and dryness.

1. Explain the rationale behind these orders.

On the second day of his hospitalization, the aide reports that Mr. Gutteman is breathing irregularly, his skin is dry and flaccid, and that she has emptied his urine reservoir several times during the day. Upon receiving this information, the physician ordered

- Blood and urine tests for presence of glucose and ketones
- Strict I&O (fluid intake and output recording)

Mr. Gutteman is found to be losing huge amounts of water in urine and the volume lost is being routinely replaced (via IV line). Mr. Gutteman's blood and urine tests are negative for glucose and ketones. Relative to these findings:

2. What would you say Mr. Gutteman's hormonal problem is and what do you think caused it?

3. Is it life threatening? (Explain your answer.)

(Answers in Appendix H)

16

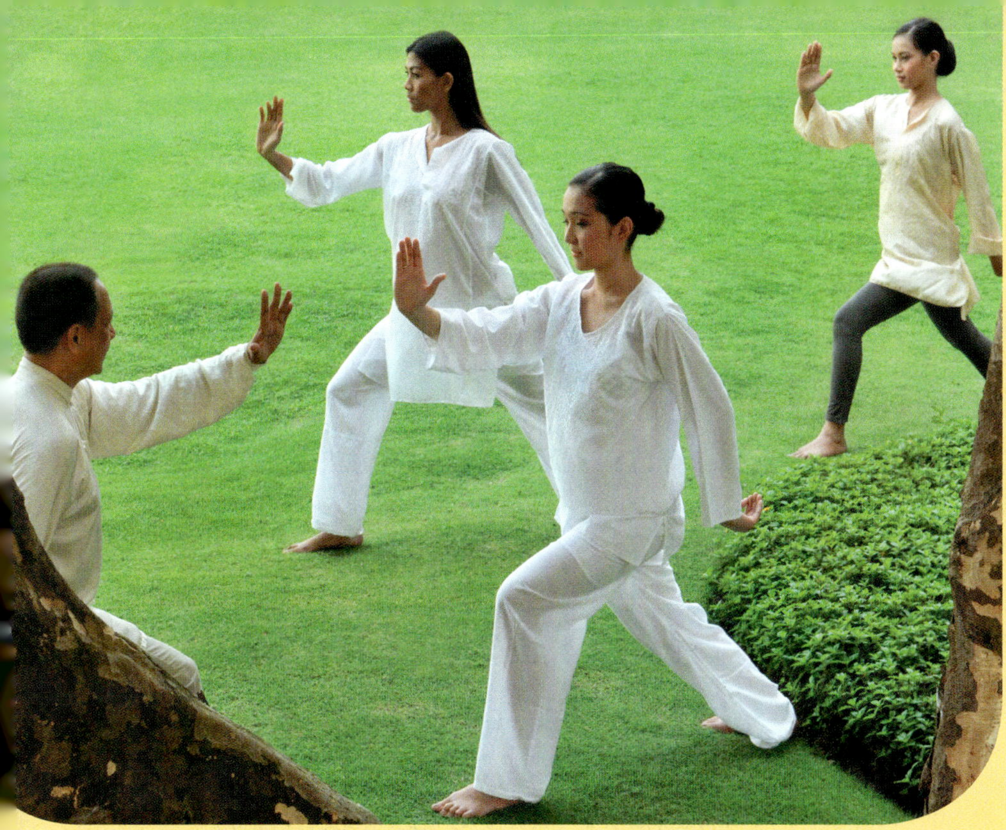

17 Blood

Blood is the river of life that surges within us, transporting nearly everything that must be carried from one place to another. Long before modern medicine, blood was viewed as magical—an elixir that held the mystical force of life—because when it drained from the body, life departed as well. Today, blood still has enormous importance in the practice of medicine. Clinicians examine it more often than any other tissue when trying to determine the cause of disease in their patients.

In this chapter, we describe the composition and functions of this life-sustaining fluid that serves as a transport "vehicle" for the organs of the cardiovascular system (*cardio* = heart, *vasc* = blood vessels). To get started, we need a brief overview of blood circulation, which is initiated by the pumping action of the heart. Blood exits the *heart* via *arteries*, which branch repeatedly until they become tiny *capillaries*. By diffusing across the capillary walls, oxygen and nutrients leave the blood and enter the body tissues, and carbon dioxide and wastes move from the tissues to the bloodstream. As oxygen-deficient blood leaves the capillary beds, it flows into *veins*, which return it to the heart. The returning

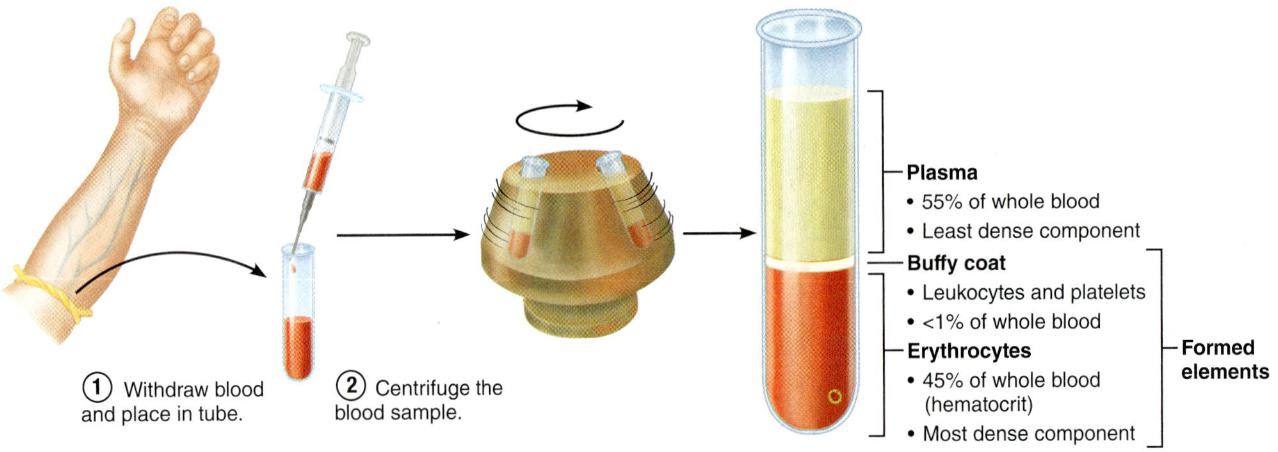

Figure 17.1 The major components of whole blood.

blood then flows from the heart to the lungs, where it picks up oxygen and then returns to the heart to be pumped throughout the body once again. Now let us look more closely at the nature of blood.

Overview: Blood Composition and Functions

✓ Describe the composition and physical characteristics of whole blood. Explain why it is classified as a connective tissue.

✓ List eight functions of blood.

Components

17

Blood is the only fluid tissue in the body. It appears to be a thick, homogeneous liquid, but the microscope reveals that it has both cellular and liquid components. Blood is a specialized connective tissue in which living blood cells, called the *formed elements*, are suspended in a nonliving fluid matrix called *plasma* (plaz′mah). Blood lacks the collagen and elastic fibers typical of other connective tissues, but dissolved fibrous proteins become visible as fibrin strands during blood clotting.

If we spin a sample of blood in a centrifuge, centrifugal force packs down the heavier formed elements and the less dense plasma remains at the top **(Figure 17.1)**. Most of the reddish mass at the bottom of the tube is *erythrocytes* (ĕ-rith′ro-sīts; *erythro* = red), the red blood cells that transport oxygen. A thin, whitish layer called the **buffy coat** is present at the erythrocyte-plasma junction. This layer contains *leukocytes* (*leuko* = white), the white blood cells that act in various ways to protect the body, and *platelets*, cell fragments that help stop bleeding.

Erythrocytes normally constitute about 45% of the total volume of a blood sample, a percentage known as the **hematocrit** (he-mat′o-krit; "blood fraction"). Normal hematocrit values vary. In healthy males the norm is 47% ± 5%; in females it is 42% ± 5%. Leukocytes and platelets contribute less than 1% of blood volume. Plasma makes up most of the remaining 55% of whole blood.

Physical Characteristics and Volume

Blood is a sticky, opaque fluid with a characteristic metallic taste. As children, we discover its saltiness the first time we stick a cut finger into our mouth. Depending on the amount of oxygen it is carrying, the color of blood varies from scarlet (oxygen rich) to dark red (oxygen poor). Blood is more dense than water and about five times more viscous, largely because of its formed elements. It is slightly alkaline, with a pH between 7.35 and 7.45.

Blood accounts for approximately 8% of body weight. Its average volume in healthy adult males is 5–6 L (about 1.5 gallons), somewhat greater than in healthy adult females (4–5 L).

Functions

Blood performs a number of functions, all concerned in one way or another with distributing substances, regulating blood levels of particular substances, or protecting the body.

Distribution

Distribution functions of blood include

- Delivering oxygen from the lungs and nutrients from the digestive tract to all body cells.
- Transporting metabolic waste products from cells to elimination sites (to the lungs to eliminate carbon dioxide, and to the kidneys to dispose of nitrogenous wastes in urine).
- Transporting hormones from the endocrine organs to their target organs.

Regulation

Regulatory functions of blood include

- Maintaining appropriate body temperature by absorbing and distributing heat throughout the body and to the skin surface to encourage heat loss.

- Maintaining normal pH in body tissues. Many blood proteins and other bloodborne solutes act as buffers to prevent excessive or abrupt changes in blood pH that could jeopardize normal cell activities. Additionally, blood acts as the reservoir for the body's "alkaline reserve" of bicarbonate ions.
- Maintaining adequate fluid volume in the circulatory system. Blood proteins prevent excessive fluid loss from the bloodstream into the tissue spaces. As a result, the fluid volume in the blood vessels remains ample to support efficient blood circulation to all parts of the body.

Protection

Protective functions of blood include

- Preventing blood loss. When a blood vessel is damaged, platelets and plasma proteins initiate clot formation, halting blood loss.
- Preventing infection. Drifting along in blood are antibodies, complement proteins, and white blood cells, all of which help defend the body against foreign invaders such as bacteria and viruses.

Blood Plasma

✓ Discuss the composition and functions of plasma.

Blood **plasma** is a straw-colored, sticky fluid (Figure 17.1). Although it is mostly water (about 90%), plasma contains over 100 different dissolved solutes, including nutrients, gases, hormones, wastes and products of cell activity, proteins, and inorganic ions (electrolytes). Electrolytes (Na^+, Cl^-, etc.) vastly outnumber the other solutes. Table 17.1 summarizes the major plasma components.

Although outnumbered by the lighter electrolytes, the heavier plasma proteins are the most abundant plasma solutes by weight, accounting for about 8% of plasma weight. Except for hormones and gamma globulins, most plasma proteins are produced by the liver. Plasma proteins serve a variety of functions, but they are *not* taken up by cells to be used as fuels or metabolic nutrients as are most other organic solutes, such as glucose, fatty acids, and amino acids.

Albumin (al-bu′min) accounts for some 60% of plasma protein. It acts as a carrier to shuttle certain molecules through the circulation, is an important blood buffer, and is the major blood protein contributing to the plasma osmotic pressure (the pressure that helps to keep water in the bloodstream).

The composition of plasma varies continuously as cells remove or add substances to the blood. However, assuming a healthy diet, plasma composition is kept relatively constant by various homeostatic mechanisms. For example, when blood protein levels drop undesirably, the liver makes more proteins. When the blood starts to become too acidic (acidosis), both the lungs and the kidneys are called into action to restore plasma's normal, slightly alkaline pH. Body organs make dozens of adjustments, day in and day out, to maintain the many plasma solutes at life-sustaining levels.

Table 17.1 Composition of Plasma

CONSTITUENT	DESCRIPTION AND IMPORTANCE
Water	90% of plasma volume; dissolving and suspending medium for solutes of blood; absorbs heat
Solutes	
Electrolytes	Most abundant solutes by number; cations include sodium, potassium, calcium, magnesium; anions include chloride, phosphate, sulfate, and bicarbonate; help to maintain plasma osmotic pressure and normal blood pH
Plasma proteins	8% (by weight) of plasma; all contribute to osmotic pressure and maintain water balance in blood and tissues; all have other functions (transport, enzymatic, etc.) as well
▪ Albumin	60% of plasma proteins; produced by liver; main contributor to osmotic pressure
▪ Globulins	36% of plasma proteins
alpha, beta	Produced by liver; most are transport proteins that bind to lipids, metal ions, and fat-soluble vitamins
gamma	Antibodies released by plasma cells during immune response
▪ Fibrinogen	4% of plasma proteins; produced by liver; forms fibrin threads of blood clot
Nonprotein nitrogenous substances	By-products of cellular metabolism, such as urea, uric acid, creatinine, and ammonium salts
Nutrients (organic)	Materials absorbed from digestive tract and transported for use throughout body; include glucose and other simple carbohydrates, amino acids (protein digestion products), fatty acids, glycerol and triglycerides (fat digestion products), cholesterol, and vitamins
Respiratory gases	Oxygen and carbon dioxide; oxygen mostly bound to hemoglobin inside RBCs; carbon dioxide transported dissolved as bicarbonate ion or CO_2, or bound to hemoglobin in RBCs
Hormones	Steroid and thyroid hormones carried by plasma proteins

☑ Check Your Understanding

1. What is the hematocrit? What is its normal value?
2. List two protective functions of blood.
3. Are plasma proteins used as fuel for body cells? Explain your answer.

For answers, see Appendix H.

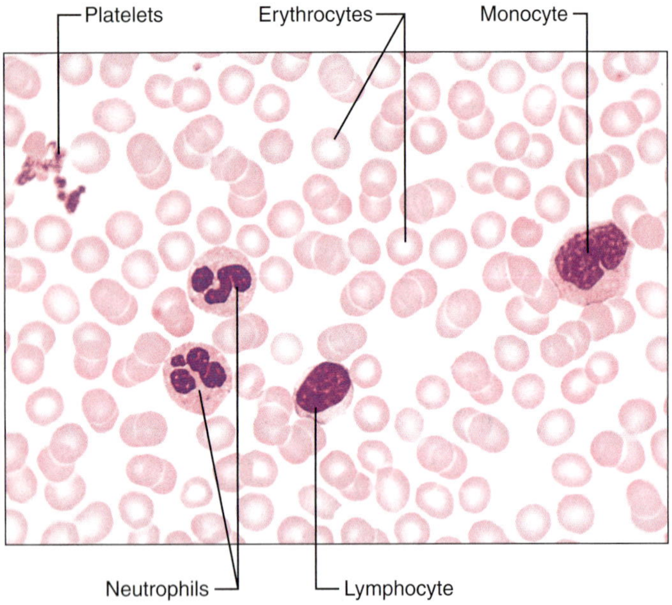

Figure 17.2 Photomicrograph of a human blood smear stained with Wright's stain. (640×)

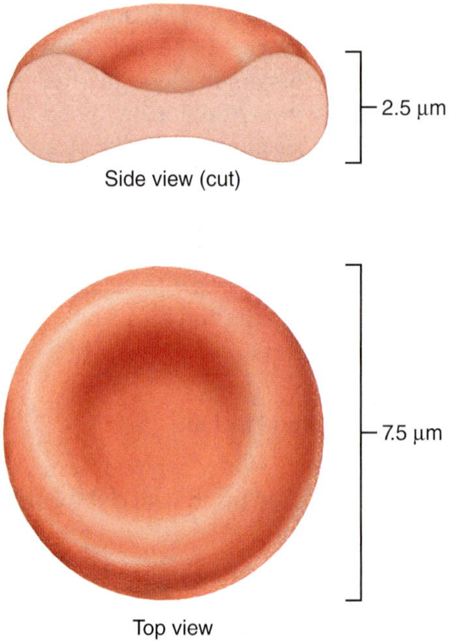

Figure 17.3 Structure of erythrocytes (red blood cells). Notice the distinctive biconcave shape.

Formed Elements

The **formed elements** of blood—*erythrocytes, leukocytes*, and *platelets*—have some unusual features.

- Two of the three are not even true cells: Erythrocytes have no nuclei or organelles, and platelets are cell fragments. Only leukocytes are complete cells.
- Most of the formed elements survive in the bloodstream for only a few days.
- Most blood cells do not divide. Instead, stem cells divide continuously in red bone marrow to replace them.

17

If you examine a stained smear of human blood under the light microscope, you will see disc-shaped red blood cells, a variety of gaudily stained spherical white blood cells, and some scattered platelets that look like debris **(Figure 17.2)**. Erythrocytes vastly outnumber the other types of formed elements. Table 17.2 on p. 644 summarizes the important characteristics of the formed elements.

Erythrocytes (Red Blood Cells)

✓ Describe the structure, function, and production of erythrocytes.

✓ Describe the chemical composition of hemoglobin.

✓ Give examples of disorders caused by abnormalities of erythrocytes. Explain what goes wrong in each disorder.

Structural Characteristics

Erythrocytes or **red blood cells (RBCs)** are small cells, about 7.5 μm in diameter **(Figure 17.3)**. Shaped like biconcave discs—flattened discs with depressed centers—they appear lighter in color at their thin centers than at their edges. Consequently, erythrocytes look like miniature doughnuts when viewed with a microscope.

Mature erythrocytes are bound by a plasma membrane, but lack a nucleus (are *anucleate*) and have essentially no organelles. In fact, they are little more than "bags" of *hemoglobin* (*Hb*), the RBC protein that functions in gas transport. Other proteins are present, such as antioxidant enzymes that rid the body of harmful oxygen radicals, but most function as structural proteins, allowing the RBC to deform yet spring back into shape.

For example, a network of proteins, especially one called *spectrin*, attached to the cytoplasmic face of RBC plasma membranes maintains the biconcave shape of an erythrocyte. The spectrin net is deformable, allowing erythrocytes to change shape as necessary—to twist, turn, and become cup shaped as they are carried passively through capillaries with diameters smaller than themselves—and then to resume their biconcave shape.

The erythrocyte is a superb example of complementarity of structure and function. It picks up oxygen in the capillaries of the lungs and releases it to tissue cells across other capillaries throughout the body. It also transports some 20% of the carbon dioxide released by tissue cells back to the lungs. Three structural characteristics contribute to erythrocyte gas transport functions:

- Its small size and biconcave shape provide a huge surface area relative to volume (about 30% more surface area than comparable spherical cells). The biconcave disc shape is ideally suited for gas exchange because no point within the cytoplasm is far from the surface.
- Discounting water content, an erythrocyte is over 97% hemoglobin, the molecule that binds to and transports respiratory gases.

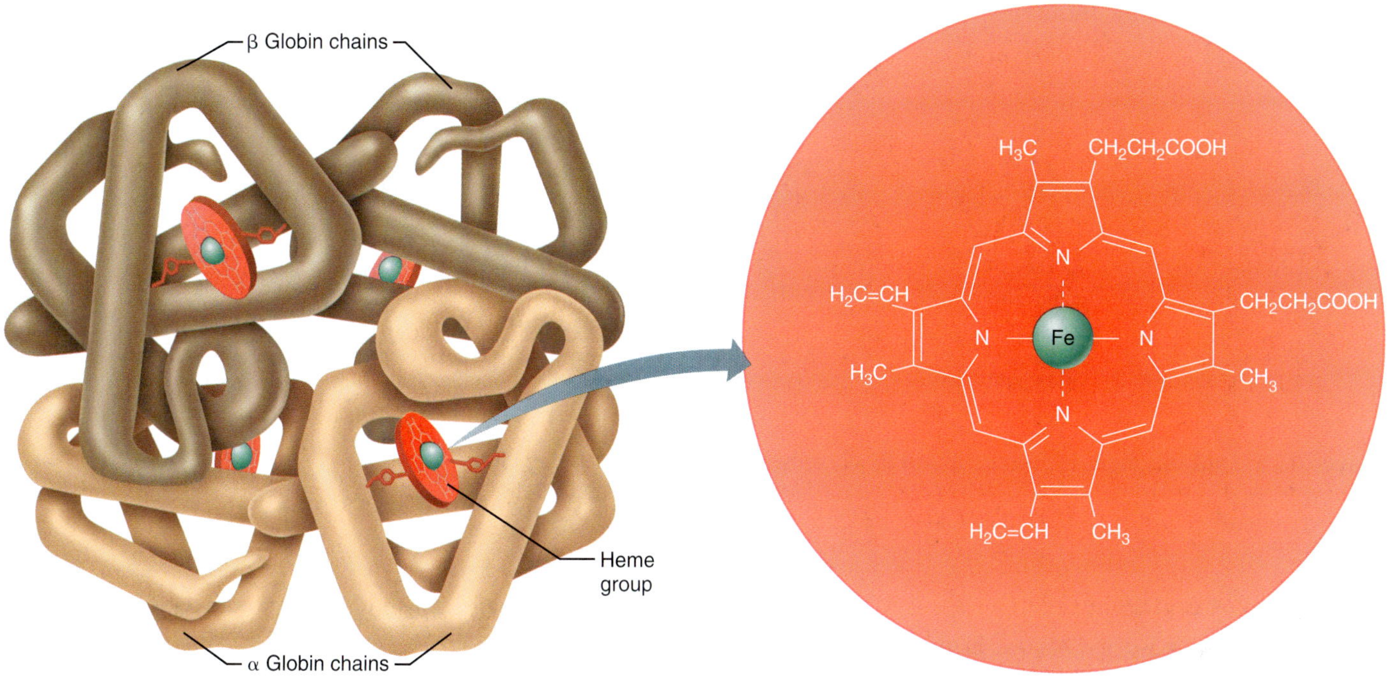

(a) Hemoglobin consists of globin (two alpha and two beta polypeptide chains) and four heme groups.

(b) Iron-containing heme pigment.

Figure 17.4 Structure of hemoglobin. Hemoglobin's structure makes it a highly efficient oxygen carrier.

- Because erythrocytes lack mitochondria and generate ATP by anaerobic mechanisms, they do not consume any of the oxygen they carry, making them very efficient oxygen transporters indeed.

Erythrocytes are the major factor contributing to blood viscosity. Women typically have a lower red blood cell count than men [4.2–5.4 million cells per microliter ($1\ \mu l = 1\ mm^3$) of blood versus 4.7–6.1 million cells/μl respectively]. When the number of red blood cells increases beyond the normal range, blood becomes more viscous and flows more slowly. Similarly, as the number of red blood cells drops below the lower end of the range, the blood thins and flows more rapidly.

Functions of Erythrocytes

Erythrocytes are completely dedicated to their job of transporting respiratory gases (oxygen and carbon dioxide). **Hemoglobin**, the protein that makes red blood cells red, binds easily and reversibly with oxygen, and most oxygen carried in blood is bound to hemoglobin. Normal values for hemoglobin are 13–18 grams per 100 milliliters of blood (g/100 ml) in adult males, and 12–16 g/100 ml in adult females.

Hemoglobin is made up of the red **heme** pigment bound to the protein **globin**. Globin consists of four polypeptide chains—two alpha (α) and two beta (β)—each binding a ringlike heme group **(Figure 17.4a)**. Each heme group bears an atom of iron set like a jewel in its center (Figure 17.4b). A hemoglobin molecule can transport four molecules of oxygen because each iron atom can combine reversibly with one molecule of oxygen. A single red blood cell contains about 250 million hemoglobin molecules, so each of these tiny cells can scoop up about 1 billion molecules of oxygen!

The fact that hemoglobin is contained in erythrocytes, rather than existing free in plasma, prevents it (1) from breaking into fragments that would leak out of the bloodstream (through porous capillary walls) and (2) from making blood more viscous and raising osmotic pressure.

Oxygen loading occurs in the lungs, and the direction of transport is from lungs to tissue cells. As oxygen-deficient blood moves through the lungs, oxygen diffuses from the air sacs of the lungs into the blood and then into the erythrocytes, where it binds to hemoglobin. When oxygen binds to iron, the hemoglobin, now called **oxyhemoglobin**, assumes a new three-dimensional shape and becomes ruby red.

In body tissues, the process is reversed. Oxygen detaches from iron, hemoglobin resumes its former shape, and the resulting **deoxyhemoglobin**, or *reduced hemoglobin*, becomes dark red. The released oxygen diffuses from the blood into the tissue fluid and then into tissue cells.

About 20% of the carbon dioxide transported in the blood combines with hemoglobin, but it binds to globin's amino acids rather than to the heme group. This formation of **carbaminohemoglobin** (kar-bam″ĭ-no-he″muh″glo′bin) occurs more readily when hemoglobin is in the reduced state (dissociated from oxygen). Carbon dioxide loading occurs in the tissues, and the direction of transport is from tissues to lungs, where carbon dioxide is eliminated from the body. We describe the loading and unloading of these respiratory gases in Chapter 22.

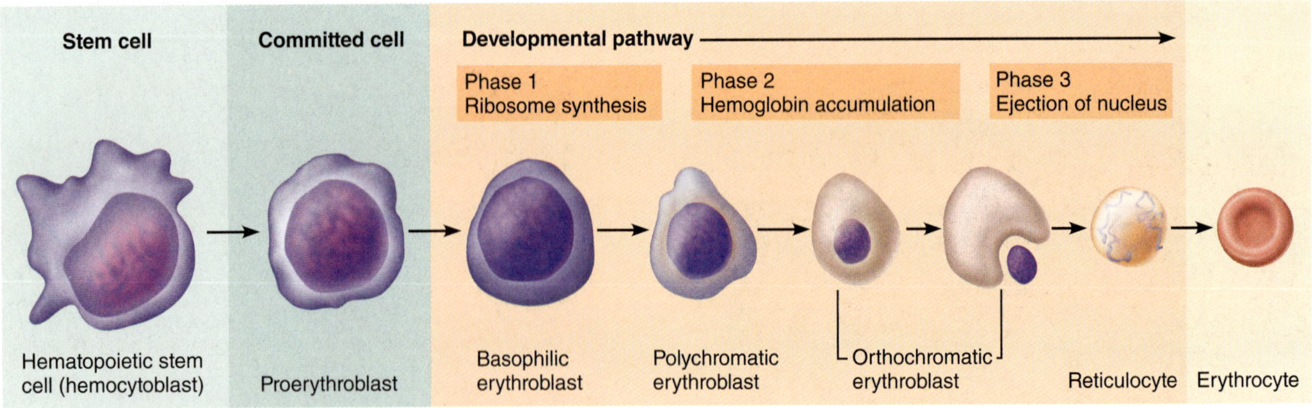

Figure 17.5 Erythropoiesis: formation of red blood cells. Reticulocytes are released into the bloodstream. The myeloid stem cell, the phase intermediate between the hematopoietic stem cell and the proerythroblast, is not illustrated.

Production of Erythrocytes

Blood cell formation is referred to as **hematopoiesis** (hem″ah-to-poi-e′sis; *hemato* = blood; *poiesis* = to make). Hematopoiesis occurs in the **red bone marrow**, which is composed largely of a soft network of reticular connective tissue bordering on wide blood capillaries called *blood sinusoids*. Within this network are immature blood cells, macrophages, fat cells, and *reticular cells* (which secrete the connective tissue fibers). In adults, red marrow is found chiefly in the bones of the axial skeleton and girdles, and in the proximal epiphyses of the humerus and femur.

The production of each type of blood cell varies in response to changing body needs and regulatory factors. As blood cells mature, they migrate through the thin walls of the sinusoids to enter the bloodstream. On average, the marrow turns out an ounce of new blood containing 100 billion new cells every day.

17

The various formed elements have different functions, but there are similarities in their life histories. All arise from the **hematopoietic stem cell**, sometimes called a *hemocytoblast* (*cyte* = cell, *blast* = bud). These undifferentiated precursor cells reside in the red bone marrow. However, the maturation pathways of the various formed elements differ, and once a cell is *committed* to a specific blood cell pathway, it cannot change. This commitment is signaled by the appearance of membrane surface receptors that respond to specific hormones or growth factors, which in turn "push" the cell toward further specialization.

Stages of Erythropoiesis Erythrocyte production, or **erythropoiesis** (ĕ-rith″ro-poi-e′sis), begins when a hematopoietic stem cell descendant called a **myeloid stem cell** transforms into a **proerythroblast** (Figure 17.5). Proerythroblasts, in turn, give rise to **basophilic erythroblasts** that produce huge numbers of ribosomes. During these first two phases, the cells divide many times. Hemoglobin is synthesized and iron accumulates as the basophilic erythroblast transforms into a **polychromatic erythroblast** and then an **orthochromatic erythroblast**. The "color" of the cell cytoplasm changes as the blue-staining ribosomes become masked by the pink color of hemoglobin. When an orthochromatic erythroblast has accumulated almost all of its hemoglobin, it ejects most of its organelles. Additionally, its nucleus degenerates and is pinched off, allowing the cell to collapse inward and eventually assume the biconcave shape. The result is the **reticulocyte** (essentially a young erythrocyte), so named because it still contains a scant *reticulum* (network) of clumped ribosomes.

The entire process from hematopoietic stem cell to reticulocyte takes about 15 days. The reticulocytes, filled almost to bursting with hemoglobin, enter the bloodstream to begin their task of oxygen transport. Usually they become fully mature erythrocytes within two days of release as their ribosomes are degraded by intracellular enzymes.

Reticulocytes account for 1–2% of all erythrocytes in the blood of healthy people. **Reticulocyte counts** provide a rough index of the *rate* of RBC formation—reticulocyte counts below or above this range indicate abnormal rates of erythrocyte formation.

Regulation and Requirements for Erythropoiesis

The number of circulating erythrocytes in a given individual is remarkably constant and reflects a balance between red blood cell production and destruction. This balance is important because having too few erythrocytes leads to tissue hypoxia (oxygen deprivation), whereas having too many makes the blood undesirably viscous.

To ensure that the number of erythrocytes in blood remains within the homeostatic range, new cells are produced at the incredibly rapid rate of more than 2 million per second in healthy people. This process is controlled hormonally and depends on adequate supplies of iron, amino acids, and certain B vitamins.

Hormonal Controls **Erythropoietin (EPO)**, a glycoprotein hormone, stimulates the formation of erythrocytes (Figure 17.6). Normally, a small amount of EPO circulates in the blood at all times and sustains red blood cell production at a basal rate. The kidneys play the major role in EPO production, although the liver also produces some. When certain kidney cells become

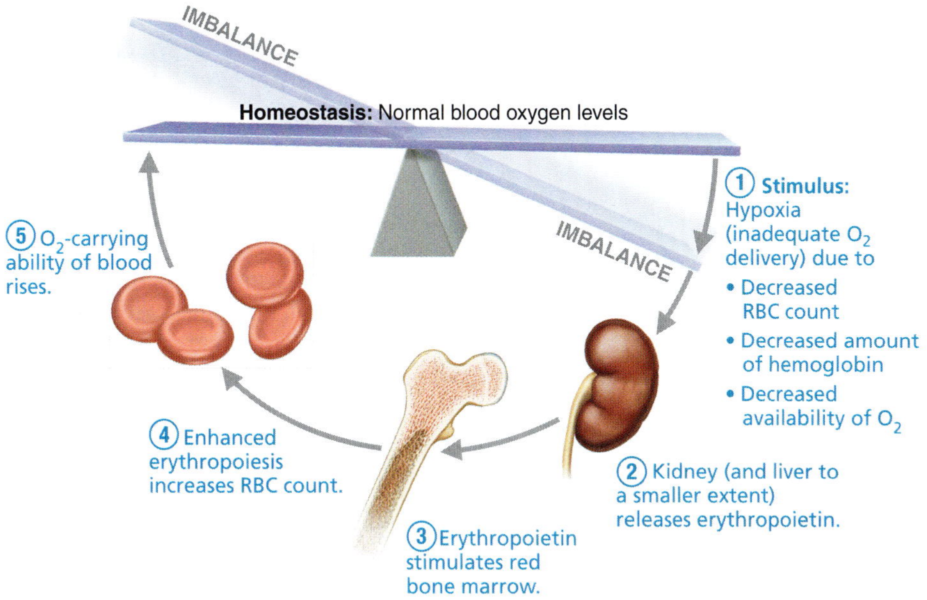

Figure 17.6 Erythropoietin mechanism for regulating erythropoiesis.

hypoxic (oxygen deficient), oxygen-sensitive enzymes are unable to carry out their normal functions of degrading an intracellular signaling molecule called hypoxia-inducible factor (HIF). As HIF accumulates, it accelerates the synthesis and release of erythropoietin.

The drop in normal blood oxygen levels that triggers EPO formation can result from

- Reduced numbers of red blood cells due to hemorrhage (bleeding) or excessive RBC destruction
- Insufficient hemoglobin per RBC (as in iron deficiency)
- Reduced availability of oxygen, as might occur at high altitudes or during pneumonia

Conversely, too many erythrocytes or excessive oxygen in the bloodstream depresses erythropoietin production. Note that it is not the number of erythrocytes in blood that controls the rate of erythropoiesis. Instead, control is based on their ability to transport enough oxygen to meet tissue demands.

Bloodborne erythropoietin stimulates red marrow cells that *are already committed* to becoming erythrocytes, causing them to mature more rapidly. One to two days after erythropoietin levels rise in the blood, the rate of reticulocyte release and the reticulocyte count rise markedly. Notice that hypoxia does not activate the bone marrow directly. Instead it stimulates the kidneys, which in turn provide the hormonal stimulus that activates the bone marrow.

Homeostatic Imbalance 17.1

Renal dialysis patients whose kidneys have failed produce too little EPO to support normal erythropoiesis. Consequently, they routinely have red blood cell counts less than half those of healthy individuals. Genetically engineered (recombinant) EPO has helped these patients immeasurably.

Unfortunately, some athletes abuse recombinant EPO—particularly professional bike racers and marathon runners seeking increased stamina and performance. However, the consequences can be deadly. By injecting EPO, healthy athletes increase their normal hematocrit from 45% to as much as 65%. Then, with the dehydration that occurs in a long race, the blood concentrates even further, becoming a thick, sticky "sludge" that can cause clotting, stroke, and heart failure. +

The male sex hormone *testosterone* also enhances the kidneys' production of EPO. Because female sex hormones do not have similar stimulatory effects, testosterone may be at least partially responsible for the higher RBC counts and hemoglobin levels seen in males. Also, a wide variety of chemicals released by leukocytes, platelets, and even reticular cells stimulates bursts of RBC production.

Dietary Requirements The raw materials required for erythropoiesis include the usual nutrients and structural materials—amino acids, lipids, and carbohydrates. Iron is essential for hemoglobin synthesis. Iron is available from the diet, and intestinal cells precisely control its absorption into the bloodstream in response to changing body stores of iron.

Approximately 65% of the body's iron supply (about 4000 mg) is in hemoglobin. Most of the remainder is stored in the liver, spleen, and (to a much lesser extent) bone marrow. Free iron ions (Fe^{2+}, Fe^{3+}) are toxic, so iron is stored inside cells as protein-iron complexes such as **ferritin** (fer′ĭ-tin) and **hemosiderin** (he″mo-sid′er-in). In blood, iron is transported loosely bound to a transport protein called **transferrin**, and developing erythrocytes take up iron as needed to form hemoglobin (Figure 17.7). Small amounts of iron are lost each day in feces, urine, and perspiration. The average daily loss of iron is 1.7 mg in women and 0.9 mg in men. In women, the menstrual flow accounts for the additional losses.

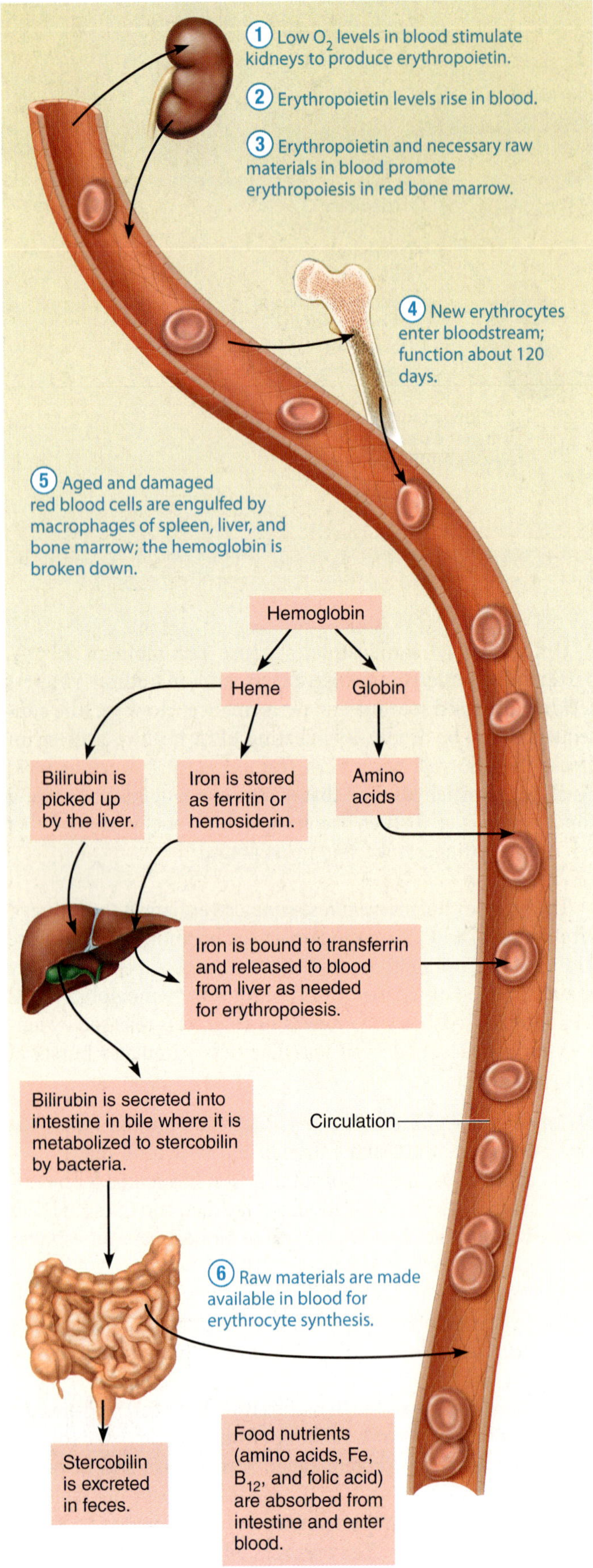

Figure 17.7 Life cycle of red blood cells.

Two B-complex vitamins—vitamin B_{12} and folic acid—are necessary for normal DNA synthesis. Even slight deficits jeopardize rapidly dividing cell populations, such as developing erythrocytes.

Fate and Destruction of Erythrocytes

Red blood cells have a useful life span of 100 to 120 days. Their anucleate condition carries with it some important limitations. Red blood cells are unable to synthesize new proteins, grow, or divide. Erythrocytes become "old" as they lose their flexibility, become increasingly rigid and fragile, and their hemoglobin begins to degenerate. They become trapped and fragment in smaller circulatory channels, particularly in those of the spleen. For this reason, the spleen is sometimes called the "red blood cell graveyard."

We will briefly describe the fate of aged and damaged erythrocytes here, but Figure 17.7 gives a more detailed account. Macrophages engulf and destroy dying erythrocytes. The heme of their hemoglobin is split off from globin. Its core of iron is salvaged, bound to protein (as ferritin or hemosiderin), and stored for reuse. The balance of the heme group is degraded to **bilirubin** (bil″ĭ-roo′bin), a yellow pigment that is released to the blood and binds to albumin for transport. Liver cells pick up bilirubin and in turn secrete it (in bile) into the intestine, where it is metabolized to *urobilinogen*. Most of this degraded pigment leaves the body in feces, as a brown pigment called *stercobilin*. The protein (globin) part of hemoglobin is metabolized or broken down to amino acids, which are released to the circulation.

Erythrocyte Disorders

Most erythrocyte disorders can be classified as anemia or polycythemia. We describe some of the many varieties and causes of these conditions next.

Anemia **Anemia** (ah-ne′me-ah; "lacking blood") is a condition in which the blood's oxygen-carrying capacity is too low to support normal metabolism. It is a *sign* of some disorder rather than a disease in itself. Its hallmark is blood oxygen levels that are inadequate to support normal metabolism. Anemic individuals are fatigued, often pale, short of breath, and chilled.

The causes of anemia can be divided into three groups: blood loss, not enough red blood cells produced, or too many of them destroyed.

- **Blood loss.** *Hemorrhagic anemia* (hem″o-raj′ik) is caused by blood loss. In acute hemorrhagic anemia, blood loss is rapid (as might follow a severe stab wound); it is treated by replacing the lost blood. Slight but persistent blood loss (due to hemorrhoids or an undiagnosed bleeding ulcer, for example) causes chronic hemorrhagic anemia. Once the primary problem is resolved, normal erythropoietic mechanisms replace the lost blood cells.
- **Not enough red blood cells produced.** A number of problems can decrease erythrocyte production. These problems range from lack of essential raw materials (such as iron) to complete and utter failure of the red bone marrow.

  Iron-deficiency anemia is generally a secondary result of hemorrhagic anemia, but it also results from inadequate

17

intake of iron-containing foods and impaired iron absorption. The erythrocytes produced, called **microcytes**, are small and pale because they cannot synthesize their normal complement of hemoglobin. The obvious treatment is to increase iron intake in diet or through iron supplements.

Pernicious anemia is an autoimmune disease that most often affects the elderly. The immune system of these individuals destroys cells of their own stomach mucosa. These cells produce a substance called **intrinsic factor** that must be present for vitamin B_{12} to be absorbed by intestinal cells. Without vitamin B_{12}, the developing erythrocytes grow but cannot divide, and large, pale cells called **macrocytes** result. Treatment involves regular intramuscular injections of vitamin B_{12} or application of a B_{12}-containing gel to the nasal lining once a week.

As you might expect, lack of vitamin B_{12} in the diet also leads to anemia. However, this is usually a problem only in strict vegetarians because meats, poultry, and fish provide ample vitamin B_{12} in the diet of nonvegetarians.

Renal anemia is caused by the lack of EPO, the hormone that controls red blood cell production. Renal anemia frequently accompanies renal disease because damaged or diseased kidneys cannot produce enough EPO. Fortunately, it can be treated with synthetic EPO.

Aplastic anemia may result from destruction or inhibition of the red marrow by certain drugs and chemicals, ionizing radiation, or viruses. In most cases, though, the cause is unknown. Because marrow destruction impairs formation of *all* formed elements, anemia is just one of its signs. Defects in blood clotting and immunity are also present. Blood transfusions provide a stopgap treatment until stem cells harvested from a donor's blood, bone marrow, or umbilical cord blood can be transplanted.

- **Too many red blood cells destroyed.** In *hemolytic anemias* (he″mo-lit′ik), erythrocytes rupture, or lyse, prematurely. Hemoglobin abnormalities, transfusion of mismatched blood, and certain bacterial and parasitic infections are possible causes. Here we focus on the hemoglobin abnormalities.

Production of abnormal hemoglobin usually has a genetic basis. Two such examples, thalassemia and sickle-cell anemia, can be serious, incurable, and sometimes fatal diseases. In both diseases the globin part of hemoglobin is abnormal and the erythrocytes produced are fragile and rupture prematurely.

Thalassemias (thal″ah-se′me-ahs; "sea blood") typically occur in people of Mediterranean ancestry, such as Greeks and Italians. One of the globin chains is absent or faulty, and the erythrocytes are thin, delicate, and deficient in hemoglobin. There are many subtypes of thalassemia, classified according to which hemoglobin chain is affected and where. They range in severity from mild to so severe that monthly blood transfusions are required.

In **sickle-cell anemia**, the havoc caused by the abnormal hemoglobin, *hemoglobin S* (*HbS*), results from a change in just one of the 146 amino acids in a beta chain of the globin molecule! (See **Figure 17.8**.) This alteration causes the beta chains to link together under low-oxygen conditions, forming stiff rods so that hemoglobin S becomes spiky and sharp. This, in turn, causes the red blood cells to become crescent shaped when they unload oxygen molecules or when the oxygen content of the blood is lower than normal, as during vigorous exercise and other activities that increase metabolic rate.

The stiff, deformed erythrocytes rupture easily and tend to dam up in small blood vessels. These events interfere with oxygen delivery, leaving the victims gasping for air and in extreme pain. Bone and chest pain are particularly severe, and infection and stroke are common sequels. Blood transfusion is still the standard treatment for an acute sickle-cell crisis, but preliminary results using inhaled nitric oxide to dilate blood vessels are promising.

Sickle-cell anemia occurs chiefly in black people who live in the malaria belt of Africa and among their descendants. It strikes nearly one of every 500 black newborns in the United States.

Why would such a dangerous genetic trait persist in a population? Globally, about 250 million people are infected with malaria and about a million die each year. While individuals with two copies of the sickle-cell gene have sickle-cell

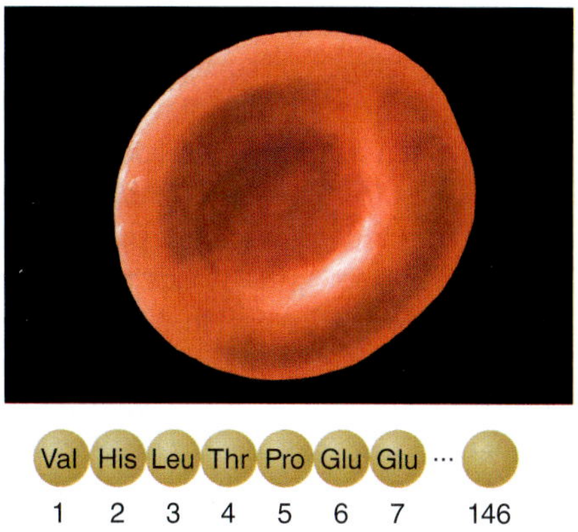

(a) Normal erythrocyte has normal hemoglobin amino acid sequence in the beta chain.

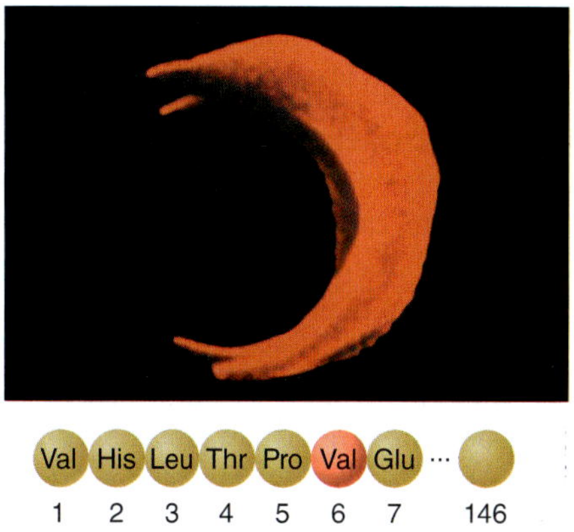

(b) Sickled erythrocyte results from a single amino acid change in the beta chain of hemoglobin.

Figure 17.8 Sickle-cell anemia. Scanning electron micrographs (4950×).

anemia, individuals with only one copy of the gene (sickle-cell trait) have a better chance of surviving malaria. Their cells only sickle under abnormal circumstances, most importantly when they are infected with malaria. Sickling reduces the malaria parasites' ability to survive and enhances macrophages' ability to destroy infected RBCs and the parasites they contain.

Several treatment approaches focus on preventing RBCs from sickling. Fetal hemoglobin (HbF) does not "sickle," even in those destined to have sickle-cell anemia. *Hydroxyurea*, a drug used to treat chronic leukemia, switches the fetal hemoglobin gene back on. This drug dramatically reduces the excruciating pain and overall severity and complications of sickle-cell anemia (by 50%). Another class of drugs reduces sickling by blocking ion channels in the RBC membrane, keeping ions and water inside the cell. Other approaches being tested include oral arginine to stimulate nitric oxide production and dilate blood vessels, stem cell transplants, and gene therapy to deliver genes for synthesizing normal beta chains.

Polycythemia **Polycythemia** (pol″e-si-the′me-ah; "many blood cells") is an abnormal excess of erythrocytes that increases blood viscosity, causing it to sludge, or flow sluggishly. *Polycythemia vera*, a bone marrow cancer, is characterized by dizziness and an exceptionally high RBC count (8–11 million cells/μl). The hematocrit may be as high as 80% and blood volume may double, causing the vascular system to become engorged with blood and severely impairing circulation. Severe polycythemia is treated by diluting blood—removing some blood and replacing it with saline.

Secondary polycythemias result when less oxygen is available or EPO production increases. The secondary polycythemia that appears in individuals living at high altitudes is a normal physiological response to the reduced atmospheric pressure and lower oxygen content of the air in such areas. RBC counts of 6–8 million/μl are common in such people.

17

Blood doping, practiced by some athletes competing in aerobic events, is artificially induced polycythemia. Some of the athlete's red blood cells are drawn off and stored. The body quickly replaces these erythrocytes because removing blood triggers the erythropoietin mechanism. Then, when the stored blood is reinfused a few days before the athletic event, a temporary polycythemia results.

Since red blood cells carry oxygen, the additional infusion should translate into increased oxygen-carrying capacity due to a higher hematocrit, and hence greater endurance and speed. Other than the risk of stroke and heart failure due to high hematocrit and high blood viscosity described earlier, blood doping seems to work. However, the practice is considered unethical and has been banned from the Olympic Games.

☑ Check Your Understanding

4. How many molecules of oxygen can each hemoglobin molecule transport? What part of the hemoglobin binds the oxygen?
5. Patients with advanced kidney disease often have anemia. Explain the connection.

For answers, see Appendix H.

Leukocytes (White Blood Cells)

✓ List the classes, structural characteristics, and functions of leukocytes.

✓ Describe how leukocytes are produced.

✓ Give examples of leukocyte disorders, and explain what goes wrong in each disorder.

General Structural and Functional Characteristics

Leukocytes (*leuko* = white), or **white blood cells (WBCs)**, are the only formed elements that are complete cells, with nuclei and the usual organelles. Accounting for less than 1% of total blood volume, leukocytes are far less numerous than red blood cells. On average, there are 4800–10,800 WBCs/μl of blood.

Leukocytes are crucial to our defense against disease. They form a mobile army that helps protect the body from damage by bacteria, viruses, parasites, toxins, and tumor cells. As such, they have special functional characteristics. Red blood cells are confined to the bloodstream, and they carry out their functions in the blood. But white blood cells are able to slip out of the capillary blood vessels—a process called **diapedesis** (di″ah-pĕ-de′sis; "leaping across")—and the circulatory system is simply their means of transport to areas of the body (mostly loose connective tissues or lymphoid tissues) where they mount inflammatory or immune responses.

As we explain in more detail in Chapter 21, the signals that prompt WBCs to leave the bloodstream at specific locations are cell adhesion molecules displayed by endothelial cells forming the capillary walls at sites of inflammation. Once out of the bloodstream, leukocytes move through the tissue spaces by **amoeboid motion** (they form flowing cytoplasmic extensions that move them along). By following the chemical trail of molecules released by damaged cells or other leukocytes, a phenomenon called **positive chemotaxis**, they pinpoint areas of tissue damage and infection and gather there in large numbers to destroy foreign substances and dead cells.

Whenever white blood cells are mobilized for action, the body speeds up their production and their numbers may double within a few hours. A *white blood cell count* of over 11,000 cells/μl is **leukocytosis**. This condition is a normal homeostatic response to an infection in the body.

Leukocytes are grouped into two major categories on the basis of structural and chemical characteristics. *Granulocytes* contain obvious membrane-bound cytoplasmic granules, and *agranulocytes* lack obvious granules. We provide general information about the various leukocytes next. More details appear in **Figure 17.9** and **Table 17.2** on p. 644.

Students are often asked to list the leukocytes in order from most abundant to least abundant. The following phrase may help you with this task: **N**ever **l**et **m**onkeys **e**at **b**ananas (neutrophils, lymphocytes, monocytes, eosinophils, basophils).

Granulocytes

Granulocytes (gran′u-lo-sīts), which include neutrophils, eosinophils, and basophils, are all roughly spherical in shape. They are larger and much shorter lived (in most cases) than

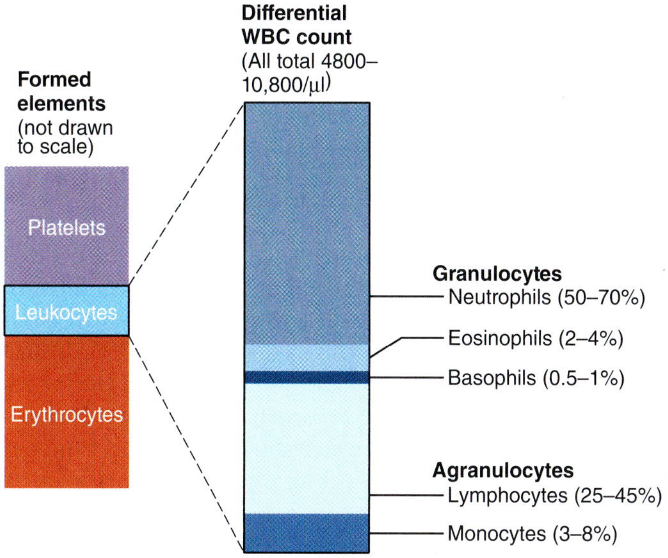

Figure 17.9 Types and relative percentages of leukocytes in normal blood. Erythrocytes comprise nearly 98% of the formed elements, and leukocytes and platelets together account for the remaining 2+%.

erythrocytes. They characteristically have lobed nuclei (rounded nuclear masses connected by thinner strands of nuclear material), and their membrane-bound cytoplasmic granules stain quite specifically with Wright's stain. Functionally, all granulocytes are phagocytes to some degree.

Neutrophils **Neutrophils** (nu′tro-filz), the most numerous white blood cells, account for 50–70% of the WBC population. Neutrophils are about twice as large as erythrocytes.

The neutrophil cytoplasm contains very fine granules (of two varieties) that are difficult to see (Table 17.2 and **Figure 17.10a**). Neutrophils get their name (literally, "neutral-loving") because their granules take up both *basic* (blue) and *acidic* (red) *dyes*. Together, the two types of granules give the cytoplasm a lilac color. Some of these granules contain hydrolytic enzymes, and are regarded as lysosomes. Others, especially the smaller granules, contain a potent "brew" of antimicrobial proteins, called **defensins**.

Neutrophil nuclei consist of three to six lobes. Because of this nuclear variability, they are often called **polymorphonuclear leukocytes** (*PMNs*) or simply *polys* (*polymorphonuclear* = many shapes of the nucleus).

Neutrophils are our body's bacteria slayers, and their numbers increase explosively during acute bacterial infections such as meningitis and appendicitis. Neutrophils are chemically attracted to sites of inflammation and are active phagocytes. They are especially partial to bacteria and some fungi, and bacterial killing is promoted by a process called a respiratory burst. In the **respiratory burst**, the cells metabolize oxygen to produce potent germ-killer oxidizing substances such as bleach and hydrogen peroxide. In addition, defensin-mediated lysis occurs when the granules containing defensins merge with a microbe-containing phagosome. The defensins form peptide "spears" that pierce holes in the membrane of the ingested "foe."

Eosinophils **Eosinophils** (e″o-sin′o-filz) account for 2–4% of all leukocytes and are approximately the size of neutrophils. Their nucleus usually resembles an old-fashioned telephone receiver—it has two lobes connected by a broad band of nuclear material (Table 17.2 and Figure 17.10b).

Large, coarse granules that stain from brick red to crimson with acid (eosin) dyes pack the cytoplasm. These granules are lysosome-like and filled with a unique variety of digestive

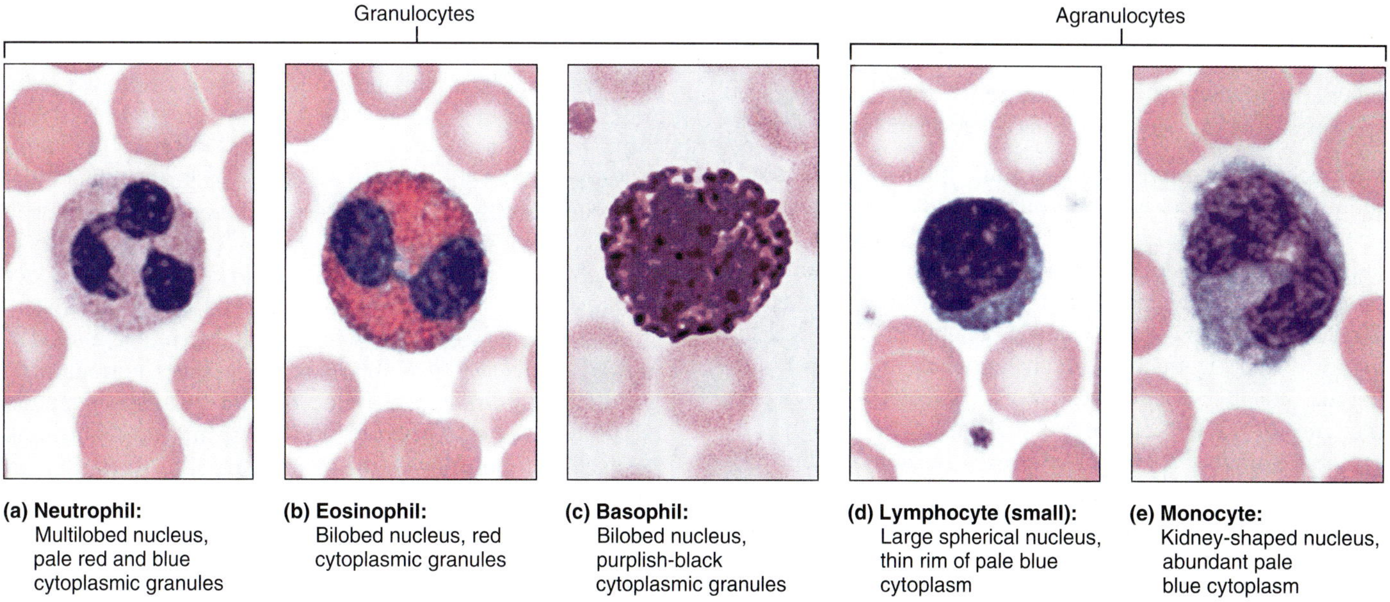

Figure 17.10 Leukocytes. In each case the leukocytes are surrounded by erythrocytes. Neutrophils, eosinophils, and basophils have visible cytoplasmic granules; lymphocytes and monocytes do not. (All 1750×, Wright's stain.)

enzymes. However, unlike typical lysosomes, they lack enzymes that specifically digest bacteria.

The most important role of eosinophils is to lead the counterattack against parasitic worms, such as flatworms (tapeworms and flukes) and roundworms (pinworms and hookworms) that are too large to be phagocytized. These worms are ingested in food (especially raw fish) or invade the body via the skin and then typically burrow into the intestinal or respiratory mucosae. Eosinophils reside in the loose connective tissues at the same body sites, and when they encounter a parasitic worm "prey," they gather around and release the enzymes from their cytoplasmic granules onto the parasite's surface, digesting it away.

Eosinophils have complex roles in many other diseases including allergies and asthma. While they contribute to the tissue damage that occurs in many immune processes, we are also beginning to recognize them as important modulators of the immune response.

Basophils **Basophils** are the rarest white blood cells, accounting for only 0.5–1% of the leukocyte population. Their cytoplasm contains large, coarse, histamine-containing granules that have an affinity for the basic dyes (*basophil* = base loving) and stain purplish-black (Figure 17.10c). *Histamine* is an inflammatory chemical that acts as a vasodilator (makes blood vessels dilate) and attracts other white blood cells to the inflamed site; drugs called antihistamines counter this effect. The deep purple nucleus is generally U or S shaped with one or two conspicuous constrictions.

Granulated cells similar to basophils, called *mast cells*, are found in connective tissues. Although mast cell nuclei tend to be more oval than lobed, the cells are similar microscopically, and both cell types bind to a particular antibody (immunoglobulin E) that causes the cells to release histamine. However, they arise from different cell lines.

17

Agranulocytes

The **agranulocytes** include lymphocytes and monocytes, WBCs that lack *visible* cytoplasmic granules. Although similar to each other structurally, they are functionally distinct and unrelated cell types. Their nuclei are typically spherical or kidney shaped.

Lymphocytes **Lymphocytes**, accounting for 25% or more of the WBC population, are the second most numerous leukocytes in the blood. When stained, a typical lymphocyte has a large, dark-purple nucleus that occupies most of the cell volume. The nucleus is usually spherical but may be slightly indented, and it is surrounded by a thin rim of pale-blue cytoplasm (Table 17.2 and Figure 17.10d). Lymphocyte diameter ranges from 5 to 17 μm, but they are often classified according to size as small (5–8 μm), medium (10–12 μm), and large (14–17 μm).

Large numbers of lymphocytes exist in the body, but relatively few (mostly the small lymphocytes) are found in the bloodstream. In fact, lymphocytes are so called because most are closely associated with lymphoid tissues (lymph nodes, spleen, etc.), where they play a crucial role in immunity. **T lymphocytes (T cells)** function in the immune response by acting directly against virus-infected cells and tumor cells. **B lymphocytes (B cells)** give rise to *plasma cells*, which produce **antibodies** (immunoglobulins) that are released to the blood. (We describe B and T lymphocyte functions in Chapter 21.)

Monocytes **Monocytes** account for 3–8% of WBCs. With an average diameter of 18 μm, they are the largest leukocytes. They have abundant pale-blue cytoplasm and a darkly staining purple nucleus, which is distinctively U or kidney shaped (Table 17.2 and Figure 17.10e).

When circulating monocytes leave the bloodstream and enter the tissues, they differentiate into highly mobile **macrophages** with prodigious appetites. Macrophages are actively phagocytic, and they are crucial in the body's defense against viruses, certain intracellular bacterial parasites, and *chronic* infections such as tuberculosis. As we explain in Chapter 21, macrophages are also important in activating lymphocytes to mount the immune response.

Production and Life Span of Leukocytes

Like erythropoiesis, **leukopoiesis**, or the production of white blood cells, is stimulated by chemical messengers. These messengers, which can act either as paracrines or hormones, are glycoproteins that fall into two families of hematopoietic factors, **interleukins** and **colony-stimulating factors**, or **CSFs**. The interleukins are numbered (e.g., IL-3, IL-5), but most CSFs are named for the leukocyte population they stimulate—for example, *granulocyte-CSF* (*G-CSF*) stimulates production of granulocytes. Hematopoietic factors, released by supporting cells of the red bone marrow and mature WBCs, not only prompt the white blood cell precursors to divide and mature, but also enhance the protective potency of mature leukocytes.

Homeostatic Imbalance 17.2

Many of the hematopoietic hormones (EPO and several of the CSFs) are used clinically. These hormones stimulate the bone marrow of cancer patients who are receiving chemotherapy (which suppresses the marrow) and of those who have received stem cell transplants, and to beef up the protective responses of AIDS patients. +

Figure 17.11 shows the pathways of leukocyte differentiation, starting with the hematopoietic stem cell that gives rise to all of the formed elements in the blood. An early branching of the pathway divides the **lymphoid stem cells**, which produce lymphocytes, from the **myeloid stem cells**, which give rise to all other formed elements. In each granulocyte line, the committed cells, called **myeloblasts** (mi'ĕ-lo-blasts"), accumulate lysosomes, becoming **promyelocytes**. The distinctive granules of each granulocyte type appear next in the **myelocyte** stage and then cell division stops. In the subsequent stage, the nuclei arc, producing the **band cell** stage. Just before granulocytes leave the marrow and enter the circulation, their nuclei constrict, beginning the process of nuclear segmentation.

The bone marrow stores mature granulocytes and usually contains about ten times more granulocytes than are found in the blood. The normal ratio of granulocytes to erythrocytes produced is about 3:1, which reflects granulocytes' much shorter life span (0.25 to 9.0 days). Most die combating invading microorganisms.

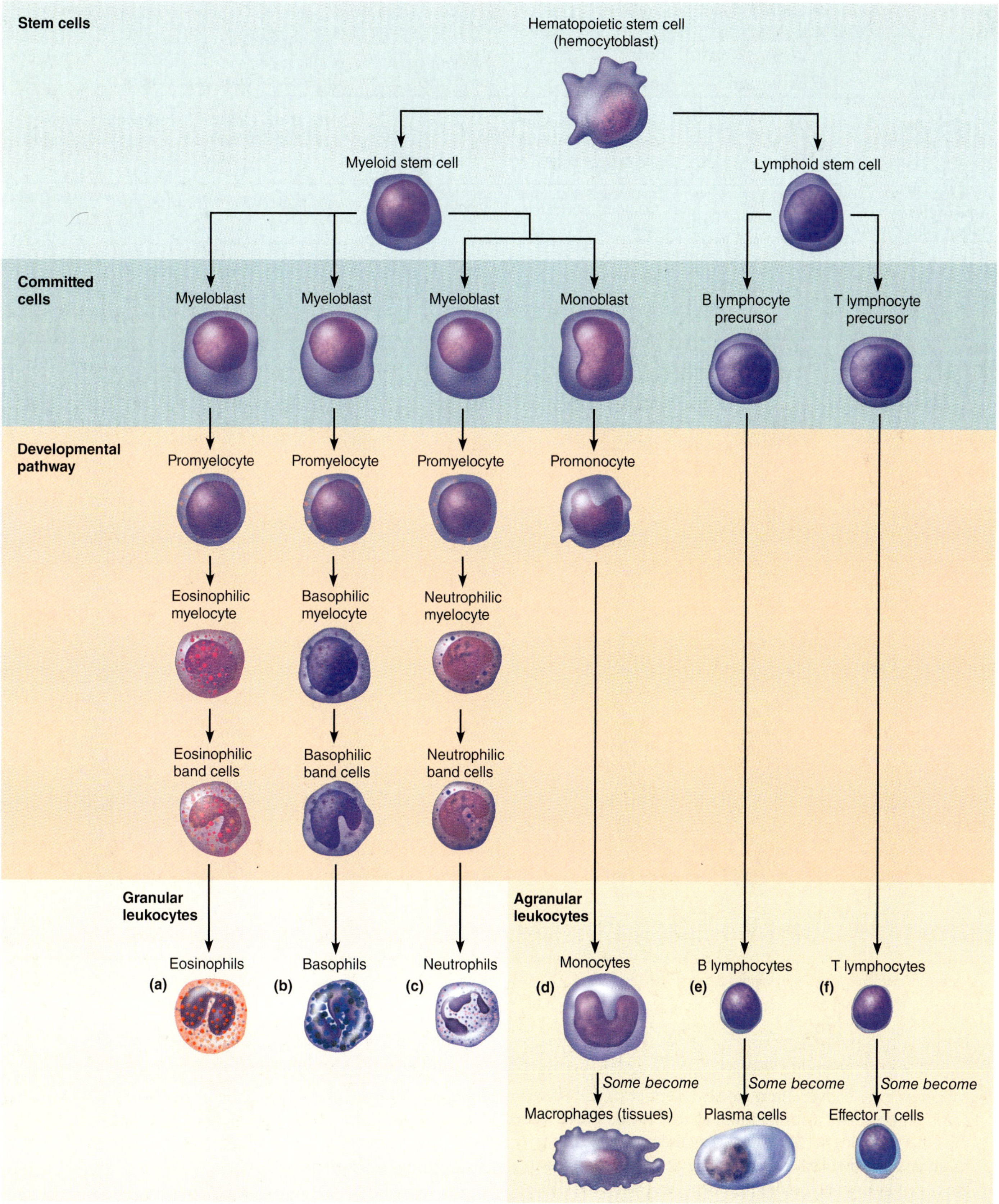

Figure 17.11 Leukocyte formation. Leukocytes arise from ancestral stem cells called hematopoietic stem cells. **(a–c)** Granular leukocytes develop via a sequence involving myeloblasts. **(d)** Monocytes, like granular leukocytes, are progeny of the myeloid stem cell and share a common precursor with neutrophils (not shown). **(e)** Only l arise via the lymphoid stem cell line

Table 17.2 Summary of Formed Elements of the Blood

CELL TYPE	ILLUSTRATION	DESCRIPTION*	CELLS/μL (mm^3) OF BLOOD	DURATION OF DEVELOPMENT (D) AND LIFE SPAN (LS)	FUNCTION
Erythrocytes (red blood cells, RBCs)	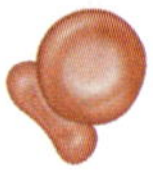	Biconcave, anucleate disc; salmon-colored; diameter 7–8 μm	4–6 million	D: about 15 days LS: 100–120 days	Transport oxygen and carbon dioxide
Leukocytes (white blood cells, WBCs)		Spherical, nucleated cells	4800–10,800		
Granulocytes					
▪ Neutrophil	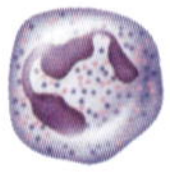	Multilobed nucleus; inconspicuous cytoplasmic granules; diameter 10–12 μm	3000–7000	D: about 14 days LS: 6 hours to a few days	Phagocytize bacteria
▪ Eosinophil	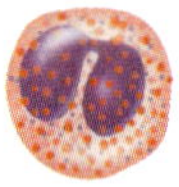	Bilobed nucleus; red cytoplasmic granules; diameter 10–14 μm	100–400	D: about 14 days LS: about 5 days	Kill parasitic worms; complex role in allergy and asthma
▪ Basophil	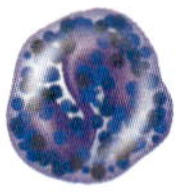	Bilobed nucleus; large purplish-black cytoplasmic granules; diameter 10–14 μm	20–50	D: 1–7 days LS: a few hours to a few days	Release histamine and other mediators of inflammation; contain heparin, an anticoagulant
Agranulocytes					
▪ Lymphocyte	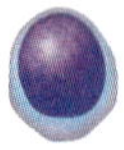	Spherical or indented nucleus; pale blue cytoplasm; diameter 5–17 μm	1500–3000	D: days to weeks LS: hours to years	Mount immune response by direct cell attack or via antibodies
▪ Monocyte	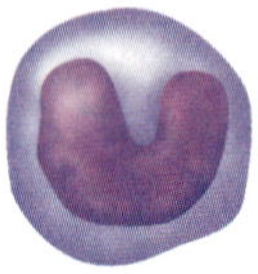	U- or kidney-shaped nucleus; gray-blue cytoplasm; diameter 14–24 μm	100–700	D: 2–3 days LS: months	Phagocytosis; develop into macrophages in the tissues
Platelets	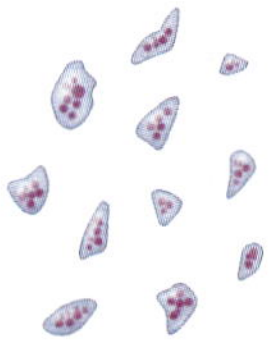	Discoid cytoplasmic fragments containing granules; stain deep purple; diameter 2–4 μm	150,000–400,000	D: 4–5 days LS: 5–10 days	Seal small tears in blood vessels; instrumental in blood clotting

*Appearance when stained with Wright's stain.

Despite their similar appearance, the two types of agranulocytes have very different lineages.

- Monocytes are derived from myeloid stem cells, and share a common precursor with neutrophils that is not shared with the other granulocytes. Cells following the monocyte line pass through the **monoblast** and **promonocyte** stages before leaving the bone marrow and becoming monocytes (Figure 17.11d).
- T and B lymphocytes are derived from **T** and **B lymphocyte precursors**, which arise from the lymphoid stem cell. The T lymphocyte precursors leave the bone marrow and travel to the thymus, where their further differentiation occurs (as we describe in Chapter 21). B lymphocyte precursors remain and mature in the bone marrow.

Monocytes may live for several months, whereas the life span of lymphocytes varies from a few hours to decades.

Leukocyte Disorders

Overproduction of abnormal leukocytes occurs in leukemia and infectious mononucleosis. At the opposite pole, **leukopenia** (loo″ko-pe′ne-ah) is an abnormally low white blood cell count (*penia* = poverty), commonly induced by drugs, particularly glucocorticoids and anticancer agents.

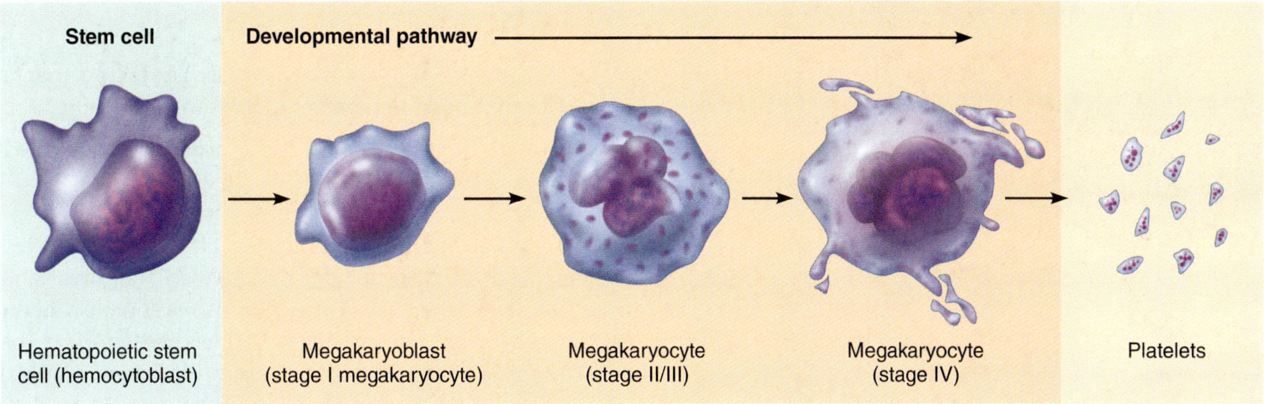

Figure 17.12 Formation of platelets. The hematopoietic stem cell gives rise to cells that undergo several mitotic divisions unaccompanied by cytoplasmic division to produce megakaryocytes. The plasma membrane of the megakaryocyte fragments, liberating the platelets. (Intermediate stages between the hematopoietic stem cell and megakaryoblast are not illustrated.)

Leukemias The term *leukemia*, literally "white blood," refers to a group of cancerous conditions involving overproduction of abnormal white blood cells. As a rule, the renegade leukocytes are members of a single *clone* (descendants of a single cell) that remain unspecialized and proliferate out of control, impairing normal red bone marrow function. The leukemias are named according to the cell type primarily involved. For example, *myeloid leukemia* involves myeloblast descendants, whereas *lymphocytic leukemia* involves the lymphocytes. Leukemia is *acute* (quickly advancing) if it derives from stem cells, and *chronic* (slowly advancing) if it involves proliferation of later cell stages.

The more serious acute forms primarily affect children. Chronic leukemia occurs more often in elderly people. Without therapy, all leukemias are fatal, and only the time course differs.

In all leukemias, cancerous leukocytes fill the red bone marrow and immature WBCs flood into the bloodstream. The other blood cell lines are crowded out, so severe anemia and bleeding problems result. Other symptoms include fever, weight loss, and bone pain. Although tremendous numbers of leukocytes are produced, they are nonfunctional and cannot defend the body in the usual way. The most common causes of death are internal hemorrhage and overwhelming infections.

Irradiation and antileukemic drugs can destroy the rapidly dividing cells and induce remissions (symptom-free periods) lasting from months to years. Stem cell transplants are used in selected patients when compatible donors are available.

Infectious Mononucleosis Sometimes called the "kissing disease," *infectious mononucleosis* is a highly contagious viral disease most often seen in young adults. Caused by the Epstein-Barr virus, its hallmark is excessive numbers of agranulocytes, many of which are atypical. The affected individual complains of being tired and achy, and has a chronic sore throat and a low-grade fever. There is no cure, but with rest the condition typically runs its course to recovery in a few weeks.

Platelets

✓ Describe the structure and function of platelets.

Platelets are not cells in the strict sense. About one-fourth the diameter of a lymphocyte, they are cytoplasmic fragments of extraordinarily large cells (up to 60 μm in diameter) called **megakaryocytes** (meg″ah-kar′e-o-sītz). In blood smears, each platelet exhibits a blue-staining outer region and an inner area containing granules that stain purple. The granules contain an impressive array of chemicals that act in the clotting process, including serotonin, Ca^{2+}, a variety of enzymes, ADP, and platelet-derived growth factor (PDGF).

Platelets are essential for the clotting process that occurs in plasma when blood vessels are ruptured or their lining is injured. By sticking to the damaged site, platelets form a temporary plug that helps seal the break. (We explain this process shortly.) Because they are anucleate, platelets age quickly and degenerate in about 10 days if they are not involved in clotting. In the meantime, they circulate freely, kept mobile but inactive by molecules (nitric oxide, prostacyclin) secreted by endothelial cells lining the blood vessels.

A hormone called **thrombopoietin** regulates the formation of platelets. Their immediate ancestral cells, the megakaryocytes, are progeny of the hematopoietic stem cell and the myeloid stem cell, but their formation is quite unusual (**Figure 17.12**). In this line, repeated mitoses of the **megakaryoblast** (also called a stage I megakaryocyte) occur, but cytokinesis does not. The final result is the mature (stage IV) megakaryocyte (literally "big nucleus cell"), a bizarre cell with a huge, multilobed nucleus and a large cytoplasmic mass.

After it forms, the megakaryocyte presses against a sinusoid (the specialized type of capillary in the red marrow) and sends cytoplasmic extensions through the sinusoid wall into the bloodstream. These extensions rupture, releasing the platelet fragments like stamps being torn from a sheet of postage

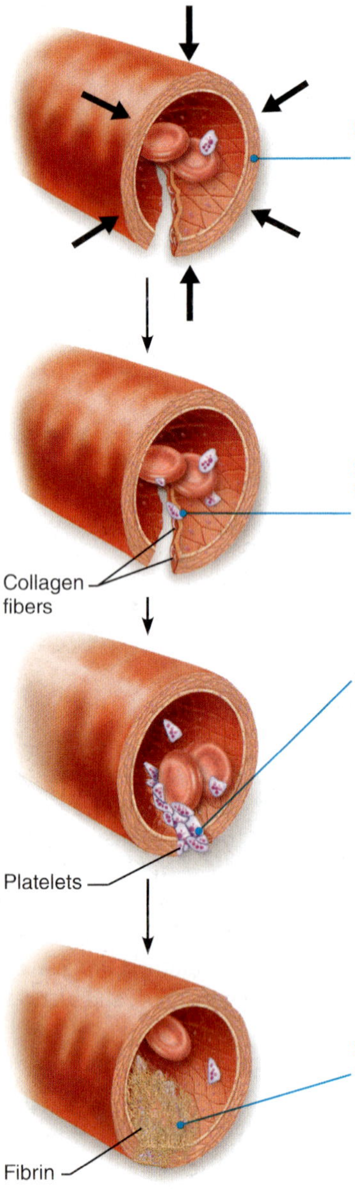

Figure 17.13 Events of hemostasis.

17

stamps and seeding the blood with platelets. The plasma membranes associated with each fragment quickly seal around the cytoplasm to form the grainy, roughly disc-shaped platelets (see Table 17.2), each with a diameter of 2–4 μm. Each microliter of blood contains 150,000 to 400,000 tiny platelets.

Check Your Understanding

6. Which WBCs turn into macrophages in tissues? Which other WBC is a voracious phagocyte?
7. Platelets are called "thrombocytes" in other animals. Which term that you've just learned relates to this name? What does this term mean?
8. Amos has leukemia. Even though his WBC count is abnormally high, Amos is prone to severe infections, bleeding, and anemia. Explain.

For answers, see Appendix H.

Hemostasis

✓ Describe the process of hemostasis. List factors that limit clot formation and prevent undesirable clotting.

✓ Give examples of hemostatic disorders. Indicate the cause of each condition.

Normally, blood flows smoothly past the intact blood vessel lining (endothelium). But if a blood vessel wall breaks, a whole series of reactions is set in motion to accomplish **hemostasis** (he″mo-sta′sis), which stops the bleeding (*stasis* = halting). Without this plug-the-hole defensive reaction, we would quickly bleed out our entire blood volume from even the smallest cuts.

The hemostasis response is fast, localized, and carefully controlled. It involves many *clotting factors* normally present in plasma as well as several substances that are released by platelets and injured tissue cells. During hemostasis, three steps occur in rapid sequence **(Figure 17.13)**: (1) vascular spasm, (2) platelet plug formation, and (3) coagulation (blood clotting). Following hemostasis, the clot retracts. It then dissolves as it is replaced by fibrous tissue that permanently prevents blood loss.

Step 1: Vascular Spasm

In the first step, the damaged blood vessels respond to injury by constricting (vasoconstriction) (Figure 17.13 (1)). Factors that trigger this **vascular spasm** include direct injury to vascular smooth muscle, chemicals released by endothelial cells and platelets, and reflexes initiated by local pain receptors. The spasm mechanism becomes more and more efficient as the amount of tissue damage increases, and is most effective in the smaller blood vessels. The spasm response is valuable because a strongly constricted artery can significantly reduce blood loss for 20–30 minutes, allowing time for the next two steps, platelet plug formation and blood clotting, to occur.

Step 2: Platelet Plug Formation

In the second step, platelets play a key role in hemostasis by aggregating (sticking together), forming a plug that temporarily seals the break in the vessel wall (Figure 17.13 (2)). They also help orchestrate subsequent events that form a blood clot.

As a rule, platelets do not stick to each other or to the smooth endothelial linings of blood vessels. Intact endothelial cells release nitric oxide and a prostaglandin called **prostacyclin** (or PGI_2). Both chemicals prevent platelet aggregation in undamaged tissue and restrict aggregation to the site of injury.

However, when the endothelium is damaged and the underlying collagen fibers are exposed, platelets adhere tenaciously to the collagen fibers. A large plasma protein called *von Willebrand factor* stabilizes bound platelets by forming a bridge between collagen and platelets. Platelets swell, form spiked processes, become stickier, and release chemical messengers including the following:

- **Adenosine diphosphate (ADP)**—a potent aggregating agent that causes more platelets to stick to the area and release their contents

Table 17.3 Blood Clotting Factors (Procoagulants)

FACTOR NUMBER	FACTOR NAME	NATURE	SOURCE	PATHWAY; FUNCTION
I	Fibrinogen	Plasma protein	Liver	Common pathway; converted to fibrin (insoluble weblike substance of clot)
II	Prothrombin	Plasma protein	Liver*	Common pathway; converted to thrombin (converts fibrinogen to fibrin)
III	Tissue factor (TF)	Plasma membrane glycoprotein	Tissue cells	Activates extrinsic pathway
IV	Calcium ions (Ca^{2+})	Inorganic ion	Plasma	Needed for essentially all stages of coagulation process; always present
V	Proaccelerin	Plasma protein	Liver, platelets	Common pathway
VI†				
VII	Proconvertin	Plasma protein	Liver*	Both extrinsic and intrinsic pathways
VIII	Antihemophilic factor (AHF)	Plasma protein	Liver, lung capillaries	Intrinsic pathway; deficiency results in hemophilia A
IX	Plasma thromboplastin component (PTC)	Plasma protein	Liver*	Intrinsic pathway; deficiency results in hemophilia B
X	Stuart factor	Plasma protein	Liver*	Common pathway
XI	Plasma thromboplastin antecedent (PTA)	Plasma protein	Liver	Intrinsic pathway; deficiency results in hemophilia C
XII	Hageman factor	Plasma protein; activated by negatively charged surfaces (e.g., glass)	Liver	Intrinsic pathway; activates plasmin; initiates clotting in vitro; activation initiates inflammation
XIII	Fibrin stabilizing factor (FSF)	Plasma protein	Liver, bone marrow	Cross-links fibrin, forming a strong, stable clot

*Synthesis requires vitamin K

†Number no longer used; substance now believed to be same as factor V

- **Serotonin** and **thromboxane A_2** (throm-boks′ān; a short-lived prostaglandin derivative)—messengers that enhance vascular spasm and platelet aggregation

As more platelets aggregate, they release more chemicals, aggregating more platelets, and so on, in a positive feedback cycle (see Figure 1.6 on p. 11). Within one minute, a platelet plug is built up, further reducing blood loss. Platelets alone are sufficient for sealing the thousands of minute rips and holes that occur unnoticed as part of the daily wear and tear in your smallest blood vessels. Because platelet plugs are loosely knit, larger breaks need additional reinforcement.

Step 3: Coagulation

The third step, **coagulation** or **blood clotting**, reinforces the platelet plug with fibrin threads that act as a "molecular glue" for the aggregated platelets (Figure 17.13 ③). The resulting blood clot (fibrin mesh) is quite effective in sealing larger breaks in a blood vessel. Blood is transformed from a liquid to a gel in a multistep process that involves a series of substances called **clotting factors**, or **procoagulants** (Table 17.3).

Most clotting factors are plasma proteins synthesized by the liver. They are numbered I to XIII according to the order of their discovery; hence, the numerical order does not reflect their reaction sequence. All (except tissue factor) normally circulate in blood in inactive form until mobilized. Although vitamin K is not directly involved in coagulation, this fat-soluble vitamin is required for synthesizing four of the clotting factors (Table 17.3).

Figure 17.14 illustrates the way clotting factors act together to form a clot. The coagulation sequence looks intimidating at first glance, but two things will help you cope with its complexity. First, realize that in most cases, *activation turns clotting factors into enzymes* by clipping off a piece of the protein, causing it to change shape. Once one clotting factor is activated, it activates the next in sequence, and so on, in a cascade. (In Figure 17.14, we use the subscript "a" to denote the activated clotting factor.) Two important exceptions to this generalization are fibrinogen and Ca^{2+}, as we will see below.

The second strategy that will help you cope is to recognize that coagulation occurs in three phases. Each phase has a specific end point, as we discuss next.

Phase 1: Two Pathways to Prothrombin Activator

Coagulation may be initiated by either the **intrinsic** or the **extrinsic pathway**. In the body, the same tissue-damaging events usually trigger both pathways. Outside the body (such as in a test tube), *only* the intrinsic pathway initiates blood clotting. Before we examine how these pathways are different, let's see what they have in common.

17

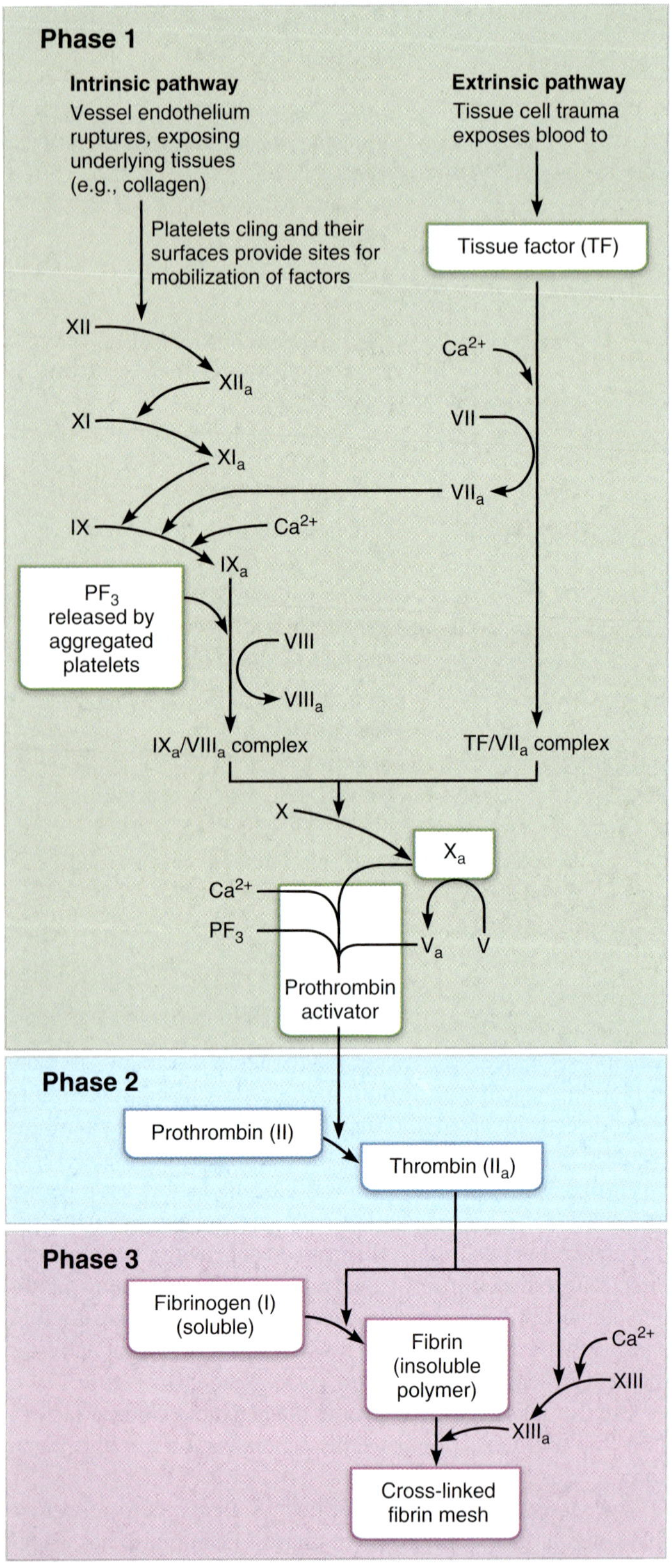

Figure 17.14 The intrinsic and extrinsic pathways of blood clotting (coagulation). The subscript "a" indicates the activated clotting factor (procoagulant).

Pivotal components in both pathways are negatively charged membranes, particularly those of platelets, that contain phosphatidylserine, also known as **PF_3** (platelet factor 3). Many intermediates of both pathways can be activated only in the presence of PF_3. The intermediate steps of each pathway *cascade* toward a common intermediate, factor X (Figure 17.14). Once factor X has been activated, it complexes with calcium ions, PF_3, and factor V to form **prothrombin activator**. This is usually the slowest step of the blood clotting process, but once prothrombin activator is present, the clot forms in 10 to 15 seconds.

The intrinsic and extrinsic pathways usually work together and are interconnected in many ways, but there are significant differences between them. The *intrinsic pathway* is

- Called *intrinsic* because the factors needed for clotting are present *within* (intrinsic to) the blood.
- Triggered by negatively charged surfaces such as activated platelets, collagen, or glass. (This is why this pathway can initiate clotting in a test tube.)
- Slower because it has many intermediate steps.

The *extrinsic pathway* is

- Called *extrinsic* because the tissue factor it requires is *outside* of blood.
- Triggered by exposing blood to a factor found in tissues underneath the damaged endothelium. This factor is called **tissue factor (TF)** or **factor III**.
- Faster because it bypasses several steps of the intrinsic pathway. In severe tissue trauma, it can form a clot in 15 seconds.

Phase 1 ends with the formation of a complex substance called *prothrombin activator.*

Phase 2: Common Pathway to Thrombin

Prothrombin activator catalyzes the conversion of a plasma protein called **prothrombin** into the active enzyme **thrombin**.

Phase 3: Common Pathway to the Fibrin Mesh

The end point of phase 3 is a *fibrin mesh* that traps blood cells and effectively seals the hole until the blood vessel can be permanently repaired. Thrombin catalyzes the transformation of the *soluble* clotting factor **fibrinogen** into **fibrin**. The fibrin molecules then polymerize (join together) to form long, hairlike, *insoluble* fibrin strands. (Notice that, unlike other clotting factors, activating fibrinogen does not convert it into an enzyme, but instead allows it to polymerize.) The fibrin strands glue the platelets together and make a web that forms the structural basis of the clot. Fibrin makes the liquid plasma become gel-like and traps formed elements that try to pass through it **(Figure 17.15)**.

In the presence of calcium ions, thrombin also activates **factor XIII (fibrin stabilizing factor)**, a cross-linking enzyme that binds the fibrin strands tightly together, forming a fibrin mesh. Cross-linking further strengthens and stabilizes the clot, effectively sealing the hole until the blood vessel can be permanently repaired.

Factors that inhibit clotting are called **anticoagulants**. Whether or not blood clots depends on a delicate balance between clotting factors and anticoagulants. Normally, anticoagulants dominate and prevent clotting, but when a vessel is ruptured, clotting factor activity in that area increases

17

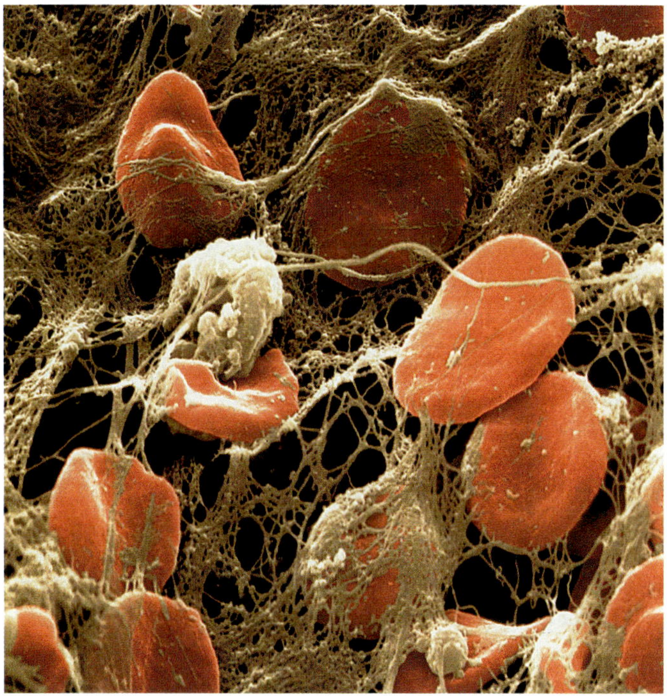

Figure 17.15 Scanning electron micrograph of erythrocytes trapped in a fibrin mesh. (2700×).

dramatically and a clot begins to form. Clot formation is normally complete within 3 to 6 minutes after blood vessel damage.

Clot Retraction and Fibrinolysis

Although the process of hemostasis is complete when the fibrin mesh is formed, there are still things that need to be done to stabilize the clot and then remove it when the injury is healed and the clot is no longer needed.

Clot Retraction

Within 30 to 60 minutes, a platelet-induced process called **clot retraction** further stabilizes the clot. Platelets contain contractile proteins (actin and myosin), and they contract in much the same manner as smooth muscle cells. As the platelets contract, they pull on the surrounding fibrin strands, squeezing **serum** (plasma minus the clotting proteins) from the mass, compacting the clot and drawing the ruptured edges of the blood vessel more closely together.

Even as clot retraction is occurring, the vessel is healing. **Platelet-derived growth factor (PDGF)** released by platelets stimulates smooth muscle cells and fibroblasts to divide and rebuild the vessel wall. As fibroblasts form a connective tissue patch in the injured area, endothelial cells, stimulated by vascular endothelial growth factor (VEGF), multiply and restore the endothelial lining.

Fibrinolysis

A clot is not a permanent solution to blood vessel injury, and a process called **fibrinolysis** removes unneeded clots when healing has occurred. This cleanup detail is crucial because small clots form continually in vessels throughout the body. Without fibrinolysis, blood vessels would gradually become completely blocked.

The critical natural "clot buster" is a fibrin-digesting enzyme called **plasmin**, which is produced when the plasma protein **plasminogen** is activated. Large amounts of plasminogen are incorporated into a forming clot, where it remains inactive until appropriate signals reach it. The presence of a clot in and around the blood vessel causes the endothelial cells to secrete **tissue plasminogen activator (tPA).** Activated factor XII and thrombin released during clotting also activate plasminogen. As a result, most plasmin activity is confined to the clot, and circulating enzymes quickly destroy any plasmin that strays into the plasma. Fibrinolysis begins within two days and continues slowly over several days until the clot finally dissolves.

Factors Limiting Clot Growth or Formation

Factors Limiting Normal Clot Growth

Once the clotting cascade has begun, it continues until a clot forms. Normally, two homeostatic mechanisms prevent clots from becoming unnecessarily large: (1) swift removal of clotting factors, and (2) inhibition of activated clotting factors. For clotting to occur in the first place, the concentration of activated clotting factors must reach certain critical levels. Clots do not usually form in rapidly moving blood because the activated clotting factors are diluted and washed away. For the same reasons, a clot stops growing when it contacts blood flowing normally.

Other mechanisms block the final step in which fibrinogen is polymerized into fibrin. They work by restricting thrombin to the clot or by inactivating it if it escapes into the general circulation. As a clot forms, almost all of the thrombin produced is bound onto the fibrin threads. This is an important safeguard because thrombin also exerts positive feedback effects on the coagulation process prior to the common pathway. Not only does it speed up the production of prothrombin activator by acting indirectly through factor V, but it also accelerates the earliest steps of the intrinsic pathway by activating platelets. By binding thrombin, fibrin effectively acts as an anticoagulant, preventing the clot from enlarging and thrombin from acting elsewhere.

Antithrombin III, a protein present in plasma, quickly inactivates any thrombin not bound to fibrin. Antithrombin III and **protein C**, another protein produced in the liver, also inhibit the activity of other intrinsic pathway clotting factors.

Heparin, the natural anticoagulant contained in basophil and mast cell granules, is also found on the surface of endothelial cells. It inhibits thrombin by enhancing the activity of antithrombin III. Like most other clotting inhibitors, heparin also inhibits the intrinsic pathway.

Factors Preventing Undesirable Clotting

As long as the endothelium is smooth and intact, platelets are prevented from clinging and piling up. Also, antithrombic substances—nitric oxide and prostacyclin—secreted by the endothelial cells normally prevent platelet adhesion. Additionally, vitamin E quinone, a molecule formed in the body when vitamin E reacts with oxygen, is a potent anticoagulant.

Disorders of Hemostasis

Blood clotting is one of nature's most elegant creations, but it sometimes goes awry. The two major disorders of hemostasis are at opposite poles. **Thromboembolic disorders** result from conditions that cause undesirable clot formation. **Bleeding disorders** arise from abnormalities that prevent normal clot formation. **Disseminated intravascular coagulation (DIC)**, which has characteristics of both types of disorder, involves both widespread clotting and severe bleeding.

Thromboembolic Disorders

Despite the body's many safeguards, undesirable intravascular clotting, called "hemostasis in the wrong place" by some, sometimes occurs.

Thrombi and Emboli A clot that develops and persists in an *unbroken* blood vessel is called a **thrombus**. If the thrombus is large enough, it may block circulation to the cells beyond the occlusion and lead to death of those tissues. For example, if the blockage occurs in the coronary circulation of the heart (coronary thrombosis), the consequences may be death of heart muscle and a fatal heart attack.

If the thrombus breaks away from the vessel wall and floats freely in the bloodstream, it becomes an **embolus** (plural: *emboli*). An embolus ("wedge") is usually no problem until it encounters a blood vessel too narrow for it to pass through. Then it becomes an **embolism**, obstructing the vessel. For example, emboli that become trapped in the lungs (pulmonary embolisms) dangerously impair the body's ability to obtain oxygen. A cerebral embolism may cause a stroke.

Conditions that roughen the vessel endothelium, such as atherosclerosis or inflammation, cause thromboembolic disease by allowing platelets to gain a foothold. Slowly flowing blood or blood stasis is another risk factor, particularly in bedridden patients and those taking a long flight without moving around. In this case, clotting factors are not washed away as usual and accumulate, allowing clots to form.

Anticoagulant Drugs A number of drugs—most importantly aspirin, heparin, and warfarin—are used clinically to prevent undesirable clotting. **Aspirin** is an antiprostaglandin drug that inhibits thromboxane A_2 formation (blocking platelet aggregation and platelet plug formation). Clinical studies of men taking low-dose aspirin (one aspirin every two days) over several years demonstrated a 50% reduction in incidence of heart attack.

Other medications that are prescribed as anticoagulants are heparin (see above) and warfarin, an ingredient in rat poison. Administered in injectable form, heparin is the anticoagulant most used in the hospital (for preoperative and postoperative heart patients and for those receiving blood transfusions). Taken orally, **warfarin** (Coumadin) is a mainstay of outpatient treatment to reduce the risk of stroke in those prone to atrial fibrillation, a condition in which blood pools in the heart. Warfarin works via a different mechanism than heparin—it interferes with the action of vitamin K in the production of some clotting factors (see Impaired Liver Function below). New on the scene is *dabigatran*, a direct inhibitor of thrombin that is a welcome alternative to warfarin.

The *Closer Look* box in Chapter 19 (pp. 700–701) describes other drugs that dissolve blood clots (such as tPA) and innovative medical techniques for treating clots.

Bleeding Disorders

Anything that interferes with the clotting mechanism can result in abnormal bleeding. The most common causes are platelet deficiency (thrombocytopenia) and deficits of some clotting factors, which can result from impaired liver function or genetic conditions such as hemophilia.

Thrombocytopenia A condition in which the number of circulating platelets is deficient, **thrombocytopenia** (throm″bo-si″to-pe′ne-ah) causes spontaneous bleeding from small blood vessels all over the body. Even normal movement leads to widespread hemorrhage, evidenced by many small purplish spots, called *petechiae* (pe-te′ke-e), on the skin.

Thrombocytopenia can arise from any condition that suppresses or destroys the red bone marrow, such as bone marrow malignancy, exposure to ionizing radiation, or certain drugs. A platelet count of under 50,000/μl of blood is usually diagnostic for this condition. Transfusions of concentrated platelets provide temporary relief from bleeding.

Impaired Liver Function When the liver is unable to synthesize its usual supply of clotting factors, abnormal and often severe bleeding occurs. The causes can range from an easily resolved vitamin K deficiency (common in newborns) to nearly total impairment of liver function (as in hepatitis or cirrhosis).

Liver cells require vitamin K to produce clotting factors. Although intestinal bacteria make some vitamin K, we obtain most of it from vegetables in our diet and dietary deficiencies are rarely a problem. However, vitamin K deficiency can occur if fat absorption is impaired, because vitamin K is a fat-soluble vitamin that is absorbed into the blood along with fats. In liver disease, the nonfunctional liver cells fail to produce not only the clotting factors, but also bile that is required to absorb fat and vitamin K.

Hemophilias The term **hemophilia** refers to several hereditary bleeding disorders that have similar signs and symptoms. *Hemophilia A* results from a deficiency of **factor VIII (antihemophilic factor)**. It accounts for 77% of cases. *Hemophilia B* results from a deficiency of factor IX. Both types are genetic conditions that occur primarily in males (X-linked conditions, discussed in Chapter 29). *Hemophilia C*, a less severe form seen in both sexes, is due to a lack of factor XI. The relative mildness of hemophilia C, compared to the A and B forms, reflects the fact that the clotting factor (factor IX) that the missing factor XI activates can also be activated by factor VII (see Figure 17.14).

Symptoms of hemophilia begin early in life. Even minor tissue trauma causes prolonged and potentially life-threatening bleeding into tissues. Commonly, the person's joints become seriously disabled and painful because of repeated bleeding into the joint cavities after exercise or trauma. Hemophilias are managed clinically by transfusions of fresh plasma or injections of the appropriate purified clotting factor. These therapies provide relief for several days but are expensive and inconvenient.

In addition, dependence on transfusions or injections has caused other problems. In the past, many hemophilia patients became infected by the hepatitis virus and, beginning in the early 1980s, by HIV, a blood-transmitted virus that depresses the immune system and causes AIDS. (See Chapter 21.) New infections are now avoided as a result of new testing methods for HIV, availability of genetically engineered clotting factors, and hepatitis vaccines.

Disseminated Intravascular Coagulation (DIC)

DIC is a situation in which widespread clotting occurs in intact blood vessels and the residual blood becomes unable to clot. Blockage of blood flow accompanied by severe bleeding follows. DIC most commonly happens as a complication of pregnancy or a result of septicemia or incompatible blood transfusions.

☑ Check Your Understanding

9. What are the three steps of hemostasis?
10. What is the key difference between fibrinogen and fibrin? Between prothrombin and thrombin? Between most factors before and after they are activated?
11. Which bleeding disorder results from not having enough platelets? From absence of clotting factor VIII?

For answers, see Appendix H.

Transfusion and Blood Replacement

✓ Describe the ABO and Rh blood groups. Explain the basis of transfusion reactions.

✓ Describe fluids used to replace blood volume and the circumstances for their use.

The human cardiovascular system minimizes the effects of blood loss by (1) reducing the volume of the affected blood vessels, and (2) stepping up the production of red blood cells. However, the body can compensate for only so much blood loss. Losing 15–30% causes pallor and weakness. Losing more than 30% of blood volume results in severe shock, which can be fatal.

Transfusing Red Blood Cells

Whole blood transfusions are routine when blood loss is rapid and substantial. In all other cases, infusions of **packed red cells** (whole blood from which most of the plasma and leukocytes have been removed) are preferred for restoring oxygen-carrying capacity. The usual blood bank procedure involves collecting blood from a donor and mixing it with an anticoagulant, such as certain citrate or oxalate salts, which prevents clotting by binding calcium ions. The shelf life of the collected blood at 4°C is about 35 days. Because blood is such a valuable commodity, it is most often separated into its component parts so that each component can be used when and where it is needed.

Human Blood Groups

People have different blood types, and transfusion of incompatible blood can be fatal. RBC plasma membranes, like those of all body cells, bear highly specific glycoproteins at their external surfaces, which identify each of us as unique from all others. These glycoprotein markers are called *antigens*. An antigen is anything the body perceives as foreign and that generates an immune response. Examples are toxins and molecules on the surfaces of bacteria, viruses, and cancer cells—and mismatched RBCs.

One person's RBC proteins may be recognized as foreign if transfused into someone with a different red blood cell type, and the transfused cells may be agglutinated (clumped together) and destroyed. Since these RBC antigens promote agglutination, they are more specifically called **agglutinogens** (ag″loo-tin′o-jenz).

At least 30 groups of naturally occurring RBC antigens (blood groups) are found in humans, and many variants occur in individual families ("private antigens") rather than in the general population. The presence or absence of various antigens allows a person's blood cells to be classified into each of these different blood groups. Antigens determining the ABO and Rh blood groups cause vigorous transfusion reactions (in which the foreign erythrocytes are destroyed) when they are improperly transfused. For this reason, blood typing for these antigens is always done before blood is transfused.

Other antigens (such as those in the MNS, Duffy, Kell, and Lewis groups) are mainly of legal or academic importance. Because these factors rarely cause transfusion reactions, blood is not specifically typed for them unless the person is expected to need several transfusions, in which case reactions are more likely to occur. Here we describe only the ABO and Rh blood groups.

ABO Blood Groups The **ABO blood groups** are based on the presence or absence of two agglutinogens, type A and type B (Table 17.4). Depending on which of these a person inherits, his or her ABO blood group will be one of the following: A, B, AB, or O. The O blood group, which has neither agglutinogen, is the most common ABO group in North America for whites, blacks, Asians, and Native Americans. AB, with both antigens, is least prevalent. The presence of either the A or the B agglutinogen results in group A or B, respectively.

Unique to the ABO blood groups is the presence in the plasma of *preformed antibodies* called **agglutinins**. The agglutinins act against RBCs carrying ABO antigens that are *not* present on a person's own red blood cells. A newborn lacks these antibodies, but they begin to appear in the plasma within two months and reach adult levels between 8 and 10 years of age. As indicated in Table 17.4, a person with neither the A nor the B antigen (group O) possesses both anti-A and anti-B antibodies, also called *a* and *b agglutinins* respectively. Those with group A blood have anti-B antibodies, while those with group B have anti-A antibodies. AB individuals have neither antibody.

Rh Blood Groups There are 52 named Rh agglutinogens, each of which is called an **Rh factor**. Only three of these, the C, D, and E antigens, are fairly common. The Rh blood typing system is so named because one Rh antigen (agglutinogen D) was originally identified in *rhesus* monkeys. Later, the same antigen was discovered in humans.

About 85% of Americans are Rh^+ (Rh positive), meaning that their RBCs carry the D antigen. As a rule, a person's ABO and Rh blood groups are reported together, for example, O^+, A^-, and so on.

Table 17.4 ABO Blood Groups

BLOOD GROUP	RBC ANTIGENS (AGGLUTINOGENS)	ILLUSTRATION	PLASMA ANTIBODIES (AGGLUTININS)	BLOOD THAT CAN BE RECEIVED	FREQUENCY (% OF U.S. POPULATION) WHITE	BLACK	ASIAN	NATIVE AMERICAN
AB	A B	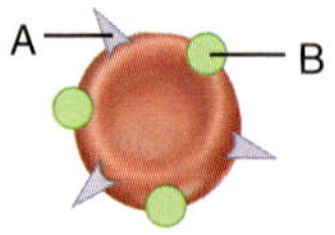	None	A, B, AB, O "Universal recipient"	4	4	5	<1
B	B	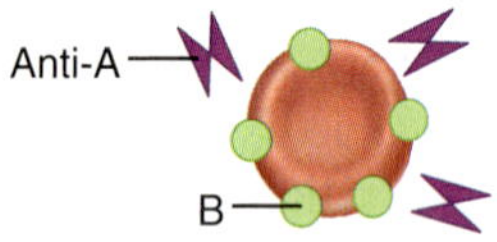	Anti-A (a)	B, O	11	20	27	4
A	A	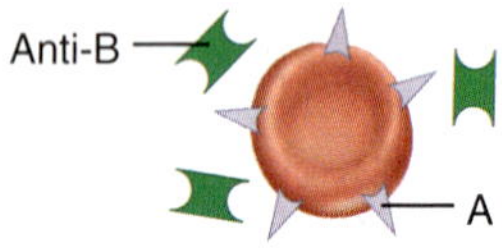	Anti-B (b)	A, O	40	27	28	16
O	None	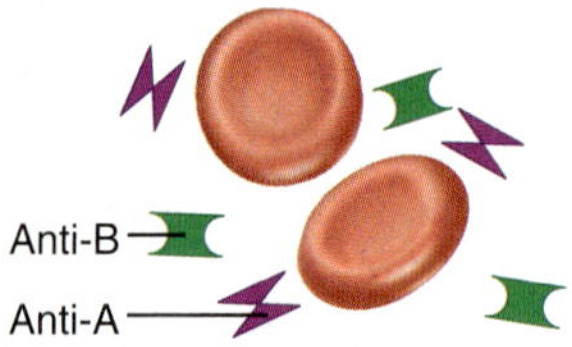	Anti-A (a) Anti-B (b)	O "Universal donor"	45	49	40	79

Unlike the ABO system antibodies, anti-Rh antibodies do not spontaneously form in the blood of Rh^- (Rh negative) individuals. However, if an Rh^- person receives Rh^+ blood, the immune system becomes sensitized and begins producing anti-Rh antibodies against the foreign antigen soon after the transfusion. Hemolysis does not occur after the first such transfusion because it takes time for the body to react and start making antibodies. But the second time, and every time thereafter, a typical transfusion reaction occurs in which the recipient's antibodies attack and rupture the donor RBCs.

Homeostatic Imbalance 17.3

An important problem related to the Rh factor occurs in pregnant Rh^- women who are carrying Rh^+ babies. The first such pregnancy usually results in the delivery of a healthy baby. But, when bleeding occurs as the placenta detaches from the uterus, the mother may be sensitized by her baby's Rh^+ antigens that pass into her bloodstream. If so, she will form anti-Rh antibodies unless treated with RhoGAM before or shortly after she has given birth. (The same precautions are taken in women who have miscarried or aborted the fetus.) RhoGAM is a serum containing anti-Rh agglutinins. By agglutinating the Rh factor, it blocks the mother's immune response and prevents her sensitization.

If the mother is not treated and becomes pregnant again with an Rh^+ baby, her antibodies will cross through the placenta and destroy the baby's RBCs, producing a condition known as **hemolytic disease of the newborn**, or **erythroblastosis fetalis**. The baby becomes anemic and hypoxic. In severe cases, brain damage and even death may result unless transfusions are done *before* birth to provide the fetus with more erythrocytes for oxygen transport. Additionally, one or two *exchange transfusions* (see Related Clinical Terms, p. 657) are done after birth. The baby's Rh^+ blood is removed, and Rh^- blood is infused. Within six weeks, the transfused Rh^- erythrocytes have been broken down and replaced with the baby's own Rh^+ cells.

Transfusion Reactions: Agglutination and Hemolysis

When mismatched blood is infused, a **transfusion reaction** occurs in which the recipient's plasma agglutinins attack the donor's red blood cells. (Note that the donor's plasma antibodies may also agglutinate the recipient's RBCs, but these antibodies are so diluted in the recipient's circulation that this does not usually present a problem.)

The initial event, agglutination of the foreign red blood cells, clogs small blood vessels throughout the body. During the next few hours, the clumped red blood cells begin to rupture or are destroyed by phagocytes, and their hemoglobin is released into the bloodstream. When the transfusion reaction is exceptionally severe, the RBCs are lysed almost immediately.

These events lead to two easily recognized problems: (1) The transfused blood cells cannot transport oxygen, and (2) the clumped red blood cells in small vessels hinder blood flow to tissues beyond those points. Less apparent, but more devastating, is the consequence of hemoglobin that escapes into the bloodstream. Circulating hemoglobin passes freely into the kidney tubules, causing cell death and renal shutdown. If shutdown is complete (acute renal failure), the recipient may die.

Transfusion reactions can also cause fever, chills, low blood pressure, rapid heartbeat, nausea, vomiting, and general toxicity, but in the absence of renal shutdown, these reactions are rarely lethal. Treatment of transfusion reactions focuses on preventing kidney damage by administering fluid and diuretics to increase urine output, diluting and washing out the hemoglobin.

As indicated in Table 17.4, group O red blood cells bear neither the A nor the B antigen, so theoretically group O is the **universal donor**. Indeed, some laboratories are developing methods to enzymatically convert other blood types to type O by clipping off the extra (A- or B-specific) sugar molecule. Since group AB plasma is devoid of antibodies to both A and B antigens, group AB people are theoretically **universal recipients** and can receive blood transfusions from any of the ABO groups. However, these classifications are misleading, because they do not take into account the other agglutinogens in blood that can trigger transfusion reactions.

The risk of transfusion reactions and transmission of life-threatening infections (particularly with HIV) from pooled blood transfusions has increased public interest in **autologous transfusions** (*auto* = self). In autologous transfusions, the patient *predonates* his or her own blood, and it is stored and immediately available if needed during an operation.

Blood Typing

It is crucial to determine the blood group of both the donor and the recipient *before* blood is transfused. **Figure 17.16** briefly outlines the general procedure for determining ABO blood type. Because it is so critical that blood groups be compatible, cross matching is also done. *Cross matching* tests whether the recipient's serum will agglutinate the donor's RBCs or the donor's serum will agglutinate the recipient's RBCs. Typing for Rh factors is done in the same manner as ABO blood typing.

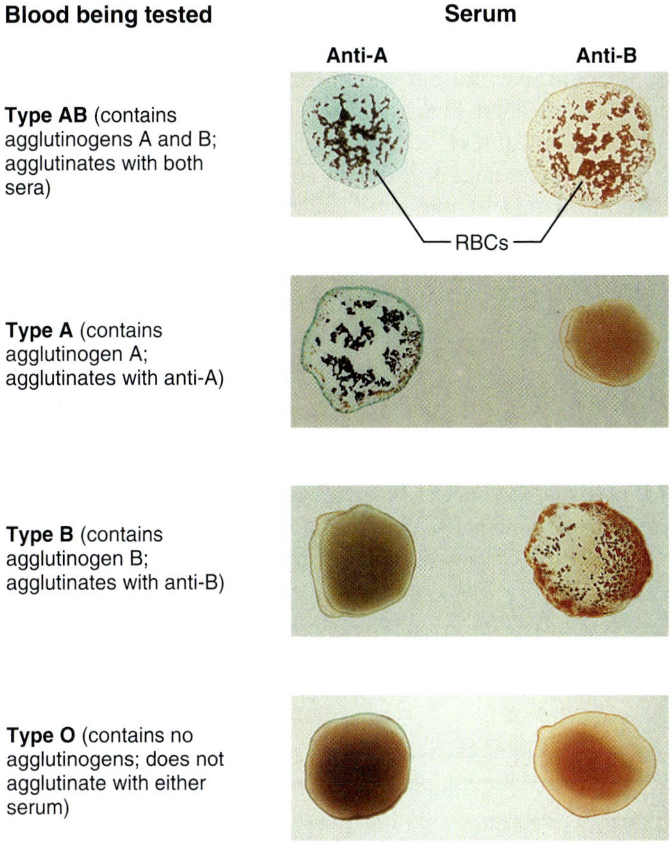

Figure 17.16 Blood typing of ABO blood types. When serum containing anti-A or anti-B agglutinins is added to a blood sample diluted with saline, agglutination will occur between the agglutinin and the corresponding agglutinogen (A or B).

Restoring Blood Volume

When a patient's blood volume is so low that death from shock is imminent, there may not be time to type blood, or appropriate whole blood may be unavailable. Such emergencies demand that blood *volume* be replaced immediately to restore adequate circulation.

Fundamentally, blood consists of proteins and cells suspended in a salt solution. Replacing lost blood volume essentially consists of replacing that isotonic salt solution. *Normal saline* or a *multiple electrolyte solution* that mimics the electrolyte composition of plasma (for example, *Ringer's solution*) are the preferred choices.

You might think that it would be important to add materials to mimic the osmotic properties of albumin in blood, and indeed this has been widely practiced. However, studies have shown that **plasma expanders** such as *purified human serum albumin, hetastarch*, and *dextran* provide no benefits over much cheaper electrolyte solutions and are actually associated with significant complications of their own. Volume replacement restores adequate circulation but cannot, of course, replace the oxygen-carrying capacity of the lost red blood cells. Research on ways to replace that capability by using artificial blood substitutes is ongoing.

Check Your Understanding

12. Nigel is told he has type B blood. Which ABO antibodies does he have in his plasma? Which agglutinogens are on his RBCs? Could he donate blood to an AB recipient? Could he receive blood from an AB donor? Explain.

For answers, see Appendix H.

Diagnostic Blood Tests

✓ Explain the diagnostic importance of blood testing.

A laboratory examination of blood yields information that can be used to evaluate a person's health. For example, in some anemias, the blood is pale and has a low hematocrit. A high fat content (*lipidemia*) gives blood plasma a yellowish hue and forecasts problems in those with heart disease. Blood glucose tests indicate how well a diabetic is controlling diet and blood sugar levels. Leukocytosis signals infections; severe infections yield larger-than-normal buffy coats in the hematocrit.

Microscopic studies of blood can reveal variations in the size and shape of erythrocytes that indicate iron deficiency or pernicious anemia. A **differential white blood cell count**, which determines the relative proportions of individual leukocyte types, is a valuable diagnostic tool. For example, a high eosinophil count may indicate a parasitic infection or an allergic response somewhere in the body.

A number of tests provide information on the status of the hemostasis system. For example, clinicians determine the **prothrombin time** to assess the ability of blood to clot, or do a **platelet count** when thrombocytopenia is suspected.

Two batteries of tests—a SMAC (SMA24, CHEM-20, or similar series) and a **complete blood count (CBC)**—are routinely ordered during physical examinations and before hospital admissions. SMAC is a blood *chemistry* profile that measures various electrolytes, glucose, and markers of liver and kidney disorders. The CBC includes counts of the different types of formed elements, the hematocrit, measurements of hemoglobin content, and size of RBCs. Together these tests provide a comprehensive picture of a person's general health in relation to normal blood values.

Appendix F lists normal values for selected blood tests.

Developmental Aspects of Blood

✓ Describe changes in the sites of blood production and in the type of hemoglobin produced after birth.

✓ Name some blood disorders that become more common with age.

Early in fetal development, blood cells form at many sites—the fetal yolk sac, liver, and spleen, among others—but by the seventh month, the red marrow has become the primary hematopoietic area and remains so (barring serious illness) throughout life. If there is a severe need for blood cell production, however, the liver and spleen may resume their fetal blood-forming roles. Additionally, inactive yellow bone marrow regions (essentially fatty tissue) may reconvert to active red marrow.

Blood cells develop from collections of mesenchymal cells, called *blood islands*, derived from the mesoderm germ layer. The fetus forms a unique hemoglobin, **hemoglobin F**, that has a higher affinity for oxygen than does adult hemoglobin (hemoglobin A). It contains two alpha and two gamma (γ) polypeptide chains per globin molecule, instead of the paired alpha and beta chains typical of hemoglobin A. After birth, the liver rapidly destroys fetal erythrocytes carrying hemoglobin F, and the baby's erythroblasts begin producing hemoglobin A.

The most common blood diseases that appear during aging are chronic leukemias, anemias, and clotting disorders. However, these and most other age-related blood disorders are usually precipitated by disorders of the heart, blood vessels, or immune system. For example, the increased incidence of leukemias in old age is believed to result from the waning efficiency of the immune system, and abnormal thrombus and embolus formation reflects atherosclerosis, which roughens the blood vessel walls.

☑ Check Your Understanding

13. Emily Wong, 17, is brought to the ER with a fever, headache, and stiff neck. You suspect bacterial meningitis. Would you expect to see an elevated neutrophil count in a differential WBC count? Explain.
14. How is hemoglobin F different from adult hemoglobin?

For answers, see Appendix H.

Blood serves as the vehicle that the cardiovascular system uses to transport substances throughout the body, so it could be considered the servant of the cardiovascular system. On the other hand, without blood, the normal functions of the heart and blood vessels are impossible. So perhaps the organs of the cardiovascular system, described in Chapters 18 and 19, are subservient to blood. The point of this circular thinking is that blood and the cardiovascular system are vitally intertwined in their common functions: to ensure that nutrients, oxygen, and other vital substances reach all tissue cells of the body and to relieve the cells of their wastes.

17

Chapter Summary

Overview: Blood Composition and Functions (pp. 632–633)

Components (p. 632)

1. Blood is composed of formed elements and plasma. The hematocrit is a measure of one formed element, erythrocytes, as a percentage of total blood volume.

Physical Characteristics and Volume (p. 632)

2. Blood is a viscous, slightly alkaline fluid representing about 8% of total body weight. Blood volume of a normal adult is about 5 L.

Functions (pp. 632–633)

3. Distribution functions include delivering oxygen and nutrients to body tissues, removing metabolic wastes, and transporting hormones.
4. Regulation functions include maintaining body temperature, constant blood pH, and adequate fluid volume.
5. Protective functions include hemostasis and prevention of infection.

Blood Plasma (p. 633)

1. Plasma is a straw-colored, viscous fluid and is 90% water. The remaining 10% is solutes, such as nutrients, respiratory gases, electrolytes, hormones, and proteins. Plasma makes up 55% of whole blood.

2. Plasma proteins, most made by the liver, include albumin, globulins, and fibrinogen. Albumin is an important blood buffer and contributes to the osmotic pressure of blood.

Formed Elements (pp. 634–646)

1. Formed elements, accounting for 45% of whole blood, are erythrocytes, leukocytes, and platelets. All formed elements arise from hematopoietic stem cells in red bone marrow.

Erythrocytes (Red Blood Cells) (pp. 634–640)

2. Erythrocytes (red blood cells, RBCs) are small, biconcave cells containing large amounts of hemoglobin. They have no nucleus and few organelles. Spectrin allows the cells to change shape as they pass through tiny capillaries.
3. Oxygen transport is the major function of erythrocytes. In the lungs, oxygen binds to iron atoms in hemoglobin molecules, producing oxyhemoglobin. In body tissues, oxygen dissociates from iron, producing deoxyhemoglobin.
4. Red blood cells begin as hematopoietic stem cells and, through erythropoiesis, proceed from the proerythroblast (committed cell) stage to the basophilic, polychromatic and orthochromatic erythroblast, and reticulocyte stages. During this process, hemoglobin accumulates and the organelles and nucleus are extruded. Differentiation of reticulocytes is completed in the bloodstream.
5. Erythropoietin and testosterone enhance erythropoiesis.
6. Iron, vitamin B_{12}, and folic acid are essential for production of hemoglobin.
7. Red blood cells have a life span of approximately 120 days. Macrophages of the spleen and liver remove old and damaged erythrocytes from the circulation. Released iron from hemoglobin is stored as ferritin or hemosiderin to be reused. The balance of the heme group is degraded to bilirubin and secreted in bile. Amino acids of globin are metabolized or recycled.

iP Respiratory System; Topic: Gas Transport, pp. 3–5, 11–17.

8. Erythrocyte disorders include anemia and polycythemia.

Leukocytes (White Blood Cells) (pp. 640–645)

9. Leukocytes are white blood cells (WBCs). All are nucleated, and all have crucial roles in defending against disease. Two main categories exist: granulocytes and agranulocytes.
10. Granulocytes include neutrophils, eosinophils, and basophils. Neutrophils are active phagocytes. Eosinophils attack parasitic worms, and their numbers increase during allergic reactions. Basophils contain histamine, which promotes vasodilation and enhances migration of leukocytes to inflammatory sites.
11. Agranulocytes have crucial roles in immunity. They include lymphocytes—the "immune cells"—and monocytes which differentiate into macrophages.
12. Leukopoiesis is directed by colony-stimulating factors and interleukins released by supporting cells of the red bone marrow and mature WBCs.
13. Leukocyte disorders include leukemias and infectious mononucleosis.

Platelets (pp. 645–646)

14. Platelets are fragments of large megakaryocytes formed in red marrow. When a blood vessel is damaged, platelets form a plug to help prevent blood loss and play a central role in the clotting cascade.

Hemostasis (pp. 646–651)

1. Hemostasis is prevention of blood loss. The three major steps of hemostasis are vascular spasm, platelet plug formation, and blood coagulation.

Vascular Spasm and Platelet Plug Formation (pp. 646–647)

2. Spasms of smooth muscle in blood vessel walls and accumulation of platelets (platelet plug) at the site of vessel injury stop or slow down blood loss temporarily until coagulation occurs.

Coagulation (pp. 647–649)

3. Coagulation of blood may be initiated by either the intrinsic or the extrinsic pathway. Platelet phospholipid (PF_3) is crucial to both pathways. Tissue factor (factor III) exposed by tissue injury allows the extrinsic pathway to bypass many steps of the intrinsic pathway. A series of activated clotting factors oversees the intermediate steps of each cascade. The pathways converge as prothrombin is converted to thrombin.

Clot Retraction and Fibrinolysis (p. 649)

4. After a clot is formed, clot retraction occurs. Serum is squeezed out and the ruptured vessel edges are drawn together. Smooth muscle, connective tissue, and endothelial cell proliferation and migration repair the injured blood vessel.
5. When healing is complete, clot digestion (fibrinolysis) occurs.

Factors Limiting Clot Growth or Formation (p. 649)

6. Abnormal expansion of clots is prevented by removal of coagulation factors in contact with rapidly flowing blood and by inhibition of activated blood factors. Prostacyclin (PGI_2) and nitric oxide secreted by the endothelial cells help prevent undesirable (unnecessary) clotting.

Disorders of Hemostasis (pp. 650–651)

7. Thromboembolic disorders involve undesirable clot formation, which can block vessels.
8. Thrombocytopenia, a deficit of platelets, causes spontaneous bleeding from small blood vessels. Hemophilia is caused by a genetic deficiency of certain coagulation factors. Liver disease can also cause bleeding disorders because many coagulation proteins are formed by the liver.
9. Disseminated intravascular coagulation (DIC) is a condition of bodywide clotting in undamaged blood vessels and subsequent hemorrhages.

Transfusion and Blood Replacement (pp. 651–653)

Transfusing Red Blood Cells (pp. 651–653)

1. Whole blood transfusions are given to replace severe and rapid blood loss. Packed RBCs are given to replace lost O_2-carrying capacity.
2. Blood group is based on agglutinogens (antigens) present on red blood cell membranes.
3. When mismatched blood is transfused, the recipient's agglutinins (plasma antibodies) clump the foreign RBCs. The clumped RBCs may block blood vessels temporarily and then are lysed. Released hemoglobin may cause renal shutdown.
4. Before whole blood can be transfused, it must be typed and cross matched to prevent transfusion reactions. The most important blood groups for which blood must be typed are the ABO and Rh groups.

Restoring Blood Volume (p. 653)

5. Plasma volume can be replaced with balanced electrolyte solutions, and these are generally preferred over plasma expanders.

Diagnostic Blood Tests (pp. 653–654)

1. Diagnostic blood tests can provide valuable information about the current status of the blood and of the body as a whole.

Developmental Aspects of Blood (p. 654)

1. Fetal hematopoietic sites include the yolk sac, liver, and spleen. By the seventh month of development, the red bone marrow is the primary blood-forming site.
2. Blood cells develop from blood islands derived from mesoderm. Fetal blood contains hemoglobin F. After birth, hemoglobin A is formed.
3. The major blood-related problems associated with aging are leukemia, anemia, and thromboembolic disease.

Review Questions

Multiple Choice/Matching

(Some questions have more than one correct answer. Select the best answer or answers from the choices given.)

1. The blood volume in an adult averages approximately **(a)** 1 L, **(b)** 3 L, **(c)** 5 L, **(d)** 7 L.
2. The hormonal stimulus that prompts red blood cell formation is **(a)** serotonin, **(b)** heparin, **(c)** erythropoietin, **(d)** thrombopoietin.
3. All of the following are true of RBCs except **(a)** biconcave disc shape, **(b)** life span of approximately 120 days, **(c)** contain hemoglobin, **(d)** contain nuclei.
4. The most numerous WBC is the **(a)** eosinophil, **(b)** neutrophil, **(c)** monocyte, **(d)** lymphocyte.
5. Blood proteins play an important part in **(a)** blood clotting, **(b)** immunity, **(c)** maintenance of blood volume, **(d)** all of the above.
6. The white blood cell that releases histamine and other inflammatory chemicals is the **(a)** basophil, **(b)** neutrophil, **(c)** monocyte, **(d)** eosinophil.
7. The blood cell that can become an antibody-secreting cell is the **(a)** lymphocyte, **(b)** megakaryocyte, **(c)** neutrophil, **(d)** basophil.
8. Which of the following does not promote multiple steps in the clotting pathway? **(a)** PF_3, **(b)** factor XI, **(c)** thrombin, **(d)** Ca^{2+}.
9. The normal pH of the blood is about **(a)** 8.4, **(b)** 7.8, **(c)** 7.4, **(d)** 4.7.
10. Suppose your blood is AB positive. This means that **(a)** agglutinogens A and B are present on your red blood cells, **(b)** there are no anti-A or anti-B antibodies in your plasma, **(c)** your blood is Rh^+, **(d)** all of the above.

Short Answer Essay Questions

11. (a) Define formed elements and list their three major categories. (b) Which is least numerous? (c) Which comprise(s) the buffy coat in a hematocrit tube?
12. Discuss hemoglobin relative to its chemical structure, its function, and the color changes it undergoes during loading and unloading of oxygen.
13. If you had a high hematocrit, would you expect your hemoglobin determination to be low or high? Why?
14. What nutrients are needed for erythropoiesis?
15. (a) Describe the process of erythropoiesis. (b) What name is given to the immature cell type released to the circulation? (c) How does it differ from a mature erythrocyte?
16. Besides the ability to move by amoeboid motion, what other physiological attributes contribute to the function of white blood cells in the body?
17. (a) If you had a severe infection, would you expect your WBC count to be closest to 5000, 10,000, or 15,000/μl? (b) What is this condition called?
18. (a) Describe the appearance of platelets and state their major function. (b) Why should platelets not be called "cells"?
19. (a) Define hemostasis. (b) List the three major phases of coagulation. Explain what initiates each phase and what the phase accomplishes. (c) In what general way do the intrinsic and extrinsic mechanisms of clotting differ? (d) Which ion is essential to virtually all stages of coagulation?
20. (a) Define fibrinolysis. (b) What is the importance of this process?
21. (a) How is clot overgrowth usually prevented? (b) List two conditions that may lead to unnecessary (and undesirable) clot formation.
22. How can liver dysfunction cause bleeding disorders?
23. (a) What is a transfusion reaction and why does it happen? (b) What are its possible consequences?
24. How can poor nutrition lead to anemia?
25. What blood-related problems are most common in the aged?

Critical Thinking and Clinical Application Questions

1. Cancer patients being treated with chemotherapeutic drugs designed to destroy rapidly dividing cells are monitored closely for changes in their red and white blood counts. Why so?
2. Mary Healy, a young woman with severe vaginal bleeding, is admitted to the emergency room. She is three months pregnant, and the physician is concerned about the volume of blood she is losing. (a) What type of transfusion will probably be given to this patient? (b) Which blood tests will be performed before starting the transfusion?
3. Alan Forsythe, a middle-aged college professor from Boston, is in the Swiss Alps studying astronomy during his sabbatical leave. He has been there for two days and plans to stay the entire year. However, he notices that he is short of breath when he walks up steps and tires easily with any physical activity. His symptoms gradually disappear, and after two months he feels fine. Upon returning to the United States, he has a complete physical exam and is told that his erythrocyte count is higher than normal. (a) Attempt to explain this finding. (b) Will his RBC count remain at this higher-than-normal level? Why or why not?
4. A young child is diagnosed as having acute lymphocytic leukemia. Her parents cannot understand why infection is a major problem for Janie when her WBC count is so high. Can you provide an explanation for Janie's parents?
5. Mrs. Ryan, a middle-aged woman, appears at the clinic complaining of multiple small hemorrhagic spots in her skin and severe nosebleeds. While taking her history, the nurse notes that Mrs. Ryan works as a rubber glue applicator at a local factory. Rubber glue contains benzene, which is known to be toxic to red marrow. Using your knowledge of physiology, explain the connection between the bleeding problems and benzene.
6. A reticulocyte count indicated that 5% of Tyler's red blood cells were reticulocytes. His blood test also indicated he had polycythemia and a hematocrit of 65%. Explain the connection between these three facts.

7. In 1998, the U.S. Food and Drug Administration approved the nation's first commercial surgical glue to control bleeding during certain surgeries. Called Tisseel, it forms a flexible mesh over an oozing blood vessel to help stem bleeding within five minutes. This sealant is made from two blood proteins that naturally cause blood to clot when they react together. Name these proteins.
8. Jenny, a healthy young woman, had a battery of tests during a physical for a new job. Her RBC count was at the higher end of the normal range at that time, but four weeks later it was substantially elevated beyond that. When asked if any circumstances had changed in her life, she admitted to taking up smoking. How might her new habit explain her higher RBC count?
9. Mr. Chu has been scheduled for surgery to have his arthritic hip replaced. His surgeon tells him he must switch from aspirin to acetaminophen for pain control before his surgery. Why?

AT THE CLINIC

Related Clinical Terms

Blood chemistry tests Chemical analysis of substances in the blood, e.g., glucose, iron, calcium, protein, bilirubin, and pH.

Blood fraction Any one of the components of whole blood that has been separated out from the other blood components, such as platelets or clotting factors.

Bone marrow biopsy A sample of red bone marrow is obtained by needle aspiration (typically from the anterior or posterior iliac crest), and examined to diagnose disorders of blood-cell formation, leukemia, various marrow infections, and anemias resulting from damage to or failure of the marrow.

Exchange transfusion A technique of removing the patient's blood and infusing donor blood until a large fraction of the patient's blood has been replaced; used to treat fetal blood incompatibilities and poisoning victims.

Hematology (hem″ah-tol′o-je) Study of blood.

Hematoma (hem″ah-to′mah) Accumulated, clotted blood in the tissues usually resulting from injury; visible as "black and blue" marks or bruises; eventually absorbed naturally unless infections develop.

Hemochromatosis (he″mo-kro″mah-to′sis) An inherited disorder of iron overload in which the intestine absorbs too much iron from the diet. The iron builds up in body tissues, where it oxidizes to form compounds that poison those organs (especially joints, liver, and pancreas).

Myeloproliferative disorder All-inclusive term for a group of proliferative disorders (disorders in which normal cell division controls are lost) including leukoerythroblastic anemia involving fibrosis of the bone marrow, polycythemia vera, and leukemia.

Plasmapheresis (plaz″mah-fĕ-re′sis) A process in which blood is removed, its plasma is separated from formed elements, and the formed elements are returned to the patient or donor. The most important application is removal of antibodies or immune complexes from the blood of individuals with autoimmune disorders (multiple sclerosis, myasthenia gravis, and others). Also used by blood banks to collect plasma for burn victims and to obtain plasma components for therapeutic use.

Septicemia (sep″tĭ-se′me-ah; *septos* = rotten) Excessive and harmful levels of bacteria or their toxins in the blood. Also called blood poisoning.

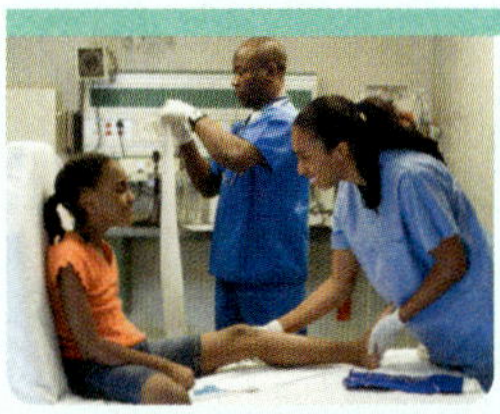

Case Study Blood

Earl Malone is a 20-year-old passenger on the bus that crashed on Route 91. Upon arrival at the scene, paramedics make the following observations:

- Right upper quadrant (abdominal) pain
- Cyanotic
- Cool and clammy skin
- Blood pressure 100/60 and falling, pulse 100

Paramedics start an IV to rapidly infuse a 0.9% sodium chloride solution (normal saline). They transport him to a small rural hospital where Mr. Malone's blood pressure continues to fall and his cyanosis worsens. The local physician begins infusing O negative packed red blood cells (PRBCs) and arranges transport by helicopter to a trauma center. She sends additional PRBC units in the helicopter for transfusion en route. After arrival at the trauma center, the following notes were added to Mr. Malone's chart:

- Abdomen firm and distended
- Blood drawn for typing and cross matching; packed A positive blood cells infused
- Emergency FAST (Focused Assessment with Sonography for Trauma) ultrasound is positive for intraperitoneal fluid

A positive FAST scan indicates intra-abdominal bleeding. Mr. Malone's condition continues to deteriorate, so he is prepared for surgery, which reveals a lacerated liver. The laceration is repaired, and Mr. Malone's vital signs stabilize.

1. Mr. Malone was going into shock because of blood loss, so paramedics infused a saline solution. Why would this help?
2. Mr. Malone was switched from saline to PRBCs. What problem does infusion of PRBCs address that the saline solution could not?
3. Why was the physician able to use O negative blood before the results of the blood type tests were obtained?
4. Mr. Malone's blood type was determined to be A positive. What plasma antibodies (agglutinins) does he have, and what type of blood can he receive?
5. What would happen if doctors had infused type B PRBCs into Mr. Malone's circulation?

(Answers in Appendix H)

17

18

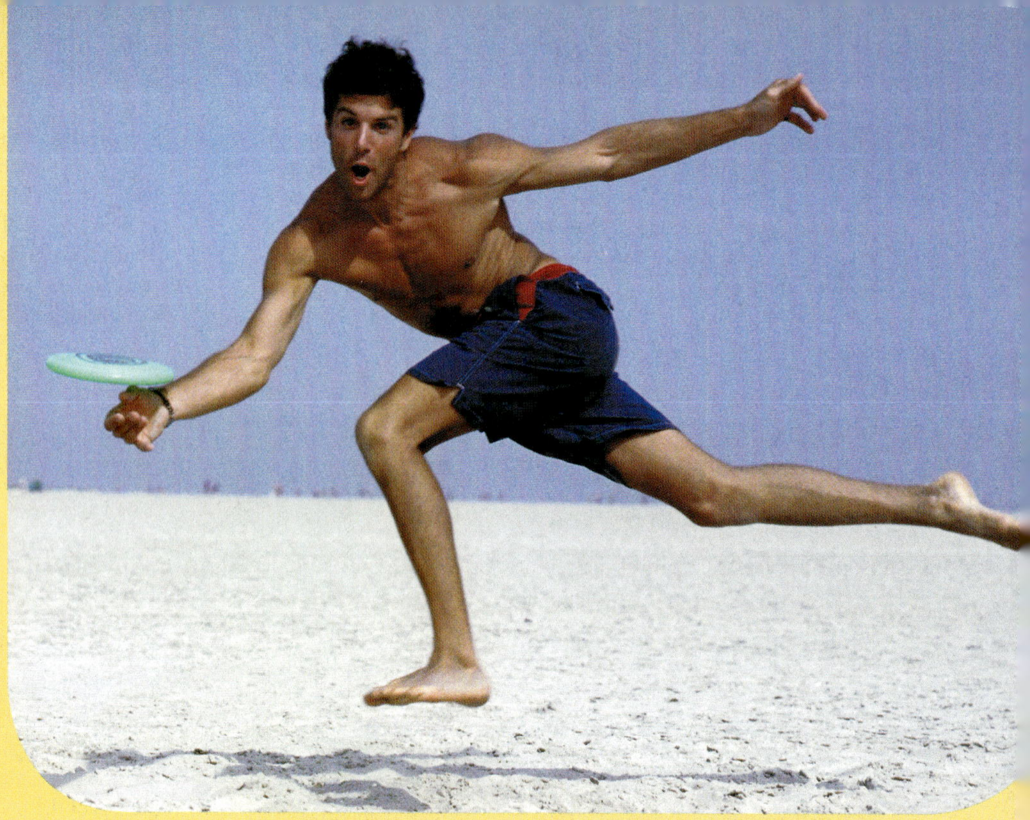

The Cardiovascular System: The Heart

Our ceaselessly beating heart has intrigued people for centuries. The ancient Greeks believed the heart was the seat of intelligence. Others thought it was the source of emotions. While these ideas have proved false, we do know that emotions affect heart rate. When your heart pounds or skips a beat, you become acutely aware of how much you depend on this dynamic organ for your very life.

Despite its vital importance, the heart does not work alone. Indeed, it is only part of the cardiovascular system, which includes the miles of blood vessels that run through your body. Day and night, tissue cells take in nutrients and oxygen and excrete wastes. Cells can make such exchanges only with their immediate environment, so some means of changing and renewing that environment is necessary to ensure a continual supply of nutrients and prevent a buildup of wastes. The cardiovascular system provides the transport system "hardware" that keeps blood continuously circulating to fulfill this critical homeostatic need.

The Pulmonary and Systemic Circuits

Stripped of its romantic cloak, the **heart** is no more than the transport system pump, and the hollow blood vessels are the delivery routes. In fact, the heart is actually two pumps side by side **(Figure 18.1)**.

- The *right side* of the heart receives oxygen-poor blood from body tissues and then pumps this blood to the lungs to pick up oxygen and dispel carbon dioxide. The blood vessels that carry blood to and from the lungs form the **pulmonary circuit** (*pulmo* = lung).
- The *left side* of the heart receives the oxygenated blood returning from the lungs and pumps this blood throughout the body to supply oxygen and nutrients to body tissues. The blood vessels that carry blood to and from all body tissues form the **systemic circuit**.

The heart has two receiving chambers, the *right atrium* and *left atrium*, that receive blood returning from the systemic and pulmonary circuits. The heart also has two main pumping chambers, the *right ventricle* and *left ventricle*, that pump blood around the two circuits. Using blood as the transport medium, the heart continually propels oxygen, nutrients, wastes, and many other substances into the interconnecting blood vessels that service body cells.

Heart Anatomy

✓ Describe the size, shape, location, and orientation of the heart in the thorax.

✓ Name the coverings of the heart.

✓ Describe the structure and function of each of the three layers of the heart wall.

Size, Location, and Orientation

The modest size and weight of the heart belie its incredible strength and endurance. About the size of a fist, the hollow, cone-shaped heart has a mass of 250 to 350 grams—less than a pound **(Figure 18.2)**.

Snugly enclosed within the **mediastinum** (me″de-ah-sti′num), the medial cavity of the thorax, the heart extends obliquely for 12 to 14 cm (about 5 inches) from the second rib to the fifth intercostal space (Figure 18.2a). As it rests on the superior surface of the diaphragm, the heart lies anterior to the vertebral column and posterior to the sternum. Approximately two-thirds of its mass lies to the left of the midsternal line; the balance projects to the right. The lungs flank the heart laterally and partially obscure it (Figure 18.2b, c).

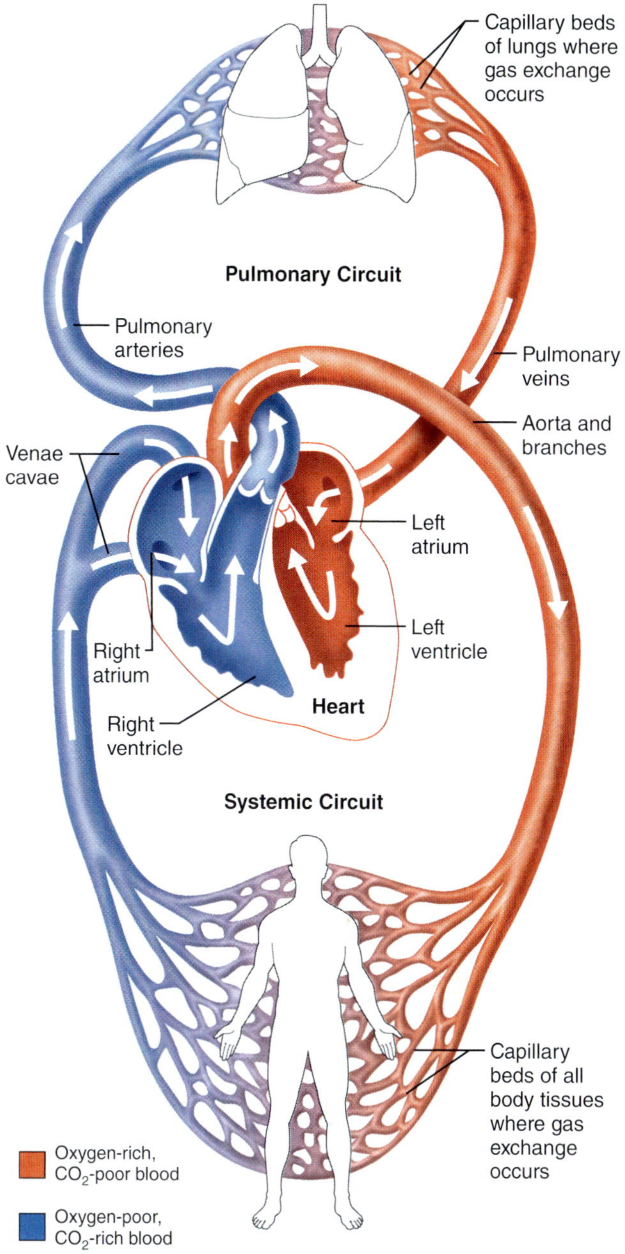

Figure 18.1 The systemic and pulmonary circuits. The right side of the heart pumps blood through the pulmonary circuit* (to the lungs and back to the left side of the heart). The left side of the heart pumps blood through the systemic circuit to all body tissues and back to the right side of the heart. The arrows indicate the direction of blood flow.

*For simplicity, the actual number of two pulmonary arteries and four pulmonary veins has been reduced to one each.

Its broad, flat **base**, or posterior surface, is about 9 cm (3.5 in) wide and directed toward the right shoulder. Its **apex** points inferiorly toward the left hip. If you press your fingers between the fifth and sixth ribs just below the left nipple, you can easily feel the **apical impulse** caused by your beating heart's apex where it touches the chest wall.

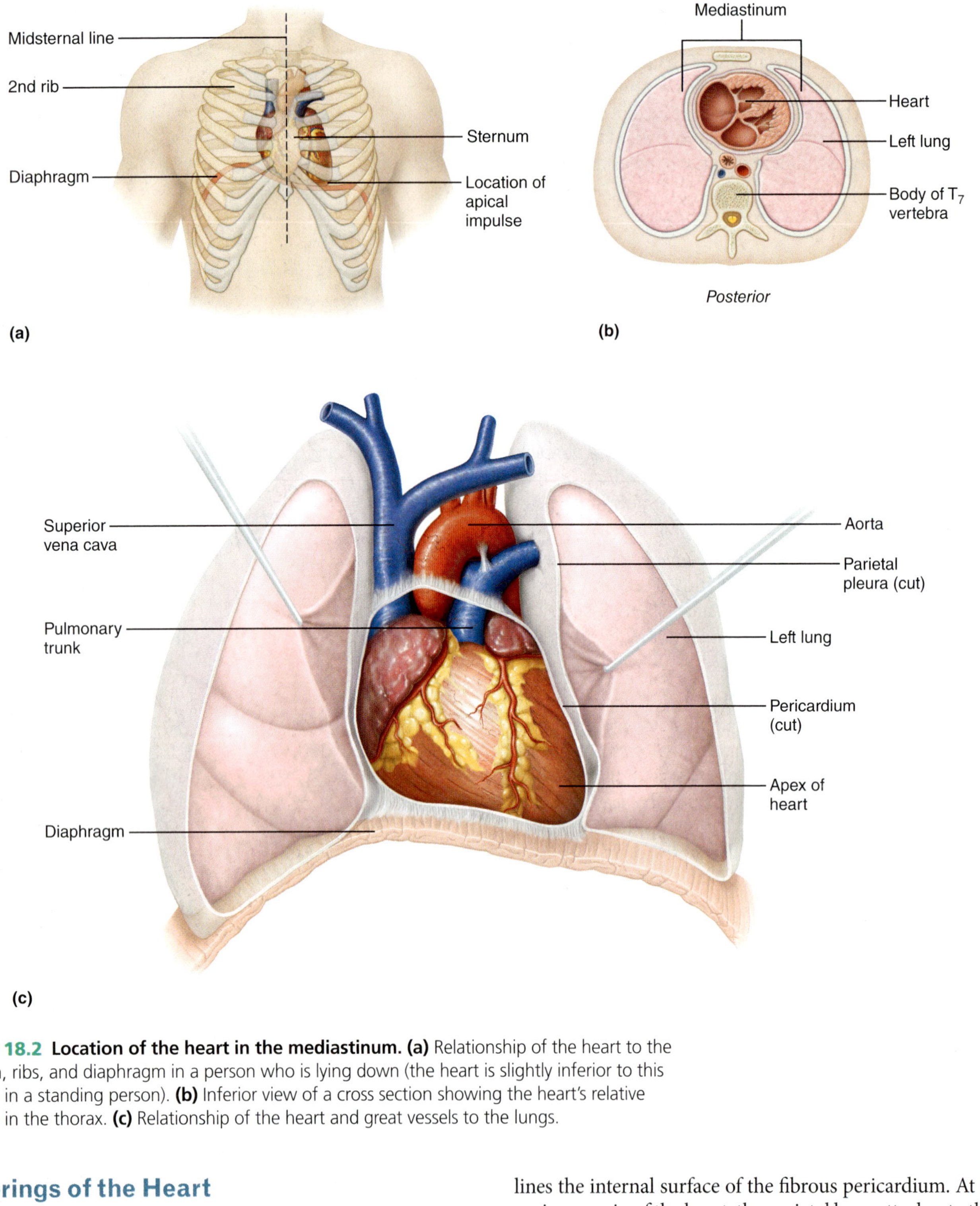

Figure 18.2 Location of the heart in the mediastinum. (a) Relationship of the heart to the sternum, ribs, and diaphragm in a person who is lying down (the heart is slightly inferior to this position in a standing person). **(b)** Inferior view of a cross section showing the heart's relative position in the thorax. **(c)** Relationship of the heart and great vessels to the lungs.

Coverings of the Heart

The heart is enclosed in a double-walled sac called the **pericardium** (per″ĭ-kar′de-um; *peri* = around, *cardi* = heart) **(Figure 18.3)**. The loosely fitting superficial part of this sac is the **fibrous pericardium**. This tough, dense connective tissue layer (1) protects the heart, (2) anchors it to surrounding structures, and (3) prevents overfilling of the heart with blood.

Deep to the fibrous pericardium is the **serous pericardium**, a thin, slippery, two-layer serous membrane that forms a closed sac around the heart (see Figure 1.10, p. 19). Its **parietal layer** lines the internal surface of the fibrous pericardium. At the superior margin of the heart, the parietal layer attaches to the large arteries exiting the heart, and then turns inferiorly and continues over the external heart surface as the **visceral layer**, also called the **epicardium** ("upon the heart"), which is an integral part of the heart wall.

Between the parietal and visceral layers is the slitlike **pericardial cavity**, which contains a film of serous fluid. The serous membranes, lubricated by the fluid, glide smoothly past one another, allowing the mobile heart to work in a relatively friction-free environment.

18

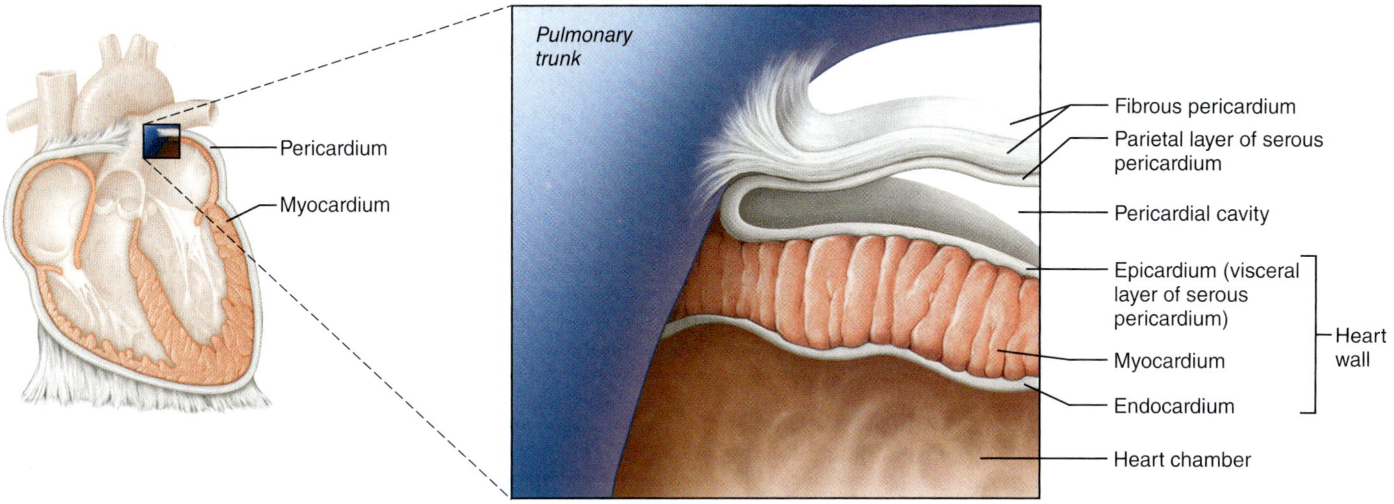

Figure 18.3 The pericardial layers and layers of the heart wall.

Homeostatic Imbalance 18.1

Pericarditis, inflammation of the pericardium, roughens the serous membrane surfaces. Consequently, as the beating heart rubs against its pericardial sac, it creates a creaking sound (*pericardial friction rub*) that can be heard with a stethoscope. Pericarditis is characterized by pain deep to the sternum. Over time, it may lead to adhesions in which the visceral and parietal pericardia stick together and impede heart activity.

In severe cases, large amounts of inflammatory fluid seep into the pericardial cavity. This excess fluid compresses the heart and limits its ability to pump blood, a condition called *cardiac tamponade* (tam″pŏ-nād′), literally, "heart plug." Physicians treat cardiac tamponade by inserting a syringe into the pericardial cavity and draining off the excess fluid. +

Layers of the Heart Wall

The heart wall, richly supplied with blood vessels, is composed of three layers: the epicardium, myocardium, and endocardium (Figure 18.3).

As we have noted, the superficial **epicardium** is the visceral layer of the serous pericardium. It is often infiltrated with fat, especially in older people.

The middle layer, the **myocardium** ("muscle heart"), is composed mainly of cardiac muscle and forms the bulk of the heart. This is the layer that contracts. In the myocardium, the branching cardiac muscle cells are tethered to one another by crisscrossing connective tissue fibers and arranged in spiral or circular *bundles* **(Figure 18.4)**. These interlacing bundles effectively link all parts of the heart together.

The connective tissue fibers form a dense network, the fibrous **cardiac skeleton**, that reinforces the myocardium internally and anchors the cardiac muscle fibers. This network of collagen and elastic fibers is thicker in some areas than others. For example, it constructs ropelike rings that provide additional support where the great vessels issue from the heart and around

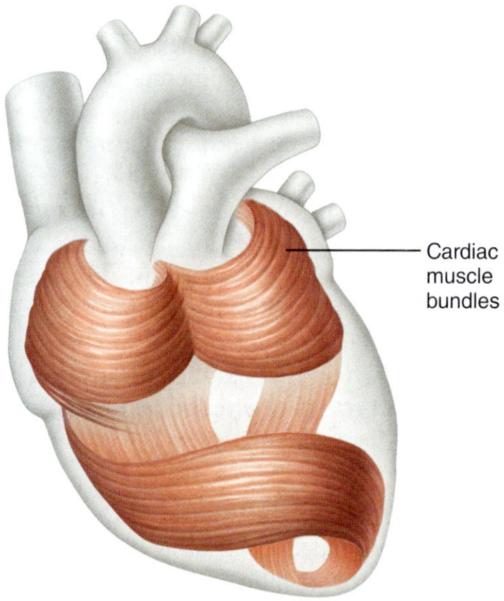

Figure 18.4 The circular and spiral arrangement of cardiac muscle bundles in the myocardium of the heart.

the heart valves (see Figure 18.6a, p. 666). Without this support, the vessels and valves might eventually become stretched because of the continuous stress of blood pulsing through them. Additionally, because connective tissue is not electrically excitable, the cardiac skeleton limits the spread of action potentials to specific pathways in the heart.

The third layer of the heart wall, the **endocardium** ("inside the heart"), is a glistening white sheet of endothelium (squamous epithelium) resting on a thin connective tissue layer. Located on the inner myocardial surface, it lines the heart chambers and covers the fibrous skeleton of the valves. The endocardium is continuous with the endothelial linings of the blood vessels leaving and entering the heart.

Check Your Understanding

1. The heart is in the mediastinum. Just what is the mediastinum?
2. From inside to outside, list the layers of the heart wall and the coverings of the heart.
3. What is the purpose of the serous fluid inside the pericardial cavity?

For answers, see Appendix H.

Chambers and Associated Great Vessels

✓ Describe the structure and functions of the four heart chambers. Name each chamber and provide the name and general route of its associated great vessel(s).

The heart has four chambers **(Figure 18.5e)**—two superior **atria** (a′tre-ah) and two inferior **ventricles** (ven′trĭ-klz). The internal partition that divides the heart longitudinally is called the **interatrial septum** where it separates the atria, and the **interventricular septum** where it separates the ventricles. The right ventricle forms most of the anterior surface of the heart. The left ventricle dominates the inferoposterior aspect of the heart and forms the heart apex.

Two grooves visible on the heart surface indicate the boundaries of its four chambers and carry the blood vessels supplying the myocardium. The **coronary sulcus** (Figure 18.5b, d), or *atrioventricular groove*, encircles the junction of the atria and ventricles like a crown (*corona* = crown). The **anterior interventricular sulcus**, cradling the anterior interventricular artery, marks the anterior position of the septum separating the right and left ventricles. It continues as the **posterior interventricular sulcus**, which provides a similar landmark on the heart's posteroinferior surface.

Atria: The Receiving Chambers

18

Except for small, wrinkled, protruding appendages called **auricles** (or′ĭ-klz; *auricle* = little ear), which increase the atrial volume somewhat, the right and left atria are remarkably free of distinguishing surface features. Internally, the right atrium has two basic parts (Figure 18.5c): a smooth-walled posterior part and an anterior portion in which bundles of muscle tissue form ridges in the walls. These muscle bundles are called **pectinate muscles** because they look like the teeth of a comb (*pectin* = comb). The posterior and anterior regions of the right atrium are separated by a C-shaped ridge called the *crista terminalis* ("terminal crest").

In contrast, the left atrium is mostly smooth and pectinate muscles are found only in the auricle. The interatrial septum bears a shallow depression, the **fossa ovalis** (o-vă′lis), that marks the spot where an opening, the *foramen ovale*, existed in the fetal heart (Figure 18.5c, e).

Functionally, the atria are receiving chambers for blood returning to the heart from the circulation (*atrium* = entryway). The atria are relatively small, thin-walled chambers because they need to contract only minimally to push blood "downstairs" into the ventricles. As a rule, they contribute little to the propulsive pumping activity of the heart.

Blood enters the *right atrium* via three veins (Figure 18.5c–e):

- The **superior vena cava** returns blood from body regions superior to the diaphragm.
- The **inferior vena cava** returns blood from body areas below the diaphragm.
- The **coronary sinus** collects blood draining from the myocardium.

Four **pulmonary veins** enter the *left atrium*, which makes up most of the heart's base. These veins, which transport blood from the lungs back to the heart, are best seen in a posterior view (Figure 18.5d).

Ventricles: The Discharging Chambers

Together the ventricles (*ventr* = underside) make up most of the volume of the heart. As already mentioned, the right ventricle forms most of the heart's anterior surface and the left ventricle dominates its posteroinferior surface. Irregular ridges of muscle called **trabeculae carneae** (trah-bek′u-le kar′ne-e; "crossbars of flesh") mark the internal walls of the ventricular chambers. Still other muscle bundles, the conelike **papillary muscles**, which play a role in valve function, project into the ventricular cavity (Figure 18.5e).

The ventricles are the discharging chambers, the actual pumps of the heart. Their walls are much more massive than the atrial walls, reflecting the difference in function between the atria and ventricles (Figure 18.5e and f). When the ventricles contract, they propel blood out of the heart into the circulation. The right ventricle pumps blood into the **pulmonary trunk**, which routes the blood to the lungs where gas exchange occurs. The left ventricle ejects blood into the **aorta** (a-or′tah), the largest artery in the body.

Heart Valves

✓ Name the heart valves and describe their location, function, and mechanism of operation.

Blood flows through the heart in one direction: from atria to ventricles and out the great arteries leaving the superior aspect of the heart. Four valves enforce this one-way traffic (Figure 18.5e and **Figure 18.6**). They open and close in response to differences in blood pressure on their two sides.

Atrioventricular (AV) Valves

The two **atrioventricular (AV) valves**, one located at each atrial-ventricular junction, prevent backflow into the atria when the ventricles contract.

- The right AV valve, the **tricuspid valve** (tri-kus′pid), has three flexible cusps (flaps of endocardium reinforced by connective tissue cores).
- The left AV valve, with two cusps, is called the **mitral valve** (mi′tral) because it resembles the two-sided bishop's miter or hat. It is sometimes called the *bicuspid valve*.

(Text continues on p. 667.)

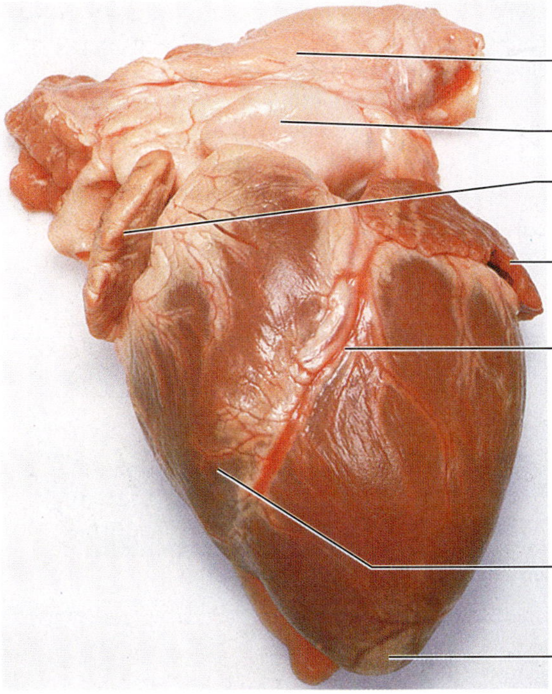

(a) Anterior aspect (pericardium removed)

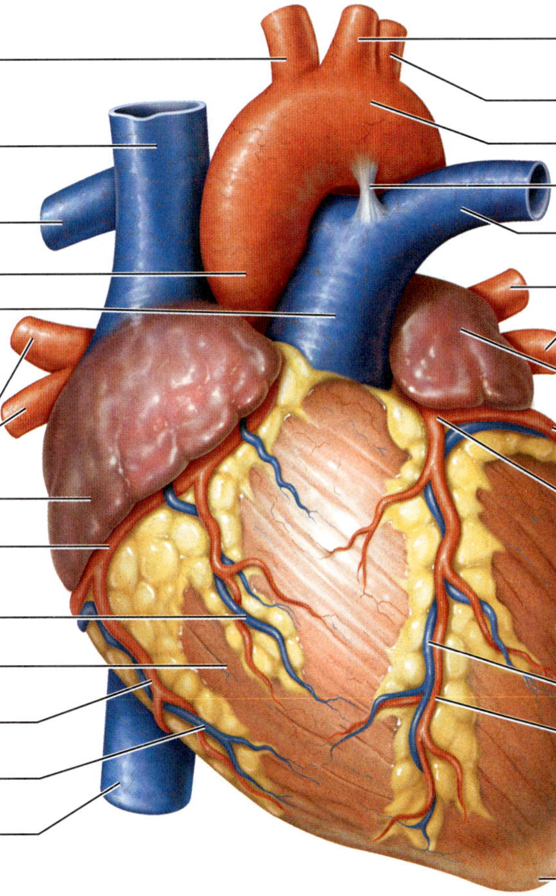

(b) Anterior view

Figure 18.5 Gross anatomy of the heart. In diagrammatic views, vessels transporting oxygen-rich blood are red; those transporting oxygen-poor blood are blue.

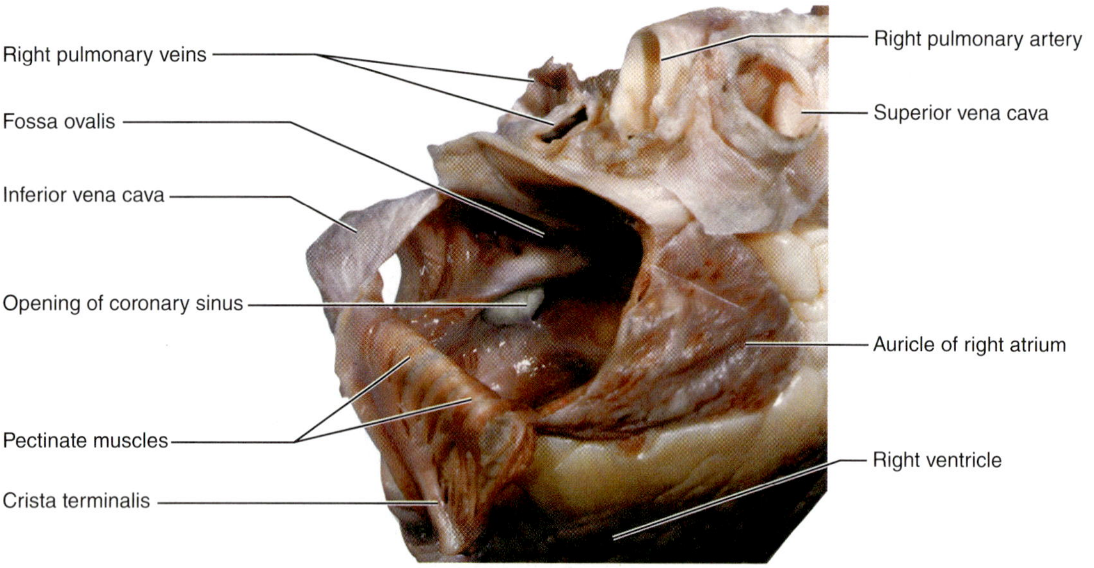

(c) Right anterior view of the internal aspect of the right atrium

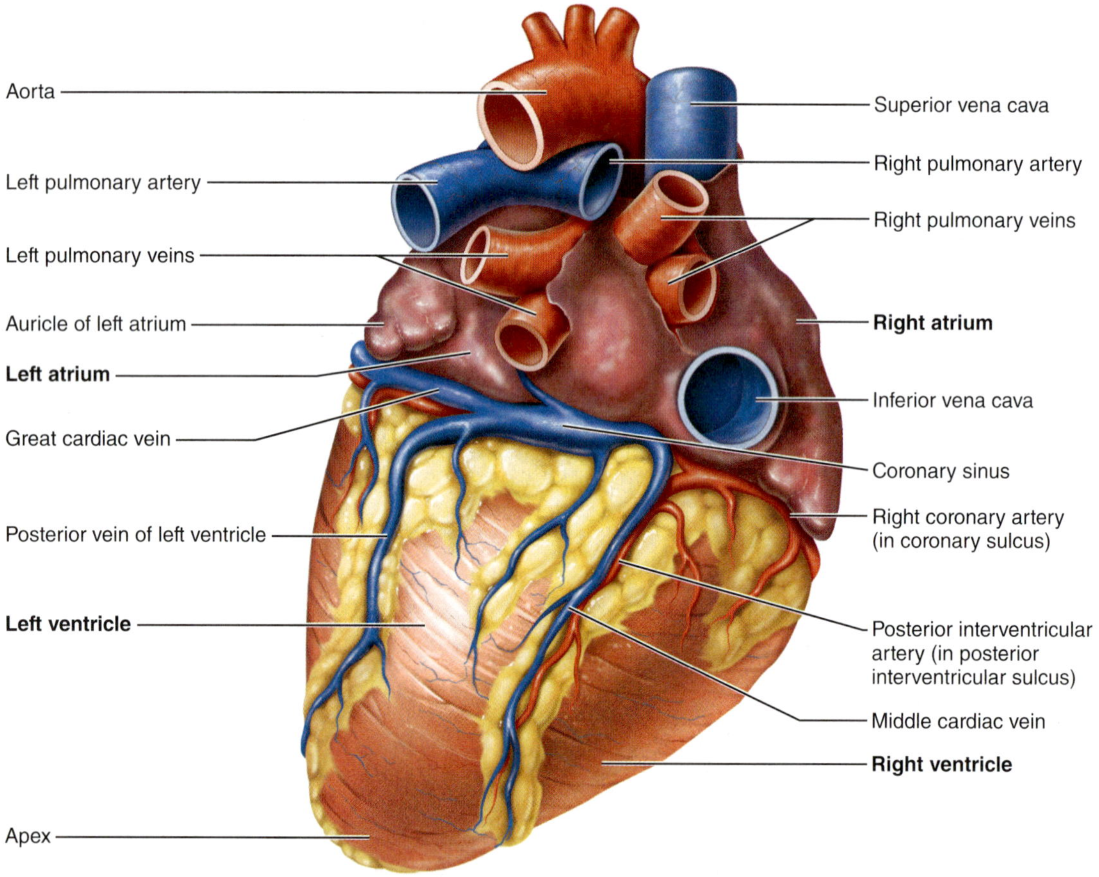

(d) Posterior surface view

Figure 18.5 *(continued)* **Gross anatomy of the heart.** In (c), the anterior wall of the atrium has been opened and folded inferiorly.

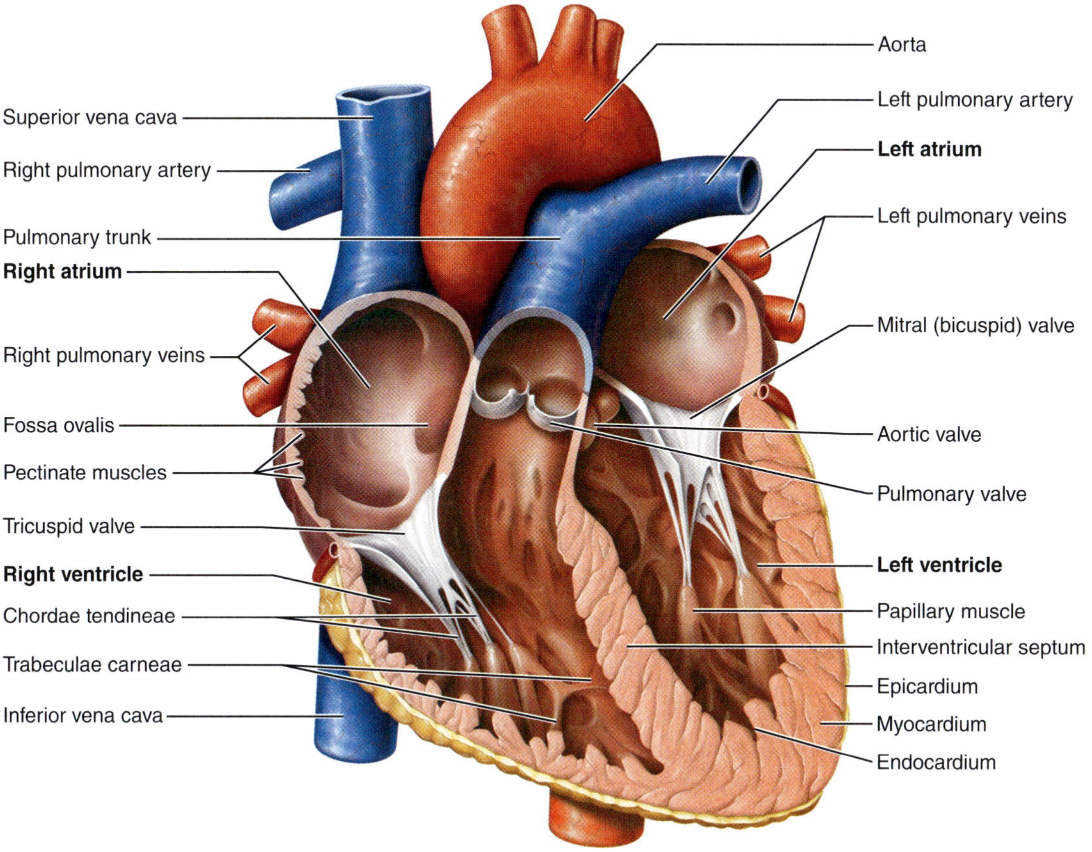

(e) Frontal section

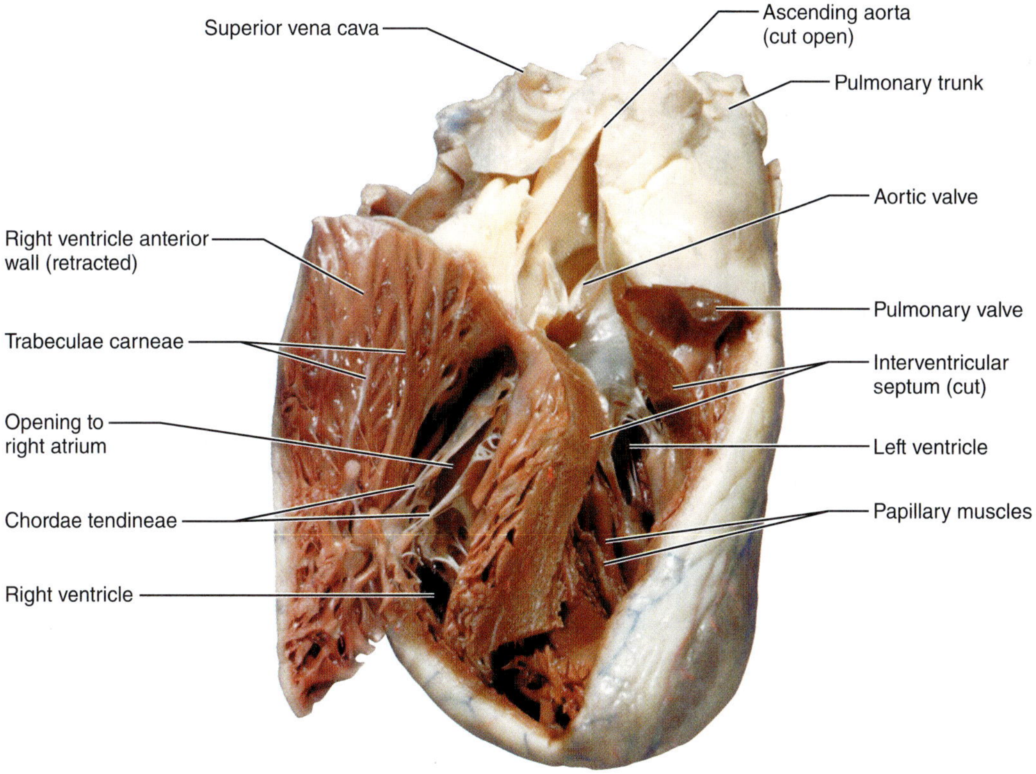

(f) Photograph; view similar to (e)

Figure 18.5 *(continued)*

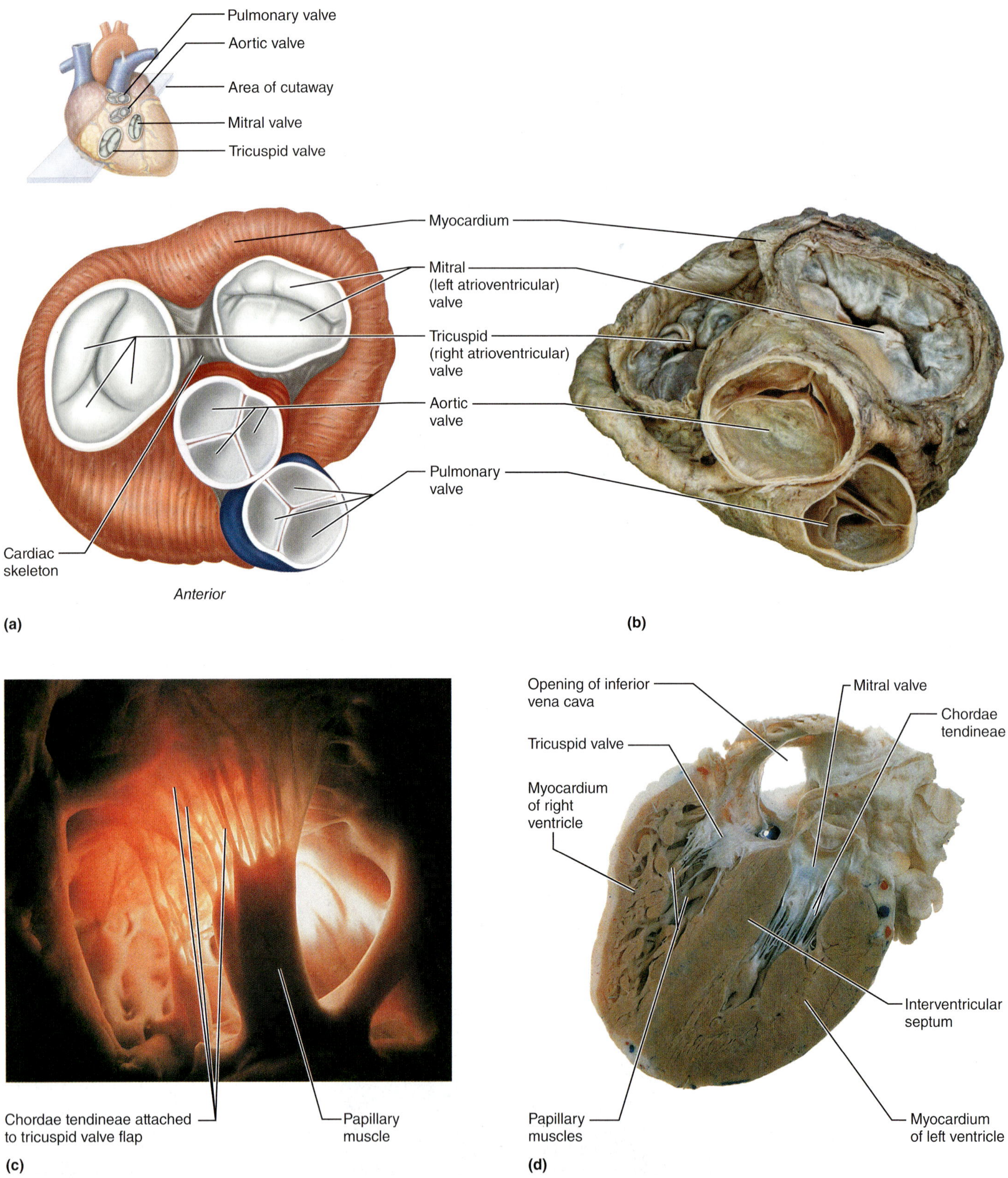

Figure 18.6 Heart valves. **(a)** Superior view of the two sets of heart valves (atria removed). The paired atrioventricular valves are located between atria and ventricles; the two semilunar valves are located at the junction of the ventricles and the arteries issuing from them. **(b)** Photograph of the heart valves, superior view. **(c)** Photograph of the tricuspid valve. This bottom-to-top view shows the valve as seen from the right ventricle. **(d)** Coronal section of the heart. (For related images, see *A Brief Atlas of the Human Body*, Figures 58 and 60.)

18

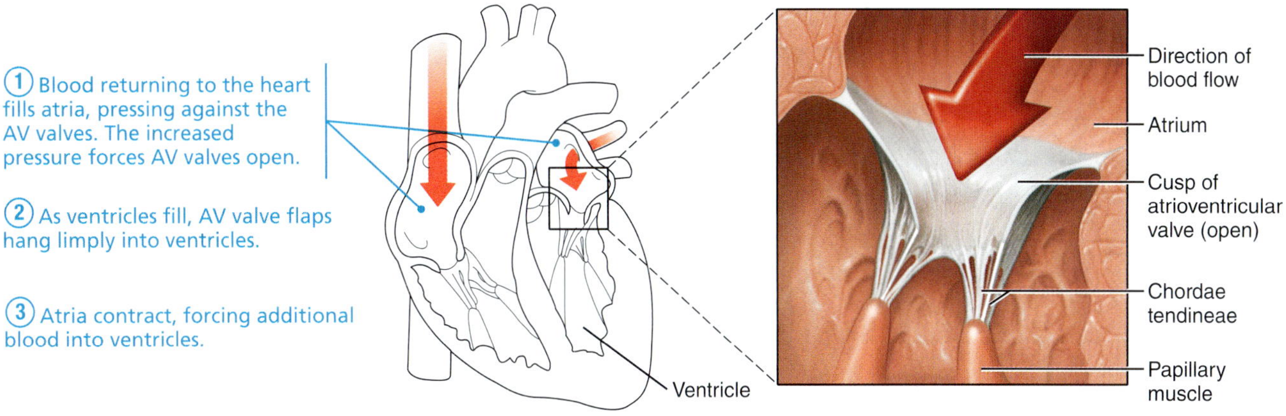

(a) AV valves open; atrial pressure greater than ventricular pressure

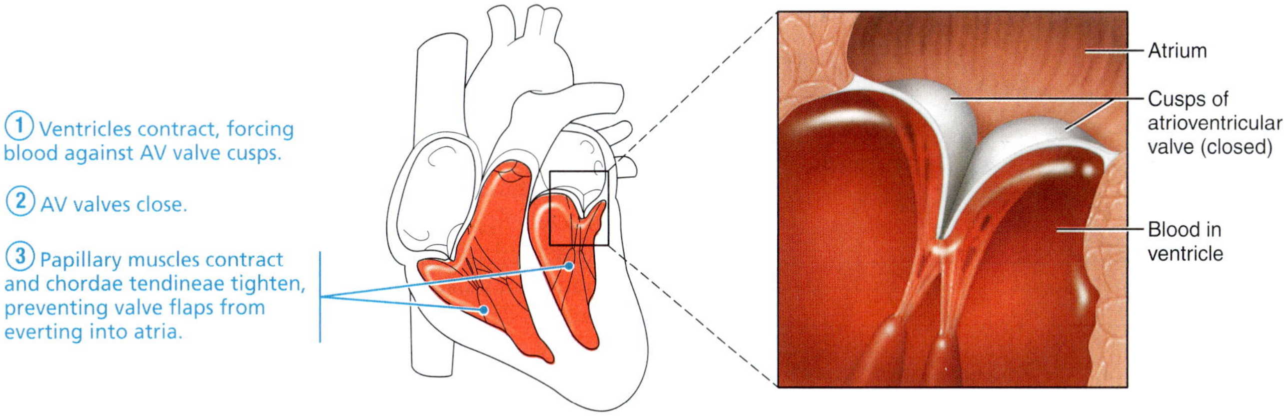

(b) AV valves closed; atrial pressure less than ventricular pressure

Figure 18.7 The atrioventricular (AV) valves.

Attached to each AV valve flap are tiny white collagen cords called **chordae tendineae** (kor′de ten″dĭ′ne-e; "tendinous cords"), "heart strings" which anchor the cusps to the papillary muscles protruding from the ventricular walls (Figure 18.6c, d).

When the heart is completely relaxed, the AV valve flaps hang limply into the ventricular chambers below and blood flows into the atria and then through the open AV valves into the ventricles **(Figure 18.7a)**. When the ventricles contract, compressing the blood in their chambers, the intraventricular pressure rises, forcing the blood superiorly against the valve flaps. As a result, the flap edges meet, closing the valve (Figure 18.7b).

The chordae tendineae and the papillary muscles serve as guy-wires that anchor the valve flaps in their *closed* position. If the cusps were not anchored, they would be blown upward (everted) into the atria, in the same way an umbrella is blown inside out by a gusty wind. The papillary muscles contract with the other ventricular musculature so that they take up the slack on the chordae tendineae as the full force of ventricular contraction hurls the blood against the AV valve flaps.

Semilunar (SL) Valves

The **aortic** and **pulmonary (semilunar, SL) valves** guard the bases of the large arteries issuing from the ventricles (aorta and pulmonary trunk, respectively) and prevent backflow into the associated ventricles. Each SL valve is fashioned from three pocketlike cusps, each shaped roughly like a crescent moon (*semilunar* = half-moon).

Like the AV valves, the SL valves open and close in response to differences in pressure. When the ventricles contract and intraventricular pressure rises above the pressure in the aorta and pulmonary trunk, the SL valves are forced open and their cusps flatten against the arterial walls as blood rushes past them **(Figure 18.8a)**. When the ventricles relax, and the blood (no longer propelled forward by ventricular contraction) flows backward toward the heart, it fills the cusps and closes the valves (Figure 18.8b).

We complete the valve story by noting what seems to be an important omission—there are no valves guarding the entrances of the venae cavae and pulmonary veins into the right and left atria, respectively. Small amounts of blood *do* spurt back into these vessels during atrial contraction, but backflow is minimal because of the inertia of the blood and because as it contracts, the atrial myocardium compresses (and collapses) these venous entry points.

Homeostatic Imbalance 18.2

Heart valves are simple devices, and the heart—like any mechanical pump—can function with "leaky" valves as long as the impairment is not too great. However, severe valve deformities can seriously hamper cardiac function.

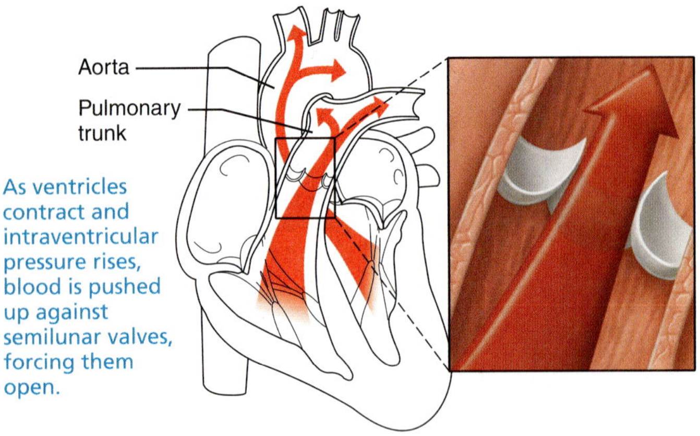

(a) Semilunar valves open

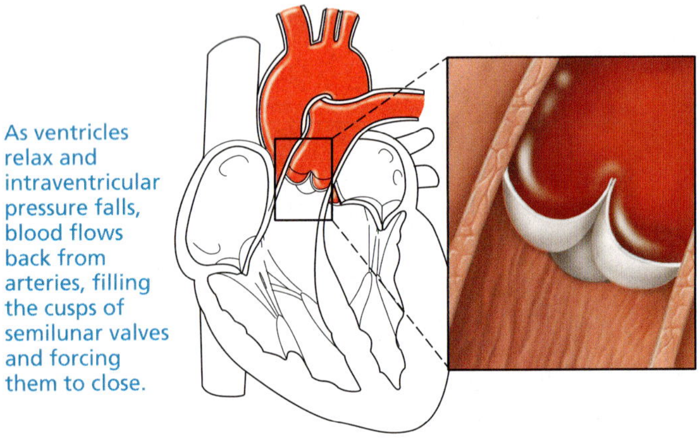

(b) Semilunar valves closed

Figure 18.8 The semilunar (SL) valves.

An *incompetent*, or *insufficient*, *valve* forces the heart to repump the same blood over and over because the valve does not close properly and blood backflows. In valvular *stenosis* ("narrowing"), the valve flaps become stiff (typically due to calcium salt deposits or scar tissue that forms following endocarditis) and constrict the opening. This stiffness compels the heart to contract more forcibly than normal. Both conditions increase the heart's workload and may weaken the heart severely over time.

The faulty valve (most often the mitral valve) can be replaced with a mechanical valve, a pig or cow heart valve chemically treated to prevent rejection, or cryopreserved valves from human cadavers. Heart valves tissue-engineered from a patient's own cells grown on a biodegradable scaffold are being developed. ✚

☑ Check Your Understanding

4. What is the function of the papillary muscles and chordae tendineae?

For answers, see Appendix H.

Pathway of Blood Through the Heart

✓ Trace the pathway of blood through the heart.

Having covered the basic anatomy of the heart, we can now follow the path that blood takes through the heart and its associated circuits. *Focus on Blood Flow Through the Heart* **(Figure 18.9)** follows a single "spurt" of blood as it passes through all four chambers of the heart and both blood circuits in its ever-repeating journey.

As you work your way through this figure, keep in mind that the left side of the heart is the *systemic circuit pump* and the right side of the heart is the *pulmonary circuit pump*. Notice how unique the pulmonary circuit is. Elsewhere in the body, veins carry relatively oxygen-poor blood to the heart, and arteries transport oxygen-rich blood from the heart. Exactly the opposite oxygenation conditions exist in veins and arteries of the pulmonary circuit.

Equal volumes of blood are pumped to the pulmonary and systemic circuits at any moment, but the two ventricles have very unequal workloads. The pulmonary circuit, served by the right ventricle, is a short, low-pressure circulation. In contrast, the systemic circuit, associated with the left ventricle, takes a long pathway through the entire body and encounters about five times as much friction, or resistance to blood flow.

This functional difference is revealed in the anatomy of the two ventricles (Figure 18.5e and **Figure 18.10**). The walls of the left ventricle are three times thicker than those of the right ventricle, and its cavity is nearly circular. The right ventricular cavity is flattened into a crescent shape that partially encloses the left ventricle, much the way a hand might loosely grasp a clenched fist. Consequently, the left ventricle can generate much more pressure than the right and is a far more powerful pump.

Coronary Circulation

✓ Name the major branches and describe the distribution of the coronary arteries.

Although the heart is more or less continuously filled with blood, this blood provides little nourishment to heart tissue. (The myocardium is too thick to make diffusion a practical means of delivering nutrients.) How, then, does the heart get nourishment? The **coronary circulation**, the functional blood supply of the heart, is the shortest circulation in the body.

Coronary Arteries

The *left* and *right coronary arteries* both arise from the base of the aorta and encircle the heart in the coronary sulcus. They provide the arterial supply of the coronary circulation **(Figure 18.11a)**.

The **left coronary artery** runs toward the left side of the heart and then divides into two major branches:

- The **anterior interventricular artery** (also known clinically as the *left anterior descending artery*) follows the anterior interventricular sulcus and supplies blood to the interventricular septum and anterior walls of both ventricles.
- The **circumflex artery** supplies the left atrium and the posterior walls of the left ventricle.

FOCUS Blood Flow Through the Heart

Figure 18.9 **The heart is a double pump, each side supplying its own circuit.**

Both sides of the heart pump at the same time, but let's follow one spurt of blood all the way through the system.

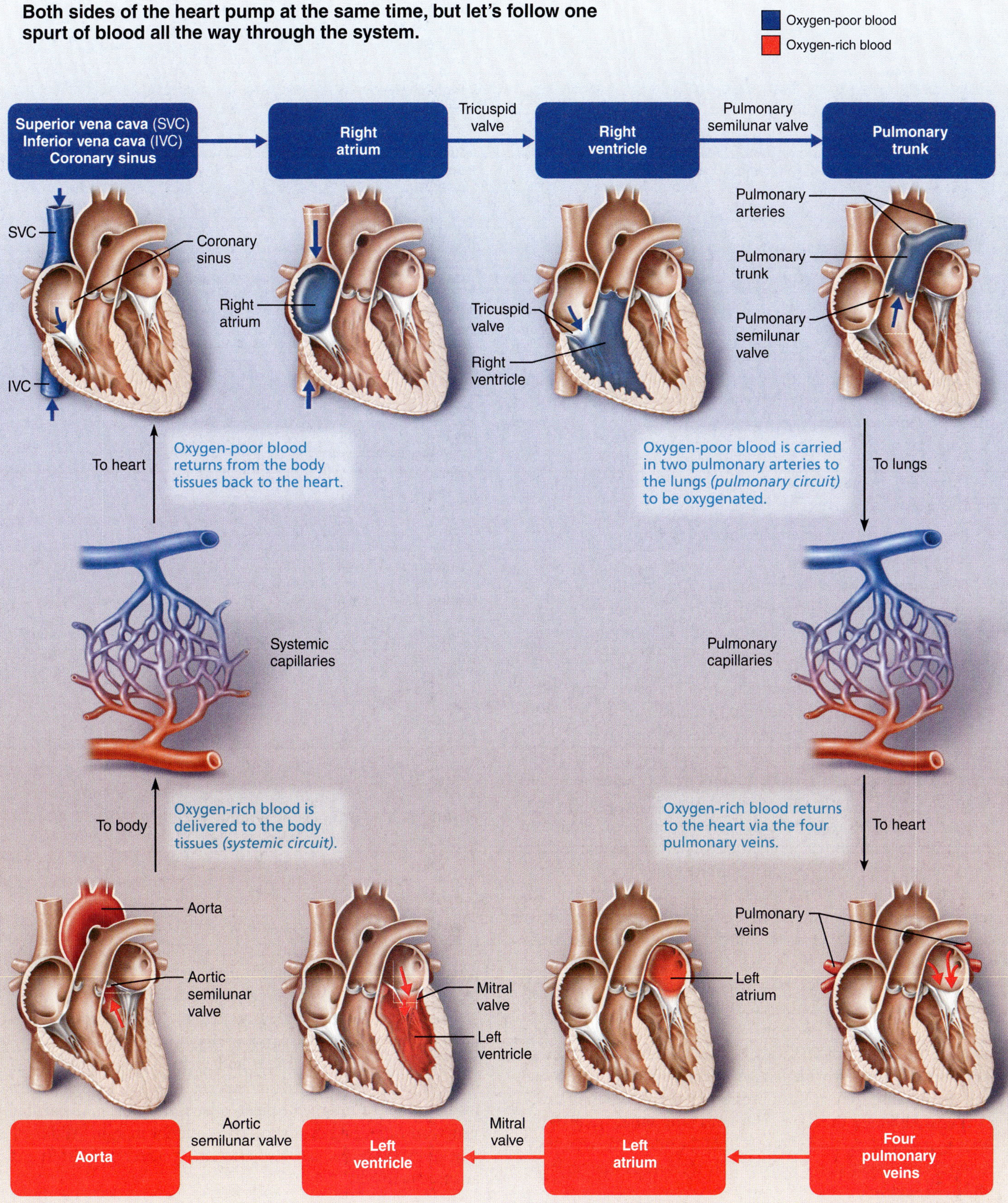

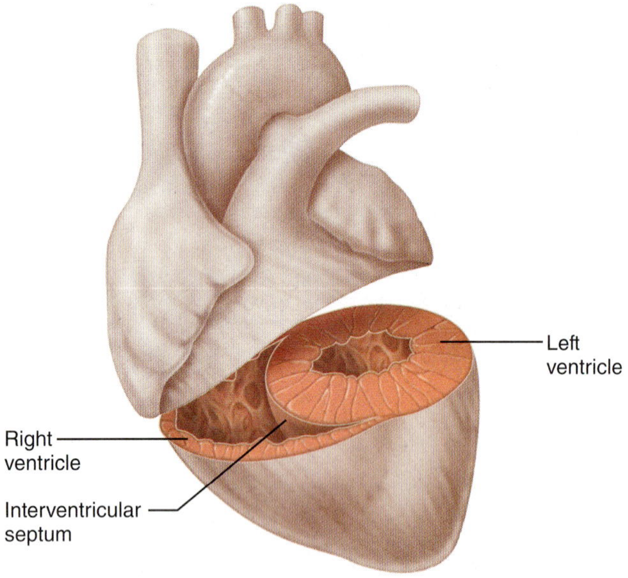

Figure 18.10 Anatomical differences between the right and left ventricles. The left ventricle has a thicker wall and its cavity is basically circular. The right ventricle cavity is crescent shaped and wraps around the left ventricle.

The **right coronary artery** courses to the right side of the heart, where it also gives rise to two branches:

- The **right marginal artery** serves the myocardium of the lateral right side of the heart.
- The **posterior interventricular artery** runs to the heart apex and supplies the posterior ventricular walls. Near the apex of the heart, this artery merges (anastomoses) with the anterior interventricular artery.

Together the branches of the right coronary artery supply the right atrium and nearly all the right ventricle.

The arterial supply of the heart varies considerably. For example, in 15% of people, the left coronary artery gives rise to *both* interventricular arteries. In about 4% of people, a single coronary artery supplies the whole heart. Additionally, there may be both right and left marginal arteries. There are many anastomoses (junctions) among the coronary arterial branches. These fusing networks provide additional (*collateral*) routes for blood delivery to the heart muscle, but are not robust enough to supply adequate nutrition when a coronary artery is suddenly occluded (blocked). Complete blockage leads to tissue death and heart attack.

The coronary arteries provide an intermittent, pulsating blood flow to the myocardium. These vessels and their main branches lie in the epicardium and send branches inward to nourish the myocardium. They deliver blood when the heart is relaxed, but are fairly ineffective when the ventricles are contracting because they are compressed by the contracting myocardium. Although the heart represents only about 1/200 of the body's weight, it requires about 1/20 of the body's blood supply. As might be expected, the left ventricle receives the most plentiful blood supply.

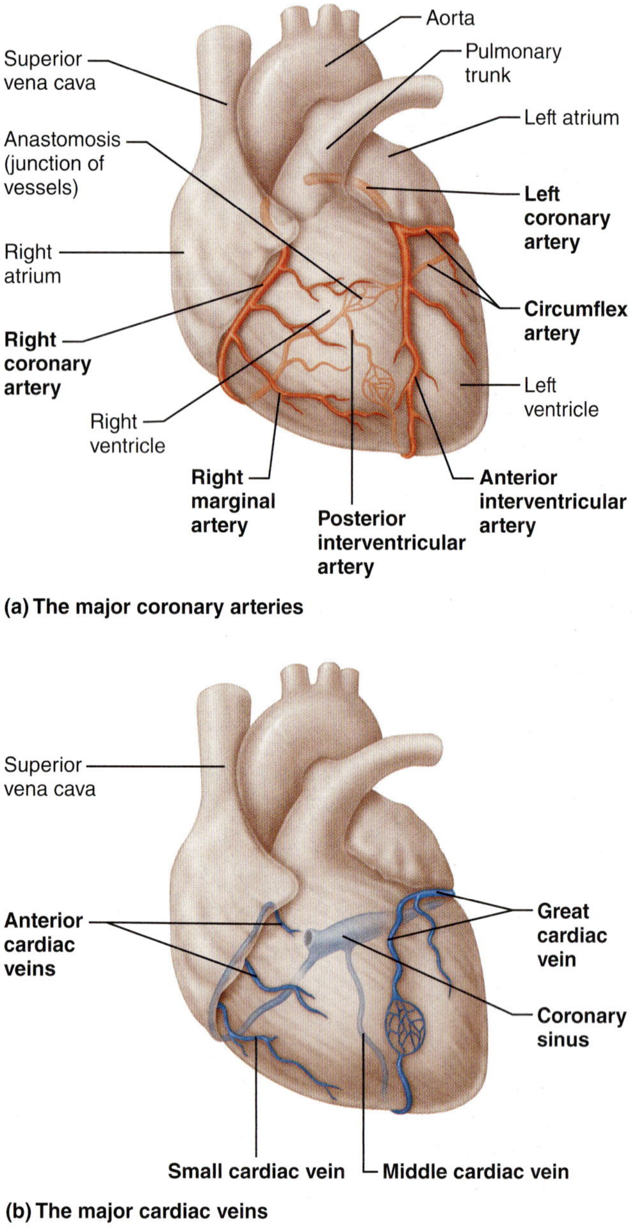

Figure 18.11 Coronary circulation. In both drawings, lighter-tinted vessels are more posterior in the heart.

Coronary Veins

After passing through the capillary beds of the myocardium, the venous blood is collected by the **cardiac veins**, whose paths roughly follow those of the coronary arteries. These veins join to form an enlarged vessel called the **coronary sinus**, which empties the blood into the right atrium. The coronary sinus is obvious on the posterior aspect of the heart (Figure 18.11b).

The sinus has three large tributaries: the **great cardiac vein** in the anterior interventricular sulcus; the **middle cardiac vein** in the posterior interventricular sulcus; and the **small cardiac vein**, running along the heart's right inferior margin. Additionally, several **anterior cardiac veins** empty directly into the right atrium anteriorly.

Homeostatic Imbalance 18.3

Blockage of the coronary arterial circulation can be serious and sometimes fatal. **Angina pectoris** (an-ji′nah pek′tor-is; "choked chest") is thoracic pain caused by a fleeting deficiency in blood delivery to the myocardium. It may result from stress-induced spasms of the coronary arteries or from increased physical demands on the heart. The myocardial cells are weakened by the temporary lack of oxygen but do not die.

Prolonged coronary blockage is far more serious because it can lead to a **myocardial infarction (MI)**, commonly called a **heart attack**, in which cells *do* die. Since adult cardiac muscle is essentially amitotic, most of the dead tissue is replaced with noncontractile scar tissue. Whether or not a person survives a myocardial infarction depends on the extent and location of the damage. Damage to the left ventricle—the systemic pump—is most serious. +

Check Your Understanding

5. Which side of the heart acts as the pulmonary pump? The systemic pump?
6. Which of the following statements are true? (a) The left ventricle wall is thicker than the right ventricle wall. (b) The left ventricle pumps blood at a higher pressure than the right ventricle. (c) The left ventricle pumps more blood with each beat than the right ventricle. Explain.
7. Name the two main branches of the right coronary artery.

For answers, see Appendix H.

Cardiac Muscle Fibers

✓ Describe the structural and functional properties of cardiac muscle, and explain how it differs from skeletal muscle.

✓ Briefly describe the events of cardiac muscle cell contraction.

Although similar to skeletal muscle, cardiac muscle displays some special anatomical features that reflect its unique blood-pumping role.

Microscopic Anatomy

Like skeletal muscle, **cardiac muscle** is striated and contracts by the sliding filament mechanism. However, in contrast to the long, cylindrical, multinucleate skeletal muscle fibers, cardiac cells are short, fat, branched, and interconnected. Each fiber contains one or at most two large, pale, *centrally* located nuclei **(Figure 18.12a)**. The intercellular spaces are filled with a loose connective tissue matrix (the *endomysium*) containing numerous capillaries. This delicate matrix is connected to the fibrous cardiac skeleton, which acts both as a tendon and as an insertion, giving the cardiac cells something to pull or exert their force against.

Skeletal muscle fibers are independent of one another both structurally and functionally. By contrast, the plasma membranes of adjacent cardiac cells interlock like the ribs of two sheets of corrugated cardboard at dark-staining junctions called **intercalated discs** (in-ter′kah-la″ted; *intercala* = insert) (Figure 18.12). Intercalated discs contain anchoring *desmosomes* and *gap junctions* (cell junctions discussed in Chapter 3). The desmosomes prevent adjacent cells from separating during contraction, and the gap junctions allow ions to pass from cell to cell, transmitting current across the entire heart. Because gap junctions electrically couple cardiac cells, the myocardium *behaves* as a single coordinated unit, or **functional syncytium** (sin-sit′e-um; *syn* = together, *cyt* = cell).

Large mitochondria account for 25–35% of the volume of cardiac cells (compared with only 2% in skeletal muscle), a characteristic that makes cardiac cells highly resistant to fatigue. Most of the remaining volume is occupied by myofibrils composed of fairly typical sarcomeres. The sarcomeres have Z discs, A bands, and I bands that reflect the arrangement of the thick (myosin) and thin (actin) filaments composing them. However, in contrast to skeletal muscle, the myofibrils of cardiac muscle cells vary greatly in diameter and branch extensively, accommodating the abundant mitochondria between them. This difference produces a banding pattern less dramatic than that seen in skeletal muscle.

The system for delivering Ca^{2+} is less elaborate in cardiac muscle cells. The T tubules are wider and fewer than in skeletal muscle and they enter the cells once per sarcomere at the Z discs. (Recall that T tubules are invaginations of the sarcolemma. In skeletal muscle, the T tubules invaginate twice per sarcomere, at the A band–I band junctions.) The cardiac sarcoplasmic reticulum is simpler and lacks the large terminal cisterns seen in skeletal muscle. Consequently, cardiac muscle fibers do not have *triads*.

Mechanism and Events of Contraction

Although both heart muscle and skeletal muscle are contractile tissues, they have three fundamental differences:

- **Means of stimulation.** Each skeletal muscle fiber must be stimulated to contract by a nerve ending, but some cardiac muscle cells are self-excitable. These cells can initiate not only their own depolarization, but that of the rest of the heart as well, in a spontaneous and rhythmic way. We describe this property, called **automaticity**, or **autorhythmicity**, in the next section.
- **Organ versus motor unit contraction.** In skeletal muscle, impulses do not spread from cell to cell. Only muscle fibers that are individually stimulated by nerve fibers contract. Skeletal muscles usually contract with only some of the muscle's motor units activated. In contrast, in cardiac muscle, either all fibers in the heart contract as a unit or the heart doesn't contract at all. This coordinated action occurs because gap junctions electrically tie all cardiac muscle cells together into a single contractile unit. Consequently, the depolarization wave travels across the heart from cell to cell via ion passage through the gap junctions.
- **Length of absolute refractory period.** Recall that the absolute refractory period is the inexcitable period when Na^+ channels are still open or inactivated. In skeletal muscle

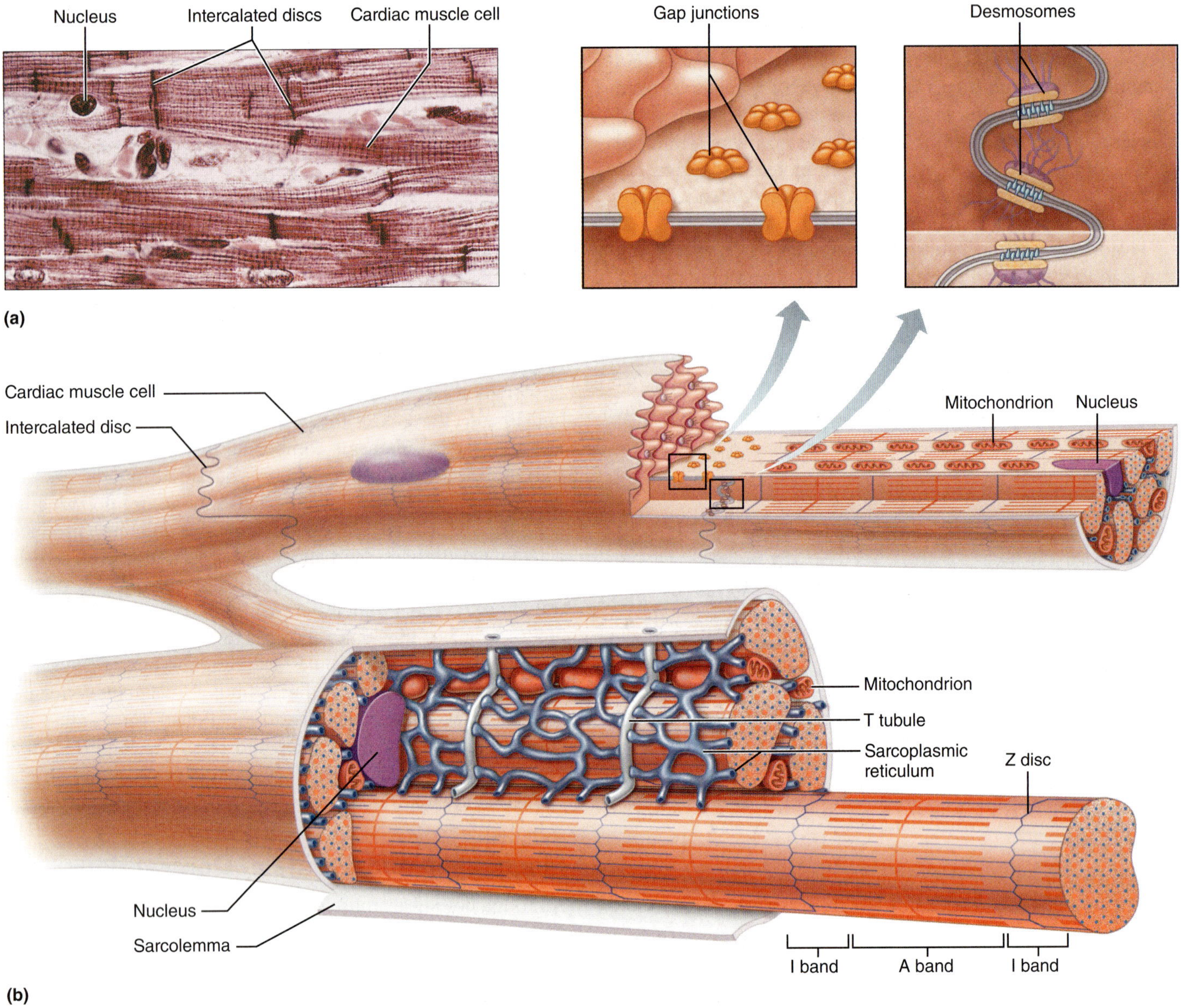

18

Figure 18.12 Microscopic anatomy of cardiac muscle. (a) Photomicrograph of cardiac muscle (600×). Notice that the cardiac muscle cells are short, branched, and striated. The dark-staining areas are intercalated discs, or junctions, between adjacent cells. **(b)** Components of intercalated discs and cardiac muscle fibers.

fibers, contractions last 15–100 ms with brief refractory periods of 1–2 ms. Contrast this to cardiac muscle cells, in which the absolute refractory period lasts over 200 ms, nearly as long as the contraction **(Figure 18.13)**. The long cardiac refractory period normally prevents tetanic contractions, which would stop the heart's pumping action.

Having probed the major differences between cardiac and skeletal muscle tissues, let's now look at their similarities. As with skeletal muscle, cardiac muscle contraction is triggered by action potentials that sweep across cell membranes. About 1% of cardiac fibers are *autorhythmic* ("self-rhythmic"), having the special ability to depolarize spontaneously and thus pace the heart. The bulk of heart muscle, however, is composed of *contractile muscle* fibers responsible for the heart's pumping activity. In these contractile muscle cells, the sequence of events leading to contraction is similar to that in skeletal muscle fibers:

1. Depolarization opens a few **fast voltage-gated Na^+ channels** in the sarcolemma, allowing extracellular Na^+ to enter. This influx initiates a positive feedback cycle that causes the rising phase of the action potential (and reversal of the membrane potential from −90 mV to nearly +30 mV; Figure 18.13 (1)). The period of Na^+ influx is very brief, because the sodium channels quickly inactivate and the Na^+ influx stops.

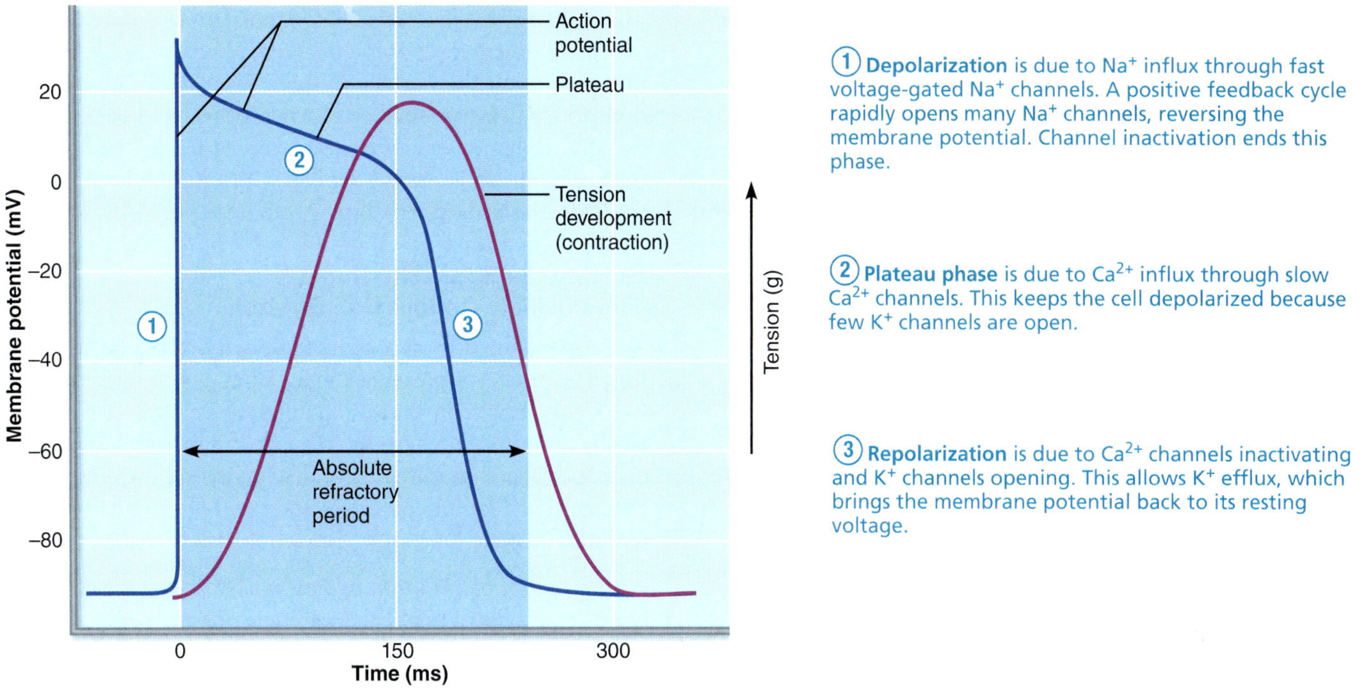

Figure 18.13 The action potential of contractile cardiac muscle cells. Relationship between the action potential, period of contraction, and absolute refractory period in a single ventricular cell.

2. Transmission of the depolarization wave down the T tubules (ultimately) causes the sarcoplasmic reticulum (SR) to release Ca^{2+} into the sarcoplasm.
3. Excitation-contraction coupling occurs as Ca^{2+} provides the signal (via troponin binding) for cross bridge activation and couples the depolarization wave to the sliding of the myofilaments.

These three steps are common to both skeletal and cardiac muscle cells (see Figure 9.11), but the two muscle types differ in how the SR is stimulated to release Ca^{2+}. Let's take a look.

Some 10–20% of the Ca^{2+} needed for the calcium pulse that triggers contraction enters the cardiac cells from the extracellular space. Once inside, it stimulates the SR to release the other 80% of the Ca^{2+} needed. Ca^{2+} is barred from entering nonstimulated cardiac fibers, but when Na^{+}-dependent membrane depolarization occurs, the voltage change also opens channels that allow Ca^{2+} to enter from the extracellular space. These channels are called **slow Ca^{2+} channels** because their opening is delayed a bit. The local influxes of Ca^{2+} through these channels trigger opening of nearby Ca^{2+}-sensitive channels in the SR tubules, which liberates bursts of Ca^{2+} ("calcium sparks") that dramatically increase the intracellular Ca^{2+} concentration.

Although Na^{+} channels have inactivated and repolarization has begun by this point, the calcium surge across the sarcolemma prolongs the depolarization potential briefly, producing a **plateau** in the action potential tracing (Figure 18.13 ②). At the same time, few K^{+} channels are open, which also prolongs the plateau and prevents rapid repolarization. As long as Ca^{2+} is entering, the cells continue to contract. Notice in Figure 18.13 that muscle tension develops during the plateau, and peaks just after the plateau ends.

Notice also that the action potential and contractile phase lasts much longer in cardiac muscle than in skeletal muscle. In skeletal muscle, the action potential typically lasts 1–2 ms and the contraction (for a single stimulus) 15–100 ms. In cardiac muscle, the action potential lasts 200 ms or more (because of the plateau), and tension development persists for 200 ms or more, providing the sustained contraction needed to eject blood from the heart.

After about 200 ms, the slope of the action potential tracing falls rapidly (Figure 18.13 ③). This repolarization results from inactivation of Ca^{2+} channels and opening of voltage-gated K^{+} channels, which allows a rapid loss of potassium from the cell that restores the resting membrane potential. During repolarization, Ca^{2+} is pumped back into the SR and the extracellular space.

18

Energy Requirements

Cardiac muscle has more mitochondria than skeletal muscle does, reflecting its greater dependence on oxygen for its energy metabolism. The heart relies almost exclusively on aerobic respiration. As a result, cardiac muscle cannot operate effectively for long without oxygen. This is in contrast to skeletal muscle, which can contract for prolonged periods by carrying out anaerobic respiration, and then restore its reserves of oxygen and fuel using excess postexercise oxygen consumption (EPOC).

Both types of muscle tissue use multiple fuel molecules, including glucose and fatty acids. But cardiac muscle is much more adaptable and readily switches metabolic pathways to use whatever nutrients are available, including lactic acid generated by skeletal muscle activity. Consequently, the real danger of an inadequate blood supply to the myocardium is not lack of nutrients, but lack of oxygen.

Homeostatic Imbalance 18.4

When a region of heart muscle is oxygen-starved (as during a heart attack), the ischemic cells (ischemic = blood deprived) begin to metabolize anaerobically, producing lactic acid. The rising H^+ level that results raises intracellular Ca^{2+}, damaging mitochondria and hindering cardiac cells' ability to produce ATP. High levels of intracellular H^+ and Ca^{2+} also cause the gap junctions (which are usually open) to close, isolating the damaged cells and forcing action potentials to find alternate routes to the cardiac cells beyond them. This may lead to fatal arrhythmias. +

Check Your Understanding

8. For each of the following, state whether it applies to skeletal muscle, cardiac muscle, or both: (a) refractory period is almost as long as the contraction; (b) source of Ca^{2+} for contraction is *only* SR; (c) AP exhibits a plateau phase; (d) has troponin; (e) has triads.
9. Cardiac muscle cannot go into tetany. Why?

For answers, see Appendix H.

Heart Physiology

Electrical Events

✓ Name the components of the conduction system of the heart, and trace the conduction pathway.

✓ Draw a diagram of a normal electrocardiogram tracing. Name the individual waves and intervals, and indicate what each represents.

✓ Name some abnormalities that can be detected on an ECG tracing.

The ability of cardiac muscle to depolarize and contract is intrinsic. In other words, it is a property of heart muscle and does not depend on the nervous system. Even if all nerve connections to the heart are severed, the heart continues to beat rhythmically, as demonstrated by transplanted hearts. Nevertheless, the healthy heart is amply supplied with autonomic nerve fibers that can alter its basic rhythm.

Setting the Basic Rhythm: The Intrinsic Conduction System

The independent, but coordinated, activity of the heart is a function of (1) the presence of gap junctions, and (2) the activity of the heart's "in-house" conduction system. The **intrinsic cardiac conduction system** consists of noncontractile cardiac cells specialized to initiate and distribute impulses throughout the heart, so that it depolarizes and contracts in an orderly, sequential manner. Let's look at how this system works.

Action Potential Initiation by Pacemaker Cells Unstimulated contractile cells of the heart (and neurons and skeletal muscle fibers) maintain a stable resting membrane potential. Unlike them, the **cardiac pacemaker cells** (or *autorhythmic cells*) making up the intrinsic conduction system have an *unstable resting potential* that continuously depolarizes, drifting slowly toward threshold. These spontaneously changing membrane potentials, called **pacemaker potentials** or **prepotentials**, initiate the action potentials that spread throughout the heart to trigger its rhythmic contractions. Let's look at the three parts of an action potential in pacemaker cells as shown in Figure 18.14.

(1) **Pacemaker potential.** The pacemaker potential is due to the special properties of the ion channels in the sarcolemma. In these cells, hyperpolarization at the end of an action potential both closes K^+ channels and opens slow Na^+ channels. The Na^+ influx alters the balance between K^+ loss and Na^+ entry, and the membrane interior becomes less and less negative (more positive).

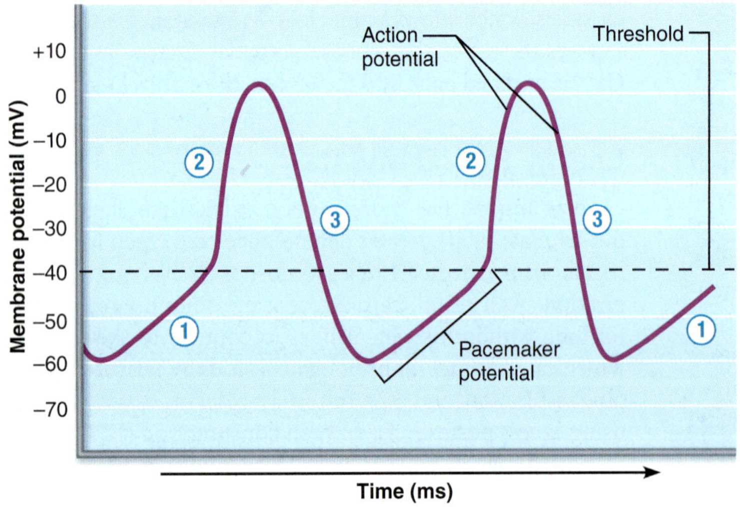

(1) Pacemaker potential This slow depolarization is due to both opening of Na^+ channels and closing of K^+ channels. Notice that the membrane potential is never a flat line.

(2) Depolarization The action potential begins when the pacemaker potential reaches threshold. Depolarization is due to Ca^{2+} influx through Ca^{2+} channels.

(3) Repolarization is due to Ca^{2+} channels inactivating and K^+ channels opening. This allows K^+ efflux, which brings the membrane potential back to its most negative voltage.

Figure 18.14 Pacemaker and action potentials of pacemaker cells in the heart.

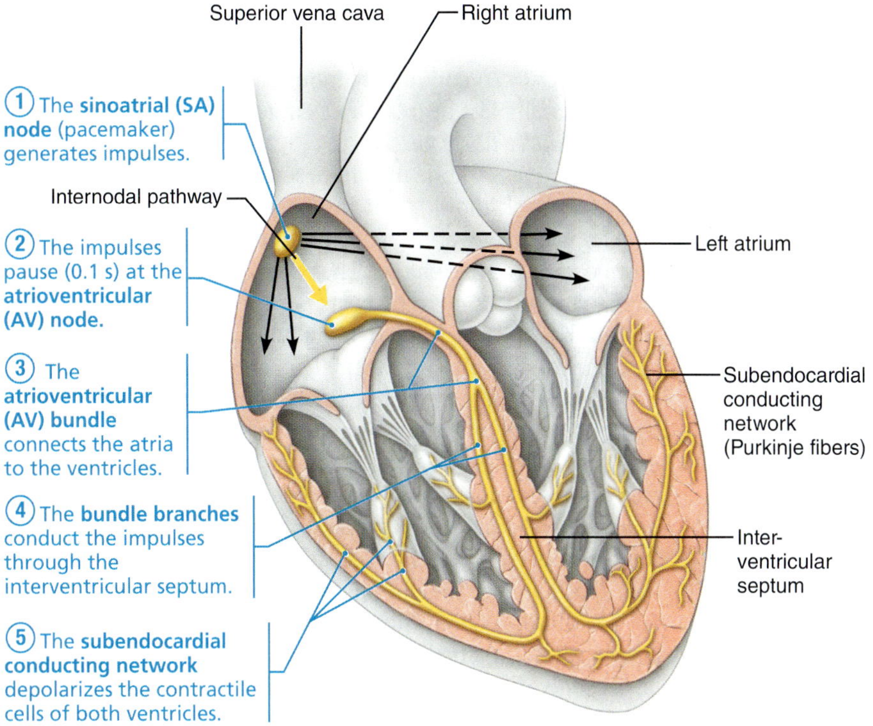

(a) Anatomy of the intrinsic conduction system showing the sequence of electrical excitation

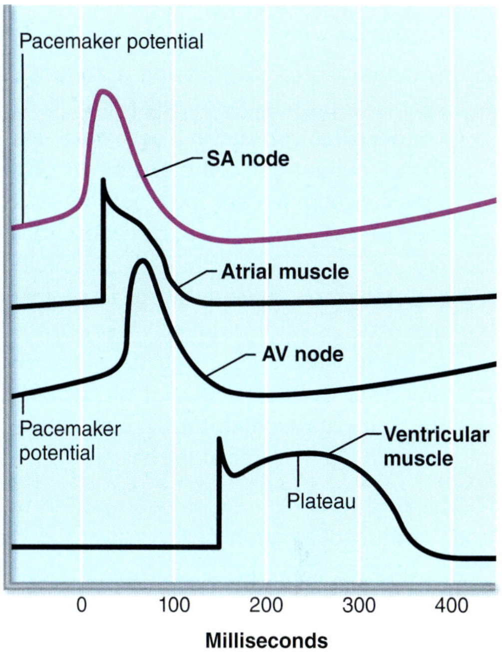

(b) Comparison of action potential shape at various locations

Figure 18.15 Intrinsic cardiac conduction system and action potential succession during one heartbeat.

② **Depolarization.** Ultimately, at threshold (approximately −40 mV), Ca^{2+} **channels** open, allowing explosive entry of Ca^{2+} from the extracellular space. As a result, in pacemaker cells, it is the influx of Ca^{2+} (rather than Na^+) that produces the rising phase of the action potential and reverses the membrane potential.

③ **Repolarization.** As in other excitable cells, the falling phase of the action potential and repolarization reflect opening of K^+ channels and K^+ efflux from the cell.

Once repolarization is complete, K^+ channels close, K^+ efflux declines, and the slow depolarization to threshold begins again.

Sequence of Excitation Cardiac pacemaker cells are found in the following areas (Figure 18.15): sinoatrial (si″no-a′tre-al) node, atrioventricular node, atrioventricular bundle, right and left bundle branches, and subendocardial conducting network (Purkinje fibers). Impulses pass across the heart in order from ① to ⑤ following the yellow pathway in **Figure 18.15a**.

① **Sinoatrial (SA) node.** The crescent-shaped **sinoatrial node** is located in the right atrial wall, just inferior to the entrance of the superior vena cava. A minute cell mass with a mammoth job, the SA node typically generates impulses about 75 times every minute. (Its inherent rate in the absence of extrinsic neural and hormonal factors is closer to 100 times per minute.) The SA node sets the pace for the heart as a whole because no other region of the conduction system or the myocardium has a faster depolarization rate. For this reason, it is the heart's **pacemaker**, and its characteristic rhythm, called **sinus rhythm**, determines heart rate.

② **Atrioventricular (AV) node.** From the SA node, the depolarization wave spreads via gap junctions throughout the atria and via the *internodal pathway* to the **atrioventricular node**, located in the inferior portion of the interatrial septum immediately above the tricuspid valve. At the AV node, the impulse is delayed for about 0.1 s, allowing the atria to respond and complete their contraction before the ventricles contract. This delay reflects the smaller diameter of the fibers here and the fact that they have fewer gap junctions for current flow. Consequently, the AV node conducts impulses more slowly than other parts of the system, just as traffic slows when cars are forced to merge from four lanes into two. Once through the AV node, the signaling impulse passes rapidly through the rest of the system.

③ **Atrioventricular (AV) bundle.** From the AV node, the impulse sweeps to the **atrioventricular bundle** (also called the **bundle of His**) in the superior part of the interventricular septum. Although the atria and ventricles abut each other, they are *not* connected by gap junctions. The AV bundle is the *only* electrical connection between them. The fibrous cardiac skeleton is nonconducting and insulates the rest of the AV junction.

④ **Right and left bundle branches.** The AV bundle persists only briefly before splitting into two pathways—the **right** and **left bundle branches**, which course along the interventricular septum toward the heart apex.

⑤ **Subendocardial conducting network.** Essentially long strands of barrel-shaped cells with few myofibrils, the **subendocardial conducting network**, also called **Purkinje fibers** (pur-kin′je), completes the pathway through the interventricular septum, penetrate into the heart apex, and then turn superiorly into the ventricular walls. The bundle branches excite the septal cells, but the bulk of ventricular depolarization depends on the large fibers of the conducting network and, ultimately, on cell-to-cell transmission of the impulse via gap junctions between the ventricular muscle cells. Because the left ventricle is much larger than the right, the subendocardial conducting network is more elaborate in that side of the heart.

The total time between initiation of an impulse by the SA node and depolarization of the last of the ventricular muscle cells is approximately 0.22 s (220 ms) in a healthy human heart.

Ventricular contraction almost immediately follows the ventricular depolarization wave. The wringing motion of contraction begins at the heart apex and moves toward the atria, following the direction of the excitation wave through the ventricle walls. This contraction ejects some of the contained blood *superiorly* into the large arteries leaving the ventricles.

The various cardiac pacemaker cells have different rates of spontaneous depolarization. The SA node normally drives the heart at a rate of 75 beats per minute. Without SA node input, the AV node would depolarize only about 50 times per minute. Without input from the AV node, the AV bundle and the subendocardial conducting network would depolarize only about 30 times per minute (though they conduct very rapidly). Note that these slower pacemakers cannot dominate the heart unless faster pacemakers stop functioning.

The cardiac conduction system coordinates and synchronizes heart activity. Without it, impulses would travel much more slowly—0.3 to 0.5 m/s as opposed to several meters per second in most parts of the conduction system. This slower rate would allow some muscle fibers to contract long before others, reducing pump effectiveness.

18

Homeostatic Imbalance 18.5

Defects in the intrinsic conduction system can cause irregular heart rhythms, or **arrhythmias** (ah-rith′me-ahz). They may also cause uncoordinated atrial and ventricular contractions, or even **fibrillation**, a condition of rapid and irregular or out-of-phase contractions in which control of heart rhythm is taken away from the SA node by rapid activity in other heart regions. The heart in fibrillation has been compared with a squirming bag of worms. Fibrillating ventricles are useless as pumps; and unless the heart is defibrillated quickly, circulation stops and brain death occurs.

Defibrillation is accomplished by electrically shocking the heart, which interrupts its chaotic twitching by depolarizing the entire myocardium. The hope is that "with the slate wiped clean" the SA node will begin to function normally and sinus rhythm will be reestablished. Implantable cardioverter defibrillators (ICDs) can continually monitor heart rhythms and slow an abnormally fast heart rate or emit an electrical shock if the heart begins to fibrillate.

A defective SA node may have several consequences. An **ectopic focus** (ek-top′ik), which is an abnormal pacemaker, may appear and take over the pacing of heart rate, or the AV node may become the pacemaker. The pace set by the AV node (**junctional rhythm**) is 40 to 60 beats per minute, slower than sinus rhythm but still adequate to maintain circulation.

Occasionally, ectopic pacemakers appear even when the SA node is operating normally. A small region of the heart becomes hyperexcitable, sometimes as a result of too much caffeine (several cups of coffee) or nicotine (excessive smoking), and generates impulses more quickly than the SA node. This leads to a *premature contraction* or **extrasystole** (ek″strah-sis′to-le) before the SA node initiates the next contraction. Then, because the heart has a longer time to fill, the next (normal) contraction is felt as a thud. As you might guess, premature *ventricular* contractions (PVCs) are most problematic.

The only route for impulse transmission from atria to ventricles is through the AV node. Thus any damage to the AV node interferes with the ability of the ventricles to receive pacing impulses, causing **heart block**. In total heart block no impulses get through and the ventricles beat at their intrinsic rate, which is too slow to maintain adequate circulation. In partial heart block, only some of the atrial impulses reach the ventricles. In both cases, artificial pacemakers are implanted to recouple the atria to the ventricles as necessary. These programmable devices speed up in response to increased physical activity just as a normal heart would, and many can send diagnostic information to the patient's doctor via telephone. ✚

Modifying the Basic Rhythm: Extrinsic Innervation of the Heart

Although the intrinsic conduction system sets the basic heart rate, fibers of the autonomic nervous system modify the marchlike beat and introduce a subtle variability from one beat to the next. The sympathetic nervous system (the "accelerator") increases both the rate and the force of heartbeat. The parasympathetic activation (the "brakes") slows the heart. We explain these neural controls later—here we discuss the anatomy of the nerve supply to the heart.

The cardiac centers are located in the medulla oblongata. The **cardioacceleratory center** projects to sympathetic neurons in the T_1–T_5 level of the spinal cord. These preganglionic neurons, in turn, synapse with postganglionic neurons in the cervical and upper thoracic sympathetic trunk **(Figure 18.16)**. From there, postganglionic fibers run through the cardiac plexus to the heart where they innervate the SA and AV nodes, heart muscle, and coronary arteries.

The **cardioinhibitory center** sends impulses to the parasympathetic dorsal vagus nucleus in the medulla, which in turn sends inhibitory impulses to the heart via branches of the vagus nerves. Most parasympathetic postganglionic motor neurons lie

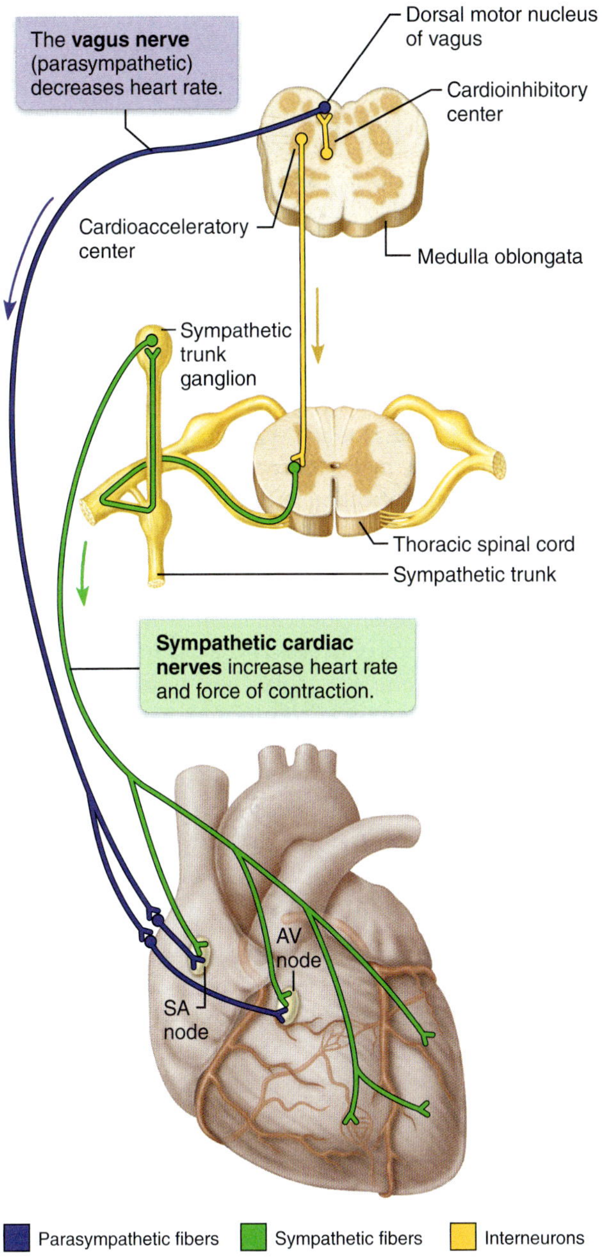

Figure 18.16 Autonomic innervation of the heart.

in ganglia in the heart wall and their fibers project most heavily to the SA and AV nodes.

Electrocardiography

The electrical currents generated in and transmitted through the heart spread throughout the body and can be detected with a device called an **electrocardiograph**. An **electrocardiogram (ECG)** is a graphic record of heart activity. An ECG is a composite of all the action potentials generated by nodal and contractile cells at a given time **(Figure 18.17)**—*not*, as sometimes assumed, a tracing of a single action potential.

To record an ECG, recording electrodes (typically 12 leads) are placed at various sites on the body surface. Three electrodes are bipolar leads that measure the voltage difference either between the arms or between an arm and a leg, and nine are unipolar leads. Together the 12 leads provide a comprehensive picture of the heart's electrical activity.

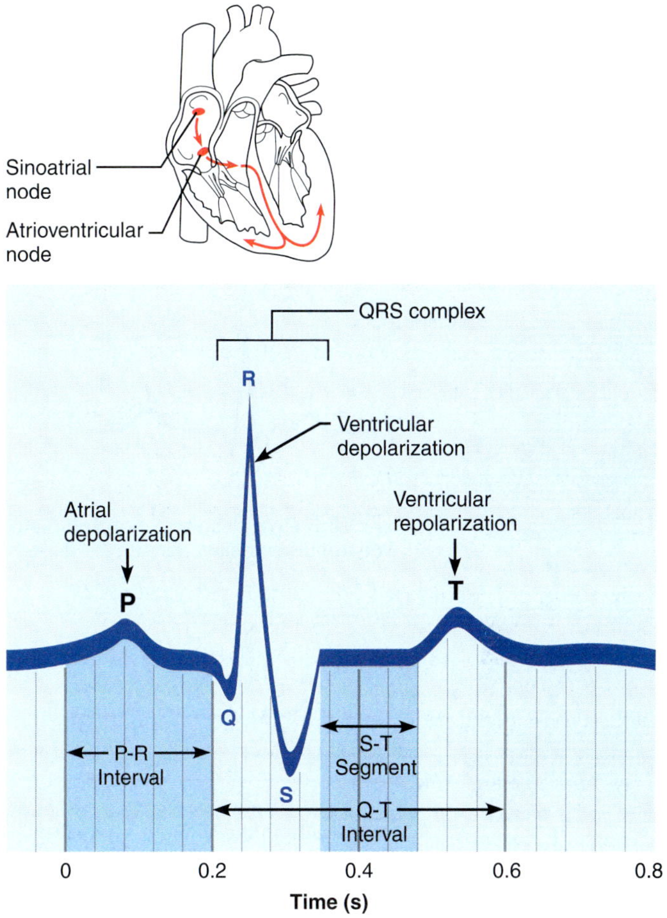

Figure 18.17 An electrocardiogram (ECG) tracing. The labels identify the three normally recognizable deflections (waves) and the important intervals.

A typical ECG has three almost immediately distinguishable waves or *deflections*: the P wave, the QRS complex, and the T wave (Figure 18.17). The first, the small **P wave**, lasts about 0.08 s and results from movement of the depolarization wave from the SA node through the atria. Approximately 0.1 s after the P wave begins, the atria contract.

The large **QRS complex** results from ventricular depolarization and precedes ventricular contraction. It has a complicated shape because the paths of the depolarization waves through the ventricular walls change continuously, producing corresponding changes in current direction. Additionally, the time required for each ventricle to depolarize depends on its size relative to the other ventricle. Average duration of the QRS complex is 0.08 s.

The **T wave,** caused by ventricular repolarization, typically lasts about 0.16 s. Repolarization is slower than depolarization, so the T wave is more spread out and has a lower amplitude (height) than the QRS complex. Because atrial repolarization takes place during the period of ventricular excitation, the wave

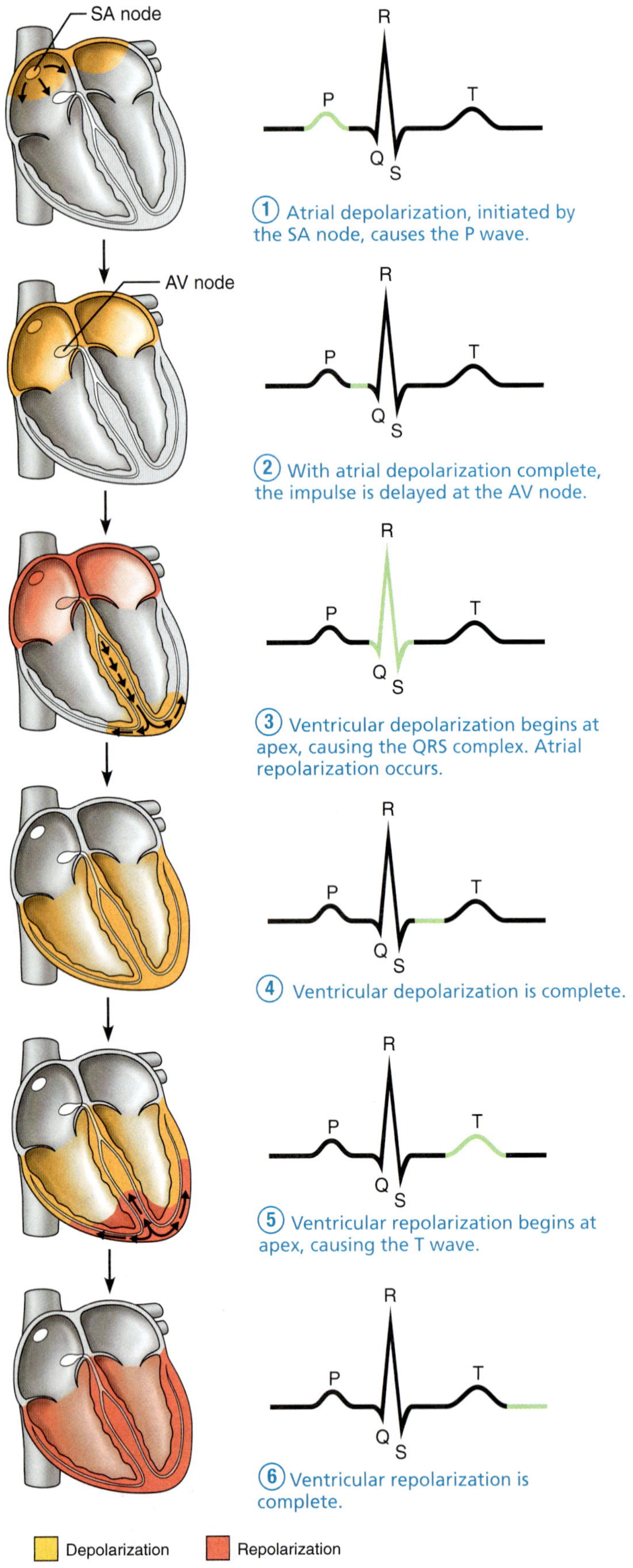

Figure 18.18 The sequence of depolarization and repolarization of the heart related to the deflection waves of an ECG tracing.

representing atrial repolarization is normally obscured by the large QRS complex being recorded at the same time.

The **P-R interval** is the time (about 0.16 s) from the beginning of atrial excitation to the beginning of ventricular excitation. If the Q wave is visible (which is often not the case), it marks the beginning of ventricular excitation, and for this reason this interval is sometimes called the **P-Q interval**. The P-R interval includes atrial depolarization (and contraction) as well as the passage of the depolarization wave through the rest of the conduction system.

During the **S-T segment** of the ECG, when the action potentials of the ventricular myocytes are in their plateau phases, the entire ventricular myocardium is depolarized. The **Q-T interval**, lasting about 0.38 s, is the period from the beginning of ventricular depolarization through ventricular repolarization.

Figure 18.18 relates the parts of an ECG to the sequence of depolarization and repolarization in the heart.

Homeostatic Imbalance 18.6

In a healthy heart, the size, duration, and timing of the deflection waves tend to be consistent. Changes in the pattern or timing of the ECG may reveal a diseased or damaged heart or problems with the heart's conduction system **(Figure 18.19)**. For example, an enlarged R wave hints of enlarged ventricles, an S-T segment that is elevated or depressed indicates cardiac ischemia, and a prolonged Q-T interval reveals a repolarization abnormality that increases the risk of ventricular arrhythmias. ✚

☑ Check Your Understanding

10. Which part of the intrinsic conduction system directly excites ventricular myocardial cells? In which direction does the depolarization wave travel across the ventricles?
11. Describe the electrical event in the heart that occurs during each of the following: (a) the QRS wave of the ECG; (b) the T wave of the ECG; (c) the P-R interval of the ECG.

For answers, see Appendix H.

Heart Sounds

✓ Describe normal heart sounds, and explain how heart murmurs differ.

Auscultating (listening to) the thorax with a stethoscope will reveal two sounds during each heartbeat. These **heart sounds**, often described as lub-dup, are associated with the heart valves closing. (The top of Figure 18.21 shows the timing of heart sounds in the cardiac cycle.)

The basic rhythm of the heart sounds is lub-dup, pause, lub-dup, pause, and so on, with the pause indicating the period when the heart is relaxing. The first sound occurs as the AV valves close. It signifies the point when ventricular pressure rises above atrial pressure (the beginning of ventricular systole, discussed in the next section). The first sound tends to be louder, longer, and more resonant than the second. The second sound occurs as the SL valves snap shut at the beginning of ventricular relaxation (diastole) resulting in a short, sharp sound.

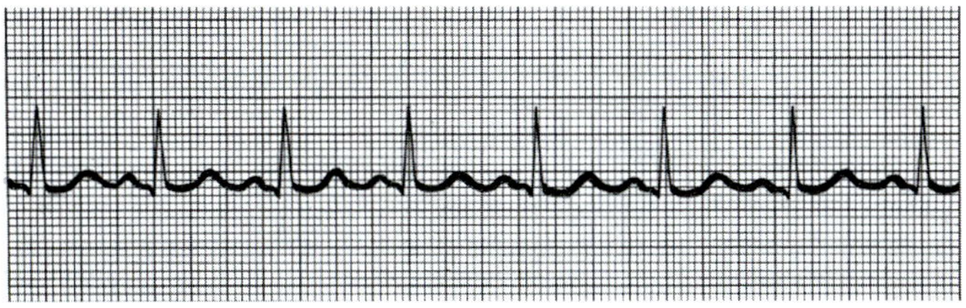

(a) Normal sinus rhythm.

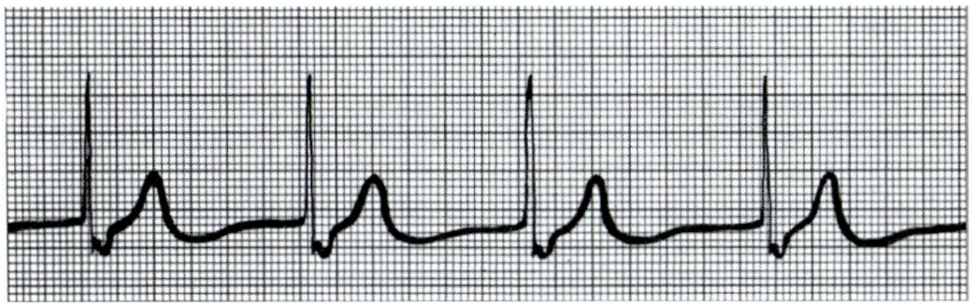

(b) Junctional rhythm. The SA node is nonfunctional, P waves are absent, and the AV node paces the heart at 40–60 beats/min.

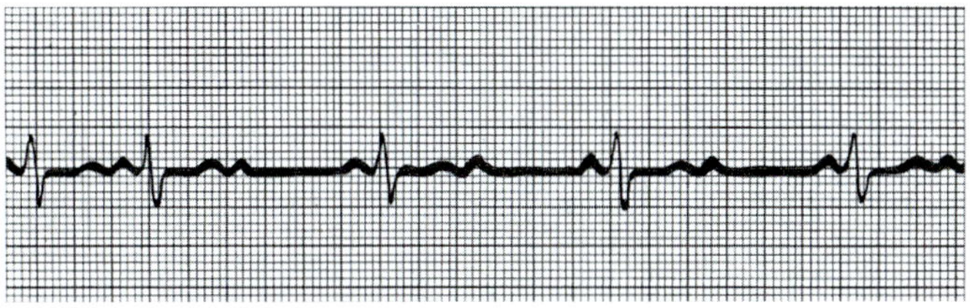

(c) Second-degree heart block. Some P waves are not conducted through the AV node; hence more P than QRS waves are seen. In this tracing, the ratio of P waves to QRS waves is mostly 2:1.

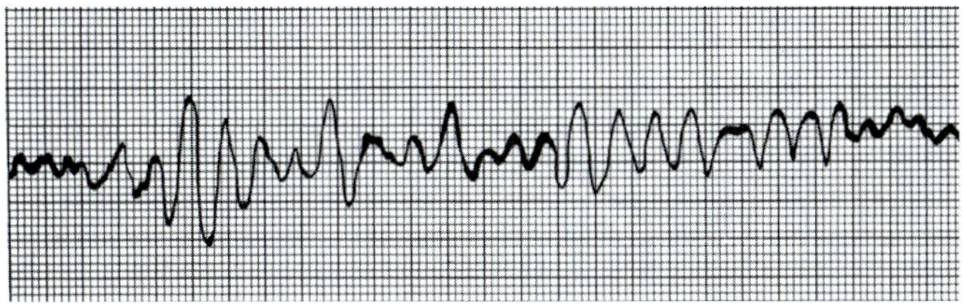

(d) Ventricular fibrillation. These chaotic, grossly irregular ECG deflections are seen in acute heart attack and electrical shock.

Figure 18.19 Normal and abnormal ECG tracings.

Because the mitral valve closes slightly before the tricuspid valve does, and the aortic SL valve generally snaps shut just before the pulmonary valve, it is possible to distinguish the individual valve sounds by auscultating four specific regions of the thorax **(Figure 18.20)**. Notice that these four points, while not directly superficial to the valves (because the sounds take oblique paths to reach the chest wall), do handily define the four corners of the normal heart. Knowing normal heart size and location is essential for recognizing an enlarged (and often diseased) heart.

Homeostatic Imbalance 18.7

Blood flows silently as long as its flow is smooth and uninterrupted. If blood strikes obstructions, however, its flow becomes turbulent and generates abnormal heart sounds, called **heart murmurs**, that can be heard with a stethoscope. Heart murmurs are fairly common in young children (and some elderly people) with perfectly healthy hearts, probably because their heart walls are relatively thin and vibrate with rushing blood.

Most often, however, murmurs indicate valve problems. An *insufficient* or *incompetent* valve fails to close completely. There is a swishing sound as blood backflows or regurgitates through the partially open valve *after* the valve has (supposedly) closed.

A *stenotic* valve fails to open completely and its narrow opening restricts blood flow *through* the valve. In a stenotic aortic valve, for instance, a high-pitched sound or click can be detected when the valve should be wide open during ventricular contraction, but is not. ✚

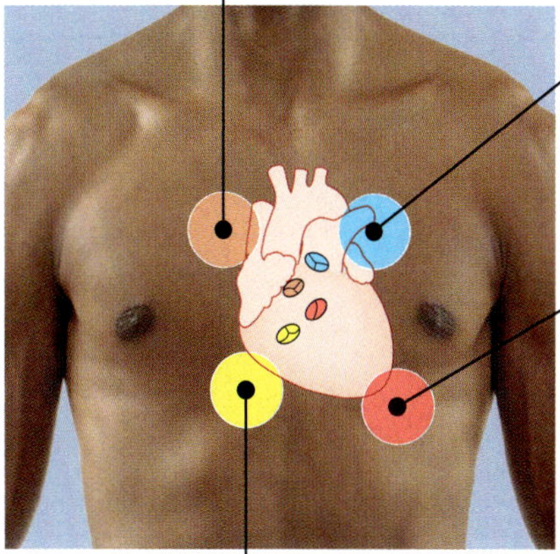

Figure 18.20 Areas of the thoracic surface where the sounds of individual valves can best be detected.

Mechanical Events: The Cardiac Cycle

✓ Describe the timing and events of the cardiac cycle.

The heart undergoes some dramatic writhing movements as it alternately contracts, forcing blood out of its chambers, and then relaxes, allowing its chambers to refill with blood. The term **systole** (sis′to-le) refers to these periods of contraction, and **diastole** (di-as′to-le) refers to those of relaxation. The **cardiac cycle** includes *all* events associated with the blood flow through the heart during one complete heartbeat—atrial systole and diastole followed by ventricular systole and diastole. These mechanical events always *follow* the electrical events seen in the ECG.

The cardiac cycle is marked by a succession of pressure and blood volume changes in the heart. Because blood circulates endlessly, we must choose an arbitrary starting point for one

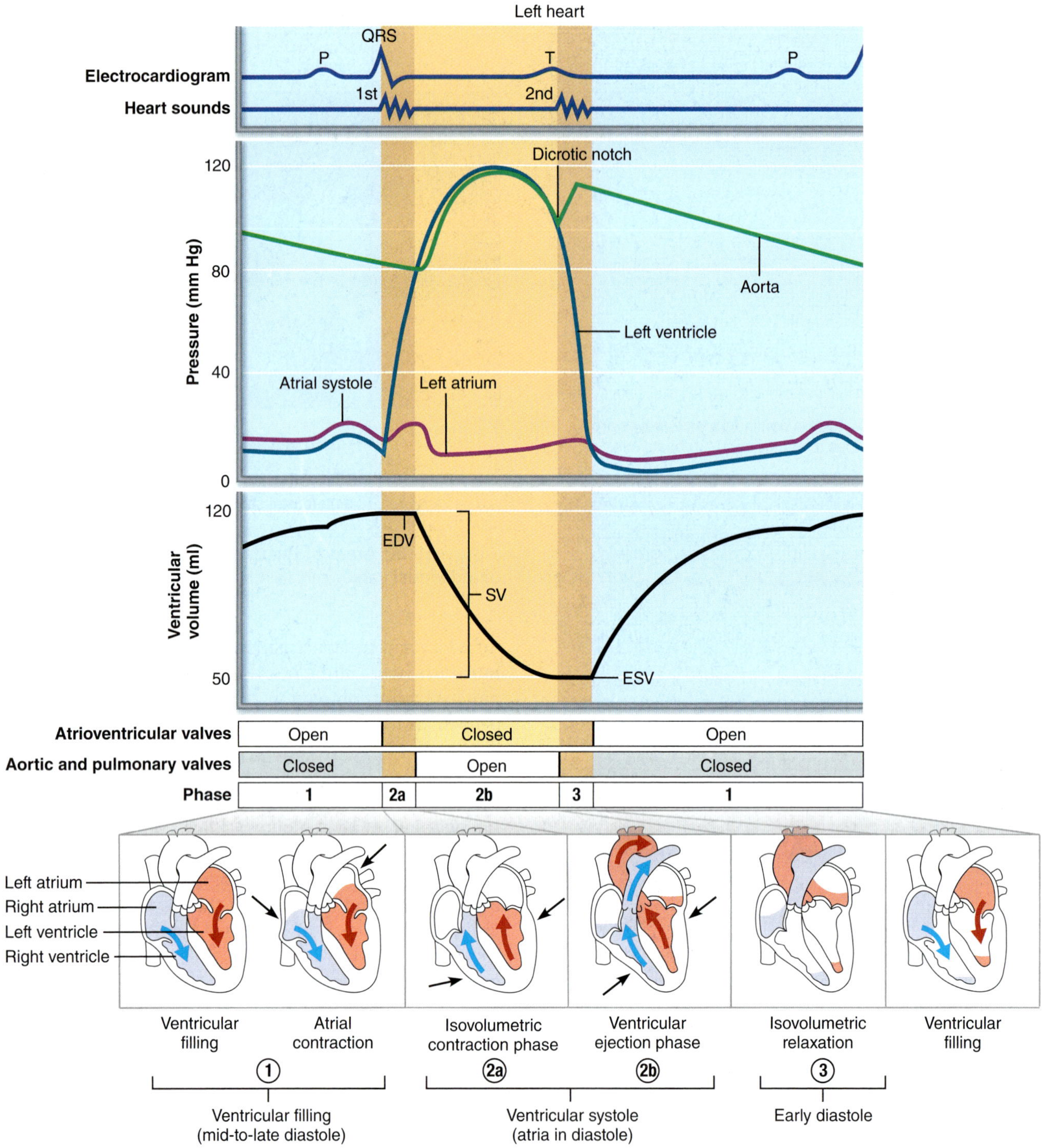

Figure 18.21 Summary of events during the cardiac cycle. An ECG tracing (*top*) correlated with graphs of pressure and volume changes (*center*) in the left side of the heart. Pressures are lower in the right side of the heart. Timing of heart sounds is also indicated. (*Bottom*) Events of phases 1 through 3 of the cardiac cycle. EDV = end diastolic volume, ESV = end systolic volume, SV = stroke volume.

turn of the cardiac cycle. As shown in **Figure 18.21**, which outlines what happens in the left side of the heart, we begin with the heart in total relaxation: Atria and ventricles are quiet, and it is mid-to-late diastole.

① **Ventricular filling: mid-to-late diastole.** Pressure in the heart is low, blood returning from the circulation is flowing passively through the atria and the open AV valves into the ventricles, and the aortic and pulmonary valves are closed. More than 80% of ventricular filling occurs during this period, and the AV valve flaps begin to drift toward the closed position. (The remaining 20% is delivered to the ventricles when the atria contract toward the end of this phase.)

Now the stage is set for atrial systole. Following depolarization (P wave of ECG), the atria contract, compressing the blood in their chambers. This causes a sudden slight rise in atrial pressure, which propels residual blood out of the atria into the ventricles. At this point the ventricles are in the last part of their diastole and have the maximum volume of blood they will contain in the cycle, an amount called the *end diastolic volume* (*EDV*). Then the atria relax and the ventricles depolarize (QRS complex). Atrial diastole persists through the rest of the cycle.

② **Ventricular systole (atria in diastole).** As the atria relax, the ventricles begin contracting. Their walls close in on the blood in their chambers, and ventricular pressure rises rapidly and sharply, closing the AV valves. The split-second period when the ventricles are completely closed chambers and the blood volume in the chambers remains constant as the ventricles contract is the **isovolumetric contraction phase** (i″so-vol″u-met′rik).

Ventricular pressure continues to rise. When it finally exceeds the pressure in the large arteries issuing from the ventricles, the isovolumetric stage ends as the SL valves are forced open and blood rushes from the ventricles into the aorta and pulmonary trunk. During this ventricular ejection phase, the pressure in the aorta normally reaches about 120 mm Hg.

③ **Isovolumetric relaxation: early diastole.** During this brief phase following the T wave, the ventricles relax. Because the blood remaining in their chambers, referred to as the *end systolic volume* (*ESV*), is no longer compressed, ventricular pressure drops rapidly and blood in the aorta and pulmonary trunk flows back toward the heart, closing the SL valves. Closure of the aortic valve raises aortic pressure briefly as backflowing blood rebounds off the closed valve cusps, an event beginning at the **dicrotic notch** shown on the pressure graph. Once again the ventricles are totally closed chambers.

All during ventricular systole, the atria have been in diastole. They have been filling with blood and the intra-atrial pressure has been rising. When blood pressure on the atrial side of the AV valves exceeds that in the ventricles, the AV valves are forced open and ventricular filling, phase ①, begins again. Atrial pressure drops to its lowest point and ventricular pressure begins to rise, completing the cycle.

Assuming the average heart beats 75 times each minute, the cardiac cycle lasts about 0.8 s, with atrial systole accounting for 0.1 s and ventricular systole 0.3 s. The remaining 0.4 s is a period of total heart relaxation, the **quiescent period**.

Notice two important points: (1) Blood flow through the heart is controlled entirely by pressure changes and (2) blood flows down a pressure gradient through any available opening. The pressure changes, in turn, reflect the alternating contraction and relaxation of the myocardium and cause the heart valves to open, which keeps blood flowing in the forward direction.

The situation in the right side of the heart is essentially the same as in the left side *except* for pressure. The pulmonary circulation is a low-pressure circulation as evidenced by the much thinner myocardium of its right ventricle. So, typical systolic and diastolic pressures for the pulmonary artery are 24 and 10 mm Hg, compared to systolic and diastolic pressures of 120 and 80 mm Hg, respectively, for the aorta. However, the two sides of the heart eject the same blood volume with each heartbeat.

Check Your Understanding

12. The second heart sound is associated with the closing of which valve(s)?
13. If the mitral valve were insufficient, would you expect to hear the murmur (of blood flowing through the valve that should be closed) during ventricular systole or diastole?
14. During the cardiac cycle, there are two periods when all four valves are closed. Name these two periods.

For answers, see Appendix H.

Cardiac Output (CO)

✓ Name and explain the effects of various factors regulating stroke volume and heart rate.

✓ Explain the role of the autonomic nervous system in regulating cardiac output.

Cardiac output (CO) is the amount of blood pumped out by *each* ventricle in 1 minute. It is the product of heart rate (HR) and stroke volume (SV). **Stroke volume** is defined as the volume of blood pumped out by one ventricle with each beat. In general, stroke volume correlates with the force of ventricular contraction.

Using normal resting values for heart rate (75 beats/min) and stroke volume (70 ml/beat), the average adult cardiac output can be computed:

$$CO = HR \times SV = \frac{75\ \text{beats}}{\text{min}} \times \frac{70\ \text{ml}}{\text{beat}}$$
$$= \frac{5250\ \text{ml}}{\text{min}} = \frac{5.25\ \text{L}}{\text{min}}$$

The normal adult blood volume is about 5 L (a little more than 1 gallon). As you can see, the entire blood supply passes through each side of the heart once each minute.

Notice that cardiac output varies directly with SV and HR. This means that CO increases when the stroke volume increases or the heart beats faster or both, and it decreases when either or both of these factors decrease.

Cardiac output is highly variable and increases markedly in response to special demands, such as running to catch a bus. **Cardiac reserve** is the difference between resting and maximal CO. In nonathletic people, cardiac reserve is typically four to five times resting CO (20–25 L/min), but CO in trained athletes during competition may reach 35 L/min (seven times resting CO).

How does the heart accomplish such tremendous increases in output? To understand this feat, let's look at how stroke volume

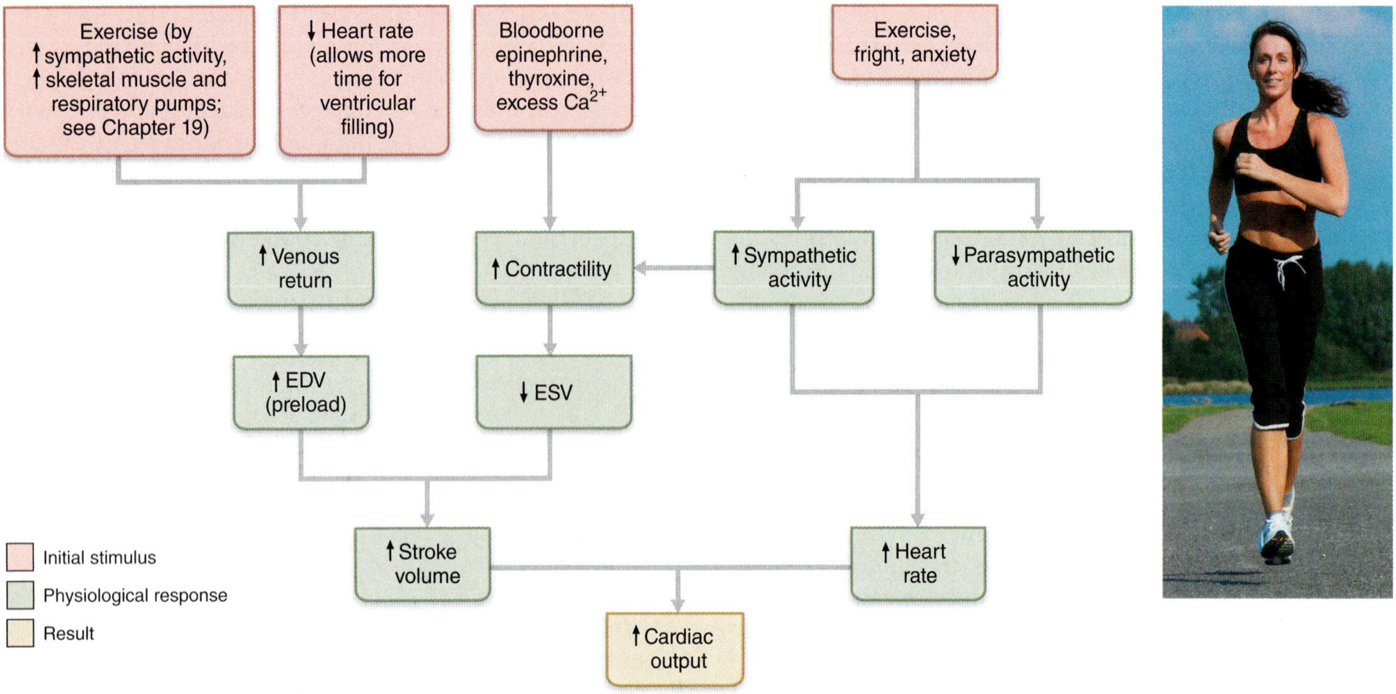

Figure 18.22 Factors involved in determining cardiac output.

and heart rate are regulated. As you read the next sections, refer to **Figure 18.22** for an overview of the factors that affect stroke volume and heart rate, and consequently, cardiac output.

Regulation of Stroke Volume

Mathematically, stroke volume (SV) represents the difference between **end diastolic volume (EDV)**, the amount of blood that collects in a ventricle during diastole, and **end systolic volume (ESV)**, the volume of blood remaining in a ventricle *after* it has contracted. The EDV, determined by how long ventricular diastole lasts and by venous pressure, is normally about 120 ml. (An increase in either factor *raises* EDV.) The ESV, determined by arterial blood pressure and the force of ventricular contraction, is approximately 50 ml. (The higher the arterial blood pressure, the higher the ESV.) To figure normal stroke volume, simply plug these values into this equation:

$$SV = EDV - ESV = \frac{120\ \text{ml}}{\text{beat}} - \frac{50\ \text{ml}}{\text{beat}} = \frac{70\ \text{ml}}{\text{beat}}$$

As you can see, each ventricle pumps out about 70 ml of blood with each beat, which is about 60% of the blood in its chambers.

So what is important here—how do we make sense out of this alphabet soup (SV, ESV, EDV)? Although many factors affect SV by altering EDV or ESV, the three most important are *preload, contractility*, and *afterload*. As we describe in detail next, preload affects EDV, whereas contractility and afterload affect the ESV.

Preload: Degree of Stretch of Heart Muscle The degree to which cardiac muscle cells are stretched just before they contract, which is called the **preload**, controls stroke volume. In a normal heart, the higher the preload, the higher the stroke volume will be. This relationship between preload and stroke volume is called the **Frank-Starling law of the heart**. Recall that at an *optimal length* of muscle fibers (and sarcomeres) (1) the maximum number of active cross bridge attachments is possible between actin and myosin, and (2) the force of contraction is maximal (see Figure 9.22, p. 302). Cardiac muscle, like skeletal muscle, exhibits a *length-tension relationship*.

Resting skeletal muscle fibers are kept near optimal length for developing maximal tension while resting cardiac cells are normally *shorter* than optimal length. As a result, stretching cardiac cells can produce dramatic increases in contractile force. The most important factor stretching cardiac muscle is **venous return**, the amount of blood returning to the heart and distending its ventricles.

Anything that increases the volume or speed of venous return, such as a slow heart rate or exercise, increases EDV and, consequently, SV and contraction force (Figure 18.22). A slow heartbeat allows more time for ventricular filling. Exercise speeds venous return because both increased sympathetic nervous system activity and the squeezing action of the skeletal muscles compress the veins, decreasing the volume of blood they contain and returning more blood to the heart. During vigorous exercise, SV may double as a result of increased venous return. Conversely, low venous return, such as might result from severe blood loss or an extremely rapid heart rate, decreases EDV, causing the heart to beat less forcefully and lowering SV.

Because the systemic and pulmonary circulations are in series, the intrinsic mechanism we just described ensures equal outputs of the two ventricles and proper distribution of blood volume between the two circuits. If one side of the heart suddenly

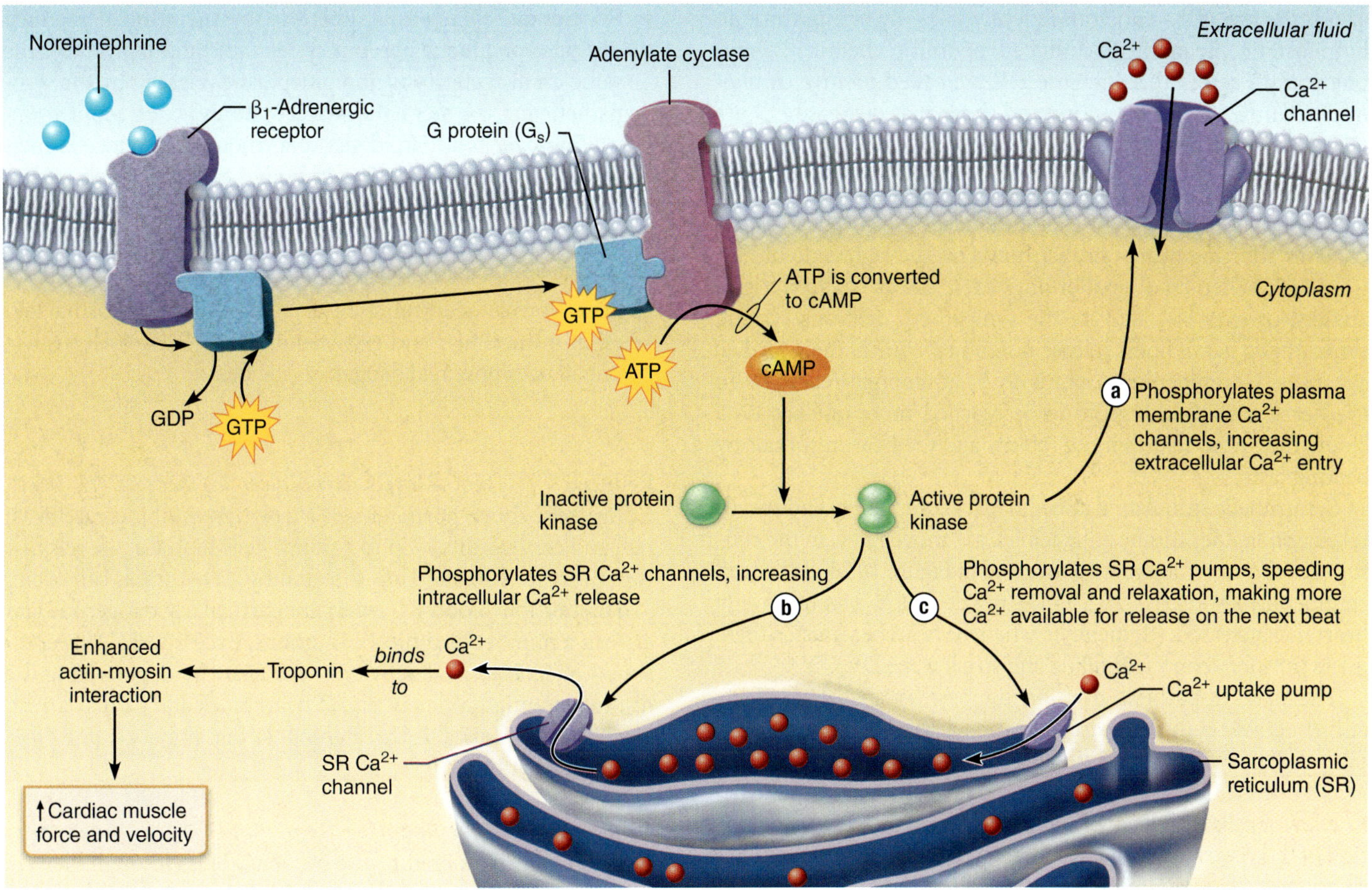

Figure 18.23 Norepinephrine increases heart contractility via a cyclic AMP second-messenger system. Cyclic AMP activates protein kinases that phosphorylate three different proteins, as shown in ⓐ, ⓑ, and ⓒ.

begins to pump more blood than the other, the increased venous return to the opposite ventricle forces that ventricle—through increased cardiac muscle stretch—to pump out an equal volume, preventing backup or accumulation of blood in the circulation.

Contractility EDV is the major *intrinsic factor* influencing SV, but *extrinsic factors* that increase heart muscle contractility can also enhance SV. **Contractility** is defined as the contractile strength achieved at a given muscle length. Note in Figure 18.22 that contractility is *independent* of muscle stretch and EDV. Contractility rises when more Ca^{2+} enters the cytoplasm from the extracellular fluid and the SR. Enhanced contractility means more blood is ejected from the heart (greater SV), hence a lower ESV.

Increased sympathetic stimulation increases contractility. As noted on p. 676, sympathetic fibers serve not only the intrinsic conduction system but the entire heart. One effect of norepinephrine or epinephrine binding is to initiate a cyclic AMP second-messenger system that increases Ca^{2+} entry, which in turn promotes more cross bridge binding and enhances ventricular contractility **(Figure 18.23)**.

A battery of other chemicals also influence contractility. Substances that increase contractility are called *positive inotropic agents* (*ino* = muscle, fiber). The hormones epinephrine, thyroxine, and glucagon; the drug digitalis; and high levels of extracellular Ca^{2+} are all positive inotropic agents. *Negative inotropic agents,* which impair or decrease contractility, include acidosis (excess H^+), rising extracellular K^+ levels, and drugs called calcium channel blockers.

Afterload: Back Pressure Exerted by Arterial Blood **Afterload** is the pressure that the ventricles must overcome to eject blood. It is essentially the back pressure that arterial blood exerts on the aortic and pulmonary valves—about 80 mm Hg in the aorta and 10 mm Hg in the pulmonary trunk.

In healthy individuals, afterload is not a major determinant of stroke volume because it is relatively constant. However, in people with hypertension (high blood pressure), afterload is important indeed because it reduces the ability of the ventricles to eject blood. Consequently, more blood remains in the heart after systole, increasing ESV and reducing stroke volume.

Regulation of Heart Rate

Given a healthy cardiovascular system, SV tends to be relatively constant. However, when blood volume drops sharply or the heart is seriously weakened, SV declines and CO is maintained by increasing HR and contractility. Temporary stressors can also influence HR—and consequently CO—by acting through homeostatic mechanisms induced neurally, chemically, and physically. Factors that increase HR are called *positive chronotropic* (*chrono* = time) factors, and those that decrease HR are *negative chronotropic* factors.

Autonomic Nervous System Regulation of Heart Rate The autonomic nervous system exerts the most important extrinsic controls affecting heart rate, as shown on the right side of Figure 18.22. When emotional or physical stressors (such as fright, anxiety, or exercise) activate the sympathetic nervous system, sympathetic nerve fibers release norepinephrine at their cardiac synapses. Norepinephrine binds to β_1-adrenergic receptors in the heart, causing threshold to be reached more quickly. As a result, the SA node fires more rapidly and the heart responds by beating faster.

Sympathetic stimulation also enhances contractility and speeds relaxation. It does this by enhancing Ca^{2+} movements in the contractile cells as we described above and in Figure 18.23. Enhanced contractility lowers ESV, so SV does not decline as it would if only heart *rate* increased. (Remember, when the heart beats faster, there is less time for ventricular filling and so a lower EDV.)

The parasympathetic division opposes sympathetic effects and effectively reduces heart rate when a stressful situation has passed. Parasympathetic-initiated cardiac responses are mediated by acetylcholine, which hyperpolarizes the membranes of its effector cells by *opening* K^+ channels. Because vagal innervation of the ventricles is sparse, parasympathetic activity has little or no effect on cardiac contractility.

Under resting conditions, both autonomic divisions continuously send impulses to the SA node of the heart, but the *dominant* influence is inhibitory. For this reason, the heart is said to exhibit **vagal tone**, and heart rate is generally slower than it would be if the vagal nerves were not innervating it. Cutting the vagal nerves results in an almost immediate increase in heart rate of about 25 beats/min, reflecting the inherent rate (100 beats/min) of the pacemaking SA node.

When sensory input from various parts of the cardiovascular system activates either division of the autonomic nervous system more strongly, the other division is temporarily inhibited. Most such sensory input is generated by *baroreceptors* which respond to changes in systemic blood pressure, as we will discuss in Chapter 19. Another example, the **atrial (Bainbridge) reflex**, is an autonomic reflex initiated by increased venous return and increased atrial filling. Stretching the atrial walls increases heart rate by stimulating both the SA node and the atrial stretch receptors. Stretch receptor activation triggers reflexive adjustments of autonomic output to the SA node, increasing heart rate.

Increased or decreased CO results in corresponding changes to systemic blood pressure, so blood pressure regulation often involves reflexive controls of heart rate. In Chapter 19 we describe in more detail neural mechanisms that regulate blood pressure.

Chemical Regulation of Heart Rate Chemicals normally present in the blood and other body fluids may influence heart rate, particularly if they become excessive or deficient.

- **Hormones.** *Epinephrine*, liberated by the adrenal medulla during sympathetic nervous system activation, produces the same cardiac effects as norepinephrine released by the sympathetic nerves: It enhances heart rate and contractility.

  Thyroxine is a thyroid gland hormone that increases metabolic rate and production of body heat. When released in large quantities, it causes a sustained increase in heart rate. Thyroxine acts directly on the heart but also *enhances* the effects of epinephrine and norepinephrine.
- **Ions.** Normal heart function depends on having normal levels of intracellular and extracellular ions. Plasma electrolyte imbalances pose real dangers to the heart.

Homeostatic Imbalance 18.8

Reduced Ca^{2+} blood levels (*hypocalcemia*) depress the heart. Conversely, above-normal levels (*hypercalcemia*) increase heart rate and contractility—up to a point. Very high Ca^{2+} levels disrupt heart function and life-threatening arrhythmias can occur.

High or low blood K^+ levels are particularly dangerous and arise in a number of clinical conditions. Excessive K^+ (*hyperkalemia*) alters electrical activity in the heart by depolarizing the resting potential, and may lead to heart block and cardiac arrest. *Hypokalemia* is also life threatening, in that the heart beats feebly and arrhythmically. ✚

Other Factors That Regulate Heart Rate Age, gender, exercise, and body temperature also influence HR, although they are less important than neural factors. Resting heart rate is fastest in the fetus (140–160 beats/min) and gradually declines throughout life. Average heart rate is faster in females (72–80 beats/min) than in males (64–72 beats/min).

Exercise raises HR by acting through the sympathetic nervous system (Figure 18.22). Exercise also increases systemic blood pressure and routes more blood to the working muscles. However, resting HR in the physically fit tends to be substantially lower than in those who are out of condition, and in trained athletes it may be as slow as 40 beats/min. We explain this apparent paradox below.

Heat increases HR by enhancing the metabolic rate of cardiac cells. This explains the rapid, pounding heartbeat you feel when you have a high fever and also accounts, in part, for the effect of exercise on HR (remember, working muscles generate heat). Cold directly decreases heart rate.

Homeostatic Imbalance 18.9

HR varies with changes in activity, but marked and persistent rate changes usually signal cardiovascular disease.

Tachycardia (tak″e-kar′de-ah; "heart hurry") is an abnormally fast heart rate (more than 100 beats/min) that may result from elevated body temperature, stress, certain drugs, or heart disease. Persistent tachycardia is considered pathological because tachycardia occasionally promotes fibrillation.

Bradycardia (brad″e-kar′de-ah; *brady* = slow) is a heart rate slower than 60 beats/min. It may result from low body temperature, certain drugs, or parasympathetic nervous activation.

It is a known, and desirable, consequence of endurance training. With physical and cardiovascular conditioning, the heart hypertrophies and SV increases, allowing a lower resting heart rate while still providing the same cardiac output. However, in poorly conditioned people persistent bradycardia may result in grossly inadequate blood circulation to body tissues, and bradycardia is often a warning of brain edema after head trauma. +

Homeostatic Imbalance of Cardiac Output

The heart's pumping action ordinarily maintains a balance between cardiac output and venous return. Were this not so, a dangerous damming up of blood (blood congestion) would occur in the veins returning blood to the heart.

In **congestive heart failure (CHF)**, the heart is such an inefficient pump that blood circulation is inadequate to meet tissue needs. This progressively worsening disorder reflects weakening of the myocardium by various conditions that damage it in different ways. Let's take a look.

- **Coronary atherosclerosis.** Coronary atherosclerosis, essentially fatty buildup that clogs the coronary arteries, impairs blood and oxygen delivery to cardiac cells. The heart becomes increasingly hypoxic and begins to contract ineffectively.
- **Persistent high blood pressure.** Normally, pressure in the aorta during diastole is 80 mm Hg, and the left ventricle exerts only slightly over that amount of force to eject blood from its chamber. When aortic diastolic blood pressure rises to 90 mm Hg or more, the myocardium must exert more force to open the aortic valve and pump out the same amount of blood. If afterload is chronically elevated, ESV rises and the myocardium hypertrophies. Eventually, the stress takes its toll and the myocardium becomes progressively weaker.
- **Multiple myocardial infarctions.** A succession of MIs (heart attacks) depresses pumping efficiency because noncontractile fibrous (scar) tissue replaces the dead heart cells.
- **Dilated cardiomyopathy (DCM)** (kar″de-o-my-ah′path-e). The cause of this condition, in which the ventricles stretch (dilate) and become flabby and the myocardium deteriorates, is often unknown. Drug toxicity (alcohol, cocaine, excess catecholamines, chemotherapeutic agents) and inflammation of the heart following an infection are implicated in some cases.

  The heart's attempts to work harder result in increasing levels of Ca^{2+} in cardiac cells. The Ca^{2+} activates calcineurin, a calcium-sensitive enzyme that initiates a cascade which switches on genes that enlarge the heart. CO is poor because ventricular contractility is impaired, and the cardiomyopathy progressively worsens.

Because the heart is a double pump, each side can initially fail independently of the other. If the left side fails, **pulmonary congestion** occurs. The right side continues to propel blood to the lungs, but the left side does not adequately eject the returning blood into the systemic circulation. Blood vessels in the lungs become engorged with blood, the pressure in them increases, and fluid leaks from the circulation into the lung tissue, causing pulmonary edema. If the congestion is untreated, the person suffocates.

If the right side of the heart fails, **peripheral congestion** occurs. Blood stagnates in body organs, and pooled fluids in the tissue spaces impair the ability of body cells to obtain adequate nutrients and oxygen and rid themselves of wastes. The resulting edema is most noticeable in the extremities (feet, ankles, and fingers).

Failure of one side of the heart puts a greater strain on the other side, and ultimately the whole heart fails. A seriously weakened, or *decompensated*, heart is irreparable. Treatment is directed primarily toward (1) removing the excess leaked fluid with *diuretics* (drugs that increase the kidneys' excretion of Na^+ and water), (2) reducing afterload with drugs that drive down blood pressure, and (3) increasing contractility with digitalis derivatives. Heart transplants and other surgical or mechanical remedies to replace damaged heart muscle provide additional hope for some cardiac patients.

☑ Check Your Understanding

15. After running to catch a bus, Josh noticed that his heart was beating faster than normally and was pounding forcefully in his chest. How did his increased HR and SV come about?
16. What problem of cardiac output might ensue if the heart beats far too rapidly for an extended period, that is, if tachycardia occurs? Why?

For answers, see Appendix H.

Developmental Aspects of the Heart

✓ Describe the development of the heart, and indicate how the fetal heart differs from the adult heart.

✓ Provide examples of age-related changes in heart function.

The human heart, derived from mesoderm and guided by powerful signaling molecules, begins as two simple endothelial tubes. They quickly fuse to form a single chamber or heart tube that is busily pumping blood by the 22nd day of gestation **(Figure 18.24)**.

Before Birth

The tube develops four slightly bulged areas that represent the earliest heart chambers. From tail to head, following the direction of blood flow, the four primitive chambers are the following (Figure 18.24b):

1. **Sinus venosus** (ven-o′sus). This chamber initially receives all the venous blood of the embryo. It will become the smooth-walled part of the right atrium and the coronary sinus. It also gives rise to the sinoatrial node, which "takes the baton" and sets heart rate early in embryonic development.
2. **Atrium.** This embryonic chamber eventually becomes the pectinate muscle–ridged parts of the atria.

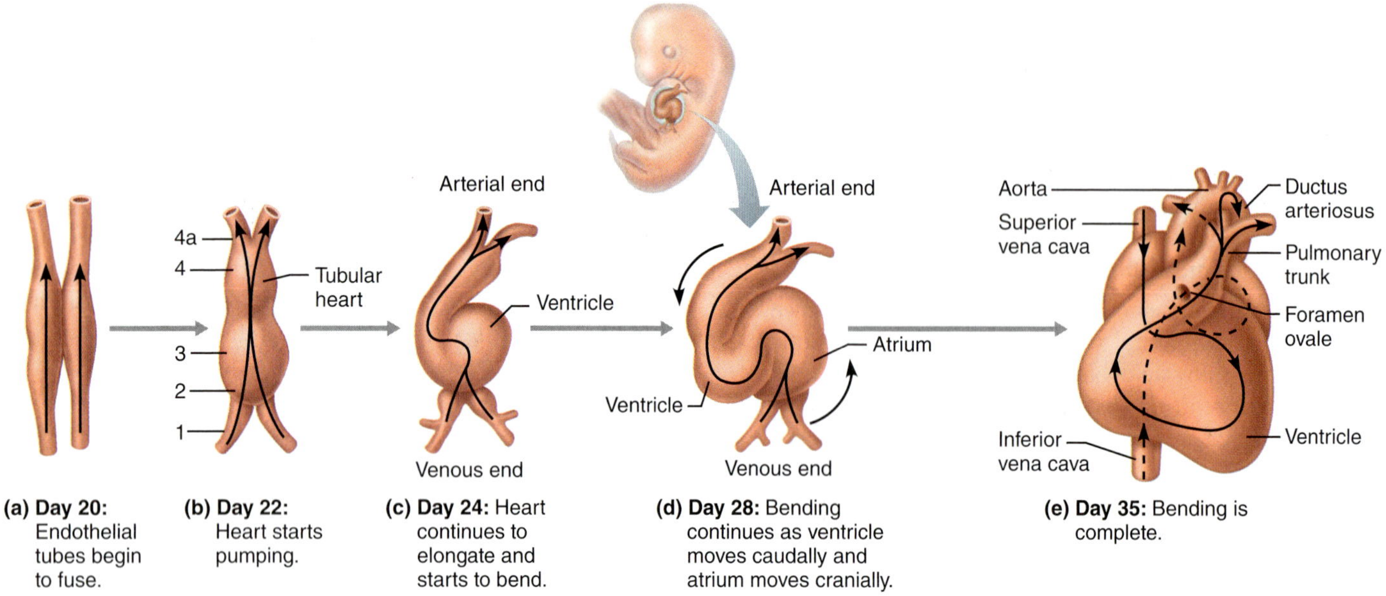

Figure 18.24 Development of the human heart. Ventral views, with the cranial direction toward the top of the figures. Arrows show the direction of blood flow. Days are approximate. **(b)** 1 is the sinus venosus; 2, the atrium; 3, the ventricle; 4, the bulbus cordis; and 4a, the truncus arteriosus.

3. **Ventricle.** The strongest pumping chamber of the early heart, the ventricle gives rise to the *left* ventricle.
4. **Bulbus cordis.** This chamber plus its cranial extension, the *truncus arteriosus* (labeled 4a in Figure 18.24b), give rise to the pulmonary trunk, the first part of the aorta, and most of the *right* ventricle.

During the next three weeks, the heart "tube" exhibits dramatic contortions as it undergoes rightward looping, and major structural changes convert it into a four-chambered organ capable of acting as a double pump—all without missing a beat! The ventricle moves caudally and the atrium cranially, assuming their adult positions. The heart divides into its four definitive chambers (via a number of stages), the midline septum forms, and the bulbus cordis splits into the pulmonary trunk and ascending aorta. After the second month, few changes other than growth occur until birth.

18

The interatrial septum of the fetal heart is incomplete. The **foramen ovale** (literally, "oval door") connects the two atria and allows blood entering the right heart to bypass the pulmonary circuit and the collapsed, nonfunctional fetal lungs (Figure 18.24e). Another lung bypass, the **ductus arteriosus**, exists between the pulmonary trunk and the aorta. At or shortly after birth, these shunts close, completing the separation between the right and left sides of the heart.

In the adult heart, the fossa ovalis reveals the position of the foramen ovale, and the **ligamentum arteriosum** is the fibrous remnant of the ductus arteriosus (see Figure 18.5b). We give a more complete description of the fetal and newborn circulation in Chapter 28 (see Figure 28.14).

Homeostatic Imbalance 18.10

Building a perfect heart is difficult. Each year about 30,000 infants are born in the U.S. with one or more of 30 different **congenital heart defects**, making them the most common of all birth defects. Some congenital heart problems are traceable to environmental influences, such as maternal infection or drug intake during month 2 when the major events of heart formation occur.

The most prevalent abnormalities produce two basic kinds of disorders in the newborn. They either (1) lead to mixing of oxygen-poor blood with oxygenated blood (so that inadequately oxygenated blood reaches the body tissues) or (2) involve narrowed valves or vessels that greatly increase the workload on the heart.

Examples of the first type of defect are *septal defects* **(Figure 18.25a)** and *patent ductus arteriosus*, in which the connection between the aorta and pulmonary trunk remains open. *Coarctation of the aorta* (Figure 18.25b) is an example of the second type of problem. *Tetralogy of Fallot* (te-tral′o-je ov fal-o′), a serious condition in which the baby becomes cyanotic within minutes of birth, encompasses both types of disorders (Figure 18.25c). Modern surgical techniques can usually correct these congenital defects. ✚

Heart Function Throughout Life

In the absence of congenital heart problems, the heart functions admirably throughout a long lifetime for most people. Homeostatic mechanisms are normally so efficient that people rarely notice when the heart is working harder.

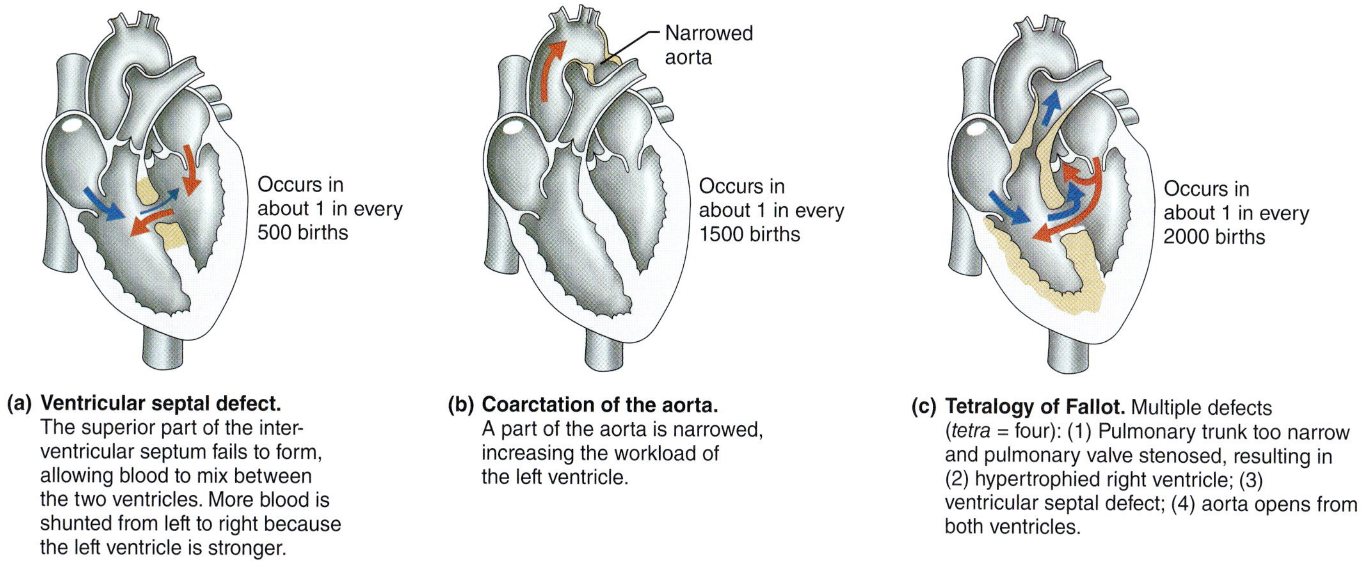

Figure 18.25 Three examples of congenital heart defects. Tan areas indicate the locations of the defects.

In people who exercise regularly and vigorously, the heart gradually adapts to the increased demand by enlarging and becoming more efficient and more powerful. Aerobic exercise also helps clear fatty deposits from blood vessel walls throughout the body, retarding atherosclerosis and coronary heart disease. Barring some chronic illnesses, this beneficial cardiac response to exercise persists into ripe old age.

The key word on benefiting from exercise is *regularity*. Regular exercise gradually enhances myocardial endurance and strength. For example, 30 minutes a day of moderately vigorous activity (brisk walking, biking, or yard work) offers significant health benefits to most adults. However, intermittent vigorous exercise, enjoyed by weekend athletes, may push an unconditioned heart beyond its ability to respond to the unexpected demands and bring on a myocardial infarction.

Because of the incredible amount of work the heart does over the course of a lifetime, certain structural changes are inevitable. Age-related changes affecting the heart include the following:

- **Valve flaps thicken and become sclerotic (stiff).** This change occurs particularly where the stress of blood flow is greatest (mitral valve). For this reason, heart murmurs are more common in elderly people.
- **Cardiac reserve declines.** Although the passing years seem to cause little change in resting heart rate, the aged heart is less able to respond to both sudden and prolonged stressors that demand increased output. In addition, the maximum HR declines as sympathetic control of the heart becomes less efficient. These changes are less of a problem in physically active seniors.
- **Cardiac muscle becomes fibrosed (scarred).** As a person ages, more and more cardiac cells die and are replaced with fibrous tissue. As a result, the heart stiffens and fills less efficiently for each heartbeat, reducing stroke volume. The nodes of the heart's conduction system may also become fibrosed, which increases the incidence of arrhythmias and other conduction problems.
- **Atherosclerosis.** The insidious progress of atherosclerosis begins in childhood, but inactivity, smoking, and stress accelerate it. The most serious consequences to the heart are hypertensive heart disease and coronary artery occlusion, both of which increase the risk of heart attack and stroke. Although the aging process itself leads to changes in blood vessel walls that promote atherosclerosis, many investigators feel that diet, not aging, is the single most important contributor to cardiovascular disease. We can lower our risk by consuming less animal fat, cholesterol, and salt.

Check Your Understanding

17. Name the two components of the fetal heart that allow blood to bypass the lungs.
18. In the past decade, many people over 70 have competed in the Ironman World Championships in Hawaii. In what way might age-related changes of the heart limit the performance of these athletes?

For answers, see Appendix H.

The heart is an exquisitely engineered double pump that operates with precision to propel blood into the large arteries leaving its chambers. However, continuous circulation of blood also depends critically on the pressure dynamics in the blood vessels. Chapter 19 considers the structure and function of these vessels and relates this information to the work of the heart to provide a complete picture of cardiovascular functioning.

Chapter Summary

MAP™ For more chapter study tools, go to the Study Area of MasteringA&P at **www.masteringaandp.com**.
There you will find:
- Interactive Physiology iP
- A&PFlix A&PFlix
- Practice Anatomy Lab PAL
- PhysioEx PEx
- Videos, Practice Quizzes and Tests, MP3 Tutor Sessions, Case Studies, and much more!

The Pulmonary and Systemic Circuits (p. 659)

1. The right side of the heart is the pulmonary circuit pump. It pumps blood through the lungs, where the blood picks up oxygen and dumps carbon dioxide. The left side of the heart is the systemic circuit pump. It pumps blood through the body's tissues, supplying them with oxygen and nutrients and removing carbon dioxide.

Heart Anatomy (pp. 659–671)

Size, Location, and Orientation (p. 659)

1. The human heart, about the size of a clenched fist, is located obliquely within the mediastinum of the thorax.

Coverings of the Heart (pp. 660–661)

2. The heart is enclosed within a double sac made up of the outer fibrous pericardium and the inner serous pericardium (parietal and visceral layers). The pericardial cavity between the serous layers contains lubricating serous fluid.

Layers of the Heart Wall (pp. 661–662)

3. Layers of the heart wall, from the interior out, are the endocardium, myocardium (reinforced by a fibrous cardiac skeleton), and epicardium (visceral layer of the serous pericardium).

18

Chambers and Associated Great Vessels (p. 662)

4. The heart has two superior atria and two inferior ventricles. Functionally, the heart is a double pump.
5. Entering the right atrium are the superior vena cava, inferior vena cava, and coronary sinus. Four pulmonary veins enter the left atrium.
6. The right ventricle discharges blood into the pulmonary trunk; the left ventricle pumps blood into the aorta.

Heart Valves (pp. 662–668)

7. The atrioventricular (AV) valves (tricuspid and mitral) prevent backflow into the atria when the ventricles are contracting; the semilunar (SL) valves (pulmonary and aortic) prevent backflow into the ventricles when the ventricles are relaxing.

Pathway of Blood Through the Heart (p. 668)

8. Oxygen-poor systemic blood enters the right atrium, passes into the right ventricle, through the pulmonary trunk to the lungs, and back to the left atrium via the pulmonary veins. Oxygen-laden blood entering the left atrium from the lungs flows into the left ventricle and then into the aorta, which provides the functional supply of all body organs. Systemic veins return the oxygen-depleted blood to the right atrium.

Coronary Circulation (pp. 668–671)

9. The right and left coronary arteries branch from the aorta and via their main branches (anterior and posterior interventricular, right marginal, and circumflex arteries) supply the heart itself. Venous blood, collected by the cardiac veins (great, middle, and small), empties into the coronary sinus.
10. Blood delivery to the myocardium occurs during heart relaxation.

iP **Cardiovascular System; Topic: Anatomy Review: The Heart, pp. 1–8.**

Cardiac Muscle Fibers (pp. 671–674)

Microscopic Anatomy (p. 671)

1. Cardiac muscle cells are branching, striated, generally uninucleate cells. They contain myofibrils consisting of typical sarcomeres.
2. Intercalated discs containing desmosomes and gap junctions connect adjacent cardiac cells. The myocardium behaves as a functional syncytium because of electrical coupling provided by gap junctions.

Mechanism and Events of Contraction (pp. 671–673)

3. As in skeletal muscle, the membrane depolarization of contractile myocytes causes opening of sodium channels and allows sodium to enter, which is responsible for the rising phase of the action potential curve. Depolarization also opens slow Ca^{2+} channels; Ca^{2+} entry prolongs the period of depolarization (creates the plateau). Ca^{2+} released by the SR and entering from the extracellular space couples the action potential to sliding of the myofilaments. Compared to skeletal muscle, cardiac muscle has a prolonged refractory period that prevents tetany.

iP **Cardiovascular System; Topic: Cardiac Action Potential, pp. 11–18.**

Energy Requirements (pp. 673–674)

4. Cardiac muscle has abundant mitochondria and depends almost entirely on aerobic respiration to form ATP.

Heart Physiology (pp. 674–685)

Electrical Events (pp. 674–678)

1. Certain noncontractile cardiac muscle cells exhibit automaticity and rhythmicity and can independently initiate action potentials. Such cells have an unstable resting potential called a pacemaker potential that gradually depolarizes, drifting toward threshold for firing. These cells compose the intrinsic conduction system of the heart.
2. The conduction system of the heart consists of the SA and AV nodes, the AV bundle and bundle branches, and the subendocardial conducting network. This system coordinates the depolarization of the heart and ensures that the heart beats as a unit. The SA node has the fastest rate of spontaneous depolarization and acts as the heart's pacemaker; it sets the sinus rhythm.
3. Defects in the intrinsic conduction system can cause arrhythmias, fibrillation, and heart block.
4. The autonomic nervous system innervates the heart. Cardiac centers in the medulla include the cardioacceleratory center, which projects to the T_1–T_5 region of the spinal cord, which in turn projects to the cervical and upper thoracic sympathetic

trunk. Postganglionic fibers innervate the SA and AV nodes and the cardiac muscle fibers. The cardioinhibitory center exerts its influence via the parasympathetic vagus nerves (X), which project to the heart wall. Most parasympathetic fibers serve the SA and AV nodes.

5. An electrocardiogram (ECG) is a graphic representation of the cardiac conduction cycle. The P wave reflects atrial depolarization. The QRS complex indicates ventricular depolarization; the T wave represents ventricular repolarization.

iP Cardiovascular System; Topic: Intrinsic Conduction System, pp. 1–7; Topic: Cardiac Action Potential, pp. 1–10.

Heart Sounds (pp. 678–679)

6. Normal heart sounds arise chiefly from turbulent blood flow during the closing of heart valves. Abnormal heart sounds, called murmurs, usually reflect valve problems.

Mechanical Events: The Cardiac Cycle (pp. 679–681)

7. A cardiac cycle consists of the events occurring during one heartbeat. During mid-to-late diastole, the ventricles fill and the atria contract. Ventricular systole consists of the isovolumetric contraction phase and the ventricular ejection phase. During early diastole, the ventricles are relaxed and are closed chambers until the atrial pressure exceeds the ventricular pressure, forcing the AV valves open. Then the cycle begins again. At a normal heart rate of 75 beats/min, a cardiac cycle lasts 0.8 s.
8. Pressure changes promote blood flow and valve opening and closing.

iP Cardiovascular System; Topic: Cardiac Cycle, pp. 1–19.

Cardiac Output (pp. 681–685)

9. Cardiac output, typically 5 L/min, is the amount of blood pumped out by each ventricle in 1 minute. Stroke volume is the amount of blood pumped out by a ventricle with each contraction. Cardiac output = heart rate × stroke volume.
10. Stroke volume depends to a large extent on the degree to which venous return stretches cardiac muscle. Approximately 70 ml, it is the difference between end diastolic volume (EDV) and end systolic volume (ESV). Anything that influences heart rate or blood volume influences venous return, hence stroke volume.
11. Activation of the sympathetic nervous system increases heart rate and contractility; parasympathetic activation decreases heart rate but has little effect on contractility. Ordinarily, the heart exhibits vagal tone.
12. Chemical regulation of the heart is effected by hormones (epinephrine and thyroxine) and ions (particularly potassium and calcium). Ion imbalances severely impair heart activity.
13. Other factors influencing heart rate are age, sex, exercise, and body temperature.
14. Congestive heart failure occurs when the pumping ability of the heart cannot provide adequate circulation to meet body needs. Right heart failure leads to systemic edema; left heart failure results in pulmonary edema.

iP Cardiovascular System; Topic: Cardiac Output, pp. 1–11.

Developmental Aspects of the Heart (pp. 685–687)

Before Birth (pp. 685–686)

1. The heart begins as a simple (mesodermal) tube that is pumping blood by the fourth week of gestation. The fetal heart has two lung bypasses: the foramen ovale and the ductus arteriosus.
2. Congenital heart defects are the most common of all birth defects. The most common of these disorders lead to inadequate oxygenation of blood or increase the workload of the heart.

Heart Function Throughout Life (pp. 686–687)

3. Age-related changes include sclerosis and thickening of the valve flaps, declines in cardiac reserve, fibrosis of cardiac muscle, and atherosclerosis.
4. Risk factors for cardiac disease include dietary factors, excessive stress, cigarette smoking, and lack of exercise.

Review Questions

Multiple Choice/Matching

(Some questions have more than one correct answer. Select the best answer or answers from the choices given.)

1. When the semilunar valves are open, which of the following are occurring? **(a)** 2, 3, 5, 6, **(b)** 1, 2, 3, 7, **(c)** 1, 3, 5, 6, **(d)** 2, 4, 5, 7.

____ (1) coronary arteries fill
____ (2) AV valves are closed
____ (3) ventricles are in systole
____ (4) ventricles are in diastole
____ (5) blood enters aorta
____ (6) blood enters pulmonary arteries
____ (7) atria contract

2. The portion of the intrinsic conduction system located in the superior interventricular septum is the **(a)** AV node, **(b)** SA node, **(c)** AV bundle, **(d)** subendocardial conducting network.
3. An ECG provides information about **(a)** cardiac output, **(b)** movement of the excitation wave across the heart, **(c)** coronary circulation, **(d)** valve impairment.
4. The sequence of contraction of the heart chambers is **(a)** random, **(b)** left chambers followed by right chambers, **(c)** both atria followed by both ventricles, **(d)** right atrium, right ventricle, left atrium, left ventricle.
5. The fact that the left ventricular wall is thicker than the right reveals that it **(a)** pumps a greater volume of blood, **(b)** pumps blood against greater resistance, **(c)** expands the thoracic cage, **(d)** pumps blood through a smaller valve.
6. The chordae tendineae **(a)** close the atrioventricular valves, **(b)** prevent the AV valve flaps from everting, **(c)** contract the papillary muscles, **(d)** open the semilunar valves.
7. In the heart, which of the following apply? **(1)** Action potentials are conducted from cell to cell across the myocardium via gap junctions, **(2)** the SA node sets the pace for the heart as a whole, **(3)** spontaneous depolarization of cardiac cells can occur in the absence of nerve stimulation, **(4)** cardiac muscle can continue to contract for long periods in the absence of oxygen. **(a)** all of the above, **(b)** 1, 3, 4, **(c)** 1, 2, 3, **(d)** 2, 3.
8. The activity of the heart depends on intrinsic properties of cardiac muscle and on neural factors. Thus, **(a)** vagus nerve stimulation of the heart reduces heart rate, **(b)** sympathetic nerve

stimulation of the heart decreases time available for ventricular filling, **(c)** sympathetic stimulation of the heart increases its force of contraction, **(d)** all of the above.

9. Freshly oxygenated blood is first received by the **(a)** right atrium, **(b)** left atrium, **(c)** right ventricle, **(d)** left ventricle.

Short Answer Essay Questions

10. Describe the location and position of the heart in the body.
11. Describe the pericardium and distinguish between the fibrous and the serous pericardia relative to histological structure and location.
12. Trace one drop of blood from the time it enters the right atrium until it enters the left atrium. What is this circuit called?
13. (a) Describe how heart contraction and relaxation influence coronary blood flow. (b) Name the major branches of the coronary arteries, and note the heart regions served by each.
14. The refractory period of cardiac muscle is much longer than that of skeletal muscle. Why is this a desirable functional property?
15. (a) Name the elements of the intrinsic conduction system of the heart in order, beginning with the pacemaker. (b) What is the important function of this conduction system?
16. Draw a normal ECG pattern. Label and explain the significance of its deflection waves.
17. Define cardiac cycle, and follow the events of one cycle.
18. What is cardiac output, and how is it calculated?
19. Discuss how the Frank-Starling law of the heart helps to explain the influence of venous return on stroke volume.
20. (a) Describe the common function of the foramen ovale and the ductus arteriosus in a fetus. (b) What problems result if these shunts remain patent (open) after birth?

Critical Thinking and Clinical Application Questions

1. A gang member was stabbed in the chest during a street fight. He was cyanotic and unconscious from lack of blood delivery to the brain. The diagnosis was cardiac tamponade. What is cardiac tamponade and how does it cause the observed symptoms?
2. You have been called upon to demonstrate the technique for listening to valve sounds. (a) Explain where you would position your stethoscope to auscultate (1) the aortic valve of a patient with severe aortic valve insufficiency and (2) a stenotic mitral valve. (b) During which period(s) would you hear these abnormal valve sounds most clearly? (During atrial diastole, ventricular systole, ventricular diastole, or atrial systole?) (c) What cues would you use to differentiate between an insufficient and a stenotic valve?
3. Florita Santos, a middle-aged woman, is admitted to the coronary care unit with a diagnosis of left ventricular failure resulting from a myocardial infarction. Her history indicated that she was aroused in the middle of the night by severe chest pain. Her skin is pale and cold, and moist sounds are heard over the lower regions of both lungs. Explain how failure of the left ventricle can cause these signs and symptoms.
4. Heather, a newborn baby, needs surgery because she was born with an aorta that arises from the right ventricle and a pulmonary trunk that issues from the left ventricle, a condition called transposition of the great vessels. What are the physiological consequences of this defect?
5. Gabriel, a heroin addict, feels tired, is weak and feverish, and has vague aches and pains. Terrified that he has AIDS, he goes to a doctor and is informed that he is suffering not from AIDS, but from a heart murmur accompanied by endocarditis. What is the most likely way that Gabriel contracted endocarditis? (Hint: See Related Clinical Terms.)
6. As Cara worked at her dissection, she became frustrated that several of the structures she had to learn about had more than one common name. Provide another name for each of these structures: (a) atrioventricular groove, (b) tricuspid valve, (c) bicuspid valve (give two synonyms), and (d) atrioventricular bundle.

AT THE CLINIC

Related Clinical Terms

Asystole (a-sis′to-le) Situation in which the heart fails to contract.

Cardiac catheterization Diagnostic procedure that involves passing a fine catheter (tubing) through a blood vessel into the heart. Oxygen content of blood, blood flow, and pressures within the heart can be measured. Findings help to detect valve problems, heart deformities, and other heart malfunctions.

Commotio cordis ("concussion of the heart") Situation in which a relatively mild blow to the chest causes heart failure and sudden death because it occurs during a vulnerable interval (2 ms) when the heart is repolarizing. Explains those rare instances when youngsters drop dead on the playing field after being hit in the chest by a ball.

Cor pulmonale (kor pul-mun-nă′le; *cor* = heart, *pulmo* = lung) A condition of right-sided heart failure resulting from elevated blood pressure in the pulmonary circuit (pulmonary hypertension). Acute cases may develop suddenly due to a pulmonary embolism; chronic cases are usually associated with chronic lung disorders such as emphysema.

Endocarditis (en″do-kar-di′tis) Inflammation of the endocardium, usually confined to the endocardium of the heart valves. Endocarditis often results from infection by bacteria that have entered the bloodstream but may result from fungal infection or an autoimmune response. Drug addicts may develop endocarditis by injecting themselves with contaminated needles.

Heart palpitation A heartbeat that is unusually strong, fast, or irregular so that the person becomes aware of it; may be caused by certain drugs, emotional pressures ("nervous heart"), or heart disorders.

Hypertrophic cardiomyopathy (HCM) The leading cause of sudden death in young athletes, this condition, which is usually inherited, causes the cardiac muscle cells to enlarge, thickening the heart wall. The heart pumps strongly but doesn't relax well during diastole when the heart is filling.

Mitral valve prolapse Valve disorder affecting up to 1% of the population; most often seen in young women. It appears to have a genetic basis resulting in abnormal chordae tendineae

Related Clinical Terms *(continued)*

or a malfunction of the papillary muscles. One or more of the mitral valve flaps become incompetent and billow into the left atrium during ventricular systole, allowing blood regurgitation. Occasionally requires valve replacement surgery.

Myocarditis (mi″o-kar-di′tis; *myo* = muscle, *card* = heart, *itis* = inflammation) Inflammation of the cardiac muscle layer (myocardium) of the heart; sometimes follows an untreated streptococcal infection in children. May weaken the heart and impair its ability to pump effectively.

Paroxysmal atrial tachycardia (PAT) Bursts of atrial contractions with little pause between them.

Ventricular tachycardia (VT or V-tac) Rapid ventricular contractions that are not coordinated with atrial activity.

Case Study Cardiovascular System: The Heart

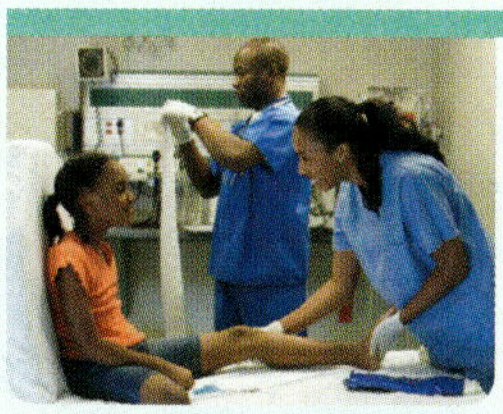

Donald Ayers, a 49-year-old male, was the driver of the bus involved in the accident on Route 91. He was brought into the ER with blunt trauma to the chest. Paramedics noted that the driver's seatbelt had broken and that he was found lying under the instrument panel. Initially unresponsive, Mr. Ayers regained consciousness and complained of chest, epigastric, and left upper quadrant pain. Examination revealed mild tachycardia (110 bpm) and a blood pressure of 105/75 mm Hg. An exam 10 minutes later showed a rapid change in blood pressure (80/55 mm Hg) and HR (130 bpm) along with muffled heart sounds, a thready (weak) pulse, and bulging neck veins. Soon after, the patient began to complain of a sudden onset of pain that radiated into his back from the injury site. The patient described the pain as "sharp, stabbing, and tearing" and it continued to increase.

1. Mr. Ayers's pulse is described as "thready." What might this indicate with respect to this patient's stroke volume?
2. Mr. Ayers's HR increased from 110 to 130 bpm. What effect will this have on his cardiac output? Explain your reasoning.

Mr. Ayers's blood pressure continued to drop, so doctors ordered a chest X ray, ECG, and spiral CT scan (a rapid CT technique). These diagnostic tests revealed four fractured ribs, an enlarged mediastinum, and pericardial effusions (fluid in the pericardium) producing cardiac tamponade.

Mr. Ayers was scheduled for emergency surgery.

3. Beginning with the concept of end diastolic volume (EDV), explain the effect that the fluid in the pericardium is having on the stroke volume of Mr. Ayers's heart.
4. Muffled heart sounds are quieter and less distinct. Explain how changes in EDV can result in muffled heart sounds.
5. The final diagnosis in this case is a dissection (tear) of the aorta. From what you know about the anatomy of the heart, where in the aorta do you think the tear is located? Explain your answer.
6. Why did Mr. Ayers's neck veins bulge?

(Answers in Appendix H)

18

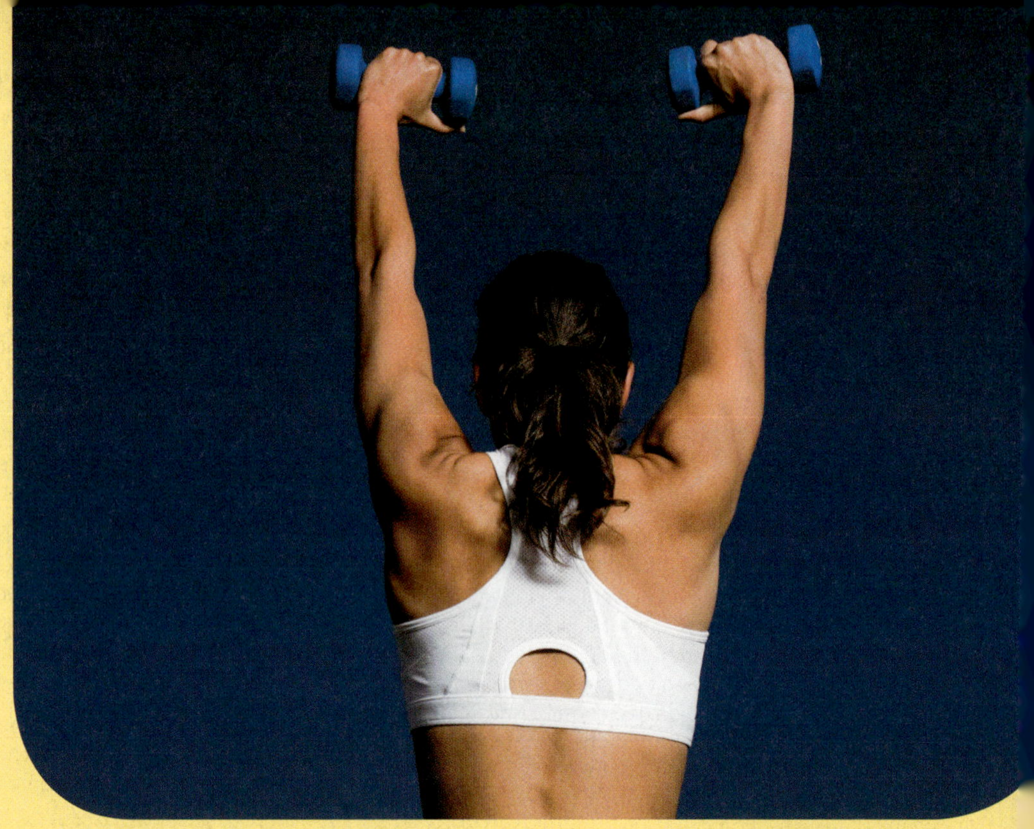

19

The Cardiovascular System: Blood Vessels

Blood vessels are sometimes compared to a system of pipes with blood circulating in them, but this analogy is only a starting point. Unlike rigid pipes, blood vessels are dynamic structures that pulsate, constrict, relax, and even proliferate. In this chapter we examine the structure and function of these important circulatory passageways.

The **blood vessels** of the body form a closed delivery system that begins and ends at the heart. The idea that blood circulates in the body dates back to the 1620s with the inspired experiments of William Harvey, an English physician. Prior to that time, people thought, as proposed by the ancient Greek physician Galen, that blood moved through the body like an ocean tide, first moving out from the heart and then ebbing back in the same vessels.

PART 1
Blood Vessel Structure and Function

The three major types of blood vessels are *arteries, capillaries,* and *veins*. As the heart contracts, it forces blood into the large arteries leaving the ventricles. The blood then moves into successively smaller arteries, finally reaching their smallest branches, the *arterioles* (ar-te′re-ōlz; "little arteries"), which feed into the capillary beds of body organs and tissues. Blood drains from the capillaries into *venules* (ven′ūlz), the smallest veins, and then on into larger and larger veins that merge to form the large veins that ultimately empty into the heart. Altogether, the blood vessels in the adult human stretch for about 100,000 km (60,000 miles) through the internal body landscape!

Arteries carry blood *away from* the heart, so they are said to "branch," "diverge," or "fork" as they form smaller and smaller divisions. **Veins**, by contrast, carry blood *toward* the heart and so are said to "join," "merge," and "converge" into the successively larger vessels approaching the heart. In the systemic circulation, arteries always carry oxygenated blood and veins always carry oxygen-poor blood. The opposite is true in the pulmonary circulation, where the arteries, still defined as the vessels leading away from the heart, carry oxygen-poor blood to the lungs, and the veins carry oxygen-rich blood from the lungs to the heart. The special umbilical vessels of a fetus also differ in the roles of veins and arteries.

Of all the blood vessels, only the capillaries have intimate contact with tissue cells and directly serve cellular needs. Exchanges between the blood and tissue cells occur primarily through the gossamer-thin capillary walls.

Structure of Blood Vessel Walls

✓ Describe the three layers that typically form the wall of a blood vessel, and state the function of each.

✓ Define vasoconstriction and vasodilation.

The walls of all blood vessels, except the very smallest, have three distinct layers, or *tunics* ("coverings"), that surround a central blood-containing space, the vessel **lumen** (**Figure 19.1**).

The innermost tunic is the **tunica intima** (in′tĭ-mah). The name is easy to remember once you know that this tunic is in *intimate* contact with the blood in the lumen. The tunica intima contains the **endothelium**, the simple squamous epithelium that lines the lumen of all vessels. The endothelium is continuous with the endocardial lining of the heart, and its flat cells fit closely together, forming a slick surface that minimizes friction as blood moves through the lumen. In vessels larger than 1 mm in diameter, a *subendothelial layer*, consisting of a basement membrane and loose connective tissue, supports the endothelium.

The middle tunic, the **tunica media** (me′de-ah), is mostly circularly arranged smooth muscle cells and sheets of elastin. The activity of the smooth muscle is regulated by sympathetic *vasomotor nerve fibers* of the autonomic nervous system and a whole battery of chemicals. Depending on the body's needs at any given moment, regulation causes either **vasoconstriction** (lumen diameter decreases as the smooth muscle contracts) or **vasodilation** (lumen diameter increases as the smooth muscle relaxes). The activities of the tunica media are critical in regulating circulatory dynamics because small changes in vessel diameter greatly influence blood flow and blood pressure. Generally, the tunica media is the bulkiest layer in arteries, which bear the chief responsibility for maintaining blood pressure and circulation.

The outermost layer of a blood vessel wall, the **tunica externa** (also called the *tunica adventitia*; ad″ven-tish′e-ah; "coming from outside"), is composed largely of loosely woven collagen fibers that protect and reinforce the vessel, and anchor it to surrounding structures. The tunica externa is infiltrated with nerve fibers, lymphatic vessels, and, in larger veins, a network of elastic fibers. In larger vessels, the tunica externa contains a system of tiny blood vessels, the **vasa vasorum** (va′sah va-sor′um)—literally, "vessels of the vessels"—that nourish the more external tissues of the blood vessel wall. The innermost (luminal) portion of the vessel obtains nutrients directly from blood in the lumen.

The three vessel types vary in length, diameter, wall thickness, and tissue makeup (see **Table 19.1** on p. 696). **Figure 19.2** summarizes how these vascular channels relate to one another and to vessels of the lymphatic system. The lymphatic system recovers fluids that leak from the circulation and is described in Chapter 20.

☑ Check Your Understanding

1. Which branch of the autonomic nervous system innervates blood vessels? Which layer of the blood vessel wall do these nerves innervate? What are the effectors (cells that carry out the response)?
2. When vascular smooth muscle contracts, what happens to the diameter of the blood vessel? What is this called?

For answers, see Appendix H.

Arterial System

✓ Compare and contrast the structure and function of the three types of arteries.

In terms of relative size and function, arteries can be divided into three groups—elastic arteries, muscular arteries, and arterioles.

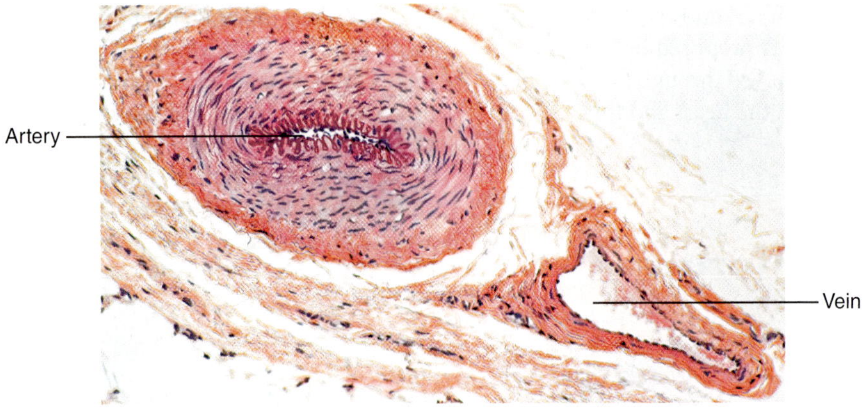

(a)

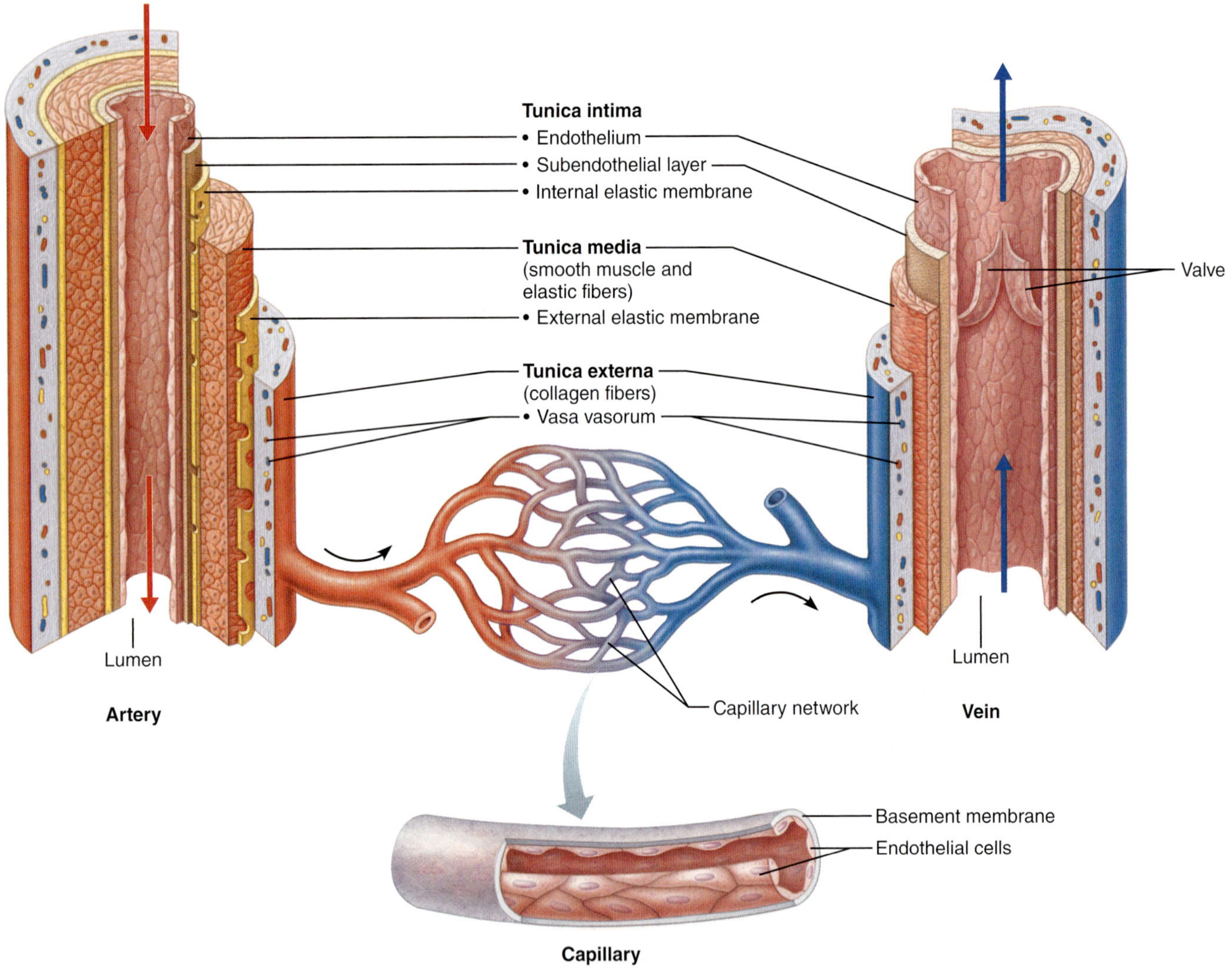

(b)

Figure 19.1 Generalized structure of arteries, veins, and capillaries. (a) Light photomicrograph of a muscular artery and the corresponding vein in cross section (100×). **(b)** Comparison of wall structure of arteries, veins, and capillaries. Note that the tunica media is thicker than the tunica externa in arteries and that the opposite is true in veins.

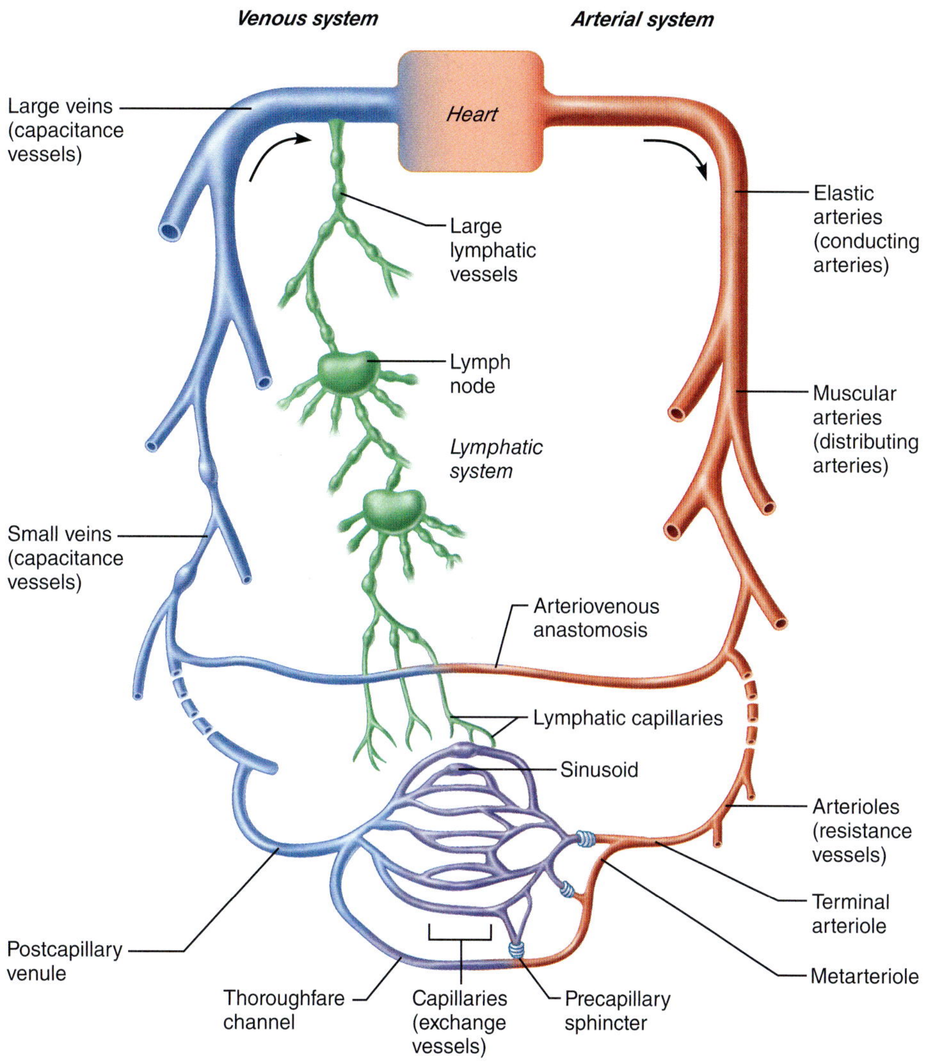

Figure 19.2 The relationship of blood vessels to each other and to lymphatic vessels. Lymphatic vessels recover excess tissue fluid and return it to the blood.

Elastic Arteries

Elastic arteries are the thick-walled arteries near the heart—the aorta and its major branches. These arteries are the largest in diameter, ranging from 2.5 cm to 1 cm, and the most elastic (Table 19.1). Because their large lumens make them low-resistance pathways that conduct blood from the heart to medium-sized arteries, elastic arteries are sometimes called *conducting arteries* (Figure 19.2).

Elastic arteries contain more elastin than any other vessel type. It is present in all three tunics, but the tunica media contains the most. There the elastin constructs concentric "holey" sheets of elastic connective tissue that look like slices of Swiss cheese sandwiched between layers of smooth muscle cells. Although elastic arteries also contain substantial amounts of smooth muscle, they are relatively inactive in vasoconstriction. Thus, in terms of function, they can be visualized as simple elastic tubes.

Elastic arteries are pressure reservoirs, expanding and recoiling as the heart ejects blood. Consequently, blood flows fairly continuously rather than starting and stopping with the pulsating rhythm of the heartbeat. If the blood vessels become hard and unyielding, as in atherosclerosis, blood flows more intermittently, similar to the way water flows through a hard rubber garden hose attached to a faucet. When the faucet is on, the high pressure makes the water gush out of the hose. But when the faucet is shut off, the water flow abruptly becomes a trickle and then stops, because the hose walls cannot recoil to keep the water under pressure. Also, without the pressure-smoothing effect of the elastic arteries, the walls of arteries throughout the body experience higher pressures. Battered by high pressures, the arteries eventually weaken and may balloon out or even burst. (These problems are discussed in *A Closer Look* on pp. 700–701.)

Table 19.1 Summary of Blood Vessel Anatomy

VESSEL TYPE/ ILLUSTRATION*	AVERAGE LUMEN DIAMETER (D) AND WALL THICKNESS (T)	*RELATIVE TISSUE MAKEUP* *Endothelium*	*Elastic Tissues*	*Smooth Muscles*	*Fibrous (Collagenous) Tissues*
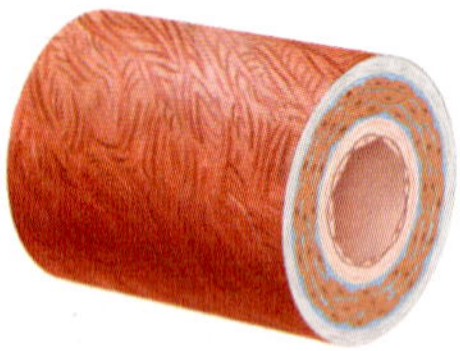 Elastic artery	D: 1.5 cm T: 1.0 mm	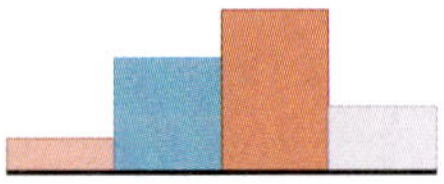			
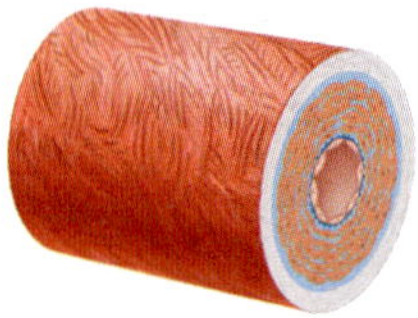 Muscular artery	D: 6.0 mm T: 1.0 mm	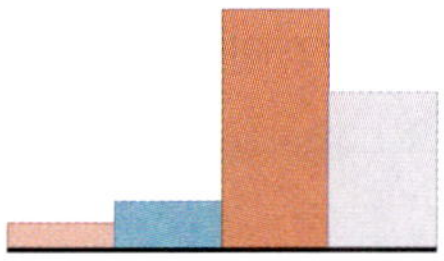			
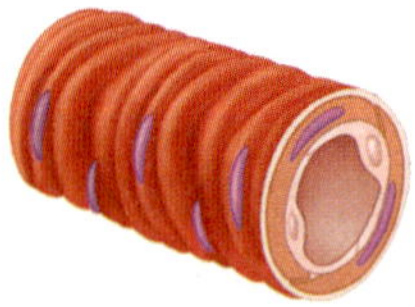 Arteriole	D: 37.0 µm T: 6.0 µm	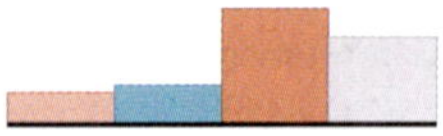			
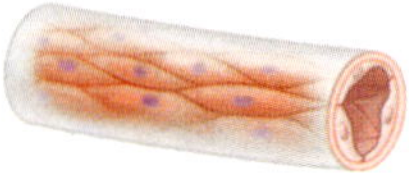 Capillary	D: 9.0 µm T: 0.5 µm				
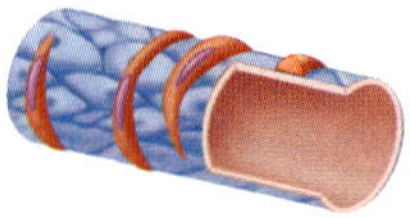 Venule	D: 20.0 µm T: 1.0 µm	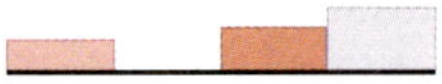			
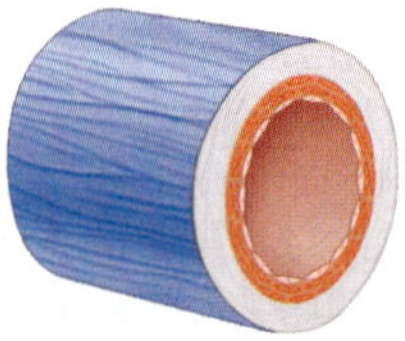 Vein	D: 5.0 mm T: 0.5 mm	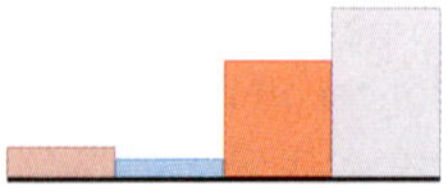			

*Size relationships are not proportional. Smaller vessels are drawn relatively larger so detail can be seen. See column 2 for actual dimensions.

Muscular Arteries

Distally the elastic arteries give way to the **muscular arteries**, which deliver blood to specific body organs (and so are sometimes called *distributing arteries*). Muscular arteries account for most of the named arteries studied in the anatomy laboratory. Their internal diameter ranges from that of a little finger to that of a pencil lead.

Proportionately, muscular arteries have the thickest tunica media of all vessels. Their tunica media contains relatively more smooth muscle and less elastic tissue than do elastic arteries (Table 19.1). For this reason, they are more active in vasoconstriction and less distensible (capable of stretching). In muscular arteries, however, there *is* an *elastic membrane* on each face of the tunica media.

Arterioles

The smallest of the arteries, **arterioles** have a lumen diameter ranging from 0.3 mm down to 10 µm. Larger arterioles have all three tunics, but their tunica media is chiefly smooth muscle with a few scattered elastic fibers. Smaller arterioles, which lead into the capillary beds, are little more than a single layer of smooth muscle cells spiraling around the endothelial lining.

As we will describe shortly, minute-to-minute blood flow into the capillary beds is determined by arteriolar diameter, which varies in response to changing neural, hormonal, and local chemical influences. When arterioles constrict, the tissues served are largely bypassed. When arterioles dilate, blood flow into the local capillaries increases dramatically.

Capillaries

✓ Describe the structure and function of a capillary bed.

The microscopic **capillaries** are the smallest blood vessels. Their exceedingly thin walls consist of just a thin tunica intima (see Figure 19.1b). In some cases, one endothelial cell forms the entire circumference of the capillary wall. At strategic locations along the outer surface of some capillaries are spider-shaped **pericytes**, smooth muscle–like cells that stabilize the capillary wall and help control capillary permeability **(Figure 19.3a).**

Average capillary length is 1 mm and average lumen diameter is 8–10 µm, just large enough for red blood cells to slip through in single file. Most tissues have a rich capillary supply, but there are exceptions. Tendons and ligaments are poorly vascularized. Cartilage and epithelia lack capillaries, but receive nutrients from blood vessels in nearby connective tissues, and the avascular cornea and lens of the eye receive nutrients from the aqueous humor.

If we compare arteries and arterioles to expressways and roads, capillaries are the back alleys and driveways that provide direct access to nearly every cell in the body. Given their location and thin walls, capillaries are ideally suited for their role—exchange of materials (gases, nutrients, hormones, and so on) between the blood and the interstitial fluid (Figure 19.2 and Table 19.1). We describe these exchanges later in this chapter. Here, we focus on capillary structure.

Types of Capillaries

Structurally, there are three types of capillaries—*continuous, fenestrated*, and *sinusoid*.

Continuous Capillaries

Continuous capillaries, abundant in the skin and muscles, are most common (Figure 19.3a). They are continuous in the sense that their endothelial cells are joined together by *tight junctions*, providing an uninterrupted lining. However, these junctions are usually incomplete and leave gaps of unjoined membrane called **intercellular clefts**, which are just large enough to allow limited passage of fluids and small solutes. Typically, the endothelial cell cytoplasm contains numerous pinocytotic vesicles that ferry fluids across the capillary wall.

Brain capillaries, however, are unique. There the tight junctions of the continuous capillaries are complete and extend around the entire perimeter of the endothelial cells, constituting the structural basis of the *blood brain barrier* that we described in Chapter 12.

Fenestrated Capillaries

Fenestrated capillaries (fen′es-tra-tid) are similar to the continuous variety except that the endothelial cells in fenestrated capillaries are riddled with oval *pores*, or *fenestrations* (*fenestra* = window) (Figure 19.3b). A delicate membrane, or diaphragm (probably condensed basal lamina material), usually covers the fenestrations. Even so, fenestrated capillaries are much more permeable to fluids and small solutes than continuous capillaries are.

Fenestrated capillaries are found wherever active capillary absorption or filtrate formation occurs. For example, fenestrated capillaries in the small intestine receive nutrients from digested food, and those in endocrine organs allow hormones rapid entry into the blood. Fenestrated capillaries with perpetually open pores occur in the kidneys, where rapid filtration of blood plasma is essential.

Sinusoid Capillaries (Sinusoids)

Sinusoid capillaries, or **sinusoids** (si′nŭ-soyds), are highly modified, leaky capillaries found only in the liver, bone marrow, spleen, and adrenal medulla. Sinusoids have large, irregularly shaped lumens and are usually fenestrated. Their endothelial lining has fewer tight junctions and larger intercellular clefts than ordinary capillaries (Figure 19.3c).

These structural adaptations allow large molecules and even blood cells to pass between the blood and surrounding tissues. In the liver, the endothelium of the sinusoids is *discontinuous* and its lining includes large **stellate macrophages** (hepatic macrophages), which remove and destroy any bacteria. In other organs, such as the spleen, phagocytes located just outside the sinusoids stick cytoplasmic extensions through the intercellular clefts into the sinusoid lumen to get at their "prey." Blood flows sluggishly through the tortuous sinusoid channels, allowing time for it to be modified in various ways.

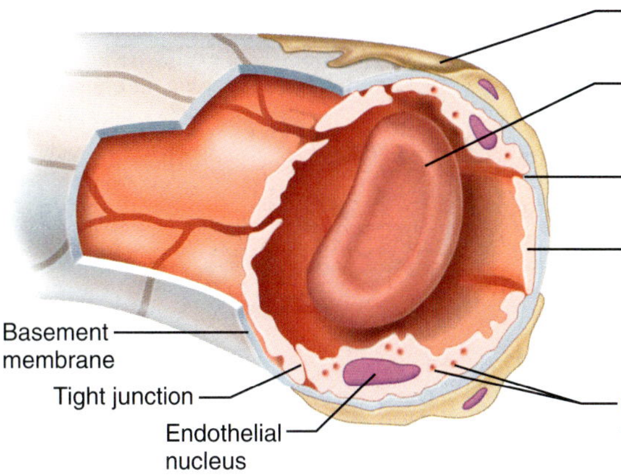

(a) Continuous capillary. Least permeable, and most common (e.g., skin, muscle).

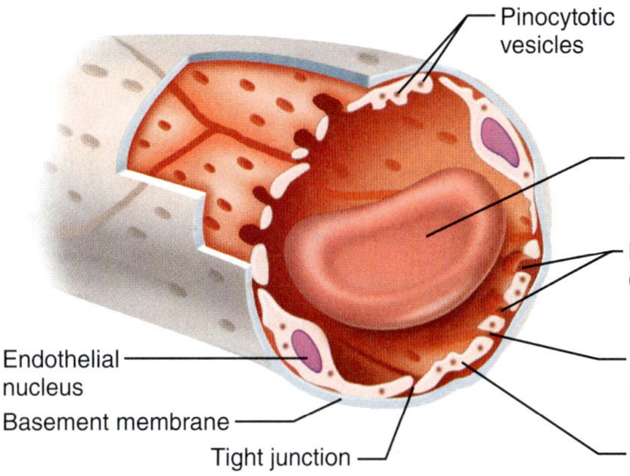

(b) Fenestrated capillary. Large fenestrations (pores) increase permeability. Occurs in areas of active absorption or filtration (e.g., kidney, small intestine).

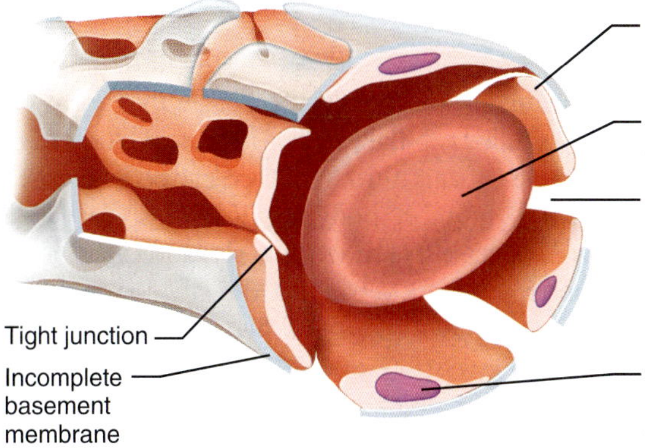

(c) Sinusoid capillary. Most permeable. Occurs in special locations (e.g., liver, bone marrow, spleen).

Figure 19.3 Capillary structure. Note that the basement membrane is incomplete only in (c) and that pericytes most often occur on continuous capillaries.

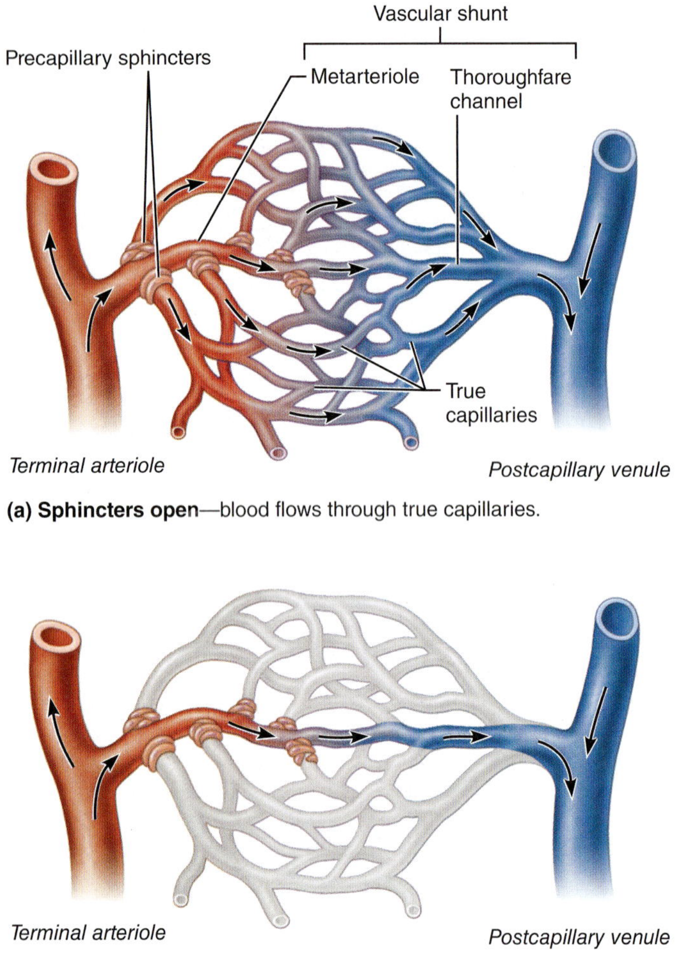

(a) Sphincters open—blood flows through true capillaries.

(b) Sphincters closed—blood flows through metarteriole–thoroughfare channel and bypasses true capillaries.

Figure 19.4 Anatomy of a capillary bed.

Capillary Beds

19

Capillaries do not function independently. Instead they form interweaving networks called **capillary beds**. The flow of blood from an arteriole to a venule—that is, through a capillary bed—is called the **microcirculation**. In most body regions, a capillary bed consists of two types of vessels: (1) a *vascular shunt* (metarteriole–thoroughfare channel), a short vessel that directly connects the arteriole and venule at opposite ends of the bed, and (2) *true capillaries*, the actual *exchange vessels* **(Figure 19.4)**.

The **terminal arteriole** feeding the bed leads into a **metarteriole** (a vessel structurally intermediate between an arteriole and a capillary), which is continuous with the **thoroughfare channel** (intermediate between a capillary and a venule). The thoroughfare channel, in turn, joins the **postcapillary venule** that drains the bed.

The **true capillaries** number 10 to 100 per capillary bed, depending on the organ or tissues served. They usually branch off the metarteriole (proximal end of the shunt) and return to the thoroughfare channel (the distal end), but occasionally they spring from the terminal arteriole and empty directly into the venule. A cuff of smooth muscle fibers, called a **precapillary sphincter**, surrounds the root of each true capillary at the metarteriole and acts as a valve to regulate blood flow into the capillary.

Blood flowing through a terminal arteriole may go either through the true capillaries or through the shunt. When the precapillary sphincters are relaxed (open), as in Figure 19.4a, blood flows through the true capillaries and takes part in exchanges with tissue cells. When the sphincters are contracted (closed), as in Figure 19.4b, blood flows through the shunts and bypasses the tissue cells.

Local chemical conditions and arteriolar vasomotor nerve fibers regulate the amount of blood entering a capillary bed. A bed may be flooded with blood or almost completely bypassed, depending on conditions in the body or in that specific organ. For example, suppose you have just eaten and are sitting relaxed, listening to your favorite musical group. Food is being digested, and blood is circulating freely through the true capillaries of your gastrointestinal organs to receive the breakdown products of digestion. Between meals, however, most of these same capillary pathways are closed.

To take another example, when you exercise vigorously, blood is rerouted from your digestive organs (food or no food) to the capillary beds of your skeletal muscles where it is more immediately needed. This rerouting helps explain why vigorous exercise right after a meal can cause indigestion or abdominal cramps.

Venous System

✓ Describe the structure and function of veins, and explain how veins differ from arteries.

Veins carry blood from the capillary beds toward the heart. Along the route, the diameter of successive venous vessels increases, and their walls gradually thicken as they progress from venules to larger and larger veins.

Venules

Capillaries unite to form **venules**, which range from 8 to 100 μm in diameter. The smallest venules, the *postcapillary venules*, consist entirely of endothelium around which pericytes congregate. Postcapillary venules are extremely porous (more like capillaries than veins in this way), and fluid and white blood cells move easily from the bloodstream through their walls. Indeed, a well-recognized sign of inflammation is adhesion of white blood cells to the postcapillary venule endothelium, followed by their migration through the wall into the inflamed tissue.

Larger venules have one or two layers of smooth muscle cells (a scanty tunica media) and a thin tunica externa as well.

Veins

Venules join to form *veins*. Veins usually have three distinct tunics, but their walls are always thinner and their lumens larger than those of corresponding arteries (see Figure 19.1 and Table 19.1). Consequently, in histological preparations, veins are usually collapsed and their lumens appear slitlike.

There is relatively little smooth muscle or elastin in the tunica media, which is poorly developed and tends to be thin even in the largest veins. The tunica externa is the heaviest wall layer. Consisting of thick longitudinal bundles of collagen fibers and elastic networks, it is often several times thicker than the tunica media. In the largest veins—the venae cavae, which return blood directly to the heart—longitudinal bands of smooth muscle make the tunica externa even thicker.

With their large lumens and thin walls, veins can accommodate a fairly large blood volume. Veins are called **capacitance vessels** and **blood reservoirs** because they can hold up to 65% of the body's blood supply at any time **(Figure 19.5)**. Even so, they are normally only partially filled.

The walls of veins can be much thinner than arterial walls without danger of bursting because the blood pressure in veins is low. However, the low-pressure condition demands several structural adaptations to ensure that veins return blood to the heart at the same rate it was pumped into the circulation. One such adaptation is their large-diameter lumens, which offer relatively little resistance to blood flow.

Venous Valves

Another adaptation is valves that prevent blood from flowing backward. **Venous valves**, formed from folds of the tunica intima, resemble the semilunar valves of the heart in both structure and function (see Figure 19.1). Venous valves are most abundant in the veins of the limbs, where gravity opposes the upward flow of blood. They are usually absent in veins of the thoracic and abdominal body cavities.

The effectiveness of venous valves is demonstrated by this simple experiment: Hang one hand by your side until the blood vessels on its dorsal aspect distend with blood. Next place two fingertips against one of the distended veins, and pressing firmly, move the superior finger proximally along the vein and then release that finger. The vein will remain collapsed (flat) despite the pull of gravity. Finally, remove your distal fingertip and watch the vein refill with blood.

Homeostatic Imbalance 19.1

Varicose veins are veins that are tortuous and dilated because of incompetent (leaky) valves. More than 15% of adults suffer from varicose veins, usually in the lower limbs.

Several factors contribute, including heredity and conditions that hinder venous return, such as prolonged standing in one position, obesity, or pregnancy. Both the "potbelly" of an overweight person and the enlarged uterus of a pregnant woman exert downward pressure on vessels of the groin, restricting return of blood to the heart. Consequently, blood pools in the lower limbs, and with time, the valves weaken and the venous walls stretch and become floppy. Superficial veins, which receive little support from surrounding tissues, are especially susceptible.

Elevated venous pressure can also cause varicose veins. For example, straining to deliver a baby or have a bowel movement raises intra-abdominal pressure, preventing blood from draining from anal veins. The resulting varicosities in the anal veins are called *hemorrhoids* (hem′ŏ-roidz). +

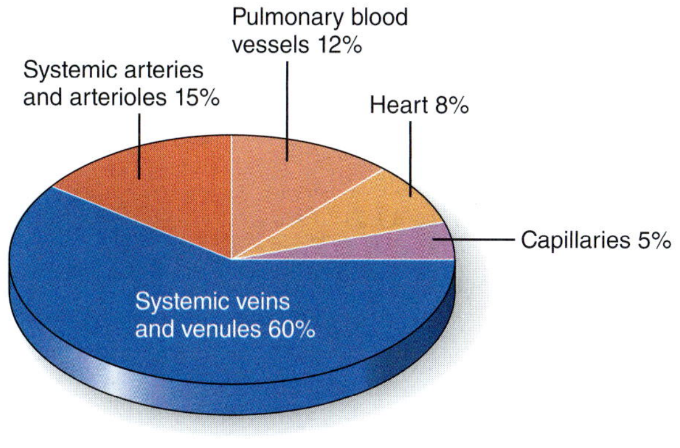

Figure 19.5 Relative proportion of blood volume throughout the cardiovascular system. The systemic veins are called capacitance vessels because they are distensible and contain a large proportion of the blood volume. Pulmonary blood vessels supply the lungs; systemic blood vessels supply the rest of the body.

Venous Sinuses

Venous sinuses, such as the *coronary sinus* of the heart and the *dural venous sinuses* of the brain, are highly specialized, flattened veins with extremely thin walls composed only of endothelium. They are supported by the tissues that surround them, rather than by any additional tunics. The dural venous sinuses, which receive cerebrospinal fluid and blood draining from the brain, are reinforced by the tough dura mater that covers the brain surface.

Vascular Anastomoses

Blood vessels form special interconnections called **vascular anastomoses** (ah-nas″to-mo′sēz; "coming together"). Most organs receive blood from more than one arterial branch, and arteries supplying the same territory often merge, forming **arterial anastomoses**. These anastomoses provide alternate pathways, called **collateral channels**, for blood to reach a given body region. If one branch is cut or blocked by a clot, the collateral channel can often provide sufficient blood to the area.

Arterial anastomoses occur around joints, where active movement may hinder blood flow through one channel. They are also common in abdominal organs, the heart, and the brain (for example, the *cerebral arterial circle* in Figure 19.22d on p. 727). Arteries that supply the retina, kidneys, and spleen either do not anastomose or have a poorly developed collateral circulation. If their blood flow is interrupted, cells supplied by such vessels die.

The metarteriole–thoroughfare channel shunts of capillary beds that connect arterioles and venules are examples of **arteriovenous anastomoses**. Veins interconnect much more freely than arteries, and **venous anastomoses** are common. (You may be able to see venous anastomoses through the skin on the dorsum of your hand.) Because venous anastomoses are abundant, an occluded vein rarely blocks blood flow or leads to tissue death.

19

Atherosclerosis? Get Out the Cardiovascular Drāno

When pipes get **clogged**, it is usually because we've dumped something down the drain that shouldn't be there—a greasy mass or a hairball. Sometimes, pipes get blocked when something is growing inside them (tree roots, for example), trapping the normal sludge coming through (see top photo). In **arteriosclerosis**, the walls of our arteries become thicker and stiffer, and **hypertension** results. In **atherosclerosis**, the most common form of arteriosclerosis, small patchy thickenings called *atheromas* form that can intrude into the vessel lumen, making it easy for **arterial spasms** or a roaming **blood clot** to close the vessel completely.

Although all arteries are susceptible to atherosclerosis, those most often affected are the aorta and the coronary and carotid arteries.

Onset and Stages

Atherosclerosis indirectly causes half of the deaths in the Western world. How does this scourge of blood vessels come about? The development of a full-blown atheroma is believed to occur in several stages.

1. **The endothelium is injured.** According to the *response to injury hypothesis*, the initial event is damage to the tunica intima caused by bloodborne chemicals, hypertension, components of cigarette smoke, or viral or bacterial infections. Researchers suspect that almost any type of chronic infection—even periodontal problems—could set the stage for atherosclerosis. How a bacterium such as *Chlamydophila pneumoniae* (found in some plaques) triggers atheroma development is not completely understood, but we know that any injury to the endothelium sets off the alarm summoning the immune system and the inflammatory process to repair the damage.
2. **Lipids accumulate and oxidize in the tunica intima.** Injured endothelial cells release chemotactic agents and growth (mitosis-inducing) factors, and begin to transport and modify lipids picked up from the blood, particularly low-density lipoproteins (LDLs) that deliver cholesterol to tissue cells via the bloodstream. This accumulated LDL oxidizes in the hostile inflammatory environment. This not only damages neighboring cells, but also acts as a chemotactic agent, attracting macrophages. Some of these macrophages become so engorged with LDLs that they are transformed into lipid-laden *foam cells*. Accumulating foam cells form a **fatty streak**, the first visible sign of an atheroma.
3. **Smooth muscle cells proliferate and a fibrous cap forms.** Smooth muscle cells migrate from the tunica media and deposit collagen and elastic fibers, thickening the intima and producing fibrous lesions with a core of dead and dying foam cells called **fibrous** or **atherosclerotic plaques**. At first the vessel walls accommodate the growing plaque by expanding outward, but eventually these fatty mounds begin to protrude into the vessel lumen, producing full-blown atherosclerosis (see bottom photo).
4. **The plaque becomes unstable.** As the plaque continues to enlarge, the cells at its center die. Calcium is deposited, and collagen fiber production by smooth muscle cells declines. Now called a **complicated plaque**, it is unstable and prone to rupture.

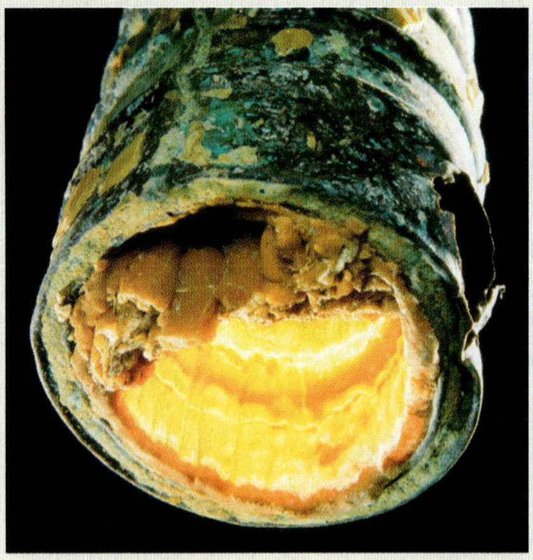

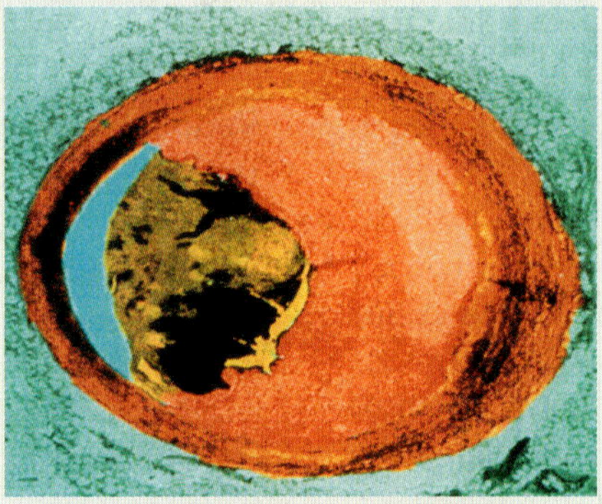

Top **A pipe clogged by accumulated deposits.** ***Bottom*** **Atherosclerotic plaques nearly close a human artery.**

Consequences

The presence of plaques stiffens artery walls and results in *hypertension*. The increased pressure stresses the plaques, making them even more unstable. Plaques also constrict the vessel and cause the arterial walls to fray and ulcerate, conditions that encourage blood sludging and backup, platelet adhesion, and thrombus formation.

Two other factors also promote thrombus formation: (1) Endothelial cells damaged by plaques release less nitric oxide and prostacyclin—chemicals that would otherwise promote vasodilation and inhibit platelet aggregation. (2) *Lipoprotein (a)*, an altered form of LDL found in some individuals, inhibits fibrinolysis by competing with plasminogen.

Plaque formation increases the risk of myocardial infarction, strokes, and aneurysms, and is responsible for the pain (angina) that occurs when heart muscle is ischemic. We often think of large complicated plaques as being the culprits for heart attacks and strokes, but plaques of any size may rupture and form a clot. At least one-third of all heart attacks are caused by plaques too small to be seen on traditional angiograms. They cause no warning symptoms, and victims appear perfectly healthy until they drop dead! One goal of current research is to find ways to identify these vulnerable plaques.

Risk Factors

Why are some of us so troubled by atherosclerosis while others are seemingly immune to its ravages? A large number of interacting risk factors determine the progress of atheroma development. Risk factors include increasing age, male sex, a family history of atherosclerosis, high blood cholesterol, hypertension, cigarette smoking, lack of exercise, diabetes, obesity, stress, and intake of trans fats.

A growing body of evidence links systemic inflammation with the formation and subsequent rupture of atherosclerotic plaques. *C-reactive protein* is a marker of systemic inflammation that is measured to predict the likelihood of future heart attacks and strokes.

Prevention and Treatment

Some risk factors are under our control. We can avoid smoking, lose weight, exercise regularly to increase blood levels of high-density lipoprotein (HDL, the "good" lipoprotein that removes cholesterol from vessel walls and carries it to the liver), and eat a healthy diet low in saturated and trans fats.

But for many of us, these measures are not enough and a pharmaceutical approach is needed. At first it was hoped that cholesterol-lowering drugs called statins would act as cardiovascular Drāno, in effect washing fatty plaques off the walls. Statins do lower LDL, but decrease plaque size by only a small amount. A significant part of their action, though, is their unexpected side benefit—anti-inflammatory activity, which appears to help stabilize existing plaques and keep them from rupturing.

The humble aspirin can also play a role. The American Heart Association recommends that people at high risk for heart attack or stroke take one baby aspirin (81 mg) daily to prevent clot formation when plaques do rupture.

Larger plaques that partially block arteries are treated in much the same way we would treat a blocked sewer pipe—dig it up and replace it or call Roto-Rooter to drill through the obstruction. In *coronary bypass surgery*, veins removed from the legs or small arteries removed from the thoracic cavity are implanted in the heart to restore myocardial circulation. In *balloon angioplasty*, a catheter with a balloon tightly packed into its tip is threaded through the vessels. When the catheter reaches the obstruction, the balloon is inflated to compress the fatty mass against the vessel wall.

Angioplasty temporarily clears the path, but *restenoses* (new blockages) often occur. *Stents*, short metal-mesh tubes that look like a ziti noodle, are inserted into the newly dilated vessels in order to hold the vessel open. Stents that slowly release drugs that inhibit smooth muscle proliferation help reduce restenosis, but these often become clogged as well. Treating the area with bursts of radiation (*brachytherapy*) can help.

When an atheroma ruptures and induces clot formation, *thrombolytic* (*clot-dissolving*) *agents* can help. A genetically engineered form of the naturally occurring *tissue plasminogen activator* (*tPA*) is injected directly into the blocked vessel. tPA restores blood flow quickly and puts an early end to many heart attacks and strokes in progress.

Of course, it's best to prevent atherosclerosis from progressing in the first place by changing our lifestyles. Americans like their burgers and butter. But if heart disease can be prevented by reversing atherosclerosis, many people with diseased arteries may be willing to trade lifelong habits for a healthy old age!

Check Your Understanding

3. Name the type of artery that matches each description: major role in dampening the pulsatile pressure of heart contractions; vasodilation or constriction determines blood flow to individual capillary beds; have the thickest tunica media relative to their lumen size.
4. Look at Figure 19.4 on p. 698 and assume that the capillary bed depicted is in your calf muscle. Which condition—(a) or (b)—would the bed be in if you were doing calf raises at the gym?
5. What is the function of venous valves? What forms the valves?
6. In the systemic circuit, which contains more blood—arteries or veins—or is it the same?

For answers, see Appendix H.

PART 2
Physiology of Circulation

Have you ever climbed a mountain? Well, get ready to climb a hypothetical mountain as you learn about circulatory dynamics. Like scaling a mountain, tackling blood pressure regulation and other topics of cardiovascular physiology is challenging while you're doing it, and exhilarating when you succeed. Let's begin the climb.

To sustain life, blood must be kept circulating. By now, you are aware that the heart is the pump, the arteries are pressure reservoirs and conduits, the arterioles are resistance vessels that control distribution, the capillaries are exchange sites, and the veins are conduits and blood reservoirs. Now for the dynamics of this system.

Introduction to Blood Flow, Blood Pressure, and Resistance

✓ Define blood flow, blood pressure, and resistance, and explain the relationships between these factors.

First we need to define three physiologically important terms—blood flow, blood pressure, and resistance—and examine how these factors relate to the physiology of blood circulation.

Definition of Terms

Blood Flow

Blood flow is the volume of blood flowing through a vessel, an organ, or the entire circulation in a given period (ml/min). If we consider the entire vascular system, blood flow is equivalent to cardiac output (CO), and under resting conditions, it is relatively constant. At any given moment, however, blood flow through *individual* body organs may vary widely according to their immediate needs.

Blood Pressure (BP)

Blood pressure (BP), the force per unit area exerted on a vessel wall by the contained blood, is expressed in millimeters of mercury (mm Hg). For example, a blood pressure of 120 mm Hg is equal to the pressure exerted by a column of mercury 120 mm high.

Unless stated otherwise, the term *blood pressure* means systemic arterial blood pressure in the largest arteries near the heart. The pressure gradient—the *differences* in blood pressure within the vascular system—provides the driving force that keeps blood moving, always from an area of higher pressure to an area of lower pressure, through the body.

Resistance

Resistance is opposition to flow and is a measure of the amount of friction blood encounters as it passes through the vessels. Because most friction is encountered in the peripheral (systemic) circulation, well away from the heart, we generally use the term **peripheral resistance**.

There are three important sources of resistance: blood viscosity, vessel length, and vessel diameter.

Blood Viscosity The internal resistance to flow that exists in all fluids is *viscosity* (vis-kos′ĭ-te) and is related to the thickness or "stickiness" of a fluid. The greater the viscosity, the less easily molecules slide past one another and the more difficult it is to get and keep the fluid moving. Blood is much more viscous than water. Because it contains formed elements and plasma proteins, it flows more slowly under the same conditions.

Blood viscosity is fairly constant, but conditions such as polycythemia (excessive numbers of red blood cells) can increase blood viscosity and, hence, resistance. On the other hand, if the red blood cell count is low, as in some anemias, blood is less viscous and peripheral resistance declines.

Total Blood Vessel Length The relationship between total blood vessel length and resistance is straightforward: the longer the vessel, the greater the resistance. For example, an infant's blood vessels lengthen as he or she grows to adulthood, and so both peripheral resistance and blood pressure increase.

19

Blood Vessel Diameter Because blood viscosity and vessel length are normally unchanging, the influence of these factors can be considered constant in healthy people. However, blood vessel diameter changes frequently and significantly alters peripheral resistance. How so? The answer lies in principles of fluid flow. Fluid close to the wall of a tube or channel is slowed by friction as it passes along the wall, whereas fluid in the center of the tube flows more freely and faster. You can verify this by watching the flow of water in a river. Water close to the bank hardly seems to move, while that in the middle of the river flows quite rapidly.

In a tube of a given size, the relative speed and position of fluid in the different regions of the tube's cross section remain constant, a phenomenon called *laminar flow* or *streamlining*. The smaller the tube, the greater the friction, because relatively more of the fluid contacts the tube wall, where its movement is impeded.

Resistance varies *inversely* with the *fourth power* of the vessel radius (one-half the diameter). This means, for example, that if the radius of a vessel doubles, the resistance drops to one-sixteenth of its original value ($r^4 = 2 \times 2 \times 2 \times 2 = 16$ and $1/r^4 = 1/16$). For this reason, the large arteries close to the heart, which do not change dramatically in diameter, contribute little to peripheral resistance. Instead, the small-diameter arterioles, which can enlarge or constrict in response to neural and chemical controls, are the major determinants of peripheral resistance.

When blood encounters either an abrupt change in vessel diameter or rough or protruding areas of the tube wall (such as the fatty plaques of atherosclerosis), the smooth laminar blood flow is replaced by *turbulent flow*, that is, irregular fluid motion where blood from the different laminae mixes. Turbulence dramatically increases resistance.

Relationship Between Flow, Pressure, and Resistance

Now that we have defined these terms, let's summarize the relationships between them.

- Blood flow (F) is *directly* proportional to the difference in blood pressure (ΔP) between two points in the circulation, that is, the blood pressure, or hydrostatic pressure, gradient. Thus, when ΔP increases, blood flow speeds up, and when ΔP decreases, blood flow declines.
- Blood flow is *inversely* proportional to the peripheral resistance (R) in the systemic circulation; if R increases, blood flow decreases.

We can express these relationships by the formula

$$F = \frac{\Delta P}{R}$$

Of these two factors influencing blood flow, R is far more important than ΔP in influencing local blood flow because R can easily be changed by altering blood vessel diameter. For example, when the arterioles serving a particular tissue dilate (thus decreasing the resistance), blood flow to that tissue increases, even though the systemic pressure is unchanged or may actually be falling.

☑ Check Your Understanding

7. List three factors that determine resistance in a vessel. Which of these factors is physiologically most important?
8. Suppose vasoconstriction decreases the diameter of a vessel to one-third its size. What happens to the rate of flow through that vessel? Calculate the expected size of the change.

For answers, see Appendix H.

Systemic Blood Pressure

✓ Describe how blood pressure differs in the arteries, capillaries, and veins.

Any fluid driven by a pump through a circuit of closed channels operates under pressure, and the nearer the fluid is to the pump, the greater the pressure exerted on the fluid. Blood flow in blood vessels is no exception, and blood flows through the blood vessels along a pressure gradient, always moving from higher- to lower-pressure areas. Fundamentally, *the pumping action of the heart generates blood flow. Pressure results when flow is opposed by resistance.*

As illustrated in **Figure 19.6**, systemic blood pressure is highest in the aorta and declines throughout the pathway to finally reach 0 mm Hg in the right atrium. The steepest drop in blood pressure occurs in the arterioles, which offer the greatest resistance to blood flow. However, as long as a pressure gradient exists, no matter how small, blood continues to flow until it completes the circuit back to the heart.

Arterial Blood Pressure

Arterial blood pressure reflects two factors: (1) how much the elastic arteries close to the heart can stretch (their *compliance* or *distensibility*) and (2) the volume of blood forced into them at any time. If the amounts of blood entering and leaving the elastic arteries in a given period were equal, arterial pressure would be constant. Instead, as Figure 19.6 reveals, blood pressure is *pulsatile*—it rises and falls in a regular fashion—in the elastic arteries near the heart.

As the left ventricle contracts and expels blood into the aorta, it imparts kinetic energy to the blood, which stretches the elastic aorta as aortic pressure reaches its peak. Indeed, if the aorta were opened during this period, blood would spurt upward 5 or 6 feet! This pressure peak generated by ventricular contraction is called the **systolic pressure** (sis-tah′lik) and averages 120 mm Hg in healthy adults. Blood moves forward into the arterial bed because the pressure in the aorta is higher than the pressure in the more distal vessels.

During diastole, the aortic valve closes, preventing blood from flowing back into the heart. The walls of the aorta (and other elastic arteries) recoil, maintaining sufficient pressure to keep the blood flowing forward into the smaller vessels. During this time, aortic pressure drops to its lowest level (approximately 70 to 80 mm Hg in healthy adults), called the **diastolic pressure** (di-as-tah′lik). You can picture the elastic arteries as pressure reservoirs that operate as auxiliary pumps to keep blood circulating throughout the period of diastole, when the heart is relaxing. Essentially, the volume and energy of blood stored in the elastic arteries during systole are given back during diastole.

The difference between the systolic and diastolic pressures is called the **pulse pressure**. It is felt as a throbbing pulsation in an artery (a *pulse*) during systole, as ventricular contraction forces blood into the elastic arteries and expands them. Increased stroke volume and faster blood ejection from the heart (a result of increased contractility) raise pulse pressure *temporarily*. Atherosclerosis chronically increases pulse pressure because the elastic arteries become less stretchy.

Because aortic pressure fluctuates up and down with each heartbeat, the important pressure figure to consider is the **mean arterial pressure (MAP)**—the pressure that propels the blood to the tissues. Diastole usually lasts longer than systole, so MAP is not simply the value halfway between systolic and diastolic pressures. Instead, it is roughly equal to the diastolic pressure plus one-third of the pulse pressure.

$$\text{MAP} = \text{diastolic pressure} + \frac{\text{pulse pressure}}{3}$$

For a person with a systolic blood pressure of 120 mm Hg and a diastolic pressure of 80 mm Hg:

$$\text{MAP} = 80 \text{ mm Hg} + \frac{40 \text{ mm Hg}}{3} = 93 \text{ mm Hg}$$

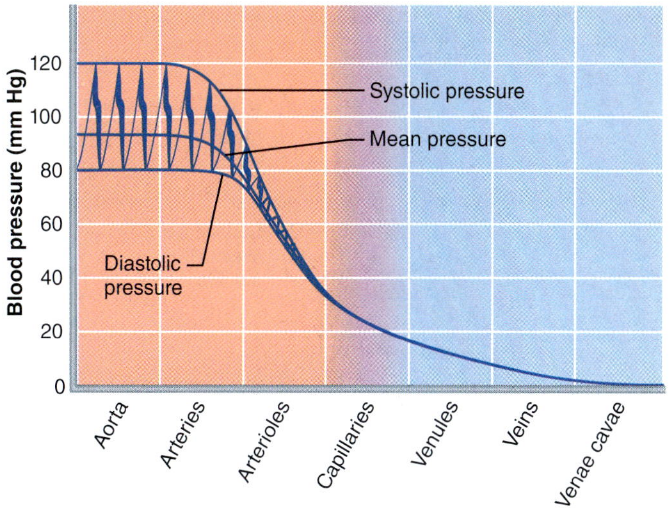

Figure 19.6 Blood pressure in various blood vessels of the systemic circulation.

MAP and pulse pressure both decline with increasing distance from the heart. The MAP loses ground to the never-ending friction between the blood and the vessel walls, and the pulse pressure is gradually phased out in the less elastic muscular arteries, where elastic rebound of the vessels ceases to occur. At the end of the arterial tree, blood flow is steady and the pulse pressure has disappeared.

Capillary Blood Pressure

As Figure 19.6 shows, by the time blood reaches the capillaries, blood pressure has dropped to approximately 35 mm Hg and by the end of the capillary beds is only around 17 mm Hg. Such low capillary pressures are desirable because (1) capillaries are fragile and high pressures would rupture them, and (2) most capillaries are extremely permeable and thus even the low capillary pressure can force solute-containing fluids (filtrate) out of the bloodstream into the interstitial space.

As we describe later in this chapter, these fluid flows are important for continuously refreshing the interstitial fluid.

19

Venous Blood Pressure

Unlike arterial pressure, which pulsates with each contraction of the left ventricle, venous blood pressure is steady and changes very little during the cardiac cycle. The pressure gradient in the veins, from venules to the termini of the venae cavae, is only about 15 mm Hg (that from the aorta to the ends of the arterioles is about 60 mm Hg).

The difference in pressure between an artery and a vein becomes very clear when the vessels are cut. If a vein is cut, the blood flows evenly from the wound, but a lacerated artery spurts blood. The very low pressure in the venous system reflects the cumulative effects of peripheral resistance, which dissipates most of the energy of blood pressure (as heat) during each circuit.

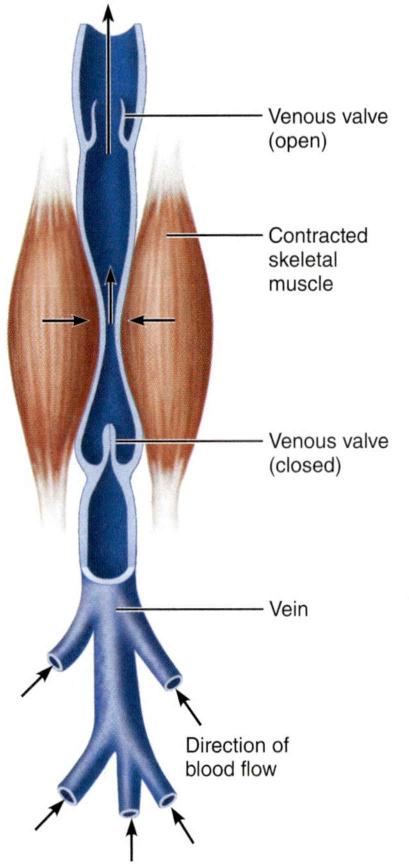

Figure 19.7 The muscular pump. When contracting skeletal muscles press against a vein, they force open the valves proximal to the area of contraction and blood is propelled toward the heart. Backflowing blood closes the valves distal to the area of contraction.

19

Despite the structural modifications of veins (large lumens and valves), venous pressure is normally too low to promote adequate venous return. For this reason, three functional adaptations are critically important to venous return:

- **The muscular pump.** The **muscular pump** consists of skeletal muscle activity. As the skeletal muscles surrounding the deep veins contract and relax, they "milk" blood toward the heart, and once blood passes each successive valve, it cannot flow back **(Figure 19.7)**. People who earn their living in "standing professions," such as hairdressers and dentists, often have swollen ankles because blood pools in their feet and legs. Indeed, standing for prolonged periods may cause fainting because skeletal muscle inactivity reduces venous return.
- **The respiratory pump.** The **respiratory pump** moves blood up toward the heart as pressure changes in the ventral body cavity during breathing. As we inhale, abdominal pressure increases, squeezing local veins and forcing blood toward the heart. At the same time, the pressure in the chest decreases, allowing thoracic veins to expand and speeding blood entry into the right atrium.
- **Sympathetic venoconstriction.** Sympathetic venoconstriction reduces the volume of blood in the veins—the capacitance vessels. As the layer of smooth muscle around the veins constricts under sympathetic control, venous volume is reduced and blood is pushed toward the heart.

All three of these functional adaptations increase venous return, which increases stroke volume (by the Frank-Starling mechanism) and therefore increases cardiac output.

Maintaining Blood Pressure

✓ List and explain the factors that influence blood pressure, and describe how blood pressure is regulated.

✓ Define hypertension. Describe its manifestations and consequences.

Maintaining a steady flow of blood from the heart to the toes is vital for organs to function properly. But making sure a person jumping out of bed in the morning does not keel over from inadequate blood flow to the brain requires the finely tuned cooperation of the heart, blood vessels, and kidneys—all supervised by the brain.

Central among the homeostatic mechanisms that regulate cardiovascular dynamics are those that maintain blood pressure, principally *cardiac output*, *peripheral resistance*, and *blood volume*. If we rearrange the formula pertaining to blood flow presented on p. 702, we can see how cardiac output (blood flow of the entire circulation) and peripheral resistance relate to blood pressure:

$$F = \Delta P/R \quad \text{or} \quad CO = \Delta P/R \quad \text{or} \quad \Delta P = CO \times R$$

Clearly, blood pressure varies *directly* with CO and *R*. Additionally, blood pressure varies directly with blood volume because CO depends on blood volume (the heart can't pump out what doesn't enter its chambers).

So in theory, a change (increase or decrease) in any of these variables would cause a corresponding change in blood pressure. However, what *really* happens in the body is that changes in one variable that threaten blood pressure homeostasis are quickly compensated for by changes in the other variables.

As we described in Chapter 18, CO is equal to *stroke volume* (ml/beat) times *heart rate* (beats/min), and normal CO is 5.0 to 5.5 L/min. **Figure 19.8** shows the main factors determining cardiac output—venous return and the neural and hormonal controls. Remember that the cardioinhibitory center in the medulla is "in charge" of heart rate most of the time and, via the parasympathetic vagus nerves, maintains the *resting heart rate*. During "resting" periods, venous return (end diastolic volume) largely controls stroke volume. During stress, the cardioacceleratory center takes over, activating the sympathetic nervous system and increasing both heart rate (by acting on the SA node) and stroke volume (by enhancing cardiac muscle contractility, which decreases end systolic volume). The enhanced CO, in turn, increases MAP.

In the following discussion we explore factors that regulate blood pressure. *Short-term regulation* by the nervous system and bloodborne hormones alters blood pressure by changing peripheral resistance and CO. *Long-term regulation* alters blood volume via the kidneys. Figure 19.11 (p. 709) summarizes the influence of nearly all of the important factors.

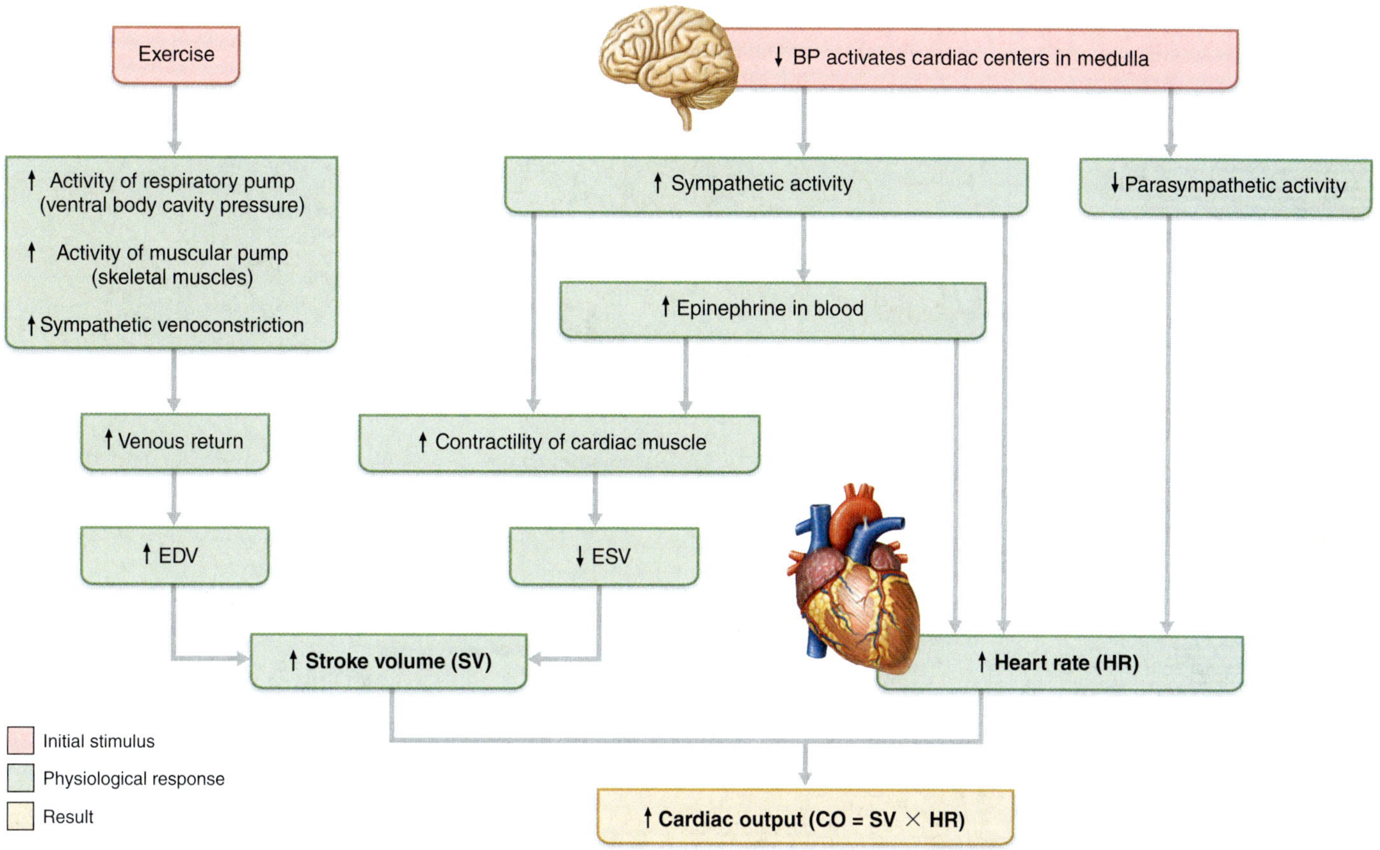

Figure 19.8 Major factors enhancing cardiac output. BP = blood pressure, EDV = end diastolic volume, ESV = end systolic volume.

Short-Term Regulation: Neural Controls

Neural controls alter both cardiac output and peripheral resistance. Neural controls of peripheral resistance are directed at two main goals:

- Maintaining adequate MAP by altering blood vessel diameter on a moment-to-moment basis. (Remember, very small changes in blood vessel diameter cause substantial changes in peripheral resistance, and hence in systemic blood pressure.) Under conditions of low blood volume, all vessels except those supplying the heart and brain are constricted to allow as much blood as possible to flow to those two vital organs.
- Altering blood distribution to respond to specific demands of various organs. For example, during exercise blood is shunted temporarily from the digestive organs to the skeletal muscles.

Most neural controls operate via reflex arcs involving *baroreceptors* and associated afferent fibers. These reflexes are integrated in the cardiovascular center of the medulla, and their output travels via autonomic fibers to the heart and vascular smooth muscle. Occasionally, inputs from *chemoreceptors* and higher brain centers also influence the neural control mechanism.

Role of the Cardiovascular Center

Several clusters of neurons in the medulla oblongata act together to integrate blood pressure control by altering cardiac output and blood vessel diameter. This **cardiovascular center** consists of the *cardiac centers* (the cardioacceleratory and cardioinhibitory centers discussed in Chapter 18), and the **vasomotor center** that controls the diameter of blood vessels.

The vasomotor center transmits impulses at a fairly steady rate along sympathetic efferents called **vasomotor fibers**. These fibers exit from the T_1 through L_2 levels of the spinal cord and innervate the smooth muscle of blood vessels, mainly arterioles. As a result, the arterioles are almost always in a state of moderate constriction, called **vasomotor tone**.

The degree of vasomotor tone varies from organ to organ. Generally, arterioles of the skin and digestive viscera receive vasomotor impulses more frequently and tend to be more strongly constricted than those of skeletal muscles. Any increase in sympathetic activity produces generalized vasoconstriction and raises blood pressure. Decreased sympathetic activity allows the vascular muscle to relax somewhat and lowers blood pressure to basal levels.

Cardiovascular center activity is modified by inputs from (1) baroreceptors (pressure-sensitive mechanoreceptors that respond to changes in arterial pressure and stretch), (2) chemoreceptors (receptors that respond to changes in blood levels of carbon dioxide, H^+, and oxygen), and (3) higher brain centers. Let's take a look.

19

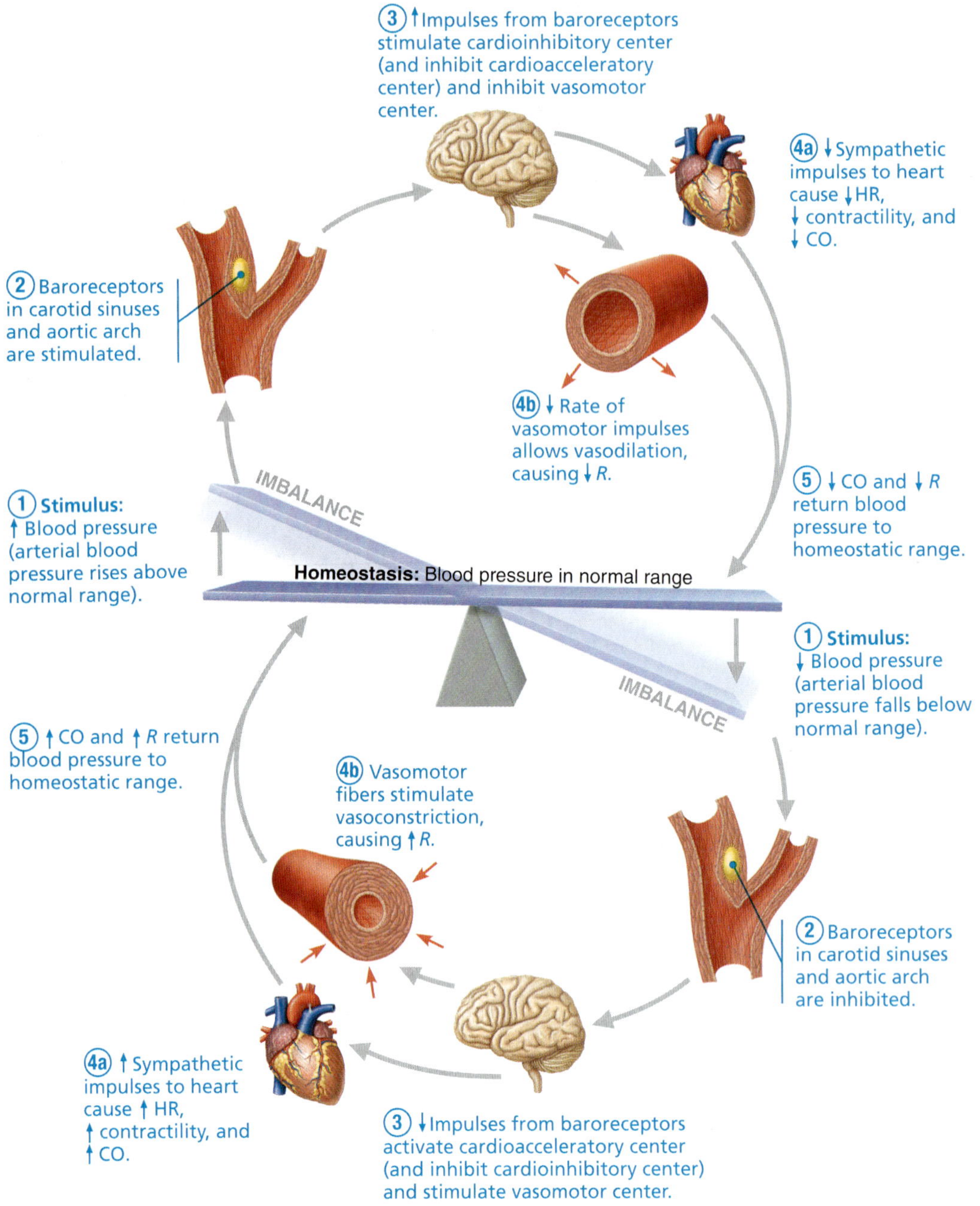

Figure 19.9 Baroreceptor reflexes that help maintain blood pressure homeostasis. CO = cardiac output; *R* = peripheral resistance; HR = heart rate; BP = blood pressure.

19

Baroreceptor Reflexes

When arterial blood pressure rises, it activates **baroreceptors**. These stretch receptors are located in the *carotid sinuses* (dilations in the internal carotid arteries, which provide the major blood supply to the brain), in the *aortic arch*, and in the walls of nearly every large artery of the neck and thorax. When stretched, baroreceptors send a rapid stream of impulses to the cardiovascular center, inhibiting the vasomotor and cardioacceleratory centers and stimulating the cardioinhibitory center. The result is a decrease in blood pressure **(Figure 19.9)**.

Three mechanisms bring this about:

- **Arteriolar vasodilation.** Decreased output from the vasomotor center allows arterioles to dilate. As peripheral resistance falls, so does MAP.
- **Venodilation.** Decreased output from the vasomotor center also allows veins to dilate, which shifts blood to the venous reservoirs. This decreases venous return and CO.
- **Decreased cardiac output.** Impulses to the cardiac centers inhibit sympathetic activity and stimulate parasympathetic activity, reducing heart rate and contractile force. As CO falls, so does MAP.

Table 19.2 Effects of Selected Hormones on Blood Pressure

HORMONE	EFFECT ON BP	VARIABLE AFFECTED	SITE OF ACTION
Epinephrine and norepinephrine (NE)	↑	↑ CO (HR and contractility)	Heart (β_1 receptors)
		↑ Peripheral resistance (vasoconstriction)	Arterioles (α receptors)
Angiotensin II	↑	↑ Peripheral resistance (vasoconstriction)	Arterioles
Atrial natriuretic peptide (ANP)	↓	↓ Peripheral resistance (vasodilation)	Arterioles
Antidiuretic hormone (ADH)	↑	↑ Peripheral resistance (vasoconstriction)	Arterioles
		↑ Blood volume (↓ water loss)	Kidney tubule cells
Aldosterone	↑	↑ Blood volume (↓ water and salt loss)	Kidney tubule cells

In the opposite situation, a decline in MAP initiates reflex vasoconstriction and increases cardiac output, bringing blood pressure back up. In this way, peripheral resistance and cardiac output are regulated in tandem to minimize changes in blood pressure.

Rapidly responding baroreceptors protect the circulation against short-term (acute) changes in blood pressure. For example, blood pressure falls (particularly in the head) when you stand up after reclining. Baroreceptors taking part in the **carotid sinus reflex** protect the blood supply to your brain, whereas those activated in the **aortic reflex** help maintain adequate blood pressure in your systemic circuit as a whole.

Baroreceptors are relatively *ineffective* in protecting us against sustained pressure changes, as evidenced by the fact that many people develop chronic hypertension. In such cases, the baroreceptors are "reprogrammed" (adapt) to monitor pressure changes at a higher set point.

Chemoreceptor Reflexes

When the carbon dioxide levels rise, or the pH falls, or oxygen content of the blood drops sharply, **chemoreceptors** in the aortic arch and large arteries of the neck transmit impulses to the cardioacceleratory center, which then increases cardiac output, and to the vasomotor center, which causes reflex vasoconstriction. The rise in blood pressure that follows speeds the return of blood to the heart and lungs.

The most prominent chemoreceptors are the *carotid* and *aortic bodies* located close by the baroreceptors in the carotid sinuses and aortic arch. Chemoreceptors play a larger role in regulating respiratory rate than blood pressure, so we consider their function in Chapter 22.

Influence of Higher Brain Centers

Reflexes that regulate blood pressure are integrated in the medulla oblongata of the brain stem. Although the cerebral cortex and hypothalamus are not involved in routine controls of blood pressure, these higher brain centers can modify arterial pressure via relays to the medullary centers.

For example, the fight-or-flight response mediated by the hypothalamus has profound effects on blood pressure. (Even the simple act of speaking can make your blood pressure jump if the person you are talking to makes you anxious.) The hypothalamus also mediates the redistribution of blood flow and other cardiovascular responses that occur during exercise and changes in body temperature.

Short-Term Regulation: Hormonal Controls

Hormones also help regulate blood pressure, both in the short term via changes in peripheral resistance and in the long term via changes in blood volume (Table 19.2). Paracrines (local chemicals), on the other hand, primarily serve to match blood flow to the metabolic need of a particular tissue. In rare instances, massive release of paracrines can affect blood pressure. We will discuss these paracrines later—here we will examine the short-term effects of hormones.

- **Adrenal medulla hormones.** During periods of stress, the adrenal gland releases **epinephrine** and **norepinephrine (NE)** to the blood. Both hormones enhance the sympathetic response by increasing cardiac output and promoting generalized vasoconstriction.
- **Angiotensin II.** When blood pressure or blood volume are low, the kidneys release renin. Renin acts as an enzyme, ultimately generating **angiotensin II** (an″je-o-ten′sin), which stimulates intense vasoconstriction, promoting a rapid rise in systemic blood pressure. It also stimulates release of aldosterone and ADH, which act in long-term regulation of blood pressure by enhancing blood volume.
- **Atrial natriuretic peptide (ANP).** The atria of the heart produce the hormone **atrial natriuretic peptide (ANP)**, which leads to a reduction in blood volume and blood pressure. As noted in Chapter 16, ANP antagonizes aldosterone and prods the kidneys to excrete more sodium and water from the body, reducing blood volume. It also causes generalized vasodilation.
- **Antidiuretic hormone (ADH).** Produced by the hypothalamus, **antidiuretic hormone** (**ADH**, also called **vasopressin**) stimulates the kidneys to conserve water. It is not usually important in short-term blood pressure regulation. However, when blood pressure falls to dangerously low levels (as during severe hemorrhage), much more ADH is released and helps restore arterial pressure by causing intense vasoconstriction.

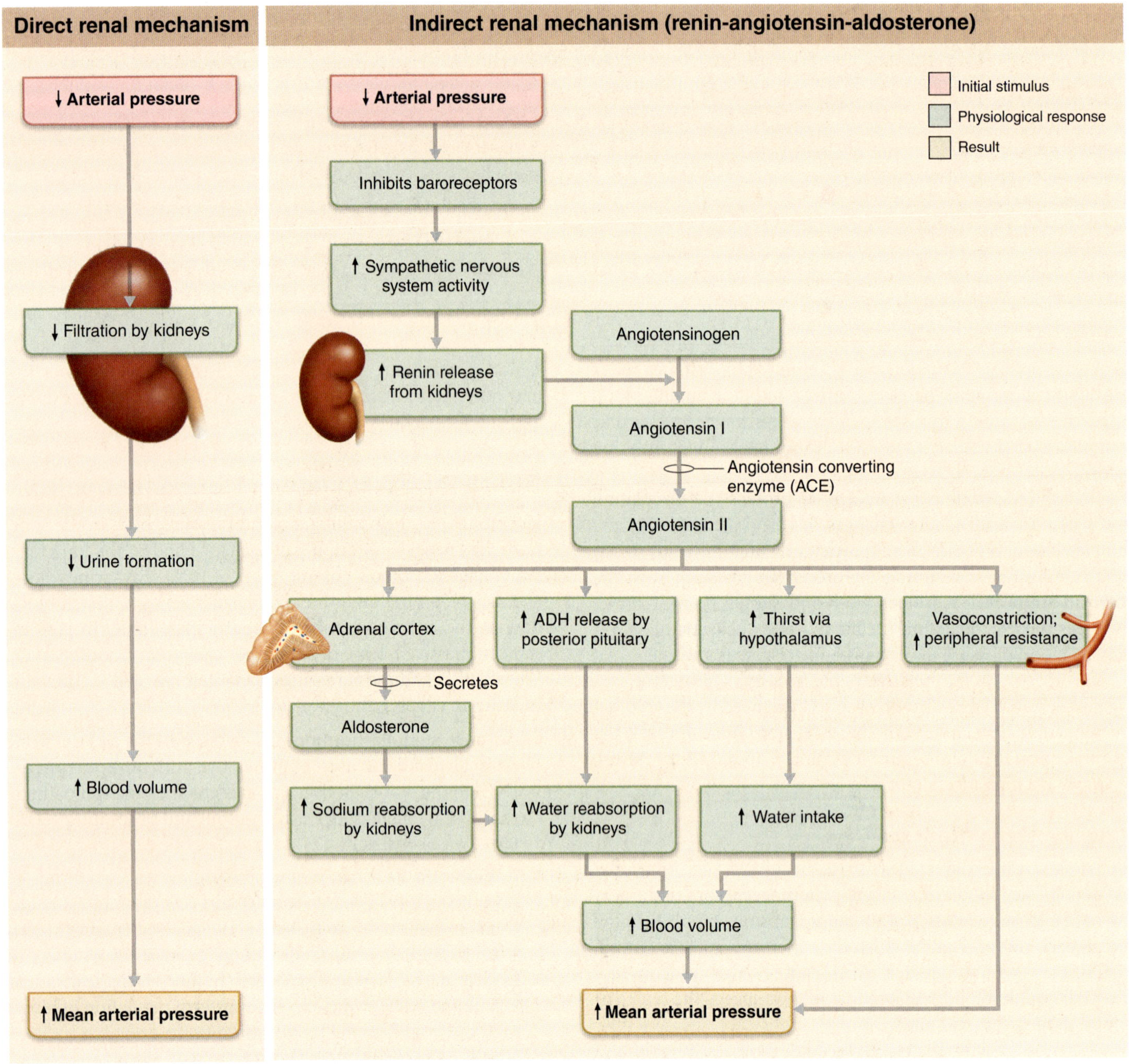

Figure 19.10 Direct and indirect (hormonal) mechanisms for renal control of blood pressure. Low blood pressure also triggers other actions not shown here that increase BP: additional mechanisms of renin release (described in Chapter 25) and short-term actions of the sympathetic nervous system.

Long-Term Regulation: Renal Mechanisms

Unlike short-term controls of blood pressure that alter peripheral resistance and cardiac output, long-term controls alter blood volume. Renal mechanisms mediate long-term regulation.

Although baroreceptors respond to short-term changes in blood pressure, they quickly adapt to prolonged or chronic episodes of high or low pressure. This is where the kidneys step in to restore and maintain blood pressure homeostasis by regulating blood volume. Although blood volume varies with age, body size, and sex, renal mechanisms usually keep it close to 5 L.

As we noted earlier, blood volume is a major determinant of cardiac output (via its influence on venous return, EDV, and stroke volume). An increase in blood volume is followed by a rise in blood pressure, and anything that increases blood volume—such as excessive salt intake, which promotes water retention—raises MAP because of the greater fluid load in the vascular tree.

By the same token, decreased blood volume translates to a fall in blood pressure. Blood loss and the garden-variety dehydration that occurs during vigorous exercise are common causes of reduced blood volume. A sudden drop in blood pressure often

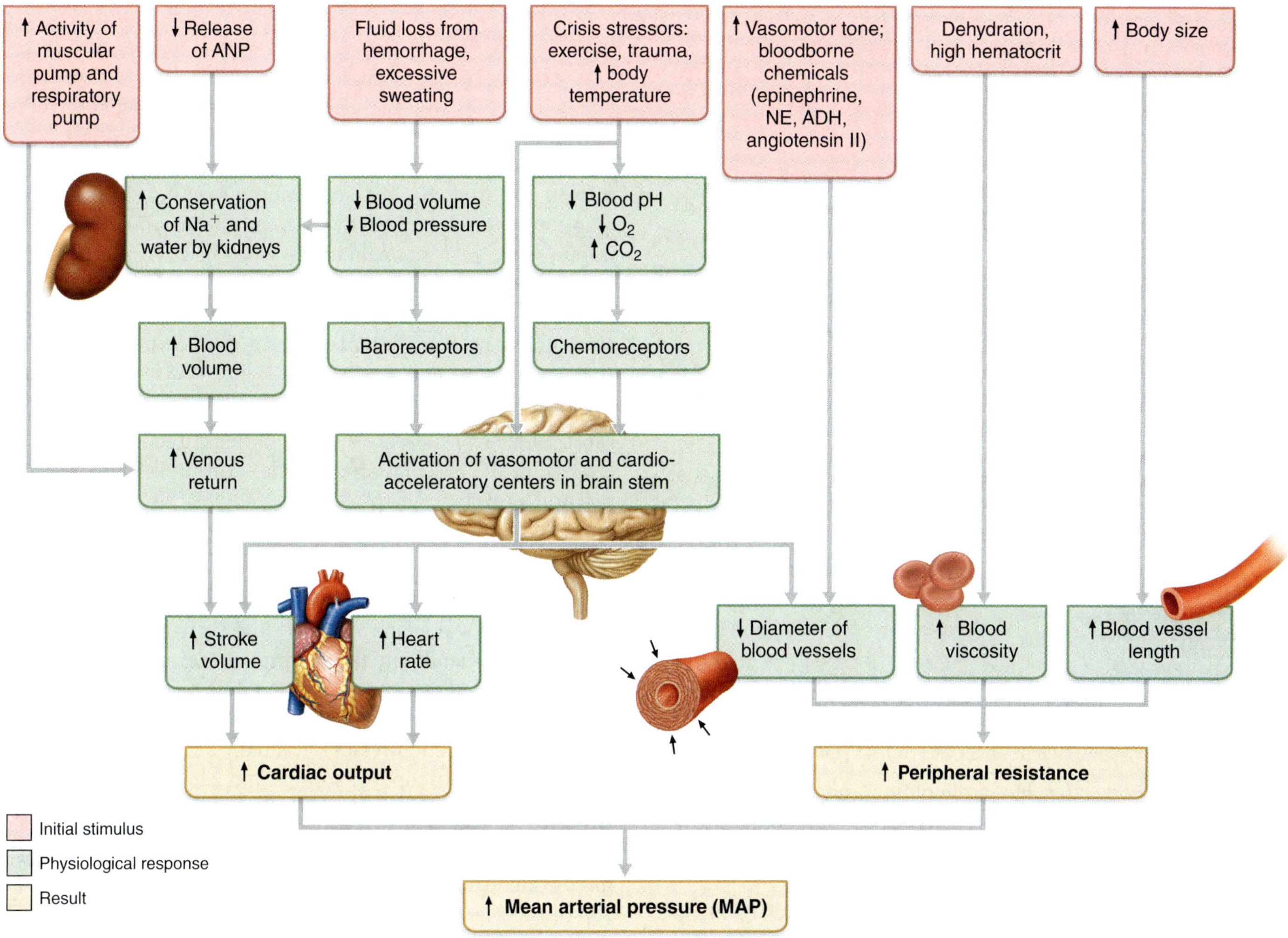

Figure 19.11 **Factors that increase MAP.**

signals internal bleeding and blood volume too low to support normal circulation.

However, these assertions—increased blood volume increases BP and decreased blood volume decreases BP—do not tell the whole story because we are dealing with a dynamic system. Increases in blood volume that raise blood pressure also stimulate the kidneys to eliminate water, which reduces blood volume and consequently blood pressure. Likewise, falling blood volume triggers renal mechanisms that increase blood volume and blood pressure. As you can see, blood pressure can be stabilized or maintained within normal limits only when blood volume is stable.

The kidneys act both directly and indirectly to regulate arterial pressure and provide the major long-term mechanisms of blood pressure control.

Direct Renal Mechanism

The *direct renal mechanism* alters blood volume independently of hormones. When either blood volume or blood pressure rises, the rate at which fluid filters from the bloodstream into the kidney tubules speeds up. In such situations, the kidneys cannot reabsorb the filtrate rapidly enough, and more of it leaves the body in urine. As a result, blood volume and blood pressure fall.

When blood pressure or blood volume is low, water is conserved and returned to the bloodstream, and blood pressure rises (**Figures 19.10** and **19.11**). As blood volume goes, so goes the arterial blood pressure.

Indirect Renal Mechanism

The kidneys can also regulate blood pressure *indirectly* via the **renin-angiotensin-aldosterone mechanism**. When arterial blood pressure declines, certain cells in the kidneys release the enzyme **renin** into the blood. Renin enzymatically cleaves **angiotensinogen**, a plasma protein made by the liver, converting it to **angiotensin I**. In turn, **angiotensin converting enzyme (ACE)** converts angiotensin I to **angiotensin II**. ACE activity is associated with the capillary endothelium in various body tissues, particularly the lungs.

Angiotensin II acts in four ways to stabilize arterial blood pressure and extracellular fluid volume (Figure 19.10).

- It stimulates the adrenal cortex to secrete **aldosterone**, a hormone that enhances renal reabsorption of sodium. As sodium moves into the bloodstream, water follows, which conserves blood volume. In addition, angiotensin II directly stimulates sodium reabsorption by the kidneys.

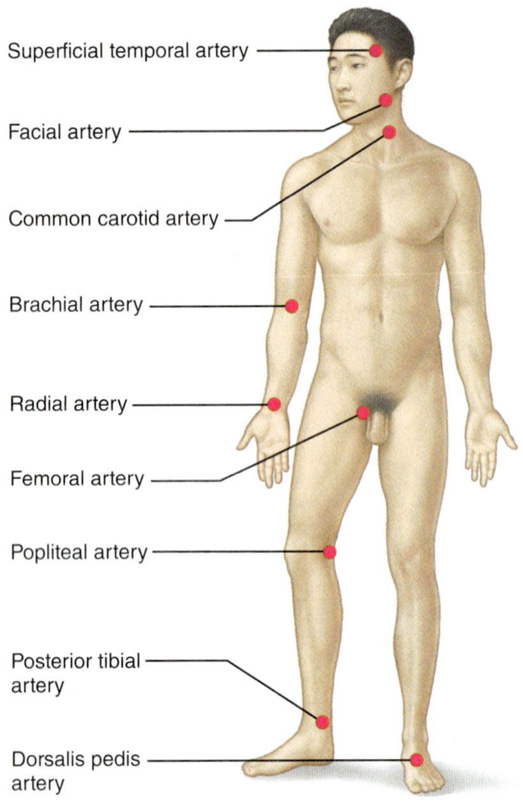

Figure 19.12 Body sites where the pulse is most easily palpated. (We discuss the specific arteries indicated on pp. 726–735.)

- It prods the posterior pituitary to release ADH, which promotes more water reabsorption by the kidneys.
- It triggers the sensation of thirst by activating the hypothalamic thirst center (see Chapter 26). This encourages water consumption, ultimately restoring blood volume and so blood pressure.
- It is a potent vasoconstrictor, increasing blood pressure by increasing peripheral resistance.

Clinical Monitoring of Circulatory Efficiency

Clinicians can assess the efficiency of a person's circulation by measuring pulse and blood pressure. These values, along with measurements of respiratory rate and body temperature, are referred to collectively as the body's **vital signs**. Let's examine how vital signs are determined or measured.

Taking a Pulse

The alternating expansion and recoil of arteries during each cardiac cycle allow us to feel a pressure wave—a **pulse**—that is transmitted through the arterial tree. You can feel a pulse in any artery that lies close to the body surface by compressing the artery against firm tissue, and this provides an easy way to count heart rate. Because it is so accessible, the point where the radial artery surfaces at the wrist, the *radial pulse*, is routinely used to take a pulse measurement, but there are several other clinically important arterial pulse points **(Figure 19.12)**.

These pulse points are also called **pressure points** because they are compressed to stop blood flow into distal tissues during hemorrhage. For example, if you seriously lacerate your hand, you can slow or stop the bleeding by compressing your radial or brachial artery.

Monitoring pulse rate is an easy way to assess the effects of activity, postural changes, and emotions on heart rate. For example, the pulse of a healthy man may be around 66 beats per minute when he is lying down, 70 when he sits up, and 80 if he suddenly stands. During vigorous exercise or emotional upset, pulse rates between 140 and 180 are not unusual because of sympathetic nervous system effects on the heart.

Measuring Blood Pressure

Most often, you measure systemic arterial blood pressure indirectly in the brachial artery of the arm by the **auscultatory method** (aw-skul′tah-to″re). The steps of this procedure are outlined next:

1. Wrap the *blood pressure cuff*, or *sphygmomanometer* (sfig″mo-mah-nom′ĕ-ter; *sphygmo* = pulse), snugly around the person's arm just superior to the elbow.
2. Inflate the cuff until the cuff pressure exceeds systolic pressure. At this point, blood flow into the arm stops and a brachial pulse cannot be felt or heard.
3. Reduce the cuff pressure gradually and listen (auscultate) with a stethoscope for sounds in the brachial artery.

The pressure read when the first soft tapping sounds are heard (the first point at which a small amount of blood is spurting through the constricted artery) is systolic pressure. As the cuff pressure is reduced further, these sounds, called the *sounds of Korotkoff*, become louder and more distinct. However, when the artery is no longer constricted and blood flows freely, the sounds can no longer be heard. The pressure at which the sounds disappear is the diastolic pressure.

Homeostatic Imbalances in Blood Pressure

Normal blood pressure for resting adults is a systolic pressure of less than 120 mm Hg and a diastolic pressure of less than 80 mm Hg. Transient elevations in blood pressure occur as normal adaptations during changes in posture, physical exertion, emotional upset, and fever. Age, sex, weight, and race also affect blood pressure. What is "normal" for you may not be normal for your grandfather or your neighbor.

Hypertension

Chronically elevated blood pressure is called **hypertension** and is characterized by a sustained increase in either systolic pressure (above 140 mm Hg) or diastolic pressure (above 90 mm Hg). The American Heart Association considers individuals to have *prehypertension* if their blood pressure values are elevated but not yet in the hypertension range. These individuals are at higher risk for developing full-blown hypertension and are often advised to change their lifestyles to reduce their risk of developing full-blown hypertension.

Chronic hypertension is a common and dangerous disease. An estimated 30% of people over age 50 are hypertensive. Although this "silent killer" is usually asymptomatic for the first 10 to 20 years, it slowly but surely strains the heart and damages the arteries. Prolonged hypertension is the major cause of heart failure, vascular disease, renal failure, and stroke. The higher the pressure, the greater the risk for these serious problems.

Because the heart is forced to pump against greater resistance, it must work harder, and over time the myocardium enlarges. When finally strained beyond its capacity, the heart weakens and its walls become flabby. Hypertension also ravages the blood vessels, accelerating the progress of atherosclerosis (see *A Closer Look* on pp. 700–701). As the vessels become increasingly blocked, blood flow to the tissues becomes inadequate and vascular complications appear in the brain, heart, kidneys, and retinas of the eyes.

Primary Hypertension Although hypertension and atherosclerosis are often linked, it is often difficult to blame hypertension on any distinct anatomical pathology. Indeed, about 90% of hypertensive people have **primary**, or **essential**, **hypertension**, for which no underlying cause has been identified. This is because primary hypertension is due to a rich interplay between your genes and a variety of environmental factors:

- **Heredity.** Hypertension runs in families. Children of hypertensive parents are twice as likely to develop hypertension as are children of normotensive parents, and more blacks than whites are hypertensive. Many of the factors listed here require a genetic predisposition, and the course of the disease varies in different population groups.
- **Diet.** Dietary factors that contribute to hypertension include high intakes of salt (NaCl), saturated fat, and cholesterol, and deficiencies in certain metal ions (K^+, Ca^{2+}, and Mg^{2+}).
- **Obesity.** Obesity causes hypertension in a number of ways that are not yet well understood. For example, adipocytes release hormones that appear to increase sympathetic tone and interfere with the ability of endothelial cells to induce vasodilation.
- **Age.** Hypertension usually appears after age 40.
- **Diabetes mellitus.**
- **Stress.** Particularly at risk are "hot reactors," people whose blood pressure zooms upward during every stressful event.
- **Smoking.** Nicotine, an important chemical in tobacco and one of the strongest toxins known, causes intense vasoconstriction not only by directly stimulating postganglionic sympathetic neurons but also by prompting release of large amounts of epinephrine and NE. Chemicals in cigarette smoke also damage the tunica intima, interfering with its ability to chemically regulate arteriolar diameter.

Primary hypertension cannot be cured, but most cases can be controlled. Restricting salt, fat, and cholesterol intake, increasing exercise and losing weight, stopping smoking, managing stress, and taking antihypertensive drugs can all help. Drugs commonly used are diuretics, beta-blockers, calcium channel blockers, angiotensin converting enzyme (ACE) inhibitors, and angiotensin II receptor blockers. Inhibiting ACE or blocking receptors for angiotensin II suppresses the renin-angiotensin-aldosterone mechanism.

Secondary Hypertension **Secondary hypertension**, which accounts for 10% of cases, is due to identifiable conditions, for example obstructed renal arteries, kidney disease, and endocrine disorders such as hyperthyroidism and Cushing's syndrome. Treatment for secondary hypertension focuses on correcting the problem that caused it.

Hypotension

In many cases, **hypotension**, or low blood pressure (below 90/60 mm Hg), simply reflects individual variations and is no cause for concern. In fact, low blood pressure is often associated with long life and an old age free of cardiovascular disease.

Hypotension is usually a concern only if it leads to inadequate blood flow to tissues. For example, hypotension may cause dizziness or fainting because of inadequate oxygen delivery to the brain. *Acute hypotension* is one of the most important signs of circulatory shock (p. 717) and a threat to patients undergoing surgery and those in intensive care units.

Orthostatic hypotension is a temporary drop in blood pressure resulting in dizziness when a person rises suddenly from a reclining or sitting position. Elderly people are prone to orthostatic hypotension because the aging sympathetic nervous system does not respond as quickly as it once did to postural changes. Blood pools briefly in the lower limbs, reducing blood pressure and consequently blood delivery to the brain. Changing position slowly gives the nervous system time to adjust and usually prevents this problem.

Occasionally, *chronic hypotension* is a sign of a serious underlying condition. Addison's disease (inadequate adrenal cortex function), hypothyroidism, or severe malnutrition can cause chronic hypotension.

19

☑ Check Your Understanding

9. Describe the baroreceptor reflex changes that occur to maintain blood pressure when you rise from a lying-down to a standing position.
10. The kidneys play an important role in maintaining MAP by influencing which variable? Explain how renal artery obstruction could cause secondary hypertension.

For answers, see Appendix H.

Blood Flow Through Body Tissues: Tissue Perfusion

✓ Explain how blood flow is regulated in the body in general and in specific organs.

Blood flow through body tissues, or **tissue perfusion**, is involved in (1) delivering oxygen and nutrients to tissue cells, and removing wastes from them, (2) exchanging gases in the lungs, (3) absorbing nutrients from the digestive tract, and (4) forming

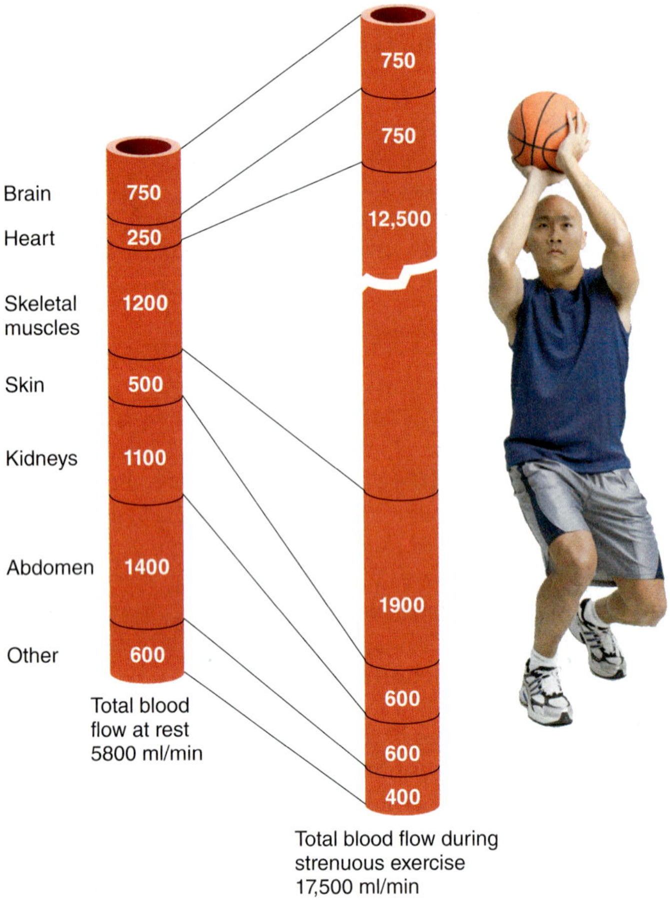

Figure 19.13 Distribution of blood flow at rest and during strenuous exercise.

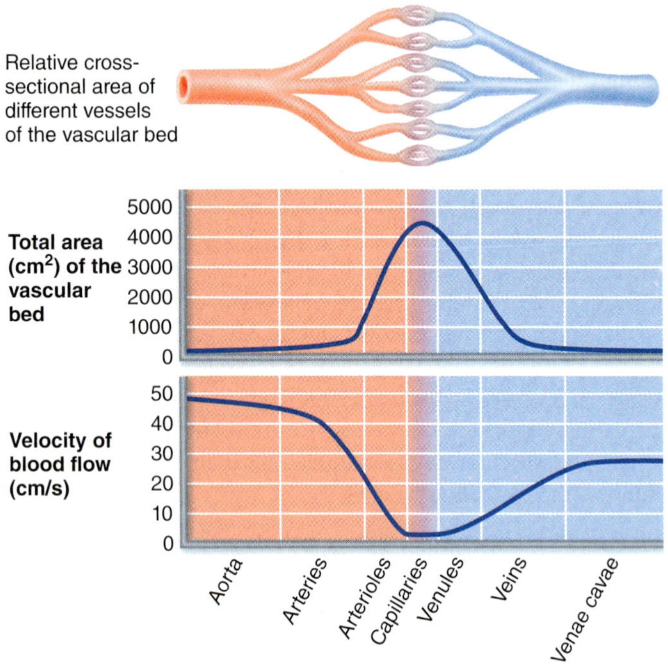

Figure 19.14 Blood flow velocity and total cross-sectional area of vessels. Various blood vessels of the systemic circulation differ in their total cross-sectional area (e.g., the cross section of all systemic capillaries combined versus the cross section of all systemic arteries combined), which affects the velocity of blood flow through them.

urine in the kidneys. The rate of blood flow to each tissue and organ is almost exactly the right amount to provide for proper function—no more, no less.

When the body is at rest, the brain receives about 13% of total blood flow, the heart 4%, kidneys 20%, and abdominal organs 24%. Skeletal muscles, which make up almost half of body mass, normally receive about 20% of total blood flow. During exercise, however, nearly all of the increased cardiac output flushes into the skeletal muscles and blood flow to the kidneys and digestive organs declines **(Figure 19.13)**.

Velocity of Blood Flow

Have you ever watched a swift river emptying into a large lake? The water's speed decreases as it enters the lake until its flow becomes almost imperceptible. This is because the total cross-sectional area of the lake is much larger than that of the river. Velocity in this case is *inversely* related to cross-sectional area. The same thing happens with blood flow inside our blood vessels.

As shown in **Figure 19.14**, the speed or velocity of blood flow changes as blood travels through the systemic circulation. It is fastest in the aorta and other large arteries (the river), slowest in the capillaries (whose large total cross-sectional area make them analogous to the lake), and then picks up speed again in the veins (the river again).

Just as in our analogy of the river and lake, blood flows fastest where the total cross-sectional area is least. As the arterial system branches, the total cross-sectional area of the vascular bed increases, and the velocity of blood flow declines proportionately. Even though the individual branches have smaller lumens, their *combined* cross-sectional areas and thus the volume of blood they can hold are much greater than that of the aorta.

For example, the cross-sectional area of the aorta is 2.5 cm^2 but the combined cross-sectional area of all the capillaries is 4500 cm^2. This difference results in fast blood flow in the aorta (40–50 cm/s) and slow blood flow in the capillaries (about 0.03 cm/s). Slow capillary flow is beneficial because it allows adequate time for exchanges between the blood and tissue cells.

As capillaries combine to form first venules and then veins, total cross-sectional area declines and velocity increases. The cross-sectional area of the venae cavae is 8 cm^2, and the velocity of blood flow varies from 10 to 30 cm/s in those vessels, depending on the activity of the skeletal muscle pump.

Autoregulation: Local Regulation of Blood Flow

As our activities change throughout the day, how does each organ or tissue manage to get the blood flow it needs? The answer is **autoregulation**, the automatic adjustment of blood flow to each tissue in proportion to the tissue's requirements at any instant. Local conditions regulate this process independent of control by nerves or hormones. MAP is the same everywhere in the body and homeostatic mechanisms adjust cardiac output as needed to maintain that constant pressure. Changes in blood flow through individual organs are controlled *intrinsically* by modifying the diameter of local arterioles feeding the capillaries.

You can compare blood flow autoregulation to water use in your home. To get water in a sink or a garden hose, you have to turn on a faucet. Whether you have several taps open or none, the pressure in the main water pipe in the street remains relatively constant, as it does in the even larger water lines closer to the pumping station. Similarly, local conditions in the arterioles feeding the capillary beds of an organ have little effect on pressure in the muscular artery feeding that organ, or in the large elastic arteries. The pumping station is, of course, the heart. The beauty of this system is that as long as the water company (circulatory feedback mechanisms) maintains a relatively constant water pressure (MAP), local demand regulates the amount of fluid (blood) delivered to various areas.

In summary, organs regulate their own blood flows by varying the resistance of their arterioles. As we describe next, these intrinsic control mechanisms may be classed as *metabolic* (chemical) or *myogenic* (physical).

Metabolic Controls

When blood flow is too low to meet a tissue's metabolic needs, oxygen levels decline and metabolic products (which act as paracrines) accumulate. These changes serve as autoregulation stimuli that lead to automatic increases in tissue blood flow.

The metabolic factors that regulate blood flow are low oxygen levels, and increases in H^+ (from CO_2 and lactic acid), K^+, adenosine, and prostaglandins. The relative importance of these factors is not clear. Many of them act directly to relax vascular smooth muscle, but some may act by causing vascular endothelial cells to release nitric oxide.

Nitric oxide (NO) is a powerful vasodilator which acts via a cyclic GMP second-messenger system. NO is quickly destroyed and its potent vasodilator effects are very brief. Even so, NO is the major player in controlling local vasodilation, often overriding sympathetic vasoconstriction when tissues need more blood flow.

The endothelium also releases potent vasoconstrictors, including the family of peptides called **endothelins**, which are among the most potent vasoconstrictors known. Normally, NO and endothelin release from endothelial cells are in a dynamic balance, but this balance tips in favor of NO when blood flow is too low for metabolic needs.

The net result of metabolically controlled autoregulation is immediate vasodilation of the arterioles serving the capillary beds of the "needy" tissues and dilation of their precapillary sphincters. Blood flow to the area rises temporarily, allowing blood to surge through the true capillaries and become available to the tissue cells.

Inflammatory chemicals (such as histamine, kinins, and prostaglandins) released in injury, infection, or allergic reactions also cause local vasodilation. Inflammatory vasodilation helps the defense mechanisms clear microorganisms and toxins from the area, and promotes healing.

Myogenic Controls

Fluctuations in systemic blood pressure would cause problems for individual organs were it not for the **myogenic responses** (*myo* = muscle; *gen* = origin) of vascular smooth muscle. Inadequate blood perfusion through an organ is quickly followed by a decline in the organ's metabolic rate and, if prolonged, organ death. Likewise, excessively high arterial pressure and tissue perfusion can be dangerous because the combination may rupture more fragile blood vessels.

Fortunately, vascular smooth muscle prevents these problems by responding directly to passive stretch (caused by increased intravascular pressure) with increased tone, which resists the stretch and causes vasoconstriction. Reduced stretch promotes vasodilation and increases blood flow into the tissue. These myogenic responses keep tissue perfusion fairly constant despite most variations in systemic pressure.

Generally, both metabolic and myogenic factors determine the final autoregulatory response of a tissue. For example, **reactive hyperemia** (hi″per-e′me-ah) refers to the dramatically increased blood flow into a tissue that occurs after the blood supply to the area has been temporarily blocked. It results both from the myogenic response and from the metabolic wastes that accumulated in the area during occlusion. **Figure 19.15** summarizes the various intrinsic (local) and extrinsic controls of arteriolar diameter.

Long-Term Autoregulation

If a tissue needs more nutrients than short-term autoregulatory mechanisms can supply, a long-term autoregulatory mechanism may develop over weeks or months to enrich local blood flow still more. The number of blood vessels in the region increases, and existing vessels enlarge. This phenomenon, called *angiogenesis*, is particularly common in the heart when a coronary vessel is partially occluded. It occurs throughout the body in people who live in high-altitude areas, where the air contains less oxygen.

Blood Flow in Special Areas

Each organ has special requirements and functions that are revealed in its pattern of autoregulation. Autoregulation in the brain, heart, and kidneys is extraordinarily efficient, maintaining adequate perfusion even when MAP fluctuates.

Skeletal Muscles

Blood flow in skeletal muscle varies with fiber type and muscle activity. Generally speaking, capillary density and blood flow are greater in red (slow oxidative) fibers than in white (fast glycolytic) fibers. Resting skeletal muscles receive about 1 L of blood per minute, and only about 25% of their capillaries are open. During rest, myogenic and general neural mechanisms predominate.

When muscles become active, blood flow increases (*hyperemia*) in direct proportion to their greater *metabolic* activity, a phenomenon called **active** or **exercise hyperemia**. This form of autoregulation occurs almost entirely in response to the decreased oxygen concentration and accumulated metabolic factors that result from the "revved-up" metabolism of working muscles.

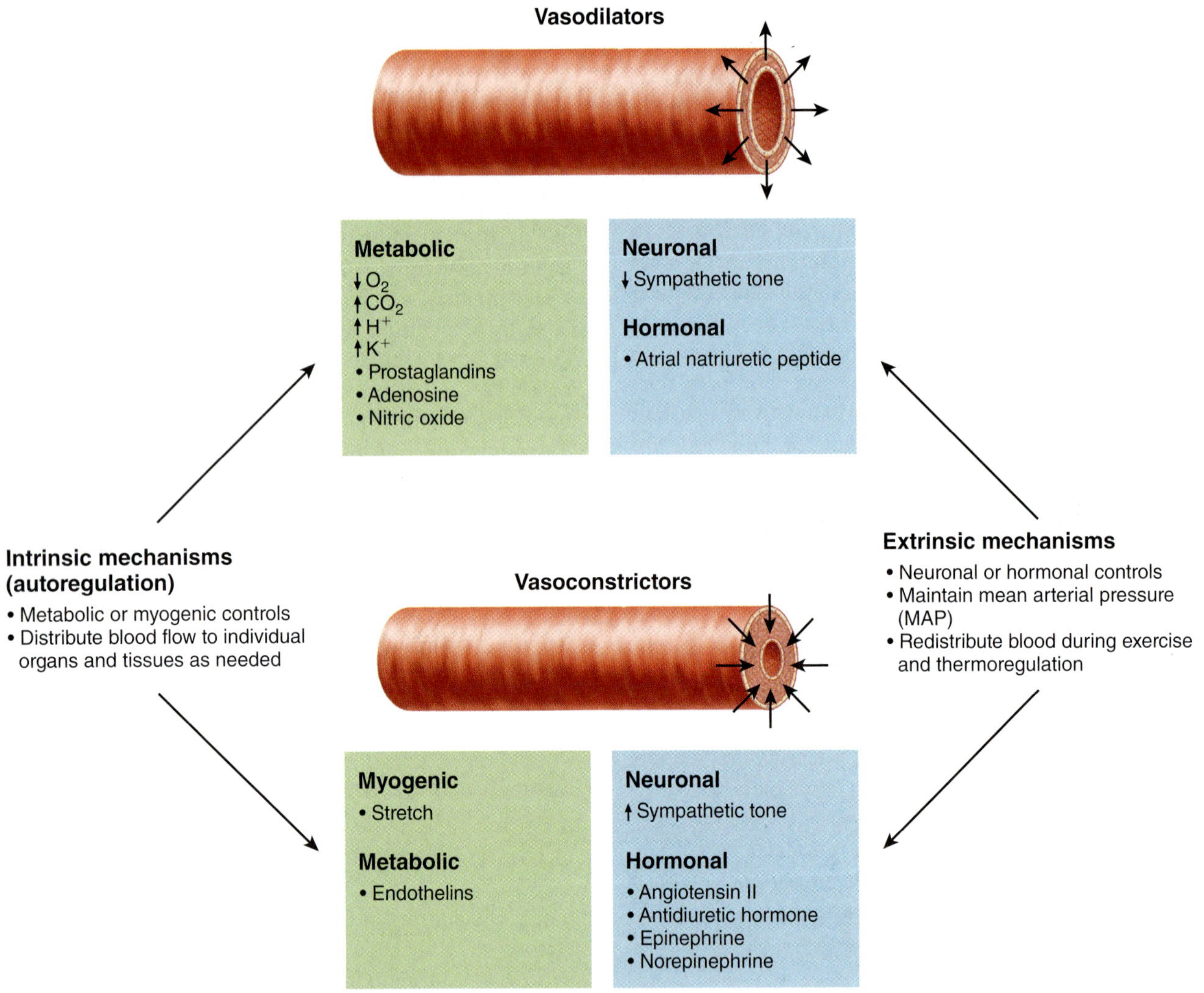

Figure 19.15 Intrinsic and extrinsic control of arteriolar smooth muscle in the systemic circulation. Epinephrine and norepinephrine constrict arteriolar smooth muscle by acting at α-adrenergic receptors. β-adrenergic receptors (causing vasodilation) are present in arterioles supplying skeletal and heart muscle, but their physiological relevance is minimal.

However, systemic adjustments mediated by the vasomotor center must also occur to ensure that blood delivery to the muscles is both faster and more abundant. During exercise, sympathetic nervous system activity increases. Norepinephrine released from sympathetic nerve endings causes vasoconstriction of the vessels of blood reservoirs such as the digestive viscera and skin, diverting blood away from these regions temporarily and ensuring that more blood reaches the muscles.

In skeletal muscles, the sympathetic nervous system and local metabolic controls have opposing effects on arteriolar diameter. During exercise, local controls *override* sympathetic vasoconstriction. Consequently, blood flow to skeletal muscles can increase tenfold or more during physical activity, as you saw in Figure 19.13, and virtually all capillaries in the active muscles open to accommodate the increased flow.

Epinephrine acting at beta (β) adrenergic receptors and acetylcholine acting at cholinergic receptors were once thought to contribute to arteriolar dilation during exercise. However, these appear to have little physiological importance in controlling human skeletal muscle blood flow.

Without question, strenuous exercise is one of the most demanding conditions the cardiovascular system faces. Ultimately, the major factor determining how long muscles can contract vigorously is the ability of the cardiovascular system to deliver adequate oxygen and nutrients and remove waste products.

The Brain

Blood flow to the brain averages 750 ml/min and is maintained at a relatively constant level. Constant cerebral blood flow is necessary because neurons are totally intolerant of ischemia. Also, the brain is unable to store essential nutrients despite being the most metabolically active organ in the body.

Cerebral blood flow is regulated by one of the body's most precise autoregulatory systems and is tailored to local neuronal need. For example, when you make a fist with your right hand, the neurons in the left cerebral motor cortex controlling that movement receive more blood than the adjoining neurons. Brain tissue is exceptionally sensitive to declining pH, and increased blood carbon dioxide levels (resulting in acidic conditions in brain tissue) cause marked vasodilation. Low blood levels of oxygen are a much less potent stimulus for autoregulation. However, very high carbon dioxide levels abolish autoregulatory mechanisms and severely depress brain activity.

Besides metabolic controls, the brain also has a myogenic mechanism that protects it from possibly damaging changes in blood pressure. When MAP declines, cerebral vessels dilate to ensure adequate brain perfusion. When MAP rises, cerebral vessels constrict, protecting the small, more fragile vessels farther along the pathway from excessive pressure. Under certain circumstances, such as brain ischemia caused by rising intracranial pressure (as with a brain tumor), the brain (via the medullary cardiovascular centers) regulates its own blood flow by triggering a rise in systemic blood pressure.

However, when systemic pressure changes are extreme, the brain becomes vulnerable. Fainting, or *syncope* (sin′cuh-pe; "cutting short"), occurs when MAP falls below 60 mm Hg. Cerebral edema is the usual result of pressures over 160 mm Hg, which dramatically increase brain capillary permeability.

The Skin

Blood flow through the skin (1) supplies nutrients to cells, (2) helps regulate body temperature, and (3) provides a blood reservoir. Autoregulation serves the first function in response to the need for oxygen, but the other two require neural intervention. The primary function of the cutaneous circulation is to help maintain body temperature, so we will concentrate on that function here.

Below the skin surface are extensive venous plexuses (networks of intertwining vessels). The blood flow through these plexuses can change from 50 ml/min to as much as 2500 ml/min, depending on body temperature. This capability reflects neural adjustments of blood flow through arterioles and through unique coiled arteriovenous anastomoses. These tiny arteriovenous shunts are located mainly in the fingertips, palms of the hands, toes, soles of the feet, ears, nose, and lips. Richly supplied with sympathetic nerve endings (unlike the shunts of most other capillary beds), they are controlled by reflexes initiated by temperature receptors or signals from higher CNS centers. The arterioles, in addition, respond to metabolic autoregulatory stimuli.

When the skin is exposed to heat, or body temperature rises for other reasons (such as vigorous exercise), the hypothalamic "thermostat" signals for reduced vasomotor stimulation of the skin vessels. As a result, warm blood flushes into the capillary beds and heat radiates from the skin surface. The arterioles dilate even more when we sweat, because an enzyme in perspiration acts on a protein in tissue fluid to produce *bradykinin*, which stimulates the vessel's endothelial cells to release the potent vasodilator NO.

When the ambient temperature is cold and body temperature drops, superficial skin vessels strongly constrict. Hence, blood almost entirely bypasses the capillaries associated with the arteriovenous anastomoses, diverting the warm blood to the deeper, more vital organs. Paradoxically, the skin may stay quite rosy because some blood gets "trapped" in the superficial capillary loops as the shunts swing into operation. The trapped blood remains red because the chilled skin cells take up less O_2.

The Lungs

Blood flow through the pulmonary circuit to and from the lungs is unusual in many ways. The pathway is relatively short, and pulmonary arteries and arterioles are structurally like veins and venules. That is, they have thin walls and large lumens. Because resistance to blood flow is low in the pulmonary arterial system, less pressure is needed to propel blood through those vessels. Consequently, arterial pressure in the pulmonary circulation is much lower than in the systemic circulation (24/10 versus 120/80 mm Hg).

In the pulmonary circulation, the autoregulatory mechanism is the *opposite* of what is seen in most tissues: Low pulmonary oxygen levels cause local vasoconstriction, and high levels promote vasodilation. While this may seem odd, it is perfectly consistent with the gas exchange role of this circulation. When the air sacs of the lungs are flooded with oxygen-rich air, the pulmonary capillaries become flushed with blood and ready to receive the oxygen load. If the air sacs are collapsed or blocked with mucus, the oxygen content in those areas is low, and blood largely bypasses those nonfunctional areas.

The Heart

Aortic pressure and the pumping activity of the ventricles influence the movement of blood through the smaller vessels of the coronary circulation. When the ventricles contract and compress the coronary vessels, blood flow through the myocardium stops. As the heart relaxes, the high aortic pressure forces blood through the coronary circulation.

Under normal circumstances, the myoglobin in cardiac cells stores sufficient oxygen to satisfy the cells' oxygen needs during systole. However, an abnormally rapid heartbeat seriously reduces the ability of the myocardium to receive adequate oxygen and nutrients during diastole.

Under resting conditions, blood flow through the heart is about 250 ml/min and is probably controlled by a myogenic mechanism. Consequently, blood flow remains fairly constant despite wide variations (50 to 140 mm Hg) in coronary perfusion pressure. During strenuous exercise, the coronary vessels dilate in response to local accumulation of vasodilators (particularly adenosine), and blood flow may increase three to four times (see Figure 19.13). Additionally, any event that decreases the oxygen content of the blood releases vasodilators that adjust the O_2 supply to the O_2 demand.

This enhanced blood flow during increased heart activity is important because under resting conditions, cardiac cells use as much as 65% of the oxygen carried to them in blood. (Most other tissue cells use about 25% of the delivered oxygen.) Consequently, increasing the blood flow is the only way to provide more oxygen to a vigorously working heart.

Check Your Understanding

11. Suppose you are in a bicycle race. What happens to the smooth muscle in the arterioles supplying your leg muscles? What is the key mechanism in this case?
12. If many arterioles in your body dilated at once, you would expect MAP to plummet. What prevents MAP from decreasing during your bicycle race?

For answers, see Appendix H.

Blood Flow Through Capillaries and Capillary Dynamics

✓ Outline factors involved in capillary dynamics, and explain the significance of each.

Blood flow through capillary networks is slow and intermittent. Intermittent flow is due to **vasomotion**, the on/off opening and closing of precapillary sphincters in response to local autoregulatory controls.

Capillary Exchange of Respiratory Gases and Nutrients

Oxygen, carbon dioxide, most nutrients, and metabolic wastes pass between the blood and interstitial fluid by diffusion. Recall that in **diffusion**, net movement always occurs along a concentration gradient—each substance moving from an area of its higher concentration to an area of its lower concentration. Hence, oxygen and nutrients pass from the blood, where their concentration is fairly high, through the interstitial fluid to the tissue cells. Carbon dioxide and metabolic wastes leave the cells, where their content is higher, and diffuse into the capillary blood.

There are four different routes across capillaries for different types of molecules, as **Figure 19.16** shows. (1) Lipid-soluble molecules, such as respiratory gases, diffuse through the lipid bilayer of the endothelial cell plasma membranes. Small water-soluble solutes, such as amino acids and sugars, pass through (2) fluid-filled intercellular capillary clefts or (3) fenestrations. (4) Some larger molecules, such as proteins, are actively transported in pinocytotic vesicles or caveolae.

As we mentioned earlier, capillaries differ in their "leakiness," or permeability. Liver capillaries, for instance, are sinusoids that allow even proteins to pass freely, whereas brain capillaries are impermeable to most substances.

Fluid Movements: Bulk Flow

While nutrient and gas exchanges are occurring across the capillary walls by diffusion, bulk fluid flows are also going on. Fluid is forced out of the capillaries through the clefts at the arterial end of the bed, but most of it returns to the bloodstream at the venous end. Though relatively unimportant to capillary exchange of nutrients and wastes, bulk flow is extremely important in determining the relative fluid volumes in the bloodstream and the interstitial space. (Approximately 20 L of fluid filter out of the capillaries each day before being returned to the blood—almost seven times the total plasma volume!)

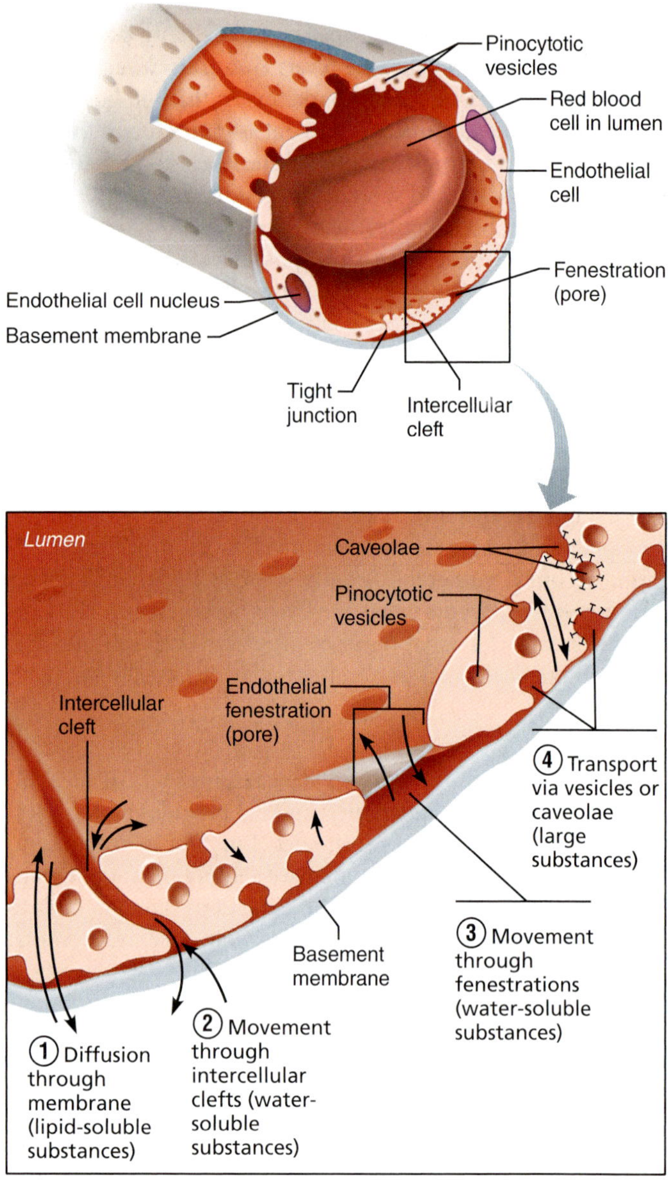

Figure 19.16 Capillary transport mechanisms. The four possible pathways or routes of transport across the endothelial cell wall of a fenestrated capillary.

As we describe next and as shown in *Focus on Bulk Flow Across Capillary Walls* **(Figure 19.17)**, the *direction and amount* of flow across capillary walls reflect the balance between two dynamic and opposing forces—hydrostatic and colloid osmotic pressures.

Hydrostatic Pressures **Hydrostatic pressure (HP)** is the force exerted by a fluid pressing against a wall. In capillaries, hydrostatic pressure is the same as *capillary blood pressure*—the pressure exerted by blood on capillary walls. **Capillary hydrostatic pressure (HP_c)** tends to force fluids through capillary walls (a process called *filtration*), leaving behind cells and most proteins. Blood pressure drops as blood flows along a capillary bed, so HP_c is higher at the arterial end of the bed (35 mm Hg) than at the venous end (17 mm Hg).

In theory, blood pressure—which forces fluid out of the capillaries—is opposed by the **interstitial fluid hydrostatic pressure (HP_{if})** acting outside the capillaries and pushing fluid in. However, there is usually very little fluid in the interstitial space, because the lymphatic vessels constantly withdraw it. HP_{if} may vary from slightly negative to slightly positive, but traditionally it is assumed to be zero.

Colloid Osmotic Pressures **Colloid osmotic pressure (OP)**, the force opposing hydrostatic pressure, is created by large nondiffusible molecules, such as plasma proteins, that are unable to cross the capillary wall. Such molecules draw water toward themselves. In other words, they encourage osmosis because the water concentration in their vicinity is lower than it is on the opposite side of the capillary wall. A quick and dirty way to remember this is "hydrostatic pressure pushes and osmotic pressure pulls (or sucks)."

The abundant plasma proteins in capillary blood (primarily albumin molecules) develop a **capillary colloid osmotic pressure (OP_c)**, also called *oncotic pressure*, of approximately 26 mm Hg. Interstitial fluid contains few proteins, so its colloid osmotic pressure **(OP_{if})** is substantially lower—from 0.1 to 5 mm Hg. Unlike HP, OP does not vary significantly from one end of the capillary bed to the other.

Hydrostatic-Osmotic Pressure Interactions We are now ready to calculate the **net filtration pressure (NFP)**, which considers all the forces acting at the capillary bed. As you work your way through the right-hand page of Figure 19.17, notice that while net *filtration* is occurring at the arteriolar end of the capillary, a negative value for NFP at the venous end of the capillary indicates that fluid is moving *into* the capillary bed (a process called *reabsorption*). As a result, net fluid flow is *out* of the circulation at the arterial ends of capillary beds and *into* the circulation at the venous ends.

However, more fluid enters the tissue spaces than returns to the blood, resulting in a net loss of fluid from the circulation of about 1.5 ml/min. Lymphatic vessels pick up this fluid and any leaked proteins and return it to the vascular system, which accounts for the relatively low levels of both fluid and proteins in the interstitial space. Were this not so, this "insignificant" fluid loss would empty your blood vessels of plasma in about 24 hours!

☑ Check Your Understanding

13. Suppose OP_{if} rises dramatically—say because of a severe bacterial infection in the surrounding tissue. (a) Predict how fluid flow will change in this situation. (b) Now calculate the NFP at the venous end of the capillary in Figure 19.17 if OP_{if} increases to 10 mm Hg. (c) In which direction does fluid flow at the venous end of the capillary now—in or out?

For answers, see Appendix H.

Circulatory Shock

✓ Define circulatory shock. List several possible causes.

Circulatory shock is any condition in which blood vessels are inadequately filled and blood cannot circulate normally. Blood flow is inadequate to meet tissue needs. If circulatory shock persists, cells die and organ damage follows.

Hypovolemic Shock

The most common form of circulatory shock is **hypovolemic shock** (hi″po-vo-le′mik; *hypo* = low, deficient; *volemia* = blood volume), which results from large-scale blood or fluid loss, as might follow acute hemorrhage, severe vomiting or diarrhea, or extensive burns. If blood volume drops rapidly, heart rate increases in an attempt to correct the problem. Thus, a weak, "thready" pulse is often the first sign of hypovolemic shock. Intense vasoconstriction also occurs, which shifts blood from the various blood reservoirs into the major circulatory channels and enhances venous return.

Blood pressure is stable at first, but eventually drops if blood loss continues. A sharp drop in blood pressure is a serious, and late, sign of hypovolemic shock. The key to managing hypovolemic shock is to replace fluid volume as quickly as possible.

Although you have not yet explored all of the body systems that respond to hypovolemic shock, acute bleeding is such a threat to life that it seems important to have a summary of its signs and symptoms and the body's attempts to restore homeostasis. **Figure 19.18** provides such a resource. Study it in part now, and in more detail later once you have studied the remaining body systems.

Vascular Shock

In **vascular shock**, blood volume is normal, but circulation is poor as a result of extreme vasodilation. A huge drop in peripheral resistance follows, as revealed by rapidly falling blood pressure.

A common cause of vascular shock is loss of vasomotor tone due to anaphylaxis (anaphylactic shock), a systemic allergic reaction in which the massive release of histamine triggers bodywide vasodilation. Two other common causes are failure of autonomic nervous system regulation (*neurogenic shock*), and septicemia (*septic shock*), a severe systemic bacterial infection (bacterial toxins are notorious vasodilators).

Transient vascular shock may occur when you sunbathe for a prolonged time. The heat of the sun on your skin dilates cutaneous blood vessels. Then, if you stand up abruptly, blood pools briefly (because of gravity) in the dilated vessels of your lower limbs rather than returning promptly to the heart. Consequently, your blood pressure falls. The dizziness you feel is a signal that your brain is not receiving enough oxygen.

Cardiogenic Shock

Cardiogenic shock, or pump failure, occurs when the heart is so inefficient that it cannot sustain adequate circulation. Its usual cause is myocardial damage, as might follow numerous myocardial infarctions (heart attacks).

☑ Check Your Understanding

14. Your neighbor, Bob, calls you because he thinks he is having an allergic reaction to a medication. You find Bob on the verge of losing consciousness and having trouble breathing. When paramedics arrive, they note his blood pressure is 63/38 and he has a rapid, thready pulse. Explain Bob's low blood pressure and rapid heart rate.

For answers, see Appendix H.

(Text continues on p. 721.)

FOCUS Bulk Flow Across Capillary Walls

Figure 19.17 Bulk fluid flow across capillary walls causes continuous mixing of fluid between the plasma and the interstitial fluid compartments, and maintains the interstitial environment.

The big picture

Fluid filters from capillaries at their arteriolar end and flows through the interstitial space. Most is reabsorbed at the venous end.

Net filtration pressure (NFP) determines the direction of fluid movement. Two kinds of pressure drive fluid flow:

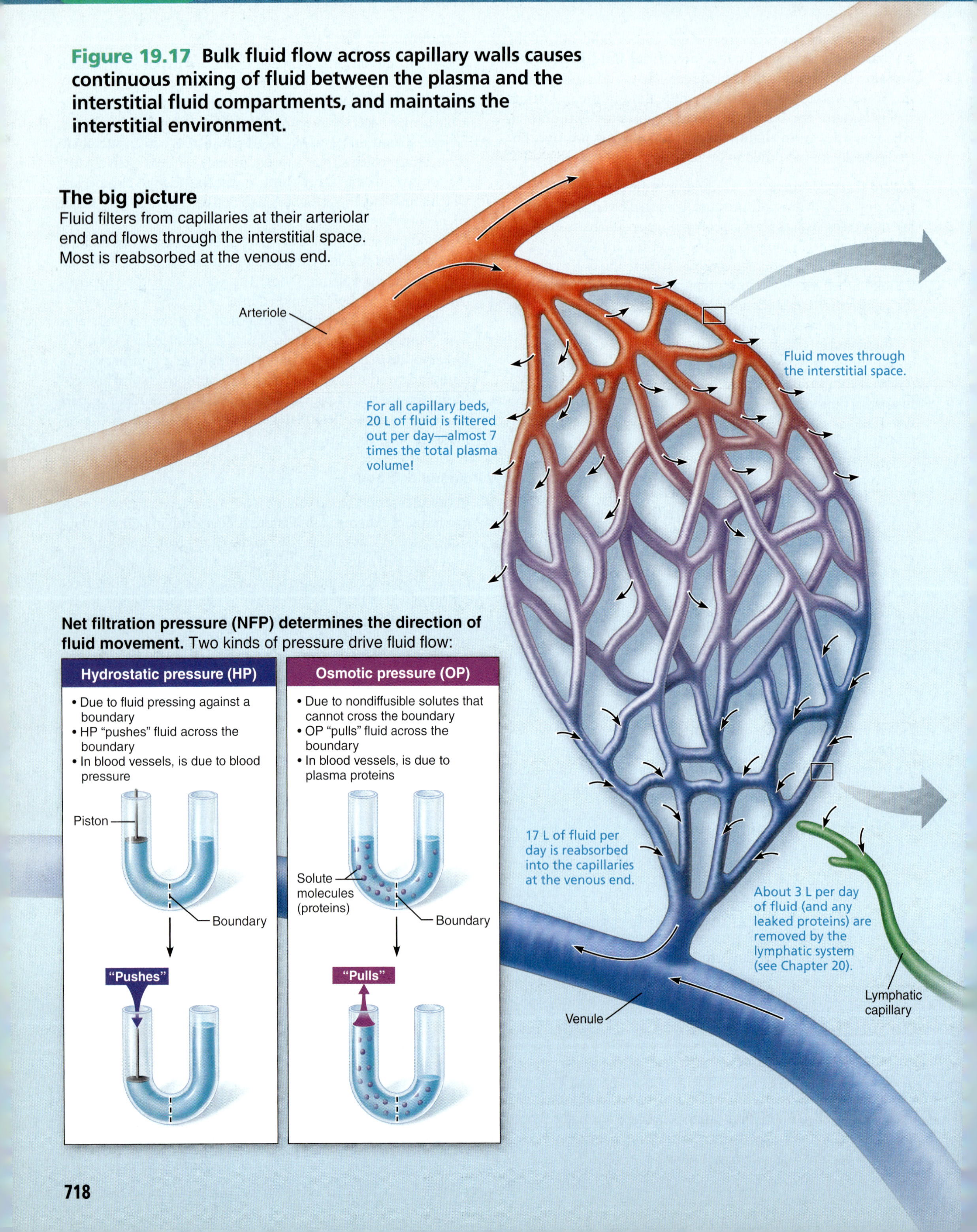

How do the pressures drive fluid flow across a capillary?

Net filtration occurs at the arteriolar end of a capillary.

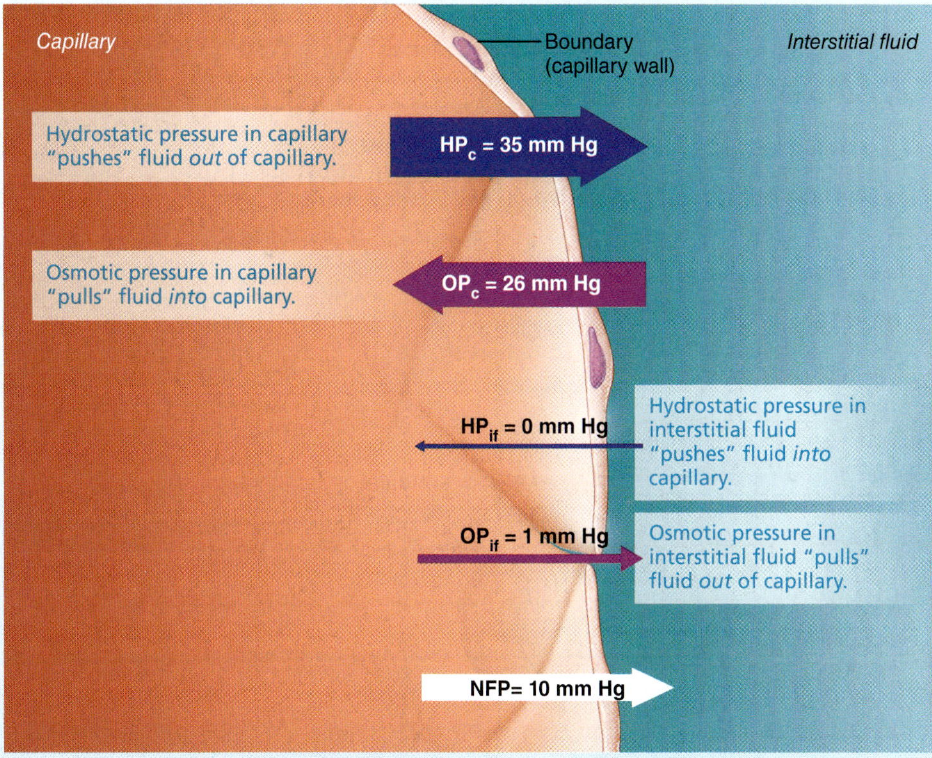

To determine the pressure driving the fluid out of the capillary at any given point, we calculate the **net filtration pressure (NFP)**—the outward pressures (HP_c and OP_{if}) minus the inward pressures (HP_{if} and OP_c). So,

$$\begin{aligned} NFP &= (HP_c + OP_{if}) - (HP_{if} + OP_c) \\ &= (35 + 1) - (0 + 26) \\ &= 10 \text{ mm Hg (net outward pressure)} \end{aligned}$$

As a result, fluid moves from the capillary into the interstitial space.

Net reabsorption occurs at the venous end of a capillary.

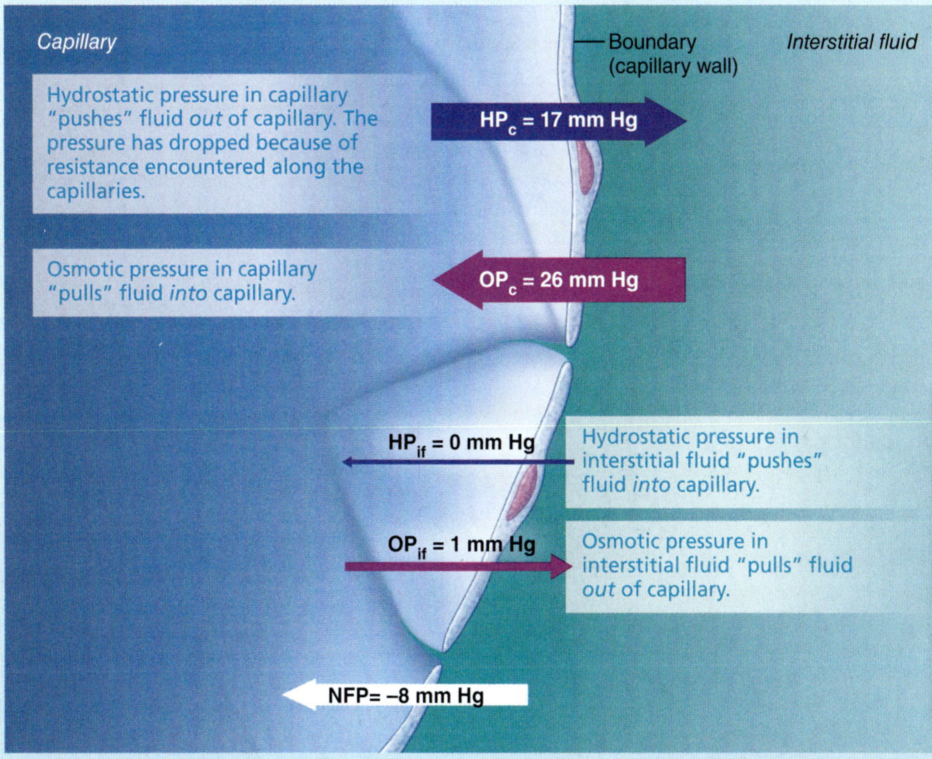

Again, we calculate the NFP:

$$\begin{aligned} NFP &= (HP_c + OP_{if}) - (HP_{if} + OP_c) \\ &= (17 + 1) - (0 + 26) \\ &= -8 \text{ mm Hg (net inward pressure)} \end{aligned}$$

Notice that the NFP at the venous end is a negative number. This means that reabsorption, not filtration, is occurring and so fluid moves from the interstitial space into the capillary.

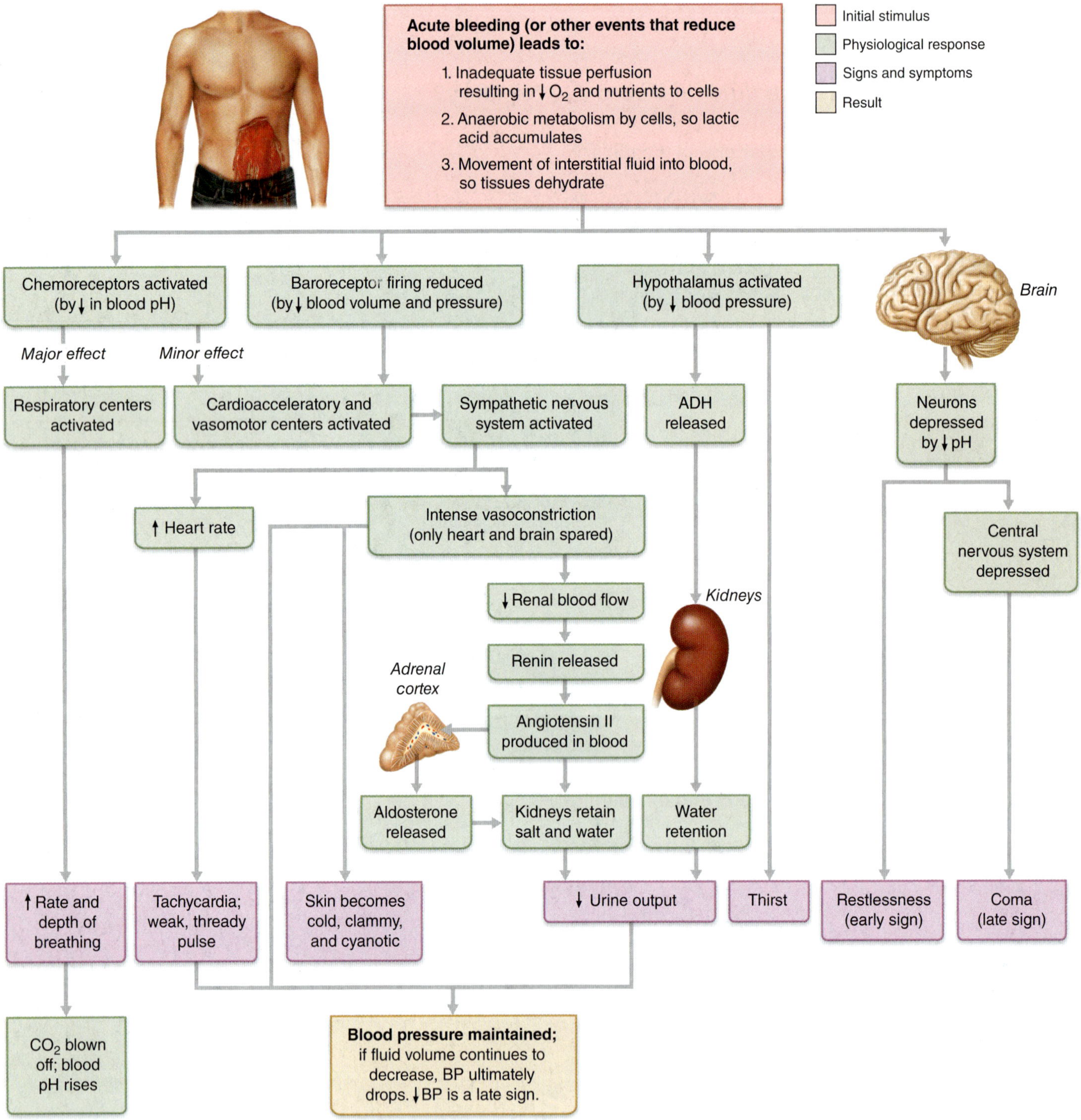

Figure 19.18 Events and signs of hypovolemic shock.

19

PART 3
Circulatory Pathways: Blood Vessels of the Body

The Two Main Circulations of the Body

✓ Trace the pathway of blood through the pulmonary circuit, and state the importance of this special circulation.

✓ Describe the general functions of the systemic circuit.

The term **vascular system** is often used to describe the body's complex network of blood vessels. However, the heart is actually a double pump that serves two distinct circulations, each with its own set of arteries, capillaries, and veins. The *pulmonary circulation* is the short loop that runs from the heart to the lungs and back to the heart. The *systemic circulation* routes blood through a long loop to all parts of the body before returning it to the heart. **Table 19.3** on pp. 722–723 shows both circuits schematically.

Systemic Arteries and Veins: Differences in Pathways and Courses

As we saw in Chapter 18, the heart pumps all of its blood into a single systemic artery—the aorta. In contrast, blood returning to the heart is delivered largely by two terminal systemic veins, the superior and inferior venae cavae. The single exception to this is the blood draining from the myocardium of the heart, which is collected by the cardiac veins and reenters the right atrium via the coronary sinus.

In addition to these differences between arteries and veins connecting to the heart, there are three important differences between systemic arteries and veins:

- **Arteries run deep while veins are both deep and superficial.** Deep veins parallel the course of the systemic arteries and both are protected by body tissues along most of their course. With a few exceptions, these veins are named identically to their companion arteries. Superficial veins run just beneath the skin and are readily seen, especially in the limbs, face, and neck. Because there are no superficial arteries, the names of the superficial veins do not correspond to the names of any of the arteries.
- **Venous pathways are more interconnected.** Unlike the fairly distinct arterial pathways, venous pathways tend to have numerous interconnections, and many veins are represented by not one but two similarly named vessels. As a result, venous pathways are more difficult to follow.
- **The brain and digestive systems have unique venous drainage systems.** Most body regions have a similar pattern for their arterial supply and venous drainage. However, the venous drainage pattern in at least two important body areas is unique. First, venous blood draining from the brain enters large *dural venous sinuses* rather than typical veins. Second, blood draining from the digestive organs enters a special subcirculation, the *hepatic portal system*, and perfuses through the liver before it reenters the general systemic circulation (see Table 19.12).

Principal Vessels of the Systemic Circulation

✓ Name and give the location of the major arteries and veins in the systemic circulation.

✓ Describe the structure and special function of the hepatic portal system.

Except for special vessels and shunts of the fetal circulation (described in Chapter 28), the principal arteries and veins of the systemic circulation are described in **Tables 19.4** through **19.13**.

Notice that by convention, oxygen-rich blood is shown red, while blood that is relatively oxygen-poor is depicted blue, regardless of vessel type. The schematic flowcharts (pipe diagrams) that accompany each table show the vessels that would be closer to the viewer in brighter, more intense colors than vessels deeper or farther from the viewer. For example, darker blue veins would be closer to the viewer than lighter blue veins in the body region shown.

(Text continues on p. 745.)

19

Table 19.3 Pulmonary and Systemic Circulations

Pulmonary Circulation

The pulmonary circulation **(Figure 19.19a)** functions only to bring blood into close contact with the alveoli (air sacs) of the lungs so that gases can be exchanged. It does not directly serve the metabolic needs of body tissues.

Oxygen-poor, dark red blood enters the pulmonary circulation as it is pumped from the right ventricle into the large **pulmonary trunk** (Figure 19.19b), which runs diagonally upward for about 8 cm and then divides abruptly to form the **right** and **left pulmonary arteries**. In the lungs, the pulmonary arteries subdivide into the **lobar arteries** (lo′bar) (three in the right lung and two in the left lung), each of which serves one lung lobe. The lobar arteries accompany the main bronchi into the lungs and then branch profusely, forming first arterioles and then the dense networks of **pulmonary capillaries** that surround and cling to the delicate air sacs. It is here that oxygen moves from the alveolar air to the blood and carbon dioxide moves from the blood to the alveolar air. As gases are exchanged and the oxygen content of the blood rises, the blood becomes bright red. The pulmonary capillary beds drain into venules, which join to form the two **pulmonary veins** exiting from each lung. The four pulmonary veins complete the circuit by unloading their precious cargo into the left atrium of the heart.

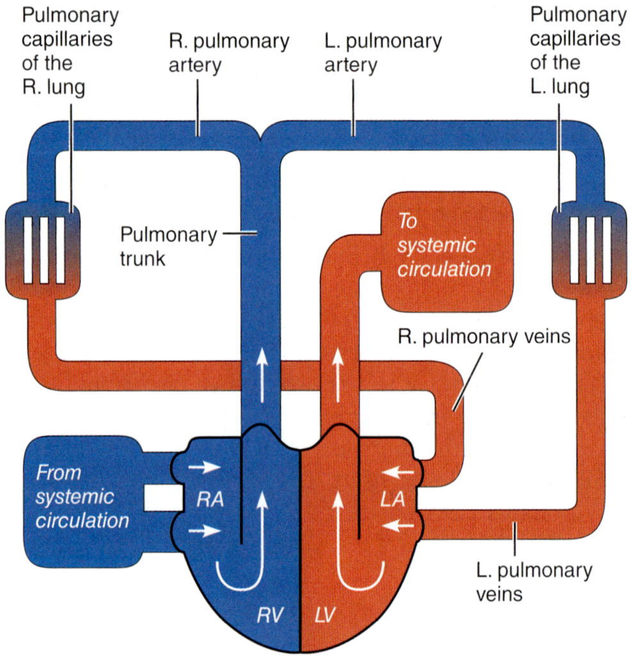

(a) Schematic flowchart.

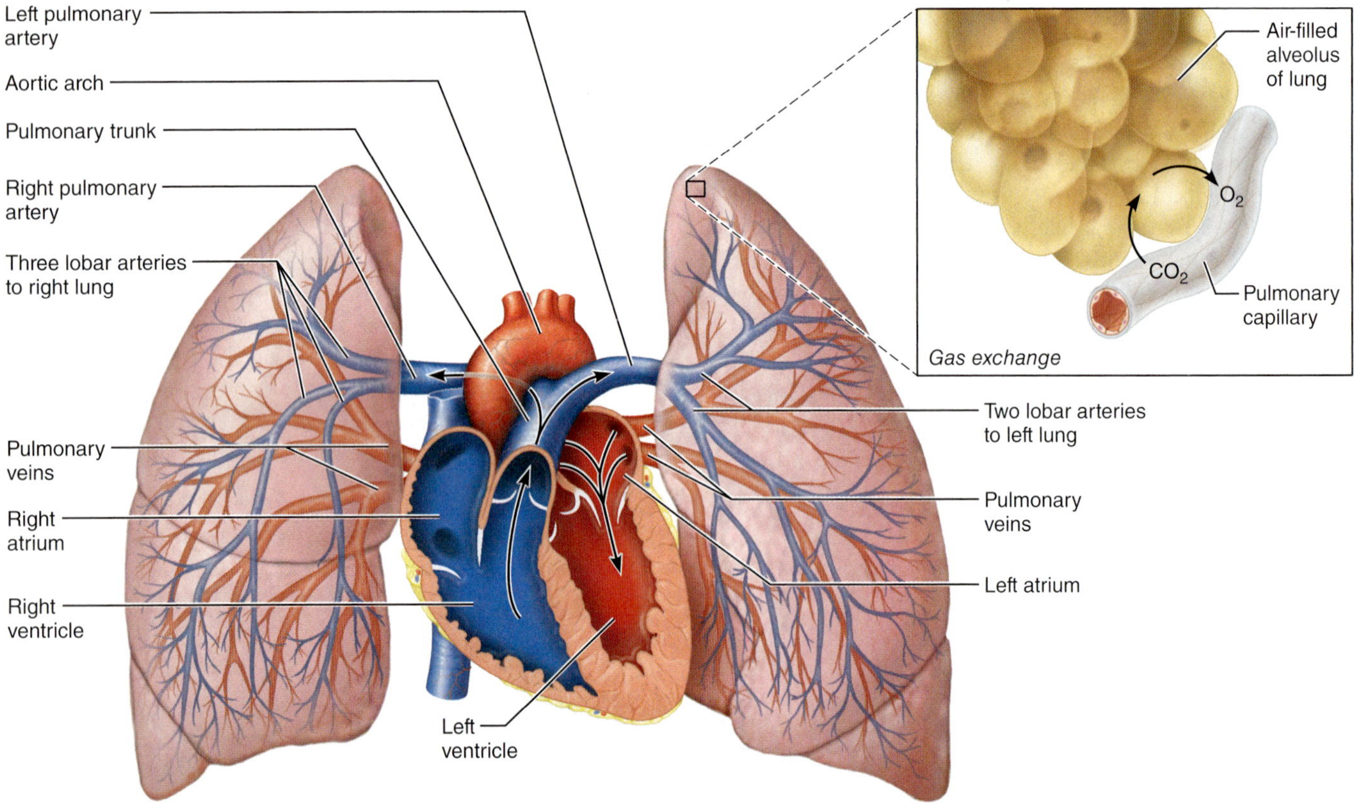

(b) Illustration. The pulmonary arterial system is shown in blue to indicate that the blood it carries is oxygen-poor. The pulmonary venous drainage is shown in red to indicate that the blood it transports is oxygen-rich.

Figure 19.19 Pulmonary circulation. RA = right atrium, RV = right ventricle, LA = left atrium, LV = left ventricle.

Table 19.3 *(continued)*

Note that any vessel with the term *pulmonary* or *lobar* in its name is part of the pulmonary circulation. All others are part of the systemic circulation.

Pulmonary arteries carry oxygen-poor, carbon dioxide–rich blood, and pulmonary veins carry oxygen-rich blood.* This is opposite to the systemic circulation, where arteries carry oxygen-rich blood and veins carry carbon dioxide–rich, relatively oxygen-poor blood.

Systemic Circulation

The systemic circulation provides the *functional blood supply* to all body tissues; that is, it delivers oxygen, nutrients, and other needed substances while carrying away carbon dioxide and other metabolic wastes. Freshly oxygenated blood* returning from the pulmonary circuit is pumped out of the left ventricle into the aorta **(Figure 19.20)**.

From the aorta, blood can take various routes, because essentially all systemic arteries branch from this single great vessel. The aorta arches upward from the heart and then curves and runs downward along the body midline to its terminus in the pelvis, where it splits to form the two large arteries serving the lower extremities. The branches of the aorta continue to subdivide to produce the arterioles and, finally, the capillaries that ramify through the organs. Venous blood draining from organs inferior to the diaphragm ultimately enters the inferior vena cava.† Except for some coronary and thoracic venous drainage (which enters the azygos system of veins), the superior vena cava drains body regions above the diaphragm. The venae cavae empty the carbon dioxide–laden blood into the right atrium of the heart.

Two important points concerning the two major circulations: (1) Blood passes from systemic veins to systemic arteries only after first moving through the pulmonary circuit (Figure 19.19a), and (2) although the entire cardiac output of the right ventricle passes through the pulmonary circulation, only a small fraction of the output of the left ventricle flows through any single organ (Figure 19.20). The systemic circulation can be viewed as multiple circulatory channels functioning in parallel to distribute blood to all body organs.

As you examine the tables that follow and locate the various systemic arteries and veins in the illustrations, be aware of cues that make your memorization task easier. In many cases, the name of a vessel reflects the body region traversed (axillary, brachial, femoral, etc.), the organ served (renal, hepatic, gonadal), or the bone followed (vertebral, radial, tibial). Also, notice that arteries and veins tend to run side by side and, in many places, they also run with nerves. Finally, be alert to the fact that the systemic vessels do not always match on the right and left sides of the body. Thus, while almost all vessels in the head and limbs are bilaterally symmetrical, some of the large, deep vessels of the trunk region are asymmetrical or unpaired.

*By convention, oxygen-rich blood is shown red and oxygen-poor blood is shown blue.

†Venous blood from the digestive viscera passes through the hepatic portal circulation (liver and associated veins) before entering the inferior vena cava.

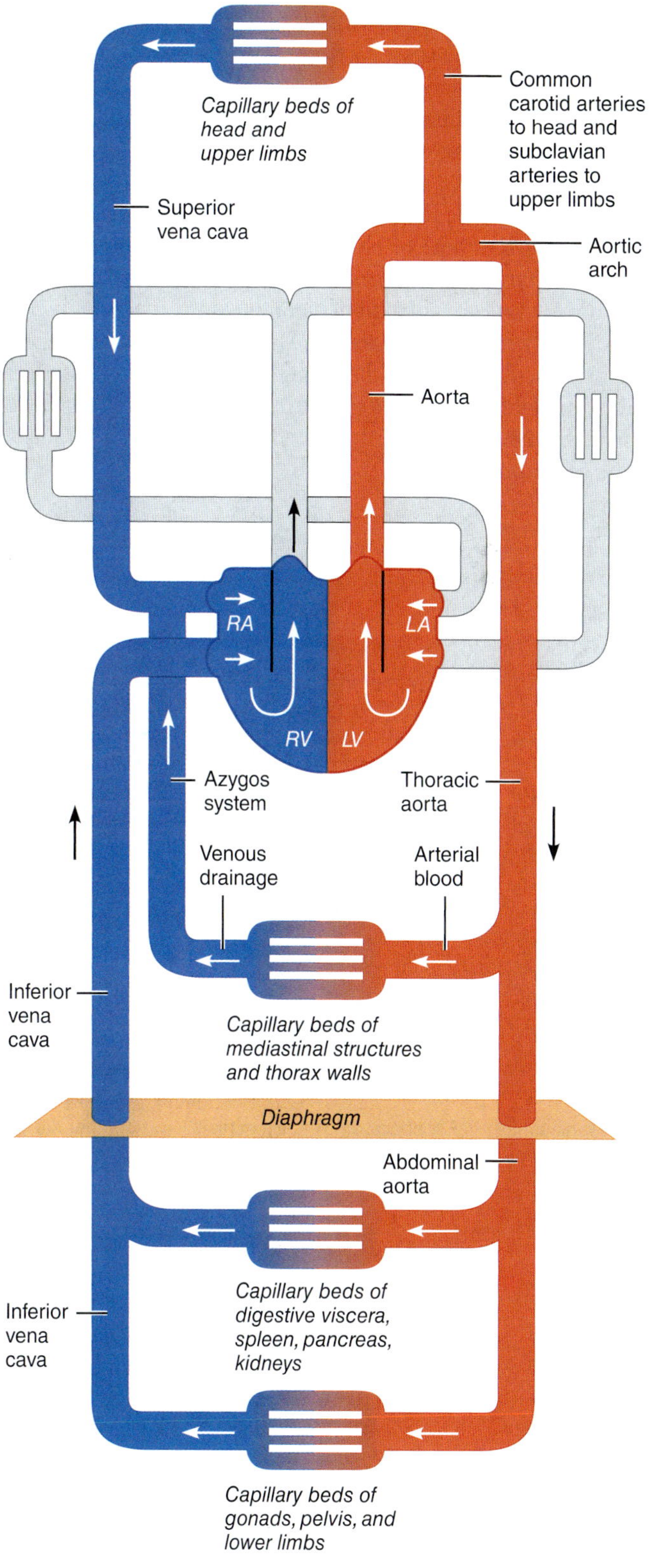

Figure 19.20 Schematic flowchart showing an overview of the systemic circulation. The pulmonary circulation is shown in gray for comparison. RA = right atrium, RV = right ventricle, LA = left atrium, LV = left ventricle.

19

Table 19.4 The Aorta and Major Arteries of the Systemic Circulation

Figure 19.21a diagrams the distribution of the aorta and major arteries of the systemic circulation in flowchart form, and Figure 19.21b illustrates them. See Tables 19.5 through 19.8 for fine points about the vessels arising from the aorta.

The **aorta** is the largest artery in the body. In adults, the aorta (a-or′tah) is approximately the size of a garden hose where it issues from the left ventricle of the heart. Its internal diameter is 2.5 cm, and its wall is about 2 mm thick. It decreases in size slightly as it runs to its terminus. The aortic valve guards the base of the aorta and prevents backflow of blood during diastole. Opposite each aortic valve cusp is an *aortic sinus*, which contains baroreceptors important in reflex regulation of blood pressure.

Different portions of the aorta are named according to shape or location. The first portion, the **ascending aorta**, runs posteriorly and to the right of the pulmonary trunk. It persists for only about 5 cm before curving to the left as the aortic arch. The only branches of the ascending aorta are the **right** and **left coronary arteries**, which supply the myocardium. The **aortic arch**, deep to the sternum, begins and ends at the sternal angle (T_4 level). Its three major branches (R to L) are: (1) the **brachiocephalic trunk** (bra′ke-o-sĕ-fal″ik; "armhead"), which passes superiorly under the right sternoclavicular joint and branches into the **right common carotid artery** (kah-rot′id) and the **right subclavian artery**, (2) the **left common carotid artery**, and (3) the **left subclavian artery**. These three vessels provide the arterial supply of the head, neck, upper limbs, and part of the thorax wall.

The **descending aorta** runs along the anterior spine. Called the **thoracic aorta** from T_5 to T_{12}, it sends off numerous small arteries to the thorax wall and viscera before piercing the diaphragm. As it enters the abdominal cavity, it becomes the **abdominal aorta**. This portion supplies the abdominal walls and viscera and ends at the L_4 level, where it splits into the **right** and **left common iliac arteries**, which supply the pelvis and lower limbs.

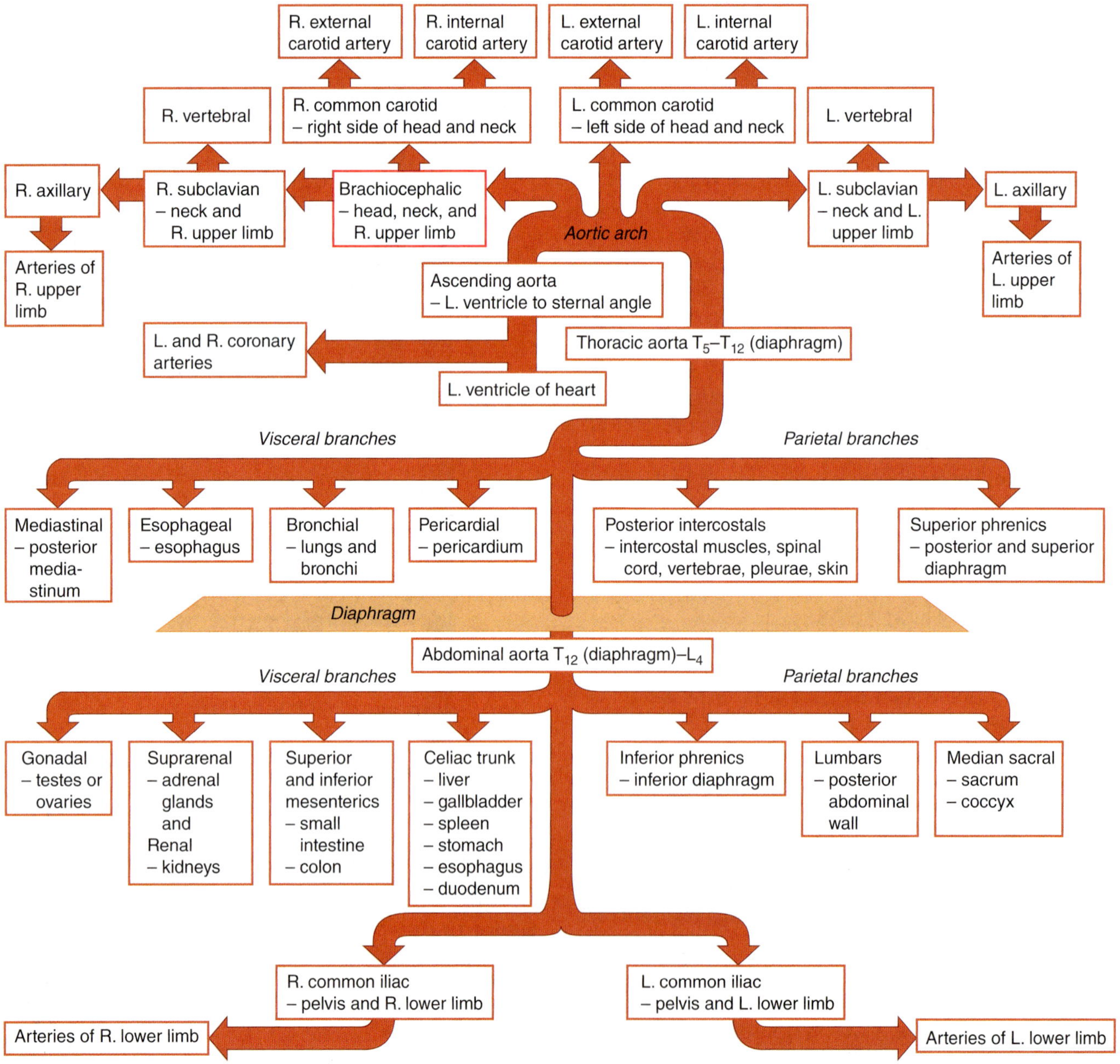

(a) Schematic flowchart

Table 19.4 *(continued)*

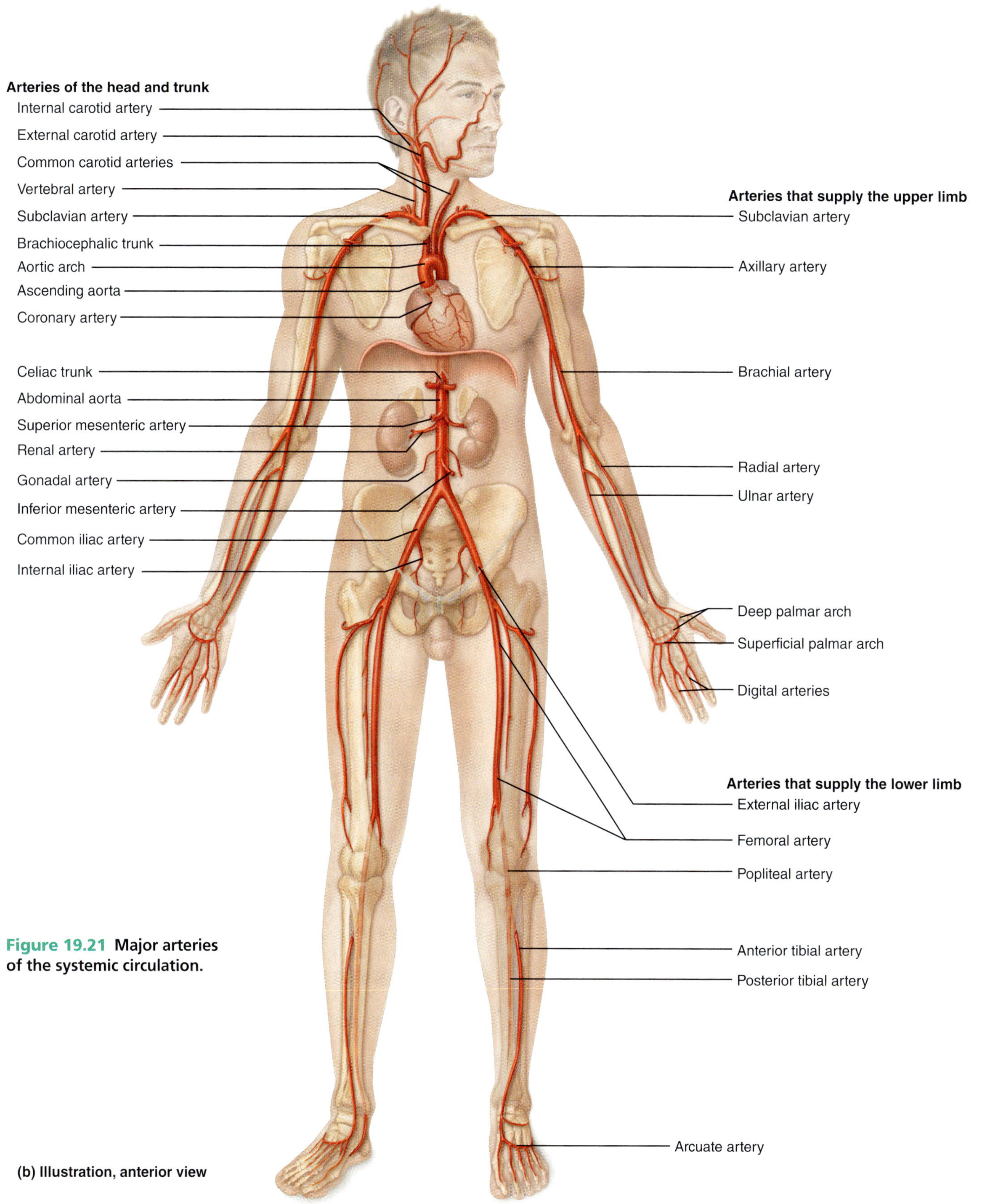

Figure 19.21 **Major arteries of the systemic circulation.**

(b) Illustration, anterior view

Table 19.5 Arteries of the Head and Neck

Four paired arteries supply the head and neck. These are the common carotid arteries, plus three branches from each subclavian artery: the vertebral arteries, the thyrocervical trunks, and the costocervical trunks **(Figure 19.22b)**. Of these, the common carotid arteries have the broadest distribution (Figure 19.22a).

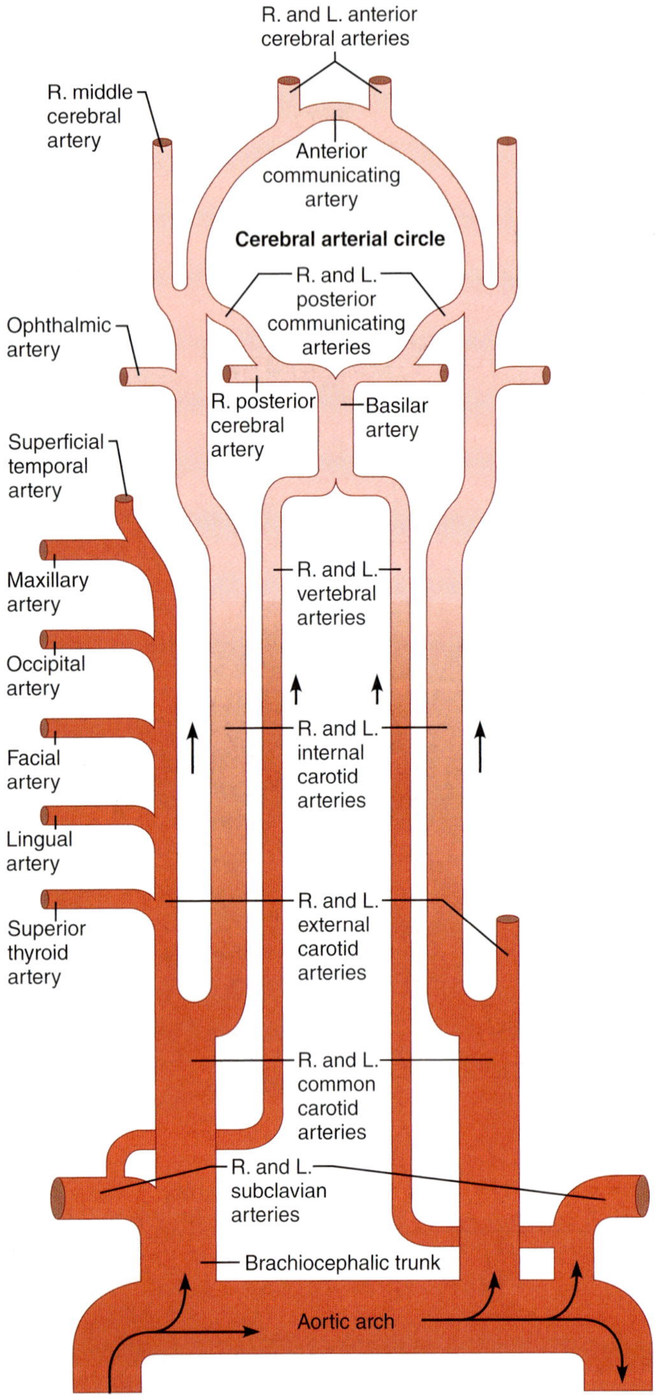

(a) Schematic flowchart

Figure 19.22 Arteries of the head, neck, and brain.

Each common carotid divides into two major branches (the internal and external carotid arteries). At the division point, each internal carotid artery has a slight dilation, the **carotid sinus**, that contains baroreceptors that assist in reflex blood pressure control. The **carotid bodies**, chemoreceptors involved in controlling respiratory rate, are located close by. Pressing on the neck in the area of the carotid sinuses can cause unconsciousness (*carot* = stupor) because the pressure created mimics high blood pressure, eliciting vasodilation, which interferes with blood delivery to the brain.

Description and Distribution

Common carotid arteries. The origins of these two arteries differ: The right common carotid artery arises from the brachiocephalic trunk; the left is the second branch of the aortic arch. The common carotid arteries ascend through the lateral neck, and at the superior border of the larynx (the level of the "Adam's apple"), each divides into its two major branches, the *external* and *internal carotid arteries*.

The **external carotid arteries** supply most tissues of the head except for the brain and orbit. As each artery runs superiorly, it sends branches to the thyroid gland and larynx **(superior thyroid artery)**, the tongue **(lingual artery)**, the skin and muscles of the anterior face **(facial artery)**, and the posterior scalp **(occipital artery)**. Each external carotid artery terminates by splitting into a **superficial temporal artery**, which supplies the parotid salivary gland and most of the scalp, and a **maxillary artery**, which supplies the upper and lower jaws and chewing muscles, the teeth, and the nasal cavity. A clinically important branch of the maxillary artery is the *middle meningeal artery* (not illustrated). It enters the skull through the foramen spinosum and supplies the inner surface of the parietal bone, squamous part of the temporal bone, and the underlying dura mater.

The larger **internal carotid arteries** supply the orbits and more than 80% of the cerebrum. They assume a deep course and enter the skull through the carotid canals of the temporal bones. Once inside the cranium, each artery gives off one main branch, the ophthalmic artery, and then divides into the anterior and middle cerebral arteries. The **ophthalmic arteries** (of-thal′mik) supply the eyes, orbits, forehead, and nose. Each **anterior cerebral artery** supplies the medial surface of the frontal and parietal lobes of the cerebral hemisphere on its side and also anastomoses with its partner on the opposite side via a short arterial shunt called the **anterior communicating artery** (Figure 19.22d). The **middle cerebral arteries** run in the lateral sulci of their respective cerebral hemispheres and supply the lateral parts of the temporal, parietal, and frontal lobes.

Vertebral arteries. The vertebral arteries spring from the subclavian arteries at the root of the neck and ascend through foramina in the transverse processes of the cervical vertebrae to enter the skull through the foramen magnum. En route, they send branches

Table 19.5 *(continued)*

to the vertebrae and cervical spinal cord and to some deep structures of the neck. Within the cranium, the right and left vertebral arteries join to form the **basilar artery** (bas′ĭ-lar), which ascends along the anterior aspect of the brain stem, giving off branches to the cerebellum, pons, and inner ear (Figure 19.22b and d). At the pons-midbrain border, the basilar artery divides into a pair of **posterior cerebral arteries**, which supply the occipital lobes and the inferior parts of the temporal lobes.

Arterial shunts called **posterior communicating arteries** connect the posterior cerebral arteries to the middle cerebral arteries anteriorly. The two posterior and single anterior communicating arteries complete the formation of an arterial anastomosis called the **cerebral arterial circle** (*circle of Willis*). This structure encircles the pituitary gland and optic chiasma and unites the brain's anterior and posterior blood supplies. It also equalizes blood pressure in the two brain areas and provides alternate routes for blood to reach the brain tissue if a carotid or vertebral artery becomes occluded.

Thyrocervical and costocervical trunks. These short vessels arise from the subclavian artery just lateral to the vertebral arteries on each side (Figures 19.22b and Figure 19.23). The thyrocervical trunk mainly supplies the thyroid gland, portions of the cervical vertebrae and spinal cord, and some scapular muscles. The costocervical trunk serves deep neck and superior intercostal muscles.

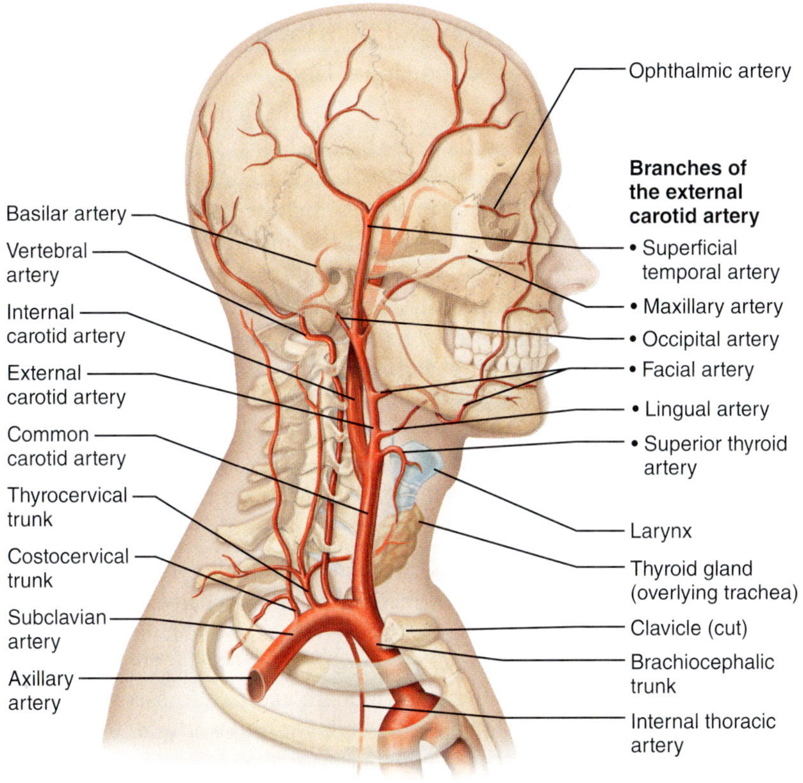

(b) Arteries of the head and neck, right aspect

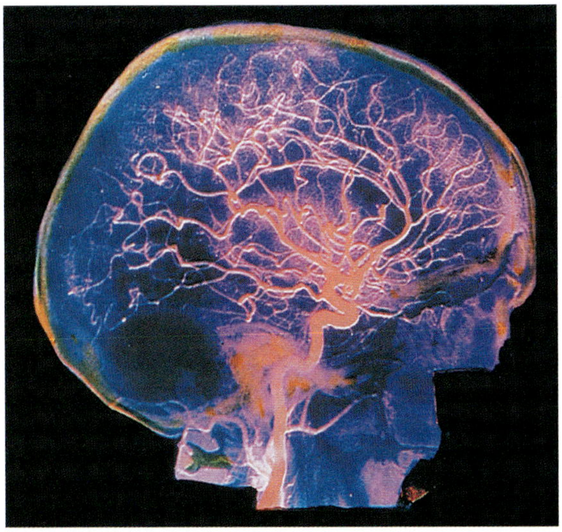

(c) Colorized arteriograph of the arterial supply of the brain

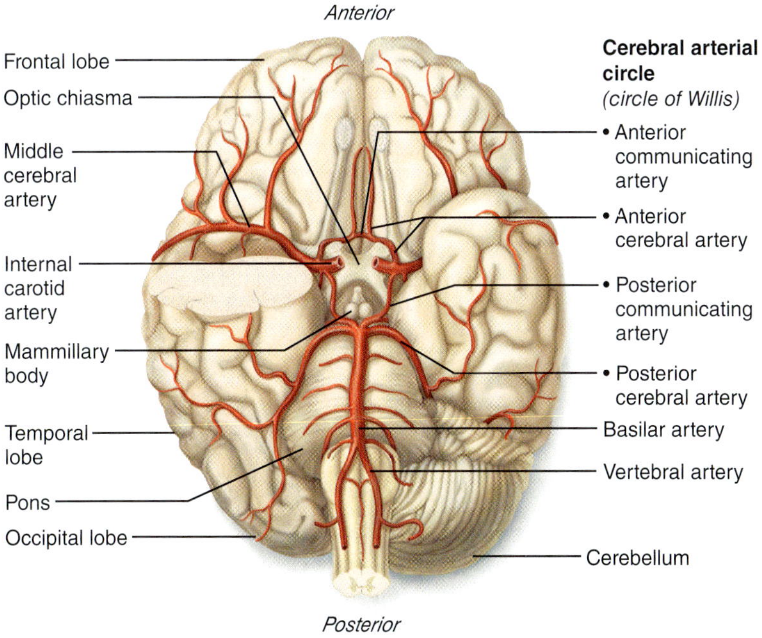

(d) Major arteries serving the brain (inferior view, right side of cerebellum and part of right temporal lobe removed)

Figure 19.22 *(continued)*

Table 19.6 Arteries of the Upper Limbs and Thorax

The upper limbs are supplied entirely by arteries arising from the **subclavian arteries** (Figure 19.23a). After giving off branches to the neck, each subclavian artery courses laterally between the clavicle and first rib to enter the axilla, where its name changes to axillary artery. The thorax wall is supplied by an array of vessels that arise either directly from the thoracic aorta or from branches of the subclavian arteries. Most visceral organs of the thorax receive their functional blood supply from small branches issuing from the thoracic aorta. Because these vessels are so small and tend to vary in number (except for the bronchial arteries), Figures 19.23a and b do not illustrate them, but several are listed at the end of this table.

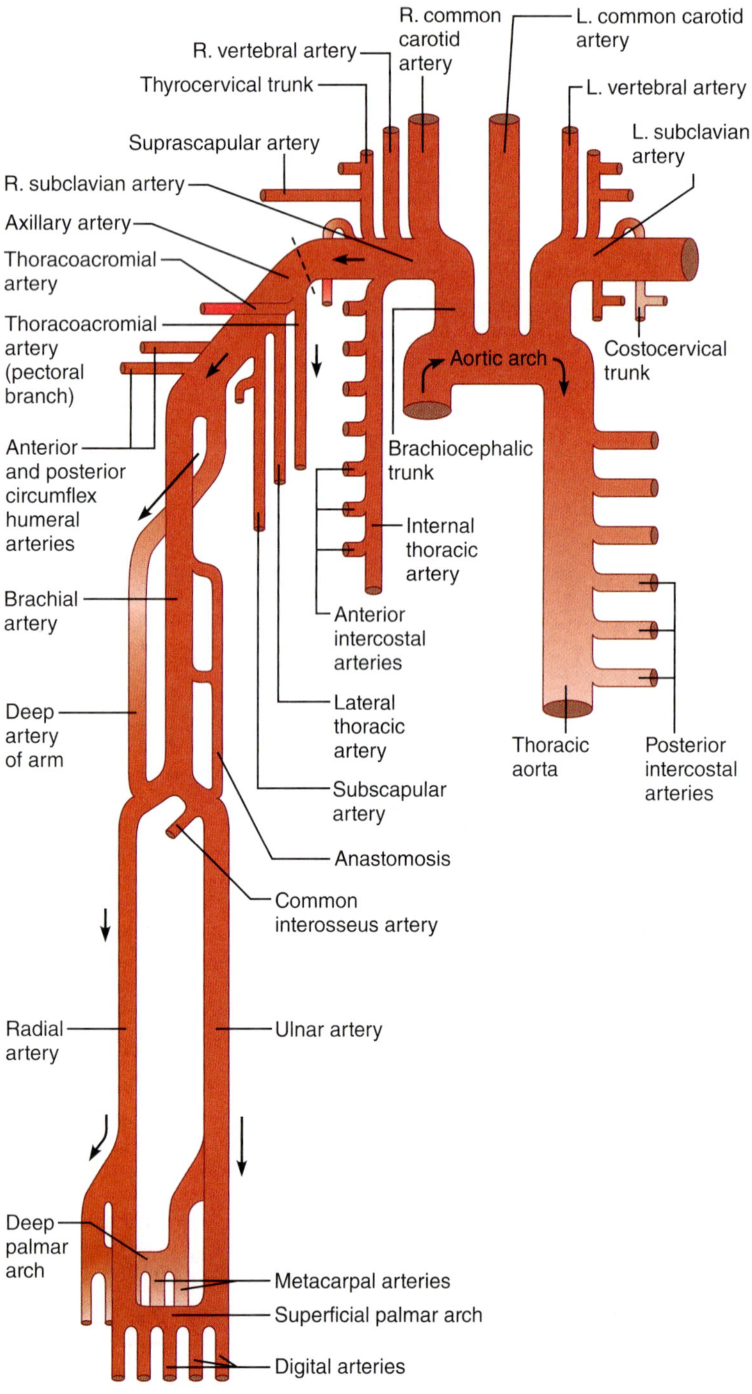

(a) Schematic flowchart

Figure 19.23 Arteries of the right upper limb and thorax.

Description and Distribution

Arteries of the Upper Limb

Axillary artery. As it runs through the axilla accompanied by cords of the brachial plexus, each axillary artery gives off branches to the axilla, chest wall, and shoulder girdle. These branches include the **thoracoacromial artery** (tho″rah-ko-ah-kro′me-al), which supplies the deltoid muscle and pectoral region; the **lateral thoracic artery**, which serves the lateral chest wall and breast; the **subscapular artery** to the scapula, dorsal thorax wall, and part of the latissimus dorsi muscle; and the **anterior** and **posterior circumflex humeral arteries**, which wrap around the humeral neck and help supply the shoulder joint and the deltoid muscle. As the axillary artery emerges from the axilla, it becomes the brachial artery.

Brachial artery. The brachial artery runs down the medial aspect of the humerus and supplies the anterior flexor muscles of the arm. One major branch, the **deep artery of the arm**, serves the posterior triceps brachii muscle. As it nears the elbow, the brachial artery gives off several small branches that contribute to an anastomosis serving the elbow joint and connecting it to the arteries of the forearm. As the brachial artery crosses the anterior midline aspect of the elbow, it provides an easily palpated pulse point (brachial pulse) (see Figure 19.12). Immediately beyond the elbow, the brachial artery splits to form the radial and ulnar arteries, which more or less follow the course of similarly named bones down the anterior forearm.

Radial artery. The radial artery runs from the median line of the cubital fossa to the styloid process of the radius. It supplies the lateral muscles of the forearm, the wrist, and the thumb and index finger. At the root of the thumb, the radial artery provides a convenient site for taking the radial pulse.

Ulnar artery. The ulnar artery supplies the medial aspect of the forearm, fingers 3–5, and the medial aspect of the index finger. Proximally, the ulnar artery gives off a short branch, the **common interosseous artery** (in″ter-os′e-us), which runs between the radius and ulna to serve the deep flexors and extensors of the forearm.

Palmar arches. In the palm, branches of the radial and ulnar arteries anastomose to form the **superficial** and **deep palmar arches**. The **metacarpal arteries** and **digital arteries** that supply the fingers arise from these palmar arches.

19

Table 19.6 *(continued)*

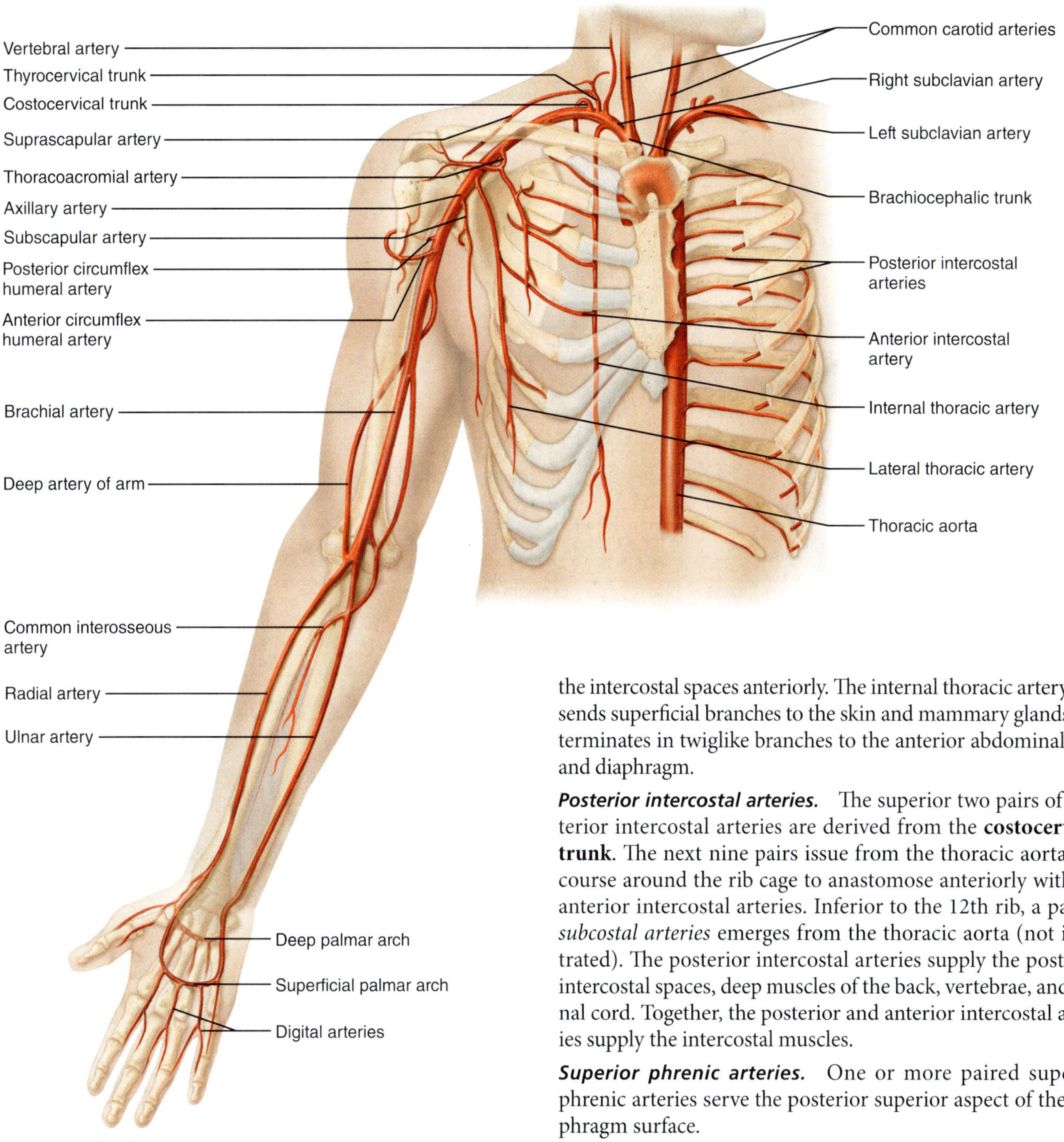

(b) Illustration, anterior view

Figure 19.23 *(continued)*

Arteries of the Thorax Wall

Internal thoracic arteries. The internal thoracic arteries (formerly called the internal mammary arteries) arise from the subclavian arteries and supply blood to most of the anterior thorax wall. Each of these arteries descends lateral to the sternum and gives off **anterior intercostal arteries**, which supply the intercostal spaces anteriorly. The internal thoracic artery also sends superficial branches to the skin and mammary glands and terminates in twiglike branches to the anterior abdominal wall and diaphragm.

Posterior intercostal arteries. The superior two pairs of posterior intercostal arteries are derived from the **costocervical trunk**. The next nine pairs issue from the thoracic aorta and course around the rib cage to anastomose anteriorly with the anterior intercostal arteries. Inferior to the 12th rib, a pair of *subcostal arteries* emerges from the thoracic aorta (not illustrated). The posterior intercostal arteries supply the posterior intercostal spaces, deep muscles of the back, vertebrae, and spinal cord. Together, the posterior and anterior intercostal arteries supply the intercostal muscles.

Superior phrenic arteries. One or more paired superior phrenic arteries serve the posterior superior aspect of the diaphragm surface.

Arteries of the Thoracic Viscera

Pericardial arteries. Several tiny branches supply the posterior pericardium.

Bronchial arteries. Two left and one right bronchial arteries supply systemic (oxygen-rich) blood to the lungs, bronchi, and pleurae.

Esophageal arteries. Four to five esophageal arteries supply the esophagus.

Mediastinal arteries. Many small mediastinal arteries serve the posterior mediastinum.

19

Table 19.7 Arteries of the Abdomen

The arterial supply to the abdominal organs arises from the abdominal aorta **(Figure 19.24a)**. Under resting conditions, about half of the entire arterial flow moves through these vessels. Except for the celiac trunk, the superior and inferior mesenteric arteries, and the median sacral artery, all are paired vessels. These arteries supply the abdominal wall, diaphragm, and visceral organs of the abdominopelvic cavity. We discuss the branches in the order of their issue.

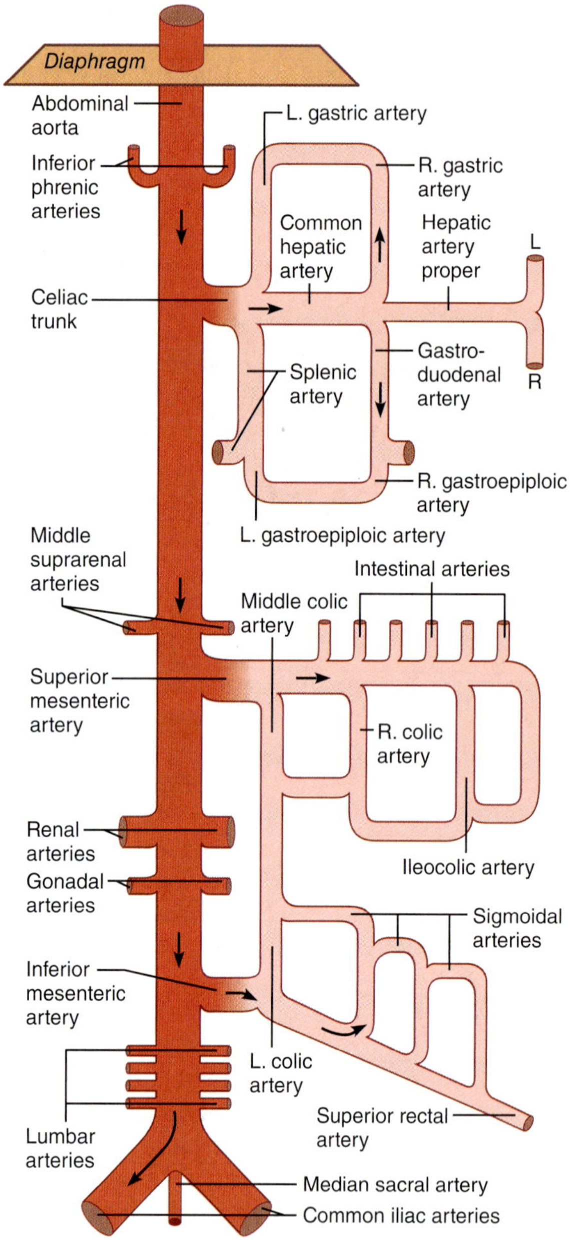

(a) Schematic flowchart.

Figure 19.24 **Arteries of the abdomen.**

Table 19.7 *(continued)*

Description and Distribution

Inferior phrenic arteries. The inferior phrenics emerge from the aorta at T_{12}, just inferior to the diaphragm (Figure 19.24c). They serve the inferior diaphragm surface.

Celiac trunk. This very large unpaired branch of the abdominal aorta divides almost immediately into three branches: the common hepatic, splenic, and left gastric arteries (Figure 19.24b). The **common hepatic artery** (hĕ-pat′ik) gives off branches to the stomach, duodenum, and pancreas. Where the **gastroduodenal artery** branches off, the common hepatic becomes the **hepatic artery proper**, which splits into right and left branches that serve the liver. As the **splenic artery** (splen′ik) passes deep to the stomach, it sends branches to the pancreas and stomach and terminates in branches to the spleen. The **left gastric artery** (*gaster* = stomach) supplies part of the stomach and the inferior esophagus. The **right** and **left gastroepiploic arteries** (gas″tro-ep″ĭ-plo′ik)—branches of the gastroduodenal and splenic arteries, respectively—serve the greater curvature of the stomach. A **right gastric artery**, which supplies the stomach's lesser curvature, may arise from the common hepatic artery or from the hepatic artery proper.

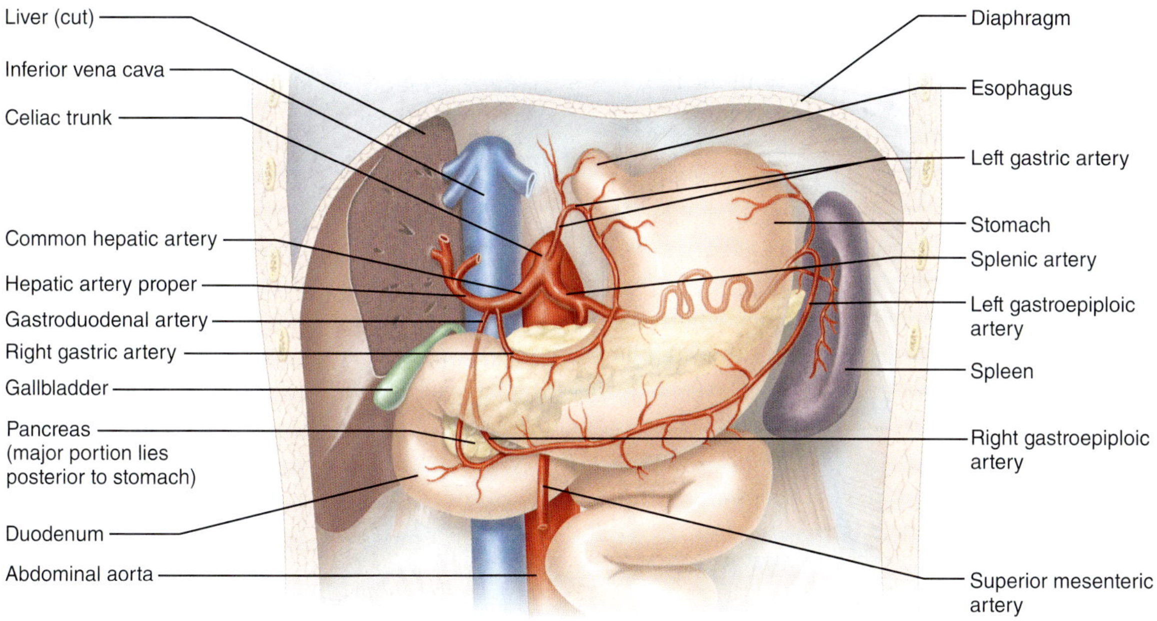

(b) The celiac trunk and its major branches. The left half of the liver has been removed.

Figure 19.24 *(continued)*

19

Table 19.7 Arteries of the Abdomen *(continued)*

Superior mesenteric artery (mes-en-ter′ik). This large, unpaired artery arises from the abdominal aorta at the L_1 level immediately below the celiac trunk (Figure 19.24d). It runs deep to the pancreas and then enters the mesentery (a drapelike membrane that supports the small intestine), where its numerous anastomosing branches serve virtually all of the small intestine via the **intestinal arteries**, and most of the large intestine—the appendix, cecum, ascending colon (via the **ileocolic** and **right colic arteries**), and part of the transverse colon (via the **middle colic artery**).

Suprarenal arteries (soo″prah-re′nal). The **middle suprarenal arteries** flank the origin of the superior mesenteric artery as they emerge from the abdominal aorta (Figure 19.24c). They supply blood to the adrenal (suprarenal) glands overlying the kidneys. The adrenal glands also receive two sets of branches not illustrated: *superior suprarenal* branches from the nearby inferior phrenic arteries, and *inferior suprarenal* branches from the nearby renal arteries.

Renal arteries. The short but wide renal arteries, right and left, issue from the lateral surfaces of the aorta slightly below the superior mesenteric artery (between L_1 and L_2). Each serves the kidney on its side.

Gonadal arteries (go-nă′dul). The paired gonadal arteries are called the **ovarian arteries** in females and the **testicular arteries** in males. The ovarian arteries extend into the pelvis to serve the ovaries and part of the uterine tubes. The much longer testicular arteries descend through the pelvis and inguinal canals to enter the scrotum, where they serve the testes.

Inferior mesenteric artery. This final major branch of the abdominal aorta is unpaired and arises from the anterior aortic surface at the L_3 level. It serves the distal part of the large intestine—from the midpart of the transverse colon to the midrectum—via its **left colic**, **sigmoidal**, and **superior rectal branches** (Figure 19.24d). Looping anastomoses between the superior and inferior mesenteric arteries help ensure that blood will continue to reach the digestive viscera in cases of trauma to one of these abdominal arteries.

Lumbar arteries. Four pairs of lumbar arteries arise from the posterolateral surface of the aorta in the lumbar region. These segmental arteries supply the posterior abdominal wall.

Median sacral artery. The unpaired median sacral artery issues from the posterior surface of the abdominal aorta at its terminus. This tiny artery supplies the sacrum and coccyx.

Common iliac arteries. At the L_4 level, the aorta splits into the right and left common iliac arteries, which supply blood to the lower abdominal wall, pelvic organs, and lower limbs (Figure 19.24c).

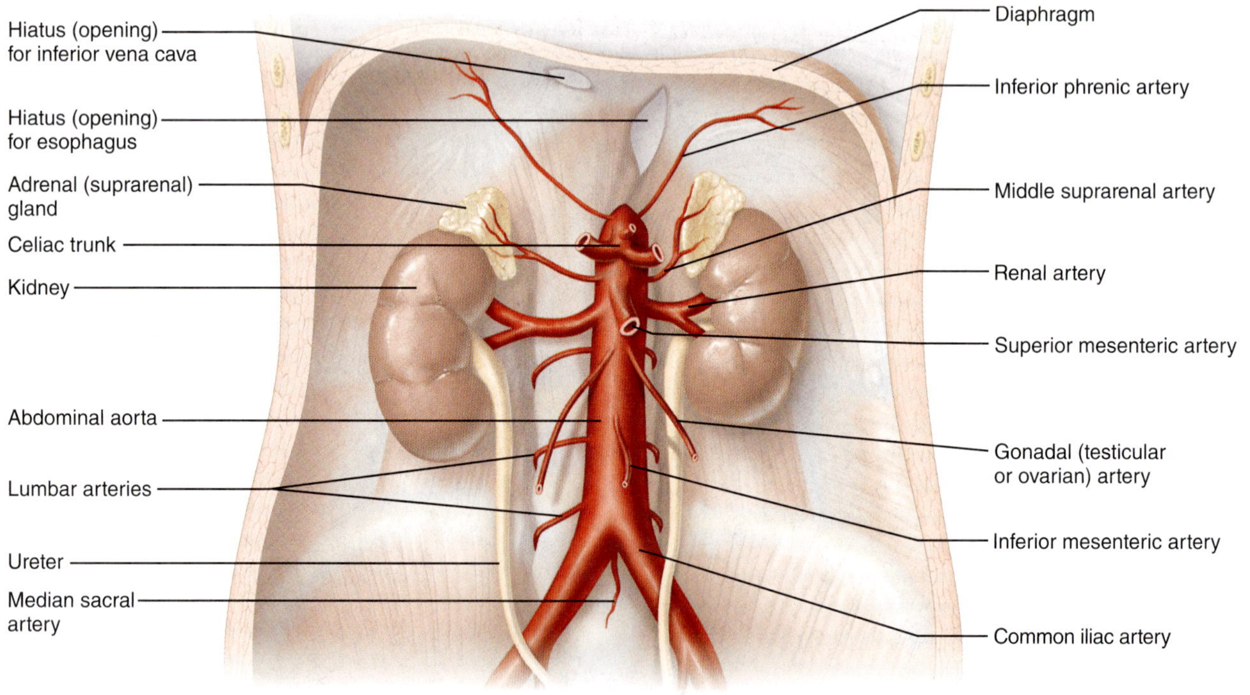

(c) Major branches of the abdominal aorta.

Figure 19.24 *(continued)* **Arteries of the abdomen.**

19

Table 19.7 *(continued)*

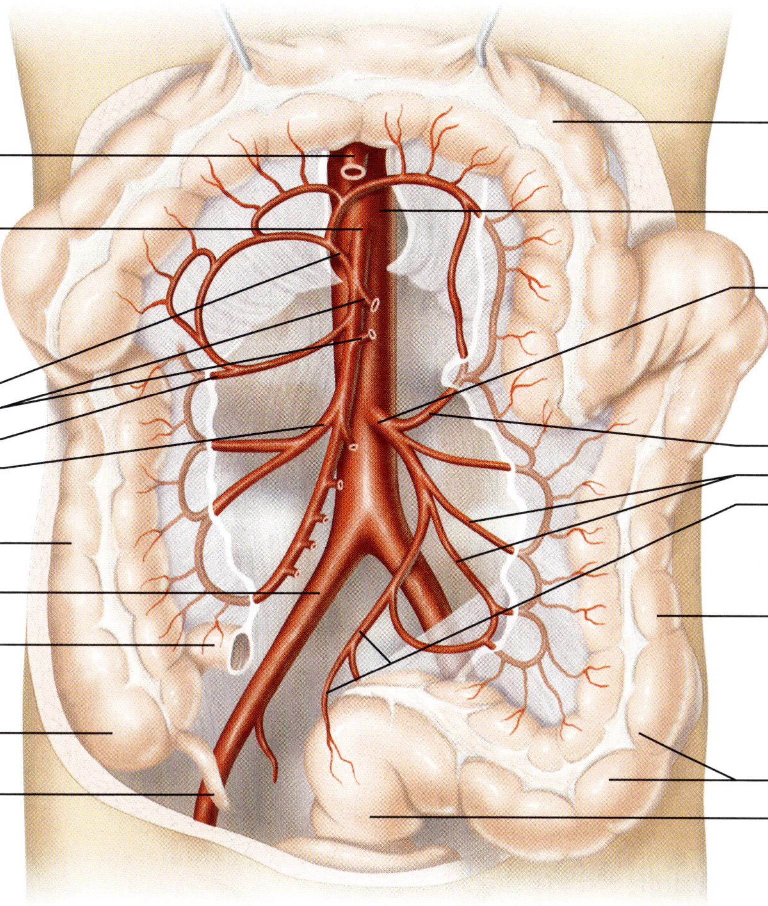

(d) Distribution of the superior and inferior mesenteric arteries. The transverse colon has been pulled superiorly.

Figure 19.24 *(continued)*

☑ Check Your Understanding

15. Which paired artery supplies most of the tissues of the head except for the brain and orbits?
16. Name the arterial anastomosis at the base of the cerebrum.
17. Name the four unpaired arteries that emerge from the abdominal aorta.

For answers, see Appendix H.

Table 19.8 Arteries of the Pelvis and Lower Limbs

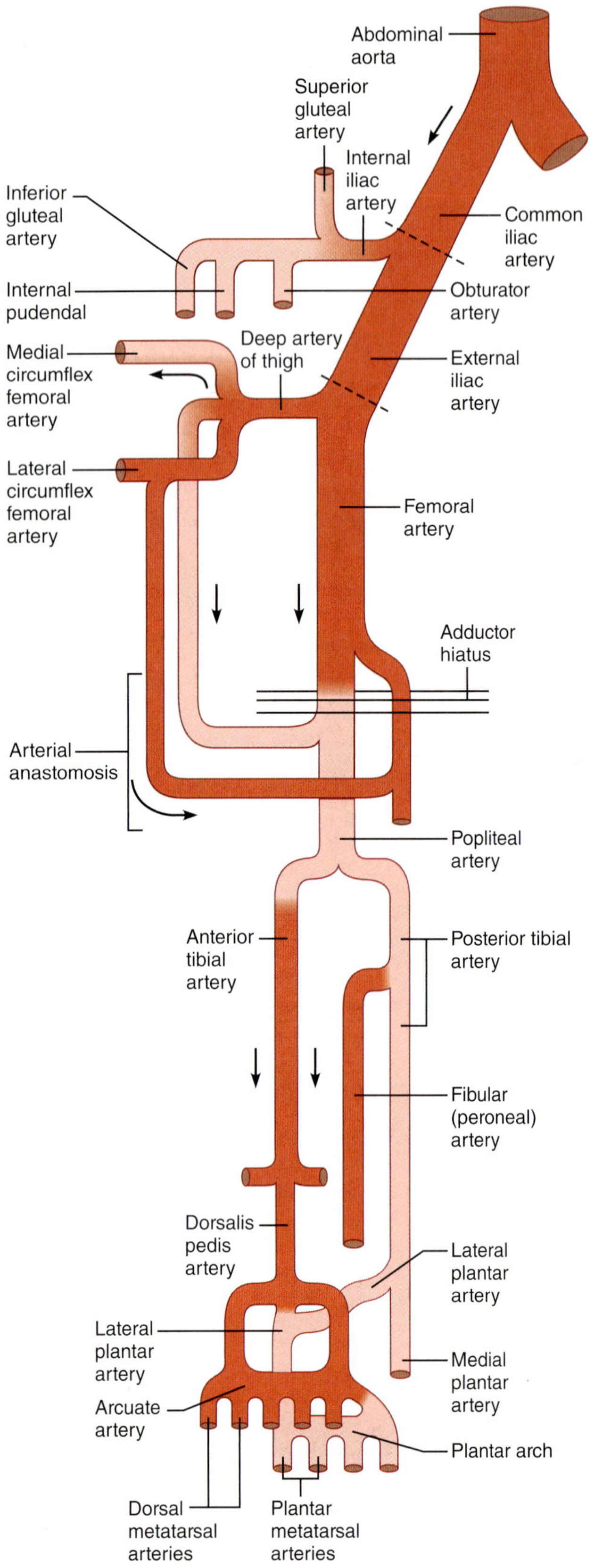

(a) Schematic flowchart

At the level of the sacroiliac joints, the **common iliac arteries** divide into two major branches, the internal and external iliac arteries **(Figure 19.25a)**. The internal iliacs distribute blood mainly to the pelvic region. The external iliacs primarily serve the lower limbs but also send branches to the abdominal wall.

Description and Distribution

Internal iliac arteries. These paired arteries run into the pelvis and distribute blood to the pelvic walls and viscera (bladder and rectum, plus the uterus and vagina in the female and the prostate and ductus deferens in the male). Additionally they serve the gluteal muscles via the **superior** and **inferior gluteal arteries**, adductor muscles of the medial thigh via the **obturator artery**, and external genitalia and perineum via the **internal pudendal artery** (not illustrated).

External iliac arteries. These arteries supply the lower limbs (Figure 19.25b). As they course through the pelvis, they give off branches to the anterior abdominal wall. After passing under the inguinal ligaments to enter the thigh, they become the femoral arteries.

Femoral arteries. As each of these arteries passes down the anteromedial thigh, it gives off several branches to the thigh muscles. The largest of the deep branches is the **deep artery of the thigh** (also called the *deep femoral artery*), which is the main supply to the thigh muscles (hamstrings, quadriceps, and adductors). Proximal branches of the deep femoral artery, the **lateral** and **medial circumflex femoral arteries**, encircle the neck of the femur. The medial circumflex artery is the major vessel to the head of the femur. If it is torn in a hip fracture, the bone tissue of the head of the femur dies. A long descending branch of the lateral circumflex artery supplies the vastus lateralis muscle. Near the knee the femoral artery passes posteriorly and through a gap in the adductor magnus muscle, the *adductor hiatus*, to enter the popliteal fossa, where its name changes to popliteal artery.

Popliteal artery. This posterior vessel contributes to an arterial anastomosis that supplies the knee region and then splits into the anterior and posterior tibial arteries of the leg.

Anterior tibial artery. The anterior tibial artery runs through the anterior compartment of the leg, supplying the extensor muscles along the way. At the ankle, it becomes the **dorsalis pedis artery**, which supplies the ankle and dorsum of the foot, and gives off a branch, the **arcuate artery**, which issues the **dorsal metatarsal arteries** to the metatarsus of the foot. The superficial dorsalis pedis ends by penetrating into the sole where it forms the medial part of the **plantar arch**. The dorsalis pedis artery provides a clinically important pulse point, the pedal pulse. If the pedal pulse is easily felt, it is fairly certain that the blood supply to the leg is good.

Figure 19.25 Arteries of the right pelvis and lower limb.

19

Table 19.8 *(continued)*

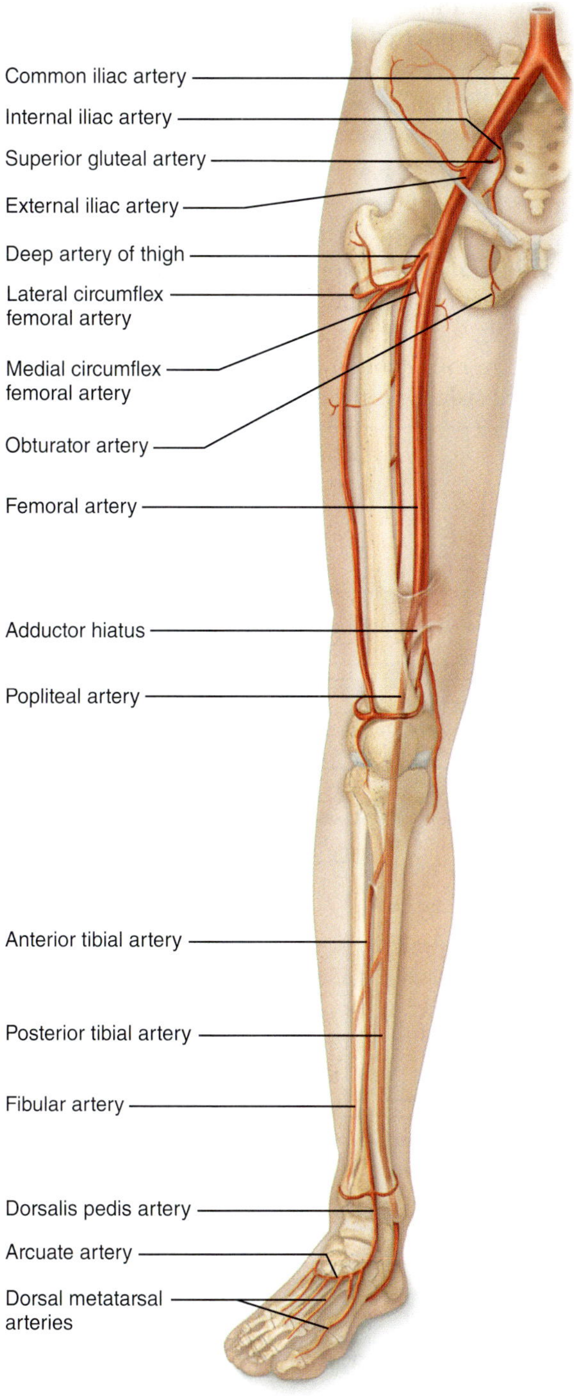

(b) Anterior view

Posterior tibial artery. This large artery courses through the posteromedial part of the leg and supplies the flexor muscles. Proximally, it gives off a large branch, the **fibular (peroneal) artery**, which supplies the lateral fibularis muscles of the leg. On the medial side of the foot, the posterior tibial artery divides into **lateral** and **medial plantar arteries** that serve the plantar surface of the foot. The lateral plantar artery forms the lateral end of the plantar arch. **Plantar metatarsal arteries** and digital arteries to the toes arise from the plantar arch.

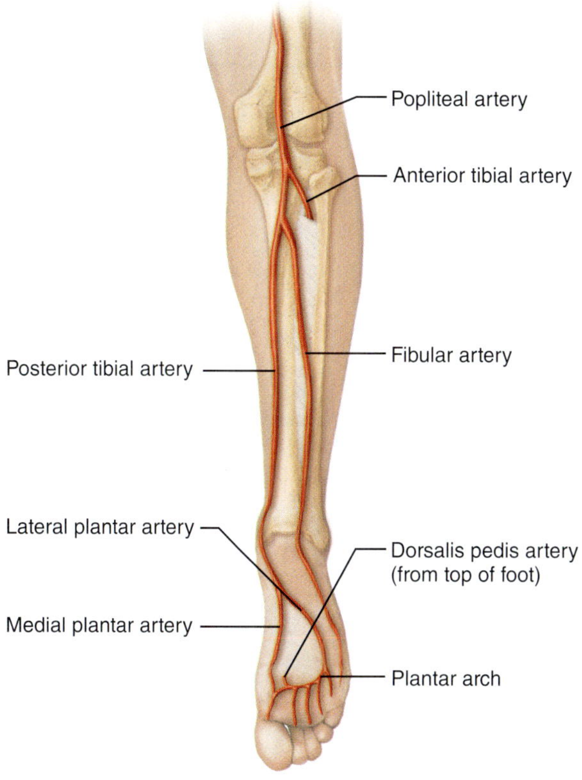

(c) Posterior view

Figure 19.25 *(continued)*

Check Your Understanding

18. You are assessing the circulation in the leg of a diabetic patient at the clinic. Name the artery you palpate in each of these three locations: behind the knee, behind the medial malleolus of the tibia, on the dorsum of the foot.

For answers, see Appendix H.

Table 19.9 The Venae Cavae and the Major Veins of the Systemic Circulation

In our survey of the systemic veins, the major tributaries (branches) of the venae cavae are noted first in **Figure 19.26**, followed by a description in Tables 19.10 through 19.13 of the venous pattern of the various body regions. Because veins run toward the heart, the most distal veins are named first and those closest to the heart last. Deep veins generally drain the same areas served by their companion arteries, so they are not described in detail.

Description and Areas Drained

Superior vena cava. This great vein receives systemic blood draining from all areas superior to the diaphragm, except the heart wall. It is formed by the union of the **right** and **left brachiocephalic veins** and empties into the right atrium (Figure 19.26b). Notice that there are two brachiocephalic veins, but only one brachiocephalic artery (trunk). Each brachiocephalic vein is formed by the joining of the **internal jugular** and **subclavian veins** on its side. In most of the flowcharts that follow, only the vessels draining blood from the right side of the body are shown (except for the azygos circulation of the thorax).

Inferior vena cava. The widest blood vessel in the body, this vein returns blood to the heart from all body regions below the diaphragm. The abdominal aorta lies directly to its left. The paired **common iliac veins** join at L_5 to form the distal end of the inferior vena cava. From this point, it courses superiorly along the anterior aspect of the spine, receiving venous blood from the abdominal walls, gonads, and kidneys. Immediately above the diaphragm, the inferior vena cava ends as it enters the inferior aspect of the right atrium.

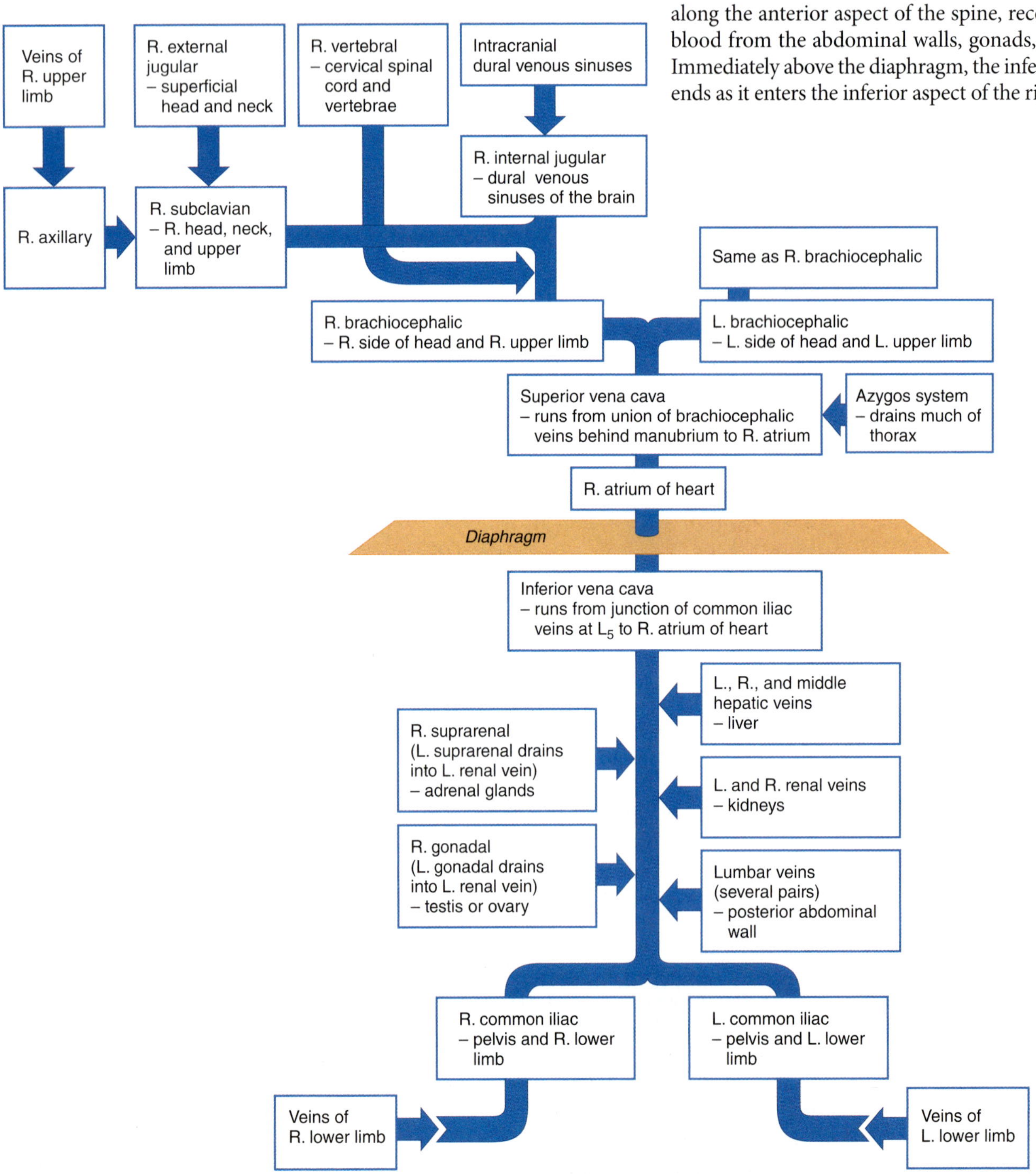

(a) Schematic flowchart

19

Table 19.9 *(continued)*

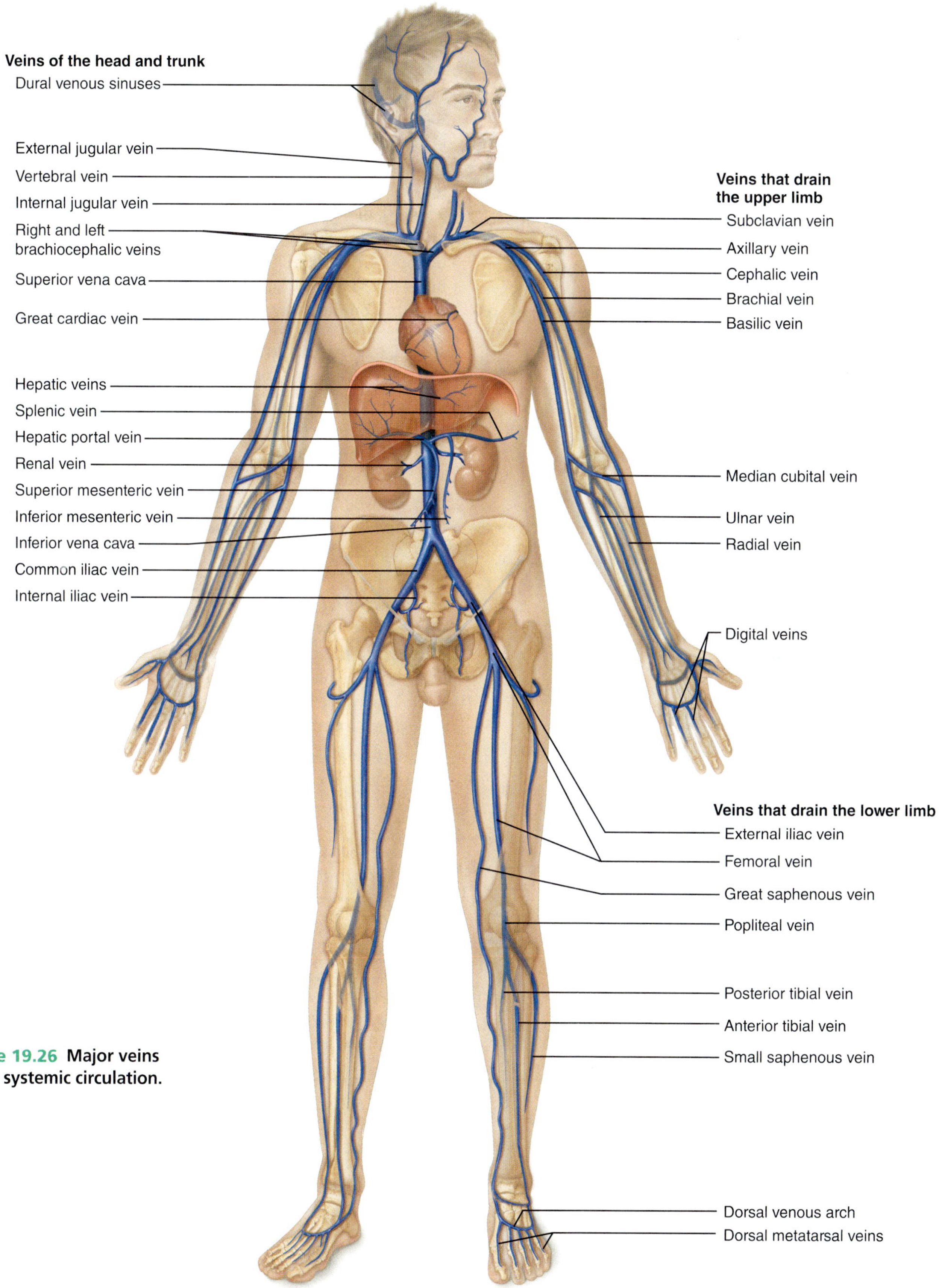

Figure 19.26 Major veins of the systemic circulation.

(b) Illustration, anterior view. The vessels of the pulmonary circulation are not shown.

Table 19.10 Veins of the Head and Neck

Three pairs of veins collect most of the blood draining from the head and neck **(Figure 19.27a)**:

- The external jugular veins, which empty into the subclavians
- The internal jugular veins
- The vertebral veins, which drain into the brachiocephalic vein

Although most extracranial veins have the same names as the extracranial arteries, their courses and interconnections differ substantially.

Most veins of the brain drain into the **dural venous sinuses**, an interconnected series of enlarged chambers located between the dura mater layers. The **superior** and **inferior sagittal sinuses** are in the falx cerebri, which dips down between the cerebral hemispheres. The inferior sagittal sinus drains into the **straight sinus** posteriorly (Figure 19.27a and c). The superior sagittal and straight sinuses then empty into the **transverse sinuses**, which run in shallow grooves on the internal surface of the occipital bone. These drain into the S-shaped **sigmoid sinuses**, which become the *internal jugular veins* as they leave the skull through the jugular foramen. The **cavernous sinuses**, which flank the sphenoid body, receive venous blood from the **ophthalmic veins** of the orbits and the facial veins, which drain the nose and upper lip area. The internal carotid artery and cranial nerves III, IV, VI, and part of V, all run *through* the cavernous sinus on their way to the orbit and face.

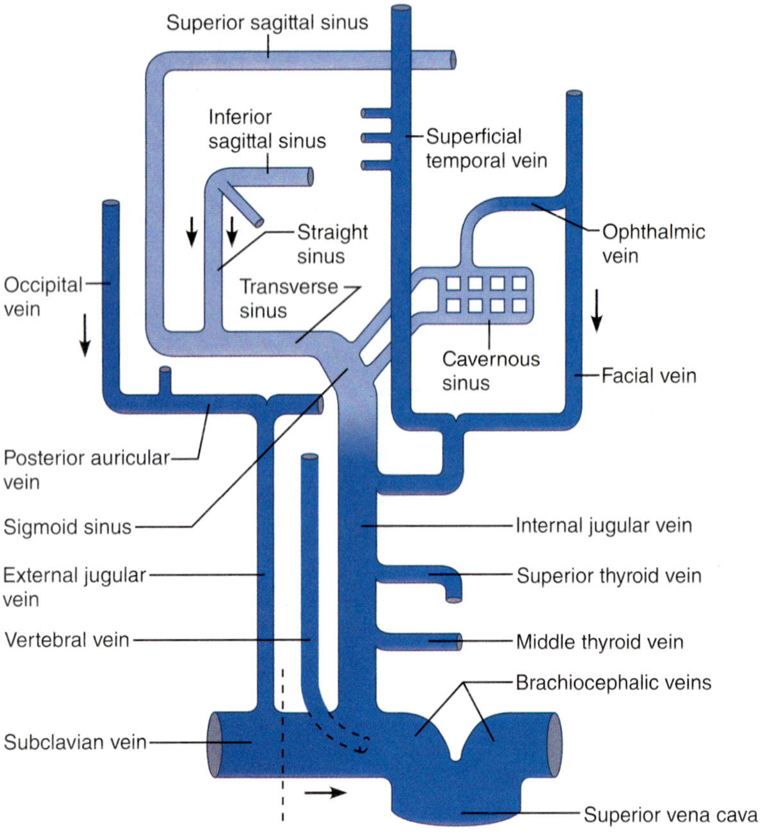

(a) Schematic flowchart

Figure 19.27 Venous drainage of the head, neck, and brain.

Description and Area Drained

External jugular veins. The right and left external jugular veins drain superficial scalp and face structures served by the external carotid arteries. However, their tributaries anastomose frequently, and some of the superficial drainage from these regions enters the internal jugular veins as well. As the external jugular veins descend through the lateral neck, they pass obliquely over the sternocleidomastoid muscles and then empty into the subclavian veins.

Vertebral veins. Unlike the vertebral arteries, the vertebral veins do not serve much of the brain. Instead they drain the cervical vertebrae, the spinal cord, and some small neck muscles. They run inferiorly through the transverse foramina of the cervical vertebrae and join the brachiocephalic veins at the root of the neck.

Internal jugular veins. The paired internal jugular veins, which receive the bulk of blood draining from the brain, are the largest of the paired veins draining the head and neck. They arise from the dural venous sinuses, exit the skull via the *jugular foramina*, and then descend through the neck alongside the internal carotid arteries. As they move inferiorly, they receive blood from some of the deep veins of the face and neck—branches of the **facial** and **superficial temporal veins** (Figure 19.27b). At the base of the neck, each internal jugular vein joins the subclavian vein on its own side to form a brachiocephalic vein. As already noted, the two brachiocephalic veins unite to form the **superior vena cava**.

19

Table 19.10 *(continued)*

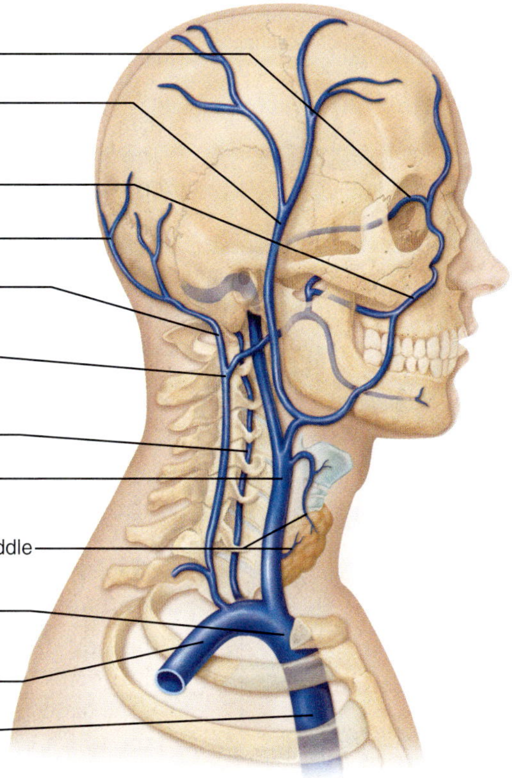

(b) Veins of the head and neck, right superficial aspect

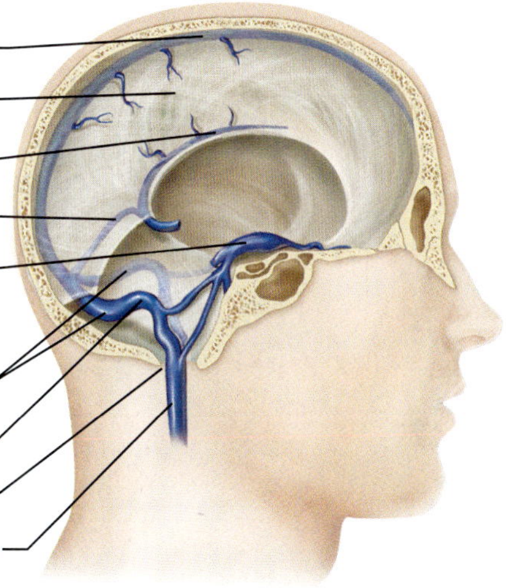

(c) Dural venous sinuses of the brain

Figure 19.27 *(continued)*

☑ Check Your Understanding

19. In what important way does the area drained by the vertebral veins differ from the area served by the vertebral arteries?

20. Which veins drain the dural venous sinuses and where do these veins terminate?

For answers, see Appendix H.

19

Table 19.11 Veins of the Upper Limbs and Thorax

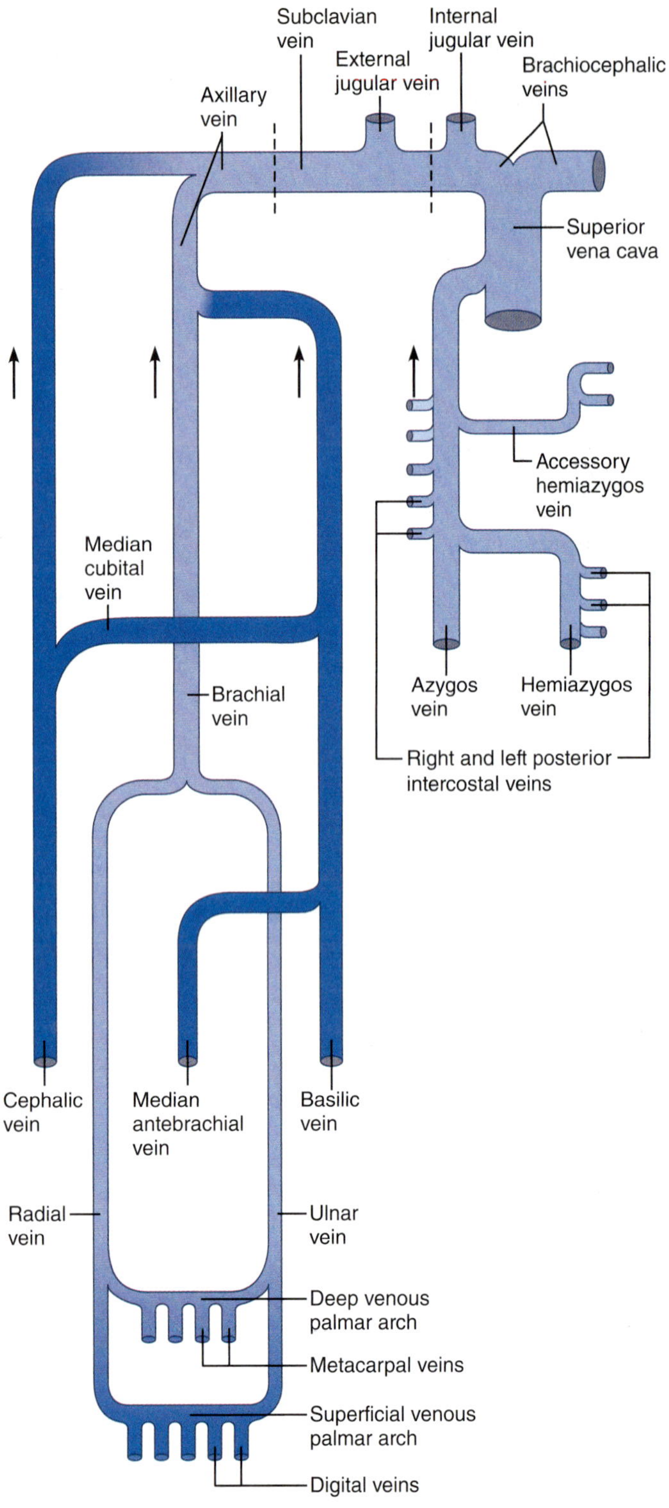

Figure 19.28 Veins of the thorax and right upper limb. For clarity, the abundant branching and anastomoses of the superficial veins are not shown.

The deep veins of the upper limbs follow the paths of their companion arteries and have the same names **(Figure 19.28a)**. However, except for the largest, most are paired veins that flank their artery. The superficial veins of the upper limbs are larger than the deep veins and are easily seen just beneath the skin. The median cubital vein, crossing the anterior aspect of the elbow, is commonly used to obtain blood samples or administer intravenous medications.

Blood draining from the mammary glands and the first two to three intercostal spaces enters the **brachiocephalic veins**. However, the vast majority of thoracic tissues and the thorax wall are drained by a complex network of veins called the **azygos system** (az′ĭ-gos). The branching nature of the azygos system provides a collateral circulation for draining the abdominal wall and other areas served by the inferior vena cava, and there are numerous anastomoses between the azygos system and the inferior vena cava.

Description and Areas Drained

Deep Veins of the Upper Limbs

The most distal deep veins of the upper limb are the radial and ulnar veins. The **deep** and **superficial venous palmar arches** of the hand empty into the **radial** and **ulnar veins** of the forearm, which then unite to form the **brachial vein** of the arm. As the brachial vein enters the axilla, it becomes the **axillary vein**, which becomes the **subclavian vein** at the level of the first rib.

Superficial Veins of the Upper Limbs

The superficial venous system begins with the *dorsal venous network* (not illustrated), a plexus of superficial veins in the dorsum of the hand. In the distal forearm, this plexus drains into two major superficial veins—the cephalic and basilic veins—which anastomose frequently as they course upward (Figure 19.28b). The **cephalic vein** bends around the radius as it travels superiorly and then continues up the lateral superficial aspect of the arm to the shoulder, where it runs in the groove between the deltoid and pectoralis muscles to join the axillary vein. The **basilic vein** courses along the posteromedial aspect of the forearm, crosses the elbow, and then joins the brachial vein in the axilla, forming the axillary vein. At the anterior aspect of the elbow, the **median cubital vein** connects the basilic and cephalic veins. The **median antebrachial vein** lies between the radial and ulnar veins in the forearm and terminates (variably) at the elbow by entering either the basilic or the cephalic vein.

The Azygos System

The azygos system consists of the following vessels, which flank the vertebral column laterally.

Azygos vein. Located against the right side of the vertebral column, the **azygos vein** (*azygos* = unpaired) originates in the abdomen, from the **right ascending lumbar vein** that drains most of the right abdominal cavity wall and from the **right posterior intercostal veins** (except the first) that drain the chest muscles. At the T_4 level, it arches over the great vessels that run to the right lung and empties into the superior vena cava.

Table 19.11 *(continued)*

Hemiazygos vein (hĕ″me-a-zi′gus; "half the azygos"). This vessel ascends on the left side of the vertebral column. Its origin, from the **left ascending lumbar vein** and the lower (9th–11th) **posterior intercostal veins**, mirrors that of the inferior portion of the azygos vein on the right. About midthorax, the hemiazygos vein passes in front of the vertebral column and joins the azygos vein.

Accessory hemiazygos vein. The accessory hemiazygos completes the venous drainage of the left (middle) thorax and can be thought of as a superior continuation of the hemiazygos vein. It receives blood from the 4th–8th posterior intercostal veins and then crosses to the right to empty into the azygos vein. Like the azygos, it receives oxygen-poor systemic blood from the bronchi of the lungs (*bronchial veins*).

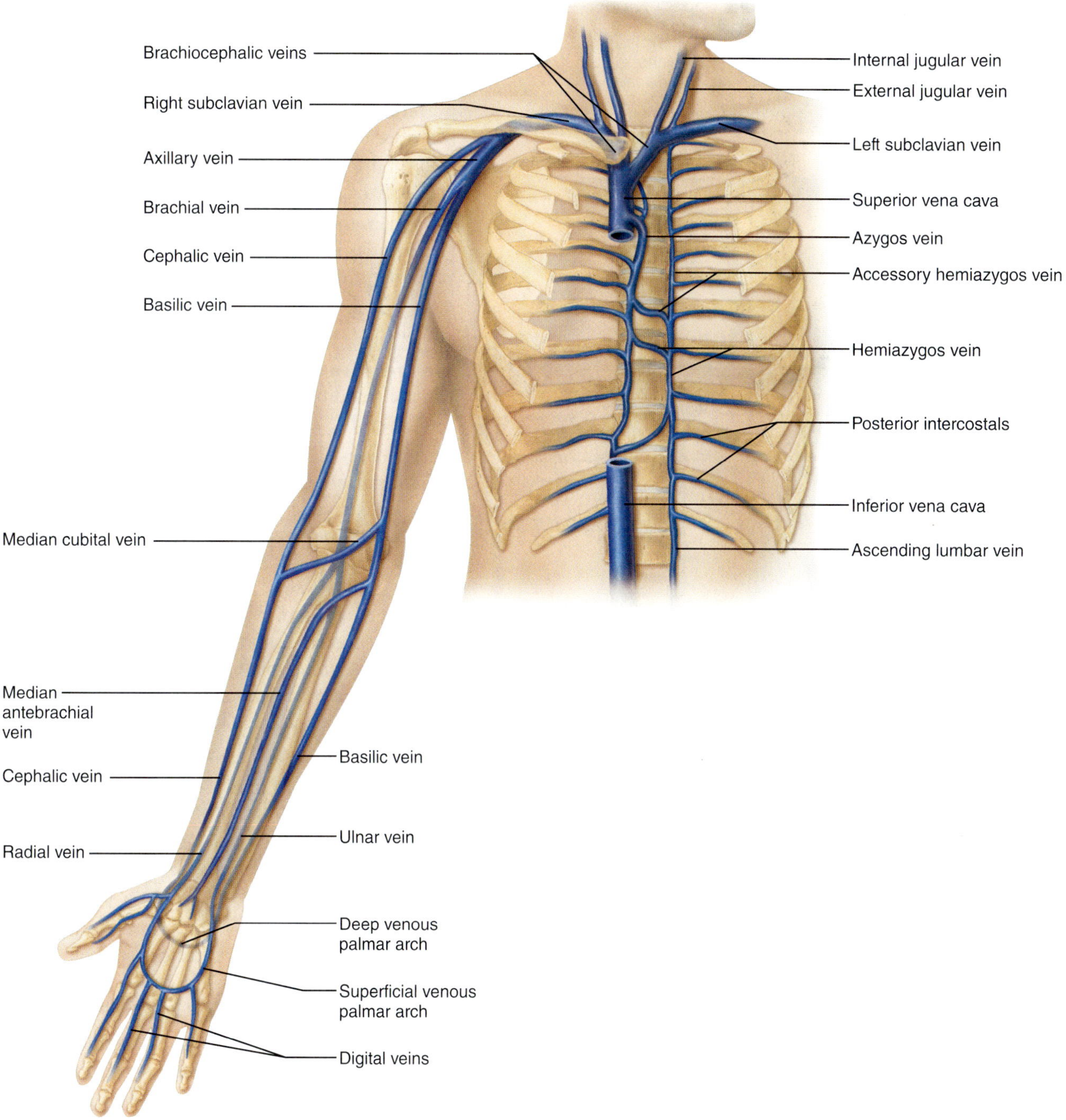

(b) Anterior view

Figure 19.28 *(continued)*

19

Table 19.12 Veins of the Abdomen

The **inferior vena cava** returns blood from the abdominopelvic viscera and abdominal walls to the heart **(Figure 19.29a)**. Most of its venous tributaries have names that correspond to the arteries serving the abdominal organs.

Veins draining the digestive viscera empty into a common vessel, the *hepatic portal vein,* which transports this venous blood into the liver before it is allowed to enter the major systemic circulation via the hepatic veins (Figure 19.29c). Such a venous system—veins connecting two capillary beds together—is called a *portal system* and always serves very specific needs. The **hepatic portal system** carries nutrient-rich blood (which may also contain toxins and microorganisms) from the digestive organs to the liver, where it can be "treated" before it reaches the rest of the body. As the blood percolates slowly through the liver sinusoid capillaries, hepatocytes process nutrients and toxins, and phagocytic cells rid the blood of bacteria and other foreign matter. The veins of the abdomen are listed in inferior to superior order.

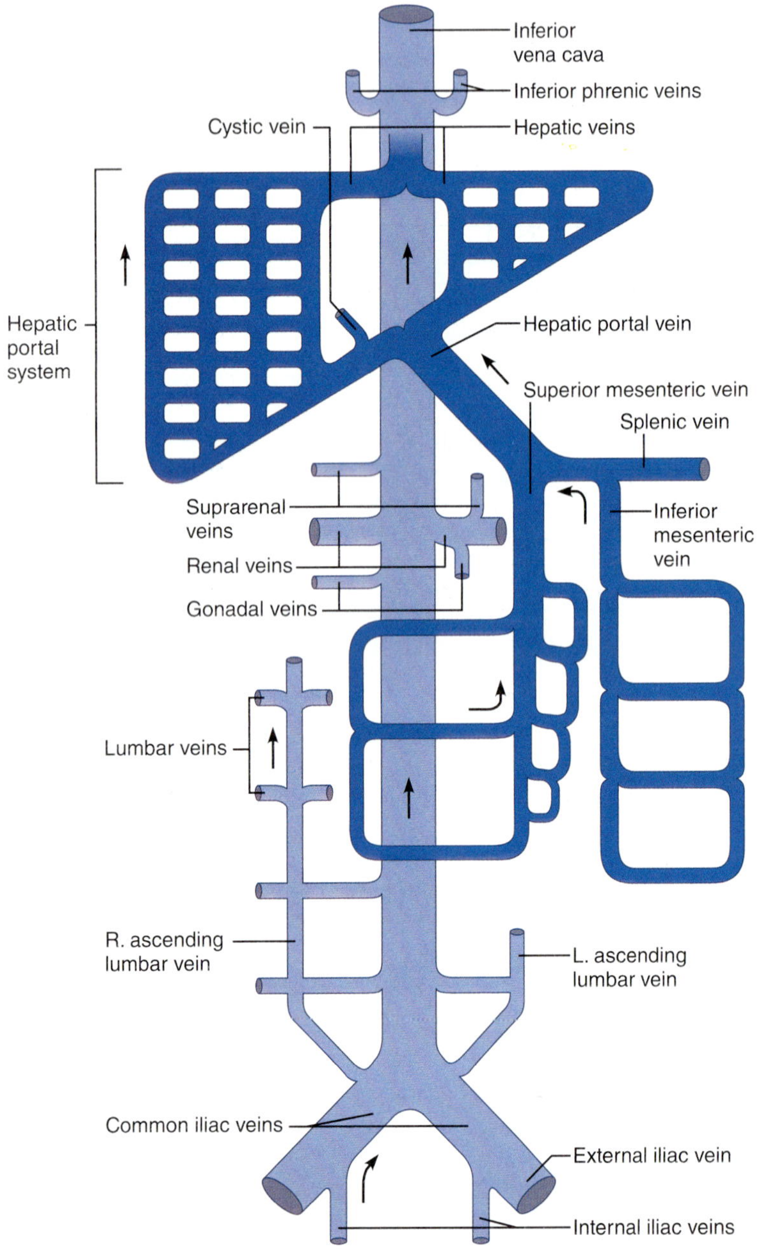

(a) Schematic flowchart.

Figure 19.29 **Veins of the abdomen.**

Description and Areas Drained

Lumbar veins. Several pairs of lumbar veins drain the posterior abdominal wall. They empty both directly into the inferior vena cava and into the ascending lumbar veins of the azygos system of the thorax.

Gonadal (testicular or ovarian) veins. The right gonadal vein drains the ovary or testis on the right side of the body and empties into the inferior vena cava. The left gonadal vein drains into the left renal vein superiorly.

Renal veins. The right and left renal veins drain the kidneys.

Suprarenal veins. The right suprarenal vein drains the adrenal gland on the right and empties into the inferior vena cava. The left suprarenal vein drains into the left renal vein.

Hepatic portal system. Like all portal systems, the hepatic portal system is a series of vessels in which two separate capillary beds lie between the arterial supply and the final venous drainage. In this case, the first capillary beds are in the stomach and intestines and drain into tributaries of the hepatic portal vein, which brings them to the second capillary bed in the liver. The short **hepatic portal vein** begins at the L_2 level. Numerous tributaries from the stomach and pancreas contribute to the hepatic portal system (Figure 19.29c), but the major vessels are as follows:

- **Superior mesenteric vein:** Drains the entire small intestine, part of the large intestine (ascending and transverse regions), and stomach.
- **Splenic vein:** Collects blood from the spleen, parts of the stomach and pancreas, and then joins the superior mesenteric vein to form the hepatic portal vein.
- **Inferior mesenteric vein:** Drains the distal portions of the large intestine and rectum and joins the splenic vein just before that vessel unites with the superior mesenteric vein to form the hepatic portal vein.

Hepatic veins. The right, left, and middle hepatic veins carry venous blood from the liver to the inferior vena cava.

Cystic veins. The cystic veins drain the gallbladder and join the portal veins in the liver.

Inferior phrenic veins. The inferior phrenic veins drain the inferior surface of the diaphragm.

Table 19.12 *(continued)*

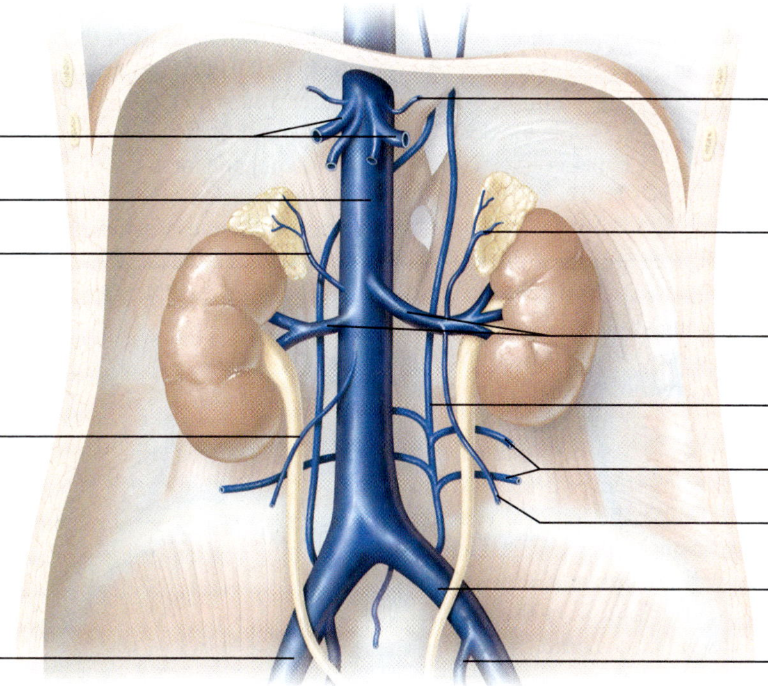

(b) Tributaries of the inferior vena cava. Venous drainage of abdominal organs not drained by the hepatic portal vein.

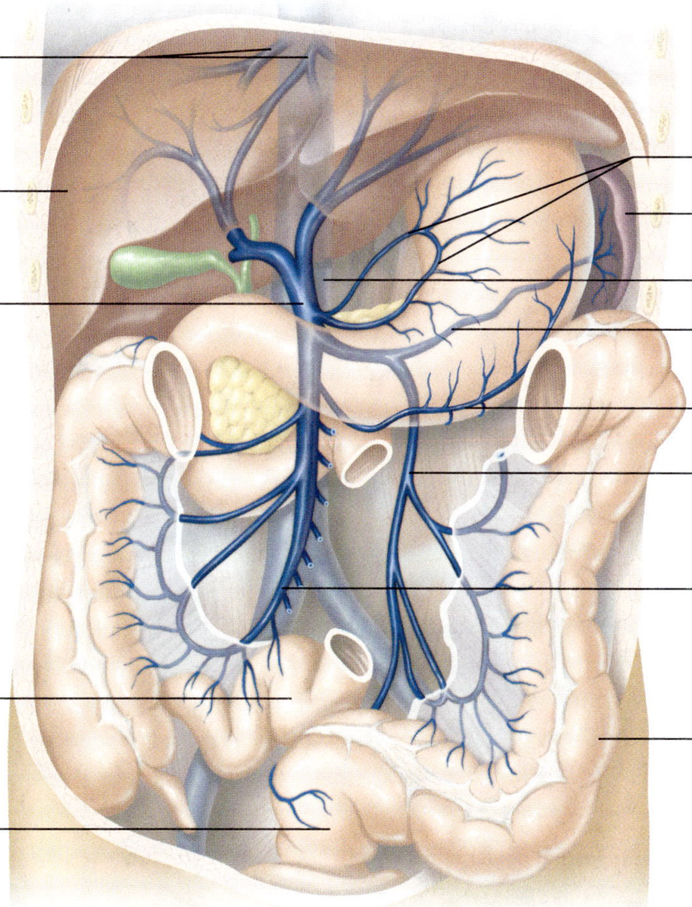

Figure 19.29 *(continued)*

(c) The hepatic portal circulation.

Table 19.13 Veins of the Pelvis and Lower Limbs

As in the upper limbs, most deep veins of the lower limbs have the same names as the arteries they accompany and many are double. Poorly supported by surrounding tissues, the two superficial saphenous veins (great and small) are common sites of varicosities. The great saphenous (*saphenous* = obvious) vein is frequently excised and used as a coronary bypass vessel.

Description and Areas Drained

Deep veins. After being formed by the union of the **medial** and **lateral plantar veins**, the **posterior tibial vein** ascends deep in the calf muscle and receives the **fibular (peroneal) vein** **(Figure 19.30)**. The **anterior tibial vein**, which is the superior continuation of the **dorsalis pedis vein** of the foot, unites at the knee with the posterior tibial vein to form the **popliteal vein**, which crosses the back of the knee. As the popliteal vein emerges from the knee, it becomes the **femoral vein**, which drains the deep structures of the thigh. The femoral vein becomes the **external iliac vein** as it enters the pelvis. In the pelvis, the external iliac vein unites with the **internal iliac vein** to form the **common iliac vein**. The distribution of the internal iliac veins parallels that of the internal iliac arteries.

Superficial veins. The **great** and **small saphenous veins** (sah-fe′nus) issue from the **dorsal venous arch** of the foot (Figure 19.30b and c). These veins anastomose frequently with each other and with the deep veins along their course. The great saphenous vein is the longest vein in the body. It travels superiorly along the medial aspect of the leg to the thigh, where it empties into the femoral vein just distal to the inguinal ligament. The small saphenous vein runs along the lateral aspect of the foot and then through the deep fascia of the calf muscles, which it drains. At the knee, it empties into the popliteal vein.

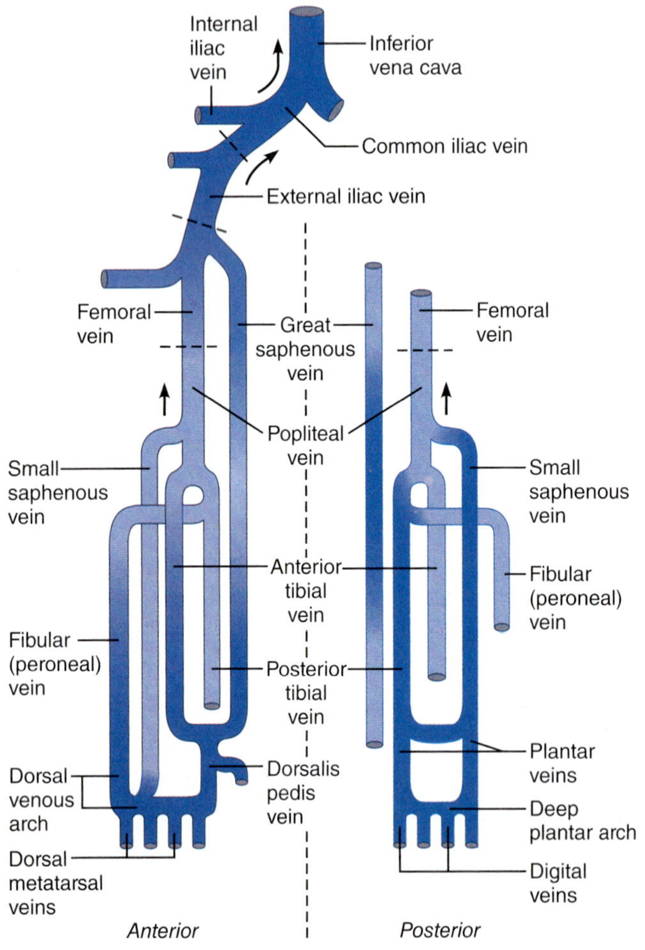

(a) Schematic flowchart of the anterior and posterior veins

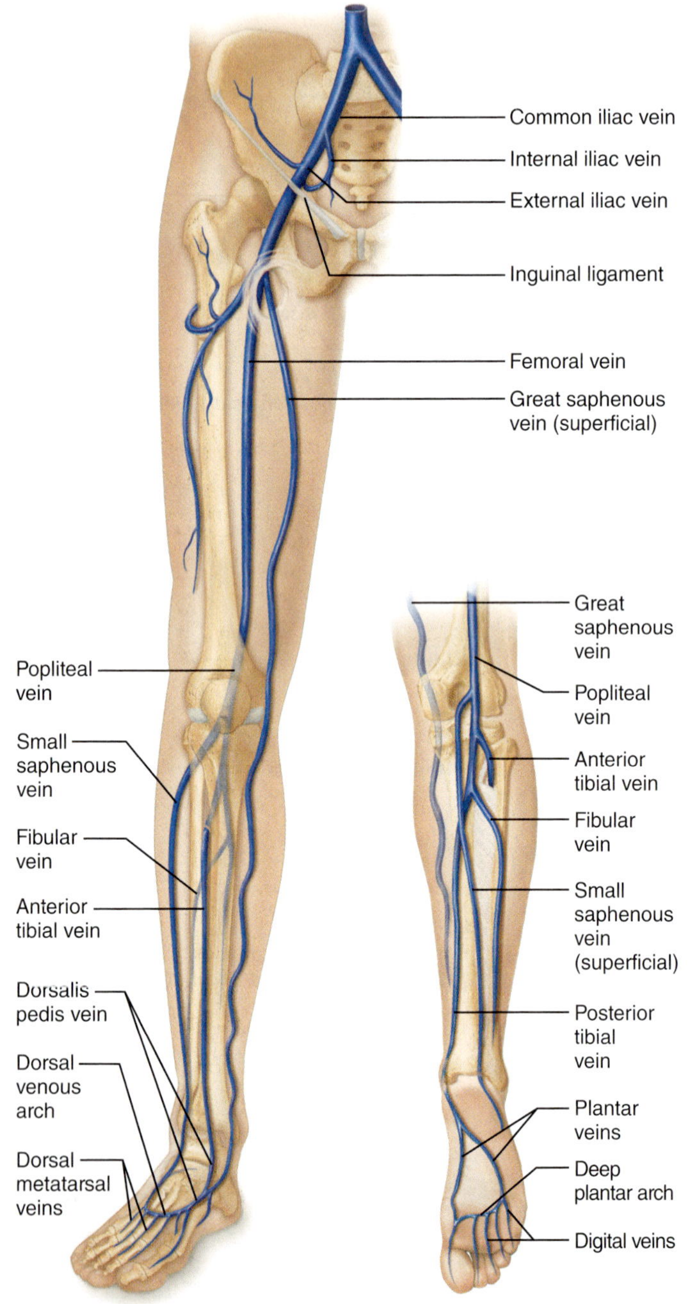

(b) Anterior view

(c) Posterior view

Figure 19.30 **Veins of the right lower limb.**

Check Your Understanding

21. What is a portal system? What is the function of the hepatic portal system?
22. Name the leg veins that often become varicosed.

For answers, see Appendix H.

Developmental Aspects of Blood Vessels

- Explain how blood vessels develop.
- Provide examples of changes that often occur in blood vessels as a person ages.

The endothelial lining of blood vessels is formed by mesodermal cells, which collect in little masses called **blood islands** throughout the microscopic embryo. These blood islands form fragile sprouting extensions that reach toward one another and toward the forming heart to lay down the rudimentary vascular tubes. Meanwhile, adjacent mesenchymal cells, stimulated by platelet-derived growth factor, surround the endothelial tubes, forming the stabilizing muscular and fibrous coats of the vessel walls.

How do blood vessels "know" where to grow? Many blood vessels simply follow the same guidance cues that nerves follow, which is why forming vessels often snuggle closely to nerves. Whether a vessel becomes an artery or a vein depends upon the local concentration of a differentiation factor called *vascular endothelial growth factor*. As noted in Chapter 18, the heart pumps blood through the rudimentary vascular system by the fourth week of development.

In addition to the fetal shunts that bypass the nonfunctional lungs (the *foramen ovale* and *ductus arteriosus*), other vascular modifications are found in the fetus. A special vessel, the *ductus venosus*, largely bypasses the liver. Also important are the *umbilical vein* and *arteries*, large vessels that circulate blood between the fetal circulation and the placenta where gas and nutrient exchanges occur with the mother's blood (see Chapter 28). Once the fetal circulatory pattern is laid down, few vascular changes occur until birth, when the umbilical vessels and shunts are occluded.

Unlike congenital heart diseases, congenital vascular problems are rare, and blood vessels are remarkably trouble-free during youth. Vessels form as needed to support body growth and wound healing, and to rebuild vessels lost each month during a woman's menstrual cycle. As we age, signs of vascular disease begin to appear. In some, the venous valves weaken, and purple, snakelike varicose veins appear. In others, more insidious signs of inefficient circulation appear: tingling fingers and toes and cramping muscles.

Although the degenerative process of atherosclerosis begins in youth, its consequences are rarely apparent until middle to old age, when it may precipitate a myocardial infarction or stroke. Until puberty, the blood vessels of boys and girls look alike, but from puberty to about age 45, women have strikingly less atherosclerosis than men because of the protective effects of estrogen. By enhancing nitric oxide production, inhibiting endothelin release, and blocking voltage-gated Ca^{2+} channels, estrogen reduces resistance to blood flow. Estrogen also stimulates the liver to produce enzymes that speed up catabolism of LDLs and increase the production of HDLs, thus reducing the risk of atherosclerosis (see *A Closer Look*).

Between the ages of 45 and 65, when estrogen production wanes in women, this "gap" between the sexes closes, and males and females above age 65 are equally at risk for cardiovascular disease. You might expect that giving postmenopausal women supplementary estrogen would maintain this protective effect. Surprisingly, clinical trials have shown that this is not the case.

Blood pressure changes with age. In a newborn baby, arterial pressure is about 90/55. Blood pressure rises steadily during childhood to finally reach the adult value (120/80). After age 40, the incidence of hypertension increases dramatically, as do associated illnesses such as heart attacks, strokes, vascular disease, and renal failure.

At least some vascular disease is a product of our modern technological culture. "Blessed" with high-protein and lipid-rich diets, empty-calorie snacks, energy-saving devices, and high-stress jobs, many of us are struck down prematurely. Lifestyle modifications—a healthy diet, regular aerobic exercise, and eliminating cigarette smoking—can help prevent cardiovascular disease. Poor diet, lack of exercise, and smoking are probably more detrimental to your blood vessels than aging itself could ever be!

Check Your Understanding

23. List three differences between systemic arteries and veins with respect to their general pathways and courses.
24. Name three fetal shunts that are occluded shortly after birth. Which structure does each shunt bypass?
25. List three common age-related vascular problems.

For answers, see Appendix H.

Now that we have described the structure and function of blood vessels, our survey of the cardiovascular system is complete. The pump, the plumbing, and the circulating fluid form a dynamic organ system that ceaselessly services every other organ system of the body, as summarized in *System Connections* on p. 746. However, our study of the circulatory system is still unfinished because we have yet to examine the lymphatic system, which acts with the cardiovascular system to ensure continuous circulation and to provide sites from which lymphocytes can police the body and provide immunity. These are the topics of Chapter 20.

Homeostatic Interrelationships Between the Cardiovascular System and Other Body Systems

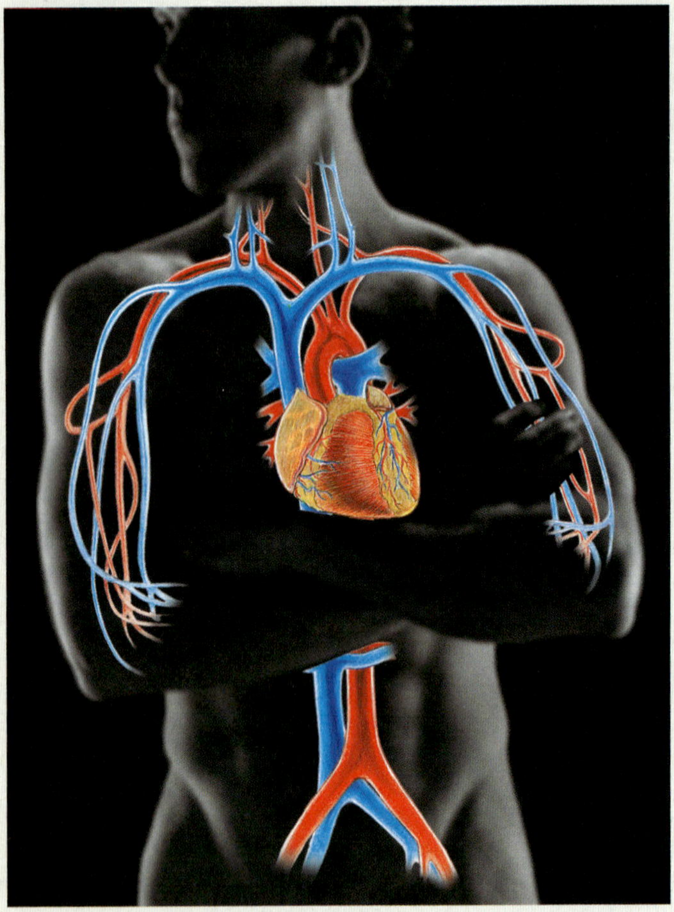

Integumentary System Chapter 5

- The cardiovascular system delivers oxygen and nutrients; carries away wastes
- The skin vasculature is an important blood reservoir and provides a site for heat loss from the body

Skeletal System Chapters 6–8

- The cardiovascular system delivers oxygen and nutrients; carries away wastes
- Bones are the sites of hematopoiesis; protect cardiovascular organs by enclosure; and provide a calcium depot

Muscular System Chapters 9–10

- The cardiovascular system delivers oxygen and nutrients; carries away wastes
- The muscle "pump" aids venous return; aerobic exercise enhances cardiovascular efficiency and helps prevent atherosclerosis

Nervous System Chapters 11–15

- The cardiovascular system delivers oxygen and nutrients; carries away wastes
- The ANS regulates cardiac rate and force; sympathetic division maintains blood pressure and controls blood flow to skin for thermoregulation

Endocrine System Chapter 16

- The cardiovascular system delivers oxygen and nutrients; carries away wastes; blood serves as a transport vehicle for hormones
- Various hormones influence blood pressure (epinephrine, ANP, angiotensin II, thyroxine, ADH); estrogen maintains vascular health in premenopausal women

Lymphatic System/Immunity Chapters 20–21

- The cardiovascular system delivers oxygen and nutrients to lymphatic organs, which house immune cells; provides transport medium for lymphocytes and antibodies; carries away wastes
- The lymphatic system picks up leaked fluid and plasma proteins and returns them to the cardiovascular system; immune cells protect cardiovascular organs from specific pathogens

Respiratory System Chapter 22

- The cardiovascular system delivers oxygen and nutrients; carries away wastes
- The respiratory system carries out gas exchange: loads oxygen and unloads carbon dioxide from the blood; respiratory "pump" aids venous return

Digestive System Chapter 23

- The cardiovascular system delivers oxygen and nutrients; carries away wastes
- The digestive system provides nutrients to the blood including iron and B vitamins essential for RBC (and hemoglobin) formation

Urinary System Chapters 25–26

- The cardiovascular system delivers oxygen and nutrients; carries away wastes; blood pressure drives filtration in the kidneys
- The urinary system helps regulate blood volume and pressure by altering urine volume and releasing renin

Reproductive System Chapter 27

- The cardiovascular system delivers oxygen and nutrients; carries away wastes
- Estrogen maintains vascular and osseous health in women

Chapter Summary

For more chapter study tools, go to the Study Area of MasteringA&P at **www.masteringaandp.com**.
There you will find:

- Interactive Physiology iP
- A&PFlix A&PFlix
- Practice Anatomy Lab PAL
- PhysioEx PEx
- Videos, Practice Quizzes and Tests, MP3 Tutor Sessions, Case Studies, and much more!

PART 1 Blood Vessel Structure and Function

1. Blood is transported throughout the body via a continuous system of blood vessels. Arteries transport blood away from the heart; veins carry blood back to the heart. Capillaries carry blood to tissue cells and are exchange sites.

Structure of Blood Vessel Walls (p. 693)

1. All blood vessels except capillaries have three layers: tunica intima, tunica media, and tunica externa. Capillary walls are composed of the tunica intima only.

Arterial System (pp. 693–696)

1. Elastic (conducting) arteries are the large arteries close to the heart that expand during systole, acting as pressure reservoirs, and then recoil during diastole to keep blood moving. Muscular (distributing) arteries carry blood to specific organs; they are less stretchy and more active in vasoconstriction. Arterioles regulate blood flow into capillary beds.
2. Atherosclerosis is a degenerative vascular disease that decreases the elasticity of arteries.

Capillaries (pp. 696–698)

1. Capillaries are microscopic vessels with very thin walls. Most exhibit intercellular clefts, which aid in the exchange between blood and interstitial fluid.
2. The most permeable capillaries are sinusoid capillaries (wide, tortuous channels). Fenestrated capillaries with pores are next most permeable. Least permeable are continuous capillaries, which lack pores.
3. Vascular shunts (metarteriole–thoroughfare channels) connect the terminal arteriole and postcapillary venule at opposite ends of a capillary bed. Most true capillaries arise from and rejoin the shunt channels. Precapillary sphincters regulate the amount of blood flowing into the true capillaries.

Venous System (pp. 698–699)

1. Veins have comparatively larger lumens than arteries, and a system of valves prevents backflow of blood.
2. Normally most veins are only partially filled; for this reason, they can serve as blood reservoirs.

Vascular Anastomoses (pp. 699–701)

1. The joining together of blood vessels to provide alternate channels in the same organ is called an anastomosis. Vascular anastomoses form between arteries, between veins, and between arterioles and venules.

iP Cardiovascular System; Topic: Anatomy Review: Blood Vessel Structure and Function, pp. 1–27.

PART 2 Physiology of Circulation

Introduction to Blood Flow, Blood Pressure, and Resistance (pp. 701–702)

1. Blood flow is the amount of blood flowing through a vessel, an organ, or the entire circulation in a given period of time. Blood pressure (BP) is the force per unit area exerted on a vessel wall by the contained blood. Resistance is opposition to blood flow; blood viscosity and blood vessel length and diameter contribute to resistance.
2. Blood flow is directly proportional to blood pressure and inversely proportional to resistance.

iP Cardiovascular System; Topic: Factors that Affect Blood Pressure, pp. 1–15.

Systemic Blood Pressure (pp. 702–704)

1. Systemic blood pressure is highest in the aorta and lowest in the venae cavae. The steepest drop in BP occurs in the arterioles, where resistance is greatest.
2. Arterial BP depends on compliance of the elastic arteries and on how much blood is forced into them. Arterial blood pressure is pulsatile, and peaks during systole; this is measured as systolic pressure. During diastole, as blood is forced distally in the circulation by the rebound of elastic arteries, arterial BP drops to its lowest value, called the diastolic pressure.
3. Pulse pressure is systolic pressure minus diastolic pressure. The mean arterial pressure (MAP) = diastolic pressure plus one-third of pulse pressure and is the pressure that keeps blood moving throughout the cardiac cycle.
4. Low capillary pressure (35 to 17 mm Hg) protects the delicate capillaries from rupture while still allowing adequate exchange across the capillary walls.
5. Venous pressure is nonpulsatile and low (declining to zero) because of the cumulative effects of resistance. Venous valves, large lumens, functional adaptations (muscular and respiratory pumps), and sympathetic nervous system activity promote venous return.

Maintaining Blood Pressure (pp. 704–711)

1. Blood pressure varies directly with CO, peripheral resistance (R), and blood volume. Vessel diameter is the major factor determining resistance, and small changes in the diameter of vessels (chiefly arterioles) significantly affect blood pressure.

iP Cardiovascular System; Topic: Measuring Blood Pressure, pp. 1–13.

2. BP is regulated by autonomic neural reflexes involving baroreceptors or chemoreceptors, the cardiovascular center (a medullary center that includes the cardiac and vasomotor centers), and autonomic fibers to the heart and vascular smooth muscle.
3. Activation of the receptors by falling BP (and to a lesser extent by a rise in blood CO_2, or falling blood pH or O_2 levels) stimulates the vasomotor center to increase vasoconstriction and the cardioacceleratory center to increase heart rate and contractility. Rising BP inhibits the vasomotor center (permitting vasodilation) and activates the cardioinhibitory center.

4. Higher brain centers (cerebrum and hypothalamus) may modify neural controls of BP via medullary centers.
5. Hormones that increase BP by promoting vasoconstriction include epinephrine and NE (these also increase heart rate and contractility), ADH, and angiotensin II (generated in response to renin release by kidney cells). Hormones that reduce BP by promoting vasodilation include atrial natriuretic peptide, which also causes a decline in blood volume.
6. The kidneys regulate blood pressure by regulating blood volume. Rising BP directly enhances filtrate formation and fluid losses in urine; falling BP causes the kidneys to retain more water, increasing blood volume.
7. Indirect renal regulation of blood volume involves the renin-angiotensin-aldosterone mechanism, a hormonal mechanism. When BP falls, the kidneys release renin, which triggers the formation of angiotensin II. Angiotensin II causes (1) release of aldosterone, stimulating salt and water retention, (2) vasoconstriction, (3) release of ADH, and (4) thirst.

iP Cardiovascular System; Topic: Blood Pressure Regulation, pp. 1–31.

8. Pulse and blood pressure measurements are used to assess cardiovascular efficiency.
9. The pulse is the alternating expansion and recoil of arterial walls with each heartbeat. Pulse points are also pressure points.
10. Blood pressure is routinely measured by the auscultatory method. Normal BP in adults is 120/80 mm Hg (systolic/diastolic).
11. Chronic hypertension (high blood pressure) is persistent BP readings of 140/90 or higher. It indicates increased peripheral resistance, which strains the heart and promotes vascular complications of other organs, particularly the eyes and kidneys. It is a major cause of myocardial infarction, stroke, and renal disease. Risk factors are high-fat, high-salt diet, obesity, diabetes mellitus, advanced age, smoking, stress, and being a member of the black race or a family with a history of hypertension.
12. Hypotension, or low blood pressure (below 90/60 mm Hg), is rarely a problem except in circulatory shock.

iP Cardiovascular System; Topic: Measuring Blood Pressure, pp. 11–12.

19

Blood Flow Through Body Tissues: Tissue Perfusion (pp. 711–720)

1. Blood flow is involved in delivering nutrients and wastes to and from cells, gas exchange, absorbing nutrients, and forming urine.
2. Blood flows fastest where the cross-sectional area of the vascular bed is least (aorta), and slowest where the total cross-sectional area is greatest (capillaries). The slow flow in capillaries allows time for nutrient-waste exchanges.
3. Autoregulation is the local adjustment of blood flow to individual organs based on their immediate requirements. It involves myogenic controls that maintain flow despite changes in blood pressure, and local chemical factors. Vasodilators include increased CO_2, H^+, and nitric oxide. Decreased O_2 concentrations also cause vasodilation. Other factors, including endothelins, decrease blood flow.

iP Cardiovascular; Topic: Autoregulation and Capillary Dynamics, pp. 1–13.

4. In most instances, autoregulation is controlled by the accumulation of local metabolites and the lack of oxygen. However, autoregulation in the brain is controlled primarily by a drop in pH and by myogenic mechanisms; and pulmonary circuit vessels dilate in response to high levels of oxygen.
5. Nutrients, gases, and other solutes smaller than plasma proteins cross the capillary wall by diffusion; larger molecules are actively transported via pinocytotic vesicles or caveolae. Water-soluble substances move through the clefts or fenestrations; fat-soluble substances pass through the lipid portion of the endothelial cell membrane.
6. Bulk flow of fluids at capillary beds determines the distribution of fluids between the bloodstream and the interstitial space. It reflects the relative effects of hydrostatic and osmotic pressures acting at the capillary (outward minus inward pressures). In general, fluid flows out of the capillary bed at the arterial end and reenters the capillary blood at the venule end.

iP Cardiovascular; Topic: Autoregulation and Capillary Dynamics, pp. 14–38.

7. Lymphatic vessels collect the small net loss of fluid and protein into the interstitial space and return it to the cardiovascular system.
8. Circulatory shock occurs when blood perfusion of body tissues is inadequate. Most cases of shock reflect low blood volume (hypovolemic shock), abnormal vasodilation (vascular shock), or pump failure (cardiogenic shock).

PART 3 Circulatory Pathways: Blood Vessels of the Body

The Two Main Circulations of the Body (p. 721)

1. The pulmonary circulation transports O_2-poor, CO_2-laden blood to the lungs for oxygenation and carbon dioxide unloading. Blood returning to the right atrium of the heart is pumped by the right ventricle to the lungs via the pulmonary trunk. Blood issuing from the lungs is returned to the left atrium by the pulmonary veins. (See Table 19.3 and Figure 19.19.)
2. The systemic circulation transports oxygenated blood from the left ventricle to all body tissues via the aorta and its branches. Venous blood returning from the systemic circuit is delivered to the right atrium via the venae cavae.

Systemic Arteries and Veins: Differences in Pathways and Courses (p. 721)

1. All arteries are deep while veins are both deep and superficial. Superficial veins tend to have numerous interconnections. Dural venous sinuses and the hepatic portal circulation are unique venous drainage patterns.

Principal Vessels of the Systemic Circulation (pp. 721–745)

1. Tables 19.3 to 19.13 and Figures 19.20 to 19.30 illustrate and describe vessels of the systemic circulation.

Developmental Aspects of Blood Vessels (p. 745)

1. The fetal vasculature develops from embryonic blood islands and mesenchyme and functions in blood delivery by the fourth week.
2. Fetal circulation differs from circulation after birth. The pulmonary and hepatic shunts and special umbilical vessels are normally occluded shortly after birth.
3. Blood pressure is low in infants and rises to adult values. Age-related vascular problems include varicose veins, hypertension, and atherosclerosis. Hypertension and associated atherosclerosis are the most important causes of cardiovascular disease in the aged.

Review Questions

Multiple Choice/Matching

(Some questions have more than one correct answer. Select the best answer or answers from the choices given.)

1. Which statement does not accurately describe veins? **(a)** Have less elastic tissue and smooth muscle than arteries, **(b)** contain more fibrous tissue than arteries, **(c)** most veins in the extremities have valves, **(d)** always carry deoxygenated blood.

2. Smooth muscle in the blood vessel wall **(a)** is found primarily in the tunica intima, **(b)** is mostly circularly arranged, **(c)** is most abundant in veins, **(d)** is usually innervated by the parasympathetic nervous system.

3. Peripheral resistance **(a)** is inversely proportional to the length of the vascular bed, **(b)** increases in anemia, **(c)** decreases in polycythemia, **(d)** is inversely related to the diameter of the arterioles.

4. Which of the following can lead to decreased venous return of blood to the heart? **(a)** an increase in blood volume, **(b)** an increase in venous pressure, **(c)** damage to the venous valves, **(d)** increased muscular activity.

5. Arterial blood pressure increases in response to **(a)** increasing stroke volume, **(b)** increasing heart rate, **(c)** atherosclerosis, **(d)** rising blood volume, **(e)** all of these.

6. Which of the following would *not* result in the dilation of the feeder arterioles and opening of the precapillary sphincters in systemic capillary beds? **(a)** a decrease in local tissue O_2 content, **(b)** an increase in local tissue CO_2, **(c)** a local increase in histamine, **(d)** a local increase in pH.

7. The structure of a capillary wall differs from that of a vein or an artery because **(a)** it has two tunics instead of three, **(b)** there is less smooth muscle, **(c)** it has a single tunic—only the tunica intima, **(d)** none of these.

8. The baroreceptors in the carotid sinus and aortic arch are sensitive to **(a)** a decrease in CO_2, **(b)** changes in arterial pressure, **(c)** a decrease in O_2, **(d)** all of these.

9. The myocardium receives its blood supply directly from the **(a)** aorta, **(b)** coronary arteries, **(c)** coronary sinus, **(d)** pulmonary arteries.

10. Blood flow in the capillaries is steady despite the rhythmic pumping of the heart because of the **(a)** elasticity of the large arteries, **(b)** small diameter of capillaries, **(c)** thin walls of the veins, **(d)** venous valves.

11. Using the letters from column B, match the artery descriptions in column A. (Note that some require more than a single choice.)

Column A	Column B
____ **(1)** unpaired branch of abdominal aorta	**(a)** right common carotid
	(b) superior mesenteric
____ **(2)** second branch of aortic arch	**(c)** left common carotid
	(d) external iliac
____ **(3)** branch of internal carotid	**(e)** inferior mesenteric
	(f) superficial temporal
____ **(4)** branch of external carotid	**(g)** celiac trunk
	(h) facial
____ **(5)** origin of femoral arteries	**(i)** ophthalmic
	(j) internal iliac

12. Tracing the blood from the heart to the right hand, we find that blood leaves the heart and passes through the aorta, the right subclavian artery, the axillary and brachial arteries, and through either the radial or ulnar artery to arrive at the hand. Which artery is missing from this sequence? **(a)** coronary, **(b)** brachiocephalic, **(c)** cephalic, **(d)** right common carotid.

13. Which of the following do not drain directly into the inferior vena cava? **(a)** inferior phrenic veins, **(b)** hepatic veins, **(c)** inferior mesenteric vein, **(d)** renal veins.

14. Suppose that at a given point along a capillary, the following forces exist: capillary hydrostatic pressure (HP_c) = 30 mm Hg, interstitial fluid hydrostatic pressure (HP_{if}) = 0 mm Hg, capillary colloid osmotic pressure (OP_c) = 25 mm Hg, and interstitial fluid colloid osmotic pressure (OP_{if}) = 2 mm Hg. The net filtration pressure at this point in the capillary is **(a)** 3 mm Hg, **(b)** −3 mm Hg, **(c)** −7 mm Hg, **(d)** 7 mm Hg.

Short Answer Essay Questions

15. How is the anatomy of capillaries and capillary beds well suited to their function?

16. Distinguish between elastic arteries, muscular arteries, and arterioles relative to location, histology, and functional adaptations.

17. Write an equation showing the relationship between peripheral resistance, blood flow, and blood pressure.

18. (a) Define blood pressure. Differentiate between systolic and diastolic blood pressure. (b) What is the normal blood pressure value for an adult?

19. Describe the neural mechanisms responsible for controlling blood pressure.

20. Explain the reasons for the observed changes in blood flow velocity in the different regions of the circulation.

21. How does the control of blood flow to the skin for the purpose of regulating body temperature differ from the control of nutrient blood flow to skin cells?

22. Describe neural and chemical (both systemic and local) effects exerted on the blood vessels when you are fleeing from a mugger. (Be careful, this is more involved than it appears at first glance.)

23. How are nutrients, wastes, and respiratory gases transported to and from the blood and tissue spaces?

24. (a) What blood vessels contribute to the formation of the hepatic portal circulation? (b) Why is a portal circulation a "strange" circulation?

25. Physiologists often consider capillaries and postcapillary venules together. (a) What functions do these vessels share? (b) Structurally, how do they differ?

Critical Thinking and Clinical Application Questions

1. Mrs. Johnson is brought to the emergency room after being involved in an auto accident. She is hemorrhaging and has a rapid, thready pulse, but her blood pressure is still within normal limits. Describe the compensatory mechanisms that act to maintain her blood pressure in the face of blood loss.

2. A 60-year-old man is unable to walk more than 100 yards without experiencing severe pain in his left leg; the pain is relieved by resting for 5–10 minutes. He is told that the arteries of his leg are becoming occluded with fatty material and is advised to have the sympathetic nerves serving that body region severed. Explain how such surgery might help to relieve this man's problem.

3. Your friend Joanie, who knows little about science, is reading a magazine article about a patient who had an "aneurysm at the base of his brain that suddenly grew much larger." The surgeons' first goal was to "keep it from rupturing," and the second goal was to "relieve the pressure on the brain stem and cranial nerves." The surgeons were able to "replace the aneurysm with a section of plastic tubing," so the patient recovered. Joanie asks you what all this means. Explain. (Hint: Check this chapter's Related Clinical Terms below.)

4. The Agawam High School band is playing some lively marches while the coaches are giving pep talks to their respective football squads. Although it is September, it is unseasonably hot (88°F/31°C) and the band uniforms are wool. Suddenly, Harry the tuba player becomes light-headed and faints. Explain his fainting in terms of vascular events.
5. When we are cold or the external temperature is low, most venous blood returning from the distal part of the arm travels in the deep veins where it picks up heat (by countercurrent exchange) from the nearby brachial artery en route. However, when we are hot, and especially during exercise, venous return from the distal arm travels in the superficial veins and those veins tend to bulge superficially in a person who is working out. Explain why venous return takes a different route in the second situation.
6. Edema (swelling due to an increase in interstitial fluid) is a common clinical problem. On one of your first days of an introductory clinical experience, you encounter four patients who all have severe edema for different reasons. Your challenge is to explain the cause of the edema. In each case, try to explain the edema in terms of either an increase or a decrease in one of the four pressures that causes bulk flow at capillaries (see Figure 19.17).
   (1) First you encounter Mrs. Taylor in the medical ward awaiting a liver transplant. What is the connection between liver failure and her edema? (Hint: Think about the liver's role in producing plasma proteins.)
   (2) Next you follow a resident to the obstetric ward, where Mrs. So is experiencing premature labor. Which of the pressures that drive bulk flow might be altered here? (Hint: What might the expanded uterus be pressing on?)
   (3) Then you are called to emergency, where Mr. Herrera is in anaphylactic shock. In anaphylactic shock, the capillaries become leaky, allowing plasma proteins that are normally kept inside the blood vessels to escape into the interstitial fluid. Which of the pressures driving bulk flow is altered in this case and in what direction is the change?
   (4) Finally, you go to the oncology ward where Mrs. O'Leary is recovering from surgery for advanced breast cancer that had infiltrated her right breast and axillary lymph nodes. All of her axillary lymph nodes were removed and unfortunately, this severed most of the lymphatic vessels draining her right arm. You notice that her right arm is quite edematous. Why? Mrs. O'Leary is given a compression sleeve to wear on this arm to help relieve the edema. Which of the pressures driving bulk flow at the capillaries will be altered by the compression sleeve?

AT THE CLINIC

Related Clinical Terms

19

Aneurysm (an′u-rizm; *aneurysm* = a widening) A balloonlike outpocketing of an artery wall that places the artery at risk for rupture; most often reflects gradual weakening of the artery by chronic hypertension or atherosclerosis. The most common sites of aneurysms are the abdominal aorta and arteries feeding the brain and kidneys.

Angiogram (an′je-o-gram″; *angio* = a vessel; *gram* = writing) Diagnostic technique involving the infusion of a radiopaque substance into the circulation for X-ray examination of specific blood vessels. The major technique for diagnosing coronary artery occlusion and risk of a heart attack.

Diuretic (*diure* = urinate) A chemical that promotes urine formation, thus reducing blood volume. Diuretic drugs are frequently prescribed to manage hypertension.

Phlebitis (flĕ-bi′tis; *phleb* = vein; *itis* = inflammation) Inflammation of a vein accompanied by painful throbbing and redness of the skin over the inflamed vessel. It is most often caused by bacterial infection or local physical trauma.

Phlebotomy (flĕ-bot′o-me; *tomy* = cut) A venous incision or puncture made for the purpose of withdrawing blood or bloodletting.

Sclerotherapy Procedure for removing varicose or spider veins. Tiny needles are used to inject hardening agents into the abnormal vein. The vein scars, closes down, and is absorbed by the body.

Thrombophlebitis Condition of undesirable intravascular clotting initiated by a roughened venous lining; often follows severe episodes of phlebitis. An ever-present danger is that the clot may detach and form an embolus.

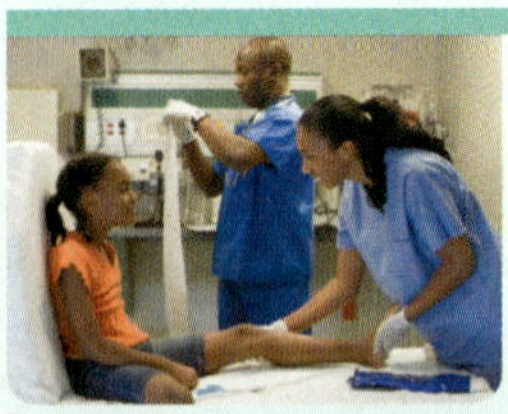

Case Study Cardiovascular System: Blood Vessels

Mr. Hutchinson, another middle-aged victim of the collision on Route 91, has a tourniquet around his thigh when admitted in an unconscious state to Noble Hospital. The emergency technician who brings him in states that his right lower limb was pinned beneath the bus for at least 30 minutes. He is immediately scheduled for surgery. Admission notes include the following:

- Multiple contusions of lower limbs
- Compound fracture of the right tibia; bone ends covered with sterile gauze
- Right leg blanched and cold, no pulse
- Blood pressure 90/48; pulse 140/min and thready; patient diaphoretic (sweaty)

1. Relative to what you have learned about tissue requirements for oxygen, what is the condition of the tissues in the right lower limb?
2. Will the fracture be attended to, or will Mr. Hutchinson's other homeostatic needs take precedence? Explain your answer choice and predict his surgical treatment.
3. What do you conclude regarding Mr. Hutchinson's cardiovascular measurements (pulse and BP), and what measures do you expect will be taken to remedy the situation before commencing surgery?

(Answers in Appendix H)

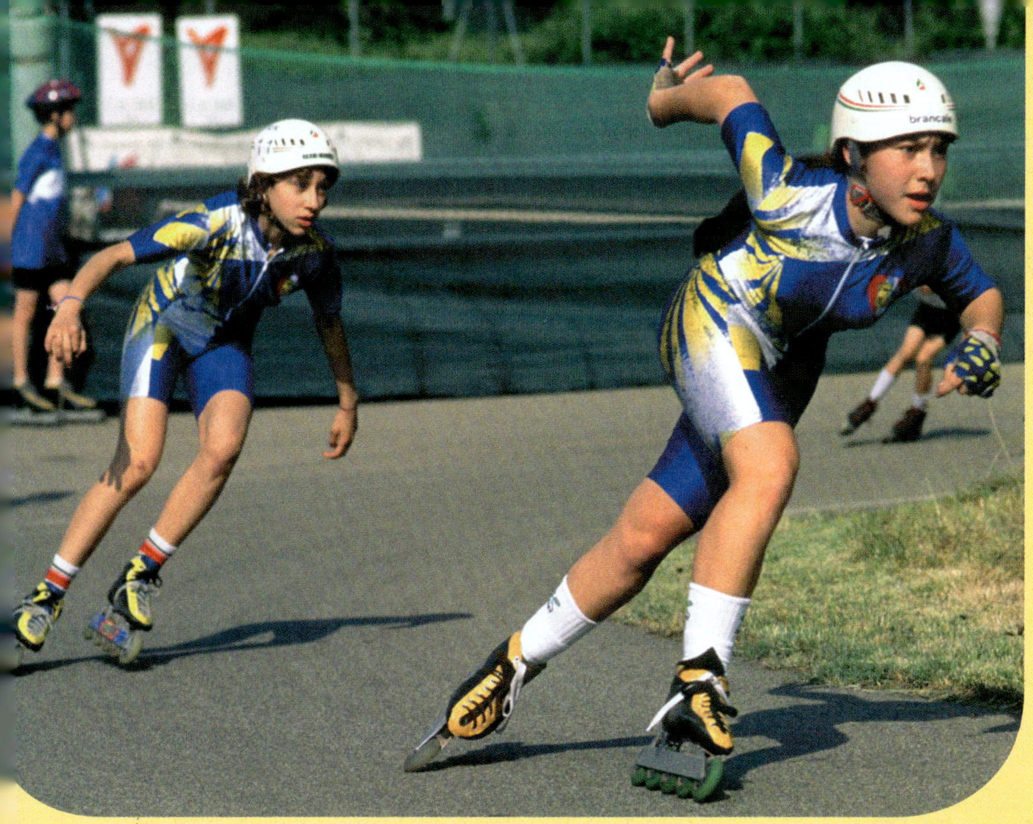

20

The Lymphatic System and Lymphoid Organs and Tissues

They can't all be superstars! When we mentally tick off the names of the body's organ systems, the lymphatic (lim-fat′ik) system and the lymphoid organs and tissues are probably not the first to come to mind. Yet if they failed their quiet background work, our cardiovascular system would stop working and our immune system would be hopelessly impaired.

This chapter is a bit unusual in that we will explore two functionally different but structurally overlapping systems, the *lymphatic system* and the *lymphoid organs and tissues*. The **lymphatic system** returns fluids that have leaked from the blood vascular system back to the blood. It actually consists of three parts:

- A meandering network of *lymphatic vessels*
- *Lymph*, the fluid contained in those vessels
- *Lymph nodes* that cleanse the lymph as it passes through them

The **lymphoid organs and tissues** provide the structural basis of the immune system. These organs and tissues house phagocytic cells and lymphocytes, which play essential roles in the body's defense mechanisms and its resistance to disease. These structures include the spleen, thymus, tonsils, and other lymphoid tissues scattered throughout the body. The lymph nodes are also part of this system, and like a keystone, they have important roles to play in both the lymphoid organs and tissues and the lymphatic system.

Let's begin by looking at the lymphatic system.

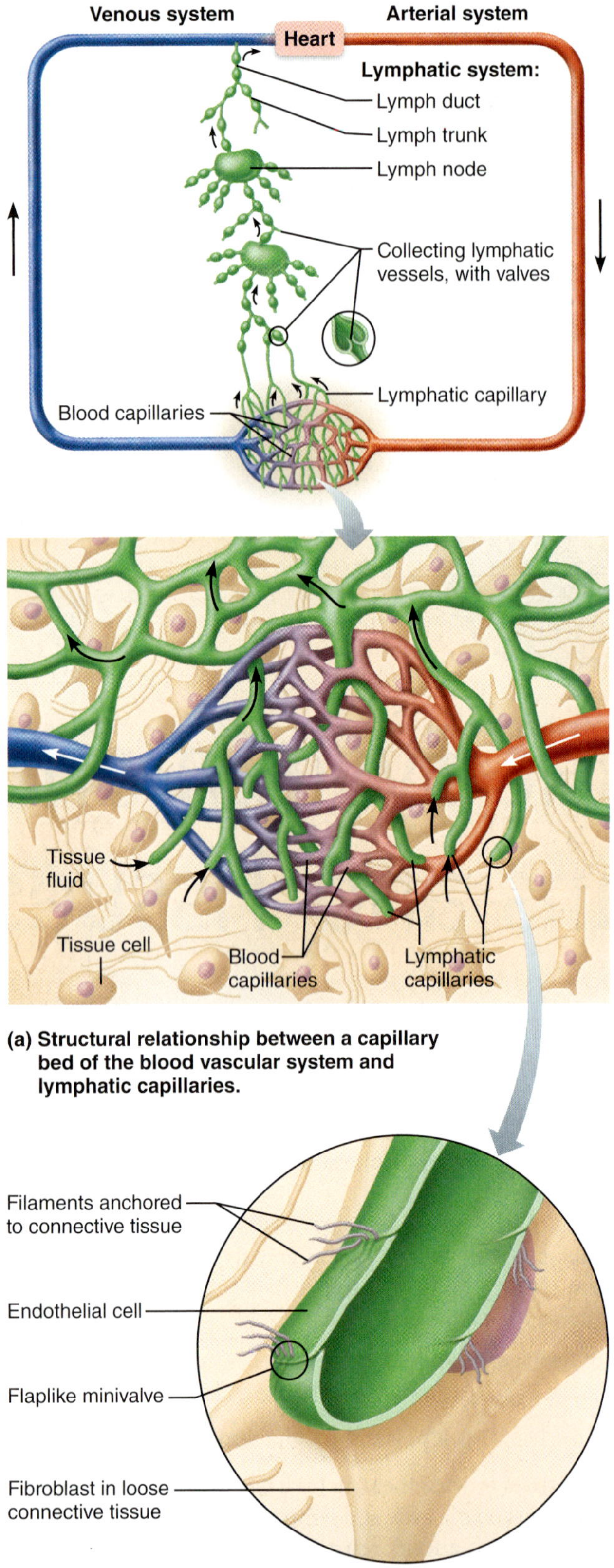

(a) Structural relationship between a capillary bed of the blood vascular system and lymphatic capillaries.

(b) Lymphatic capillaries are blind-ended tubes in which adjacent endothelial cells overlap each other, forming flaplike minivalves.

Figure 20.1 Distribution and special features of lymphatic capillaries. Arrows in (a) indicate direction of fluid movement.

Lymphatic System

✓ List the functions of the lymphatic vessels.

✓ Describe the structure and distribution of lymphatic vessels.

✓ Describe the source of lymph and mechanism(s) of lymph transport.

As blood circulates through the body, nutrients, wastes, and gases are exchanged between the blood and the interstitial fluid. As we explained in *Focus on Bulk Flow Across Capillaries* (Figure 19.17 on pp. 718–719), the hydrostatic and colloid osmotic pressures operating at capillary beds force fluid out of the blood at the arterial ends of the beds ("upstream") and cause most of it to be reabsorbed at the venous ends ("downstream"). The fluid that remains behind in the tissue spaces, as much as 3 L daily, becomes part of the interstitial fluid.

This leaked fluid, plus any plasma proteins that escape from the bloodstream, must somehow be returned to the blood to ensure that the cardiovascular system has sufficient blood volume to operate properly. This problem of circulatory dynamics is resolved by the **lymphatic vessels**, or **lymphatics**, elaborate networks of drainage vessels that collect the excess protein-containing interstitial fluid and return it to the bloodstream. Once interstitial fluid enters the lymphatic vessels, it is called **lymph** (*lymph* = clear water).

Distribution and Structure of Lymphatic Vessels

The lymphatic vessels form a one-way system in which lymph flows only toward the heart.

Lymphatic Capillaries

The transport of lymph begins in microscopic blind-ended **lymphatic capillaries (Figure 20.1a)**. These capillaries weave between the tissue cells and blood capillaries in the loose connective tissues of the body. Lymphatic capillaries are widespread, but they are absent from bones and teeth, bone marrow, and the entire central nervous system (where the excess tissue fluid drains into the cerebrospinal fluid).

Although similar to blood capillaries, lymphatic capillaries are so remarkably permeable that they were once thought to be open at one end like a straw. We now know that they owe their permeability to two unique structural modifications:

- The endothelial cells forming the walls of lymphatic capillaries are not tightly joined. Instead, the edges of adjacent cells overlap each other loosely, forming easily opened, flaplike *minivalves* (Figure 20.1b).
- Collagen filaments anchor the endothelial cells to surrounding structures so that any increase in interstitial fluid volume opens the minivalves, rather than causing the lymphatic capillaries to collapse.

So, what we have is a system analogous to one-way swinging doors in the lymphatic capillary wall. When fluid pressure in the interstitial space is greater than the pressure in the lymphatic capillary, the minivalve flaps gape open, allowing fluid to enter the lymphatic capillary. However, when the pressure is greater

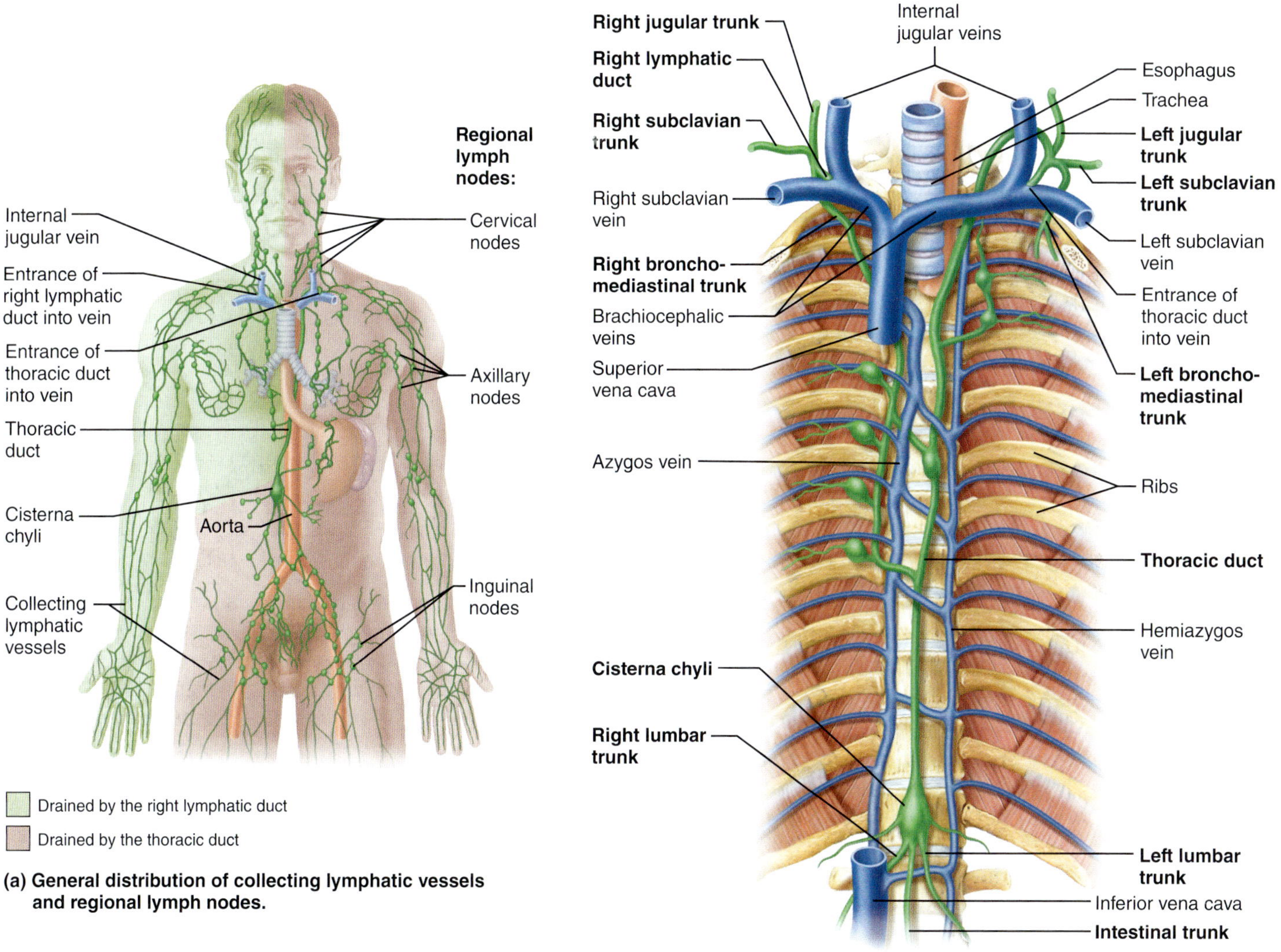

(a) General distribution of collecting lymphatic vessels and regional lymph nodes.

(b) Major lymphatic trunks and ducts in relation to veins and surrounding structures. Anterior view of thoracic and abdominal wall.

Figure 20.2 The lymphatic system.

20

inside the lymphatic capillary, it forces the endothelial minivalve flaps shut, preventing lymph from leaking back out as the pressure moves it along the vessel.

Proteins in the interstitial space are unable to enter blood capillaries, but they enter lymphatic capillaries easily. In addition, when tissues become inflamed, lymphatic capillaries develop openings that permit uptake of even larger particles such as cell debris, pathogens (disease-causing microorganisms such as bacteria and viruses), and cancer cells. The pathogens can then use the lymphatics to travel throughout the body. This threat to the body is partly resolved by the fact that the lymph "detours" through the lymph nodes, where it is cleansed of debris and "examined" by cells of the immune system.

A special set of lymphatic capillaries called **lacteals** (lak′te-alz) transports absorbed fat from the small intestine to the bloodstream. Lacteals are so called because of the milky white lymph that drains through them (*lact* = milk). This fatty lymph, called **chyle** ("juice"), drains from the fingerlike villi of the intestinal mucosa.

Larger Lymphatic Vessels

From the lymphatic capillaries, lymph flows through successively larger and thicker-walled channels—first collecting vessels, then trunks, and finally the largest of all, the ducts (Figure 20.1). The **collecting lymphatic vessels** have the same three tunics as veins, but the collecting vessels have thinner walls and more internal valves, and they anastomose more. In general, lymphatics in the skin travel along with superficial *veins*, while the deep lymphatic vessels of the trunk and digestive viscera travel with the deep *arteries*. The exact anatomical distribution of lymphatic vessels varies greatly between individuals, even more than it does for veins.

The largest collecting vessels unite to form **lymphatic trunks**, which drain fairly large areas of the body. The major trunks, named mostly for the regions from which they drain lymph, are the paired **lumbar**, **bronchomediastinal**, **subclavian**, and **jugular trunks**, and the single **intestinal trunk** (**Figure 20.2b**).

Lymph is eventually delivered to one of two large *ducts* in the thoracic region. The **right lymphatic duct** drains lymph from the right upper limb and the right side of the head and thorax (Figure 20.2a). The much larger **thoracic duct** receives lymph from the rest of the body. It arises anterior to the first two lumbar vertebrae as an enlarged sac, the **cisterna chyli** (sis-ter′nah ki′li), that collects lymph from the two large lumbar trunks that drain the lower limbs and from the intestinal trunk that drains the digestive organs. As the thoracic duct runs superiorly, it receives lymphatic drainage from the left side of the thorax, left upper limb, and the left side of the head. Each terminal duct empties its lymph into the venous circulation at the junction of the internal jugular vein and subclavian vein on its own side of the body (Figure 20.2b).

Homeostatic Imbalance 20.1

Like the larger blood vessels, the larger lymphatics receive their nutrient blood supply from a branching vasa vasorum. When lymphatic vessels are severely inflamed, the related vessels of the vasa vasorum become congested with blood. As a result, the pathway of the associated superficial lymphatics becomes visible through the skin as red lines that are tender to the touch. This unpleasant condition is called *lymphangitis* (lim″fan-ji′tis; *angi* = vessel). +

Lymph Transport

The lymphatic system lacks an organ that acts as a pump. Under normal conditions, lymphatic vessels are low-pressure conduits, and the same mechanisms that promote venous return in blood vessels act here as well—the milking action of active skeletal muscles, pressure changes in the thorax during breathing, and valves to prevent backflow. Lymphatic vessels are usually bundled together in connective tissue sheaths along with blood vessels, and pulsations of nearby arteries also promote lymph flow. In addition to these mechanisms, smooth muscle in the walls of all but the smallest lymphatic vessels contracts rhythmically, helping to pump the lymph along.

Even so, lymph transport is sporadic and slow. Movement of adjacent tissues is extremely important in propelling lymph through the lymphatics. When physical activity or passive movements increase, lymph flows much more rapidly (balancing the greater rate of fluid loss from the blood in such situations). For this reason, it is a good idea to immobilize a badly infected body part to hinder flow of inflammatory material from that region.

Homeostatic Imbalance 20.2

Anything that prevents the normal return of lymph to the blood—such as when tumors block the lymphatics or lymphatics are removed during cancer surgery—results in short-term but severe localized edema (*lymphedema*). Usually, however, the vessels remaining in the area grow and drainage is reestablished. +

To summarize, the lymphatic vessels:

- Return excess tissue fluid to the bloodstream
- Return leaked proteins to the blood
- Carry absorbed fat from the intestine to the blood (through lacteals)

Check Your Understanding

1. What is lymph? Where does it come from?
2. Name two lymphatic ducts and indicate the body regions usually drained by each.
3. What is the driving force for lymph movement?

For answers, see Appendix H.

Lymphoid Cells and Tissues

✓ Describe the basic structure and cellular population of lymphoid tissue. Differentiate between diffuse and follicular lymphoid tissues.

In order to understand the role of the lymphoid organs in the body, let's investigate their components—lymphoid cells and lymphoid tissues—before considering the organs themselves.

Lymphoid Cells

The lymphoid cells consist of immune system cells found in lymphoid tissues together with the supporting cells that form the "scaffolding" of those tissues.

Lymphocytes, the main warriors of the immune system, arise in red bone marrow (along with other formed elements). They then mature into one of the two main varieties of lymphocytes—**T cells (T lymphocytes)** or **B cells (B lymphocytes)**—that protect the body against antigens. (*Antigens* are anything that provokes an immune response, such as bacteria and their toxins, viruses, mismatched RBCs, or cancer cells.) Activated T cells manage the immune response, and some of them directly attack and destroy infected cells. B cells protect the body by producing **plasma cells**, daughter cells that secrete antibodies into the blood (or other body fluids). Antibodies mark antigens for destruction by phagocytes or other means. Chapter 21 explores the roles of the lymphocytes in immunity.

Macrophages play a crucial role in body protection and the immune response by phagocytizing foreign substances and by helping to activate T cells. So, too, do the spiny-looking **dendritic cells** that capture antigens and bring them back to the lymph nodes.

Last but not least are the **reticular cells**, fibroblast-like cells that produce the reticular fiber **stroma** (stro′mah), which is the network that supports the other cell types in lymphoid organs and tissues (**Figure 20.3**).

Lymphoid Tissue

Lymphoid tissue is an important component of the immune system, mainly because it (1) houses and provides a proliferation site for lymphocytes and (2) furnishes an ideal surveillance vantage point for lymphocytes and macrophages.

Lymphoid tissue, largely composed of a type of loose connective tissue called **reticular connective tissue**, dominates all the lymphoid organs except the thymus. Macrophages live on the fibers of the reticular connective tissue network. Huge numbers of lymphocytes squeeze through the walls of postcapillary

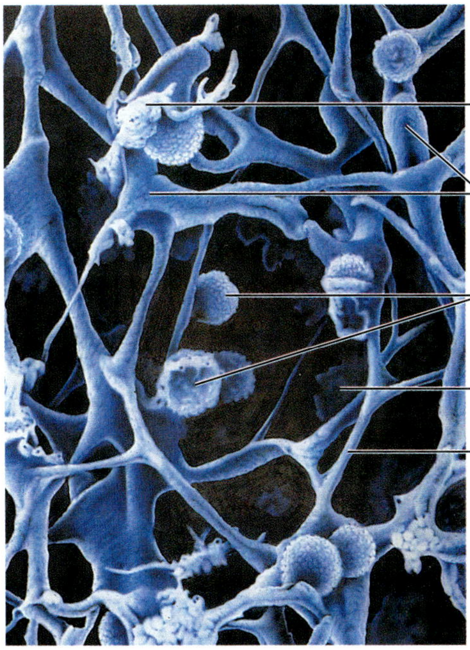

Figure 20.3 Reticular connective tissue in a human lymph node. Scanning electron micrograph (690×).

venules coursing through this network and temporarily occupy its spaces (Figure 20.3). Then, they leave to patrol the body again. The cycling of lymphocytes between the circulatory vessels, lymphoid tissues, and loose connective tissues of the body ensures that lymphocytes reach infected or damaged sites quickly.

Lymphoid tissue comes in various "packages," such as diffuse lymphoid tissue and lymphoid follicles.

- **Diffuse lymphoid tissue**—a loose arrangement of lymphoid cells and some reticular fibers—is found in virtually every body organ. Larger collections appear in the lamina propria of mucous membranes such as those lining the digestive tract.
- **Lymphoid follicles (lymphoid nodules)** are solid, spherical bodies consisting of tightly packed lymphoid cells and reticular fibers. Follicles often have lighter-staining **germinal centers** where proliferating B cells predominate. These centers enlarge dramatically when the B cells are dividing rapidly and producing plasma cells. In many cases, the follicles form part of larger lymphoid organs, such as lymph nodes. However, isolated aggregations of lymphoid follicles occur in the intestinal wall as Peyer's patches (aggregated lymphoid nodules) and in the appendix (see p. 759).

Lymph Nodes

✓ Describe the general location, histological structure, and functions of lymph nodes.

The principal lymphoid organs in the body are the **lymph nodes**, which cluster along the lymphatic vessels of the body. There are hundreds of these small organs, but because they are usually embedded in connective tissue, they are not ordinarily visible. Large clusters of lymph nodes occur near the body surface in the inguinal, axillary, and cervical regions, places where the collecting lymphatic vessels converge to form trunks (see Figure 20.2a).

Lymph nodes have two basic functions, both concerned with body protection:

- **Filtration.** As lymph is transported back to the bloodstream, the lymph nodes act as lymph "filters." Macrophages in the nodes remove and destroy microorganisms and other debris that enter the lymph from the loose connective tissues, preventing them from being delivered to the blood and spreading to other parts of the body.
- **Immune system activation.** Lymph nodes and other lymphoid organs are strategically located sites where lymphocytes encounter antigens and are activated to mount an attack against them. Let's look at how the structure of a lymph node supports its defensive functions.

Structure of a Lymph Node

Lymph nodes vary in shape and size, but most are bean shaped and less than 2.5 cm (1 inch) in length. Each node is surrounded by a dense fibrous **capsule** from which connective tissue strands called **trabeculae** extend inward to divide the node into a number of compartments **(Figure 20.4)**. The node's internal framework, or stroma, of reticular fibers physically supports its ever-changing population of lymphocytes.

A lymph node has two histologically distinct regions, the **cortex** and the **medulla**. The superficial part of the cortex contains densely packed follicles, many with germinal centers heavy with dividing B cells. Dendritic cells nearly encapsulate the follicles and abut the deeper part of the cortex, which primarily houses T cells in transit. The T cells circulate continuously between the blood, lymph nodes, and lymph, performing their surveillance role.

Medullary cords are thin inward extensions from the cortical lymphoid tissue, and contain both types of lymphocytes. Throughout the node are **lymph sinuses**, large lymph capillaries spanned by crisscrossing reticular fibers. Numerous macrophages reside on these reticular fibers and phagocytize foreign matter in the lymph as it flows by in the sinuses. Additionally, some of the lymph-borne antigens in the percolating lymph leak into the surrounding lymphoid tissue, where they activate lymphocytes to mount an immune attack against them.

Circulation in the Lymph Nodes

Lymph enters the convex side of a lymph node through a number of **afferent lymphatic vessels**. It then moves through a large, baglike sinus, the **subcapsular sinus**, into a number of smaller sinuses that cut through the cortex and enter the medulla. The lymph meanders through these **medullary sinuses** and finally exits the node at its **hilum** (hi′lum), the indented region on the concave side, via **efferent lymphatic vessels**.

There are fewer efferent vessels draining the node than afferent vessels feeding it, so the flow of lymph through the node

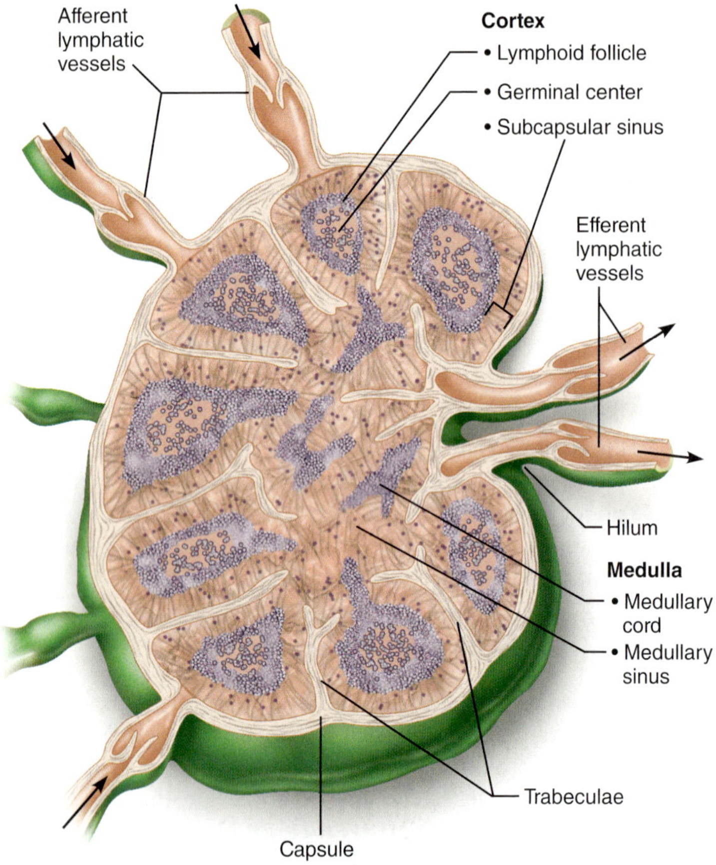

(a) Longitudinal view of the internal structure of a lymph node and associated lymphatics

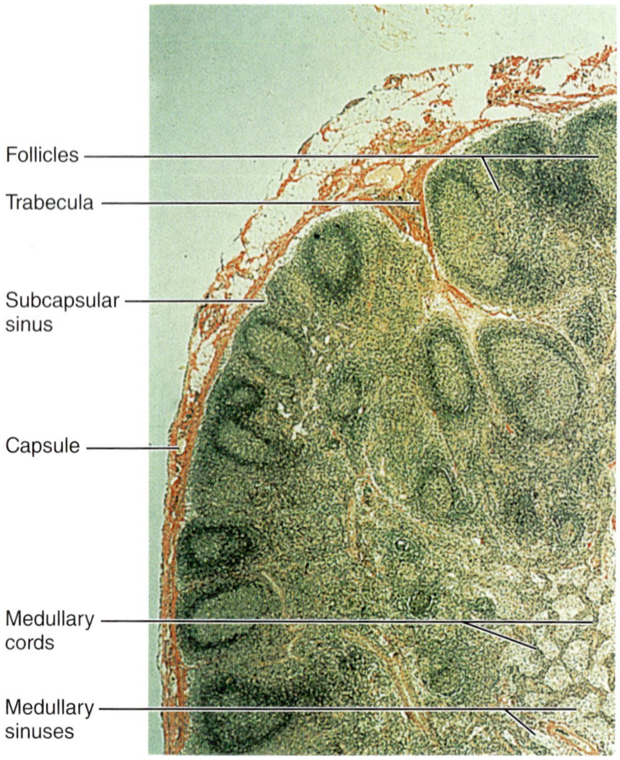

(b) Photomicrograph of part of a lymph node (72×)

Figure 20.4 Lymph node. In (a), notice that several afferent lymphatics converge on its convex side, whereas fewer efferent lymphatics exit at its hilum.

20

stagnates somewhat, allowing time for the lymphocytes and macrophages to carry out their protective functions. Lymph passes through several nodes before it is completely cleansed.

Homeostatic Imbalance 20.3

Sometimes lymph nodes are overwhelmed by the agents they are trying to destroy. For example, when large numbers of bacteria are trapped in the nodes, the nodes become inflamed, swollen, and tender to the touch, a condition often referred to (erroneously) as swollen "glands." Such infected lymph nodes are called *buboes* (bu′bōz). (Buboes are the most obvious symptom of bubonic plague, the "Black Death" that killed much of Europe's population in the late Middle Ages.)

Lymph nodes can also become secondary cancer sites, particularly when metastasizing cancer cells enter lymphatic vessels and become trapped there. Cancer-infiltrated lymph nodes are swollen but usually not painful, a fact that helps distinguish cancerous nodes from those infected by microorganisms. ✚

Check Your Understanding

4. What is a lymphoid follicle? What type of lymphocyte predominates in follicles, especially in their germinal centers?

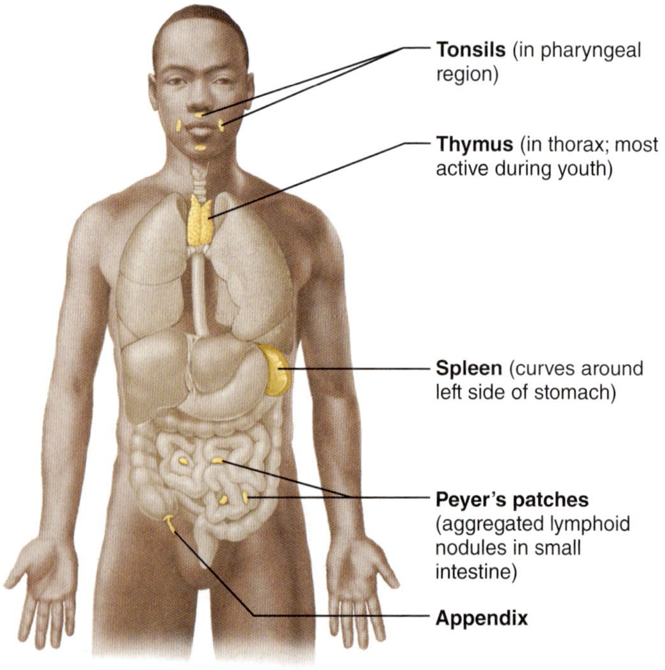

Figure 20.5 Lymphoid organs.

5. What is the benefit of having fewer efferent than afferent lymphatics in lymph nodes?

For answers, see Appendix H.

Other Lymphoid Organs

✓ Name and describe the other lymphoid organs of the body. Compare and contrast them with lymph nodes, structurally and functionally.

Lymph nodes are just one example of the many types of **lymphoid organs**, or aggregates of lymphoid tissue, in the body. Others are the spleen, thymus, tonsils, and Peyer's patches (aggregated lymphoid nodules) of the small intestine **(Figure 20.5)**, as well as bits of lymphoid tissue scattered in the connective tissues.

What do all these organs have in common? Except for the thymus, all are composed of reticular connective tissue. Although all lymphoid organs help protect the body, only the lymph nodes filter lymph. The other lymphoid organs and tissues typically have efferent lymphatics draining them, but lack afferent lymphatics.

Spleen

The soft, blood-rich **spleen** is about the size of a fist and is the largest lymphoid organ. Located in the left side of the abdominal cavity just beneath the diaphragm, it curls around the anterior aspect of the stomach (Figure 20.5 and **Figure 20.6**). It is served by the large *splenic artery* and *vein*, which enter and exit the *hilum* on its slightly concave anterior surface.

The spleen provides a site for lymphocyte proliferation and immune surveillance and response. But perhaps even more

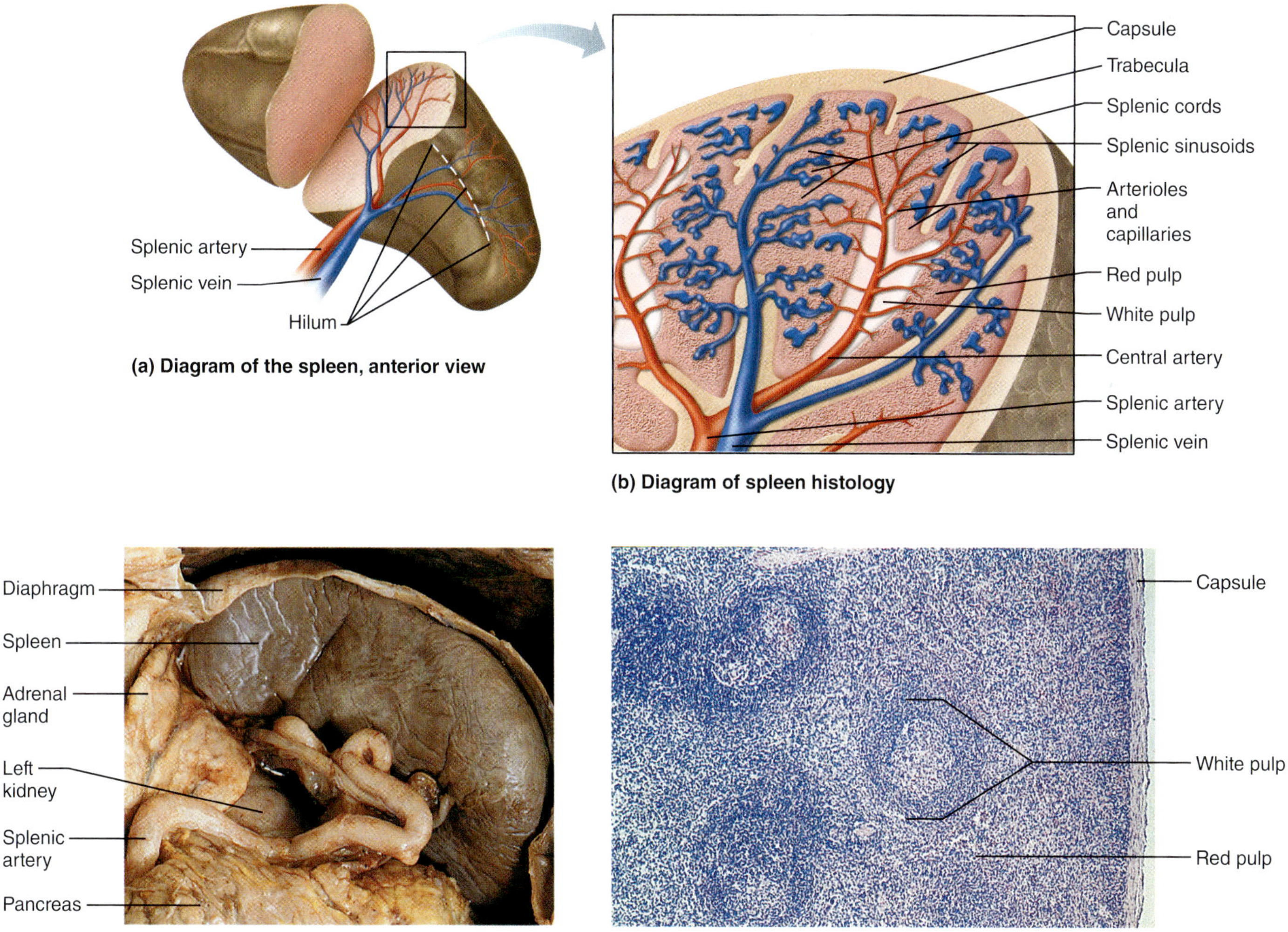

(a) Diagram of the spleen, anterior view

(b) Diagram of spleen histology

(c) Photograph of the spleen in its normal position in the abdominal cavity, anterior view.

(d) Photomicrograph of spleen tissue (30×). The white pulp, a lymphoid tissue with many lymphocytes, is surrounded by red pulp containing abundant erythrocytes.

Figure 20.6 The spleen. (For a related image, see *A Brief Atlas of the Human Body*, Plate 39.)

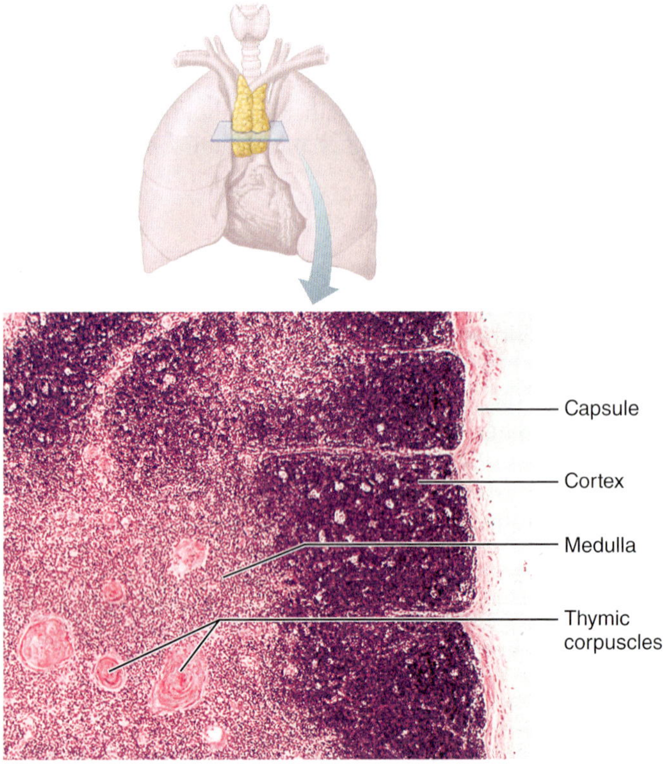

Figure 20.7 The thymus. The photomicrograph of a portion of the thymus shows part of a lobule with cortical and medullary regions (85×).

important are its blood-cleansing functions. Besides extracting aged and defective blood cells and platelets from the blood, its macrophages remove debris and foreign matter from blood flowing through its sinuses. The spleen also performs three additional, and related, functions. The spleen:

- Stores some of the breakdown products of red blood cells for later reuse (for example, it salvages iron for making hemoglobin). It releases other breakdown products to the blood for processing by the liver.
- Stores blood platelets and monocytes for release into the blood when needed.
- May be a site of erythrocyte production in the fetus (a capability that normally ceases before birth).

20

Like lymph nodes, the spleen is surrounded by a fibrous capsule and has trabeculae that extend inward. Histologically, the spleen consists of two components: white pulp and red pulp.

- **White pulp** is where immune functions take place, so it is composed mostly of lymphocytes suspended on reticular fibers. The white pulp clusters or forms "cuffs" around central arteries (small branches of the splenic artery) in the organ and forms what appear to be islands in a sea of red pulp.
- **Red pulp** is where worn-out red blood cells and bloodborne pathogens are destroyed, so it contains huge numbers of erythrocytes and the macrophages that engulf them. It is essentially all splenic tissue that is not white pulp. It consists of **splenic cords**, regions of reticular connective tissue, that separate the blood-filled **splenic sinusoids** (venous sinuses).

The names of the pulp regions reflect their appearance in fresh spleen tissue rather than their staining properties. Indeed, as you can see in the photomicrograph in Figure 20.6d, the white pulp sometimes appears darker than the red pulp due to the darkly staining nuclei of the densely packed lymphocytes.

Homeostatic Imbalance 20.4

Because the spleen's capsule is relatively thin, a direct blow or severe infection may cause it to rupture, spilling blood into the peritoneal cavity. Once, *splenectomy* (surgical removal of the ruptured spleen) was the standard treatment and thought necessary to prevent life-threatening hemorrhage and shock. However, surgeons have discovered that, if left alone, the spleen can often repair itself and so the frequency of emergency splenectomies has decreased dramatically at major trauma centers. If the spleen must be removed, the liver and bone marrow take over most of its functions. In children younger than 12, the spleen will regenerate if a small part of it is left in the body. ✚

Thymus

The bilobed **thymus** (thi′mus) has important functions primarily during the early years of life. It is found in the inferior neck and extends into the superior thorax, where it partially overlies the heart deep to the sternum (see Figure 20.5 and **Figure 20.7**). In the thymus, T lymphocyte precursors mature to become immunocompetent lymphocytes. In other words, the thymus is where T lymphocytes become able to defend us against specific pathogens in the immune response.

Prominent in newborns, the thymus continues to increase in size during the first year, when it is highly active. After puberty, it starts to atrophy gradually and by old age it has been replaced almost entirely by fibrous and fatty tissue and is difficult to distinguish from surrounding connective tissue. Even though it atrophies, the thymus continues to produce immunocompetent cells as we age, although at a declining rate.

To understand thymic histology, it helps to compare the thymus to a cauliflower head—the flowerets represent *thymic lobules*, each containing an outer cortex and an inner medulla (Figure 20.7). Most thymic cells are lymphocytes. In the cortical regions the rapidly dividing lymphocytes are densely packed, with a few macrophages scattered among them.

The lighter-staining medullary areas contain fewer lymphocytes plus some bizarre structures called **thymic corpuscles**. Consisting of concentric whorls of keratinized epithelial cells, they were thought to be sites of T cell destruction. Recent evidence suggests that thymic corpuscles are involved in the development of *regulatory T cells*, a class of T lymphocytes that are important for preventing autoimmune responses.

The thymus differs from other lymphoid organs in three important ways:

- The thymus has no follicles because it lacks B cells.
- The thymus is the only lymphoid organ that does not *directly* fight antigens. Instead, the thymus functions strictly as

a maturation site for T lymphocyte precursors. These precursors must be kept isolated from foreign antigens to prevent their premature activation. In fact, there is a *blood thymus barrier* that keeps bloodborne antigens out of the thymus.

- The stroma of the thymus consists of epithelial cells rather than reticular fibers. These epithelial cells provide the physical and chemical environment in which T lymphocytes mature.

Mucosa-Associated Lymphoid Tissue (MALT)

Mucosa-associated lymphoid tissues (**MALT**) are a set of distributed lymphoid tissues strategically located in mucous membranes throughout the body (see Figure 4.11 on p. 141 to review mucous membranes). MALT helps protect us from the never-ending onslaught of pathogens that seek to enter our bodies. Here we will consider the largest collections of MALT—the tonsils, Peyer's patches, and appendix. In addition to these large named collections, MALT also occurs in the mucosa of the respiratory and genitourinary organs as well as the rest of the digestive tract.

Tonsils

The **tonsils** form a ring of lymphoid tissue around the entrance to the pharynx (throat), where they appear as swellings of the mucosa (**Figure 20.8** and Figure 22.3). The tonsils are named according to location.

- The paired **palatine tonsils** are located on either side at the posterior end of the oral cavity. These are the largest tonsils and the ones most often infected.
- The **lingual tonsil** is the collective term for a lumpy collection of lymphoid follicles at the base of the tongue.
- The **pharyngeal tonsil** (referred to as the *adenoids* if enlarged) is in the posterior wall of the nasopharynx.
- The tiny **tubal tonsils** surround the openings of the auditory tubes into the pharynx.

The tonsils gather and remove many of the pathogens entering the pharynx in food or in inhaled air.

The lymphoid tissue of the tonsils contains follicles with obvious germinal centers surrounded by diffusely scattered lymphocytes. The tonsils are not fully encapsulated, and the epithelium overlying them invaginates deep into their interior, forming blind-ended **tonsillar crypts** (Figure 20.8). The crypts trap bacteria and particulate matter, and the bacteria work their way through the mucosal epithelium into the lymphoid tissue, where most are destroyed. It seems a bit dangerous to "invite" infection this way, but this strategy produces a wide variety of immune cells that have a "memory" for the trapped pathogens. In other words, the body takes a calculated risk early on (during childhood) for the benefits of heightened immunity and better health later.

Peyer's Patches

Peyer's patches (pi′erz), or **aggregated lymphoid nodules**, are large clusters of lymphoid follicles, structurally similar to the tonsils. They are located in the wall of the distal portion of the small intestine (Figure 20.5 and **Figure 20.9**).

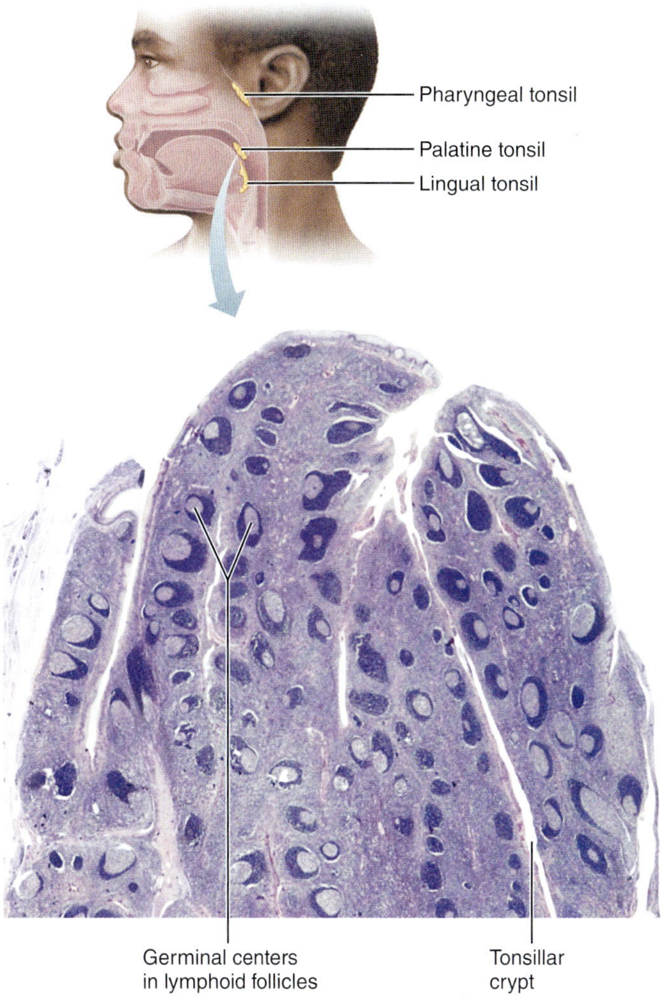

Figure 20.8 Histology of the palatine tonsil. The exterior surface of the tonsil is covered by stratified squamous epithelium, which invaginates deeply to form tonsillar crypts (10×).

Appendix

The **appendix** is a tubular offshoot of the first part of the large intestine and contains a high concentration of lymphoid follicles. Like Peyer's patches, the appendix is in an ideal position (1) to destroy bacteria (which are present in large numbers in the intestine) before these pathogens can breach the intestinal wall, and (2) to generate many "memory" lymphocytes for long-term immunity.

Developmental Aspects of the Lymphatic System and Lymphoid Organs and Tissues

✓ Outline the development of the lymphatic system and the lymphoid organs and tissues.

By the fifth week of embryonic development, the beginnings of the lymphatic vessels and the main clusters of lymph nodes are apparent. These arise as **lymph sacs** that bud from developing veins.

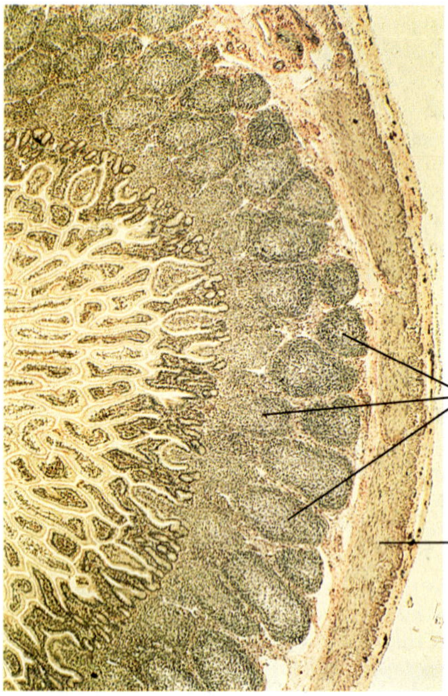

Figure 20.9 Peyer's patch (aggregated lymphoid nodules). Cross section of wall of the ileum of the small intestine (20×).

The first of these, the *jugular lymph sacs*, arise at the junctions of the internal jugular and subclavian veins and form a branching system of lymphatic vessels throughout the thorax, upper extremities, and head. The two main connections of the jugular lymph sacs to the venous system are retained and become the right lymphatic duct and, on the left, the superior part of the thoracic duct. Caudally the elaborate system of abdominal lymphatics buds largely from the primitive inferior vena cava. The lymphatics of the pelvic region and lower extremities form from sacs on the iliac veins.

Except for the thymus, which is an endodermal derivative, the lymphoid organs develop from mesodermal mesenchymal cells that migrate to particular body sites and develop into reticular tissue. The thymus, the first lymphoid organ to appear, forms as an outgrowth of the lining of the primitive pharynx. It then detaches and migrates caudally to the thorax where it becomes infiltrated with lymphocyte precursors derived from hematopoietic tissues elsewhere in the embryo's body.

Except for the spleen and tonsils, the lymphoid organs are poorly developed before birth. Shortly after birth, they become heavily populated by lymphocytes, and their development parallels the maturation of the immune system.

☑ Check Your Understanding

6. What is MALT? List several components of MALT.
7. List several functions of the spleen.
8. Which lymphoid organ develops first?

For answers, see Appendix H.

Although the functions of the lymphatic vessels and lymphoid organs overlap, each helps maintain body homeostasis in unique ways, as summarized in *System Connections*. The lymphatic vessels help maintain blood volume. The macrophages of lymphoid organs remove and destroy foreign matter in lymph and blood. Additionally, lymphoid organs and tissues provide sites from which the immune system can be mobilized. In Chapter 21, we continue this story as we examine the inflammatory and immune responses that allow us to resist a constant barrage of pathogens.

Chapter Summary

20

MAP™ For more chapter study tools, go to the Study Area of MasteringA&P at **www.masteringaandp.com**.

There you will find:

- Interactive Physiology iP
- A&PFlix A&PFlix
- Practice Anatomy Lab PAL
- PhysioEx PEx
- Videos, Practice Quizzes and Tests, MP3 Tutor Sessions, Case Studies, and much more!

1. Lymphatic vessels, lymph nodes, and lymph make up the lymphatic system. Lymphatic vessels return fluids that have leaked from the blood vascular system back to the blood. Lymphoid organs and tissues protect the body by removing foreign material from the lymph and blood streams, and provide a site for immune surveillance.

Lymphatic System (pp. 752–754)

Distribution and Structure of Lymphatic Vessels (pp. 752–754)

1. Lymphatic vessels form a one-way network—lymphatic capillaries, collecting vessels, trunks, and ducts—in which fluid flows only toward the heart. The right lymphatic duct drains lymph from the right arm and right side of the upper body; the thoracic duct receives lymph from the rest of the body. These ducts empty into the blood vascular system at the junction of the internal jugular and subclavian veins in the neck.
2. Lymphatic capillaries are exceptionally permeable, admitting proteins and particulate matter from the interstitial space.
3. Pathogens and cancer cells may spread through the body via the lymphatic stream.

Lymph Transport (pp. 754)

4. The flow of lymphatic fluid is slow; it is maintained by skeletal muscle contraction, pressure changes in the thorax, and contractions of the lymphatic vessels. Valves prevent backflow.

iP Immune System; Topic: Anatomy Review, pp. 7–9.

Homeostatic Interrelationships Between the Lymphatic System/Immunity and Other Body Systems

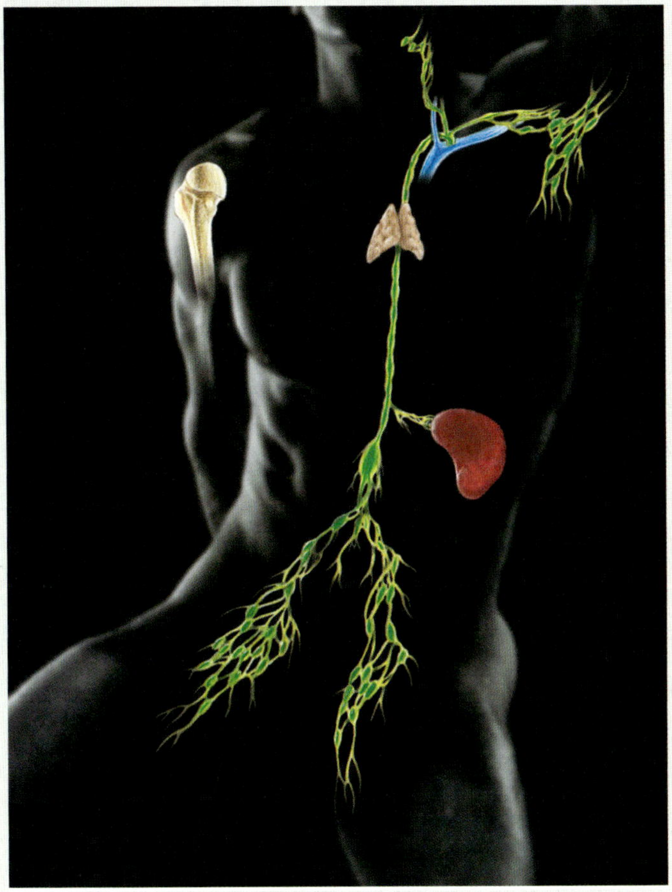

Nervous System Chapters 11–15

- Lymphatic vessels pick up leaked plasma fluid and proteins in PNS structures; immune cells protect PNS structures from specific pathogens
- The nervous system innervates larger lymphatics; opiate neuropeptides influence immune functions; the brain helps regulate immune response

Endocrine System Chapter 16

- Lymphatic vessels pick up leaked fluids and proteins; lymph helps distribute hormones; immune cells protect endocrine organs
- Stress hormones depress immune activity; the thymus produces hormones and paracrines that are involved in the maturation of T cells

Cardiovascular System Chapters 17–19

- Lymphatic vessels pick up leaked plasma and proteins; spleen removes and destroys aged RBCs and debris, and stores iron and platelets; immune cells protect cardiovascular organs from specific pathogens
- Blood is the source of lymph; lymphatics develop from veins; blood circulates immune elements

Respiratory System Chapter 22

- Lymphatic vessels pick up leaked fluids and proteins from respiratory organs; immune cells protect respiratory organs from specific pathogens; the tonsils and plasma cells in the respiratory mucosa (which secrete the antibody IgA) prevent pathogen invasion
- The lungs provide O_2 needed by lymphoid/immune cells and eliminate CO_2; the pharynx houses the tonsils; respiratory "pump" aids lymph flow

Digestive System Chapter 23

- Lymphatic vessels pick up leaked fluids and proteins from digestive organs; lymph transports some products of fat digestion to the blood; lymphoid follicles in the intestinal wall prevent invasion of pathogens
- The digestive system digests and absorbs nutrients needed by cells of lymphoid organs; gastric acidity inhibits pathogens' entry into blood

Urinary System Chapters 25–26

- Lymphatic vessels pick up leaked fluid and proteins from urinary organs; immune cells protect urinary organs from specific pathogens
- Urinary system eliminates wastes and maintains homeostatic balances of water, pH, and electrolytes in the blood for lymphoid/immune cell functioning; urine flushes some pathogens out of the urinary tract

Reproductive System Chapter 27

- Lymphatic vessels pick up leaked fluid and proteins; immune cells protect against pathogens
- Reproductive organs' hormones may influence immune functioning; acidity of vaginal secretions is bacteriostatic

Integumentary System Chapter 5

- Lymphatic vessels pick up leaked plasma fluid and proteins from the dermis; lymphocytes in lymphoid organs and tissues enhance the skin's protective role by defending against specific pathogens via the immune response
- The skin's keratinized epithelium provides a mechanical barrier to pathogens; epithelial dendritic cells and dermal macrophages act as antigen presenters in the immune response; acid pH of skin secretions inhibits growth of bacteria on the skin

Skeletal System Chapters 6–8

- Lymphatic vessels pick up leaked plasma fluid and proteins from the periostea; immune cells protect bones from pathogens
- The bones house hematopoietic tissue which produces the lymphocytes (and macrophages) that populate lymphoid organs and provide immunity

Muscular System Chapters 9–10

- Lymphatic vessels pick up leaked fluids and proteins; immune cells protect muscles from pathogens
- The skeletal muscle "pump" aids the flow of lymph; shivering produces heat at the beginning of a fever

Lymphoid Cells and Tissues (pp. 754–755)

Lymphoid Cells (p. 754)

1. The cells in lymphoid tissues include lymphocytes (cells called T cells or B cells), plasma cells (antibody-producing offspring of B cells), macrophages and dendritic cells (cells that capture antigens and initiate an immune response), and reticular cells that form the lymphoid tissue stroma.

Lymphoid Tissue (pp. 754–755)

2. Lymphoid tissue is reticular connective tissue. It houses macrophages and a continuously changing population of lymphocytes. It is an important element of the immune system.
3. Lymphoid tissue may be diffuse or packaged into dense follicles. Follicles often display germinal centers (areas where B cells are proliferating).

iP Immune System; Topic: Anatomy Review, pp. 4–5

Lymph Nodes (pp. 755–757)

1. Lymph nodes, the principal lymphoid organs, are clustered along lymphatic vessels. Lymph nodes filter lymph and help activate the immune system.

Structure of a Lymph Node (p. 755)

2. Each lymph node has a fibrous capsule, a cortex, and a medulla. The cortex contains mostly lymphocytes, which act in immune responses; the medulla contains macrophages, which engulf and destroy viruses, bacteria, and other foreign debris, as well as lymphocytes and plasma cells.

Circulation in the Lymph Nodes (pp. 755–757)

3. Lymph enters the lymph nodes via afferent lymphatic vessels and exits via efferent vessels. There are fewer efferent vessels; therefore, lymph flow stagnates within the lymph node, allowing time for its cleansing.

iP Immune System; Topic: Anatomy Review, pp. 10–12.

Other Lymphoid Organs (pp. 757–759)

1. Unlike lymph nodes, the spleen, thymus, tonsils, and Peyer's patches do not filter lymph. Most lymphoid organs contain both macrophages and lymphocytes.

Spleen (pp. 757–758)

2. The spleen provides a site for lymphocyte proliferation and immune function, and destroys aged or defective red blood cells and bloodborne pathogens. It also stores and releases the breakdown products of hemoglobin as necessary, stores platelets, and acts as a hematopoietic site in the fetus.

Thymus (pp. 758–759)

3. The thymus is most functional during youth. The thymus provides the environment in which T lymphocytes mature and become immunocompetent.

Mucosa-Associated Lymphoid Tissue (MALT) (p. 759)

4. Peyer's patches of the intestinal wall, lymphoid follicles of the appendix, tonsils of the pharynx and oral cavity, and follicles in the genitourinary and respiratory tract mucosae are known as MALT (mucosa-associated lymphoid tissue). They prevent pathogens in these passages from penetrating the mucous membrane lining.

iP Immune System; Topic: Anatomy Review, pp. 13–14, 16–20.

Developmental Aspects of the Lymphatic System and Lymphoid Organs and Tissues (pp. 759–760)

1. Lymphatics develop as outpocketings of developing veins. The thymus develops from endoderm; the other lymphoid organs derive from mesenchymal cells of mesoderm.
2. The thymus is the first lymphoid organ to develop.
3. Lymphoid organs are populated by lymphocytes, which arise from hematopoietic tissue.

20

Review Questions

Multiple Choice/Matching

(Some questions have more than one correct answer. Select the best answer or answers from the choices given.)

1. Lymphatic vessels **(a)** serve as sites for immune surveillance, **(b)** filter lymph, **(c)** transport leaked plasma proteins and fluids to the cardiovascular system, **(d)** are represented by vessels that resemble arteries, capillaries, and veins.
2. The saclike initial portion of the thoracic duct is the **(a)** lacteal, **(b)** right lymphatic duct, **(c)** cisterna chyli, **(d)** lymph sac.
3. Entry of lymph into the lymphatic capillaries is promoted by which of the following? **(a)** one-way minivalves formed by overlapping endothelial cells, **(b)** the respiratory pump, **(c)** the skeletal muscle pump, **(d)** greater fluid pressure in the interstitial space.
4. The structural framework of lymphoid organs is **(a)** areolar connective tissue, **(b)** hematopoietic tissue, **(c)** reticular tissue, **(d)** adipose tissue.
5. Lymph nodes are densely clustered in all of the following body areas *except* **(a)** the brain, **(b)** the axillae, **(c)** the groin, **(d)** the cervical region.
6. The germinal centers in lymph nodes are largely sites of **(a)** macrophages, **(b)** proliferating B lymphocytes, **(c)** T lymphocytes, **(d)** all of these.
7. The red pulp areas of the spleen are sites of **(a)** splenic sinusoids, macrophages, and red blood cells, **(b)** clustered lymphocytes, **(c)** connective tissue septa.
8. The lymphoid organ that functions primarily during youth and then begins to atrophy is the **(a)** spleen, **(b)** thymus, **(c)** palatine tonsils, **(d)** bone marrow.
9. Collections of lymphoid tissue (MALT) that guard mucosal surfaces include all of the following except **(a)** appendix follicles, **(b)** the tonsils, **(c)** Peyer's patches, **(d)** the thymus.

Short Answer Essay Questions

10. Compare and contrast blood, interstitial fluid, and lymph.
11. Compare the structure and functions of a lymph node to those of the spleen.
12. (a) Which anatomical characteristic ensures that the flow of lymph through a lymph node is slow? (b) Why is this desirable?
13. There are no lymphatic arteries. Why isn't this a problem?

Critical Thinking and Clinical Application Questions

1. Mrs. Jackson, a 59-year-old woman, has undergone a left radical mastectomy (removal of the left breast and left axillary lymph nodes and vessels). Her left arm is severely swollen and painful, and she is unable to raise it to more than shoulder height. (a) Explain her signs and symptoms. (b) Can she expect to have relief from these symptoms in time? How so?
2. A friend tells you that she has tender, swollen "glands" along the left side of the front of her neck. You notice that she has a bandage on her left cheek that is not fully hiding a large infected cut there. Exactly what are her swollen "glands," and how did they become swollen?
3. Once almost a rite of childhood, tonsillectomy (surgical removal of the tonsils) is now rarely performed. Similarly, while ruptured spleens were once routinely removed, they are now conserved whenever possible. Why should these lymphoid organs be preserved when possible?

AT THE CLINIC

Related Clinical Terms

Elephantiasis (el″lĕ-fan-ti′ah-sis) Typically a tropical disease in which the lymphatics (particularly those of the lower limbs and scrotum) become clogged with parasitic roundworms, an infectious condition called filariasis. Swelling (due to edema) reaches enormous proportions.

Hodgkin's lymphoma A malignancy of lymphoid tissue; symptoms include swollen, nonpainful lymph nodes, fatigue, and often intermittent fever and night sweats. Characterized by presence of giant malignantly transformed B cells called Reed-Sternberg cells. Infection with Epstein-Barr virus (see mononucleosis below) and genetic susceptibility appear to be predisposing factors. Treated with chemotherapy and radiation; high cure rate.

Lymphadenopathy (lim-fad″ĕ-nop′ah-the; *adeno* = a gland; *pathy* = disease) Any disease of the lymph nodes.

Lymphangiography (lim-fan″je-og′rah-fe) Diagnostic procedure in which the lymphatic vessels are injected with radiopaque dye and then visualized with X rays.

Lymphoma Any neoplasm (tumor) of the lymphoid tissue, whether benign or malignant.

Mononucleosis A viral disease common in adolescents and young adults; symptoms include fatigue, fever, sore throat, and swollen lymph nodes. Caused by the Epstein-Barr virus, which is transmitted in saliva ("kissing disease") and specifically attacks B lymphocytes. This attack leads to a massive activation of T lymphocytes, which in turn attack the virus-infected B cells. Large numbers of oversized T lymphocytes circulate in the bloodstream. (These lymphocytes were originally misidentified as monocytes: *mononucleosis* = a condition of monocytes.) Usually lasts four to six weeks.

Non-Hodgkin's lymphoma Includes all cancers of lymphoid tissues except Hodgkin's lymphoma. Involves uncontrolled multiplication and metastasis of undifferentiated lymphocytes, with swelling of the lymph nodes, spleen, and Peyer's patches; other organs may eventually become involved. The seventh most common cancer. A rapidly progressing type, which primarily affects young people, grows quickly but responds to chemotherapy; up to a 75% remission rate. A slowly progressing type, which affects the elderly, resists chemotherapy and so is often fatal.

Sentinel node The first node that receives lymph drainage from a body area suspected of being cancerous. When examined for presence of cancer cells, this node gives the best indication of whether metastasis through the lymphatic vessels has occurred.

Splenomegaly (sple″no-meg′ah-le; *mega* = big) Enlargement of the spleen due to accumulation of infectious microorganisms; typically caused by septicemia, mononucleosis, malaria, or leukemia.

Tonsillitis (ton″sĭ-li′tis; *itis* = inflammation) Inflammation of the tonsils, typically due to bacterial infection. Tonsils become red, swollen, and sore.

Case Study Lymphatic System/Immunity

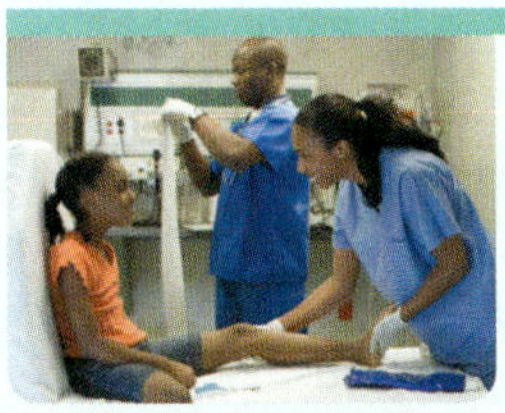

Back to following the progress of Mr. Hutchinson, we learn that the routine complete blood count (CBC) performed on admission reveals that his leukocyte count is dangerously low and follow-up lab tests show that his lymphocytes are deficient. One day postsurgery, he complains of pain in his right ring finger (that hand had a crush injury). When examined, the affected finger and the dorsum of the right hand are edematous, and red streaks radiate superiorly on his right forearm. Higher-than-normal doses of antibiotics are prescribed, and a sling is applied to the affected arm. Nurses are instructed to wear gloves and gown when giving Mr. Hutchinson his care.

Relative to these observations:

1. What do the red streaks emanating from the bruised finger indicate? What would you conclude his problem was if there were no red streaks but the right arm was very edematous?
2. Why is it important that Mr. Hutchinson not move the affected arm excessively (i.e., why was the sling ordered)?
3. How might the low lymphocyte count, megadoses of antibiotics, and orders for additional clinical staff protection be related?
4. Do you predict that Mr. Hutchinson's recovery will be uneventful or problematic? Why?

(Answers in Appendix H)

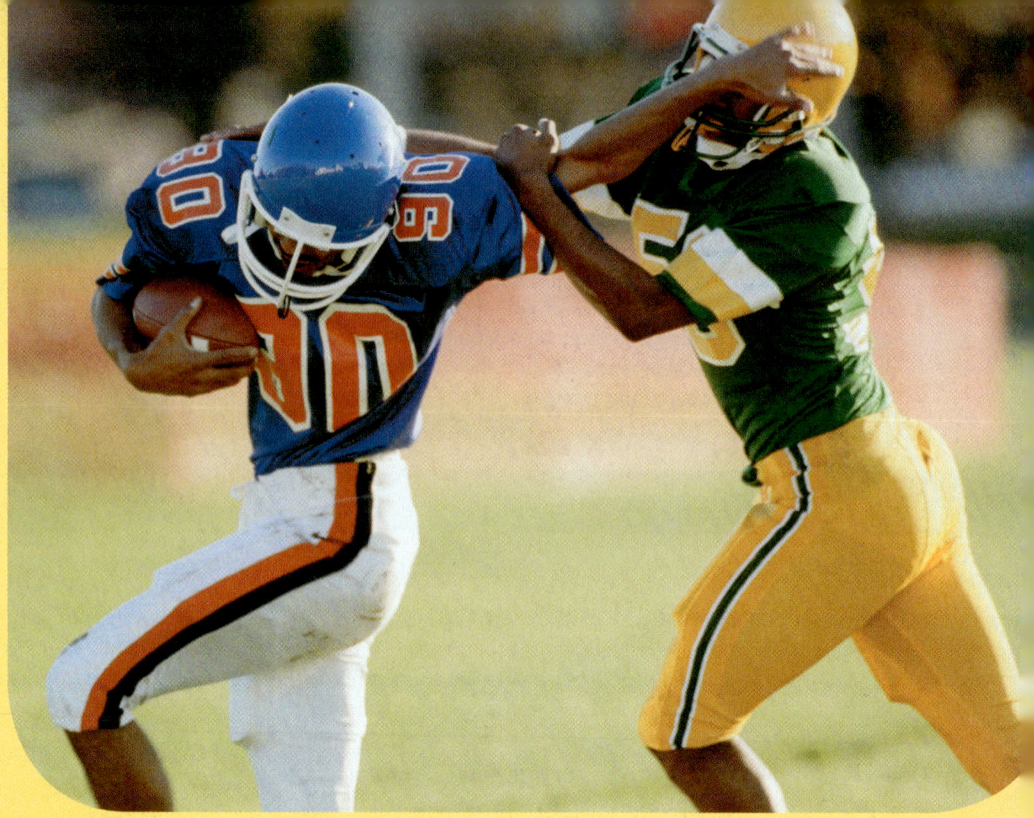

21

The Immune System: Innate and Adaptive Body Defenses

Every second of every day, armies of hostile bacteria, fungi, and viruses swarm on our skin and yet we stay amazingly healthy most of the time. The body has evolved a single-minded approach to such foes—if you're not with us, you're against us! To implement that stance, it relies heavily on two intrinsic defense systems that act both independently and cooperatively to provide resistance to disease, or **immunity** (*immun* = free).

1. The **innate (nonspecific) defense system**, like a lowly foot soldier, is always prepared, responding within minutes to protect the body from all foreign substances. This system has two "barricades." The *first line of defense* is the external body membranes—intact skin and mucosae. The *second line of defense*, called into action whenever the first line has been penetrated, relies on internal defenses such as antimicrobial proteins, phagocytes, and other cells to inhibit the invaders' spread throughout the body. The hallmark of the second line of defense is inflammation.

2. The **adaptive (specific) defense system** is more like an elite fighting force equipped with high-tech weapons to attack *particular* foreign substances. The adaptive defense response, which provides the body's *third line of defense*, takes considerably more time to mount than the innate defense response.

Although we consider them separately, the innate and adaptive systems always work hand in hand. An overview of these two systems is shown in **Figure 21.1**. Small portions of this diagram will reappear in subsequent figures to let you know which part of the immune system we're dealing with.

Although certain organs of the body (notably lymphoid organs) are intimately involved in the immune response, the **immune system** is a *functional system* rather than an organ system in an anatomical sense. Its "structures" are a diverse array of molecules plus trillions of immune cells (especially lymphocytes) that inhabit lymphoid tissues and circulate in body fluids.

Once, the term *immune system* was equated with the adaptive defense system only. However, we now know that the innate and adaptive defenses are deeply intertwined. Specifically:

- The innate and adaptive systems release and recognize many of the same defensive molecules.
- The innate responses are not as nonspecific as once thought. Indeed, they have specific pathways to target certain foreign substances.
- Proteins released during innate responses alert cells of the adaptive system to the presence of specific foreign molecules in the body.

When the immune system is operating effectively, it protects the body from most infectious microorganisms, cancer cells, and (unfortunately) transplanted organs and grafts. It does this both directly, by cell attack, and indirectly, by releasing mobilizing chemicals and protective antibody molecules.

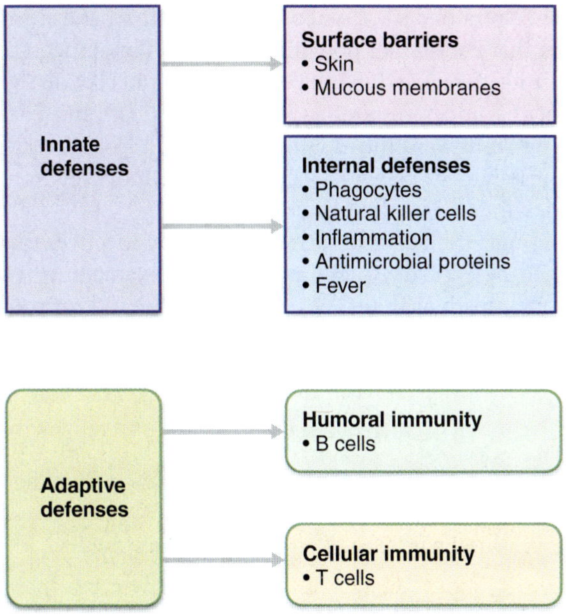

Figure 21.1 Overview of innate and adaptive defenses. Humoral immunity (primarily involving B lymphocytes) and cellular immunity (involving T lymphocytes) are distinct but overlapping areas of adaptive immunity. For simplicity, the many interactions between innate and adaptive defenses are not shown here.

PART 1
Innate Defenses

Because the innate defenses are part and parcel of our anatomy, you could say we come fully equipped with innate defenses. The mechanical barriers that cover body surfaces and the cells and chemicals that act on the initial internal battlefronts are in place at birth, ready to ward off invading **pathogens** (harmful or disease-causing microorganisms).

Many times, our innate defenses alone ward off infection by destroying pathogens. In other cases, the adaptive immune system is called into action to reinforce and enhance the innate defenses. Either way, the innate defenses reduce the workload of the adaptive system by preventing the entry and spread of microorganisms in the body.

Surface Barriers: Skin and Mucosae

✓ Describe surface membrane barriers and their protective functions.

The body's first line of defense—the *skin* and the *mucous membranes*, along with the secretions these membranes produce—is highly effective. As long as the epidermis is unbroken, this heavily keratinized epithelial membrane is a formidable physical barrier to most microorganisms that swarm on the skin. Keratin is also resistant to most weak acids and bases and to bacterial enzymes and toxins. Intact mucosae provide similar mechanical barriers within the body. Recall that mucous membranes line all body cavities that open to the exterior: the digestive, respiratory, urinary, and reproductive tracts.

Besides serving as physical barriers, skin and mucous membranes produce a variety of protective chemicals:

- **Acid.** The acidity of skin, vaginal, and stomach secretions—the *acid mantle*—inhibits bacterial growth.
- **Enzymes.** *Lysozyme*—found in saliva, respiratory mucus, and lacrimal fluid of the eye—destroys bacteria. Protein-digesting enzymes in the stomach kill many different microorganisms.
- **Mucin.** *Mucin* dissolved in water forms thick, sticky mucus that lines the digestive and respiratory passageways. This mucus traps many microorganisms. In contrast, the mucin in watery saliva traps microorganisms and washes them out of the mouth into the stomach where they are digested.
- **Defensins.** Mucous membranes and skin secrete small amounts of broad-spectrum antimicrobial peptides called *defensins*. Defensin output increases dramatically in response to inflammation when surface barriers are breached. Using various mechanisms, such as disruption of microbial membranes, defensins help to control bacterial and fungal colonization in the exposed areas.
- **Other chemicals.** In the skin, some lipids in sebum and *dermcidin* in eccrine sweat are toxic to bacteria.

The respiratory tract mucosae also have structural modifications that counteract potential invaders. Tiny mucus-coated hairs inside the nose trap inhaled particles, and cilia on the mucosa of the upper respiratory tract sweep dust- and bacteria-laden mucus toward the mouth, preventing it from entering the lower respiratory passages, where the warm, moist environment provides an ideal site for bacterial growth.

Although the surface barriers are quite effective, they are breached by everyday nicks and cuts, for example, when you brush your teeth or shave. When this happens and microorganisms invade deeper tissues, your *internal* innate defenses—the second line of defense—come into play.

Check Your Understanding

1. What distinguishes the innate defense system from the adaptive defense system?
2. What is the first line of defense against disease?

For answers, see Appendix H.

Internal Innate Defenses: Cells and Chemicals

✓ Explain the importance of phagocytosis and natural killer cells in innate body defense.

The body uses an enormous number of nonspecific cellular and chemical means to protect itself, including phagocytes, natural killer cells, antimicrobial proteins, and fever. The inflammatory response enlists macrophages, mast cells, all types of white blood cells, and dozens of chemicals that kill pathogens and help repair tissue. These protective tactics identify potentially harmful substances by recognizing (binding tightly to) surface carbohydrates present on infectious organisms (bacteria, viruses, and fungi) but not on human cells.

21

Phagocytes

Pathogens that get through the skin or mucosae into the underlying connective tissue are confronted by *phagocytes* (*phago* = eat). **Neutrophils**, the most abundant type of white blood cell, become phagocytic on encountering infectious material in the tissues. However, the most voracious phagocytes are **macrophages** ("big eaters"), which derive from white blood cells called **monocytes** that leave the bloodstream, enter the tissues, and develop into macrophages.

Free macrophages wander throughout the tissue spaces in search of cellular debris or "foreign invaders." *Fixed macrophages*, like *stellate macrophages* in the liver, are permanent residents of particular organs. Whatever their mobility, all macrophages are similar structurally and functionally.

Phagocytosis

A phagocyte engulfs particulate matter much the way an amoeba ingests a food particle. Flowing cytoplasmic extensions bind to the particle and then pull it inside, enclosed within a membrane-lined vesicle **(Figure 21.2a)**. The resulting **phagosome** then fuses with a *lysosome* to form a **phagolysosome** (steps ①–③ in Figure 21.2b).

Phagocytic attempts are not always successful. In order for a phagocyte to ingest a pathogen, the phagocyte must first *adhere* or cling to that pathogen, a feat made possible by recognizing the pathogen's carbohydrate "signature." Many bacteria have external capsules that conceal their carbohydrate signatures, allowing them to elude capture because phagocytes cannot bind to them.

Our immune systems get around this problem by coating pathogens with **opsonins**. Opsonins are complement proteins (discussed shortly) or antibodies that provide "handles" to which phagocyte receptors can bind. Any pathogen can be coated with opsonins, a process called **opsonization** ("to make tasty"), which greatly accelerates phagocytosis of that pathogen.

Generally, neutrophils and macrophages kill ingested prey by acidifying the phagolysosome and digesting its contents with lysosomal enzymes. However, some pathogens such as the tuberculosis bacillus and certain parasites are resistant to lysosomal enzymes and can even multiply within the phagolysosome. In this case, other immune cells called helper T cells release chemicals that stimulate the macrophage, activating additional enzymes that produce a lethal **respiratory burst**. The respiratory burst promotes killing of pathogens by:

- Liberating a deluge of highly destructive free radicals (including superoxide)
- Producing oxidizing chemicals (H_2O_2 and a substance identical to household bleach)
- Increasing the phagolysosome's pH and osmolarity, which activates other protein-digesting enzymes that digest the invader

Neutrophils also pierce the pathogen's membrane by using *defensins*, the antimicrobial peptides we mentioned earlier.

When phagocytes are unable to ingest their targets (because of size, for example), they can release their toxic chemicals into the extracellular fluid. Whether killing ingested or extracellular targets, neutrophils rapidly destroy themselves in the process, whereas macrophages are more robust and can go on to kill another day.

Natural Killer (NK) Cells

Natural killer (NK) cells, which "police" the body in blood and lymph, are a unique group of defensive cells that can lyse and kill cancer cells and virus-infected body cells before the adaptive immune system is activated. Sometimes called the "pit bulls" of the defense system, NK cells are part of a small group of *large granular lymphocytes*.

Unlike lymphocytes of the adaptive immune system, which only recognize and react against *specific* virus-infected or tumor cells, NK cells are far less picky. They can eliminate a variety of infected or cancerous cells by detecting general abnormalities such as the lack of "self" cell-surface proteins called MHC, described on p. 774. The name "natural" killer cells reflects their nonspecificity.

NK cells are not phagocytic. They kill by directly contacting the target cell, inducing it to undergo apoptosis (programmed cell death). This is the same killing method used by cytotoxic

Innate defenses → Internal defenses

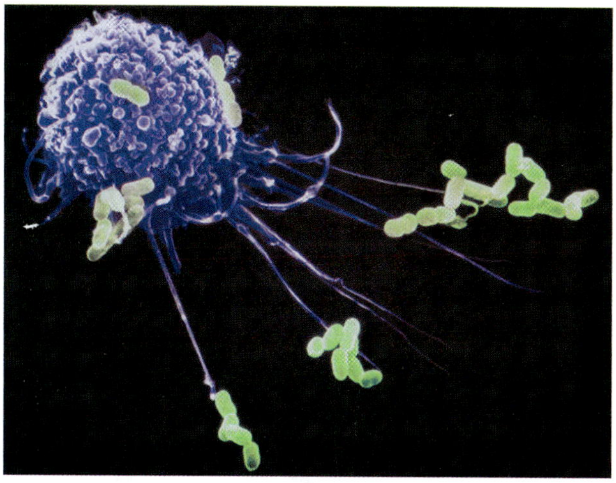

(a) A macrophage (purple) uses its cytoplasmic extensions to pull rod-shaped bacteria (green) toward it. Scanning electron micrograph (4800×).

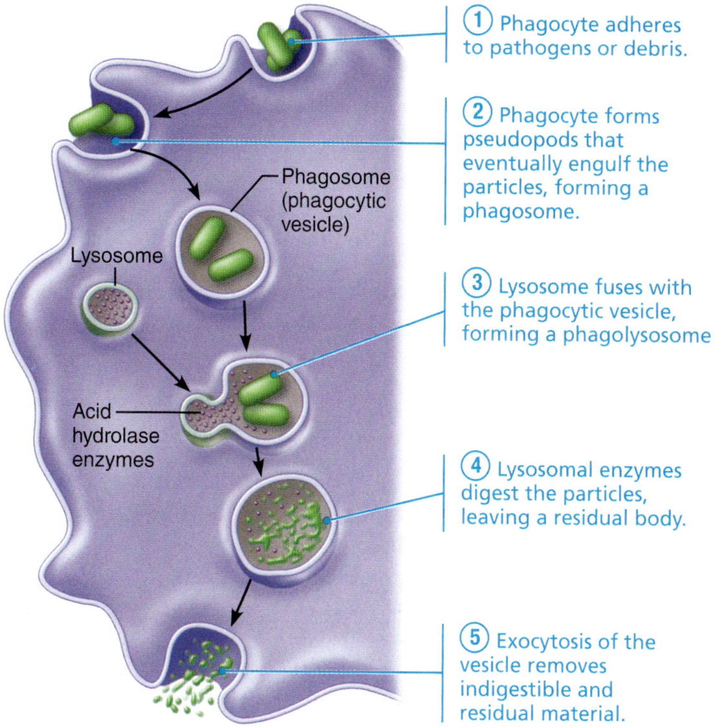

(b) Events of phagocytosis.

Figure 21.2 Phagocytosis.

T cells (described fully on p. 789). NK cells also secrete potent chemicals that enhance the inflammatory response.

Inflammation: Tissue Response to Injury

✓ Describe the inflammatory process. Identify several inflammatory chemicals and indicate their specific roles.

The **inflammatory response** is triggered whenever body tissues are injured by physical trauma (a blow), intense heat, irritating chemicals, or infection by viruses, fungi, or bacteria. The inflammatory response has several beneficial effects. It:

- Prevents the spread of damaging agents to nearby tissues
- Disposes of cell debris and pathogens
- Alerts the adaptive immune system
- Sets the stage for repair

The four *cardinal signs* of short-term, or acute, inflammation are *redness, heat* (*inflam* = set on fire), *swelling*, and *pain*. Some authorities consider *impaired function* to be a fifth cardinal sign. For instance, movement in an inflamed joint may be hampered temporarily, forcing it to rest, which aids healing. Figure 21.3 summarizes the inflammatory process and shows how these cardinal signs come about.

Inflammatory Chemical Release

The inflammatory process begins with a chemical "alarm"—a flood of inflammatory chemicals released into the extracellular fluid. Inflammatory chemicals are released by injured or stressed tissue cells, and immune cells. They can also be formed from proteins circulating in the blood. For example, **mast cells**, a key component of the inflammatory response, release the potent inflammatory chemical **histamine** (his′tah-mēn).

Macrophages (and cells of certain boundary tissues such as epithelial cells lining the gastrointestinal and respiratory tracts) have special membrane receptors that allow them to recognize invaders and sound a chemical alarm. These surface membrane receptors, called **Toll-like receptors (TLRs)**, play a central role in triggering immune responses. There are 11 types of human TLRs, each recognizing a particular class of attacking microbe. For example, one type responds to a glycolipid in cell walls of the tuberculosis bacterium and another to a component of gram-negative bacteria such as *Salmonella*. Once activated, a TLR triggers the release of inflammatory chemicals called *cytokines*.

Other inflammatory chemicals include **kinins** (ki′ninz), **prostaglandins** (pros″tah-glan′dinz), and **complement**. All inflammatory chemicals dilate local arterioles and make local capillaries leakier, as we discuss next. In addition, many attract leukocytes to the injured area and some have individual inflammatory roles as well (Table 21.1).

Vasodilation and Increased Vascular Permeability

Vasodilation accounts for two of the cardinal signs of inflammation. The *redness* and *heat* of an inflamed region are both due to local **hyperemia** (congestion with blood) that occurs when local arterioles dilate.

21

Innate defenses → Internal defenses

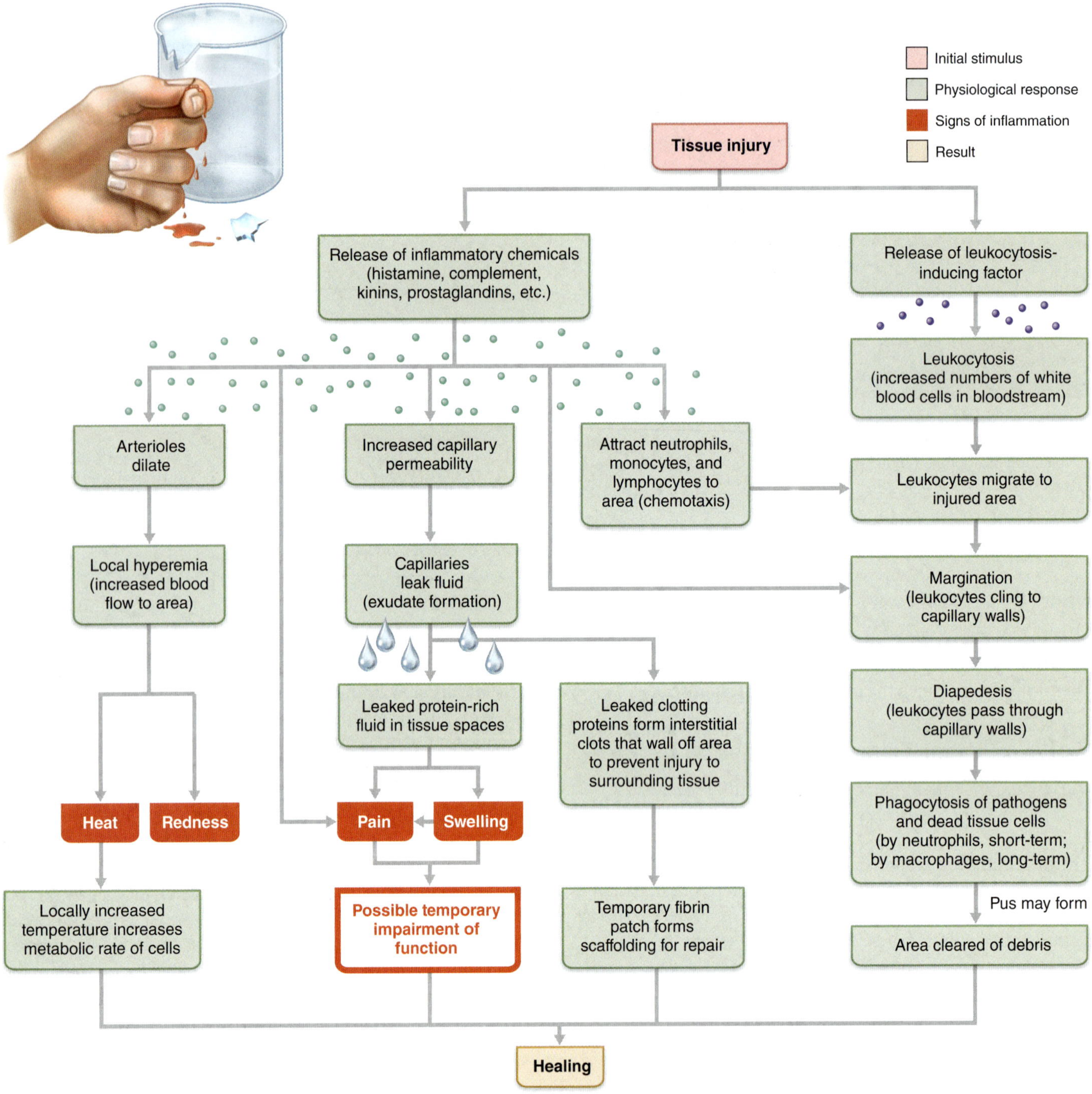

Figure 21.3 Inflammation: flowchart of events. The four cardinal signs of acute inflammation are shown in red boxes, as is impaired function, which in some cases constitutes a fifth cardinal sign.

Inflammatory chemicals also increase the permeability of local capillaries. Consequently, **exudate**—fluid containing clotting factors and antibodies—seeps from the blood into the tissue spaces. This exudate causes the local *swelling*, also called edema, that presses on adjacent nerve endings, contributing to a sensation of *pain*. Pain also results from the release of bacterial toxins, and the sensitizing effects of released prostaglandins and kinins. Aspirin and some other anti-inflammatory drugs produce their analgesic (pain-reducing) effects by inhibiting prostaglandin synthesis.

Although edema may seem detrimental, it isn't. The surge of protein-rich fluids into the tissue spaces sweeps foreign material into lymphatic vessels for processing in the lymph nodes. It also

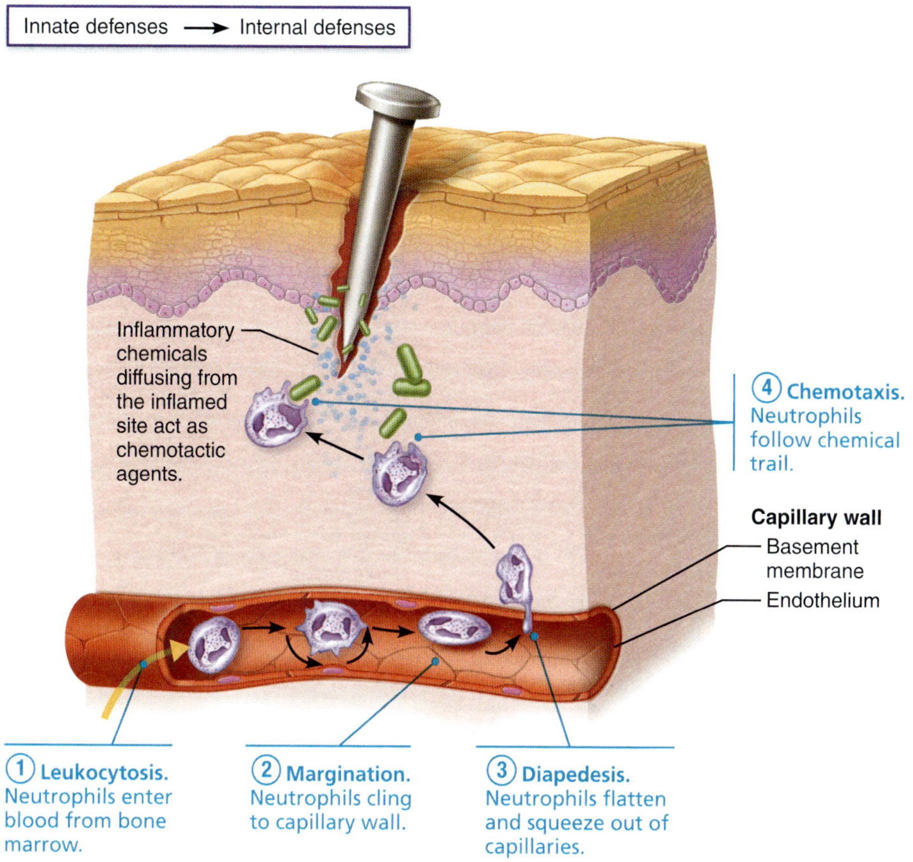

Figure 21.4 **Phagocyte mobilization.**

delivers important proteins such as complement and clotting factors to the interstitial fluid (Figure 21.3).

The clotting factors form a gel-like fibrin mesh (a clot) that acts as a scaffold for permanent repair. The mesh also isolates the injured area and prevents bacteria and other harmful agents from spreading. Walling off the injured area is such an important defense strategy that some bacteria (such as *Streptococcus*) have evolved enzymes that break down the clot, allowing them to invade surrounding tissues.

Phagocyte Mobilization

Soon after inflammation begins, phagocytes flood the damaged area. Neutrophils lead, followed by macrophages. If pathogens provoked the inflammation, a group of plasma proteins known as complement is activated and elements of adaptive immunity (lymphocytes and antibodies) also arrive at the injured site. **Figure 21.4** illustrates the four steps in which phagocytes are mobilized to infiltrate the injured site.

1. **Leukocytosis.** Injured cells release chemicals called **leukocytosis-inducing factors**. In response, neutrophils enter blood from red bone marrow and within a few hours, the number of neutrophils in blood increases four- to fivefold. This **leukocytosis,** the increase in white blood cells (WBCs), is characteristic of inflammation.
2. **Margination.** Inflamed endothelial cells sprout cell adhesion molecules (CAMs) that signal "this is the place." As neutrophils encounter these CAMs, they slow and roll along the surface, eventually achieving an initial foothold. When activated by inflammatory chemicals, CAMs on neutrophils bind tightly to endothelial cells. **Margination** refers to this phenomenon of phagocytes clinging to the inner walls (margins) of the capillaries and postcapillary venules.
3. **Diapedesis.** Continued chemical signaling prompts the neutrophils to flatten and squeeze between the endothelial cells of the capillary walls—a process called **diapedesis**.
4. **Chemotaxis.** Inflammatory chemicals act as homing devices, or more precisely **chemotactic agents**. Neutrophils and other WBCs migrate up the gradient of chemotactic agents to the site of injury (positive **chemotaxis**). Within an hour after the inflammatory response has begun, neutrophils have collected at the site and are devouring any foreign material present.

As the body's counterattack continues, monocytes follow neutrophils into the injured area. Monocytes are fairly poor phagocytes, but within 12 hours of leaving the blood and entering the tissues, they swell and develop large numbers of lysosomes, becoming macrophages with insatiable appetites. These late-arriving macrophages replace the neutrophils on the battlefield.

Macrophages are the central actors in the final disposal of cell debris as an acute inflammation subsides, and they predominate at sites of prolonged, or *chronic*, inflammation. The ultimate goal of an inflammatory response is to clear the injured area of pathogens, dead tissue cells, and any other debris

Table 21.1 Inflammatory Chemicals

CHEMICAL	SOURCE	PHYSIOLOGICAL EFFECTS
Histamine	Granules of mast cells and basophils. Released in response to mechanical injury, presence of certain microorganisms, and chemicals released by neutrophils.	Promotes vasodilation of local arterioles. Increases permeability of local capillaries, promoting formation of exudate.
Kinins (bradykinin and others)	A plasma protein, kininogen, is cleaved by the enzyme kallikrein found in plasma, urine, saliva, and in lysosomes of neutrophils and other types of cells. Cleavage releases active kinin peptides.	Same as for histamine. Also induce chemotaxis of leukocytes and prompt neutrophils to release lysosomal enzymes, thereby enhancing generation of more kinins. Induce pain.
Prostaglandins	Fatty acid molecules produced from arachidonic acid found in all cell membranes; generated by enzymes of neutrophils, basophils, mast cells, and others.	Same as for histamine. Also induce neutrophil chemotaxis. Induce pain.
Complement	See Table 21.2 below.	
Cytokines	See Table 21.6 (p. 790).	

Table 21.2 Summary of Innate Body Defenses

CATEGORY/ASSOCIATED ELEMENTS	PROTECTIVE MECHANISM
First Line of Defense: Surface Membrane Barriers	
Intact skin epidermis	Forms mechanical barrier that prevents entry of pathogens and other harmful substances into body
▪ Acid mantle of skin	Skin secretions (sweat and sebum) make epidermal surface acidic, which inhibits bacterial growth; also contain various bactericidal chemicals
▪ Keratin	Provides resistance against acids, alkalis, and bacterial enzymes
Intact mucous membranes	Form mechanical barrier that prevents entry of pathogens
▪ Mucus	Traps microorganisms in respiratory and digestive tracts
▪ Nasal hairs	Filter and trap microorganisms in nasal passages
▪ Cilia	Propel debris-laden mucus away from nasal cavity and lower respiratory passages
▪ Gastric juice	Contains concentrated hydrochloric acid and protein-digesting enzymes that destroy pathogens in stomach
▪ Acid mantle of vagina	Inhibits growth of most bacteria and fungi in female reproductive tract
▪ Lacrimal secretion (tears); saliva	Continuously lubricate and cleanse eyes (tears) and oral cavity (saliva); contain lysozyme, an enzyme that destroys microorganisms
▪ Urine	Normally acid pH inhibits bacterial growth; cleanses the lower urinary tract as it flushes from the body
Second Line of Defense: Innate Cellular and Chemical Defenses	
Phagocytes	Engulf and destroy pathogens that breach surface membrane barriers; macrophages also contribute to adaptive immune responses
Natural killer (NK) cells	Promote apoptosis (cell suicide) by directly attacking virus-infected or cancerous body cells; recognize general abnormalities rather than specific antigens; do not form memory cells
Inflammatory response	Prevents injurious agents from spreading to adjacent tissues, disposes of pathogens and dead tissue cells, and promotes tissue repair; released inflammatory chemicals attract phagocytes (and other immune cells) to the area
Antimicrobial proteins	
▪ Interferons (α, β, γ)	Proteins released by virus-infected cells and certain lymphocytes; act as chemical messengers to protect uninfected tissue cells from viral takeover; mobilize immune system
▪ Complement	A group of bloodborne proteins that, when activated, lyse microorganisms, enhance phagocytosis by opsonization, and intensify inflammatory and other immune responses
Fever	Systemic response initiated by pyrogens; high body temperature inhibits microbes from multiplying and enhances body repair processes

so that tissue can be repaired. Once this is accomplished, healing usually occurs quickly.

Homeostatic Imbalance 21.1

In severely infected areas, the battle takes a considerable toll on both sides, and creamy yellow **pus** (a mixture of dead or dying neutrophils, broken-down tissue cells, and living and dead pathogens) may accumulate in the wound. If the inflammatory mechanism fails to clear the area of debris, collagen fibers may be laid down, which walls off the sac of pus, forming an *abscess*. The abscess may need to be surgically drained before healing can occur.

Some bacteria, such as tuberculosis bacilli, resist digestion by the macrophages that engulf them. They escape the effects of prescription antibiotics by remaining snugly enclosed within their macrophage hosts. In such cases, *infectious granulomas* form. These tumorlike growths contain a central region of infected macrophages surrounded by uninfected macrophages and an outer fibrous capsule.

A person may harbor pathogens walled off in granulomas for years without displaying any symptoms. However, if the person's resistance to infection is ever compromised, the bacteria may be activated and break free, leading to clinical disease symptoms. +

Antimicrobial Proteins

✓ Name the body's antimicrobial substances and describe their function.

A variety of **antimicrobial proteins** enhance our innate defenses by attacking microorganisms directly or by hindering their ability to reproduce. The most important antimicrobial proteins are interferons and complement proteins (Table 21.2).

Interferons

Viruses—essentially nucleic acids surrounded by a protein envelope—lack the cellular machinery to generate ATP or synthesize proteins. They do their "dirty work" in the body by invading tissue cells and taking over the cellular metabolic machinery needed to reproduce themselves.

Infected cells can do little to save themselves, but some can secrete small proteins called **interferons (IFNs)** (in″ter-fēr′onz) to help protect cells that have not yet been infected. The IFNs diffuse to nearby cells, which they stimulate to synthesize proteins that "interfere" with viral replication in still-healthy cells by blocking protein synthesis and degrading viral RNA (Figure 21.5). Because IFN protection is not *virus-specific*, IFNs produced against a particular virus protect against other viruses, too.

The IFNs are a family of immune modulating proteins produced by a variety of body cells, each having a slightly different physiological effect. IFN alpha (α) and beta (β) have the antiviral effects that we've just described and also activate NK cells. Another interferon, IFN gamma (γ), or immune interferon, is secreted by lymphocytes and has widespread immune mobilizing effects, such as activating macrophages. Because both macrophages and NK cells can also act directly against cancerous cells, the interferons have an indirect role in fighting cancer. Genetically engineered IFNs have found a niche in treating several

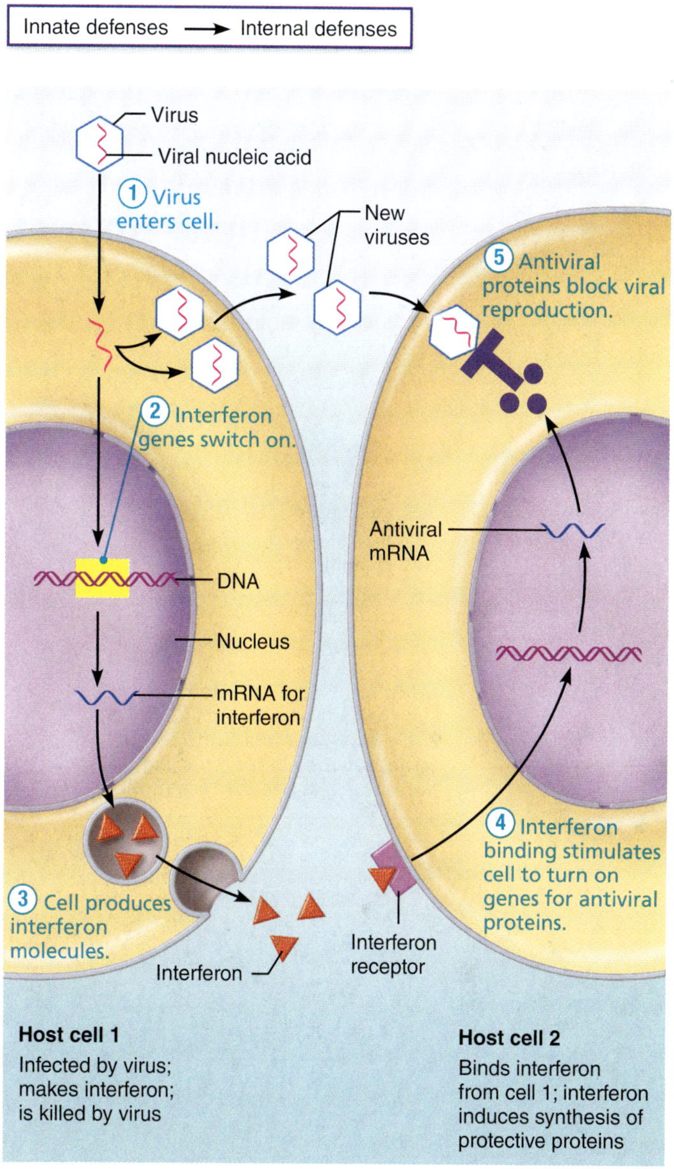

Figure 21.5 The interferon mechanism against viruses.

disorders including hepatitis C, genital warts, multiple sclerosis, and hairy cell leukemia.

Complement

The term **complement system**, or simply **complement**, refers to a group of at least 20 plasma proteins that normally circulate in the blood in an inactive state. These proteins include C1 through C9, factors B, D, and P, plus several regulatory proteins.

Complement provides a major mechanism for destroying foreign substances in the body. Its activation unleashes inflammatory chemicals that amplify virtually all aspects of the inflammatory process. Activated complement also lyses and kills certain bacteria and other cell types. (Luckily our own cells are equipped with proteins that normally inhibit complement activation.) Although complement is a nonspecific defensive mechanism, it "complements" (enhances) the effectiveness of *both* innate and adaptive defenses.

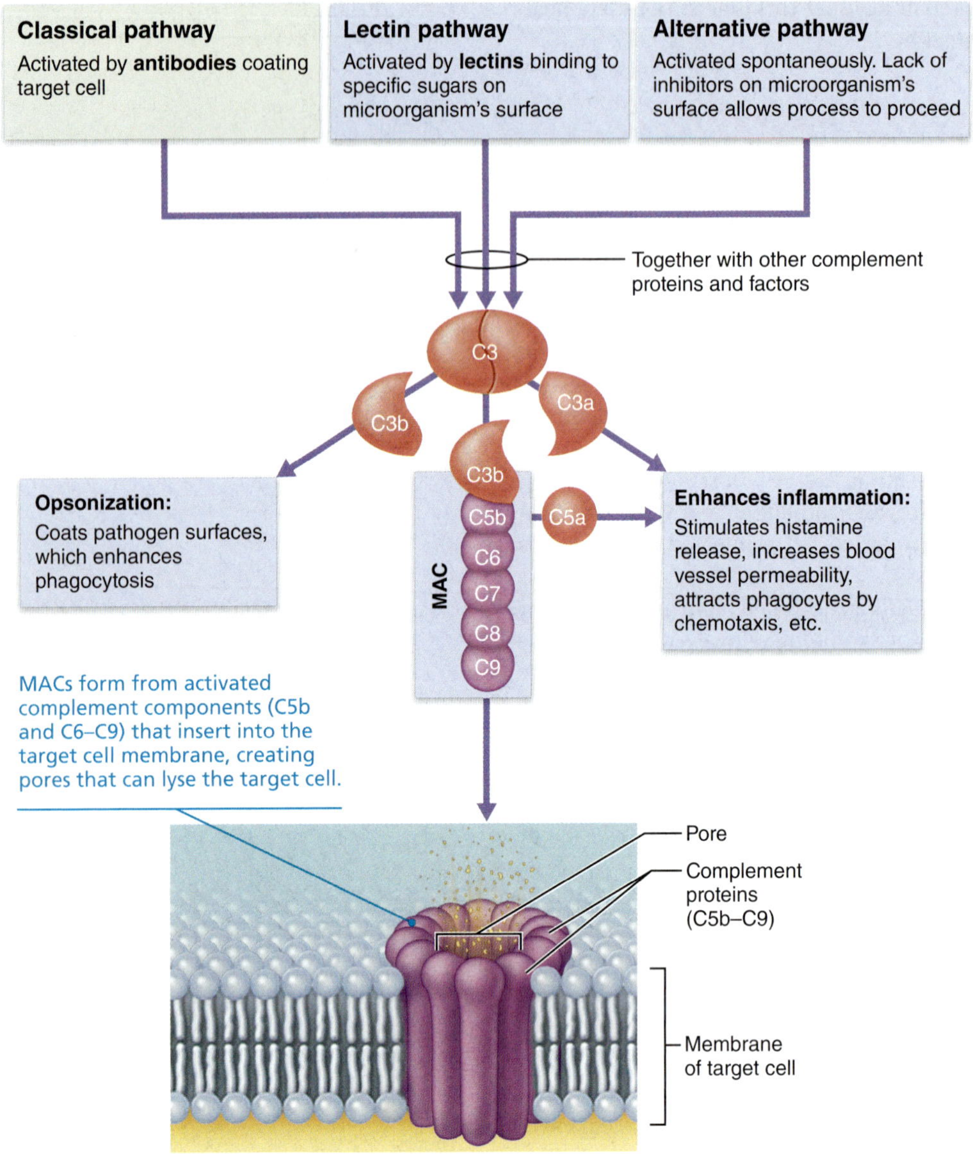

Figure 21.6 Complement activation. All three pathways that activate complement converge at C3. C3 splits into two active pieces: C3a and C3b, which enhance inflammation and act as opsonins. In certain target cells (mostly bacteria), C3b also activates other complement proteins that can form a membrane attack complex (MAC).

Figure 21.6 outlines the three pathways by which complement can be activated.

- The **classical pathway** involves *antibodies*, water-soluble protein molecules that the adaptive immune system produces to fight off foreign invaders. When antibodies bind to pathogens, they can also bind complement components. This double binding, called *complement fixation*, is the first step in this complement activation pathway. (We describe this in more detail on p. 782.)
- The **lectin pathway** involves *lectins*, water-soluble protein molecules that the innate immune system produces to recognize foreign invaders. When lectins bind specific sugars on the surface of microorganisms, they can then bind and activate complement.
- The **alternative pathway** is triggered when spontaneously activated C3 and other complement factors interact on the surface of microorganisms. These microorganisms lack the complement activation inhibitors our own cells have.

Like the blood clotting cascade, complement activation by any of these pathways involves a cascade in which proteins are activated in an orderly sequence—each step catalyzing the next. The three pathways converge at C3, which cleaves into C3a and C3b. This event initiates a common terminal pathway that enhances inflammation, promotes phagocytosis, and can cause cell lysis.

Cell lysis begins when C3b binds to the target cell's surface and triggers the insertion of a group of complement proteins called **MAC (membrane attack complex)** into the cell's membrane. MAC forms and stabilizes a hole in the membrane that allows a massive influx of water, lysing the target cell.

The C3b molecules that coat the microorganism provide "handles" that receptors on macrophages and neutrophils can adhere to, allowing them to engulf the particle more rapidly. As noted earlier, this process is called *opsonization*. C3a and other cleavage products formed during complement fixation amplify the inflammatory response by stimulating mast cells and basophils to release histamine and by attracting neutrophils and other inflammatory cells to the area.

Fever

✓ Explain how fever helps protect the body.

Inflammation is a localized response to infection, but sometimes the body's response to the invasion of microorganisms is more widespread. **Fever**, or abnormally high body temperature, is a systemic response to invading microorganisms.

Fever is an adaptive response that seems to benefit the body. When leukocytes and macrophages are exposed to foreign substances in the body, they release chemicals called **pyrogens** (*pyro* = fire). These pyrogens act on the body's thermostat—a cluster of neurons in the hypothalamus—raising the body's temperature above normal [37°C (98.6°F)].

Fever causes the liver and spleen to sequester iron and zinc, making them less available to support bacterial growth. Additionally, fever increases the metabolic rate of tissue cells in general, speeding up repair processes.

Check Your Understanding

3. What is opsonization and how does it help phagocytes? Give an example of a molecule that acts as an opsonin.
4. Under what circumstances might NK cells kill our own cells?
5. What are the cardinal signs of inflammation and what causes them?

For answers, see Appendix H.

PART 2
Adaptive Defenses

Most of us would find it wonderfully convenient if we could walk into a single clothing store and buy a complete wardrobe—hat to shoes—that fits perfectly regardless of any special figure problems. We know that such a service would be next to impossible to find. And yet, we take for granted our **adaptive immune system**, the body's built-in *specific defensive system* that stalks and eliminates with nearly equal precision almost any type of pathogen that intrudes into the body.

When it operates effectively, the adaptive immune system protects us from a wide variety of infectious agents, as well as from abnormal body cells. When it fails, or is disabled, devastating diseases such as cancer and AIDS result. The activity of the adaptive immune system tremendously amplifies the inflammatory response and is responsible for most complement activation.

At first glance, the adaptive system seems to have a major shortcoming. Unlike the innate system, which is always ready and able to react, the adaptive system must "meet" or be primed by an initial exposure to a specific foreign substance (antigen). Only then can it protect the body against that substance, and this priming takes precious time.

Experiments in the late 1800s revealed the basis of this specific immunity. Researchers demonstrated that animals surviving a serious bacterial infection have protective factors (the proteins we now call *antibodies*) in their blood that defend against future attacks by the same pathogen. Furthermore, researchers found that if antibody-containing serum from the surviving animals was injected into animals that had not been exposed to the pathogen, the injected animals would also be protected. These landmark experiments were exciting because they revealed three important aspects of the adaptive immune response:

- **It is specific.** It recognizes and targets *particular* pathogens or foreign substances that initiate the immune response.
- **It is systemic.** Immunity is not restricted to the initial infection site.
- **It has "memory."** After an initial exposure, it recognizes and mounts even stronger attacks on previously encountered pathogens.

At first antibodies were thought to be the sole artillery of the adaptive immune system. Then, in the mid-1900s researchers discovered that injecting antibody-containing serum did *not* always protect the recipient from diseases the serum donor had survived. In such cases, however, injecting the donor's lymphocytes *did* provide immunity. As the pieces fell into place, researchers recognized two separate but overlapping arms of adaptive immunity, each using a variety of attack mechanisms that vary with the intruder.

Humoral immunity (hu′mor-ul), also called **antibody-mediated immunity**, is provided by antibodies present in the body's "humors," or fluids (blood, lymph, etc.). Though they are produced by lymphocytes, antibodies circulate freely in the blood and lymph, where they bind primarily to *extracellular* targets—bacteria, bacterial toxins, and free viruses—inactivating them temporarily and marking them for destruction by phagocytes or complement.

When lymphocytes themselves rather than antibodies defend the body, the immunity is called **cellular** or **cell-mediated immunity** because living cells provide the protection. Cellular immunity also has *cellular* targets—virus-infected or parasite-infected tissue cells, cancer cells, and cells of foreign grafts. The lymphocytes act against such targets either *directly*, by killing the infected cells, or *indirectly*, by releasing chemicals that enhance the inflammatory response or activate other lymphocytes or macrophages.

Before we describe the humoral and cellular responses, let's first consider the *antigens* that trigger the activity of the remarkable cells involved in adaptive immunity.

Antigens

✓ Define antigen and describe how antigens affect the adaptive defenses.

✓ Define complete antigen, hapten, and antigenic determinant.

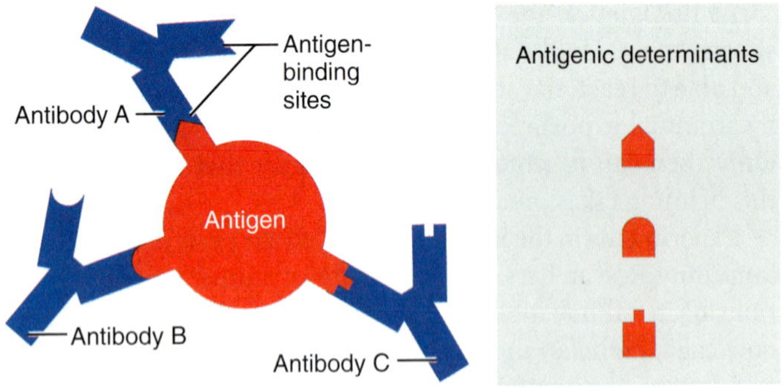

Figure 21.7 Most antigens have several different antigenic determinants. Antibodies (and related receptors on lymphocytes) bind to small areas on the antigen surface called antigenic determinants. In this example, three different types of antibodies react with different antigenic determinants on the same antigen molecule.

Antigens (an′tĭ-jenz) are substances that can mobilize the adaptive defenses and provoke an immune response. They are the ultimate targets of all adaptive immune responses. (*Antigen* is a contraction of "*anti*body *gen*erating"—the result of mobilizing one branch of adaptive immunity.) Most antigens are large, complex molecules (both natural and synthetic) that are not normally present in the body. Consequently, as far as our immune system is concerned, they are intruders, or **nonself**.

Complete Antigens and Haptens

Antigens can be *complete* or *incomplete*. **Complete antigens** have two important functional properties:

- **Immunogenicity**, which is the ability to stimulate specific lymphocytes to proliferate (multiply).
- **Reactivity**, which is the ability to react with the activated lymphocytes and the antibodies released by immunogenic reactions.

21

An almost limitless variety of foreign molecules can act as complete antigens, including virtually all foreign proteins, many large polysaccharides, and some lipids and nucleic acids. Of these, proteins are the strongest antigens. Pollen grains and microorganisms—such as bacteria, fungi, and virus particles—are all immunogenic because their surfaces bear many different foreign macromolecules.

As a rule, small molecules—such as peptides, nucleotides, and many hormones—are not immunogenic. But if they link up with the body's own proteins, the adaptive immune system may recognize the *combination* as foreign and mount an attack that is harmful rather than protective. (We describe these reactions, called *hypersensitivities*, later in the chapter.) In such cases, the troublesome small molecule is called a **hapten** (hap′ten; *haptein* = grasp) or **incomplete antigen**. Unless attached to protein carriers, haptens have reactivity but not immunogenicity. Besides certain drugs (particularly penicillin), chemicals that act as haptens are found in poison ivy, animal dander, detergents, cosmetics, and a number of common household and industrial products.

Antigenic Determinants

The ability of a molecule to act as an antigen depends on both its size and its complexity. Only certain parts of the antigen, called **antigenic determinants**, are immunogenic. Free antibodies or lymphocyte receptors bind to these antigenic determinants in much the same manner that an enzyme binds to a substrate.

Most naturally occurring antigens have a variety of antigenic determinants on their surfaces, some more potent than others in provoking an immune response (**Figure 21.7**). Different lymphocytes "recognize" different antigenic determinants, so a single antigen may mobilize several lymphocyte populations and stimulate formation of many kinds of antibodies.

Large proteins have hundreds of chemically different antigenic determinants, which accounts for their high immunogenicity and reactivity. However, large simple molecules such as plastics, which have many identical, regularly repeating units (and so are not chemically complex), have little or no immunogenicity. Such substances are used to make artificial implants because the substances are not seen as foreign and rejected by the body.

Self-Antigens: MHC Proteins

A huge variety of protein molecules dot the external surfaces of all our cells. Assuming your immune system has been properly "programmed," your **self-antigens** are not foreign or antigenic to you, but they are strongly antigenic to other individuals. (This is the basis of transfusion reactions and graft rejection.)

Among the cell surface proteins that identify a cell as *self* is a group of glycoproteins called **MHC proteins**. Genes of the **major histocompatibility complex (MHC)** code for these proteins. Because millions of combinations of these genes are possible, it is unlikely that any two people except identical twins have the same MHC proteins. Each MHC protein has a deep groove that holds a peptide, either a self-antigen or a foreign antigen. As we will describe shortly, T lymphocytes can only bind antigens that are presented (displayed to them) on MHC proteins.

☑ Check Your Understanding

6. Name three key characteristics of adaptive immunity.
7. What is the difference between a complete antigen and a hapten?
8. What marks a cell as "self" as opposed to "nonself"?

For answers, see Appendix H.

Cells of the Adaptive Immune System: An Overview

✓ Compare and contrast the origin, maturation process, and general function of B and T lymphocytes.

✓ Define immunocompetence and self-tolerance, and describe their development in B and T lymphocytes.

✓ Name several antigen-presenting cells and describe their roles in adaptive defenses.

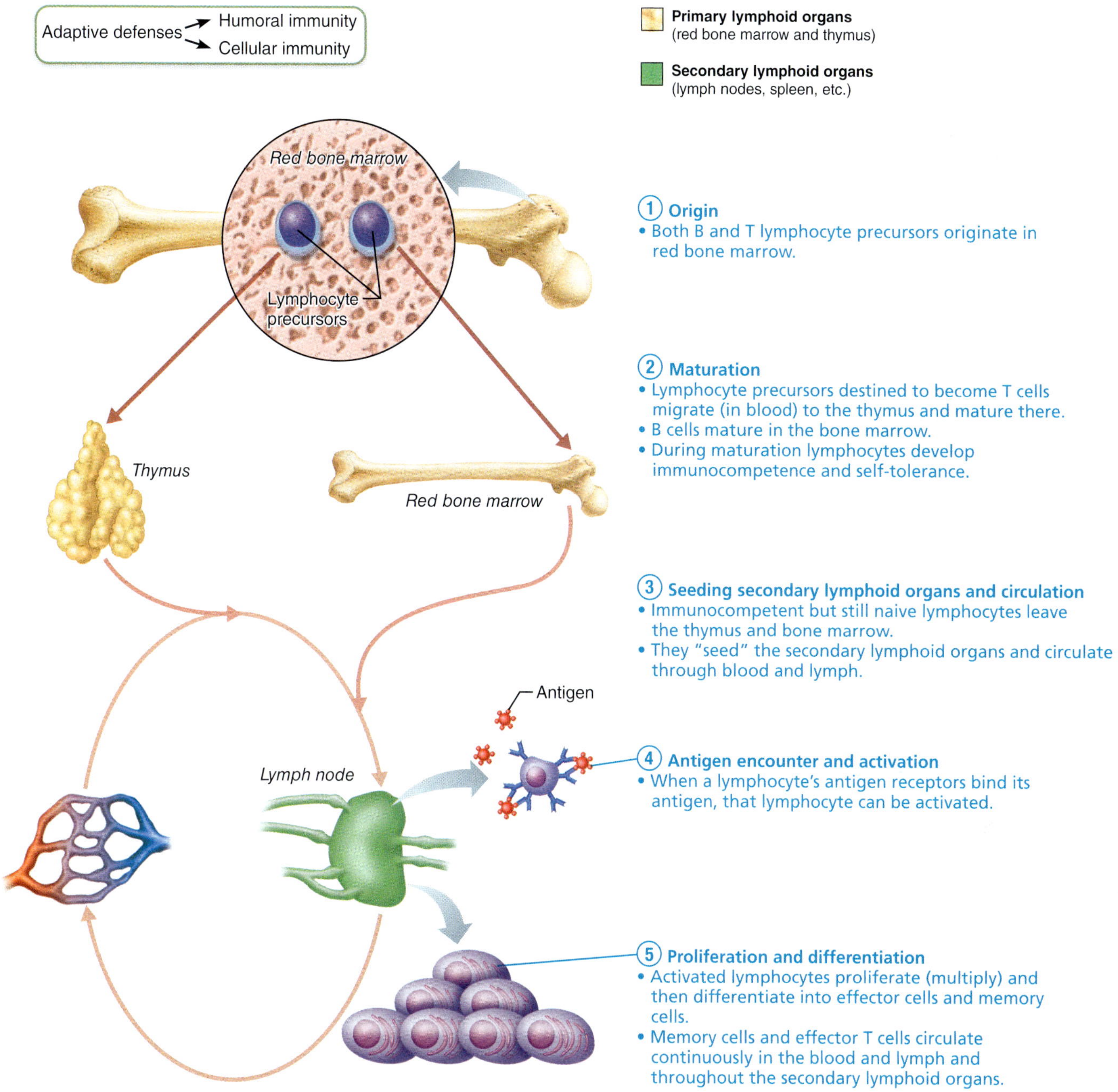

Figure 21.8 Lymphocyte development, maturation, and activation.

The adaptive immune system involves three crucial types of cells: two distinct populations of lymphocytes, plus *antigen-presenting cells* (*APCs*).

- **B lymphocytes (B cells)** oversee humoral immunity.
- **T lymphocytes (T cells)** are non-antibody-producing lymphocytes that constitute the cellular arm of adaptive immunity.
- APCs do not respond to specific antigens as lymphocytes do. Instead, they play essential auxiliary roles.

Lymphocytes

Despite their differences, B and T lymphocytes share a common pattern of development and common steps in their life cycles. Let's take a look.

Lymphocyte Development, Maturation, and Activation

The development, maturation, and activation of B and T cells share the five general steps shown in **Figure 21.8**.

Origin (Figure 21.8 ①) Like all blood cells, lymphocytes originate in red bone marrow from hematopoietic stem cells.

Maturation (Figure 21.8 ②) Lymphocytes are "educated" (go through a rigorous selection process) as they mature. The aim of this education is twofold:

- **Immunocompetence.** Each lymphocyte must become able (competent) to recognize its one specific antigen by binding to it. This ability is called **immunocompetence**. When B or T cells become immunocompetent, they display a unique type

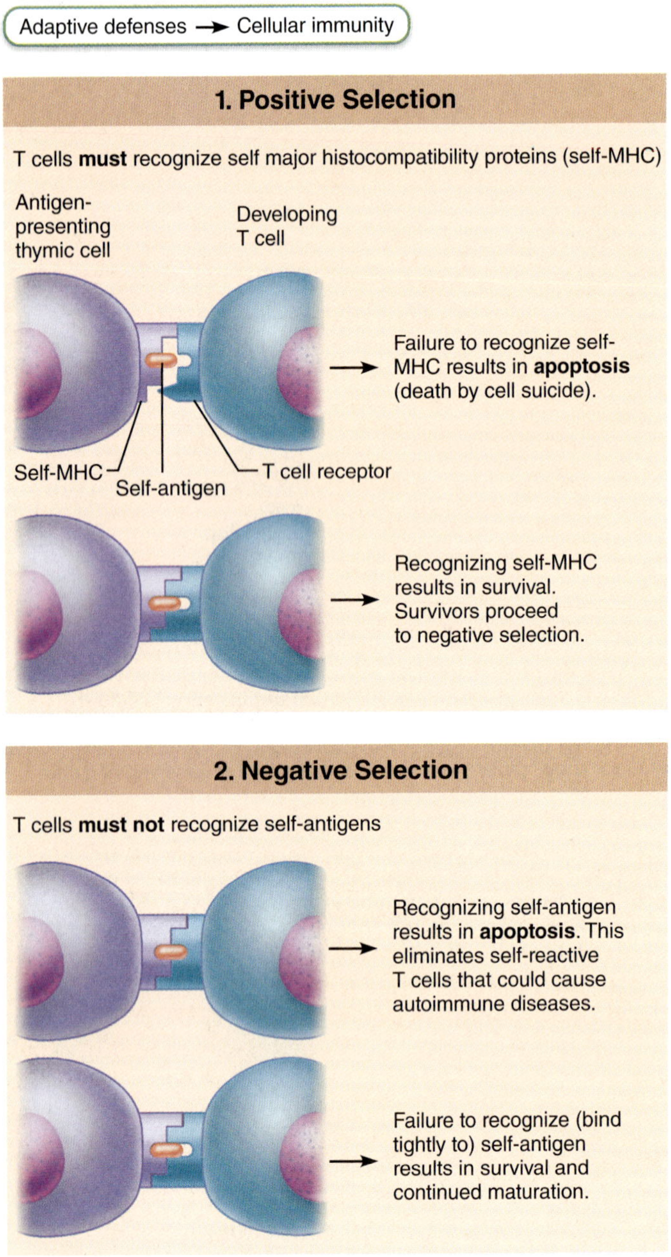

Figure 21.9 T cell education in the thymus.

of receptor on their surface. These receptors (some 10^5 per cell) enable the lymphocyte to recognize and bind a specific antigen. Once these receptors appear, the lymphocyte is committed to react to one (and only one) distinct antigenic determinant because *all* of its antigen receptors are the same. The receptors on B cells are in fact membrane-bound antibodies. The receptors on T cells are not antibodies but are products of the same gene superfamily and have similar functions.

- **Self-tolerance.** Each lymphocyte must be relatively unresponsive to self-antigens so that it does not attack the body's own cells. This is called **self-tolerance**.

B and T cells acquire immunocompetence and self-tolerance in different parts of the body. T cells undergo this two- to three-day maturation process in the thymus. B cells become immunocompetent and self-tolerant in the bone marrow. The lymphoid organs where the lymphocytes become immunocompetent—thymus and bone marrow—are called **primary lymphoid organs**. All other lymphoid organs are referred to as **secondary lymphoid organs**.

The selection process (education) that lymphocytes undergo is best understood in T cells, so we will explore it first. T cell education consists of positive and negative selection **(Figure 21.9)**, both of which occur in the thymus.

1. **Positive selection** is the first of two tests a developing T lymphocyte must pass. It ensures that *only* T cells that are able to recognize self-MHC proteins survive. Remember that T cells cannot bind antigens unless the antigens are presented on self-MHC proteins. T cells that are unable to recognize self-MHC are eliminated by apoptosis.
2. **Negative selection**, the second test, ensures that T cells do not recognize self-antigens displayed on self-MHC. If they do, they are eliminated by apoptosis. Negative selection is the basis for immunologic self-tolerance, making sure that T cells don't attack the body's own cells, which would cause autoimmune disorders.

This education of T cells is expensive indeed—only about 2% of T cells survive it and continue to become successful immunocompetent, self-tolerant T cells.

Less is known about the factors that control B cell maturation, but a similar selection process is thought to occur in the bone marrow. B cells that successfully make antigen receptors are positively selected and those whose antigen receptors are self-reactive are eliminated (*clonal deletion*). However, selection is not perfect for either B or T cells—some self-reactive lymphocytes survive.

Seeding Secondary Lymphoid Organs and Circulation (Figure 21.8 ③) Immunocompetent B and T cells that have not yet been exposed to antigen are called **naive**. Naive B cells and T cells are exported from the primary lymphoid organs to seed (colonize) the secondary lymphoid organs—lymph nodes, spleen, and so on—where they are likely to encounter antigens.

Lymphocytes, especially the T cells (which account for 65–85% of bloodborne lymphocytes), circulate continuously throughout the body. Circulating greatly increases a lymphocyte's chance of coming into contact with antigens located in different parts of the body, as well as with huge numbers of macrophages and other lymphocytes. For example, a T cell circulates through lymph and blood and back to a lymph node about once a day. Although lymphocyte circulation appears to be random, lymphocyte movement into the tissues is highly specific, regulated by homing signals (CAMs) displayed on vascular endothelial cells.

Antigen Encounter and Activation (Figure 21.8 ④) The first encounter between an immunocompetent but naive lymphocyte and an invading antigen usually takes place in a lymph node or the spleen, but it may happen in any secondary lymphoid organ. Immune cells in lymph nodes are in a strategic position to encounter a large variety of antigens because lymphatic capillaries pick up proteins and pathogens from nearly all body tissues.

When an antigen binds to the particular lymphocyte that has a receptor for it, the antigen selects that lymphocyte for further development. This is called **clonal selection**. If the proper signals (which we describe later) are present, the selected lymphocyte will activate to complete its differentiation.

Proliferation and Differentiation (Figure 21.8 (5)) Once activated, the lymphocyte rapidly proliferates to form an army of cells all exactly like itself and bearing the same antigen-specific receptors. This army of identical cells, all descended from the *same* ancestor cell, is called a **clone**.

Most members of the clone become **effector cells**, the cells that actually do the work of fighting infection. A few members of the clone become **memory cells** that are able to respond quickly after any subsequent encounter with the same antigen. B and T memory cells and effector T cells circulate throughout the body on continuous patrol.

Generation of Antigen Receptor Diversity in Lymphocytes

We know that lymphocytes become immunocompetent *before* meeting the antigens they may later attack. *Our genes, not antigens we encounter, determine which specific foreign substances our immune system will be able to recognize and resist.* In other words, the immune cell receptors represent our genetically acquired knowledge of the microbes that are likely to be in our environment. An antigen simply determines which existing T or B cells will proliferate and mount the attack against it.

Only some of the antigens our lymphocytes are programmed to resist will ever invade our bodies. Consequently, only some members of our army of immunocompetent cells are mobilized in our lifetime. The others are forever idle.

Our lymphocytes make up to a billion different types of antigen receptors. These receptors, like all other proteins, are specified by genes, so you might think that an individual must have billions of genes. Not so; each body cell only contains about 25,000 genes that code for all the proteins the cell must make.

How can a limited number of genes generate a seemingly limitless number of different antigen receptors? Molecular genetic studies have shown that the genes that dictate the structure of each antigen receptor are not present as such in lymphocyte stem cells. Instead of a complete set of "antigen receptor genes," stem cells contain a few hundred genetic bits and pieces that can be thought of as a "Lego set" for antigen receptor genes. As each lymphocyte becomes immunocompetent, these gene segments are shuffled and combined in different ways, a process called *somatic recombination*. The information of the newly assembled genes is then expressed as the surface receptors of B and T cells and as the antibodies later released by the B cell's "offspring."

Antigen-Presenting Cells (APCs)

Antigen-presenting cells (APCs) engulf antigens and then present fragments of them, like signal flags, on their own surfaces where T cells can recognize them. Naive T cells can only be activated by antigens that are presented to them on MHC proteins by APCs. In other words, APCs *present antigens* to the cells that will deal with the antigens. The major types of cells acting as APCs are *dendritic cells*, *macrophages*, and *B lymphocytes*.

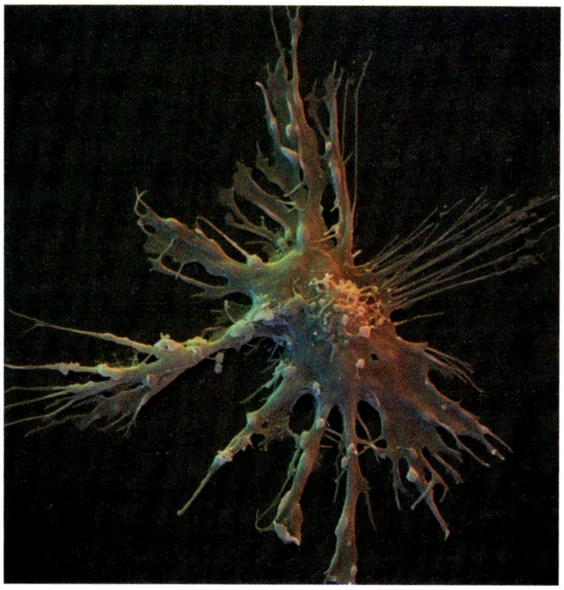

Figure 21.10 Dendritic cell. Scanning electron micrograph (1050×).

Dendritic Cells

Dendritic cells are found at the body's frontiers (skin, for example) where they act as mobile sentinels. With their long, wispy extensions, dendritic cells are very efficient antigen catchers **(Figure 21.10)**. Once they have internalized antigens by phagocytosis, they enter nearby lymphatics to get to a lymph node where they will present the antigens to T cells.

Migration of dendritic cells to secondary lymphoid organs is now recognized as the most important way of ensuring that lymphocytes encounter invading antigens. Indeed, dendritic cells are the most effective antigen presenter known—it's their only job. This early alert spares the body a good deal of tissue damage that might otherwise occur.

Dendritic cells are one of the key links between innate and adaptive immunity. They initiate adaptive immune responses tailored to the type of pathogen they have encountered.

Macrophages

Macrophages are widely distributed throughout the lymphoid organs and connective tissues. Although macrophages, like dendritic cells, can activate naive T cells, macrophages often present antigens to T cells for another reason—to be activated themselves. Certain effector T cells release chemicals that prod macrophages to become *activated macrophages*, true "killers" that are insatiable phagocytes and secrete bactericidal chemicals.

B Lymphocytes

Unlike dendritic cells and macrophages, B cells do not activate naive T cells. Instead, they present antigens to a certain kind of T cell (called a helper T cell) in order to obtain "help" in their own activation. We will discuss this more on p. 787.

Adaptive defenses → Humoral immunity

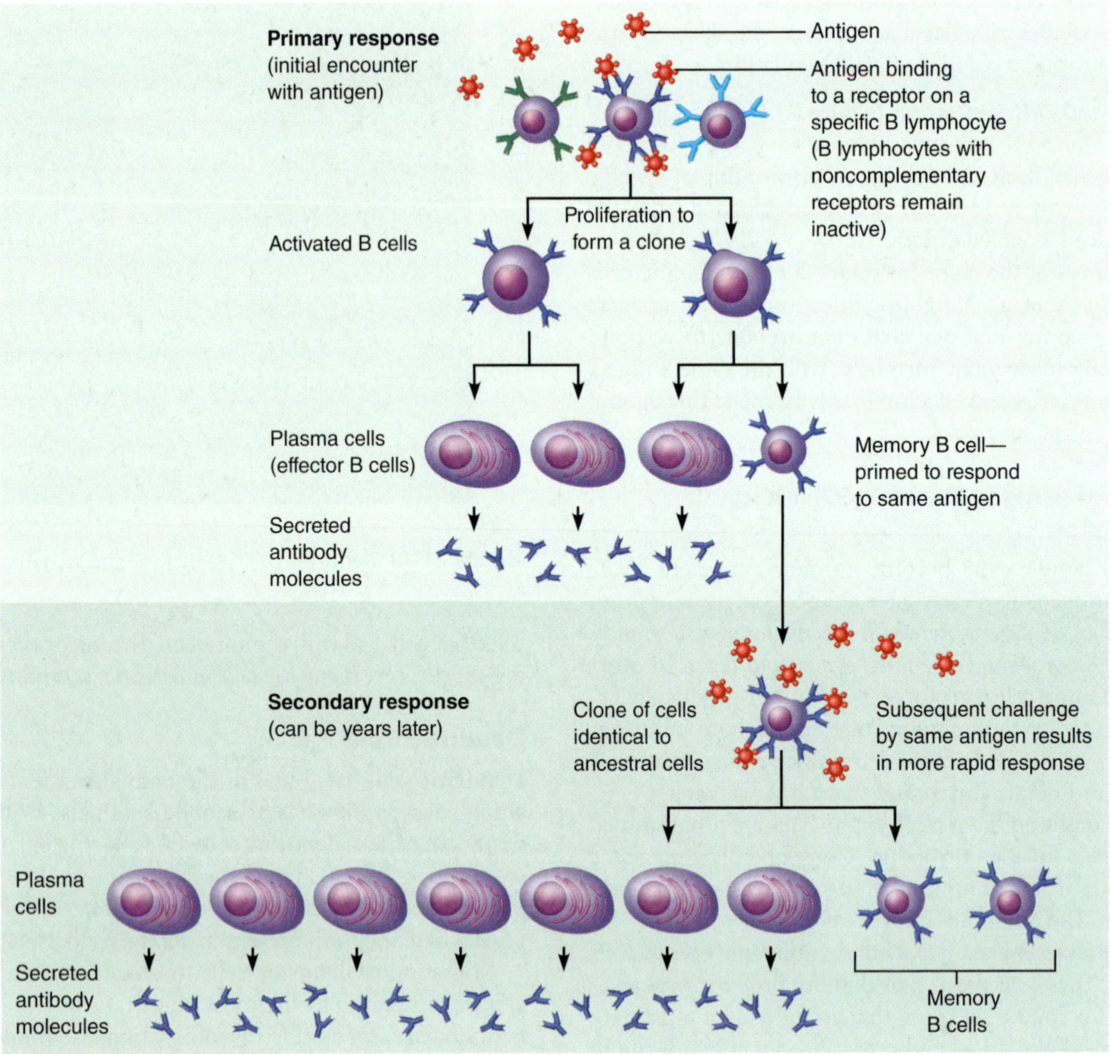

Figure 21.11 Clonal selection of a B cell.

Check Your Understanding

9. What event (or observation) signals that a B or T cell has achieved immunocompetence?
10. Which of the following T cells would survive education in the thymus? (a) one that recognizes neither MHC nor self-antigen, (b) one that recognizes both MHC and self-antigen, (c) one that recognizes MHC but not self-antigen, (d) one that recognizes self-antigen but not MHC.
11. Name three different APCs. Which is most important for T lymphocyte activation?
12. In clonal selection, "who" does the selecting? What is being selected?

For answers, see Appendix H.

In summary, the two-fisted adaptive immune system uses lymphocytes, APCs, and specific molecules to identify and destroy all substances—both living and nonliving—that are in the body but not recognized as self. The system's response to such threats depends on the ability of its cells to (1) recognize antigens by binding to them and (2) communicate with one another so that the whole system mounts a response specific to those antigens. As you will see, interactions between various lymphocytes, and between lymphocytes and APCs, underlie virtually all phases of the adaptive immune response.

Table 21.3 outlines major similarities and differences between B and T lymphocytes. This will help orient you as you delve into the details of humoral and cellular immunity.

Humoral Immune Response

- ✓ Define humoral immunity.
- ✓ Describe the process of clonal selection of a B cell.
- ✓ Recount the roles of plasma cells and memory cells in humoral immunity.

Table 21.3 Overview of B and T Lymphocytes

	B LYMPHOCYTES	T LYMPHOCYTES
Type of immune response	Humoral	Cellular
Antibody secretion	Yes	No
Primary targets	Extracellular pathogens (e.g., bacteria, fungi, parasites, some viruses in extracellular fluid)	Intracellular pathogens (e.g., virus-infected cells) and cancer cells
Site of origin	Red bone marrow	Red bone marrow
Site of maturation	Red bone marrow	Thymus
Effector cells	Plasma cells	Cytotoxic T (T_C) cells Helper T (T_H) cells Regulatory T (T_{Reg}) cells
Memory cell formation	Yes	Yes

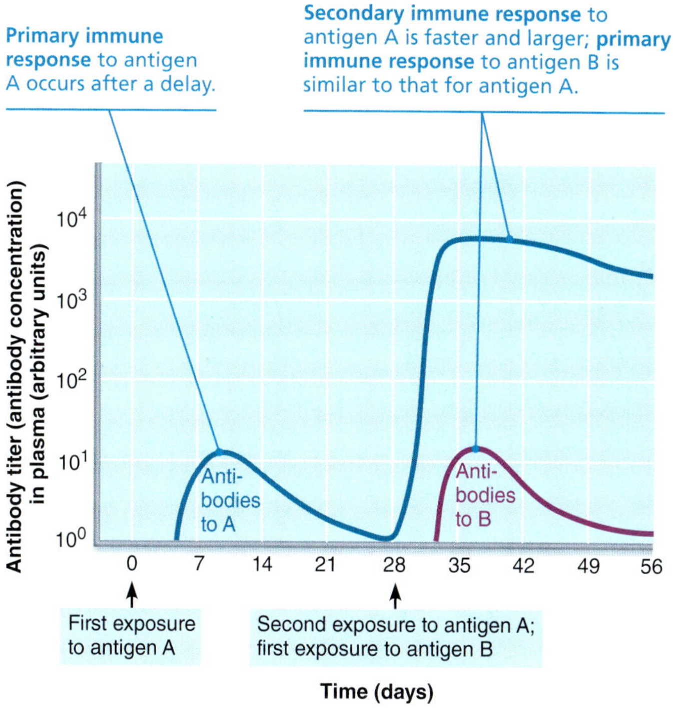

Figure 21.12 Primary and secondary humoral responses. The primary response to antigen A generates memory cells that give rise to the enhanced secondary response to antigen A. The response to antigen B is independent of the response to antigen A.

Now that you understand the common steps in lymphocyte maturation and activation, let's examine how this basic pattern applies to B lymphocytes. When a B cell encounters its antigen, that antigen provokes the *humoral immune response*, in which antibodies specific for that antigen are made.

Activation and Differentiation of B Cells

An immunocompetent but naive B lymphocyte is *activated* when matching antigens bind to its surface receptors and cross-link adjacent receptors together. Antigen binding is quickly followed by receptor-mediated endocytosis of the cross-linked antigen-receptor complexes. As we described previously, this is called *clonal selection* and is followed by proliferation and differentiation into effector cells **(Figure 21.11)**. (As we will see shortly, interactions with T cells are usually required to help B cells achieve full activation.)

Most cells of the clone differentiate into **plasma cells**, the antibody-secreting *effector cells* of the humoral response. Plasma cells develop the elaborate internal machinery (largely rough endoplasmic reticulum) needed to secrete antibodies at the unbelievable rate of about 2000 molecules per second. Each plasma cell functions at this breakneck pace for 4 to 5 days and then dies. The secreted antibodies, each with the same antigen-binding properties as the receptor molecules on the surface of the parent B cell, circulate in the blood or lymph. There they bind to free antigens and mark them for destruction by other innate or adaptive mechanisms.

Clone cells that do not become plasma cells become long-lived **memory cells**. They can mount an almost immediate humoral response if they encounter the same antigen again in the future (Figure 21.11, bottom).

Immunological Memory

The cellular proliferation and differentiation we have just described constitute the **primary immune response**, which occurs on first exposure to a particular antigen. The primary response typically has a lag period of 3 to 6 days after the antigen encounter. This lag period mirrors the time required for the few B cells specific for that antigen to proliferate (about 12 generations) and for their offspring to differentiate into plasma cells. After the mobilization period, plasma antibody levels rise, reach peak levels in about 10 days, and then decline **(Figure 21.12)**.

If (and when) someone is reexposed to the same antigen, whether it's the second or twenty-second time, a **secondary immune response** occurs. Secondary immune responses are faster, more prolonged, and more effective, because the immune system has already been primed to the antigen, and sensitized memory cells are already "on alert." These memory cells provide what is commonly called **immunological memory**.

Within hours after recognizing the "old enemy" antigen, a new army of plasma cells is being generated. Within 2 to 3 days the antibody concentration in the plasma, called the *antibody titer*, rises steeply to reach much higher levels than in the primary response. Secondary response antibodies not only bind with greater affinity (more tightly), but their blood levels remain high for weeks to months. (When the appropriate chemical signals are present, plasma cells can keep functioning for much longer than the 4 to 5 days seen in primary responses.) Memory cells persist

21

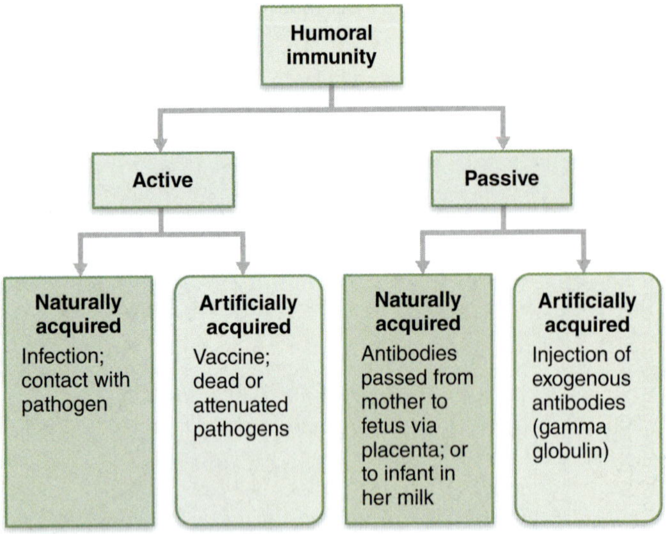

Figure 21.13 Active and passive humoral immunity. Active immunity establishes immunological memory; passive immunity never does.

for long periods in humans and many retain their capacity to produce powerful secondary humoral responses for life.

The same general events occur in the cellular immune response: A primary response sets up a pool of effector cells (in this case, T cells) and generates memory cells that can then mount secondary responses.

Active and Passive Humoral Immunity

✓ Compare and contrast active and passive humoral immunity.

21

When your B cells encounter antigens and produce antibodies against them, you are exhibiting **active humoral immunity**. Active immunity is acquired in two ways **(Figure 21.13)**. It is (1) *naturally acquired* when you get a bacterial or viral infection, during which time you may develop symptoms of the disease and suffer a little (or a lot), and (2) *artificially acquired* when you receive **vaccines**. Indeed, once researchers realized that secondary responses are so much more vigorous than primary responses, the race was on to develop vaccines to "prime" the immune response by providing a first encounter with the antigen.

Most vaccines contain pathogens that are dead or *attenuated* (living, but extremely weakened), or their components. Vaccines provide two benefits:

- They spare us most of the symptoms and discomfort of the disease that would otherwise occur during the primary response.
- Their weakened antigens provide functional antigenic determinants that are both immunogenic and reactive.

Vaccine *booster shots*, which may intensify the immune response at later encounters with the same antigen, are also available.

Vaccines have wiped out smallpox and have substantially lessened the illness caused by such former childhood killers as whooping cough, polio, and measles. Although vaccines have dramatically reduced hepatitis B, tetanus, influenza, and pneumonia in adults, immunization of adults in the U.S. has a much lower priority than that of children. As a result more than 65,000 Americans die each year from vaccine-preventable infections.

Conventional vaccines have shortcomings. In extremely rare cases, vaccines have caused the very disease they are trying to prevent because the attenuated virus wasn't weakened enough. In some individuals, contaminating proteins (for example, egg albumin) cause allergic responses to the vaccine. The new "naked DNA" antiviral vaccines, blasted into the skin with a gene gun, and *edible* vaccines taken orally appear to circumvent these problems, but are not always effective.

Passive humoral immunity differs from active immunity, both in the antibody source and in the degree of protection it provides (Figure 21.13). Instead of being made by your plasma cells, ready-made antibodies are introduced into your body. As a result, your B cells are not challenged by antigens, immunological memory does not occur, and the protection provided by the "borrowed" antibodies ends when they naturally degrade in the body.

Passive immunity is conferred *naturally* on a fetus or infant when the mother's antibodies cross the placenta or are ingested with the mother's milk. For several months after birth, the baby is protected from all the antigens to which the mother has been exposed.

Passive immunity can also be conferred *artificially* by administering exogenous antibodies (from outside your own body) as *gamma globulin*, harvested from the plasma of an immune donor. Exogenous antibodies are used to prevent hepatitis A and treat poisonous snake bites (antivenom), botulism, rabies, and tetanus (antitoxin) because these rapidly fatal diseases would kill a person before active immunity could be established. The donated antibodies provide immediate protection, but their effect is short-lived (two to three weeks).

☑ Check Your Understanding

13. Why is the secondary response to an antigen so much faster than the primary response?
14. How do vaccines protect against common childhood illnesses such as chicken pox, measles, and mumps?

For answers, see Appendix H.

Antibodies

✓ Describe the structure of an antibody monomer, and name the five classes of antibodies.

✓ Explain the function(s) of antibodies and describe clinical uses of monoclonal antibodies.

Antibodies, also called **immunoglobulins (Igs)** (im″u-no-glob′u-linz), constitute the **gamma globulin** part of blood proteins. As we mentioned earlier, antibodies are proteins secreted in response to an antigen by effector B cells called plasma cells, and the antibodies bind specifically with that antigen. They are formed in response to an incredible number of different antigens.

Despite their variety, all antibodies can be grouped into one of five Ig classes, each slightly different in structure and function.

Adaptive defenses → Humoral immunity

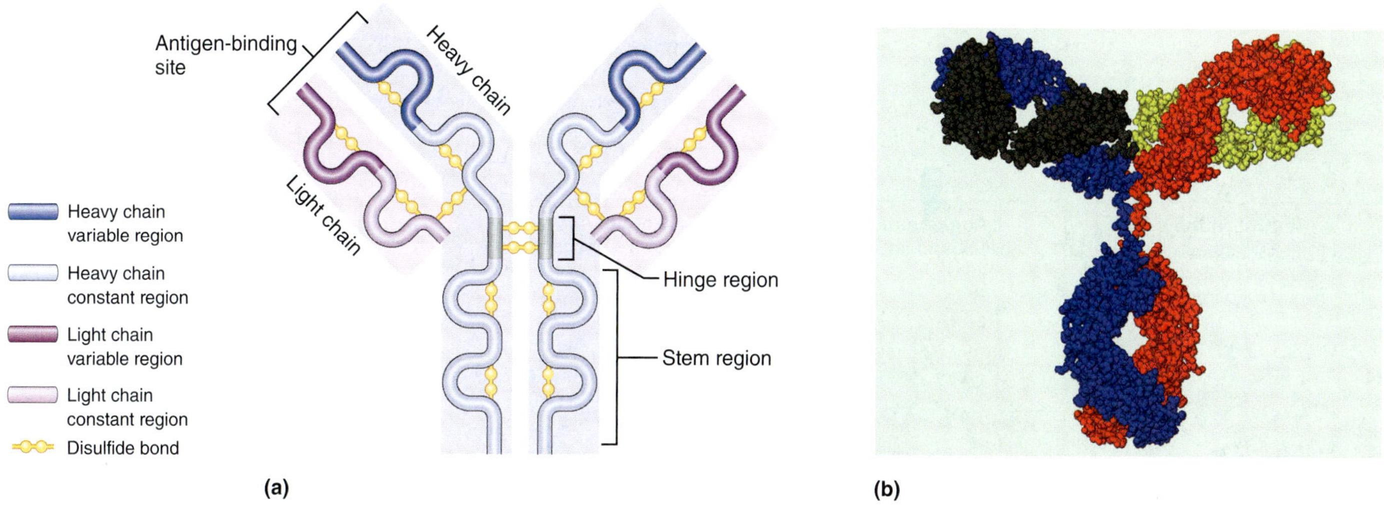

Figure 21.14 Antibody structure. (a) Schematic antibody structure (based on IgG) consists of four polypeptides—two short *light chains* and two long *heavy chains* joined together by disulfide bonds (S–S). Each chain has a V (variable) region (which differs in antibodies from different cells) and a C (constant) region (essentially identical in different antibodies of the same class). Together, the variable regions form the antigen-binding sites—two per antibody monomer. **(b)** Computer-generated image of antibody structure.

Before seeing how these Ig classes differ from one another, let's look at how all antibodies are alike.

Basic Antibody Structure

Regardless of its class, each antibody consists of four looping polypeptide chains linked together by disulfide (sulfur-to-sulfur) bonds. The four chains combined form a molecule, called an **antibody monomer** (mon′o-mer), with two identical halves. The molecule as a whole is T or Y shaped **(Figure 21.14)**.

Two of the chains, called the **heavy (H) chains**, are identical to each other (blue chains in Figure 21.14a). The other two chains, called the **light (L) chains** (pink), are also identical to each other, but they are only about half as long as each H chain. The heavy chains have a flexible *hinge* region at their approximate "middles." The "loops" on each chain are created by disulfide bonds that cause the intervening parts of the polypeptide chains to loop out.

Each chain forming an antibody has a **variable (V) region** at one end and a **constant (C) region** at the other end. Antibodies responding to different antigens have very different V regions, but their C regions are the same (or nearly so) in all antibodies of a given class. In each arm of the monomer, the V regions of the heavy and light chains combine to form an **antigen-binding site** shaped to "fit" a specific antigenic determinant. Consequently, each antibody monomer has two such antigen-binding regions.

The C regions that form the *stem* of the antibody monomer determine the antibody class and serve common functions in all antibodies: These are the *effector regions* of the antibody that dictate (1) the cells and chemicals of the body the antibody can bind to, and (2) how the antibody class functions to eliminate antigens. For example, some antibodies fix complement, some circulate in blood while others are found primarily in body secretions, some cross the placental barrier, and so on.

Antibody Classes

The five major immunoglobulin classes are designated IgM, IgA, IgD, IgG, and IgE, on the basis of the C regions in their heavy chains. (Remember the name MADGE to recall the five Ig types.)

The antibodies of each class have different characteristics, biological roles, and locations in the body, as shown in **Table 21.4**. IgM in plasma is huge compared to the other antibodies. It is constructed from five Y-shaped units, or *monomers*, linked together to form a *pentamer* (*penta* = five). IgA occurs in both monomer and *dimer* (two linked monomers) forms. IgD, IgG, and IgE are monomers and have the same basic Y-shaped structure.

A single B cell can switch from making one class of antibody to another, thereby producing two or more different antibody classes having the same antigen specificity. For example, the first antibody released in the primary response is IgM, and then later plasma cells begin to secrete IgG. During secondary responses, almost all of the Ig protein is IgG.

Antibody Targets and Functions

Though antibodies themselves cannot destroy antigens, they can inactivate antigens and tag them for destruction **(Figure 21.15)**. The common event in all antibody-antigen interactions is formation of **antigen-antibody** (or **immune**) **complexes**. Defensive mechanisms used by antibodies include neutralization, agglutination, precipitation, and complement fixation, with the first two most important.

21

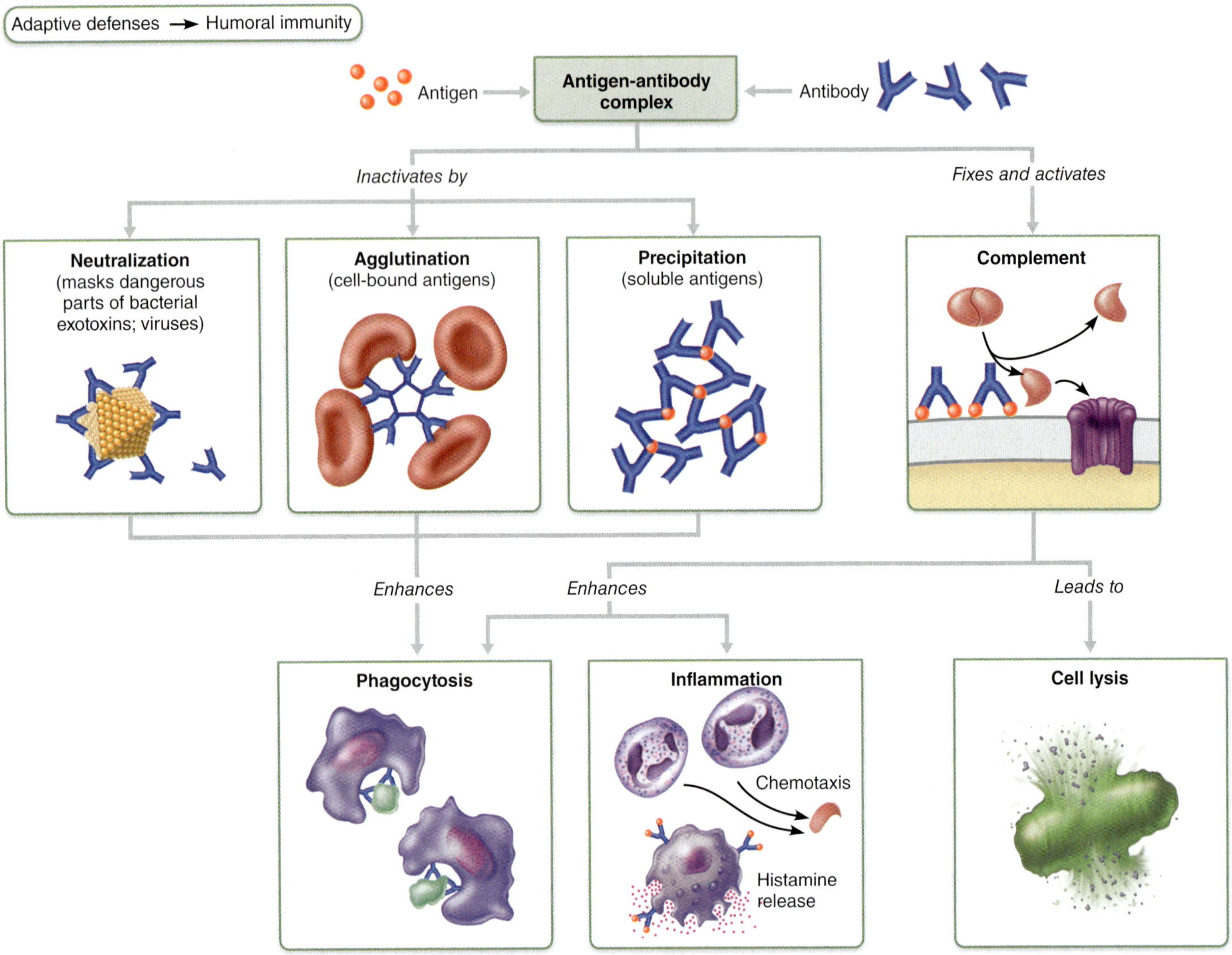

Figure 21.15 Mechanisms of antibody action. Antibodies act against free viruses, red blood cell antigens, bacterial toxins, intact bacteria, fungi, and parasitic worms.

21

Neutralization **Neutralization**, the simplest defensive mechanism, occurs when antibodies block specific sites on viruses or bacterial exotoxins (toxic chemicals secreted by bacteria). As a result, the virus or exotoxin cannot bind to receptors on tissue cells. Phagocytes eventually destroy the antigen-antibody complexes.

Agglutination Because antibodies have more than one antigen-binding site, they can bind to the same determinant on more than one antigen at a time. Consequently, antigen-antibody complexes can be cross-linked into large lattices. When cell-bound antigens are cross-linked, the process causes clumping, or **agglutination**, of the foreign cells. IgM, with 10 antigen-binding sites, is an especially potent agglutinating agent (see Table 21.4). Recall from Chapter 17 that agglutination occurs when mismatched blood is transfused (the foreign red blood cells clump) and is the basis of tests used for blood typing.

Precipitation In **precipitation**, soluble molecules (instead of cells) are cross-linked into large complexes that settle out of solution. Like agglutinated bacteria, precipitated antigen molecules are much easier for phagocytes to capture and engulf than are freely moving antigens.

Complement Fixation and Activation Complement fixation and activation is the chief antibody defense used against cellular antigens, such as bacteria or mismatched red blood cells. When several antibodies bind close together on the same cell, the complement-binding sites on their stem regions align. This triggers complement fixation into the antigenic cell's surface, followed by cell lysis.

Additionally, as we described earlier, molecules released during complement activation tremendously amplify the inflammatory response and promote phagocytosis via opsonization. This sets into motion a positive feedback cycle that enlists more and more defensive elements.

A quick and dirty way to remember how antibodies work is to remember they have a PLAN of action—**p**recipitation, **l**ysis (by complement), **a**gglutination, and **n**eutralization.

Table 21.4 Immunoglobulin Classes*

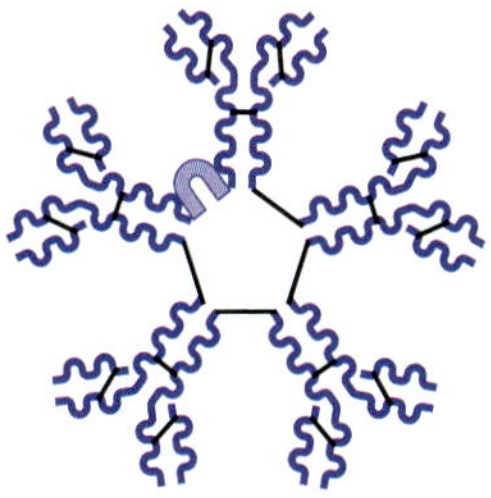 IgM (pentamer)	▪ The first immunoglobulin class secreted by plasma cells during the primary response. (This fact is diagnostically useful because presence of IgM in plasma usually indicates current infection by the pathogen eliciting IgM's formation.) ▪ Readily fixes and activates complement. ▪ Exists in monomer and pentamer (five united monomers) forms. ▪ The monomer serves as an antigen receptor on the B cell surface. ▪ The pentamer (illustrated) circulates in blood plasma. ▪ Numerous antigen-binding sites make it a potent agglutinating agent.
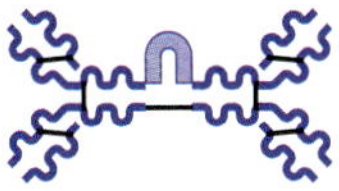 IgA (dimer)	▪ The dimer (illustrated), referred to as **secretory IgA**, is found in body secretions such as saliva, sweat, intestinal juice, and milk. ▪ Secretory IgA helps stop pathogens from attaching to epithelial cell surfaces (including mucous membranes and the epidermis). ▪ The monomer exists in limited amounts in plasma.
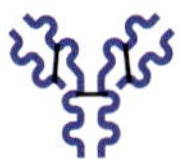 IgD (monomer)	▪ Found on the B cell surface. ▪ Functions as a B cell antigen receptor (as does IgM).
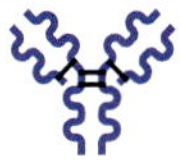 IgG (monomer)	▪ The most abundant antibody in plasma, accounting for 75–85% of circulating antibodies. ▪ The main antibody of both secondary and late primary responses. ▪ Readily fixes and activates complement. ▪ Protects against bacteria, viruses, and toxins circulating in blood and lymph. ▪ Crosses the placenta and confers passive immunity from the mother to the fetus.
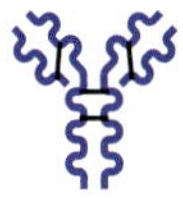 IgE (monomer)	▪ Stem end binds to mast cells or basophils. Antigen binding to its receptor end triggers these cells to release histamine and other chemicals that mediate inflammation and an allergic reaction. ▪ Secreted by plasma cells in skin, mucosae of the gastrointestinal and respiratory tracts, and tonsils. ▪ Only traces of IgE are found in plasma. ▪ Levels rise during severe allergic attacks or chronic parasitic infections of the gastrointestinal tract.

*Key characteristics are listed in blue type.

Homeostatic Imbalance 21.2

Around the world, billions of people are infected by parasitic worms such as *Ascaris* and *Schistosoma*. These large pathogens are difficult for our immune systems to deal with and "PLAN" is insufficient.

Nevertheless, antibodies still play a critical role in the worm's destruction. IgE antibodies coat the surface of parasitic worms, marking them for destruction by eosinophils. When eosinophils encounter antibody-coated worms, they bind to the exposed stems of the IgE. This triggers the eosinophils to release the toxic contents of their large cytoplasmic granules all over their prey. ✚

Monoclonal Antibodies as Clinical and Research Tools

In addition to their role in providing passive immunity, commercially prepared antibodies are essential in research, clinical testing, and treatment. **Monoclonal antibodies**, produced by descendants of a single cell, are pure antibody preparations specific for a single antigenic determinant.

Monoclonal antibodies are made by fusing tumor cells and B lymphocytes. The resulting cell hybrids, called **hybridomas** (hi″brĭ-do′mahz), have desirable traits of both parent cells. Like tumor cells, hybridomas proliferate indefinitely in culture, and like B cells, they produce a single type of antibody.

Monoclonal antibodies are used to diagnose pregnancy, certain sexually transmitted diseases, some cancers, hepatitis, and rabies. These monoclonal antibody tests are more specific, sensitive, and rapid than other tests. Monoclonal antibodies are also used to treat leukemia and lymphomas, cancers that are present in the circulation and so are easily accessible to injected antibodies. They also serve as "guided missiles" to deliver anticancer drugs only to cancerous tissue, and to treat certain autoimmune diseases (as we will discuss later).

Summary of Antibody Actions

At the most basic level, the race between antibody production and pathogen multiplication determines whether or not you become sick. Remember, however, that forming antigen-antibody complexes does *not* destroy the antigens. Instead, it prepares them for destruction by innate defenses.

Antibodies produced by plasma cells are in many ways the simplest, most versatile ammunition of the immune response. Nevertheless, they provide only partial immunity. Their prey are *extracellular pathogens*—intact bacteria, free viruses, and soluble foreign molecules—in other words, pathogens that are free in body secretions and tissue fluid and circulating in blood and lymph. Antibodies never invade solid tissues unless a lesion is present.

Until recently, the accepted dogma was that antibodies *only* act extracellularly. Remarkably, we now know that antibodies can act intracellularly as well. Antibodies that are attached to a virus before that virus infects a cell can "hang on" to the virus as it slips inside the cell. There, the antibodies activate intracellular mechanisms that destroy the virus. Even so, antibodies are not very effective against pathogens like viruses and tuberculosis bacilli that quickly slip inside body cells to multiply there. For

21

these intracellular pathogens, the cellular arm of adaptive immunity comes into play.

Check Your Understanding

15. Which class of antibody is most abundant in blood? Which is secreted first in a primary immune response? Which is most abundant in secretions?
16. List four ways in which antibodies can bring about destruction of a pathogen.

For answers, see Appendix H.

Cellular Immune Response

✓ Define cellular immunity and describe the process of activation and clonal selection of T cells.

✓ Describe the roles of different types of T cells.

T cells are best suited for cell-to-cell interactions. When antigens are presented to a T lymphocyte, they provoke a cellular immune response. Some activated T cells directly kill body cells infected by viruses or bacteria; abnormal or cancerous body cells; and cells of infused or transplanted foreign tissues. Other T cells release chemicals that regulate the immune response.

The T cells that mediate cellular immunity are a diverse lot, much more complex than B cells in both classification and function. There are two major populations of T cells based on which of two structurally related *cell differentiation glycoproteins*—CD4 or CD8—a mature T cell displays. The CD4 and CD8 glycoproteins are surface receptors but are distinct from the T cell antigen receptors. They play a role in interactions between T cells and other cells.

When activated, CD4 and CD8 cells differentiate into the three major kinds of *effector cells* of cellular immunity **(Figure 21.16)**.

- **CD4 cells** usually become *helper T cells* (T_H) that help activate B cells, other T cells, and macrophages, and direct the adaptive immune response.
- **CD8 cells** become *cytotoxic T cells* (T_C) that destroy any cells in the body that harbor anything foreign.
- Some CD4 cells become *regulatory T cells* (T_{Reg}), which moderate the immune response.

Activated CD4 and CD8 cells can also become memory T cells. We will provide details of T cells' roles shortly. Note that the names of the effector cells (helper, cytotoxic, regulatory) are reserved for *activated* T cells, while naive T cells are simply called CD4 or CD8 cells.

MHC Proteins and Antigen Presentation

Unlike B cells and antibodies, T cells cannot "see" either free antigens or antigens that are in their natural state. T cells can recognize and respond only to *processed* fragments of protein antigens displayed on surfaces of body cells (APCs and others).

Antigen presentation is necessary for both activation of naive T cells and the normal functioning of effector T cells. The cell surface proteins on which antigens are presented to T cells are called MHC proteins. As you might guess, we need to understand how these critical players in antigen presentation work before we can understand how T cells work. There are two classes of MHC proteins—class I MHC proteins and class II MHC proteins.

Class I MHC Proteins

Class I MHC proteins are found on the surface of virtually *all* body cells except red blood cells. Each class I MHC protein has a groove that holds an antigen—a protein fragment 8 or 9 amino acids long.

Where do these protein fragments come from? All antigens displayed on class I MHC proteins are **endogenous antigens**—fragments of proteins synthesized *inside the cell*. In a healthy cell, endogenous antigens are all self-antigens, generally bits of digested cellular proteins. But in an infected cell, endogenous antigens may also include fragments of foreign antigens that are synthesized within the infected cell but "belong to" the pathogen. In a cancerous cell, endogenous antigens can include altered cancer proteins.

As proteases (protein-digesting enzymes) degrade cytoplasmic proteins as part of their natural recycling, a random sample of the resulting protein fragments is transported into the endoplasmic reticulum. Inside the ER, these peptides bind to newly synthesized class I MHC proteins. Transport vesicles then export the "loaded" class I MHC proteins to the cell surface.

Class I MHC proteins are crucial for both activating naive CD8 cells and "informing" cytotoxic T cells that infectious microorganisms are hiding in body cells. Without them, viruses and certain bacteria that thrive in cells could multiply unnoticed and unbothered.

When class I MHC proteins display fragments of our own proteins (self-antigens), cytotoxic T cells passing by get the signal "Leave this cell alone, it's ours!" and ignore them. But when class I MHC proteins display foreign antigens, they "sound a molecular alarm" that signals invasion. In this signaling, the class I MHC proteins both (1) act as antigen holders and (2) form the self part of the self-nonself complexes that cytotoxic T cells must recognize in order to kill.

Class II MHC Proteins

Unlike the widely distributed class I MHC proteins, the second type of MHC protein is less widespread. **Class II MHC proteins** are typically found *only on the surfaces of cells that present antigens to CD4 cells*: dendritic cells, macrophages, and B cells. Like their class I MHC counterparts, class II MHC proteins are synthesized at the ER and bind to peptide fragments. However, the peptides they bind are longer (14–17 amino acids) and come from **exogenous antigens**—antigens from *outside* the cell that have been engulfed by the cell that displays them.

The engulfed exogenous antigens are broken down by proteases inside a phagolysosome. Vesicles from the ER containing class II MHC proteins fuse with the phagolysosome, and the antigen fragments bind to the groove of the MHC proteins. The vesicle is then exported to the cell surface, where the class II MHC protein displays its prize for CD4 cells to recognize.

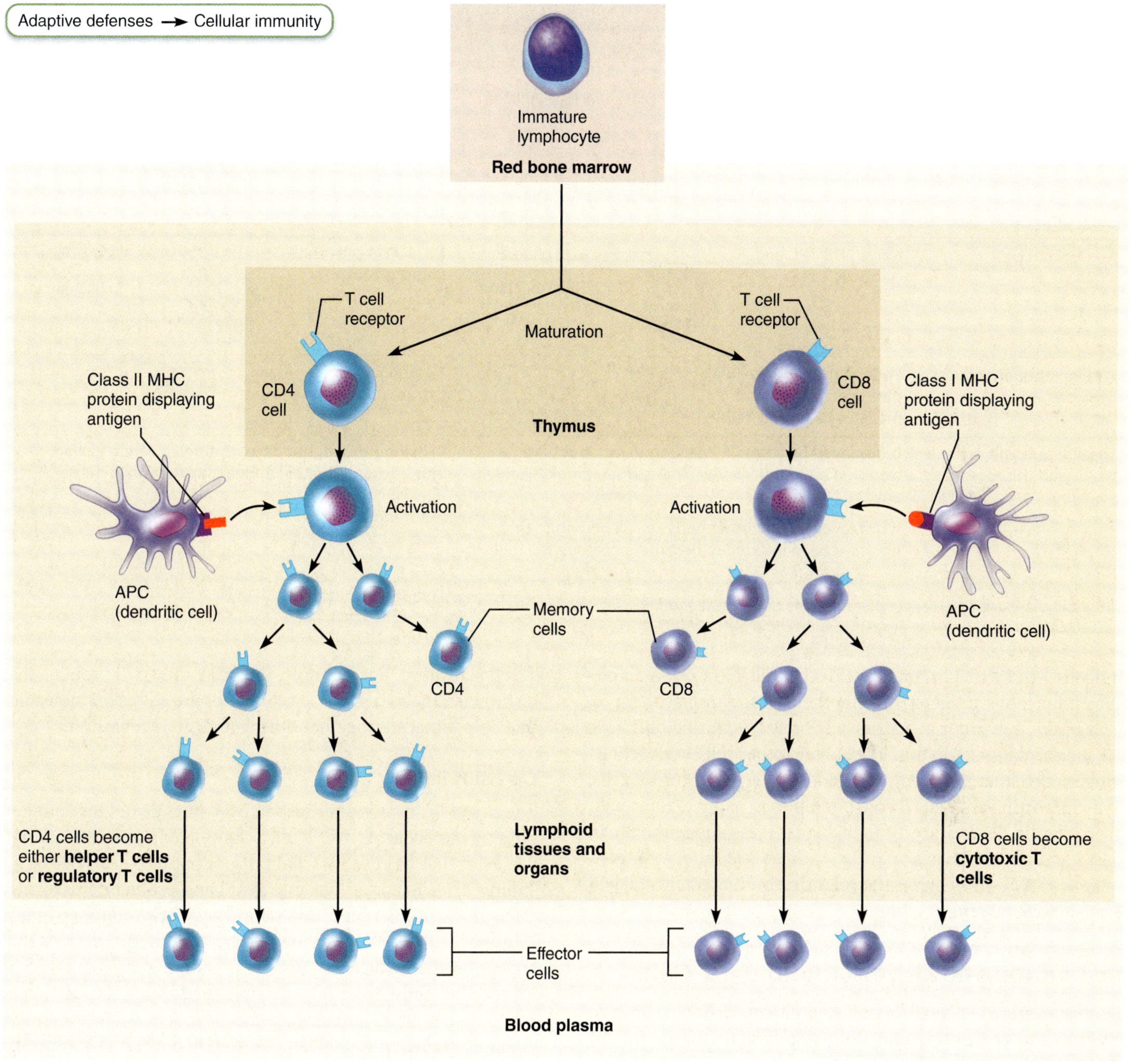

Figure 21.16 Major types of T cells.

Class II MHC proteins loaded with foreign antigens generally signal CD4 cells that help is required. It's as if they are showing the CD4 cells what the foreign invader "looks like." Most often, the result is that the CD4 cell will help mount a defense against the antigen.

MHC Restriction

CD4 and CD8 cells have different requirements for the class of MHC protein that presents antigens to them. This constraint, acquired during the education process in the thymus, is called *MHC restriction*.

- CD4 cells (that usually become helper T cells) are restricted to binding antigens only on class II MHC proteins, which are typically displayed on antigen-presenting cell (APC) surfaces.
- CD8 cells (that become cytotoxic T cells) are activated by antigen fragments on class I MHC proteins, also found on the surface of APCs. Once activated, cytotoxic T cells look for this same antigen presented on class I MHC proteins located on any cell in the body.

The MHC restriction for CD8 cells presents a problem for APCs. As a rule, class I MHC proteins display endogenous

Table 21.5 Role of MHC Proteins in Cellular Immunity

	CLASS I	CLASS II
Displayed by	All nucleated cells 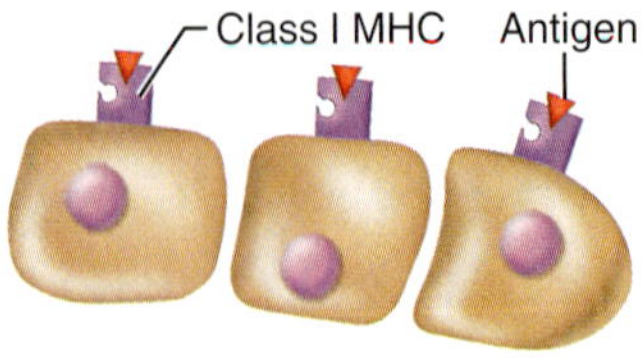	APCs (dendritic cells, macrophages, B cells) 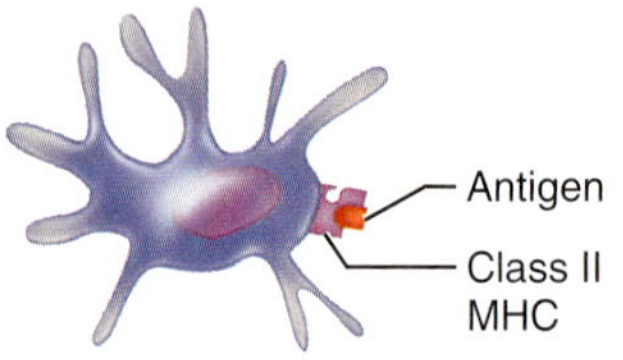
Recognized by	Naive CD8 cells and cytotoxic T cells 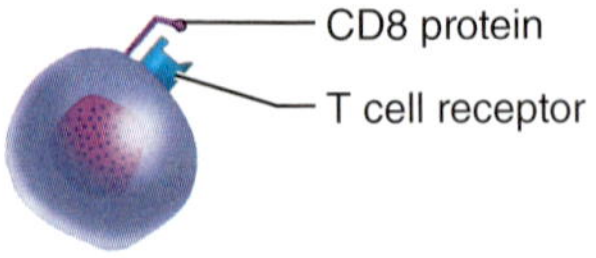	Naive CD4 cells and helper T cells 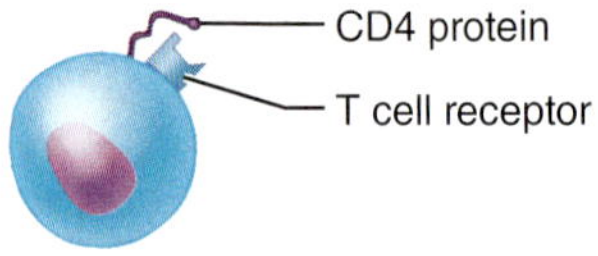
Foreign antigens on MHC are	Endogenous (intracellular pathogens or proteins made by cancerous cells)* 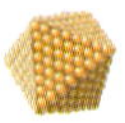	Exogenous (phagocytized extracellular pathogens) 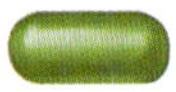
Foreign antigens on MHC send this message	**If displayed by an APC:** "I belong to self, but have captured a foreign invader. This is what it looks like. Kill any cell that displays it." **If displayed by any other body cell:** "I belong to self, but have been invaded or become cancerous. Kill me!"	"I belong to self, but have captured a foreign invader. This is what it looks like. Help me mount a defense against it."

*Dendritic cells are an exception because they can present *another cell's* endogenous antigens on their class I MHC proteins to activate CD8 cells.

antigens—those that originate inside that cell. How do APCs obtain endogenous antigens from another cell and display them on class I MHCs in order to activate CD8 cells? Dendritic cells have the special ability to do this. They obtain other cells' endogenous antigens by either engulfing dying virus-infected or tumor cells, or by importing antigens through temporary gap junctions with infected cells. Dendritic cells then display these antigens on *both* class I and class II MHCs.

Table 21.5 summarizes the roles that MHC proteins play in T cell activation and function.

Activation and Differentiation of T Cells

T cell activation is actually a two-step process involving antigen binding and co-stimulation. Both steps usually occur on the surface of the same APC, and both steps are required for *clonal selection*.

Antigen Binding

This first step mostly entails what we have already described: T cell antigen receptors **(TCRs)** bind to an antigen-MHC complex on the surface of an APC. Like B cell receptors, a TCR has variable and constant regions, but it consists of two rather than four polypeptide chains.

As you will recall from our discussion of T cell education, TCRs must perform *double recognition*: They must recognize both MHC (self-antigen) and the foreign antigen it displays. The TCR that recognizes (by binding) the nonself-self complex triggers multiple intracellular signaling pathways that lead to T cell activation. Other T cell surface proteins also play a role in T cell activation. For example, the CD4 and CD8 proteins that distinguish the two major T cell groups are adhesion molecules that help bind cells together during antigen recognition.

Co-stimulation

The story isn't over yet because step 2 comes next. Once antigen binding has occurred, the T cell is stimulated but is still "idling," like a car that has been started but not put into gear. Before an "idling" T cell can be "put into gear" and proliferate to form a clone, it must also bind one or more **co-stimulatory signals** **(Figure 21.17 (2b))**. These signals are yet other molecules that appear on the surfaces of APCs in tissues that are damaged or invaded by pathogens. For example, dendritic cells and macrophages sprout *B7 proteins* on their surfaces when the innate defenses are being mobilized. The binding of B7 to its specific receptor on a T cell is a crucial co-stimulatory signal.

What happens if a T cell binds to antigen without receiving the co-stimulatory signal? In this case, the T cell becomes tolerant to that antigen and is unable to divide or secrete cytokines. This state of unresponsiveness to antigen is called **anergy**.

The two-signal sequence acts as a kind of "double-handshake," a safeguard to prevent the immune system from destroying healthy cells. Without this safeguard, class I MHC proteins, which occur on all body cells and which display peptides from within the cell, could activate cytotoxic T cells, leading to widespread damage of healthy cells.

The important thing to understand is that along with antigen binding, co-stimulation is crucial for T cell activation. To go back to our idling car analogy, the car will not go anywhere unless it has both (1) been started and (2) put into gear.

Proliferation and Differentiation

Once activated by antigen binding and co-stimulation, a T cell enlarges and proliferates. Cytokines (which we will discuss next) released by APCs or T cells themselves promote this process. Cells of the resulting clone differentiate to perform functions according to their T cell class. This primary response peaks within a week of exposure to the triggering antigen. A period of apoptosis then occurs between days 7 and 30, during which time the activated T cells die off and effector activity wanes as the amount of antigen declines.

This wholesale disposal of T cells has a critical protective role because activated T cells are potential hazards. They produce huge amounts of inflammatory cytokines, which contribute to infection-driven hyperplasia, and may promote cancer in chronically inflamed tissue. Additionally, once they've done their job, the effector T cells are unnecessary and thus disposable. Thousands of clone members become memory T cells, persisting perhaps for life, and providing a reservoir of T cells that can later mediate secondary responses to the same antigen.

Cytokines

The chemical messengers involved in cellular immunity belong to a group of molecules called **cytokines**, a general term for mediators that influence cell development, differentiation, and responses in the immune system. Cytokines include interferons and interleukins. In **Table 21.6** on p. 790, you can see some of the large variety of these molecules and their myriad effects on target cells.

Cytokines include hormone-like or paracrine-like glycoproteins released by a variety of cells. As we mentioned previously, some cytokines promote T cell proliferation. For example, **interleukin 1 (IL-1)**, released by macrophages, stimulates T cells to liberate **interleukin 2 (IL-2)** and to synthesize more IL-2 receptors. IL-2 is a key growth factor. Acting on the cells that release it (as well as other T cells), it sets up a positive feedback cycle that encourages activated T cells to divide even more rapidly.

Additionally, all activated T cells secrete one or more other cytokines that help amplify and regulate a variety of adaptive and innate immune responses. Some (such as *tumor necrosis factor*) are cell toxins. Others (e.g., *gamma interferon*) enhance the killing power of macrophages; and still others are inflammatory chemicals.

☑ Check Your Understanding

17. Class II MHC proteins display what kind of antigens? What class of T cell recognizes antigens bound to class II MHC? What types of cells display these proteins?
18. What happens when antigens are bound in the absence of co-stimulators?

For answers, see Appendix H.

Roles of Specific Effector T Cells

✓ Describe T cell functions in the body.

Adaptive defenses → Cellular immunity

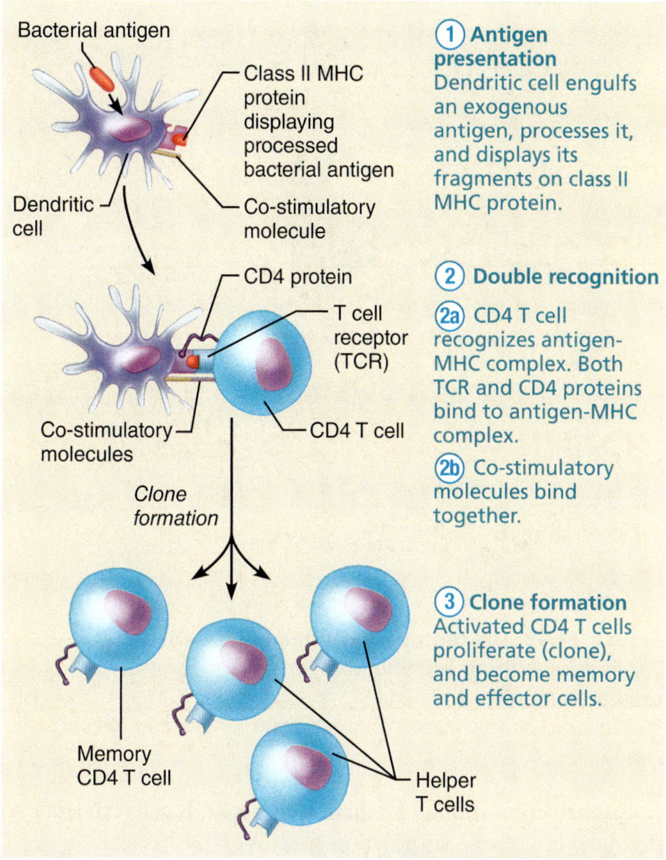

Figure 21.17 Clonal selection of T cells involves simultaneous recognition of self and nonself. Activation of CD4 cells is shown here, but activation of CD8 cells is similar.

Activated T cells (like B cells) can become either effector cells or memory cells. Next, we will focus on the three major groups of effector T cells: helper, cytotoxic, and regulatory T cells. (There are other minor "oddball" populations, but we will not consider them here).

Helper T Cells

Helper T (T_H) cells play a central role in adaptive immunity, mobilizing both its humoral and cellular arms **(Figure 21.18)**. Once activated by APC presentation of antigen, T_H cells help activate B and T cells, and induce B and T cells to proliferate. In fact, without the help of "director" T_H cells, there is *no* adaptive immune response. Their cytokines furnish the chemical help needed to recruit other immune cells.

Activation of B Cells Helper T cells interact directly with B cells displaying antigen fragments bound to class II MHC receptors (Figure 21.18a). Whenever a T_H cell binds to a B cell, the T_H cell releases cytokines that prod the B cells into dividing more rapidly. Then, like the boss of an assembly line, the T_H

Adaptive defenses → Humoral immunity / Cellular immunity

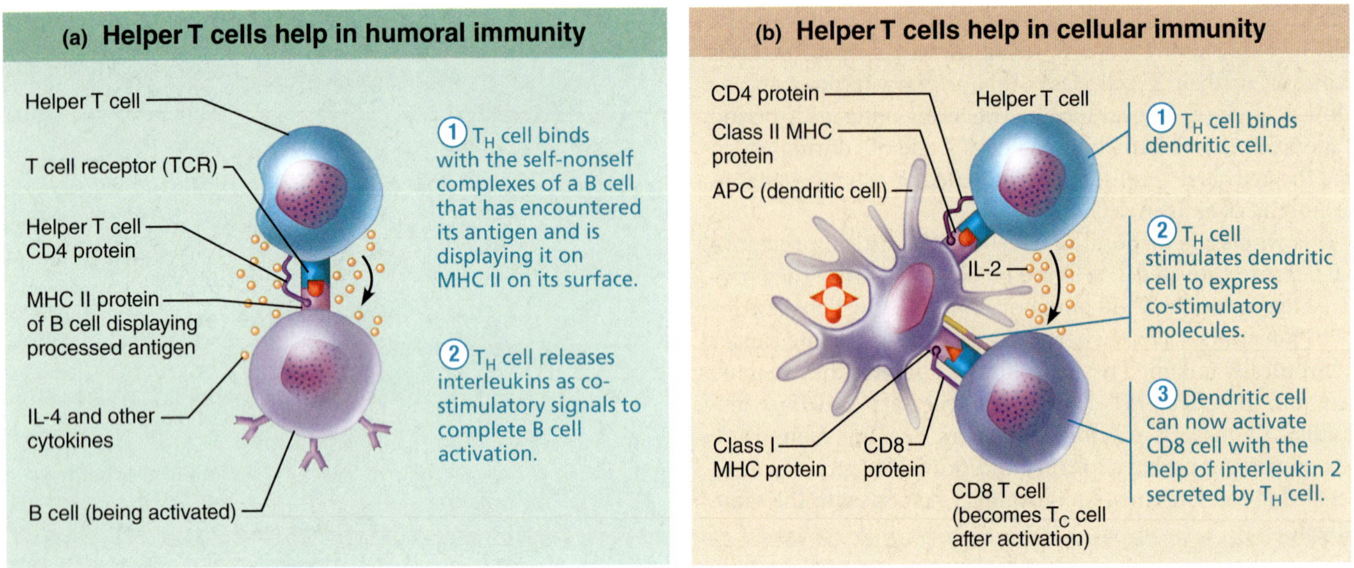

Figure 21.18 The central role of helper T cells in mobilizing both humoral and cellular immunity. (a) T_H and B cells usually must interact directly for full B cell activation. **(b)** In response to T_H cell binding, dendritic cells express co-stimulatory molecules required to activate CD8 T cells. (Some types of antigens induce these co-stimulatory molecules themselves, in which case T_H cell help may not be needed.) The T_H cell also produces interleukin 2, which causes the CD8 cell to proliferate and differentiate into a T_C cell.

cell signals for antibody formation to begin. B cells continue to divide as long as T_H stimulation continues. In this way, helper T cells help unleash the protective potential of B cells.

B cells may be activated solely by binding to certain antigens called **T cell–independent antigens**. However, T cell-independent antigen responses tend to be weak and short-lived. Most antigens are **T cell–dependent antigens** that require T cell help to activate the B cells to which they bind.

21

Activation of CD8 Cells Like B cells, CD8 cells usually require help from T_H cells to activate into destructive cytotoxic T cells. As shown in Figure 21.18b, T_H cells cause dendritic cells to express on their surfaces the co-stimulatory molecules required to activate CD8 cells.

Amplification of Innate Defenses T_H cells also amplify the responses of the innate immune system. For example, they activate macrophages to become more potent killers. The cytokines released by T_H cells not only mobilize lymphocytes and macrophages but also attract other types of white blood cells into the area and tremendously amplify innate defenses. As the released chemicals summon more and more cells into the battle, the immune response gains momentum, and the sheer number of immune elements overwhelms the antigens.

Subsets of T_H Cells It is interesting, but not surprising, that different subsets of helper T cells exist. The subset that develops during T_H cell differentiation depends on the type of antigen and the site at which it is encountered as well as the cytokine exposure of the differentiating T_H cell.

- *T_H1 cells* stimulate inflammation, activate macrophages, and promote differentiation of cytotoxic T cells. In other words, they mediate most aspects of cellular immunity.
- *T_H2 cells* mainly defend against parasitic worms. They mobilize eosinophils to the battlefield and activate immune responses that depend on B cells and antibody formation. They are also the cells that promote allergies.
- *T_H17 cells* link together adaptive and innate immunity by releasing IL-17, which promotes inflammatory responses against extracellular microbes and may underlie most autoimmune diseases.

Cytotoxic T Cells

Cytotoxic T (T_C) cells (activated CD8 cells) are the only T cells that can directly attack and kill other cells. T_C cells roam the body, circulating in and out of the blood and lymph and through lymphoid organs in search of body cells displaying antigens that the T_C cells recognize. Their main targets are virus-infected cells, but they also attack tissue cells infected by certain intracellular bacteria or parasites, cancer cells, and foreign cells introduced into the body by blood transfusions or organ transplants.

Before the onslaught can begin, the cytotoxic T cell must "dock" on the target cell by binding to a self-nonself complex. Remember, all body cells display class I MHC antigens, so T_C cells can destroy all infected or abnormal body cells. The attack on foreign human cells, such as those of a graft, is more difficult to explain because here *all* of the antigens are nonself. However,

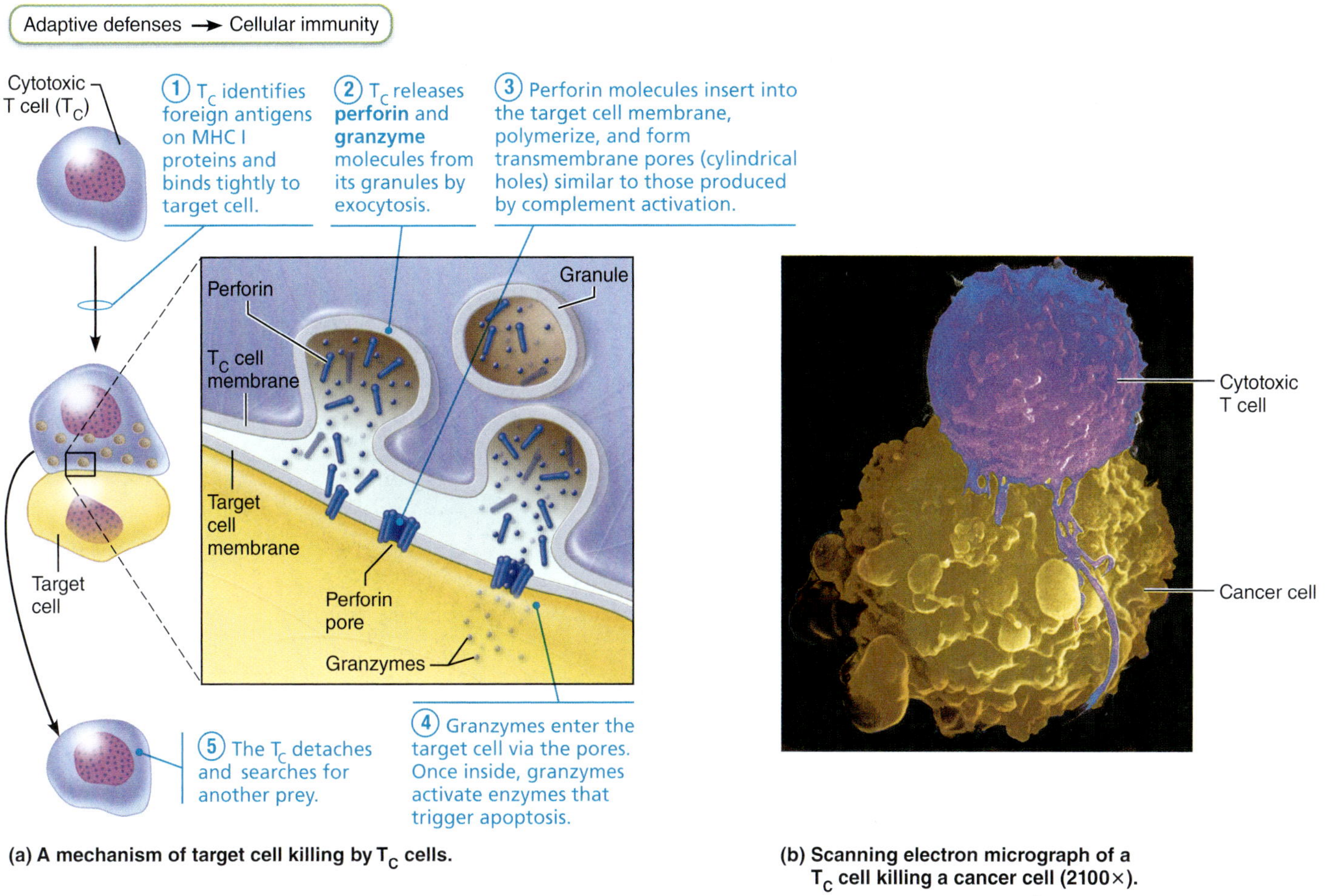

Figure 21.19 Cytotoxic T cells attack infected and cancerous cells. MHC proteins and T cell receptors not shown.

apparently the T_C cells sometimes "see" the foreign class I MHC antigens as a combination of self class I MHC protein bound to foreign antigen.

Once cytotoxic T cells recognize their targets, how do they deliver a **lethal hit**? There are two major mechanisms. One involves **perforins** and **granzymes** (**Figure 21.19**). The other involves binding to a specific membrane receptor on the target cell that stimulates the target cell to undergo apoptosis.

NK cells, introduced earlier, use the same key mechanisms to kill their target cells. NK cells, however, do not look for foreign antigen displayed on class I MHC proteins. Instead they search for other signs of abnormality, including the *lack* of class I MHC or the presence of antibodies coating the target cell. Stressed cells also often express different surface markers (such as some belonging to a family called MIC), which can activate NK cells. In short, NK cells stalk abnormal or foreign cells in the body that T_C cells can't "see."

NK cells and T_C lymphocytes roam the body, adhering to and crawling over the surfaces of other cells, examining them for markers they might recognize, a process called **immune surveillance**. NK cells check to make sure each cell has "identity flags" (class I MHC proteins *inhibit* NK cell attack), whereas T_C cells check the "identity flags" to see if they look the way they are supposed to (foreign antigens *stimulate* T_C cell attack).

Regulatory T Cells

While T_H cells help activate adaptive immune responses, related T cells called **regulatory T (T_{Reg}) cells** dampen the immune response. They act either by direct contact or by releasing inhibitory cytokines such as IL-10 and TGF-β.

T_{Reg} cells are important in preventing autoimmune reactions because they suppress self-reactive lymphocytes in the periphery—that is, outside the lymphoid organs. T_{Reg} cells and their subpopulations are currently hot research topics. For example, researchers hope to use them to induce tolerance to transplanted tissue and to lessen the severity of autoimmune diseases.

■ ■ ■

In summary, each type of T cell has unique roles to play in the immune response, yet is intimately intertwined with other immune cells and elements. **Table 21.7** on p. 792 summarizes the

21

Table 21.6 Selected Cytokines

CYTOKINE	FUNCTION IN IMMUNE RESPONSE
Interferons (IFNs)	
▪ Alpha (α) and beta (β)	Secreted by many cells. Have antiviral effects; activate NK cells.
▪ Gamma (γ)	Secreted by lymphocytes. Activates macrophages; stimulates synthesis and expression of more class I and II MHC proteins; promotes differentiation of T_H cells into T_H1.
Interleukins (ILs)	
▪ IL-1	Secreted by activated macrophages. Promotes inflammation and T cell activation; causes fever (acts as a pyrogen that resets the thermostat of the hypothalamus).
▪ IL-2	Secreted by T_H cells. Stimulates T and B cell proliferation, T_{Reg} cell development, and NK cell activation.
▪ IL-4	Secreted by some T_H cells. Promotes differentiation to T_H2; promotes B cell activation; switches antibody production to IgE.
▪ IL-5	Secreted by some T_H cells and mast cells. Attracts and activates eosinophils; causes plasma cells to secrete IgA antibodies.
▪ IL-10	Secreted by macrophages, T_H, and T_{Reg} cells. Inhibits macrophages and dendritic cells; turns down cellular and innate immune response.
▪ IL-12	Secreted by dendritic cells and macrophages. Stimulates T_C and NK cell activity; promotes T_H1 differentiation.
▪ IL-17	Secreted by T_H17 cells. Important in innate and adaptive immunity and recruiting neutrophils. Involved in inflammation in many autoimmune diseases.
Suppressor factors	A generic term for a number of cytokines that suppress the immune system, for example TGF-β and IL-10.
Transforming growth factor beta (TGF-β)	A suppressor factor similar to IL-10; stimulates T_{Reg} and T_H17 cell development.
Tumor necrosis factors (TNFs)	Produced by lymphocytes and in large amounts by macrophages. Promote inflammation; enhance phagocyte chemotaxis and nonspecific killing; slow tumor growth by selectively damaging tumor blood vessels; promote cell death by apoptosis.

cells and molecules of the adaptive immune response. **Figure 21.20** gives an overview of the entire primary immune response, both innate and adaptive. The lesson to take away with you is that without helper T cells, *there is no adaptive immune response* because the helper cells direct or help complete the activation of both B cells and T cells. Their crucial role in immunity is painfully evident when they are destroyed, as in AIDS (see p. 793).

21

Organ Transplants and Prevention of Rejection

✓ Describe the four varieties of grafts.

✓ Indicate the tests ordered before an organ transplant is done, and methods used to prevent transplant rejection.

Organ transplants, a viable treatment option for many patients with end-stage cardiac or renal disease, have been done with mixed success for over 50 years. Immune rejection presents a particular problem when the goal is to provide such patients with functional organs from a living or recently deceased donor.

There are four varieties of grafts:

- **Autografts** are tissue grafts transplanted from one body site to another in the *same person*.
- **Isografts** are grafts donated to a patient by a *genetically identical individual*, the only example being identical twins.
- **Allografts** are grafts transplanted from individuals who are *not genetically identical* but belong to the *same* species.
- **Xenografts** are grafts *taken from another animal species*, such as transplanting a baboon heart into a human.

Transplant success depends on the similarity of the tissues because NK cells, macrophages, antibodies, and especially T cells act vigorously to destroy any foreign tissue. Autografts and isografts are the ideal donor tissues. Given an adequate blood supply and no infection, they are almost always successful because the MHC proteins are identical.

Successful xenografts from genetically engineered animals are still just a promise on the horizon. Consequently, the type most frequently used is also the most problematic: the allograft. The organ is usually obtained from a living human donor (in the case of kidney, liver, or bone marrow) or harvested from a human donor who has just died (heart or lung).

Before an allograft is attempted, the ABO and other blood group antigens of donor and recipient must be determined, because these antigens are also present on most body cells. Next, recipient and donor tissues are typed to determine their MHC antigen match. MHC variation among human tissues is tremendous, so matching all MHC antigens is impossible. In general, however, the closer the match, the less likely is rejection.

Following surgery the patient is treated with *immunosuppressive therapy*. This involves drugs of the following categories: (1) corticosteroid drugs to suppress inflammation;

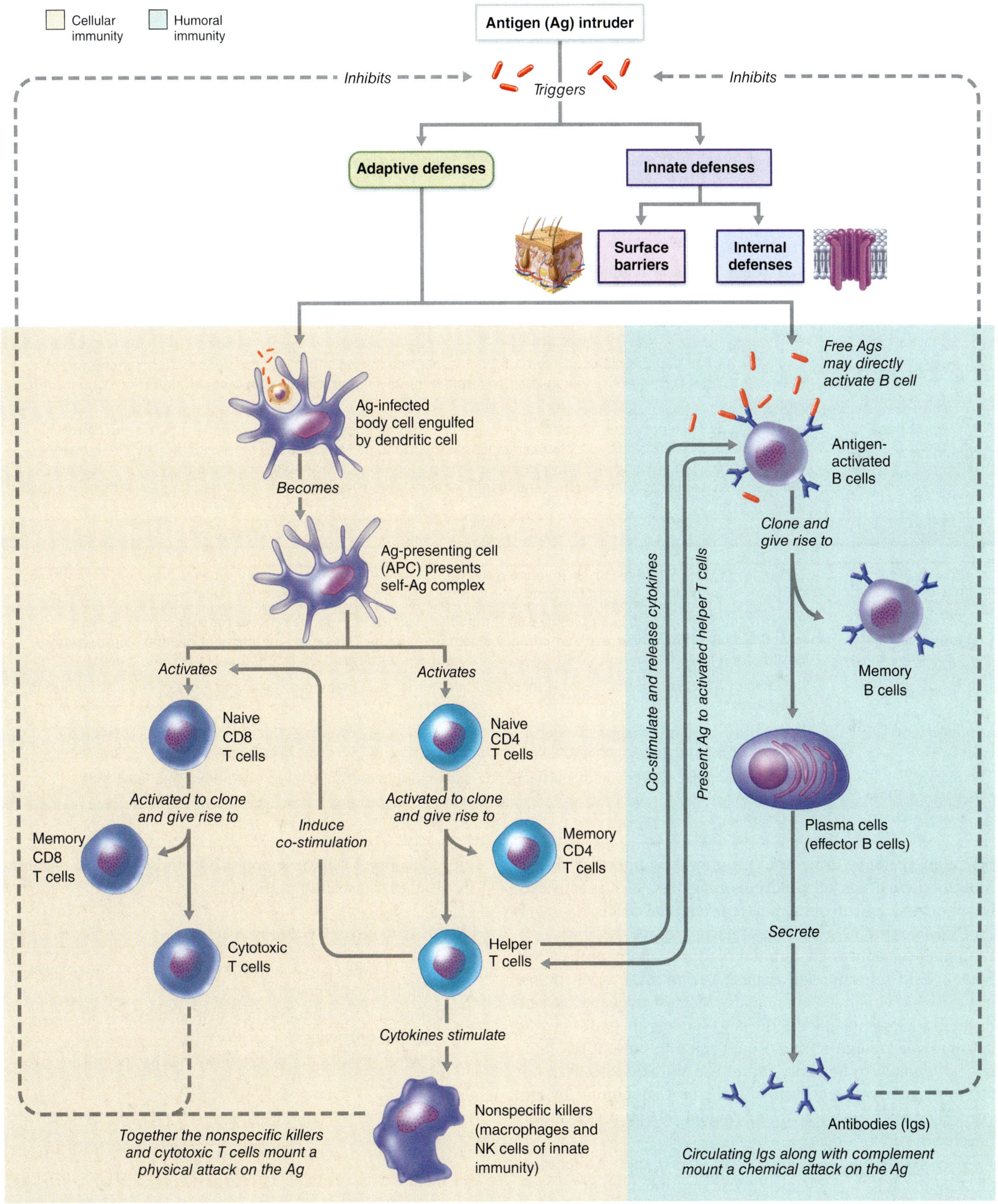

Figure 21.20 Simplified summary of the primary immune response. Co-stimulation usually requires direct cell-cell interactions; cytokines enhance these and many other events. Although complement, NK cells, and phagocytes are innate defenses, they are enlisted in the fight by cytokines. (For simplicity, only B cell receptors are illustrated.)

Table 21.7 Cells and Molecules of the Adaptive Immune Response

ELEMENT	FUNCTION IN IMMUNE RESPONSE
Cells	
B cell	Lymphocyte that matures in bone marrow. Induced to replicate by antigen binding, usually followed by helper T cell interactions in lymphoid tissues. Its progeny (clone members) form plasma cells and memory cells.
Plasma cell	Antibody-producing "machine"; produces huge numbers of antibodies (immunoglobulins) with the same antigen specificity. An effector B cell.
Helper T cell (T_H)	An effector CD4 T cell central to both humoral and cellular immunity. It stimulates production of cytotoxic T cells and plasma cells to fight invaders, activates macrophages, and acts both directly and indirectly by releasing cytokines. Three major subsets (T_H1, T_H2, and T_H17).
Cytotoxic T cell (T_C)	An effector CD8 T cell. Activation usually requires helper T cell involvement. Its specialty is killing virus-invaded body cells and cancer cells; also involved in rejection of foreign tissue grafts.
Regulatory T cell (T_{Reg})	Slows or stops activity of immune system. Important in controlling autoimmune diseases; several different populations exist.
Memory cell	Descendant of activated B cell or any class of T cell; generated during initial immune response (primary response). May exist in body for years after, enabling it to respond quickly and efficiently to subsequent infections or encounters with same antigen.
Antigen-presenting cell (APC)	Any of several cell types (dendritic cell, macrophage, B cell) that engulfs and digests antigens that it encounters, then presents parts of them on its plasma membrane (bound to an MHC protein) for recognition by T cells bearing receptors for the same antigen. This function, antigen presentation, is essential for activation of T cells and normal cell-mediated responses. Macrophages and dendritic cells also release chemicals (cytokines) that activate many other immune cells.
Molecules	
Antigen	Substance capable of provoking an immune response. Typically a large, complex molecule (e.g., protein or modified protein) not normally present in the body.
Antibody (immunoglobulin or Ig)	Protein produced by B cell or by plasma cell. Antibodies produced by plasma cells are released into body fluids (blood, lymph, saliva, mucus, etc.), where they attach to antigens. This causes complement fixation, neutralization, precipitation, or agglutination, which "marks" the antigens for destruction by phagocytes or complement.
Perforins, granzymes	Released by T_C cells. Perforins create large pores in the target cell's membrane, allowing entry of apoptosis-inducing granzymes.
Complement	Group of bloodborne proteins activated after binding to antibody-covered antigens or certain molecules on the surface of microorganisms; enhances inflammatory response and lyses some microorganisms.
Cytokines	Small proteins that act as chemical messengers between various parts of the immune system. See Table 21.6.

21

(2) antiproliferative drugs, and (3) immunosuppressant drugs. Many of these drugs kill rapidly dividing cells (such as activated lymphocytes), and all of them have severe side effects.

The major problem with immunosuppressive therapy is that the patient's suppressed immune system cannot protect the body against other foreign agents. As a result, overwhelming bacterial and viral infection remains the most frequent cause of death in transplant patients. The key to successful graft survival is to provide enough immunosuppression to prevent rejection but not enough to be toxic, and to use antibiotics to keep infections under control. Even with the best conditions, by ten years after receiving a transplant, roughly 50% of patients have rejected the donor organ.

Many research projects are seeking ways to induce tolerance. One approach is to create a **chimeric immune system** (*chimer* = monster) by temporarily suppressing the recipient's bone marrow and then dousing it with bone marrow from the same donor as the new organ in the hope that this combined immune system will treat the transplanted organ as self. Another approach tries to harness the body's own tolerance-inducing cells, the regulatory T cells, to suppress only those immune reactions that lead to transplant rejection.

☑ Check Your Understanding

19. Which type of T cell is the most important in both cellular and humoral immunity? Why?
20. Describe the killing mechanism of cytotoxic T cells that involves perforins.
21. Which proteins must be carefully matched before an organ transplant?

For answers, see Appendix H.

Homeostatic Imbalances of Immunity

✓ Give examples of immunodeficiency diseases and of hypersensitivity states.

✓ Cite factors involved in autoimmune disease.

Certain circumstances can cause the immune system to weaken, fail, or act in a way that damages the body. Most such problems can be classified as immunodeficiencies, autoimmune diseases, or hypersensitivities.

Immunodeficiencies

An **immunodeficiency** is a congenital or acquired condition that impairs the production or function of immune cells or certain molecules, such as complement or antibodies.

The most devastating *congenital immunodeficiencies* are a group of related disorders called **severe combined immunodeficiency (SCID) syndromes**, which result from various genetic defects that produce a marked deficit of B and T cells. One SCID defect, for example, results in a defective *adenosine deaminase* (*ADA*) enzyme. Without normal ADA activity, metabolites that are lethal to T cells accumulate in the body.

Children afflicted with SCID have little or no protection against disease-causing organisms of any type. Interventions must begin in the first months of life because minor infections easily shrugged off by most children cause SCID victims to become deathly ill. Untreated, this condition is fatal, but successful transplants of matched donor hematopoietic stem cells dramatically improve survival rates. Genetic engineering techniques using viruses to carry corrected genes into the victim's own hematopoietic stem cells can also help.

There are various *acquired immunodeficiencies*. For example, *Hodgkin's lymphoma*, a cancer of the B cells, can lead to immunodeficiency by depressing lymph node cells. Immunosuppressive drugs used in transplantation and certain drugs used to treat cancer also suppress the immune system.

HIV and AIDS

The most devastating of the acquired immunodeficiencies is **acquired immune deficiency syndrome (AIDS)**, which cripples the immune system by interfering with the activity of helper T cells.

First identified in the United States in 1981 among homosexual men and intravenous drug users, AIDS is characterized by severe weight loss, night sweats, swollen lymph nodes, and increasingly frequent opportunistic infections, including a rare type of pneumonia called *pneumocystis pneumonia*, and the bizarre malignancy *Kaposi's sarcoma*, a cancer of the blood vessels evidenced by purple skin lesions. The course of AIDS is often grim, finally ending in complete debilitation and death from cancer or overwhelming infection.

Biology of HIV AIDS is caused by the **human immunodeficiency virus (HIV)**, a virus transmitted in body secretions—especially blood, semen, and vaginal secretions. HIV commonly enters the body via blood transfusions or blood-contaminated needles and during sexual intercourse. It is also present in saliva and tears, and there are documented cases of transmission by oral sex. An infected mother can also transmit the virus to her fetus.

HIV destroys T_H cells, depressing cellular immunity. Although B cells and T_C cells initially mount a vigorous response to viral exposure, over time a profound deficit of B cell and T_C cell function develops. The whole immune system is turned topsy-turvy.

The virus multiplies steadily in the lymph nodes throughout most of the asymptomatic period, which averages ten years in the absence of treatment. Symptoms appear when the lymph nodes can no longer contain the virus and the immune system collapses. The virus also invades the brain (which accounts for the dementia some AIDS patients develop).

HIV targets CD4 cells via their CD4 surface proteins. Researchers have identified an HIV envelope glycoprotein complex (gp120/gp41) that fits into the CD4 receptor like a plug fits into a socket. Once these and other proteins have connected, the virus fuses with the target cell.

Once inside, HIV "sets up housekeeping," using the viral enzyme *reverse transcriptase* to produce DNA from its (viral) RNA. This DNA copy, now called a *provirus*, inserts itself into the target cell's DNA and directs the cell to crank out new copies of viral RNA and proteins so that the virus can multiply and infect other cells.

Although T_H cells are the main HIV targets, other body cells displaying CD4 proteins (macrophages, monocytes, and dendritic cells) are also at risk. The HIV reverse transcriptase enzyme is not very accurate and produces errors rather frequently, causing HIV's relatively high mutation rate and its changing resistance to drugs.

Epidemiology The years since 1981 have witnessed a global AIDS epidemic. Currently, about 33 million people are living with HIV worldwide, almost 90% of them in the developing countries of Asia and sub-Saharan Africa. Half of the victims are women, indicating that in the hardest hit regions, most HIV transmission occurs via heterosexual contacts.

More than 1 million Americans are now infected with HIV. Of these, a quarter don't even know they are infected, either because anti-HIV antibodies are not yet detectable in their blood (this may take as long as six months after infection), or because they have not been tested.

The "face of AIDS" is changing too. Homosexual men still account for the bulk of cases transmitted by sexual contact in the U.S., but more and more heterosexuals are contracting this disease. Particularly disturbing is the number of diagnosed cases among teenagers and young adults—AIDS is the sixth leading killer of Americans ages 25 to 44.

Treatment and Prevention No cure for AIDS has yet been found. Fortunately, a number of antiviral drugs are available, and these fall into four broad classes.

- *Fusion inhibitors* prevent the virus from entering the cell in the first place.
- *Integrase inhibitors* block the virus from integrating its genetic information into the host's DNA.
- *Reverse transcriptase inhibitors* and *protease inhibitors* inhibit important viral enzymes needed for viral replication after the virus has entered the target cell.

Combination therapy using several drugs at once delivers a one-two punch to the virus. It delays drug resistance and causes the *viral load* (amount of HIV virus per milliliter of blood) to plummet while boosting the number of T_H cells. Sadly, even combination drug therapies fail as the virus becomes resistant.

For years, the long-term goal has been to develop a vaccine to prevent HIV infection. Unfortunately, out of the numerous vaccine trials to date, only one has had even modest success, and this goal remains a long way away. In the meantime, barrier methods such as latex condoms remain the prevention method of choice. For those women who cannot always insist on condom use, a new antiretroviral vaginal gel can reduce infection risk by about 50%.

Autoimmune Diseases

Occasionally the immune system loses its ability to distinguish friend (self) from foe (foreign antigens). When this happens, the artillery of the immune system, like friendly fire, turns against itself. The body produces antibodies (*autoantibodies*) and cytotoxic T cells that destroy its own tissues. This puzzling phenomenon is called **autoimmunity**. If a disease state results, it is referred to as **autoimmune disease**.

Some 5% of adults in North America—two-thirds of them women—are afflicted with an autoimmune disease. You have already encountered examples of autoimmune diseases in earlier chapters, and you will encounter more later on. Some important autoimmune diseases are:

- *Rheumatoid arthritis*, which systematically destroys joints (see pp. 270–271)
- *Myasthenia gravis*, which impairs communication between nerves and skeletal muscles (see p. 286)
- *Multiple sclerosis*, which destroys the myelin of the white matter of the brain and spinal cord (see pp. 405–406)
- *Graves' disease*, which prompts the thyroid gland to produce excessive amounts of thyroxine (see p. 610) and causes the eyeballs to protrude more anteriorly
- *Type 1 (insulin-dependent) diabetes mellitus*, which destroys pancreatic beta cells, resulting in a deficit of insulin and inability to use carbohydrates (see p. 620)
- *Systemic lupus erythematosus (SLE)*, a systemic disease that particularly affects the kidneys, heart, lungs, and skin (see Related Clinical Terms, p. 800)
- *Glomerulonephritis*, which damages the kidney's filtration membrane and severely impairs renal function (see p. 988)

Treatment of Autoimmune Diseases

The most widely used treatments for autoimmune conditions suppress the entire immune system—for example, anti-inflammatory drugs such as corticosteroids. Newer treatments seek to target specific aspects of the immune response. Fortunately, the immune system offers many potential targets because it is so complex. Two widely used therapeutic approaches involve:

- Blocking the actions of various cytokines using antibodies against them or their receptors
- Blocking the co-stimulatory molecules required to activate effector cells

Approaches still being developed include reestablishing self-tolerance by:

- Activating regulatory T cells
- Inducing self-tolerance using vaccines
- Destroying self-reactive immune cells by directing antibodies against them

The biggest challenge is selectively blocking autoimmune responses without blocking responses necessary to combat infection.

Failure of Self-Tolerance

Every autoimmune disease represents a failure of self-tolerance. How does this happen? As you recall, lymphocytes undergo an extensive education in the bone marrow or thymus that weeds out self-reactive cells. This weeding is thorough, but not too thorough, since there are pathogens that look somewhat like self. Weakly self-reactive lymphocytes that can detect these pathogens are allowed into the periphery, where they may cause autoimmune disease if they become activated.

Recall that activation of a T cell requires a co-stimulatory signal on an APC (see p. 786), and these co-stimulatory signals are only present if the APC has received "danger" signals alerting it to damage or invasion. This is an important safety check that generally keeps both humoral and cellular immunity under control. In addition, regulatory T (T_{Reg}) cells inhibit autoimmune reactions.

Normally, these mechanisms are sufficient, but sometimes self-reactive lymphocytes slip out of control. One of the following conditions or events may trigger this:

- **Foreign antigens resemble self-antigens.** If the determinants on a self-antigen resemble those on a foreign antigen, antibodies made against the foreign antigen can cross-react with the self-antigen. In the age-old disease *rheumatic fever*, for instance, antibodies produced during a streptococcal infection react with heart antigens, causing lasting damage to the heart muscle and valves, as well as to joints and kidneys.
- **New self-antigens appear.** Self-proteins not previously exposed to the immune system may appear in the circulation. They may be generated by (1) gene mutations that cause new proteins to appear at the external cell surface, (2) changes in the structure of self-antigens as a result of hapten attachment or infectious damage, or (3) novel self-antigens, normally hidden behind barriers such as the blood brain barrier, that are released by trauma. These newly generated proteins then become immune system targets.

Hypersensitivities

Hypersensitivities result when the immune system damages tissue as it fights off a perceived threat (such as pollen or animal dander) that would otherwise be harmless to the body. People rarely die of hypersensitivities. They just make you miserable.

The different types of hypersensitivity reactions are distinguished by (1) their time course, and (2) whether they involve antibodies or T cells. Antibody-associated reactions cause *immediate* and *subacute hypersensitivities*. T cells cause *delayed hypersensitivities*.

Immediate Hypersensitivities

Immediate hypersensitivities, also called **acute** or **type I hypersensitivities**, are simply what most of us would call **allergies** (*allo* = altered; *erg* = reaction). An **allergen** is an antigen that causes an allergic reaction. Allergic reactions begin within seconds after contact with the allergen and last about half an hour.

The initial meeting with an allergen produces no symptoms but it sensitizes the person. APCs digest the allergen and present its fragments to CD4 cells as usual. In susceptible individuals, an abnormally large number of these CD4 cells differentiate into IL-4-secreting T_H2 cells. IL-4 stimulates B cells to mature into IgE-secreting plasma cells, which spew out huge amounts of antibody specific for that allergen. When the IgE molecules attach to *mast cells* and *basophils*, sensitization is complete.

Later encounters with the same allergen trigger an allergic reaction, in which the allergen promptly binds and cross-links the IgE antibodies on the surfaces of the mast cells and basophils. This event induces an enzymatic cascade. Mast cells and basophils release a flood of *histamine* and other inflammatory chemicals that together induce the inflammatory response typical of allergy **(Figure 21.21)**.

Allergic reactions may be local or systemic (bodywide). Mast cells are abundant in connective tissues of the skin and beneath the mucosa of respiratory passages and the gastrointestinal tract, and these areas are common sites of local allergic reactions.

Histamine causes blood vessels to dilate and become leaky, and is largely to blame for the best recognized symptoms of allergy: runny nose, itching reddened skin (hives), and watery eyes. When the allergen is inhaled, symptoms of *asthma* appear because smooth muscle in the walls of the bronchioles contracts, constricting those small passages and restricting air flow. When the allergen is ingested in food or via drugs, gastrointestinal discomfort (cramping, vomiting, or diarrhea) occurs. Over-the-counter antiallergy drugs contain antihistamines that counteract these effects.

The systemic response known as **anaphylactic shock** is fairly rare. It typically occurs when the allergen directly enters the blood and circulates rapidly through the body—for example, a bee sting, spider bite, or injection of a foreign substance (such as penicillin or other drugs that act as haptens).

The mechanism of anaphylactic shock is essentially the same as that of local responses, but when mast cells and basophils are enlisted throughout the body, the outcome is life threatening. The bronchioles constrict (and the tongue may swell), making it difficult to breathe, and the sudden vasodilation and fluid loss from the bloodstream may cause circulatory collapse (hypotensive shock) and death within minutes. Epinephrine is the drug of choice to reverse these histamine-mediated effects.

Subacute Hypersensitivities

Like the immediate types, **subacute hypersensitivities** are caused by antibodies (IgG and IgM rather than IgE). However,

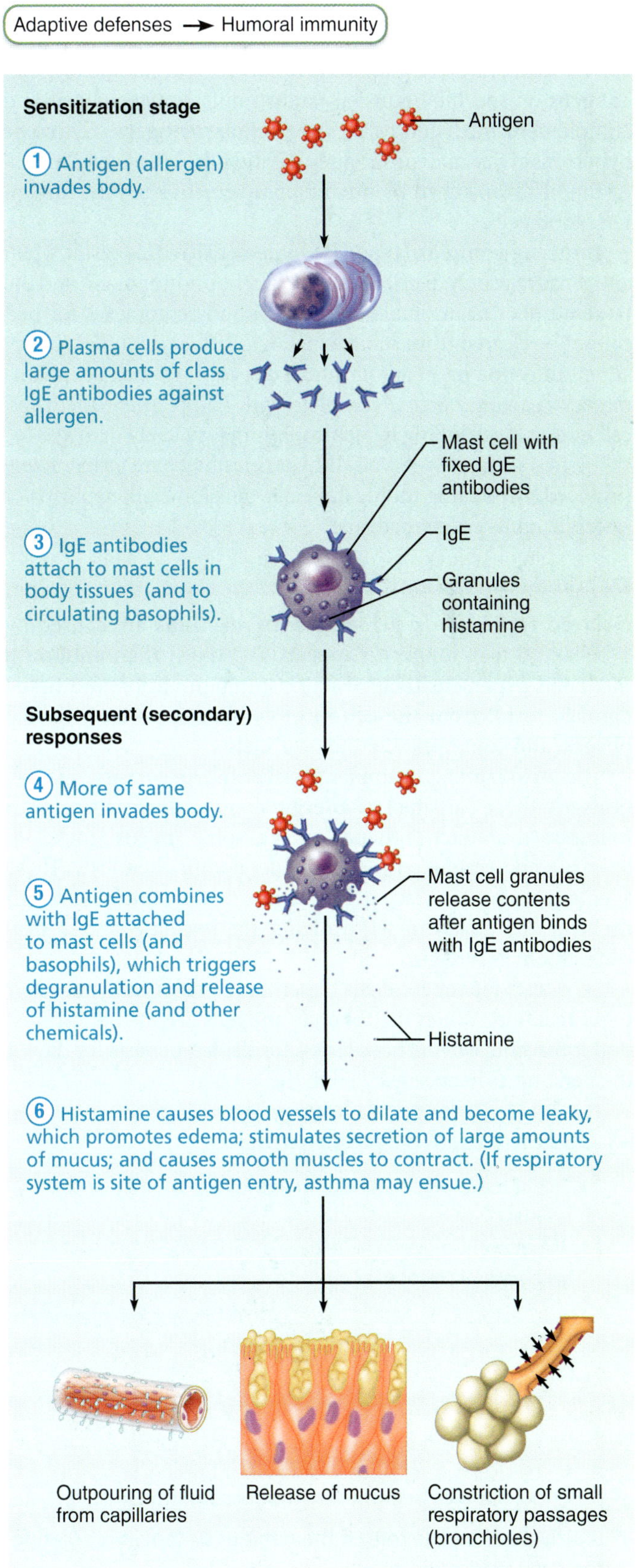

Figure 21.21 Mechanism of an acute allergic (immediate hypersensitivity) response.

21

their onset is slower (1–3 hours after antigen exposure) and the reaction lasts longer (10–15 hours).

Cytotoxic (type II) reactions occur when antibodies bind to antigens on specific body cells and stimulate phagocytosis and complement-mediated lysis of the cellular antigens. Cytotoxic hypersensitivity may occur after a patient has received a transfusion of mismatched blood and complement lyses the foreign red blood cells.

Immune-complex (type III) hypersensitivities result when antigens are widely distributed through the body or blood and the huge number of insoluble antigen-antibody complexes formed cannot be cleared from a particular area. (This may reflect a persistent infection or an autoimmune disease.) An intense inflammatory reaction occurs, complete with complement-mediated cell lysis and cell killing by neutrophils that severely damages local tissues. Examples of type III hypersensitivity are *farmer's lung* (induced by inhaling moldy hay) and the glomerulonephritis of systemic lupus erythematosus.

Delayed Hypersensitivities

Delayed (type IV) hypersensitivity reactions are caused by T cells and take longer to appear (1–3 days) than antibody-mediated hypersensitivity reactions. Inflammation and tissue damage result from the action of cytokine-activated macrophages, and sometimes cytotoxic T cells.

The most familiar examples of delayed hypersensitivity reactions are those classified as **allergic contact dermatitis** which follow skin contact with poison ivy, some metals (nickel in jewelry), and certain cosmetic and deodorant chemicals. These agents act as haptens (see p. 774), and after they diffuse through the skin and attach to self-proteins, the immune system perceives them as foreign.

Skin tests for tuberculosis depend on a delayed hypersensitivity reaction. When the tubercle antigens are introduced just under the skin, a small hard lesion forms that persists for days if the person has been sensitized to the antigen.

21

☑ Check Your Understanding

22. What makes HIV particularly hard for the immune system to defeat?
23. What event triggers the release of histamine from mast cells in an allergic response?

For answers, see Appendix H.

Developmental Aspects of the Immune System

✓ Describe changes in immunity that occur with aging.

✓ Briefly describe the role of the nervous system in regulating the immune response.

Stem cells of the immune system originate in the liver and spleen during weeks 1–9 of embryonic development. Later the bone marrow becomes the predominant source of stem cells, and it persists in this role into adult life. As we have seen, the lymphocyte precursors develop self-tolerance and immunocompetence in their "programming organs" (thymus and bone marrow) and then populate other lymphoid tissues.

The newborn's immune system depends primarily on antibodies, and hence on T_H2 lymphocytes. The T_H1 system is educated and gets stronger as a result of encounters with microbes—both harmful and harmless. If such exposure and education does not occur, immune balance is upset and the T_H2 system flourishes, causing the immune system to teeter toward allergies. Unhappily, the desire to keep our children squeaky clean with antibiotics that kill off both harmful and harmless bacteria may derail normal immune development.

A wide variety of factors outside the immune system influence immune function. For example:

- *Nervous system.* The study of psychoneuroimmunology—a brain-twisting term coined to describe links between the brain and the immune system—helps explain how depression, emotional stress, and grief can impair the immune response.
- *Diet.* Recently, researchers have discovered that vitamin D is required for activation of CD8 cells to become T_C cells. This may explain the finding of a clinical trial in which vitamin D supplements reduced the incidence of seasonal influenza in children. On the other hand, vitamin D deficiency has been linked with autoimmune diseases such as multiple sclerosis.

The immune system normally serves us very well until late in life. Then its efficiency begins to wane, and its ability to fight infection declines. Old age is also accompanied by greater susceptibility to both immunodeficiency and autoimmune diseases. The greater incidence of cancer in the elderly may also reflect the progressive failure of the immune system. We do not know why the immune system begins to fail, but we do know that the thymus begins to atrophy after puberty and the production of naive T and B cells declines with age, possibly because progenitor cells reach the limits of their ability to divide.

■ ■ ■

Our amazingly diverse adaptive defenses are regulated by cellular interactions and a flood of chemicals. T cells and antibodies make perfect partners. Antibodies respond swiftly to toxins and molecules on the outer surfaces of foreign organisms, and T cells destroy foreign antigens hidden inside cells and our own cells that have become mutinous (cancer cells). The innate immune system exhibits a different arsenal for body defense, an arsenal that is simpler perhaps and more easily understood. The innate and adaptive defenses are tightly interlocked, each providing what the other cannot and amplifying each other's effects.

Chapter Summary

For more chapter study tools, go to the Study Area of MasteringA&P at **www.masteringaandp.com**.
There you will find:
- Interactive Physiology iP
- A&PFlix A&PFlix
- Practice Anatomy Lab PAL
- PhysioEx PEx
- Videos, Practice Quizzes and Tests, MP3 Tutor Sessions, Case Studies, and much more!

PART 1 Innate Defenses

Surface Barriers: Skin and Mucosae (pp. 765–766)

1. Skin and mucous membranes constitute the first line of defense. Their role is to prevent pathogens from entering the body. Protective membranes line all body cavities and organs exposed to the exterior.
2. Surface membranes provide mechanical barriers to pathogens. Some have structural modifications and produce secretions that enhance their defensive effects: The skin's acidity, lysozyme, mucus, keratin, and ciliated cells are examples.

iP = IP Immune System; Topic: Innate Host Defenses, pp. 3–5.

Internal Innate Defenses: Cells and Chemicals (pp. 766–773)

1. The innate cellular and chemical defenses provide the body's second line of defense.

Phagocytes (p. 766)

2. Phagocytes (macrophages, neutrophils, and the like) engulf and destroy pathogens that breach epithelial barriers. This process is facilitated when opsonins (antibodies or complement to which the phagocyte's receptors can bind) attach to the pathogen's surface. The respiratory burst enhances cell killing.

Natural Killer Cells (pp. 766–767)

3. Natural killer (NK) cells are large granular lymphocytes that act nonspecifically to kill virus-infected and cancerous cells.

Inflammation: Tissue Response to Injury (pp. 767–771)

4. The inflammatory response prevents the spread of harmful agents, disposes of pathogens and dead tissue cells, and promotes healing. Exudate forms; protective leukocytes enter the area; fibrin walls off the area; and tissue repair occurs.
5. The cardinal signs of inflammation are swelling, redness, heat, and pain. These result from inflammatory chemicals that induce vasodilation and make blood vessels more permeable. Impaired function may be a fifth cardinal sign.

Antimicrobial Proteins (pp. 771–773)

6. Interferons are a group of related proteins synthesized by virus-infected cells and certain immune cells that prevent viruses from multiplying in other body cells.
7. Activation of complement (a group of plasma proteins) on the membrane of a foreign cell promotes phagocytosis of that cell, enhances inflammation, and sometimes causes lysis of the target cell.

Fever (p. 773)

8. Fever enhances the body's fight against pathogens by increasing metabolism, which speeds up defensive actions and repair processes, and by prompting the liver and spleen to sequester iron and zinc needed for bacterial multiplication.

iP Immune System; Topic: Innate Host Defenses, pp. 6–23.

PART 2 Adaptive Defenses

1. The adaptive immune system recognizes something as foreign and acts to immobilize, neutralize, or remove it. The adaptive immune response is antigen-specific, systemic, and has memory. It provides the body's third line of defense.

iP Immune System; Topic: Immune System Overview, p. 7.

Antigens (pp. 773–774)

1. Antigens are substances capable of generating an immune response.

Complete Antigens and Haptens (p. 774)

2. Complete antigens have both immunogenicity and reactivity. Incomplete antigens or haptens must combine with a body protein before becoming immunogenic.

Antigenic Determinants (p. 774)

3. Antigenic determinants are the portions of antigen molecules that are recognized as foreign. Most antigens have many such sites.

Self-Antigens: MHC Proteins (p. 774)

4. Major histocompatibility complex (MHC) proteins are membrane-bound glycoproteins that mark our cells as "self."

iP Immune System; Topic: Immune System Overview, p. 8; Topic: Cellular Immunity, pp. 5–8.

Cells of the Adaptive Immune System: An Overview (pp. 774–778)

Lymphocytes (pp. 775–777)

1. Lymphocytes arise from hematopoietic stem cells of the bone marrow and are educated to develop immunocompetence and self-tolerance. T cells are educated in the thymus and provide cellular immunity. B cells are educated in the bone marrow and provide humoral immunity. Immunocompetence is signaled by the appearance of antigen-specific receptors on the surface of the lymphocyte. Immunocompetent lymphocytes seed the secondary lymphoid organs, where the antigen encounter occurs, and circulate between the blood, lymph, and lymphoid organs. When naive lymphocytes encounter their antigen, clonal selection, proliferation, and differentiation occur. Most of the clone members become effector cells, but some become memory cells.
2. In both B and T lymphocytes, antigen receptor diversity is generated by shuffling gene fragments.

Antigen-Presenting Cells (pp. 777–778)

3. Antigen-presenting cells (APCs) include dendritic cells, macrophages, and B lymphocytes. They internalize antigens and present antigenic determinants on their surfaces for recognition by T cells.

21

iP Immune System; Topic: Common Characteristics of B and T Lymphocytes, pp. 8–13.

Humoral Immune Response (pp. 778–784)

Activation and Differentiation of B Cells (p. 779)

1. When B cells are activated, most of the clone members become effector cells called plasma cells, which secrete antibodies. This is the primary adaptive immune response.

Immunological Memory (pp. 779–780)

2. Other clone members become memory B cells, capable of mounting a rapid attack against the same antigen in subsequent encounters (secondary immune responses). The memory B cells provide humoral immunological memory.

Active and Passive Humoral Immunity (p. 780)

3. Active humoral immunity is acquired during an infection or via vaccination and provides immunological memory. Passive immunity is conferred when a donor's antibodies are injected into the bloodstream, or when the mother's antibodies cross the placenta. Its protection is short-lived; immunological memory is not established.

Antibodies (pp. 780–784)

4. The antibody monomer consists of four polypeptide chains, two heavy and two light. Each chain has both a constant and a variable region. Constant regions determine antibody function and class. Variable regions enable the antibody to recognize its specific antigen.
5. Five classes of antibodies exist: IgM, IgA, IgD, IgG, and IgE. They differ structurally and functionally.
6. Antibody functions include complement fixation and antigen neutralization, precipitation, and agglutination.
7. Monoclonal antibodies are pure preparations of a single antibody type useful in diagnostic tests and treating some types of cancer.

iP Immune System; Topic: Common Characteristics of B and T Lymphocytes, pp. 14–15; Topic: Humoral Immunity, pp. 3–14.

Cellular Immune Response (pp. 784–792)

MHC Proteins and Antigen Presentation (pp. 784–786)

1. MHC proteins present antigens to T cells. Class I MHC proteins are found on all nucleated cells, but class II MHC proteins are found only on APCs.

Activation and Differentiation of T Cells (pp. 786–787)

2. Immunocompetent CD4 and CD8 T cells are activated by binding to an antigen-MHC complex on the surface of an APC. A co-stimulatory signal is also essential. The resulting clone members differentiate into either the appropriate effector T cells that mount the primary immune response (e.g., helper or cytotoxic T cells) or memory T cells.
3. The immune response is enhanced by cytokines such as interleukin 1 released by macrophages, and interleukin 2, gamma interferon, and others released by activated T cells.

Roles of Specific Effector T Cells (pp. 787–790)

4. Helper T cells are required for full activation of most B and T cells, activate macrophages, and release essential cytokines. Cytotoxic T cells directly attack and kill infected cells and cancer cells. Regulatory T (T_{Reg}) cells help to maintain tolerance.

Organ Transplants and Prevention of Rejection (pp. 790–792)

5. Cell-mediated responses reject grafts and foreign organ transplants unless the recipient is immunosuppressed. Infections are major complications in such patients.

iP Immune System; Topic: Cellular Immunity, pp. 3–4, 11–14.

Homeostatic Imbalances of Immunity (pp. 792–796)

Immunodeficiencies (pp. 793–794)

1. Immunodeficiency diseases include acquired immune deficiency syndrome (AIDS), caused by HIV, and severe combined immunodeficiency (SCID) syndromes. Overwhelming infections are fatal because the immune system is unable to combat them.

Autoimmune Diseases (p. 794)

2. Autoimmune disease occurs when the body regards its own tissues as foreign and mounts an immune attack against them. Examples include rheumatoid arthritis and multiple sclerosis.

Hypersensitivities (pp. 794–796)

3. Hypersensitivity is an abnormally intense reaction to an otherwise harmless antigen. Immediate hypersensitivities (allergies) are mounted by IgE antibodies. Subacute hypersensitivities, involving both antibodies and complement, include antibody-mediated cytotoxic and immune-complex hypersensitivities. Cell-mediated hypersensitivity is called delayed hypersensitivity.

Developmental Aspects of the Immune System (p. 796)

1. Development of the immune response occurs around the time of birth. The ability of the immune system to recognize foreign substances is genetically determined.
2. The nervous system plays an important role in regulating immune responses. Emotional stress impairs immune function.
3. With aging, the immune system becomes less responsive. The elderly more often suffer from immune deficiency, autoimmune diseases, and cancer.

21

Review Questions

Multiple Choice/Matching

(Some questions have more than one correct answer. Select the best answer or answers from the choices given.)

1. All of the following are considered innate body defenses *except* **(a)** complement, **(b)** phagocytosis, **(c)** antibodies, **(d)** lysozyme, **(e)** inflammation.
2. The process by which neutrophils squeeze through capillary walls in response to inflammatory signals is called **(a)** diapedesis, **(b)** chemotaxis, **(c)** margination, **(d)** opsonization.
3. Antibodies released by plasma cells are involved in **(a)** humoral immunity, **(b)** immediate hypersensitivity reactions, **(c)** autoimmune disorders, **(d)** all of the above.

4. Which of the following antibodies can fix complement? **(a)** IgA, **(b)** IgD, **(c)** IgE, **(d)** IgG, **(e)** IgM.
5. Which antibody class is abundant in body secretions? **(a)** IgA, **(b)** IgD, **(c)** IgE, **(d)** IgG, **(e)** IgM.
6. Small molecules that must combine with large proteins to become immunogenic are called **(a)** complete antigens, **(b)** kinins, **(c)** antigenic determinants, **(d)** haptens.
7. Lymphocytes that develop immunocompetence in the bone marrow are **(a)** T lymphocytes, **(b)** B lymphocytes, **(c)** NK cells, **(d)** B and T lymphocytes.
8. Cells that can directly attack target cells include all of the following *except* **(a)** macrophages, **(b)** cytotoxic T cells, **(c)** helper T cells, **(d)** natural killer cells.
9. Which of the following is not involved in the activation of a B cell? **(a)** antigen, **(b)** helper T cell, **(c)** cytokine, **(d)** cytotoxic T cell.
10. The cell type most often invaded by HIV is a(n) **(a)** eosinophil, **(b)** cytotoxic T cell, **(c)** natural killer cell, **(d)** helper T cell, **(e)** B cell.
11. Complement fixation promotes all of the following except **(a)** cell lysis, **(b)** inflammation, **(c)** opsonization, **(d)** interferon release, **(e)** chemotaxis of neutrophils and other cells.
12. Using the letters from column B, match the cell description in column A. (Note that all require more than a single choice.)

Column A	Column B
____ **(1)** phagocyte	**(a)** natural killer cell
____ **(2)** releases histamine	**(b)** neutrophil
____ **(3)** releases perforins	**(c)** dendritic cell
____ **(4)** lymphocyte	**(d)** mast cell
____ **(5)** effector cells of adaptive immunity	**(e)** cytotoxic T cell
	(f) B cell
____ **(6)** antigen-presenting cell	**(g)** macrophage
	(h) helper T cell
	(i) basophil

Short Answer Essay Questions

13. Besides acting as mechanical barriers, the skin epidermis and mucosae of the body have other attributes that contribute to their protective roles. Cite the common body locations and the importance of mucus, lysozyme, keratin, acid pH, and cilia.
14. Explain why attempts at phagocytosis are not always successful; cite factors that increase the likelihood of success.
15. What is complement? How does it cause bacterial lysis? What are some of the other roles of complement?
16. Interferons are referred to as antiviral proteins. What stimulates their production, and how do they protect uninfected cells? Which cells of the body secrete interferons?
17. Differentiate between humoral and cellular adaptive immunity.
18. Although the adaptive immune system has two arms, it has been said, "no T cells, no immunity." Explain.
19. Define immunocompetence and self-tolerance. How is self-tolerance achieved?
20. Differentiate between a primary and a secondary immune response. Which is more rapid and why?
21. Define antibody. Using an appropriately labeled diagram, describe the structure of an antibody monomer. Indicate and label variable and constant regions, heavy and light chains.
22. What is the role of the variable regions of an antibody? Of the constant regions?
23. Name the five antibody classes and describe where each is most likely to be found in the body.
24. How do antibodies help defend the body?
25. Do vaccines produce active or passive humoral immunity? Explain your answer. Why is passive immunity less satisfactory?
26. Describe the process of activation of a CD4 T cell.
27. Describe the specific roles of helper, regulatory, and cytotoxic T cells in normal cellular immunity.
28. Name several cytokines and describe their role in the immune response.
29. Define hypersensitivity. List three types of hypersensitivity reactions. For each, note whether antibodies or T cells are involved and provide two examples.
30. What events can result in autoimmune disease?
31. What accounts for the declining efficiency of the immune system with age?

Critical Thinking and Clinical Application Questions

1. Jenny, a 6-year-old child who has been raised in a germ-free environment from birth, is a victim of one of the most severe examples of an abnormal immune system. Jenny also suffers from cancer caused by the Epstein-Barr virus. Relative to this case: **(a)** What is the usual fate of children with Jenny's condition and similar circumstances if no treatment is attempted? **(b)** Why is Jenny's brother chosen as the hematopoietic stem cell donor? **(c)** Why is her physician planning to use umbilical cord blood as a source of stem cells for transplant if her brother's stem cells fail (what are the hoped-for results)? **(d)** Attempt to explain Jenny's cancer. **(e)** What similarities and dissimilarities exist between Jenny's illness and AIDS?
2. Some people with a deficit of IgA exhibit recurrent respiratory tract infections. Explain this observation.
3. Capillary permeability increases and plasma proteins leak into the interstitial fluid as part of the inflammatory process. Why is this desirable?
4. Costanza was picking grapes in her father's arbor when she felt a short prickling pain in her finger. She ran crying to her father, who removed an insect stinger and calmed her with a glass of lemonade. Twenty minutes later Costanza's finger was red, swollen, and throbbing where she had been stung. What type of immune response was she exhibiting? What treatment would relieve her discomfort?
5. Caroline, a pregnant 29-year-old, has been HIV-positive for at least 10 years, dating back to when she was homeless and injecting heroin on a regular basis. While she currently has no symptoms of AIDS, she is taking several medications and is worried about the possibility that her baby might be infected. How do you think the HIV virus might be transferred from a mother to her offspring? Which of Caroline's cells are infected by the virus and why is the viral attack on these cells so devastating? Why is Caroline taking medication even though she has no symptoms? What types of medications might she be taking and how do they affect the virus and its replication?

AT THE CLINIC

Related Clinical Terms

Congenital thymic aplasia An immune deficiency disease in which the thymus fails to develop. Affected individuals have no T cells, hence little or no immune protection; fetal thymic and bone marrow transplants have been helpful in some cases.

Eczema (ek′zĕ-mah) A clinical term for several conditions that cause "weeping" skin lesions and intense itching. One common cause, *atopic dermatitis*, has a strong familial predisposition, has features of immediate hypersensitivity, and usually begins in the first five years of life. Recent research suggests the underlying defect may be increased leakiness of the skin.

Hashimoto's thyroiditis An autoimmune disease in which both B and T lymphocytes attack the thyroid gland. It is the most common cause of hypothyroidism, affecting mostly middle-aged and elderly women. Genetic factors associated with this autoimmune disease (certain MHC variants) make individuals susceptible to environmental triggers (possibly iodine, irradiation, or trauma).

Immunization The process of rendering a subject immune (by vaccination or injecting antiserum).

Immunology The study of immunity.

Immunopathology Disease of the immune system.

Septic shock (sepsis) A dangerous condition in which the inflammatory response goes out of control. Kills 200,000 people a year in the U.S. Results from especially severe bacterial infections or more ordinary infections that grow rapidly worse in patients with weakened defenses, such as the hospitalized elderly recovering from surgery. In an inflammatory response, neutrophils and other white blood cells secrete cytokines that increase capillary permeability. In sepsis, continued cytokine release makes capillaries so leaky that the bloodstream is depleted of fluid. Blood pressure falls and the body organs shut down, causing death in 50% of cases. Sepsis has proven difficult to control and its incidence remains high.

Systemic lupus erythematosus (SLE) (er″ĭ-the″mah-to′sus) A systemic autoimmune disorder that occurs mainly in young females. Diagnosis is helped by finding antinuclear (anti-DNA) antibodies in the patient's blood. DNA–anti-DNA complexes (typical of type III hypersensitivity) localize in the kidneys (the capillary filters, or glomeruli), blood vessels, brain, and synovial membranes of joints. This results in glomerulonephritis, vascular problems, loss of memory and mental sharpness, and painful arthritis. Reddened skin lesions, particularly a "butterfly rash" (the sign of the wolf, or *lupus*) on the face, are common.

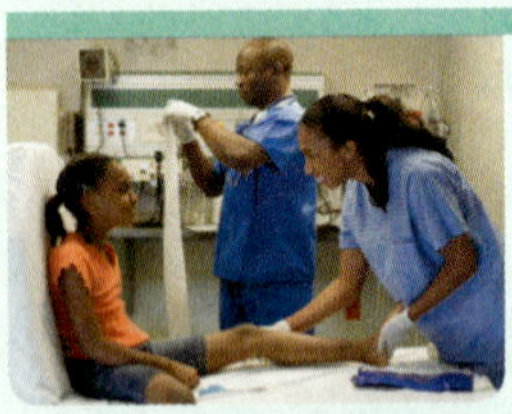

Case Study Immune System

Remember Mr. Ayers, the bus driver from Chapter 18? When we last saw him, he was headed for surgery. Although his dissected aorta was repaired, by the time surgical exposure and blood vessel clamping had been achieved, the dissection had extended up into the origin of his left common carotid artery. As a result, a clot formed that caused a massive stroke. Unfortunately, this left him with severe and permanent brain damage, and he was declared brain dead.

A discussion of Mr. Ayers's situation with his family confirmed his status as an organ donor. The organ recovery coordinator evaluated Mr. Ayers's suitability as a candidate for organ donation. Tissue typing (histocompatibility) tests were conducted, and the results were entered into the UNOS (United Network for Organ Sharing) database. Two potential recipients were identified. Mr. Ayers's right kidney was given in transplantation to a 35-year-old man, and his left kidney was given to a 27-year-old woman. Following surgery, both recipients were placed on immunosuppressive drug therapy.

1. In organ transplants, the transplanted organ is referred to as a graft. What type of graft is represented by the two kidneys that Mr. Ayers has donated?
2. Tissue typing characterizes the class I and II MHC proteins. What is an MHC protein?
3. What is the difference between class I and class II MHC proteins?
4. Why is the matching of the MHC molecules and the tissue compatibility so important in this case?
5. Why were the recipients of the two kidneys put on immunosuppressive drug therapy?

(Answers in Appendix H)

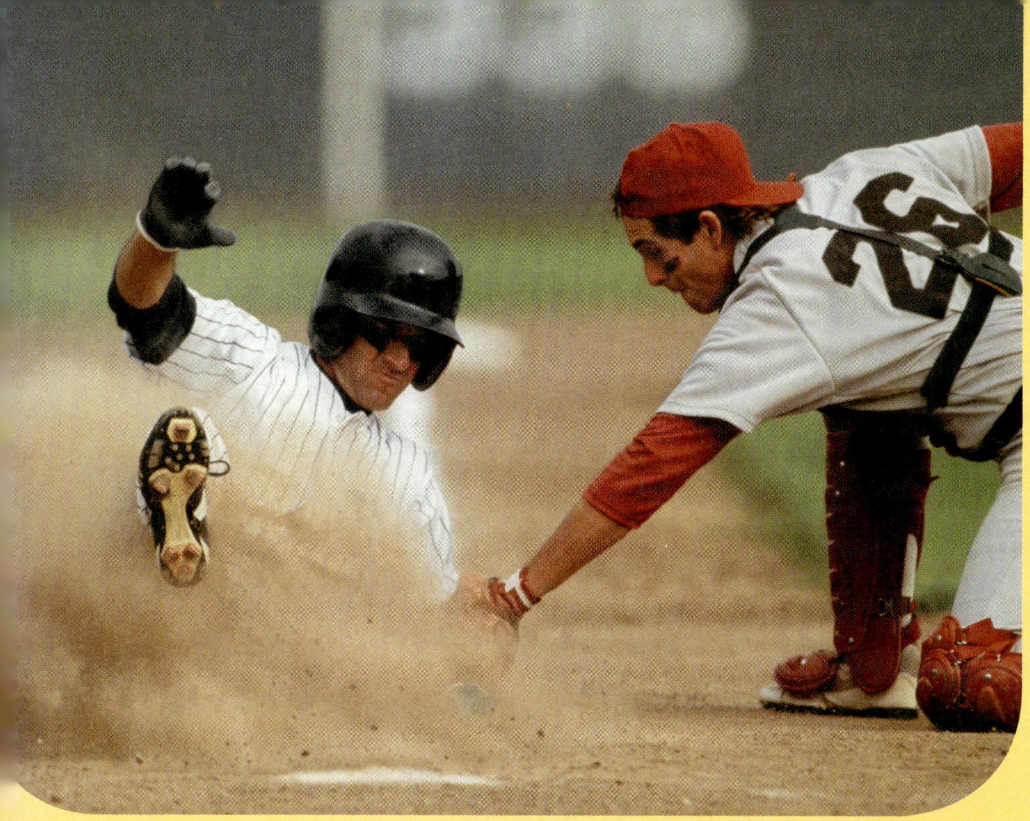

22

The Respiratory System

Far from self-sustaining, our bodies depend on the external environment, both as a source of substances we need to survive and as a catch basin for wastes. Our trillions of cells require a continuous supply of oxygen to carry out their vital functions. We can live without food or water for days, but we cannot do without oxygen for even a little while.

As cells use oxygen, they give off carbon dioxide, a waste product the body must get rid of. They also generate dangerous free radicals, the inescapable by-products of living in a world full of oxygen.

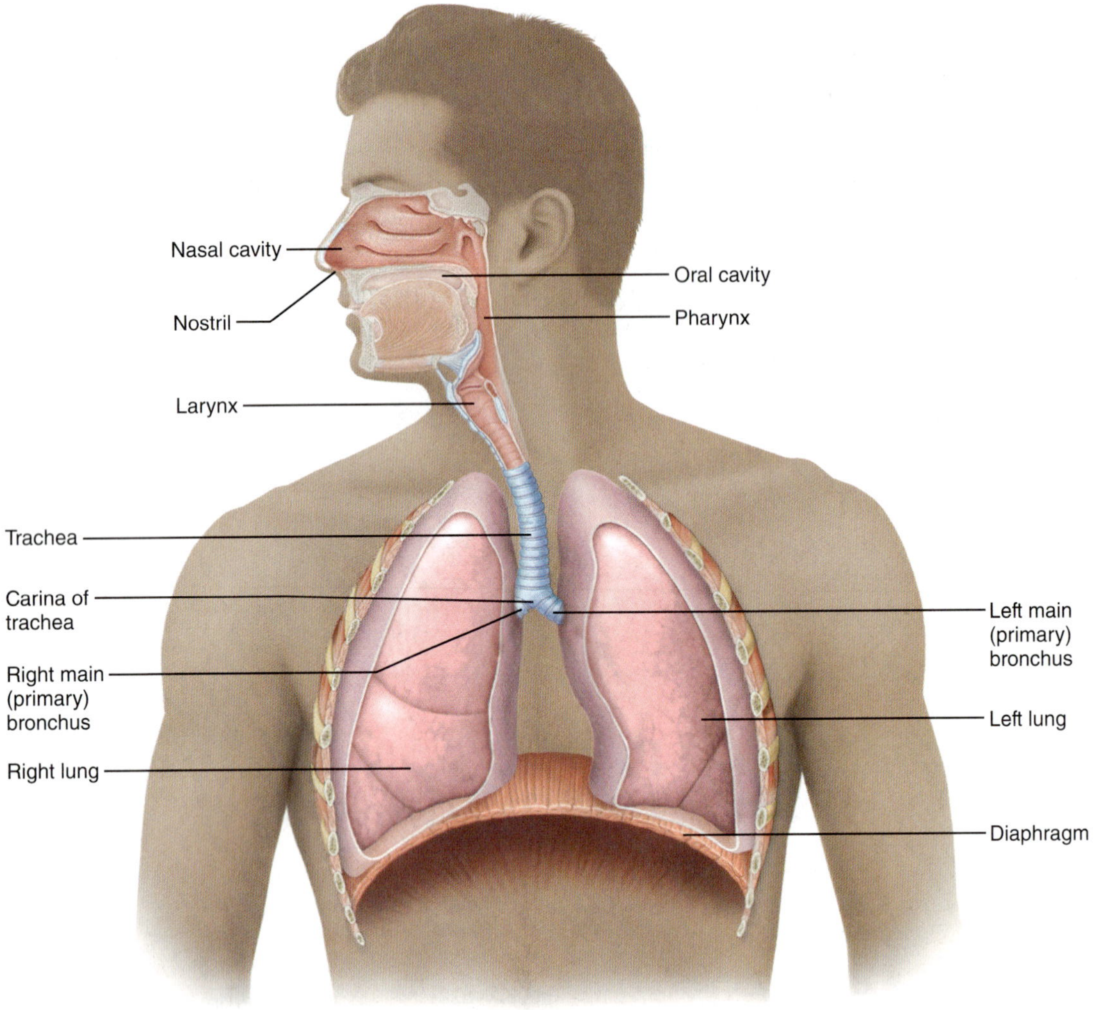

Figure 22.1 The major respiratory organs in relation to surrounding structures.

22

The major function of the **respiratory system** is to supply the body with oxygen and dispose of carbon dioxide. To accomplish this function, at least four processes, collectively called **respiration**, must happen:

1. **Pulmonary ventilation** (commonly called breathing): Air is moved into and out of the lungs (during *inspiration* and *expiration*) so the gases there are continuously changed and refreshed.
2. **External respiration:** Oxygen diffuses from the lungs to the blood, and carbon dioxide diffuses from the blood to the lungs.
3. **Transport of respiratory gases:** Oxygen is transported from the lungs to the tissue cells of the body, and carbon dioxide is transported from the tissue cells to the lungs. The cardiovascular system accomplishes this transport using blood as the transporting fluid.
4. **Internal respiration:** Oxygen diffuses from blood to tissue cells, and carbon dioxide diffuses from tissue cells to blood.

The respiratory system is responsible for only the first two processes **(Figure 22.1)**, but it cannot accomplish its primary goal of obtaining oxygen and eliminating carbon dioxide unless the third and fourth processes also occur. As you can see, the respiratory and circulatory systems are closely coupled, and if either system fails, the body's cells begin to die from oxygen starvation.

The actual use of oxygen and production of carbon dioxide by tissue cells, known as cellular respiration, is the cornerstone of all energy-producing chemical reactions in the body. We discuss *cellular respiration*, which is not a function of the respiratory system, in the metabolism section of Chapter 24.

Because it moves air, the respiratory system is also involved with the sense of smell and with speech.

Functional Anatomy of the Respiratory System

✓ Identify the organs forming the respiratory passageway(s) in descending order until you reach the alveoli.

✓ Describe the location, structure, and function of each of the following: nose, paranasal sinuses, pharynx, and larynx.

✓ List and describe several protective mechanisms of the respiratory system.

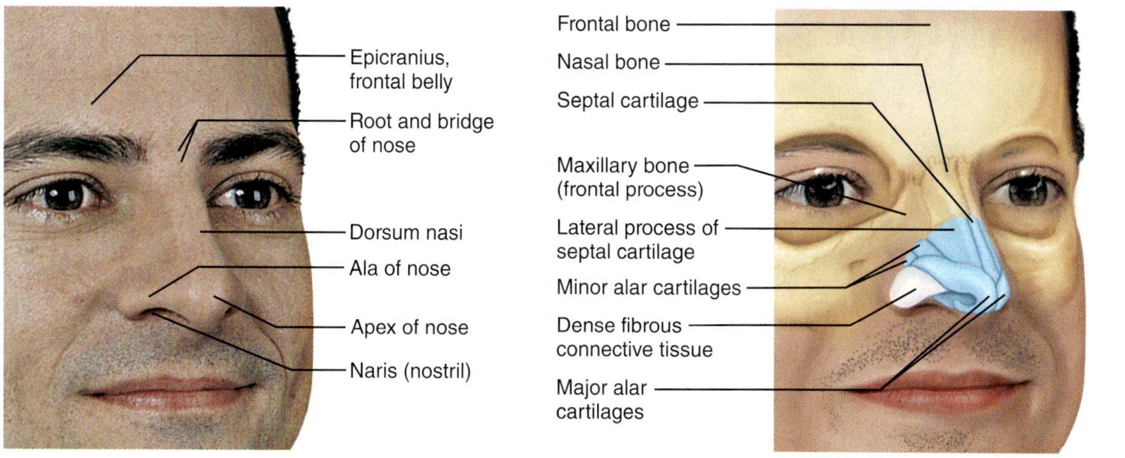

(a) Surface anatomy **(b) External skeletal framework**

Figure 22.2 The external nose.

The respiratory system (Figure 22.1) includes the *nose, nasal cavity*, and *paranasal sinuses*; the *pharynx*; the *larynx*; the *trachea*; the *bronchi* and their smaller branches; and the *lungs*, which contain tiny air sacs called *alveoli*. Functionally, the system consists of two zones.

- The **respiratory zone**, the actual site of gas exchange, is composed of the respiratory bronchioles, alveolar ducts, and alveoli, all microscopic structures.
- The **conducting zone** includes all other respiratory passageways, which provide fairly rigid conduits for air to reach the gas exchange sites. The conducting zone organs also cleanse, humidify, and warm incoming air. As a result, air reaching the lungs has fewer irritants (dust, bacteria, etc.) than when it entered the body, and it is warm and damp, like the air of the tropics.

Table 22.1 summarizes the functions of the major organs of the respiratory system. In addition to these organs, some authorities also include the respiratory muscles (diaphragm, etc.) as part of this system. Although we will consider how these skeletal muscles bring about the volume changes that promote ventilation, we continue to classify them as part of the *muscular system*.

The Nose and Paranasal Sinuses

The nose is the only externally visible part of the respiratory system. Unlike the eyes and lips, facial features often referred to poetically, the nose is usually an irreverent target. We are urged to keep our nose to the grindstone and keep it out of other people's business. Considering its important functions, however, it deserves more esteem. The nose (1) provides an airway for respiration, (2) moistens and warms entering air, (3) filters and cleans inspired air, (4) serves as a resonating chamber for speech, and (5) houses the olfactory (smell) receptors.

The structures of the nose are divided into the *external nose* and the internal *nasal cavity* for ease of consideration.

External Nose

The surface features of the external nose include the *root* (area between the eyebrows), *bridge*, and *dorsum nasi* (anterior margin), the latter terminating in the *apex* (tip of the nose) **(Figure 22.2a)**. The external openings of the nose, the **nostrils** or **nares** (na′rēz), are bounded laterally by the flared *alae*.

The skeletal framework of the external nose is fashioned by the nasal and frontal bones superiorly (forming the bridge and root, respectively), the maxillary bones laterally, and flexible plates of hyaline cartilage (the alar and septal cartilages, and the lateral processes of the septal cartilage) inferiorly (Figure 22.2b). Noses vary a great deal in size and shape, largely because of differences in nasal cartilages. The skin covering the nose's anterior and lateral aspects is thin and contains many sebaceous glands.

Nasal Cavity

The internal **nasal cavity** lies in and posterior to the external nose. During breathing, air enters the cavity by passing through the *nostrils* or *nares* (Figure 22.2a and **Figure 22.3b**). The nasal cavity is divided by a midline **nasal septum**, formed anteriorly by the septal cartilage and posteriorly by the vomer bone and perpendicular plate of the ethmoid bone (see Figure 7.13b, p. 214). The nasal cavity is continuous posteriorly with the nasal portion of the pharynx through the **posterior nasal apertures**, also called the *choanae* (ko-a′ne; "funnels").

The roof of the nasal cavity is formed by the ethmoid and sphenoid bones of the skull. The floor is formed by the *palate*, which separates the nasal cavity from the oral cavity below. Anteriorly, where the palate is supported by the palatine bones and processes of the maxillary bones, it is called the **hard palate**. The unsupported posterior portion is the muscular **soft palate**.

The part of the nasal cavity just superior to the nostrils, called the **nasal vestibule**, is lined with skin containing sebaceous and sweat glands and numerous hair follicles. The hairs, or **vibrissae** (vi-bris′e; *vibro* = to quiver), filter coarse particles (dust, pollen) from inspired air. The rest of the nasal cavity is lined with two types of mucous membrane.

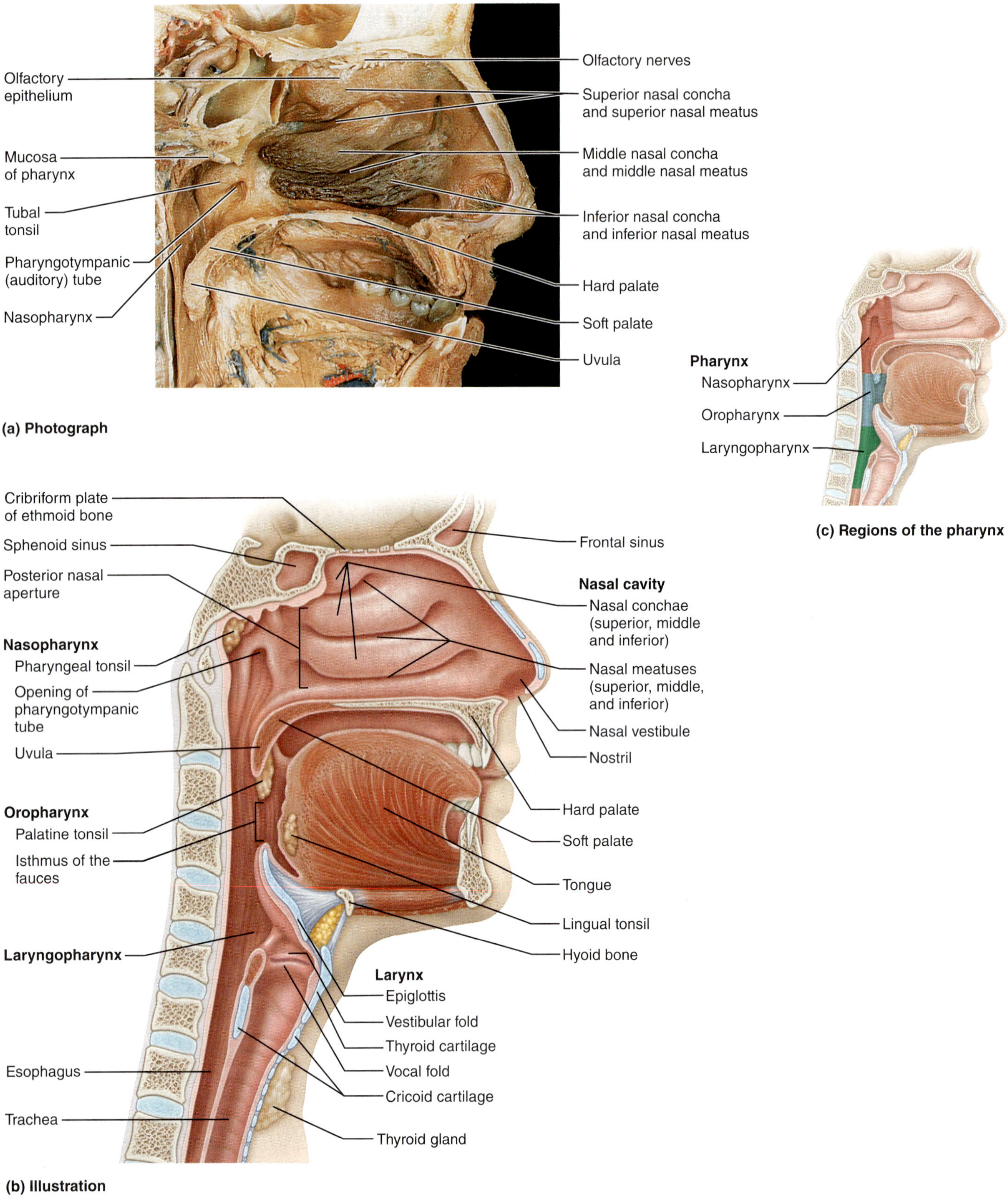

Figure 22.3 The upper respiratory tract. Midsagittal section of the head and neck. (For a related image, see *A Brief Atlas of the Human Body*, Figure 47.)

Table 22.1 Principal Organs of the Respiratory System

STRUCTURE	DESCRIPTION, GENERAL AND DISTINCTIVE FEATURES	FUNCTION
Nose (external nose and nasal cavity)	Jutting external portion is supported by bone and cartilage. Internal nasal cavity is divided by midline nasal septum and lined with mucosa.	Produces mucus; filters, warms, and moistens incoming air; resonance chamber for speech
	Roof of nasal cavity contains olfactory epithelium.	Receptors for sense of smell
Paranasal sinuses	Mucosa-lined, air-filled cavities in cranial bones surrounding nasal cavity.	Same as for nasal cavity except no receptors for smell; also lighten skull
Pharynx	Passageway connecting nasal cavity to larynx and oral cavity to esophagus. Three subdivisions: nasopharynx, oropharynx, and laryngopharynx.	Passageway for air and food
	Houses tonsils (lymphoid tissue masses involved in protection against pathogens).	Facilitates exposure of immune system to inhaled antigens
Larynx	Connects pharynx to trachea. Has framework of cartilage and dense connective tissue. Opening (glottis) can be closed by epiglottis or vocal folds.	Air passageway; prevents food from entering lower respiratory tract
	Houses vocal folds (true vocal cords).	Voice production
Trachea	Flexible tube running from larynx and dividing inferiorly into two main bronchi. Walls contain C-shaped cartilages that are incomplete posteriorly where connected by trachealis.	Air passageway; cleans, warms, and moistens incoming air
Bronchial tree	Consists of right and left main bronchi, which subdivide within the lungs to form lobar and segmental bronchi and bronchioles. Bronchiolar walls lack cartilage but contain complete layer of smooth muscle. Constriction of this muscle impedes expiration.	Air passageways connecting trachea with alveoli; cleans, warms, and moistens incoming air
Alveoli	Microscopic chambers at termini of bronchial tree. Walls of simple squamous epithelium overlie thin basement membrane. External surfaces are intimately associated with pulmonary capillaries.	Main sites of gas exchange
	Special alveolar cells produce surfactant.	Reduces surface tension; helps prevent lung collapse
Lungs	Paired composite organs that flank mediastinum in thorax. Composed primarily of alveoli and respiratory passageways. Stroma is fibrous elastic connective tissue, allowing lungs to recoil passively during expiration.	House respiratory passages smaller than the main bronchi
Pleurae	Serous membranes. Parietal pleura lines thoracic cavity; visceral pleura covers external lung surfaces.	Produce lubricating fluid and compartmentalize lungs

- The small patch of **olfactory mucosa** lines the slitlike superior region of the nasal cavity and contains smell receptors in its **olfactory epithelium** (see p. 565).
- The **respiratory mucosa** lines most of the nasal cavity. The respiratory mucosa is a pseudostratified ciliated columnar epithelium, containing scattered *goblet cells*, that rests on a lamina propria richly supplied with seromucous *nasal glands*.

Seromucous nasal glands contain mucus-secreting mucus cells and serous cells that secrete a watery fluid containing enzymes. Each day, these glands secrete about a quart (a liter) of mucus containing *lysozyme*, an antibacterial enzyme. The sticky mucus traps inspired dust, bacteria, and other debris, while lysozyme attacks and chemically destroys bacteria. The epithelial cells of the respiratory mucosa also secrete *defensins*, natural antibiotics that help kill invading microbes. Additionally, the high water content of the mucus film humidifies incoming air.

The ciliated cells of the respiratory mucosa create a gentle current that moves the sheet of contaminated mucus posteriorly toward the throat, where it is swallowed and digested. We are usually unaware of this important action of our nasal cilia, but when exposed to cold air they become sluggish, allowing mucus to accumulate in the nasal cavity and dribble out the nostrils. This, along with the fact that water vapor in expired air tends to condense at lower temperatures, explains why you have a "runny" nose on a crisp wintry day.

The nasal mucosa is richly supplied with sensory nerve endings, and contact with irritating particles (dust, pollen, and the like) triggers a sneeze reflex. The sneeze forces air outward in a violent burst—a crude but effective way to expel irritants.

Rich plexuses of capillaries and thin-walled veins underlie the nasal epithelium and warm incoming air as it flows across the mucosal surface. When the inspired air is cold, the vascular plexus becomes engorged with blood, intensifying the air-heating process. Because these blood vessels are abundant and located superficially, nosebleeds are common and often profuse.

Nasal Conchae Protruding medially from each lateral wall of the nasal cavity are three scroll-like mucosa-covered projections, the *superior*, *middle*, and *inferior nasal conchae* (kong′ke)

(Figure 22.3). The groove inferior to each concha is a *nasal meatus* (me-a′tus).

The curved conchae greatly increase the mucosal surface area exposed to air and enhance air turbulence in the cavity. The gases in inhaled air swirl through the twists and turns, deflecting heavier, nongaseous particles onto the mucus-coated surfaces, where they become trapped. As a result, few particles larger than 6 μm make it past the nasal cavity.

The conchae and nasal mucosa not only function during inhalation to filter, heat, and moisten the air, but also act during exhalation to reclaim this heat and moisture. In other words, inspired air cools the conchae, then during exhalation these cooled conchae precipitate moisture and extract heat from the humid air flowing over them. This reclamation process minimizes the amount of moisture and heat lost from the body through breathing, helping us to survive in dry and cold climates.

Paranasal Sinuses

The nasal cavity is surrounded by a ring of **paranasal sinuses** (Figure 22.3b). They are located in the frontal, sphenoid, ethmoid, and maxillary bones (see Figure 7.14, p. 215). The sinuses lighten the skull, and together with the nasal cavity they warm and moisten the air. The mucus they produce ultimately flows into the nasal cavity, and the suctioning effect created by nose blowing helps drain the sinuses.

Homeostatic Imbalance 22.1

Cold viruses, streptococcal bacteria, and various allergens can cause *rhinitis* (ri-ni′tis), inflammation of the nasal mucosa accompanied by excessive mucus production, nasal congestion, and postnasal drip. The nasal mucosa is continuous with the mucosa of the respiratory tract, explaining the typical nose to throat to chest progression of colds. Because the mucosa extends tentacle-like into the nasolacrimal (tear) ducts and paranasal sinuses, nasal cavity infections often spread to those regions, causing **sinusitis** (inflamed sinuses).

When mucus or infectious materials block the passageways connecting the sinuses to the nasal cavity, the air in the sinus cavities is absorbed. The result is a partial vacuum and a *sinus headache* localized over the inflamed areas. ✚

The Pharynx

The funnel-shaped **pharynx** (far′ingks) connects the nasal cavity and mouth superiorly to the larynx and esophagus inferiorly. Commonly called the *throat*, the pharynx vaguely resembles a short length of garden hose as it extends for about 13 cm (5 inches) from the base of the skull to the level of the sixth cervical vertebra (Figure 22.1).

From superior to inferior, the pharynx is divided into three regions—the *nasopharynx*, *oropharynx*, and *laryngopharynx* (Figure 22.3c). The muscular pharynx wall is composed of skeletal muscle throughout its length (see Table 10.3, pp. 334–335). However, the cellular composition of its mucosa varies from one pharyngeal region to another.

The Nasopharynx

The **nasopharynx** is posterior to the nasal cavity, inferior to the sphenoid bone, and superior to the level of the soft palate. Because it lies above the point where food enters the body, it serves *only* as an air passageway. During swallowing, the soft palate and its pendulous *uvula* (u′vu-lah; "little grape") move superiorly, an action that closes off the nasopharynx and prevents food from entering the nasal cavity. (When we giggle, this sealing action fails and fluids being swallowed can end up spraying out the nose.)

The nasopharynx is continuous with the nasal cavity through the posterior nasal apertures (Figure 22.3b). Its pseudostratified ciliated epithelium takes over the job of propelling mucus where the nasal mucosa leaves off. High on its posterior wall is the **pharyngeal tonsil** (far-rin′je-al) (or *adenoids*), which traps and destroys pathogens entering the nasopharynx in air.

Homeostatic Imbalance 22.2

Infected and swollen adenoids block air passage in the nasopharynx, making it necessary to breathe through the mouth. As a result, the air is not properly moistened, warmed, or filtered before reaching the lungs. When the adenoids are chronically enlarged, both speech and sleep may be disturbed. ✚

The *pharyngotympanic* (*auditory*) *tubes*, which drain the middle ear cavities and allow middle ear pressure to equalize with atmospheric pressure, open into the lateral walls of the nasopharynx (Figure 22.3a). A ridge of pharyngeal mucosa posterior to each of these openings constitutes the *tubal tonsil*. Its strategic location helps protect the middle ear against infections likely to spread from the nasopharynx.

The Oropharynx

The **oropharynx** lies posterior to the oral cavity and is continuous with it through an archway called the **isthmus of the fauces** (faw′sēz; "throat") (Figure 22.3b). Because the oropharynx extends inferiorly from the level of the soft palate to the epiglottis, both swallowed food and inhaled air pass through it.

As the nasopharynx blends into the oropharynx, the epithelium changes from pseudostratified columnar to a more protective stratified squamous epithelium. This structural adaptation accommodates the increased friction and chemical trauma (characteristic of hot and spicy foods) accompanying food passage.

The paired **palatine tonsils** lie embedded in the lateral walls of the oropharyngeal mucosa just posterior to the oral cavity. The **lingual tonsil** covers the posterior surface of the tongue.

The Laryngopharynx

Like the oropharynx above it, the **laryngopharynx** (lah-ring″go-far′ingks) serves as a passageway for food and air and is lined with a stratified squamous epithelium. It lies directly posterior to the upright epiglottis and extends to the larynx, where the respiratory and digestive pathways diverge. At that point the laryngopharynx is continuous with the esophagus posteriorly.

The esophagus conducts food and fluids to the stomach; air enters the larynx anteriorly. During swallowing, food has the "right of way," and air passage temporarily stops.

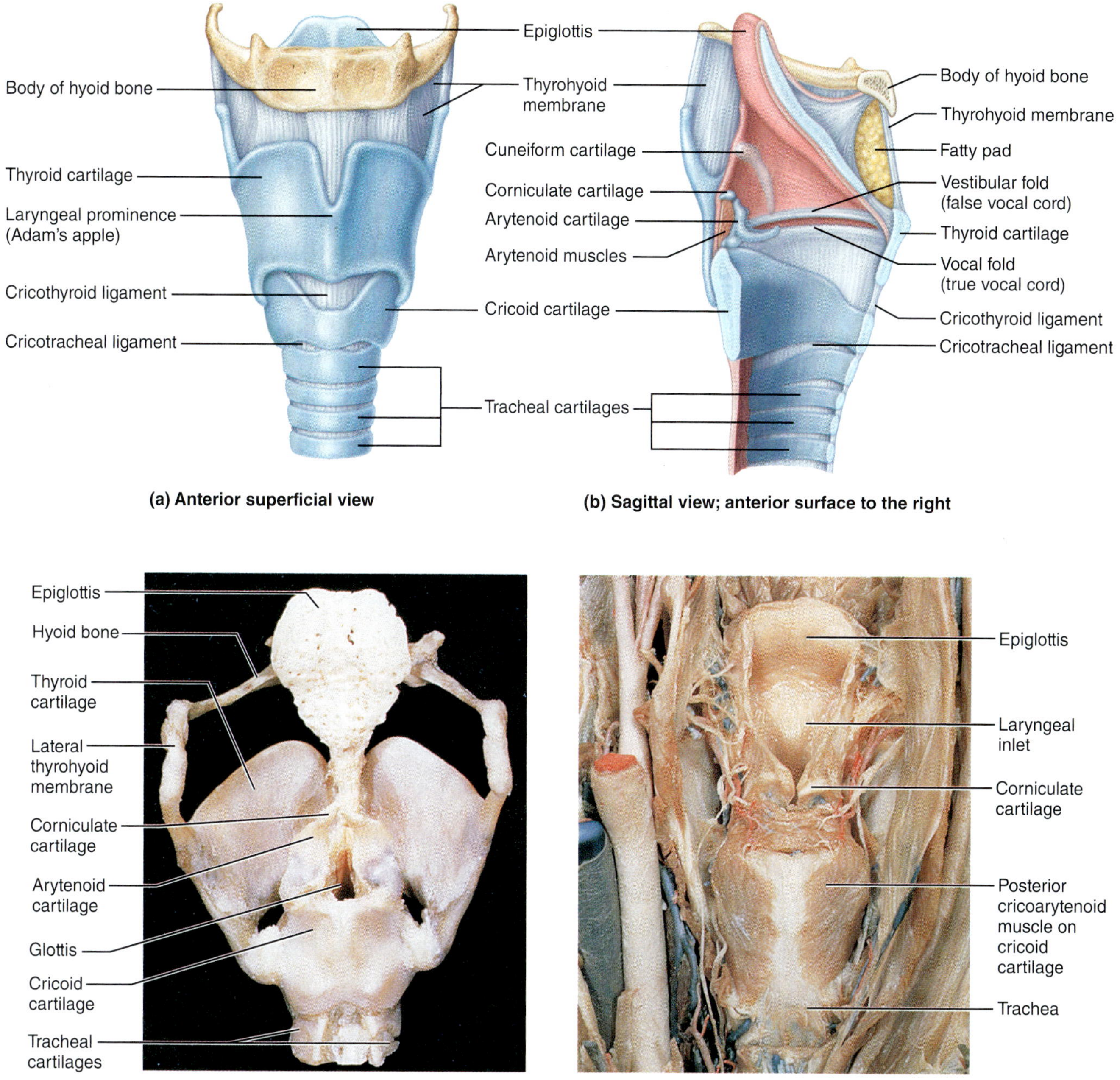

(a) Anterior superficial view

(b) Sagittal view; anterior surface to the right

(c) Photograph of cartilaginous framework of the larynx, posterior view

(d) Photograph of posterior aspect

Figure 22.4 **The larynx.**

The Larynx

Basic Anatomy

The **larynx** (lar′ingks), or voice box, extends for about 5 cm (2 inches) from the level of the third to the sixth cervical vertebra. Superiorly it attaches to the hyoid bone and opens into the laryngopharynx. Inferiorly it is continuous with the trachea (Figure 22.3b).

The larynx has three functions. Its two main tasks are to provide a *patent* (open) airway and to act as a switching mechanism to route air and food into the proper channels. Because the larynx houses the vocal folds (vocal cords), its third function is voice production.

The framework of the larynx is an intricate arrangement of nine cartilages connected by membranes and ligaments **(Figure 22.4)**. Except for the epiglottis, all laryngeal cartilages are hyaline cartilages.

The large, shield-shaped **thyroid cartilage** is formed by the fusion of two cartilage plates. The midline **laryngeal prominence** (lah-rin′je-al), which marks the fusion point, is obvious externally as the *Adam's apple*. The thyroid cartilage is typically

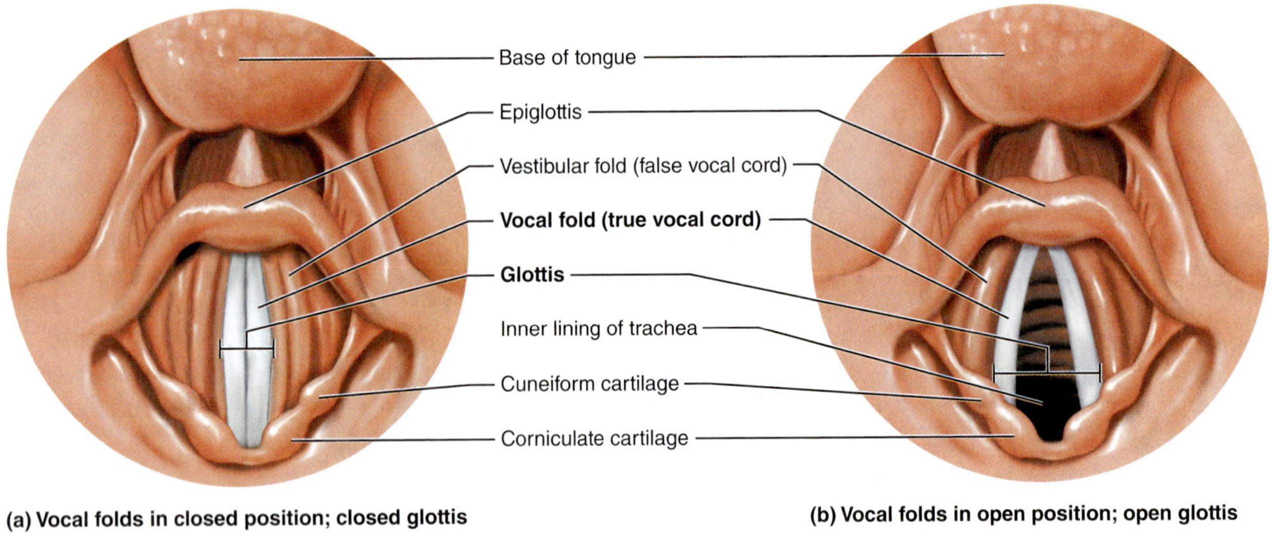

Figure 22.5 Movements of the vocal folds. Drawings of superior views of the larynx and vocal folds, as if looking at a patient's larynx through a laryngoscope.

larger in males than in females because male sex hormones stimulate its growth during puberty. Inferior to the thyroid cartilage is the ring-shaped **cricoid cartilage** (kri′koid), perched atop and anchored to the trachea inferiorly.

Three pairs of small cartilages—**arytenoid** (ar″ĭ-te′noid), **cuneiform** (ku-ne′ĭ-form), and **corniculate cartilages**—form part of the lateral and posterior walls of the larynx. The most important of these are the pyramid-shaped arytenoid cartilages, which anchor the vocal folds.

Epiglottis The ninth cartilage, the flexible, spoon-shaped **epiglottis** (ep″ĭ-glot′is; "above the glottis"), is composed of elastic cartilage and is almost entirely covered by a taste bud–containing mucosa. The epiglottis extends from the posterior aspect of the tongue to its anchoring point on the anterior rim of the thyroid cartilage (Figure 22.4b and c).

22

When only air is flowing into the larynx, the inlet to the larynx is wide open and the free edge of the epiglottis projects upward. During swallowing, the larynx is pulled superiorly and the epiglottis tips to cover the laryngeal inlet. Because this action keeps food out of the lower respiratory passages, the epiglottis has been called the guardian of the airways. Anything other than air entering the larynx initiates the cough reflex to expel the substance. This protective reflex does not work when we are unconscious, so it is never a good idea to administer liquids when attempting to revive an unconscious person.

Vocal Folds Lying under the laryngeal mucosa on each side are the **vocal ligaments**, which attach the arytenoid cartilages to the thyroid cartilage. These ligaments, composed largely of elastic fibers, form the core of mucosal folds called the **vocal folds**, or **true vocal cords**, which appear pearly white because they lack blood vessels **(Figure 22.5)**.

The vocal folds vibrate, producing sounds as air rushes up from the lungs. The vocal folds and the medial opening between them through which air passes are called the **glottis**. Superior to the vocal folds is a similar pair of mucosal folds called the **vestibular folds**, or **false vocal cords.** These play no direct part in sound production but help to close the glottis when we swallow.

Epithelium of Larynx Stratified squamous epithelium lines the superior portion of the larynx, an area subject to food contact. Below the vocal folds the epithelium is a pseudostratified ciliated columnar type that filters dust. The power stroke of its cilia is directed upward toward the pharynx to continually move mucus *away* from the lungs. We help move mucus up and out of the larynx when we "clear our throat."

Voice Production

Speech involves the intermittent release of expired air as the glottis opens and closes. The length of the vocal folds and the size of the glottis change with the action of the intrinsic laryngeal muscles that clothe the cartilages. Most of these muscles move the arytenoid cartilages. As the length and tension of the vocal folds change, the pitch of the sound varies. Generally, the tenser the vocal folds, the faster they vibrate and the higher the pitch.

As a boy's larynx enlarges during puberty, his vocal folds become longer and thicker. Because this causes them to vibrate more slowly, his voice becomes deeper. Until the young man learns to control his newly enlarged vocal folds, his voice "cracks."

Loudness of the voice depends on the force with which the airstream rushes across the vocal folds. The greater the force, the stronger the vibration and the louder the sound. The vocal folds do not move at all when we whisper, but they vibrate vigorously when we yell. The muscles of the chest, abdomen, and back provide the power for the airstream.

The vocal folds actually produce buzzing sounds. The perceived quality of the voice depends on the coordinated activity of many structures above the glottis. For example, the entire length of the pharynx acts as a resonating chamber, to amplify and enhance the sound quality. The oral, nasal, and sinus cavities also contribute to vocal resonance. In addition, good enunciation depends on muscles in the pharynx, tongue, soft palate, and lips that "shape" sound into recognizable consonants and vowels.

Homeostatic Imbalance 22.3

Inflammation of the vocal folds, or **laryngitis**, causes the vocal folds to swell, interfering with their vibration. This changes the vocal tone, causing hoarseness, or in severe cases limiting us to a whisper. Laryngitis is most often caused by viral infections, but may also be due to overusing the voice, very dry air, bacterial infections, tumors on the vocal folds, or inhalation of irritating chemicals. +

Sphincter Functions of the Larynx

Under certain conditions, the vocal folds act as a sphincter that prevents air passage. During abdominal straining associated with defecation, the glottis closes to prevent exhalation and the abdominal muscles contract, causing the intra-abdominal pressure to rise. These events, collectively known as **Valsalva's maneuver**, help empty the rectum and can also splint (stabilize) the body trunk when lifting a heavy load.

The Trachea

The **trachea** (tra′ke-ah), or *windpipe*, descends from the larynx through the neck and into the mediastinum. It ends by dividing into the two main bronchi at midthorax (see Figure 22.1). In humans, it is 10–12 cm (about 4 inches) long and 2 cm (3/4 inch) in diameter, and very flexible and mobile. Interestingly, early anatomists mistook the trachea for a rough-walled artery (*trachea* = rough).

The tracheal wall consists of several layers that are common to many tubular body organs—the *mucosa, submucosa*, and *adventitia*—plus a layer of hyaline cartilage **(Figure 22.6)**. The **mucosa** has the same goblet cell–containing pseudostratified epithelium that occurs throughout most of the respiratory tract. Its cilia continually propel debris-laden mucus toward the pharynx. This epithelium rests on a fairly thick lamina propria that has a rich supply of elastic fibers.

Homeostatic Imbalance 22.4

Smoking inhibits and ultimately destroys cilia. Without ciliary activity, coughing is the only way to prevent mucus from accumulating in the lungs. For this reason, smokers with respiratory congestion should avoid medications that inhibit the cough reflex. +

The **submucosa**, a connective tissue layer deep to the mucosa, contains seromucous glands that help produce the mucus "sheets" within the trachea. The submucosa is supported by 16 to 20 C-shaped rings of hyaline cartilage encased by the **adventitia**, the outermost layer of connective tissue (Figure 22.6).

The trachea's elastic elements make it flexible enough to stretch and move inferiorly during inspiration and recoil during expiration, but the cartilage rings prevent it from collapsing and keep the airway patent despite the pressure changes that occur during breathing. The open posterior parts of the cartilage rings, which abut the esophagus (Figure 22.6a), are connected by smooth muscle fibers of the **trachealis** and by soft connective tissue. Because this portion of the tracheal wall is flexible, the esophagus can expand anteriorly as swallowed food passes through it.

Contraction of the trachealis muscle decreases the trachea's diameter, causing expired air to rush upward from the lungs with greater force. This action helps expel mucus from the trachea when we cough by accelerating the exhaled air to speeds of 100 mph!

The last tracheal cartilage is expanded, and a spar of cartilage, called the **carina** (kar-ri′nah; "keel"), projects posteriorly from its inner face, marking the point where the trachea branches into the two *main bronchi*. The mucosa of the carina is highly sensitive and violent coughing is triggered when a foreign object makes contact with it.

By the time incoming air reaches the end of the trachea, it is warm, cleansed of most impurities, and saturated with water vapor.

Homeostatic Imbalance 22.5

Tracheal obstruction is life threatening. Many people have suffocated after choking on a piece of food that suddenly closed off their trachea. The **Heimlich maneuver**, a procedure in which air in the victim's lungs is used to "pop out," or expel, an obstructing piece of food, has saved many people from becoming victims of "café coronaries." The maneuver is simple to learn and easy to do. However, it is best learned by demonstration because cracked ribs are a distinct possibility when it is done incorrectly. +

22

Check Your Understanding

1. Air moving from the nose to the trachea passes by a number of structures. List (in order) as many of these structures as you can.
2. Which structure seals the larynx when we swallow?
3. Which structural features of the trachea allow it to expand and contract, yet keep it from collapsing?

For answers, see Appendix H.

The Bronchi and Subdivisions

✓ Distinguish between conducting and respiratory zone structures.

✓ Describe the makeup of the respiratory membrane, and relate structure to function.

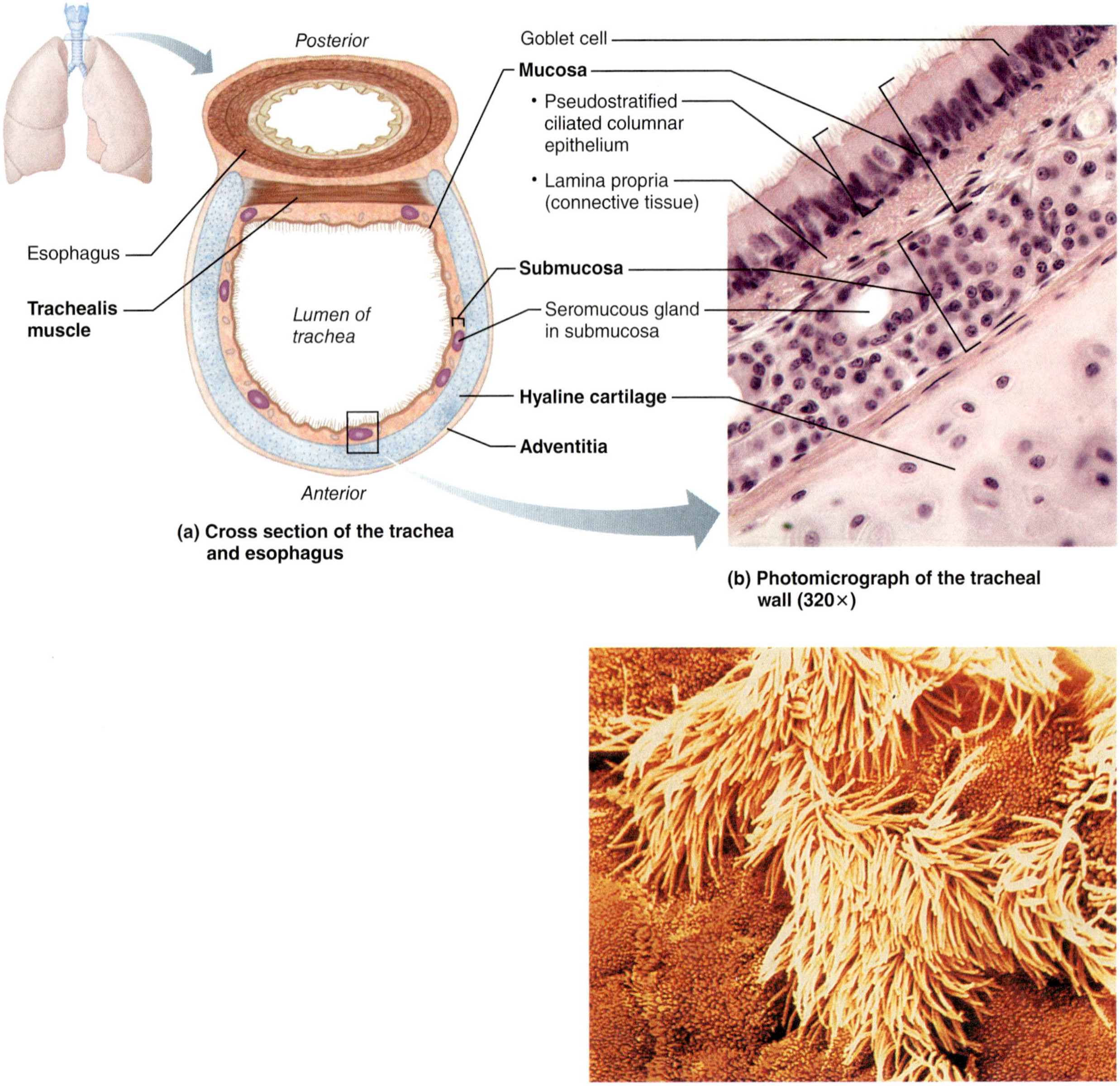

(a) Cross section of the trachea and esophagus

(b) Photomicrograph of the tracheal wall (320×)

(c) Scanning electron micrograph of cilia in the trachea (2500×)

Figure 22.6 Tissue composition of the tracheal wall. In the scanning electron micrograph in (c), the cilia appear as yellow, grasslike projections. Mucus-secreting goblet cells (orange) with short microvilli are interspersed between the ciliated cells.

The air passageways in the lungs branch and branch again, about 23 times overall, in a pattern often called the **bronchial tree (Figure 22.7)**. At the tips of the bronchial tree, conducting zone structures give way to respiratory zone structures **(Figure 22.8)**.

Conducting Zone Structures

The trachea divides to form the **right** and **left main (primary) bronchi** (brong′ki) approximately at the level of T_7 in an erect (standing) person. Each bronchus runs obliquely in the mediastinum before plunging into the medial depression (hilum) of the lung on its own side (Figure 22.7). The right main bronchus is wider, shorter, and more vertical than the left. Consequently, it is more common for an inhaled foreign object to get stuck there.

Once inside the lungs, each main bronchus subdivides into **lobar (secondary) bronchi**—three on the right and two on the left—each supplying one lung lobe. The lobar bronchi branch into third-order **segmental (tertiary) bronchi**, which divide repeatedly into smaller and smaller bronchi (fourth-order, fifth-order, etc.). Passages smaller than 1 mm in diameter are called **bronchioles** ("little bronchi"), and the tiniest of these, the **terminal bronchioles**, are less than 0.5 mm in diameter.

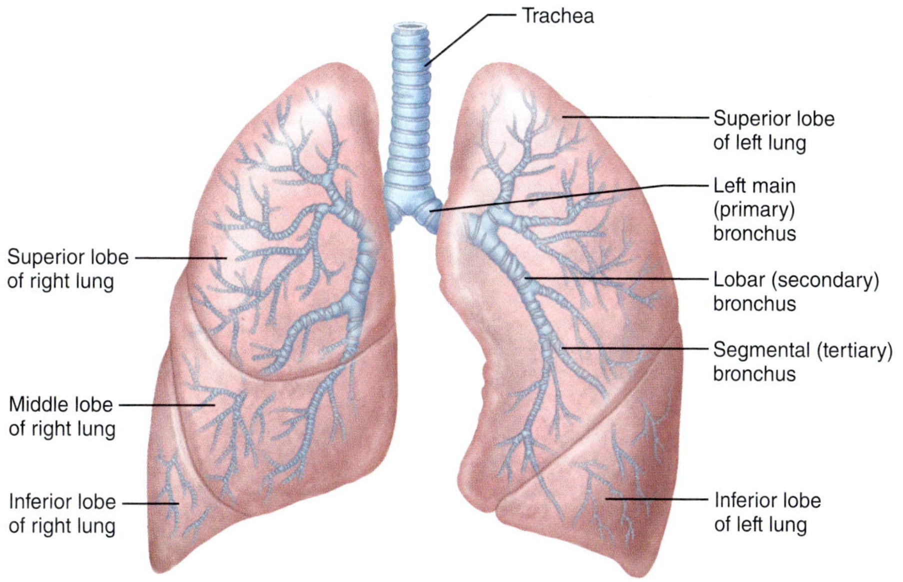

Figure 22.7 Conducting zone passages. The air pathway inferior to the larynx consists of the trachea and the main, lobar, and segmental bronchi, which branch into the smaller bronchi and bronchioles until reaching the terminal bronchioles of the lungs.

The tissue composition of the walls of the main bronchi mimics that of the trachea. However, as the conducting tubes become smaller, the following structural changes occur:

- **Support structures change.** Irregular *plates* of cartilage replace the cartilage rings, and by the time the bronchioles are reached, the tube walls no longer contain supportive cartilage. However, the tube walls throughout the bronchial tree contain elastic fibers.
- **Epithelium type changes.** The mucosal epithelium thins as it changes from pseudostratified columnar to columnar and then to cuboidal in the terminal bronchioles. Mucus-producing cells and cilia are sparse in the bronchioles. For this reason, most airborne debris found at or below the level of the bronchioles must be removed by macrophages in the alveoli.
- **Amount of smooth muscle increases.** The relative amount of smooth muscle in the tube walls increases as the passageways become smaller. A complete layer of circular smooth muscle in the bronchioles and the lack of supporting cartilage (which would hinder constriction) allows the bronchioles to provide substantial resistance to air passage under certain conditions (as we will describe later).

Respiratory Zone Structures

Defined by the presence of thin-walled air sacs called **alveoli** (al-ve′o-li; *alveol* = small cavity), the respiratory zone begins as the terminal bronchioles feed into **respiratory bronchioles** within the lung (Figure 22.8). Protruding from these smallest bronchioles are scattered alveoli. The respiratory bronchioles lead into winding **alveolar ducts**, whose walls consist of diffusely arranged rings of smooth muscle cells, connective tissue fibers, and outpocketing alveoli. The alveolar ducts lead into terminal clusters of alveoli called **alveolar sacs** or **alveolar saccules**.

Many people mistakenly equate alveoli, the site of gas exchange, with alveolar sacs, but they are not the same thing. The alveolar sac is analogous to a bunch of grapes, and the alveoli are the individual grapes. The 300 million or so gas-filled alveoli in the lungs account for most of our lung volume and provide a tremendous surface area for gas exchange.

The Respiratory Membrane The walls of the alveoli are composed primarily of a single layer of squamous epithelial cells, called **type I alveolar cells**, surrounded by a flimsy basement membrane. The thinness of their walls is hard to imagine, but a sheet of tissue paper is 15 times thicker!

The external surfaces of the alveoli are densely covered with a "cobweb" of pulmonary capillaries **(Figure 22.9)**. Together, the capillary and alveolar walls and their fused basement membranes form the **respiratory membrane**, a 0.5-μm-thick *blood air barrier* that has blood flowing past on one side and gas on the other (Figure 22.9c). Gas exchanges occur readily by simple diffusion across the respiratory membrane—O_2 passes from the alveolus into the blood, and CO_2 leaves the blood to enter the gas-filled alveolus.

Scattered amid the squamous type I alveolar cells that form the major part of the alveolar walls are cuboidal type II alveolar cells (Figure 22.9c). **Type II alveolar cells** secrete a fluid containing a detergent-like substance called *surfactant* that coats the gas-exposed alveolar surfaces. (We describe surfactant's role in reducing the surface tension of the alveolar fluid later in this chapter.) Type II alveolar cells also secrete a number of antimicrobial proteins that are important elements of innate immunity.

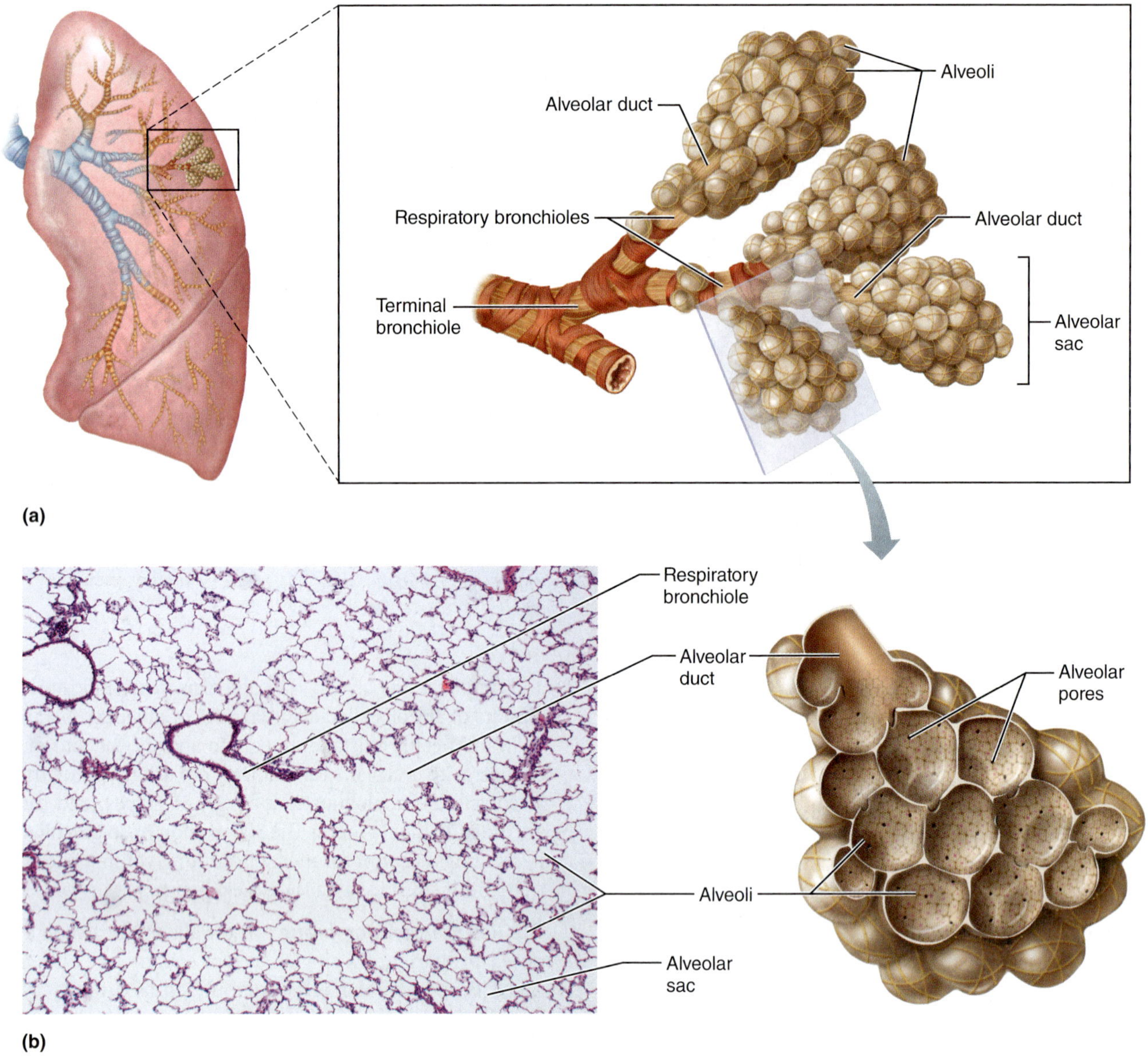

Figure 22.8 Respiratory zone structures. (a) Diagrammatic view of respiratory bronchioles, alveolar ducts, alveolar sacs, and alveoli. **(b)** Photomicrograph of a section of human lung, showing the respiratory structures that form the final divisions of the bronchial tree (80×). Notice the thinness of the alveolar walls.

The alveoli have three other significant features: (1) They are surrounded by fine elastic fibers of the same type that surround the entire bronchial tree. (2) Open **alveolar pores** connecting adjacent alveoli allow air pressure throughout the lung to be equalized and provide alternate air routes to any alveoli whose bronchi have collapsed due to disease. (3) Remarkably efficient **alveolar macrophages** crawl freely along the internal alveolar surfaces.

Although huge numbers of infectious microorganisms are continuously carried into the alveoli, alveolar surfaces are usually sterile. Because the alveoli are "dead ends," aged and dead macrophages must be prevented from accumulating in them. Most macrophages simply get swept up by the ciliary current of superior regions and carried passively to the pharynx. In this manner, we clear and swallow over 2 million alveolar macrophages per hour!

The Lungs and Pleurae

✓ Describe the gross structure of the lungs and pleurae.

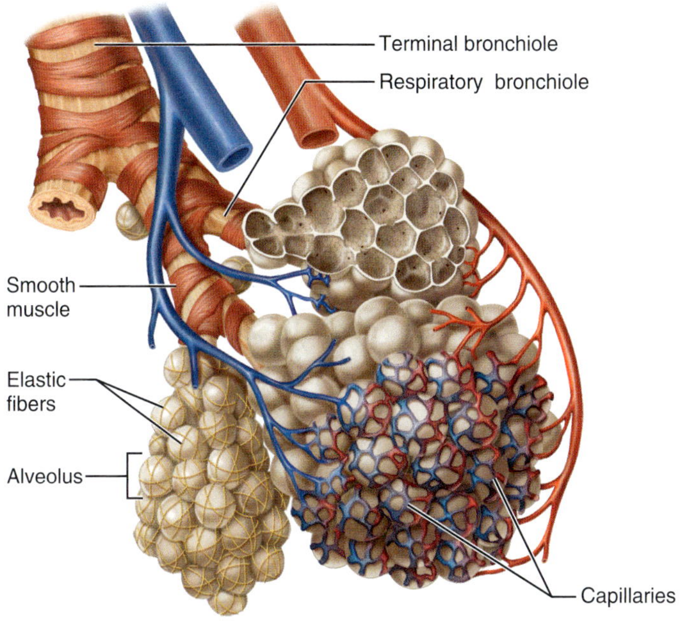

(a) Diagrammatic view of capillary-alveoli relationships

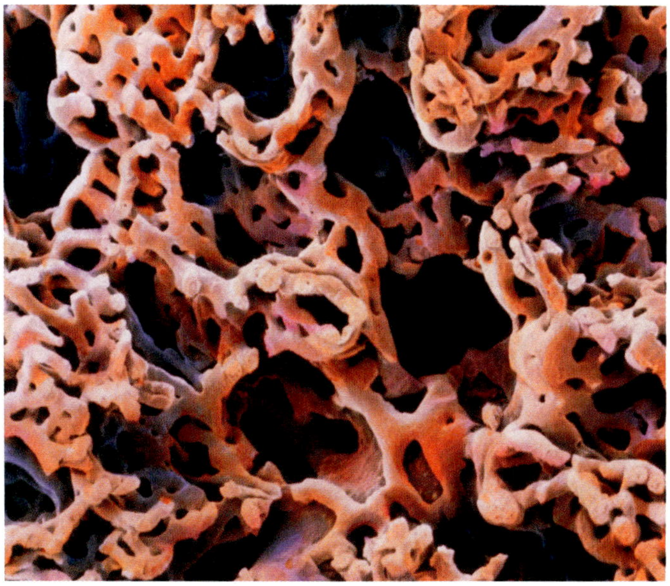

(b) Scanning electron micrograph of pulmonary capillary casts (70x)

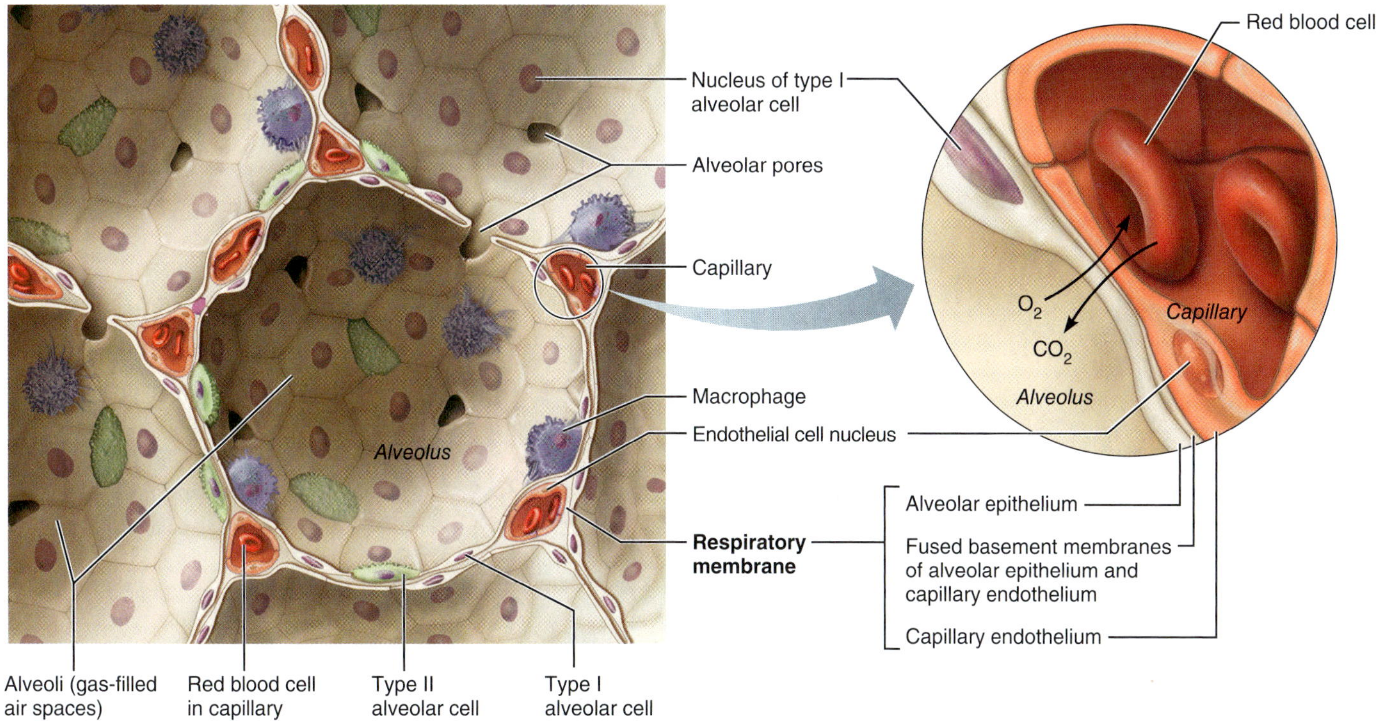

(c) Detailed anatomy of the respiratory membrane

Figure 22.9 Alveoli and the respiratory membrane. Elastic fibers and capillaries surround all alveoli, but for clarity they are shown only on some alveoli in (a). In (b), the tissue forming the alveoli has been removed. Only the capillary network remains.

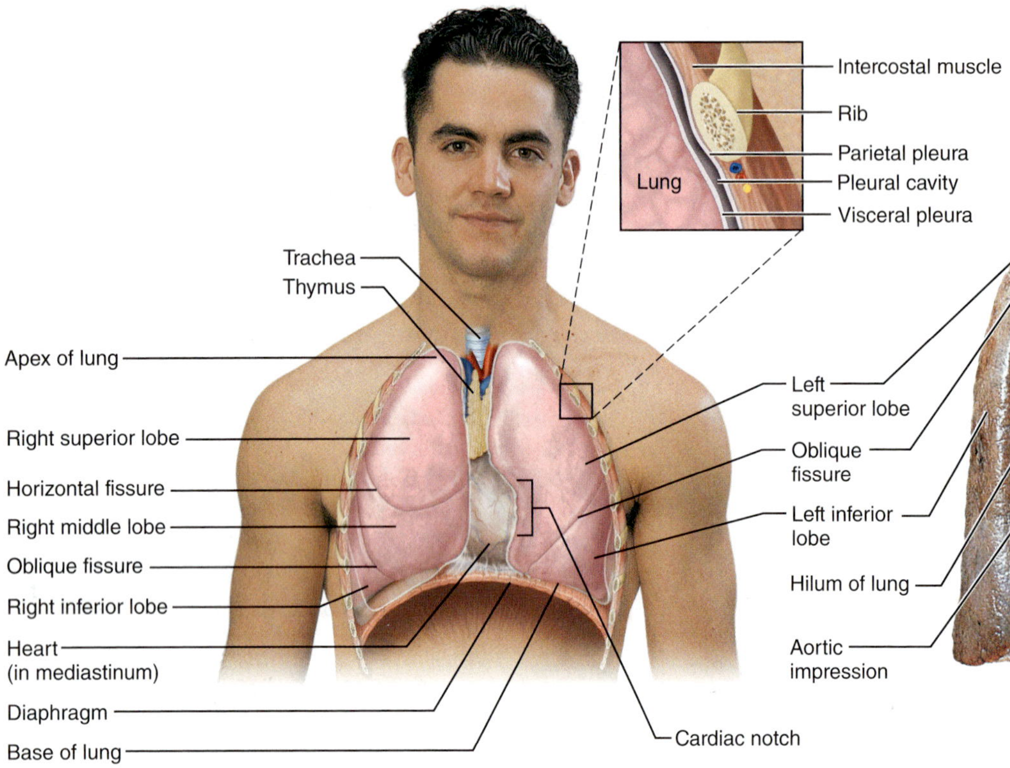

(a) Anterior view. The lungs flank mediastinal structures laterally.

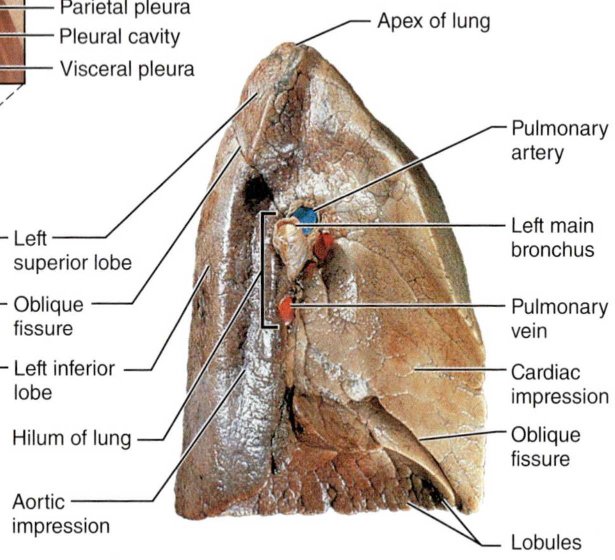

(b) Photograph of medial view of the left lung.

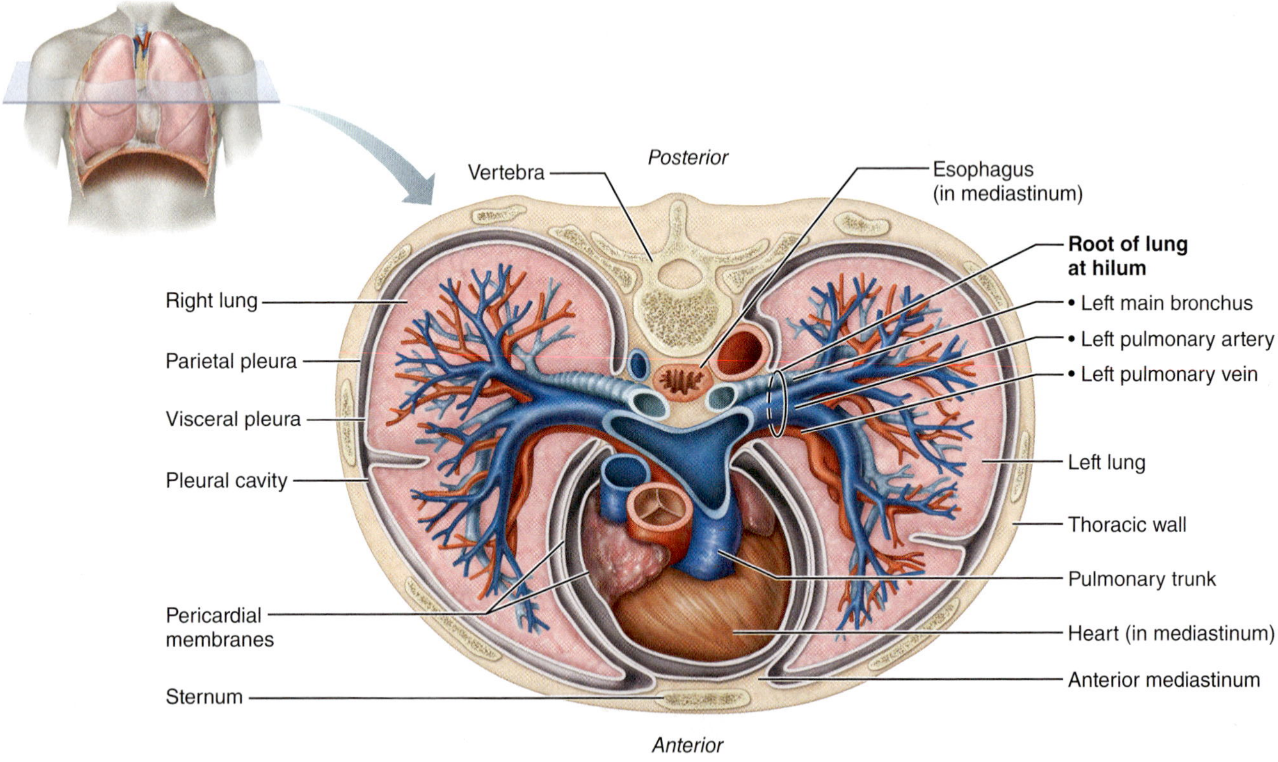

(c) Transverse section through the thorax, viewed from above. Lungs, pleural membranes, and major organs in the mediastinum are shown.

Figure 22.10 Anatomical relationships of organs in the thoracic cavity. In (c), the size of the pleural cavity is exaggerated for clarity.

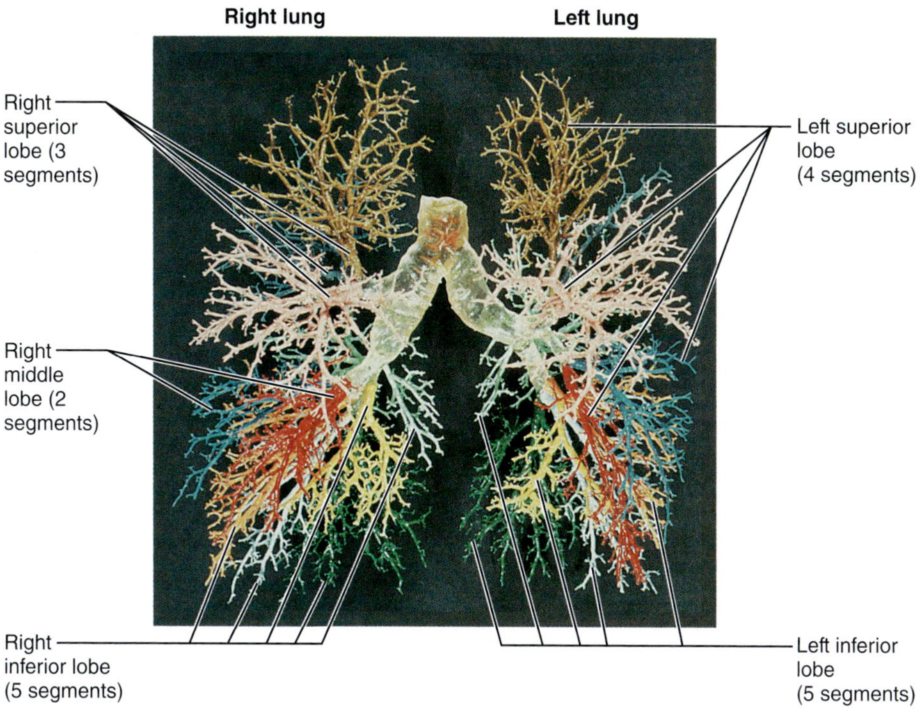

Figure 22.11 A cast of the bronchial tree. The individual bronchopulmonary segments have been painted different colors.

The paired **lungs** occupy all of the thoracic cavity except the mediastinum, which houses the heart, great blood vessels, bronchi, esophagus, and other organs **(Figure 22.10)**.

Gross Anatomy of the Lungs

Each cone-shaped lung is surrounded by pleurae and connected to the mediastinum by vascular and bronchial attachments, collectively called the lung **root**. The anterior, lateral, and posterior lung surfaces lie in close contact with the ribs and form the continuously curving **costal surface**. Just deep to the clavicle is the **apex**, the narrow superior tip of the lung. The concave, inferior surface that rests on the diaphragm is the **base**.

On the mediastinal surface of each lung is an indentation, the **hilum**, through which pulmonary and systemic blood vessels, bronchi, lymphatic vessels, and nerves enter and leave the lungs. Each main bronchus plunges into the hilum on its own side and begins to branch almost immediately. All conducting and respiratory passageways distal to the main bronchi are found in the lungs.

The two lungs differ slightly in shape and size because the apex of the heart is slightly to the left of the median plane. The left lung is smaller than the right, and the **cardiac notch**—a concavity in its medial aspect—is molded to and accommodates the heart (Figure 22.10a). The left lung is subdivided into superior and inferior **lobes** by the *oblique fissure*, whereas the right lung is partitioned into superior, middle, and inferior lobes by the *oblique* and *horizontal fissures*.

Each lobe contains a number of pyramid-shaped **bronchopulmonary segments** separated from one another by connective tissue septa. The right lung has 10 bronchopulmonary segments, but the left lung is more variable and consists of 8 to 10 segments **(Figure 22.11)**. Each segment is served by its own artery and vein and receives air from an individual segmental (tertiary) bronchus.

The bronchopulmonary segments are clinically important because pulmonary disease is often confined to one or a few segments. Their connective tissue partitions allow diseased segments to be surgically removed without damaging neighboring segments or impairing their blood supply.

The smallest subdivisions of the lung visible with the naked eye are the **lobules**, which appear at the lung surface as hexagons ranging from the size of a pencil eraser to the size of a penny (Figure 22.10b). A large bronchiole and its branches serve each lobule. In most city dwellers and in smokers, the connective tissue that separates the individual lobules is blackened with carbon.

As we mentioned earlier, the lungs consist largely of air spaces. The balance of lung tissue, or its **stroma** (literally "mattress" or "bed"), is mostly elastic connective tissue. As a result, the lungs are soft, spongy, elastic organs that together weigh just over 1 kg (2.2 lb). The elasticity of healthy lungs reduces the work of breathing, as we will describe shortly.

Blood Supply and Innervation of the Lungs

The lungs are perfused by two circulations, the pulmonary and the bronchial, which differ in size, origin, and function.

Pulmonary Circulation of the Lungs Systemic venous blood that is to be oxygenated in the lungs is delivered by the **pulmonary arteries**, which lie anterior to the main bronchi (Figure 22.10c). In the lungs, the pulmonary arteries branch profusely along with the bronchi and finally feed into the **pulmonary capillary networks** surrounding the alveoli (see Figure 22.9a).

22

The **pulmonary veins** convey the freshly oxygenated blood from the respiratory zone of the lungs to the heart. Their tributaries course back to the hilum both with the corresponding bronchi and in the connective tissue septa separating the bronchopulmonary segments.

The pulmonary circuit is a low-pressure, high-volume circulation. Because *all* of the body's blood passes through the lungs about once each minute, the lung capillary endothelium is an ideal location for enzymes that act on materials in the blood. Examples include *angiotensin converting enzyme*, which activates an important blood pressure hormone, and enzymes that inactivate certain prostaglandins.

Bronchial Circulation of the Lungs In contrast to the pulmonary circulation, the **bronchial arteries** provide oxygenated systemic blood to lung tissue. The bronchial arteries arise from the aorta, enter the lungs at the hilum, and then run along the branching bronchi. They provide a high-pressure, low-volume supply of oxygenated blood to all lung tissues except the alveoli. The tiny bronchial veins drain some systemic venous blood from the lungs, but there are multiple anastomoses between the two circulations, and most venous blood returns to the heart via the pulmonary veins.

Innervation of the Lungs The lungs are innervated by parasympathetic and sympathetic motor fibers, and visceral sensory fibers. These nerve fibers enter each lung through the **pulmonary plexus** on the lung root and run along the bronchial tubes and blood vessels in the lungs. Parasympathetic fibers cause the air tubes to constrict, whereas sympathetic fibers dilate them.

The Pleurae

The **pleurae** (ploo′re; "sides") form a thin, double-layered serosa. The layer called the **parietal pleura** covers the thoracic wall and superior face of the diaphragm (Figure 22.10a, c). It continues around the heart and between the lungs, forming the lateral walls of the mediastinal enclosure and snugly enclosing the lung root. From here, the pleura extends as the layer called the **visceral pleura** to cover the external lung surface, dipping into and lining its fissures.

22

The pleurae produce **pleural fluid**, which fills the slitlike **pleural cavity** between them. This lubricating secretion allows the lungs to glide easily over the thorax wall during our breathing movements. Although the pleurae slide easily across each other, the surface tension of the pleural fluid strongly resists their separation. Consequently, the lungs cling tightly to the thorax wall and expand and recoil passively as the volume of the thoracic cavity alternately increases and decreases during breathing.

The pleurae also help divide the thoracic cavity into three chambers—the central mediastinum and the two lateral pleural compartments, each containing a lung. This compartmentalization helps prevent one mobile organ (for example, the lung or heart) from interfering with another. It also limits the spread of local infections.

Homeostatic Imbalance 22.6

Pleurisy (ploo′rĭ-se), inflammation of the pleurae, often results from pneumonia. Inflamed pleurae become rough, resulting in friction and stabbing pain with each breath. As the disease progresses, the pleurae may produce excessive amounts of fluid. This increased fluid relieves the pain caused by pleural surfaces rubbing together, but may exert pressure on the lungs and hinder breathing movements.

Other fluids that may accumulate in the pleural cavity include blood (leaked from damaged blood vessels) and blood filtrate (the watery fluid that oozes from the lung capillaries when left-sided heart failure occurs). The general term for fluid accumulation in the pleural cavity is *pleural effusion*. +

Check Your Understanding

4. What features of the alveoli and their respiratory membranes suit them to their function of exchanging gases by diffusion?
5. A 3-year-old boy is brought to the emergency department after aspirating (inhaling) a peanut. Bronchoscopy confirms the suspicion that the peanut is lodged in a bronchus and then it is successfully extracted. Which main bronchus was the peanut most likely to be in? Why?
6. The lungs are perfused by two different circulations. Name these circulations and indicate their roles in the lungs.

For answers, see Appendix H.

Mechanics of Breathing

Breathing, or **pulmonary ventilation**, consists of two phases: **inspiration**, the period when air flows into the lungs, and **expiration**, the period when gases exit the lungs.

Pressure Relationships in the Thoracic Cavity

✓ Explain the functional importance of the partial vacuum that exists in the intrapleural space.

Before we discuss the breathing process, it is important to understand that *respiratory pressures are always described relative to* **atmospheric pressure (P_{atm})**, which is the pressure exerted by the air (gases) surrounding the body. At sea level, atmospheric pressure is 760 mm Hg (the pressure exerted by a column of mercury 760 mm high). This pressure can also be expressed in atmosphere units: atmospheric pressure = 760 mm Hg = 1 atm.

A negative respiratory pressure in any respiratory area indicates that the pressure in that region is lower than atmospheric pressure. For instance, a respiratory pressure of −4 mm Hg indicates a pressure that is lower than atmospheric pressure by 4 mm Hg (760 − 4 = 756 mm Hg). In this case, 756 mm Hg is the absolute pressure in that region. A positive respiratory pressure is higher than atmospheric pressure, and zero respiratory pressure is equal to atmospheric pressure. Now we are ready to examine the pressure relationships that normally exist in the thoracic cavity.

Intrapulmonary Pressure (P_{pul})

The **intrapulmonary** (intra-alveolar) **pressure** (**P_{pul}**) is the pressure in the alveoli. Intrapulmonary pressure rises and falls with the phases of breathing, but it *always* equalizes with the atmospheric pressure eventually **(Figure 22.12)**.

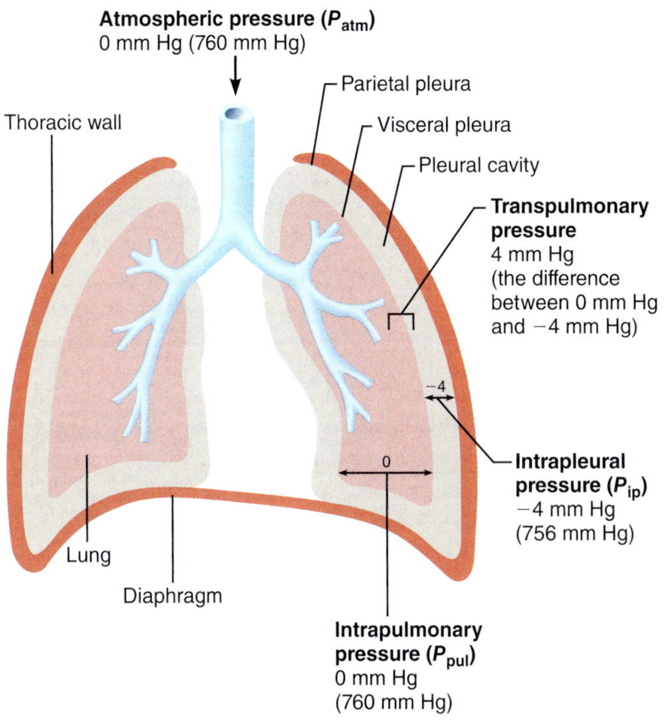

Figure 22.12 Intrapulmonary and intrapleural pressure relationships. Values shown are pressures relative to atmospheric pressure (760 mm Hg at sea level). Absolute pressures are given in parentheses. These pressures are at the end of a normal expiration. For illustration, the size of the pleural cavity has been greatly exaggerated.

Intrapleural Pressure (P_{ip})

The pressure in the pleural cavity, the **intrapleural pressure (P_{ip})**, also fluctuates with breathing phases, but is always about 4 mm Hg less than P_{pul}. That is, P_{ip} is *always* negative relative to P_{pul}.

What causes this negative intrapleural pressure? To answer this question, let's examine the forces that exist in the thorax. First of all, we know there are opposing forces. Two forces act to pull the lungs (visceral pleura) away from the thorax wall (parietal pleura) and cause the lungs to collapse:

- **The lungs' natural tendency to recoil.** Because of their elasticity, lungs always assume the smallest size possible.
- **The surface tension of the alveolar fluid.** The molecules of the fluid lining the alveoli attract each other. This produces *surface tension* that constantly acts to draw the alveoli to their smallest possible dimension.

However, these lung-collapsing forces are opposed by the natural elasticity of the chest wall, a force that tends to pull the thorax outward and enlarge the lungs. So which force wins? In a healthy person, the answer is neither, because of the strong adhesive force between the parietal and visceral pleurae. Pleural fluid secures the pleurae together in the same way a drop of water holds two glass slides together. The pleurae slide from side to side easily, but they remain closely apposed, and separating them requires extreme force. The net result of the dynamic interplay between these forces is a negative P_{ip}.

The amount of pleural fluid in the pleural cavity must remain minimal to maintain a negative P_{ip}. The pleural fluid is actively pumped out of the pleural cavity into the lymphatics continuously. If it wasn't, fluid would accumulate in the intrapleural space (remember, fluids move from high to low pressure), producing a positive pressure in the pleural cavity.

We cannot overemphasize the importance of negative pressure in the intrapleural space and the tight coupling of the lungs to the thorax wall. Any condition that equalizes P_{ip} with the intrapulmonary (or atmospheric) pressure causes *immediate lung collapse*. It is the **transpulmonary pressure**—the difference between the intrapulmonary and intrapleural pressures ($P_{pul} - P_{ip}$)—that keeps the air spaces of the lungs open or, phrased another way, keeps the lungs from collapsing. Moreover, *the size of the transpulmonary pressure determines the size of the lungs* at any time—the greater the transpulmonary pressure, the larger the lungs.

Homeostatic Imbalance 22.7

Atelectasis (at″ĕ-lik′tah-sis), or lung collapse, occurs when a bronchiole becomes plugged (as may follow pneumonia). Its associated alveoli then absorb all of their air and collapse. Atelectasis can also occur when air enters the pleural cavity either through a chest wound or a rupture of the visceral pleura, which allows air from the respiratory tract to enter the pleural cavity.

The presence of air in the pleural cavity is referred to as a **pneumothorax** (nu″mo-tho′raks; "air thorax"), and is reversed by drawing air out of the intrapleural space with chest tubes. This procedure allows the pleurae to heal and the lung to reinflate and resume normal function. Note that because the lungs are in separate cavities, one lung can collapse without interfering with the other. +

Pulmonary Ventilation

- ✓ Relate Boyle's law to events of inspiration and expiration.
- ✓ Explain the relative roles of the respiratory muscles and lung elasticity in producing the volume changes that cause air to flow into and out of the lungs.

Pulmonary ventilation, consisting of inspiration and expiration, is a mechanical process that depends on volume changes in the thoracic cavity. A rule to keep in mind throughout the following discussion is that *volume changes* lead to *pressure changes*, and pressure changes lead to the *flow of gases* to equalize the pressure.

Boyle's law gives the relationship between the pressure and volume of a gas: At constant temperature, the pressure of a gas varies inversely with its volume. That is,

$$P_1V_1 = P_2V_2$$

where P is the pressure of the gas, V is its volume, and subscripts 1 and 2 represent the initial and resulting conditions respectively.

Gases always *fill* their container. Consequently, in a large container, the molecules in a given amount of gas will be far apart and the pressure will be low. But if the volume of the container is reduced, the gas molecules will be forced closer together and the pressure will rise.

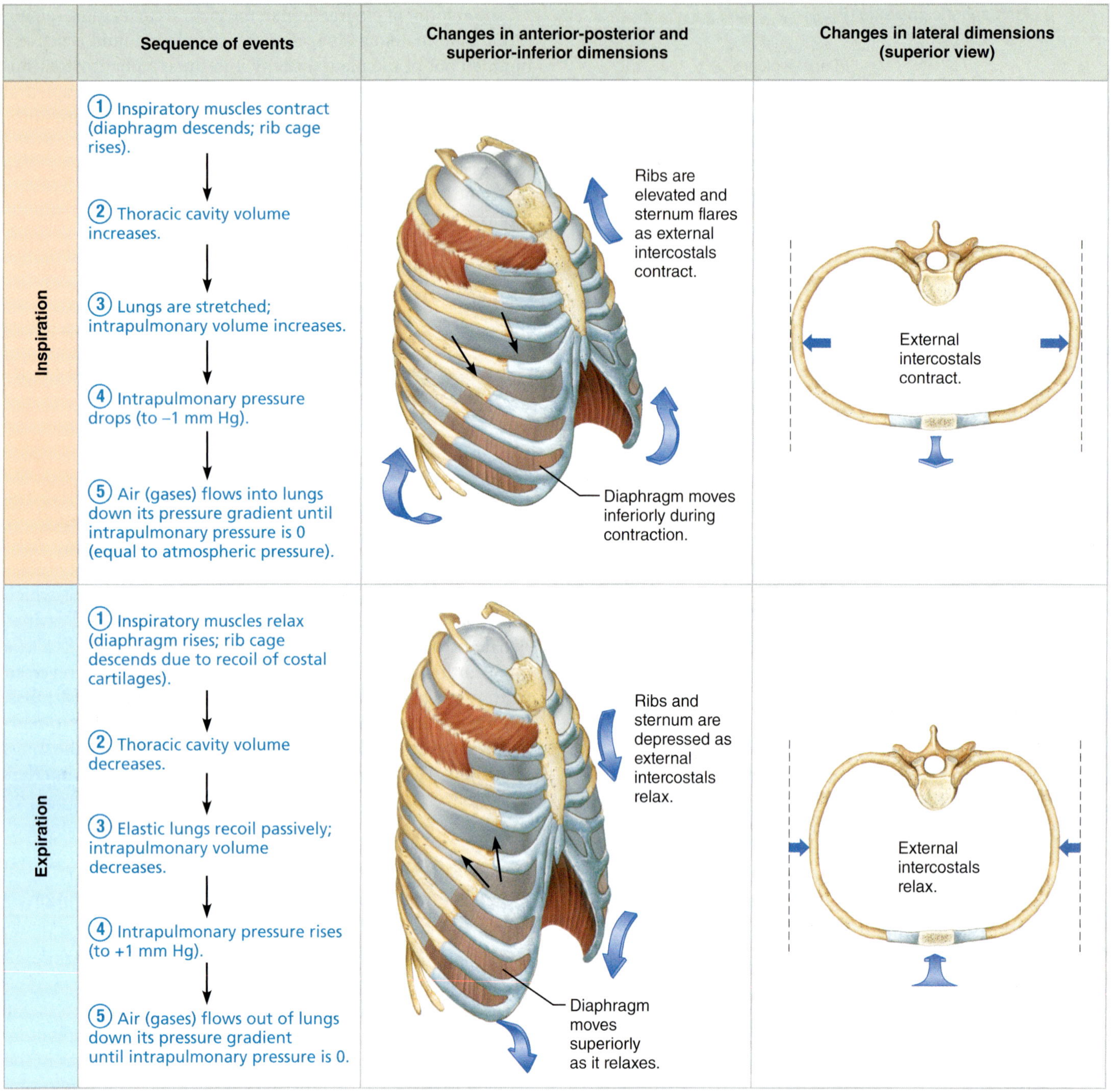

Figure 22.13 Changes in thoracic volume and sequence of events during inspiration and expiration. The sequence of events in the left column includes volume changes during inspiration (top) and expiration (bottom). The lateral views in the middle column show changes in the superior-inferior dimension (as the diaphragm alternately contracts and relaxes, see black arrows) and in the anterior-posterior dimension (as the external intercostal muscles alternately contract and relax). The superior views of transverse thoracic sections in the right column show lateral dimension changes resulting from alternate contraction and relaxation of the external intercostal muscles.

A good example is an inflated automobile tire. The tire is hard and strong enough to bear the weight of a car because air is compressed to about one-third of its atmospheric volume inside the tire, providing high pressure. Now let's see how this relates to inspiration and expiration.

Inspiration

Visualize the thoracic cavity as a gas-filled box with a single entrance at the top, the tubelike trachea. The volume of this box is changeable and can be increased by enlarging all of its dimensions, thereby decreasing the gas pressure inside it. This drop in

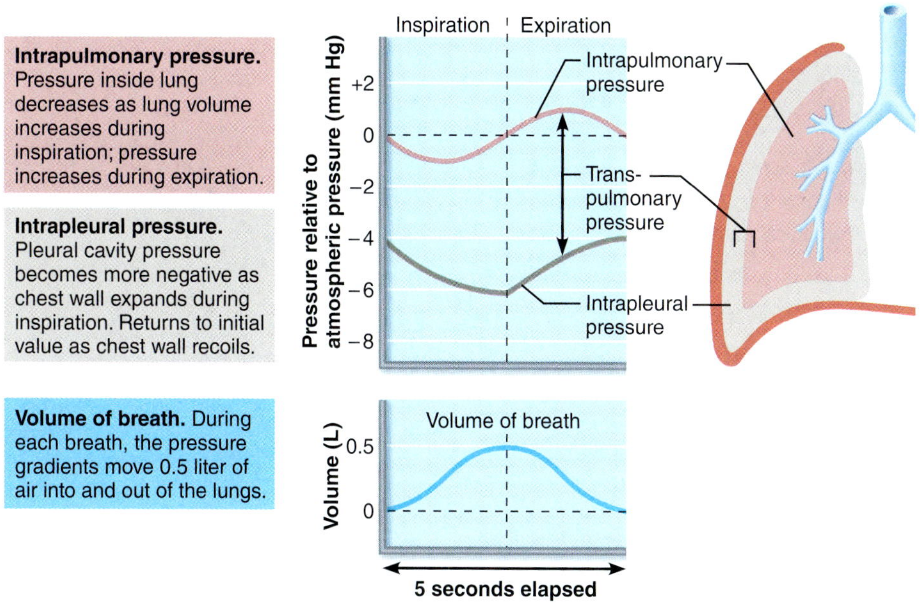

Figure 22.14 Changes in intrapulmonary and intrapleural pressures during inspiration and expiration. Notice that normal atmospheric pressure (760 mm Hg) is given a value of 0 on the scale.

pressure causes air to rush into the box from the atmosphere, because gases always flow down their pressure gradients.

The same thing happens during normal quiet inspiration, when the **inspiratory muscles**—the diaphragm and external intercostal muscles—are activated. Here's how quiet inspiration works:

- **Action of the diaphragm.** When the dome-shaped diaphragm contracts, it moves inferiorly and flattens out (**Figure 22.13**, top). As a result, the superior-inferior dimension (height) of the thoracic cavity increases.
- **Action of the intercostal muscles.** When the external intercostal muscles contract, they lift the rib cage and pull the sternum superiorly (Figure 22.13, top). Because the ribs curve downward as well as forward around the chest wall, the broadest lateral and anteroposterior dimensions of the rib cage are normally directed obliquely downward. But when the ribs are raised and drawn together, they swing outward, expanding the diameter of the thorax both laterally and in the anteroposterior plane. This is much like the action that occurs when a curved bucket handle is raised—it moves outward as it moves upward.

Although these actions expand the thoracic dimensions by only a few millimeters along each plane, this is enough to increase thoracic volume by almost 500 ml—the usual volume of air that enters the lungs during a normal quiet inspiration. Of the two types of inspiratory muscles, the diaphragm is far more important in producing these volume changes that lead to normal quiet inspiration.

As the thoracic dimensions increase during inspiration, the lungs are stretched and the intrapulmonary volume increases. As a result, P_{pul} drops about 1 mm Hg relative to P_{atm}. Anytime the intrapulmonary pressure is less than the atmospheric pressure ($P_{pul} < P_{atm}$), air rushes into the lungs along the pressure gradient. Inspiration ends when $P_{pul} = P_{atm}$. During the same period, P_{ip} declines to about −6 mm Hg relative to P_{atm} **(Figure 22.14)**.

During the *deep* or *forced inspirations* that occur during vigorous exercise and in some chronic obstructive pulmonary diseases, accessory muscles further increase thoracic volume. Several muscles, including the scalenes and sternocleidomastoid muscles of the neck and the pectoralis minor of the chest, raise the ribs even more than during quiet inspiration. Additionally, the back extends as the erector spinae muscles straighten the thoracic curvature.

Expiration

In healthy individuals, quiet expiration is a passive process that depends more on lung elasticity than on muscle contraction. As the inspiratory muscles relax and resume their resting length, the rib cage descends and the lungs recoil (Figure 22.13, bottom). As a result, both the thoracic and intrapulmonary volumes decrease. This volume decrease compresses the alveoli, and P_{pul} rises to about 1 mm Hg above atmospheric pressure (Figure 22.14). When $P_{pul} > P_{atm}$, the pressure gradient forces gases to flow out of the lungs.

Forced expiration is an active process produced by contracting abdominal wall muscles, primarily the oblique and transversus muscles. These contractions (1) increase the intra-abdominal pressure, which forces the abdominal organs superiorly against the diaphragm, and (2) depress the rib cage. The internal intercostal muscles also help depress the rib cage and decrease thoracic volume.

To precisely regulate air flow from the lungs, it is necessary to control the accessory muscles of expiration. For instance, the ability of a trained vocalist to hold a musical note depends on the coordinated activity of several muscles normally used in forced expiration.

☑ Check Your Understanding

7. What is the driving force for pulmonary ventilation?
8. What causes the intrapulmonary pressure to decrease during inspiration?
9. What causes the partial vacuum (negative pressure) inside the pleural cavity? What happens to a lung if air enters the pleural cavity? What is the clinical name for this condition?

For answers, see Appendix H.

Physical Factors Influencing Pulmonary Ventilation

✓ List several physical factors that influence pulmonary ventilation.

As we have seen, the lungs are stretched during inspiration and recoil passively during expiration. The inspiratory muscles consume energy to enlarge the thorax. Energy is also used to overcome various factors that hinder air passage and pulmonary ventilation. We examine these factors next.

Airway Resistance

The major *nonelastic* source of resistance to gas flow is friction, or drag, encountered in the respiratory passageways. The following equation gives the relationship between gas flow (F), pressure (P), and resistance (R):

$$F = \frac{\Delta P}{R}$$

Notice that the factors determining gas flow in the respiratory passages and blood flow in the cardiovascular system are equivalent. The amount of gas flowing into and out of the alveoli is directly proportional to ΔP, the *difference* in pressure, or pressure gradient, between the external atmosphere and the alveoli.

Normally, very small differences in pressure produce large changes in the volume of gas flow. The average pressure gradient during normal quiet breathing is 2 mm Hg or less, and yet it is sufficient to move 500 ml of air in and out of the lungs with each breath.

But, as the equation also indicates, gas flow changes *inversely* with resistance. In other words, gas flow decreases as resistance increases. As in the cardiovascular system, resistance in the respiratory tree is determined mostly by the diameters of the conducting tubes. However, as a rule, airway resistance is insignificant for two reasons:

- Airway diameters in the first part of the conducting zone are huge, relative to the low viscosity of air.
- As the airways get progressively smaller, there are progressively more branches. As a result, although individual bronchioles are tiny, there are an enormous number of them in parallel, so the total cross-sectional area is huge.

Consequently, the greatest resistance to gas flow occurs in the medium-sized bronchi **(Figure 22.15)**. At the terminal bronchioles, gas flow stops and diffusion takes over as the main force driving gas movement, so resistance is no longer an issue.

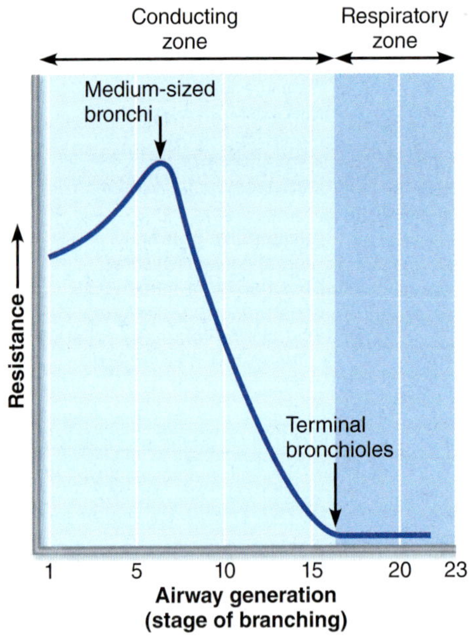

Figure 22.15 Resistance in respiratory passageways. Airway resistance peaks in the medium-sized bronchi and then declines sharply as the total cross-sectional area of the airways increases rapidly.

Homeostatic Imbalance 22.8

Smooth muscle of the bronchiolar walls is exquisitely sensitive to neural controls and certain chemicals. For example, inhaled irritants activate a reflex of the parasympathetic division of the nervous system that causes vigorous constriction of the bronchioles and dramatically reduces air passage. During an acute *asthma attack*, histamine and other inflammatory chemicals can cause such strong bronchoconstriction that pulmonary ventilation almost completely stops, regardless of the pressure gradient. Conversely, epinephrine released during sympathetic nervous system activation or administered as a drug dilates bronchioles and reduces airway resistance. Local accumulations of mucus, infectious material, or solid tumors in the passageways are important sources of airway resistance in those with respiratory disease.

Whenever airway resistance rises, breathing movements become more strenuous, but such compensation has its limits. When the bronchioles are severely constricted or obstructed, even the most magnificent respiratory efforts cannot restore ventilation to life-sustaining levels. +

Alveolar Surface Tension

At any gas-liquid boundary, the molecules of the liquid are more strongly attracted to each other than to the gas molecules. This unequal attraction produces a state of tension at the liquid surface, called **surface tension**, that (1) draws the liquid molecules

22

closer together and reduces their contact with the dissimilar gas molecules, and (2) resists any force that tends to increase the surface area of the liquid.

Water is composed of highly polar molecules and has a very high surface tension. As the major component of the liquid film that coats the alveolar walls, water is always acting to reduce the alveoli to their smallest possible size, as we noted earlier.

If the film were pure water, the alveoli would collapse between breaths. But the alveolar film also contains **surfactant** (ser-fak′tant), a detergent-like complex of lipids and proteins produced by the type II alveolar cells. Surfactant decreases the cohesiveness of water molecules, much the way a laundry detergent reduces the attraction of water for water, allowing water to interact with and pass through fabric. As a result, the surface tension of alveolar fluid is reduced, and less energy is needed to overcome those forces to expand the lungs and discourage alveolar collapse. Breaths that are deeper than normal stimulate type II cells to secrete more surfactant.

Homeostatic Imbalance 22.9

When too little surfactant is present, surface tension can collapse the alveoli. Once this happens, the alveoli must be completely reinflated during each inspiration, an effort that uses tremendous amounts of energy. This is the problem faced by newborns with **infant respiratory distress syndrome (IRDS)**, a condition peculiar to premature babies. Since fetal lungs do not produce adequate amounts of surfactant until the last two months of development, babies born prematurely often are unable to keep their alveoli inflated between breaths.

IRDS is treated by spraying natural or synthetic surfactant into the newborn's respiratory passageways. In addition, devices that maintain positive airway pressure throughout the respiratory cycle can keep the alveoli open between breaths. Severe cases require mechanical ventilators.

Many IRDS survivors suffer from *bronchopulmonary dysplasia*, a chronic lung disease, during childhood and beyond. This condition is believed to result from inflammatory injury caused by mechanically ventilating the premature newborn's delicate respiratory zone structures. ✚

Lung Compliance

Healthy lungs are unbelievably stretchy, and this distensibility is called **lung compliance**. Specifically, lung compliance (C_L) is a measure of the change in lung volume (ΔV_L) that occurs with a given change in transpulmonary pressure [$\Delta(P_{pul} - P_{ip})$]. This relationship is stated as

$$C_L = \frac{\Delta V_L}{\Delta(P_{pul} - P_{ip})}$$

The more a lung expands for a given rise in transpulmonary pressure, the greater its compliance. Said another way, the higher the lung compliance, the easier it is to expand the lungs at any given transpulmonary pressure.

Lung compliance is determined largely by two factors: (1) distensibility of the lung tissue and (2) alveolar surface tension. Because lung distensibility is generally high and surfactant keeps alveolar surface tension low, healthy lungs tend to have high compliance, which favors efficient ventilation.

Any decrease in the natural resilience of the lungs diminishes lung compliance. Chronic inflammation, or infections such as tuberculosis, can cause nonelastic scar tissue to replace normal lung tissue (*fibrosis*). Decreased production of surfactant can also impair lung compliance. The lower the lung compliance, the more energy is needed just to breathe.

Since the lungs are contained within the thoracic cavity, we also need to consider the compliance (distensibility) of the thoracic wall. Factors that reduce the compliance of the thoracic wall hinder lung expansion. The total compliance of the respiratory system is comprised of lung compliance and thoracic wall compliance.

Homeostatic Imbalance 22.10

Deformities of the thorax, ossified costal cartilages (common during old age), and paralyzed intercostal muscles all hinder thoracic expansion, reducing total respiratory compliance. ✚

Respiratory Volumes and Pulmonary Function Tests

- ✓ Explain and compare the various lung volumes and capacities.
- ✓ Define dead space.
- ✓ Indicate types of information that can be gained from pulmonary function tests.

The amount of air flushed in and out of the lungs depends on the conditions of inspiration and expiration. Consequently, several respiratory volumes can be described. Specific combinations of these respiratory volumes, called *respiratory capacities*, are measured to gain information about a person's respiratory status.

Respiratory Volumes

The four **respiratory volumes** of interest are tidal, inspiratory reserve, expiratory reserve, and residual. The values recorded in **Figure 22.16a** (and used in the following text) represent normal values for a healthy 20-year-old male weighing about 70 kg (155 lb). Figure 22.16b provides average values for males and females.

During normal quiet breathing, about 500 ml of air moves into and then out of the lungs with each breath. This respiratory volume is the **tidal volume (TV)**. The amount of air that can be inspired forcibly beyond the tidal volume (2100 to 3200 ml) is the **inspiratory reserve volume (IRV)**.

The **expiratory reserve volume (ERV)** is the amount of air—normally 1000 to 1200 ml—that can be expelled from the lungs after a normal tidal volume expiration. Even after the most strenuous expiration, about 1200 ml of air remains in the lungs; this is the **residual volume (RV)**, which helps to keep the alveoli patent (open) and prevent lung collapse.

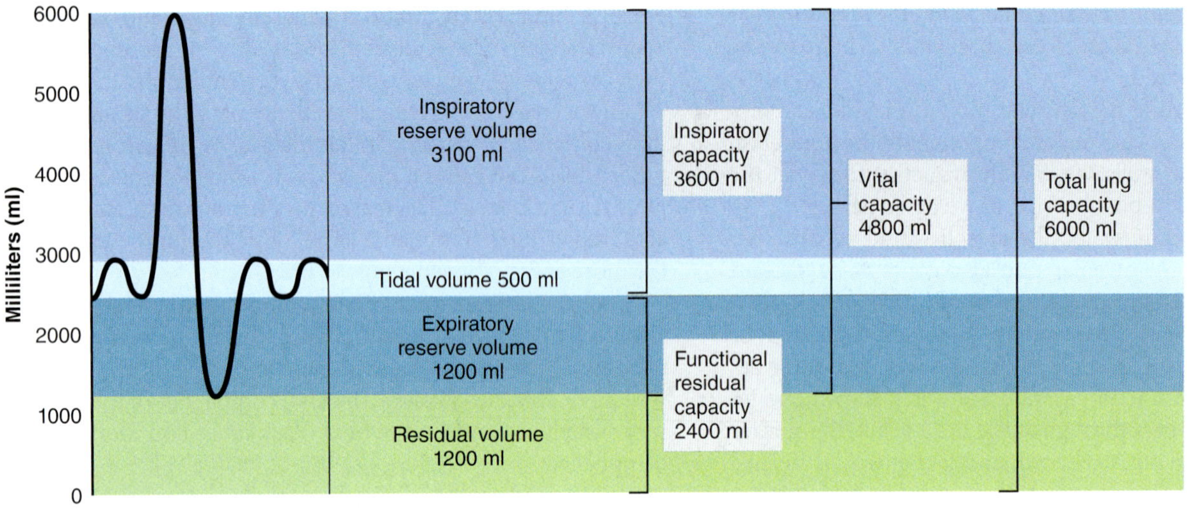

(a) Spirographic record for a male

	Measurement	Adult male average value	Adult female average value	Description
Respiratory volumes	Tidal volume (TV)	500 ml	500 ml	Amount of air inhaled or exhaled with each breath under resting conditions
	Inspiratory reserve volume (IRV)	3100 ml	1900 ml	Amount of air that can be forcefully inhaled after a normal tidal volume inspiration
	Expiratory reserve volume (ERV)	1200 ml	700 ml	Amount of air that can be forcefully exhaled after a normal tidal volume expiration
	Residual volume (RV)	1200 ml	1100 ml	Amount of air remaining in the lungs after a forced expiration
Respiratory capacities	Total lung capacity (TLC)	6000 ml	4200 ml	Maximum amount of air contained in lungs after a maximum inspiratory effort: TLC = TV + IRV + ERV + RV
	Vital capacity (VC)	4800 ml	3100 ml	Maximum amount of air that can be expired after a maximum inspiratory effort: VC = TV + IRV + ERV
	Inspiratory capacity (IC)	3600 ml	2400 ml	Maximum amount of air that can be inspired after a normal tidal volume expiration: IC = TV + IRV
	Functional residual capacity (FRC)	2400 ml	1800 ml	Volume of air remaining in the lungs after a normal tidal volume expiration: FRC = ERV + RV

22

(b) Summary of respiratory volumes and capacities for males and females

Figure 22.16 Respiratory volumes and capacities. Idealized spirographic record of respiratory volumes in (a) is for a healthy young 70-kg adult male.

Respiratory Capacities

The **respiratory capacities** include inspiratory, functional residual, vital, and total lung capacities (Figure 22.16). The respiratory capacities always consist of two or more lung volumes.

- **Inspiratory capacity (IC)** is the total amount of air that can be inspired after a normal tidal volume expiration, so it is the sum of TV and IRV.
- **Functional residual capacity (FRC)** represents the amount of air remaining in the lungs after a normal tidal volume expiration and is the combined RV and ERV.
- **Vital capacity (VC)** is the total amount of exchangeable air. It is the sum of TV, IRV, and ERV. In healthy young males, VC is approximately 4800 ml.
- **Total lung capacity (TLC)** is the sum of all lung volumes and is normally around 6000 ml.

As indicated in Figure 22.16b, lung volumes and capacities (with the possible exception of TV) tend to be smaller in women than in men because of women's smaller size.

Dead Space

Some of the inspired air fills the conducting respiratory passageways and never contributes to gas exchange in the alveoli. The volume of these conducting zone conduits, which make up the **anatomical dead space**, typically amounts to about 150 ml. (The rule of thumb is that the anatomical dead space volume in a healthy young adult is equal to 1 ml per pound of ideal body weight.) This means that if TV is 500 ml, only 350 ml of it is

Table 22.2 Effects of Breathing Rate and Depth on Alveolar Ventilation of Three Hypothetical Patients

BREATHING PATTERN OF HYPOTHETICAL PATIENT	DEAD SPACE VOLUME (DSV)	TIDAL VOLUME (TV)	RESPIRATORY RATE*	MINUTE VENTILATION (MVR)	ALVEOLAR VENTILATION (AVR)	% EFFECTIVE VENTILATION (AVR/MVR)
I—Normal rate and depth	150 ml	500 ml	20/min	10,000 ml/min	7000 ml/min	70%
II—Slow, deep breathing	150 ml	1000 ml	10/min	10,000 ml/min	8500 ml/min	85%
III—Rapid, shallow breathing	150 ml	250 ml	40/min	10,000 ml/min	4000 ml/min	40%

*Respiratory rate values are artificially adjusted to provide equivalent minute ventilation as a baseline for comparing alveolar ventilation.

involved in alveolar ventilation. The remaining 150 ml of the tidal breath is in the anatomical dead space.

If some alveoli cease to act in gas exchange (due to alveolar collapse or obstruction by mucus, for example), the **alveolar dead space** is added to the anatomical dead space. The sum of the nonuseful volumes is the **total dead space**.

Pulmonary Function Tests

The various lung volumes and capacities are often abnormal in people with pulmonary disorders. The original clinical measuring tool, a **spirometer** (spi-rom′ĕ-ter), was a cumbersome instrument utilizing a hollow bell inverted over water. Now patients simply blow into a small electronic measuring device.

Spirometry is most useful for evaluating losses in respiratory function and for following the course of certain respiratory diseases. It cannot provide a specific diagnosis, but it can distinguish between *obstructive pulmonary disease* involving increased airway resistance (such as chronic bronchitis) and *restrictive diseases* involving reduced total lung capacity. (These changes might be due to diseases such as tuberculosis, or to fibrosis due to exposure to certain environmental agents such as asbestos). In obstructive diseases, TLC, FRC, and RV may increase because the lungs hyperinflate, whereas in restrictive diseases, VC, TLC, FRC, and RV decline because lung expansion is limited.

We can obtain more information by assessing the *rate* at which gas moves into and out of the lungs.

- **Forced vital capacity (FVC)** measures the amount of gas expelled when a subject takes a deep breath and then forcefully exhales maximally and as rapidly as possible.
- **Forced expiratory volume (FEV)** determines the amount of air expelled during specific time intervals of the FVC test.

For example, the volume exhaled during the first second is FEV_1. Those with healthy lungs can exhale about 80% of the FVC within 1 second. Those with obstructive pulmonary disease exhale considerably less than 80% of the FVC within 1 second, while those with restrictive disease can exhale 80% or more of FVC in 1 second even though their FVC is reduced.

Alveolar Ventilation

The **minute ventilation** is the total amount of gas that flows into or out of the respiratory tract in 1 minute. During normal quiet breathing, the minute ventilation in healthy people is about 6 L/min (500 ml per breath multiplied by 12 breaths per minute). During vigorous exercise, the minute ventilation may reach 200 L/min.

Minute ventilation values provide a rough yardstick for assessing respiratory efficiency, but the **alveolar ventilation rate (AVR)** is a better index of effective ventilation. The AVR takes into account the volume of air wasted in the dead space and measures the flow of fresh gases in and out of the alveoli during a particular time interval. We can compute AVR using this equation:

$$\underset{\text{(ml/min)}}{\text{AVR}} = \underset{\text{(breaths/min)}}{\text{frequency}} \times \underset{\text{(ml/breath)}}{(\text{TV} - \text{dead space})}$$

In healthy people, AVR is usually about 12 breaths per minute times the difference of 500 − 150 ml per breath, or 4200 ml/min.

Because anatomical dead space is constant in a particular individual, increasing the volume of each inspiration (breathing depth) enhances AVR and gas exchange more than raising the respiratory rate. AVR drops dramatically during rapid shallow breathing because most of the inspired air never reaches the exchange sites. Furthermore, as tidal volume approaches the dead space value, effective ventilation approaches zero, regardless of how fast a person is breathing. Table 22.2 summarizes the effects of breathing rate and breathing depth on alveolar ventilation for three hypothetical patients.

Nonrespiratory Air Movements

Many processes other than breathing move air into or out of the lungs, and these processes may modify the normal respiratory rhythm. Most of these **nonrespiratory air movements** result from reflex activity, but some are produced voluntarily. Table 22.3 describes the most common of these movements.

☑ Check Your Understanding

10. Resistance in the airways is typically low. Why? (Give at least two reasons.)
11. Premature infants often lack adequate surfactant. How does this affect their ability to breathe?
12. Explain why slow, deep breaths ventilate the alveoli more effectively than do rapid, shallow breaths.

For answers, see Appendix H.

Table 22.3 Nonrespiratory Air (Gas) Movements

MOVEMENT	MECHANISM AND RESULT
Cough	Taking a deep breath, closing glottis, and forcing air superiorly from lungs against glottis; glottis opens suddenly and a blast of air rushes upward. Can dislodge foreign particles or mucus from lower respiratory tract and propel them superiorly.
Sneeze	Similar to a cough, except that expelled air is directed through nasal cavity as well as through oral cavity; depressed uvula routes air upward through nasal cavity. Clears upper respiratory passages.
Crying	Inspiration followed by releasing air in a number of short expirations. Primarily an emotionally induced mechanism.
Laughing	Essentially same as crying in terms of air movements produced. Also an emotionally induced response.
Hiccups	Sudden inspirations resulting from spasms of diaphragm; believed to be initiated by irritation of diaphragm or phrenic nerves, which serve diaphragm. Sound occurs when inspired air hits vocal folds of closing glottis.
Yawn	Very deep inspiration, taken with jaws wide open; not believed to be triggered by levels of oxygen or carbon dioxide in blood. Ventilates all alveoli (not the case in normal quiet breathing).

Gas Exchanges Between the Blood, Lungs, and Tissues

- ✓ State Dalton's law of partial pressures and Henry's law.
- ✓ Describe how atmospheric and alveolar air differ in composition, and explain these differences.
- ✓ Relate Dalton's and Henry's laws to events of external and internal respiration.

As you've discovered, during *external respiration* oxygen enters and carbon dioxide leaves the blood in the lungs by diffusion. At the body tissues, where the process is called *internal respiration*, the same gases move in opposite directions, also by diffusion. To understand these processes, let's examine the physical properties of gases and consider the composition of alveolar gas.

22

Basic Properties of Gases

Beyond Boyle's law, two more gas laws provide most of the information we need—*Dalton's law of partial pressures* reveals how a gas behaves when it is part of a mixture of gases, and *Henry's law* helps us understand how gases move into and out of solution.

Dalton's Law of Partial Pressures

Dalton's law of partial pressures states that the total pressure exerted by a mixture of gases is the sum of the pressures exerted independently by each gas in the mixture. Further, the pressure exerted by each gas—its **partial pressure**—is directly proportional to the percentage of that gas in the gas mixture.

As indicated in Table 22.4, nitrogen makes up about 79% of air, and the partial pressure of nitrogen P_{N_2} is 78.6% × 760 mm Hg, or 597 mm Hg. Oxygen, which accounts for nearly 21% of air, has a partial pressure P_{O_2} of 159 mm Hg (20.9% × 760 mm Hg). Together nitrogen and oxygen contribute about 99% of the total atmospheric pressure. Air also contains 0.04% carbon dioxide, up to 0.5% water vapor, and insignificant amounts of inert gases (such as argon and helium).

At high altitudes, where the atmosphere is less influenced by gravity, partial pressures decline in direct proportion to the decrease in atmospheric pressure. For example, at 10,000 feet above sea level where the atmospheric pressure is 523 mm Hg, P_{O_2} is 110 mm Hg.

Moving in the opposite direction, atmospheric pressure increases by 1 atm (760 mm Hg) for each 33 feet of descent (in water) below sea level. At 99 feet below sea level, the total pressure exerted on the body is equivalent to 4 atm, or 3040 mm Hg, and the partial pressure exerted by each component gas is also quadrupled.

Henry's Law

Henry's law states that when a gas is in contact with a liquid, the gas will dissolve in the liquid in proportion to its partial pressure. Accordingly, the greater the concentration of a particular gas in the gas phase, the more and the faster that gas will go into solution in the liquid.

At equilibrium, the partial pressures in the gas and liquid phases are the same. If, however, the partial pressure of the gas later becomes greater in the liquid than in the adjacent gas phase, some of the dissolved gas molecules will reenter the gaseous phase. So the direction and amount of movement of a gas are determined by its partial pressure in the two phases. This flexible situation is exactly what occurs when gases are exchanged in the lungs and tissues. For example, when P_{CO_2} in the pulmonary capillaries is higher than in the lungs, CO_2 diffuses out of the blood and enters the air in the alveoli.

How much of a gas will dissolve in a liquid at any given partial pressure also depends on the *solubility* of the gas in the liquid and the *temperature* of the liquid. The gases in air have very different solubilities in water (and in blood plasma). Carbon dioxide is most soluble. Oxygen is only 1/20 as soluble as CO_2, and N_2 is only half as soluble as O_2. For this reason, at a given partial pressure, much more CO_2 than O_2 dissolves in water, and practically no N_2 goes into solution.

When a liquid's temperature rises, gas solubility decreases. Think of club soda, which is produced by forcing CO_2 gas to dissolve in water under high pressure. If you take the cap off a bottle of club soda and leave it in the fridge, it will slowly go flat. But if you leave it at room temperature, it will very quickly go flat. In both cases, you end up with plain water—all the CO_2 gas has escaped from solution.

Table 22.4 Comparison of Gas Partial Pressures and Approximate Percentages in the Atmosphere and in the Alveoli

	ATMOSPHERE (SEA LEVEL)		ALVEOLI	
GAS	APPROXIMATE PERCENTAGE	PARTIAL PRESSURE (mm Hg)	APPROXIMATE PERCENTAGE	PARTIAL PRESSURE (mm Hg)
N_2	78.6	597	74.9	569
O_2	20.9	159	13.7	104
CO_2	0.04	0.3	5.2	40
H_2O	0.46	3.7	6.2	47
	100.0%	760	100.0%	760

Hyperbaric oxygen chambers provide clinical applications of Henry's law. These chambers contain O_2 gas at pressures higher than 1 atm and are used to force greater-than-normal amounts of O_2 into the blood of patients suffering from carbon monoxide poisoning (see p. 829) or tissue damage following radiation therapy. Hyperbaric therapy is also used to treat individuals with gas gangrene, because the anaerobic bacteria causing this infection cannot live in the presence of high O_2 levels.

Scuba diving provides another illustration of Henry's law. If divers rise rapidly from the depths, dissolved nitrogen forms bubbles in their blood, causing "the bends."

Homeostatic Imbalance 22.11

Although breathing O_2 gas at 2 atm is not a problem for short periods, **oxygen toxicity** develops rapidly when P_{O_2} is greater than 2.5–3 atm. Excessively high O_2 concentrations generate huge amounts of harmful free radicals, resulting in profound CNS disturbances, coma, and death. ✚

Composition of Alveolar Gas

As shown in Table 22.4, the gaseous makeup of the atmosphere is quite different from that in the alveoli. The atmosphere is almost entirely O_2 and N_2; the alveoli contain more CO_2 and water vapor and much less O_2. These differences reflect the effects of:

- Gas exchanges occurring in the lungs (O_2 diffuses from the alveoli into the pulmonary blood and CO_2 diffuses in the opposite direction)
- Humidification of air by conducting passages
- The mixing of alveolar gas that occurs with each breath. Because only 500 ml of air enter with each tidal inspiration, gas in the alveoli is actually a mixture of newly inspired gases and gases remaining in the respiratory passageways between breaths.

The alveolar partial pressures of O_2 and CO_2 are easily changed by increasing breathing depth and rate. A high AVR brings more O_2 into the alveoli, increasing alveolar P_{O_2} and rapidly eliminating CO_2 from the lungs.

External Respiration

During external respiration (pulmonary gas exchange), dark red blood flowing through the pulmonary circuit is transformed into the scarlet river that is returned to the heart for distribution by systemic arteries to all body tissues. This color change is due to O_2 uptake and binding to hemoglobin in red blood cells (RBCs), but CO_2 exchange (unloading) is occurring equally fast.

The following three factors influence external respiration:

- Thickness and surface area of the respiratory membrane
- Partial pressure gradients and gas solubilities
- Ventilation-perfusion coupling that matches alveolar ventilation with pulmonary blood perfusion

Let's look at these factors one by one.

Thickness and Surface Area of the Respiratory Membrane

In healthy lungs, the respiratory membrane is only 0.5 to 1 μm thick, and gas exchange is usually very efficient.

Homeostatic Imbalance 22.12

The effective thickness of the respiratory membrane increases dramatically if the lungs become waterlogged and edematous, as in pneumonia or left heart failure (see p. 685). Under such conditions, even the 0.75 s that red blood cells spend in transit through the pulmonary capillaries may not be enough for adequate gas exchange, and body tissues suffer from oxygen deprivation. ✚

The greater the surface area of the respiratory membrane, the more gas can diffuse across it in a given time period. In healthy lungs, the alveolar surface area is enormous. Spread flat, the total gas exchange surface of these tiny sacs in an adult male's lungs is about 90 m^2—approximately 40 times greater than the surface area of his skin!

Homeostatic Imbalance 22.13

Certain pulmonary diseases drastically reduce the alveolar surface area. For instance, in emphysema the walls of adjacent alveoli break down and the alveolar chambers enlarge. Tumors,

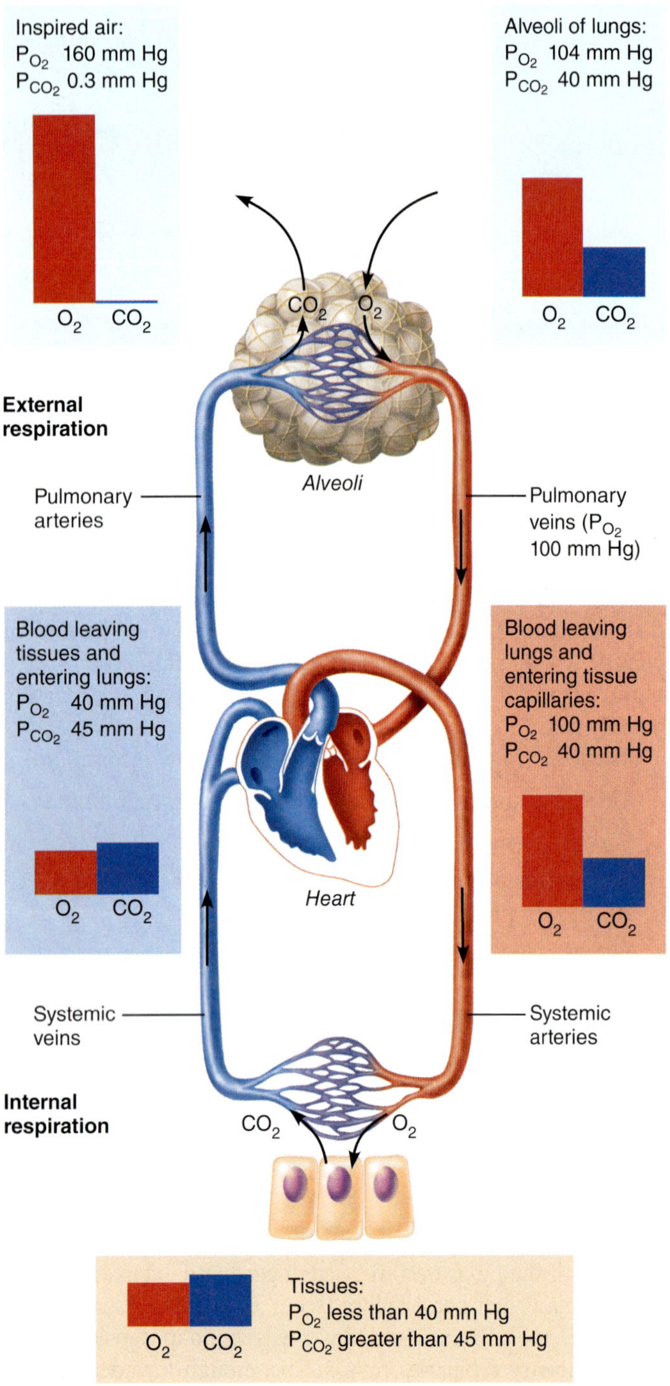

Figure 22.17 Partial pressure gradients promoting gas movements in the body. Top: Gradients promoting O_2 and CO_2 exchange across the respiratory membrane in the lungs. Bottom: Gradients promoting gas movements across systemic capillary membranes in body tissues. (Note that the small decrease in P_{O_2} in blood leaving lungs is due to partial dilution of pulmonary capillary blood with less oxygenated blood.)

mucus, or inflammatory material also reduce surface area by blocking gas flow into the alveoli. ✚

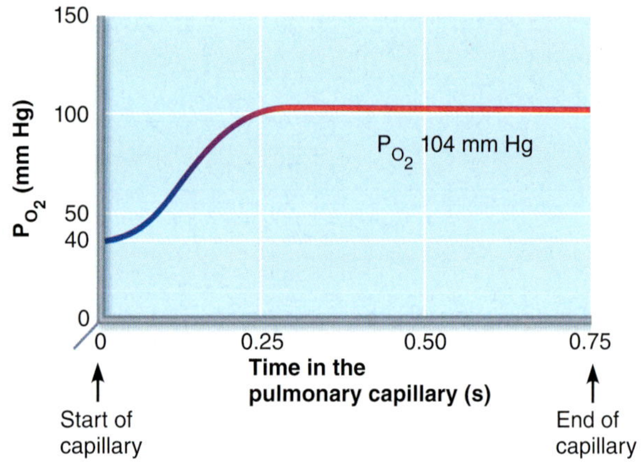

Figure 22.18 Oxygenation of blood in the pulmonary capillaries at rest. Note that the time from blood entering the pulmonary capillaries (indicated by 0) until the P_{O_2} is 104 mm Hg is approximately 0.25 second.

Partial Pressure Gradients and Gas Solubilities

Partial pressure gradients of O_2 and CO_2 drive the diffusion of these gases across the respiratory membrane. A steep oxygen partial pressure gradient exists across the respiratory membrane because the P_{O_2} of deoxygenated blood in the pulmonary arteries is only 40 mm Hg, as opposed to a P_{O_2} of approximately 104 mm Hg in the alveoli. As a result, O_2 diffuses rapidly from the alveoli into the pulmonary capillary blood **(Figure 22.17)**.

Equilibrium—that is, a P_{O_2} of 104 mm Hg on both sides of the respiratory membrane—usually occurs in 0.25 second, which is about one-third of the time a red blood cell spends in a pulmonary capillary **(Figure 22.18)**. The lesson here is that blood can flow through the pulmonary capillaries three times as quickly and still be adequately oxygenated.

Carbon dioxide diffuses in the opposite direction along a much gentler partial pressure gradient of about 5 mm Hg (45 mm Hg to 40 mm Hg) until equilibrium occurs at 40 mm Hg. Expiration then gradually expels carbon dioxide from the alveoli.

Even though the O_2 pressure gradient for oxygen diffusion is much steeper than the CO_2 gradient, equal amounts of these gases are exchanged. Why? The reason is because CO_2 is 20 times more soluble in plasma and alveolar fluid than O_2.

Ventilation-Perfusion Coupling

For optimal gas exchange, there must be a close match, or coupling, between *ventilation* (the amount of gas reaching the alveoli), and *perfusion* (the blood flow in pulmonary capillaries). Both are controlled by local autoregulatory mechanisms that continuously respond to local conditions:

- P_{O_2} controls perfusion by changing *arteriolar* diameter.
- P_{CO_2} controls ventilation by changing *bronchiolar* diameter.

Influence of Local P_{O_2} on Perfusion We begin with perfusion because we introduced its autoregulatory control in Chapter 19. If alveolar ventilation is inadequate, local P_{O_2} is low because

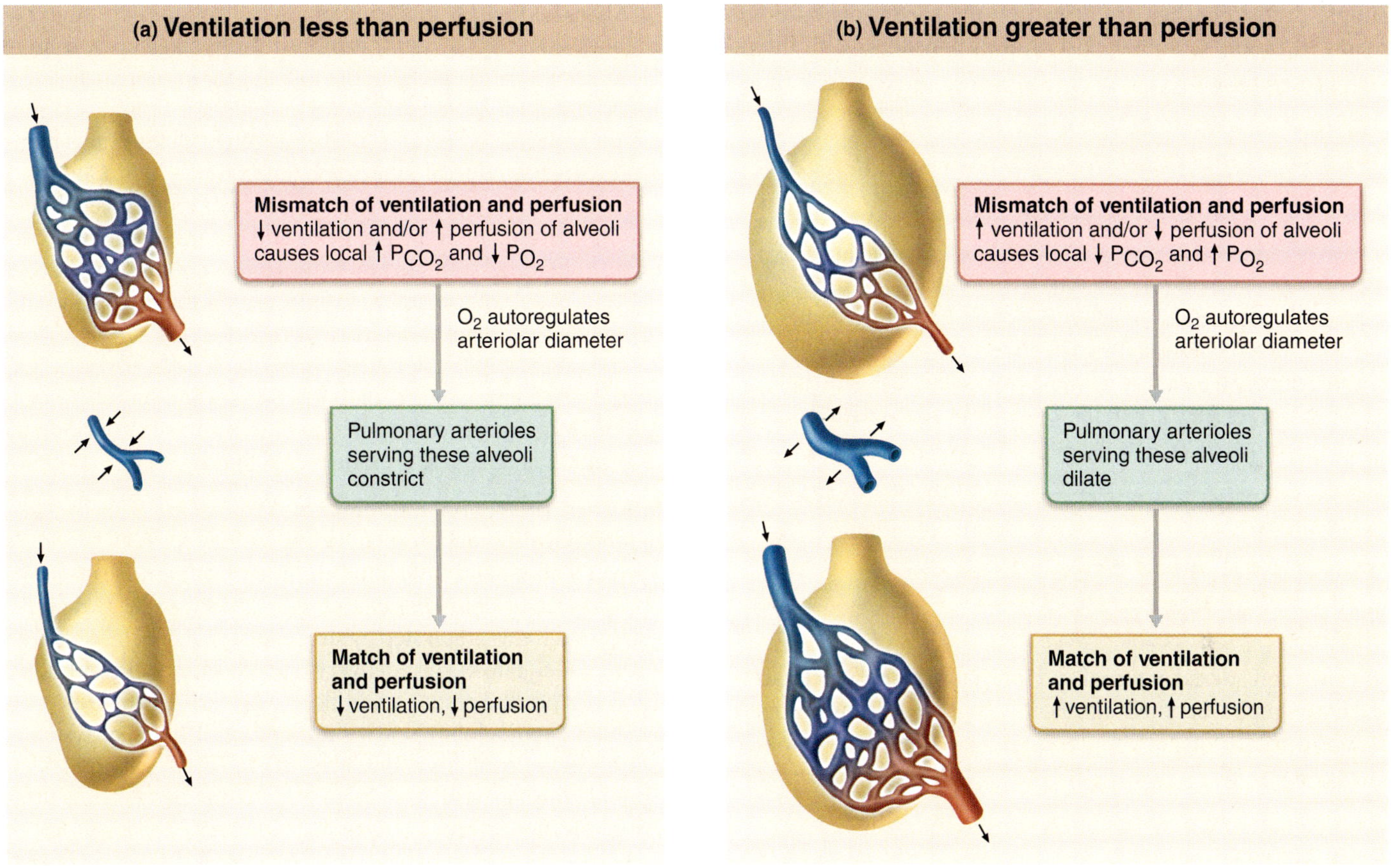

Figure 22.19 Ventilation-perfusion coupling. Autoregulatory events result in local matching of blood flow (perfusion) through the pulmonary capillaries with the amount of alveolar ventilation.

blood takes O_2 away more quickly than ventilation can replenish it **(Figure 22.19a)**. As a result, the terminal arterioles constrict, redirecting blood to respiratory areas where P_{O_2} is high and oxygen pickup is more efficient.

In alveoli where ventilation is maximal, high P_{O_2} dilates pulmonary arterioles and blood flow into the associated pulmonary capillaries increases (Figure 22.19b). Notice that the autoregulatory mechanism controlling pulmonary vascular muscle is the opposite of the mechanism controlling arterioles in the systemic circulation.

Influence of Local P_{CO_2} on Ventilation Bronchioles servicing areas where alveolar CO_2 levels are high dilate, allowing CO_2 to be eliminated from the body more rapidly. Bronchioles serving areas where P_{CO_2} is low constrict.

Balancing Ventilation and Perfusion The changing diameter of local bronchioles and arterioles synchronizes alveolar ventilation and pulmonary perfusion. Poor alveolar ventilation results in low oxygen and high carbon dioxide levels in the alveoli. Consequently, pulmonary arterioles constrict and airways dilate, bringing blood flow and air flow into closer physiological match. High P_{O_2} and low P_{CO_2} in the alveoli cause bronchioles serving the alveoli to constrict, and promote flushing of blood into the pulmonary capillaries.

Although these homeostatic mechanisms provide appropriate conditions for efficient gas exchange, they never completely balance ventilation and perfusion in every alveolus due to other factors. In particular, (1) gravity causes regional variations in both blood and air flow in the lungs, and (2) the occasional alveolar duct plugged with mucus creates unventilated areas. These factors, together with blood shunted from the bronchial veins, account for the slight drop in P_{O_2} from alveolar air (104 mm Hg) to pulmonary venous blood (100 mm Hg), as shown in Figure 22.17.

Internal Respiration

Internal respiration involves capillary gas exchange in body tissues. In internal respiration, the partial pressure and diffusion gradients are reversed from the situation we have just described for external respiration and pulmonary gas exchange. However, the factors promoting gas exchanges between systemic capillaries and tissue cells are essentially identical to those acting in the lungs (see Figure 22.17).

Tissue cells continuously use O_2 for their metabolic activities and produce CO_2. Because P_{O_2} is always lower in tissues than it is in systemic arterial blood (40 mm Hg versus 100 mm Hg), O_2 moves rapidly from blood into tissues until equilibrium is reached. At the same time, CO_2 moves quickly along its pressure gradient into blood. As a result, venous blood draining the tissue capillary beds and returning to the heart has a P_{O_2} of 40 mm Hg and a P_{CO_2} of 45 mm Hg.

In summary, the gas exchanges that occur between blood and alveoli and between blood and tissue cells take place by simple diffusion. They are driven by the partial pressure gradients of O_2 and CO_2 that exist on the opposite sides of the exchange membranes.

Check Your Understanding

13. You are given a sealed container of water and air. The P_{CO_2} and P_{O_2} in the air are both 100 mm Hg. What are the P_{CO_2} and P_{O_2} in the water? Which gas has more molecules dissolved in the water? Why?
14. P_{O_2} in the alveoli is about 56 mm Hg lower than in the inspired air. Explain this difference.
15. Suppose a patient is receiving oxygen by mask. Are the arterioles leading into the O_2-enriched alveoli dilated or constricted? What is the advantage of this response?

For answers, see Appendix H.

Transport of Respiratory Gases by Blood

We have considered external and internal respiration consecutively to emphasize their similarities, but keep in mind that it is blood that transports O_2 and CO_2 between these two exchange sites.

Oxygen Transport

✓ Describe how oxygen is transported in blood, and explain how temperature, pH, BPG, and P_{CO_2} affect oxygen loading and unloading.

Molecular oxygen is carried in blood in two ways: bound to hemoglobin within red blood cells and dissolved in plasma. Oxygen is poorly soluble in water, so only about 1.5% of the oxygen transported is carried in the dissolved form. Indeed, if this were the *only* means of oxygen transport, a P_{O_2} of 3 atm or a cardiac output of 15 times normal would be required to provide the oxygen levels needed by body tissues! Hemoglobin, of course, solves this problem—98.5% of the oxygen is carried from lungs to tissues in a loose chemical combination with hemoglobin.

22

Association of Oxygen and Hemoglobin

As we described in Chapter 17, hemoglobin (Hb) is composed of four polypeptide chains, each bound to an iron-containing heme group (see Figure 17.4). Because the iron atoms bind oxygen, each hemoglobin molecule can combine with four molecules of O_2, and oxygen loading is rapid and reversible.

The hemoglobin-oxygen combination, called **oxyhemoglobin** (ok″sĭ-he″mo-glo′bin), is written **HbO_2**. Hemoglobin that has released oxygen is called **reduced hemoglobin**, or **deoxyhemoglobin**, and is written **HHb**. A single reversible equation describes the loading and unloading of O_2:

$$HHb + O_2 \underset{\text{Tissues}}{\overset{\text{Lungs}}{\rightleftharpoons}} HbO_2 + H^+$$

After the first O_2 molecule binds to iron, the Hb molecule changes shape. As a result, it more readily takes up two more O_2 molecules, and uptake of the fourth is even more facilitated. When one, two, or three oxygen molecules are bound, a hemoglobin molecule is *partially saturated*. When all four of its heme groups are bound to O_2, the hemoglobin is *fully saturated*.

By the same token, unloading of one oxygen molecule enhances the unloading of the next, and so on. In this way, the *affinity* (binding strength) of hemoglobin for oxygen changes with the extent of oxygen saturation, and both loading and unloading of oxygen are very efficient.

The rate at which Hb reversibly binds or releases O_2 is regulated by P_{O_2}, temperature, blood pH, P_{CO_2}, and blood concentration of an organic chemical called BPG. These factors interact to ensure that adequate O_2 is delivered to tissue cells.

Influence of P_{O_2} on Hemoglobin Saturation The **oxygen-hemoglobin dissociation curve** shows how local P_{O_2} controls oxygen loading and unloading from hemoglobin. *Focus on the Oxygen-Hemoglobin Dissociation Curve* **(Figure 22.20)** walks you through this graph step by step, explaining how hemoglobin ensures adequate oxygen delivery under a variety of conditions.

Under normal resting conditions (P_{O_2} = 100 mm Hg), arterial blood hemoglobin is 98% saturated, and 100 ml of systemic arterial blood contains about 20 ml of O_2. This *oxygen content* of arterial blood is written as 20 vol % (volume percent). As arterial blood flows through systemic capillaries, it releases about 5 ml of O_2 per 100 ml of blood, yielding an Hb saturation of 75% and an O_2 content of 15 vol % in venous blood. This means that substantial amounts of O_2 are normally still available in venous blood (the *venous reserve*), which can be used if needed.

The nearly complete saturation of Hb in arterial blood explains why breathing deeply increases both the alveolar and arterial blood P_{O_2} but causes very little increase in the O_2 saturation of hemoglobin. Remember, P_{O_2} measurements indicate only the amount of O_2 dissolved in plasma, not the amount bound to hemoglobin. However, P_{O_2} values are a good index of lung function, and when arterial P_{O_2} is significantly less than alveolar P_{O_2} some degree of respiratory impairment exists.

Influence of Other Factors on Hemoglobin Saturation Temperature, blood pH, P_{CO_2}, and the amount of BPG in the blood all influence hemoglobin saturation at a given P_{O_2}. Red blood cells (RBCs) produce BPG (2,3-bisphosphoglycerate) as they break down glucose by the anaerobic process called glycolysis. BPG binds reversibly with hemoglobin, and its levels rise when oxygen levels are chronically low.

All of these factors influence Hb saturation by modifying hemoglobin's three-dimensional structure, thereby changing its affinity for O_2. Generally speaking, an *increase* in temperature, P_{CO_2}, H^+, or BPG levels in blood lowers Hb's affinity for O_2, enhancing oxygen unloading from the blood. This is shown by the rightward shift of the oxygen-hemoglobin dissociation curve in **Figure 22.21** on p. 832. (The purple lines represent normal body conditions, and the red lines show the shift to the right.)

Conversely, a *decrease* in any of these factors increases hemoglobin's affinity for oxygen, decreasing oxygen unloading. This change shifts the dissociation curve to the left (as the blue lines show in Figure 22.21).

If you give a little thought to how these factors are related, you'll realize that they all tend to be highest in the systemic capillaries, where oxygen unloading is the goal. As cells metabolize glucose and use O_2, they release CO_2, which increases the P_{CO_2} and H^+ levels in capillary blood. Both declining blood pH (acidosis) and increasing P_{CO_2} weaken the Hb-O_2 bond, a phenomenon called the **Bohr effect**. This enhances oxygen unloading where it is most needed.

Additionally, heat is a by-product of metabolic activity, and active tissues are usually warmer than less active ones. A rise in temperature affects hemoglobin's affinity for O_2 both directly and indirectly (via its influence on RBC metabolism and BPG synthesis). Collectively, these factors see to it that Hb unloads much more O_2 in the vicinity of hard-working tissue cells.

Homeostatic Imbalance 22.14

Inadequate oxygen delivery to body tissues is called **hypoxia** (hi-pok′se-ah). Hypoxia is more visible in fair-skinned people because their skin and mucosae take on a bluish cast (become *cyanotic*) when Hb saturation falls below 75%. In dark-skinned individuals, this color change can be observed only in the mucosae and nail beds.

Hypoxia is classified based on cause:

- **Anemic hypoxia** reflects poor O_2 delivery resulting from too few RBCs or from RBCs that contain abnormal or too little Hb.
- **Ischemic (stagnant) hypoxia** results from impaired or blocked blood circulation. Congestive heart failure may cause bodywide ischemic hypoxia, whereas emboli or thrombi block oxygen delivery only to tissues distal to the obstruction.
- **Histotoxic hypoxia** occurs when body cells are unable to use O_2 even though adequate amounts are delivered. Metabolic poisons, such as cyanide, can cause histotoxic hypoxia.
- **Hypoxemic hypoxia** is indicated by reduced arterial P_{O_2}. Possible causes include disordered or abnormal ventilation-perfusion coupling, pulmonary diseases that impair ventilation, and breathing air containing scant amounts of O_2.
- **Carbon monoxide poisoning** is a unique type of hypoxemic hypoxia, and a leading cause of death from fire. Carbon monoxide (CO) is an odorless, colorless gas that competes vigorously with O_2 for heme binding sites. Moreover, because Hb's affinity for CO is more than 200 times greater than its affinity for oxygen, CO is a highly successful competitor. Even at minuscule partial pressures, carbon monoxide can displace oxygen.

  CO poisoning is particularly dangerous because it does not produce the characteristic signs of hypoxia—cyanosis and respiratory distress. Instead the victim is confused and has a throbbing headache. In rare cases, fair skin becomes cherry red (the color of the Hb-CO complex), which the eye of the beholder interprets as a healthy "blush." Patients with CO poisoning are given hyperbaric therapy (if available) or 100% O_2 until the CO has been cleared from the body. ✚

Carbon Dioxide Transport

✓ Describe carbon dioxide transport in the blood.

Normally active body cells produce about 200 ml of CO_2 each minute—exactly the amount excreted by the lungs. Blood transports CO_2 from the tissue cells to the lungs in three forms (**Figure 22.22** on p. 833):

1. **Dissolved in plasma** (7–10%). The smallest amount of CO_2 is transported simply dissolved in plasma.
2. **Chemically bound to hemoglobin** (just over 20%). Dissolved CO_2 is bound and carried in the RBCs as **carbaminohemoglobin** (kar-bam″ĭ-no-he″mo-glo′bin):

$$CO_2 + Hb \rightleftharpoons \underset{\text{carbaminohemoglobin}}{HbCO_2}$$

   This reaction is rapid and does not require a catalyst. Carbon dioxide transport in RBCs does not compete with oxyhemoglobin transport because carbon dioxide binds directly to the amino acids of globin (not to the heme).

   CO_2 loading and unloading are directly influenced by the P_{CO_2} and the degree of Hb oxygenation. Carbon dioxide rapidly dissociates from hemoglobin in the lungs, where the P_{CO_2} of alveolar air is lower than that in blood. Carbon dioxide readily binds with hemoglobin in the tissues, where the P_{CO_2} is higher than that in blood. Deoxygenated hemoglobin combines more readily with carbon dioxide than does oxygenated hemoglobin, as we will see in the discussion of the Haldane effect below.
3. **As bicarbonate ions in plasma** (about 70%). Most carbon dioxide molecules entering the plasma quickly enter RBCs, where the reactions that prepare carbon dioxide for transport as **bicarbonate ions (HCO_3^-)** in plasma mostly occur. As illustrated in Figure 22.22a, when dissolved CO_2 diffuses into RBCs, it combines with water, forming carbonic acid (H_2CO_3). H_2CO_3 is unstable and dissociates into hydrogen ions and bicarbonate ions:

$$\underset{\text{carbon dioxide}}{CO_2} + \underset{\text{water}}{H_2O} \rightleftharpoons \underset{\text{carbonic acid}}{H_2CO_3} \rightleftharpoons \underset{\text{hydrogen ion}}{H^+} + \underset{\text{bicarbonate ion}}{HCO_3^-}$$

   Although this reaction also occurs in plasma, it is thousands of times faster in RBCs because they (and not plasma) contain **carbonic anhydrase** (kar-bon′ik an-hi′drās), an enzyme that reversibly catalyzes the conversion of carbon dioxide and water to carbonic acid. Hydrogen ions released during the reaction (as well as CO_2 itself) bind to Hb, triggering the Bohr effect. In this way CO_2 loading enhances O_2 release. Because of the buffering effect of Hb, the liberated H^+ causes little change in pH under resting conditions. As a result, blood becomes only slightly more acidic (the pH declines from 7.4 to 7.34) as it passes through the tissues.

(Text continues on p. 832.)

Figure 22.20 The amount of oxygen carried by hemoglobin depends on the P_{O_2} (the amount of oxygen) available locally. This relationship ensures optimal oxygen pickup and delivery.

The oxygen-hemoglobin dissociation curve will help you understand how the properties of hemoglobin (Hb) affect oxygen binding in the lungs and oxygen release in the tissues.

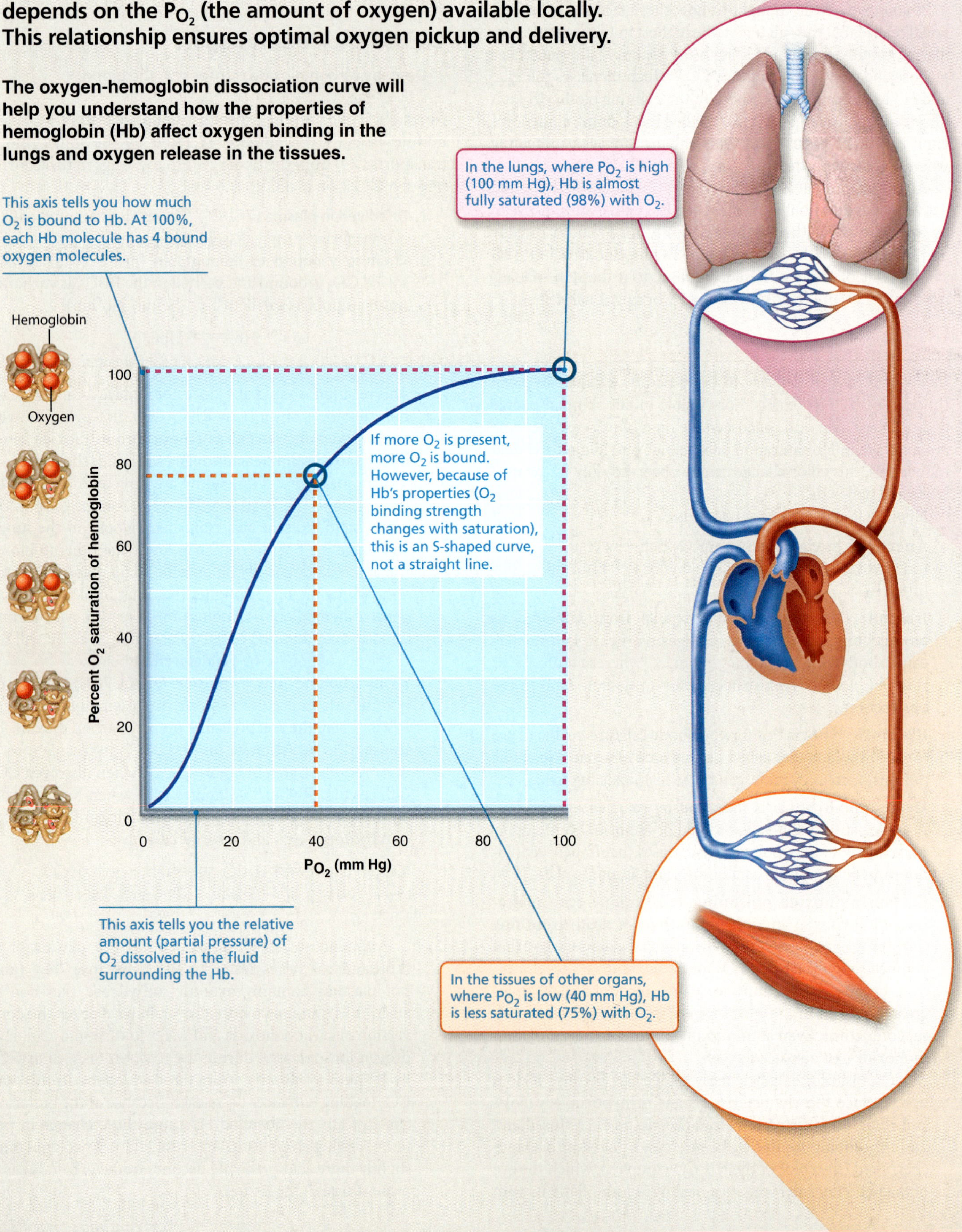

In the lungs

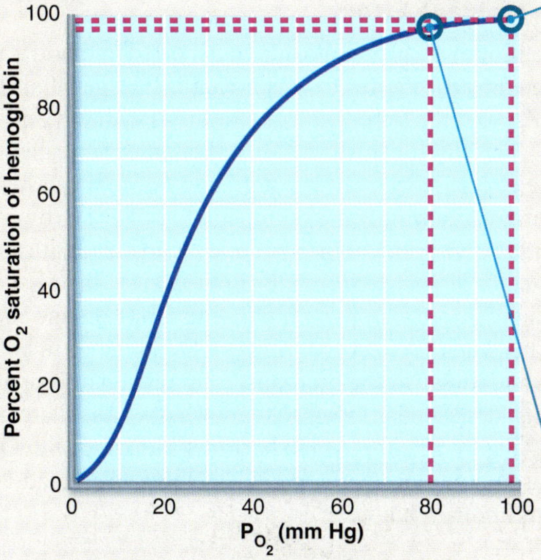

At sea level, there is lots of O_2. At a P_{O_2} in the lungs of 100 mm Hg, Hb is 98% saturated.

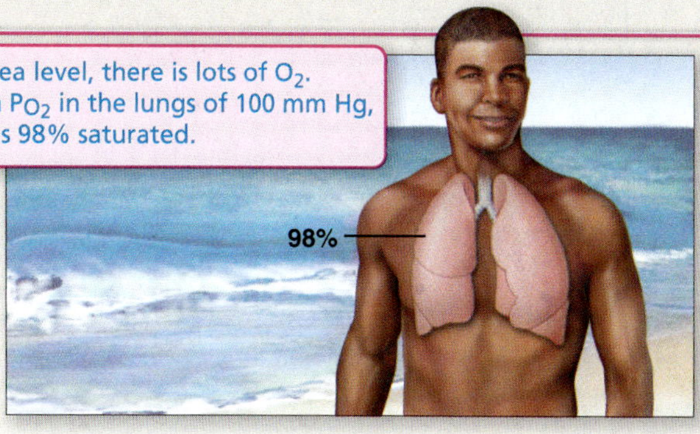

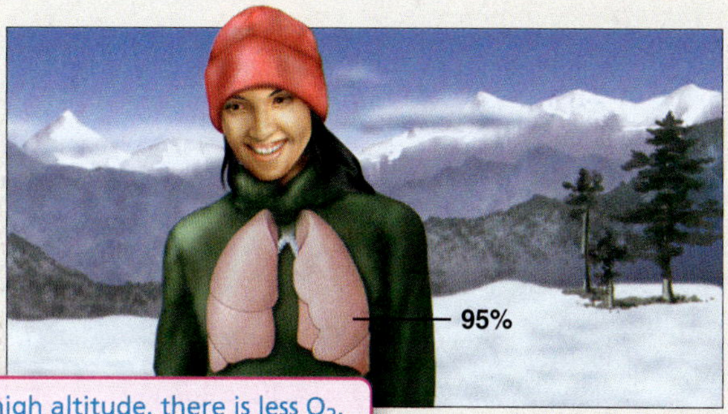

At high P_{O_2}, large changes in P_{O_2} cause only small changes in Hb saturation. Notice that the curve is relatively flat here. Hb's properties produce a *safety margin* that ensures that Hb is almost fully saturated even with a substantial P_{O_2} decrease. As a result, Hb remains saturated even at high altitude or with lung disease.

At high altitude, there is less O_2. At a P_{O_2} in the lungs of only 80 mm Hg, Hb is still 95% saturated.

In the tissues

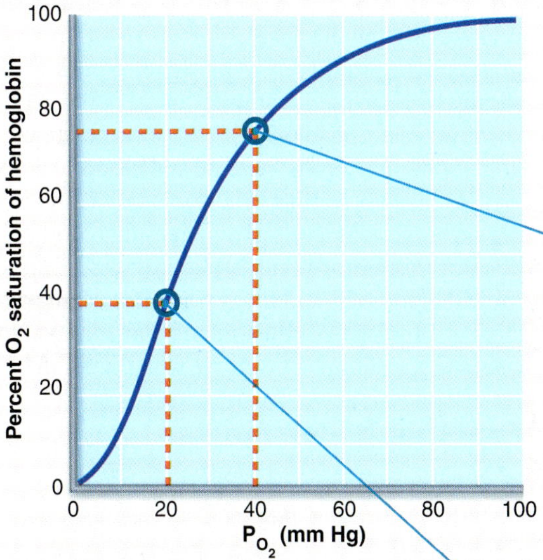

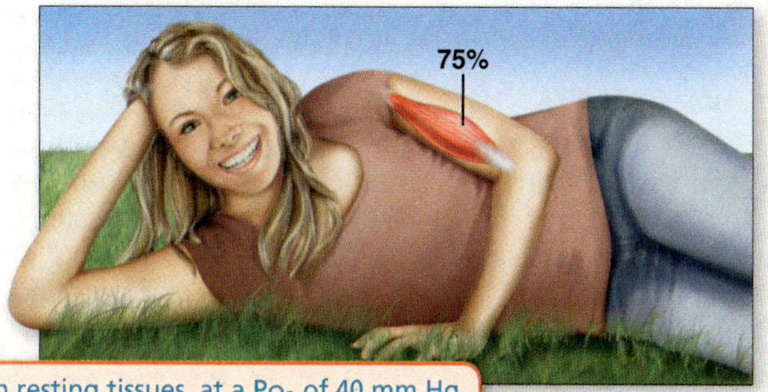

In resting tissues, at a P_{O_2} of 40 mm Hg, Hb is 75% saturated—only 23% of O_2 carried by Hb is released.

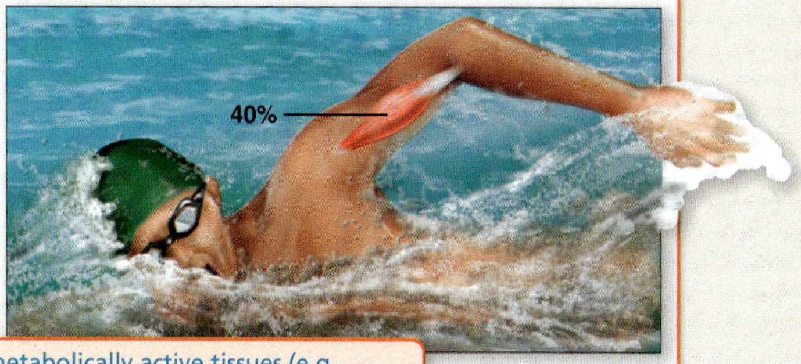

At low P_{O_2}, large changes in P_{O_2} cause large changes in Hb saturation. Tissues other than lungs have a low P_{O_2} because they consume O_2. Notice that the curve is relatively steep at low P_{O_2}. Hb's properties ensure that oxygen is delivered where it is most needed—when tissues need more, they get more.

In metabolically active tissues (e.g., exercising muscle), the P_{O_2} is even lower. At a P_{O_2} of 20 mm Hg, Hb is only 40% saturated—an additional 35% of O_2 has been unloaded for tissue use.

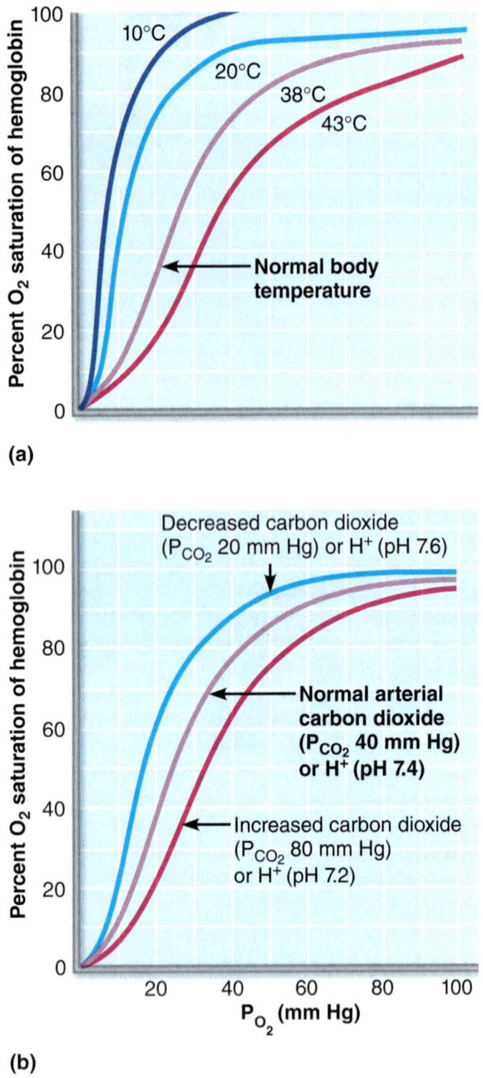

Figure 22.21 Effect of temperature, P_{CO_2}, and blood pH on the oxygen-hemoglobin dissociation curve. Oxygen unloading is enhanced at conditions of **(a)** increased temperature, **(b)** increased P_{CO_2}, and/or hydrogen ion concentration (decreased pH), causing the dissociation curve to shift to the right. This response is called the Bohr effect.

Once generated, HCO_3^- moves quickly from the RBCs into the plasma, where it is carried to the lungs. To counterbalance the rapid outrush of these anions from the RBCs, chloride ions (Cl^-) move from the plasma into the RBCs. This ion exchange process, called the **chloride shift**, occurs via facilitated diffusion through a RBC membrane protein.

In the lungs, the process is reversed (Figure 22.22b). As blood moves through the pulmonary capillaries, its P_{CO_2} declines from 45 mm Hg to 40 mm Hg. For this to occur, CO_2 must first be freed from its "bicarbonate housing." HCO_3^- reenters the RBCs (and Cl^- moves into the plasma) and binds with H^+ to form carbonic acid. Carbonic anhydrase then splits carbonic acid to release CO_2 and water. This CO_2, along with that released from hemoglobin and from solution in plasma, then diffuses along its partial pressure gradient from the blood into the alveoli.

The Haldane Effect

The amount of carbon dioxide transported in blood is markedly affected by the degree to which blood is oxygenated. The lower the P_{O_2} and the lower the Hb saturation with oxygen, the more CO_2 that blood can carry. This phenomenon, called the **Haldane effect**, reflects the greater ability of reduced hemoglobin to form carbaminohemoglobin and to buffer H^+ by combining with it. As CO_2 enters the systemic bloodstream, it causes more oxygen to dissociate from Hb (Bohr effect). The dissociation of O_2 allows more CO_2 to combine with Hb (Haldane effect).

The Haldane effect encourages CO_2 exchange in both the tissues and lungs. In the pulmonary circulation, the situation that we just described is reversed—uptake of O_2 facilitates release of CO_2 (Figure 22.22b). As Hb becomes saturated with O_2, the H^+ released combines with HCO_3^-, helping to unload CO_2 from the pulmonary blood.

Influence of CO_2 on Blood pH

Typically, the H^+ released during carbonic acid dissociation is buffered by Hb or other proteins within the RBCs or in plasma. The HCO_3^- generated in the red blood cells diffuses into the plasma, where it acts as the *alkaline reserve* part of the blood's carbonic acid–bicarbonate buffer system.

The **carbonic acid–bicarbonate buffer system** is very important in resisting shifts in blood pH, as shown in the equation in point 3 concerning CO_2 transport (p. 829). For example, if the hydrogen ion concentration in blood begins to rise, excess H^+ is removed by combining with HCO_3^- to form carbonic acid (a weak acid). If H^+ concentration in blood drops below desirable levels, carbonic acid dissociates, releasing hydrogen ions and lowering the pH again.

Changes in respiratory rate or depth can alter blood pH dramatically by altering the amount of carbonic acid in blood. Slow, shallow breathing allows CO_2 to accumulate in blood. As a result, carbonic acid levels increase and blood pH drops. Conversely, rapid, deep breathing quickly flushes CO_2 out of blood, reducing carbonic acid levels and increasing blood pH.

In this way, respiratory ventilation provides a fast-acting system to adjust blood pH (and P_{CO_2}) when it is disturbed by metabolic factors. Respiratory adjustments play a major role in the acid-base balance of the blood, as we will discuss in Chapter 26.

☑ Check Your Understanding

16. Rapidly metabolizing tissues generate large amounts of CO_2 and H^+. How does this affect O_2 unloading? What is this effect called?
17. List the three ways CO_2 is transported in blood and state approximate percentages of each.
18. What is the relationship between CO_2 and pH in the blood? Explain.

For answers, see Appendix H.

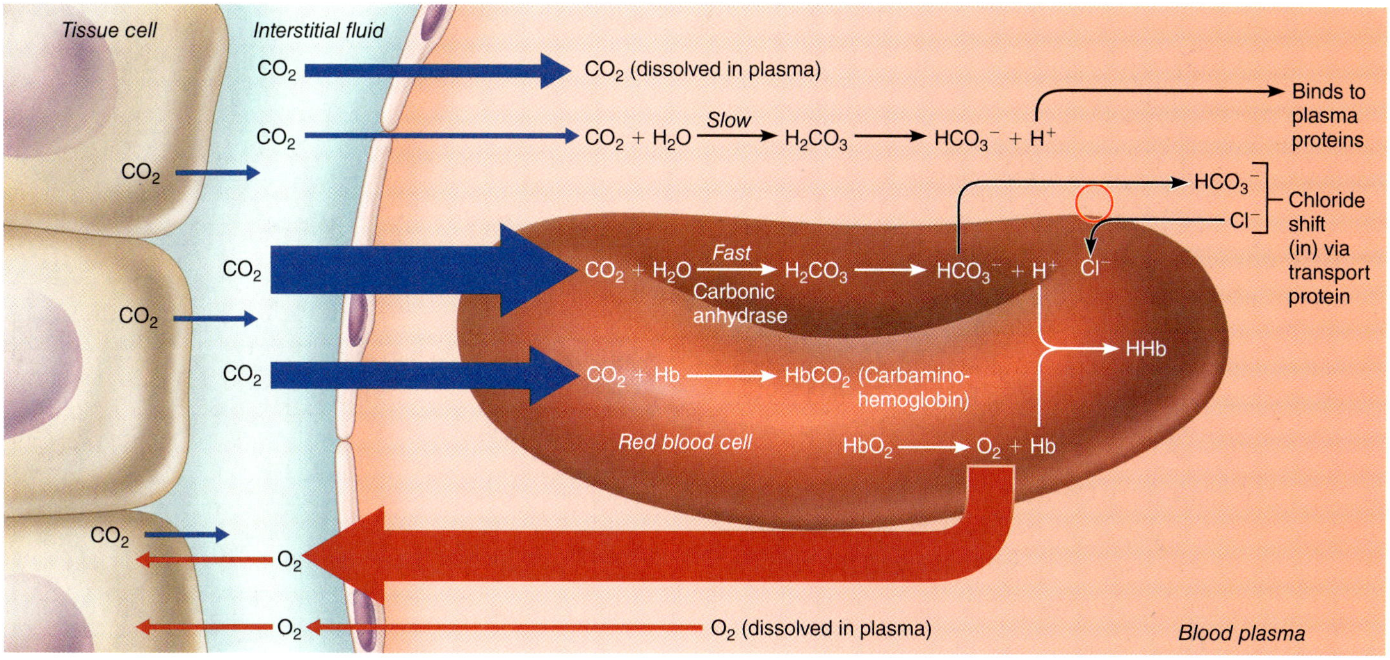

(a) Oxygen release and carbon dioxide pickup at the tissues

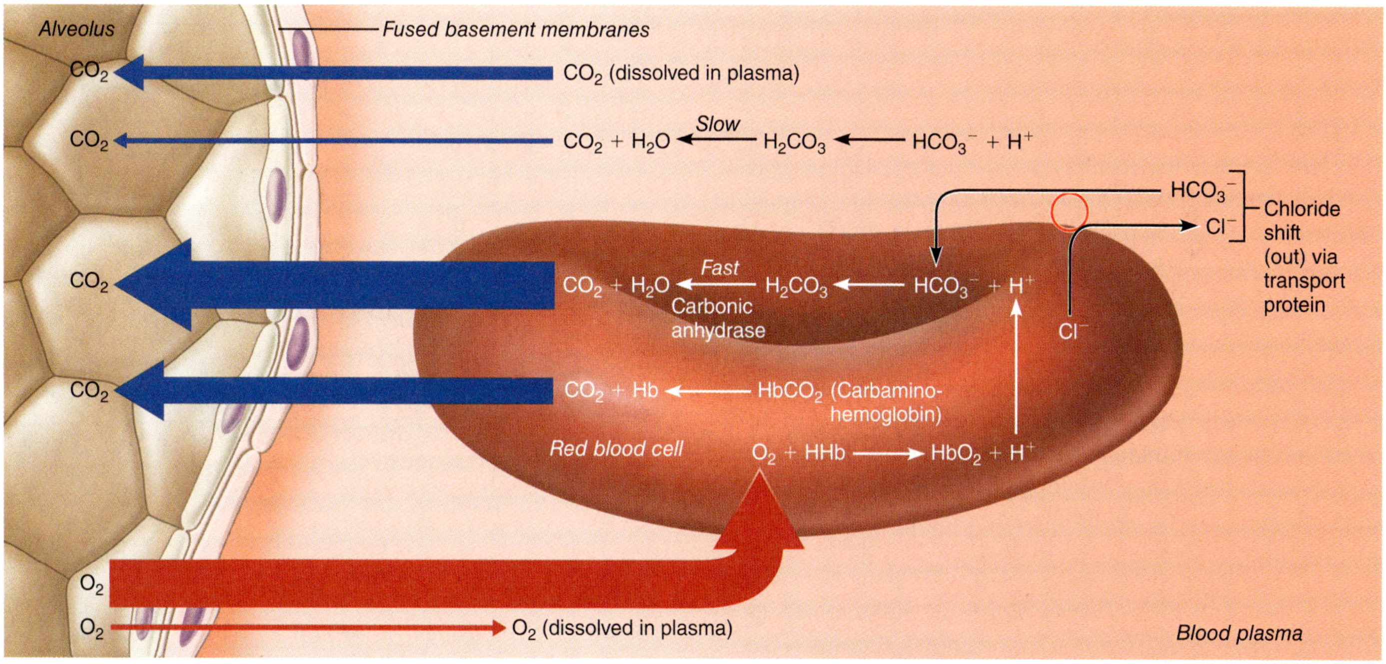

(b) Oxygen pickup and carbon dioxide release in the lungs

Figure 22.22 Transport and exchange of CO_2 and O_2. Relative sizes of the transport arrows indicate the proportionate amounts of O_2 and CO_2 moved by each method. (H_2CO_3 = carbonic acid, HCO_3^- = bicarbonate, HHb = reduced hemoglobin, HbO_2 = oxyhemoglobin.)

22

Control of Respiration

Although our tidelike breathing seems so beautifully simple, its control is more complex than you might think. Higher brain centers, chemoreceptors, and other reflexes all modify the basic respiratory rhythms generated in the brain stem.

Neural Mechanisms

✓ Describe the neural controls of respiration.

Control of respiration primarily involves neurons in the reticular formation of the medulla and pons. Because the medulla sets the respiratory rhythm, we will begin there.

Medullary Respiratory Centers

Clustered neurons in two areas of the medulla oblongata appear to be critically important in respiration **(Figure 22.23)**. These are:

- The **ventral respiratory group (VRG)**, a network of neurons that extends in the ventral brain stem from the spinal cord to the pons-medulla junction
- The **dorsal respiratory group (DRG)**, located dorsally near the root of cranial nerve IX

Ventral Respiratory Group (VRG) The VRG appears to be a rhythm-generating and integrative center. It contains groups of neurons that fire during inspiration and others that fire during expiration in a dance of mutual inhibition.

When its inspiratory neurons fire, a burst of impulses travels along the **phrenic** and **intercostal nerves** to excite the diaphragm and external intercostal muscles, respectively (Figure 22.23). As a result, the thorax expands and air rushes into the lungs. When the VRG's expiratory neurons fire, the output stops, and expiration occurs passively as the inspiratory muscles relax and the lungs recoil.

22

This cyclic on/off activity of the inspiratory and expiratory neurons repeats continuously and produces a respiratory rate of 12–15 breaths per minute, with inspiratory phases lasting about 2 seconds followed by expiratory phases lasting about 3 seconds. This normal respiratory rate and rhythm is called **eupnea** (ūp-ne′ah; *eu* = good, *pne* = breath).

During severe hypoxia, VRG networks generate gasping (perhaps in a last-ditch effort to restore O_2 to the brain). Respiration stops when a certain cluster of VRG neurons is completely suppressed, as by an overdose of morphine or alcohol.

Dorsal Respiratory Group (DRG) Until recently, it was thought that the DRG acts as an inspiratory center, performing many of the tasks now known to be performed by the VRG. In almost all mammals, including humans, the DRG integrates input from peripheral stretch and chemoreceptors (which we will describe shortly) and communicates this information to the VRG. It may seem surprising, but many of the details of this system so essential to life are still being worked out.

Pontine Respiratory Centers

Although the VRG generates the basic respiratory rhythm, the *pontine respiratory centers* influence and modify the activity of medullary neurons. For example, pontine centers appear to smooth out the transitions from inspiration to expiration, and vice versa. When lesions are made in its superior region, inspirations become very prolonged, a phenomenon called *apneustic breathing*.

The **pontine respiratory group** and other pontine centers transmit impulses to the VRG of the medulla (Figure 22.23). This input modifies and fine-tunes the breathing rhythms generated by the VRG during certain activities such as vocalization, sleep, and exercise. As you would expect from these functions,

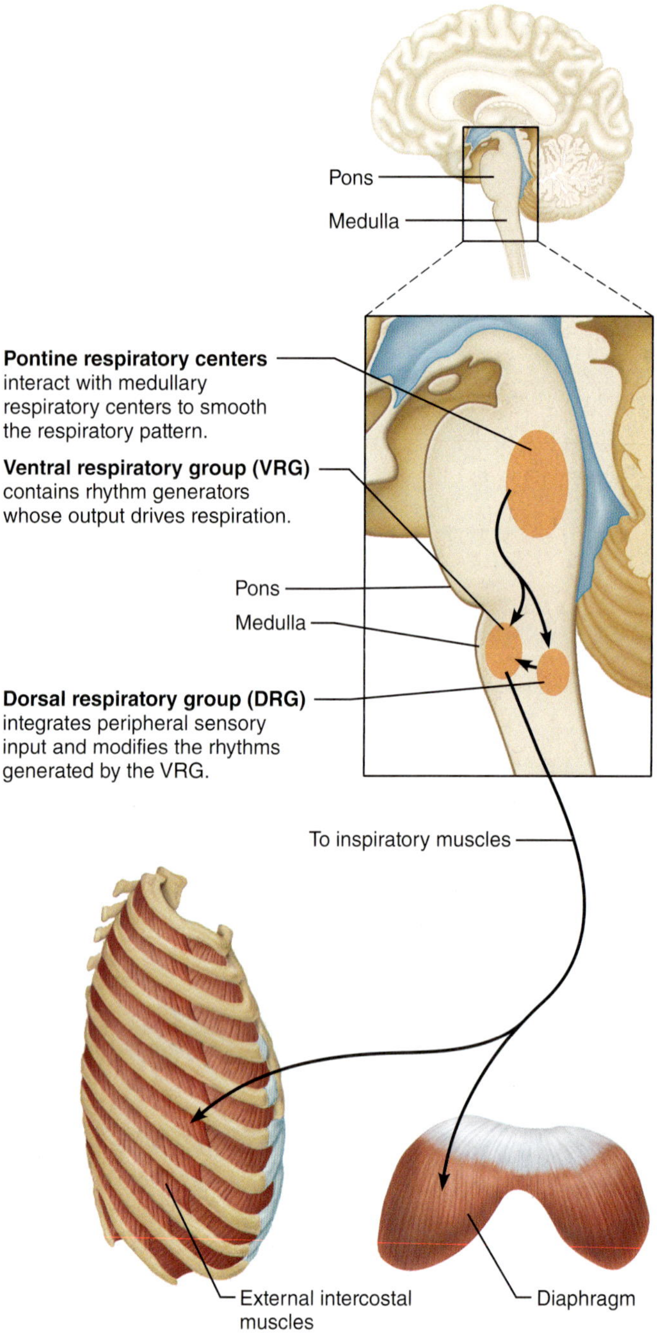

Figure 22.23 Locations of respiratory centers and their postulated connections. The efferent pathway shown here is incomplete. Medullary neurons communicate with lower motor neurons in the spinal cord, but these are omitted for simplicity.

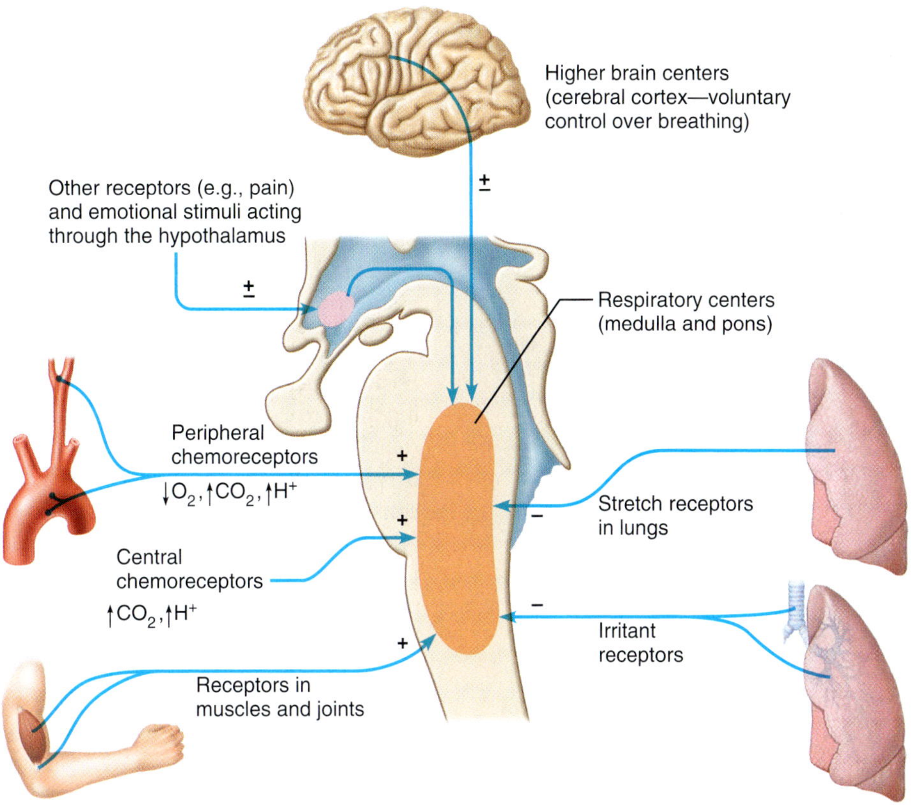

Figure 22.24 Neural and chemical influences on brain stem respiratory centers. Excitatory influences (+) increase the frequency of impulses sent to the muscles of respiration and recruit additional motor units, resulting in deeper, faster breathing. Inhibitory influences (−) have the reverse effect. In some cases, the impulses may be excitatory or inhibitory (±), depending on which receptors or brain regions are activated. The cerebral cortex also directly innervates respiratory muscle motor neurons (not shown).

the pontine respiratory centers, like the DRG, receive input from higher brain centers and from various sensory receptors in the periphery.

Generation of the Respiratory Rhythm

There is little question that breathing is rhythmic, but we still cannot fully explain the origin of its rhythm. One hypothesis is that there are *pacemaker neurons,* which have intrinsic (automatic) rhythmicity like the pacemaker cells found in the heart. Pacemaker-like activity has been demonstrated in certain VRG neurons, but suppressing their activity does not abolish breathing.

This leads us to the second (and more widely accepted) hypothesis: Normal respiratory rhythm results from reciprocal inhibition of interconnected neuronal networks in the medulla. Rather than a single set of pacemaker neurons, there are two sets that inhibit each other and cycle their activity to generate the rhythm.

Factors Influencing Breathing Rate and Depth

✓ Compare and contrast the influences of arterial pH, arterial partial pressures of oxygen and carbon dioxide, lung reflexes, volition, and emotions on respiratory rate and depth.

Inspiratory depth is determined by how actively the respiratory center stimulates the motor neurons serving the respiratory muscles. The greater the stimulation, the greater the number of motor units excited and the greater the force of respiratory muscle contractions. Respiratory rate is determined by how long the inspiratory center is active or how quickly it is switched off.

Changing body demands can modify depth and rate of breathing. The respiratory centers in the medulla and pons are sensitive to both excitatory and inhibitory stimuli. We describe these stimuli next and they are summarized in **Figure 22.24**.

22

Chemical Factors

Among the factors that influence breathing rate and depth, the most important are changing levels of CO_2, O_2, and H^+ in arterial blood. Sensors responding to such chemical fluctuations, called **chemoreceptors**, are found in two major body locations:

- **Central chemoreceptors** are located throughout the brain stem, including the ventrolateral medulla.
- **Peripheral chemoreceptors** are found in the aortic arch and carotid arteries.

Influence of P_{CO_2} Of all the chemicals influencing respiration, CO_2 is the most potent and the most closely controlled. Normally, arterial P_{CO_2} is 40 mm Hg and is maintained within ±3 mm Hg of

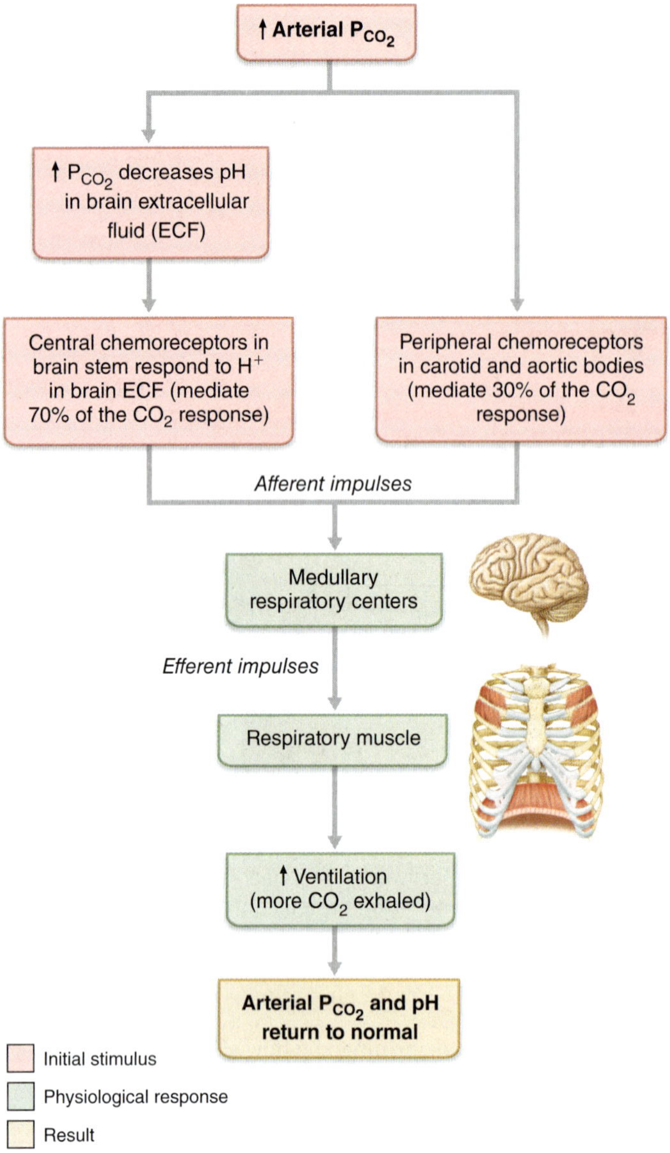

Figure 22.25 Changes in P_{CO_2} and blood pH regulate ventilation by a negative feedback mechanism.

this level by an exquisitely sensitive homeostatic mechanism that is mediated mainly by the effect of rising CO_2 levels on the central chemoreceptors of the brain stem (Figure 22.25).

As P_{CO_2} levels rise in the blood, a condition referred to as **hypercapnia** (hi″per-kap′ne-ah), CO_2 accumulates in the brain. As CO_2 accumulates, it is hydrated to form carbonic acid. The acid dissociates, H^+ is liberated, and the pH drops. This is the same reaction that occurs when CO_2 enters RBCs (see p. 829).

The increase in H^+ excites the central chemoreceptors, which make abundant synapses with the respiratory regulatory centers. As a result, the depth and rate of breathing increase. This enhanced alveolar ventilation quickly flushes CO_2 out of the blood, raising blood pH.

An elevation of only 5 mm Hg in arterial P_{CO_2} doubles alveolar ventilation, even when arterial O_2 levels and pH haven't changed. When P_{O_2} and pH are below normal, the response to elevated P_{CO_2} is even greater. Increased ventilation is normally self-limiting, ending when homeostatic blood P_{CO_2} levels are restored.

Notice that while rising blood CO_2 levels act as the initial stimulus, it is rising levels of H^+ generated within the brain that prod the central chemoreceptors into increased activity. (CO_2 readily diffuses across the blood brain barrier between the brain and the blood, but H^+ does not.) In the final analysis, control of breathing during rest is aimed primarily at *regulating the H^+ concentration in the brain.*

Homeostatic Imbalance 22.15

Hyperventilation is an increase in the rate and depth of breathing that exceeds the body's need to remove CO_2. A person experiencing an anxiety attack may hyperventilate involuntarily. As they blow off CO_2, the low CO_2 levels in the blood (**hypocapnia**) constrict cerebral blood vessels. This reduces brain perfusion, producing cerebral ischemia that causes dizziness or fainting. Earlier symptoms of hyperventilation are tingling and involuntary muscle spasms (tetany) in the hands and face caused by blood Ca^{2+} levels falling as pH rises.

The symptoms of hyperventilation may be averted by breathing into a paper bag. The air being inspired from the bag is expired air, rich in carbon dioxide, which causes carbon dioxide to be retained in the blood. ✚

When P_{CO_2} is abnormally low, respiration is inhibited and becomes slow and shallow. In fact, periods of **apnea** (breathing cessation) may occur until arterial P_{CO_2} rises and again stimulates respiration.

Sometimes swimmers voluntarily hyperventilate so they can hold their breath longer during swim meets. This is dangerous. Blood O_2 content rarely drops much below 60% of normal during regular breath-holding, because as P_{O_2} drops, P_{CO_2} rises enough to make breathing unavoidable. However, strenuous hyperventilation can lower P_{CO_2} so much that a lag period occurs before P_{CO_2} rebounds enough to stimulate respiration again. This lag may allow oxygen levels to fall well below 50 mm Hg, causing the swimmer to black out (and perhaps drown) before he or she has the urge to breathe.

Influence of P_{O_2} The peripheral chemoreceptors—found in the **aortic bodies** of the aortic arch and in the **carotid bodies** at the bifurcation of the common carotid arteries—contain cells sensitive to arterial O_2 levels (Figure 22.26). The main oxygen sensors are in the carotid bodies.

Under normal conditions, declining P_{O_2} has only a slight effect on ventilation, mostly limited to enhancing the sensitivity of peripheral receptors to increased P_{CO_2}. Arterial P_{O_2} must drop *substantially*, to at least 60 mm Hg, before O_2 levels become a major stimulus for increased ventilation.

This is not as strange as it may appear. Remember, there is a huge reservoir of O_2 bound to Hb, and Hb remains almost entirely saturated unless or until the P_{O_2} of alveolar gas and arterial blood falls below 60 mm Hg. The brain stem centers then begin to suffer from O_2 starvation, and their activity is depressed. At the same time, the peripheral chemoreceptors become excited and stimulate the respiratory centers to increase ventilation, even if P_{CO_2} is normal. In this way, the peripheral chemoreceptor system can maintain ventilation even though the brain stem centers are depressed by hypoxia.

Influence of Arterial pH Changes in arterial pH can modify respiratory rate and rhythm even when CO_2 and O_2 levels are normal. Because H^+ does not cross the blood brain barrier, the increased ventilation that occurs in response to falling arterial pH is mediated through the peripheral chemoreceptors.

Although changes in P_{CO_2} and H^+ concentration are interrelated, they are distinct stimuli. A drop in blood pH may reflect CO_2 retention, but it may also result from metabolic causes, such as accumulation of lactic acid during exercise or of fatty acid metabolites (ketone bodies) in patients with poorly controlled diabetes mellitus. Regardless of cause, as arterial pH declines, respiratory system controls attempt to compensate and raise the pH. They do this by increasing respiratory rate and depth to eliminate CO_2 (and carbonic acid) from the blood.

Summary of Interactions of P_{CO_2}, P_{O_2}, and Arterial pH Although every cell in the body must have O_2 to live, the body's need to rid itself of CO_2 is the most important stimulus for breathing in a healthy person. However, CO_2 does not act in isolation, and various chemical factors enforce or inhibit one another's effects. These interactions are summarized here:

- *Rising CO_2 levels are the most powerful respiratory stimulant.* As CO_2 is hydrated in brain tissue, liberated H^+ acts directly on the central chemoreceptors, causing a reflexive increase in breathing rate and depth. Low P_{CO_2} levels depress respiration.
- *Under normal conditions, blood P_{O_2} affects breathing only indirectly by influencing peripheral chemoreceptor sensitivity to changes in P_{CO_2}.* Low P_{O_2} augments P_{CO_2} effects, and high P_{O_2} levels diminish the effectiveness of CO_2 stimulation.
- *When arterial P_{O_2} falls below 60 mm Hg, it becomes the major stimulus for respiration, and ventilation is increased via reflexes initiated by the peripheral chemoreceptors.* This may increase O_2 loading into the blood, but it also causes hypocapnia (low P_{CO_2} blood levels) and an increase in blood pH, both of which inhibit respiration.
- *Changes in arterial pH resulting from CO_2 retention or metabolic factors act indirectly through the peripheral chemoreceptors to alter ventilation, which in turn modifies arterial P_{CO_2} and pH.* Arterial pH does not influence the central chemoreceptors directly.

Influence of Higher Brain Centers

Hypothalamic Controls Acting through the hypothalamus and the rest of the limbic system, strong emotions and pain send signals to the respiratory centers, modifying respiratory rate and depth. For example, have you ever touched something cold and clammy and gasped? That response was mediated through the hypothalamus. So too is the breath holding that occurs when we are angry and the increased respiratory rate that occurs when we are excited. A rise in body temperature raises the respiratory rate, while a drop in body temperature produces the opposite effect. Sudden chilling (a dip in the North Atlantic Ocean in late October) can stop your breathing (apnea)—or at the very least, leave you gasping.

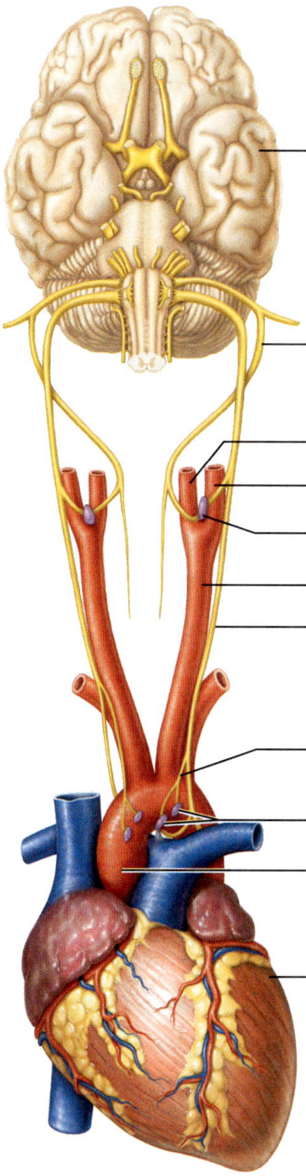

Figure 22.26 Location and innervation of the peripheral chemoreceptors in the carotid and aortic bodies.

Cortical Controls Although the brain stem respiratory centers normally regulate breathing involuntarily, we can also exert conscious (voluntary) control over the rate and depth of our breathing. We can choose to hold our breath or take an extra-deep breath, for example. During voluntary control, the cerebral motor cortex sends signals to the motor neurons that stimulate the respiratory muscles, bypassing the medullary centers.

Our ability to voluntarily hold our breath is limited, however, because the brain stem respiratory centers automatically reinitiate breathing when the blood concentration of CO_2 reaches critical levels. That explains why drowning victims typically have water in their lungs.

Pulmonary Irritant Reflexes

The lungs contain receptors that respond to an enormous variety of irritants. When activated, these receptors communicate with the respiratory centers via vagal nerve afferents. Accumulated mucus, inhaled debris such as dust, or noxious fumes stimulate receptors in the bronchioles that promote reflex constriction of those air passages. The same irritants stimulate a cough in the trachea or bronchi, and stimulate a sneeze in the nasal cavity.

The Inflation Reflex

The visceral pleurae and conducting passages in the lungs contain numerous stretch receptors that are vigorously stimulated when the lungs are inflated. These receptors signal the medullary respiratory centers via afferent fibers of the vagus nerves, sending inhibitory impulses that end inspiration and allow expiration to occur.

As the lungs recoil, the stretch receptors become quiet, and inspiration is initiated once again. This reflex, called the **inflation reflex**, or **Hering-Breuer reflex** (her′ing broy′er), is thought to be more a protective response (to prevent the lungs from being stretched excessively) than a normal regulatory mechanism.

☑ Check Your Understanding

19. Which brain stem respiratory area is thought to generate the respiratory rhythm?
20. Which chemical factor in blood normally provides the most powerful stimulus to breathe? Which chemoreceptors are most important for this response?

For answers, see Appendix H.

Respiratory Adjustments

22

✓ Compare and contrast the hyperpnea of exercise with hyperventilation.

✓ Describe the process and effects of acclimatization to high altitude.

Exercise

Respiratory adjustments during exercise are geared both to intensity and duration of the exercise. Working muscles consume tremendous amounts of O_2 and produce large amounts of CO_2, so ventilation can increase 10- to 20-fold during vigorous exercise. Increased ventilation in response to metabolic needs is called **hyperpnea** (hi″perp-ne′ah).

How does hyperpnea differ from hyperventilation? The respiratory changes in hyperpnea do not alter blood O_2 and CO_2 levels significantly. By contrast, hyperventilation is excessive ventilation, and is characterized by low P_{CO_2} and alkalosis.

Exercise-enhanced ventilation does *not* appear to be prompted by rising P_{CO_2} and declining P_{O_2} and pH in the blood for two reasons. First, ventilation increases abruptly as exercise begins, followed by a gradual increase, and then a steady state of ventilation. When exercise stops, there is an initial small but abrupt decline in ventilation rate, followed by a gradual decrease to the pre-exercise value. Second, although venous levels change, arterial P_{CO_2} and P_{O_2} levels remain surprisingly constant during exercise. In fact, P_{CO_2} may fall below normal and P_{O_2} may rise slightly because the respiratory adjustments are so efficient.

Our present understanding of the mechanisms that produce these observations is sketchy, but the most accepted explanation is as follows.

The abrupt increase in ventilation that occurs as exercise begins reflects interaction of three neural factors:

1. Psychological stimuli (our conscious anticipation of exercise)
2. Simultaneous cortical motor activation of skeletal muscles and respiratory centers
3. Excitatory impulses reaching respiratory centers from proprioceptors in moving muscles, tendons, and joints

The subsequent gradual increase and then plateauing of respiration probably reflect the rate of CO_2 delivery to the lungs (the "CO_2 flow"). The small but abrupt decrease in ventilation that occurs as exercise ends reflects the three neural factors listed above being shut off. The subsequent gradual decline to baseline ventilation likely reflects a gradual decline in CO_2 flow after exercise ends.

The rise in lactic acid levels during exercise results from anaerobic respiration. However, it is *not* a result of inadequate respiratory function, because alveolar ventilation and pulmonary perfusion are as well matched during exercise as during rest (hemoglobin remains fully saturated). Rather, it reflects cardiac output limitations or inability of the skeletal muscles to further increase their oxygen consumption.

In light of this fact, the practice of inhaling pure O_2 by mask, used by some football players to replenish their "oxygen-starved" bodies as quickly as possible, is useless. The panting athlete *does* need more oxygen, but inspiring extra oxygen will not help, because the shortage is in the muscles—not the lungs.

High Altitude

Most people live between sea level and an altitude of approximately 2400 m (8000 feet). In this range, differences in atmospheric pressure are not great enough to cause healthy people any problems when they spend brief periods in the higher-altitude areas.

However, if you travel quickly from sea level to elevations above 8000 ft, where atmospheric pressure and P_{O_2} are lower, your body responds with symptoms of *acute mountain sickness (AMS)*—headaches, shortness of breath, nausea, and dizziness. AMS is common in travelers to ski resorts such as Vail, Colorado (8120 ft), and Brian Head, Utah (a heart-pounding 9600 ft). In severe cases of AMS, lethal pulmonary and cerebral edema may occur.

When you move on a *long-term* basis from sea level to the mountains, your body makes respiratory and hematopoietic adjustments via an adaptive response called **acclimatization**. As we have already explained, decreases in arterial P_{O_2} cause the peripheral chemoreceptors to become more responsive to increases in P_{CO_2}, and a substantial decline in P_{O_2} directly stimulates them. As a result, ventilation increases as the brain attempts to restore gas exchange to previous levels.

Within a few days, the minute ventilation stabilizes at a level 2–3 L/min higher than the sea level rate. Increased ventilation also reduces arterial CO_2 levels, so the P_{CO_2} of individuals living at high altitudes is typically below 40 mm Hg (its value at sea level).

High-altitude conditions always result in lower-than-normal hemoglobin saturation levels because less O_2 is available to be loaded. For example, at about 19,000 ft above sea level, O_2 saturation of arterial blood is only 67% (compared to nearly 98% at sea level). But Hb unloads only 20–25% of its oxygen at sea level, which means that even at the reduced saturations at high altitudes, the O_2 needs of the tissues are still met under resting conditions.

Additionally, at high altitudes hemoglobin's affinity for O_2 is reduced because BPG concentrations increase. This releases more O_2 to the tissues during each circulatory round.

Although body tissues at high altitude receive adequate oxygen under normal conditions, problems arise when all-out efforts are demanded of the cardiovascular and respiratory systems (as athletes discovered during the 1968 Summer Olympics on the high mesa of Mexico City, at 7370 ft). Unless a person is fully acclimatized, such conditions almost guarantee that body tissues will become severely hypoxic.

When blood O_2 levels decline, the kidneys produce more erythropoietin, which stimulates bone marrow production of RBCs (see Chapter 17, p. 636). This phase of acclimatization, which occurs slowly, provides long-term compensation for living at high altitudes.

☑ Check Your Understanding

21. An injured soccer player arrives by ambulance in the emergency room. She is in obvious distress, breathing rapidly. Her blood P_{CO_2} is 26 mm Hg and pH is 7.5. Is she suffering from hyperventilation or hyperpnea? Explain.
22. What long-term adjustments does the body make when living at high altitude?

For answers, see Appendix H.

Homeostatic Imbalances of the Respiratory System

✓ Compare the causes and consequences of chronic bronchitis, emphysema, asthma, tuberculosis, and lung cancer.

The respiratory system is particularly vulnerable to infectious diseases because it is wide open to airborne pathogens. We considered many of these conditions, such as rhinitis and laryngitis, earlier in the chapter.

Here we turn our attention to the most disabling respiratory disorders: *chronic obstructive pulmonary disease (COPD), asthma, tuberculosis,* and *lung cancer*. COPD and lung cancer

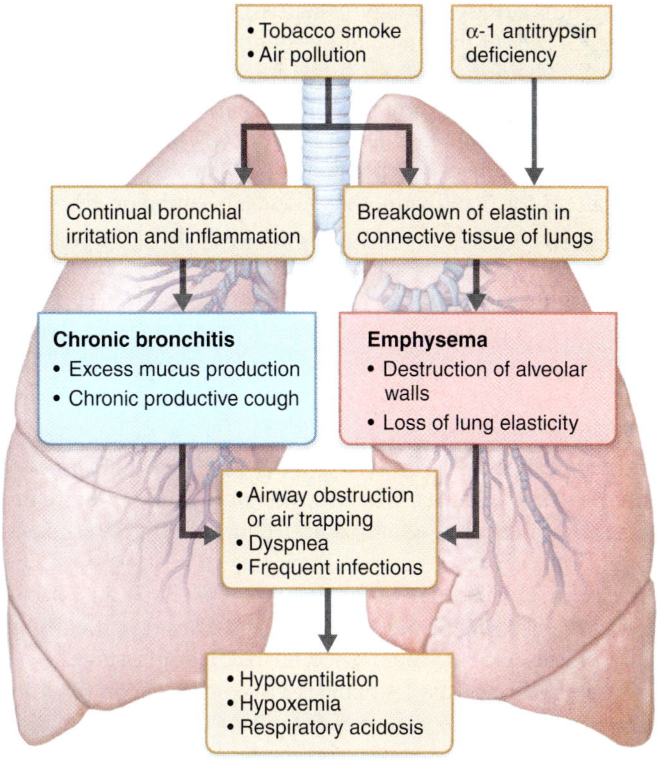

Figure 22.27 The pathogenesis of COPD.

are living proof of the devastating effects of tobacco smoke on the body. Long known to promote cardiovascular disease, smoking is perhaps even more effective at destroying the lungs.

Chronic Obstructive Pulmonary Disease (COPD)

The **chronic obstructive pulmonary diseases (COPD)**, exemplified best by emphysema and chronic bronchitis, are a major cause of disability and death in North America. The key physiological feature of these diseases is an irreversible decrease in the ability to force air out of the lungs. Other features they share in common **(Figure 22.27)**:

- More than 80% of patients have a history of smoking.
- **Dyspnea** (disp-ne′ah), difficult or labored breathing often referred to as "air hunger," gets progressively worse.
- Coughing and frequent pulmonary infections are common.
- Most COPD victims develop respiratory failure manifested as **hypoventilation** (insufficient ventilation in relation to metabolic needs, causing them to retain CO_2), respiratory acidosis, and hypoxemia.

Emphysema

Emphysema is distinguished by permanent enlargement of the alveoli, accompanied by destruction of the alveolar walls. Invariably the lungs lose their elasticity. This has three important consequences: (1) Accessory muscles must be enlisted to breathe, and victims are perpetually exhausted because breathing requires 15–20% of their total body energy supply (as opposed to 5% in healthy individuals). (2) For complex reasons, the bronchioles open during inspiration but collapse during expiration, trapping huge volumes of air in the alveoli. This hyperinflation leads to development of a permanently expanded "barrel chest" and flattens the diaphragm, thus reducing ventilation efficiency. (3) Damage to the pulmonary capillaries as the alveolar walls disintegrate increases resistance in the pulmonary circuit, forcing the right ventricle to overwork and consequently become enlarged. In addition to smoking, hereditary factors (e.g., alpha-1 antitrypsin deficiency) cause emphysema in some patients.

Chronic Bronchitis

In **chronic bronchitis**, inhaled irritants lead to chronic production of excessive mucus. The mucosae of the lower respiratory passageways become inflamed and fibrosed. These responses obstruct the airways, severely impairing lung ventilation and gas exchange. Pulmonary infections are frequent because bacteria thrive in the stagnant pools of mucus. However, the degree of dyspnea is usually moderate compared to emphysema.

As with emphysema, smoking is a major risk factor. Environmental pollution also promotes chronic bronchitis.

COPD: Symptoms and Treatments

In the clinical setting you might see two very different patterns that represent the extremes of patients with COPD. One pattern has traditionally been called the "pink puffer": These patients work so hard to maintain adequate ventilation that they lose weight, becoming thin but still having nearly normal blood gases. In contrast, "blue bloaters," commonly of stocky build, become sufficiently hypoxic that they are obviously cyanotic. The hypoxia causes constriction of pulmonary blood vessels, leading to pulmonary hypertension and right-sided heart failure.

22

Traditionally, "pink puffers" were associated with emphysema while "blue bloaters" were associated with chronic bronchitis. As usual, things are not that clear-cut. It turns out that patients with the same underlying disease can display either of these clinical patterns, and this may depend on a third factor—the strength of their innate respiratory drive. Most COPD patients fall between these two clinical extremes.

COPD is routinely treated with bronchodilators and corticosteroids in aerosol form (inhalers). Severe dyspnea and hypoxia mandate oxygen use. For a few patients, surgical treatment for COPD, called *lung volume reduction surgery*, may be beneficial. In this procedure, part of the grossly enlarged lungs is removed to give the remaining lung tissue room to expand. While this surgery does not prolong life, it can offer certain COPD patients better quality of life, although at a high cost.

COPD patients in acute respiratory distress are commonly given oxygen. Oxygen must be administered with care, however. In some of these patients, giving pure oxygen can increase the blood P_{CO_2} (and lower blood pH) to life-threatening levels. Why does this happen? First, oxygen dilates pulmonary arterioles, increasing perfusion and worsening an already poor ventilation-perfusion mismatch. Second, oxygen drives more CO_2 off of hemoglobin (the Haldane effect), dumping it into alveoli from which it cannot be removed because of the underlying disease. The solution is to use the minimum concentration of oxygen that relieves the patient's hypoxia.

Asthma

Asthma is characterized by episodes of coughing, dyspnea, wheezing, and chest tightness—alone or in combination. A sense of panic accompanies most acute attacks. Although sometimes classed with COPD because it is an obstructive disorder, asthma is marked by acute episodes followed by symptom-free periods—that is, the obstruction is *reversible*.

The cause of asthma has been hard to pin down. Initially it was viewed as a consequence of bronchospasms triggered by various factors such as cold air, exercise, or allergens. However, bronchoconstriction has relatively little effect on air flow through normal lungs. Researchers have found that in allergic asthma (the most common kind), active inflammation of the airways comes first. The inflammation is an immune response controlled by T_H2 cells, a subset of T lymphocytes. By secreting certain interleukins, T_H2 cells stimulate the production of IgE and recruit inflammatory cells (notably eosinophils) to the site.

Once someone has allergic asthma, the inflammation persists even during symptom-free periods and makes the airways hypersensitive. (The most common triggers are in the home—the allergens from dust mites, cockroaches, cats, dogs, and fungi.) Once the airway walls are thickened with inflammatory exudate, the effect of bronchospasm is vastly magnified and can dramatically reduce air flow.

About one in ten people in North America suffer from asthma—children more than adults. Over the past 20 years, the number of cases has risen dramatically, an increase which may now be plateauing.

While asthma remains a major health problem, better treatment options have reduced the number of asthma-related deaths. Instead of merely treating the symptoms with fast-acting bronchodilators, we now treat the underlying inflammation using inhaled corticosteroids. Newer approaches limit airway inflammation by using antileukotrienes and antibodies against the patient's own IgE class of antibodies.

Tuberculosis (TB)

Tuberculosis (TB), the infectious disease caused by the bacterium *Mycobacterium tuberculosis*, is spread by coughing and primarily enters the body in inhaled air. TB mostly affects the lungs but can spread through the lymphatics to other organs.

One-third of the world's population is infected, but most people never develop active TB because a massive inflammatory and immune response usually contains the primary infection in fibrous, or calcified, nodules (tubercles) in the lungs. However, the bacteria survive in the nodules and when the person's immunity is weakened, they may break out and cause symptomatic TB. Symptoms include fever, night sweats, weight loss, racking cough, and coughing up blood.

During the mid-1980s, there was an alarming increase in TB due to TB-infected HIV patients. This trend has now been brought under control and TB rates in the U.S. are again decreasing.

However, deadly strains of drug-resistant (even multidrug-resistant) TB can develop when treatment is incomplete or inadequate. Resistant strains are found elsewhere in the world and have appeared in North America.

Homeless shelters, with their densely packed populations, are ideal breeding grounds for drug-resistant strains. The TB bacterium grows slowly and drug therapy entails a 12-month course of antibiotics. The transient nature of shelter populations makes it difficult to track TB patients and ensure they take their medications for the full 12 months. The threat of TB epidemics is so real that health centers in some cities are detaining such patients against their will for as long as it takes to complete a cure.

Lung Cancer

Lung cancer is the leading cause of cancer death for both men and women in North America, killing more people every year than breast, prostate, and colorectal cancer combined. This is tragic, because lung cancer is largely preventable—nearly 90% of cases result from smoking.

The cure rate for lung cancer is notoriously low, with most victims dying within one year of diagnosis. The five-year survival rate is about 17%. Because lung cancer is aggressive and metastasizes rapidly and widely, most cases are not diagnosed until they are well advanced.

Lung cancer appears to follow closely the oncogene-activating steps outlined in *A Closer Look* in Chapter 4. Ordinarily, nasal hairs, sticky mucus, and cilia do a fine job of protecting the lungs from chemical and biological irritants, but when a person smokes, these defenses are overwhelmed and eventually stop functioning. In particular, smoking paralyzes the cilia that clear mucus from the airways, allowing irritants and pathogens to accumulate. The "cocktail" of free radicals and other carcinogens in tobacco smoke eventually translates into lung cancer.

The three most common types of lung cancer are:

- **Adenocarcinoma** (about 40% of cases), which originates in peripheral lung areas as solitary nodules that develop from bronchial glands and alveolar cells.
- **Squamous cell carcinoma** (25–30%), which arises in the epithelium of the bronchi or their larger subdivisions and tends to form masses that may cavitate (hollow out) and bleed.
- **Small cell carcinoma** (about 20%), round lymphocyte-sized cells that originate in the main bronchi and grow aggressively in small grapelike clusters within the mediastinum. Metastasis from the mediastinum is especially rapid. Some small cell carcinomas cause additional problems because they produce certain hormones. For example, some secrete ACTH (leading to Cushing's syndrome) or ADH (resulting in the syndrome of inappropriate ADH secretion, or SIADH; see p. 601).

Because lung cancers metastasize aggressively and early, the key to survival is early detection. A recent study of heavy smokers showed that using helical CT scans instead of standard chest X rays improved tumor detection and reduced mortality by 20%. A promising screening test for lung cancer that is still in development is a simple breath test using a detector made of gold nanoparticles.

If the cancer has not metastasized before it is discovered, complete removal of the diseased lung has the greatest potential for prolonging life and providing a cure. With metastatic lung cancer, radiation therapy and chemotherapy are the only options, but these have low success rates.

Fortunately, there are several new therapies on the horizon. These include (1) antibodies that target specific growth factors or other molecules required by the tumor or that deliver toxic agents directly to the tumor, (2) cancer vaccines to stimulate the immune system to fight the tumor, and (3) various forms of gene therapy to replace the defective genes that make tumor cells divide continuously. As clinical trials progress, we will learn which of these approaches is most effective.

Developmental Aspects of the Respiratory System

✓ Trace the embryonic development of the respiratory system.

✓ Describe normal changes that occur in the respiratory system from infancy to old age.

Because embryos develop in a cephalocaudal (head-to-tail) direction, the upper respiratory structures appear first. By the fourth week of development, two thickened plates of ectoderm, the **olfactory placodes** (plak′ōds), are present on the anterior aspect of the head (**Figure 22.28**). These quickly invaginate to form **olfactory pits** that form the nasal cavities. The olfactory pits then extend posteriorly to connect with the developing pharynx, which forms at the same time from the endodermal germ layer.

The epithelium of the lower respiratory organs develops as an outpocketing of the foregut endoderm, which becomes the pharyngeal mucosa. This protrusion, called the **laryngotracheal bud**, is present by the fifth week of development. The proximal part of the bud forms the tracheal lining, and its distal end splits and forms the mucosae of the bronchi and all their subdivisions, including (eventually) the lung alveoli. Mesoderm covers these endoderm-derived linings and forms the walls of the respiratory passageways and the stroma of the lungs.

By 28 weeks, the respiratory system has developed sufficiently to allow a baby born prematurely to breathe on its own. As we noted earlier, infants born before this time often exhibit infant respiratory distress syndrome resulting from inadequate surfactant production.

During fetal life, the lungs are filled with fluid and the placenta makes all respiratory exchanges. Vascular shunts cause circulating blood to largely bypass the lungs (see Chapter 28). At birth, the respiratory passageways fill with air. As the P_{CO_2} in the baby's blood rises, the respiratory centers are excited,

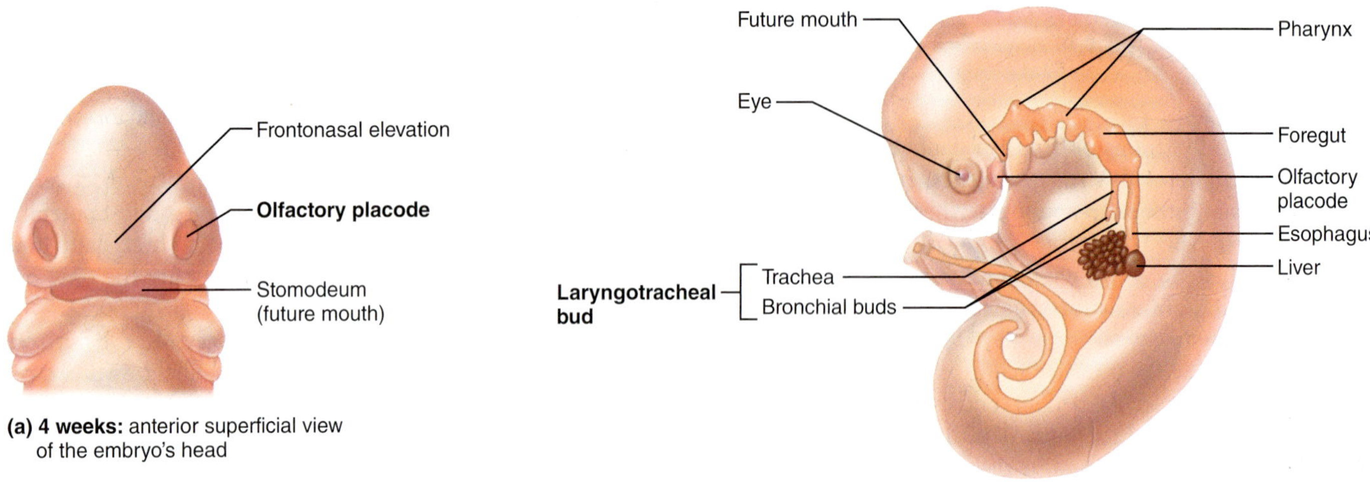

(a) 4 weeks: anterior superficial view of the embryo's head

(b) 5 weeks: left lateral view of the developing lower respiratory passageway mucosae

Figure 22.28 Embryonic development of the respiratory system.

causing the baby to take its first breath. The alveoli inflate and begin to function in gas exchange, but it is nearly two weeks before the lungs are fully inflated.

Homeostatic Imbalance 22.16

Important birth defects of the respiratory system include *cleft palate* (described in Chapter 7) and cystic fibrosis. **Cystic fibrosis (CF)**, the most common lethal genetic disease in North America, strikes in one out of every 2400 births. In CF, abnormally viscous mucus clogs the respiratory passages, providing a breeding ground for airborne bacteria and predisposing the child to respiratory infections.

At the root of CF is a faulty gene that codes for the *CFTR* (cystic fibrosis transmembrane conductance regulator) *protein.* The normal CFTR protein works as a membrane channel to control Cl^- flow in and out of cells. In one common mutation, CFTR lacks a critical amino acid and so does not fold correctly. As a result, it gets "stuck" in the endoplasmic reticulum, is marked for degradation, and never reaches the plasma membrane to perform its normal role. Consequently, less Cl^- is secreted and less water follows, resulting in the thick mucus typical of CF.

This thick mucus forms a perfect harbor for bacterial infection. By early adulthood, 80% of patients are colonized by *Pseudomonas aeruginosa*, which causes chronic inflammation and triggers the disabled cells to churn out a thick sludge of abnormal mucus. Repeated cycles of infection and inflammation eventually result in extensive tissue damage that can be treated only by a lung transplant.

Defects in the CFTR protein can affect other organ systems, too. The ducts of the pancreas become clogged with secretions, impairing food digestion. Obstructed reproductive ducts render 97% of males with CF infertile. Characteristically, sweat glands of CF patients produce extremely salty perspiration.

Conventional therapy for CF has included mucus-dissolving drugs, "clapping" the chest to loosen the thick mucus, and antibiotics to prevent infection. The goal of CF research is to restore normal salt and water movements by (1) introducing normal CFTR genes into respiratory tract mucosa cells, (2) prodding another channel protein to take over the duties of transporting Cl^-, and (3) developing techniques to free the CFTR protein from the ER. A novel and surprisingly simple approach involves inhaling hypertonic saline droplets. This draws water into the mucus, making it more liquid. Alone or in combination, these therapies provide new hope to patients with CF. ✚

The respiratory rate is highest in newborn infants (40–80 breaths per minute). At five years of age it is around 25 per minute, and in adults it is between 12 and 18 per minute. In old age, the rate often increases again.

At birth, only about one-sixth of the final number of alveoli are present. The lungs continue to mature and form more alveoli until young adulthood. However, if a person begins smoking in the early teens, the lungs never completely mature, and those additional alveoli are lost forever.

In infants, the ribs take a nearly horizontal course. For this reason, infants rely almost entirely on descent of the diaphragm to increase thoracic volume for inspiration. By the second year, the ribs are more obliquely positioned, and the adult form of breathing is established.

The maximum amount of oxygen we can use during aerobic metabolism, $\dot{V}_{O_2max}$, declines about 9% per decade in inactive people beginning in their mid-20s. In those who remain active, $\dot{V}_{O_2max}$ still declines but much less. As we age, the thoracic wall becomes more rigid and the lungs gradually lose their elasticity, decreasing the ability to ventilate the lungs. Vital capacity declines by about one-third by age 70. Blood O_2 levels decline slightly, and many old people tend to become hypoxic during sleep and exhibit *sleep apnea* (they stop breathing temporarily during sleep).

Homeostatic Interrelationships Between the Respiratory System and Other Body Systems

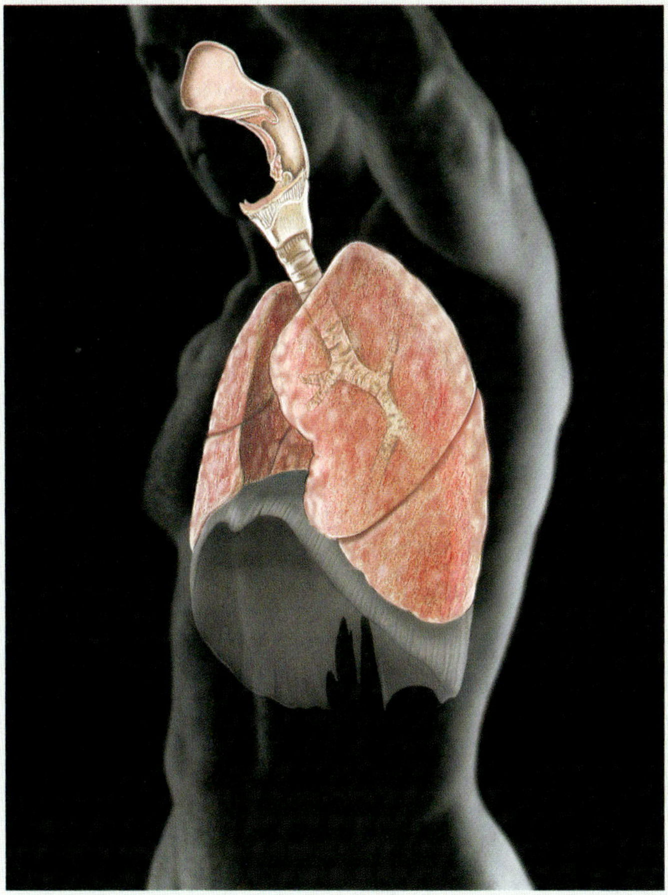

Nervous System Chapters 11–15

- Respiratory system provides oxygen needed for normal neuronal activity and disposes of carbon dioxide
- Medullary and pontine centers regulate respiratory rate and depth; stretch receptors in lungs and chemoreceptors provide feedback

Endocrine System Chapter 16

- Respiratory system provides oxygen and disposes of carbon dioxide; angiotensin converting enzyme in lungs converts angiotensin I to angiotensin II
- Epinephrine dilates the bronchioles; testosterone promotes laryngeal enlargement in pubertal males; glucocorticoids promote surfactant production

Cardiovascular System Chapters 17–19

- Respiratory system provides oxygen and disposes of carbon dioxide; carbon dioxide present in blood as HCO_3^- and H_2CO_3 contributes to blood buffering
- Blood is the transport medium for respiratory gases

Lymphatic System/Immunity Chapters 20–21

- Respiratory system provides oxygen and disposes of carbon dioxide; tonsils in pharynx house immune cells
- Lymphatic system helps to maintain blood volume required for respiratory gas transport; immune system protects respiratory organs from bacteria, bacterial toxins, viruses, protozoa, fungi, and cancer

Digestive System Chapter 23

- Respiratory system provides oxygen and disposes of carbon dioxide
- Digestive system provides nutrients needed by respiratory system organs

Urinary System Chapters 25–26

- Respiratory system provides oxygen and disposes of carbon dioxide to provide short-term pH homeostasis
- Kidneys dispose of metabolic wastes of respiratory system organs (other than carbon dioxide) and maintain long-term pH homeostasis

Reproductive System Chapter 27

- Respiratory system provides oxygen and disposes of carbon dioxide

Integumentary System Chapter 5

- Respiratory system provides oxygen and disposes of carbon dioxide
- Skin protects respiratory system organs by forming surface barriers

Skeletal System Chapters 6–8

- Respiratory system provides oxygen and disposes of carbon dioxide
- Bones protect lungs and bronchi by enclosure

Muscular System Chapters 9–10

- Respiratory system provides oxygen needed for muscle activity and disposes of carbon dioxide
- Activity of the diaphragm and intercostal muscles essential for producing volume changes that lead to pulmonary ventilation; regular exercise increases respiratory efficiency

The number of glands in the nasal mucosa decreases as does blood flow to this mucosa. For this reason, the nose dries and produces a thick mucus that makes us want to clear our throat. Additionally, many of the respiratory system's protective mechanisms become less effective with age. Mucosal cilia are less active, and the macrophages in the lungs become sluggish. The net result is that the elderly are more at risk for respiratory tract infections, particularly pneumonia and influenza.

Check Your Understanding

23. What distinguishes the obstruction in asthma from that in chronic bronchitis?
24. What is the underlying defect in cystic fibrosis?
25. List two reasons for the decline in vital capacity seen with age.

For answers, see Appendix H.

Lungs, bronchial tree, heart, and connecting blood vessels—together, these organs fashion a remarkable system that oxygenates blood, removes carbon dioxide, and ensures that all tissue cells have access to these services. Although the cooperation of the respiratory and cardiovascular systems is obvious, all organ systems depend on the functioning of the respiratory system, as summarized in *System Connections* on p. 843.

Chapter Summary

MAP™ For more chapter study tools, go to the Study Area of MasteringA&P at **www.masteringaandp.com**.
There you will find:

- Interactive Physiology iP
- A&PFlix A&PFlix
- Practice Anatomy Lab PAL
- PhysioEx PEx
- Videos, Practice Quizzes and Tests, MP3 Tutor Sessions, Case Studies, and much more!

1. Respiration involves four processes: pulmonary ventilation, external respiration, transport of respiratory gases in the blood, and internal respiration. Both the respiratory system and the cardiovascular system are involved in respiration.

Functional Anatomy of the Respiratory System (pp. 802–816)

1. Respiratory system organs are divided functionally into conducting zone structures (nose to terminal bronchioles), which filter, warm, and moisten incoming air; and respiratory zone structures (respiratory bronchioles to alveoli), where gas exchanges occur.

The Nose and Paranasal Sinuses (pp. 803–806)

2. The nose provides an airway for respiration; warms, moistens, and cleanses incoming air; and houses the olfactory receptors.
3. Bone and cartilage plates shape the external nose. The nasal cavity, which opens to the exterior, is divided by the nasal septum. Paranasal sinuses and nasolacrimal ducts drain into the nasal cavities.

The Pharynx (p. 806)

4. The pharynx extends from the base of the skull to the level of C_6. The nasopharynx is an air conduit; the oropharynx and laryngopharynx are common passageways for food and air. Tonsils are found in the oropharynx and nasopharynx.

The Larynx (pp. 807–809)

5. The larynx, or voice box, contains the vocal folds (cords). It also provides a patent airway and serves as a switching mechanism to route food and air into the proper channels.
6. The epiglottis prevents food or liquids from entering the respiratory channels during swallowing.

The Trachea (p. 809)

7. The trachea extends from the larynx to the main bronchi. C-shaped cartilage rings reinforce the trachea and keep the trachea patent. Its mucosa is ciliated.

The Bronchi and Subdivisions (pp. 809–812)

8. The right and left main bronchi run into their respective lungs, within which they subdivide into smaller and smaller passageways.
9. The terminal bronchioles lead into respiratory zone structures: respiratory bronchioles, alveolar ducts, alveolar sacs, and finally alveoli. Gas exchange occurs in the alveoli, across the respiratory membrane.
10. As the respiratory conduits become smaller, the amount of cartilage decreases and is finally lost; the mucosa thins, and smooth muscle in the walls increases.

iP Respiratory System; Topic: Anatomy Review: Respiratory Structures, p. 6.

The Lungs and Pleurae (pp. 812–816)

11. The lungs, the paired organs of gas exchange, flank the mediastinum in the thoracic cavity. Each is suspended in pleurae via its root and has a base, an apex, and medial and costal surfaces. The right lung has three lobes; the left has two.
12. The lungs are primarily air passageways/chambers, supported by an elastic connective tissue stroma.
13. The pulmonary arteries carry deoxygenated blood returned from the systemic circulation to the lungs, where gas exchange occurs. The pulmonary veins return newly oxygenated (and most bronchial venous) blood back to the heart to be distributed throughout the body. The bronchial arteries provide the nutrient blood supply of the lungs.
14. The parietal pleura lines the thoracic wall and mediastinum; the visceral pleura covers external lung surfaces. Pleural fluid reduces friction during breathing movements.

iP Respiratory System; Topic: Anatomy Review: Respiratory Structures, pp. 1–5.

Mechanics of Breathing (pp. 816–824)

Pressure Relationships in the Thoracic Cavity (pp. 816–817)

1. Intrapulmonary pressure is the pressure within the alveoli. Intrapleural pressure is the pressure within the pleural

cavity; normally it is negative relative to intrapulmonary pressures.

iP Respiratory System; Topic: Pulmonary Ventilation, pp. 7–9.

Pulmonary Ventilation (pp. 817–820)

2. Gases travel from an area of higher pressure to an area of lower pressure.
3. Inspiration occurs when the diaphragm and external intercostal muscles contract, increasing the dimensions (and volume) of the thorax. As the intrapulmonary pressure drops, air rushes into the lungs until the intrapulmonary and atmospheric pressures are equalized.
4. Expiration is largely passive, occurring as the inspiratory muscles relax and the lungs recoil. When intrapulmonary pressure exceeds atmospheric pressure, gases flow from the lungs.

iP Respiratory System; Topic: Pulmonary Ventilation, pp. 3–6, 11–13.

Physical Factors Influencing Pulmonary Ventilation (pp. 820–821)

5. Friction in the air passageways causes resistance, which decreases air passage and causes breathing movements to become more strenuous. The greatest resistance to air flow occurs in the midsize bronchi.
6. Surface tension of alveolar fluid acts to reduce alveolar size and collapse the alveoli. Surfactant reduces this tendency.
7. Premature infants have problems keeping their lungs inflated owing to the lack of surfactant in their alveoli, resulting in infant respiratory distress syndrome (IRDS). Surfactant formation begins late in fetal development.
8. Total respiratory compliance depends on elasticity of lung tissue and flexibility of the bony thorax. When compliance is impaired, inspiration becomes more difficult.

iP Respiratory System; Topic: Pulmonary Ventilation, pp. 14–18.

Respiratory Volumes and Pulmonary Function Tests (pp. 821–823)

9. The four respiratory volumes are tidal, inspiratory reserve, expiratory reserve, and residual. The four respiratory capacities are vital, functional residual, inspiratory, and total lung. Spirometry measures respiratory volumes and capacities.
10. Anatomical dead space is the air-filled volume (about 150 ml) of the conducting passageways. If alveoli become nonfunctional in gas exchange, their volume is added to the anatomical dead space, and the sum is the total dead space.
11. The FVC and FEV tests, which determine the rate at which VC air can be expelled, are particularly valuable in distinguishing between obstructive and restrictive disease.
12. Alveolar ventilation is the best index of ventilation efficiency because it accounts for anatomical dead space.

$$\text{AVR} = (\text{TV} - \text{dead space}) \times \text{respiratory rate}$$

Nonrespiratory Air Movements (pp. 823–824)

13. Nonrespiratory air movements are voluntary or reflex actions that clear the respiratory passageways or express emotions.

Gas Exchanges Between the Blood, Lungs, and Tissues (pp. 824–828)

Basic Properties of Gases (pp. 824–825)

1. Dalton's law states that each gas in a mixture of gases exerts pressure in proportion to its percentage in the total mixture.
2. Henry's law states that the amount of gas that will dissolve in a liquid is proportional to the partial pressure of that gas. Other important factors are the solubility of the gas in the liquid and the temperature of the liquid.

iP Respiratory System; Topic: Gas Exchange, pp. 1–6.

Composition of Alveolar Gas (p. 825)

3. Alveolar gas contains more carbon dioxide and water vapor and considerably less oxygen than atmospheric air.

External Respiration (pp. 825–827)

4. External respiration is the process of gas exchange that occurs in the lungs. Oxygen enters the pulmonary capillaries; carbon dioxide leaves the blood and enters the alveoli. Factors influencing this process include the partial pressure gradients, the thickness of the respiratory membrane, surface area available, and ventilation-perfusion coupling (matching alveolar ventilation with pulmonary perfusion).

Internal Respiration (pp. 827–828)

5. Internal respiration is the gas exchange that occurs between the systemic capillaries and the tissues. Carbon dioxide enters the blood, and oxygen leaves the blood and enters the tissues.

iP Respiratory System; Topic: Gas Exchange, pp. 6–11, 15–16.

Transport of Respiratory Gases by Blood (pp. 828–833)

Oxygen Transport (pp. 828–829)

1. Molecular oxygen is carried bound to hemoglobin in the red blood cells. The amount of oxygen bound to hemoglobin depends on the P_{O_2} and P_{CO_2} of blood, blood pH, the presence of BPG, and temperature. A small amount of oxygen gas is transported dissolved in plasma.
2. Hypoxia occurs when inadequate amounts of oxygen are delivered to body tissues. When this occurs, the skin and mucosae may become cyanotic.

Carbon Dioxide Transport (pp. 829–833)

3. CO_2 is transported in the blood dissolved in plasma, chemically bound to hemoglobin, and (primarily) as bicarbonate ions in plasma. Loading and unloading of O_2 and CO_2 are mutually beneficial.
4. Accumulating CO_2 lowers blood pH; depletion of CO_2 from blood raises blood pH.

iP Respiratory System; Topic: Gas Transport, pp. 1–15.

Control of Respiration (pp. 834–838)

Neural Mechanisms (pp. 834–835)

1. Medullary respiratory centers are the ventral and dorsal respiratory groups. The ventral respiratory group is likely responsible for the rhythmicity of breathing.
2. The pontine respiratory centers influence the activity of the medullary respiratory centers.

Factors Influencing Breathing Rate and Depth (pp. 835–838)

3. Important chemical factors modifying baseline respiratory rate and depth are arterial levels of CO_2, H^+, and O_2.
4. An increasing arterial P_{CO_2} level (hypercapnia) is the most powerful respiratory stimulant. It acts (via release of H^+ in brain tissue) on central chemoreceptors to cause a reflexive increase in the rate and depth of breathing.

5. Hypocapnia depresses respiration and results in decreased ventilation and, possibly, apnea.
6. Arterial P_{O_2} levels below 60 mm Hg strongly stimulate peripheral chemoreceptors.
7. Decreased pH and a decline in blood P_{O_2} act on peripheral chemoreceptors and enhance the response to CO_2.
8. Emotions, pain, body temperature changes, and other stressors can alter respiration by acting through hypothalamic centers. Respiration can also be controlled voluntarily for short periods.
9. Dust, mucus, fumes, and pollutants initiate pulmonary irritant reflexes.
10. The inflation (Hering-Breuer) reflex is a protective reflex initiated by extreme overinflation of the lungs; it acts to terminate inspiration.

iP Respiratory System; Topic: Control of Respiration, pp. 6–14.

Respiratory Adjustments (pp. 838–839)

Exercise (p. 838)

1. As exercise begins, there is an abrupt increase in ventilation (hyperpnea) followed by a more gradual increase. When exercise stops, there is an abrupt decrease in ventilation followed by a gradual decline to baseline values.
2. P_{O_2}, P_{CO_2}, and blood pH remain quite constant during exercise and hence do not appear to account for changes in ventilation. Inputs from higher centers and proprioceptors may contribute.

High Altitude (pp. 838–839)

3. At high altitudes, arterial P_{O_2} and hemoglobin saturation levels fall because of the decrease in atmospheric pressure compared to sea level. Increased ventilation helps restore P_{O_2} to physiological levels.
4. Long-term acclimatization involves increased erythropoiesis.

Homeostatic Imbalances of the Respiratory System (pp. 839–841)

1. Two major respiratory disorders are COPD (emphysema and chronic bronchitis) and lung cancer; smoking is a significant cause. A third major disorder is asthma. Multidrug-resistant tuberculosis may become a major public health problem.

Chronic Obstructive Pulmonary Disease (pp. 839–840)

22

2. COPD is characterized by an irreversible decrease in the ability to force air out of the lungs.
3. In emphysema, alveoli enlarge permanently and disintegrate. The lungs lose their elasticity, and expiration becomes an active process.
4. Chronic bronchitis is characterized by excessive mucus production in the lower respiratory passageways, which severely impairs ventilation and gas exchange.

Asthma (p. 840)

5. Asthma is a reversible obstructive condition caused by an immune response that causes its victims to wheeze and gasp for air as their inflamed respiratory passages constrict. It is marked by acute episodes and symptom-free periods.

Tuberculosis (TB) (pp. 840–841)

6. Tuberculosis, an infectious disease caused by an airborne bacterium, mainly affects the lungs. Although most infected individuals remain asymptomatic by walling off the bacteria in nodules (tubercles), symptoms appear when immunity is depressed. Some patients' failure to complete drug therapy has produced multidrug-resistant TB strains.

Lung Cancer (p. 841)

7. Lung cancer, promoted by free radicals and other carcinogens, is extremely aggressive and metastasizes rapidly.

Developmental Aspects of the Respiratory System (pp. 841–844)

1. The superior respiratory system mucosa develops from the invagination of the ectodermal olfactory placodes. The mucosa of the inferior passageways develops from an outpocketing of the endodermal foregut lining. Mesoderm forms the walls of the respiratory conduits and the lung stroma.
2. Cystic fibrosis (CF), the most common fatal hereditary disease in North America, results from an abnormal CFTR protein that fails to form a chloride channel. The result is thick mucus, which clogs respiratory passages and invites infection.
3. With age, the thorax becomes more rigid, the lungs become less elastic, and vital capacity declines. In addition, sleep apnea becomes more common, and respiratory system protective mechanisms are less effective.

Review Questions

Multiple Choice/Matching

(Some questions have more than one correct answer. Select the best answer or answers from the choices given.)

1. Cutting the phrenic nerves will result in **(a)** air entering the pleural cavity, **(b)** paralysis of the diaphragm, **(c)** stimulation of the diaphragmatic reflex, **(d)** paralysis of the epiglottis.
2. Which of the following laryngeal cartilages is/are not paired? **(a)** epiglottis, **(b)** arytenoid, **(c)** cricoid, **(d)** cuneiform, **(e)** corniculate.
3. Under ordinary circumstances, the inflation reflex is initiated by **(a)** noxious chemicals, **(b)** the ventral respiratory group, **(c)** overinflation of the alveoli and bronchioles, **(d)** the pontine respiratory centers.
4. The detergent-like substance that keeps the alveoli from collapsing between breaths because it reduces the surface tension of the water film in the alveoli is called **(a)** lecithin, **(b)** bile, **(c)** surfactant, **(d)** reluctant.
5. Which of the following determines the direction of gas movement? **(a)** solubility in water, **(b)** partial pressure gradient, **(c)** temperature, **(d)** molecular weight and size of the gas molecule.
6. When the inspiratory muscles contract, **(a)** the size of the thoracic cavity increases in diameter, **(b)** the size of the thoracic cavity increases in length, **(c)** the volume of the thoracic cavity decreases, **(d)** the size of the thoracic cavity increases in both length and diameter.

7. The nutrient blood supply of the lungs is provided by **(a)** the pulmonary arteries, **(b)** the aorta, **(c)** the pulmonary veins, **(d)** the bronchial arteries.
8. Oxygen and carbon dioxide are exchanged in the lungs and through all cell membranes by **(a)** active transport, **(b)** diffusion, **(c)** filtration, **(d)** osmosis.
9. Which of the following would not normally be treated by 100% oxygen therapy? (Choose all that apply.) **(a)** anoxia, **(b)** carbon monoxide poisoning, **(c)** respiratory crisis in an emphysema patient, **(d)** eupnea.
10. Most oxygen carried in the blood is **(a)** in solution in the plasma, **(b)** combined with plasma proteins, **(c)** chemically combined with the heme in red blood cells, **(d)** in solution in the red blood cells.
11. Which of the following has the greatest stimulating effect on the respiratory centers in the brain? **(a)** oxygen, **(b)** carbon dioxide, **(c)** calcium, **(d)** willpower.
12. In mouth-to-mouth artificial respiration, the rescuer blows air from his or her own respiratory system into that of the victim. Which of the following statements are correct?
    (1) Expansion of the victim's lungs is brought about by blowing air in at higher than atmospheric pressure (positive-pressure breathing).
    (2) During inflation of the lungs, the intrapleural pressure increases.
    (3) This technique will not work if the victim has a hole in the chest wall, even if the lungs are intact.
    (4) Expiration during this procedure depends on the elasticity of the alveolar and thoracic walls.
    (a) all of these, **(b)** 1, 2, 4, **(c)** 1, 2, 3, **(d)** 1, 4.
13. A baby holding its breath will **(a)** have brain cells damaged because of low blood oxygen levels, **(b)** automatically start to breathe again when the carbon dioxide levels in the blood reach a high enough value, **(c)** suffer heart damage because of increased pressure in the carotid sinus and aortic arch areas, **(d)** be called a "blue baby."
14. Under ordinary circumstances, which of the following blood components is of no physiological significance? **(a)** bicarbonate ions, **(b)** carbaminohemoglobin, **(c)** nitrogen, **(d)** chloride.
15. Damage to which of the following would most likely result in cessation of breathing? **(a)** the pontine respiratory group, **(b)** the ventral respiratory group of the medulla, **(c)** the stretch receptors in the lungs, **(d)** the dorsal respiratory group of the medulla.
16. The bulk of carbon dioxide is carried **(a)** chemically combined with the amino acids of hemoglobin as carbaminohemoglobin in the red blood cells, **(b)** as the ion HCO_3^- in the plasma after first entering the red blood cell, **(c)** as carbonic acid in the plasma, **(d)** chemically combined with the heme portion of Hb.

Short Answer Essay Questions

17. Trace the route of air from the nares to an alveolus. Name subdivisions of organs where applicable, and differentiate between conducting and respiratory zone structures.
18. (a) Why is it important that the trachea is reinforced with cartilage rings? (b) Why is it advantageous that the rings are incomplete posteriorly?
19. Briefly explain the anatomical "reason" why most men have deeper voices than boys or women.
20. The lungs are mostly passageways and elastic tissue. (a) What is the role of the elastic tissue? (b) Of the passageways?
21. Describe the functional relationships between volume changes and gas flow into and out of the lungs.
22. Discuss how airway resistance, lung compliance, and alveolar surface tension influence pulmonary ventilation.
23. (a) Differentiate clearly between minute respiratory volume and alveolar ventilation rate. (b) Which provides a more accurate measure of ventilatory efficiency, and why?
24. State Dalton's law of partial pressures and Henry's law.
25. (a) Define hyperventilation. (b) If you hyperventilate, do you retain or expel more carbon dioxide? (c) What effect does hyperventilation have on blood pH?
26. Describe age-related changes in respiratory function.

Critical Thinking and Clinical Application Questions

1. Harry, the swimmer with the fastest time on the Springfield College swim team, routinely hyperventilates before a meet, as he says, "to sock some more oxygen into my lungs so I can swim longer without having to breathe." First of all, what basic fact about oxygen loading has Harry forgotten (a lapse leading to false thinking)? Second, how is Harry jeopardizing not only his time but his life?
2. A member of the "Blues" gang was rushed into an emergency room after receiving a knife wound in the left side of his thorax. The diagnosis was pneumothorax and a collapsed lung. Explain exactly (a) why the lung collapsed, and (b) why only one lung (not both) collapsed.
3. A surgeon removed three adjacent bronchopulmonary segments from the left lung of a patient with TB. Almost half of the lung was removed, yet there was no severe bleeding, and relatively few blood vessels had to be cauterized (closed off). Why was the surgery so easy to perform?
4. After a week of scuba diving in the Bahamas, Mary Ann boards an airplane. During her flight home, she develops aching joints, nausea, and dyspnea, which resolve upon landing. During the flight, the cabin pressure was equivalent to an altitude of 8000 feet. Explain her problems.

AT THE CLINIC

Related Clinical Terms

Adenoidectomy (adenotonsillectomy) Surgical removal of an infected pharyngeal tonsil (adenoids).

Adult respiratory distress syndrome (ARDS) A dangerous lung condition that can develop after severe illness or injury to the body. Neutrophils leave the body's capillaries in large numbers and then secrete chemicals that increase capillary permeability. The capillary-rich lungs are heavily affected. As the lungs fill with fluid, the patient suffocates. Even with mechanical ventilation, ARDS is hard to control and often lethal.

Aspiration (as″pĭ-ra′shun) (1) Inhaling or drawing something into the lungs or respiratory passages. Pathological aspiration—drawing vomit or excessive mucus into the lungs—may occur when a person is unconscious or anesthetized; turning the head to one side is preventive. (2) Withdrawing fluid by suction (use

Related Clinical Terms *(continued)*

of an aspirator); done during surgery to keep an area free of blood or other body fluids; mucus is aspirated from the trachea of tracheotomy patients.

Bronchoscopy (*scopy* = viewing) Use of a viewing tube inserted through the nose or mouth to examine the internal surface of the main bronchi in the lung. Forceps attached to the tip of the tube can remove trapped objects or take samples of mucus for examination.

Cheyne-Stokes breathing (chān′stōks) Abnormal breathing pattern sometimes seen just before death (the "death rattle") and in people with combined neurological and cardiac disorders. It consists of bursts of tidal volume breaths (increasing and then decreasing in depth) alternating with periods of apnea. Trauma and hypoxia of the brain stem centers, as well as P_{CO_2} imbalances between arterial blood and brain, may be causative factors.

Deviated septum Condition in which the nasal septum takes a more lateral course than usual and may obstruct breathing; often manifests in old age or from nose trauma.

Endotracheal tube A thin plastic tube threaded into the trachea through the nose or mouth; used to deliver oxygen to patients who are breathing inadequately, in a coma, or under anesthesia.

Epistaxis (ep″ĭ-stak′sis; *epistazo* = to bleed at the nose) Nosebleed; commonly follows trauma to the nose or excessive nose blowing. Most nasal bleeding is from the highly vascularized anterior septum and can be stopped by pinching the nostrils closed or packing them with cotton.

Nasal polyps Mushroomlike benign growths of the nasal mucosa; sometimes caused by infections, but most often cause is unknown. May block air flow.

Orthopnea (or″thop-ne′ah; *ortho* = straight, upright) Inability to breathe in the horizontal (lying down) position.

Otorhinolaryngology (o″to-ri″no-lar″in-gol′o-je; *oto* = ear; *rhino* = nose) Branch of medicine that deals with diagnosis and treatment of diseases of the ears, nose, and throat.

Pneumonia Infectious inflammation of the lungs, in which fluid accumulates in the alveoli; the eighth most common cause of death in the United States. Most of the more than 50 varieties of pneumonia are viral or bacterial.

Pulmonary embolism Obstruction of the pulmonary artery or one of its branches by an embolus (most often a blood clot that has been carried from the lower limbs and through the right side of the heart into the pulmonary circulation). Symptoms are chest pain, productive bloody cough, tachycardia, and rapid, shallow breathing. Can cause sudden death unless treated quickly; usual treatment is oxygen by mask, pain relievers, and anticoagulant drugs. Severe cases may also require clot busters (thrombolytic drugs).

Stuttering A problem of voice production in which the first syllable of words is repeated in "machine-gun" fashion. Primarily a problem with neural control of the larynx and other voice-producing structures. Many stutterers become fluent when whispering or singing, both of which involve a change in the manner of vocalization.

Sudden infant death syndrome (SIDS) Unexpected death of an apparently healthy infant during sleep. Commonly called crib death, SIDS is one of the most frequent causes of death in infants under 1 year old. Believed to be a problem of immaturity of the respiratory control centers. Most cases occur in infants placed in a prone position (on their abdomen) to sleep—a position that may result in hypoxia and hypercapnia due to rebreathing exhaled (CO_2-rich) air. Since 1992, a campaign recommending placing infants on their back to sleep has lowered the incidence of SIDS in the U.S. by 40% or more.

Tracheotomy (tra″ke-ot′o-me) Surgical opening of the trachea; done to provide an alternate route for air to reach the lungs when more superior respiratory passageways are obstructed (as by food or a crushed larynx).

22

Case Study Respiratory System

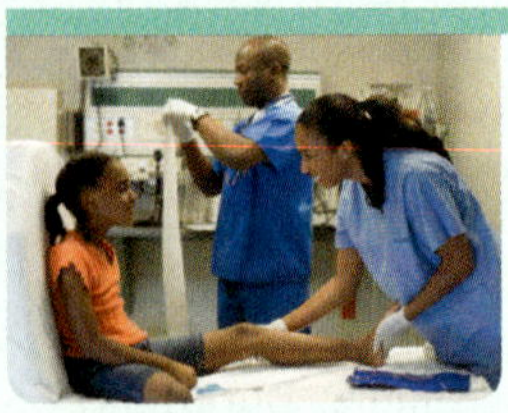

Barbara Joley was in the bus that was hit broadside. When she was freed from the wreckage, she was deeply cyanotic and her respiration had stopped. Her heart was still beating, but her pulse was fast and thready. The emergency medical technician reported that when Barbara was found, her head was cocked at a peculiar angle and it looked like she had a fracture at the level of the C_2 vertebra. The following questions refer to these observations.

1. How might the "peculiar" head position explain Barbara's cessation of breathing?
2. What procedures (do you think) the emergency personnel should have initiated immediately?
3. Why is Barbara cyanotic? Explain cyanosis.
4. Assuming that Barbara survives, how will her accident affect her lifestyle in the future?

Barbara survived transport to the hospital and notes recorded at admission included the following observations.

- Right thorax compressed; ribs 7 to 9 fractured
- Right lung atelectasis

Relative to these notes:

5. What is atelectasis and why is only the right lung affected?
6. How do the recorded injuries relate to the atelectasis?
7. What treatment will be done to reverse the atelectasis? What is the rationale for this treatment?

(Answers in Appendix H)

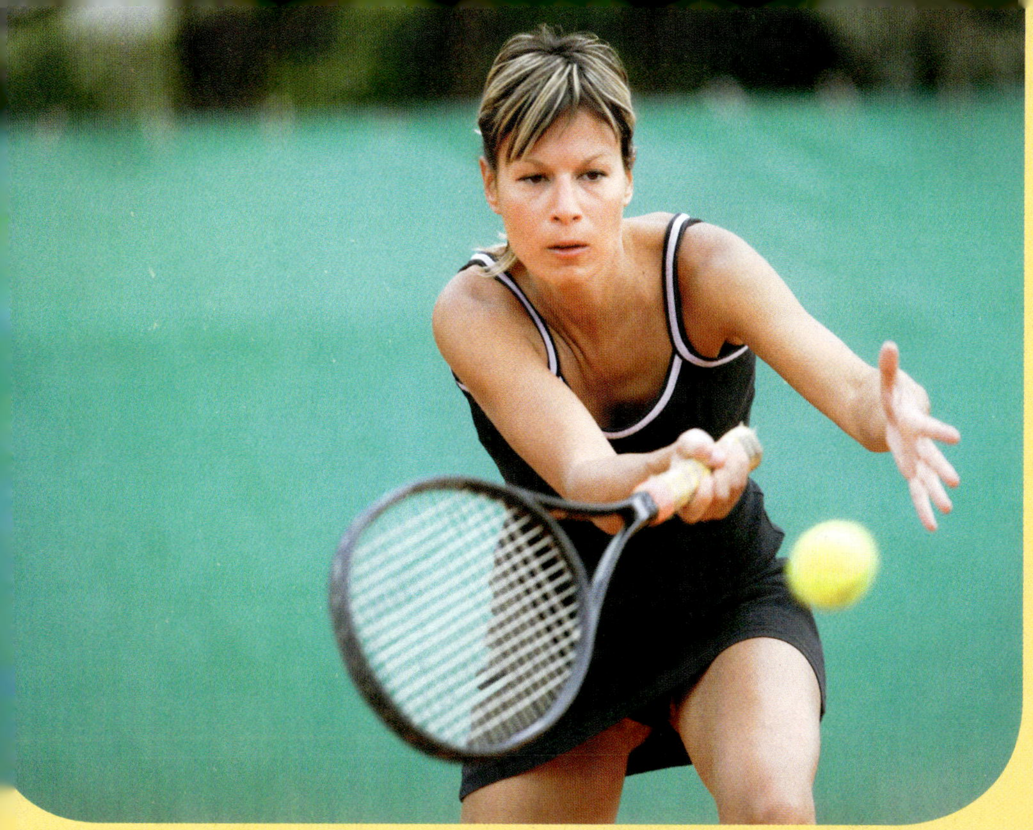

23

The Digestive System

Children are fascinated by the workings of the digestive system. They relish crunching a potato chip, delight in making "mustaches" with milk, and giggle when their stomach "growls." As adults, we know that a healthy digestive system is essential to life, because it converts foods into the raw materials that build and fuel our body's cells. Specifically, the **digestive system** takes in food, breaks it down into nutrient molecules, absorbs these molecules into the bloodstream, and then rids the body of the indigestible remains.

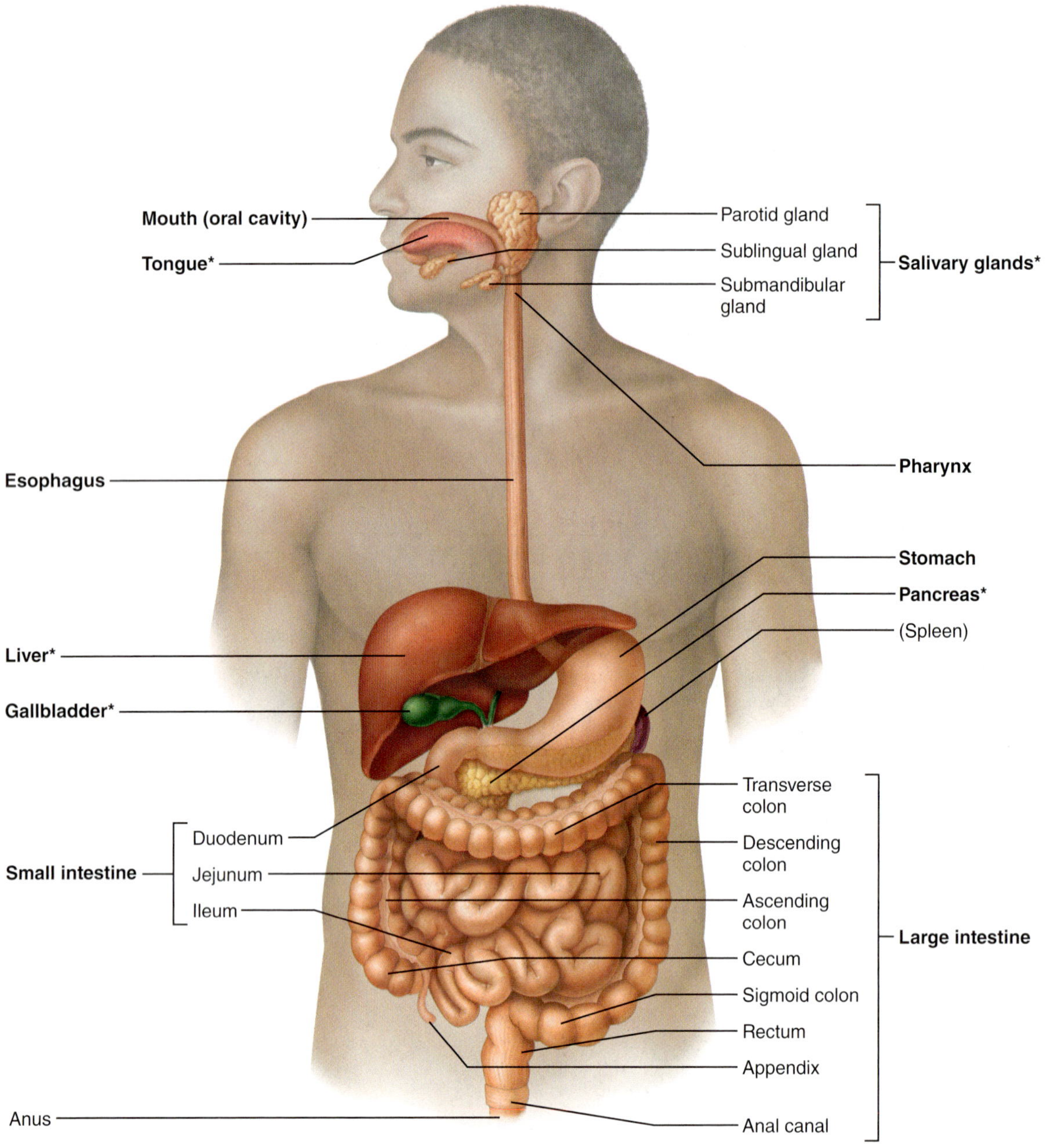

Figure 23.1 Alimentary canal and related accessory digestive organs. Organs with asterisks are accessory organs. Those without asterisks are alimentary canal organs (except the spleen, a part of the lymphatic system). (For a related image, see *A Brief Atlas of the Human Body*, Figure 64a.)

23

PART 1
Overview of the Digestive System

✓ Describe the function of the digestive system, and differentiate between organs of the alimentary canal and accessory digestive organs.

The organs of the digestive system fall into two main groups: (1) those of the *alimentary canal* (al″ĭ-men′tar-e; *aliment* = nourish) and (2) *accessory digestive organs* **(Figure 23.1)**.

The **alimentary canal**, also called the **gastrointestinal (GI) tract** or gut, is the continuous muscular tube that winds through the body from the mouth to the anus. It **digests** food—breaks it down into smaller fragments (*digest* = dissolve)—and **absorbs** the digested fragments through its lining into the blood.

The organs of the alimentary canal are the *mouth, pharynx, esophagus, stomach, small intestine,* and *large intestine.* The large intestine leads to the terminal opening, or *anus.* In a cadaver, the alimentary canal is approximately 9 m (about 30 ft) long, but in a living person, it is considerably shorter because of its muscle tone. Food material in this tube is technically outside the body because the canal is open to the external environment at both ends.

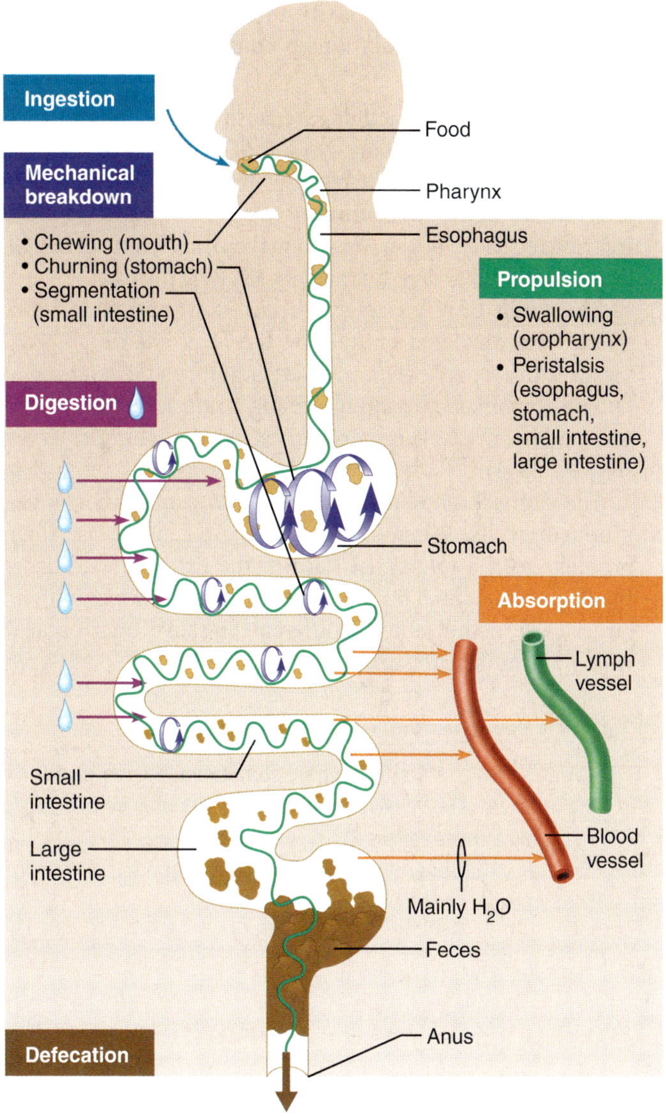

Figure 23.2 Gastrointestinal tract activities. Note that sites of digestion produce enzymes or receive enzymes or other secretions made by accessory organs outside the alimentary canal.

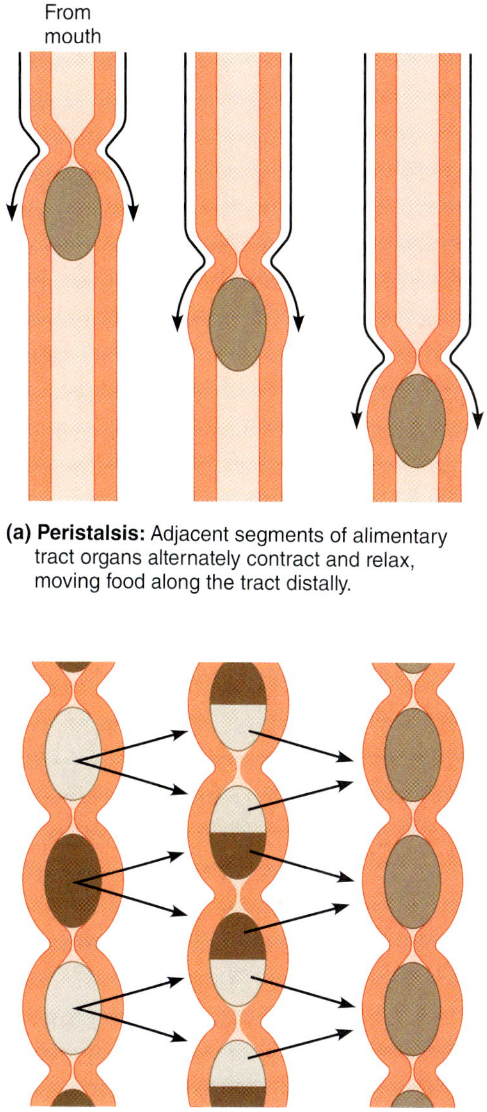

(a) Peristalsis: Adjacent segments of alimentary tract organs alternately contract and relax, moving food along the tract distally.

(b) Segmentation: Nonadjacent segments of alimentary tract organs alternately contract and relax, moving food forward then backward. Food mixing and slow food propulsion occur.

Figure 23.3 Peristalsis and segmentation.

The **accessory digestive organs** are the *teeth*, *tongue*, *gallbladder*, and a number of large digestive glands—the *salivary glands*, *liver*, and *pancreas*. The teeth and tongue are in the mouth, or oral cavity, while the digestive glands and gallbladder lie outside the GI tract and connect to it by ducts. The accessory digestive glands produce a variety of secretions that help break down foodstuffs.

Digestive Processes

✓ List and define the major processes occurring during digestive system activity.

We can view the digestive tract as a "disassembly line" in which food becomes less complex at each step of processing and its nutrients become available to the body. The processing of food by the digestive system involves six essential activities **(Figure 23.2)**:

1. **Ingestion** is simply taking food into the digestive tract, usually via the mouth.
2. **Propulsion**, which moves food through the alimentary canal, includes *swallowing*, which is initiated voluntarily, and *peristalsis* (per″ĭ-stal′sis), an involuntary process. **Peristalsis** (*peri* = around; *stalsis* = constriction), the major means of propulsion, involves alternating waves of contraction and relaxation of muscles in the organ walls **(Figure 23.3a)**. Its main effect is to squeeze food along the tract, but some mixing occurs as well. In fact, peristaltic waves are so powerful that, once swallowed, food and fluids will reach your stomach even if you stand on your head.
3. **Mechanical breakdown** increases the surface area of ingested food, physically preparing it for digestion by enzymes. Mechanical processes include chewing, mixing food with saliva by the tongue, churning food in the

23

stomach, and **segmentation**, or rhythmic local constrictions of the small intestine (Figure 23.3b). Segmentation mixes food with digestive juices and makes absorption more efficient by repeatedly moving different parts of the food mass over the intestinal wall. Although mechanical breakdown is sometimes referred to as *mechanical digestion*, historically the term digestion applies only to chemical breakdown processes that utilize enzymes.

4. **Digestion** involves a series of catabolic steps in which enzymes secreted into the lumen (cavity) of the alimentary canal break down complex food molecules to their chemical building blocks.
5. **Absorption** is the passage of digested end products (plus vitamins, minerals, and water) from the lumen of the GI tract through the mucosal cells by active or passive transport into the blood or lymph.
6. **Defecation** eliminates indigestible substances from the body via the anus in the form of feces.

Some of these processes are the job of a single organ. For example, only the mouth ingests and only the large intestine defecates. But most digestive system activities require the cooperation of several organs and occur bit by bit as food moves along the tract as described later.

☑ Check Your Understanding

1. Name one organ of the alimentary canal found in the thorax. Name three organs located in the abdominal cavity.
2. What is the usual site of ingestion?
3. Which digestive system activity actually moves nutrients from the outside to the inside of the body?

For answers, see Appendix H.

23

Basic Functional Concepts

✓ Describe stimuli and controls of digestive activity.

A theme we have stressed in this book is the body's efforts to maintain a constant internal environment. Most organ systems respond to changes in that environment either by attempting to restore some plasma variable to its former levels or by changing their own function.

The digestive system, however, creates an optimal environment for its functioning in the lumen of the GI tract, an area that is actually *outside* the body. Essentially all digestive tract regulatory mechanisms control luminal conditions so that food breakdown and absorption can occur there as effectively as possible.

Two facts apply to these regulatory mechanisms:

- **Digestive activity is provoked by a range of mechanical and chemical stimuli.** Sensors involved in controlling GI tract activity are located in the walls of the tract organs. These sensors respond to several stimuli, most importantly stretching of the organ by food in the lumen, osmolarity (solute concentration) and pH of the contents, and the presence of substrates and end products of digestion. When stimulated, these receptors initiate reflexes that (1) activate or inhibit glands that secrete digestive juices into the lumen or hormones into the blood or (2) stimulate smooth muscle of the GI tract walls to mix lumen contents and move them along the tract.
- **Controls of digestive activity are both intrinsic and extrinsic.** Many of the controlling systems of the digestive tract are *intrinsic*—"in-house" nerve plexuses and hormone-producing cells. The so-called **gut brain** consisting of enteric nerve plexuses spreads like chicken wire along the entire length of the GI tract and regulates digestive activity all along the tract.

  Two kinds of reflex activity occur, short and long. *Short reflexes* are mediated entirely by the local *enteric* or "gut" plexuses in response to stimuli arising in the GI tract. *Long reflexes* are initiated by stimuli arising inside or outside the GI tract and involve CNS centers and extrinsic autonomic nerves (Figure 23.4).

  The stomach and small intestine also contain hormone-producing cells. When stimulated, these cells release their products to the interstitial fluid in the extracellular space. Blood and interstitial fluid distribute these hormones to their target cells in the same or different digestive tract organs, which they induce to secrete or contract.

☑ Check Your Understanding

4. When sensors in the GI tract are stimulated, they respond via reflexes. What types of digestive activity may be put into motion via those reflexes?
5. The term "gut brain" does not really mean there is a brain in the digestive system. What does it refer to?

For answers, see Appendix H.

Digestive System Organs: Relationships

Relationship of the Digestive Organs to the Peritoneum

✓ Describe the location and function of the peritoneum.

✓ Define retroperitoneal and name the retroperitoneal organs of the digestive system.

Most digestive system organs reside in the abdominopelvic cavity. Recall from Chapter 1 that all ventral body cavities contain slippery *serous membranes*. The **peritoneum** of the abdominopelvic cavity is the most extensive of these membranes (Figure 23.5a). The **visceral peritoneum** covers the external surfaces of most digestive organs and is continuous with the **parietal peritoneum** that lines the body wall (see Figure 23.30d, p. 889). Between the two peritoneums is the **peritoneal cavity**, a slitlike potential space containing a slippery fluid secreted by the serous membranes. The serous fluid lubricates the mobile digestive organs, allowing them to glide easily across one another and along the body wall as they carry out their activities.

A **mesentery** (mes′en-ter″e) is a double layer of peritoneum—a sheet of two serous membranes fused back to back—that extends to the digestive organs from the body wall. Mesenteries provide routes for blood vessels, lymphatics, and nerves to reach

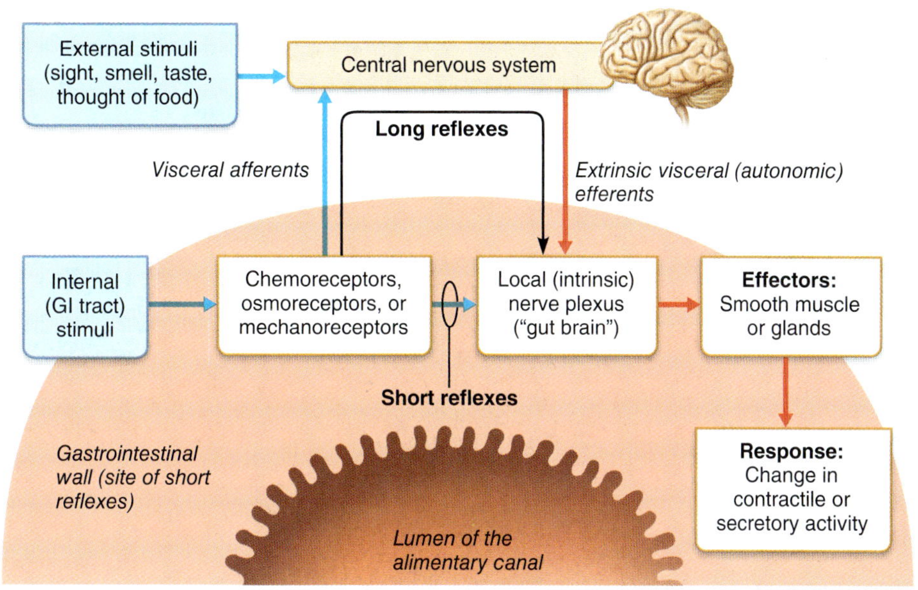

Figure 23.4 Neural reflex pathways initiated by stimuli inside or outside the gastrointestinal tract.

the digestive viscera; hold organs in place; and store fat. In most places the mesentery is *dorsal* and attaches to the posterior abdominal wall, but there are *ventral* mesenteries too, such as the one that extends from the liver to the anterior abdominal wall (Figure 23.5a). Some digestive organ mesenteries have specific names (such as the *omenta*), or are called "ligaments" (even though these peritoneal folds are nothing like the fibrous ligaments that connect bones).

Not all alimentary canal organs are suspended by a mesentery. For example, during development, some regions of the small intestine adhere to the dorsal abdominal wall (Figure 23.5b). In so doing, they lose their mesentery and come to lie posterior to the peritoneum. These organs, which include most of the pancreas and duodenum (the first part of the small intestine), and parts of the large intestine, are called **retroperitoneal organs** (*retro* = behind). By contrast, digestive organs (like the stomach) that keep their mesentery and remain in the peritoneal cavity are called **intraperitoneal** or **peritoneal organs**.

Homeostatic Imbalance 23.1

Peritonitis is inflammation of the peritoneum. It can arise from a piercing abdominal wound, a perforating ulcer that leaks stomach juices into the peritoneal cavity, or poor sterile technique during abdominal surgery. However, most commonly it results from a burst appendix that sprays bacteria-containing

23

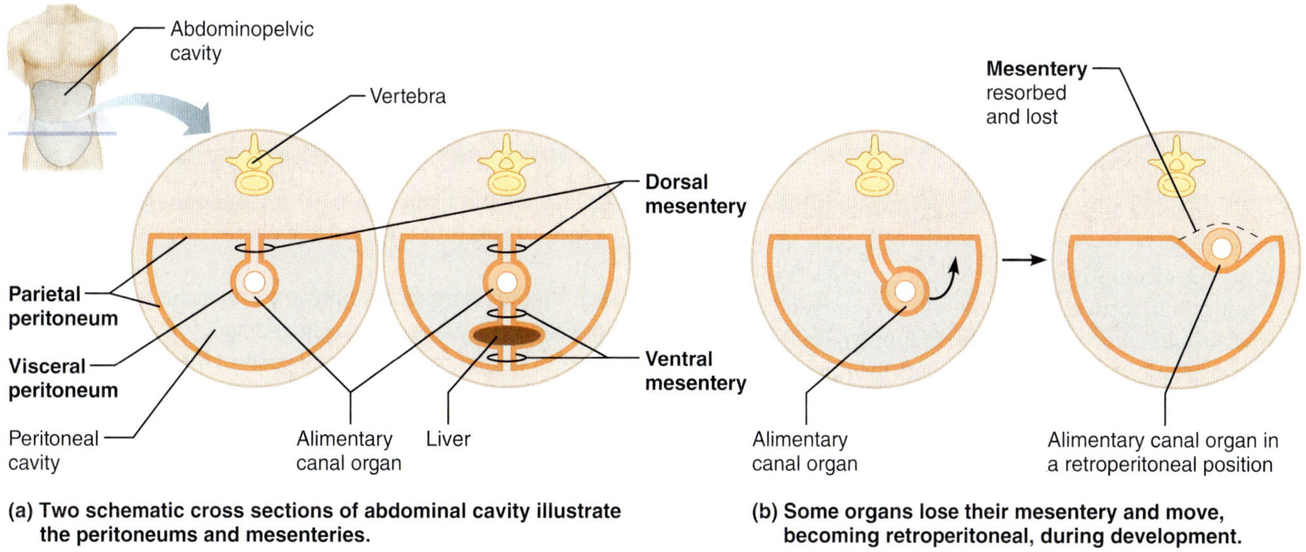

Figure 23.5 The peritoneum and the peritoneal cavity. Note that the peritoneal cavity is much smaller than depicted here.

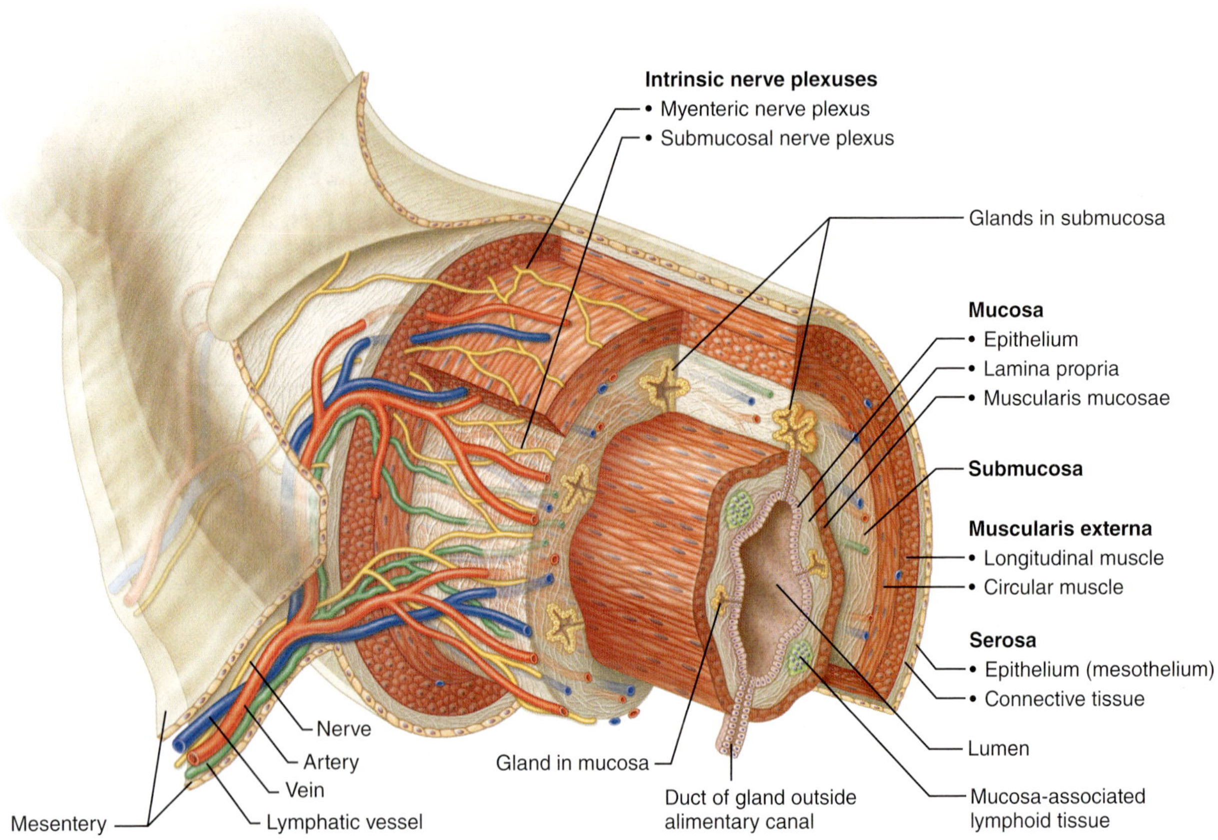

Figure 23.6 Basic structure of the alimentary canal. Its four basic layers are the mucosa, submucosa, muscularis externa, and serosa.

feces all over the peritoneum. In peritonitis, the peritoneal coverings tend to stick together around the infection site. This localizes the infection, providing time for macrophages to prevent the inflammation from spreading.

If peritonitis becomes widespread within the peritoneal cavity, it is dangerous and often lethal. Treatment includes removing as much infectious debris as possible and administering megadoses of antibiotics. +

Blood Supply: The Splanchnic Circulation

✓ Define splanchnic circulation.

✓ Indicate the importance of the hepatic portal system.

The **splanchnic circulation** includes those arteries that branch off the abdominal aorta to serve the digestive organs and the *hepatic portal circulation*. The arterial supply—the branches of the celiac trunk that serve the spleen, liver, and stomach, and the mesenteric arteries that serve the small and large intestines (see pp. 875 and 887)—normally receives one-quarter of the cardiac output. This percentage increases after a meal. The hepatic portal circulation (pp. 742–743) collects nutrient-rich venous blood draining from the digestive viscera and delivers it to the liver.

☑ Check Your Understanding

6. How does the location of the visceral peritoneum differ from that of the parietal peritoneum?
7. Of the following organs, which is/are retroperitoneal? Stomach, pancreas, liver.
8. What name is given to the venous portion of the splanchnic circulation?

For answers, see Appendix H.

Histology of the Alimentary Canal

✓ Describe the tissue composition and general function of each of the four layers of the alimentary canal.

Each digestive organ has only a share of the work of digestion. Consequently, it helps to consider structural characteristics that promote similar functions in all parts of the alimentary canal before we consider the functional anatomy of each digestive organ.

From the esophagus to the anal canal, the walls of the alimentary canal have the same four basic layers, or *tunics—mucosa, submucosa, muscularis externa*, and *serosa* **(Figure 23.6)**. Each layer contains a predominant tissue type that plays a specific role in food breakdown.

The Mucosa

The **mucosa**, or **mucous membrane**—the innermost layer—is a moist epithelial membrane that lines the alimentary canal lumen from mouth to anus. Its major functions are to:

- *Secrete* mucus, digestive enzymes, and hormones
- *Absorb* the end products of digestion into the blood
- *Protect* against infectious disease

The mucosa in a particular region of the GI tract may perform one or all three of these functions.

More complex than most other mucosae in the body, the typical digestive mucosa consists of three sublayers: (1) a lining epithelium, (2) a lamina propria, and (3) a muscularis mucosae. Except for that of the mouth, esophagus, and anus where it is stratified squamous, the **epithelium** of the mucosa is a *simple columnar epithelium* rich in mucus-secreting cells. The slippery mucus it produces protects certain digestive organs from being digested by enzymes working within their cavities and eases food passage along the tract. In the stomach and small intestine, the mucosa also contains both enzyme-synthesizing and hormone-secreting cells. In such sites, the mucosa is a diffuse kind of endocrine organ as well as part of the digestive organ.

The **lamina propria** (*proprius* = one's own), which underlies the epithelium, is loose areolar connective tissue. Its capillaries nourish the epithelium and absorb digested nutrients. Its isolated lymphoid follicles, part of **MALT** (the mucosa-associated lymphoid tissue described on p. 759), help defend us against bacteria and other pathogens, which have rather free access to our digestive tract. Particularly large collections of lymphoid follicles occur within the pharynx (as the tonsils) and in the appendix.

External to the lamina propria is the **muscularis mucosae**, a scant layer of smooth muscle cells that produces local movements of the mucosa. In the small intestine, this muscle layer's tone throws the mucosa into a series of small folds that immensely increase its surface area.

The Submucosa

The **submucosa**, just external to the mucosa, is areolar connective tissue containing a rich supply of blood and lymphatic vessels, lymphoid follicles, and nerve fibers which supply the surrounding tissues of the GI tract wall. Its abundant elastic fibers enable the stomach to regain its normal shape after temporarily storing a large meal.

The Muscularis Externa

Surrounding the submucosa is the **muscularis externa**, also simply called the **muscularis**. This layer is responsible for segmentation and peristalsis. It typically has an inner *circular layer* and an outer *longitudinal layer* of smooth muscle cells (see Figures 4.9c and 23.6). In several places along the tract, the circular layer thickens, forming *sphincters* that act as valves to control food passage from one organ to the next and prevent backflow.

The Serosa

The **serosa**, the outermost layer of the intraperitoneal organs, is the *visceral peritoneum*. In most alimentary canal organs, it is formed of areolar connective tissue covered with *mesothelium*, a single layer of squamous epithelial cells (see Figures 4.8a and 4.3a, respectively).

In the esophagus, which is located in the thoracic instead of the abdominopelvic cavity, the serosa is replaced by an **adventitia** (ad″ven-tish′e-ah), ordinary fibrous connective tissue that binds the esophagus to surrounding structures. Retroperitoneal organs have *both* a serosa (on the side facing the peritoneal cavity) and an adventitia (on the side abutting the dorsal body wall).

Enteric Nervous System of the Alimentary Canal

As we noted earlier, the alimentary canal has its own in-house nerve supply, staffed by the so-called **enteric neurons** (*enter* = gut), which communicate widely with one another to regulate digestive system activity. These semiautonomous enteric neurons constitute the bulk of the two major *intrinsic nerve plexuses* (ganglia interconnected by unmyelinated fiber tracts) found in the walls of the alimentary canal: the submucosal and myenteric nerve plexuses (Figure 23.6).

The **submucosal nerve plexus** occupies the submucosa whereas the large **myenteric nerve plexus** (mi-en-ter′ik; "intestinal muscle") lies between the circular and longitudinal muscle layers of the muscularis externa. Enteric neurons of these plexuses provide the major nerve supply to the GI tract wall and control GI tract motility (motion). Control of the patterns of segmentation and peristalsis is largely automatic, involving pacemaker cells and local reflex arcs between enteric neurons in the same or different organs.

The enteric nervous system is also linked to the central nervous system by (1) afferent visceral fibers and (2) sympathetic and parasympathetic branches (motor fibers) of the autonomic nervous system that enter the intestinal wall and synapse with neurons in the intrinsic plexuses. Hence, extrinsic controls—exerted by autonomic fibers via long reflex arcs—also regulate digestive activity (see Figure 23.4). Generally speaking, parasympathetic inputs enhance digestive activities, whereas sympathetic impulses inhibit them.

But the largely independent enteric ganglia are much more than just way stations for the autonomic nervous system. Indeed, the enteric nervous system contains over 100 million neurons, more than the entire spinal cord.

Check Your Understanding

9. Name the layers of the alimentary canal from the inside out.
10. Jerry has been given a drug that inhibits parasympathetic stimulation of his digestive tract. Should he "eat hearty" or temporarily refrain from eating, and why?

For answers, see Appendix H.

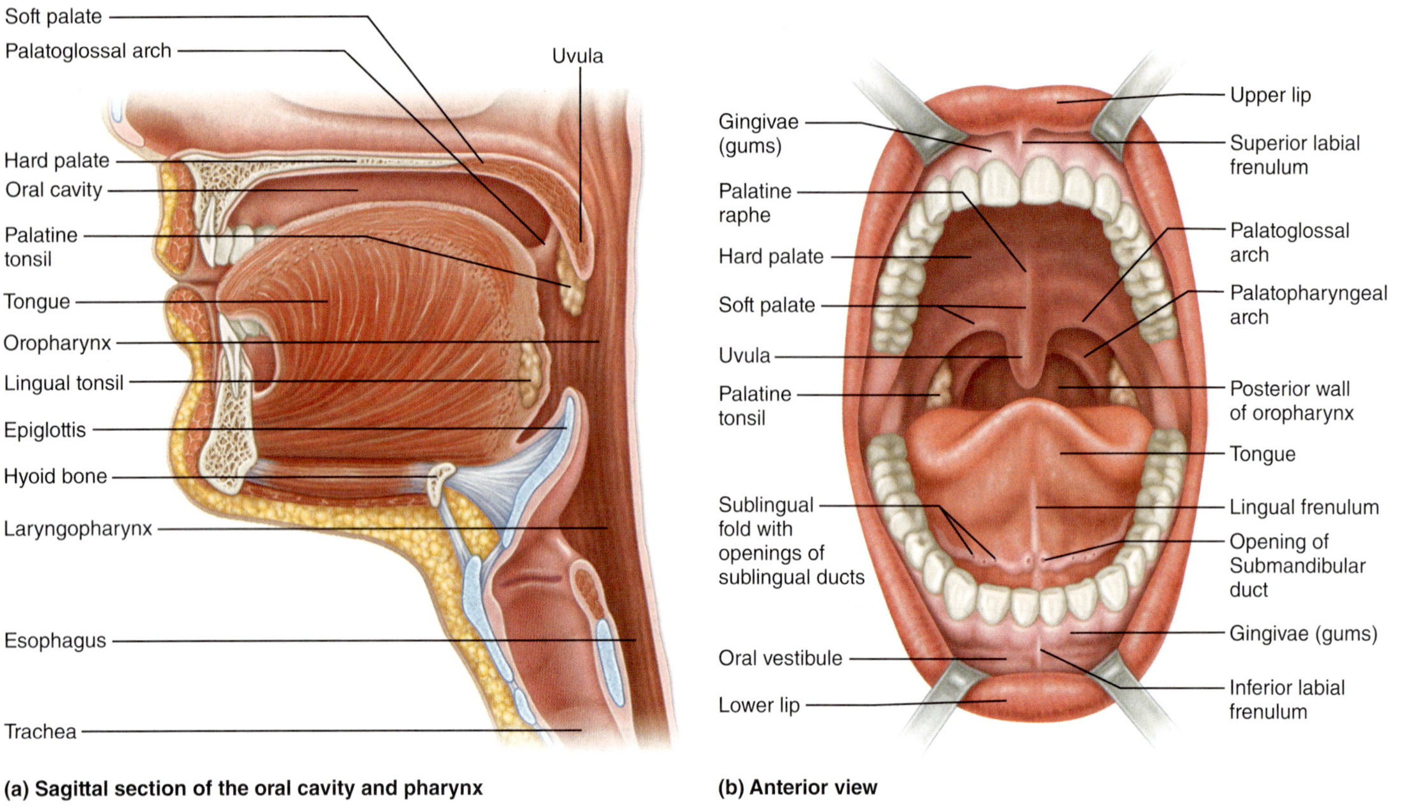

Figure 23.7 **Anatomy of the oral cavity (mouth).**

23

PART 2
Functional Anatomy of the Digestive System

Now that we have summarized some points that unify the digestive system organs, let's consider the special structural and functional capabilities of each organ of this system. Figure 23.1 shows most of these organs in their normal body positions, so you may find it helpful to refer back to that illustration from time to time as you read the following sections.

The Mouth and Associated Organs

- ✓ Describe the gross and microscopic anatomy and the basic functions of the mouth, pharynx, and esophagus.
- ✓ Describe the composition and functions of saliva, and explain how salivation is regulated.
- ✓ Explain the dental formula and differentiate clearly between deciduous and permanent teeth.

The mouth is the only part of the alimentary canal involved in ingestion. However, most digestive functions associated with the mouth reflect the activity of the related accessory organs, such as teeth, salivary glands, and tongue. In the mouth we chew food and mix it with saliva containing enzymes that begin the process of digestion. The mouth also begins the propulsive process of swallowing, which carries food through the pharynx and esophagus to the stomach.

The Mouth

The **mouth** is also called the **oral cavity**, or *buccal cavity* (buk′al). Its boundaries are the lips anteriorly, cheeks laterally, palate superiorly, and tongue inferiorly **(Figure 23.7)**. Its anterior opening is the **oral orifice**. Posteriorly, the oral cavity is continuous with the *oropharynx*.

The walls of the mouth are lined with a thick stratified squamous epithelium (see Figure 4.3e) which withstands considerable friction. The epithelium on the gums, hard palate, and dorsum of the tongue is slightly keratinized for extra protection against abrasion during eating. Like all moist surface linings, the oral mucosa responds to injury by producing antimicrobial peptides called *defensins,* which helps to explain how the mouth—a site teeming with disease-causing microbes—remains so remarkably healthy.

The Lips and Cheeks

The **lips** (**labia**) and the **cheeks**, which help keep food between the teeth when we chew, are composed of a core of skeletal muscle covered externally by skin. The *orbicularis oris muscle* forms the fleshy lips; the cheeks are formed largely by the *buccinators*. The recess bounded externally by the lips and cheeks and internally by the gums and teeth is the **oral vestibule** ("porch"). The area that lies within the teeth and gums is the **oral cavity proper.** The **labial frenulum** (fren′u-lum) is a median fold that joins the internal aspect of each lip to the gum (Figure 23.7b).

The Palate

The **palate**, forming the roof of the mouth, has two distinct parts: the hard palate anteriorly and the soft palate posteriorly (Figure 23.7). The **hard palate** is underlain by the palatine bones and the palatine processes of the maxillae, and it forms a rigid surface against which the tongue forces food during chewing. The mucosa on either side of its *raphe* (ra′fe), a midline ridge, is slightly corrugated, which helps create friction.

The **soft palate** is a mobile fold formed mostly of skeletal muscle that rises reflexively to close off the nasopharynx when we swallow.

- To demonstrate this action, try to breathe and swallow at the same time.

Laterally, the soft palate is anchored to the tongue by the **palatoglossal arches** and to the wall of the oropharynx by the more posterior **palatopharyngeal arches**. These two paired folds form the boundaries of the **fauces** (faw′sēz; *fauc* = throat), the arched area of the oropharynx that contains the palatine tonsils. Projecting downward from the free edge of the soft palate is the fingerlike **uvula** (u′vu-lah).

The Tongue

The **tongue** occupies the floor of the mouth (Figure 23.7). The tongue is composed of interlacing bundles of skeletal muscle fibers, and during chewing, it grips the food and constantly repositions it between the teeth. The tongue also mixes food with saliva forming it into a compact mass called a **bolus** (bo′lus; "a lump"), and then initiates swallowing by pushing the bolus posteriorly into the pharynx. The versatile tongue also helps us form consonants (k, d, t, and so on) when we speak.

The tongue has both intrinsic and extrinsic skeletal muscle fibers. The **intrinsic muscles** are confined in the tongue and are not attached to bone. Their muscle fibers, which run in several different planes, allow the tongue to change its shape (but not its position), becoming thicker, thinner, longer, or shorter as needed for speech and swallowing.

The **extrinsic muscles** extend to the tongue from their points of origin on bones of the skull or the soft palate, as described in Chapter 10 (see Table 10.2 and Figure 10.8). The extrinsic muscles alter the tongue's position. They protrude it, retract it, and move it from side to side. The tongue has a median septum of connective tissue, and each half contains identical muscle groups. A fold of mucosa called the **lingual frenulum** secures the tongue to the floor of the mouth and limits its posterior movements.

Homeostatic Imbalance 23.2

Children born with an extremely short lingual frenulum are often referred to as "tongue-tied" because restricted tongue movement distorts speech. This congenital condition, called *ankyloglossia* ("fused tongue"), is corrected surgically by snipping the frenulum. ✚

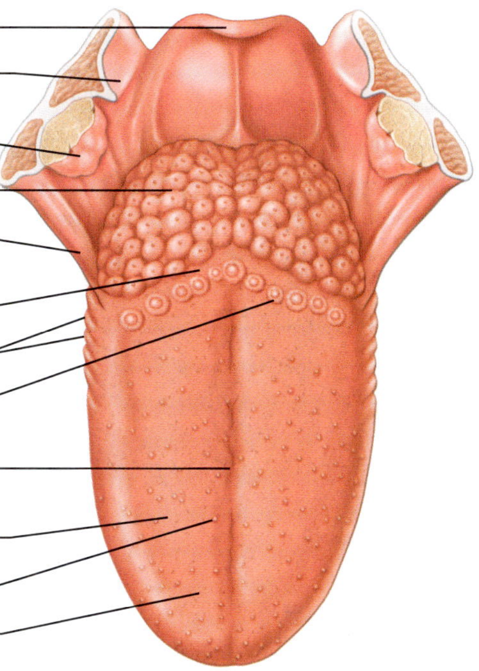

Figure 23.8 Dorsal surface of the tongue, and the tonsils.

The superior tongue surface bears papillae, peglike projections of the underlying mucosa **(Figure 23.8)**. The conical **filiform papillae** roughen the tongue surface, helping us lick semisolid foods (such as ice cream) and providing friction for manipulating foods. These papillae, the smallest and most numerous type, align in parallel rows on the tongue dorsum. They contain keratin, which stiffens them and gives the tongue its whitish appearance. The mushroom-shaped **fungiform papillae** are scattered widely over the tongue surface. Each has a vascular core that gives it a reddish hue. Ten to twelve large **vallate papillae** are located in a V-shaped row at the back of the tongue. They resemble the fungiform papillae but have an additional surrounding furrow. Pleatlike **foliate papillae** are located on the lateral aspects of the posterior tongue.

The fungiform, vallate, and foliate papillae house taste buds, but those on the foliate papillae function in taste primarily in infancy and early childhood. Serous cells just beneath the foliate and vallate papillae secrete *lingual lipase,* a fat-digesting enzyme that operates in the acid environment of the stomach.

Immediately posterior to the vallate papillae is the **terminal sulcus**, a groove that distinguishes the portion of the tongue that lies in the oral cavity (its body) from its posterior portion in the oropharynx (its root). The mucosa covering the root of the tongue lacks papillae, but it is still bumpy because of the nodular *lingual tonsil*, which lies just deep to its mucosa (Figure 23.8).

☑ Check Your Understanding

11. How does the oral vestibule differ from the oral cavity proper?
12. Which structure forms the roof of the mouth?
13. Besides preparing food for swallowing, the tongue has another role. What is it?

For answers, see Appendix H.

23

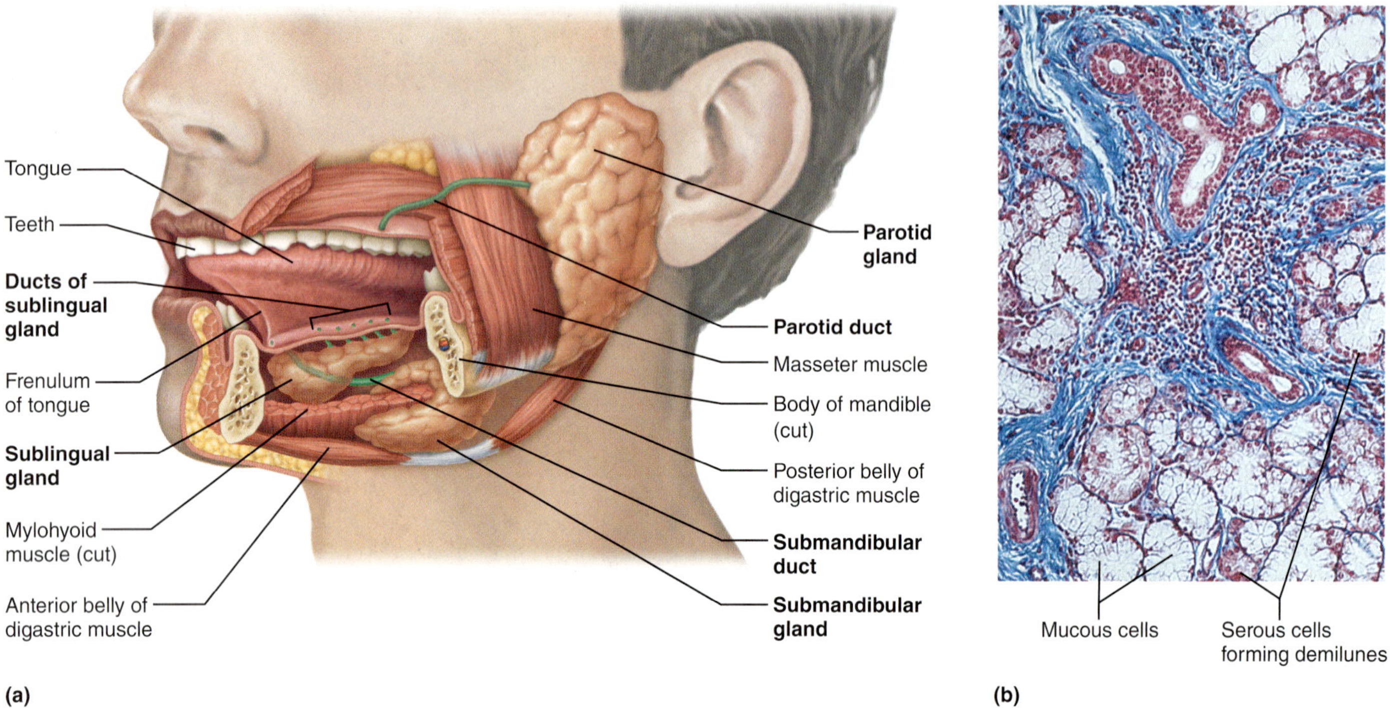

Figure 23.9 The salivary glands. (a) The parotid, submandibular, and sublingual glands associated with the left aspect of the oral cavity. **(b)** Photomicrograph of the sublingual gland (150×), which is a mixed salivary gland. Mucus-producing cells stain light blue and serous-secreting units stain purple. The serous cells sometimes form demilunes around the bases of the mucous cells.

The Salivary Glands

A number of glands associated with the oral cavity secrete **saliva**. Saliva:

- Cleanses the mouth
- Dissolves food chemicals so they can be tasted
- Moistens food and helps compact it into a bolus
- Contains enzymes that begin the chemical breakdown of starchy foods

23

Most saliva is produced by the **major** or **extrinsic salivary glands** that lie outside the oral cavity and empty their secretions into it. **Minor** or **intrinsic salivary glands** (buccal glands and others) scattered throughout the oral cavity mucosa augment the output slightly.

The major salivary glands are paired compound tubuloalveolar glands that develop from the oral mucosa and remain connected to it by ducts **(Figure 23.9a)**. The large, roughly triangular **parotid gland** (pah-rot′id; *par* = near, *otid* = the ear) lies anterior to the ear between the masseter muscle and the skin. Its prominent duct parallels the zygomatic arch, pierces the buccinator muscle, and opens into the vestibule next to the second upper molar.

Branches of the facial nerve run through the parotid gland on their way to the muscles of facial expression. For this reason, surgery on this gland can result in facial paralysis.

Homeostatic Imbalance 23.3

Mumps, a common children's disease, is an inflammation of the parotid glands caused by the mumps virus (*myxovirus*), which spreads from person to person in saliva. If you check the location of the parotid glands in Figure 23.9a, you can understand why people with mumps complain that it hurts to open their mouth or chew. Other signs and symptoms include moderate fever and pain when swallowing acid foods (pickles, grapefruit juice, etc.). Mumps in adult males carries a 25% risk of infecting the testes too, leading to sterility. +

About the size of a walnut, the **submandibular gland** lies along the medial aspect of the mandibular body. Its duct runs beneath the mucosa of the oral cavity floor and opens at the base of the lingual frenulum (see Figure 23.7b). The small, almond-shaped **sublingual gland** lies anterior to the submandibular gland under the tongue and opens via 10–20 ducts into the floor of the mouth (Figure 23.9a).

The salivary glands are composed of two types of secretory cells: serous and mucous (Figure 23.9b). **Serous cells** produce a watery secretion containing enzymes, ions, and a tiny bit of mucin, whereas **mucous cells** produce **mucus**, a stringy, viscous solution. The parotid and submandibular glands contain mostly serous cells. Buccal glands have approximately equal numbers of serous and mucous cells. The sublingual glands contain mostly mucous cells.

Composition of Saliva

Saliva is largely water—97 to 99.5%—and therefore is hypo-osmotic. Its osmolarity depends on the specific glands that are active and the stimulus for salivation. As a rule, saliva is slightly acidic (pH 6.75 to 7.00), but its pH may vary. Its solutes include electrolytes (Na^+, K^+, Cl^-, PO_4^{3-}, and HCO_3^-); the digestive enzymes salivary amylase and lingual lipase (both optimally active at an acid pH); the proteins mucin, lysozyme, and IgA; and metabolic wastes (urea and uric acid). When dissolved in water, the glycoprotein *mucin* forms thick mucus that lubricates the oral cavity and hydrates foodstuffs.

Saliva protects against microorganisms because it contains (1) *IgA antibodies*; (2) *lysozyme*, a bactericidal enzyme that inhibits bacterial growth in the mouth and may help prevent tooth decay; and (3) *defensins* (see p. 641). Besides acting as a local antibiotic, defensins function as cytokines to call defensive cells (lymphocytes, neutrophils, etc.) into the mouth for battle.

In addition to these three protectors, the friendly bacteria that live on the back of the tongue promote the conversion of food-derived nitrates in saliva into *nitric oxide* (NO) in an acid environment. This transformation occurs around the gums, where acid-producing bacteria tend to cluster, and in the hydrochloric acid–rich secretions of the stomach. The highly toxic nitric oxide is believed to be bactericidal in these locations.

Control of Salivation

The minor salivary glands secrete saliva continuously in amounts just sufficient to keep the mouth moist. But when food enters the mouth, the major glands are activated and copious amounts of saliva pour out. The average output of saliva is about 1500 ml per day, but can be much higher when salivary glands are appropriately stimulated.

Salivation is controlled primarily by the parasympathetic division of the autonomic nervous system. When we ingest food, chemoreceptors and mechanoreceptors in the mouth send signals to the **salivatory nuclei** in the brain stem (pons and medulla). As a result, parasympathetic nervous system activity increases. Impulses sent via motor fibers in the *facial* (VII) and *glossopharyngeal* (IX) *nerves* dramatically increase the output of watery (serous), enzyme-rich saliva.

The chemoreceptors are activated most strongly by acidic substances such as vinegar and citrus juice. The mechanoreceptors are activated by virtually any mechanical stimulus in the mouth—even chewing rubber bands.

Sometimes just the sight or smell of food is enough to get the juices flowing. The mere thought of hot fudge sauce on peppermint ice cream will make many a mouth water! Irritation of the lower GI tract by bacterial toxins, spicy foods, or hyperacidity also increases salivation. This response may help wash away or neutralize the irritants.

In contrast to parasympathetic controls, the sympathetic division (specifically fibers in T_1–T_3) causes release of a thick, mucin-rich saliva. Strong activation of the sympathetic division constricts blood vessels serving the salivary glands and almost completely inhibits saliva release, causing a dry mouth (*xerostomia*; *xero* = dry). Dehydration also inhibits salivation because low blood volume reduces filtration pressure at capillary beds.

Homeostatic Imbalance 23.4

Anything that inhibits saliva secretion promotes tooth decay and makes it difficult to talk and eat. Decomposing food particles accumulate and bacteria flourish, resulting in *halitosis* (hal″ĭ-to′sis; "bad breath"). The odor is caused mainly by the metabolic activity of anaerobic protein-digesting bacteria at the back of the tongue that yields hydrogen sulfide (rotten egg smell), and methyl mercaptan (also in feces), cadaverine (associated with rotting corpses), and other smelly chemicals. ✚

Check Your Understanding

14. What is the importance of the serous portion of saliva?
15. Name three antimicrobial substances found in saliva.

For answers, see Appendix H.

The Teeth

The **teeth** lie in sockets (alveoli) in the gum-covered margins of the mandible and maxilla. The role of the teeth in food processing needs little introduction. We *masticate*, or chew, by opening and closing our jaws and moving them from side to side while using our tongue to move the food between our teeth. In the process, the teeth tear and grind the food, physically breaking it down into smaller fragments.

Dentition and the Dental Formula

Ordinarily by age 21, two sets of teeth, the **primary** and **permanent dentitions**, have formed **(Figure 23.10)**. The primary dentition consists of the **deciduous teeth** (de-sid′u-us; *decid* = falling off), also called **milk** or **baby teeth**. The first teeth to appear, at about age 6 months, are the lower central incisors. Additional pairs of teeth erupt at one- to two-month intervals until about 24 months, when all 20 milk teeth have emerged.

As the deep-lying **permanent teeth** enlarge and develop, the roots of the milk teeth are resorbed from below, causing them to loosen and fall out between ages 6 and 12. Generally, all the permanent teeth but the third molars have erupted by the end of adolescence. The third molars, also called *wisdom teeth*, emerge between ages 17 and 25. There are usually 32 permanent teeth in a full set, but sometimes the wisdom teeth never erupt or are completely absent.

Homeostatic Imbalance 23.5

When a tooth remains embedded in the jawbone, it is said to be *impacted*. Impacted teeth can cause a good deal of pressure and pain and must be removed surgically. Wisdom teeth are most commonly involved. ✚

Teeth are classified according to their shape and function as incisors, canines, premolars, and molars (Figure 23.10). The chisel-shaped **incisors** are adapted for cutting or nipping off

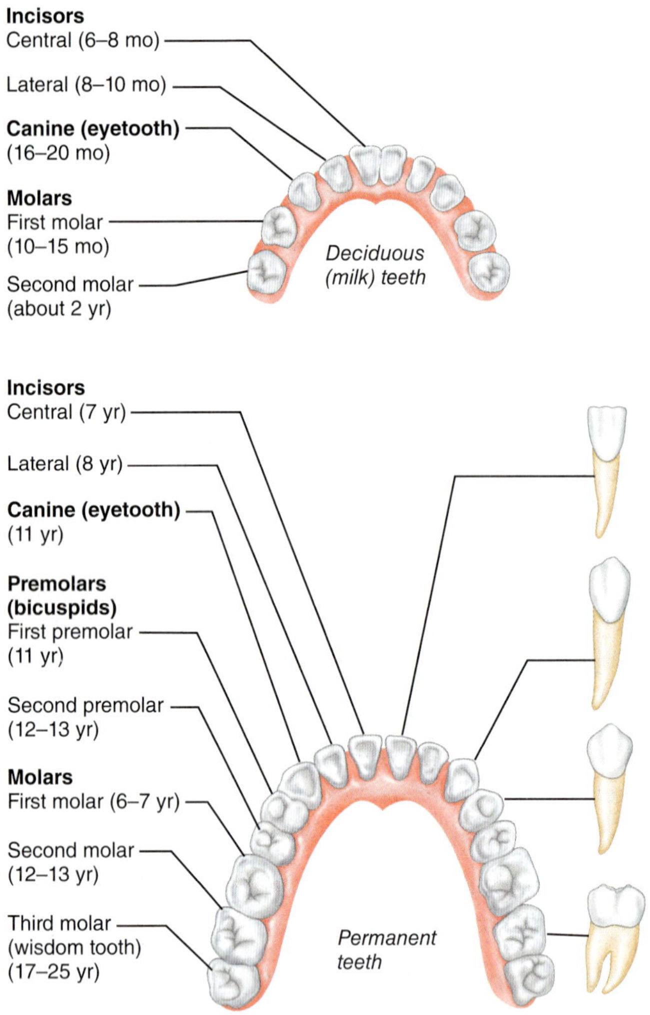

Figure 23.10 Human dentition. Teeth of the lower jaw: the deciduous and permanent sets. Approximate age at which tooth erupts is shown in parentheses. The shapes of individual teeth are shown on the right.

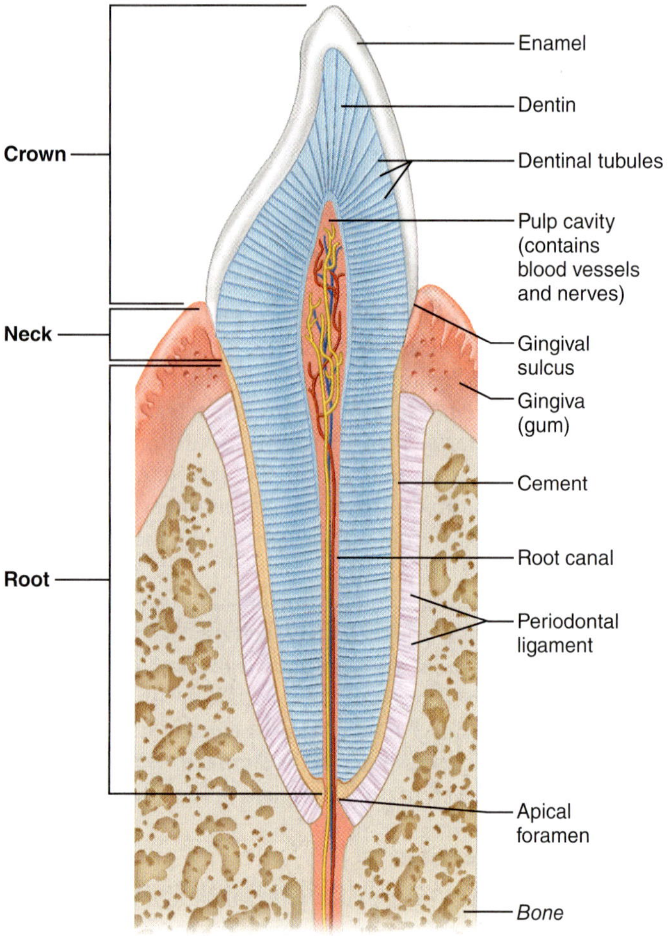

Figure 23.11 Longitudinal section of a canine tooth within its bony socket (alveolus).

pieces of food. The conical or fanglike **canines** (cuspids or eyeteeth) tear and pierce. The **premolars** (bicuspids) and **molars** have broad crowns with rounded cusps (tips) best suited for grinding or crushing. The molars, with four or five cusps, are the best grinders. During chewing, the upper and lower molars repeatedly lock together, an action that generates tremendous crushing forces.

The **dental formula** is a shorthand way of indicating the numbers and relative positions of the different types of teeth. This formula is written as a ratio, uppers over lowers, for *one-half* of the mouth. Since the other side is a mirror image, we obtain total dentition by multiplying the dental formula by 2.

The primary dentition consists of two incisors (I), one canine (C), and two molars (M) on each side of each jaw, and its dental formula is written as

$$\frac{\text{2I, 1C, 2M (upper jaw)}}{\text{2I, 1C, 2M (lower jaw)}} \times 2 \quad \text{(20 teeth)}$$

Similarly, the permanent dentition [two incisors, one canine, two premolars (PM), and three molars] is

$$\frac{\text{2I, 1C, 2PM, 3M}}{\text{2I, 1C, 2PM, 3M}} \times 2 \quad \text{(32 teeth)}$$

Tooth Structure

Each tooth has two major regions: the crown and the root **(Figure 23.11)**. The enamel-covered **crown** is the exposed part of the tooth above the **gingiva** (jin′jĭ-vah), or **gum**, which surrounds the tooth like a tight collar. **Enamel**, a brittle ceramic-like material thick as a dime, directly bears the force of chewing. The hardest substance in the body, it is heavily mineralized with calcium salts, and its densely packed hydroxyapatite (mineral) crystals are oriented in force-resisting columns perpendicular to the tooth's surface. The cells that produce enamel degenerate when the tooth erupts; consequently, decayed or cracked areas of enamel will not heal and must be artificially filled.

The **root** is the portion of the tooth embedded in the jawbone. Canine teeth, incisors, and premolars have one root, although the first upper premolars commonly have two. The first two upper molars have three roots, while the corresponding lower molars have two. The root pattern of the third molar varies, but a fused single root is most common.

A constricted tooth region called the **neck** connects the crown and root. **Cement**, a calcified connective tissue, covers the outer surface of the root and attaches the tooth to the thin **periodontal ligament** (per″e-o-don′tal; "around the tooth"). This ligament anchors the tooth in the bony socket (alveolus) of the jaw, forming a fibrous joint called a *gomphosis*. Where the gingiva borders on a tooth, it dips downward to form a shallow groove called the *gingival sulcus*.

In youth, the gingiva adheres tenaciously to the enamel covering the crown. But as the gums recede with age, the gingiva adheres to the more sensitive cement covering the superior region of the root. As a result, teeth *appear* to get longer in old age—hence the expression "long in the tooth."

Dentin, a protein-rich bonelike material, underlies the enamel cap and forms the bulk of a tooth. More resilient than enamel, dentin acts as a shock absorber during biting and chewing. Dentin surrounds a central **pulp cavity** containing a number of soft tissue structures (connective tissue, blood vessels, and nerve fibers) collectively called **pulp**. Pulp supplies nutrients to the tooth tissues and provides tooth sensation. Where the pulp cavity extends into the root, it becomes the **root canal**. At the proximal end of each root canal is an **apical foramen** that allows blood vessels, nerves, and other structures to enter the pulp cavity.

The teeth are served by the superior and inferior alveolar nerves, branches of the trigeminal nerve (see Table 13.2, p. 496). The superior and inferior alveolar arteries, branches of the maxillary artery (see Figure 19.22b, p. 727), supply blood.

Dentin contains unique radial striations called *dentinal tubules* (Figure 23.11). Each tubule contains an elongated process of an **odontoblast** (o-don′to-blast; "tooth former"), the cell type that secretes and maintains the dentin. The odontoblasts line the pulp cavity just deep to the dentin. Dentin forms throughout adult life and gradually encroaches on the pulp cavity. New dentin can also be laid down fairly rapidly to compensate for tooth damage or decay.

Enamel, dentin, and cement are all calcified and resemble bone (to differing extents), but they differ from bone because they are avascular. Enamel differs from cement and dentin because it lacks collagen and is almost entirely mineral.

Homeostatic Imbalance 23.6

A blow to the jaw can result in death of a tooth's nerve. If local swelling pinches off the blood supply to the tooth, the nerve dies and the tooth darkens. Typically, bacteria infect the pulp sometime later and must be removed by *root canal therapy*. After the cavity is sterilized and filled with inert material, the tooth is capped (covered with an artificial crown). +

Tooth and Gum Disease

Dental caries (kār′ēz; "rottenness"), or **cavities**, result from bacterial action that gradually demineralizes enamel and underlying dentin. Decay begins when **dental plaque** (a film of sugar, bacteria, and other mouth debris) adheres to the teeth. Bacterial metabolism of the trapped sugars produces acids, which dissolve the calcium salts of the teeth. Once the salts are leached out, enzymes released by the bacteria readily digest the remaining organic matrix of the tooth. Frequent brushing and daily flossing help prevent caries by removing plaque.

More serious than tooth decay is the effect of unremoved plaque on the gums. As dental plaque accumulates, it calcifies, forming **calculus** (kal′ku-lus; "stone") or tartar. These stony-hard deposits disrupt the seal between gingivae and teeth, deepening the sulcus and putting the gums at risk for infection by pathogenic anaerobic bacteria. In the early stages of such an infection, called **gingivitis** (jin″jĭ-vi′tis), the gums are red, sore, swollen, and may bleed.

Gingivitis is reversible if the calculus is removed, but if it is neglected the bacteria eventually form pockets of infection which become inflamed. Neutrophils and immune system cells attack not only the intruders but also body tissues, carving deep pockets around the teeth, destroying the periodontal ligament, and activating osteoclasts which dissolve the bone. This serious condition, **periodontal disease** or **periodontitis**, affects up to 95% of all people over age 35 and accounts for 80–90% of tooth loss in adults.

Tooth loss from periodontitis is not inevitable. Even advanced periodontitis can be treated by scraping the teeth, cleaning the infected pockets, cutting the gums to shrink the pockets, and following up with anti-inflammatory and antibiotic therapy. These treatments alleviate the bacterial infestations and encourage the surrounding tissues to reattach to the teeth and bone. Clinical treatment is followed up by a home regimen of consistent brushing, flossing, and hydrogen peroxide rinses.

Periodontal disease may jeopardize more than just teeth. Some contend that it increases the risk of heart disease and stroke in at least two ways: (1) the chronic inflammation promotes atherosclerotic plaque, and (2) bacteria entering the blood from infected gums stimulate the formation of clots that clog coronary and cerebral arteries. Risk factors for periodontal disease include smoking, diabetes mellitus, and oral (tongue or lip) piercing.

Check Your Understanding

16. Seven-year-old Tina ran to her daddy to show him her lower central incisor which she had wiggled until it "fell out." Is this a primary or permanent tooth? What name is given to teeth that (according to Tina) fall out?
17. Which tooth substance is harder than bone? Which tooth region includes nervous tissue and blood vessels?
18. Which teeth are the "grinders"?

For answers, see Appendix H.

The Pharynx

From the mouth, food passes posteriorly into the **oropharynx** and then the **laryngopharynx** (see Figure 23.7a), both common passageways for food, fluids, and air. (The nasopharynx has no digestive role.)

The histology of the pharyngeal wall resembles that of the oral cavity. The mucosa contains a friction-resistant stratified

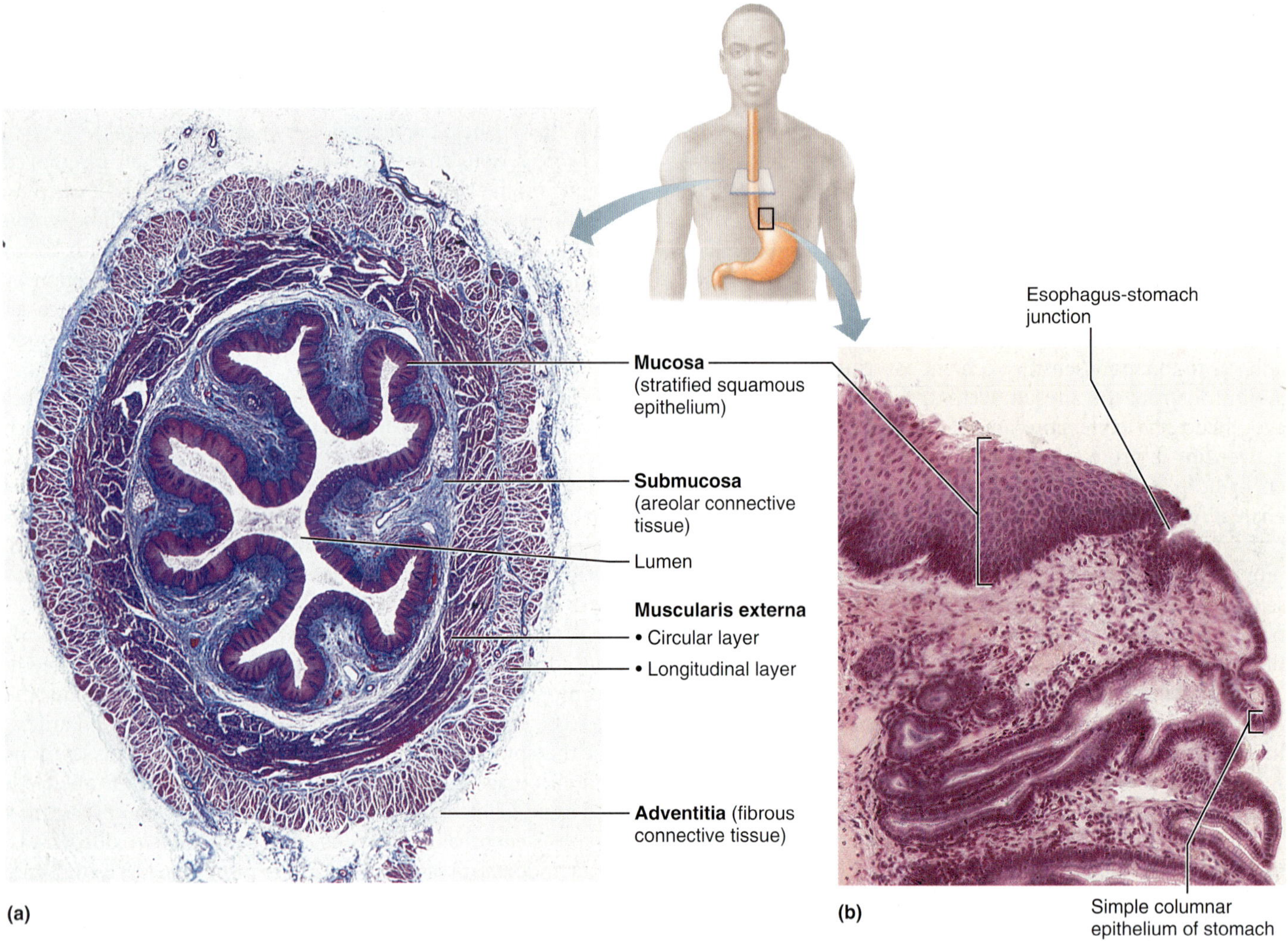

Figure 23.12 Microscopic structure of the esophagus. (a) Cross-sectional view of the esophagus taken from the region close to the stomach junction (10×). The muscularis is composed of smooth muscle. **(b)** Longitudinal section through the esophagus-stomach junction (130×). Notice the abrupt transition from the stratified squamous epithelium of the esophagus (top) to the simple columnar epithelium of the stomach (bottom).

23

squamous epithelium well supplied with mucus-producing glands. The external muscle layer consists of two *skeletal muscle* layers. The cells of the inner layer run longitudinally. Those of the outer layer, the *pharyngeal constrictor* muscles, encircle the wall like three stacked fists (see Figure 10.9c). Contractions of these muscles propel food into the esophagus below.

The Esophagus

The **esophagus** (ĕ-sof′ah-gus; "carry food") is a muscular tube about 25 cm (10 inches) long and is collapsed when not involved in food propulsion **(Figure 23.12)**. After food moves through the laryngopharynx, it is routed into the esophagus posteriorly as the epiglottis closes off the larynx to incoming food.

As shown in Figure 23.1, the esophagus takes a fairly straight course through the mediastinum of the thorax. It pierces the diaphragm at the **esophageal hiatus** (hi-a′tus; "gap") to enter the abdomen. It joins the stomach at the **cardial orifice** within the abdominal cavity. The cardial orifice is surrounded by the **gastroesophageal** or **cardiac sphincter** (gas″tro-ĕ-sof″ah-je′al), which is a *physiological* sphincter (see Figure 23.13). That is, it acts as a sphincter, but the only structural evidence of this sphincter is a slight thickening of the circular smooth muscle at that point. The muscular diaphragm, which surrounds this sphincter, helps keep it closed when food is not being swallowed. Mucous cells on both sides of the sphincter help protect the esophagus from reflux of stomach acid.

Homeostatic Imbalance 23.7

Heartburn, the first symptom of *gastroesophageal reflux disease* (*GERD*), is the burning, radiating substernal pain that occurs when stomach acid regurgitates into the esophagus. Symptoms are so similar to those of a heart attack that many first-time sufferers of heartburn are rushed to the emergency room. Heartburn is most likely when a person has eaten or drunk to excess, and in conditions that force abdominal contents superiorly, such as extreme obesity, pregnancy, and running, which splashes stomach contents upward with each step (runner's reflux).

Heartburn is also common in those with a **hiatal hernia**, a structural abnormality (most often due to abnormal relaxation or weakening of the gastroesophageal sphincter) in which the superior part of the stomach protrudes slightly above the diaphragm. Since the diaphragm no longer reinforces the sphincter, gastric juice may enter the esophagus, particularly when lying down. If the episodes are frequent and prolonged, *esophagitis* (inflammation of the esophagus) and *esophageal ulcers* may result. An even more threatening sequel is esophageal cancer. These consequences can usually be prevented or managed by avoiding late-night snacks and using antacid preparations. +

Unlike the mouth and pharynx, the esophagus wall has all four of the basic alimentary canal layers described earlier. Some features of interest:

- The esophageal mucosa contains a *nonkeratinized* stratified squamous epithelium. At the esophagus-stomach junction, that abrasion-resistant epithelium changes abruptly to the simple columnar epithelium of the stomach, which is specialized for secretion (Figure 23.12b).
- When the esophagus is empty, its mucosa and submucosa are thrown into longitudinal folds (Figure 23.12a). When food is in transit in the esophagus, these folds flatten out.
- The submucosa contains mucus-secreting *esophageal glands*. As a bolus moves through the esophagus, it compresses these glands, causing them to secrete mucus that "greases" the esophageal walls and aids food passage.
- The muscularis externa is skeletal muscle in its superior third, a mixture of skeletal and smooth muscle in its middle third, and entirely smooth muscle in its inferior third.
- Instead of a serosa, the esophagus has a fibrous adventitia composed entirely of connective tissue, which blends with surrounding structures along its route.

Check Your Understanding

19. To which two organ systems does the pharynx belong?
20. How is the muscularis externa of the esophagus unique in the body?
21. What is the functional significance of the epithelial change seen at the esophagus-stomach junction?

For answers, see Appendix H.

Digestive Processes: Mouth to Esophagus

✓ Describe the mechanisms of chewing and swallowing.

The mouth and its accessory digestive organs are involved in most digestive processes. The mouth (1) ingests, (2) begins mechanical breakdown by chewing, (3) initiates propulsion by swallowing, and (4) starts the chemical breakdown (digestion) of polysaccharides.

Except for a few drugs that are absorbed through the oral mucosa (for example, nitroglycerine used to alleviate the pain of angina), essentially no absorption occurs in the mouth.

In contrast to the multifunctional mouth, the pharynx and esophagus merely serve as conduits to pass food from the mouth to the stomach. Their single digestive system function is food propulsion, accomplished by swallowing.

Since we cover digestion in a special physiology section later in the chapter, we will discuss only the mechanical processes of chewing and swallowing food here.

Mastication (Chewing)

As food enters the mouth, its mechanical breakdown begins with **mastication**, or chewing. The cheeks and closed lips hold food between the teeth, the tongue mixes food with saliva to soften it, and the teeth cut and grind solid foods into smaller morsels.

Mastication is partly voluntary and partly reflexive. We voluntarily put food into our mouths and contract the muscles that close our jaws. The pattern and rhythm of continued jaw movements are controlled mainly by stretch reflexes and in response to pressure inputs from receptors in the cheeks, gums, and tongue, but they can also be voluntary if desired.

Deglutition (Swallowing)

To send food on its way from the mouth, it is first compacted by the tongue into a bolus and is then swallowed. **Deglutition** (deg″loo-tish′un), or swallowing, is a complicated process that involves coordinated activity of over 22 separate muscle groups. It has two major phases, the buccal and the pharyngeal-esophageal.

The **buccal phase** occurs in the mouth and is voluntary. In the buccal phase, we place the tip of the tongue against the hard palate, and then contract the tongue to force the bolus into the oropharynx (**Figure 23.13** (1)). As food enters the pharynx and stimulates tactile receptors there, it passes out of our control and into the realm of involuntary reflex activity.

Triggered by that "bit of saliva" or food reaching receptors in the posterior pharynx, the involuntary **pharyngeal-esophageal phase** of swallowing is controlled by the swallowing center located in the brain stem (medulla and lower pons). Various cranial nerves, most importantly the vagus nerves, transmit motor impulses from the swallowing center to the muscles of the pharynx and esophagus. Once food enters the pharynx, respiration is momentarily inhibited and all routes except the desired one into the digestive tract are blocked off (Figure 23.13 (2)): The tongue blocks off the mouth. The soft palate rises to close off the nasopharynx. The larynx rises so that the epiglottis covers its opening into the respiratory passageways, and the upper esophageal sphincter relaxes.

Wavelike peristaltic contractions create pressure waves that propel food through the pharynx and into the esophagus (Figure 23.13 (3)–(5)). Solid foods pass from the oropharynx to the stomach in about 8 seconds, and fluids, aided by gravity, pass

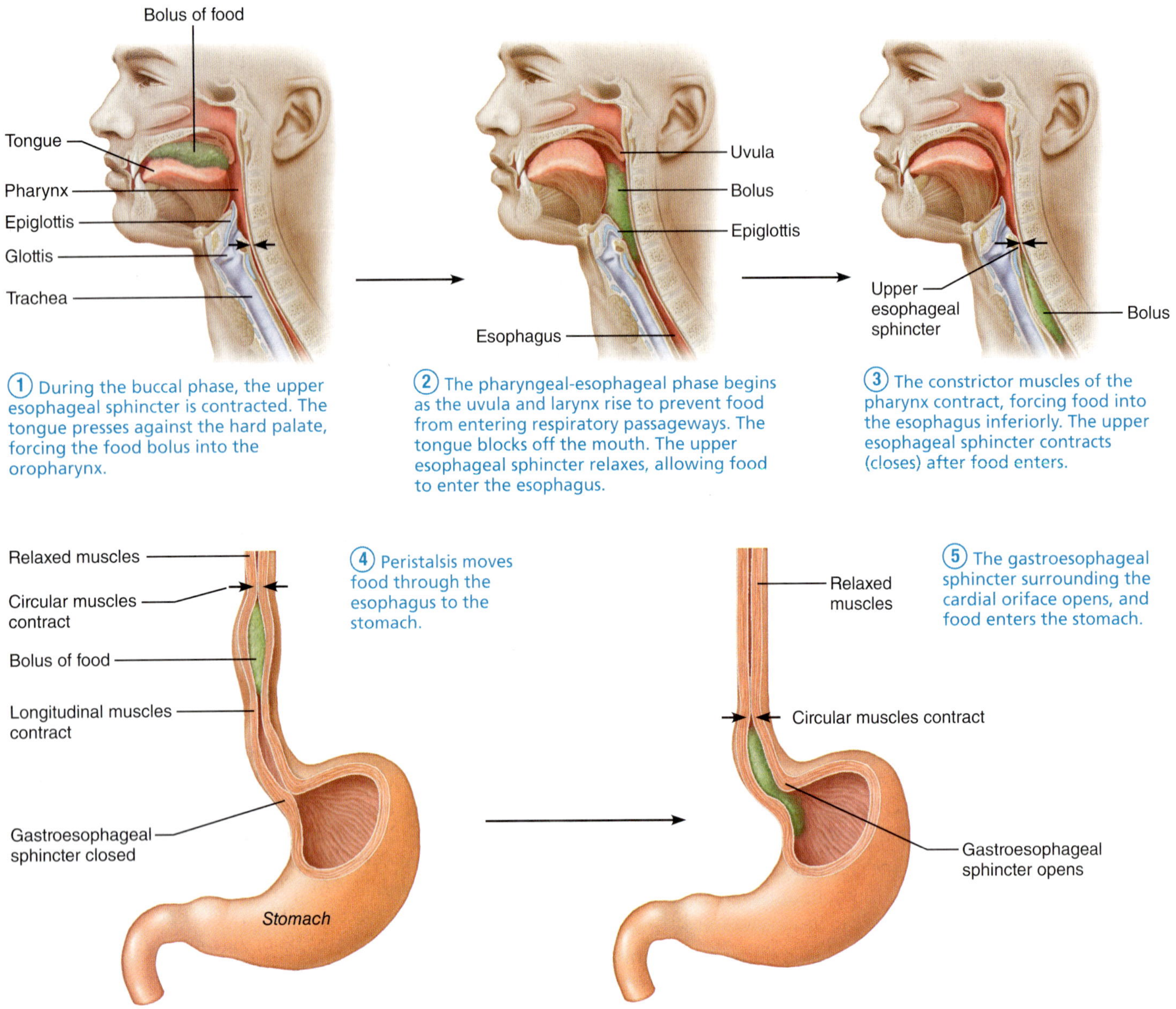

Figure 23.13 Deglutition (swallowing). The process of swallowing consists of a voluntary (buccal) phase (step ①) and an involuntary (pharyngeal-esophageal) phase (steps ②–⑤).

in 1 to 2 seconds. Just before the peristaltic wave (and food) reaches the end of the esophagus, the gastroesophageal sphincter relaxes reflexively to allow food to enter the stomach. After food entry, that sphincter closes, preventing regurgitation.

If we talk or inhale while swallowing, the various protective mechanisms may be short-circuited and food may enter the respiratory passageways instead. This event typically triggers the cough reflex to expel the food.

☑ Check Your Understanding

22. What role does the tongue play in swallowing?
23. How are the respiratory passages blocked during swallowing?

For answers, see Appendix H.

The Stomach

✓ Identify structural modifications of the wall of the stomach that enhance the digestive process.

✓ Name the cell types responsible for secreting the various components of gastric juice and indicate the importance of each component in stomach activity.

✓ Describe stomach structure and indicate changes in the basic alimentary canal structure that aid its digestive function.

Below the esophagus, the GI tract expands to form the **stomach** (see Figure 23.1), a temporary "storage tank" where chemical breakdown of proteins begins and food is converted to a creamy paste called **chyme** (kīm; "juice"). The stomach lies in the upper

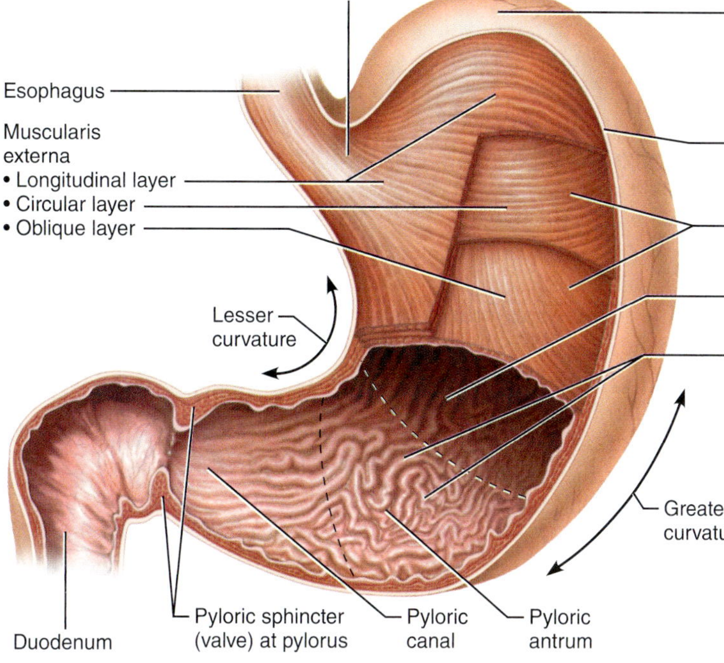

(a)

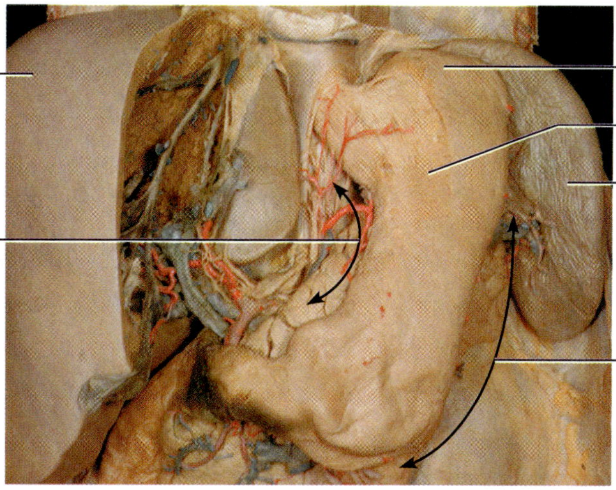

(b)

Figure 23.14 Anatomy of the stomach. (a) Gross internal anatomy (frontal section). **(b)** Photograph of external aspect of stomach. (For a related image, see *A Brief Atlas of the Human Body*, Figure 69a.)

left quadrant of the peritoneal cavity, nearly hidden by the liver and diaphragm. Though relatively fixed at both ends, the stomach is quite movable in between. It tends to lie high and run horizontally in short, stout people (a steer-horn stomach) and is often elongated vertically in tall, thin people (a J-shaped stomach).

Gross Anatomy

The adult stomach varies from 15 to 25 cm (6 to 10 inches) long, but its diameter and volume depend on how much food it contains. An empty stomach has a volume of about 50 ml and a cross-sectional diameter only slightly larger than the large intestine, but when it is really distended it can hold about 4 L (1 gallon) of food and may extend nearly to the pelvis! When empty, the stomach collapses inward, throwing its mucosa (and submucosa) into large, longitudinal folds called **rugae** (roo′ge; *ruga* = wrinkle, fold).

Figure 23.14a shows the major regions of the stomach. The small **cardial part**, or **cardia** ("near the heart"), surrounds the cardial orifice through which food enters the stomach from the esophagus. The **fundus** is the stomach's dome-shaped part, tucked beneath the diaphragm, that bulges superolaterally to the cardia. The **body**, or the midportion of the stomach, is continuous inferiorly with the funnel-shaped **pyloric part**. The wider and more superior area of the pyloric part, the **pyloric antrum** (*antrum* = cave) narrows to form the **pyloric canal**, which terminates at the **pylorus**. The pylorus is continuous with the duodenum through the **pyloric sphincter** or **valve**, which controls stomach emptying (*pylorus* = gatekeeper).

The convex lateral surface of the stomach is its **greater curvature**, and its concave medial surface is the **lesser curvature**. Extending from these curvatures are two mesenteries, called *omenta* (o-men′tah), that help tether the stomach to other digestive organs and the body wall (see Figure 23.30, p. 889). The **lesser omentum** runs from the liver to the lesser curvature of the stomach, where it becomes continuous with the visceral peritoneum covering the stomach. The **greater omentum** drapes inferiorly from the greater curvature of the stomach to cover the coils of the small intestine. It then runs dorsally and superiorly, wrapping the spleen and the transverse portion of the large intestine before blending with the *mesocolon*, a dorsal mesentery that secures the large intestine to the parietal peritoneum of the posterior abdominal wall.

The greater omentum is riddled with fat deposits (*oment* = fatty skin) that give it the appearance of a lacy apron. It also contains large collections of lymph nodes. The immune cells and macrophages in these nodes "police" the peritoneal cavity and intraperitoneal organs.

The stomach is served by the autonomic nervous system. Sympathetic fibers from thoracic splanchnic nerves are relayed through the celiac plexus. Parasympathetic fibers are supplied by the vagus nerve. The arterial supply of the stomach is provided by branches (gastric and splenic) of the celiac trunk (see Figure 19.24). The corresponding veins are part of the hepatic portal system and ultimately drain into the hepatic portal vein (see Figure 19.29c).

Microscopic Anatomy

The stomach wall contains the four tunics typical of most of the alimentary canal, but its muscularis and mucosa are modified for the special roles of the stomach. Besides the usual circular and longitudinal layers of smooth muscle, the muscularis externa has an incomplete innermost layer of smooth muscle fibrils that runs *obliquely* (Figure 23.14a and **Figure 23.15a**). This arrangement allows the stomach not only to mix, churn, and move food along the tract (the job of the circular and longitudinal muscle layers), but also to pummel the food, physically breaking it down into smaller fragments and ramming it into the small intestine. (The oblique fibers accomplish the ramming by jackknifing the stomach into a V shape, which provides a propulsive action in the pyloric part.)

The lining epithelium of the stomach mucosa is a simple columnar epithelium composed entirely of mucous cells. They produce a cloudy, protective two-layer coat of alkaline mucus in which the surface layer consists of viscous, insoluble mucus that traps a layer of bicarbonate-rich fluid beneath it. This otherwise smooth lining is dotted with millions of deep **gastric pits**, which lead into tubular **gastric glands** that produce the stomach secretion called **gastric juice** (Figure 23.15).

The cells forming the walls of the gastric pits are primarily mucous cells, but those composing the gastric glands vary in different stomach regions. For example, the cells in the glands of the cardia and pylorus primarily secrete mucus, whereas cells of the pyloric antrum produce mucus and several hormones including most of the stimulatory hormone called gastrin.

Types of Gland Cells

Glands of the stomach fundus and body, where most digestion occurs, are substantially larger and produce the majority of the stomach secretions. The glands in these regions contain a variety of secretory cells, including mucous neck, parietal, chief, and enteroendocrine cells.

Mucous Neck Cells **Mucous neck cells**, scattered in the "neck" and more basal regions of the glands, produce a thin, soluble mucus quite different from that secreted by the mucous cells of the surface epithelium (Figure 23.15b). It is not yet understood what special function this *acidic* mucus performs.

Parietal Cells **Parietal cells**, found mainly in the more apical region of the glands scattered among the chief cells (described next), simultaneously secrete *hydrochloric acid* (*HCl*) and *intrinsic factor* (Figure 23.15b, c). Although parietal cells appear oval when viewed with a light microscope, they actually have three prongs that bear dense microvilli (they look like fuzzy pitchforks!). This structure provides a huge surface area for secreting H^+ and Cl^- into the stomach lumen.

HCl makes the stomach contents extremely acidic (pH 1.5–3.5), a condition necessary for activation and optimal activity of protein-digesting enzyme **pepsin**. The acidity also helps digest food by denaturing proteins and breaking down cell walls of plant foods, and is harsh enough to kill many of the bacteria ingested with foods. Intrinsic factor is a glycoprotein required for vitamin B_{12} absorption in the small intestine.

Chief Cells **Chief cells** occur mainly in the basal regions of the gastric glands. The cuboidal chief cells produce *pepsinogen* (pep-sin′o-jen), the inactive form of the pepsin. When these cells are stimulated, the first pepsinogen molecules they release are activated by HCl encountered in the apical region of the gland (Figure 23.15c). But once pepsin is present, it also catalyzes the conversion of pepsinogen to pepsin. The activation process involves removing a small peptide fragment from pepsinogen, causing it to change shape and expose its active site. This positive feedback process is limited only by the amount of pepsinogen present.

Chief cells also secrete lipases (fat-digesting enzymes). Formerly thought to be insignificant in fat digestion, these gastric lipases now appear to account for about 15% of overall GI lipolysis.

Enteroendocrine Cells **Enteroendocrine cells** (en″ter-o-en′do-krin; "gut endocrine"), typically located deep in the gastric glands (Figure 23.15b, c), release a variety of chemical messengers directly into the interstitial fluid of the lamina propria. Some of these, for example **histamine** and **serotonin**, act locally as paracrines. Others, such as **somatostatin**, act both as paracrines locally and as

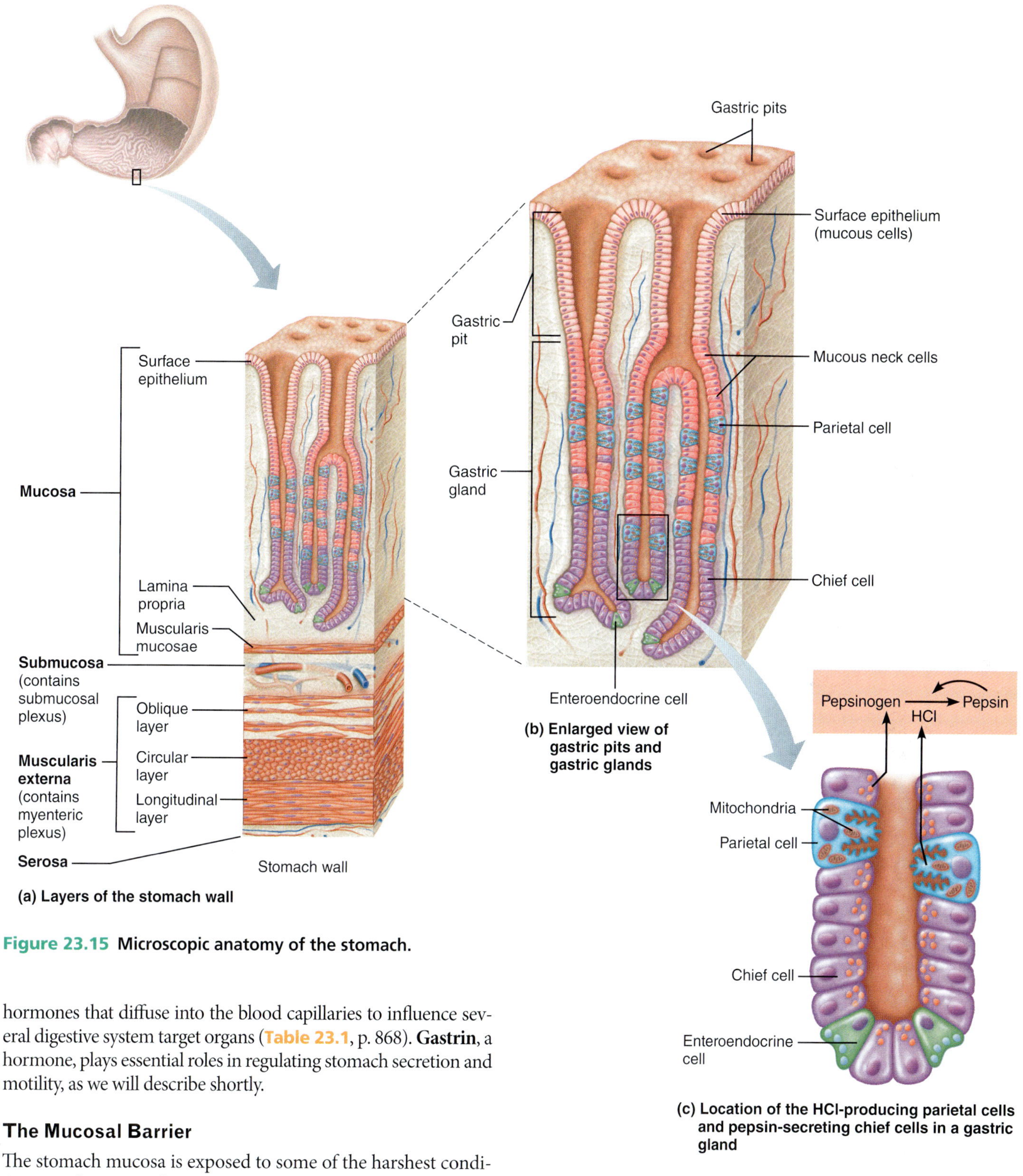

Figure 23.15 **Microscopic anatomy of the stomach.**

hormones that diffuse into the blood capillaries to influence several digestive system target organs (Table 23.1, p. 868). **Gastrin**, a hormone, plays essential roles in regulating stomach secretion and motility, as we will describe shortly.

The Mucosal Barrier

The stomach mucosa is exposed to some of the harshest conditions in the entire digestive tract. Gastric juice is corrosively acidic (the H^+ concentration in the stomach can be 100,000 times that found in blood), and its protein-digesting enzymes can digest the stomach itself.

However, the stomach is not a passive victim of its formidable environment. It mounts an aggressive counterattack to protect itself, producing the **mucosal barrier**. Three factors create this barrier:

- *A thick coating of bicarbonate-rich mucus* builds up on the stomach wall.
- *The epithelial cells of the mucosa are joined together by tight junctions* that prevent gastric juice from leaking into underlying tissue layers.
- *Damaged epithelial mucosal cells are shed and quickly replaced* by division of *undifferentiated stem cells* that reside where the

Table 23.1 Hormones and Paracrines That Act in Digestion*

HORMONE	SITE OF PRODUCTION	STIMULUS FOR PRODUCTION	TARGET ORGAN	ACTIVITY
Cholecystokinin (CCK)	Duodenal mucosa	Fatty chyme (also partially digested proteins)	Stomach	▪ Inhibits stomach's secretory activity
			Liver/pancreas	▪ Potentiates secretin's actions on these organs
			Pancreas	▪ Increases output of enzyme-rich pancreatic juice
			Gallbladder	▪ Stimulates organ to contract and expel stored bile
			Hepatopancreatic sphincter	▪ Relaxes sphincter to allow entry of bile and pancreatic juice into duodenum
Gastric inhibitory peptide (GIP) (or glucose-dependent insulinotropic peptide)	Duodenal mucosa	Fatty chyme	Stomach	▪ Inhibits HCl production (minor effect)
			Pancreas (beta cells)	▪ Stimulates insulin release
Gastrin	Stomach mucosa (G cells)	Food (particularly partially digested proteins) in stomach (chemical stimulation); acetylcholine released by nerve fibers	Stomach (parietal cells)	▪ Increases HCl secretion ▪ Stimulates gastric emptying (minor effect)
			Small intestine	▪ Stimulates contraction of intestinal muscle
			Ileocecal valve	▪ Relaxes ileocecal valve
			Large intestine	▪ Stimulates mass movements
Histamine	Stomach mucosa	Food in stomach	Stomach	▪ Activates parietal cells to release HCl
Intestinal gastrin	Duodenal mucosa	Acidic and partially digested foods in duodenum	Stomach	▪ Stimulates gastric glands and motility
Motilin	Duodenal mucosa	Fasting; periodic release every 1½-2 hours by neural stimuli	Proximal duodenum	▪ Stimulates migrating motor complex
Secretin	Duodenal mucosa	Acidic chyme (also partially digested proteins and fats)	Stomach	▪ Inhibits gastric gland secretion and gastric motility during gastric phase of secretion
			Pancreas	▪ Increases output of pancreatic juice rich in bicarbonate ions; potentiates CCK's action
			Liver	▪ Increases bile output
Serotonin	Stomach mucosa	Food in stomach	Stomach	▪ Causes contraction of stomach muscle
Somatostatin	Stomach mucosa; duodenal mucosa	Food in stomach; stimulation by sympathetic nerve fibers	Stomach	▪ Inhibits gastric secretion of all products
			Pancreas	▪ Inhibits secretion
			Small intestine	▪ Inhibits GI blood flow; thus inhibits intestinal absorption
			Gallbladder and liver	▪ Inhibits contraction and bile release
Vasoactive intestinal peptide (VIP)	Enteric neurons	Chyme containing partially digested foods	Small intestine	▪ Stimulates buffer secretion ▪ Dilates intestinal capillaries ▪ Relaxes intestinal smooth muscle
			Pancreas	▪ Increases secretion
			Stomach	▪ Inhibits acid secretion

*Except for somatostatin, all of these polypeptides also stimulate the growth (particularly of the mucosa) of the organs they affect.

23

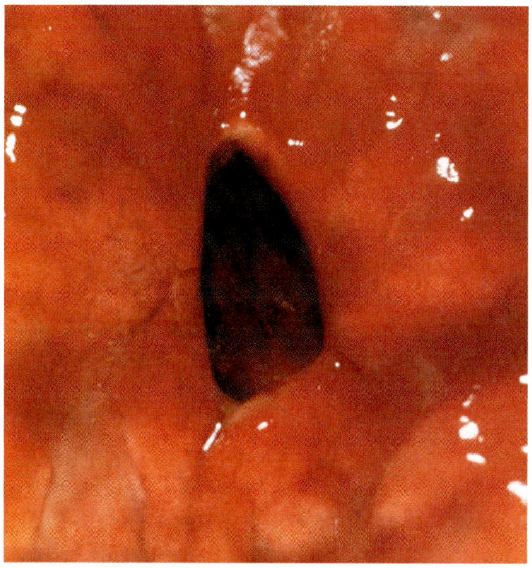

(a) A gastric ulcer lesion

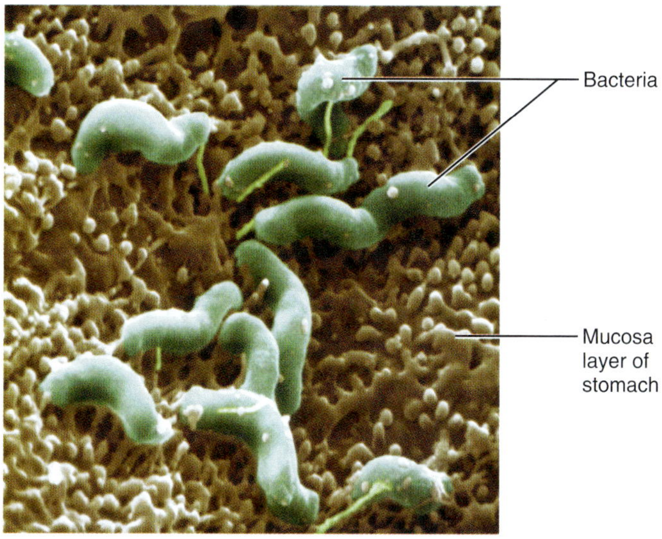

(b) *H. pylori* bacteria

Figure 23.16 Photographs of a gastric ulcer and the *H. pylori* bacteria that most commonly cause it.

gastric pits join the gastric glands. The stomach surface epithelium of mucous cells is completely renewed every three to six days, but the more sheltered glandular cells deep within the gastric glands have a much longer life span.

Homeostatic Imbalance 23.8

Anything that breaches the gel-like mucosal barrier causes inflammation of the stomach wall, a condition called *gastritis*. Persistent damage to the underlying tissues can promote **peptic ulcers**, specifically called **gastric ulcers** when they are erosions of the stomach wall **(Figure 23.16a)**. The most distressing symptom of gastric ulcers is gnawing epigastric pain that seems to bore through to your back. The pain typically occurs 1–3 hours after eating and is often relieved by eating again. The danger posed by ulcers is perforation of the stomach wall, leading to peritonitis and, perhaps, massive hemorrhage.

For years, ulcers were blamed on factors that increased HCl production or reduced mucus secretion, including aspirin and nonsteroidal anti-inflammatory drugs (NSAIDs such as ibuprofen), smoking, spicy food, alcohol, coffee, and stress. Although acid conditions *are* necessary for ulcers to form, acidity in itself is not sufficient to cause them. Ninety percent of recurrent ulcers are the work of a certain strain of acid-resistant, corkscrew-shaped *Helicobacter pylori* bacteria (Figure 23.16b), which burrow like a drill bit through the mucus and destroy the protective mucosal layer, leaving denuded areas. Even more troubling are studies that link this bacterium to some stomach cancers.

More than half of the population harbors *H. pylori*, but these pathological effects occur in only 10–20% of infected individuals. The antimicrobial activity of gastric mucin appears to protect most of us from *H. pylori*'s invasive attacks.

A breath test can easily detect the presence of *H. pylori*. A simple two-week-long course of antibiotics kills the embedded bacteria, promotes healing of the ulcers, and prevents recurrence. For active ulcers, a blocker for H_2 (histamine) receptors may also help because it inhibits HCl secretion by blocking histamine's effects.

The relatively few peptic ulcers not caused by *H. pylori* generally result from long-term use of NSAIDs. In such noninfectious cases, H_2-receptor blocker drugs such as cimetidine (Tagamet) and ranitidine (Zantac) are the therapy of choice. ✚

Check Your Understanding

24. What structural modification of the stomach wall underlies the stomach's ability to mechanically break down food?
25. Two substances secreted by cells of the gastric glands are needed to produce the active protein-digesting enzyme pepsin. What are these substances and which cells secrete them?
26. Which protective substances or activities make up the so-called mucosal barrier?

For answers, see Appendix H.

Digestive Processes in the Stomach

✓ Explain how gastric secretion and stomach motility are regulated.

✓ Define and account for the alkaline tide.

Except for ingestion and defecation, the stomach is involved in the whole "menu" of digestive activities. Besides serving as a holding area for ingested food, the stomach continues the demolition job begun in the oral cavity by further degrading food both physically and chemically. It then delivers chyme, the product of its activity, into the small intestine.

Protein digestion begins in the stomach and is the main type of enzymatic breakdown that occurs there. HCl produced by stomach glands denatures dietary proteins in preparation for enzymatic digestion. (The unfolded amino acid chain is more accessible to the enzymes.)

The most important protein-digesting enzyme produced by the gastric mucosa is pepsin. In infants, however, the stomach glands also secrete **rennin**, an enzyme that acts on milk protein (casein), converting it to a curdy substance that looks like soured milk. Additionally, lingual lipase released by the minor salivary glands may digest some triglycerides in the stomach for a short time before the lipase itself is digested.

Two common lipid-soluble substances—alcohol and aspirin—pass easily through the stomach mucosa into the blood. Alcohol and aspirin may cause gastric bleeding, so these substances should be avoided by people with gastric ulcers.

Despite the obvious benefits of preparing food to enter the intestine, the only stomach function essential to life is secretion of intrinsic factor. **Intrinsic factor** is required for intestinal absorption of vitamin B_{12}, needed to produce mature erythrocytes. In its absence, *pernicious anemia* results. However, if vitamin B_{12} is administered by injection, individuals can survive with minimal digestive problems even after total gastrectomy (stomach removal). **Table 23.2** (p. 885) summarizes the stomach's activities.

Since we describe digestion and absorption later, here we will focus on events that regulate (1) secretory activity of the gastric glands and (2) stomach motility and emptying.

Regulation of Gastric Secretion

Both neural and hormonal mechanisms control gastric secretion. Under normal conditions the gastric mucosa pours out as much as 3 L of gastric juice—an acid brew so potent it can dissolve nails—every day.

Both long (vagus nerve–mediated) and short (local enteric) nerve reflexes provide nervous control (see Figure 23.4, p. 853). When the vagus nerves stimulate the stomach, secretory activity of virtually all of its glands increases. (By contrast, activation of sympathetic nerves depresses secretory activity.) Hormonal control of gastric secretion is largely the province of gastrin, which stimulates secretion of enzymes and HCl, and of hormones produced by the small intestine, which are mostly gastrin antagonists.

23

Stimuli acting at three distinct sites—the head, stomach, and small intestine—provoke or inhibit gastric secretions. Accordingly, the three phases of gastric secretion are called the *cephalic, gastric*, and *intestinal phases* **(Figure 23.17)**. The effector site is the stomach in all cases and, once initiated, one or all three phases may be occurring at the same time.

Phase 1: Cephalic (Reflex)

The **cephalic**, or **reflex**, **phase** of gastric secretion occurs *before* food enters the stomach (Figure 23.17). Only a few minutes long, this phase is triggered by the aroma, taste, sight, or thought of food, and it gets the stomach ready for its upcoming digestive chore.

Sensory inputs from olfactory receptors and taste buds are relayed to the hypothalamus. The hypothalamus, in turn, stimulates the vagal nuclei of the medulla oblongata, which transmits motor impulses via the vagus nerves to parasympathetic enteric ganglia. Enteric ganglionic neurons then stimulate the stomach glands.

The enhanced secretory activity that results when we see or think of food is a *conditioned reflex* and occurs only when we like or want the food. If we are depressed or have no appetite, this part of the cephalic reflex is suppressed.

Phase 2: Gastric

Once food reaches the stomach, local neural and hormonal mechanisms initiate the **gastric phase** (Figure 23.17). This phase lasts three to four hours and provides about two-thirds of the gastric juice released.

Stimuli and Inhibitors The most important stimuli are distension, peptides, and low acidity. Stomach distension activates stretch receptors and initiates both local (myenteric) reflexes and long (vagovagal) reflexes. In the long type of reflex, impulses travel to the medulla and then back to the stomach via vagal fibers. Both types of reflexes lead to acetylcholine (ACh) release, which in turn stimulates the output of more gastric juice.

Though neural influences initiated by stomach distension are important, the hormone gastrin probably plays a greater role in stimulating stomach gland secretion during the gastric phase. Chemical stimuli provided by partially digested proteins, caffeine, and rising pH directly activate gastrin-secreting enteroendocrine cells called **G cells** in the stomach antrum. Gastrin stimulates the release of enzymes, but its main target is the HCl-secreting parietal cells, which it prods to spew out even more HCl. Highly acidic (pH below 2) gastric contents *inhibit* gastrin secretion—a situation that commonly occurs between meals.

When protein foods are in the stomach, the pH of the gastric contents generally rises because proteins act as buffers to tie up H^+. The rise in pH stimulates gastrin secretion and subsequently HCl release, which in turn provides the acidic conditions needed to digest proteins. The more protein in the meal, the greater the amount of gastrin and HCl released. As proteins are digested, the gastric contents gradually become more acidic, which again inhibits the gastrin-secreting cells. This negative feedback mechanism helps maintain optimal pH and working conditions for gastric enzymes.

The neural reflexes already described also activate G cells. Stress, fear, anxiety, or anything that triggers the fight-or-flight response inhibits gastric secretion because the sympathetic division overrides parasympathetic controls of digestion (Figure 23.17).

Control of the HCl-secreting parietal cells is multifaceted. It is stimulated by three chemicals, all of which bind to G protein–coupled receptors on the parietal cell's membrane and work through second-messenger systems. *ACh* released by parasympathetic nerve fibers and *gastrin* secreted by G cells bring about their effects by increasing intracellular Ca^{2+} levels. *Histamine*, released by the so-called *enterochromaffin-like* (ECL) cells mainly in response to gastrin, acts through cyclic AMP (cAMP).

When only one of the three chemicals binds to parietal cells, HCl secretion is scanty, but when all three bind, HCl pours forth. As we noted earlier, antihistamines, such as cimetidine, which bind to and block the H_2 (histamine) receptors of parietal

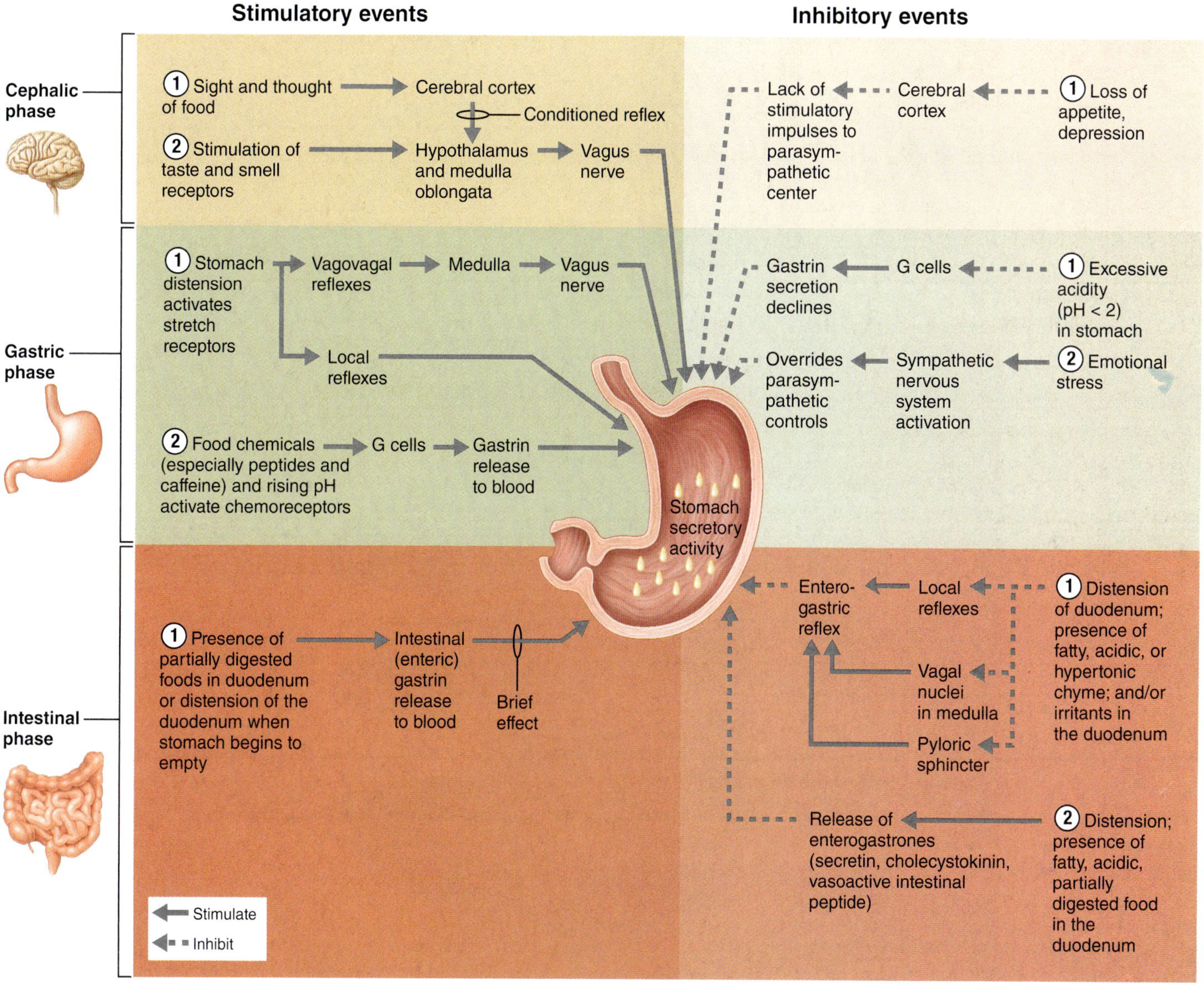

Figure 23.17 Neural and hormonal mechanisms that regulate release of gastric juice. Stimulatory factors are shown on the left; inhibitory factors are shown on the right.

cells, are used to treat gastric ulcers due to hyperacidity. So, as you might guess, histamine is the major player here.

HCl Formation The process of HCl formation within the parietal cells is complicated, but it appears to go something like this (Figure 23.18): When parietal cells are appropriately stimulated, H^+ is actively pumped into the stomach lumen against a tremendous concentration gradient by H^+-K^+ ATPases in exchange for K^+ ions that move into the cell. K^+ then cycles back into the lumen via K^+ channels. Chloride ions (Cl^-) follow H^+ into the lumen to maintain an electrical balance in the stomach, completing the process of HCl secretion. The Cl^- is obtained from blood plasma, while H^+ comes from the breakdown of carbonic acid (formed by the combination of carbon dioxide and water) within the parietal cell:

$$CO_2 + H_2O \rightarrow H_2CO_3 \rightarrow H^+ + HCO_3^-$$

As H^+ is pumped from the cell and HCO_3^- (bicarbonate ion) accumulates within the cell, HCO_3^- is ejected through the basolateral cell membrane into the capillary blood. As a result, blood draining from the stomach is more alkaline than the blood serving it. This phenomenon is called the **alkaline tide**. Notice that a HCO_3^--Cl^- antiporter in the basolateral membrane moves HCO_3^- and Cl^- in opposite directions, and this is how the Cl^- moves into the lumen as the chloride part of the HCl product. K^+ and Cl^- move into the stomach lumen by diffusing through membrane channels.

Phase 3: Intestinal

The **intestinal phase** of gastric secretion has two components—stimulatory and inhibitory (see Figure 23.17). The excitatory aspect is set into motion as partially digested food fills the initial part (duodenum) of the small intestine. This stimulates

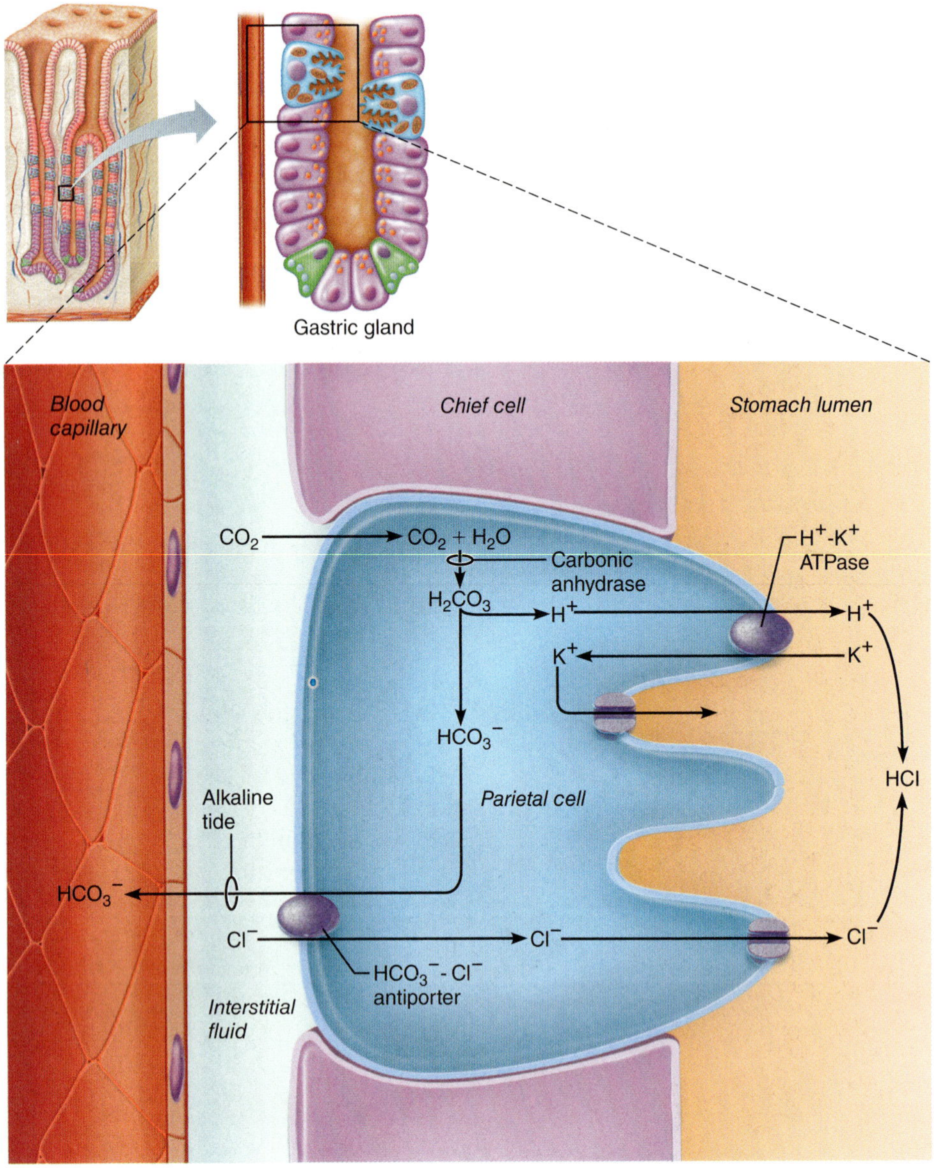

Figure 23.18 Mechanism of HCl secretion by parietal cells. H^+ and HCO_3^- (bicarbonate ions) are generated from the dissociation of carbonic acid (H_2CO_3) within the parietal cell. As H^+-K^+ ATPase pumps H^+ into the lumen, K^+ enters the cell. Meanwhile, the HCO_3^--Cl^- antiporter transports HCO_3^- into the interstitial space in exchange for chloride ions (Cl^-), establishing the alkaline tide. Cl^- and K^+ then diffuse into the lumen through membrane channels.

intestinal mucosal cells to release **intestinal (enteric) gastrin**, a hormone that encourages the gastric glands to continue their secretory activity. This stimulatory effect is brief because as the intestine distends with chyme containing large amounts of H^+, fats, partially digested proteins, and various irritating substances, the inhibitory component is triggered in the form of the **enterogastric reflex**.

The enterogastric reflex is actually a trio of reflexes that (1) inhibit the vagal nuclei in the medulla, (2) inhibit local reflexes, and (3) activate sympathetic fibers that cause the pyloric sphincter to tighten and prevent further food entry into the small intestine. As a result, gastric secretory activity declines. These "brakes" on gastric activity protect the small intestine from excessive acidity and match the small intestine's processing abilities to the amount of chyme entering it.

If pushed beyond its capacity to accept chyme, the small intestine's refusal is quick and recognizable—nausea and vomiting. This phenomenon, called the *dumping syndrome*, is an unpleasant experience in many who have had their stomach volume reduced in order to lose weight (see p. 943).

In addition, the factors we just named trigger the release of several intestinal hormones, collectively called **enterogastrones**. They include **secretin** (se-kre′tin), **cholecystokinin (CCK)** (ko″le-sis″to-ki′nin), and **vasoactive intestinal peptide (VIP)**. All of these hormones inhibit gastric secretion when the stomach is very active and also play other roles (see Table 23.1).

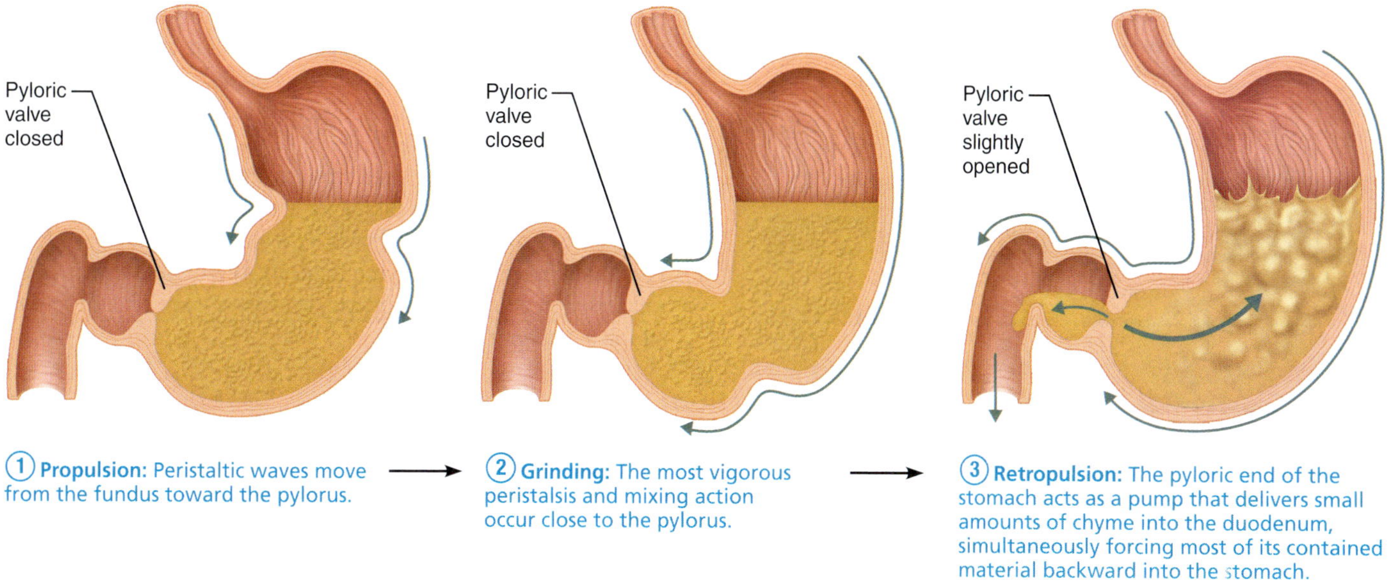

Figure 23.19 Peristaltic waves in the stomach.

Regulation of Gastric Motility and Emptying

Stomach contractions not only accommodate its filling and cause its emptying, but they also compress, knead, and mix the food with gastric juice to produce chyme. The processes of mechanical breakdown and propulsion are inseparable in the stomach due to a unique type of peristalsis.

Response of the Stomach to Filling

The stomach stretches to accommodate incoming food, but internal stomach pressure remains constant until about 1.5 L of food have been ingested. Thereafter, the pressure rises. The relatively unchanging pressure in a filling stomach is due to two factors:

- **Receptive relaxation** of smooth muscle in the stomach fundus and body which occurs both in anticipation of and in response to food moving through the esophagus and into the stomach. The swallowing center of the brain stem coordinates this process, which is mediated by the vagus nerves acting on serotonin- and NO-releasing enteric neurons.
- **Gastric accommodation**, which is an example of smooth muscle *plasticity*. It is the intrinsic ability of visceral smooth muscle to exhibit the *stress-relaxation response*, in other words, it can stretch without greatly increasing its tension and contracting expulsively. As we described in Chapter 9, this capability is very important in hollow organs, like the stomach, that must serve as temporary reservoirs.

Gastric Contractile Activity

As in the esophagus, the stomach exhibits peristalsis. After a meal, peristalsis begins near the gastroesophageal sphincter, where it produces gentle rippling movements of the thin stomach wall. But as the contractions approach the pylorus, where the stomach musculature is thicker, they become much more powerful. Consequently, the contents of the fundus and body (food storage area) remain relatively undisturbed, while foodstuffs in and around the pyloric antrum receive a truly lively pummeling and mixing.

The pyloric part of the stomach, which holds about 30 ml of chyme, acts as a dynamic filter that allows only liquids and small particles to pass through the barely open pyloric valve. Normally, each peristaltic wave reaching the pyloric muscle squirts 3 ml or less of chyme into the small intestine. Because the contraction also *closes* the valve, which is normally partially relaxed, the rest (about 27 ml) is propelled backward into the stomach, where it is mixed further (**Figure 23.19**). This back-and-forth pumping action (retropulsion) effectively breaks up solids in the gastric contents.

Although the intensity of the stomach's peristaltic waves can be modified, their rate is constant—always around three per minute. This contractile rhythm is set by *enteric pacemaker cells*, muscle-like noncontractile cells formerly called *interstitial cells of Cajal* (kă-hal′). Located in the longitudinal smooth muscle layer, the pacemaker cells depolarize and repolarize spontaneously three times each minute, establishing the so-called *cyclic slow waves* of the stomach, or its **basic electrical rhythm (BER)**. Since gap junctions couple the pacemakers electrically to the rest of the smooth muscle sheet, their "beat" is transmitted efficiently and quickly to the entire muscularis.

The pacemakers set the maximum frequency of contraction, but they do not initiate the contractions or regulate their force. Instead, they generate subthreshold depolarization waves, which are then "ignited" (enhanced by further depolarization and brought to threshold) by neural and hormonal factors.

The same factors that increase the strength of stomach contractions also enhance gastric secretions. Distension of the stomach wall by food activates stretch receptors and gastrin-secreting cells, both of which ultimately stimulate gastric

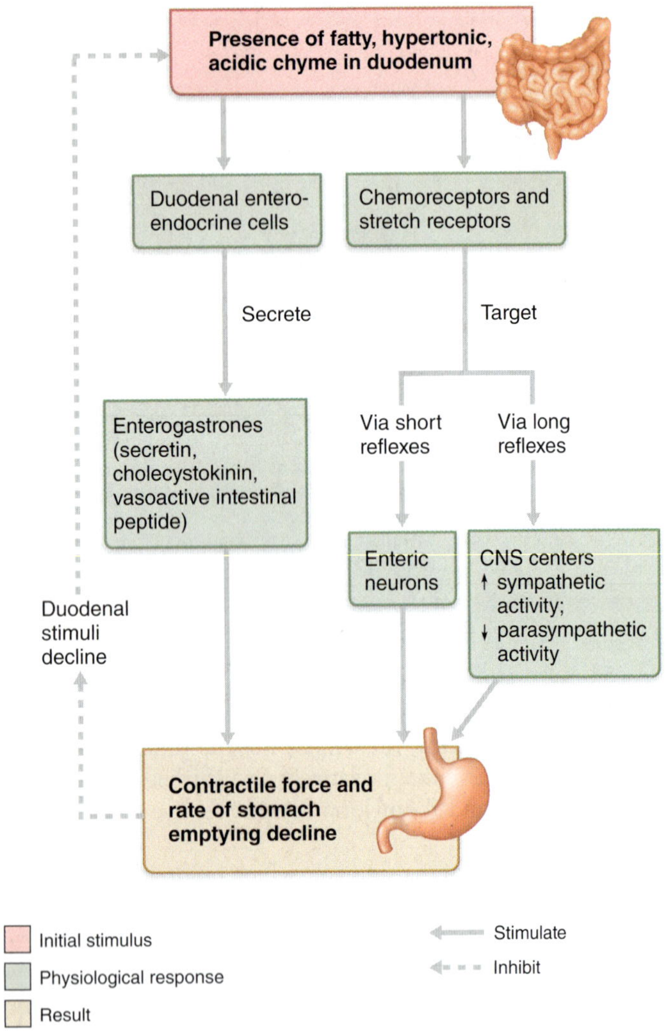

Figure 23.20 Neural and hormonal factors that inhibit gastric emptying. These controls ensure that the food is well liquefied in the stomach and prevent the small intestine from being overwhelmed.

23

smooth muscle and increase gastric motility. For this reason, the more food there is in the stomach, the more vigorous the stomach mixing and emptying movements will be—within certain limits—as we describe next.

Regulation of Gastric Emptying

The stomach usually empties completely within four hours after a meal. However, the larger the meal (the greater the stomach distension) and the more liquid its contents, the faster the stomach empties. Fluids pass quickly through the stomach. Solids linger, remaining until they are well mixed with gastric juice and converted to the liquid state.

The rate of gastric emptying also depends as much—and perhaps more—on the contents of the duodenum as on what is happening in the stomach. The stomach and duodenum act in tandem like a "coupled meter" that functions at less than full capacity. As chyme enters the duodenum, receptors in its wall respond to chemical signals and to stretch, initiating the enterogastric reflex and the hormonal (enterogastrone) mechanisms that inhibit acid and pepsin secretion as we described earlier. These mechanisms inhibit gastric secretion and prevent further duodenal filling by reducing the force of pyloric contractions **(Figure 23.20)**.

A carbohydrate-rich meal moves through the duodenum rapidly, but fats form an oily layer at the top of the chyme and are digested more slowly by enzymes acting in the intestine. For this reason, when chyme entering the duodenum is fatty, reflexes slow stomach emptying, and food may remain in the stomach six hours or more.

Homeostatic Imbalance 23.9

Vomiting, or **emesis**, is an unpleasant experience that empties the stomach by a different route. Many factors signal the stomach to "launch lunch," but the most common are extreme stretching of the stomach or intestine or irritants such as bacterial toxins, excessive alcohol, spicy foods, and certain drugs.

Bloodborne molecules and sensory impulses stream from the irritated sites to the **emetic center** (e-met′ik) of the medulla where they initiate a number of motor responses. Before vomiting, an individual typically feels nauseated, is pale, and salivates excessively. A deep inspiration directly precedes vomiting. The diaphragm and abdominal wall muscles contract, increasing intra-abdominal pressure, the gastroesophageal sphincter relaxes, and the soft palate rises to close off the nasal passages. As a result, the stomach (and perhaps duodenal) contents are forced upward through the esophagus and pharynx and out the mouth.

Excessive vomiting can cause dehydration and severely disrupt the body's electrolyte and acid-base balance. Since large amounts of HCl are lost in vomitus, the blood becomes alkaline as the stomach attempts to replace its lost acid. ✚

☑ Check Your Understanding

27. Name the three phases of gastric secretion.
28. How does the presence of food in the small intestine inhibit gastric secretion and motility?
29. How does the pH of venous blood leaving the stomach change during a meal?

For answers, see Appendix H.

The Small Intestine and Associated Structures

✓ Identify and describe structural modifications of the wall of the small intestine that enhance the digestive process.

✓ Differentiate between the roles of the various cell types of the intestinal mucosa.

✓ Describe the function of intestinal hormones and paracrines.

In the small intestine, usable food is finally prepared for its journey into the cells of the body. However, this vital function cannot happen without the aid of secretions from the liver (bile)

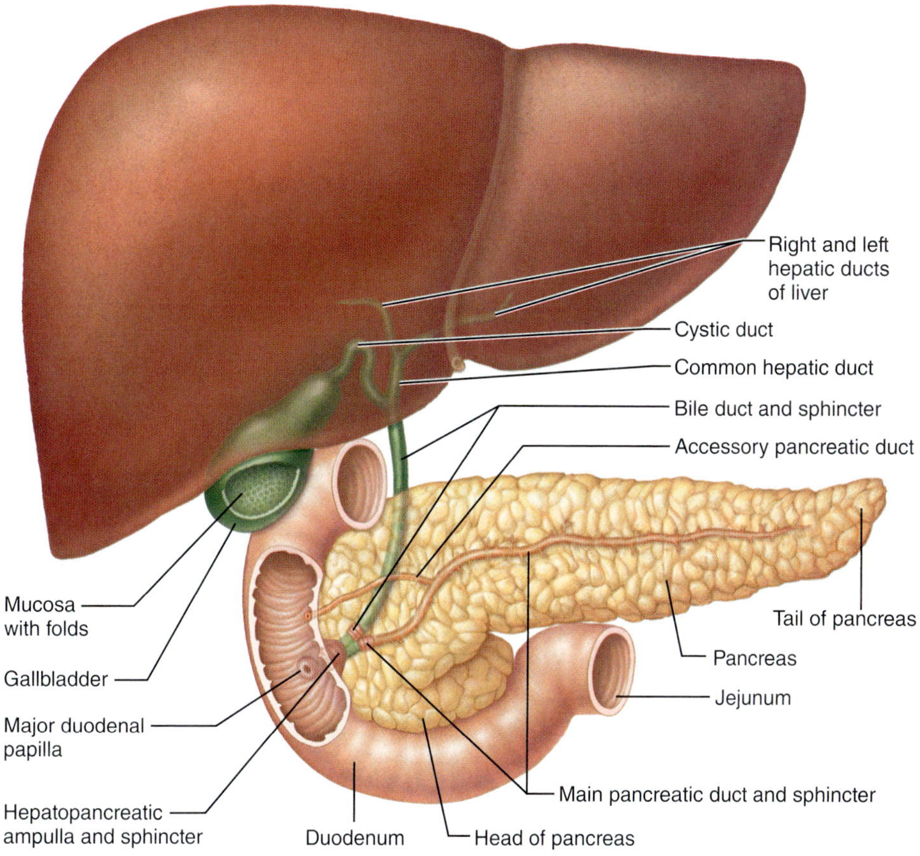

Figure 23.21 The duodenum of the small intestine, and related organs. Ducts from the pancreas, gallbladder, and liver empty into the duodenum.

and pancreas (digestive enzymes). We will also consider these accessory organs in this section.

The Small Intestine

The **small intestine** is the body's major digestive organ. Within its twisted passageways, digestion is completed and virtually all absorption occurs.

Gross Anatomy

The small intestine is a convoluted tube extending from the pyloric sphincter to the **ileocecal valve (sphincter)** (il″e-o-se′kal) where it joins the large intestine. It is the longest part of the alimentary canal, but is only about half the diameter of the large intestine, ranging from 2.5 to 4 cm (1–1.6 inches). Although 6–7 m long (approximately 20 ft, the height of a two-story building) in a cadaver, the small intestine is only 2–4 m (7–13 ft) long during life because of muscle tone.

The small intestine has three subdivisions: the duodenum, which is mostly retroperitoneal, and the jejunum and ileum, both intraperitoneal organs (see Figure 23.1). The relatively immovable **duodenum** (du″o-de′num; "twelve finger widths long"), which curves around the head of the pancreas, is about 25 cm (10 inches) long **(Figure 23.21)**. Although it is the shortest intestinal subdivision, the duodenum has the most features of interest.

The bile duct, delivering bile from the liver, and the main pancreatic duct, carrying pancreatic juice from the pancreas, unite in the wall of the duodenum in a bulblike point called the **hepatopancreatic ampulla** (hep″ah-to-pan″kre-at′ik am-pul′ah; *ampulla* = flask). The ampulla opens into the duodenum via the volcano-shaped **major duodenal papilla**. A smooth muscle valve called the **hepatopancreatic sphincter** controls the entry of bile and pancreatic juice.

The **jejunum** (jĕ-joo′num; "empty"), about 2.5 m (8 ft) long, extends from the duodenum to the ileum. The **ileum** (il′e-um; "twisted"), approximately 3.6 m (12 ft) in length, joins the large intestine at the ileocecal valve. The jejunum and ileum hang in sausagelike coils in the central and lower part of the abdominal cavity, suspended from the posterior abdominal wall by the fan-shaped *mesentery* (see Figure 23.30). The large intestine encircles these more distal parts of the small intestine.

Nerve fibers serving the small intestine include parasympathetics from the vagus and sympathetics from the thoracic splanchnic nerves, both relayed through the superior mesenteric (and celiac) plexus.

The arterial supply is primarily from the superior mesenteric artery (pp. 732–733). The veins parallel the arteries and typically drain into the superior mesenteric vein. From there, the nutrient-rich venous blood from the small intestine drains into the hepatic portal vein, which carries it to the liver.

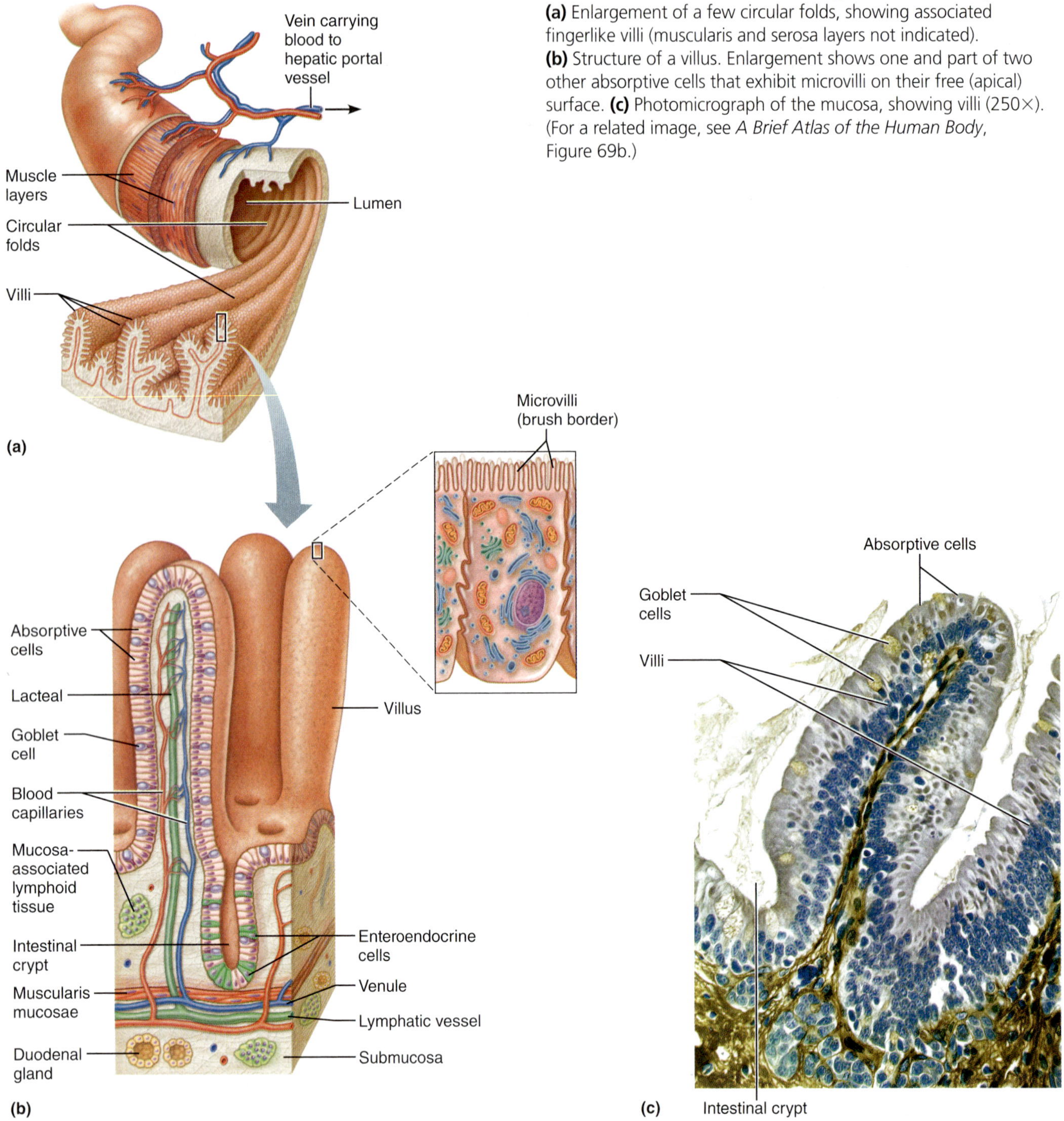

Figure 23.22 Structural modifications of the small intestine that increase its surface area for digestion and absorption. **(a)** Enlargement of a few circular folds, showing associated fingerlike villi (muscularis and serosa layers not indicated). **(b)** Structure of a villus. Enlargement shows one and part of two other absorptive cells that exhibit microvilli on their free (apical) surface. **(c)** Photomicrograph of the mucosa, showing villi (250×). (For a related image, see *A Brief Atlas of the Human Body*, Figure 69b.)

Microscopic Anatomy

Modifications for Absorption The small intestine is highly adapted for absorbing nutrients. Its length alone provides a huge surface area, and its wall has three structural modifications—circular folds, villi, and microvilli—that amplify its absorptive surface enormously (by a factor of more than 600 times). In fact, the intestinal surface area is about equal to 200 square meters, the size of a singles tennis court! Most absorption occurs in the proximal part of the small intestine, so these specializations decrease in number toward its distal end.

The **circular folds** are deep, permanent folds of the mucosa and submucosa **(Figure 23.22a)**. Nearly 1 cm tall, these folds force chyme to spiral through the lumen, slowing its movement and allowing time for full nutrient absorption.

Villi (vil′i; "tufts of hair") are fingerlike projections of the mucosa, over 1 mm high, that give it a velvety texture, much like the soft nap of a towel (Figure 23.22). The villi are large and leaflike in the duodenum (the intestinal site of most active absorption) and gradually narrow and shorten along the length of the small intestine. The epithelial cells of the villi (called *enterocytes*) are chiefly absorptive columnar cells. In the core of each villus is a dense capillary bed and a wide lymphatic capillary called a **lacteal** (lak′te-al). Digested foodstuffs are absorbed through the epithelial cells into both the capillary blood and the lacteal.

The exceptionally long, densely packed **microvilli** of the absorptive cells of the mucosa give the mucosal surface a fuzzy appearance called the **brush border** (Figure 23.22b enlargement and **Figure 23.23**). The plasma membranes of the microvilli bear enzymes referred to as **brush border enzymes**, which complete the digestion of carbohydrates and proteins in the small intestine.

Histology of the Small Intestine Wall Externally the subdivisions of the small intestine appear to be nearly identical, but their internal and microscopic anatomies reveal some important differences. The four tunics typical of the GI tract are also seen here, but the mucosa and submucosa are modified to reflect the intestine's functions in the digestive pathway.

The epithelium of the villus mucosa is largely simple columnar *absorptive cells* bound by tight junctions and richly endowed with microvilli. These cells bear the primary responsibility for absorbing nutrients and electrolytes. The epithelium also has many mucus-secreting *goblet cells*. Between the villi, the mucosa is studded with *pits* that lead into tubular glands called **intestinal crypts** (see Figure 23.22b, c).

Crypt epithelial cells are primarily secretory cells that secrete *intestinal juice*, a watery mixture that contains mucus and serves as a carrier fluid for absorbing nutrients from chyme. Scattered through the crypt epithelium are *enteroendocrine cells*, the source of the enterogastrones—secretin and cholecystokinin to name two—and T cells called *intraepithelial lymphocytes* (*IELs*), which represent an important immunological defensive component.

Deep in the crypts are specialized secretory cells called *Paneth cells*, which fortify the small intestine's defenses by releasing antimicrobial agents such as defensins and *lysozyme*, an antibacterial enzyme. These secretions destroy certain bacteria and help to determine which bacteria colonize the intestinal lumen. The crypts decrease in number along the length of the small intestine, but the goblet cells become more abundant.

The various epithelial cells arise from continuously dividing stem cells at the base of the crypts. As the daughter cells gradually migrate up the villi, they differentiate, becoming specialized cell types—absorptive cells, goblet cells, and enteroendocrine cells. The fourth differentiated cell type is the Paneth cells, which remain at the base of the crypts. The other three types undergo apoptosis and are shed from the villus tips, renewing the villus epithelium every two to four days.

Homeostatic Imbalance 23.10

Treatments for cancer, such as radiation therapy and chemotherapy, preferentially target rapidly dividing cells. They kill cancer cells, but also nearly obliterate the rapidly dividing GI tract epithelium. Many patients suffer nausea, vomiting, and diarrhea after each treatment. ✚

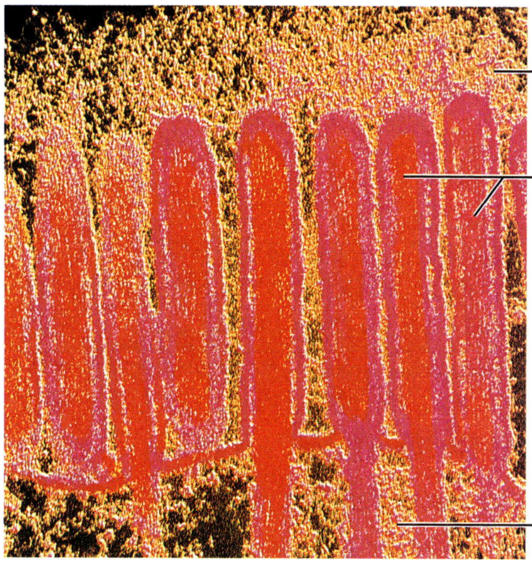

Figure 23.23 Microvilli of the small intestine. False-color electron micrograph. Microvilli (28,000×) of absorptive cells appear as red projections from the surface of the absorptive cell. Yellow granules are mucus granules.

The mucosa contains both individual follicles and *aggregated lymphoid nodules*, the latter called **Peyer's patches** (pi′erz). Peyer's patches are primarily located in the lamina propria but occasionally protrude into the submucosa below. Their increasing abundance toward the distal end of the small intestine reflects the fact that this region of the small intestine contains huge numbers of bacteria that must be prevented from entering the bloodstream.

The lymphoid tissue of the mucosa also contains proliferating B lymphocytes that leave the intestine, enter the blood, and then home in on the intestinal lamina propria. There, in their new home, they release immunoglobin A (IgA), which helps protect against intestinal pathogens (see p. 783).

The submucosa is typical areolar connective tissue. Elaborate mucus-secreting **duodenal glands** in the submucosa of the duodenum produce an alkaline (bicarbonate-rich) mucus that helps neutralize acidic chyme moving in from the stomach. When this protective mucus barrier is inadequate, the intestinal wall erodes and *duodenal ulcers* result.

The muscularis is typical and bilayered. Except for the bulk of the duodenum, which is retroperitoneal and has an adventitia, visceral peritoneum (serosa) covers the external intestinal surface.

Intestinal Juice: Composition and Control

The intestinal glands normally secrete 1 to 2 L of intestinal juice daily. The major stimulus for its production comes from hypertonic or acidic chyme, which cause distension or irritation of the intestinal mucosa.

Normally, intestinal juice is slightly alkaline (7.4–7.8), and isotonic with blood plasma. Intestinal juice is largely water but also contains some mucus, which is secreted both by the duodenal glands and by goblet cells of the mucosa. Intestinal juice is enzyme-poor because intestinal enzymes are limited to the bound enzymes of the brush border.

Check Your Understanding

30. What common advantage do circular folds, villi, and microvilli provide to the digestive process? Which of these modifications causes chyme to spiral through the lumen and slows its passage?
31. What are brush border enzymes?
32. What is a lacteal and what is its function?
33. Name three secretory products that help protect the intestinal mucosa from bacterial damage.

For answers, see Appendix H.

The Liver and Gallbladder

- ✓ Describe the histologic anatomy of the liver.
- ✓ State the role of bile in digestion.
- ✓ Describe the role of the gallbladder.

The *liver* and *gallbladder* are accessory organs associated with the small intestine. The liver, one of the body's most important organs, has many metabolic and regulatory roles. However, its *digestive* system function is to produce bile for export to the duodenum. Bile is a fat emulsifier that breaks down fats into tiny particles to make them more readily digestible. We will describe this process when we discuss the digestion and absorption of fats later in the chapter. Although the liver also processes nutrient-laden venous blood delivered to it from the digestive organs, this is a metabolic rather than a digestive role (see Chapter 24.) The gallbladder is chiefly a storage organ for bile.

Gross Anatomy of the Liver

The ruddy, blood-rich **liver** is the largest gland in the body, weighing about 1.4 kg (3 lb) in the average adult. Shaped like a wedge, it occupies most of the right hypochondriac and epigastric regions (see Figure 1.12), extending farther to the right of the body midline than to the left. Located under the diaphragm, the liver lies almost entirely within the rib cage, which provides some protection (see Figure 23.1 and **Figure 23.24**).

23

The liver has four primary lobes. The largest, the *right lobe*, is visible on all liver surfaces and separated from the smaller *left lobe* by a deep fissure (Figure 23.24a). The posteriormost *caudate lobe* and the *quadrate lobe*, which lies inferior to the left lobe, are visible in an inferior view of the liver (Figure 23.24b).

A mesentery, the **falciform ligament**, separates the right and left lobes anteriorly and suspends the liver from the diaphragm and anterior abdominal wall. Running along the inferior edge of the falciform ligament is the **round ligament**, or **ligamentum teres** (te′rēz; "round"), a fibrous remnant of the fetal umbilical vein. Except for the superiormost liver area (the *bare area*), which touches the diaphragm, the entire liver is enclosed by the visceral peritoneum.

As we mentioned earlier, a ventral mesentery, the lesser omentum, anchors the liver to the lesser curvature of the stomach (see Figure 23.30b). The **hepatic artery** and the **hepatic portal vein**, which enter the liver at the **porta hepatis** ("gateway to the liver"), and the common hepatic duct, which runs inferiorly from the liver, all travel through the lesser omentum to reach their destinations. The gallbladder rests in a recess on the inferior surface of the right liver lobe (Figure 23.24b).

The traditional scheme of defining liver lobes (outlined above) has been criticized because it is based on superficial features of the liver. Hepatic surgeons prefer to discuss the liver in terms of eight segments based on its internal anatomy relative to its vascular and biliary supply. This system permits them to remove sections while encountering the fewest major vascular structures and the lowest risk.

Bile leaves the liver through several bile ducts that ultimately fuse to form the large **common hepatic duct**, which travels downward toward the duodenum. Along its course, that duct fuses with the **cystic duct** draining the gallbladder to form the **bile duct** (see Figure 23.21).

Microscopic Anatomy of the Liver

The liver is composed of sesame seed–sized structural and functional units called **liver lobules**. Each lobule is a roughly hexagonal (six-sided) structure consisting of plates of *liver cells*, or **hepatocytes** (hep′ah-to-sīts), organized like bricks in a garden wall **(Figure 23.25)**. The hepatocyte plates radiate outward from a **central vein** running in the longitudinal axis of the lobule. To make a rough model of a liver lobule, open a thick paperback book until its two covers meet: The pages represent the plates of hepatocytes and the hollow cylinder formed by the rolled spine represents the central vein.

If you keep in mind that the liver's main function is to filter and process the nutrient-rich blood delivered to it, its histology makes a lot of sense. At each of the six corners of a lobule is a **portal triad** (*portal tract* region), so named because it contains three basic structures (Figure 23.25c):

- A branch of the *hepatic artery* (supplying oxygen-rich arterial blood to the liver)
- A branch of the *hepatic portal* vein (carrying venous blood laden with nutrients from the digestive viscera)
- A *bile duct*

Between the hepatocyte plates are enlarged, heavily fenestrated **liver sinusoids**. Blood from both the hepatic portal vein and the hepatic artery percolates from the triad regions through these sinusoids and empties into the central vein. From the central veins blood eventually enters the hepatic veins, which drain the liver, and empties into the inferior vena cava. Forming part of the sinusoid walls are star-shaped **stellate macrophages**, also called **hepatic macrophages** (Figure 23.25c). They remove debris such as bacteria and worn-out blood cells from the blood as it flows past.

The versatile hepatocytes have large amounts of both rough and smooth ER, Golgi apparatus, peroxisomes, and mitochondria. Equipped in this way, the hepatocytes can secrete or generate some 900 ml of bile daily. The hepatocytes also:

- Process bloodborne nutrients in various ways (e.g., they store glucose as glycogen and use amino acids to make plasma proteins)
- Store fat-soluble vitamins
- Play important roles in detoxification, such as ridding the blood of ammonia by converting it to urea (Chapter 24)

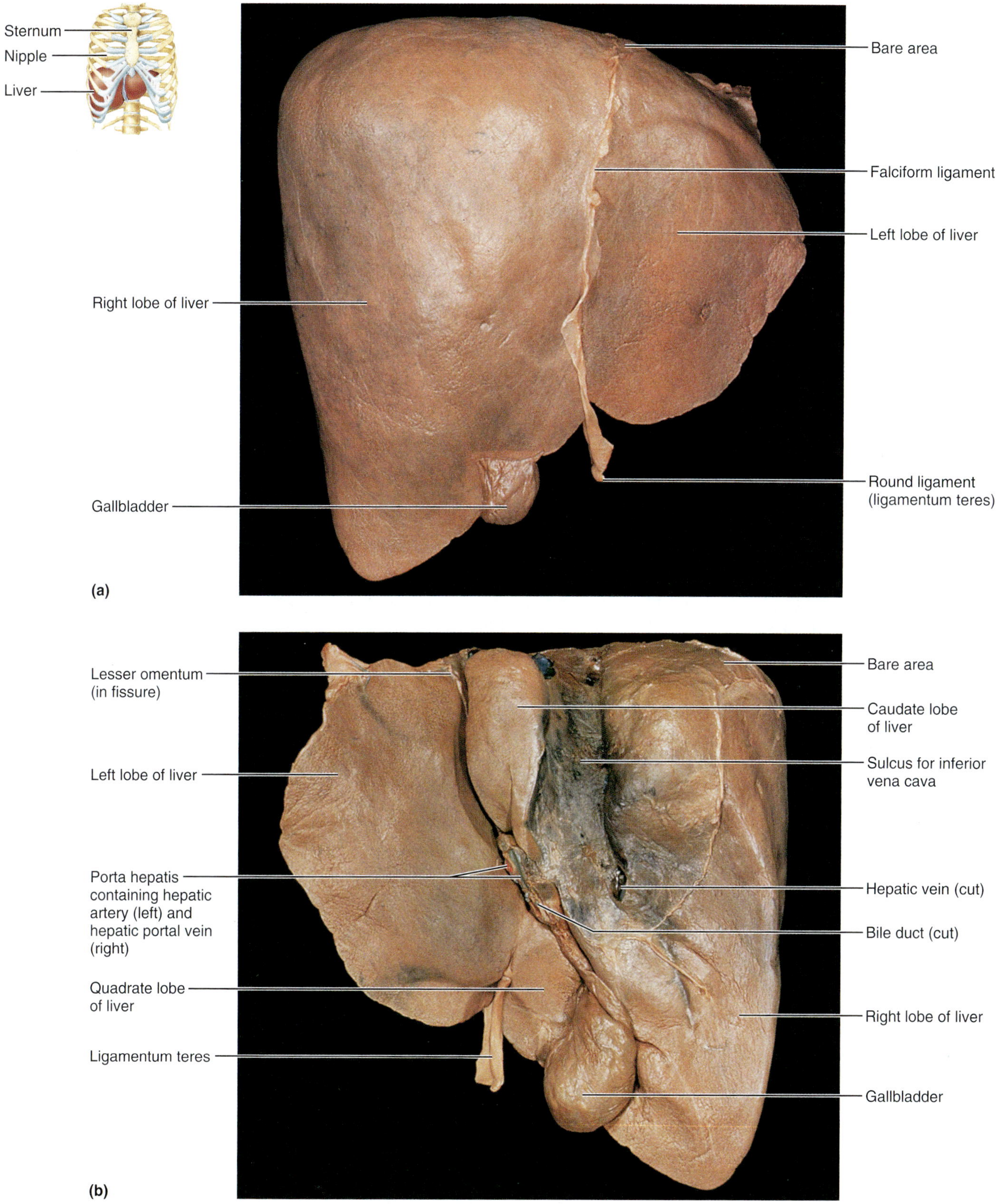

Figure 23.24 Gross anatomy of the human liver. (a) Anterior view of the liver. **(b)** Posteroinferior aspect of the liver. In this view a group of fissures separate the four liver lobes. The porta hepatis is a deep fissure that contains the hepatic portal vein, hepatic artery, common hepatic duct, and lymphatics. (For related images, see *A Brief Atlas of the Human Body*, Figures 64 and 65.)

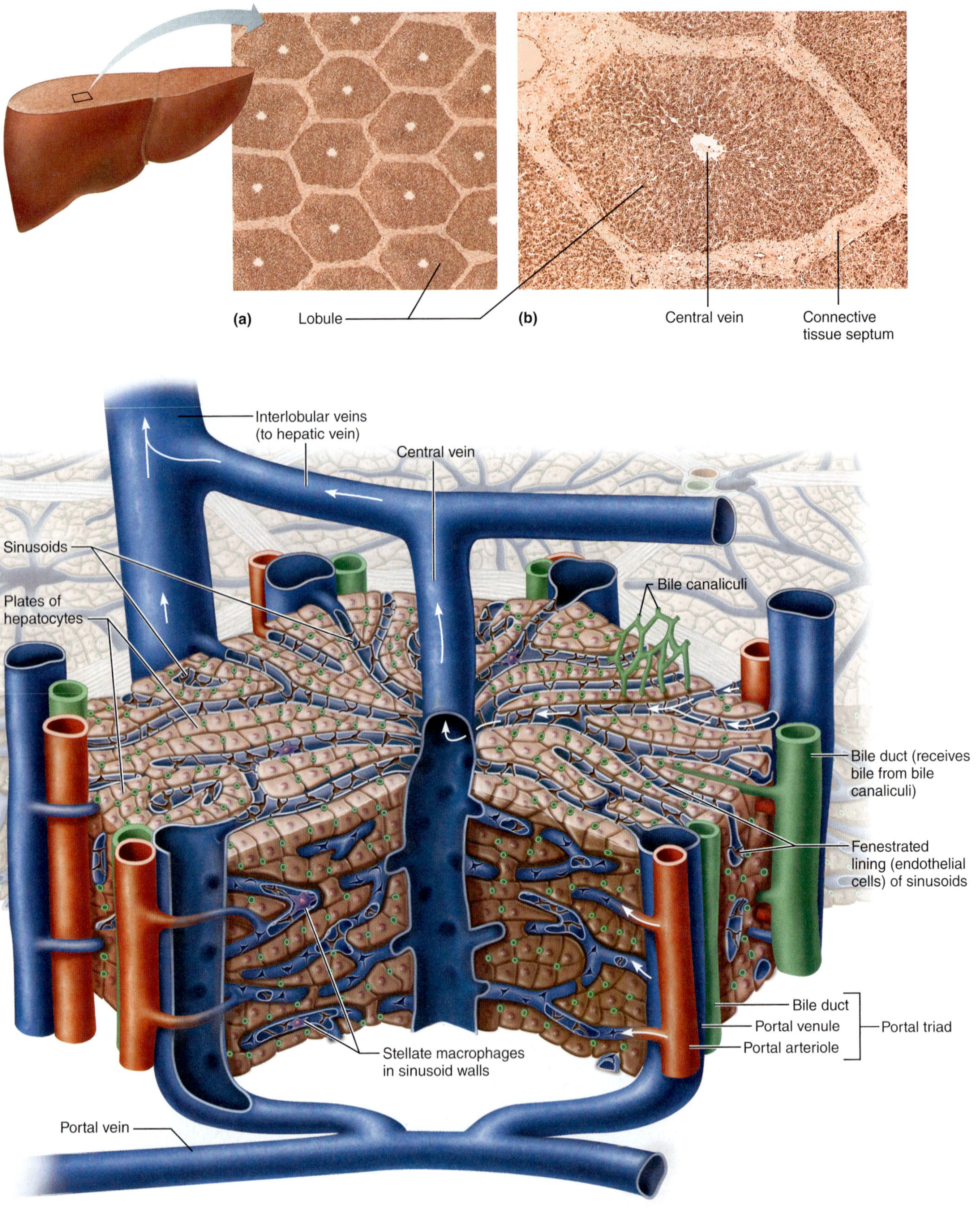

Figure 23.25 Microscopic anatomy of the liver. (a) Classic lobular pattern of a pig liver. **(b)** Enlarged view of one liver lobule. **(c)** Three-dimensional representation of a small portion of one liver lobule, showing the structure of sinusoids. Arrows indicate the direction of blood flow.

Thanks to these various jobs, blood leaving the liver contains fewer nutrients and waste materials than the blood that entered it.

The regenerative capacity of the liver is exceptional. It can regenerate to its former size in 6–12 months even after surgical removal or loss of 80% of its mass. When the liver is injured, hepatocytes secrete *growth factors* that prompt endothelial cells lining the sinusoids to proliferate and release other growth factors. These, in turn, prompt the hepatocytes to multiply and replace dead and dying liver tissue.

Secreted bile flows through tiny canals, called **bile canaliculi** (kan″ah-lik′u-li; "little canals"), that run between adjacent hepatocytes toward the bile duct branches in the portal triads (Figure 23.25c). Although most illustrations show the canaliculi as discrete tubular structures (shown here in green), their walls are actually formed by the apical membranes of adjoining hepatocytes. Notice that blood and bile flow in opposite directions in the liver lobule. Bile entering the bile ducts eventually leaves the liver via the common hepatic duct to travel toward the duodenum.

Homeostatic Imbalances of the Liver

Hepatitis (hep″ah-ti′tis), or inflammation of the liver, is most often due to viral infection. So far six hepatitis-causing viruses have been identified, from A to F. Two of these (HVA and HVE) are transmitted enterically (acquired through eating contaminated food), and the infections they cause tend to be self-limiting. Those transmitted via blood—most importantly HVB and HVC—are linked to chronic hepatitis and liver cirrhosis (see discussion below). HVD is a mutated virus that needs HVB to be infectious. So far, little is known about HVF. Nonviral causes of acute hepatitis include drug toxicity and wild mushroom poisoning.

In the United States, over 40% of hepatitis cases are due to HVB, which is transmitted via blood transfusions, contaminated needles, or sexual contact. A serious problem in its own right, hepatitis B carries with it a greater menace—an elevated risk of liver cancer. However, childhood immunization using vaccines produced in bacteria is sweeping the feet out from under HVB, and the incidence of acute hepatitis from this strain has fallen dramatically since its peak in 1985.

Hepatitis A, commonly called infectious hepatitis and accounting for about 32% of cases, is a more benign form frequently observed in day-care centers. It is transmitted via sewage-contaminated food, raw shellfish, water, and by the feces-mouth route, which explains why it is important for restaurant employees to scrub their hands after using the washroom. The highly successful HepA vaccine helps prevent hepatitis A infection and shedding of the virus in feces.

Hepatitis E is transmitted in a way similar to hepatitis A. It causes waterborne epidemics, largely in developing countries, and is a major cause of death (up to 25%) in pregnant women. It is relatively insignificant in the United States.

Hepatitis C has emerged as the most important liver disease in the United States because it produces persistent or chronic liver infections (as opposed to acute infections). More than 4 million Americans are infected and over 10,000 die annually due to sequels of HVC infection. However, the life-threatening C form of hepatitis is now being successfully treated by combination drug therapy entailing weekly injections of interferon and ribavirin (Rebetol), an oral antiviral drug.

Cirrhosis (sĭr-ro′sis; "orange colored") is a progressive chronic inflammation of the liver that typically results from severe chronic hepatitis or chronic alcoholism. The damaged hepatocytes regenerate, but the liver's connective (scar) tissue regenerates faster. As a result, the liver becomes fatty and fibrous, depressing its activity. The scar tissue obstructs blood flow throughout the hepatic portal system, causing **portal hypertension**.

Some veins of the portal system anastomose with veins that drain into the venae cavae (*portal-caval anastomoses*). However, these connecting veins are small and tend to burst when forced to carry large volumes of blood. Signs of their failure include vomiting blood, and a snakelike network of distended veins surrounding the navel. This network is called *caput medusae* (kap′ut mĕ-du′se; "medusa head") after a monster in Greek mythology whose hair was made of writhing snakes. Other complications due to portal hypertension include esophageal varices (swollen veins in the esophagus) and ascites (accumulated fluid in the peritoneal cavity.)

Liver transplants are the only clinically proven effective treatment for patients with end-stage liver disease. The one- and five-year survival rate of such transplants is approximately 90% and 75%, respectively. However, donor organs are scarce and many patients die while waiting for a suitable organ.

Composition of Bile

Bile is a yellow-green, alkaline solution containing bile salts, bile pigments, cholesterol, triglycerides, phospholipids (lecithin and others), and a variety of electrolytes. Of these, *only* bile salts and phospholipids aid the digestive process.

Bile salts, primarily cholic and chenodeoxycholic acids, are cholesterol derivatives. Their role is to *emulsify* fats—break them down into smaller pieces and distribute them throughout the watery intestinal contents, just as a dish detergent breaks up a pool of fat drippings in a roasting pan. Bile salts physically separate large fat globules entering the small intestine into millions of smaller, more accessible fatty droplets that provide large surface areas for the fat-digesting enzymes to work on. Bile salts also facilitate fat and cholesterol absorption (discussed later). In addition, they help solubilize cholesterol, both that contained in bile and that entering the small intestine in food.

Many substances secreted in bile leave the body in feces, but bile salts are not among them. Instead, a recycling mechanism called the *enterohepatic circulation* conserves bile salts. In this process, bile salts are (1) reabsorbed into the blood by the ileum, (2) returned to the liver via the hepatic portal blood, and then (3) resecreted in newly formed bile. This pool of bile salts recirculates two or three times for a single meal.

The chief bile pigment is **bilirubin** (bil″ĭ-roo′bin), a waste product of the heme of hemoglobin formed during the breakdown of worn-out erythrocytes (see Chapter 17). The globin and iron parts of hemoglobin are saved and recycled, but bilirubin is absorbed from the blood by liver cells, excreted into bile, and metabolized in the small intestine by resident bacteria. One of its breakdown

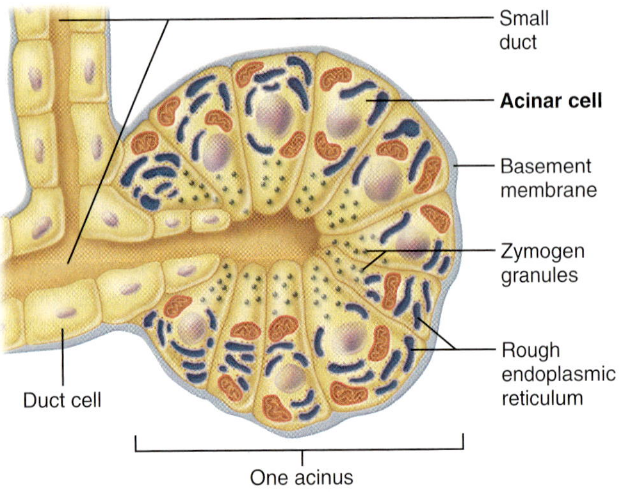

(a)

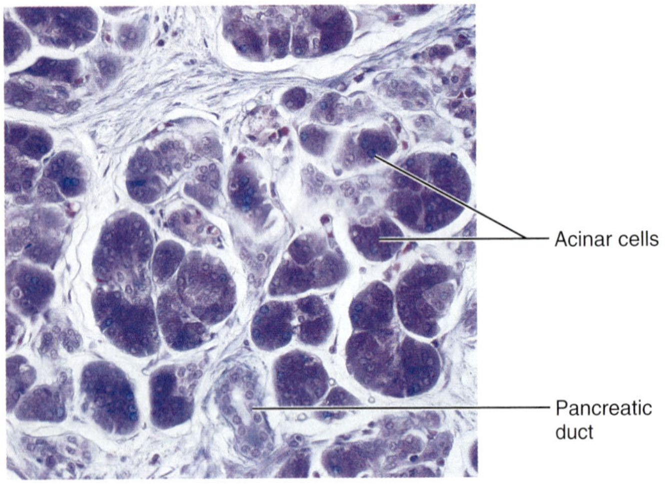

(b)

Figure 23.26 Structure of the enzyme-producing tissue of the pancreas. (a) Schematic view of one acinus (a secretory unit). The acinar cells contain abundant zymogen (enzyme-containing) granules and dark-staining rough ER (typical of gland cells producing large amounts of protein for export). **(b)** Photomicrograph of pancreatic acinar tissue (155×).

products, *stercobilin* (ster′ko-bi″lin), gives feces a brown color. In the absence of bile, feces are gray-white and have fatty streaks because essentially no fats are digested or absorbed.

The Gallbladder

The gallbladder is a thin-walled green muscular sac about 10 cm (4 inches) long. The size of a kiwi fruit, it snuggles in a shallow fossa on the inferior surface of the liver (see Figures 23.1 and 23.24) from which its rounded fundus protrudes.

The gallbladder stores bile that is not immediately needed for digestion and concentrates it by absorbing some of its water and ions. When empty, its mucosa is thrown into honeycomb-like folds (see Figure 23.21) that, like the rugae of the stomach, allow the organ to expand as it fills. Its muscular wall contracts to expel bile into the *cystic duct*. From there bile flows into the bile duct. The gallbladder, like most of the liver, is covered by visceral peritoneum.

Homeostatic Imbalance 23.11

Bile is the major vehicle for excreting cholesterol from the body, and bile salts keep the cholesterol dissolved within bile. Too much cholesterol or too few bile salts allows the cholesterol to crystallize, forming **gallstones** or *biliary calculi* (bil′e-a″re kal′ku-li), which obstruct the flow of bile from the gallbladder. When the gallbladder or its duct contracts, the sharp crystals cause agonizing pain that radiates to the right thoracic region.

Gallstones are easy to diagnose because they show up well with ultrasound imaging. Treatments for gallstones include dissolving the crystals with drugs, pulverizing them with ultrasound vibrations (lithotripsy), vaporizing them with lasers, and the classical treatment, surgically removing the gallbladder. When the gallbladder is removed, the bile duct enlarges to assume the bile-storing role.

Bile duct blockage prevents both bile salts and bile pigments from entering the intestine. As a result, yellow bile pigments accumulate in blood and eventually are deposited in the skin, causing it to become yellow, or *jaundiced*. Jaundice caused by blocked ducts is called *obstructive jaundice*, but jaundice may also reflect liver disease (in which the liver is unable to carry out its normal metabolic duties). ✚

Check Your Understanding

34. What is a portal triad?
35. What is the importance of the enterohepatic circulation?
36. What is the role of the stellate macrophages of the liver?

For answers, see Appendix H.

The Pancreas

✓ State the role of pancreatic juice in digestion.

The **pancreas** (pan′kre-as; *pan* = all, *creas* = flesh, meat) is a soft, tadpole-shaped gland that extends across the abdomen from its *tail* (abutting the spleen) to its *head*, which is encircled by the C-shaped duodenum (see Figures 23.1 and 23.21). Most of the pancreas is retroperitoneal and lies deep to the greater curvature of the stomach.

An accessory digestive organ, the pancreas is important to the digestive process because it produces enzymes that break down all categories of foodstuffs. This exocrine product, called **pancreatic juice**, drains from the pancreas into the duodendum via the centrally located **main pancreatic duct**. The pancreatic duct generally fuses with the bile duct just as it enters the duodenum (at the hepatopancreatic ampulla). A smaller *accessory pancreatic duct* empties directly into the duodenum just proximal to the main duct.

Within the pancreas are the **acini** (as′ĭ-ni; singular: acinus), clusters of secretory acinar cells surrounding ducts **(Figure 23.26a)**. These cells are full of rough endoplasmic reticulum and exhibit deeply staining **zymogen granules** (zi′mo-jen; "fermenting") containing the inactive digestive enzymes (proenzymes) they manufacture.

Scattered amid the acini are the lightly staining *pancreatic islets*. These mini-endocrine glands release insulin and glucagon, hormones that play an important role in carbohydrate metabolism (see Chapter 16).

Composition of Pancreatic Juice

Approximately 1200 to 1500 ml of clear pancreatic juice is produced daily. It consists mainly of water, and contains enzymes and electrolytes (primarily bicarbonate ions). The acinar cells produce the enzyme-rich component of pancreatic juice. The epithelial cells lining the smallest pancreatic ducts release the bicarbonate ions that make it alkaline (about pH 8).

Normally, the amount of HCl produced in the stomach is exactly balanced by the amount of bicarbonate (HCO_3^-) secreted by the pancreas, and as HCO_3^- is secreted into the pancreatic juice, H^+ enters the blood. Consequently, the pH of venous blood returning to the heart remains relatively unchanged because acidic blood draining from the pancreas neutralizes the alkaline blood draining from the stomach.

The high pH of pancreatic fluid helps neutralize acid chyme entering the duodenum and provides the optimal environment for intestinal and pancreatic enzymes. Like pepsin of the stomach, pancreatic *proteases* (protein-digesting enzymes) are produced and released in inactive forms, which are activated in the duodenum, where they do their work. This protects the pancreas from digesting itself.

For example, within the duodenum, **enteropeptidase** (formerly called *enterokinase*), an intestinal brush border protease, activates *trypsinogen* to **trypsin**. Trypsin, in turn, activates more trypsinogen and two other pancreatic proteases (*procarboxypeptidase* and *chymotrypsinogen*) to their active forms, **carboxypeptidase** (kar-bok″se-pep′tĭ-dās) and **chymotrypsin** (ky″mo-trip′sin), respectively **(Figure 23.27)**.

Other pancreatic enzymes—**amylase**, **lipases**, and **nucleases**—are secreted in active form, but require that ions or bile be present in the intestinal lumen for optimal activity.

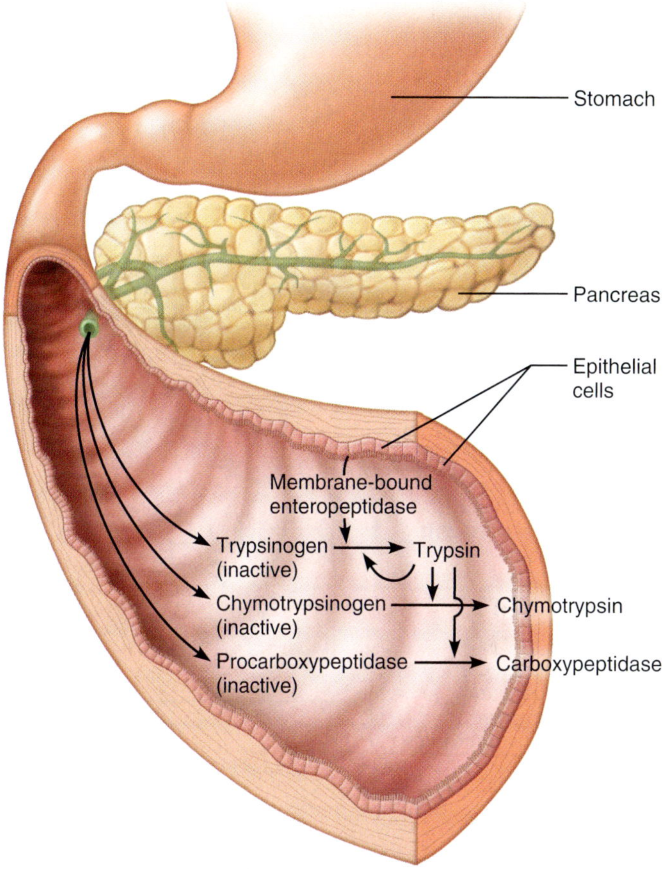

Figure 23.27 Activation of pancreatic proteases in the small intestine. Pancreatic proteases are secreted in an inactive form and are activated in the duodenum.

Check Your Understanding

37. What do zymogen granules contain?

38. What is the functional difference between pancreatic acini and islets?

For answers, see Appendix H.

Regulation of Bile and Pancreatic Secretion and Entry into the Small Intestine

✓ Describe how bile and pancreatic juice secretion into the small intestine are regulated.

The same factors—hormones and neural stimuli—that regulate the secretion of bile and pancreatic juice also regulate their release to the small intestine. There they "do their business" in food digestion. The hormones include cholecystokinin and secretin.

Bile salts themselves are the major stimulus for enhanced bile secretion **(Figure 23.28)**. After a fatty meal, when the enterohepatic circulation is returning large amounts of bile salts to the liver, its output of bile rises dramatically. *Secretin*, released by intestinal cells exposed to fatty chyme, also stimulates liver cells to secrete bile.

When no digestion is occurring, the hepatopancreatic sphincter (guarding the entry of bile and pancreatic juice into the duodenum) is closed and the released bile backs up the cystic duct into the gallbladder, where it is stored until needed. Although the liver makes bile continuously, bile does not usually enter the small intestine until the gallbladder contracts.

The major stimulus for gallbladder contraction is *cholecystokinin*, which is released to the blood when acidic, fatty chyme enters the duodenum (Figure 23.28). Besides causing the gallbladder to contract, CCK (1) stimulates secretion of pancreatic juice and (2) relaxes the hepatopancreatic sphincter so that bile and pancreatic juice can enter the duodenum.

Both secretin and cholecystokinin prompt the pancreas to secrete its juice. Secretin, released in response to the presence of HCl in the intestine, mainly targets the pancreatic duct cells,

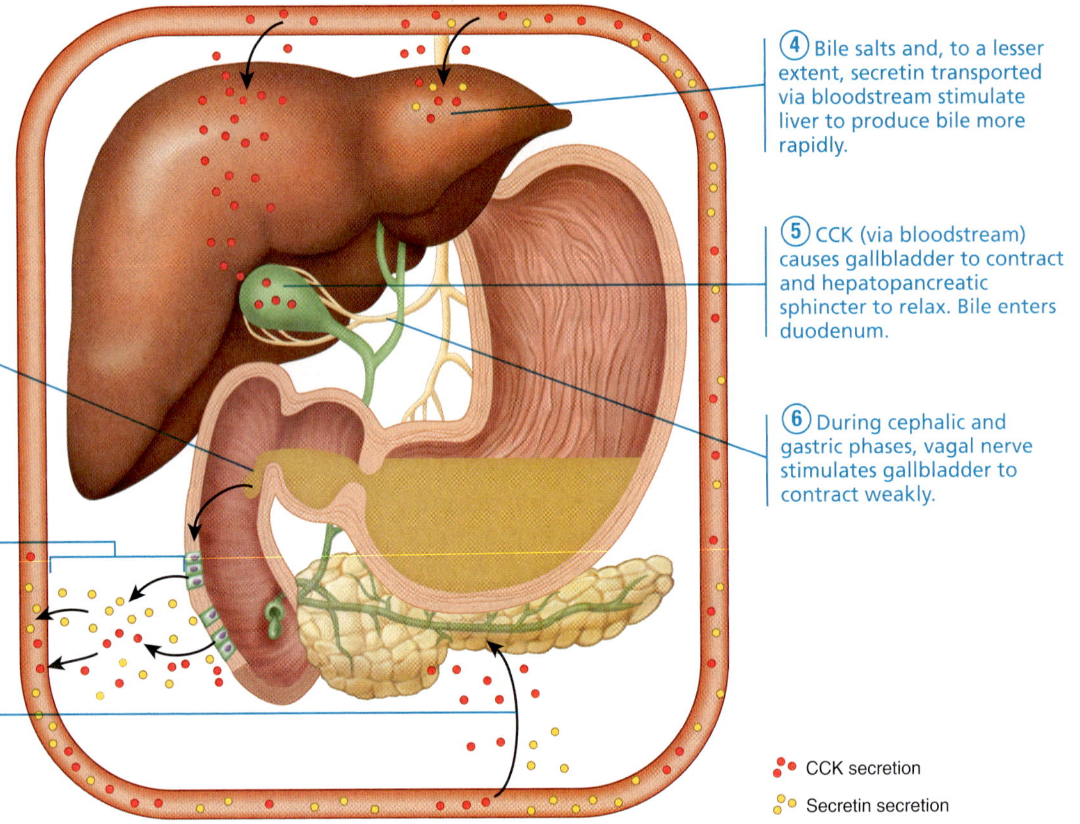

Figure 23.28 Mechanisms promoting secretion and release of bile and pancreatic juice. When digestion is not occurring, bile is stored and concentrated in the gallbladder. Acidic fatty chyme entering the small intestine initiates several mechanisms that accelerate the output of pancreatic juice and bile, and cause the gallbladder to contract and the hepatopancreatic sphincter to relax. This allows bile and pancreatic juice to enter the small intestine. The single most important stimulus for bile secretion is an increased level of bile salts in the enterohepatic circulation.

23

resulting in a watery *bicarbonate-rich* pancreatic juice. CCK, released in response to proteins and fats in chyme, stimulates the acini to release *enzyme-rich* pancreatic juice, and potentiates the effect of secretin. Table 23.1 summarizes CCK and the other digestive hormones and paracrines (p. 868).

Parasympathetic impulses delivered by vagus nerve fibers are a minor stimulus for gallbladder contraction. Vagal stimulation also prompts the release of pancreatic juice, mainly during the cephalic and gastric phases of gastric secretion.

☑ Check Your Understanding

39. What is the makeup of the fluid in the pancreatic duct? In the cystic duct? In the bile duct?
40. What stimulates CCK release and what are its effects on the digestive process?

For answers, see Appendix H.

Digestive Processes in the Small Intestine

By the time food reaches the small intestine it is unrecognizable, but still far from being digested. Carbohydrates and proteins are partially degraded, but fat digestion has only begun. The process of digestion accelerates during the chyme's tortuous three- to six-hour journey through the small intestine, and it is here that most of the water and virtually all nutrients are absorbed. Like the stomach, the small intestine plays no part in ingestion or defecation.

Requirements for Optimal Intestinal Digestive Activity

Although a primary function of the small intestine is to break down chyme chemically, intestinal juice provides little of what is needed to perform this function. Most of the substances required for digestion—bile, digestive enzymes (except for the brush border enzymes), and bicarbonate ions (to provide the proper pH for enzymatic catalysis)—are *imported* from the liver and pancreas. Hence, anything that impairs liver or pancreatic function or delivery of their juices to the small intestine severely hinders our ability to digest food and absorb nutrients. The other primary function of the small intestine—absorption—is efficiently accomplished by its absorptive cells with their rich crop of apical microvilli.

Optimal digestive activity in the small intestine also depends on a slow, measured delivery of chyme from the stomach. Why is this so? Entering chyme is usually hypertonic. For this reason, if large amounts of chyme were rushed into the small intestine,

Table 23.2 Overview of the Functions of the Gastrointestinal Organs

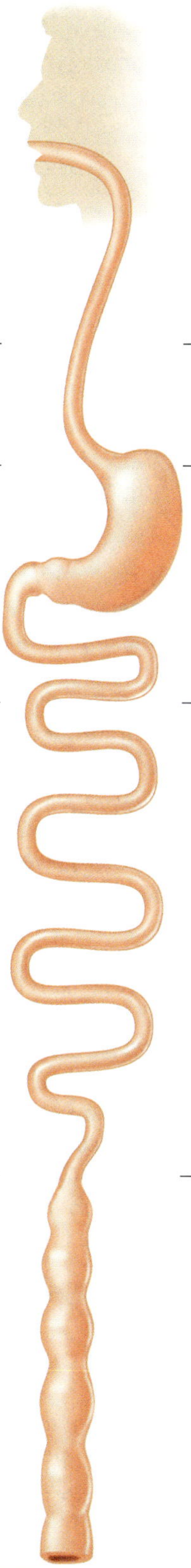

ORGAN	MAJOR FUNCTIONS*	COMMENTS/ADDITIONAL FUNCTIONS
Mouth and associated accessory organs	Ingestion: food is voluntarily placed into oral cavity Propulsion: voluntary (buccal) phase of deglutition (swallowing) initiated by tongue; propels food into pharynx Mechanical breakdown: mastication (chewing) by teeth and mixing movements by tongue Digestion: salivary amylase in saliva, produced by salivary glands, begins chemical breakdown of starch	Mouth serves as a receptacle; most functions performed by associated accessory organs. Mucus in saliva helps dissolve foods so they can be tasted and moistens food so that tongue can compact it into a bolus that can be swallowed. Saliva cleanses and lubricates oral cavity and teeth.
Pharynx and esophagus	Propulsion: peristaltic waves move food bolus to stomach, thus accomplishing involuntary (pharyngeal-esophageal) phase of deglutition	Primarily food chutes; mucus produced helps to lubricate food passageways.
Stomach	Mechanical breakdown and propulsion: peristaltic waves mix food with gastric juice and propel it into the duodenum Digestion: pepsin begins the digestion of proteins Absorption: absorbs a few fat-soluble substances (aspirin, alcohol, some drugs)	Also stores food until it can be moved into the duodenum. Hydrochloric acid produced is a bacteriostatic agent and activates protein-digesting enzymes. Mucus produced helps lubricate and protect stomach from self-digestion. Intrinsic factor produced is required for intestinal absorption of vitamin B_{12}.
Small intestine and associated accessory organs (liver, gallbladder, pancreas)	Mechanical breakdown and propulsion: segmentation by smooth muscle of the small intestine continually mixes contents with digestive juices and, along with short-distance peristaltic waves, moves food along tract, allowing sufficient time for digestion and absorption Digestion: digestive enzymes delivered from pancreas and brush border enzymes attached to microvilli membranes complete digestion of all classes of foods Absorption: breakdown products of carbohydrate, protein, fat, and nucleic acid digestion, plus vitamins, electrolytes, and water, are absorbed by active and passive mechanisms	Small intestine is highly modified for digestion and absorption (circular folds, villi, and microvilli). Alkaline mucus produced by intestinal glands and bicarbonate-rich juice ducted in from pancreas help neutralize acidic chyme and provide proper environment for enzymatic activity. Bile produced by liver emulsifies fats and enhances (1) fat digestion and (2) absorption of fatty acids, monoglycerides, cholesterol, phospholipids, and fat-soluble vitamins. Gallbladder stores and concentrates bile, releasing it to small intestine in response to hormonal signals.
Large intestine	Digestion: some remaining food residues are digested by enteric bacteria (which also produce vitamin K and some B vitamins) Absorption: absorbs most remaining water, electrolytes (largely NaCl), and vitamins produced by bacteria Propulsion: propels feces toward rectum by haustral churning and mass movements Defecation: reflex triggered by rectal distension; eliminates feces from body	Temporarily stores and concentrates residues until defecation can occur. Copious mucus produced by goblet cells eases passage of feces through colon.

*The colored boxes beside the functions correspond to the color coding of digestive functions (gastrointestinal tract activities) illustrated in Figure 23.2.

Table 23.3 Control of Small Intestinal Motility

PHASE	STIMULUS	MECHANISM	EFFECT ON MOTILITY
Gastric 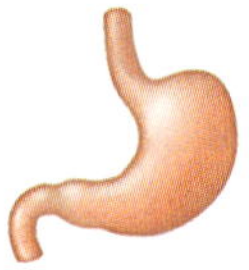	↑ Gastric motility and emptying	Long neural reflexes (gastroileal reflex)	↑ Activity in ileum
		Gastrin	↑ Segmenting movements in ileum; relaxes ileocecal sphincter
Intestinal 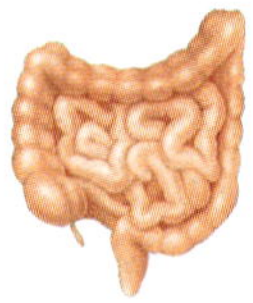	Distension of small intestine	Long and short neural reflexes	↑ Strength of segmentation
	Reduced intestinal volume; fasting	Long and short neural reflexes; initiated by ↑ blood levels of motilin	Initiates migrating motor complex (peristalsis); repeats until next meal

the osmotic water loss from the blood into the intestinal lumen would result in dangerously low blood volume. Additionally, the low pH of entering chyme must be adjusted upward and the chyme must be well mixed with bile and pancreatic juice for digestion to continue. These modifications take time, and the pumping action of the stomach pylorus carefully controls food movement into the small intestine (see pp. 873–874 and Figure 23.19) to prevent the duodenum from being overwhelmed.

Since we cover the actual chemistry of digestion and absorption in detail later, here we will examine how the motility of the small intestine mixes and propels food and how this motility is regulated.

Motility of the Small Intestine

Intestinal smooth muscle mixes chyme thoroughly with bile and pancreatic and intestinal juices, and moves food residues through the ileocecal valve into the large intestine. In contrast to the peristaltic waves of the stomach, *segmentation* is the most common motion of the small intestine.

Segmentation If we examine the small intestine with X-ray fluoroscopy after it is "loaded" with a meal, it looks like the intestinal contents are being massaged—alternately contracting and relaxing rings of smooth muscle simply move the chyme backward and forward a few centimeters at a time (see Figure 23.3b). As with stomach peristalsis, intrinsic pacemaker cells in the circular smooth muscle layer initiate these segmenting movements. However, unlike the stomach pacemakers, which have only one rhythm, the pacemakers in the duodenum depolarize more frequently than those in the ileum. As a result, segmentation also moves intestinal contents slowly and steadily toward the ileocecal valve at a rate that allows ample time to complete digestion and absorption.

The intensity of segmentation is altered by long and short reflexes, which parasympathetic activity enhances and sympathetic activity decreases, and by hormones (Table 23.3). The more intense the contractions, the greater the mixing, but the basic contractile rhythms of the various intestinal regions remain unchanged.

Migrating Motor Complex True peristalsis occurs late in the intestinal phase only after most nutrients have been absorbed. At this point, segmenting movements wane and the duodenal mucosa begins to release the hormone *motilin*.

As motilin blood levels rise, peristaltic waves are initiated in the proximal duodenum every 90 to 120 minutes and sweep slowly along the intestine, moving 50–70 cm (about 2 ft) before dying out. Each successive wave begins a bit more distally, a pattern of peristaltic activity called the **migrating motor complex (MMC)**. A complete "trip" from duodenum to ileum takes about two hours. The process then repeats itself, sweeping the last remnants of the meal plus bacteria, sloughed-off mucosal cells, and other debris into the large intestine.

This "housekeeping" function prevents bacteria in the large intestine from entering the small intestine. As food again enters the stomach with the next meal, segmentation replaces peristalsis.

The local enteric neurons of the GI tract wall coordinate these intestinal motility patterns and a variety of effects occur depending on which neurons are activated or inhibited. For example, an ACh-releasing (cholinergic) sensory neuron in the small intestine, once activated, may simultaneously send messages to several different interneurons in the myenteric plexus that regulate peristalsis. As a result, the proximal area constricts and forces chyme along the tract, as the lumen of the distal part of the intestine enlarges to receive it.

Ileocecal Control Most of the time, the ileocecal sphincter is closed. However, two mechanisms—one neural and the other hormonal—cause it to relax and allow food residues to enter the cecum when ileal motility increases:

- The **gastroileal reflex** (gas″tro-il′e-ul), a long reflex triggered by stomach activity, increases the force of segmentation in the ileum and relaxes the sphincter.
- Gastrin released by the stomach increases the motility of the ileum and relaxes the ileocecal sphincter.

Once the chyme has passed through, it exerts backward pressure that closes the valve's flaps, preventing regurgitation into the ileum. This reflex sweeps the contents of the previous meal completely out of the stomach and small intestine as the next meal is eaten.

Check Your Understanding

41. Distension of the stomach and duodenal walls have different effects on stomach secretory activity. What are these effects?
42. Which is more important in moving food along the small intestine—peristalsis or segmentation?
43. What is the MMC and why is it important?

For answers, see Appendix H.

The Large Intestine

✓ List the major functions of the large intestine.

✓ Describe the regulation of defecation.

The **large intestine** frames the small intestine on three sides and extends from the ileocecal valve to the anus (see Figure 23.1). Its diameter, at about 7 cm, is greater than that of the small intestine (hence, *large* intestine), but it is much shorter (1.5 m versus 6 m). Its major digestive functions are to absorb most of the remaining water from indigestible food residues (delivered to it in a fluid state), store the residues temporarily, and then eliminate them from the body as semisolid **feces** (fe′sēz). It also absorbs metabolites produced by resident bacteria as they avidly ferment carbohydrates not absorbed in the small intestine.

Gross Anatomy

The large intestine exhibits three features not seen elsewhere—teniae coli, haustra, and epiploic appendages. Except for its terminal end, the longitudinal muscle layer of its muscularis is mostly reduced to three bands of smooth muscle called **teniae coli** (ten′ne-e ko′li; "ribbons of the colon"). Their tone puckers the wall of the large intestine into pocketlike sacs called **haustra** (haw′strah; "to draw up"; singular: *haustrum*). Another obvious feature of the large intestine is its **epiploic appendages** (ep″ĭ-plo′ik; "membrane covered"), which are small fat-filled pouches of visceral peritoneum that hang from the surface of the large intestine **(Figure 23.29a)**. Their significance is not known.

Subdivisions of the Large Intestine

The large intestine has the following subdivisions: cecum, appendix, colon, rectum, and anal canal. The saclike **cecum** (se′kum; "blind pouch"), which lies below the ileocecal valve in the right iliac fossa, is the first part of the large intestine (Figure 23.29a).

Attached to the posteromedial surface of the cecum is the blind, wormlike **appendix**. The appendix contains masses of lymphoid tissue, and as part of MALT (see p. 759) it plays an important role in body immunity. Additionally, it serves as a storehouse of bacteria and recolonizes the gut when needed. However, the appendix has an important structural shortcoming—its twisted structure provides an ideal location for enteric bacteria to accumulate and multiply.

Homeostatic Imbalance 23.12

Acute inflammation of the appendix, or **appendicitis**, results from a blockage (often by feces) that traps infectious bacteria in its lumen. Unable to empty its contents, the appendix swells, squeezing off venous drainage, which may lead to ischemia and necrosis (death and decay) of the appendix. If the appendix ruptures, feces containing bacteria spray over the abdominal contents, causing *peritonitis*.

The symptoms of appendicitis vary, but the first symptom is usually pain in the umbilical region. Loss of appetite, nausea and vomiting, and pain relocalization to the lower right abdominal quadrant follow. Immediate surgical removal of the appendix (appendectomy) is the accepted treatment. Appendicitis is most common during adolescence, when the entrance to the appendix is at its widest. ✚

The **colon** has several distinct regions. Proximally, as the **ascending colon**, it travels up the right side of the abdominal cavity to the level of the right kidney. Here it makes a right-angle turn—the **right colic (hepatic) flexure**—and travels across the abdominal cavity as the **transverse colon**. Directly anterior to the spleen, it bends acutely at the **left colic (splenic) flexure** and descends down the left side of the posterior abdominal wall as the **descending colon**. Inferiorly, it enters the pelvis, where it becomes the S-shaped **sigmoid colon**.

The colon is retroperitoneal, except for its transverse and sigmoid parts. These parts are intraperitoneal and anchored to the posterior abdominal wall by mesentery sheets called **mesocolons (Figure 23.30c, d)**.

In the pelvis, at the level of the third sacral vertebra, the sigmoid colon joins the **rectum**, which runs posteroinferiorly just in front of the sacrum. The position of the rectum allows a number of pelvic organs (e.g., the prostate of males) to be examined digitally (with a finger) through the anterior rectal wall. This is called a **rectal exam**.

Despite its name (*rectum* = straight), the rectum has three lateral curves or bends, represented internally as three transverse folds called **rectal valves** (Figure 23.29b). These valves stop feces from being passed along with gas (flatus).

The **anal canal**, the last segment of the large intestine, lies in the perineum, entirely external to the abdominopelvic cavity. About 3 cm long, it begins where the rectum penetrates the levator ani muscle of the pelvic floor and opens to the body exterior at the **anus**. The anal canal has two sphincters, an involuntary **internal anal sphincter** composed of smooth muscle (part of the muscularis), and a voluntary **external anal sphincter** composed of skeletal muscle. The sphincters, which act rather like purse strings to open and close the anus, are ordinarily closed except during defecation.

Microscopic Anatomy

The wall of the large intestine differs in several ways from that of the small intestine. The large intestine *mucosa* is simple columnar epithelium except in the anal canal. Because most food is absorbed before reaching the large intestine, there are no circular folds, no villi, and virtually no cells that secrete digestive

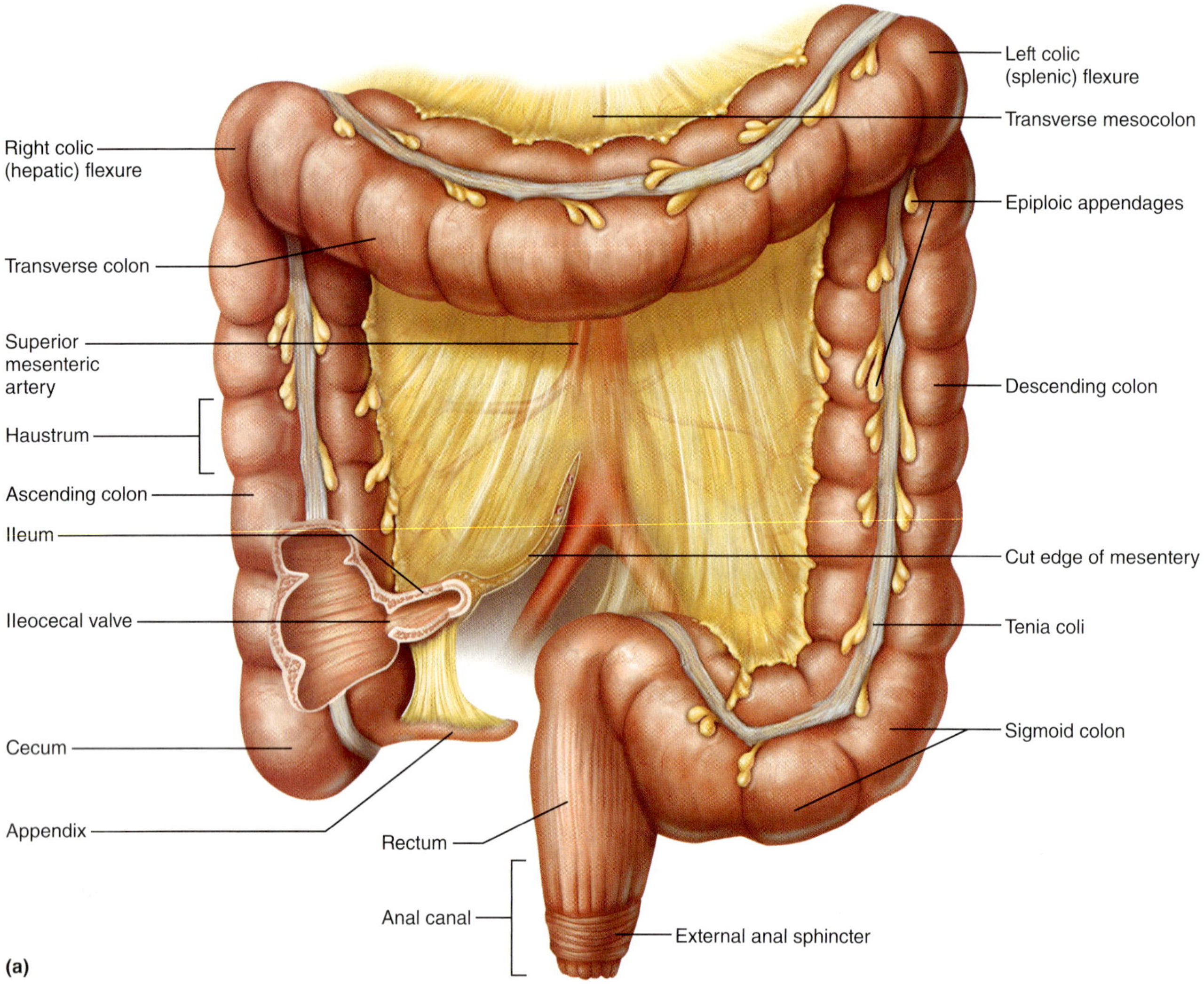

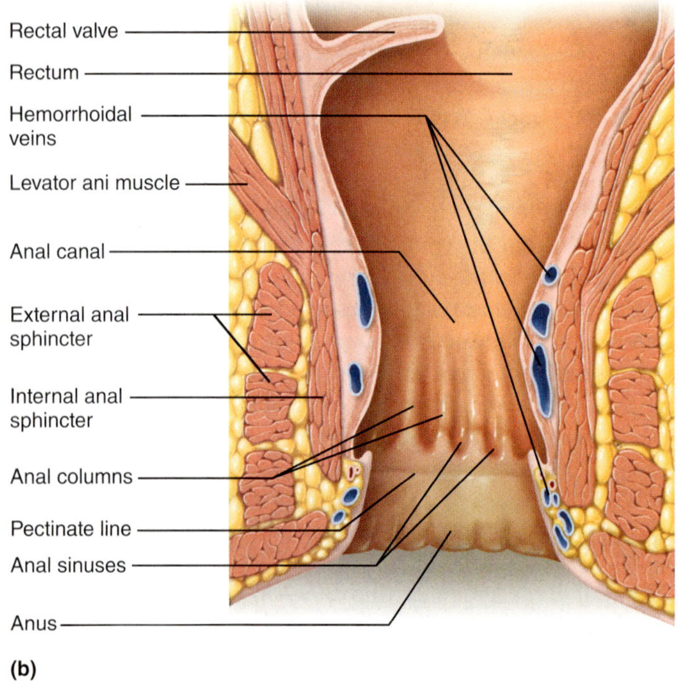

Figure 23.29 Gross anatomy of the large intestine. **(a)** Diagrammatic view. **(b)** Structure of the anal canal.

enzymes. However, its mucosa is thicker, its abundant crypts are deeper, and the crypts contain tremendous numbers of goblet cells. Mucus produced by goblet cells eases the passage of feces and protects the intestinal wall from irritating acids and gases released by resident bacteria.

The mucosa of the anal canal, a stratified squamous epithelium, merges with the true skin surrounding the anus and is quite different from the mucosa in the rest of the colon, reflecting the greater abrasion that this region receives. Superiorly, it hangs in long ridges or folds called **anal columns. Anal sinuses**, recesses between the anal columns, exude mucus when compressed by feces, which aids in emptying the anal canal (Figure 23.29b).

The horizontal, tooth-shaped line that parallels the inferior margins of the anal sinuses is called the *pectinate line*. Superior to this line, visceral sensory fibers innervate the mucosa, which is relatively insensitive to pain. The area inferior to the pectinate line is very sensitive to pain, a reflection of the somatic sensory fibers serving it.

Two superficial venous plexuses are associated with the anal canal, one with the anal columns and the other with the anus

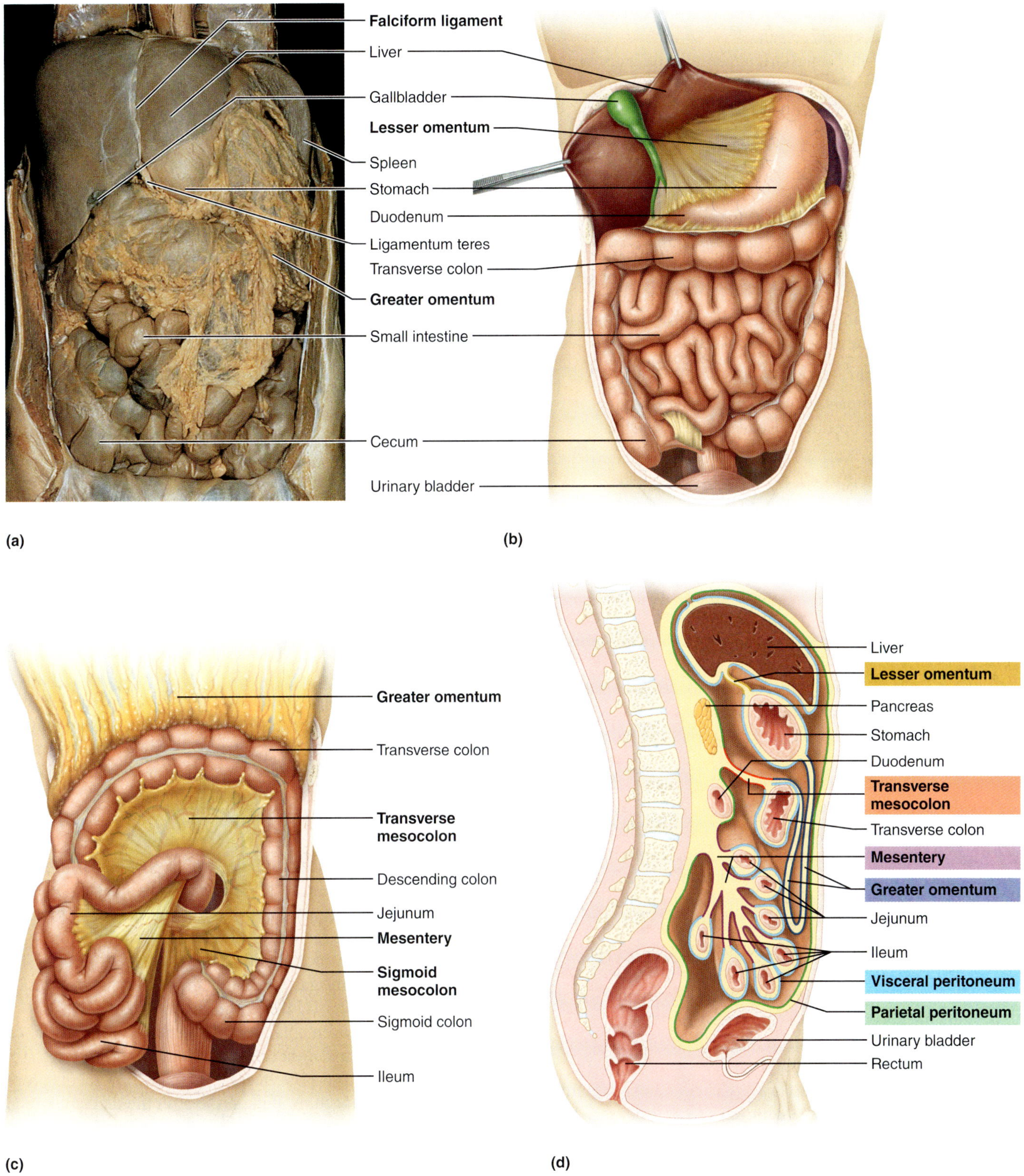

Figure 23.30 Mesenteries of the abdominal digestive organs. (a) The greater omentum, a dorsal mesentery, is shown in its normal position covering the abdominal viscera. **(b)** The liver and gallbladder have been reflected superiorly to reveal the lesser omentum, a ventral mesentery attaching the liver to the lesser curvature of the stomach. **(c)** The greater omentum has been reflected superiorly to reveal the mesentery attachments of the small and large intestine. **(d)** Sagittal section of the abdominopelvic cavity of a male. Mesentery labels appear in colored boxes.

itself. If these (hemorrhoidal) veins become inflamed, itchy varicosities called *hemorrhoids* result.

The rectum and anal canal lack teniae coli and haustra. However, the rectum's muscularis muscle layers are complete and well developed, consistent with its role in generating strong contractions to expel feces.

Bacterial Flora

Although most bacteria entering the cecum from the small intestine are dead (killed by lysozyme, defensins, HCl, and protein-digesting enzymes), some are still "alive and kicking." Together with bacteria that enter the GI tract via the anus, these constitute the **bacterial flora** of the large intestine, an astonishing 10 million discrete types. These bacteria:

- Colonize the colon
- Synthesize B complex vitamins and some of the vitamin K the liver needs to produce several clotting proteins
- Metabolize some host-derived molecules (mucin, heparin, and hyaluronic acid)
- Ferment some of the indigestible carbohydrates (cellulose, xylan, and others), releasing irritating acids and a mixture of gases (including dimethyl sulfide, H_2, N_2, CH_4, and CO_2)

Some of these gases, such as dimethyl sulfide, are quite odorous (smelly). About 500 ml of gas (flatus) is produced each day, much more when we eat certain carbohydrate-rich foods (such as beans).

Although the huge intestinal population of bacteria would seem to be enough inhabitants, the feces also have others, including viruses and protozoans. Of these, at least 20 are known pathogens.

Most enteric bacteria coexist peacefully with their host as long as they remain in the gut lumen. An elegant system keeps the bacteria from breaching the mucosal barrier. The epithelial cells of the gut mucosa respond to specific bacterial components by releasing chemicals that recruit immune cells, particularly dendritic cells, into the mucosa. The dendritic cells pry open tight junctions between the epithelial cells and send extensions into the lumen to sample the microbial antigens. They then migrate to the nearby lymphoid follicles (MALT) within the gut mucosa where they present the antigens to T cells. As a result, an IgA antibody–mediated response restricted to the gut lumen is triggered that prevents the bacteria from straying into tissues deep to the mucosa where they might elicit a much more widespread systemic response.

23

Though beneficial in most ways, the coexistence of enteric bacteria with our immune system does sometimes fail. When that happens, the painful and debilitating conditions known as inflammatory bowel disease (see Related Clinical Terms, p. 905) may result.

Digestive Processes in the Large Intestine

What is finally delivered to the large intestine contains few nutrients, but it still has 12 to 24 hours more to spend there. Except for a small amount of digestion of that residue by the enteric bacteria, no further food breakdown occurs in the large intestine.

The large intestine harvests vitamins made by the bacterial flora and reclaims most of the remaining water and some of the electrolytes (particularly sodium and chloride). However, nutrient absorption is not its *major* function. As mentioned, the primary concerns of the large intestine are propulsive activities that force fecal material toward the anus and eliminate it from the body (defecation).

Homeostatic Imbalance 23.13

The large intestine is important for our comfort, but it is not essential for life. If the colon is removed, as may be necessitated by colon cancer, the terminal ileum is brought out to the abdominal wall in a procedure called an *ileostomy* (il″e-os′to-me). From there food residues are eliminated into a sac attached to the abdominal wall. Another surgical technique, ileoanal juncture, links the ileum directly to the anal canal. +

Motility of the Large Intestine

The large intestine musculature is inactive much of the time, but pressure in the ileum terminus opens the ileocecal sphincter and then closes it, preventing backward movement of the chyme. When presented with food residue the colon becomes motile, but its contractions are sluggish or short-lived. The movements most seen in the colon are **haustral contractions**, slow segmenting movements lasting about one minute that occur every 30 minutes or so.

These contractions, which occur mainly in the ascending and transverse colon, reflect local controls of smooth muscle within the walls of the individual haustra. As a haustrum fills with food residue, the distension stimulates its muscle to contract, which propels the luminal contents into the next haustrum. These movements also mix the residue, which aids in water absorption.

Mass movements (also called mass peristalsis) are long, slow-moving, but powerful contractile waves that move over large areas of the colon three or four times daily and force the contents toward the rectum. Typically, they occur during or just after eating, which indicates that the presence of food in the stomach activates the gastroileal reflex in the small intestine and the propulsive **gastrocolic reflex** in the colon.

Segmenting movements in the descending and sigmoid colon promote the final desiccation (drying out) of the feces. This part of the colon also stores feces until mass movements propel the feces into the rectum. Bulk, or fiber, in the diet strengthens colon contractions and softens the feces, allowing the colon to act like a well-oiled machine.

Homeostatic Imbalance 23.14

When the diet lacks bulk and the volume of residues in the colon is small, the colon narrows and its contractions become more powerful, increasing the pressure on its walls. This promotes formation of **diverticula** (di″ver-tik′u-lah), small herniations of the mucosa through the colon walls.

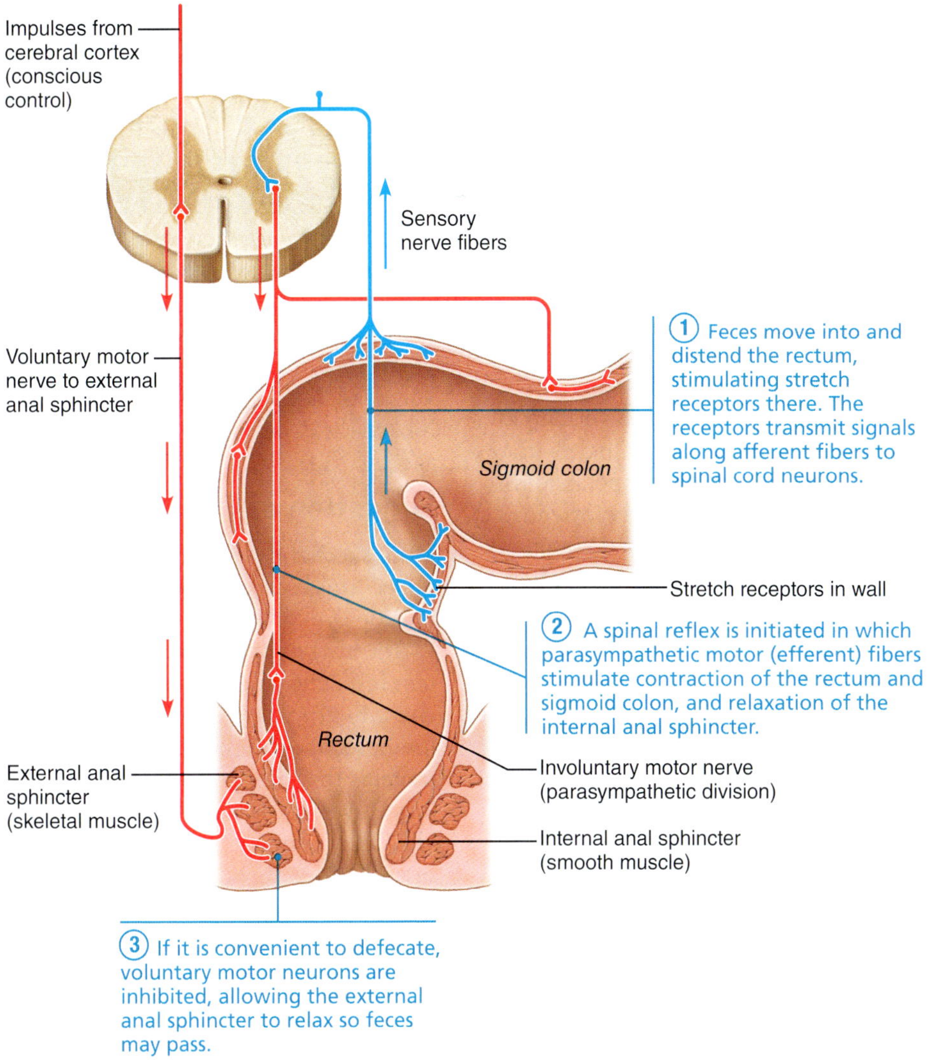

Figure 23.31 Defecation reflex.

This condition, called **diverticulosis**, most commonly occurs in the sigmoid colon, and affects over half of people over age 70. In about 20% of cases, diverticulosis progresses to **diverticulitis**, in which the diverticula become inflamed and may rupture, leaking into the peritoneal cavity, which can be life threatening. Foods and products that make feces bulkier help prevent diverticulitis.

Irritable bowel syndrome (*IBS*) is a functional GI disorder not explained by anatomical or biochemical abnormalities. Affected individuals have recurring (or persistent) abdominal pain that is relieved by defecation, changes in the consistency (watery to stonelike) and frequency of their stools, and varying complaints of bloating, flatulence, nausea, and depression. Stress is a common precipitating factor, and stress management is an important aspect of treatment. ✚

The semisolid feces delivered to the rectum, also called the stool, contain undigested food residues, mucus, sloughed-off epithelial cells, millions of bacteria, and just enough water to allow their smooth passage. Of the 500 ml or so of food residue entering the cecum daily, approximately 150 ml becomes feces.

Defecation

The rectum is usually empty, but when mass movements force feces into it, stretching of the rectal wall initiates the **defecation reflex**. This parasympathetic reflex, mediated by the spinal cord, causes the sigmoid colon and the rectum to contract, and the internal anal sphincter to relax (**Figure 23.31** (1) and (2)). As feces are forced into the anal canal, messages reach the brain allowing us to decide whether the external (voluntary) anal sphincter should open or remain constricted to stop passage of feces temporarily (Figure 23.31 (3)).

If defecation is delayed, the reflex contractions end within a few seconds and the rectal walls relax. The next mass movement initiates the defecation reflex again—and so on, until the person chooses to defecate or the urge becomes irresistible.

During defecation, the muscles of the rectum contract to expel the feces. We aid this process voluntarily by closing the glottis and contracting our diaphragm and abdominal wall muscles to increase the intra-abdominal pressure (a procedure called *Valsalva's maneuver*). We also contract the levator ani muscle (pp. 344–345), which lifts the anal canal superiorly. This lifting action leaves the feces below the anus—and outside the body. Involuntary or automatic defecation (fecal incontinence) occurs in infants because they have not yet gained control of their external anal sphincter. It also occurs in those with spinal cord transections.

Homeostatic Imbalance 23.15

Watery stools, or **diarrhea**, result from any condition that rushes food residue through the large intestine before that organ has had sufficient time to absorb the remaining water. Causes include irritation of the colon by bacteria or, less commonly, prolonged physical jostling of the digestive viscera (occurs in marathon runners). Prolonged diarrhea may result in dehydration and electrolyte imbalance (acidosis and loss of potassium).

Conversely, when food remains in the colon for extended periods, too much water is absorbed and the stool becomes hard and difficult to pass. This condition, called **constipation**, may result from lack of fiber in the diet, improper bowel habits (failing to heed the "call"), lack of exercise, emotional stress, or laxative abuse. +

Check Your Understanding

44. What propulsive movements are unique to the large intestine?
45. What is the result of stimulation of stretch receptors in the rectal walls?
46. In what ways are enteric bacteria important to our nutrition?

For answers, see Appendix H.

PART 3
Physiology of Digestion and Absorption

23

- ✓ List the enzymes involved in digestion; name the foodstuffs on which they act.
- ✓ List the end products of protein, fat, carbohydrate, and nucleic acid digestion.
- ✓ Describe the process by which breakdown products of foodstuffs are absorbed in the small intestine.

So far in this chapter, we have examined the structure and function of the organs that make up the digestive system. Now let's investigate the chemical processing (enzymatic breakdown) and absorption of each class of foodstuffs as it moves through the GI tract. As you read along, you may find it helpful to refer to the summary in **Figure 23.32**.

Digestion

After foodstuffs have spent even a short time in the stomach, they are unrecognizable. Nonetheless, they are still mostly the foods that that we ingested—carbohydrates, proteins, fats and so on. Mechanical breakdown has only changed their appearance. By contrast, digestion breaks down ingested foods into their chemical building blocks, which are very different molecules chemically.

Mechanism of Digestion: Enzymatic Hydrolysis

Digestion is a catabolic process that breaks down large food molecules to *monomers* (chemical building blocks) small enough to be absorbed by the GI tract lining. Digestion is accomplished by enzymes secreted into the lumen of the alimentary canal by intrinsic and accessory glands. Recall that enzymatic breakdown of any food molecule is **hydrolysis** (hi-drol′ĭ-sis) because it involves adding a water molecule to each molecular bond to be broken (lysed).

Digestion of Carbohydrates

Monosaccharides (simple sugars), the monomers of carbohydrates, are absorbed without further ado. Only three monosaccharides are common in our diet: *glucose*, *fructose*, and *galactose*.

The more complex carbohydrates that our digestive system is able to break down to monosaccharides are the disaccharides *sucrose* (table sugar), *lactose* (milk sugar), and *maltose* (grain sugar), and the polysaccharides *glycogen* and *starch*. The proteins that transport the monosaccharides into the cells are located very close to the disaccharidase enzymes on the microvilli. They combine with the monosaccharides as soon as the disaccharides are broken down. Because the intestine can absorb only monosaccharides, all dietary carbohydrates must be digested to monosaccharides to be absorbed.

In the average diet, most (up to 60%) digestible carbohydrates are in the form of starch, with smaller amounts of disaccharides and monosaccharides. Humans lack enzymes capable of breaking down most other polysaccharides, such as cellulose. As a result, indigestible polysaccharides do not nourish us but they do help move food along the GI tract by providing bulk, or fiber.

Digestion of starch (and perhaps glycogen) begins in the mouth (Figure 23.32). **Salivary amylase**, present in saliva, splits starch into *oligosaccharides*, smaller fragments of two to eight linked glucose molecules. Salivary amylase works best in the slightly acid to neutral environment (pH of 6.75–7.00) maintained in the mouth by the buffering effects of bicarbonate and phosphate ions in saliva. Starch digestion continues until amylase is inactivated by stomach acid and broken apart by the stomach's protein-digesting enzymes. Generally speaking, the larger the meal, the longer amylase continues to work in the stomach because foodstuffs in its relatively immobile fundus are poorly mixed with gastric juices.

Starchy foods and other digestible carbohydrates that escape being broken down by salivary amylase are acted on by **pancreatic amylase** in the small intestine. About 10 minutes after entering the small intestine, starch is entirely converted to various oligosaccharides, mostly maltose.

Intestinal brush border enzymes further digest these products to monosaccharides. The most important brush border enzymes are **dextrinase** and **glucoamylase**, which act on oligosaccharides composed of more than three simple sugars, and **maltase**, **sucrase**, and **lactase**, which hydrolyze maltose, sucrose, and lactose respectively into their constituent monosaccharides.

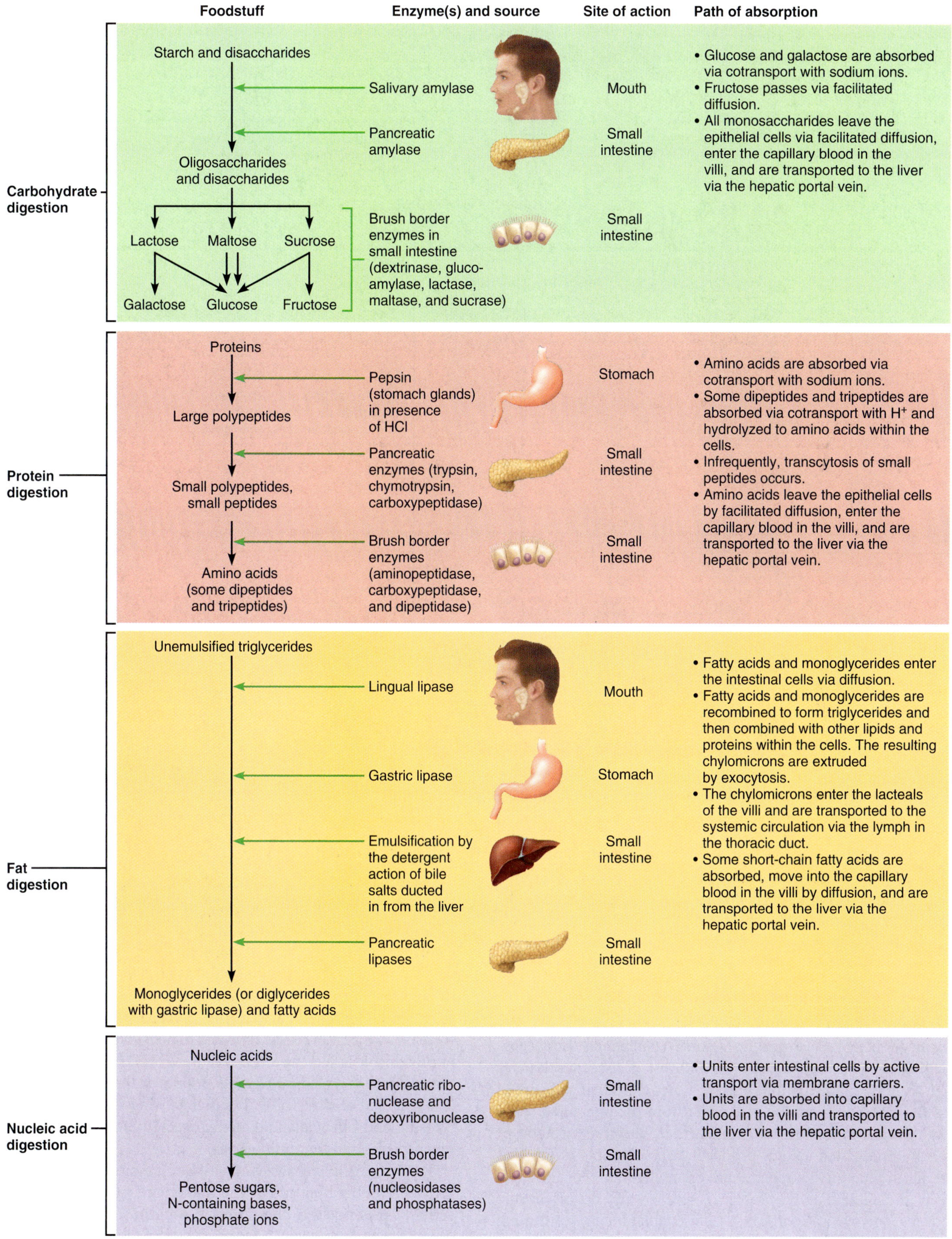

Figure 23.32 Flowchart of digestion and absorption of foodstuffs.

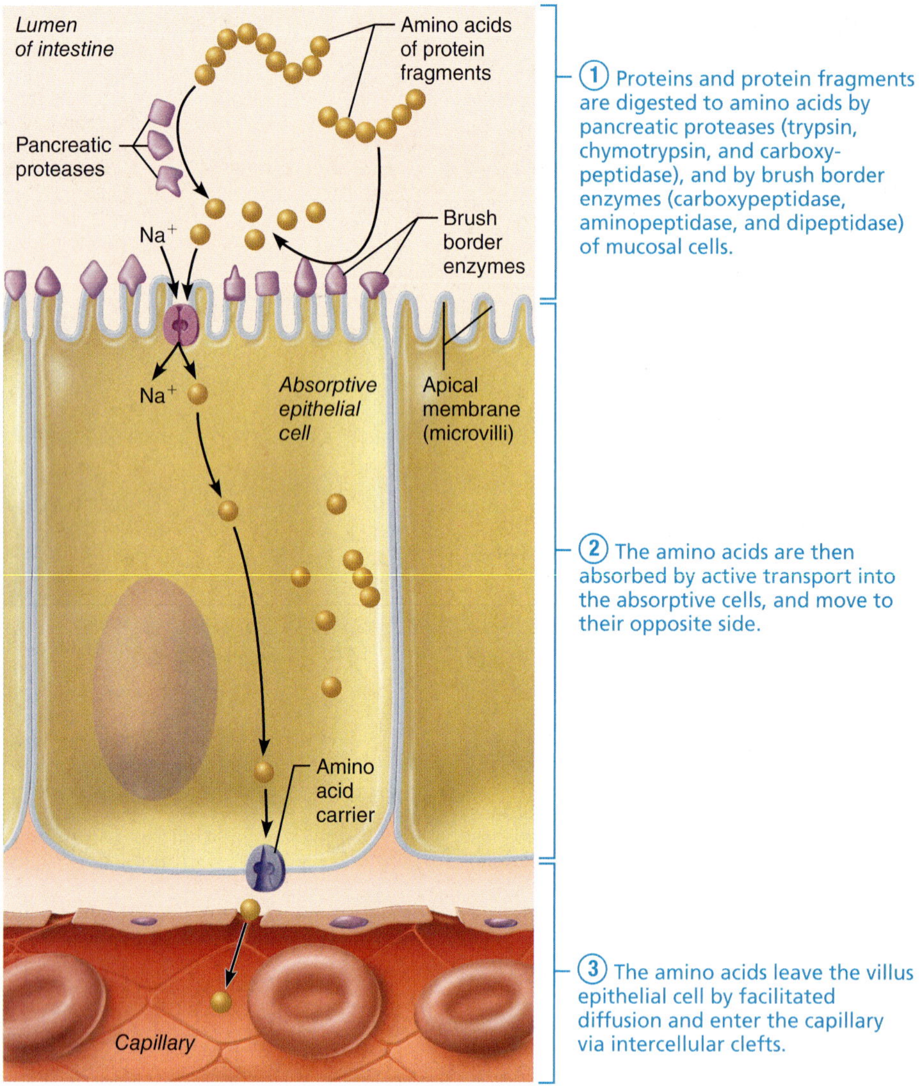

Figure 23.33 Protein digestion and absorption in the small intestine.

23

Because the colon does not secrete digestive enzymes, digestion *officially ends* in the small intestine. As noted earlier, however, resident colon bacteria do break down and metabolize the residual complex carbohydrates and some proteins further, adding much to their own nutrition but essentially nothing to ours.

Homeostatic Imbalance 23.16

In some people, intestinal lactase is present at birth but then becomes deficient due to genetic factors. When people with *lactose intolerance* consume lactose, the undigested disaccharides create osmotic gradients that prevent water from being absorbed in the intestines and also pull water from the interstitial space into the intestines. The result is diarrhea. Bacterial metabolism of the undigested solutes produces large amounts of gas that result in bloating, flatulence, and cramping pain. For the most part, the solution to this problem is simple—add lactase enzyme "drops" to your milk or take a lactase tablet before consuming milk products. ✚

Digestion of Proteins

Proteins digested in the GI tract include not only dietary proteins (typically about 125 g per day), but also 15–25 g of enzyme proteins secreted into the GI tract lumen by its various glands and (probably) an equal amount of protein derived from sloughed and disintegrating mucosal cells. Healthy individuals digest much of this protein all the way to its **amino acid** monomers.

Protein digestion begins in the stomach when pepsinogen secreted by the chief cells is activated to **pepsin** (actually a group of protein-digesting enzymes) (Figure 23.32). Pepsin functions optimally in the acidic pH range found in the stomach: 1.5–2.5. It preferentially cleaves bonds involving the amino acids tyrosine and phenylalanine, breaking the proteins down into polypeptides and free amino acids.

Pepsin, which hydrolyzes 10–15% of ingested protein, is inactivated by the high pH in the duodenum, so its proteolytic activity is restricted to the stomach. **Rennin** (the enzyme that coagulates milk protein) is not produced in adults.

Protein fragments entering the small intestine are greeted by a host of proteolytic enzymes (**Figure 23.33** ①). **Trypsin** and **chymotrypsin** secreted by the pancreas cleave the proteins into smaller peptides, which in turn become the grist for other enzymes. The pancreatic and brush border enzyme **carboxypeptidase** splits off one amino acid at a time from the end of the polypeptide chain that bears the carboxyl group. Other brush border enzymes such as **aminopeptidase** and **dipeptidase** liberate the final amino acid products. Aminopeptidase digests a protein, one amino acid at a time, by working from the amine end.

Both carboxypeptidase and aminopeptidase can independently dismantle a protein, but the teamwork between these enzymes and between trypsin and chymotrypsin, which attack the more internal parts of the protein, speeds up the process tremendously.

Digestion of Lipids

Triglycerides (neutral fats) are the most abundant fats in the diet. The small intestine is the primary site of lipid digestion because the pancreas is the major source of fat-digesting enzymes, or **lipases** (see Figure 23.32).

Because triglycerides and their breakdown products are insoluble in water, fats need special "pretreatment" with bile salts to be digested and absorbed in the watery environment of the small intestine. In aqueous solutions, triglycerides aggregate to form large fat globules, and only the triglyceride molecules at the surfaces of such fatty masses are accessible to the water-soluble lipase enzymes. However, this problem is quickly resolved because as the fat globules enter the duodenum, they are coated with detergent-like bile salts.

Bile salts have both nonpolar and polar regions. Their nonpolar (hydrophobic) parts cling to the fat molecules, and their polar (ionized hydrophilic) parts allow them to repel each other and interact with water. As a result, fatty droplets are pulled off the large fat globules, forming a stable *emulsion*—an aqueous suspension of fatty droplets, each about 1 mm in diameter (**Figure 23.34** ①).

Emulsification does *not* break chemical bonds. It just reduces the attraction between fat molecules so they can be more widely dispersed. This process vastly increases the number of triglyceride molecules exposed to the pancreatic lipases. Without bile, lipids could not be completely digested during the time food spends in the small intestine.

The pancreatic lipases catalyze the breakdown of fats by cleaving off two of the fatty acid chains, yielding free **fatty acids** and **monoglycerides**—glycerol with one fatty acid chain attached (Figure 23.34 ②). Fat-soluble vitamins that ride with fats require no digestion.

Digestion of Nucleic Acids

The nuclei of the cells of ingested foods contain DNA and RNA. **Pancreatic nucleases** in pancreatic juice hydrolyze the nucleic acids to their **nucleotide** monomers. Intestinal brush border enzymes (**nucleosidases** and **phosphatases**) then break the nucleotides apart to release their free bases, pentose sugars, and phosphate ions (see Figure 23.32).

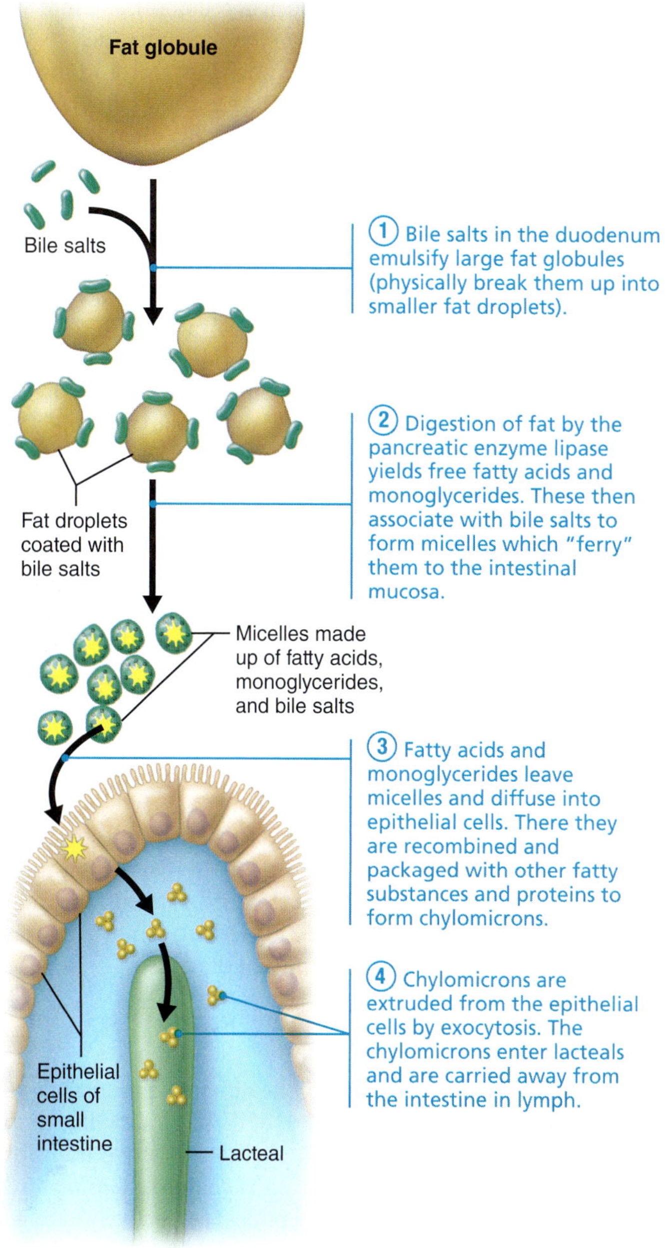

Figure 23.34 Emulsification, digestion, and absorption of fats.

Absorption

There is much more flowing through the alimentary tube than food monomers. Indeed, up to 10 L of food, drink, and GI secretions enter the alimentary canal daily, but only 1 L or less reaches the large intestine. Virtually all of the foodstuffs, 80% of the electrolytes, and most of the water (remember water follows salt) are absorbed in the small intestine. Although absorption occurs all along the length of the small intestine, most of it is completed by the time chyme reaches the ileum.

The major absorptive role of the ileum is to reclaim bile salts to be recycled back to the liver for resecretion. It is virtually impossible to exceed the absorptive capacity of the human gut, and at the end of the ileum, all that remains is some water, indigestible food materials (largely plant fibers such as cellulose), and millions of bacteria. This debris is passed on to the large intestine.

To understand absorption, remember that the fluid mosaic structure of the plasma membrane dictates that nonpolar substances, which can dissolve in the lipid core of the membrane, can be absorbed passively, and that polar substances must be absorbed by carrier mechanisms. Most nutrients are absorbed through the mucosa of the intestinal villi by *active transport* processes driven directly or indirectly (secondarily) by metabolic energy (ATP). They then enter the capillary blood in the villus to be transported in the hepatic portal vein to the liver. The exception is some lipid digestion products, which are absorbed passively by diffusion and then enter the lacteal in the villus to be carried via lymphatic fluid to the blood.

Because tight junctions join the epithelial cells of the intestinal mucosa at their apical surfaces, substances cannot move *between* cells for the most part. Consequently, materials must pass through the epithelial cells and into the interstitial fluid abutting their basolateral membranes to enter the blood capillaries.

As we describe the absorption of each nutrient class, you may want to refer to the absorption summary on the right-hand side of Figure 23.32 (p. 893).

Carbohydrate Absorption

Glucose and galactose, liberated by the breakdown of starch and disaccharides, are shuttled by secondary active transport with Na^+ into the epithelial cells **(Figure 23.35)**. They then move out of these cells by facilitated diffusion and pass into the capillaries via intercellular clefts. By contrast, fructose moves entirely by facilitated diffusion (to enter and exit the cells).

Protein Absorption

23

Several types of carriers transport the different amino acids resulting from protein digestion. Most of these carriers, like those for glucose and galactose, are coupled to the active transport of sodium (see Figure 23.33 ②). Short chains of two or three amino acids (dipeptides and tripeptides, respectively) are actively absorbed by H^+-dependent cotransport. They are digested to their amino acids within the epithelial cells. The amino acids enter the capillary blood by diffusion (Figure 23.33 ③).

Homeostatic Imbalance 23.17

Whole proteins are not usually absorbed, but in rare cases intact proteins are taken up by endocytosis and released on the opposite side of the epithelial cell by exocytosis. This process is most common in newborn infants, reflecting the immaturity of their intestinal mucosa (gastric acid secretion does not reach normal levels until weeks after birth, and the mucosa is leakier than it is later.) Absorption of whole proteins accounts for many early food allergies: The immune system "sees" the intact proteins as antigenic and mounts an attack. These allergies usually disappear as the mucosa matures.

This mechanism may also provide a route for IgA antibodies in breast milk to reach an infant's bloodstream. These antibodies confer some passive immunity on the infant, providing temporary protection against antigens to which the mother has been sensitized. +

Lipid Absorption

Just as bile salts accelerate lipid digestion, they are also essential for the absorption of its end products. As the water-insoluble products of fat digestion—the monoglycerides and free fatty acids—are liberated by lipase activity, they quickly become associated with bile salts and *lecithin* (a phospholipid found in bile) to form micelles (Figure 23.34 ②). **Micelles** (mi-selz′) are collections of fatty elements clustered together with bile salts in such a way that the polar (hydrophilic) ends of the molecules face the water and the nonpolar portions form the core. Also nestled in the hydrophobic core are cholesterol molecules and fat-soluble vitamins. Although micelles are similar to emulsion droplets, they are much smaller "vehicles" and easily diffuse between microvilli to come into close contact with the apical cell surface.

Upon reaching the epithelial cells, the various lipid substances leave the micelles and move through the lipid phase of the plasma membrane by simple diffusion (Figure 23.34 ③). Without the micelles, the lipids will simply float on the surface of the chyme (like oil on water), inaccessible to the absorptive surfaces of the epithelial cells. Generally, fat absorption is completed in the ileum, but in the absence of bile (as might occur when a gallstone blocks the cystic duct) it happens so slowly that most of the fat passes into the large intestine and is lost in feces.

Once the free fatty acids and monoglycerides enter the epithelial cells, the smooth ER converts them back into triglycerides. The triglycerides are then combined with lecithin and other phospholipids and cholesterol, and coated with a "skin" of proteins to form water-soluble lipoprotein droplets called **chylomicrons** (ki″lo-mi′kronz). These are dispatched to the Golgi apparatus where they are processed for extrusion from the cell. This series of events is quite different from the absorption of amino acids and simple sugars, which pass through the epithelial cells unchanged.

The milky-white chylomicrons are too large to pass through either the plasma membrane of the epithelial cell or the basement membrane of a blood capillary. Instead, the chylomicron-containing vesicles migrate to the basolateral membrane and are extruded by exocytosis (Figure 23.34 ④). They then enter the more permeable lacteals. Thus, most fat enters the lymphatic stream for distribution in the lymph. Eventually the chylomicrons are emptied into the venous blood in the neck region via the thoracic duct, which drains the digestive viscera.

While in the bloodstream, the triglycerides of the chylomicrons are hydrolyzed to free fatty acids and glycerol by **lipoprotein lipase**, an enzyme associated with capillary endothelium. The fatty acids and glycerol can then pass through the capillary walls to be used by tissue cells for energy or stored as fats in adipose tissue. Liver cells then combine the residual chylomicron material with proteins, and these "new" lipoproteins are used to transport cholesterol in the blood.

Passage of short-chain fatty acids is quite different from what we have just described. These fat breakdown products do not depend on the presence of bile salts or micelles and are not recombined to form triglycerides within the intestinal cells. They simply diffuse into the portal blood for distribution.

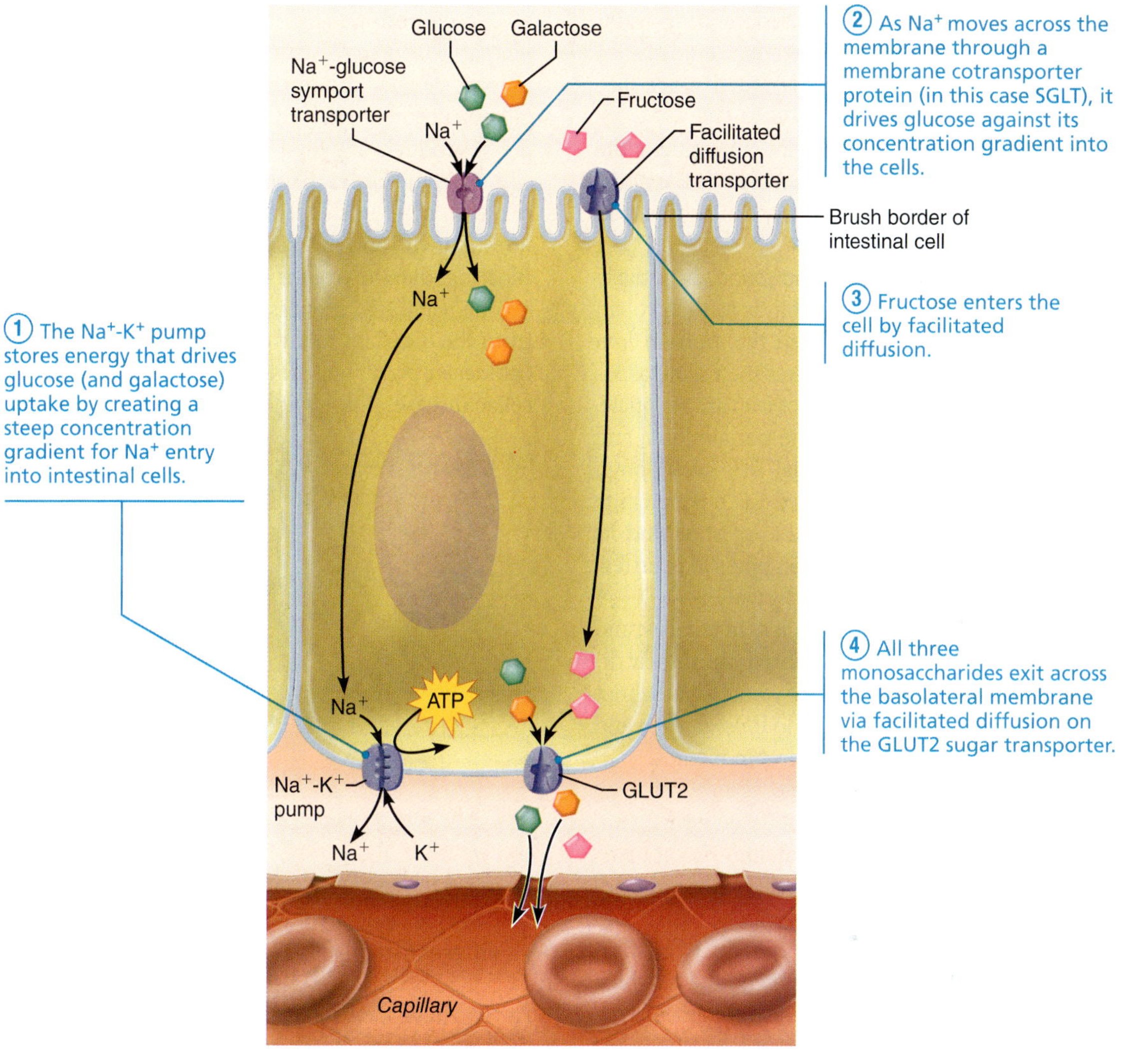

Figure 23.35 **Absorption of monosaccharides.**

Nucleic Acid Absorption

Special carriers in the epithelium of the villi actively transport the breakdown products of nucleic acid digestion—pentose sugars, nitrogenous bases, and phosphate ions—across the epithelium. These then enter the blood.

Vitamin Absorption

The small intestine absorbs dietary vitamins, and the large intestine absorbs some of the K and B vitamins made by its enteric bacterial "guests." As we already noted, fat-soluble vitamins (A, D, E, and K) dissolve in dietary fats, become incorporated into the micelles, and move across the villus epithelium passively (by diffusion). It follows that gulping pills containing fat-soluble vitamins without simultaneously eating some fat-containing food results in little or no absorption of these vitamins.

Most water-soluble vitamins (B vitamins and vitamin C) are absorbed easily by diffusion or via specific active or passive transporters. The exception is vitamin B_{12}, which is a very large, charged molecule. *Intrinsic factor*, produced by the stomach, binds to vitamin B_{12}. The vitamin B_{12}–intrinsic factor complex then binds to specific mucosal receptor sites in the terminal ileum, which trigger its active uptake by endocytosis.

Electrolyte Absorption

Absorbed electrolytes come from both ingested foods and gastrointestinal secretions. Most ions are actively absorbed along the entire length of the small intestine. But absorption of iron and calcium is largely limited to the duodenum.

As we mentioned earlier, absorption of sodium ions in the small intestine is coupled to active absorption of glucose and amino acids. For the most part, anions passively follow the electrical potential established by sodium transport. In other words, Na^+ is actively pumped out of the epithelial cells by a Na^+-K^+ pump after entering those cells. Chloride ions are also transported actively, and in the terminus of the small intestine HCO_3^- is actively secreted into the lumen in exchange for Cl^-.

Potassium ions move across the intestinal mucosa passively by facilitated diffusion (or via leaky tight junctions) in response to changing osmotic gradients. As water is absorbed from the lumen, rising potassium levels in chyme create a concentration gradient for its absorption. Anything that interferes with water absorption (resulting in diarrhea) not only reduces potassium absorption but also "pulls" K^+ from the interstitial space into the intestinal lumen.

For most nutrients, the amount *reaching* the intestine is the amount absorbed, regardless of the nutritional state of the body. In contrast, absorption of iron and calcium is intimately related to the body's need for them at the time.

Ionic iron, essential for hemoglobin production, is actively transported into the mucosal cells, where it binds to the protein **ferritin** (fer′ĭ-tin). This phenomenon is called the *mucosal iron barrier*. The intracellular iron-ferritin complexes then serve as local storehouses for iron. When body reserves of iron are adequate, little (only 10–20%) is allowed to pass into the portal blood, and most of the stored iron is lost as the epithelial cells later slough off. However, when iron reserves are depleted (as during acute or chronic hemorrhage), iron uptake from the intestine and its release to the blood accelerate. In the blood, iron binds to **transferrin**, a plasma protein that transports it in the circulation.

Menstrual bleeding is a major route of iron loss in females, and premenopausal women require about 50% more iron in their diets. Additionally, the intestinal epithelial cells of women have about four times as many iron transport proteins as do those of men and little iron is lost from the body other than that lost in menses.

Calcium absorption is closely related to blood levels of ionic calcium. The active form of **vitamin D** promotes active calcium absorption. Decreased blood levels of ionic calcium prompt *parathyroid hormone* (*PTH*) release from the parathyroid glands. Besides facilitating the release of calcium ions from bone matrix and enhancing the reabsorption of calcium by the kidneys, PTH stimulates activation of vitamin D to calcitriol by the kidneys, which in turn accelerates calcium ion absorption in the small intestine.

23

Water Absorption

Approximately 9 L of water, mostly derived from GI tract secretions, enter the small intestine daily. Water is the most abundant substance in chyme, and 95% of it is absorbed in the small intestine by osmosis. Most of the rest is absorbed in the large intestine, leaving only about 0.1 L to soften the feces.

The normal rate of water absorption is 300 to 400 ml per hour. Water moves freely in both directions across the intestinal mucosa, but *net osmosis* occurs whenever a concentration gradient is established by the active transport of solutes (particularly Na^+) into the mucosal cells. In this way, water uptake is effectively coupled to solute uptake and, in turn, affects the absorption of substances that normally pass by diffusion. As water moves into mucosal cells, these substances follow along their concentration gradients.

Malabsorption of Nutrients

Malabsorption, or impaired nutrient absorption, has many and varied causes. It can result from anything that interferes with the delivery of bile or pancreatic juice to the small intestine. Factors that damage the intestinal mucosa (severe bacterial infections and some antibiotics) or reduce its absorptive surface area are also common causes.

A common malabsorption syndrome is *gluten-sensitive enteropathy* or *celiac disease*, which affects one in 100 people. This chronic genetic condition is caused by an immune reaction to gluten, a protein plentiful in all grains but corn and rice. Breakdown products of gluten interact with molecules of the immune system in the GI tract, forming complexes. These complexes activate T cells, which then attack the intestinal lining, damaging intestinal villi and reducing the surface area of the brush border. Bloating, diarrhea, pain, and malnutrition result.

The usual treatment is to eliminate gluten-containing grains from the diet. Not many children can envision a world without cookies or pizza, but these are just two of the foods people with celiac disease must avoid.

☑ Check Your Understanding

47. What type of chemical reaction is the basis of all enzymatic food breakdown?
48. Fill in the blank: Amylase is to starch as ___ is to fats.
49. What is the role of bile salts in the digestive process? In absorption?

For answers, see Appendix H.

Developmental Aspects of the Digestive System

✓ Describe embryonic development of the digestive system.

✓ Describe abnormalities of the gastrointestinal tract at different stages of life.

As we have described many times before, the very young embryo is flat and consists of three germ layers. From top to bottom, they are ectoderm, mesoderm, and endoderm. This flattened cell mass soon folds to form a cylindrical body, and its internal cavity becomes the cavity of the alimentary canal, which is initially closed at both ends.

The epithelial lining of the developing alimentary canal, or **primitive gut**, forms from endoderm **(Figure 23.36a)**. The rest of the wall arises from mesoderm. The anteriormost endoderm (that of the foregut) touches a depressed area of the surface ectoderm called the **stomodeum** (sto″mo-de′um; "on the way to becoming the mouth"). The two membranes fuse, forming the **oral membrane** which soon breaks through to form the opening of the mouth. Similarly, the end of the hindgut fuses with an ectodermal depression, the **proctodeum** (*procto* = anus), to form the **cloacal membrane** (*cloaca* = sewer), which then breaks through to form the anus.

By week 5, the alimentary canal is a continuous "tube" extending from mouth to anus and opens to the external environment at each end. Shortly after, the glandular organs (salivary glands, liver with gallbladder, and pancreas) bud out from the mucosa at various points (Figure 23.36b). These glands retain their connections, which become ducts leading into the digestive tract.

Homeostatic Imbalance 23.18

The digestive system is susceptible to many congenital defects that interfere with feeding. The most common are **cleft palate**,

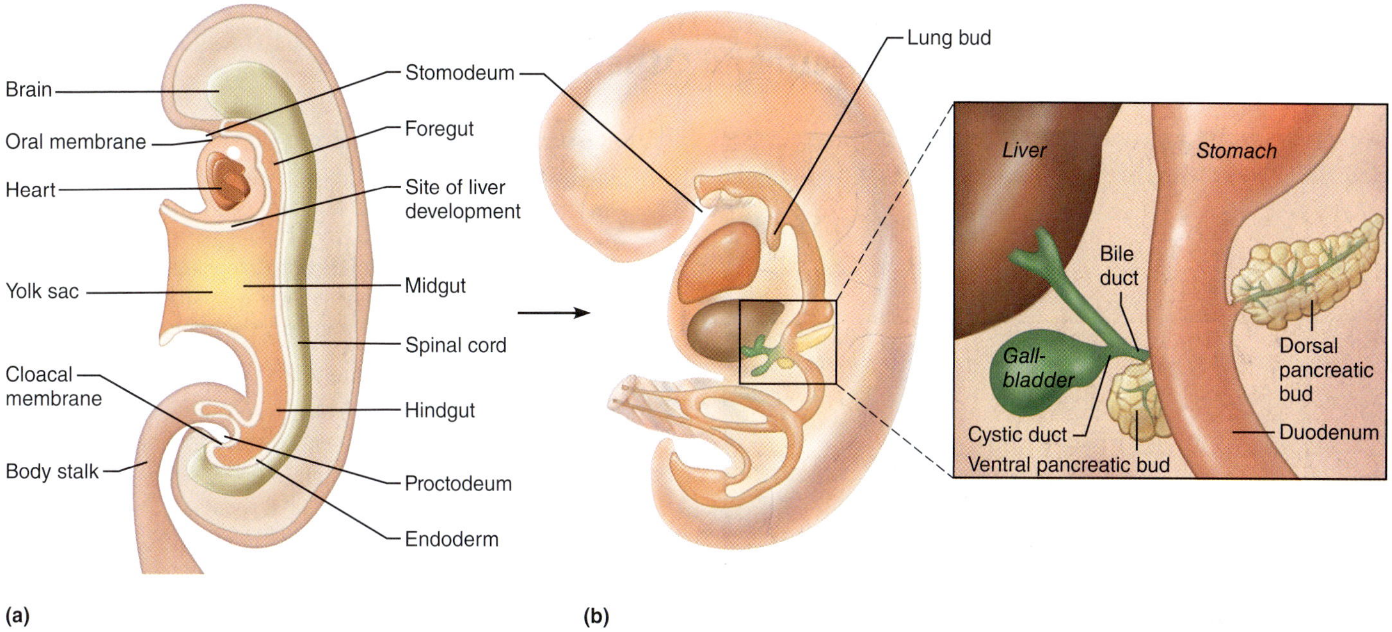

Figure 23.36 Embryonic development of the digestive system. (a) Three-week-old embryo. The endoderm has folded, and the foregut and hindgut have formed. (The midgut is still open and continuous with the yolk sac.) **(b)** By five weeks of development, the accessory organs are budding out from the endodermal layer, as shown in the enlargement.

in which the palatine bones or palatine processes of the maxillae (or both) fail to fuse, and **cleft lip**, which often occur together. Of the two, cleft palate is far more serious because the child is unable to suck properly.

Another common defect is *tracheoesophageal fistula*, in which there is an opening between the esophagus and the trachea, and the esophagus often lacks a connection to the stomach. The baby chokes and becomes cyanotic during feedings because food enters the respiratory passageways. Surgery can usually correct these defects.

Cystic fibrosis (described in more detail in Chapter 22, p. 842) primarily affects the lungs, but it also impairs the activity of the pancreas. In this genetic disease, the mucous glands produce abnormally thick mucus, which blocks ducts and passageways of organs. Blockage of the pancreatic duct prevents pancreatic juice from reaching the small intestine. This impairs the digestion of chyme, and most fats and fat-soluble vitamins are not digested or absorbed. Consequently the stools are bulky and fat laden. The pancreatic problems can be handled by administering pancreatic enzymes with meals. +

During fetal life, the developing infant receives all of its nutrients through the placenta. Nonetheless, the fetal GI tract is "trained" in utero for future food digestion as the fetus naturally swallows some of the surrounding amniotic fluid. This fluid contains several chemicals that stimulate GI maturation, including gastrin and epidermal growth factor.

Digestive System After Birth

Feeding is a newborn baby's most important activity, and several reflexes enhance the infant's ability to obtain food: The *rooting reflex* helps the infant find the nipple, and the *sucking reflex* helps the baby hold onto the nipple and swallow.

Newborn babies tend to double their birth weight within six months, and their caloric intake and food processing ability are extraordinary. For example, a 6-week-old infant weighing about 4 kg (less than 9 lb) drinks about 600 ml of milk daily. A 65-kg adult (143 lb) would have to drink 10 L of milk to ingest a corresponding volume of fluid! However, the stomach of a newborn infant is very small, so feeding must be frequent (every 3–4 hours). Peristalsis is inefficient, and vomiting is not unusual. As the teeth break through the gums, the infant progresses to solid foods and is usually eating an adult diet by the age of 2 years.

As a rule, the digestive system operates throughout childhood and adulthood with relatively few problems. However, contaminated food or extremely spicy or irritating foods sometimes cause **gastroenteritis** (gas″tro-en″tě-ri′tis), inflammation of the GI tract. Ulcers and gallbladder problems—inflammation or **cholecystitis** (ko″le-sis-ti′tis), and gallstones—are problems of middle age.

Aging and the Digestive System

During old age, GI tract activity declines. Fewer digestive juices are produced, absorption is less efficient, and peristalsis slows. The result is less frequent bowel movements and, often, constipation. Taste and smell are less acute, and periodontal disease often develops. Many elderly people live alone or on a reduced income. These factors, along with increasing physical disability, tend to make eating less appealing, and many of our elderly citizens are poorly nourished.

Diverticulosis, fecal incontinence, and cancer of the GI tract are fairly common problems of the aged. Stomach and colon cancers rarely have early signs, and often metastasize

Homeostatic Interrelationships Between the Digestive System and Other Body Systems

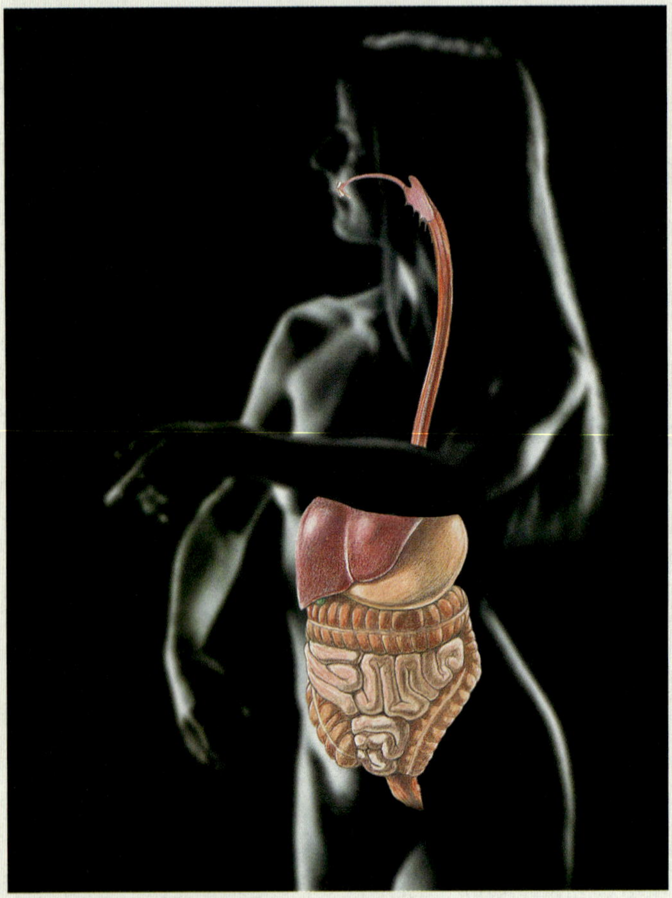

Integumentary System Chapter 5

- Digestive system provides nutrients needed for energy, growth, and repair; supplies fats that provide insulation in the dermis and subcutaneous tissue
- The skin synthesizes vitamin D needed for calcium absorption from the intestine; protects by enclosure

Skeletal System Chapters 6–8

- Digestive system provides nutrients needed for energy, growth, and repair; absorbs calcium needed for bone salts
- Skeletal system protects some digestive organs by bone; cavities store some nutrients (e.g., calcium, fats)

Muscular System Chapters 9–10

- Digestive system provides nutrients needed for energy, growth, and repair; liver removes lactic acid, resulting from muscle activity, from the blood
- Skeletal muscle activity increases motility of GI tract

Nervous System Chapters 11–15

- Digestive system provides nutrients needed for normal neural functioning; nutrient signals influence neural regulation of satiety
- Neural controls of digestive function; in general, parasympathetic fibers accelerate and sympathetic fibers inhibit digestive activity; reflex and voluntary controls of defecation

Endocrine System Chapter 16

- Liver removes hormones from blood, ending their activity; digestive system provides nutrients needed for energy, growth, and repair; pancreas, stomach, and small intestine have hormone-producing cells
- Hormones and paracrines help regulate digestive function

Cardiovascular System Chapters 17–19

- Digestive system provides nutrients to heart and blood vessels; absorbs iron needed for hemoglobin synthesis; absorbs water necessary for normal plasma volume; liver secretes bilirubin resulting from hemoglobin breakdown in bile and stores iron for reuse
- Cardiovascular system transports nutrients absorbed by alimentary canal to all tissues of body; distributes hormones of the digestive tract

Lymphatic System/Immunity Chapters 20–21

- Digestive system provides nutrients for normal functioning; lysozyme of saliva and HCl of stomach provide nonspecific protection against bacteria
- Lacteals drain fatty lymph from digestive tract organs and convey it to blood; Peyer's patches and lymphoid tissue in mesentery house macrophages and immune cells that protect digestive tract organs against infection; plasma cells provide IgA in digestive tract secretions

Respiratory System Chapter 22

- Digestive system provides nutrients needed for energy metabolism, growth, and repair
- Respiratory system provides oxygen to and disposes of carbon dioxide produced by digestive system organs

Urinary System Chapters 25–26

- Digestive system provides nutrients for energy, growth, and repair
- Kidneys transform vitamin D to its active form, which is needed for calcium absorption

Reproductive System Chapter 27

- Digestive system provides nutrients for energy, growth, and repair and extra nutrition needed to support fetal growth (making them inoperable) before a person seeks medical attention. Should metastasis occur, secondary cancer of the liver is almost guaranteed because of the "detour" the splanchnic venous blood takes through the liver via the hepatic portal circulation.

However, when detected early, most GI tract cancers are treatable. The best advice is to have regular dental and medical checkups. Most oral cancers are detected during routine dental examinations, 50% of all rectal cancers can be felt digitally, and nearly 80% of colon cancers can be seen and removed during a colonoscopy.

Until now it was believed that most colorectal cancers derive from initially benign, knobby mucosal tumors called polyps. However, flat pancake-like growths which blend in with the surrounding tissue are more common in Americans than originally thought and are 10 times more likely to be cancerous than polyps. Researchers believe that the flat growths represent a separate pathway to colon cancer. This information will likely have a big impact on gastroenterology and scheduling of tests for colon cancer. Currently recommendations are to have an occult blood examination once a year and a colonoscopy at 3- to 10-year intervals depending on prior findings.

Check Your Understanding

50. From which germ layer does the digestive system mucosa develop?
51. How does cystic fibrosis interfere with the digestive process?
52. Why are colon and stomach cancers so dangerous?

For answers, see Appendix H.

As summarized in *System Connections*, the digestive system keeps the blood well supplied with the nutrients needed by all body tissues to fuel their energy needs and to synthesize new proteins for growth and maintenance of health. Now we are ready to examine how body cells use these nutrients, the topic of Chapter 24.

Chapter Summary

For more chapter study tools, go to the Study Area of MasteringA&P at **www.masteringaandp.com**. There you will find:

- Interactive Physiology iP
- A&PFlix A&PFlix
- Practice Anatomy Lab PAL
- PhysioEx PEx
- Videos, Practice Quizzes and Tests, MP3 Tutor Sessions, Case Studies, and much more!

PART 1 Overview of the Digestive System

1. The digestive system includes organs of the alimentary canal (mouth, pharynx, esophagus, stomach, small and large intestines) and accessory digestive system organs (teeth, tongue, salivary glands, liver, gallbladder, and pancreas).

Digestive Processes (pp. 851–852)

1. Digestive system activities include six processes: ingestion (food intake); propulsion (movement of food through the tract); mechanical breakdown (processes that physically mix or break foods down into smaller fragments); digestion (food breakdown by enzymatic action); absorption (transport of products of digestion through the intestinal mucosa into the blood); and defecation (elimination of the undigested residues [feces] from the body).

Basic Functional Concepts (p. 852)

1. The digestive system controls the environment within its lumen to ensure optimal conditions for digestion and absorption of foodstuffs.
2. Receptors and hormone-secreting cells in the alimentary canal wall respond to stretch and chemical signals that result in stimulation or inhibition of GI secretory activity or motility. The alimentary canal has an intrinsic nerve supply.

iP Digestive System; Topic: Control of the Digestive System, pp. 1, 3, 4–5, 8.

Digestive System Organs: Relationships (pp. 852–855)

1. The parietal and visceral layers of the peritoneum are continuous with one another via several extensions (mesenteries, falciform ligament, lesser and greater omenta), and are separated by a potential space containing serous fluid, which decreases friction during organ activity.
2. The digestive viscera are served by the splanchnic circulation, consisting of arterial branches of the celiac trunk and aorta and the hepatic portal circulation.
3. All organs of the GI tract have the same basic pattern of tissue layers in their walls; all have a mucosa, submucosa, muscularis, and serosa (or adventitia). Intrinsic nerve plexuses (enteric nervous system) are found within the wall.

PART 2 Functional Anatomy of the Digestive System

The Mouth and Associated Organs (pp. 856–861)

1. Food enters the GI tract via the mouth, which is continuous with the oropharynx posteriorly. The boundaries of the mouth are the lips and cheeks, palate, and tongue.
2. The oral mucosa is stratified squamous epithelium, an adaptation seen where abrasion occurs.
3. The tongue is mucosa-covered skeletal muscle. Its intrinsic muscles allow it to change shape; its extrinsic muscles allow it to change position.
4. Saliva is produced by many minor salivary glands and three pairs of major salivary glands—parotid, submandibular, and sublingual—that secrete their product into the mouth via ducts. Largely water, saliva also contains ions, proteins, metabolic wastes, lysozyme, defensins, IgA, salivary amylase, and mucin.
5. Saliva moistens and cleanses the mouth; moistens foods, aiding their compaction; dissolves food chemicals to allow for taste; and begins digestion of starch (salivary amylase). Saliva output is increased by parasympathetic reflexes initiated by activation of chemical and pressure receptors in the mouth and by conditioned reflexes. The sympathetic nervous system depresses salivation.

6. The 20 deciduous teeth begin to be shed at the age of 6 and are gradually replaced during childhood and adolescence by the 32 permanent teeth.
7. Teeth are classed as incisors, canines, premolars, and molars. Each tooth has an enamel-covered crown and a cement-covered root. The bulk of the tooth is dentin, which surrounds the central pulp cavity. A periodontal ligament secures the tooth to the bony alveolus.

The Pharynx (pp. 861–862)

1. Food propelled from the mouth passes through the oropharynx and laryngopharynx. The mucosa of the pharynx is stratified squamous epithelium; skeletal muscles in its wall (constrictor muscles) move food toward the esophagus.

The Esophagus (pp. 862–863)

1. The esophagus extends from the laryngopharynx and joins the stomach at the cardial orifice, which is surrounded by the gastroesophageal sphincter.
2. The esophageal mucosa is stratified squamous epithelium. Its muscularis is skeletal muscle superiorly and changes to smooth muscle inferiorly. It has an adventitia rather than a serosa.

Digestive Processes: Mouth to Esophagus (pp. 863–864)

1. The mouth and associated accessory organs accomplish food ingestion and mechanical breakdown (chewing and mixing), initiate the digestion of starch (salivary amylase), and propel food into the pharynx (buccal phase of swallowing).
2. Teeth masticate food. Chewing is initiated voluntarily and then controlled reflexively.
3. The tongue mixes food with saliva, compacts it into a bolus, and initiates swallowing (the buccal phase). The pharynx and esophagus are primarily food conduits that conduct food to the stomach by peristalsis. The swallowing center in the medulla and pons controls this phase reflexively. When the peristaltic wave approaches the gastroesophageal sphincter, the sphincter relaxes to allow food to enter the stomach.

iP Digestive System; Topic: Motility, pp. 3–5.

The Stomach (pp. 864–874)

23

1. The J-shaped stomach lies in the upper left quadrant of the abdomen. Its major regions are the cardia, fundus, body, and pyloric part. When empty, its internal surface exhibits rugae.
2. The stomach muscularis contains a third (oblique) layer of smooth muscle that allows it to churn and mix food.
3. The stomach mucosa is simple columnar epithelium dotted with gastric pits that lead into gastric glands. Secretory cells in the gastric glands include pepsinogen-producing chief cells; parietal cells, which secrete hydrochloric acid and intrinsic factor; mucous neck cells, which produce mucus; and enteroendocrine cells, which secrete hormones.
4. The mucosal barrier, which protects the stomach from self-digestion and HCl, reflects the fact that the mucosal cells are connected by tight junctions, secrete a thick mucus, and are quickly replaced when damaged.
5. Protein digestion is initiated in the stomach by activated pepsin and requires acidic conditions (provided by HCl). Few substances are absorbed in the stomach.
6. Both nervous and hormonal factors control gastric secretory activity. The three phases of gastric secretion are cephalic, gastric, and intestinal. Most food-related stimuli acting on the head and stomach (cephalic and gastric, respectively) stimulate gastric secretion. Most stimuli acting on the small intestine trigger the enterogastric reflex and release of secretin and CCK, both of which inhibit gastric secretory activity. Sympathetic activity also inhibits gastric secretion.
7. Mechanical breakdown in the stomach is triggered by stomach distension and coupled to food propulsion and stomach emptying. Food movement into the duodenum is controlled by the pylorus and feedback signals from the small intestine. Pacemaker cells in the smooth muscle sheet set the maximal rate of peristalsis.

iP Digestive System; Topic: Control of the Digestive System, pp. 3, 5–6, 8.

The Small Intestine and Associated Structures (pp. 874–887)

1. The small intestine is the major digestive and absorptive organ. It extends from the pyloric sphincter to the ileocecal valve. Its three subdivisions are the duodenum, jejunum, and ileum. The bile duct and pancreatic duct join to form the hepatopancreatic ampulla and empty their secretions into the duodenum through the hepatopancreatic sphincter.
2. Circular folds, villi, and microvilli increase the intestinal surface area for digestion and absorption.
3. The duodenal submucosa contains elaborate mucus-secreting duodenal glands. The mucosa of the ileum contains Peyer's patches (lymphoid follicles). The duodenum is covered not with a serosa but an adventitia.
4. Intestinal juice is largely water and relatively enzyme-poor. The major stimuli for its release are stretch and chemicals.
5. The liver is a lobed organ overlying the stomach. Its digestive role is to produce bile, which it secretes into the common hepatic duct.
6. The structural and functional units of the liver are the liver lobules. Blood flowing to the liver via the hepatic artery and hepatic portal vein flows into its sinusoids, from which stellate macrophages remove debris and hepatocytes remove nutrients. Hepatocytes store glucose as glycogen, use amino acids to make plasma proteins, and detoxify metabolic wastes and drugs.
7. Bile is made continuously by the hepatocytes. Bile salts and secretin stimulate bile production.
8. The gallbladder, a muscular sac that lies beneath the right liver lobe, stores and concentrates bile.
9. Bile contains electrolytes, a variety of fatty substances, bile salts, and bile pigments in an aqueous medium. Bile salts are emulsifying agents; they disperse fats and form water-soluble micelles, which solubilize the products of fat digestion.
10. Cholecystokinin released by the small intestine stimulates the gallbladder to contract and the hepatopancreatic sphincter to relax, allowing bile (and pancreatic juice) to enter the duodenum.
11. The pancreas is retroperitoneal between the spleen and small intestine. Its exocrine product, pancreatic juice, is carried to the duodenum via the pancreatic duct.
12. Pancreatic juice is a HCO_3^--rich fluid containing enzymes that digest all categories of foods. Intestinal hormones and the vagus nerves control secretion of pancreatic juice.

iP Digestive System; Topic: Secretion, pp. 11–14.

13. Mechanical breakdown and propulsion in the small intestine mix chyme with digestive juices and bile and force the residues, largely by segmentation, through the ileocecal valve. Pacemaker cells set the rate of segmentation. Ileocecal valve opening is controlled by the gastroileal reflex and gastrin.

The Large Intestine (pp. 887–892)

1. The subdivisions of the large intestine are the cecum (and appendix), colon (ascending, transverse, descending, and sigmoid portions), rectum, and anal canal. It opens to the body exterior at the anus.

2. The longitudinal muscle in the muscularis is reduced to three bands (teniae coli), which pucker its wall, producing haustra. The mucosa of most of the large intestine is simple columnar epithelium containing abundant goblet cells.
3. The major functions of the large intestine are absorption of water, some electrolytes, and vitamins made by enteric bacteria, and defecation (evacuation of food residues from the body).
4. The defecation reflex is triggered when feces enter the rectum. It involves parasympathetic reflexes leading to contraction of the rectal walls and is aided by Valsalva's maneuver.

iP Digestive System; Topic: Anatomy Review, pp. 3–5.

PART 3 Physiology of Digestion and Absorption

Digestion (pp. 892–895)

1. Digestion is accomplished by hydrolysis, catalyzed by enzymes.
2. Most digestion is done in the small intestine by intestinal (brush border) enzymes and, more importantly, by pancreatic enzymes. Alkaline pancreatic juice neutralizes the acidic chyme and provides the proper environment for operation of the enzymes. Both pancreatic juice (the main source of lipases) and bile are necessary for fat breakdown.

Absorption (pp. 895–898)

1. Virtually all of the foodstuffs and most of the water and electrolytes are absorbed in the small intestine. Most nutrients are absorbed by active transport processes, except for fat digestion products, fat-soluble vitamins, and most water-soluble vitamins (which are absorbed by diffusion).
2. Fat breakdown products are solubilized by bile salts (in micelles), resynthesized to triglycerides in the intestinal mucosal cells, and combined with other lipids and protein as chylomicrons that enter the lacteals. Other absorbed substances enter the villus blood capillaries and are transported to the liver via the hepatic portal vein.

Developmental Aspects of the Digestive System (pp. 898–901)

1. The glandular accessory organs (salivary glands, liver, pancreas, and gallbladder) form from outpocketings of the foregut endoderm. The mucosa of the alimentary canal develops from the endoderm, which folds to form a tube. The remaining three tunics of the alimentary canal wall are formed by mesoderm.
2. Important congenital abnormalities of the digestive tract include cleft palate/lip, tracheoesophageal fistula, and cystic fibrosis. All interfere with normal nutrition.
3. Various inflammations plague the digestive system throughout life. Appendicitis is common in adolescents, gastroenteritis and food poisoning can occur at any time (given the proper irritating factors), and ulcers and gallbladder problems increase in middle age.
4. The efficiency of all digestive system processes declines in the elderly, and periodontal disease is common. Diverticulosis, fecal incontinence, and GI tract cancers such as stomach and colon cancer appear with increasing frequency in an aging population.

Review Questions

Multiple Choice/Matching

(Some questions have more than one correct answer. Select the best answer or answers from the choices given.)

1. The peritoneal cavity **(a)** is the same thing as the abdominopelvic cavity, **(b)** is filled with air, **(c)** like the pleural and pericardial cavities is a potential space containing serous fluid, **(d)** contains the pancreas and all of the duodenum.
2. Obstruction of the hepatopancreatic sphincter impairs digestion by reducing the availability of **(a)** bile and HCl, **(b)** HCl and intestinal juice, **(c)** pancreatic juice and intestinal juice, **(d)** pancreatic juice and bile.
3. The action of an enzyme is influenced by **(a)** its chemical surroundings, **(b)** its specific substrate, **(c)** the presence of needed cofactors or coenzymes, **(d)** all of these.
4. Carbohydrates are acted on by **(a)** peptidases, trypsin, and chymotrypsin, **(b)** amylase, maltase, and sucrase, **(c)** lipases, **(d)** peptidases, lipases, and galactase.
5. The parasympathetic nervous system influences digestion by **(a)** relaxing smooth muscle, **(b)** stimulating peristalsis and secretory activity, **(c)** constricting sphincters, **(d)** none of these.
6. The digestive juice product containing enzymes capable of digesting all four major foodstuff categories is **(a)** pancreatic, **(b)** gastric, **(c)** salivary, **(d)** biliary.
7. The vitamin associated with calcium absorption is **(a)** A, **(b)** K, **(c)** C, **(d)** D.
8. Someone has eaten a meal of buttered toast, cream, and eggs. Which of the following would you expect to happen? **(a)** Compared to the period shortly after the meal, gastric motility and secretion of HCl decrease when the food reaches the duodenum; **(b)** gastric motility increases even as the person is chewing the food (before swallowing); **(c)** fat will be emulsified in the duodenum by the action of bile; **(d)** all of these.
9. The site of production of cholecystokinin is **(a)** the stomach, **(b)** the small intestine, **(c)** the pancreas, **(d)** the large intestine.
10. Which of the following is not characteristic of the colon? **(a)** It is divided into ascending, transverse, and descending portions; **(b)** it contains abundant bacteria, some of which synthesize certain vitamins; **(c)** it is the main absorptive site; **(d)** it absorbs much of the water and salts remaining in the wastes.
11. The gallbladder(**a)** produces bile, **(b)** is attached to the pancreas, **(c)** stores and concentrates bile, **(d)** produces secretin.
12. The sphincter between the stomach and duodenum is **(a)** the pyloric sphincter, **(b)** the gastroesophageal sphincter, **(c)** the hepatopancreatic sphincter, **(d)** the ileocecal sphincter.

In items 13–17, trace the path of a single protein molecule that has been ingested.

13. The protein molecule will be digested by enzymes made by **(a)** the mouth, stomach, and colon, **(b)** the stomach, liver, and small intestine, **(c)** the small intestine, mouth, and liver, **(d)** the pancreas, stomach, and small intestine.
14. The protein molecule must be digested before it can be transported to and utilized by the cells because **(a)** protein is only useful directly, **(b)** protein has a low pH, **(c)** proteins in the circulating blood produce an adverse osmotic pressure, **(d)** the protein is too large to be readily absorbed.
15. The products of protein digestion enter the bloodstream largely through cells lining **(a)** the stomach, **(b)** the small intestine, **(c)** the large intestine, **(d)** the bile duct.

16. Before the blood carrying the products of protein digestion reaches the heart, it first passes through capillary networks in **(a)** the spleen, **(b)** the lungs, **(c)** the liver, **(d)** the brain.
17. Having passed through the regulatory organ selected above, the products of protein digestion are circulated throughout the body. They will enter individual body cells by **(a)** active transport, **(b)** diffusion, **(c)** osmosis, **(d)** phagocytosis.

Short Answer Essay Questions

18. Make a simple line drawing of the organs of the alimentary canal and label each organ. Then add three labels to your drawing—salivary glands, liver, and pancreas—and use arrows to show where each of these organs empties its secretions into the alimentary canal.
19. Sara was on a diet but she could not eat less and kept claiming her stomach had a mind of its own. She was joking, but indeed, there is a "gut brain" called the enteric nervous system. Is it part of the parasympathetic and sympathetic nervous system? Explain.
20. Name the layers of the alimentary canal wall. Note the tissue composition and major function of each layer.
21. What is a mesentery? Mesocolon? Greater omentum?
22. Name the six functional activities of the digestive system.
23. (a) Describe the boundaries of the oral cavity. (b) Why do you suppose its mucosa is stratified squamous epithelium rather than the more typical simple columnar epithelium?
24. (a) What is the normal number of permanent teeth? Of deciduous teeth? (b) What substance covers the tooth crown? Its root? (c) What substance makes up the bulk of a tooth? (d) What and where is pulp?
25. Describe the two phases of swallowing, noting the organs involved and the activities that occur.
26. Describe the role of these cells found in gastric glands: parietal, chief, mucous neck, and enteroendocrine.
27. Describe the regulation of the cephalic, gastric, and intestinal phases of gastric secretion.
28. (a) What is the relationship between the cystic, common hepatic, bile, and pancreatic ducts? (b) What is the point of fusion of the bile and pancreatic ducts called?
29. Explain why fatty stools result from the absence of bile or pancreatic juice.
30. Indicate the function of the stellate macrophages and the hepatocytes of the liver.
31. What are (a) brush border enzymes? (b) chylomicrons?
32. Activation of pancreatic enzymes in the small intestine is a good example of the wisdom of the body. How so?
33. Name one inflammatory condition of the digestive system particularly common to adolescents, two common in middle age, and one common in old age.
34. What are the effects of aging on digestive system activity?

Critical Thinking and Clinical Application Questions

1. You are a research assistant at a pharmaceutical company. Your group has been asked to develop an effective laxative that (1) provides bulk and (2) is nonirritating to the intestinal mucosa. Explain why these requests are important by describing what would happen if the opposite conditions were present.
2. After a heavy meal rich with fried foods, Debby Collins, an overweight 45-year-old woman, was rushed to the emergency room with severe spasmodic pains in her epigastric region that radiated to the right side of her rib cage. She indicated that the attack came on suddenly, and her abdomen was found to be tender to the touch and somewhat rigid. What do you think is this patient's problem and why is her pain discontinuous (colicky)? What are the treatment options and what might happen if the problem is not resolved?
3. A baby is admitted to the hospital with a history of diarrhea and watery feces occurring over the last three days. The baby has sunken fontanelles, indicating extreme dehydration. Tests indicate that the baby has a bacterium-induced colitis, and antibiotics are prescribed. Because of the baby's loss of intestinal juices, do you think that his blood pH would indicate acidosis or alkalosis? Explain your reasoning.
4. Gary Francis, a middle-aged salesman, complains of a burning pain in the "pit of his stomach," usually beginning about two hours after eating and abating after drinking a glass of milk. When asked to indicate the site, he points to his epigastric region. The GI tract is examined by X-ray fluoroscopy. A gastric ulcer is visualized, and drug therapy using an antibiotic-bismuth approach is recommended. (a) Why is this treatment suggested? (b) What are the possible consequences of nontreatment?
5. Dr. Dolan used an endoscope to view Mr. Habib's colon. He noted the presence of several polyps and removed them during the same procedure. What is an endoscope? Why did Dr. Dolan opt to remove the polyps immediately?
6. Mr. Holden has had severe diarrhea all day and is severely weakened. Explain why his nurse is concerned about his present condition.
7. What is the protective value of having several sets of tonsils at the oral entry to the pharynx?

AT THE CLINIC

Related Clinical Terms

Achalasia A disorder in which swallowing is hindered or prevented. Botox injections can relax the esophageal sphincter.

Ascites (ah-si'tēz; *asci* = bag, bladder) Abnormal accumulation of fluid within the peritoneal cavity; if excessive, causes visible bloating of the abdomen. May result from portal hypertension caused by liver cirrhosis or by heart or kidney disease.

Barrett's esophagus A pathological change in the epithelium of the lower esophagus from stratified squamous to a columnar epithelium. A possible sequel to untreated chronic gastroesophageal reflux due to hiatal hernia, it predisposes the individual to aggressive esophageal cancer (adenocarcinoma).

Bruxism (bruck'sizm) Grinding or clenching of teeth, usually at night during sleep in response to stress. Can wear down and crack the teeth.

Bulimia (bu-lim'e-ah; *bous* = ox; *limos* = hunger) Binge-purge behavior—episodes of massive overeating followed by some method of purging (self-induced vomiting, taking laxatives or diuretics, or excessive exercise). Most common in women of high school or college age and in high school males in certain athletic activities (wrestling). Rooted in a pathological fear of being fat, and a need for control; provides a means of handling stress and depression. Consequences include eroded tooth enamel, stomach

Related Clinical Terms *(continued)*

trauma or rupture (from vomiting), and severe electrolyte disturbances which impair heart activity. Therapy includes hospitalization to control behavior, and nutritional counseling.

Dysphagia (dis-fa′je-ah; *dys* = difficult, abnormal; *phag* = eat) Difficulty swallowing; usually due to obstruction or physical trauma to the esophagus.

Endoscopy (en-dos′ko-pe; *endo* = within, inside; *scopy* = viewing) Visual examination of a ventral body cavity or the interior of a visceral organ with a flexible tubelike device called an endoscope, which contains a light source and a lens. A general term for a colonoscopy (viewing the colon), sigmoidoscopy (viewing the sigmoid colon), etc.

Enteritis (*enteron* = intestine) Inflammation of the intestine, especially the small intestine.

Hemochromatosis (he″mo-kro″mah-to′sis; *hemo* = blood; *chroma* = color; osis = condition of) A disorder in iron metabolism due to excessive/prolonged iron intake or a breakdown of the mucosal iron barrier; excess iron is deposited in the tissues, increasing skin pigmentation and the risk of hepatic cancer and liver cirrhosis. Also called *bronze diabetes* and *iron storage disease.*

Ileus (il′e-us) A condition in which all GI tract movement stops and the gut appears to be paralyzed. Can result from electrolyte imbalances and blockade of parasympathetic impulses by drugs (such as those commonly used during abdominal surgery); usually reversed when these interferences end. The reappearance of intestinal sounds (gurgling, etc.) indicates restoration of motility.

Inflammatory bowel disease (IBD) A noncontagious, periodic inflammation of the intestinal wall now understood to be an abnormal immune and inflammatory response to bacterial antigens that normally occur in the intestine. Linked to a newly discovered T_H cell (T_H17), certain cytokines, and a deficit of antimicrobial substances normally secreted by the gut mucosa (lysozyme, defensins, and others). Afflicts up to two of every 1000 people. Symptoms include cramping, diarrhea, weight loss, and intestinal bleeding. Two subtypes occur: (1) Crohn's disease, a syndrome characterized by relapsing and remitting periods, is more serious, with deep ulcers and fissures developing along the whole intestine, but mostly in the terminal ileum. (2) Ulcerative colitis is characterized by a shallow inflammation of the large-intestinal mucosa, mainly in the rectum. Both types are treated with a special diet, reducing stress, antibiotics, and anti-inflammatory and immunosuppressant drugs. Extremely severe cases of ulcerative colitis are treated by colectomy (removal of a portion of the colon).

Laparoscopy (lap″ah-ros′ko-pe; *lapar* = the flank; *scopy* = observation) Examination of the peritoneal cavity and its organs with an endoscope inserted through the anterior abdominal wall. Often used to assess the condition of the digestive organs and the pelvic reproductive organs of females.

Orthodontics (or″tho-don′tiks; *ortho* = straight) Branch of dentistry that prevents and corrects misaligned teeth.

Pancreatitis (pan″kre-ah-ti′tis) A rare but extremely serious inflammation of the pancreas. May result from excessively high levels of fat in the blood or excessive alcohol ingestion, but most often results when a gallstone blocks the bile duct and pancreatic enzymes are activated in the pancreatic duct, causing the pancreatic tissue and duct to be digested (literally, eating from within). This painful condition can lead to nutritional deficiencies because pancreatic enzymes are essential to food digestion in the small intestine.

Peptic ulcers Term referring to gastric and duodenal ulcers.

Proctology (prok-tol′o-je; *procto* = rectum, anus; *logy* = study of) Branch of medicine dealing with treatment of diseases of the colon, rectum, and anus.

Pyloric stenosis (pi-lor′ik stě-no′sis; *stenosis* = narrowing, constriction) Congenital abnormality in which the pyloric sphincter is abnormally constricted. There is usually no problem until the baby begins to take solid food, and then projectile vomiting begins. Corrected surgically.

Vagotomy (va-got′o-me) Cutting or severing of the vagus nerve to decrease secretion of gastric juice in those with peptic ulcers that do not respond to medication.

Xerostomia (ze″ro-sto′me-ah; *zer* = dry, *stom* = mouth) Extreme dryness of the mouth; can be caused by cysts that block salivary glands or autoimmune invasion of the salivary glands or ducts (Sjögren's syndrome).

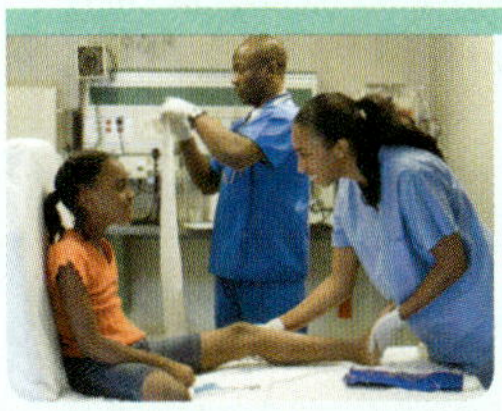

Case Study Digestive System

Remember Mr. Gutteman, the gentleman who was dehydrating? It seems that his tremendous output of urine was only one of his current problems. Today, he complains of a headache, gnawing epigastric pain, and "the runs" (diarrhea). To pinpoint the problem, he is asked the following questions.

- Have you had these symptoms previously? (Response: "Yes, but never this bad.")
- Are you allergic to any foods? (Response: "Shellfish doesn't like me and milk gives me the runs.")

As a result of his responses, a lactose-free diet is ordered for Mr. Gutteman instead of the regular diet originally prescribed.

1. Why is the new diet prescribed? (What is believed to be his problem?)

Mr. Gutteman's problem continues despite the diet change. In fact, the frequency of diarrhea increases and by the end of the next day, he is complaining of severe abdominal pain. Again, he is asked some questions to probe his condition. One is whether he has traveled outside the country recently. He has not, reducing the possibility of infection with *Shigella* bacteria, which is associated with poor sanitation. Other questions:

- Do you drink alcohol and how much? (Response: "Little or none.")
- Have you recently eaten raw eggs or a salad containing mayonnaise at a gathering? (Response: "No.")
- Are there certain foods that seem to precipitate these attacks? (Response: "Yes, when I have coffee and a sandwich.")

2. On the basis of these responses, what do you think Mr. Gutteman's diarrhea stems from? How will it be diagnosed and treated?

(Answers in Appendix H)

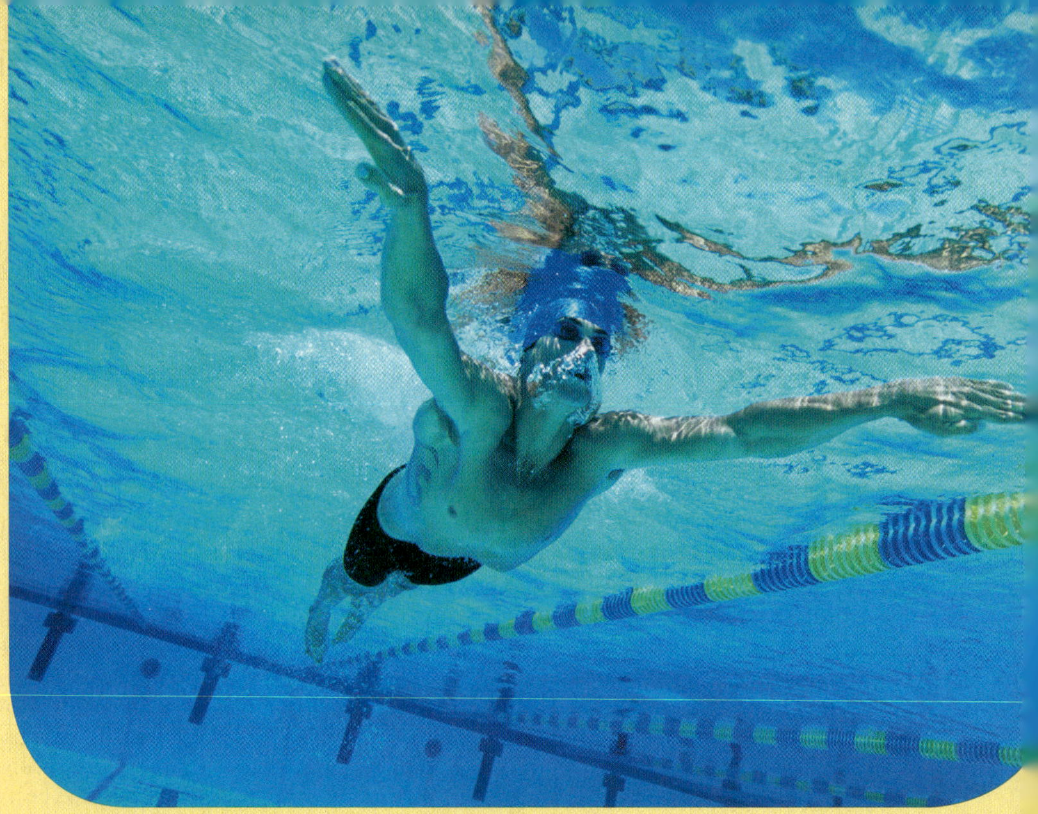

24

Nutrition, Metabolism, and Body Temperature Regulation

Are you a food lover? We are too. In fact, most people fall into one of two camps—those who live to eat and those who eat to live. The saying "you are what you eat" is true in that part of the food we eat is converted to our living flesh. In other words, our bodies use some nutrients to build cell structures, replace worn-out parts, and synthesize functional molecules. However, most nutrients we ingest are used as metabolic fuel. That is, they are oxidized and transformed to ATP, the chemical energy form used by cells.

The energy value of foods is measured in **kilocalories** (kcal) or "large calories" (C). One kilocalorie is the amount of heat energy needed to raise the temperature of 1 kilogram of water 1°C (1.8°F). This unit is the "calorie" that dieters count so conscientiously.

In Chapter 23, we talked about how foods are digested and absorbed, but what happens to these foods once they enter the blood? Why do we need bread, meat, and fresh vegetables? Why does everything we eat seem to turn to fat? In this chapter we will answer these questions as we examine both the nature of nutrients and their metabolic roles.

Diet and Nutrition

✓ Define nutrient, essential nutrient, and calorie.

✓ List the six major nutrient categories. Note important sources and main cellular uses.

A **nutrient** is a substance in food the body uses to promote normal growth, maintenance, and repair. The nutrients needed for health divide neatly into six categories. Three of these—carbohydrates, lipids, and proteins—are **major nutrients** that make up the bulk of what we eat. The fourth and fifth categories, vitamins and minerals, though equally crucial for health, are required in only minute amounts.

In a strict sense, water, which accounts for about 60% by volume of the food we eat, is also a major nutrient. We described its importance in the body in Chapter 2, so here we consider only the five nutrient categories listed above.

Most foods offer a combination of nutrients. A balanced diet of foods from each of the different food groups normally guarantees adequate amounts of all the needed nutrients.

In 1992, the U.S. Department of Agriculture released a food guide pyramid in which four food groups were stacked horizontally in the shape of a pyramid. Since then, several alternative versions have made an appearance claiming to be more healthy nutritionwise and focusing on exercise as an aid to good health.

The version put out in 1992 by Walter Willett, called the **Healthy Eating Pyramid** (Figure 24.1a), looks at six major food groups, subdividing some of them further. It uses the traditional (horizontal) orientation of food groups; emphasizes eating whole-grain foods and lots of fruits and vegetables; and recommends substituting plant oils for animal fats and restricting red meat, sweets, and starchy foods.

Fresh out of the oven in 2011 is **MyPlate** a food guide with a completely new symbol—a round dinner plate. Put out by the USDA, it shows food categories in healthy proportions in sections of a place setting rather than as segments of a pyramid (Figure 24.1b). The fact that each food group is shown as part of a single meal suggests how consumers might plan their meals relative to amounts and variety of foods selected from each food group. Occupying half the plate are fruits and vegetables (more vegetable than fruit). These are balanced in the other half by grains and proteins (more grain than protein). A glass represents dairy, the fifth food group. Links provide details on

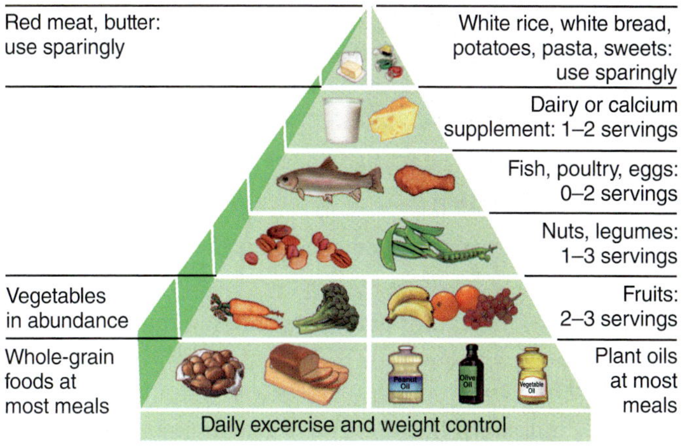

(a) Healthy Eating Pyramid

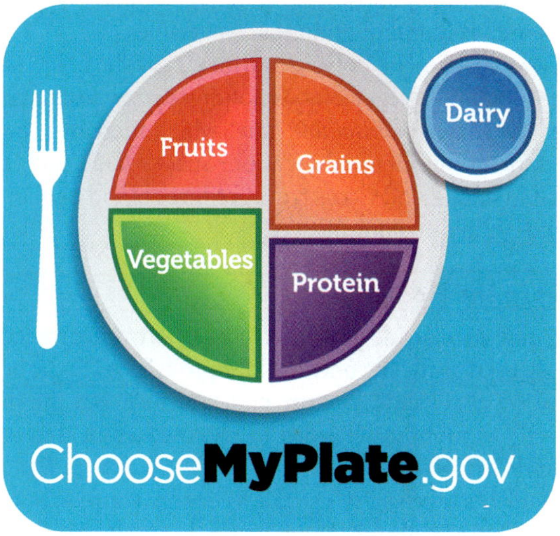

(b) USDA's MyPlate

Figure 24.1 Two visual food guides.

healthy choices in each food group. You can personalize the MyPlate diet by age, sex, and activity level by going to the MyPlate website (www.choosemyplate.gov).

To be perfectly honest, nutrition advice is constantly in flux and often mired in the self-interest of food companies. Nonetheless, basic dietary principles have not changed in years and are not in dispute: Eat less overall; eat plenty of fruits, vegetables, and whole grains; avoid junk food; and exercise regularly.

The ability of cells, especially liver cells, to convert one type of molecule to another is truly remarkable. These interconversions allow the body to use a wide range of foods and to adjust to varying food intakes. But there are limits to our ability to conjure up new molecules from old.

At least 45 and possibly 50 molecules, called **essential nutrients**, cannot be made fast enough to meet the body's needs, so our diet must provide them. As long as we ingest all the essential nutrients, the body can synthesize the hundreds of additional molecules required for life and good health. While "essential" is a standard way to describe the chemicals that must be obtained from outside sources, this term is misleading because both essential and nonessential nutrients are equally vital for normal functioning.

Carbohydrates

✓ Distinguish between simple and complex carbohydrate sources.

✓ Indicate the major uses of carbohydrates in the body.

Dietary Sources

Except for milk sugar (lactose) and negligible amounts of glycogen in meats, all the carbohydrates we ingest are derived from plants. Sugars (monosaccharides and disaccharides) come from fruits, sugar cane, sugar beets, honey, and milk. The polysaccharide starch is found in grains and vegetables.

Two varieties of polysaccharides provide fiber. Cellulose, plentiful in most vegetables, is not digested by humans but provides roughage, or *insoluble fiber*, which increases the bulk of the stool and facilitates defecation. *Soluble fiber*, such as pectin found in apples and citrus fruits, reduces blood cholesterol levels, a desirable goal for most of us.

Uses in the Body

The monosaccharide **glucose** is *the* carbohydrate molecule ultimately used as fuel by body cells to produce ATP. Carbohydrate digestion also yields fructose and galactose, but the liver converts these monosaccharides to glucose before they enter the general circulation.

Many body cells also use fats as energy sources, but neurons and red blood cells rely almost entirely on glucose for their energy needs. Because even a temporary shortage of blood glucose can severely depress brain function and lead to neuron death, the body carefully monitors and regulates blood glucose levels. Any glucose in excess of what is needed for ATP synthesis is converted to glycogen or fat and stored for later use.

Other uses of monosaccharides are meager. Small amounts of pentose sugars are used to synthesize nucleic acids, and a variety of sugars are attached to externally facing plasma membrane proteins and lipids.

Dietary Requirements

The low-carbohydrate diet of the Inuit (Eskimos) and the high-carbohydrate diet of peoples in the Far East indicate that humans can be healthy even with wide variations in carbohydrate intake. The minimum requirement for carbohydrates is not known, but 100 grams per day is presumed to be the smallest amount needed to maintain adequate blood glucose levels. The recommended dietary allowance (130 g/day) is based on the amount needed to fuel the brain, not the total amount needed to supply all daily activities.

The recommended intake to maintain health is 45–65% of total calorie intake, with the emphasis on *complex* carbohydrates (whole grains and vegetables), rather than simple carbohydrates (monosaccharides and disaccharides). When less than 50 grams per day are consumed, tissue proteins and fats are used for energy fuel.

American adults typically consume about 46% of dietary food energy in the form of carbohydrates. Because starchy foods (rice, pasta, breads) cost less than meat and other high-protein foods, carbohydrates make up an even greater percentage of the diet in low-income groups. Highly processed carbohydrate foods such as candy and soft drinks provide concentrated energy sources only—so-called "empty calories." Eating refined, sugary foods instead of the more complex carbohydrates may cause nutritional deficiencies as well as obesity. **Table 24.1** lists other possible consequences of excessive intake of carbohydrates.

Lipids

✓ Indicate uses of lipids in the body.

✓ Distinguish between saturated, unsaturated, and trans fatty acid sources.

Dietary Sources

The most abundant dietary lipids are triglycerides, also called neutral fats (Chapter 2). We eat saturated fats in animal products such as meat and dairy foods, in a few tropical plant products such as coconut, and in hydrogenated oils (trans fats) such as margarine and solid shortenings used in baking. Unsaturated fats are present in seeds, nuts, olive oil, and most vegetable oils. Fats are digested to monoglycerides and fatty acids, and then reconverted to triglycerides for transport in the lymph.

Major sources of cholesterol are egg yolk, meats and organ meats, shellfish, and milk products. However, it is estimated that the liver produces about 85% of blood cholesterol regardless of dietary intake.

The liver is also adept at converting one fatty acid to another, but it cannot synthesize *linoleic acid* (lin″o-le′ik), a fatty acid component of *lecithin* (les′ĭ-thin). For this reason, linoleic acid, an omega-6 fatty acid, is an *essential fatty acid* that must be ingested. Linolenic acid, an omega-3 fatty acid, may also be essential. Fortunately, most vegetable oils contain both linoleic and linolenic acids.

Uses in the Body

Fats have fallen into disfavor, particularly among those for whom the "battle of the bulge" is constant. But fats make foods tender, flaky, or creamy, and make us feel full and satiated (satisfied). Furthermore, dietary fats *are* essential for several reasons:

- Fats help the body absorb fat-soluble vitamins.
- Triglycerides are the major energy fuel of hepatocytes and skeletal muscle.
- Phospholipids are an integral component of myelin sheaths and cellular membranes.
- Fatty deposits in adipose tissue provide (1) a protective cushion around body organs, (2) an insulating layer beneath the skin, and (3) an easy-to-store concentrated source of energy fuel.
- *Prostaglandins* (pros″tah-glan′dinz), regulatory molecules formed from linoleic acid via arachidonic acid (ah″rah-kĭ-don′ik), play a role in smooth muscle contraction, control of blood pressure, and inflammation.

Table 24.1 Summary of Carbohydrate, Lipid, and Protein Nutrients

FOOD SOURCES	RECOMMENDED DAILY ALLOWANCE (RDA) FOR ADULTS	PROBLEMS	
		EXCESSES	DEFICITS
Carbohydrates			
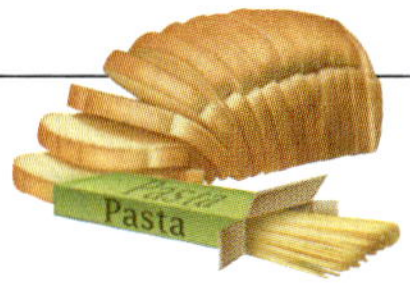			
Total Digestible ▪ **Complex carbohydrates** (starches): bread, cereal, crackers, flour, pasta, rice, potatoes ▪ **Simple carbohydrates (sugars):** carbonated drinks, candy, fruit, ice cream, pudding, young (immature) vegetables	130 g 45–65% of total caloric intake	Obesity; diabetes mellitus; nutritional deficits; dental caries; gastrointestinal irritation; elevated triglycerides in plasma	Tissue wasting (in extreme deprivation); metabolic acidosis resulting from accelerated fat use for energy
Total Fiber	25–30 g		
Lipids			
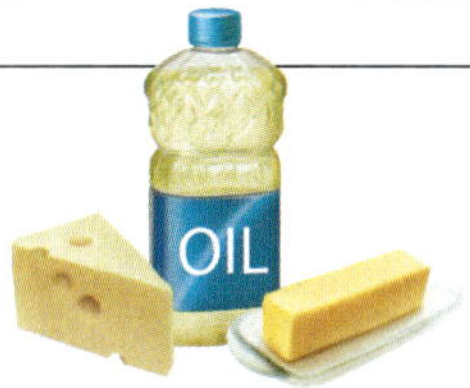			
Total	65 g 20–35% of total caloric intake	Obesity and increased risk of cardiovascular disease (particularly if excesses of saturated and trans fat)	Weight loss; fat stores and tissue proteins catabolized to provide metabolic energy; problems controlling heat loss (due to depletion of subcutaneous fat)
▪ **Animal sources:** lard, meat, poultry, eggs, milk, milk products	20 g		
▪ **Plant sources:** chocolate; corn, soy, cottonseed, olive oils; coconut; corn; peanuts	11–17 g		
▪ **Essential fatty acids:** fish oil, corn, cottonseed, soy oils; wheat germ; vegetable shortenings	1.1–1.6 g	Excess dietary intake of omega-3 fatty acid may increase risk of stroke	Poor growth; skin lesions (eczema-like); depression
▪ **Cholesterol and trans fatty acids:** organ meats (liver, kidneys, brains), egg yolks, fish roe; smaller concentrations in milk products and meat	Not determined	Increased levels of blood cholesterol and low-density lipoproteins, correlated with increased risk of cardiovascular disease	Increased risk of stroke (CVA) in susceptible individuals
Proteins			
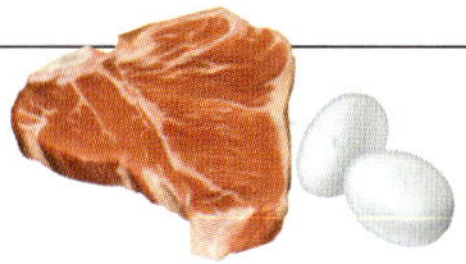			
▪ **Complete proteins:** eggs, milk, milk products, meat (fish, poultry, pork, beef, lamb), soybeans ▪ **Incomplete proteins:** legumes (lima beans, kidney beans, lentils); nuts and seeds; grains and cereals; vegetables	0.8 g/kg body weight 12–20% of total caloric intake	Obesity; enhanced calcium excretion and bone loss; high cholesterol levels in blood; kidney stones	Profound weight loss and tissue wasting; retarded growth in children; anemia; edema (due to deficits of plasma proteins) During pregnancy: miscarriage or premature birth

Unlike triglycerides, cholesterol is not used for energy. It is important as a stabilizing component of plasma membranes and is the precursor from which bile salts, steroid hormones, and other essential molecules are formed.

Dietary Requirements

Fats represent over 40% of the calories in the typical American diet. There are no precise recommendations on amount or type of dietary fats, but the American Heart Association suggests:

- Fats should represent 30% or less of total caloric intake.
- Saturated fats should be limited to 10% or less of total fat intake.
- Daily cholesterol intake should be no more than 300 mg (the amount in one egg yolk).

The goal of these recommendations is to keep total blood cholesterol below 200 mg/dl. Because a diet high in saturated fats and cholesterol may contribute to cardiovascular disease, these are wise guidelines. Table 24.1 summarizes sources of the various lipid classes and consequences of deficiency or excessive intake.

Fat Substitutes

In an attempt to reduce fat intake without losing fat's appetizing aspects, many people have turned to fat substitutes. Perhaps the oldest fat substitute is air (beaten into a product to make it fluffy). Other fat substitutes are modified starches and gums, and milk whey protein. Except for those based on dietary fibers (gums), these products are metabolized and provide calories. One of the newest substitutes, Olestra, a fat-based product made from cottonseeds, is not metabolized because it is not digested or absorbed.

Most fat substitutes have two drawbacks: (1) They don't stand up to the intense heat needed to fry foods, and (2) although manufacturers claim otherwise, they don't taste nearly as good as the "real thing." The ones that are not absorbed tend to cause flatus (gas) or diarrhea, and may interfere with absorption of fat-soluble drugs, vitamins, and beta-carotene, a precursor of vitamin A.

Proteins

✓ Distinguish between nutritionally complete and incomplete proteins.

✓ Indicate uses of proteins in the body.

✓ Define nitrogen balance and indicate possible causes of positive and negative nitrogen balance.

Dietary Sources

Animal products contain the highest-quality proteins, in other words, those with the greatest amount and best ratios of *essential amino acids* **(Figure 24.2)**. Proteins in eggs, milk, fish, and most meats are **complete proteins** that meet all the body's amino acid requirements for tissue maintenance and growth (Table 24.1). Legumes (beans and peas), nuts, and cereals are protein-rich, but their proteins are nutritionally incomplete because they are low in one or more of the essential amino acids. The exception to this generalization is soybeans, plant-derived complete proteins.

Strict vegetarians must carefully plan their diets to obtain all the essential amino acids and prevent protein malnutrition. When ingested together, cereal grains and legumes provide all the essential amino acids (Figure 24.2b). Some combination of these foods is found in the diets of all cultures (for instance, the rice and beans seen on nearly every plate in a Mexican restaurant). For nonvegetarians, grains and legumes are useful as partial substitutes for more expensive animal proteins.

Uses in the Body

Proteins are important structural materials of the body, including, for example, keratin in skin, collagen and elastin in connective tissues, and muscle proteins. In addition, functional proteins such as enzymes and some hormones regulate an incredible variety of body functions. Whether amino acids are used to synthesize new proteins or burned for energy depends on a number of factors:

- **The all-or-none rule.** All amino acids needed to make a particular protein must be present in a cell at the same time and in sufficient amounts. If one is missing, the protein cannot be made. Because essential amino acids cannot be stored, those not used immediately to build proteins are oxidized for energy or converted to carbohydrates or fats.
- **Adequacy of caloric intake.** For optimal protein synthesis, the diet must supply sufficient carbohydrate or fat calories for ATP production. When it doesn't, dietary and tissue proteins are used for energy.
- **Nitrogen balance.** In healthy adults the rate of protein synthesis equals the rate of protein breakdown and loss, a homeostatic state called **nitrogen balance**. The body is in nitrogen balance when the amount of nitrogen ingested in proteins equals the amount excreted in urine and feces.

  The body is in *positive nitrogen balance* when the amount of protein incorporated into tissue is greater than the amount being broken down and used for energy—the normal situation in growing children and pregnant women. A positive balance also occurs when tissues are being repaired following illness or injury.

  In *negative nitrogen balance*, protein breakdown for energy exceeds the amount of protein being incorporated into tissues. This occurs during physical and emotional stress (for example, infection, injury, or burns), when the quality or quantity of dietary protein is poor, or during starvation.
- **Hormonal controls.** Certain hormones, called *anabolic hormones*, accelerate protein synthesis and growth. The effects of these hormones vary continually throughout life. For example, *pituitary growth hormone* stimulates tissue growth during childhood and conserves protein in adults, and the *sex hormones* trigger the growth spurt of adolescence. Other hormones, such as the adrenal *glucocorticoids* released dur-

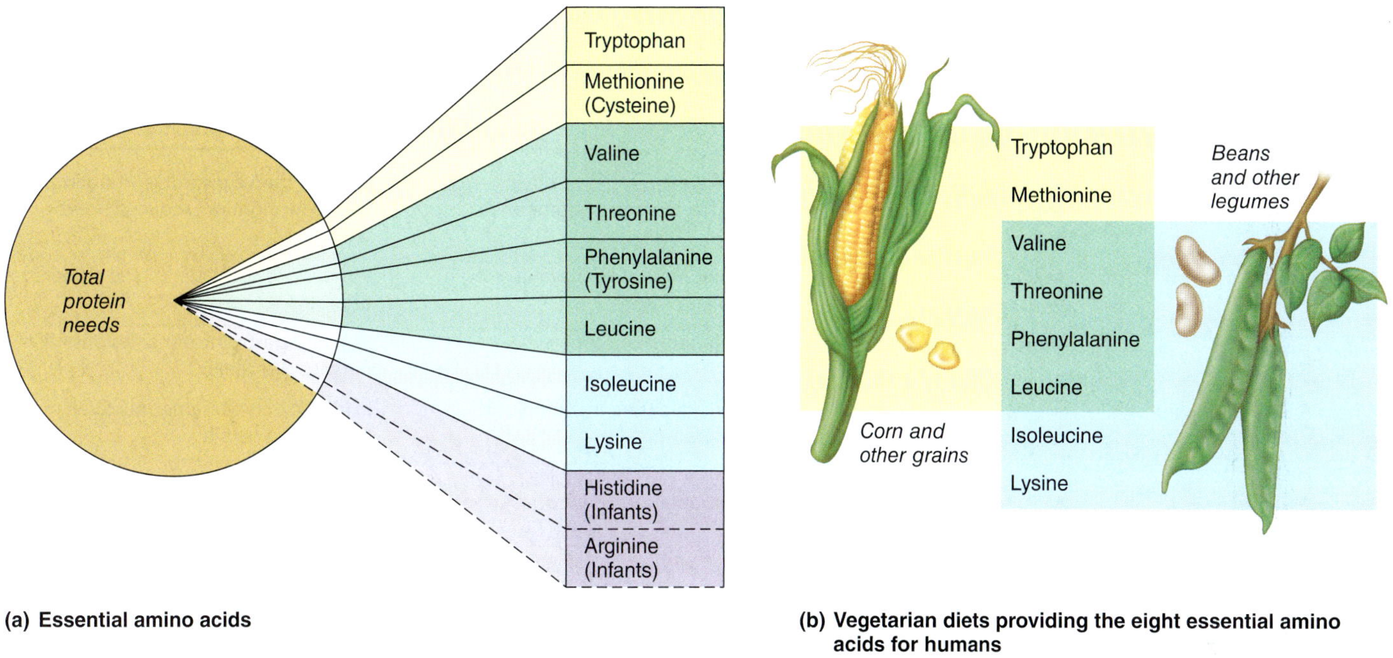

Figure 24.2 Essential amino acids. For protein synthesis to occur, 10 essential amino acids must be readily available and in the correct proportions. **(a)** Relative amounts of the essential amino acids and total proteins needed by adults. Notice that the essential amino acids represent only a small percentage of the total recommended protein intake. Histidine and arginine, graphed with dashed lines, are essential in infants but not in adults. Amino acids shown in parentheses are not essential but can substitute in part for methionine and phenylalanine. **(b)** Vegetarian diets must be carefully constructed to provide all essential amino acids. A meal of corn and beans fills the bill: Corn provides the essential amino acids not in beans and vice versa.

ing stress, enhance protein breakdown and conversion of amino acids to glucose.

Dietary Requirements

Besides supplying essential amino acids, dietary proteins furnish the raw materials for making nonessential amino acids and various nonprotein nitrogen-containing substances. The amount of protein a person needs reflects his or her age, size, metabolic rate, and current state of nitrogen balance. As a rule of thumb, nutritionists recommend a daily intake of 0.8 g per kilogram of body weight. A small serving of fish and a glass of milk supply about 30 g of protein.

Most Americans eat far more protein than they need. Prolonged high protein consumption may lead to bone loss. This may occur because metabolizing sulfur-containing amino acids makes the blood more acidic and calcium is pulled from the bones to buffer these acids.

☑ Check Your Understanding

1. What are the six major nutrients?
2. Why is it important to include cellulose in a healthy diet even though we do not digest it?
3. How does the body use triglycerides? Cholesterol?
4. John eats nothing but baked bean sandwiches. Is he getting all the essential amino acids he needs in this restricted diet?

For answers, see Appendix H.

Vitamins

✓ Distinguish between fat- and water-soluble vitamins, and list the vitamins in each group.

✓ For each vitamin, list important sources, body functions, and important consequences of its deficit or excess.

Vitamins (*vita* = life) are potent organic compounds needed in minute amounts for growth and good health. Unlike other organic nutrients, vitamins are not used for energy and do not serve as building blocks, but they are crucial in helping the body use those nutrients that do. Without vitamins, all the carbohydrates, proteins, and fats we eat would be useless.

Most vitamins function as **coenzymes** (or parts of coenzymes), which act with an enzyme to accomplish a particular chemical task. For example, the B vitamins act as coenzymes when glucose is oxidized for energy. We will describe the roles of some vitamins in the metabolism discussion later in this chapter.

Most vitamins are not made in the body, so we must ingest them in foods or vitamin supplements. The exceptions are vitamin D made in the skin, and small amounts of B vitamins and vitamin K synthesized by intestinal bacteria. In addition, the body can convert *beta-carotene* (kar′o-tēn), the orange pigment in carrots and other foods, to vitamin A. (For this reason, beta-carotene and substances like it are called *provitamins*.)

Vitamins are found in all major food groups, but no one food contains all the required vitamins. A balanced diet is the best way to ensure a full vitamin complement.

Table 24.2 Vitamin Requirements of Humans

VITAMIN	MAJOR DIETARY SOURCES	MAJOR FUNCTIONS IN THE BODY	SYMPTOMS OF DEFICIENCY OR EXTREME EXCESS
Water-Soluble Vitamins			
Vitamin B_1 (thiamine)	Pork, legumes, peanuts, whole grains	Coenzyme used in removing CO_2 from organic compounds	Beriberi (nerve disorders—tingling, poor coordination, reduced heart function)
Vitamin B_2 (riboflavin)	Dairy products, meats, enriched grains, vegetables	Component of coenzymes FAD and FMN	Skin lesions such as cracks at corners of mouth
Niacin (B_3)	Nuts, meats, grains	Component of coenzyme NAD^+	Skin and gastrointestinal lesions, nervous disorders **Liver damage**
Vitamin B_6 (pyridoxine)	Meats, vegetables, whole grains	Coenzyme used in amino acid metabolism	Irritability, convulsions, muscular twitching, anemia **Unstable gait, numb feet, poor coordination**
Pantothenic acid (B_5)	Most foods: meats, dairy products, whole grains, etc.	Component of coenzyme A	Fatigue, numbness, tingling of hands and feet
Folic acid (folacin) (B_9)	Green vegetables, oranges, nuts, legumes, whole grains	Coenzyme in nucleic acid and amino acid metabolism	Anemia, birth defects **May mask deficiency of vitamin B_{12}**
Vitamin B_{12}	Meats, eggs, dairy products	Coenzyme in nucleic acid metabolism; maturation of red blood cells	Anemia, nervous system disorders (numbness, loss of balance)
Biotin	Legumes, other vegetables, meats	Coenzyme in synthesis of fat, glycogen, and amino acids	Scaly skin inflammation, neuromuscular disorders
Vitamin C (ascorbic acid)	Fruits and vegetables, especially citrus fruits, broccoli, cabbage, tomatoes, green peppers	Used in collagen synthesis (such as for bone, cartilage, gums); antioxidant; aids in detoxification; improves iron absorption	Scurvy (degeneration of skin, teeth, blood vessels), weakness, delayed wound healing, impaired immunity **Gastrointestinal upset**
Fat-Soluble Vitamins			
Vitamin A (retinol)	Provitamin A (beta-carotene) in deep green and orange vegetables and fruits; retinol in dairy products	Component of visual pigments; maintenance of epithelial tissues; antioxidant; helps prevent damage to cell membranes	Blindness and increased death rate **Headache, irritability, vomiting, hair loss, blurred vision, liver and bone damage**
Vitamin D	Dairy products, egg yolk; also made in human skin in presence of sunlight	Aids in absorption and use of calcium and phosphorus; promotes bone growth	Rickets (bone deformities) in children, bone softening in adults **Brain, cardiovascular, and kidney damage**
Vitamin E (tocopherol)	Vegetable oils, nuts, seeds	Antioxidant; helps prevent damage to cell membranes	Degeneration of the nervous system
Vitamin K (phylloquinone)	Green vegetables, tea; also made by colon bacteria	Important in blood clotting	Defective blood clotting **Liver damage and anemia**

Source: From Jane B. Reece, CAMPBELL BIOLOGY, 9th Edition, © 2011. Reprinted by permission of Pearson Education, Inc., Upper Saddle River, N. J.

Initially vitamins were given letter designations that indicated the order of their discovery. Although more chemically descriptive names have been assigned to them, this earlier terminology is still commonly used.

Vitamins are either water soluble or fat soluble. **Water-soluble** vitamins—the B-complex vitamins and vitamin C—are absorbed along with water from the gastrointestinal tract. (The exception is vitamin B_{12}: To be absorbed, it must bind to intrinsic factor, a stomach secretion.) The body's lean tissue stores insignificant amounts of water-soluble vitamins, and any ingested amounts not used within an hour or so are excreted in urine. Consequently, health problems resulting from excessive levels of these vitamins are rare.

Fat-soluble vitamins (A, D, E, and K) bind to ingested lipids and are absorbed along with their digestion products. Anything that interferes with fat absorption also interferes with the uptake of fat-soluble vitamins. Except for vitamin K, fat-soluble vitamins are stored in the body, and pathologies due to fat-soluble vitamin toxicity, particularly excess vitamin A, are well documented clinically.

As we describe in the next section, metabolism uses oxygen, and during these reactions some potentially harmful free radicals are generated. Vitamins C, E, and A (in the form of its dimer beta-carotene) and the mineral selenium are *antioxidants* that neutralize tissue-damaging free radicals. The whole story of how antioxidants interact in the body is still murky, but chemists propose that, much like a bucket brigade, they pass the dangerous free electron from one molecule to the next, until a chemical such as glutathione finally absorbs it and the body flushes it out in urine. Broccoli, cabbage, cauliflower, and brussels sprouts are all good sources of vitamins A and C.

The notion that megadoses of vitamin supplements are the road to eternal youth and glowing health is useless at best—and at worst, may cause serious health problems, particularly in the case of fat-soluble vitamins. Table 24.2 contains an overview of the roles of vitamins in the body.

Minerals

- ✓ List minerals essential for health.
- ✓ Indicate important dietary sources of minerals and describe how each is used.

The body requires moderate amounts of seven **minerals** (calcium, phosphorus, potassium, sulfur, sodium, chlorine, magnesium) and trace amounts of about a dozen others (Table 24.3). Minerals make up about 4% of the body by weight, with calcium and phosphorus (as bone salts) accounting for about three-quarters of this amount.

Minerals, like vitamins, are not used for fuel but work with other nutrients to ensure a smoothly functioning body. Incorporating minerals into structures makes them stronger. For example, calcium, phosphorus, and magnesium salts harden the teeth and strengthen the skeleton.

Most minerals are ionized in body fluids or bound to organic compounds to form phospholipids, hormones, and various functional proteins. For example, iron is essential to the oxygen-binding heme of hemoglobin, and sodium and chloride ions are the major electrolytes in blood. The amount of a particular mineral in the body gives very few clues to its importance in body function. For example, just a few milligrams of iodine (required for thyroid hormone synthesis) can make a critical difference to health.

A fine balance between uptake and excretion is crucial for retaining needed amounts of minerals while preventing toxic overload. Sodium present in virtually all natural and minimally processed foods poses little or no health risk. However, the large amounts added to processed foods and sprinkled on prior to eating may contribute to fluid retention and high blood pressure. This is particularly true in American blacks, whose kidneys have a greater tendency to retain salt than do those of American whites.

Fats and sugars are practically devoid of minerals, and highly refined cereals and grains are poor sources. The most mineral-rich foods are vegetables, legumes, milk, and some meats.

☑ Check Your Understanding

5. Vitamins are not used for energy fuels. What are they used for?
6. Which B vitamin requires the help of a product made in the stomach to be absorbed? What is that gastric product?
7. Which mineral is essential for thyroxine synthesis? For making bones hard? For hemoglobin synthesis?

For answers, see Appendix H.

Overview of Metabolic Reactions

- ✓ Define metabolism. Explain how catabolism and anabolism differ.
- ✓ Define oxidation and reduction and indicate the importance of these reactions in metabolism.
- ✓ Indicate the role of coenzymes used in cellular oxidation reactions.
- ✓ Explain the difference between substrate-level phosphorylation and oxidative phosphorylation.

Once inside body cells, nutrients become involved in an incredible variety of biochemical reactions known collectively as **metabolism** (*metabol* = change). During metabolism, substances are constantly built up and torn down. Cells use energy to extract more energy from foods, and then use some of this extracted energy to drive their activities. Even at rest, the body uses energy on a grand scale.

Anabolism and Catabolism

Metabolic processes are either *anabolic* (synthetic, building up) or *catabolic* (degradative, tearing down). **Anabolism** (ah-nab′o-lizm) is the general term for all reactions that build larger molecules or structures from smaller ones, such as the bonding together of amino acids to build proteins. **Catabolism** (kah-tab′o-lizm) refers to all processes that break down complex structures to simpler ones—for example, the hydrolysis of foods in the digestive tract.

In the group of catabolic reactions collectively called **cellular respiration**, food fuels, particularly glucose, are broken down in cells and some of the energy released is captured to form ATP, the cells' energy currency. ATP then serves as the "chemical drive shaft" that links energy-releasing catabolic reactions to cellular work.

Recall from Chapter 2 that reactions driven by ATP are coupled. ATP is never hydrolyzed directly. Instead enzymes shift its high-energy phosphate groups to other molecules, which are then said to be **phosphorylated** (fos″for′ĭ-la-ted). Phosphorylation primes a molecule to change in a way that increases its activity, produces motion, or does work. For example, phosphorylation activates many regulatory enzymes that catalyze key steps in metabolic pathways.

Three major stages are involved in processing energy-containing nutrients in the body (Figure 24.3). (Note that the blue arrows in the figure represent catabolic reactions and the purple arrows represent anabolic reactions.)

- *Stage 1* is digestion in the gastrointestinal tract, which we described in Chapter 23. The absorbed nutrients are then transported in blood to the tissue cells.

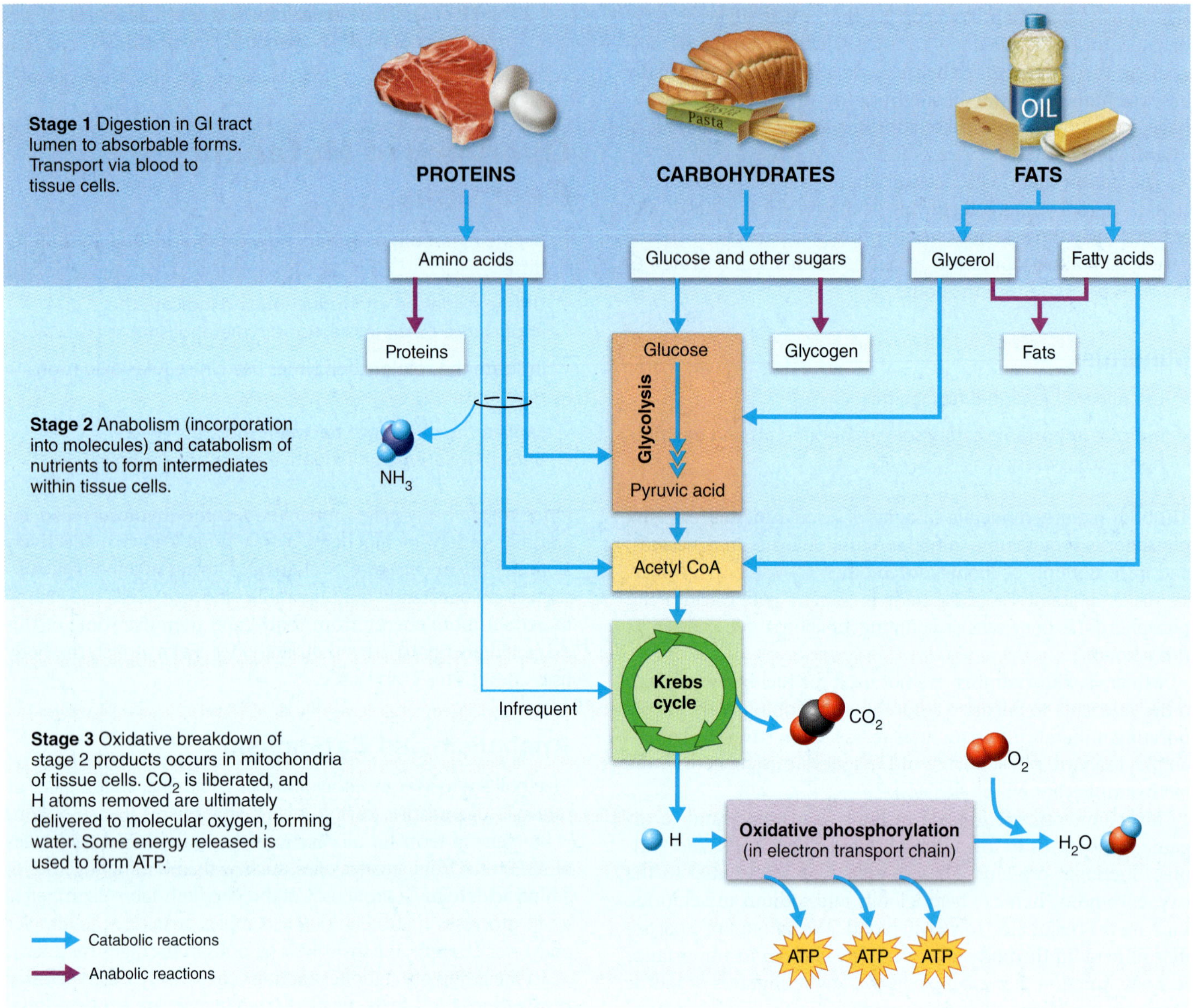

24

Figure 24.3 Three stages of metabolism of energy-containing nutrients.

- *Stage 2* occurs in the tissue cells. Newly delivered nutrients are either built into lipids, proteins, and glycogen by anabolic pathways or broken down by catabolic pathways to *pyruvic acid* (pi-roo′vik) and *acetyl CoA* (as′ĕ-til ko-a′) in the cell cytoplasm. Notice in Figure 24.3 that a major catabolic pathway of stage 2 is *glycolysis*, which we will discuss later in this chapter.
- *Stage 3*, which occurs in the mitochondria, is almost entirely catabolic. It requires oxygen, and completes the breakdown of foods, producing carbon dioxide and water and harvesting large amounts of ATP. As Figure 24.3 shows, the *Krebs cycle* and *oxidative phosphorylation* are key pathways in stage 3. We will discuss both later.

The primary function of *cellular respiration*, which consists of the glycolysis of stage 2 and all events of stage 3, is to generate ATP, which traps some of the chemical energy of the original food molecules in its own high-energy bonds. The body can also store energy in fuels, such as glycogen and fats, and mobilize these stores later to produce ATP for cellular use.

You do not need to memorize Figure 24.3, but you may want to refer to it often as a cohesive summary of nutrient processing and metabolism in the body.

Oxidation-Reduction Reactions and the Role of Coenzymes

Many of the reactions that take place within cells are **oxidation reactions**. *Oxidation* was originally defined as the combination of oxygen with other elements, seen in the rusting of iron (the slow formation of iron oxide) and the burning of wood. In burning, oxygen combines rapidly with carbon, producing carbon dioxide, water, and an enormous amount of energy, which is liberated as heat and light.

Table 24.3 Mineral Requirements of Humans

MINERAL	MAJOR DIETARY SOURCES	MAJOR FUNCTIONS IN THE BODY	SYMPTOMS OF DEFICIENCY*
Greater Than 200 mg per Day Required			
Calcium (Ca)	Dairy products, dark green vegetables, legumes	Bone and tooth formation, blood clotting, nerve and muscle function	Retarded growth, possibly loss of bone mass
Phosphorus (P)	Dairy products, meats, grains	Bone and tooth formation, acid-base balance, nucleotide synthesis	Weakness, loss of minerals from bone, calcium loss
Sulfur (S)	Proteins from many sources	Component of certain amino acids	Symptoms of protein deficiency
Potassium (K)	Meats, dairy products, many fruits and vegetables, grains	Acid-base balance, water balance, nerve function	Muscular weakness, paralysis, nausea, heart failure
Chlorine (Cl)	Table salt	Acid-base balance, formation of gastric juice, nerve function, osmotic balance	Muscle cramps, reduced appetite
Sodium (Na)	Table salt	Acid-base balance, water balance, nerve function	Muscle cramps, reduced appetite
Magnesium (Mg)	Whole grains, green leafy vegetables	Cofactor; ATP bioenergetics	Nervous system disturbances
Trace Amounts Required			
Iron (Fe)	Meats, eggs, legumes, whole grains, green leafy vegetables	Component of hemoglobin and of electron carriers in energy metabolism; enzyme cofactor	Iron-deficiency anemia, weakness, impaired immunity
Fluorine (F)	Drinking water, tea, seafood	Maintenance of tooth (and probably bone) structure	Higher frequency of tooth decay
Zinc (Zn)	Meats, seafood, grains	Component of certain digestive enzymes and other proteins	Growth failure, skin abnormalities, reproductive failure, impaired immunity
Copper (Cu)	Seafood, nuts, legumes, organ meats	Enzyme cofactor in iron metabolism, melanin synthesis, electron transport	Anemia, cardiovascular abnormalities
Manganese (Mn)	Nuts, grains, vegetables, fruits, tea	Enzyme cofactor	Abnormal bone and cartilage
Iodine (I)	Seafood, dairy products, iodized salt	Component of thyroid hormones	Goiter (enlarged thyroid)
Cobalt (Co)	Meats and dairy products	Component of vitamin B_{12}	None, except as B_{12} deficiency
Selenium (Se)	Seafood, meats, whole grains	Enzyme cofactor; antioxidant functioning in close association with vitamin E	Muscle pain, possibly heart muscle deterioration
Chromium (Cr)	Brewer's yeast, liver, seafood, meats, some vegetables	Involved in glucose and energy metabolism	Impaired glucose metabolism
Molybdenum (Mo)	Legumes, grains, some vegetables	Enzyme cofactor	Disorder in excretion of nitrogen-containing compounds

*All of these minerals are also harmful when consumed in excess.

Source: From Jane B. Reece, CAMPBELL BIOLOGY, 9th Edition, © 2011. Reprinted by permission of Pearson Education, Inc., Upper Saddle River, N. J.

24

Later it was discovered that oxidation also occurs when hydrogen atoms are *removed* from compounds, so the definition was expanded to its current form: *Oxidation is the gain of oxygen or the loss of hydrogen.* As explained in Chapter 2, whichever way oxidation occurs, the oxidized substance always *loses* (or nearly loses) electrons as they move to (or toward) a substance that more strongly attracts them.

To explain this loss of electrons, let's review the consequences of different electron-attracting abilities of atoms (see pp. 31–35). Consider a molecule made up of a hydrogen atom plus some other kinds of atoms. Hydrogen is very electropositive, so its lone electron usually spends more time orbiting the other atoms of the molecule. But when a hydrogen *atom* is removed, its electron goes with it, and the molecule as a whole loses that electron. Conversely, oxygen is very electron-hungry (electronegative), so when oxygen binds with other atoms the shared electrons spend more time in oxygen's vicinity. Again, the molecule as a whole loses electrons.

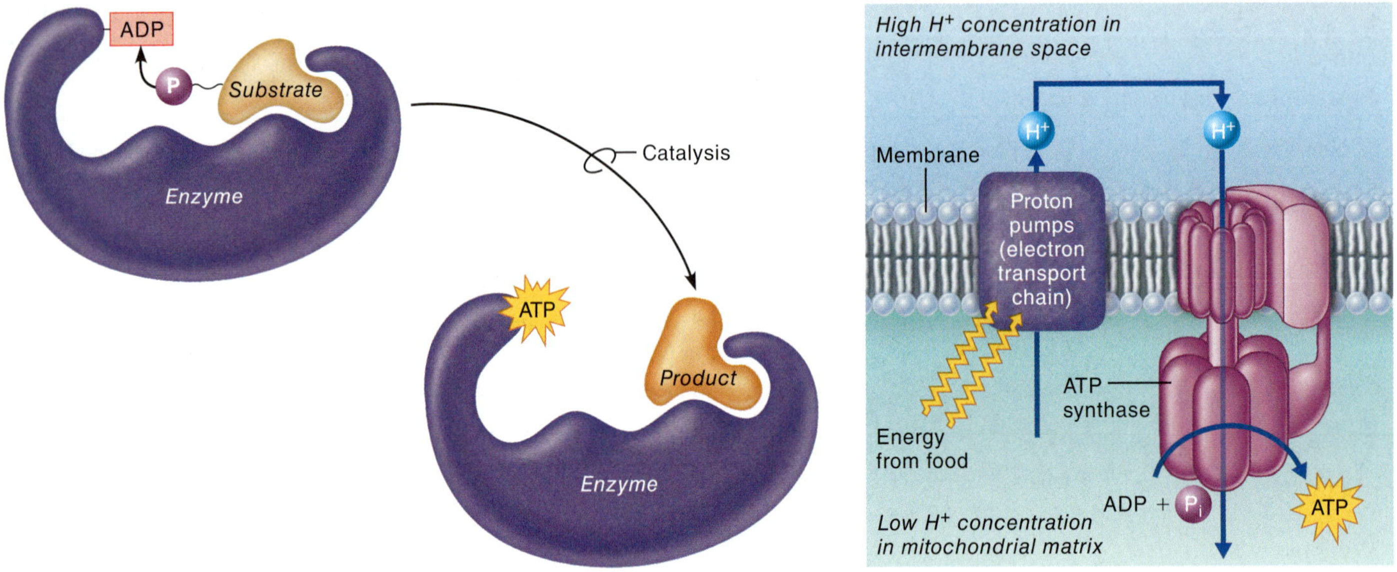

(a) Substrate-level phosphorylation

(b) Oxidative phosphorylation

Figure 24.4 Mechanisms of phosphorylation. (a) Substrate-level phosphorylation occurs when a high-energy phosphate group is transferred directly from a substrate to ADP to form ATP. This reaction occurs both in the cytosol and in the mitochondrial matrix. **(b)** Oxidative phosphorylation, which occurs in mitochondria, is carried out by electron transport proteins that act as proton "pumps" to create a proton gradient across the inner mitochondrial membranes. The source of energy for this pumping is energy released when food molecules are oxidized. As the protons flow passively back into the mitochondrial matrix through ATP synthase, some of this gradient energy is captured and used to bind phosphate groups to ADP.

As you will soon see, essentially all oxidation of food fuels involves the step-by-step removal of pairs of hydrogen atoms (and also pairs of electrons) from the substrate molecules, eventually leaving only carbon dioxide (CO_2). Molecular oxygen (O_2) is the final electron acceptor. It combines with the removed hydrogen atoms at the very end of the process, to form water (H_2O).

Whenever one substance loses electrons (is oxidized), another substance gains them (is reduced). For this reason, oxidation and reduction are coupled reactions and we speak of **oxidation-reduction (redox) reactions**. The key understanding about redox reactions is that "oxidized" substances *lose* energy and "reduced" substances *gain* energy as energy-rich electrons are transferred from one substance to the next. Consequently, as food fuels are oxidized, their energy is transferred to a "bucket brigade" of other molecules and ultimately to ADP to form energy-rich ATP.

Like all other chemical reactions in the body, redox reactions are catalyzed by enzymes. Those that catalyze redox reactions in which hydrogen atoms are removed are called **dehydrogenases** (de-hi′dro-jen-ās″ez), while enzymes catalyzing the transfer of oxygen are **oxidases**.

Most of these enzymes require the help of a specific coenzyme, typically derived from one of the B vitamins. Although the enzymes catalyze the removal of hydrogen atoms to oxidize a substance, they cannot *accept* the hydrogen (hold on or bond to it). Their *coenzymes*, however, can act as hydrogen (or electron) acceptors, becoming reduced each time a substrate is oxidized.

Two very important coenzymes of the oxidative pathways are **nicotinamide adenine dinucleotide (NAD^+)** (nik″o-tin′ah-mīd), based on *niacin*, and **flavin adenine dinucleotide (FAD)**, derived from *riboflavin*. The oxidation of succinic acid to fumaric acid and the simultaneous reduction of FAD to $FADH_2$, an example of a coupled redox reaction, is

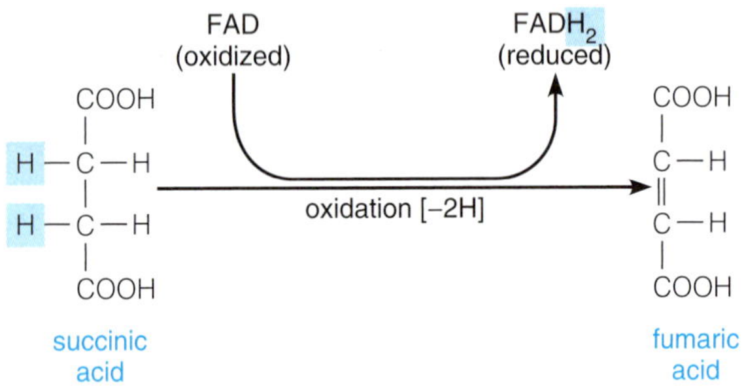

ATP Synthesis

How do our cells capture some of the energy liberated during cellular respiration to make ATP molecules? There appear to be two mechanisms—substrate-level phosphorylation and oxidative phosphorylation.

Substrate-level phosphorylation occurs when high-energy phosphate groups are transferred directly from phosphorylated substrates (metabolic intermediates such as glyceraldehyde 3-phosphate) to ADP (**Figure 24.4a**). Essentially, this process occurs because the high-energy bonds attaching the phosphate groups to the substrates are even more unstable than those in ATP. ATP is synthesized by this route twice during glycolysis, and once during each turn of the Krebs cycle. The enzymes catalyzing

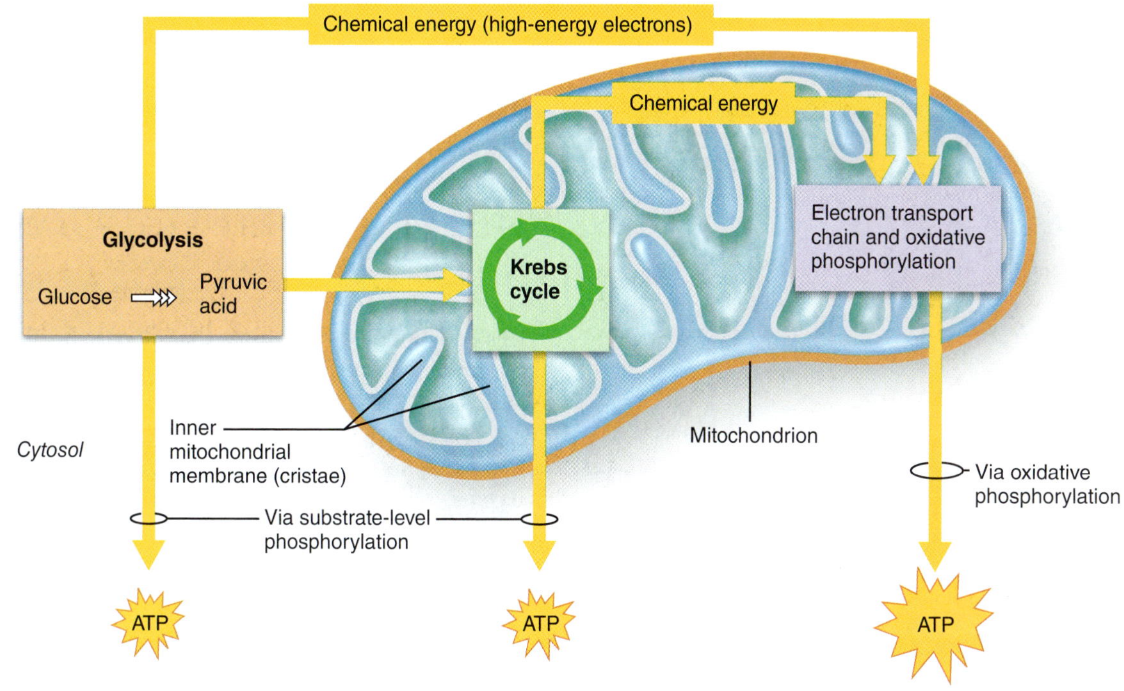

(1) Glycolysis, in the cytosol, breaks down each glucose molecule into two molecules of pyruvic acid.

(2) The pyruvic acid then enters the mitochondrial matrix, where the Krebs cycle decomposes it to CO_2. During glycolysis and the Krebs cycle, substrate-level phosphorylation forms small amounts of ATP.

(3) Energy-rich electrons picked up by coenzymes are transferred to the electron transport chain, built into the cristae membrane. The electron transport chain carries out oxidative phosphorylation, which accounts for most of the ATP generated by cellular respiration.

Figure 24.5 During cellular respiration, ATP is formed in the cytosol and in the mitochondria.

substrate-level phosphorylations are located in both the cytosol (where glycolysis occurs) and in the watery matrix inside the mitochondria (where the Krebs cycle takes place) **(Figure 24.5)**.

Oxidative phosphorylation is more complicated, but it also releases most of the energy that is eventually captured in ATP bonds during cellular respiration. Oxidative phosphorylation, which is carried out by electron transport proteins forming part of the inner mitochondrial membranes, is an example of a chemiosmotic process. **Chemiosmotic processes** couple the movement of substances across membranes to chemical reactions.

In this case, some of the energy released during the oxidation of food fuels (the "chemi" part of chemiosmotic) is used to pump (*osmo* = push) protons (H^+) across the inner mitochondrial membrane into the intermembrane space (Figure 24.4b). This creates a steep concentration gradient for protons across the membrane. Then, when H^+ flows back across the membrane (through a membrane channel protein called *ATP synthase*), some of this gradient energy is captured and used to attach phosphate groups to ADP.

☑ Check Your Understanding

8. What is a redox reaction?
9. How are anabolism and catabolism linked by ATP?
10. What is the energy source for the proton pumps of oxidative phosphorylation?

For answers, see Appendix H.

Metabolism of Major Nutrients

Carbohydrate Metabolism

✓ Summarize important events and products of glycolysis, the Krebs cycle, and electron transport.

✓ Define glycogenesis, glycogenolysis, and gluconeogenesis.

The story of carbohydrate metabolism is really a tale of glucose metabolism because all food carbohydrates are eventually transformed to glucose. Glucose enters tissue cells by facilitated diffusion, a process that is greatly enhanced by insulin. Immediately after entering a cell, glucose is phosphorylated to *glucose-6-phosphate* by transfer of a phosphate group to its sixth carbon during a coupled reaction with ATP:

$$\text{Glucose} + \text{ATP} \rightarrow \text{glucose-6-PO}_4 + \text{ADP}$$

Most body cells lack the enzymes needed to reverse this reaction, so it effectively traps glucose inside the cells. Because

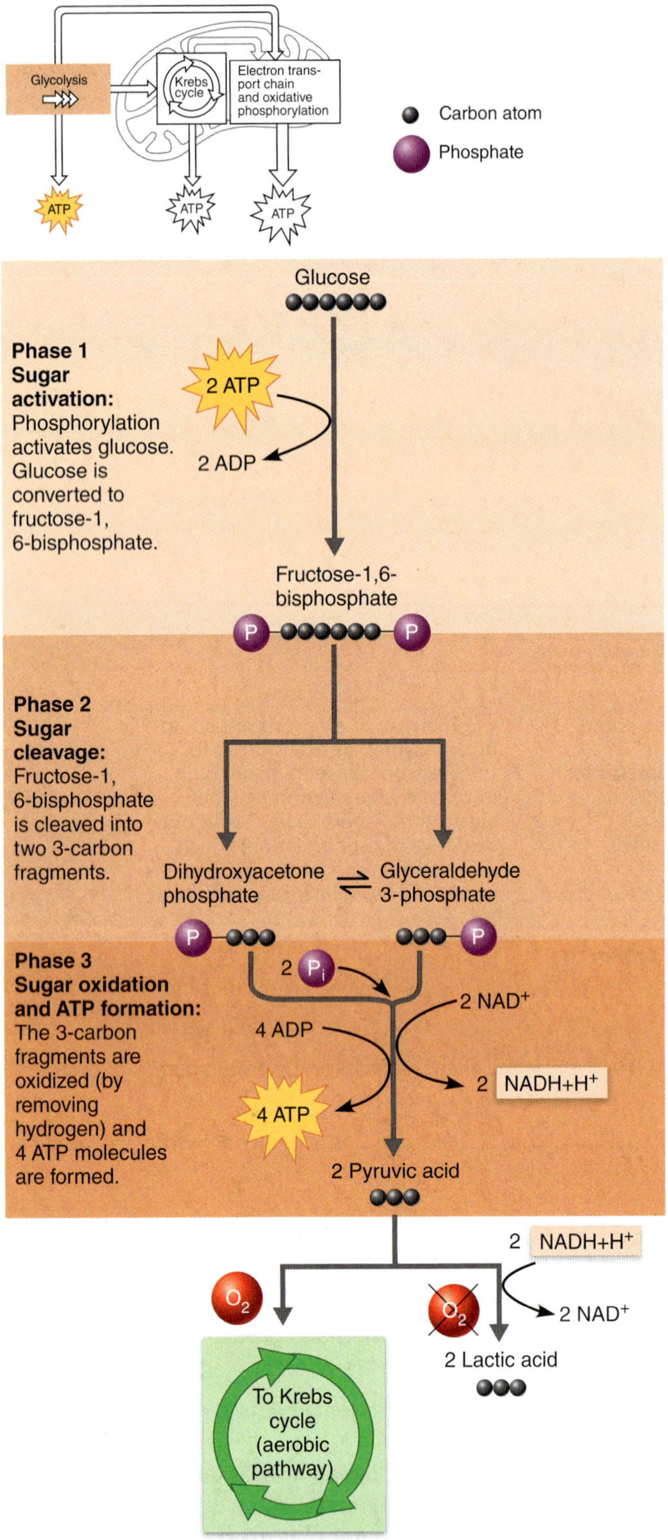

Figure 24.6 The three major phases of glycolysis. The fate of pyruvic acid depends on whether or not molecular O_2 is available.

glucose-6-phosphate is a *different* molecule from simple glucose, the reaction also keeps intracellular glucose levels low, maintaining a concentration gradient for glucose entry. Only intestinal mucosa cells, kidney tubule cells, and liver cells have the enzymes needed to reverse this phosphorylation reaction, which reflects their central roles in glucose uptake *and* release. The catabolic and anabolic pathways for carbohydrates all begin with glucose-6-phosphate.

Oxidation of Glucose

Glucose is the pivotal fuel molecule in the oxidative (ATP-producing) pathways. Glucose is catabolized via the reaction

$$\underset{\text{glucose}}{C_6H_{12}O_6} + \underset{\text{oxygen}}{6O_2} \rightarrow \underset{\text{water}}{6H_2O} + \underset{\text{carbon dioxide}}{6CO_2} + 32\ \text{ATP} + \text{heat}$$

This equation gives few hints that glucose breakdown is complex and involves three of the pathways featured in Figures 24.3 and 24.5:

1. Glycolysis (color-coded orange throughout the chapter)
2. The Krebs cycle (color-coded green)
3. The electron transport chain and oxidative phosphorylation (color-coded lavender)

These metabolic pathways occur in a definite order, and we will consider them sequentially.

Glycolysis Also called the *glycolytic pathway*, **glycolysis** (gli-kol′ĭ-sis; "sugar splitting") occurs in the cytosol of cells. This pathway, a series of ten chemical steps, converts glucose to two *pyruvic acid* molecules. All steps are fully reversible except the first, during which glucose entering the cell is phosphorylated to glucose-6-phosphate.

Glycolysis is an *anaerobic process* (an-a′er-ōb-ik; *an* = without, *aero* = air). Although this term is sometimes mistakenly interpreted to mean the pathway occurs only in the absence of oxygen, it actually means that glycolysis *does not use oxygen and occurs whether or not oxygen is present.*

The three major phases of the glycolytic pathway shown in **Figure 24.6** are described below. Appendix D shows the complete glycolytic pathway.

Phase 1. Sugar activation. In phase 1, glucose is phosphorylated and converted to fructose-6-phosphate, which is then phosphorylated again. These three steps use two ATP molecules (which are recouped later) and yield fructose-1,6-bisphosphate. The two separate reactions of the sugar with ATP provide the *activation energy* needed to prime the later stages of the pathway, so phase 1 is sometimes called the *energy investment phase.* (Recall the importance of activation energy in preparing substances to react, as described in Chapter 2.)

Phase 2. Sugar cleavage. During phase 2, fructose-1,6-bisphosphate is split into two 3-carbon fragments that exist (reversibly) as one of two isomers: glyceraldehyde (glis″er-al′dĕ-hīd) 3-phosphate or dihydroxyacetone (dī″hi-drok″se-as′ĕ-tōn) phosphate.

Phase 3. Sugar oxidation and ATP formation. In phase 3, actually consisting of six steps, two major events happen. First, the two 3-carbon fragments are oxidized by the removal of hydrogen, which NAD^+ picks up. In this way, some of glucose's energy is transferred to NAD^+. Second, inorganic phosphate groups (P_i) are attached to each oxidized fragment by high-energy bonds. Later, when these terminal phosphates are cleaved off, enough energy is captured to form four ATP molecules. As we noted earlier, formation of ATP this way is called *substrate-level phosphorylation*.

The final products of glycolysis are two molecules of **pyruvic acid** and two molecules of reduced NAD^+ (which is NADH + H^+). There is a net gain of two ATP molecules per glucose molecule. Four ATPs are produced, but remember that two are consumed in phase 1 to "prime the pump." Each pyruvic acid molecule has the formula $C_3H_4O_3$, and glucose is $C_6H_{12}O_6$. Between them the two pyruvic acid molecules have lost four hydrogen atoms, which are now bound to two molecules of NAD^+. NAD carries a positive charge (NAD^+), so when it accepts a hydrogen pair, NADH + H^+ is the resulting reduced product. Although a small amount of ATP has been harvested, the other two products of glucose oxidation (H_2O and CO_2) have yet to appear.

The fate of pyruvic acid, which still contains most of glucose's chemical energy, depends on the availability of oxygen at the time the pyruvic acid is produced. Because the supply of NAD^+ is limited, glycolysis can continue only if the reduced coenzymes (NADH + H^+) formed during glycolysis are relieved of their extra hydrogen. Only then can they continue to act as hydrogen acceptors.

When oxygen is readily available, this is no problem. NADH + H^+ delivers its burden of hydrogen atoms to the enzymes of the electron transport chain in the mitochondria, which deliver them to O_2, forming water. However, when oxygen is not present in sufficient amounts, as might occur during strenuous exercise, NADH + H^+ unloads its hydrogen atoms *back onto pyruvic acid*, reducing it. This addition of two hydrogen atoms to pyruvic acid yields **lactic acid** (see bottom right of Figure 24.6). Some of this lactic acid diffuses out of the cells and is transported to the liver for processing.

When oxygen is again available, lactic acid is oxidized back to pyruvic acid and enters the **aerobic pathways** (the oxygen-requiring Krebs cycle and electron transport chain within the mitochondria), and is completely oxidized to water and carbon dioxide. The liver may also convert lactic acid all the way back to glucose-6-phosphate (reverse glycolysis) and then store it as glycogen, or free it of its phosphate and release it to the blood if blood sugar levels are low.

Except for red blood cells (which typically carry out *only* glycolysis), prolonged anaerobic metabolism ultimately results in acid-base problems. Consequently, *totally* anaerobic conditions resulting in lactic acid formation provide only a temporary route for rapid ATP production. Totally anaerobic conditions can go on without tissue damage for the longest periods in skeletal muscle, for much shorter periods in cardiac muscle, and almost not at all in the brain. Although glycolysis generates ATP rapidly, each glucose molecule yields only 2 ATP as compared to the 30 to 32 ATP when a glucose molecule is completely oxidized.

Krebs Cycle Named after its discoverer Hans Krebs, the **Krebs cycle** is the next stage of glucose oxidation. The Krebs cycle, which occurs in the mitochondrial matrix, is fueled largely by pyruvic acid produced during glycolysis and by fatty acids resulting from fat breakdown.

Because pyruvic acid is a charged molecule, it must enter the mitochondrion by active transport with the help of a transport protein. Once in the mitochondrion, the first order of business is a **transitional phase** that converts pyruvic acid to acetyl CoA. This occurs via a three-step process (**Figure 24.7**, top):

1. **Decarboxylation.** In this step, one of pyruvic acid's carbons is removed and released as carbon dioxide gas, a process called **decarboxylation**. CO_2 diffuses out of the cells into the blood to be expelled by the lungs. This is the first time that CO_2 is released during cellular respiration.
2. **Oxidation.** The remaining 2C fragment (acetic acid) is oxidized by removing hydrogen atoms, which are picked up by NAD^+.
3. **Formation of acetyl CoA.** Acetic acid is combined with *coenzyme A* to produce the reactive final product, **acetyl coenzyme A (acetyl CoA)**. Coenzyme A is a sulfur-containing coenzyme derived from vitamin B_5.

Acetyl CoA is now ready to enter the Krebs cycle and be broken down completely by mitochondrial enzymes. Coenzyme A shuttles the 2-carbon acetic acid to an enzyme that condenses it with a 4-carbon acid called **oxaloacetic acid** (ok″sah-lo″ah-sēt′ik) to produce the 6-carbon **citric acid**. Because citric acid is the first substrate of the cycle, biochemists prefer to call the Krebs cycle the **citric acid cycle**.

As the cycle moves through its eight successive steps, the atoms of citric acid are rearranged to produce different intermediate molecules, most called **keto acids** (Figure 24.7). The acetic acid that enters the cycle is broken apart carbon by carbon (decarboxylated) and oxidized, simultaneously generating NADH + H^+ and $FADH_2$. At the end of the cycle, acetic acid has been totally disposed of and oxaloacetic acid, the *pickup molecule*, is regenerated.

What are the products of the Krebs cycle? Because two *decarboxylations* and four *oxidations* occur, the products are two CO_2 molecules and four molecules of reduced coenzymes (3 NADH + H^+ and 1 $FADH_2$). The addition of water at certain steps accounts for some of the released hydrogen. One molecule of ATP is formed (via substrate-level phosphorylation) during each turn of the cycle. The detailed events of each of the eight steps of the Krebs cycle are described in Appendix D.

Now let's back up and account for the pyruvic acid molecules entering the mitochondria. We need to consider the products of both the transitional phase and the Krebs cycle itself. Altogether, each pyruvic acid yields three CO_2 molecules and five molecules of reduced coenzymes—1 $FADH_2$ and 4 NADH + H^+ (equal to removing 10 hydrogen atoms). The products of glucose oxidation in the Krebs cycle are twice that (remember 1 glucose = 2 pyruvic acids): six CO_2, ten molecules of reduced coenzymes, and two ATP molecules.

Notice that it is these Krebs cycle reactions that produce the CO_2 evolved during glucose oxidation. The reduced coenzymes, which carry their extra electrons in high-energy linkages, must now be oxidized if the Krebs cycle and glycolysis are to continue.

Although glycolysis is exclusive to carbohydrate oxidation, breakdown products of carbohydrates, fats, and proteins can feed into the Krebs cycle to be oxidized for energy. On the other hand, some Krebs cycle intermediates can be siphoned off to make fatty acids and nonessential amino acids. Thus, the Krebs cycle is a source of building materials for anabolic reactions, as well as the final common pathway for oxidizing food fuels.

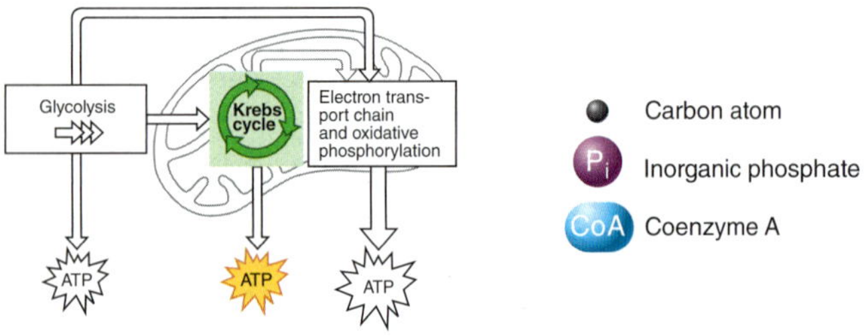

Figure 24.7 Simplified version of the Krebs (citric acid) cycle. During each turn of the cycle, two carbon atoms are removed from the substrates as CO_2 (decarboxylation reactions); four oxidations by removal of hydrogen atoms occur, producing four molecules of reduced coenzymes (3 NADH + H^+ and 1 $FADH_2$); and one ATP is synthesized by substrate-level phosphorylation. An additional decarboxylation and an oxidation reaction occur in the transitional phase (at top) that converts pyruvic acid, the product of glycolysis, to acetyl CoA, the molecule that enters the Krebs cycle pathway.

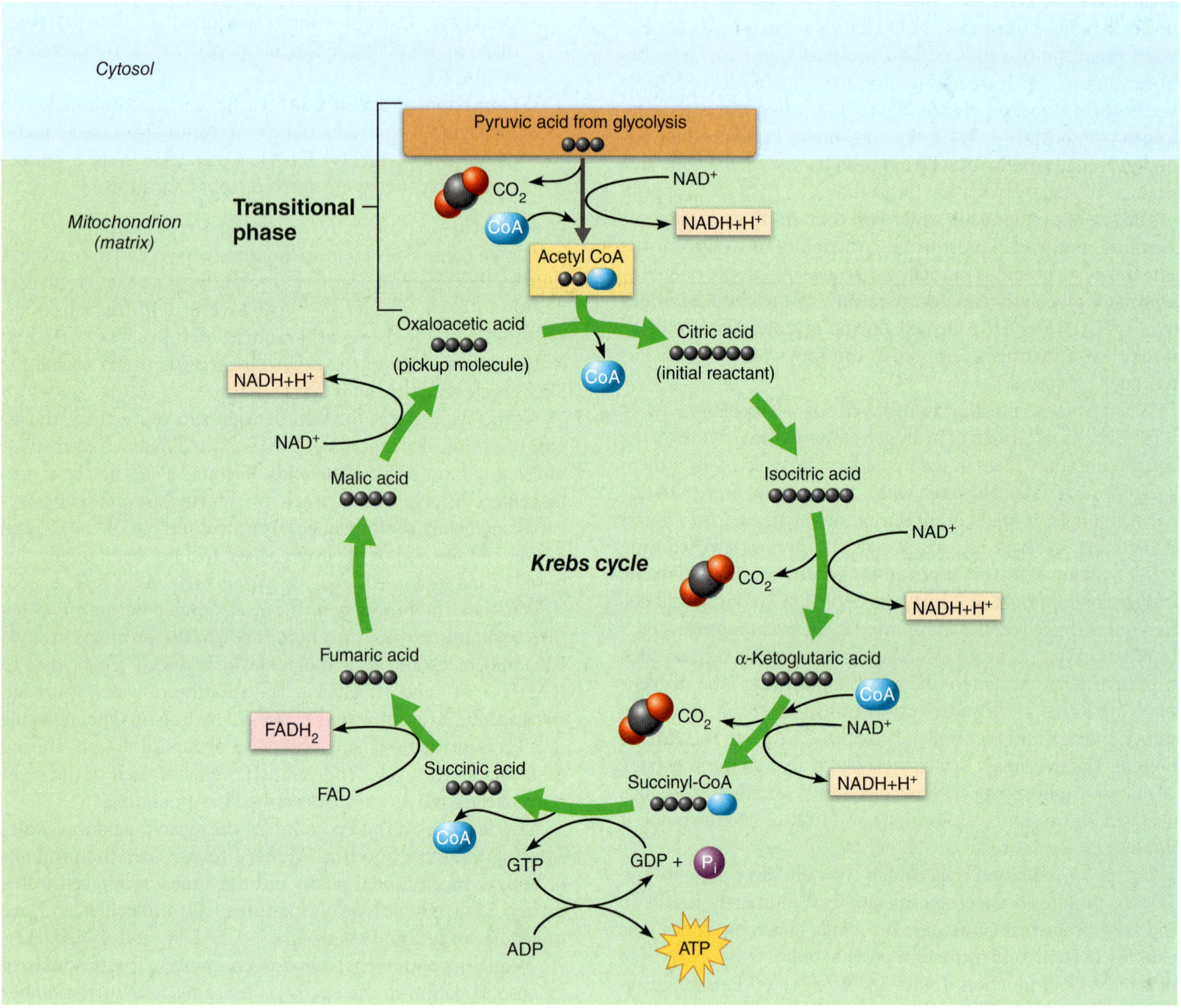

Electron Transport Chain and Oxidative Phosphorylation Like glycolysis, none of the reactions of the Krebs cycle use oxygen directly. This is the exclusive function of the **electron transport chain**, which carries out the final catabolic reactions that occur on the mitochondrial cristae. However, because the reduced coenzymes produced in the Krebs cycle are the substrates for the electron transport chain, these two pathways are coupled, and both are *aerobic*, meaning they require oxygen.

In the electron transport chain, the hydrogens removed during the oxidation of food fuels are combined with O_2 to form water, and the energy released during those reactions is harnessed to attach P_i groups to ADP, forming ATP. As we noted earlier, this type of phosphorylation process is called *oxidative phosphorylation*. Let's peek under the hood of a cell's power plant and see how this rather complicated process works.

Most components of the electron transport chain are proteins that are bound to metal atoms (known as *cofactors*). These proteins vary in composition and form multiprotein complexes that are firmly embedded in the inner mitochondrial membrane as shown in *Focus on Oxidative Phosphorylation* **(Figure 24.8)**. For

FOCUS Oxidative Phosphorylation

Figure 24.8 Oxidative phosphorylation has two phases:
Phase 1: The electron transport chain creates a proton (H^+) gradient across the inner mitochondrial membrane using high-energy electrons removed from food fuels.
Phase 2: Chemiosmosis uses the energy of the proton gradient to synthesize ATP.

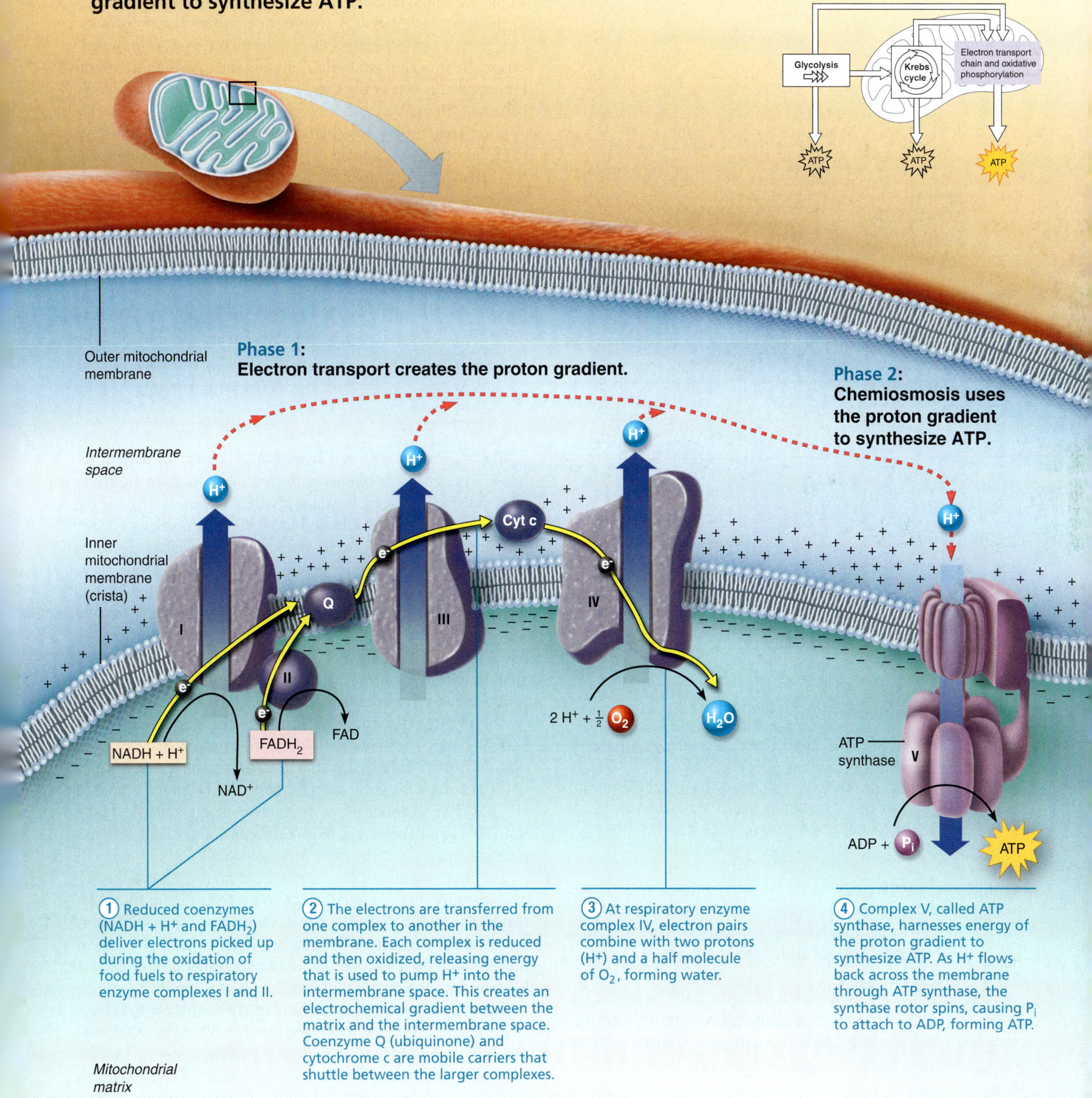

(1) Reduced coenzymes ($NADH + H^+$ and $FADH_2$) deliver electrons picked up during the oxidation of food fuels to respiratory enzyme complexes I and II.

(2) The electrons are transferred from one complex to another in the membrane. Each complex is reduced and then oxidized, releasing energy that is used to pump H^+ into the intermembrane space. This creates an electrochemical gradient between the matrix and the intermembrane space. Coenzyme Q (ubiquinone) and cytochrome c are mobile carriers that shuttle between the larger complexes.

(3) At respiratory enzyme complex IV, electron pairs combine with two protons (H^+) and a half molecule of O_2, forming water.

(4) Complex V, called ATP synthase, harnesses energy of the proton gradient to synthesize ATP. As H^+ flows back across the membrane through ATP synthase, the synthase rotor spins, causing P_i to attach to ADP, forming ATP.

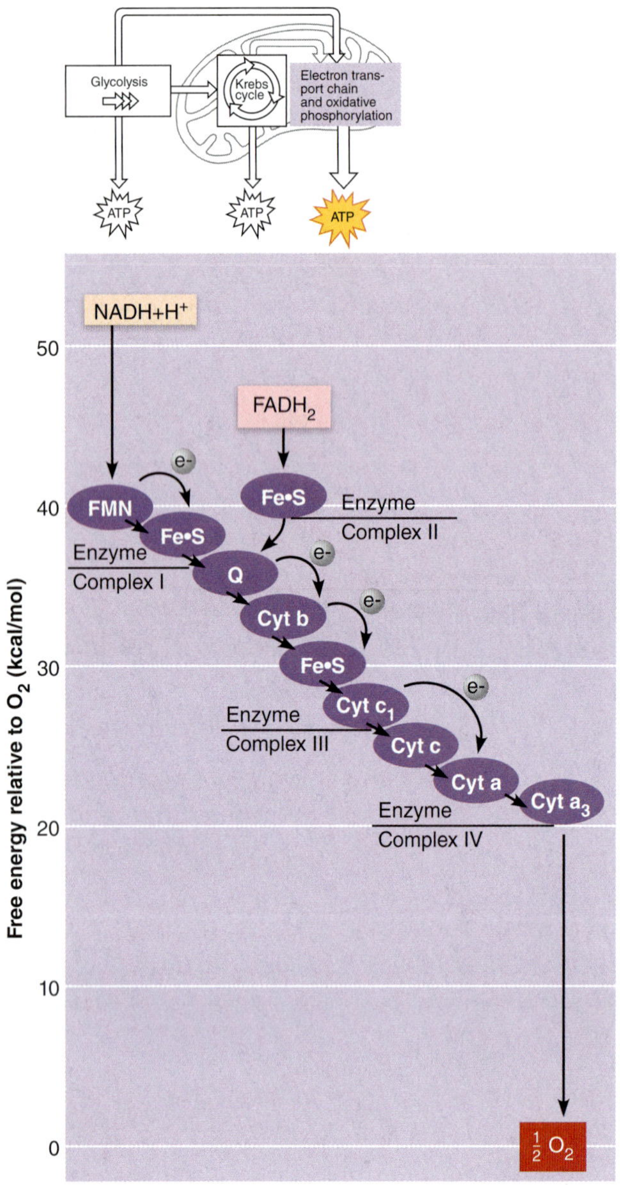

Figure 24.9 Electronic energy gradient in the electron transport chain. Each member of the chain (respiratory enzyme complex) alternates between a reduced state and an oxidized state. A complex becomes reduced by accepting electrons from its "uphill" neighbor and then reverts to its oxidized form as it passes electrons to its "downhill" neighbor. The electron transport chain breaks up the overall energy drop into smaller steps.

example, some of the proteins, the **flavins**, contain flavin mononucleotide (FMN) derived from the vitamin riboflavin, and others contain both sulfur (S) and iron (Fe). Most of these proteins, however, are brightly colored iron-containing pigments called **cytochromes** (si′to-krōmz; *cyto* = cell, *chrom* = color), including complexes III and IV depicted in Figure 24.8. Neighboring carriers are clustered together to form four **respiratory enzyme complexes** that are alternately reduced and oxidized as they pick up electrons and pass them on to the next complex in the sequence.

As Figure 24.8 shows, the first such complex accepts hydrogen atoms from NADH + H^+, oxidizing it to NAD^+. $FADH_2$ transfers its hydrogen atoms slightly farther along the chain to the small complex II. The hydrogen atoms that the reduced coenzymes deliver to the electron transport chain are quickly split into protons (H^+) plus electrons. The electrons are shuttled along the inner mitochondrial membrane from one complex to the next, losing energy with each transfer. The protons escape into the watery matrix, only to be picked up and "pumped" across the inner mitochondrial membrane into the intermembrane space by one of the three major respiratory enzyme complexes (I, III, or IV).

Ultimately the electron pairs are delivered to half a molecule of O_2 (in other words, to an oxygen atom), creating oxygen ions (O^-) that strongly attract H^+ and form water, as indicated by the reaction

$$2H^+ + 2e^- + \tfrac{1}{2}O_2 \rightarrow H_2O$$

Virtually all the water resulting from glucose oxidation is formed during oxidative phosphorylation. Because NADH + H^+ and $FADH_2$ are oxidized as they release their burden of picked-up hydrogen atoms, the net reaction for the electron transport chain is

$$\underset{\text{reduced coenzyme}}{\text{Coenzyme-2H}} + \tfrac{1}{2}O_2 \rightarrow \underset{\text{oxidized coenzyme}}{\text{coenzyme}} + H_2O$$

The transfer of electrons from NADH + H^+ to oxygen releases large amounts of energy. If hydrogen combined directly with molecular oxygen, the energy would be released in one big burst and most of it would be lost to the environment as heat. Instead, energy is released in many small steps as the electrons stream from one electron acceptor to the next.

Each successive carrier has a greater affinity for electrons than those preceding it. For this reason, the electrons cascade "downhill" from NADH + H^+ to progressively lower energy levels until they are finally delivered to oxygen, which has the greatest affinity of all for electrons. You could say that oxygen "pulls" the electrons down the chain **(Figure 24.9)**.

The electron transport chain functions as an energy converter by using the stepwise release of electronic energy to pump protons from the matrix into the intermembrane space. Because the inner mitochondrial membrane is nearly impermeable to H^+, this chemiosmotic process creates an **electrochemical proton (H^+) gradient** across that membrane, a gradient that has potential energy and the capacity to do work.

The proton gradient (1) creates a pH gradient, with the H^+ concentration in the matrix much lower than that in the intermembrane space; and (2) generates a voltage across the membrane that is negative on the matrix side and positive between the mitochondrial membranes. Both conditions strongly attract H^+ back into the matrix. But how can they get there?

The only areas of the membrane freely permeable to H^+ are large enzyme-protein complexes (complex V) called **ATP synthases**. These complexes, which populate the inner mitochondrial membrane **(Figure 24.10)**, lay claim to being nature's

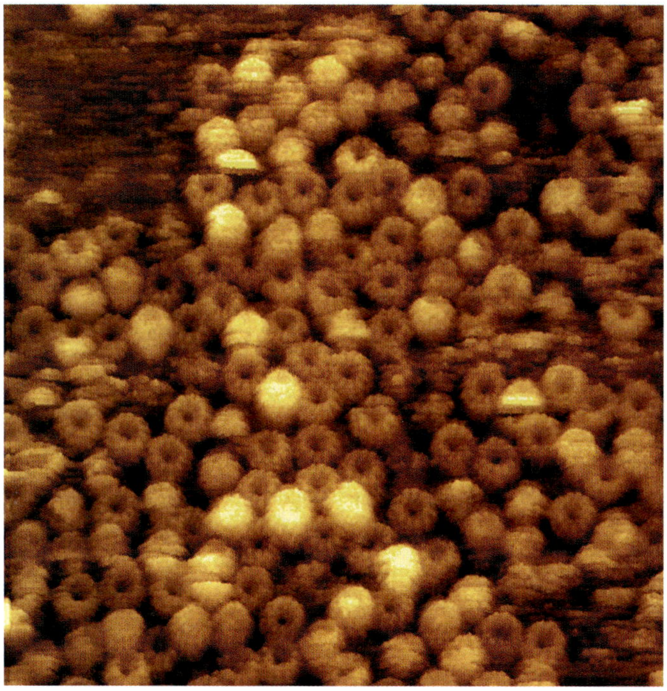

Figure 24.10 Atomic force microscopy reveals the structure of energy-converting ATP synthase rotor rings.

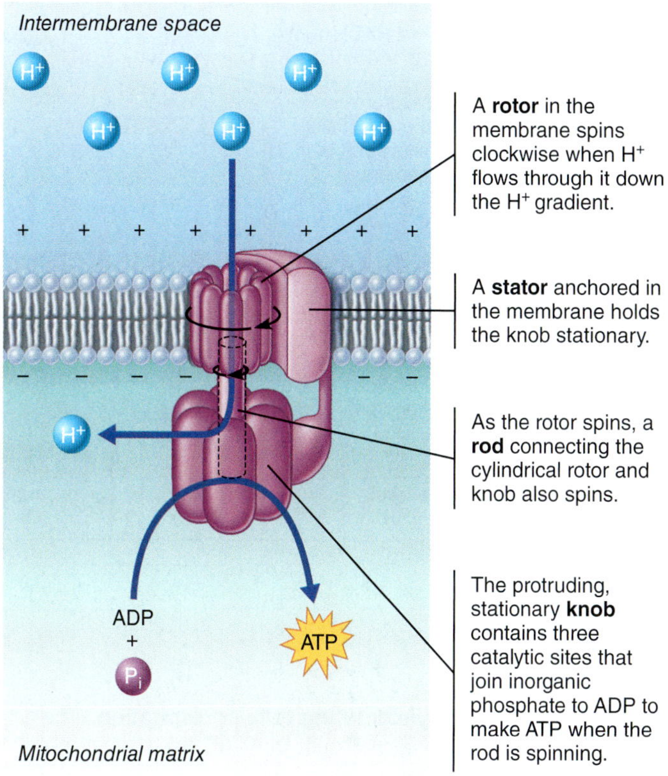

Figure 24.11 Structure and function of ATP synthase.

smallest rotary motors. As the protons take this "route" they create an electrical current, and ATP synthase harnesses this electrical energy to catalyze attachment of a phosphate group to ADP to form ATP **(Figure 24.11)**. The enzyme's subunits appear to work together like gears. As the ATP synthase core rotates, ADP and inorganic phosphate are pulled in and ATP is churned out, completing the process of oxidative phosphorylation.

How exactly does ATP synthase work? Studies of its molecular structure are providing answers. The enzyme complex consists of two major linked parts: (1) a *rotor* embedded in the inner mitochondrial membrane (Figure 24.11), and (2) a *knob* extending into the mitochondrial matrix, which is stabilized by a *stator* anchored in the membrane. A rod connects the rotor and the knob. The current created by the downhill flow of H^+ causes the rotor and rod to rotate, just as flowing water turns a water wheel. This rotation activates catalytic sites in the knob where ADP and P_i are combined to make ATP.

Notice something here: The ATP synthase works like an ion pump running in reverse. Recall from Chapter 3 that ion pumps use ATP as their energy source to transport ions against an electrochemical gradient. Here we have ATP synthases using the energy of a proton gradient to power ATP synthesis.

The proton gradient also supplies energy to pump needed metabolites (ADP, pyruvic acid, inorganic phosphate) and calcium ions across the relatively impermeable inner mitochondrial membrane. The outer membrane is freely permeable to these substances, so no "help" is needed there. The supply of energy from oxidation is not limitless however, so when more of the gradient energy is used to drive these transport processes, less is available to make ATP.

Homeostatic Imbalance 24.1

Studies of metabolic poisons support the chemiosmotic model of oxidative phosphorylation. For example, cyanide (the gas used in gas chambers) disrupts oxidative phosphorylation by binding to cytochrome oxidase and blocking electron flow from complex IV to oxygen (see Figure 24.9). Poisons called "uncouplers" abolish the proton gradient by making the inner mitochondrial membrane permeable to H^+. Consequently, although the electron transport chain continues to deliver electrons to oxygen at a furious pace and oxygen consumption rises, no ATP is made.+

When ADP enters the mitochondrial matrix, it stimulates the production of ATP. As ADP is transported in, ATP moves out in a coupled transport process.

Summary of ATP Production The average person at rest uses energy at the rate of roughly 100 kcal/hour, which is equal to 116 watts, or slightly more than that of a standard lightbulb. This may seem a tiny amount, but from a biochemical standpoint it places a staggering power demand on our mitochondria. Luckily, they are up to the task.

When O_2 is present, cellular respiration is remarkably efficient. Of the 686 kcal of energy present in 1 mole of glucose, as much as 262 kcal can be captured in ATP bonds. (The rest is liberated as heat.) This corresponds to an energy capture of about 38%, making cells far more efficient than any man-made machines, which capture only 10–30% of the energy available to them.

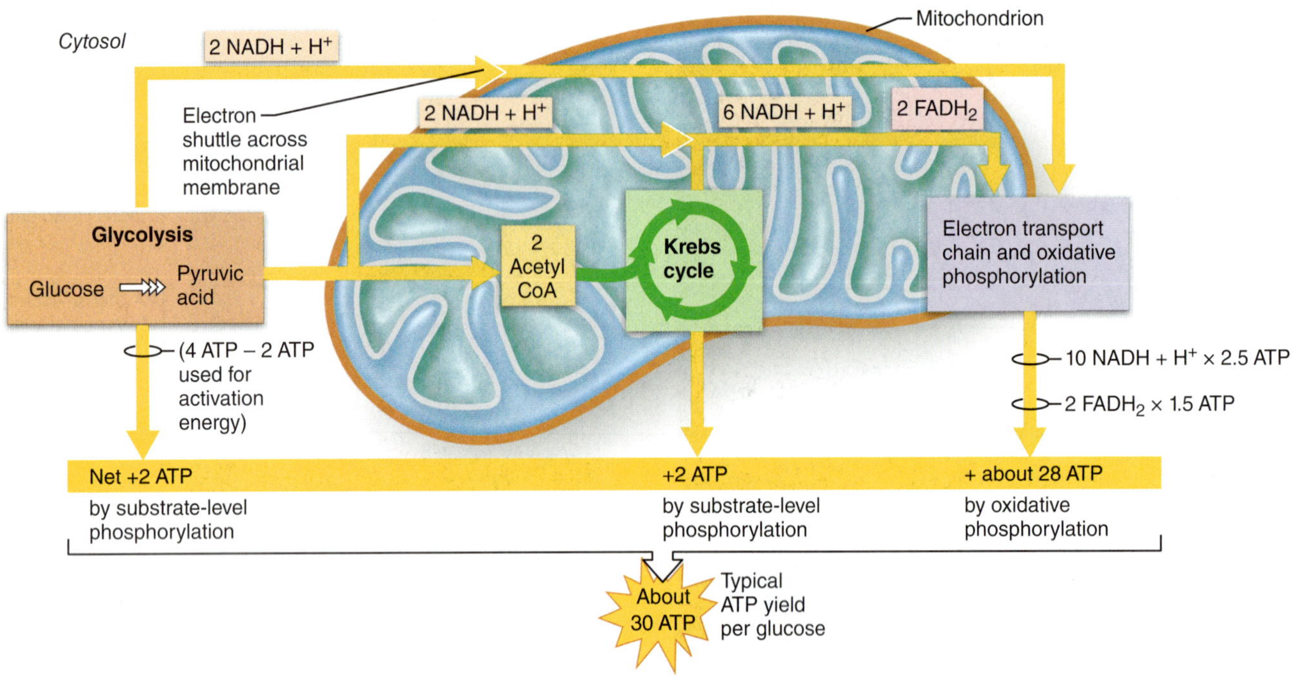

Figure 24.12 Energy yield during cellular respiration. (The typical energy yield of 30 ATP per glucose takes into account the 2 ATP used for shuttling NADH + H^+ to the electron transport chain.)

During cellular respiration, most energy flows in this sequence:

Glucose → NADH + H^+ → electron transport chain → proton gradient energy → ATP

Let's do a little bookkeeping to summarize the net energy gain from one glucose molecule. First, we tally the results of substrate-level phosphorylation, giving us a net gain of 4 ATP produced directly by substrate-level phosphorylations (2 during glycolysis and 2 during the Krebs cycle). Next we must calculate the much greater number of ATP molecules produced by oxidative phosphorylation **(Figure 24.12)**.

24

For each NADH + H^+ that transfers a pair of high-energy electrons to the electron transport chain, the proton gradient generates about 2½ ATP molecules. The oxidation of $FADH_2$ is less efficient because it doesn't donate electrons to the "top" of the electron transport chain as does NADH + H^+, but to a lower energy level (at complex II). So, for each 2 H delivered by $FADH_2$, just about 1½ ATP molecules are produced.

Now let's tally the results of oxidative phosphorylation. The 2 NADH + H^+ generated during glycolysis yield 5 ATP molecules. The 8 NADH + H^+ and the 2 $FADH_2$ produced during the Krebs cycle are "worth" 20 and 3 ATP respectively.

Overall, complete oxidation of 1 glucose molecule to CO_2 and H_2O by both substrate-level phosphorylation and oxidative phosphorylation yields a maximum of 32 molecules of ATP (Figure 24.12). However, there is uncertainty about the energy yield of reduced NAD^+ that glycolysis generates *outside* the mitochondria. The crista membrane is not permeable to reduced NAD^+ generated in the cytosol, so NADH + H^+ formed during glycolysis uses a *shuttle molecule* to deliver its extra electron pair to the electron transport chain. It appears that cells using the malate/aspartate shuttle harvest the whole 2½ ATP from oxidation of reduced NAD^+, but in cells using a different shuttle (the glycerol phosphate shuttle for example) the shuttle has an energy cost. At present, the consensus is that the net energy yield for reoxidation of reduced NAD^+ in this case is probably the same as for $FADH_2$, that is, 1½ ATP per electron pair.

So, if we deduct 2 ATP to cover the "fare" for the shuttle, our bookkeeping comes up with a grand total of 30 ATP per glucose as the typical energy yield. (Actually our figures are probably still too high because, as mentioned earlier, the proton gradient energy is also used to do other work and the electron transport chain may not work at maximum capacity all of the time.)

☑ Check Your Understanding

11. Briefly, how do substrate-level and oxidative phosphorylation differ?
12. What happens in the glycolytic pathway if oxygen and pyruvic acid are absent and NADH + H^+ cannot transfer its "picked-up" hydrogen to pyruvic acid?
13. What two major kinds of chemical reactions occur in the Krebs cycle, and how are these reactions indicated symbolically?

For answers, see Appendix H.

Glycogenesis, Glycogenolysis, and Gluconeogenesis

Although most glucose is used to generate ATP molecules, unlimited amounts of glucose do *not* result in unlimited ATP synthesis, because cells cannot store large amounts of ATP.

When more glucose is available than can immediately be oxidized, rising intracellular ATP concentrations eventually inhibit glucose catabolism and cause glucose to be stored as glycogen or fat. Because the body can store much more fat than glycogen, fats account for 80–85% of stored energy.

Glycogenesis When high ATP levels begin to "turn off" glycolysis, glucose molecules are combined in long chains to form glycogen, the animal carbohydrate storage product. This process is called **glycogenesis** (*glyco* = sugar; *genesis* = origin) (**Figure 24.13**, right side).

Glycogenesis begins as glucose entering cells is phosphorylated to glucose-6-phosphate and then converted to its isomer, *glucose-1-phosphate*. The terminal phosphate group is cleaved off as the enzyme *glycogen synthase* catalyzes the attachment of glucose to the growing glycogen chain. Liver and skeletal muscle cells are most active in glycogen synthesis and storage.

Glycogenolysis On the other hand, when blood glucose levels drop, glycogen lysis (splitting) occurs. This process is known as **glycogenolysis** (gli″ko-jĕ-nol′ĭ-sis) (Figure 24.13, left side). The enzyme *glycogen phosphorylase* oversees phosphorylation and cleavage of glycogen to release glucose-1-phosphate, which is then converted to glucose-6-phosphate, a form that can enter the glycolytic pathway to be oxidized for energy.

In muscle cells and most other cells, the glucose-6-phosphate resulting from glycogenolysis is trapped because it cannot cross the cell membrane. However, hepatocytes (and some kidney and intestinal cells) contain *glucose-6-phosphatase*, an enzyme that removes the terminal phosphate, producing free glucose. Because glucose can then readily diffuse from the cell into the blood, the liver can use its glycogen stores to provide blood sugar for other organs when blood glucose levels drop. Liver glycogen is also an important energy source for skeletal muscles that have depleted their own glycogen reserves.

Athletes and Carbohydrates A common misconception is that athletes need to eat large amounts of protein to improve their performance and maintain muscle mass. Actually, a diet rich in complex carbohydrates results in more glycogen storage in muscle, and is more effective than high-protein meals for sustaining intense muscle activity.

Notice that the emphasis is on *complex* carbohydrates. Eating a candy bar before an athletic event to provide "quick" energy does more harm than good because it stimulates insulin secretion, which favors glucose use and retards fat use at a time when fat use should be maximal. Building muscle protein or avoiding its loss requires not only extra protein, but also extra (protein-sparing) complex carbohydrate calories to meet the greater energy needs of increasingly massive muscles.

Endurance athletes—long-distance runners in particular—are well aware of the practice of glycogen loading, popularly called "carbo loading," for endurance events. Carbo loading "tricks" the muscles into storing more glycogen than they normally would. It generally involves eating a carbohydrate-rich diet (75% of energy intake) for three to four days before an endurance event while decreasing activity. This practice increases muscle glycogen stores to as much as twice the normal amount.

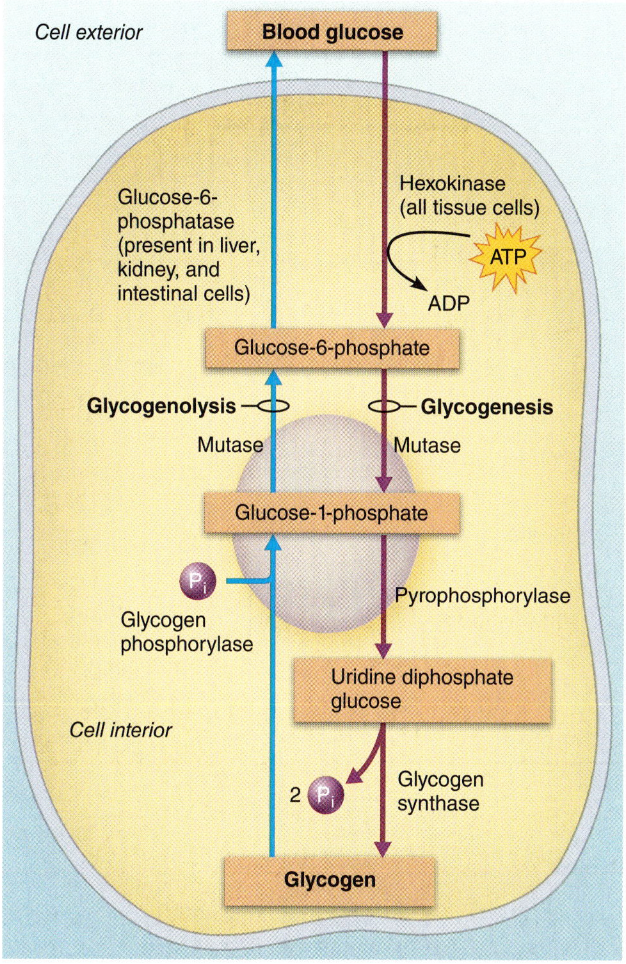

Figure 24.13 Glycogenesis and glycogenolysis. When glucose supplies exceed demands, glycogenesis (conversion of glucose to glycogen) occurs. Falling blood glucose levels stimulate glycogenolysis (breakdown of glycogen to release glucose).

Carbo loading is standard practice among marathon runners and distance cyclists, because studies have shown that it improves performance and endurance.

Gluconeogenesis When too little glucose is available to stoke the "metabolic furnace," glycerol and amino acids are converted to glucose. **Gluconeogenesis**, the process of forming new (*neo*) glucose from *noncarbohydrate* molecules, occurs in the liver.

Gluconeogenesis takes place when dietary sources and glucose reserves have been used up and blood glucose levels are beginning to drop. Gluconeogenesis protects the body, especially the nervous system, from the damaging effects of low blood sugar (*hypoglycemia*) by ensuring that ATP synthesis can continue.

☑ Check Your Understanding

14. What name is given to the chemical reaction in which glycogen is broken down to its glucose subunits?
15. What does carbo loading accomplish?

For answers, see Appendix H.

24

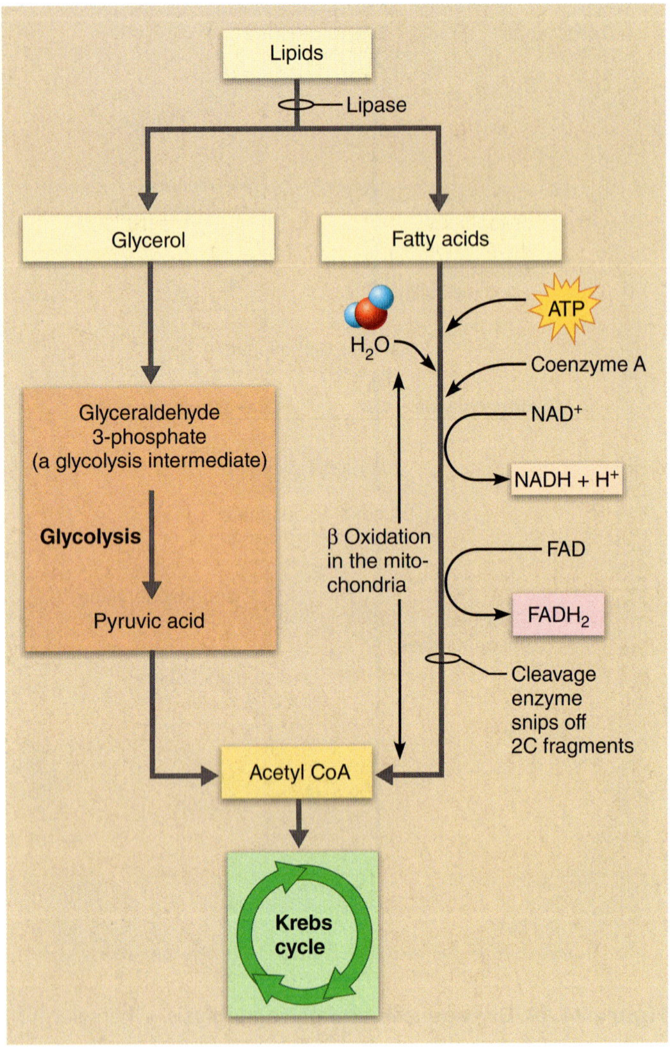

Figure 24.14 Initial phase of lipid oxidation. Glycerol is converted to a glycolysis intermediate, and completes the glycolytic pathway through pyruvic acid to acetyl CoA. The fatty acids undergo beta (β) oxidation in which they are activated by a coupled reaction with ATP, combined with coenzyme A, and then oxidized twice (reducing NAD^+ and FAD). The acetyl CoA created in β oxidation is cleaved off and the process begins again.

Lipid Metabolism

✓ Describe the process by which fatty acids are oxidized for energy.

✓ Define ketone bodies, and indicate the stimulus for their formation.

Fats are the body's most concentrated source of energy. They contain very little water, and the energy yield from fat catabolism is approximately twice that from either glucose or protein catabolism—9 kcal per gram of fat versus 4 kcal per gram of carbohydrate or protein. Most products of fat digestion are transported in lymph in the form of fatty-protein droplets called *chylomicrons* (see Chapter 23). Eventually, enzymes on capillary endothelium hydrolyze the lipids in the chylomicrons, and the resulting fatty acids and glycerol are taken up by body cells and processed in various ways.

Oxidation of Glycerol and Fatty Acids

Of the various lipids, only triglycerides are routinely oxidized for energy. Their catabolism involves the separate oxidation of their two different building blocks: glycerol and fatty acid chains **(Figure 24.14)**.

Most body cells easily convert glycerol to glyceraldehyde 3-phosphate, a glycolysis intermediate that eventually enters the Krebs cycle. Glyceraldehyde is equal to half a glucose molecule, and ATP energy harvest from its complete oxidation is approximately half that of glucose (15 ATP/glycerol).

Beta oxidation, the initial phase of fatty acid oxidation, occurs in the mitochondria. The net result is that the fatty acid chains are broken apart into two-carbon *acetic acid* fragments, and coenzymes (FAD and NAD^+) are reduced (Figure 24.14, right side). Each acetic acid molecule is fused to coenzyme A, forming acetyl CoA. The term "beta oxidation" reflects the fact that the carbon in the beta (third) position is oxidized during the process and in each case the fatty acid is cleaved between the alpha and beta carbons. Oxaloacetic acid then picks up acetyl CoA, which enters the aerobic pathways to be oxidized to CO_2 and H_2O.

Notice that unlike glycerol, which enters the glycolytic pathway, acetyl CoA resulting from fatty acid breakdown *cannot* be used for gluconeogenesis. Why? This is because the metabolic pathway is irreversible past pyruvic acid.

Lipogenesis

There is a continuous turnover of triglycerides in adipose tissue. New fats are "put in the larder" for later use, while stored fats are broken down and released to the blood. That bulge of fatty tissue you see today does *not* contain the same fat molecules it did a month ago.

Glycerol and fatty acids from dietary fats not immediately needed for energy are recombined into triglycerides and stored. About 50% ends up in subcutaneous tissue, and the balance is stockpiled in other fat depots of the body.

Triglyceride synthesis, or **lipogenesis**, occurs when cellular ATP and glucose levels are high (**Figure 24.15**, magenta arrows). Excess ATP also leads to an accumulation of acetyl CoA and glyceraldehyde 3-PO_4, two intermediates of glucose metabolism that would otherwise feed into the Krebs cycle. But when these two metabolites are present in excess, they are channeled into triglyceride synthesis pathways.

Acetyl CoA molecules are condensed together, forming fatty acid chains that grow two carbons at a time. (This accounts for the fact that almost all fatty acids in the body contain an even number of carbon atoms.) Because acetyl CoA, an intermediate in glucose catabolism, is also the *starting point* for fatty acid synthesis, glucose is easily converted to fat. Glyceraldehyde 3-PO_4 is converted to glycerol, which is condensed with fatty acids to form triglycerides. Consequently, even with a low-fat diet, carbohydrate intake can provide *all the raw materials* needed to make triglycerides. When blood

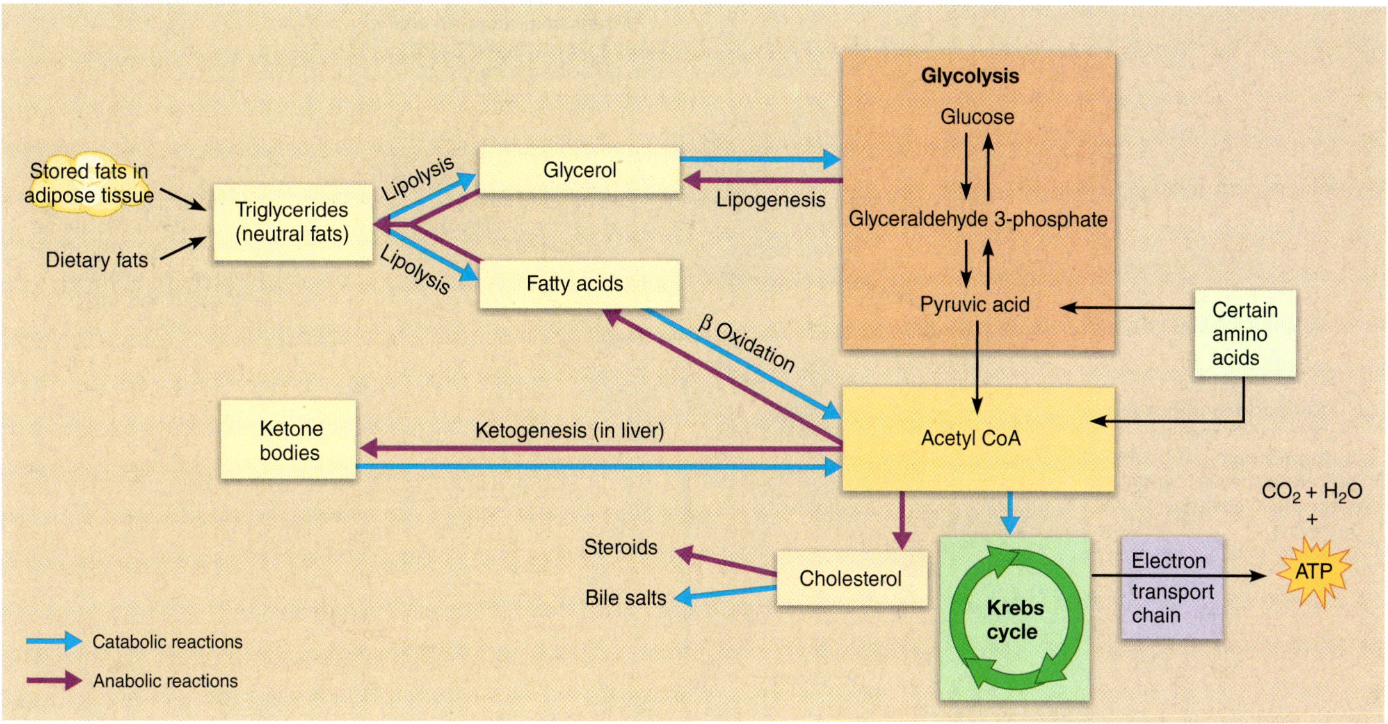

Figure 24.15 Metabolism of triglycerides. When needed for energy, fats enter catabolic pathways. Glycerol enters the glycolytic pathway and beta oxidation breaks down the fatty acids to acetyl CoA, which enters the Krebs cycle. When fats are to be synthesized (lipogenesis) and stored, the intermediates are drawn from glycolysis and the Krebs cycle in a reversal of the processes noted above. Excess dietary fats are stored in adipose tissue. When triglycerides are the primary energy source, the liver releases their breakdown products in the form of ketone bodies. Excessive amounts of carbohydrates and amino acids are also converted to triglycerides (lipogenesis).

sugar is high, lipogenesis is the major activity in adipose tissues and is also an important liver function.

Lipolysis

Lipolysis (lĭ-pol′ĭ-sis; "fat splitting"), the breakdown of stored fats into glycerol and fatty acids, is essentially lipogenesis in reverse (Figure 24.15, blue arrows). The fatty acids and glycerol are released to the blood, helping to ensure that body organs have continuous access to fat fuels for aerobic respiration. (The liver, cardiac muscle, and resting skeletal muscles actually prefer fatty acids as an energy fuel.)

The adage "Fats burn in the flame of carbohydrates" becomes clear when carbohydrate intake is inadequate. Under such conditions, lipolysis accelerates as the body attempts to fill the fuel gap with fats. However, the ability of acetyl CoA to enter the Krebs cycle depends on the availability of oxaloacetic acid to act as the pickup molecule (see Figure 24.7). When carbohydrates are deficient, oxaloacetic acid is converted to glucose (to fuel the brain). Without oxaloacetic acid, fat oxidation is incomplete, and acetyl CoA accumulates.

Via a process called **ketogenesis**, the liver converts acetyl CoA molecules to **ketone bodies**, or **ketones**, which are released into the blood. Ketone bodies include acetoacetic acid, β-hydroxybutyric acid, and acetone. (The *keto acids* cycling through the Krebs cycle and the *ketone bodies* resulting from fat metabolism are quite different and should not be confused.)

Homeostatic Imbalance 24.2

When ketone bodies accumulate in the blood, *ketosis* results and large amounts of ketone bodies are excreted in the urine. Ketosis is a common consequence of starvation, unwise dieting (too little carbohydrate), and diabetes mellitus.

Because most ketone bodies are organic acids, ketosis leads to *metabolic acidosis*. The body's buffer systems cannot tie up the acids (ketones) fast enough, and blood pH drops to dangerously low levels. The person's breath smells fruity as acetone vaporizes from the lungs, and breathing becomes more rapid as the respiratory system tries to reduce blood carbonic acid by blowing off CO_2 to force the blood pH up. In severe untreated cases, the person may become comatose or even die as the acid pH depresses the nervous system. ✚

Synthesis of Structural Materials

All body cells use phospholipids and cholesterol to build their membranes. Phospholipids are important components of the myelin sheaths of neurons, and the ovaries, testes, and adrenal cortex use cholesterol to synthesize their steroid hormones. In addition, the liver:

- Synthesizes lipoproteins to transport cholesterol, fats, and other substances in the blood
- Synthesizes cholesterol from acetyl CoA
- Uses cholesterol to form bile salts

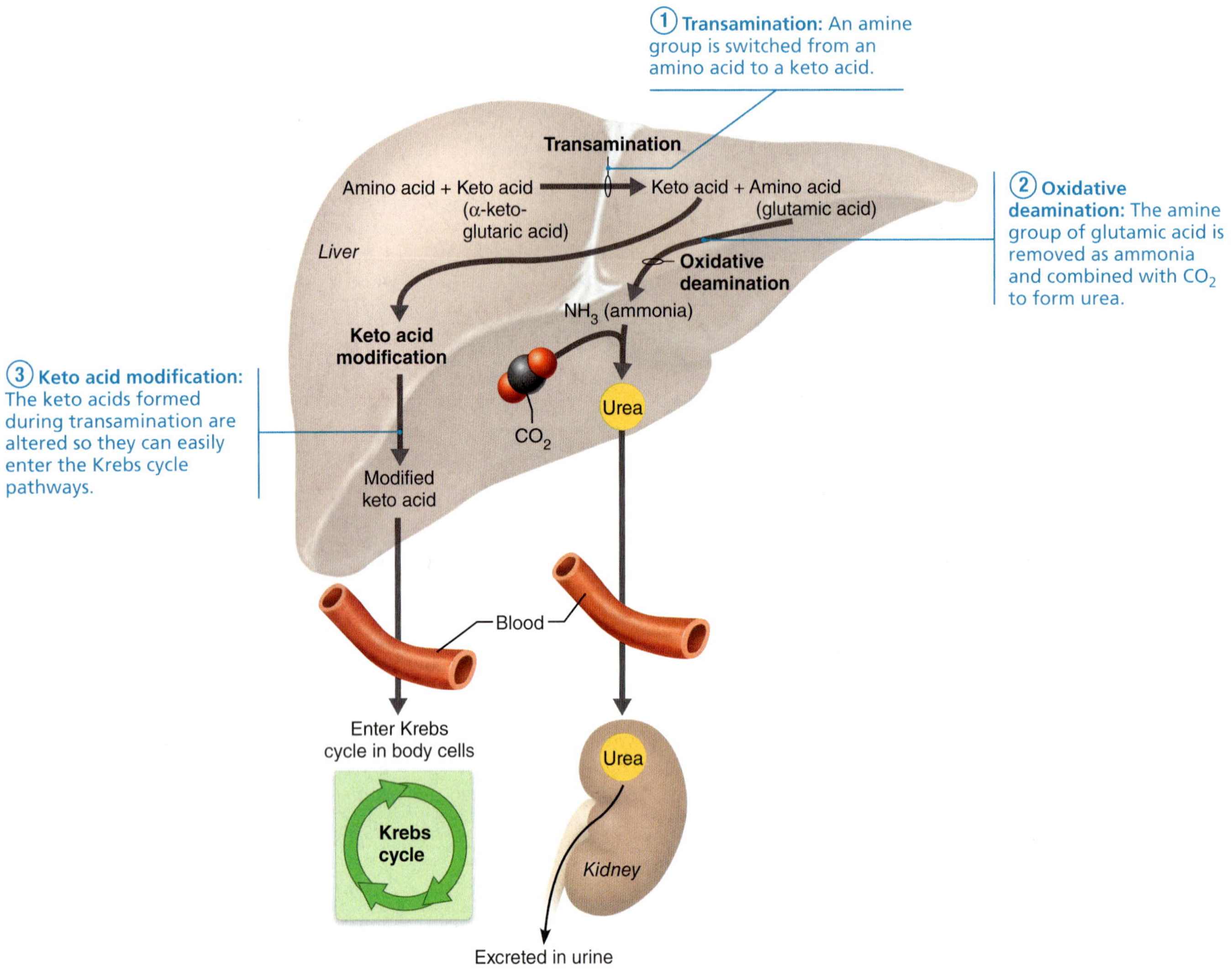

Figure 24.16 Transamination, oxidative deamination, and keto acid modification: processes that occur when amino acids are utilized for energy.

24

Check Your Understanding

16. Which part of triglyceride molecules enters the glycolytic pathway?
17. What is the central molecule in fat metabolism?
18. What are the products of beta oxidation?

For answers, see Appendix H.

Protein Metabolism

✓ Describe how amino acids are metabolized for energy.

✓ Describe the need for protein synthesis in body cells.

Like all other biological molecules, proteins have a limited life span and must be broken down and replaced before they deteriorate. As proteins are broken down, their amino acids are recycled and used to build new proteins or modified to form a different N-containing compound. Cells take up newly ingested amino acids from the blood by active transport processes and use them to *replace* tissue proteins at the rate of about 100 grams each day.

Although popular opinion has it that excess protein can be stored by the body, nothing is farther from the truth. When more protein is available than is needed for anabolic purposes, amino acids are oxidized for energy or converted to fat for future energy needs.

Oxidation of Amino Acids

Before amino acids can be oxidized for energy, they must be *deaminated*, that is, their amine group (NH_2) must be removed. (In sulfur-containing amino acids, such as methionine and cysteine, sulfur is released prior to deamination.) The resulting molecule is then converted to pyruvic acid or to one of the keto acid intermediates in the Krebs cycle [acetyl CoA, alpha (α) ketoglutaric acid, succinyl CoA, fumaric acid, or oxaloacetic acid].

The key molecule in these conversions is the nonessential amino acid *glutamic acid* (gloo-tam′ik). As **Figure 24.16** shows, the following events occur:

Table 24.4 Thumbnail Summary of Metabolic Reactions

Carbohydrates	
Cellular respiration	Reactions that together complete the oxidation of glucose, yielding CO_2, H_2O, and ATP
Glycolysis	Converts glucose to pyruvic acid
Glycogenesis	Polymerizes glucose to form glycogen
Glycogenolysis	Hydrolyzes glycogen to glucose monomers
Gluconeogenesis	Forms glucose from noncarbohydrate precursors
Krebs cycle	Completely breaks down pyruvic acid to CO_2, yielding small amounts of ATP and reduced coenzymes
Electron transport chain	Splits H removed during oxidations to H^+ and e^- and creates a proton gradient used to bond ADP to P_i (forming ATP)
Lipids	
Beta oxidation	Converts fatty acids to acetyl CoA
Lipolysis	Breaks down lipids to fatty acids and glycerol
Lipogenesis	Forms lipids from acetyl CoA and glyceraldehyde phosphate
Proteins	
Transamination	Transfers an amine group from an amino acid to α-ketoglutaric acid, thereby transforming α-ketoglutaric acid to glutamic acid
Oxidative deamination	Removes an amine group from glutamic acid as ammonia and regenerates α-ketoglutaric acid (the liver converts NH_3 to urea)

1. **Transamination** (trans″am-ĭ-na′shun). A number of amino acids can transfer their amine group to α-ketoglutaric acid (a Krebs cycle keto acid), thereby transforming α-ketoglutaric acid to glutamic acid. In the process, the original amino acid becomes a keto acid (that is, it has an oxygen atom where the amine group formerly was). This reaction is fully reversible.
2. **Oxidative deamination.** In the liver, the amine group of glutamic acid is removed as **ammonia (NH_3)**, and α-ketoglutaric acid is regenerated. The liberated NH_3 molecules are combined with CO_2, yielding **urea** and water. The urea is released to the blood and excreted from the body in urine. Because ammonia is toxic to body cells, the ease with which glutamic acid funnels amine groups into the **urea cycle** is extremely important. This cycle rids the body not only of NH_3 produced during oxidative deamination, but also of bloodborne NH_3 produced by intestinal bacteria.
3. **Keto acid modification.** The goal of amino acid degradation is to produce molecules that can be oxidized in the Krebs cycle or converted to glucose. Keto acids resulting from transamination are altered as necessary to produce metabolites that can enter the Krebs cycle. The most important of these metabolites are pyruvic acid, acetyl CoA, α-ketoglutaric acid, and oxaloacetic acid (see Figure 24.7). Because the reactions of glycolysis are reversible, deaminated amino acids that are converted to pyruvic acid can be reconverted to glucose and contribute to gluconeogenesis.

Protein Synthesis

Amino acids are the most important anabolic nutrients. Not only do they form all protein structures, but they form the bulk of the body's functional molecules as well. As we described in Chapter 3, protein synthesis occurs on ribosomes, where ribosomal enzymes oversee the formation of peptide bonds linking the amino acids together into protein polymers. Hormones (growth hormone, thyroxine, sex hormones, and others) precisely control the amount and type of protein synthesized, and protein anabolism reflects hormonal balance at each stage of life.

During your lifetime, your cells will synthesize 225–450 kg (about 500–1000 lb) of proteins, depending on your size. However, you do not need to consume anywhere near that amount of protein because the body easily forms nonessential amino acids by siphoning keto acids from the Krebs cycle and transferring amine groups to them. Most of these transformations occur in the liver, which provides nearly all the nonessential amino acids needed to produce the relatively small amount of protein that the body synthesizes each day.

However, as noted earlier, a complete set of amino acids must be present for protein synthesis to take place, so the diet must provide all essential amino acids. If some are lacking, the rest are oxidized for energy even though they may be needed for anabolism. In such cases, body protein is broken down to supply the essential amino acids needed, and negative nitrogen balance results.

To review the various metabolic reactions described so far, consult Table 24.4.

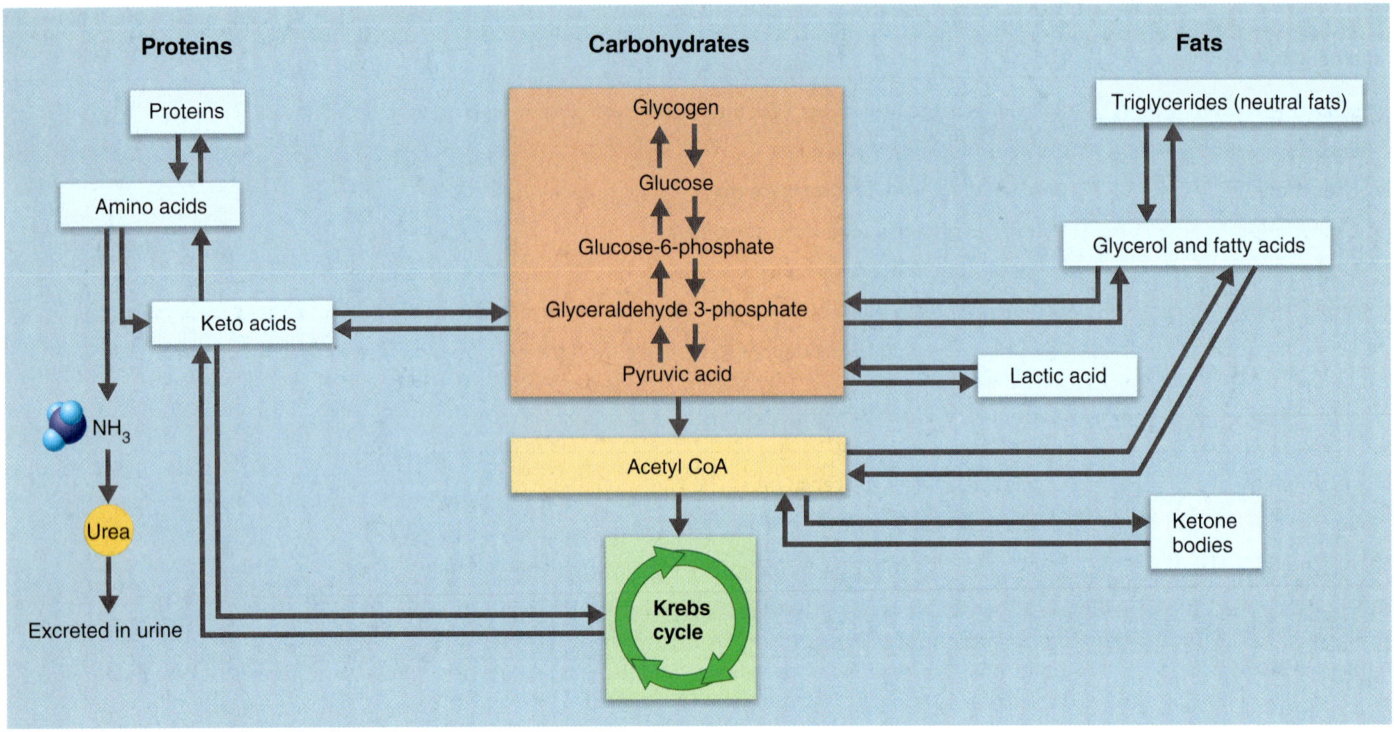

Figure 24.17 Interconversion of carbohydrates, fats, and proteins. The liver, adipose tissue, and skeletal muscles are the primary effectors determining the amounts and direction of the conversions shown from one nutrient pool to another.

Check Your Understanding

19. What does the liver use as its substrates when it synthesizes nonessential amino acids?
20. What happens to the ammonia removed from amino acids when they are used for energy fuel?

For answers, see Appendix H.

24

Metabolic States of the Body

✓ Explain the concept of amino acid or carbohydrate-fat pools, and describe pathways by which substances in these pools can be interconverted.

✓ Summarize important events of the absorptive and postabsorptive states, and explain how these events are regulated.

Catabolic-Anabolic Steady State of the Body

Now that we have examined metabolism at cellular levels, let's step back to look at the body as a system that deploys metabolic processes to provide fuel. Your body exists in a *dynamic catabolic-anabolic state*, that is, its organic molecules are continuously broken down and rebuilt—frequently at a head-spinning rate.

The body draws on its **nutrient pools**—stores of amino acids, carbohydrates, and fats—to meet its varying needs **(Figure 24.17)**. These pools are interconvertible because their pathways are linked by key intermediates. The liver, adipose tissue, and skeletal muscles are the primary effector organs or tissues determining the amounts and direction of the conversions shown in the figure.

The **amino acid pool** is the body's total supply of free amino acids. Our bodies lose small amounts of amino acids and proteins daily in urine and in sloughed hairs and skin cells. Typically, we replace these lost molecules via our diet. Otherwise, amino acids arising from tissue breakdown return to the pool. This pool is the source of amino acids used to synthesize proteins and form amino acid derivatives. In addition, as we described above, gluconeogenesis can convert deaminated amino acids to glucose. Not all events of amino acid metabolism occur in all cells. For example, *only* the liver forms urea. Nonetheless, the concept of a common amino acid pool is valid because all cells are connected by the blood.

Because carbohydrates are easily and frequently converted to fats, the **carbohydrate** and **fat pools** are usually considered together. There are two major differences between the carbohydrate-fat pool and the amino acid pool:

- Fats and carbohydrates are oxidized directly to produce cellular energy, whereas amino acids can be used to supply energy *only after being converted to a carbohydrate intermediate* (a keto acid).
- Excess carbohydrate and fat can be stored as such, whereas excess amino acids are *not* stored as protein. Instead, they are oxidized for energy or converted to fat or glycogen for storage.

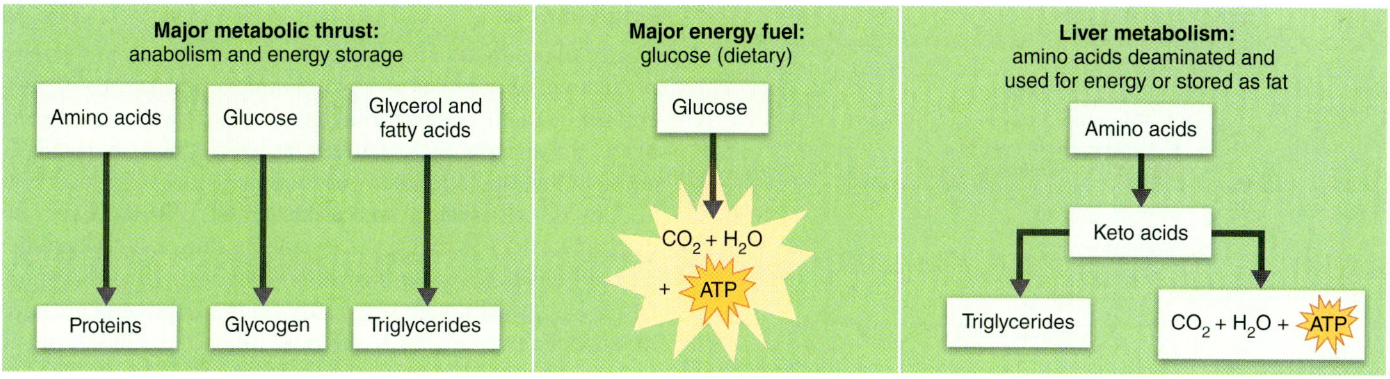

(a) Major events of the absorptive state

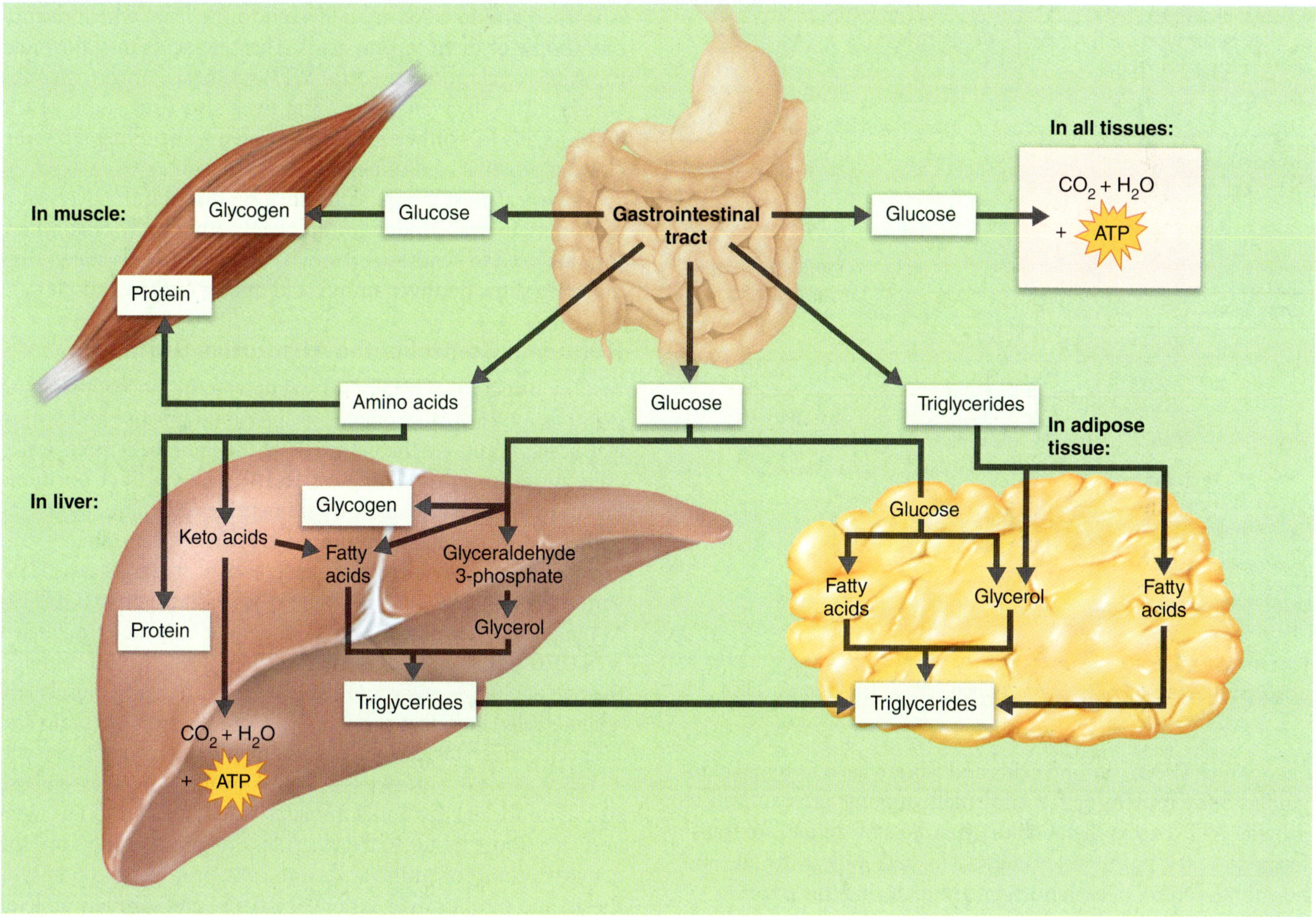

(b) Principal pathways of the absorptive state

Figure 24.18 Major events and principal metabolic pathways of the absorptive state. Although not indicated in (b), amino acids are also taken up by tissue cells and used for protein synthesis, and fats (triglycerides) are the primary energy fuel of muscle, liver cells, and adipose tissue.

Metabolic controls act to equalize blood concentrations of energy sources between two nutritional states—the *absorptive state* and the *postabsorptive state*. People who eat "three squares" a day are in the absorptive state for the four hours during and after each meal and in the postabsorptive state in the late morning, late afternoon, and all night.

Absorptive State

The absorptive state, or *fed state*, is the time during and shortly after eating, when nutrients are flushing into the blood from the GI tract. During the absorptive state anabolism exceeds catabolism and nutrients are stored **(Figure 24.18)**. Glucose is the major

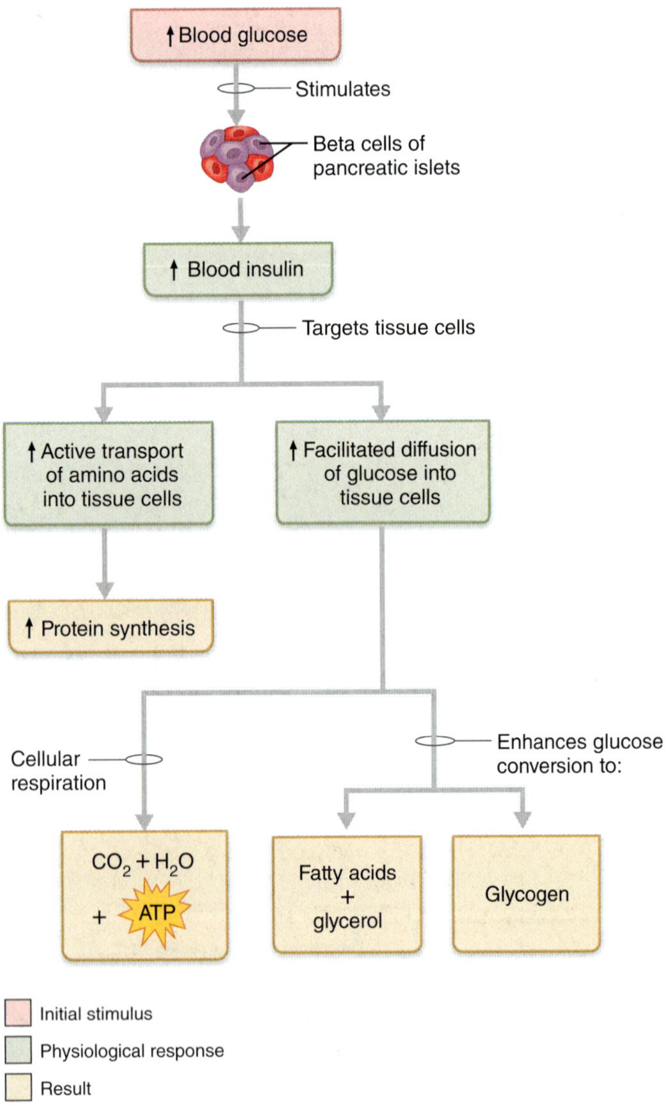

Figure 24.19 Insulin directs nearly all events of the absorptive state. (Note: Not all effects shown occur in all cells.)

energy fuel. Dietary amino acids and fats are used to remake degraded body protein or fat, and small amounts are oxidized to provide ATP. Excess metabolites, regardless of source, are transformed to fat if not used for anabolism. Let's look at the fate and hormonal control of each nutrient group during this phase.

Carbohydrates

Absorbed monosaccharides are delivered directly to the liver, where fructose and galactose are converted to glucose. Glucose, in turn, is released to the blood or converted to glycogen and fat. Glycogen formed in the liver is stored there, but most fat synthesized there is packaged with proteins as *very low density lipoproteins* (*VLDLs*) and released to the blood to be picked up by adipose tissues for storage.

Bloodborne glucose not sequestered by the liver enters body cells to be metabolized for energy. Excess glucose is stored in skeletal muscle cells as glycogen or in adipose cells as fat.

Triglycerides

Nearly all products of fat digestion enter the lymph in the form of chylomicrons, which are hydrolyzed to fatty acids and glycerol before they can pass through the capillary walls. *Lipoprotein lipase*, the enzyme that catalyzes fat hydrolysis, is particularly active in the capillaries of muscle and fat tissues.

Adipose cells, skeletal and cardiac muscle cells, and liver cells use triglycerides as their primary energy source, but when dietary carbohydrates are limited, other cells begin to oxidize more fat for energy. Although some fatty acids and glycerol are used for anabolic purposes by tissue cells, most enter adipose tissue to be reconverted to triglycerides and stored.

Amino Acids

Absorbed amino acids are delivered to the liver, which deaminates some of them to keto acids. The keto acids may flow into the Krebs cycle to be used for ATP synthesis, or they may be converted to liver fat stores. The liver also uses some of the amino acids to synthesize plasma proteins, including albumin, clotting proteins, and transport proteins.

However, most amino acids flushing through the liver sinusoids remain in the blood for uptake by other body cells, where they are used to synthesize proteins. Figure 24.18 has been simplified to show nonliver amino acid uptake only by muscle.

Hormonal Control of the Absorptive State

Insulin directs essentially all events of the absorptive state **(Figure 24.19)**. After a meal, rising blood glucose and amino acid levels stimulate the beta cells of the pancreatic islets to secrete more insulin (see Figure 16.19). The GI tract hormone glucose-dependent insulinotropic peptide (GIP) and parasympathetic stimulation also promote the release of insulin.

Insulin binds to membrane receptors of its target cells. This stimulates the translocation of the glucose transporter (GLUT4) to the plasma membrane, which enhances the carrier-mediated facilitated diffusion of glucose into those cells. Within minutes, the rate of glucose entry into tissue cells (particularly muscle and adipose cells) increases about 20-fold. The exception is brain and liver cells, which take up glucose whether or not insulin is present.

Once glucose enters tissue cells, insulin enhances glucose oxidation for energy and stimulates its conversion to glycogen and, in adipose tissue, to triglycerides. Insulin also "revs up" the active transport of amino acids into cells, promotes protein synthesis, and inhibits liver export of glucose and virtually all liver enzymes that promote gluconeogenesis.

As you can see, insulin is a **hypoglycemic hormone** (hi″po-gli-se′mik). It sweeps glucose out of the blood into tissue cells, lowering blood glucose levels. It also enhances glucose oxidation or storage while inhibiting any process that might raise blood glucose levels.

Homeostatic Imbalance 24.3

Diabetes mellitus is a disorder of inadequate insulin production or abnormal insulin receptors. Without insulin or receptors that "recognize" it, glucose is unavailable to most body cells.

Blood glucose levels remain high, and large amounts of glucose are excreted in urine. Metabolic acidosis, protein wasting, and weight loss occur as large amounts of fats and tissue proteins are used for energy. (Chapter 16 describes diabetes mellitus in more detail.) +

Postabsorptive State

The postabsorptive state, or *fasting state,* is the period when the GI tract is empty and body reserves are broken down to supply energy. Net synthesis of fat, glycogen, and proteins ends, and catabolism of these substances begins to occur **(Figure 24.20a)**.

The primary goal during the postabsorptive state is to maintain blood glucose levels within the homeostatic range (70–110 mg of glucose per 100 ml). Remember that constant blood glucose is important because the brain almost always uses glucose as its energy source. Most events of the postabsorptive state either make glucose available to the blood or save glucose for the organs that need it most by using fats for energy.

Sources of Blood Glucose

So where does blood glucose come from in the postabsorptive state? Sources include stored glycogen in the liver and skeletal muscles, tissue proteins, and, in limited amounts, fats (Figure 24.20b).

1. **Glycogenolysis in the liver.** The liver's glycogen stores (about 100 g) are the first line of glucose reserves. They are mobilized quickly and efficiently and can maintain blood sugar levels for about four hours during the postabsorptive state.
2. **Glycogenolysis in skeletal muscle.** Glycogen stores in skeletal muscle are approximately equal to those of the liver. Before liver glycogen is exhausted, glycogenolysis begins in skeletal muscle (and to a lesser extent in other tissues). However, the glucose produced is not released to the blood because, unlike the liver, skeletal muscle lacks the enzymes needed to dephosphorylate glucose. Instead, glucose is partly oxidized to pyruvic acid (or, during anaerobic conditions, lactic acid), which enters the blood, is reconverted to glucose by the liver, and is released to the blood again. Thus, skeletal muscle contributes to blood glucose homeostasis indirectly, via liver mechanisms.
3. **Lipolysis in adipose tissues and the liver.** Adipose and liver cells produce glycerol by lipolysis, and the liver converts the glycerol to glucose (gluconeogenesis) and releases it to the blood. Because acetyl CoA, a product of the beta oxidation of fatty acids, is produced beyond the *reversible* steps of glycolysis, fatty acids *cannot* be used to bolster blood glucose levels.
4. **Catabolism of cellular protein.** Tissue proteins become the major source of blood glucose during prolonged fasting when glycogen and fat stores are nearly exhausted. Cellular amino acids are deaminated and converted to glucose in the liver. During fasts lasting several weeks, the kidneys also carry out gluconeogenesis and contribute as much glucose to the blood as the liver.

Even during prolonged fasting or starvation, the body sets priorities. Muscle proteins are the first to go (to be catabolized). Movement is not nearly as important as maintaining wound healing and the immune response. But as long as life continues, so does the body's ability to produce the ATP needed to drive life processes.

Of course there are limits to the amount of tissue protein that can be catabolized before the body stops functioning. The heart is almost entirely muscle protein, and when it is severely catabolized, the result is death. In general, the amount of fat the body contains determines the time a person can survive without food.

Glucose Sparing

Even collectively, all of the manipulations aimed at increasing blood glucose are not enough to supply energy for prolonged fasting. Luckily, the body can adapt to burn more fats and proteins, which enter the Krebs cycle along with glucose breakdown products. The increased use of noncarbohydrate fuel molecules (especially triglycerides) to conserve glucose is called **glucose sparing**.

As the body progresses from the absorptive to the postabsorptive state, the brain continues to take its share of blood glucose, but virtually every other organ switches to fatty acids as its major energy source, sparing glucose for the brain. During this transition phase, lipolysis begins in adipose tissues. Tissue cells pick up released fatty acids and oxidize them for energy. In addition, the liver oxidizes fats to ketone bodies and releases them to the blood for use by tissue cells.

If fasting continues for longer than four or five days, the brain too begins to use large quantities of ketone bodies as well as glucose as its energy fuel. The brain's ability to use an alternative fuel source has survival value—much less tissue protein has to be ravaged to form glucose.

Hormonal and Neural Controls of the Postabsorptive State

The sympathetic nervous system interacts with several hormones to control events of the postabsorptive state. Consequently, regulation of this state is much more complex than that of the absorptive state when a single hormone, insulin, holds sway.

An important trigger for initiating postabsorptive events is reduced insulin release, which occurs as blood glucose levels drop. Falling insulin levels inhibit all insulin-induced cellular responses. Interestingly, drinking moderate amounts of beer, wine, or gin before or during a meal improves the body's use of insulin. That is, it lowers blood glucose without increasing insulin release. The advantage of this is obvious because although blood glucose naturally spikes after a meal, prolonged elevation can increase the risk of diabetes mellitus and heart disease.

Declining glucose levels also stimulate the alpha cells of the pancreatic islets to release the insulin antagonist **glucagon**. Like other hormones acting during the postabsorptive state, glucagon is a **hyperglycemic hormone**—it raises blood glucose levels.

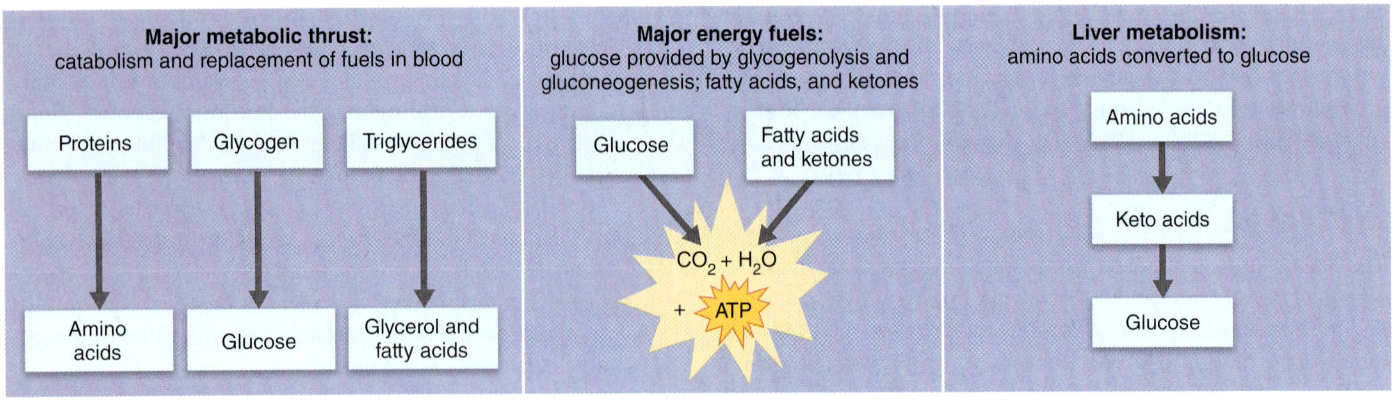

(a) Major events of the postabsorptive state

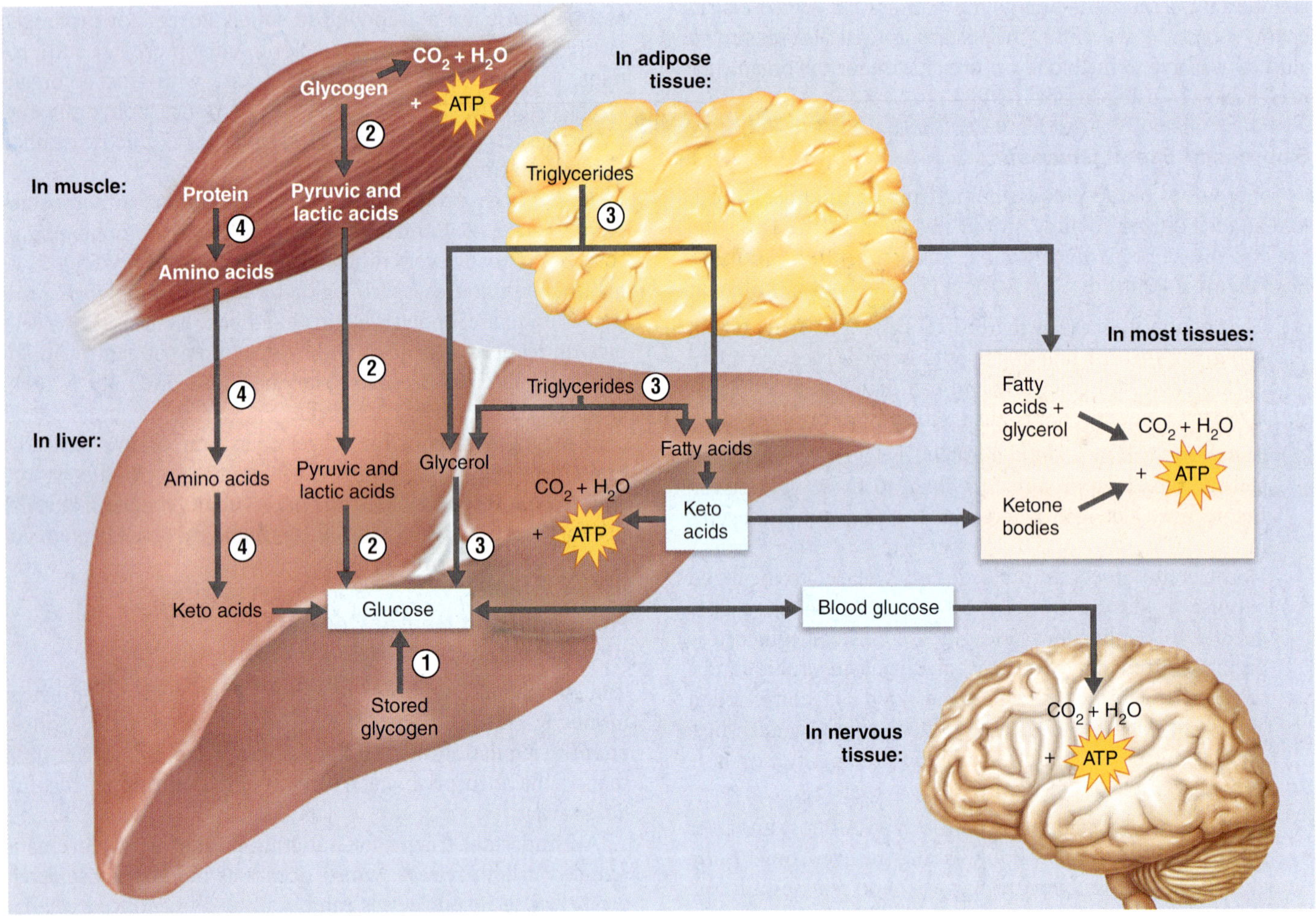

(b) Principal pathways of the postabsorptive state

Figure 24.20 Major events and principal metabolic pathways of the postabsorptive state.

Glucagon targets the liver and adipose tissue **(Figure 24.21)**. Hepatocytes respond by accelerating glycogenolysis and gluconeogenesis. Adipose cells mobilize their fatty stores (lipolysis) and release fatty acids and glycerol to the blood. In this way, glucagon "refurbishes" blood energy sources by enhancing *both* glucose and fatty acid levels. Under certain hormonal conditions and persistent low glucose levels or prolonged fasting, most of the fat mobilized is converted to ketone bodies. Glucagon release is inhibited after the next meal or whenever blood glucose levels rise and insulin secretion begins again.

So far, the picture is pretty straightforward. Increasing blood glucose levels trigger insulin release, which "pushes" glucose out of blood and into cells. This drop in blood glucose stimulates secretion of glucagon, which "pulls" glucose from the cells into blood. However, there is more than a push-pull mechanism here because rising amino acid levels in the blood stimulate the release of both insulin and glucagon.

This effect is insignificant when we eat a balanced meal, but it has an important adaptive role when we eat a high-protein, low-carbohydrate meal. In this instance, the stimulus for insulin release is strong, and if it were not counterbalanced, the brain might be damaged by the abrupt onset of hypoglycemia as glucose rushes out of the blood. Simultaneous release of glucagon modulates the effects of insulin and helps stabilize blood glucose levels.

The sympathetic nervous system also plays a crucial role in supplying fuel quickly when blood glucose levels drop suddenly. Adipose tissue is well supplied with sympathetic fibers, and epinephrine released by the adrenal medulla in response to sympathetic activation acts on the liver, skeletal muscle, and adipose tissues. Together, these stimuli mobilize fat and promote glycogenolysis—essentially the same effects prompted by glucagon.

Injury, anxiety, or any other stressor that mobilizes the fight-or-flight response will trigger this control pathway, as does exercise. During exercise, large amounts of fuels must be made available for muscles, and the metabolic profile is essentially the same as that of a fasting person when glucagon and the sympathetic nervous system are in control except that the facilitated diffusion of glucose into muscle is enhanced. (The mechanism of this enhancement is not yet understood.)

In addition to glucagon and epinephrine, a number of other hormones—including growth hormone (GH), thyroxine, sex hormones, and corticosteroids—influence metabolism and nutrient flow. Prolonged fasting or rapid declines in blood glucose levels enhance growth hormone (GH) secretion, which exerts important anti-insulin effects. For example, GH reduces the ability of insulin to promote glucose uptake in fat and muscle.

However, the release and activity of most of these hormones are not specifically related to absorptive or postabsorptive metabolic events. Table 24.5 summarizes typical metabolic effects of various hormones.

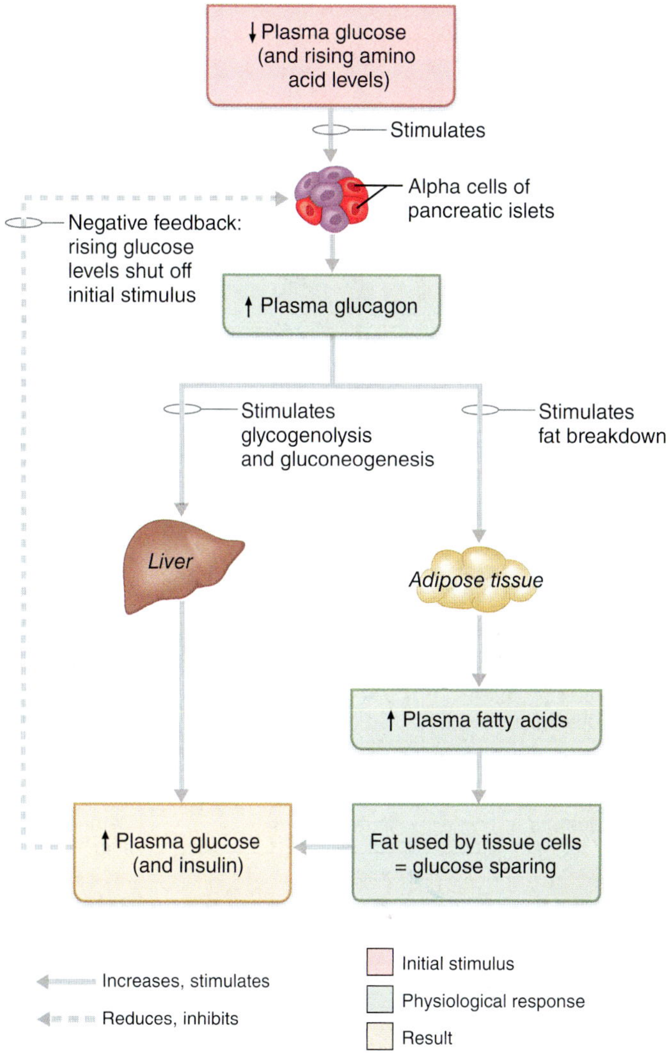

Figure 24.21 Glucagon is a hyperglycemic hormone that stimulates a rise in blood glucose levels. The dashed arrow indicates negative feedback control exerted by rising plasma glucose levels on glucagon secretion.

☑ Check Your Understanding

21. Which three organs or tissues are the primary effector organs determining the amounts and directions of interconversions in the nutrient pools?
22. Generally speaking, what kinds of reactions and events characterize the absorptive state? The postabsorptive state?
23. Which hormone is glucagon's main antagonist?
24. Which event increases both glucagon and insulin release?

For answers, see Appendix H.

The Metabolic Role of the Liver

✓ Describe several metabolic functions of the liver.

✓ Differentiate between LDLs and HDLs relative to their structures and major roles in the body.

One of the most biochemically complex organs in the body, the liver processes nearly every class of nutrients and plays a major role in regulating plasma cholesterol levels. In a pinch, mechanical contraptions can stand in for a failed heart, lungs, or kidney, but the only thing that can do the versatile liver's work is a hepatocyte.

The hepatocytes carry out some 500 or more intricate metabolic functions. A description of all of these functions is well beyond the scope of this text, but Table 24.6 provides a brief summary.

Cholesterol Metabolism and Regulation of Blood Cholesterol Levels

Cholesterol has received little attention in this discussion so far, primarily because it is not used as an energy source. It serves instead as the structural basis of bile salts, steroid hormones, and vitamin D and is a major component of plasma membranes.

Table 24.5 Summary of Normal Hormonal Influences on Metabolism

HORMONE'S EFFECTS	INSULIN	GLUCAGON	EPINEPHRINE	GROWTH HORMONE	THYROXINE	CORTISOL	TESTOSTERONE
Stimulates glucose uptake by cells	✓				✓		
Stimulates amino acid uptake by cells	✓			✓			
Stimulates glucose catabolism for energy	✓				✓		
Stimulates glycogenesis	✓						
Stimulates lipogenesis and fat storage	✓						
Inhibits gluconeogenesis	✓						
Stimulates protein synthesis (anabolic)	✓			✓	✓		✓
Stimulates glycogenolysis		✓	✓				
Stimulates lipolysis and fat mobilization		✓	✓	✓	✓	✓	
Stimulates gluconeogenesis		✓	✓	✓		✓	
Stimulates protein breakdown (catabolic)						✓	

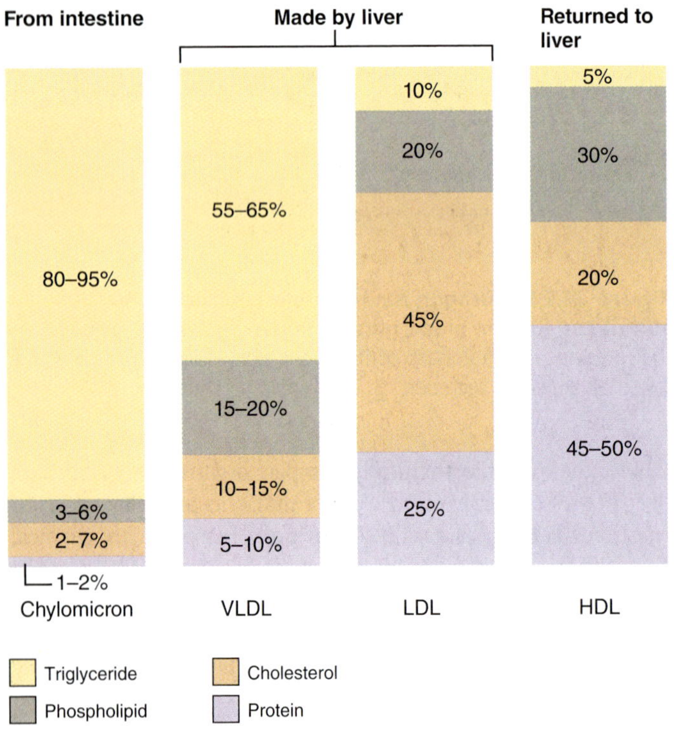

Figure 24.22 Approximate composition of lipoproteins that transport lipids in body fluids. VLDL = very low density lipoprotein, LDL = low-density lipoprotein, HDL = high-density lipoprotein.

About 15% of blood cholesterol comes from the diet. The liver—and to a lesser extent other body cells, particularly intestinal cells—make the other 85% from acetyl CoA. Cholesterol is lost from the body when it is catabolized and secreted in bile salts, which are eventually excreted in feces.

Cholesterol Transport

Because triglycerides and cholesterol are insoluble in water, they do not circulate free in the blood. Instead, they are transported to and from tissue cells bound to small lipid-protein complexes called **lipoproteins**. These complexes solubilize the hydrophobic lipids, and contain signals that regulate lipid entry and exit at specific target cells.

Lipoproteins vary in their relative fat-protein composition, but they all contain triglycerides, phospholipids, and cholesterol in addition to protein **(Figure 24.22)**. In general, the higher the percentage of lipid in the lipoprotein, the lower its density; and the greater the proportion of protein, the higher its density. On this basis, there are **very low density lipoproteins (VLDLs), low-density lipoproteins (LDLs),** and **high-density lipoproteins (HDLs)**. *Chylomicrons*, which transport absorbed lipids from the GI tract, are a separate class and have the lowest density of all.

The liver is the primary source of VLDLs, which transport triglycerides from the liver to peripheral (nonliver) tissues, mostly to *adipose tissues*. Once the triglycerides are unloaded, the residues are converted to LDLs, which are cholesterol-rich. The job of the LDLs is to transport cholesterol to *peripheral tissues*, making it available to tissue cells to synthesize membranes or hormones, and to store it for later use. Docking of LDL to the LDL receptor triggers receptor-mediated endocytosis of the entire particle.

The major function of HDLs, which are particularly rich in phospholipids and proteins, is to scoop up and transport excess cholesterol *from peripheral tissues to the liver*, where it is broken down and becomes part of bile. The liver makes the protein envelopes of the HDL particles and then ejects them into the bloodstream in collapsed form, rather like deflated beach balls. Once in the blood, these still-incomplete HDL particles

Table 24.6 Summary of Metabolic Functions of the Liver

METABOLIC PROCESSES TARGETED	FUNCTIONS
Carbohydrate Metabolism	
Particularly important in maintaining blood glucose homeostasis	▪ Converts galactose and fructose to glucose ▪ Stores glucose as glycogen when blood glucose levels are high; in response to hormonal controls, performs glycogenolysis and releases glucose to blood ▪ Gluconeogenesis: converts amino acids and glycerol to glucose when glycogen stores are exhausted and blood glucose levels are falling ▪ Converts glucose to fats for storage
Fat Metabolism	
Although most cells are capable of some fat metabolism, liver bears the major responsibility	▪ Primary body site of beta oxidation (breakdown of fatty acids to acetyl CoA) ▪ Converts excess acetyl CoA to ketone bodies for release to tissue cells ▪ Stores fats ▪ Forms lipoproteins for transport of fatty acids, fats, and cholesterol in blood ▪ Synthesizes cholesterol from acetyl CoA; catabolizes cholesterol to bile salts, which are secreted in bile
Protein Metabolism	
Without liver metabolism of proteins, severe survival problems ensue: many essential clotting proteins would not be made, and ammonia would not be disposed of, for example	▪ Deaminates amino acids for their conversion to glucose or for ATP synthesis; amount of deamination that occurs outside the liver is unimportant ▪ Forms urea for removal of ammonia from body; inability to perform this function (e.g., in cirrhosis or hepatitis) allows ammonia to accumulate in the blood ▪ Forms most plasma proteins (exceptions are gamma globulins and some hormones and enzymes); plasma protein depletion causes rapid mitosis of the hepatocytes and actual growth of liver, which is coupled with increased synthesis of plasma proteins until blood values are again normal ▪ Transamination: interconversion of nonessential amino acids; amount that occurs outside liver is inconsequential
Vitamin/Mineral Storage	
	▪ Stores vitamin A (1–2 years' supply) ▪ Stores sizable amounts of vitamins D and B_{12} (1–4 months' supply) ▪ Stores iron; other than iron bound to hemoglobin, most of body's supply is stored in liver as ferritin
Biotransformation Functions	
	▪ Metabolizes alcohol and drugs by inactivating them for excretion by the kidneys, and performs reactions that may result in products which are more active, changed in activity, or less active ▪ Processes bilirubin resulting from RBC breakdown and excretes bile pigments in bile ▪ Metabolizes bloodborne hormones to forms that can be excreted in urine

fill with cholesterol picked up from tissue cells and "pulled" from artery walls. HDL also provides the steroid-producing organs, like the ovaries and adrenal glands, with their raw material (cholesterol).

Recommended Total Cholesterol, HDL, and LDL Levels

For adults, the recommended total cholesterol level is 200 mg/dl of blood (or substantially lower). Blood cholesterol levels above 200 mg/dl have been linked to atherosclerosis, which clogs the arteries and causes strokes and heart attacks. However, it is not enough to simply measure total cholesterol. The form in which cholesterol is transported in the blood is more important clinically.

As a rule, high levels of HDLs are considered *good* because the transported cholesterol is destined for degradation (think H for healthy). HDL levels above 60 are thought to protect against heart disease, and levels below 40 are considered undesirable. In the United States, HDL levels average 40–50 in males and 50–60 in women.

High LDL levels (130 or above) are considered *bad* (think L for lousy) because when LDLs are excessive, potentially lethal cholesterol deposits are laid down in the artery walls. The goal for LDL levels is 100 or less, but new guidelines for those at risk for cardiac disease recommend 70 mg/dl or less. A good rule of thumb is that HDL levels can't be too high and LDL levels can't be too low.

Factors Regulating Blood Cholesterol Levels

A negative feedback loop partially adjusts the amount of cholesterol produced by the liver according to the amount of cholesterol in the diet. A high cholesterol intake inhibits its synthesis by the liver, but it is not a one-to-one relationship because the liver produces a certain basal amount of cholesterol (about 85% of desirable values) even when dietary intake is high. Conversely, severely restricting dietary cholesterol, although helpful, does not markedly reduce blood cholesterol levels.

However, the relative amounts of saturated and unsaturated fatty acids in the diet do have an important effect on blood cholesterol levels. Saturated fatty acids *stimulate liver synthesis* of cholesterol and *inhibit its excretion* from the body. In contrast, unsaturated (mono- and polyunsaturated) fatty acids (found in olive oil and in most vegetable oils, respectively) *enhance excretion* of cholesterol and its catabolism to bile salts, thereby reducing total cholesterol levels.

The unhappy exception to this good news about unsaturated fats concerns **trans fats**, "healthy" oils that have been hardened by hydrogenation to make them more solid, such as some margarines. Trans fats actually have a worse effect on blood cholesterol levels than saturated fats do. The trans fatty acids spark a greater increase in LDLs and a greater reduction in HDLs, producing the unhealthiest ratio of total cholesterol to HDL.

The unsaturated omega-3 fatty acids found in especially large amounts in some cold-water fish (such as salmon) lower the proportions of both saturated fats and cholesterol. The omega-3 fatty acids make blood platelets less sticky, thus helping prevent spontaneous clotting that can block blood vessels. They also appear to lower blood pressure, even in people with normal blood pressure. In those with moderate to high cholesterol levels, replacing lipid- and cholesterol-rich animal proteins in the diet with soy protein helps lower blood cholesterol.

Factors other than diet also influence blood cholesterol levels. For example, cigarette smoking and stress lower HDL levels, whereas regular aerobic exercise and estrogen lower LDL levels and increase HDL levels. Interestingly, body shape provides clues to risky blood levels of cholesterol and fats. "Apples" (people with upper body and abdominal fat, seen more often in men) tend to have higher levels of cholesterol and LDLs than "pears" (whose fat is localized in the hips and thighs, a pattern more common in women).

Most cells other than liver and intestinal cells obtain the bulk of the cholesterol they need for membrane synthesis from the blood. When a cell needs cholesterol, it makes membrane receptor proteins for LDL. LDL binds to the receptors, is engulfed in coated pits by endocytosis, and within 15 minutes the endocytotic vesicles fuse with lysosomes, where the cholesterol is freed for use. When excessive cholesterol accumulates in a cell, it inhibits both the cell's own cholesterol synthesis and its synthesis of LDL receptors.

Homeostatic Imbalance 24.4

Previously, high cholesterol and LDL:HDL ratios were considered the most valid predictors of risk for atherosclerosis, cardiovascular disease, and heart attack. However, almost half of those who get heart disease have normal cholesterol levels, while others with poor lipid profiles remain free of heart problems. Presently, LDL levels and assessments of other cardiovascular disease risk factors are believed to be more accurate indicators of whether treatment is needed, and many physicians recommend dietary changes regardless of total cholesterol or HDL levels.

Cholesterol-lowering drugs such as *statins* are routinely prescribed for people with LDL levels over 130. It is estimated that more than 10 million Americans are now taking statins. +

Check Your Understanding

25. If you had your choice, would you prefer to have high blood levels of HDLs or LDLs? Explain your answer.
26. What is the maximum recommended cholesterol level for adults?
27. What are trans fats and how do they affect LDL and HDL levels?

For answers, see Appendix H.

Energy Balance

✓ Explain what is meant by body energy balance.

✓ Describe several theories of food intake regulation.

When any fuel is burned, it consumes oxygen and liberates heat. The "burning" of food fuels by our cells is no exception. As we described in Chapter 2, energy can be neither created nor destroyed—only converted from one form to another. If we apply this principle (actually the *first law of thermodynamics*) to cell metabolism, it means that bond energy released as foods are catabolized must be precisely balanced by the total energy output of the body. For this reason, a dynamic balance exists between the body's energy intake and energy output:

$$\text{Energy intake} = \underset{\text{(heat + work + energy storage)}}{\text{energy output}}$$

Energy intake is the energy liberated during food oxidation. (Undigested foods are not part of the equation because they contribute no energy.) **Energy output** includes energy (1) immediately lost as heat (about 60% of the total), (2) used to do work (driven by ATP), and (3) stored as fat or glycogen. Because losses of organic molecules in urine, feces, and perspiration are very small in healthy people, they are usually ignored in calculating energy output.

A close look at this situation reveals that *nearly all the energy derived from foodstuffs is eventually converted to heat.* Heat is lost during every cellular activity—when ATP bonds are formed and when they are cleaved to do work, as muscles contract, and through friction as blood flows through blood vessels. Though cells cannot use this energy to do work, the heat warms the tissues and blood and helps maintain the homeostatic body temperature that allows metabolic reactions to occur efficiently. Energy storage is an important part of the equation only during periods of growth and net fat deposit.

When energy intake and energy output are balanced, body weight remains stable. When they are not, weight is either gained or lost. Unhappily for many people, the body's weight-controlling systems appear to be designed more to protect us against weight loss than weight gain.

Obesity

How fat is too fat? What distinguishes a person who is obese from one who is merely overweight? Let's take a look.

The bathroom scale, though it helps to determine degrees of overweight, is an inaccurate guide because body weight tells little of body composition. Dense bones and well-developed muscles can make a fit, healthy person technically overweight. Arnold Schwarzenegger, for example, has tipped the scales at a hefty 257 lb.

The official medical measure of obesity and body fatness is the **body mass index (BMI)**, an index of a person's weight relative to height. To estimate BMI, multiply weight in pounds by 705 and then divide by your height in inches squared:

$$\text{BMI} = \text{wt(lb)} \times 705/\text{ht(inches)}^2$$

Overweight is defined by a BMI between 25 and 30 and carries some health risk. Obesity is a BMI greater than 30 and has a markedly increased health risk.

The most common view of obesity is that it is a condition of excessive triglyceride storage. We bewail our inability to rid ourselves of fat, but the real problem is that we keep refilling the storehouses by downing too many calories. A body fat content of 18–20% of body weight (males and females respectively) is deemed normal for adults.

However it's defined, obesity is perplexing and poorly understood, and the economic toll of obesity-related disease is staggering. Chronic low-grade systemic inflammation accompanies obesity and contributes to insulin resistance and type 2 diabetes mellitus. People who are obese also have a higher incidence of atherosclerosis, hypertension, heart disease, and osteoarthritis.

The U.S. is big and getting bigger, at least around its middle. Two out of three adults are overweight. Of that number, one out of three is obese and one in twelve has diabetes. U.S. kids are getting fatter too: 20 years ago, 5% were overweight; today over 15% are and more are headed that way. Furthermore, because kids are opting for video games and nachos instead of tag or touch football and an apple, their general cardiovascular fitness is declining as well and health risks associated with excess weight start frighteningly early. *A Closer Look* on pp. 942–943 discusses weight-control methods used by some obese people.

Regulation of Food Intake

Control of food intake poses difficult questions to researchers. For example, what type of receptor could sense the body's total calorie content and alert us to start eating or put down that fork? Despite heroic research efforts, no such single receptor type has been found.

It has been known for some time that the hypothalamus, particularly its *arcuate nucleus* (*ARC*) and two other areas—the *lateral hypothalamic area* (*LHA*) and the *ventromedial nucleus* (*VMN*)—release several peptides that influence feeding behavior. Most importantly, this influence ultimately reflects the activity of two distinct sets of neurons—one set that promotes hunger and the other that causes satiety:

- The NPY/AgRP group of ARC releases neuropeptide Y (NPY) and agouti-related peptides, which collectively enhance appetite by stimulating the orexin-releasing second-order neurons of the LHA (**Figure 24.23**, right side).
- The other neuron group in ARC consists of the POMC/CART neurons, which suppress appetite by releasing the peptides pro-opiomelanocortin (POMC) and cocaine- and amphetamine-regulated transcript (CART). POMC and CART act on the ventromedial nucleus, causing its neurons to release CRH (corticotropin-releasing hormone), an important appetite suppressor.

Current theories of how feeding behavior and hunger are regulated focus on several factors, most importantly (1) neural signals from the digestive tract, (2) bloodborne signals related to body energy stores, and (3) hormones. To a smaller degree, body temperature and psychological factors also play a role.

All these factors appear to operate through feedback signals to the feeding centers of the brain. Brain receptors include thermoreceptors, chemoreceptors (for glucose, insulin, and others), and receptors that respond to a number of specific peptides (leptin, neuropeptide Y, and others). The hypothalamic nuclei play an essential role in regulating hunger and satiety, but brain stem areas are also involved. Sensors in peripheral locations have also been suggested, with the liver and gut itself (alimentary canal) the prime candidates. Controls of food intake come in two varieties—short term and long term.

Short-Term Regulation of Food Intake

Short-term regulation of appetite and feeding behavior involves neural signals from the GI tract, blood levels of nutrients, and GI tract hormones. For the most part, the short-term signals target hypothalamic centers via the solitary tract (and nucleus) of the brain stem (Figure 24.23).

Neural Signals from the Digestive Tract One way the brain evaluates the contents of the gut depends on vagal nerve fibers that carry on a two-way conversation between gut and brain. For example, clinical tests show that ingesting protein produces a 30–40% larger and longer response in vagal afferents than ingesting the same amount of glucose. Furthermore, activating stretch receptors ultimately inhibits appetite, because GI tract distension sends signals along vagus nerve afferents that suppress the appetite-enhancing or hunger center. Using these signals, together with others it receives, the brain can decode what is eaten and how much.

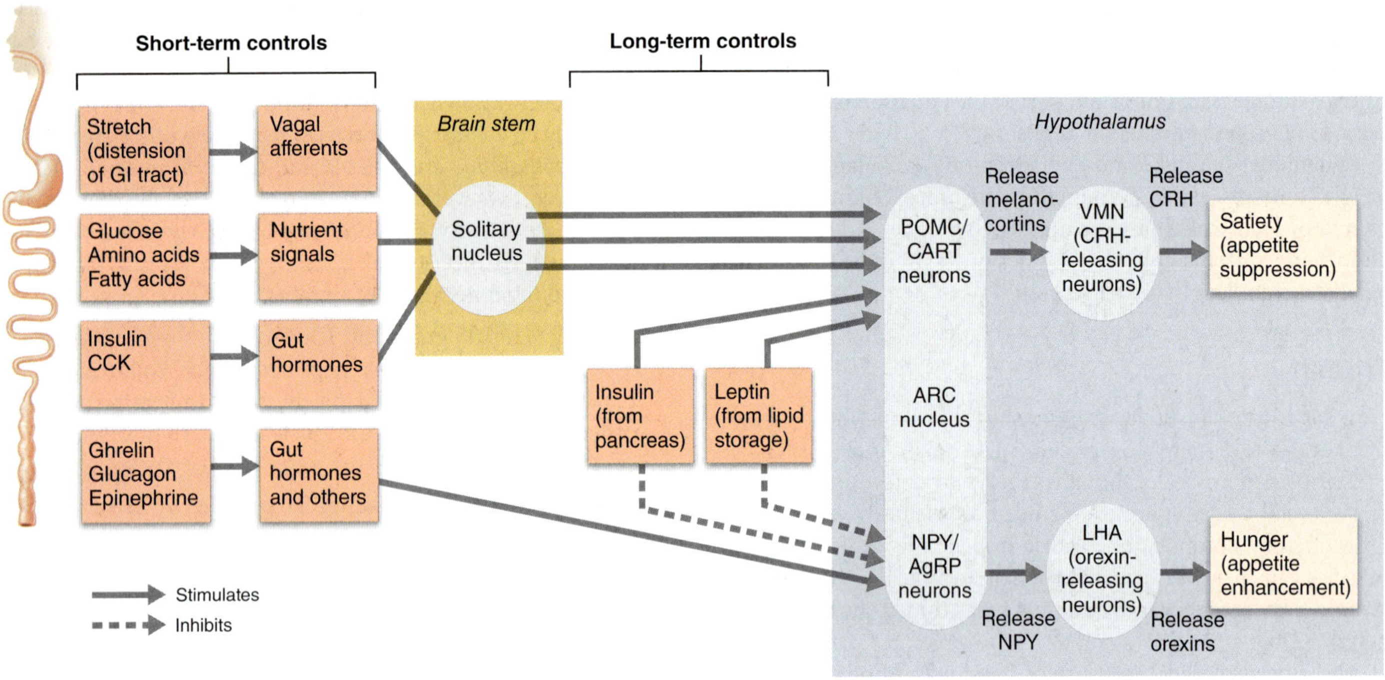

Figure 24.23 Model for hypothalamic command of appetite and food intake. The arcuate nucleus (ARC) of the brain contains two sets of neurons with opposing effects. Activating the NPY and orexin neurons enhances appetite, whereas activating POMC/CART neurons has the opposite effect. These centers connect with interneurons in other brain centers, and signals are transmitted through the brain stem to the body. Many appetite-regulating hormones act through the ARC, though they may also exert direct effects on other brain centers. (AgRP = agouti-related peptide, ARC = arcuate nucleus, CART = cocaine- and amphetamine-regulated transcript, CCK = cholecystokinin, CRH = corticotropin-releasing hormone, LHA = lateral hypothalamic area, NPY = neuropeptide Y, POMC = pro-opiomelanocortin, VMN = ventromedial nucleus)

Nutrient Signals Related to Energy Stores Blood levels of glucose, amino acids, and fatty acids provide information to the brain that may help adjust energy intake to energy output. For example, nutrient signals that indicate fullness or satiety include:

- *Rising blood glucose levels.* When we eat, rising blood glucose levels ultimately depress eating (Figure 24.23). During fasting and hypoglycemia, this signal is absent, resulting in hunger and "turning on" food-seeking behavior.

  The brain shows other responses to glucose and high-caloric food as well. When we ingest sugar, the brain's reward (pleasure) system "gives off fireworks" in the form of rising dopamine levels to a greater or lesser degree. Perhaps this response is the genesis of overeating (hedonistic) behavior.
- *Elevated blood levels of amino acids* depress eating, but the precise mechanism is unknown.
- *Blood concentrations of fatty acids* provide a mechanism for controlling hunger. The larger the amount of fatty acids in the blood, the more eating behavior is inhibited.

Hormones Gut hormones, including insulin and cholecystokinin (CCK) released during food absorption, act as satiety signals to depress hunger. Cholecystokinin, which blocks the appetite-inducing effect of NPY, is most important.

In contrast, glucagon and epinephrine levels rise during fasting and stimulate hunger. Ghrelin (Ghr), produced by the stomach, is a powerful appetite stimulant. In fact, ghrelin appears to be the "dinner bell" or trigger for initiating a meal. Its level peaks just before mealtime, signaling the brain that it is time to eat, and then the level troughs out after the meal.

Long-Term Regulation of Food Intake

A key component of the long-term controls of feeding behavior is the hormone **leptin** ("thin"). Secreted exclusively by adipose cells in response to an increase in body fat mass, leptin indicates the body's total energy stores in fat tissue. (Thus adipose tissue acts as a "Fat-o-Stat" that sends chemical messages to the brain in the form of leptin.)

When levels of leptin rise in the blood, it binds to receptors in ARC that specifically (1) suppress the release of neuropeptide Y and (2) stimulate the expression of CART. NPY is the most potent appetite stimulant known. By blocking its release, leptin prevents the release of the appetite-enhancing orexins from the LHA. This decreases appetite and food intake, eventually promoting weight loss.

When fat stores shrink, leptin blood levels drop, an event that exerts opposite effects on the two sets of ARC neurons. Consequently, appetite and food intake increase, and (eventually) weight gain occurs.

Initially it seemed that leptin was the magic bullet that obesity researchers were looking for, but their hopes were soon dashed. Rising leptin levels do promote weight loss, but only to a certain point. Furthermore, individuals who are obese have higher-than-normal leptin blood levels, but for some unknown reason, they are resistant to its action. Now the consensus is that leptin's main role is to protect against weight loss in times of nutritional deprivation.

Although leptin has received the most attention as a long-term appetite and metabolism regulator, there are several other players. Insulin, like leptin, inhibits NPY release in non-insulin-resistant individuals, but its effect is less potent.

Additional Regulatory Factors

There is no easy answer to explain how body weight is regulated, but theories abound. Rising ambient temperature discourages food seeking, whereas cold temperature activates the hunger center. Depending on the individual, stress may increase or decrease food-seeking behavior, but chronic stress in combination with a junk food (high-fat and -sugar) diet promotes sharply increased release of NPY.

Psychological factors are thought to be important in people who are obese, but even when psychological factors contribute to obesity, individuals do not continue to gain weight endlessly. Controls still operate but at a higher set-point weight. Certain adenovirus infections, sleep deprivation, and even the composition of gut bacteria are additional factors that may affect a person's fat mass and weight regulation, according to some clinical studies.

Whew! How does all this information fit together? So far we only have bits and pieces of the story, but Figure 24.23 shows the best current model based on animal studies.

Check Your Understanding

28. What three groups of stimuli influence short-term regulation of feeding behavior?
29. What is the most important long-term regulator of feeding behavior and appetite?

For answers, see Appendix H.

Metabolic Rate and Heat Production

✓ Define basal metabolic rate and total metabolic rate. Name factors that influence each.

The body's rate of energy output, the **metabolic rate**, is the total heat produced by all the chemical reactions and mechanical work of the body. We can measure metabolic rate directly or indirectly. In the *direct method*, a person enters a chamber called a **calorimeter** and water circulating around the chamber absorbs heat liberated by the body. The rise in water temperature is directly related to the heat produced by the person's body. The *indirect method* uses a **respirometer** to measure oxygen consumption, which is directly proportional to heat production. For each liter of oxygen used, the body produces about 4.8 kcal of heat.

Basal Metabolic Rate (BMR)

Because many factors influence metabolic rate, it is usually measured under standardized conditions. The person is in a postabsorptive state (has not eaten for at least 12 hours), is reclining, and is mentally and physically relaxed. The temperature of the room is a comfortable 20–25°C. The measurement obtained under these circumstances, the **basal metabolic rate (BMR)**, reflects the energy the body needs to perform only its most essential activities, such as breathing and maintaining resting levels of organ function. Although named the *basal* metabolic rate, this measurement is *not* the lowest metabolic state of the body. That situation occurs during sleep, when skeletal muscles are completely relaxed.

The BMR, often referred to as the "energy cost of living," is reported in kilocalories per square meter of body surface per hour (kcal/m^2/h). A 70-kg adult has a BMR of approximately 66 kcal/h. You can approximate your BMR by multiplying weight in kilograms (2.2 lb = 1 kg) by 1 if you are male and by 0.9 if you are female.

Several factors influence BMR, including body surface area, age, gender, body temperature, stress, and the hormone thyroxine.

Body Surface Area BMR is related to overall weight and size, but the critical factor is body surface area. As the ratio of body surface area to body volume increases, heat loss to the environment increases and the metabolic rate must be higher to replace the lost heat. For this reason, if two people weigh the same, the taller or thinner person will have the higher BMR.

Age and Gender In general, the younger the person, the higher the BMR. Children and adolescents require large amounts of energy for growth. In old age, BMR declines dramatically as skeletal muscles begin to atrophy. (This helps explain why elderly people who fail to reduce their caloric intake gain weight.)

Gender also plays a role. Metabolic rate is disproportionately higher in males than in females, because males typically have more muscle, which is very active metabolically even during rest. Fatty tissue, present in greater relative amounts in females, is metabolically more sluggish than muscle.

Body Temperature Body temperature and BMR tend to rise and fall together. Fever markedly increases metabolic rate above basal levels.

Stress Whether physical or emotional, stress increases BMR by mobilizing the sympathetic nervous system. As norepinephrine and epinephrine (released by adrenal medullary cells) flood into the blood, they raise BMR primarily by stimulating fat catabolism.

Thyroxine The amount of **thyroxine** produced by the thyroid gland is probably the most important hormonal factor in determining BMR. For this reason, thyroxine has been dubbed the "metabolic hormone." Its direct effect on most body cells (except brain cells) is to increase O_2 consumption and heat production, presumably by accelerating the use of ATP to operate the sodium-potassium pump. As ATP reserves decline, cellular respiration accelerates. Thus, the more thyroxine produced, the higher the BMR.

Homeostatic Imbalance 24.5

Hyperthyroidism causes a host of problems resulting from the excessive BMR it produces. The body catabolizes stored fats and tissue proteins and, despite increased hunger and food intake,

A CLOSER LOOK

Obesity: Magical Solution Wanted

Fat—unwanted, **unloved**, and yet often overabundant. Besides the **physical toll**, the **social stigma** and economic disadvantages of obesity are legendary. A fat person pays higher insurance premiums, is discriminated against in the job market, has fewer clothing choices, and endures frequent humiliation throughout life.

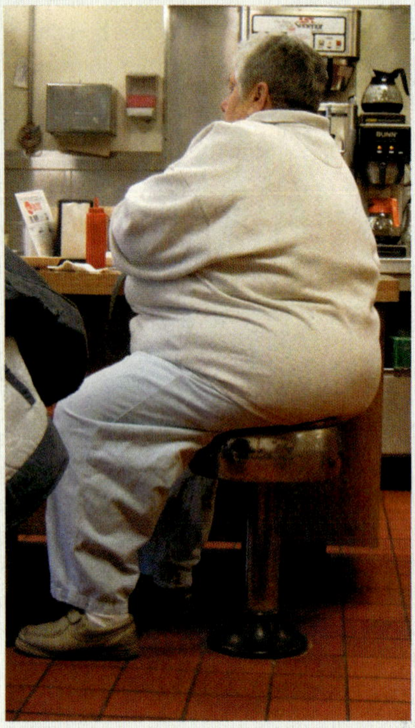

What Causes Obesity?

It's a fair bet that few people choose to become obese. So what causes it? Some possibilities are:

1. **Overeating during childhood promotes adult obesity.** Some believe that the "clean your plate" order sets the stage for adult obesity by increasing the number of adipose cells formed during childhood. The more adipose cells there are, the more fat can be stored.
2. **Obese people are more fuel efficient and more effective "fat storers."** Although it is often assumed that people who are obese eat more, this is not necessarily true—many actually eat less than people of normal weight. When yo-yo dieters lose weight, their metabolic rate falls sharply. But, when they subsequently gain weight, their metabolic rate temporarily increases like a furnace being stoked. Each successive weight loss occurs more slowly, but they regain weight three times as fast.

   Furthermore, fats pack more wallop per calorie (are more fattening) than proteins or carbohydrates because of the way the body processes them. If we ingest 100 excess carbohydrate calories, 23 are used in metabolic processing and 77 are stored. However, if the 100 excess calories come from fat, only 3 calories are "burned" and the rest (97) are stored.

   These facts apply to everyone, but when you are obese the picture is even bleaker. "Fat" fat cells of overweight people:

   - Sprout more alpha receptors, which favor fat accumulation.
   - Send different molecular messages than "thin" fat cells. They spew out inflammatory cytokines (tumor necrosis factor and others) that can promote insulin resistance and they release less adiponectin, a hormone that improves the action of insulin in glucose uptake and storage.
   - Have exceptionally efficient lipoprotein lipases, which unload fat from the blood (usually to fat cells).

   Although it would appear that the so-called satiety chemicals (hormones and others) should prevent massive fat deposit, this seems not to be the case in obese people. It may be that excess weight promotes not only insulin resistance but leptin resistance as well.
3. **Genetic predisposition.** Morbid obesity is the destiny of those inheriting two obesity genes. These people, given extra calories, will always lay them down as fat, as opposed to those that lay down more muscle with some of the excess. However, a true genetic predisposition for "fatness" appears to account for only about 5% of obese Americans.
4. **Viral infection.** Surprisingly, a recent study has shown a link between obesity and infection with a particular cold virus (adenovirus 360). The virus has been shown to increase the number and fat content of adipocytes in laboratory animals, but further studies are needed to determine if there is a true cause-effect relationship in humans.

Treatments—The Bad and the Good

Some so-called treatments for obesity are almost more dangerous than the disease itself. Unfortunate strategies include the following.

1. **"Water pills."** Diuretics prompt the kidneys to excrete more water and may cause a few pounds of weight loss for a few hours. They can also cause serious dehydration and electrolyte imbalance.
2. **Diets.** Diet products and books sell well, but do they work and are they safe? There is a long-standing duel between those promoting low-carbohydrate (high-protein and -fat) regimens such as the Atkins and South Beach diets, and those espousing the traditional low-fat (high–complex carbohydrates) diet.

   Clinical studies show that people on the low-carbohydrate diets lose weight more quickly at first, but plateau at 6 months. They seem to preferentially lose fat from the body trunk, a weight distribution pattern (the

24

the person often loses weight. Bones weaken and muscles, including the heart, begin to atrophy.

In contrast, *hypothyroidism* results in slowed metabolism, obesity, and diminished thought processes. ✚

Physical Training Surprisingly, physical training has little effect on BMR. Although it would appear that athletes, especially those with greatly enhanced muscle mass, should have much higher BMRs than nonathletes, there is little difference between those of the same gender and body surface area.

Total Metabolic Rate (TMR)

The **total metabolic rate (TMR)** is the rate of kilocalorie consumption needed to fuel *all* ongoing activities—involuntary "apple") associated with heart disease and diabetes mellitus. (This propensity to these diseases, called "metabolic syndrome," appears to be due to the large amounts of inflammatory cytokines released by visceral fat cells.) When dieting continued for a year, those on the low-fat diets lost just as much weight as did those on the low-carbohydrate diets. Although there was concern that the low-carbohydrate diets would promote undesirable plasma cholesterol and lipid values, for the most part this has not been the case.

Diets that have users counting the glycemic indexes of the food they eat, such as the New Glucose Revolution diet, distinguish between good carbs (whole grains, nonstarchy vegetables and fruits) and bad carbs (starches, sugary foods, refined grains). Many physicians approve.

The oldie-but-goodie Weight Watchers diet, which has dieters counting points, still works and allows virtually any food choice as long as the allowed point count isn't exceeded.

Some over-the-counter liquid high-protein diets contain such poor-quality (incomplete) protein that they are actually dangerous. The worst are those that contain collagen protein instead of milk or soybean sources.

3. **Surgery.** Sometimes sheer desperation prompts surgical solutions: reducing stomach volume by banding; gastric bypass surgery, which may involve stomach stapling and intestinal bypass surgery, or the more radical biliopancreatic diversion (BPD); and liposuction (removing fat by suctioning).

   BPD rearranges the digestive tract. The surgeon removes up to two-thirds of the stomach and cuts the small intestine in half, suturing one portion to the stomach opening. This diverts pancreatic juice and bile away from the "new intestine," so far fewer nutrients and no fats are absorbed. Patients can eat anything they want without gaining weight, but exceeding the stomach capacity leads to the dumping syndrome (nausea and vomiting).

   Many BPD procedures have been remarkably effective at promoting weight loss and restoring health. Blood pressure returns to normal in many who were originally hypertensive, and sleep apnea is reduced. Additionally, up to 86% of patients with long-standing type 2 diabetes mellitus find they are suddenly diabetes free or demonstrate a dramatic improvement in their regulation of the disease within weeks after the procedure. This result may prove to be the single greatest benefit of BPD.

   Liposuction reshapes the body by suctioning off fat deposits, but it is not a good choice for losing weight. It carries all the risks of surgery, and unless eating habits change, fat depots elsewhere in the body overfill.

4. **Gastrointestinal liners.** A GI liner, which prevents food from contacting the first 20 inches or so of the intestinal wall, is inserted endoscopically through the mouth. Nutrients are still absorbed beyond the liner but in obviously reduced amounts. This device seems to help some obese individuals lose weight.

5. **Diet drugs and weight-loss supplements.** Currently popular weight-loss drugs include phentermine, phendimetrazine, diethylpropion, and orlistat. Phentermine is one-half of the former fen-phen (Redux) combination that caused heart problems, deaths, and litigation for its producer in the 1990s. It acts by increasing sympathetic nervous system activity, which raises blood pressure and heart rate and decreases hunger. Phendimetrazine and diethylpropion have amphetamine-like effects, stimulating the central nervous system to increase heart rate and blood pressure and decrease hunger.

   Orlistat (Xenical) interferes with pancreatic lipase so that part of the fat eaten is not digested or absorbed, which also interferes with the absorption of fat-soluble vitamins. It is effective as a weight-loss agent, but its side effects (diarrhea and anal leakage) are unpleasant to say the least. It also carries the risk of severe liver injury.

   Currently a number of drugs are being developed that act at several different CNS sites, including neuropeptide Y inhibitors.

   Several over-the-counter weight-loss supplements that claim to increase metabolism and burn calories have proved to be very dangerous. For example:

   - Capsules containing usnic acid, a chemical found in some lichens, damages hepatocytes and has led to liver failure in a few cases.
   - Ephedra-containing supplements are notorious—over 100 deaths and 16,000 cases of problems including strokes, seizures, and headaches have been reported.

   When it comes to supplements, the burden of proof is on the U.S. FDA to show that the product is unsafe. For this reason, the true extent of problems caused by weight-loss supplements is not known—while the worst cases attract attention, less serious ones go unreported or undiagnosed.

So are there any good treatments for obesity? To be absolutely honest—not yet. However, animal studies have shown that activating brown fat counteracts weight gain and type 2 diabetes. The possibility that activated brown adipose tissue could deter or reverse obesity is definitely worth exploring.

At present, the only realistic way to lose weight is to take in fewer calories and increase physical activity. Fidgeting helps and so does resistance exercise, which increases muscle mass. Physical exercise depresses appetite and increases metabolic rate not only during activity but also for some time after. The only way to keep the weight off is to make dietary and exercise changes lifelong habits.

and voluntary. BMR accounts for a surprisingly large part of TMR. For example, a woman whose total energy needs per day are about 2000 kcal may spend 1400 kcal or so supporting vital body activities.

Skeletal muscles make up nearly half of body mass, so skeletal muscle activity causes the most dramatic short-term changes in TMR. Even slight increases in muscular work can cause remarkable leaps in TMR and heat production. When a well-trained athlete exercises vigorously for several minutes, TMR may increase 20-fold and remain elevated for several hours after exercise stops.

Food ingestion also induces a rapid increase in TMR. This effect, called **food-induced thermogenesis**, is greatest when proteins and alcohol are ingested. The heightened metabolic

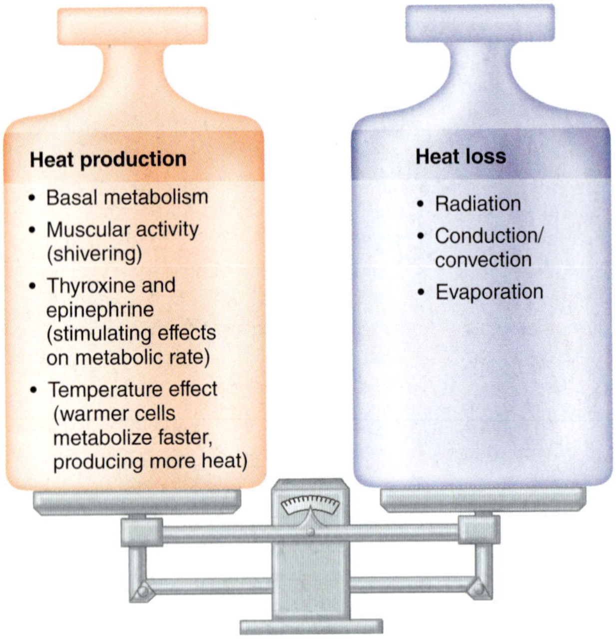

Figure 24.24 Body temperature remains constant as long as heat production and heat loss are balanced.

activity of the liver during such periods probably accounts for the bulk of additional energy use. In contrast, fasting or very low caloric intake depresses TMR and results in a slower breakdown of body reserves.

Check Your Understanding

30. Which of the following contributes to a person's BMR? Kidney function, breathing, jogging, eating, fever.
31. Samantha is tall and slim, but athletic and well toned. Her friend Ginger is short and stocky, bordering on obese. Which would be expected to have a greater BMR, relatively speaking?

For answers, see Appendix H.

24

Regulation of Body Temperature

✓ Distinguish between core and shell body temperature.

✓ Describe how body temperature is regulated, and indicate the common mechanisms regulating heat production/retention and heat loss from the body.

As shown in **Figure 24.24**, body temperature represents the balance between heat production and heat loss. All body tissues produce heat, but those most active metabolically produce the greatest amounts. When the body is at rest, most heat is generated by the liver, heart, brain, kidneys, and endocrine organs, with the inactive skeletal muscles accounting for only 20–30%.

This situation changes dramatically with even slight changes in muscle tone. When we are cold, shivering helps warm us up, and during vigorous exercise, skeletal muscles can produce 30 to 40 times more heat than the rest of the body. A change in muscle activity is one of the most important means of modifying body temperature.

Body temperature averages 37°C ± 0.5°C (98.6°F) and is usually maintained within the range 35.8–38.2°C (96–101°F), despite considerable change in external (air) temperature. A healthy individual's body temperature fluctuates approximately 1°C (1.8°F) in 24 hours, lowest in early morning and highest in late afternoon or early evening.

The adaptive value of temperature homeostasis becomes apparent when we consider how temperature affects enzymatic activity. At normal body temperature, conditions are optimal for enzymatic activity. Rising body temperature accelerates enzymatic catalysis: With each rise of 1°C, the rate of chemical reactions increases about 10%. If temperature rises above the homeostatic range, neurons are depressed and proteins begin to denature. Children below the age of 5 go into convulsions when body temperature reaches 41°C (106°F), and 43°C (about 109°F) appears to be the absolute limit for life.

In contrast, most body tissues can withstand marked reductions in temperature if other conditions are carefully controlled. This fact underlies the use of body cooling during open heart surgery when the heart must be stopped. Low body temperature reduces metabolic rate (and consequently nutrient requirements of body tissues and the heart), allowing more time for surgery without incurring tissue damage.

Core and Shell Temperatures

Different body regions have different resting temperatures. The body's **core** (organs within the skull and the thoracic and abdominal cavities) has the highest temperature and its **shell** (essentially the skin) has the lowest temperature in most circumstances. Of the two body sites used routinely to obtain body temperature clinically, the rectum typically has a temperature about 0.4°C (0.7°F) higher than the mouth and is a better indicator of core temperature.

It is core temperature that is precisely regulated. Blood serves as the major *agent of heat exchange* between the core and shell. Whenever the shell is warmer than the external environment, the body loses heat as warm blood is allowed to flush into skin capillaries. On the other hand, when heat must be conserved, blood largely bypasses the skin. This reduces heat loss and allows the shell temperature to fall toward that of the environment.

For this reason, core temperature stays relatively constant, but the temperature of the shell may fluctuate substantially, for example, between 20°C (68°F) and 40°C (104°F), as it adapts to changes in body activity and external temperature. (You really *can* have cold hands and a warm heart.)

Mechanisms of Heat Exchange

Heat exchange between our skin and the external environment works in the same way as heat exchange between inanimate objects **(Figure 24.25)**. It helps to think of an object's temperature—whether that object is a radiator or your skin—as a guide to its heat content (think "heat concentration"). Then just remember that heat always flows down its concentration gradient from a warmer region to a cooler region. The body uses four mechanisms of heat transfer—radiation, conduction, convection, and evaporation.

Radiation **Radiation** is the loss of heat in the form of infrared waves (thermal energy). Any object that is warmer than objects in its environment—for example, a radiator and (usually) the body—will transfer heat to those objects. Under normal conditions, close to half of your body heat loss occurs by radiation.

Because radiant energy flows from warmer to cooler, radiation explains why a cold room warms up shortly after it fills with people (the "body heat furnace," so to speak). Your body also gains heat by radiation, as demonstrated by the way your skin warms when you sunbathe.

Conduction **Conduction** transfers heat from a warmer object to a cooler one when the two are in direct contact with each other. For example, when you step into a hot tub, some of the heat of the water transfers to your skin, and warm buttocks transfer heat to the seat of a chair by conduction.

Convection **Convection** is the process that occurs because warm air expands and rises and cool air, being denser, falls. Consequently, the warmed air enveloping the body is continually replaced by cooler air molecules. Convection substantially enhances heat transfer from the body surface to the air because the cooler air absorbs heat by conduction more rapidly than the already-warmed air.

Together, conduction and convection account for 15–20% of heat loss to the environment. These processes are enhanced by anything that moves air more rapidly across the body surface, such as wind or a fan, in other words, by *forced convection*.

Evaporation The fourth mechanism by which the body loses heat is **evaporation**. Water evaporates because its molecules absorb heat from the environment and become energetic enough—in other words, vibrate fast enough—to escape as a gas, which we know as water vapor. The heat absorbed by water during evaporation is called **heat of vaporization**. The evaporation of water from body surfaces removes large amounts of body heat. Every gram of water that evaporates removes about 0.58 kcal of heat from the body.

There is a basal level of body heat loss due to the continuous evaporation of water from the lungs and oral mucosa, and through the skin. The unnoticeable water loss occurring via these routes is called **insensible water loss**, and the accompanying heat loss is **insensible heat loss**. Insensible heat loss dissipates about 10% of the basal heat production of the body and is a constant not subject to body temperature controls. When necessary, however, the body's control mechanisms do initiate heat-promoting activities to counterbalance this insensible heat loss.

Evaporative heat loss becomes an active or *sensible* process when body temperature rises and sweating produces increased amounts of water for vaporization. Extreme emotional states activate the sympathetic nervous system, causing body temperature to rise by one degree or so, and vigorous exercise can raise body temperature as much as 2–3°C (3.6–5.4°F). Vigorous muscular activity can produce and evaporate 1–2 L/h of perspiration, removing 600–1200 kcal of heat from the body each hour. This is more than 30 times the amount of heat lost via insensible heat loss!

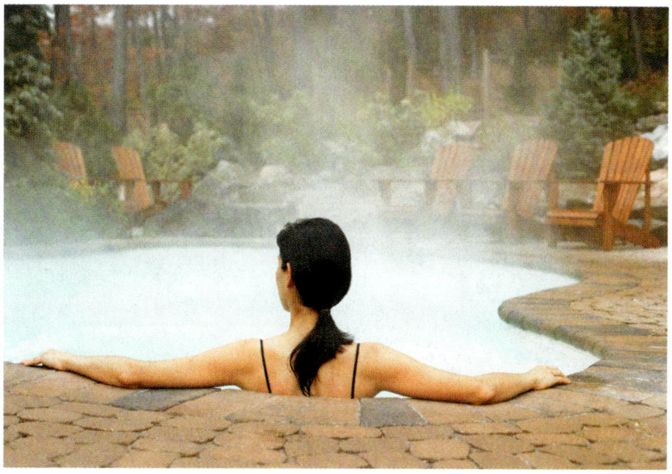

Figure 24.25 Mechanisms of heat exchange. A woman enjoying a hot tub illustrates several mechanisms of heat exchange between the body and its environment. (1) Conduction: Heat transfers from the hot water to the skin. (2) Radiation: Heat transfers from the exposed part of the body to the cooler air. (3) Convection: Warmed air moves away from the body via breezes. There may also be (4) evaporation of perspiration: Excess body heat is carried away.

Homeostatic Imbalance 24.6

When sweating is heavy and prolonged, especially in untrained individuals, losses of water and NaCl may cause painful muscle spasms called *heat cramps*. The solution is simple: Drink fluids. +

Role of the Hypothalamus

Although other brain regions contribute, the hypothalamus, particularly its *preoptic* region, is the main integrating center for thermoregulation. Together the **heat-loss center** (located more anteriorly) and the **heat-promoting center** make up the brain's **thermoregulatory centers**.

The hypothalamus receives afferent input from (1) **peripheral thermoreceptors** located in the shell (the skin), and (2) **central thermoreceptors** sensitive to blood temperature and located in the body core including the anterior portion of the hypothalamus. Much like a thermostat, the hypothalamus responds to this input by reflexively initiating appropriate heat-promoting or heat-loss activities.

The central thermoreceptors are more critically located than the peripheral ones, but varying inputs from the shell probably alert the hypothalamus of the need to prevent temperature changes in the core. In other words, they allow the hypothalamus to anticipate changes to be made.

Heat-Promoting Mechanisms

When the external temperature is low or blood temperature falls for any reason, the heat-promoting center is activated. It triggers one or more of the following four mechanisms to maintain or increase core body temperature (Figure 24.26, bottom).

1. **Constriction of cutaneous blood vessels.** Activation of the sympathetic vasoconstrictor fibers serving the blood

24

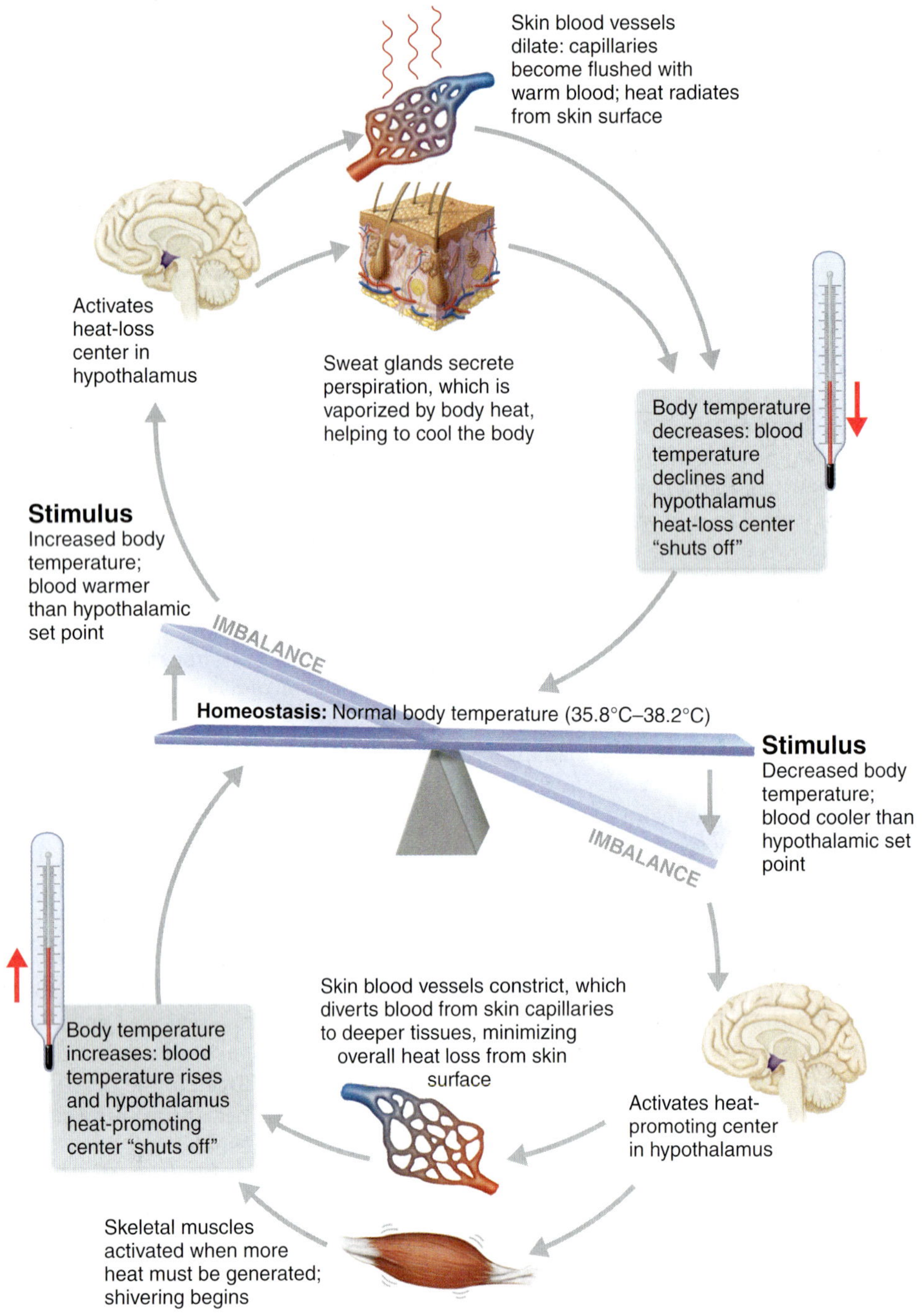

Figure 24.26 Mechanisms of body temperature regulation.

vessels of the skin causes strong vasoconstriction. This restricts blood to deep body areas and largely bypasses the skin. Because a layer of insulating subcutaneous (fatty) tissue separates the skin from deeper organs, this reduces heat loss from the shell dramatically and lowers shell temperature toward that of the external environment.

Homeostatic Imbalance 24.7

Restricting blood flow to the skin is not a problem for a brief period, but if it is prolonged (as during exposure to very cold weather), skin cells deprived of oxygen and nutrients begin to die. This extremely serious condition is *frostbite*. ✚

2. **Shivering.** Shivering—involuntary shuddering contractions—is triggered when brain centers controlling muscle tone are activated and muscle tone reaches sufficient levels to alternately stimulate stretch receptors in antagonistic muscles. Shivering raises body temperature because skeletal muscle activity produces large amounts of heat.
3. **Increase of metabolic rate.** Cold stimulates the adrenal medulla to release epinephrine and norepinephrine in response to sympathetic nerve stimuli, elevating the

metabolic rate and enhancing heat production. This mechanism, called **chemical (nonshivering) thermogenesis**, occurs in infants. Recently, deposits of brown adipose tissue, a special kind of adipose tissue that dissipates energy by producing heat by this mechanism, have also been demonstrated in adult humans.

4. **Enhanced thyroxine release.** When environmental temperature decreases gradually, as in the transition from summer to winter, the hypothalamus of infants releases *thyrotropin-releasing hormone*. This hormone activates the anterior pituitary to release *thyroid-stimulating hormone*, which induces the thyroid to liberate more thyroid hormone to the blood. Because thyroid hormone raises metabolic rate, body heat production rises. Adults do not show a similar TSH response to cold exposure.

Besides these involuntary adjustments, we humans make a number of *behavioral modifications* to prevent overcooling of our body core:

- Putting on more or warmer clothing to restrict heat loss (hat, gloves, and "insulated" outer garments)
- Drinking hot fluids
- Changing posture to reduce exposed body surface area (hunching over or clasping the arms across the chest)
- Increasing physical activity to generate more heat (jumping up and down, clapping the hands)

Heat-Loss Mechanisms

Heat-loss mechanisms protect the body from excessively high temperatures. Most heat loss occurs through the skin via radiation, conduction, convection, and evaporation.

How do heat-exchange mechanisms help us lose heat? The answer is quite simple. Whenever core body temperature rises above normal, it inhibits the hypothalamic heat-promoting center. At the same time, it activates the heat-loss center and triggers one or both of the following (Figure 24.26, top):

1. **Dilation of cutaneous blood vessels.** Inhibiting the vasomotor fibers serving blood vessels of the skin allows the vessels to dilate. As the blood vessels swell with warm blood, the shell loses heat by radiation, conduction, and convection.
2. **Enhanced sweating.** If the body is extremely overheated or if the environment is so hot—over 33°C (about 92°F)—that heat cannot be lost by other means, evaporation becomes necessary. Sympathetic fibers activate the sweat glands to spew out large amounts of perspiration. Evaporation of perspiration is an efficient means of ridding the body of surplus heat as long as the air is dry.

However, when the relative humidity is high, evaporation occurs much more slowly. In such cases, the heat-liberating mechanisms cannot work well, and we feel miserable and irritable. Behavioral or voluntary measures commonly taken to reduce body heat in such circumstances include

- Reducing activity ("laying low")
- Seeking a cooler environment (a shady spot) or using a device to increase convection (a fan) or cooling (an air conditioner)
- Wearing light-colored, loose clothing that reflects radiant energy. (This is actually cooler than being nude because bare skin absorbs most of the radiant energy striking it.)

Homeostatic Imbalance 24.8

Overexposure to a hot and humid environment makes normal heat-loss processes ineffective. The resulting **hyperthermia** (elevated body temperature) depresses the hypothalamus. At a core temperature of around 41°C (105°F), heat-control mechanisms are suspended, creating a vicious *positive feedback cycle*. Increasing temperatures increase the metabolic rate, which increases heat production. The skin becomes hot and dry and, as the temperature continues to spiral upward, multiple organ damage becomes a distinct possibility, including brain damage. This condition, called **heat stroke**, can be fatal unless corrective measures are initiated immediately (immersing the body in cool water and administering fluids).

The terms *heat exhaustion* and *exertion-induced heat exhaustion* are often used to describe the heat-associated extreme sweating and collapse of an individual during or following vigorous physical activity. This condition, evidenced by elevated body temperature and mental confusion and/or fainting, is due to dehydration and consequent low blood pressure. In contrast to heat stroke, heat-loss mechanisms are still functional in heat exhaustion. However, heat exhaustion can rapidly progress to heat stroke if the body is not cooled and rehydrated promptly.

Hypothermia (hi″po-ther′me-ah) is low body temperature resulting from prolonged uncontrolled exposure to cold. Vital signs (respiratory rate, blood pressure, and heart rate) decrease as cellular enzymes become sluggish. Drowsiness sets in and, oddly, the person becomes comfortable even though previously he or she felt extremely cold. Shivering stops at a core temperature of 30–32°C (87–90°F) when the body has exhausted its heat-generating capabilities. Uncorrected, hypothermia progresses to coma and finally death (by cardiac arrest), when body temperatures approach 21°C (70°F). +

Fever

Fever is *controlled hyperthermia*. Most often, it results from infection somewhere in the body, but it may be caused by cancer, allergic reactions, or CNS injuries.

Whatever the cause, macrophages and other cells release cytokines, originally called *pyrogens* (literally, "fire starters"), at least two of which are now known to be interleukins. These chemicals act on the hypothalamus, causing release of prostaglandins which reset the hypothalamic thermostat to a higher-than-normal temperature, so that heat-promoting mechanisms kick in. As a result of vasoconstriction, heat loss from the body surface declines, the skin cools, and shivering begins to generate heat. These "chills" are a sure sign body temperature is rising.

The temperature rises until it reaches the new setting, and then is maintained at that setting until natural body defenses or medications reverse the disease process. Chemical messengers called *cryogens* (vasopressin and others) prevent fever from becoming excessive and reset the thermostat to a lower (or normal) level. Then, heat-loss mechanisms swing into action.

Sweating begins and the skin becomes flushed and warm. Physicians have long recognized these signs as signals that body temperature is falling (aah, she has passed the crisis). As we explained in Chapter 21, fever speeds healing by increasing the metabolic rate, and it also appears to inhibit bacterial growth.

☑ Check Your Understanding

32. What is the body's core?
33. Cindy is flushed and her teeth are chattering even though her bedroom temperature is 72°F. Why do you think this is happening?
34. How does convection differ from conduction in causing heat loss?

For answers, see Appendix H.

Developmental Aspects of Nutrition and Metabolism

✓ Describe the effects of inadequate protein intake on the fetal nervous system.

✓ Describe the cause and consequences of the low metabolic rate typical of the elderly.

✓ List ways that medications commonly used by aged people may influence their nutrition and health.

Good nutrition is essential in utero, as well as throughout life. If the mother is ill nourished, the development of her infant is affected. Most serious is the lack of adequate calories, proteins, and vitamins needed for fetal tissue growth, especially brain growth. Additionally, inadequate nutrients during the first three years after birth will lead to mental deficits or learning disorders because brain growth continues during this time. Proteins are needed for muscle and bone growth, and calcium is required for strong bones. Although anabolic processes are less critical after growth is completed, sufficient nutrients are still essential to maintain normal tissue replacement and metabolism.

Homeostatic Imbalance 24.9

There are many inborn errors of metabolism (or genetic disorders), but perhaps the two most common are *cystic fibrosis* (see Chapter 22) and *phenylketonuria* (*PKU*) (fen″il-ke″to-nu′re-ah).

In PKU, tissue cells are unable to use the amino acid phenylalanine (fen″il-al′ah-nēn), which is present in all protein foods. The defect involves a deficiency of the enzyme that converts phenylalanine to tyrosine. Phenylalanine cannot be metabolized, so it and its deaminated products accumulate in the blood and act as neurotoxins that cause brain damage and retardation within a few months. These consequences are uncommon today because most states require a urine or blood test to identify affected newborns, and these children are put on a low-phenylalanine diet. Expectant women with PKU are sometimes encouraged to follow a controlled phenylalanine diet during their pregnancy.

There are a number of other enzyme defects, classified according to the impaired process as carbohydrate, lipid, or mineral metabolic disorders. The carbohydrate deficit *galactosemia* results from an abnormality in or lack of the liver enzymes needed to transform galactose to glucose. Galactose accumulates in the blood and leads to mental deficits.

In the carbohydrate disorder *glycogen storage disease*, glycogen synthesis is normal, but one of the enzymes needed to convert it back to glucose is missing. As excessive amounts of glycogen are stored, its storage organs (liver and skeletal muscles) become glutted with glycogen and enlarge tremendously. ✚

With the exception of *type 1 diabetes mellitus*, children free of genetic disorders rarely exhibit metabolic problems. However, by middle age and particularly old age, *type 2 diabetes mellitus* becomes a major problem, particularly in people who are obese.

Metabolic rate declines throughout the life span. In old age, muscle and bone wasting and declining efficiency of the endocrine system take their toll. Because many elderly are also less active, the metabolic rate is sometimes so low that it becomes nearly impossible to obtain adequate nutrition without gaining weight. The elderly also use more medications than any other group, at a time of life when the liver has become less efficient in its detoxifying duties.

Many drugs and popular remedies influence nutrition. For example:

- Some diuretics prescribed for congestive heart failure or hypertension (to flush fluids out of the body) can cause severe hypokalemia by promoting excessive loss of potassium.
- Some antibiotics—for example, sulfa drugs, tetracycline, and penicillin—interfere with food digestion and absorption. They may also cause diarrhea, further decreasing absorption.
- Although physicians discourage its use because it interferes with absorption of fat-soluble vitamins, mineral oil is still a popular laxative with the elderly.
- About half the elderly in the U.S. consume alcohol. When it is substituted for food, nutrient stores can be depleted. Excessive alcohol intake leads to absorption problems, certain vitamin and mineral deficiencies, deranged metabolism, and damage to the liver and pancreas.

Although malnutrition and a waning metabolic rate present problems to some elderly, certain nutrients—notably glucose—appear to contribute to the aging process in all of us. Nonenzymatic reactions (the so-called *browning reactions*) between glucose and proteins, long known to discolor and toughen foods, may have the same effects on body proteins. When enzymes attach sugars to proteins, they do so at specific sites and the glycoproteins produced play well-defined roles in the body. By contrast, nonenzymatic binding of glucose to proteins (a process that increases with age) is haphazard and eventually causes cross-links between proteins. This type of binding probably contributes to lens clouding, and the general tissue stiffening and loss of elasticity so common in the aged.

Check Your Understanding

35. List at least two reasons that metabolic rate declines in old age.
36. List two types of drugs or over-the-counter products that can interfere with the nutrition of elderly people.

For answers, see Appendix H.

Nutrition is one of the most overlooked areas in clinical medicine. Yet, what we eat and drink influences nearly every phase of metabolism and plays a major role in our overall health. Now that we have examined the fates of nutrients in body cells, we are ready to study the urinary system, the organ system that works tirelessly to rid the body of nitrogen wastes resulting from metabolism and to maintain the purity of our internal fluids.

Chapter Summary

MAP™ For more chapter study tools, go to the Study Area of MasteringA&P at **www.masteringaandp.com**.
There you will find:
- Interactive Physiology iP
- A&PFlix A&PFlix
- Practice Anatomy Lab PAL
- PhysioEx PEx
- Videos, Practice Quizzes and Tests, MP3 Tutor Sessions, Case Studies, and much more!

Diet and Nutrition (pp. 907–913)

1. Nutrients include water, carbohydrates, lipids, proteins, vitamins, and minerals. The bulk of the organic nutrients is used as fuel to produce cellular energy (ATP). The energy value of foods is measured in kilocalories (kcal).
2. Essential nutrients are those that are inadequately synthesized by body cells and must be ingested in the diet.

Carbohydrates (p. 908)

3. Carbohydrates are obtained primarily from plant products. Absorbed monosaccharides other than glucose are converted to glucose by the liver.
4. Monosaccharides are used primarily for cellular fuel. Small amounts are used for nucleic acid synthesis and to add sugar residues to plasma membranes.
5. Recommended carbohydrate intake for adults is 45–65% of daily caloric intake.

Lipids (pp. 908–910)

6. Most dietary lipids are triglycerides. The primary sources of saturated fats are animal products, tropical oils, and hydrogenated oils; unsaturated fats are present in plant products, nuts, and cold-water fish. The major sources of cholesterol are egg yolk, meats, and milk products.
7. Linoleic and linolenic acids are essential fatty acids.
8. Triglycerides provide reserve energy, cushion body organs, and insulate the body. Phospholipids are used to synthesize plasma membranes and myelin. Cholesterol is used in plasma membranes and is the structural basis of vitamin D, steroid hormones, and bile salts.
9. Fat intake should represent 30% or less of caloric intake, and saturated and trans fats should be replaced by mono- and polyunsaturated fats if possible.

Proteins (pp. 910–911)

10. Animal products provide high-quality complete protein containing all 10 essential amino acids. Most plant products lack one or more of the essential amino acids.
11. Amino acids are the structural building blocks of the body and of important regulatory molecules.
12. Protein synthesis can and will occur if all essential amino acids are present and sufficient carbohydrate (or fat) calories are available to produce ATP. Otherwise, amino acids will be burned for energy.
13. Nitrogen balance occurs when protein synthesis equals protein loss.
14. A dietary intake of 0.8 g of protein per kg of body weight is recommended for most healthy adults.

Vitamins (pp. 911–913)

15. Vitamins are organic compounds needed in minute amounts. Most act as coenzymes. The richest sources are whole grains, vegetables, legumes, and fruit.
16. Except for vitamin D and the K and B vitamins made by enteric bacteria, vitamins are not made in the body.
17. Water-soluble vitamins (B and C) are not stored to excess in the body. Fat-soluble vitamins include vitamins A, D, E, and K; all but vitamin K are stored and can accumulate to toxic amounts.

Minerals (p. 913)

18. Besides calcium, phosphorus, potassium, sulfur, sodium, chloride, and magnesium, the body requires trace amounts of at least a dozen other minerals.
19. Minerals are not used for energy. Some are used to mineralize bone; others are bound to organic compounds or exist as ions in body fluids, where they play various roles in cell processes and metabolism.
20. Mineral uptake and excretion are carefully regulated to prevent mineral toxicity. The richest sources of minerals are some meats, vegetables, nuts, and legumes.

Overview of Metabolic Reactions (pp. 913–917)

1. Metabolism encompasses all chemical reactions necessary to maintain life. Metabolic processes are either anabolic or catabolic.
2. Cellular respiration refers to catabolic processes during which energy is released and some is captured in ATP bonds.
3. Energy is released when organic compounds are oxidized. Cellular oxidation is accomplished primarily by removing hydrogen (electrons). When molecules are oxidized, others are simultaneously reduced by accepting hydrogen (or electrons).
4. Most enzymes catalyzing oxidation-reduction reactions require coenzymes as hydrogen acceptors. Two important coenzymes in these reactions are NAD^+ and FAD.
5. In animal cells, the two mechanisms of ATP synthesis are substrate-level phosphorylation and oxidative phosphorylation.

iP Muscular System; Topic: Muscle Metabolism, pp. 3–8.

24

Metabolism of Major Nutrients (pp. 917–930)

Carbohydrate Metabolism (pp. 917–925)

1. Carbohydrate metabolism is essentially glucose metabolism.
2. Phosphorylation of glucose on entry into cells effectively traps it in most tissue cells.
3. Glucose is oxidized to carbon dioxide and water via three successive pathways: glycolysis, Krebs cycle, and electron transport chain. Some ATP is harvested in each pathway, but the bulk is captured in the electron transport chain.
4. Glycolysis is a reversible pathway in which glucose is converted to two pyruvic acid molecules; two molecules of reduced NAD^+ are formed, and there is a net gain of 2 ATP. Under aerobic conditions, pyruvic acid enters the Krebs cycle; under anaerobic conditions, it is reduced to lactic acid.
5. The Krebs cycle is fueled by pyruvic acid (and fatty acids). To enter the cycle, pyruvic acid is converted to acetyl CoA. The acetyl CoA is then oxidized and decarboxylated. Complete oxidation of two pyruvic acid molecules yields 6 CO_2, 8 NADH + H^+, 2 $FADH_2$, and a net gain of 2 ATP. Much of the energy originally present in the bonds of pyruvic acid is now present in the reduced coenzymes.
6. In the electron transport chain, (a) reduced coenzymes are oxidized by delivering hydrogen to a series of oxidation-reduction acceptors; (b) hydrogen is split into hydrogen ions and electrons (as electrons run downhill from acceptor to acceptor, the energy released is used to pump H^+ into the mitochondrial intermembrane space, which creates an electrochemical proton gradient); (c) the energy stored in the electrochemical proton gradient drives H^+ back through ATP synthase, which uses the energy to form ATP; (d) H^+ and electrons are combined with oxygen to form water.
7. For each glucose molecule oxidized to carbon dioxide and water, there is a net gain of 32 ATP: 4 ATP from substrate-level phosphorylation and 28 ATP from oxidative phosphorylation. The shuttle for reduced NAD^+ produced in the cytosol may use 2 ATP of that amount.
8. When cellular ATP reserves are high, glucose catabolism is inhibited and glucose is converted to glycogen (glycogenesis) or to fat (lipogenesis). Much more fat than glycogen is stored.
9. When blood glucose levels begin to fall, glycogenolysis occurs, in which glycogen stores are converted to glucose. The liver can also perform gluconeogenesis, the formation of glucose from noncarbohydrate (fat or protein) molecules.

24

iP Muscular System; Topic: Muscle Metabolism, pp. 10–22.

Lipid Metabolism (pp. 926–928)

10. End products of lipid digestion (and cholesterol) are transported in blood in the form of chylomicrons.
11. Glycerol is converted to glyceraldehyde 3-phosphate and enters the Krebs cycle or is converted to glucose.
12. Fatty acids are oxidized by beta oxidation into acetic acid fragments. These are bound to coenzyme A and enter the Krebs cycle as acetyl CoA. Dietary fats not needed for energy or structural materials are stored in adipose tissue.
13. There is a continual turnover of fats in fat depots. Breakdown of fats to fatty acids and glycerol is called lipolysis.
14. When excessive amounts of fats are used, the liver converts acetyl CoA to ketone bodies and releases them to the blood. Excessive levels of ketone bodies (ketosis) lead to metabolic acidosis.
15. All cells use phospholipids and cholesterol to build their plasma membranes. The liver forms many functional molecules from lipids.

Protein Metabolism (pp. 928–930)

16. To be oxidized for energy, amino acids are converted to keto acids that can enter the Krebs cycle. This involves transamination, oxidative deamination, and keto acid modification.
17. Amine groups removed during deamination (as ammonia) are combined with carbon dioxide by the liver to form urea. Urea is excreted in urine.
18. Deaminated amino acids may also be converted to fatty acids and glucose.
19. Amino acids are the body's most important building blocks. Nonessential amino acids are made in the liver by transamination.
20. In adults, most protein synthesis serves to replace tissue proteins and to maintain nitrogen balance.
21. Protein synthesis requires the presence of all 10 essential amino acids. If any are lacking, amino acids are used as energy fuels.

Metabolic States of the Body (pp. 930–935)

Catabolic-Anabolic Steady State of the Body (pp. 930–931)

1. The amino acid pool provides amino acids for synthesis of proteins and amino acid derivatives, ATP synthesis, and energy storage. To be stored, amino acids are first deaminated and then converted to fats or glycogen.
2. The carbohydrate-fat pool primarily provides fuels for ATP synthesis and other molecules that can be stored as energy reserves.
3. The nutrient pools are connected by the bloodstream; fats, carbohydrates, and proteins may be interconverted via common intermediates.

Absorptive State (pp. 931–933)

4. During the absorptive state (during and shortly after a meal), glucose is the major energy source; needed structural and functional molecules are made; excess carbohydrates, fats, and amino acids are stored as glycogen and fat.
5. Events of the absorptive state are controlled by insulin, which enhances the entry of glucose (and amino acids) into cells and accelerates its use for ATP synthesis or storage as glycogen or fat.

Postabsorptive State (pp. 933–935)

6. The postabsorptive state is the period when bloodborne fuels are provided by breakdown of energy reserves. Glucose is made available to the blood by glycogenolysis, lipolysis, and gluconeogenesis. Glucose sparing begins. During prolonged fasting, the brain also begins to metabolize ketone bodies.
7. Events of the postabsorptive state are controlled largely by glucagon and the sympathetic nervous system, which mobilize glycogen and fat reserves and trigger gluconeogenesis.

The Metabolic Role of the Liver (pp. 935–938)

1. The liver is the body's main metabolic organ and it plays a crucial role in processing (or storing) virtually every nutrient group. It helps maintain blood energy sources, metabolizes hormones, and detoxifies drugs and other substances.

Cholesterol Metabolism and Regulation of Blood Cholesterol Levels (pp. 935–938)

2. The liver synthesizes cholesterol, catabolizes cholesterol and secretes it in the form of bile salts, and makes lipoproteins. The liver makes a basal amount of cholesterol (85%) even when dietary cholesterol intake is excessive.

3. LDLs transport triglycerides and cholesterol from the liver to the tissues, whereas HDLs transport cholesterol from the tissues to the liver (for catabolism and elimination).
4. Excessively high LDL levels are implicated in atherosclerosis, cardiovascular disease, and stroke.

Energy Balance (pp. 938–948)

1. Body energy intake (derived from food oxidation) is precisely balanced by energy output (heat, work, and energy storage). Eventually, all of the energy intake is converted to heat.

Obesity (p. 939)

2. When energy balance is maintained, weight remains stable. When excess amounts of energy are stored, the result is obesity (condition of excessive fat storage resulting in a BMI above 30).

Regulation of Food Intake (pp. 939–941)

3. The hypothalamus (particularly its arcuate nucleus) and other brain centers are involved in regulating eating behavior.
4. Factors thought to be involved in regulating food intake include (a) neural signals from the gut to the brain; (b) nutrient signals related to total energy storage; (c) plasma concentrations of hormones that control events of the absorptive and postabsorptive states, and hormones that provide feedback signals to brain feeding centers (leptin appears to exert the main long-term controls of appetite and energy metabolism); (d) body temperature, psychological factors, and others.

Metabolic Rate and Heat Production (pp. 941–944)

5. Energy used by the body per hour is the metabolic rate.
6. Basal metabolic rate (BMR), reported in $kcal/m^2/h$, is the measurement obtained when the person is at comfortable room temperature, supine, relaxed, and in the postabsorptive state. BMR indicates energy needed to drive only the resting body processes.
7. Factors influencing metabolic rate include body surface area, age and gender, body temperature, stress, and thyroxine; also the specific dynamic action of foods, and muscular activity.

Regulation of Body Temperature (pp. 944–948)

8. Body temperature reflects the balance between heat production and heat loss and is normally 37°C ($\pm$ 0.5°C), which is optimal for physiological activities.
9. At rest, most body heat is produced by the liver, heart, brain, kidneys, and endocrine organs. Activation of skeletal muscles causes dramatic increases in body heat production.
10. The body core (organs within the skull and the ventral body cavity) generally has the highest temperature. The shell (the skin) is the heat-exchange surface, and is usually coolest.
11. Blood serves as the major heat-exchange agent between the core and the shell. When skin capillaries are flushed with blood and the skin is warmer than the environment, the body loses heat. When blood is withdrawn to deep organs, heat loss from the shell is inhibited.
12. Heat-exchange mechanisms include radiation, conduction, convection, and evaporation. Evaporation, the conversion of water to water vapor, requires the absorption of heat. For each gram of water vaporized, about 0.6 kcal of heat is absorbed.
13. The hypothalamus acts as the body's thermostat. Its heat-promotion and heat-loss centers receive inputs from peripheral and central thermoreceptors, integrate these inputs, and initiate responses leading to heat loss or heat promotion.
14. Heat-promoting mechanisms include constriction of skin vasculature, and shivering. If environmental cold is prolonged, the thyroid gland may be stimulated to release more thyroxine.
15. When heat must be removed from the body, dermal blood vessels dilate, allowing heat loss through radiation, conduction, and convection. When greater heat loss is mandated (or the environmental temperature is so high that radiation and conduction are ineffective), sweating is initiated. Evaporation of perspiration is an efficient means of heat loss as long as the humidity is low.
16. Profuse sweating can lead to heat exhaustion, indicated by a rise in temperature, a drop in blood pressure, and collapse. When the body cannot rid itself of surplus heat, body temperature rises to the point where all thermoregulatory mechanisms become ineffective—a potentially lethal condition called heat stroke.
17. Fever is controlled hyperthermia, which follows thermostat resetting to higher levels by prostaglandins and initiation of heat-promotion mechanisms, evidenced by the chills. When the disease process is reversed, heat-loss mechanisms are initiated.

Developmental Aspects of Nutrition and Metabolism (pp. 948–949)

1. Good nutrition is essential for normal fetal development and normal growth during childhood.
2. Inborn errors of metabolism include cystic fibrosis, PKU, glycogen storage disease, galactosemia, and many others. Hormonal disorders, such as lack of insulin or thyroid hormone, may also lead to metabolic abnormalities. Diabetes mellitus is the most significant metabolic disorder in middle-aged and older adults.
3. In old age, metabolic rate declines as enzyme and endocrine systems become less efficient and skeletal muscles atrophy. Reduced caloric needs make it difficult to obtain adequate nutrition without becoming overweight.
4. Elderly individuals ingest more medications than any other age group, and many of these drugs negatively affect their nutrition.

Review Questions

Multiple Choice/Matching

(Some questions have more than one correct answer. Select the best answer or answers from the choices given.)

1. Which of the following reactions would liberate the most energy? **(a)** complete oxidation of a molecule of sucrose to CO_2 and water, **(b)** conversion of a molecule of ADP to ATP, **(c)** respiration of a molecule of glucose to lactic acid, **(d)** conversion of a molecule of glucose to carbon dioxide and water.
2. The formation of glucose from glycogen is **(a)** gluconeogenesis, **(b)** glycogenesis, **(c)** glycogenolysis, **(d)** glycolysis.
3. The net gain of ATP from the complete metabolism (aerobic) of glucose is closest to **(a)** 2, **(b)** 30, **(c)** 3, **(d)** 4.

4. Which of the following best defines cellular respiration? **(a)** intake of carbon dioxide and output of oxygen by cells, **(b)** excretion of waste products, **(c)** inhalation of oxygen and exhalation of carbon dioxide, **(d)** oxidation of substances by which energy is released in usable form to the cells.
5. What is formed during aerobic respiration when electrons are passed down the electron transport chain? **(a)** oxygen, **(b)** water, **(c)** glucose, **(d)** $NADH + H^+$.
6. Metabolic rate is relatively low in **(a)** youth, **(b)** physical exercise, **(c)** old age, **(d)** fever.
7. In a temperate climate under ordinary conditions, the greatest loss of body heat occurs through **(a)** radiation, **(b)** conduction, **(c)** evaporation, **(d)** none of the above.
8. Which of the following is not a function of the liver? **(a)** glycogenolysis and gluconeogenesis, **(b)** synthesis of cholesterol, **(c)** detoxification of alcohol and drugs, **(d)** synthesis of glucagon, **(e)** deamination of amino acids.
9. Amino acids are essential (and important) to the body for all the following except **(a)** production of some hormones, **(b)** production of antibodies, **(c)** formation of most structural materials, **(d)** as a source of quick energy.
10. A person has been on a hunger strike for seven days. Compared to normal, he has **(a)** increased release of fatty acids from adipose tissue, and ketosis, **(b)** elevated glucose concentration in the blood, **(c)** increased plasma insulin concentration, **(d)** increased glycogen synthase (enzyme) activity in the liver.
11. Transamination is a chemical process by which **(a)** protein is synthesized, **(b)** an amine group is transferred from an amino acid to a keto acid, **(c)** an amine group is cleaved from the amino acid, **(d)** amino acids are broken down for energy.
12. Three days after removing the pancreas from an animal, the researcher finds a persistent increase in **(a)** acetoacetic acid concentration in the blood, **(b)** urine volume, **(c)** blood glucose, **(d)** all of the above.
13. Hunger, appetite, obesity, and physical activity are interrelated. Thus, **(a)** hunger sensations arise primarily from the stimulation of receptors in the stomach and intestinal tract in response to the absence of food in these organs; **(b)** obesity, in most cases, is a result of the abnormally high enzymatic activity of the fat-synthesizing enzymes in adipose tissue; **(c)** in all cases of obesity, the energy content of the ingested food has exceeded the energy expenditure of the body; **(d)** in a normal individual, increasing blood glucose concentration increases hunger sensations.
14. Body temperature regulation is **(a)** influenced by temperature receptors in the skin, **(b)** influenced by the temperature of the blood perfusing the heat regulation centers of the brain, **(c)** subject to both neural and hormonal control, **(d)** all of the above.
15. Which of the following yields the greatest caloric value per gram? **(a)** fats, **(b)** proteins, **(c)** carbohydrates, **(d)** all are equal in caloric value.

Short Answer Essay Questions

16. What is cellular respiration? What is the common role of FAD and NAD^+ in cellular respiration?
17. Describe the site, major events, and outcomes of glycolysis.
18. Pyruvic acid is a product of glycolysis, but it is not the substance that joins with the pickup molecule to enter the Krebs cycle. What is that substance?
19. Define glycogenesis, glycogenolysis, gluconeogenesis, and lipogenesis. Which is (are) likely to be occurring (a) shortly after a carbohydrate-rich meal, (b) just before waking up in the morning?
20. What is the harmful result when excessive amounts of fats are burned for energy? Name two conditions that might lead to this result.
21. Make a flowchart that indicates the pivotal intermediates through which glucose can be converted to fat.
22. Distinguish between the role of HDLs and that of LDLs.
23. List some factors that influence plasma cholesterol levels. Also list the sources and fates of cholesterol in the body.
24. What is meant by "body energy balance," and what happens if the balance is not precise?
25. Explain the effect of the following on metabolic rate: thyroxine levels, eating, body surface area, muscular exercise, emotional stress, starvation.
26. Explain the terms "core" and "shell" relative to body temperature balance. What serves as the heat-transfer agent from one to the other?
27. Compare and contrast mechanisms of heat loss with mechanisms of heat promotion, and explain how these mechanisms determine body temperature.

Critical Thinking and Clinical Application Questions

1. Calculate the number of ATP molecules that can be harvested during the complete oxidation of an 18-carbon fatty acid. (Take a deep breath and think about it—you can do it.)
2. Every year dozens of elderly people are found dead in their unheated apartments and listed as victims of hypothermia. What is hypothermia, and how does it kill? Why are the elderly more susceptible to hypothermia than the young?
3. Frank Moro has been diagnosed as having severe atherosclerosis and high blood cholesterol levels. He is told that he is at risk for a stroke or a heart attack. First, what foods would you suggest that he avoid like the plague? What foods would you suggest he add or substitute? What activities would you recommend?
4. In the 1940s, some physicians prescribed low doses of a chemical called dinitrophenol (DNP) to help patients lose weight. This drug therapy was abandoned after a few patients died. DNP uncouples the chemiosmotic machinery. Explain how this causes weight loss.
5. While attempting to sail solo from Los Angeles to Tahiti, Simon encountered a storm that marooned him on an uninhabited island. He was able, using his ingenuity and a pocket knife, to obtain plenty of fish to eat, and roots were plentiful. However, the island was barren of fruits and soon his gums began to bleed and he started to develop several infections. Analyze his problem.
6. Gregor, a large beefy man, came home from the doctor's office and complained to his wife that his blood tests "were bad." He told her that the doctor said he would have to give up some of his steaks and butter. He went on to mourn the fact that he would have to start eating more cottage cheese and olive oil instead. What kind of problem was revealed by his "bad" blood tests? How should his wife respond to his choice of food substitutes and why? What foods should she suggest?

AT THE CLINIC

Related Clinical Terms

Appetite A desire for food. A psychological phenomenon dependent on memory and associations, as opposed to hunger, which is a physiological need to eat.

Familial hypercholesterolemia (hi″per-ko-les″ter-ol-e′me-ah). An inherited condition in which the LDL receptors are absent or abnormal, the uptake of cholesterol by tissue cells is blocked, and the total concentration of cholesterol (and LDLs) in the blood is enormously elevated. Atherosclerosis develops at an early age, heart attacks begin in the third or fourth decade, and most die by age 60 from coronary artery disease. Treatment entails dietary modifications, exercise, and cholesterol-reducing drugs.

Kwashiorkor (kwash″e-or′kor) Severe protein and calorie deficiency which is particularly devastating in children, resulting in mental retardation and failure to grow. A consequence of malnutrition or starvation, it is characterized by a bloated abdomen because the amount of plasma proteins is inadequate to keep fluid in the bloodstream. Skin lesions and infections are likely.

Marasmus (mah-raz′mus) Protein-calorie malnutrition, accompanied by progressive wasting. Often due to ingesting food of very poor quality. Growth for age is severely stunted.

Pica (pi′kah) Craving and eating substances not normally considered nutrients, such as clay, cornstarch, or dirt.

Skin-fold test Clinical test of body fatness. A skin fold in the back of the arm or below the scapula is measured with a caliper. A fold over 1 inch in thickness indicates excess fat. Also called the fat-fold test.

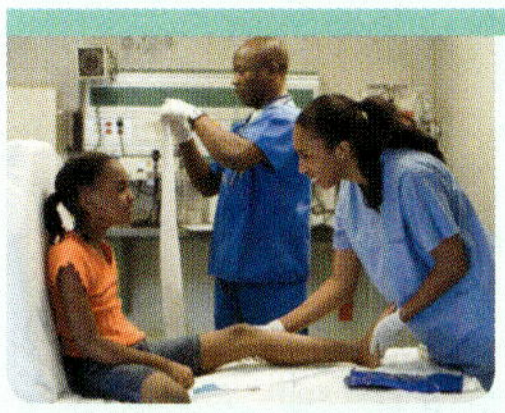

Case Study Nutrition and Metabolism

Kyle Boulard, a 35-year-old male, is believed to be one of the primary causes of the accident on Route 91. Passengers on the bus reported that Mr. Boulard was clearly intoxicated when he boarded the bus. According to these reports, Mr. Boulard behaved erratically, appeared disoriented, and left his seat and staggered down the aisle. Just prior to the accident, he had stumbled into the driver's compartment. Paramedics found Mr. Boulard in a disoriented state when they arrived on the scene, but noted only minor injuries. A "fruity acetone combined with alcohol" smell was noted on his breath. What follows is a summary of the notable test results:

General	Blood	Urine
BP: 95/58	pH: 7.1	Odor: "fruity acetone"
HR: 110	Glucose: 345 mg/dl	pH: 4.3
	Ketone bodies: 22 mg/dl	Glucose: strongly positive
	Blood alcohol: 110 mg/dl	

1. Urine glucose is usually negative. Using the information in Appendix F, look up normal values for blood pH, blood glucose, blood ketone bodies, and urine pH, and identify whether each test result is normal or abnormal.
2. A "fruity acetone combined with alcohol" smell was detected in Mr. Boulard's breath, and in his urine. Which substance is producing the "fruity acetone" smell?
3. Where in the body are ketone bodies produced? What energy source does the body use to produce these substances?
4. The production of large amounts of ketone bodies is often seen when glucose is not readily available as an energy source (e.g., in starvation). In Mr. Boulard's case, large amounts of glucose are in the blood. Explain why his body is producing ketones in the presence of such large amounts of glucose.
5. Explain how the pH of Mr. Boulard's blood and urine is related to the ketone bodies measured in each of these fluids.

(Answers in Appendix H)

24

25

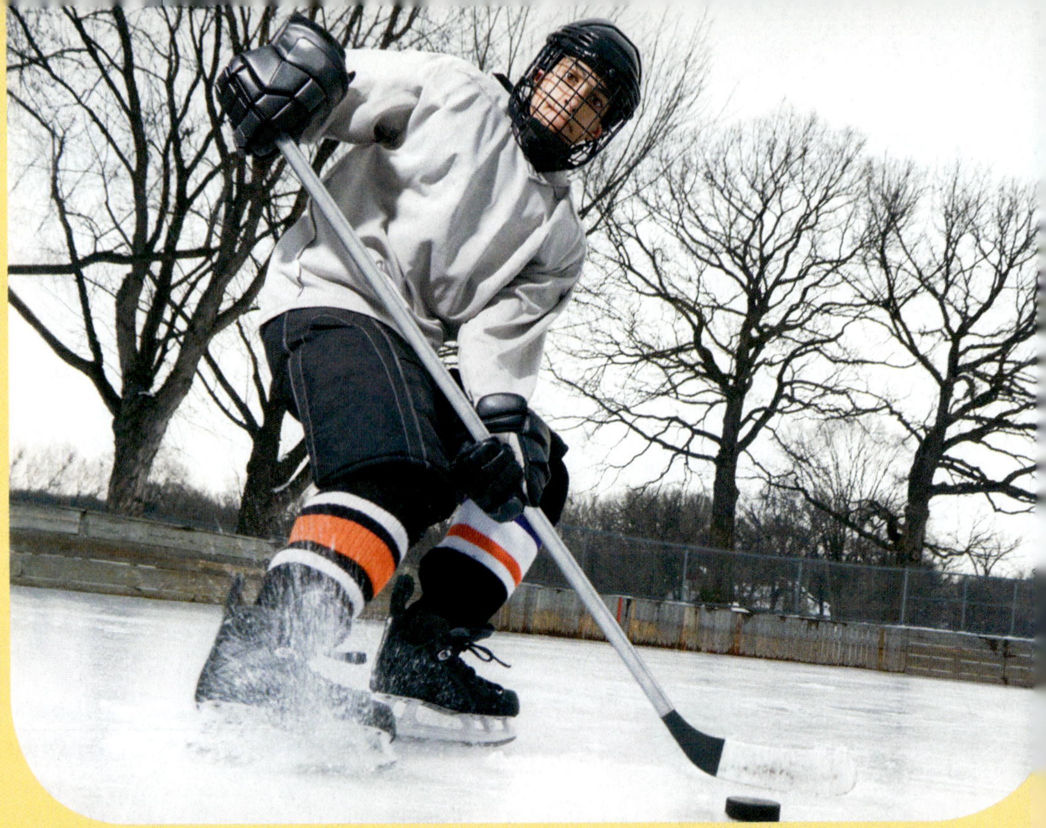

The Urinary System

Every day the kidneys filter nearly 200 liters of fluid from our bloodstream, allowing toxins, metabolic wastes, and excess ions to leave the body in urine while returning needed substances to the blood. Much like a water purification plant that keeps a city's water drinkable and disposes of its wastes, the kidneys are usually unappreciated until they malfunction and body fluids become contaminated.

The kidneys perform a chemical balancing act that would be tricky even for the best chemical engineer. They maintain the body's internal environment by:

- Regulating the total volume of water in the body and the total concentration of solutes in that water (osmolality).
- Regulating the concentrations of the various ions in the extracellular fluids. (Even relatively small changes in some ion concentrations such as K^+ can be fatal.)
- Ensuring long-term acid-base balance.
- Excreting metabolic wastes and foreign substances such as drugs or toxins.

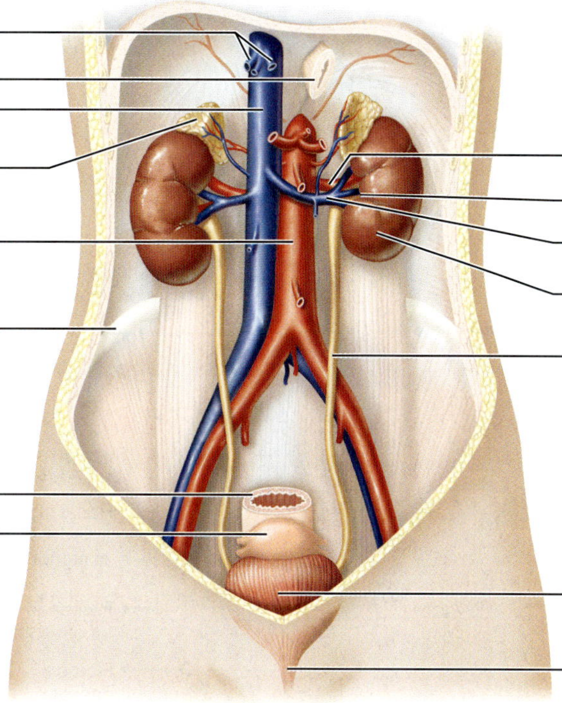

Figure 25.1 The urinary system. Anterior view of the female urinary organs. (Most unrelated abdominal organs have been omitted.)

- Producing *erythropoietin* and *renin* (re′nin; *ren* = kidney), important molecules for regulating red blood cell production and blood pressure, respectively.
- Converting vitamin D to its active form.
- Carrying out gluconeogenesis during prolonged fasting (see p. 924).

The urine-forming kidneys are crucial components of the **urinary system** **(Figure 25.1)**. The urinary system also includes:

- *Ureters*—paired tubes that transport urine from the kidneys to the urinary bladder
- *Urinary bladder*—a temporary storage reservoir for urine
- *Urethra*—a tube that carries urine from the bladder to the body exterior

Kidney Anatomy

✓ Describe the gross anatomy of the kidney and its coverings.

Location and External Anatomy

The bean-shaped kidneys lie in a retroperitoneal position (between the dorsal body wall and the parietal peritoneum) in the *superior* lumbar region **(Figure 25.2)**. Extending approximately from T_{12} to L_3, the kidneys receive some protection from the lower part of the rib cage (Figure 25.2b). The right kidney is crowded by the liver and lies slightly lower than the left.

An adult's kidney has a mass of about 150 g (5 ounces) and its average dimensions are 11 cm long, 6 cm wide, and 3 cm thick—about the size of a large bar of soap. The lateral surface is convex. The medial surface is concave and has a vertical cleft called the **renal hilum** that leads into an internal space within the kidney called the *renal sinus.* The ureter, renal blood vessels, lymphatics, and nerves all join each kidney at the hilum and occupy the sinus. Atop each kidney is an *adrenal* (or *suprarenal*) *gland*, an endocrine gland that is functionally unrelated to the kidney.

Three layers of supportive tissue surround each kidney (Figure 25.2a). From superficial to deep, these are:

- The **renal fascia**, an outer layer of dense fibrous connective tissue that anchors the kidney and the adrenal gland to surrounding structures
- The **perirenal fat capsule**, a fatty mass that surrounds the kidney and cushions it against blows
- The **fibrous capsule**, a transparent capsule that prevents infections in surrounding regions from spreading to the kidney

25

Homeostatic Imbalance 25.1

The kidneys' fatty encasement holds them in their normal body position. If the amount of fatty tissue dwindles (as with extreme emaciation or rapid weight loss), one or both kidneys may drop to a lower position, an event called *renal ptosis* (to′sis; "a fall"). Renal ptosis may cause a ureter to become kinked, causing urine to back up and exert pressure on kidney tissue. Backup of urine from ureteral obstruction or other causes is called

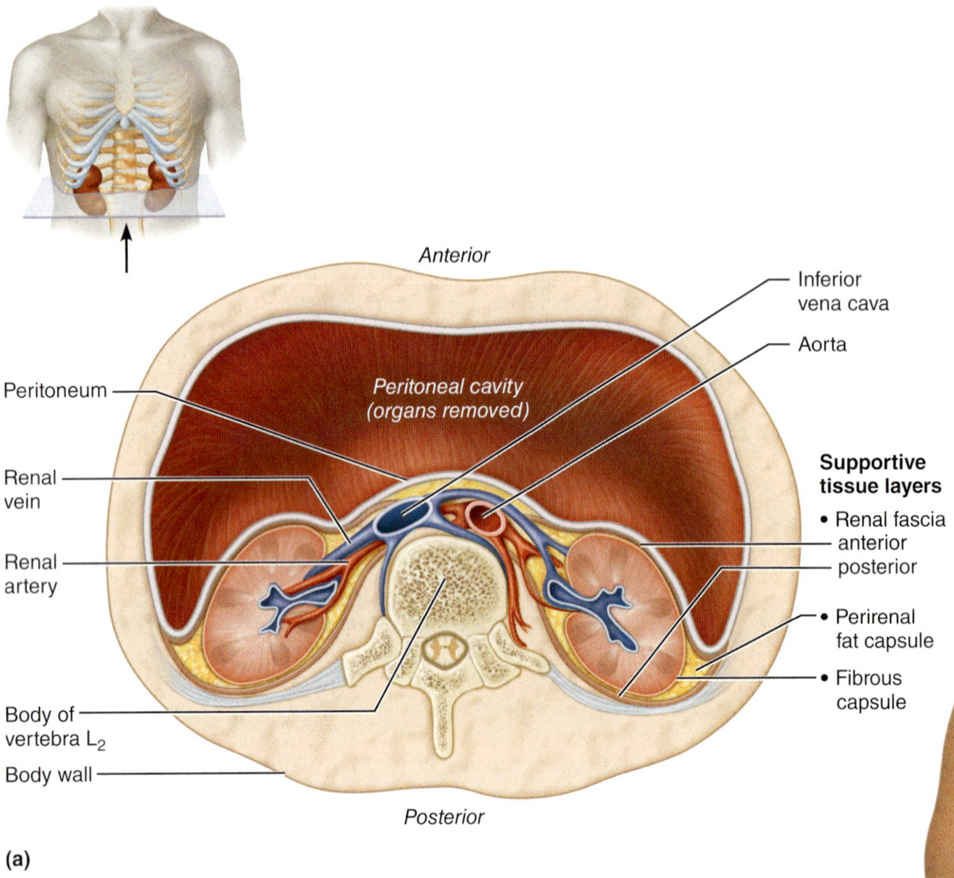

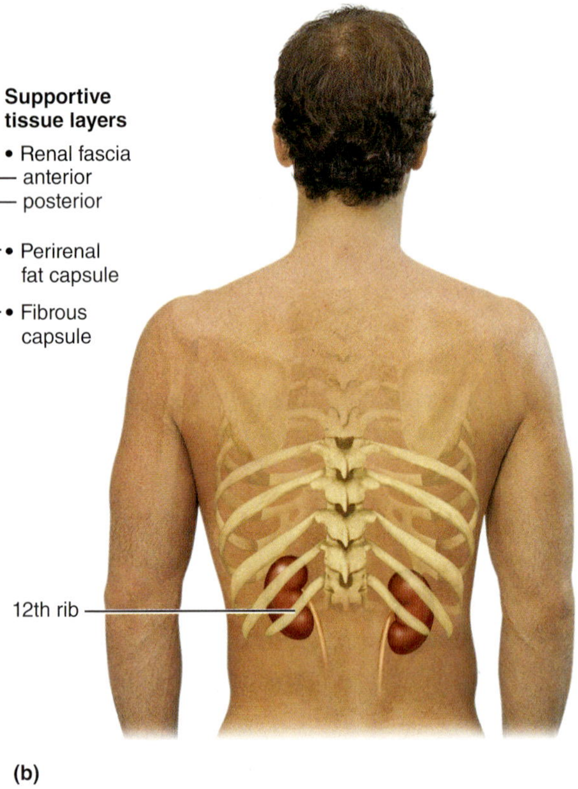

Figure 25.2 Position of the kidneys against the posterior body wall. (a) Cross section viewed from inferior direction. Note the retroperitoneal position and the supportive tissue layers of the kidney. **(b)** Posterior in situ view showing relationship of the kidneys to the 12th ribs.

hydronephrosis (hi″dro-nĕ-fro′sis; "water in the kidney"). Hydronephrosis can severely damage the kidney, leading to necrosis (tissue death) and renal failure. ✚

Internal Gross Anatomy

A frontal section through a kidney reveals three distinct regions: *cortex*, *medulla*, and *pelvis* **(Figure 25.3)**. The most superficial region, the **renal cortex**, is light-colored and has a granular appearance. Deep to the cortex is the darker, reddish-brown **renal medulla**, which exhibits cone-shaped tissue masses called **medullary** or **renal pyramids**. The broad *base* of each pyramid faces toward the cortex, and its apex, or *papilla* ("nipple"), points internally. The pyramids appear striped because they are formed almost entirely of parallel bundles of microscopic urine-collecting tubules and capillaries. The **renal columns**, inward extensions of cortical tissue, separate the pyramids. Each pyramid and its surrounding cortical tissue constitutes one of approximately eight **lobes** of a kidney.

The **renal pelvis**, a funnel-shaped tube, is continuous with the ureter leaving the hilum. Branching extensions of the pelvis form two or three **major calyces** (ka′lih-sēz; singular: calyx). Each major calyx subdivides to form several **minor calyces**, cup-shaped areas that enclose the papillae.

The calyces collect urine, which drains continuously from the papillae, and empty it into the renal pelvis. The urine then flows through the renal pelvis and into the ureter, which moves it to the bladder to be stored. The walls of the calyces, pelvis, and ureter contain smooth muscle that contracts rhythmically to propel urine by peristalsis.

Homeostatic Imbalance 25.2

Pyelitis (pi″ĕ-li′tis) is an infection of the renal pelvis and calyces. Infections or inflammations that affect the entire kidney are *pyelonephritis* (pi″ĕ-lo-nĕ-fri′tis). Kidney infections in females are usually caused by fecal bacteria that spread from the anal region to the urinary tract. Less often they result from bloodborne

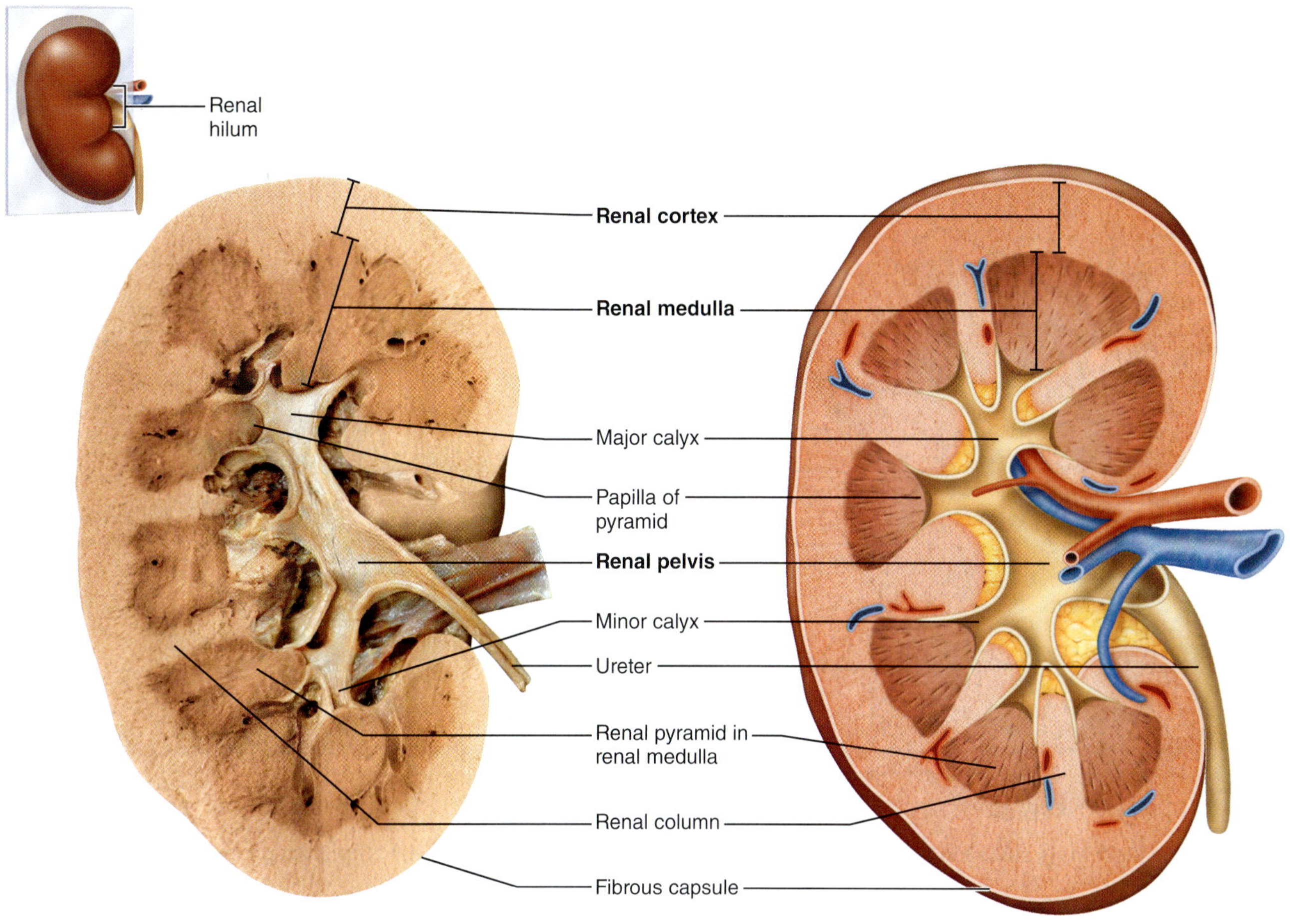

(a) Photograph of right kidney, frontal section **(b) Diagrammatic view**

Figure 25.3 Internal anatomy of the kidney. Frontal sections. (For a related image, see *A Brief Atlas of the Human Body*, Figure 71.)

bacteria (traveling from other infected sites) that lodge and multiply in a kidney.

In severe cases of pyelonephritis, the kidney swells, abscesses form, and the pelvis fills with pus. Untreated, the kidney may be severely damaged, but antibiotic therapy can usually treat the infection successfully. ✚

Blood and Nerve Supply

✓ Trace the blood supply through the kidney.

The kidneys continuously cleanse the blood and adjust its composition, so it is not surprising that they have a rich blood supply. Under normal resting conditions, the large **renal arteries** deliver one-fourth of the total cardiac output (about 1200 ml) to the kidneys each minute.

The renal arteries exit at right angles from the abdominal aorta, and the right renal artery is longer than the left because the aorta lies to the left of the midline. As each renal artery approaches a kidney, it divides into five **segmental arteries** **(Figure 25.4)**. Within the renal sinus, each segmental artery branches further to form several **interlobar arteries**.

At the cortex-medulla junction, the interlobar arteries branch into the **arcuate arteries** (ar′ku-āt) that arch over the bases of the medullary pyramids. Small **cortical radiate arteries** (also called *interlobular arteries*) radiate outward from the arcuate arteries to supply the cortical tissue. More than 90% of the blood entering the kidney perfuses the renal cortex.

Afferent arterioles branching from the cortical radiate arteries begin a complex arrangement of microscopic blood vessels. These vessels are key elements of kidney function, and we will examine them in the next section when we describe the nephron.

Veins pretty much trace the pathway of the arterial supply in reverse (Figure 25.4). Blood leaving the renal cortex drains sequentially into the **cortical radiate, arcuate, interlobar**, and finally **renal veins**. (There are no segmental veins.) The renal veins exit from the kidneys and empty into the inferior vena cava. Because the inferior vena cava lies to the right of the vertebral column, the left renal vein is about twice as long as the right.

The **renal plexus**, a variable network of autonomic nerve fibers and ganglia, provides the nerve supply of the kidney and its ureter. An offshoot of the celiac plexus, the renal plexus is largely supplied by sympathetic fibers from the most inferior thoracic and first lumbar splanchnic nerves, which course along with the renal

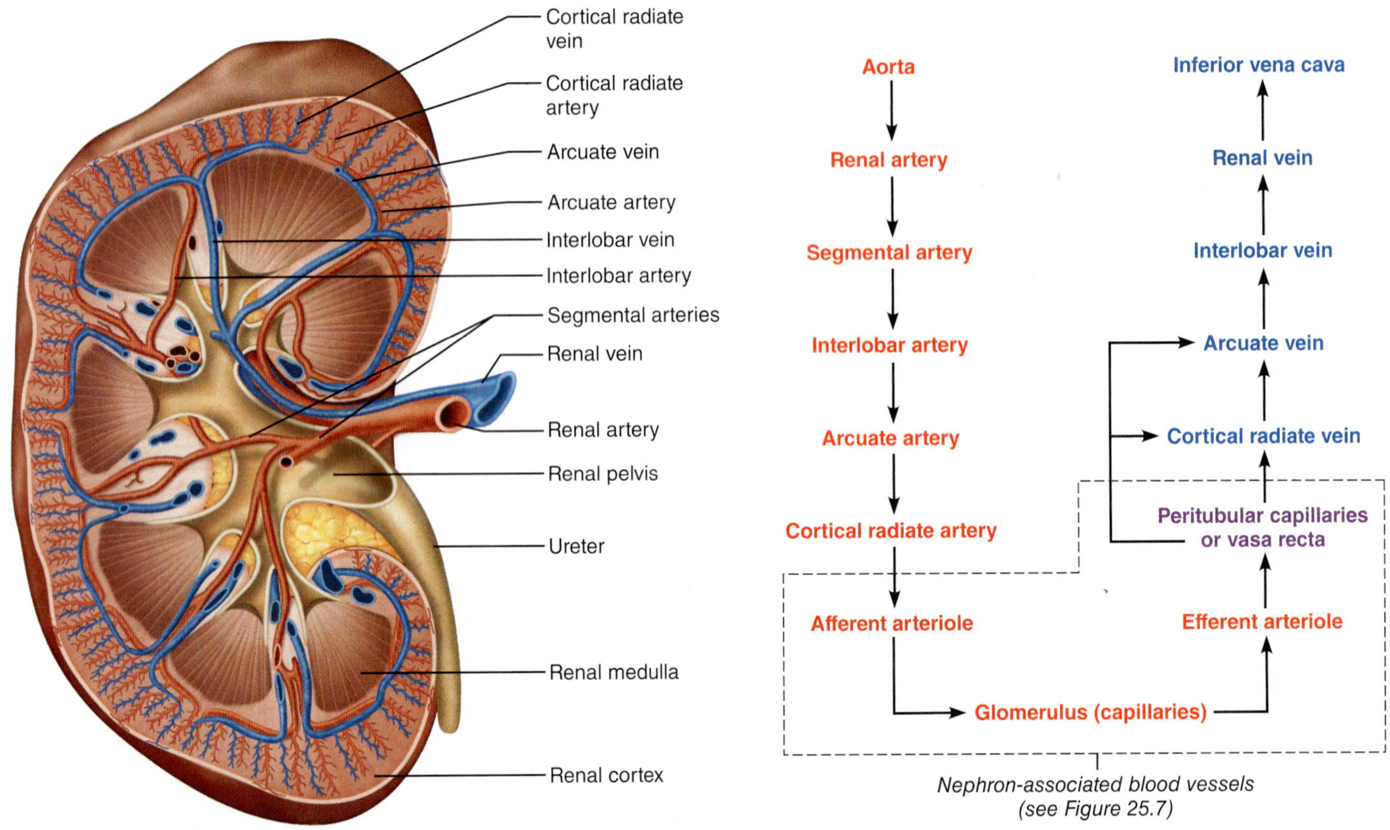

(a) Frontal section illustrating major blood vessels

(b) Path of blood flow through renal blood vessels

Figure 25.4 Blood vessels of the kidney.

artery to reach the kidney. These sympathetic vasomotor fibers regulate renal blood flow by adjusting the diameter of renal arterioles and also influence the formation of urine by the nephron.

25

☑ Check Your Understanding

1. Roger is hit in the lower back by an errant baseball. What protects his kidneys from this mechanical trauma?
2. From inside to outside, list the three layers of supportive tissue that surround each kidney. Where is the parietal peritoneum in relation to these layers?
3. The lumen of the ureter is continuous with a space inside the kidney. This space has branching extensions. What are the names of this space and its extensions?

For answers, see Appendix H.

Nephrons

✓ Describe the anatomy of a nephron.

Nephrons (nef′ronz) are the structural and functional units of the kidneys. Each kidney contains over 1 million of these tiny blood-processing units, which carry out the processes that form urine **(Figure 25.5)**. In addition, there are thousands of *collecting ducts*, each of which collects fluid from several nephrons and conveys it to the renal pelvis.

Each nephron consists of a *renal corpuscle* and a *renal tubule*. All of the renal corpuscles are located in the renal cortex, while the renal tubules begin in the cortex and then pass into the medulla before returning to the cortex.

Renal Corpuscle

Each **renal corpuscle** consists of a tuft of capillaries called a **glomerulus** (glo-mer′u-lus; *glom* = ball of yarn) and a cup-shaped hollow structure called the **glomerular capsule** (or **Bowman's capsule**). The glomerular capsule completely surrounds the glomerulus, much as a well-worn baseball glove encloses a ball, and is continuous with its renal tubule.

Glomerulus The endothelium of the glomerular capillaries is *fenestrated* (penetrated by many pores), which makes these capillaries exceptionally porous. This property allows large amounts of solute-rich but virtually protein-free fluid to pass from the blood into the glomerular capsule. This plasma-derived fluid or **filtrate** is the raw material that the renal tubules process to form urine.

Glomerular Capsule The glomerular capsule has an external parietal layer and a visceral layer that clings to the glomerular capillaries.

- The *parietal layer* is simple squamous epithelium (Figures 25.5, 25.8, and 25.10a). This layer contributes to the capsule structure but plays no part in forming filtrate.

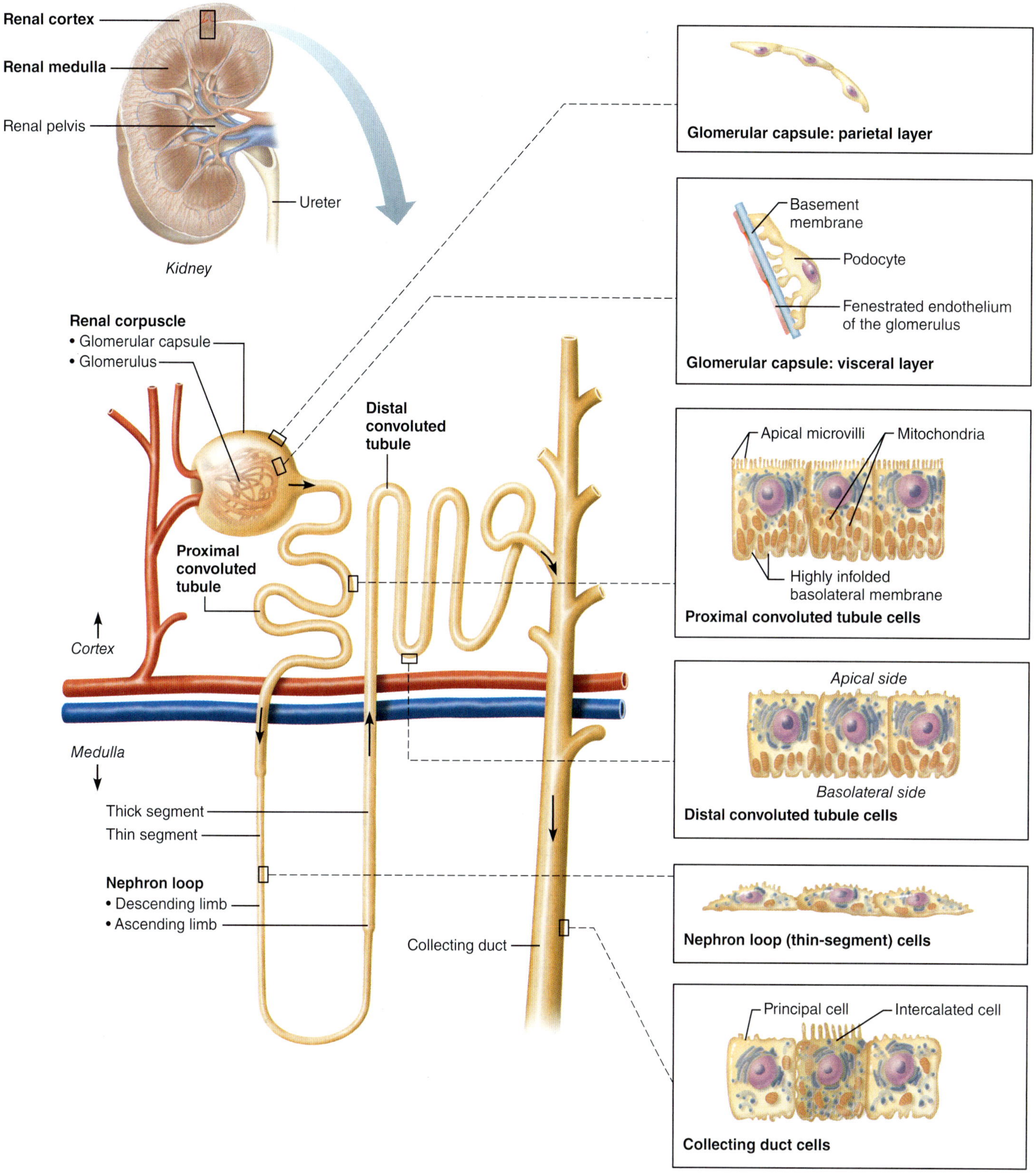

Figure 25.5 Location and structure of nephrons. Schematic view of a nephron depicting the structural characteristics of epithelial cells forming its various regions.

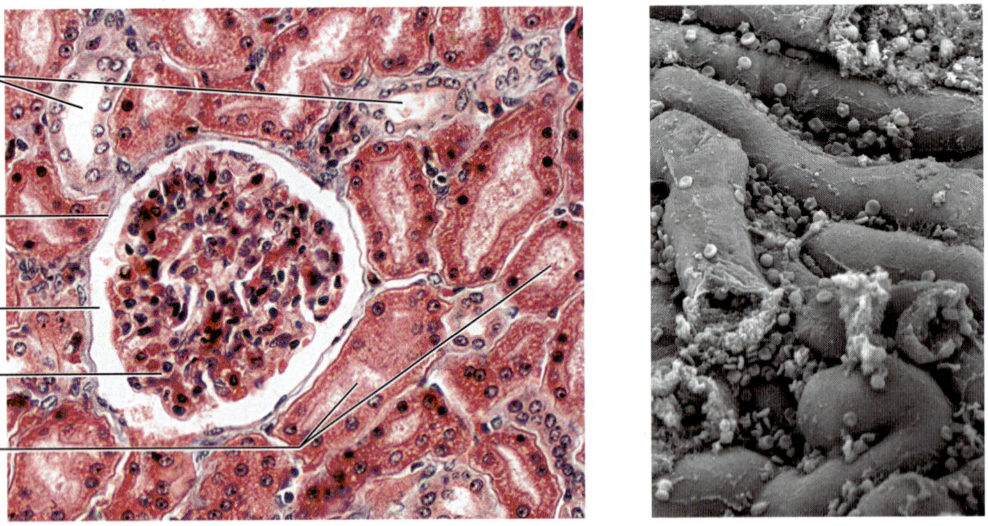

(a) Photomicrograph of renal cortical tissue (180×)

(b) Scanning electron micrograph of renal tubules (250×)

Figure 25.6 **Renal cortical tissue.**

- The *visceral layer*, which clings to the glomerular capillaries, consists of highly modified, branching epithelial cells called **podocytes** (pod′o-sīts; "foot cells") (see Figure 25.10a and b). The octopus-like podocytes terminate in **foot processes**, which interdigitate as they cling to the basement membrane of the glomerulus. The clefts or openings between the foot processes are called **filtration slits**. Through these slits, filtrate enters the **capsular space** inside the glomerular capsule.

We describe the *filtration membrane*, the filter that lies between the blood in the glomerulus and the filtrate in the capsular space, on p. 965.

25

Renal Tubule and Collecting Duct

The **renal tubule** is about 3 cm (1.2 inches) long and has three major parts. It leaves the glomerular capsule as the elaborately coiled *proximal convoluted tubule*, drops into a hairpin loop called the *nephron loop*, and then winds and twists again as the *distal convoluted tubule* before emptying into a collecting duct. The terms *proximal* and *distal* indicate the relationship of the convoluted tubules to the renal corpuscle—filtrate from the renal corpuscle passes through the proximal convoluted tubule first and then the distal convoluted tubule, which is thus "further away" from the renal corpuscle. The meandering nature of the renal tubule increases its length and enhances its filtrate processing capabilities.

Throughout their length, the renal tubule and collecting duct consist of a single layer of polar epithelial cells on a basement membrane. However, each region has a unique histology that reflects its role in processing filtrate.

Proximal Convoluted Tubule (PCT) The walls of the **proximal convoluted tubule** are formed by cuboidal epithelial cells with large mitochondria, and their apical (luminal) surfaces bear dense microvilli (Figure 25.5 and **Figure 25.6**). Just as in the intestine, this *brush border* dramatically increases the surface area and capacity for reabsorbing water and solutes from the filtrate and secreting substances into it.

Nephron Loop The U-shaped **nephron loop** (formerly called the *loop of Henle*) has **descending** and **ascending limbs**. The proximal part of the descending limb is continuous with the proximal tubule and its cells are similar. The rest of the descending limb, called the *descending thin limb*, consists of a simple squamous epithelium. The epithelium becomes cuboidal or even low columnar in the ascending part of the nephron loop, which is therefore called the *thick ascending limb*. In most nephrons, the entire ascending limb is thick but in some nephrons, the thin segment extends around the bend as the *ascending thin limb*. The thick and thin parts of the nephron loop are also referred to as thick and thin segments.

Distal Convoluted Tubule (DCT) The epithelial cells of the **distal convoluted tubule**, like those of the PCT, are cuboidal and confined to the cortex, but they are thinner and almost entirely lack microvilli (Figure 25.5).

Collecting Duct Each **collecting duct** contains two cell types. The more numerous *principal cells* have sparse, short microvilli and are responsible for maintaining the body's water and Na^+ balance. The *intercalated cells* are cuboidal cells with abundant microvilli. There are two varieties of intercalated cells (types A and B), and each plays a role in maintaining the acid-base balance of the blood.

Each collecting duct receives filtrate from many nephrons. The collecting ducts run through the medullary pyramids, giving them their striped appearance. As the collecting ducts approach the renal pelvis, they fuse together and deliver urine into the minor calyces via papillae of the pyramids.

Classes of Nephrons

Nephrons are generally divided into two major groups, cortical and juxtamedullary **(Figure 25.7a)**.

- **Cortical nephrons** account for 85% of the nephrons in the kidneys. Except for small parts of their nephron loops that dip into the outer medulla, they are located entirely in the cortex.

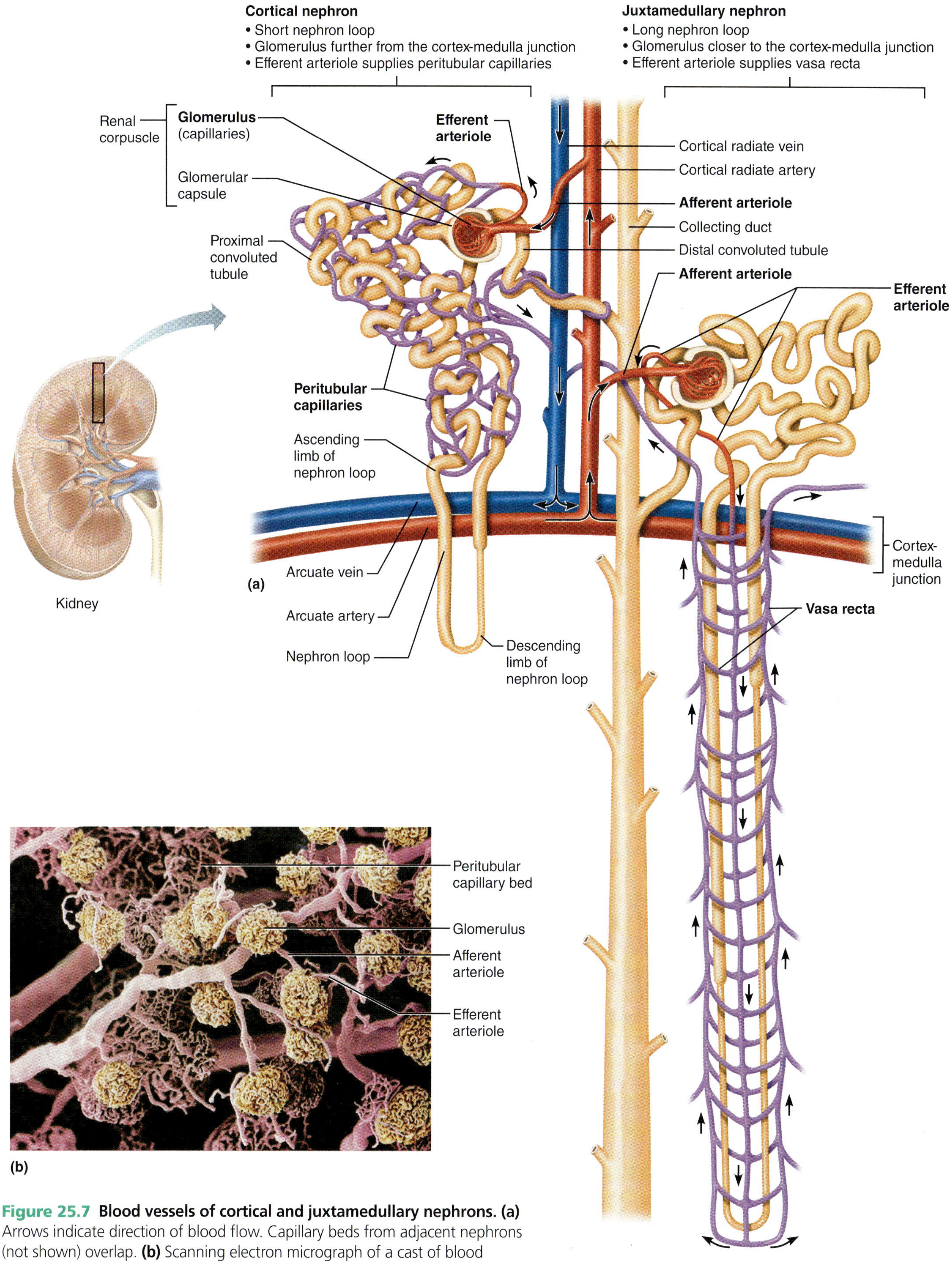

(b)

Figure 25.7 Blood vessels of cortical and juxtamedullary nephrons. (a) Arrows indicate direction of blood flow. Capillary beds from adjacent nephrons (not shown) overlap. **(b)** Scanning electron micrograph of a cast of blood vessels associated with nephrons (60×). View looking down onto the cortex.

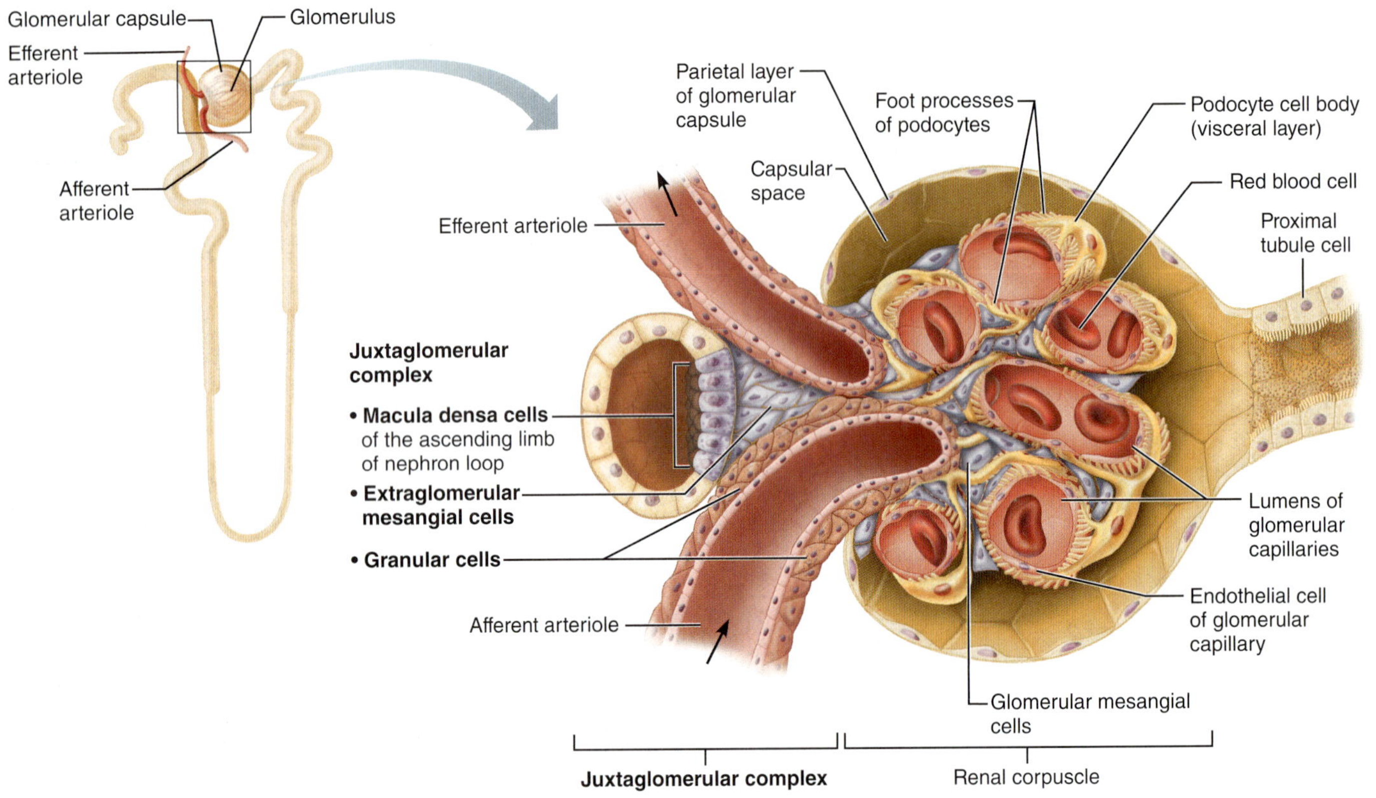

Figure 25.8 Juxtaglomerular complex (JGC) of a nephron. Mesangial cells that surround the glomerular capillaries (glomerular mesangial cells) are not part of the JGC.

- **Juxtamedullary nephrons** (juks″tah-mĕ′dul-ah-re) originate close to (*juxta* = near to) the cortex-medulla junction, and they play an important role in the kidneys' ability to produce concentrated urine. They have long nephron loops that deeply invade the medulla, and their ascending limbs have both thin and thick segments.

25

Nephron Capillary Beds

The renal tubule of every nephron is closely associated with two capillary beds: the *glomerulus* and the *peritubular capillaries* (Figure 25.7). In addition, juxtamedullary nephrons are associated with special capillaries called the *vasa recta.*

Glomerulus The glomerulus, in which the capillaries run in parallel, is specialized for filtration. It differs from all other capillary beds in the body in that it is both fed and drained by arterioles—the **afferent arteriole** and **efferent arteriole**, respectively. This arrangement maintains the high pressure in the glomerulus that is needed for filtration, a process we discuss on p. 965. Filtration produces a large amount of fluid, most (99%) of which is reabsorbed by the renal tubule cells and returned to the blood in the peritubular capillary beds.

The afferent arterioles arise from the *cortical radiate arteries* that run through the renal cortex. The efferent arterioles feed into either the peritubular capillaries or the vasa recta.

Peritubular Capillaries The **peritubular capillaries** cling closely to adjacent renal tubules and empty into nearby venules. Because they arise from the high-resistance efferent arterioles, they only experience low pressure. As a result, these low-pressure, porous capillaries readily absorb solutes and water from the tubule cells as these substances are reclaimed from the filtrate. Renal tubules are closely packed together, so the peritubular capillaries of each nephron absorb substances from several adjacent nephrons.

Vasa Recta Notice in Figure 25.7a that the efferent arterioles serving the juxtamedullary nephrons tend *not* to break up into meandering peritubular capillaries. Instead they form bundles of long straight vessels called **vasa recta** (va′sah rek′tah; "straight vessels") that extend deep into the medulla paralleling the longest nephron loops. The thin-walled vasa recta play an important role in forming concentrated urine, as we will describe shortly.

In summary, the nephrons have two functionally different capillary beds separated by efferent arterioles. The first capillary bed (the glomerulus) produces the filtrate. The second (a combination of peritubular capillaries and vasa recta) reclaims most of that filtrate.

Juxtaglomerular Complex (JGC)

Each nephron has a **juxtaglomerular complex** (JGC) (juks″ tah-glo-mer′u-lar), a region where the most distal portion of the ascending limb of the nephron loop lies against the afferent arteriole feeding the glomerulus (and sometimes the efferent arteriole) **(Figure 25.8)**. Both the ascending limb and the afferent arteriole are modified at the point of contact.

The JGC includes three populations of cells that help regulate the rate of filtrate formation and systemic blood pressure.

- The **macula densa** (mak′u-lah den′sah; "dense spot") is a group of tall, closely packed cells in the ascending limb of the nephron loop that lies adjacent to the granular cells (Figure 25.8). The macula densa cells are chemoreceptors that monitor the NaCl content of the filtrate entering the distal convoluted tubule.
- **Granular cells** [also called *juxtaglomerular (JG) cells*] are in the arteriolar walls. They are enlarged smooth muscle cells with prominent secretory granules containing the enzyme *renin* (see p. 621). Granular cells act as mechanoreceptors that sense the blood pressure in the afferent arteriole.
- *Extraglomerular mesangial cells* lie between the arteriole and tubule cells, and are interconnected by gap junctions. These cells may pass regulatory signals between macula densa and granular cells.

We discuss the physiological role of the JGC in the next section.

Check Your Understanding

4. Name the tubular components of a nephron in the order that filtrate passes through them.
5. What are the structural differences between juxtamedullary and cortical nephrons?
6. What type of capillaries are the glomerular capillaries? What is their function?

For answers, see Appendix H.

Kidney Physiology: Mechanisms of Urine Formation

If you had to design a system to chemically balance and cleanse the blood, how would you do it? Conceptually, it's really very simple. The body solves this problem in the following way. First, it "dumps" cell- and protein-free blood into a separate "waste container." From this container, it reclaims everything the body needs to keep (which is almost everything filtered). Finally, the kidney selectively adds specific things to the container, fine-tuning the body's chemical balance. Anything left in the container becomes urine. This is basically how nephrons work.

Urine formation and the adjustment of blood composition involve three processes (**Figure 25.9**):

1. **Glomerular filtration.** *Glomerular filtration* ("dumping into the waste container") takes place in the renal corpuscle and produces a cell- and protein-free filtrate.
2. **Tubular reabsorption.** *Tubular reabsorption* ("reclaiming what the body needs to keep") is the process of selectively moving substances from the filtrate back into the blood. It takes place in the renal tubules and collecting ducts. Tubular reabsorption reclaims almost everything filtered—all of the glucose and amino acids, and some 99% of the water, salt, and other components. Anything that is *not* reabsorbed becomes urine.

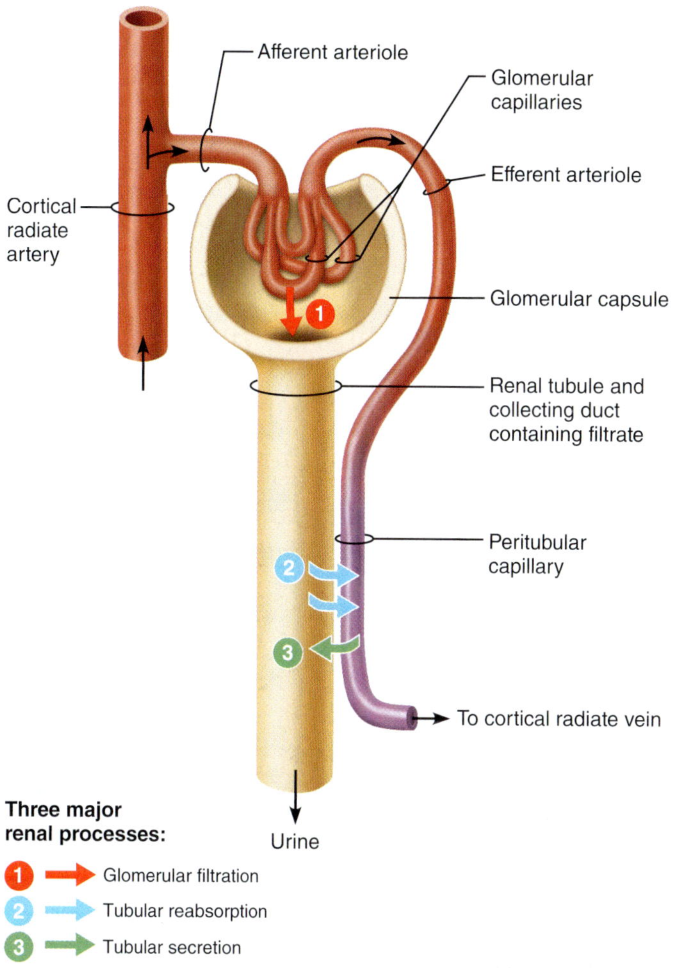

Figure 25.9 A schematic, uncoiled nephron showing the three major renal processes that adjust plasma composition. Each kidney actually has more than a million nephrons acting in parallel.

3. **Tubular secretion.** *Tubular secretion* ("selectively adding to the waste container") is the process of selectively moving substances from the blood into the filtrate. Like tubular reabsorption, it occurs along the length of the tubule and collecting duct.

The kidneys process an enormous volume of blood each day. Of the approximately 1200 ml of blood that passes through the glomeruli each minute, some 650 ml is plasma, and about one-fifth of this (120–125 ml) is forced into the glomerular capsules as filtrate. This is equivalent to filtering your entire plasma volume more than 60 times each day! Considering the magnitude of their task, it is not surprising that the kidneys (which account for only 1% of body weight) consume 20–25% of all oxygen used by the body at rest.

Filtrate and urine are quite different. Filtrate contains everything found in blood plasma except proteins. **Urine** contains unneeded substances such as excess salts and metabolic wastes. The kidneys process about 180 L (47 gallons!) of blood-derived fluid daily. Of this amount, less than 1% (1.5 L) typically leaves the body as urine; the rest returns to the circulation.

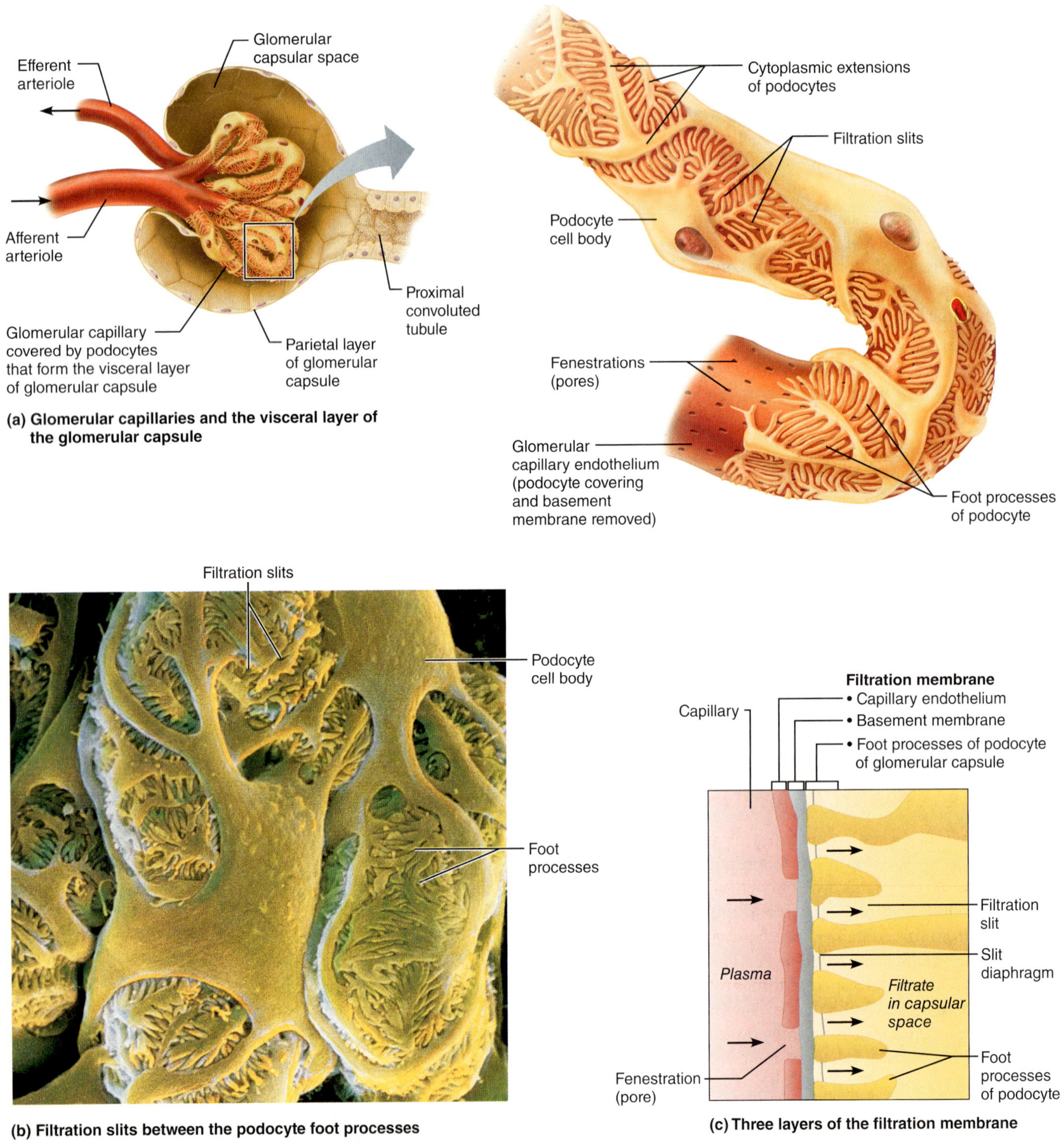

Figure 25.10 The filtration membrane. (a) The visceral (inner) layer of the glomerular capsule consists of podocytes that surround the glomerular capillaries. Some podocytes and the basement membrane have been removed to show the fenestrations (pores) in the underlying capillary wall. **(b)** Scanning electron micrograph of the visceral layer (6000×). **(c)** Diagram of a section through the filtration membrane showing all three structural elements.

Urine Formation, Step 1: Glomerular Filtration

✓ Describe the forces (pressures) that promote or counteract glomerular filtration.

✓ Compare the intrinsic and extrinsic controls of the glomerular filtration rate.

Glomerular filtration is a passive process in which hydrostatic pressure forces fluids and solutes through a membrane. The glomeruli can be viewed as simple mechanical filters because filtrate formation does not directly consume metabolic energy. Let's first look at the structure of the filtration membrane and then see how it works.

The Filtration Membrane

The **filtration membrane** lies between the blood and the interior of the glomerular capsule. It is a porous membrane that allows free passage of water and solutes smaller than plasma proteins. As **Figure 25.10c** shows, its three layers are:

1. **Fenestrated endothelium of the glomerular capillaries.** The fenestrations (capillary pores) allow all blood components except blood cells to pass through.
2. **Basement membrane.** The basement membrane lies between the other two layers and is composed of their fused basal laminae. It forms a physical barrier that blocks all but the smallest proteins while still permitting most other solutes to pass. The glycoproteins of the gel-like basement membrane give it a negative charge. As a result, the basement membrane electrically repels many negatively charged macromolecular anions such as plasma proteins, reinforcing the blockade based on molecular size.
3. **Foot processes of podocytes of the glomerular capsule.** The visceral layer of the glomerular capsule is made of podocytes that have filtration slits between their foot processes. If any macromolecules manage to make it through the basement membrane, *slit diaphragms*—thin membranes that extend across the filtration slits—prevent almost all of them from traveling farther.

Macromolecules that get "hung up" in the filtration membrane are engulfed by specialized pericytes called *glomerular mesangial cells* (Figure 25.8).

Molecules smaller than 3 nm in diameter—such as water, glucose, amino acids, and nitrogenous wastes—pass freely from the blood into the glomerular capsule. As a result, these substances usually have similar concentrations in the blood and the glomerular filtrate. Larger molecules pass with greater difficulty, and those larger than 5 nm are generally barred from entering the tubule. Keeping the plasma proteins *in* the capillaries maintains the colloid osmotic (oncotic) pressure of the glomerular blood, preventing the loss of all its water to the capsular space. The presence of proteins or blood cells in the urine usually indicates a problem with the filtration membrane.

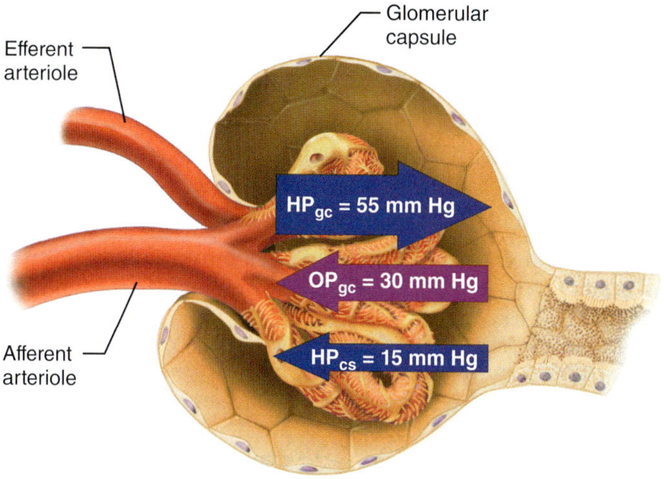

NFP = Net filtration pressure
= outward pressures − inward pressures
= $(HP_{gc}) - (HP_{cs} + OP_{gc})$
= (55) − (15 + 30)
= 10 mm Hg

Figure 25.11 Forces determining net filtration pressure (NFP). The pressure values cited in the diagram are approximate. HP_{gc} = hydrostatic pressure of glomerular capillaries, OP_{gc} = osmotic pressure of glomerular capillaries, HP_{cs} = hydrostatic pressure of capsular space.

Pressures That Affect Filtration

The principles that govern filtration from the glomerulus are the same as those that govern filtration from any capillary bed. *Focus on Bulk Flow Across Capillary Walls* (Figure 19.17 on p. 718) shows filtration in normal capillary beds. **Figure 25.11** applies these principles to the glomerular capillaries of the nephron.

Outward Pressures Outward pressures promote filtrate formation.

- The **hydrostatic pressure in glomerular capillaries (HP_{gc})** is essentially glomerular blood pressure. It is the chief force pushing water and solutes out of the blood and across the filtration membrane. The blood pressure in the glomerulus is extraordinarily high (approximately 55 mm Hg compared to an average of 26 mm Hg or so in other capillary beds) and it remains high across the entire capillary bed. This is because the glomerular capillaries are drained by a high-resistance efferent arteriole whose diameter is smaller than the afferent arteriole that feeds them. As a result, filtration occurs along the entire length of each glomerular capillary and reabsorption does not occur as it would in other capillary beds.
- Theoretically, the *colloid osmotic pressure in the capsular space* of the glomerular capsule would "pull" filtrate into the tubule. However, this pressure is essentially zero because virtually no proteins enter the capsule, so we will not consider it further.

25

Inward Pressures Two inward forces inhibit filtrate formation by opposing HP_{gc}.

- The **hydrostatic pressure in the capsular space (HP_{cs})** is the pressure exerted by filtrate in the glomerular capsule. HP_{cs} is much higher than hydrostatic pressure surrounding most capillaries because filtrate is confined in a small space with a narrow outlet.
- The **colloid osmotic pressure in glomerular capillaries (OP_{gc})** is the pressure exerted by the proteins in the blood.

As shown in Figure 25.11, the above pressures determine the **net filtration pressure (NFP)**. NFP largely determines the glomerular filtration rate, which we consider next.

Glomerular Filtration Rate (GFR)

The **glomerular filtration rate** is the volume of filtrate formed each minute by the combined activity of all 2 million glomeruli of the kidneys. GFR is directly proportional to each of the following factors:

- **Net filtration pressure.** NFP is the main controllable factor. Of the pressures determining NFP, the most important is hydrostatic pressure in the glomerulus. This pressure can be controlled by changing the diameter of the afferent (and sometimes the efferent) arterioles, as we will see shortly.
- **Total surface area available for filtration.** Glomerular capillaries have a huge surface area (collectively equal to the surface area of the skin). Glomerular mesangial cells surrounding these capillaries can fine-tune GFR by contracting to adjust the total surface area available for filtration.
- **Filtration membrane permeability.** Glomerular capillaries are thousands of times more permeable than other capillaries because of their fenestrations.

25

The huge surface area and high permeability of the filtration membrane explain how the relatively modest 10 mm Hg NFP can produce huge amounts of filtrate. Furthermore, the NFP in the glomerulus favors filtration over the entire length of the capillary, unlike other capillary beds where filtration occurs only at the arteriolar end and reabsorption occurs at the venous end. As a result, the adult kidneys produce about 180 L of filtrate daily, in contrast to the 2 to 4 L formed daily by all other capillary beds combined. This 180 L of filtrate per day translates to the normal GFR of 120–125 ml/min.

Regulation of Glomerular Filtration

GFR is tightly regulated to serve two crucial and sometimes opposing needs. The kidneys need a relatively constant GFR to make filtrate and do their job maintaining extracellular homeostasis. On the other hand, the body as a whole needs a constant blood pressure, and this is closely tied to GFR in the following way: Assuming nothing else changes, an increase in GFR increases urine output, which reduces blood volume and blood pressure. The opposite holds true for a decrease in GFR.

Two types of controls serve these two different needs. *Intrinsic controls* (*renal autoregulation*) act locally within the kidney to maintain GFR, while *extrinsic controls* by the nervous and endocrine systems maintain blood pressure. In extreme changes of blood pressure (mean arterial pressure less than 80 or greater than 180 mm Hg), extrinsic controls take precedence over intrinsic controls in an effort to prevent damage to the brain and other crucial organs.

GFR can be controlled by changing a single variable—glomerular hydrostatic pressure. All major control mechanisms act primarily to change this one variable. If the glomerular hydrostatic pressure rises, NFP rises and so does GFR. If the glomerular hydrostatic pressure falls by as little as 18%, GFR drops to zero. Clearly hydrostatic pressure in the glomerulus must be tightly controlled. Let's see how the intrinsic and extrinsic mechanisms accomplish this feat.

Intrinsic Controls: Renal Autoregulation By adjusting its own resistance to blood flow, a process called **renal autoregulation**, the kidney can maintain a nearly constant GFR despite fluctuations in systemic arterial blood pressure. Renal autoregulation uses two different mechanisms: (1) a *myogenic mechanism* and (2) a *tubuloglomerular feedback mechanism* (**Figure 25.12**, left side).

1. **Myogenic mechanism.** The **myogenic mechanism** (mi″o-jen′ik) reflects a property of vascular smooth muscle—it contracts when stretched and relaxes when not stretched. Rising systemic blood pressure stretches vascular smooth muscle in the arteriolar walls, causing the afferent arterioles to constrict. This constriction restricts blood flow into the glomerulus and prevents glomerular blood pressure from rising to damaging levels. Declining systemic blood pressure causes dilation of afferent arterioles and raises glomerular hydrostatic pressure. Both responses help maintain normal NFP and GFR.
2. **Tubuloglomerular feedback mechanism.** Autoregulation by the flow-dependent **tubuloglomerular feedback mechanism** is "directed" by the *macula densa cells* of the *juxtaglomerular complex* (see Figure 25.8). These cells, located in the walls of the ascending limb of the nephron loop, respond to filtrate NaCl concentration (which varies directly with filtrate flow rate). When GFR increases, there is not enough time for reabsorption and the concentration of NaCl in the filtrate remains high. The macula densa cells respond to high levels of NaCl in filtrate by releasing vasoconstrictor chemicals (ATP and others) that cause intense constriction of the afferent arteriole, reducing blood flow into the glomerulus. This drop in blood flow decreases the NFP and GFR, slowing the flow of filtrate and allowing more time for filtrate processing (NaCl reabsorption).

   On the other hand, the low NaCl concentration of slowly flowing filtrate inhibits ATP release from macula densa cells, causing vasodilation of the afferent arterioles (Figure 25.12). This allows more blood to flow into the glomerulus, thus increasing NFP and GFR.

Autoregulatory mechanisms maintain a relatively constant GFR over an arterial pressure range from about 80 to 180 mm Hg. Consequently, normal day-to-day changes in our blood pressure (such as during exercise, sleep, or changes in posture)

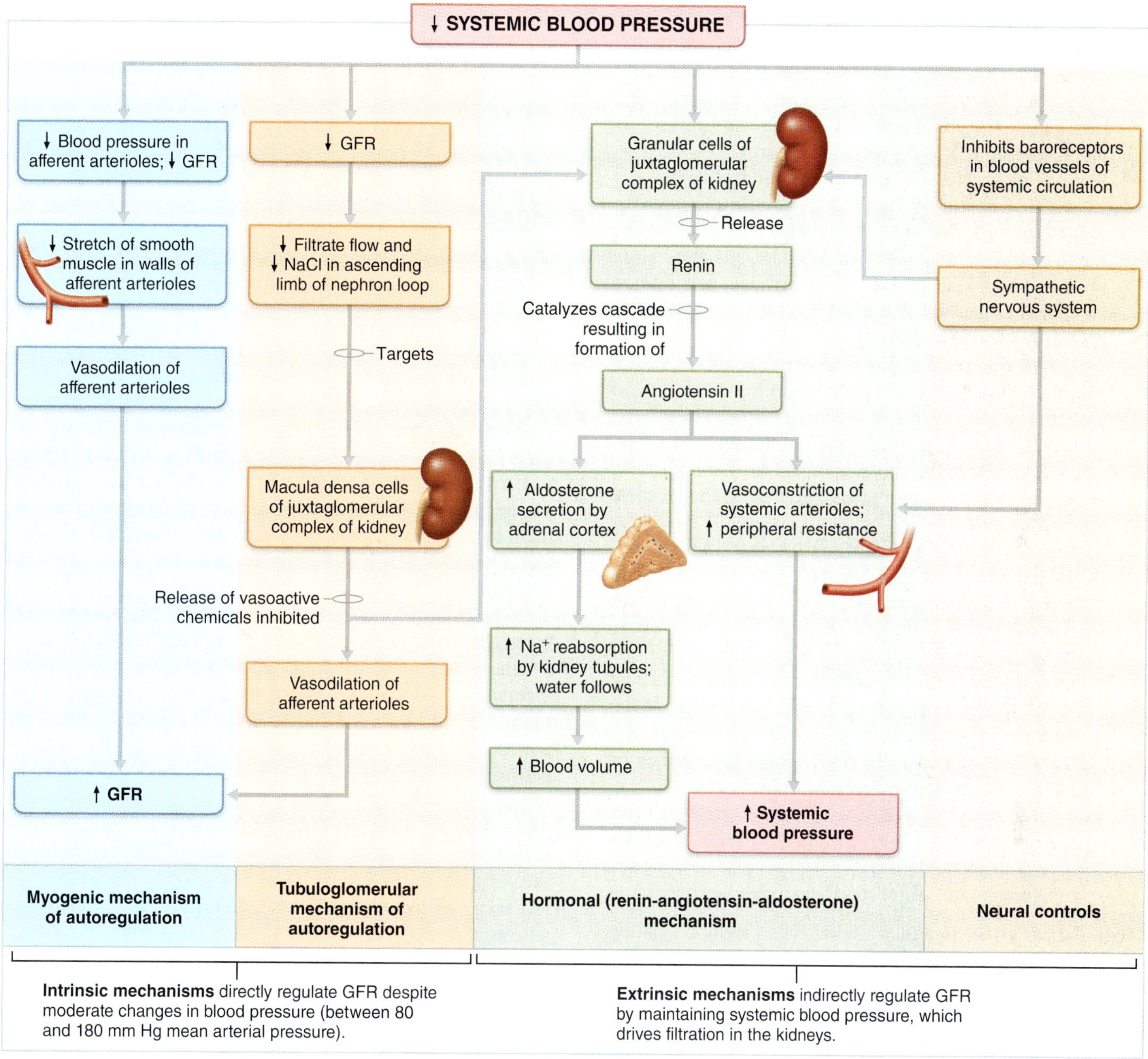

Figure 25.12 Physiological mechanisms regulating glomerular filtration rate (GFR) in the kidneys. (Note that while the extrinsic controls are aimed at maintaining blood pressure, they also maintain GFR since bringing blood pressure back up allows the kidneys to maintain GFR.)

do not cause large changes in water and solute excretion. However, the intrinsic controls cannot handle extremely low systemic blood pressure, such as might result from serious hemorrhage (*hypovolemic shock*). Once the mean arterial pressure drops below 80 mm Hg, autoregulation ceases and extrinsic controls take over.

Extrinsic Controls: Neural and Hormonal Mechanisms The purpose of the extrinsic controls regulating the GFR is to maintain systemic blood pressure (Figure 25.12, right side).

1. **Sympathetic nervous system controls.** Neural renal controls serve the needs of the body as a whole—sometimes to the detriment of the kidneys. When the volume of the extracellular fluid is normal and the sympathetic nervous system is at rest, the renal blood vessels are dilated and renal autoregulation mechanisms prevail. However, when the extracellular fluid volume is extremely low (as in hypovolemic shock during severe hemorrhage) it is necessary to shunt blood to vital organs and neural controls may override autoregulatory mechanisms. This could reduce renal blood flow to the point of damaging the kidneys.

   When blood pressure falls, norepinephrine released by sympathetic nerve fibers (and epinephrine released by the adrenal medulla) causes vascular smooth muscle to constrict, increasing peripheral resistance and bringing blood pressure back up toward normal. This is the baroreceptor reflex we discussed in Chapter 19. As part of this reflex, the afferent arterioles also constrict. Constriction of the afferent arterioles decreases GFR and so helps restore blood volume and blood pressure to normal.

2. **Renin-angiotensin-aldosterone mechanism.** As we discussed in Chapter 19 (p. 709), the **renin-angiotensin-aldosterone mechanism** is the body's main mechanism for increasing blood pressure. Without adequate blood pressure (as might be due to hemorrhage, dehydration, etc.), glomerular filtration is not possible, so this mechanism regulates GFR indirectly.

   Low blood pressure causes the granular cells of the juxtaglomerular complex to release **renin** by one or more of three pathways:
   - *Direct stimulation of granular cells.* As part of the baroreceptor reflex, renal sympathetic nerves activate β_1-adrenergic receptors that cause the granule cells to release renin.
   - *Stimulation of the granular cells by input from activated macula densa cells.* Low blood pressure or vasoconstriction of the afferent arterioles by the sympathetic nervous system reduces GFR, slowing down the flow of filtrate through the renal tubules. When macula densa cells sense the low NaCl concentration of this sluggishly flowing filtrate, they signal the granular cells to release renin. They may signal by releasing less ATP (also thought to be the tubuloglomerular feedback messenger), by releasing *more* of the prostaglandin PGE_2, or both.
   - *Reduced stretch of granular cells.* Granular cells act as mechanoreceptors. A drop in mean arterial blood pressure reduces the tension in the granular cells' plasma membranes and stimulates them to release more renin.

Other Factors Affecting GFR Renal cells produce a battery of chemicals, many of which act as paracrines (local signaling molecules) affecting renal arterioles. These include *adenosine* and *prostaglandin E_2 (PGE_2)*; adenosine can be produced extracellularly from released ATP. In addition, the kidney makes its own locally acting *angiotensin II* that reinforces the effects of hormonal angiotensin II described in Chapter 19 (p. 707).

25

Homeostatic Imbalance 25.3

Abnormally low urinary output (less than 50 ml/day), called *anuria* (ah-nu′re-ah), may indicate that glomerular blood pressure is too low to cause filtration. Renal failure and anuria can also result from situations in which the nephrons stop functioning, including acute nephritis, transfusion reactions, and crush injuries. +

☑ Check Your Understanding

7. Extrinsic and intrinsic controls of GFR serve two different purposes. What are they?
8. Calculate net filtration pressure given the following values: glomerular hydrostatic pressure = 50 mm Hg, blood colloid osmotic pressure = 25 mm Hg, capsular hydrostatic pressure = 20 Hg.
9. Which of the pressures that determine NFP is regulated by both intrinsic and extrinsic controls of GFR?

For answers, see Appendix H.

Urine Formation, Step 2: Tubular Reabsorption

✓ Describe the mechanisms underlying water and solute reabsorption from the renal tubules into the peritubular capillaries.

✓ Describe how sodium and water reabsorption are regulated in the distal tubule and collecting duct.

Our total plasma volume filters into the renal tubules about every 22 minutes, so all our plasma would drain away as urine in less than 30 minutes were it not for **tubular reabsorption**, which quickly reclaims most of the tubule contents and returns them to the blood. Tubular reabsorption is a selective *transepithelial process* that begins as soon as the filtrate enters the proximal tubules.

To reach the blood, reabsorbed substances follow either the *transcellular* or *paracellular route* **(Figure 25.13)**. In the transcellular route, transported substances move through the *apical membrane*, the cytosol, and the *basolateral membrane* of the tubule cell and then the endothelium of the peritubular capillaries. Movement of substances in the paracellular route—*between* the tubule cells—is limited by the tight junctions connecting these cells. In the proximal nephron, however, these tight junctions are "leaky" and allow water and some important ions (Ca^{2+}, Mg^{2+}, K^+, and some Na^+) to pass through the paracellular route.

Given healthy kidneys, virtually all organic nutrients such as glucose and amino acids are completely reabsorbed to maintain or restore normal plasma concentrations. On the other hand, the reabsorption of water and many ions is continuously regulated and adjusted in response to hormonal signals. Depending on the substances transported, the reabsorption process may be *active* or *passive*. **Active tubular reabsorption** requires ATP either directly (primary active transport) or indirectly (secondary active transport; see Figure 3.11, p. 75) for at least one of its steps. **Passive tubular reabsorption** encompasses diffusion, facilitated diffusion, and osmosis—processes in which substances move down their electrochemical gradients.

The transport mechanisms that are so important for kidney cell function are the same ones used by all other cells. You may wish to review these basic transport mechanisms on pp. 67–79 to refresh your memory.

Tubular Reabsorption of Sodium

Sodium ions are the single most abundant cation in the filtrate, and about 80% of the energy used for active transport is devoted to reabsorbing them. Sodium reabsorption is almost always active and via the transcellular route. Let's begin with the ATP-driven step.

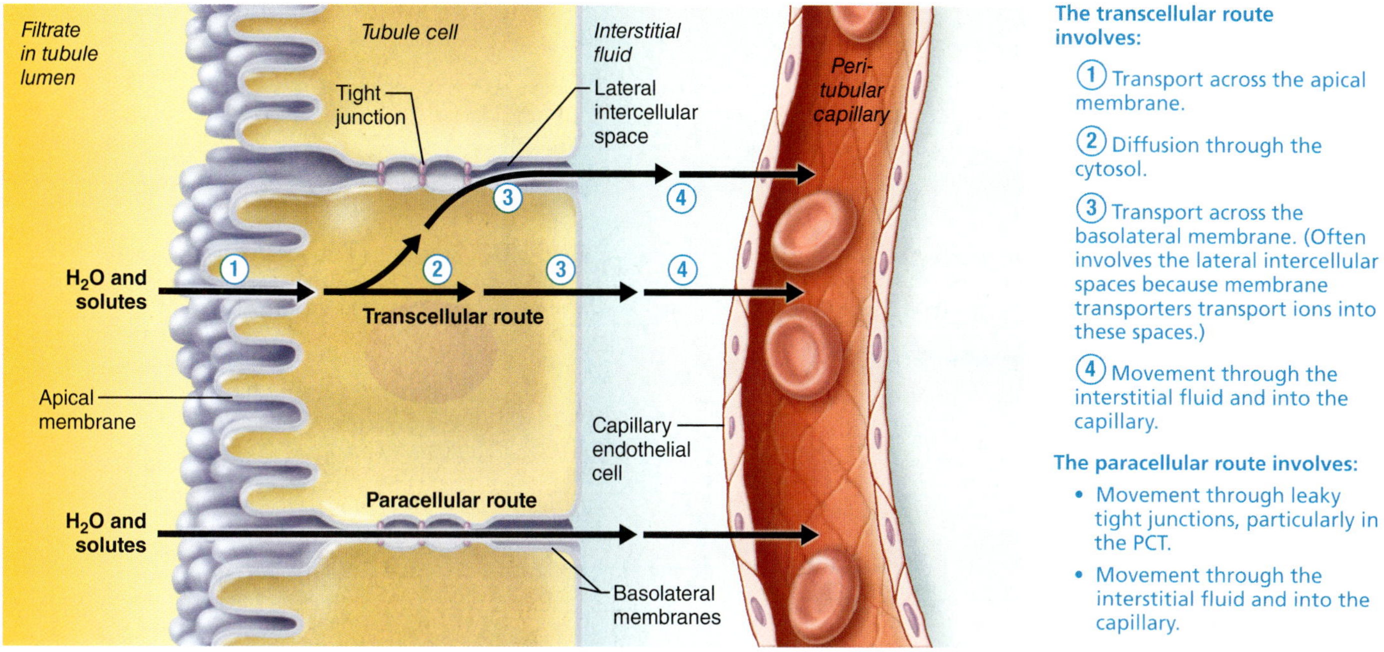

Figure 25.13 Transcellular and paracellular routes of tubular reabsorption. Generally, water and solutes move into the peritubular capillaries through intercellular clefts. For simplicity, transporters, ion channels, intercellular clefts, and aquaporins are not depicted.

Sodium Transport Across the Basolateral Membrane Na^+ is actively transported out of the tubule cell by *primary active transport*—a Na^+-K^+ ATPase pump in the basolateral membrane (**Figure 25.14** ①). From there, the bulk flow of water sweeps Na^+ into adjacent peritubular capillaries. This bulk flow of water and solutes into the peritubular capillaries is rapid because the blood there has low hydrostatic pressure and high osmotic pressure (remember, most proteins remain in the blood instead of filtering out into the tubule).

Sodium Transport Across the Apical Membrane Active pumping of Na^+ from the tubule cells results in a strong electrochemical gradient that favors its entry at the apical face via *secondary active transport* (symport or antiport) carriers (Figure 25.14 ②, ③) or via facilitated diffusion through channels (not illustrated). This occurs because (1) the pump maintains the intracellular Na^+ concentration at low levels, and (2) the K^+ pumped into the tubule cells almost immediately diffuses out into the interstitial fluid via leakage channels, leaving the interior of the tubule cell with a net negative charge.

Because each tubule segment plays a slightly different role in reabsorption, the precise mechanism by which Na^+ is reabsorbed at the apical membrane varies.

Tubular Reabsorption of Nutrients, Water, and Ions

The reabsorption of Na^+ by primary active transport provides the energy and the means for reabsorbing almost every other substance, including water.

Secondary Active Transport Substances reabsorbed by *secondary active transport* (the "push" comes from the gradient created by Na^+-K^+ pumping at the basolateral membrane) include glucose, amino acids, some ions, and vitamins. In nearly all these cases, an apical carrier moves Na^+ down its concentration gradient as it cotransports (symports) another solute (Figure 25.14 ③). Cotransported solutes move across the basolateral membrane by facilitated diffusion via other transport proteins (not shown) before moving into the peritubular capillaries.

Passive Tubular Reabsorption of Water The movement of Na^+ and other solutes establishes a strong osmotic gradient, and water moves by osmosis into the peritubular capillaries. Transmembrane proteins called **aquaporins** aid this process by acting as water channels across cell membranes (Figure 25.14 ④).

In continuously water-permeable regions of the renal tubules, such as the PCT, aquaporins are always present in the tubule cell membranes. Their presence "obliges" the body to absorb water in the proximal nephron regardless of its state of over- or underhydration. This water flow is referred to as **obligatory water reabsorption**.

Aquaporins are virtually absent in the apical membranes of the collecting duct unless antidiuretic hormone (ADH) is present. Water reabsorption that depends on ADH is called **facultative water reabsorption**.

Passive Tubular Reabsorption of Solutes As water leaves the tubules, the concentration of solutes in the filtrate increases and, if able, they too follow their concentration gradients into the peritubular capillaries. This phenomenon—solutes following solvent—explains the passive reabsorption of a number of solutes present in the filtrate, such as lipid-soluble substances, certain ions, and some urea (Figure 25.14 ⑤, ⑥). It also explains in

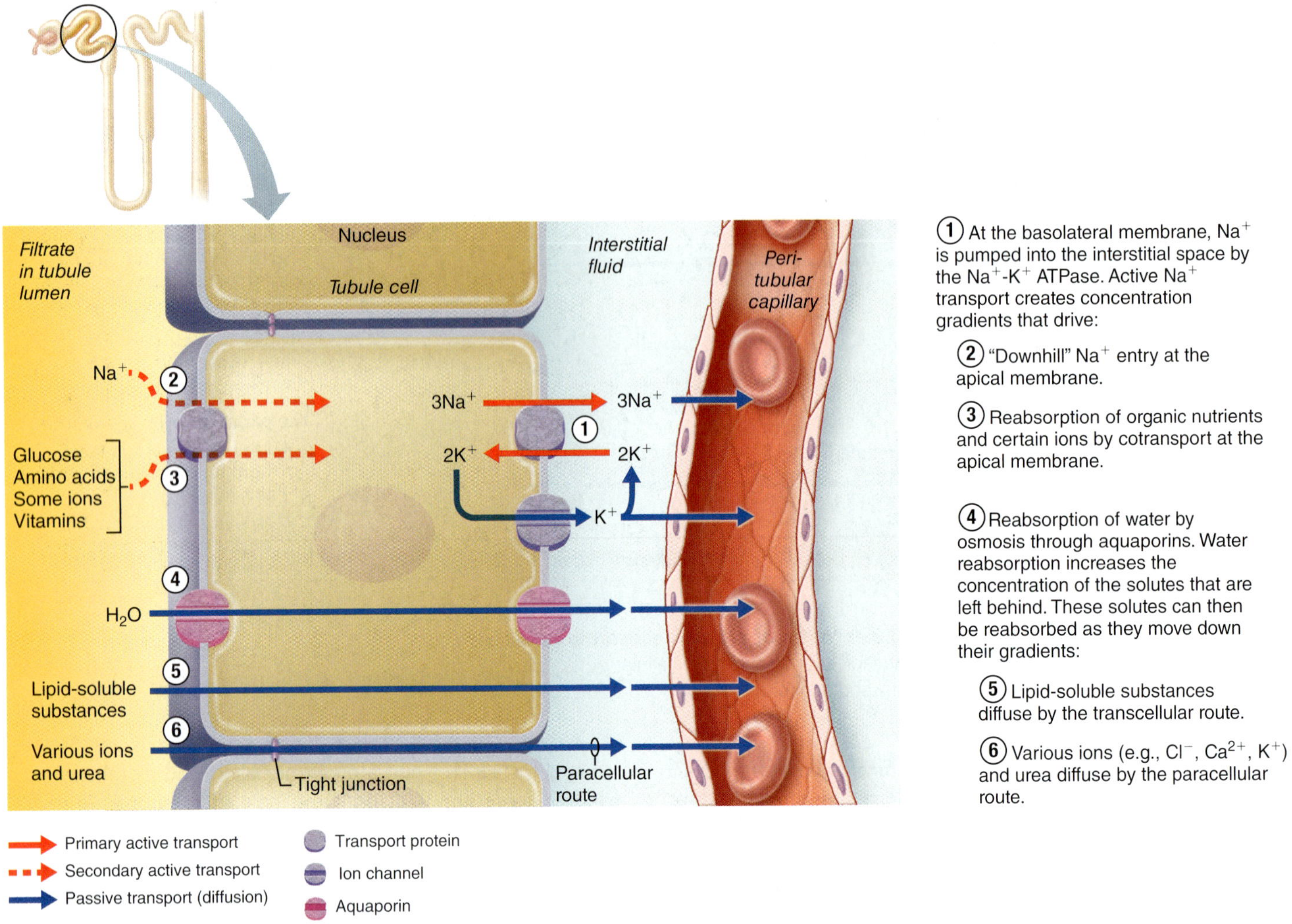

Figure 25.14 Reabsorption by PCT cells. Though not illustrated here, most organic nutrients reabsorbed in the PCT move through the basolateral membrane by facilitated diffusion. Microvilli have been omitted for simplicity.

part why lipid-soluble drugs and environmental pollutants are difficult to excrete: Since lipid-soluble compounds can generally pass through membranes, they will follow their concentration gradients and be reabsorbed, even if this is not "desirable."

As Na^+ ions move through the tubule cells into the peritubular capillary blood, they also establish an electrical gradient that favors passive reabsorption of anions (primarily Cl^-) to restore electrical neutrality in the filtrate and plasma.

Transport Maximum

The transcellular transport systems for the various solutes are quite specific and *limited.* There is a **transport maximum (T_m)** for nearly every substance that is reabsorbed using a transport protein in the membrane. The T_m (reported in mg/min) reflects the number of transport proteins in the renal tubules available to ferry a particular substance. In general, there are plenty of transporters (and therefore high T_m values) for substances such as glucose that need to be retained, and few or no transporters for substances of no use to the body.

When the transporters are saturated—that is, all bound to the substance they transport—the excess is excreted in urine. This is what happens in individuals who become hyperglycemic because of uncontrolled diabetes mellitus. As plasma levels of glucose approach and exceed 180 mg/dl, the glucose T_m is exceeded and large amounts of glucose may be lost in the urine even though the renal tubules are still functioning normally.

Reabsorptive Capabilities of the Renal Tubules and Collecting Ducts

Table 25.1 compares the reabsorptive abilities of various regions of the renal tubules and collecting ducts.

Proximal Convoluted Tubule The entire renal tubule is involved in reabsorption to some degree, but the PCT cells are by far the most active "reabsorbers" and the events just described occur mainly in this tubular segment. Normally, the PCT reabsorbs *all* of the glucose and amino acids in the filtrate and 65% of the Na^+ and water. The bulk of the electrolytes are reabsorbed

Table 25.1 Reabsorption Capabilities of Different Segments of the Renal Tubules and Collecting Ducts

TUBULE SEGMENT	SUBSTANCE REABSORBED	MECHANISM
Proximal Convoluted Tubule (PCT)		
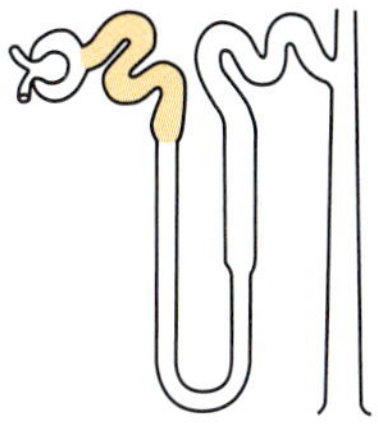	Sodium ions (Na^+)	Primary active transport via basolateral Na^+-K^+ pump; crosses apical membrane through channels, symporters, or antiporters
	Virtually all nutrients (glucose, amino acids, vitamins, some ions)	Secondary active transport with Na^+
	Cl^-, K^+, Mg^{2+}, Ca^{2+}, and other ions	Passive paracellular diffusion driven by electrochemical gradient
	HCO_3^-	Secondary active transport linked to H^+ secretion and Na^+ reabsorption (see Chapter 26)
	Water	Osmosis; driven by solute reabsorption (obligatory water reabsorption)
	Lipid-soluble solutes	Passive diffusion driven by the concentration gradient created by reabsorption of water
	Urea	Primarily passive paracellular diffusion driven by chemical gradient
Nephron Loop		
Descending limb	Water	Osmosis
Ascending limb	Na^+, Cl^-, K^+	Secondary active transport of Cl^-, Na^+, and K^+ via Na^+-K^+-$2Cl^-$ cotransporter in thick portion; paracellular diffusion; Na^+-H^+ antiport
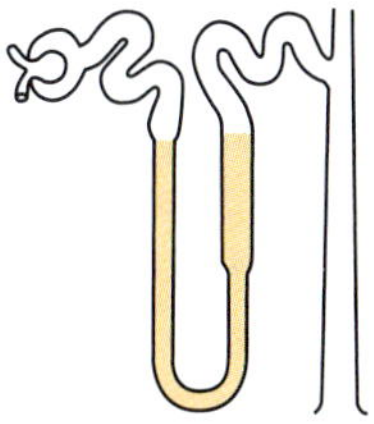	Ca^{2+}, Mg^{2+}	Passive paracellular diffusion driven by electrochemical gradient
Distal Convoluted Tubule (DCT)		
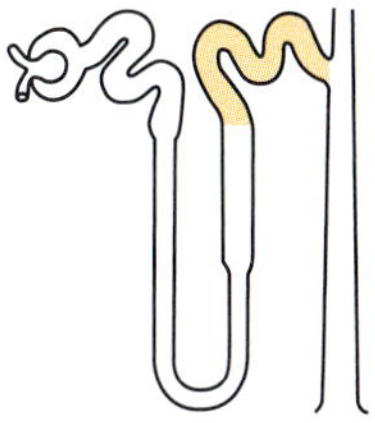	Na^+, Cl^-	Primary active Na^+ transport at basolateral membrane; secondary active transport at apical membrane via Na^+-Cl^- symporter and channels; aldosterone-regulated at distal portion
	Ca^{2+}	Passive uptake via PTH-modulated channels in apical membrane; primary and secondary active transport (antiport with Na^+) in basolateral membrane
Collecting Duct		
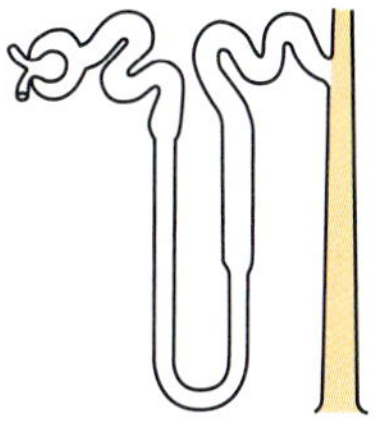	Na^+, K^+, HCO_3^-, Cl^-	Primary active transport of Na^+ (requires aldosterone); passive paracellular diffusion of some Cl^-; cotransport of Cl^- and HCO_3^-; K^+ is both reabsorbed and secreted (aldosterone dependent), usually resulting in net K^+ secretion
	Water	Osmosis; controlled (facultative) water reabsorption; ADH required to insert aquaporins
	Urea	Facilitated diffusion in response to concentration gradient in the deep medulla region; recycles and contributes to medullary osmotic gradient

by the time the filtrate reaches the nephron loop. Nearly all of the uric acid and about half of the urea are reabsorbed in the proximal tubule, but both are later secreted back into the filtrate.

Nephron Loop Beyond the PCT, the permeability of the tubule epithelium changes dramatically. Here, for the first time, water reabsorption is not coupled to solute reabsorption. Water can leave the descending limb of the nephron loop but *not* the ascending limb, where aquaporins are scarce or absent in the tubule cell membranes. For reasons that we will explain shortly, these permeability differences play a vital role in the kidneys' ability to form dilute or concentrated urine.

The rule for water is that it leaves the descending (but not the ascending) limb of the nephron loop. The opposite is true for solutes. Virtually no solute reabsorption occurs in the descending limb, but solutes are reabsorbed both actively and passively in the ascending limb.

In the thin segment of the ascending limb, Na^+ moves passively down the concentration gradient created by water reabsorption. In the thick ascending limb, a Na^+-K^+-$2Cl^-$ symporter is the main means of Na^+ entry at the apical surface. A Na^+-K^+ ATPase operates at the basolateral membrane to create the ionic gradient that drives the symporter. The thick ascending limb also has Na^+-H^+ antiporters. In addition, some 50% of Na^+ passes via the paracellular route in this region.

Distal Convoluted Tubule and Collecting Duct While reabsorption in the PCT and nephron loop does not vary with the body's needs, reabsorption in the DCT and collecting duct is fine-tuned by hormones. Because most of the filtered water and solutes have been reabsorbed by the time the DCT is reached, only a small amount of the filtered load is subject to this fine tuning (e.g., about 10% of the originally filtered NaCl and 25% of the water). We introduce hormones that act at the DCT and collecting duct here but discuss them in more detail in Chapter 26.

- **Antidiuretic hormone (ADH).** As its name reveals, ADH inhibits *diuresis* (di″u-re′sis), or urine output. ADH makes the principal cells of the collecting ducts more permeable to water by causing aquaporins to be inserted into their apical membranes. The amount of ADH determines the number of aquaporins, and thus the amount of water that is reabsorbed there. When the body is overhydrated, extracellular fluid osmolality decreases, decreasing ADH secretion by the posterior pituitary (see p. 599) and making the collecting ducts relatively impermeable to water. ADH also increases urea reabsorption by the collecting ducts, as we will describe later.
- **Aldosterone.** Aldosterone fine-tunes reabsorption of the remaining Na^+. Decreased blood volume or blood pressure, or high extracellular K^+ concentration (hyperkalemia), can cause the adrenal cortex to release aldosterone to the blood. Except for hyperkalemia (which *directly* stimulates the adrenal cortex to secrete aldosterone), these conditions promote the renin-angiotensin-aldosterone mechanism (see Figure 25.12).

  Aldosterone targets the principal cells of the collecting ducts and cells of the distal portion of the DCT (prodding them to synthesize and retain more apical Na^+ and K^+ channels, and more basolateral Na^+-K^+ ATPases). As a result, little or no Na^+ leaves the body in urine. In the absence of aldosterone, these segments reabsorb much less Na^+ and about 2% of Na^+ filtered daily can be lost—an amount incompatible with life.

  Physiologically, aldosterone's role is to increase blood volume, and therefore blood pressure, by enhancing Na^+ reabsorption. In general, water follows Na^+ if aquaporins are present. Aldosterone also reduces blood K^+ concentrations because aldosterone-induced reabsorption of Na^+ is coupled to K^+ secretion in the principal cells of the collecting duct. That is, as Na^+ enters the cell, K^+ moves into the lumen.

25

- **Atrial natriuretic peptide (ANP).** In contrast to aldosterone, which acts to conserve Na^+, ANP reduces blood Na^+, thereby decreasing blood volume and blood pressure. Released by cardiac atrial cells when blood volume or blood pressure is elevated, ANP exerts several effects that lower blood Na^+ content, including direct inhibition of Na^+ reabsorption at the collecting ducts.
- **Parathyroid hormone (PTH).** Acting primarily at the DCT, PTH increases the reabsorption of Ca^{2+}.

Urine Formation, Step 3: Tubular Secretion

✓ Describe the importance of tubular secretion and list several substances that are secreted.

The most important way to clear plasma of unwanted substances is to simply not reabsorb them from the filtrate. Another way is **tubular secretion**—essentially, reabsorption in reverse. Tubular secretion moves *selected* substances (such as H^+, K^+, NH_4^+, creatinine, and certain organic acids and bases) from the peritubular capillaries through the tubule cells into the filtrate. Also, some substances (such as HCO_3^-) that are synthesized in the tubule cells are secreted.

The urine eventually excreted contains *both filtered and secreted substances.* With one major exception (K^+), the PCT is the main site of secretion, but the cortical parts of the collecting ducts are also active **(Figure 25.15)**.

Tubular secretion is important for

- *Disposing of substances, such as certain drugs and metabolites, that are tightly bound to plasma proteins.* Because plasma proteins are generally not filtered, the substances they bind are not filtered and so must be secreted.
- *Eliminating undesirable substances or end products that have been reabsorbed by passive processes.* Urea and uric acid, two nitrogenous wastes, are both handled in this way. Urea handling in the nephron is complicated and will be discussed on p. 976, but the net effect is that 40–50% of the urea in the filtrate is excreted.
- *Ridding the body of excess K^+.* Because virtually all K^+ present in the filtrate is reabsorbed in the PCT and ascending nephron loop, nearly all K^+ in urine comes from aldosterone-driven active tubular secretion into the late DCT and collecting ducts.
- *Controlling blood pH.* When blood pH drops toward the acidic end of its homeostatic range, the renal tubule cells actively secrete more H^+ into the filtrate and retain and generate more HCO_3^- (a base). As a result, blood pH rises and the urine drains off the excess H^+. Conversely, when blood pH approaches the alkaline end of its range, Cl^- is reabsorbed instead of HCO_3^-, which is allowed to leave the body in urine. We will discuss the kidneys' role in pH homeostasis in more detail in Chapter 26.

Figure 25.15 summarizes tubular reabsorption and secretion in the various parts of the nephron and collecting duct.

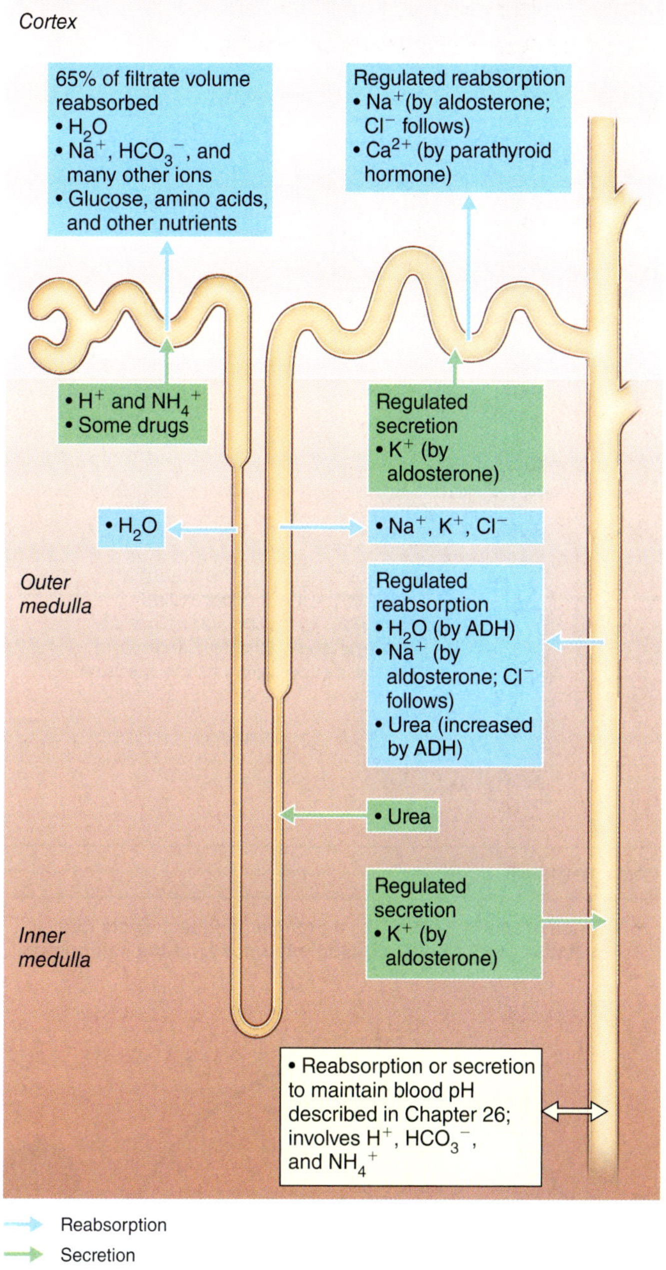

Figure 25.15 Summary of tubular reabsorption and secretion. The various regions of the renal tubule carry out reabsorption and secretion and maintain a gradient of osmolality within the medullary interstitial fluid. Color gradients represent varying osmolality at different points in the interstitial fluid.

☑ Check Your Understanding

10. In which part of the nephron does most reabsorption occur?
11. How are primary and secondary active transport processes (both shown in Figure 25.14) different?
12. How does the movement of Na^+ drive the reabsorption of water and solutes?
13. List several substances that are secreted into the kidney tubules.

For answers, see Appendix H.

Regulation of Urine Concentration and Volume

✓ Describe the mechanisms responsible for the medullary osmotic gradient.

✓ Explain formation of dilute versus concentrated urine.

From day to day, and even hour to hour, our intake and loss of fluids can vary dramatically. For example, when you run on a hot summer day, you dehydrate as you rapidly lose fluid as sweat. On the other hand, if you drink a pitcher of lemonade while sitting on the porch, you overhydrate. In response, the kidneys make adjustments to keep the solute concentration of body fluids constant at about 300 mOsm, the normal osmotic concentration of blood plasma. Maintaining constant osmolality of extracellular fluids is crucial for preventing cells, particularly in the brain, from shrinking or swelling from the osmotic movement of water.

Recall from Chapter 3 (p. 72) that a solution's osmolality is the concentration of solute particles per kilogram of water. Because 1 osmol (equivalent to 1 mole of particles) is a fairly large unit, the milliosmol (mOsm) (mil″e-oz′mōl), equal to 0.001 osmol, is generally used. In the discussion that follows, we use mOsm to indicate mOsm/kg.

The kidneys keep the solute load of body fluids constant by regulating urine concentration and volume. When you dehydrate, your kidneys produce a small volume of concentrated urine. When you overhydrate, your kidneys produce a large volume of dilute urine.

The kidneys accomplish this feat using countercurrent mechanisms. In the kidneys, the term *countercurrent* means that fluid flows in opposite directions through adjacent segments of the same tube connected by a hairpin turn* (see Figure 25.16). This arrangement makes it possible to exchange materials between the two segments.

Two types of countercurrent mechanisms determine urine concentration and volume:

- The **countercurrent multiplier** is the interaction between the flow of filtrate through the ascending and descending limbs of the long nephron loops of juxtamedullary nephrons.
- The **countercurrent exchanger** is the flow of blood through the ascending and descending portions of the vasa recta.

These countercurrent mechanisms establish and maintain an osmotic gradient extending from the cortex through the depths of the medulla. This gradient—the **medullary osmotic gradient**—allows the kidneys to vary urine concentration dramatically.

How do the kidneys form the osmotic gradient? *Focus on the Medullary Osmotic Gradient* **(Figure 25.16)** explores the answer to this question.

*The term "countercurrent" is commonly misunderstood to mean that the direction of fluid flow in the nephron loops is opposite that of the blood in the vasa recta. In fact, there is no one-to-one relationship between individual nephron loops and capillaries of the vasa recta as might be suggested by two-dimensional diagrams such as Figure 25.16. Instead, there are many tubules and capillaries packed together. Each tubule is surrounded by many blood vessels, whose flow is not necessarily counter to flow in that tubule (see Figure 25.7).

(Text continues on p. 976.)

25

Figure 25.16 Juxtamedullary nephrons create an osmotic gradient within the renal medulla that allows the kidney to produce urine of varying concentration.

The three key players and their orientation in the osmotic gradient:

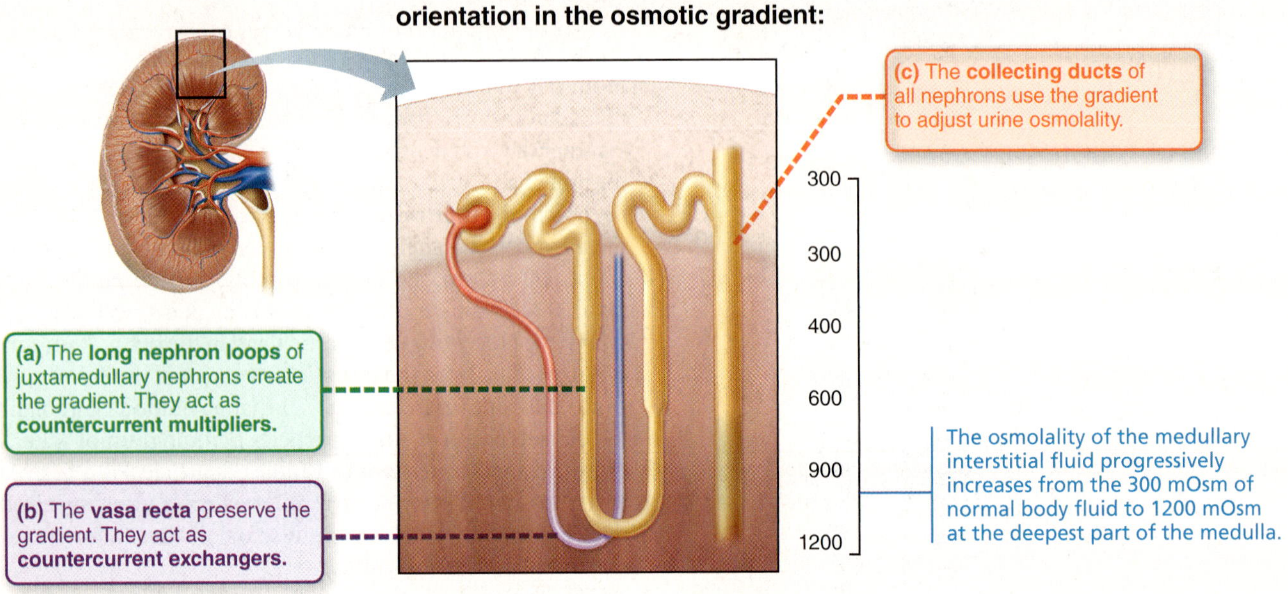

(a) Long nephron loops of juxtamedullary nephrons create the gradient.

The countercurrent multiplier depends on three properties of the nephron loop to establish the osmotic gradient.

These properties establish a positive feedback cycle that uses the flow of fluid to multiply the power of the salt pumps.

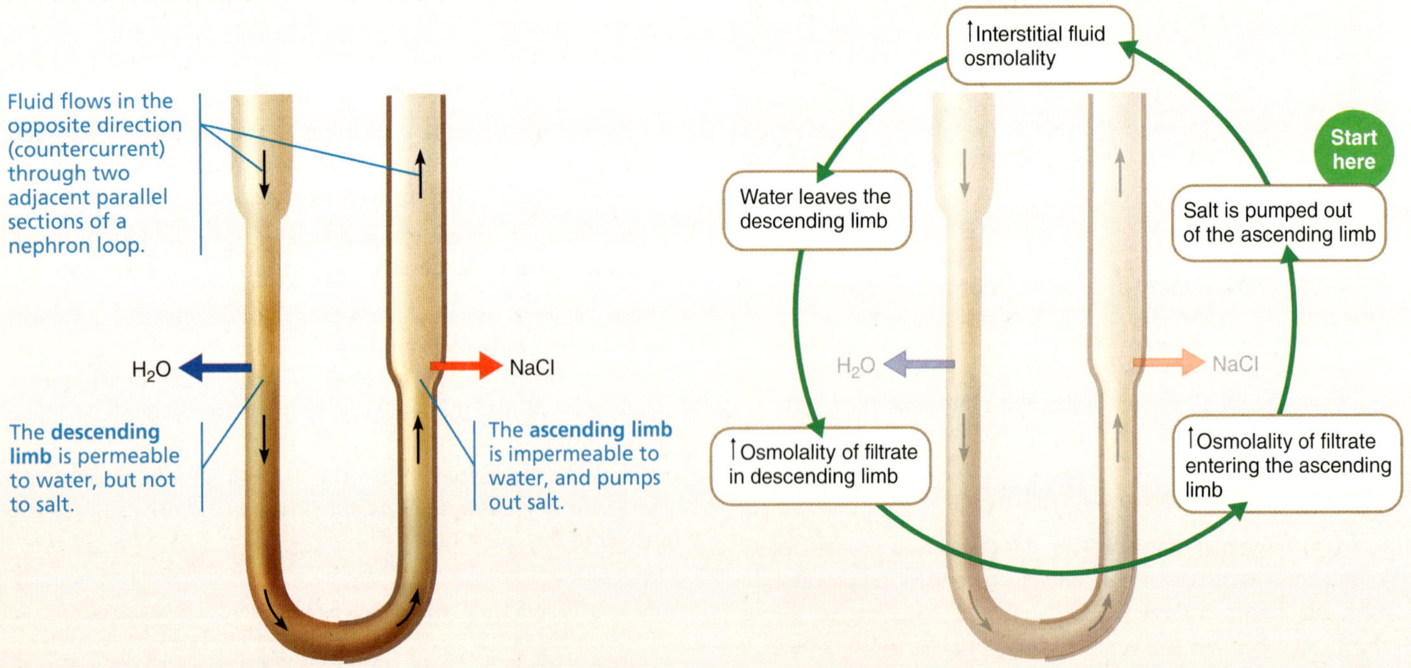

(a) *(continued)* **As water and solutes are reabsorbed, the loop first concentrates the filtrate, then dilutes it.**

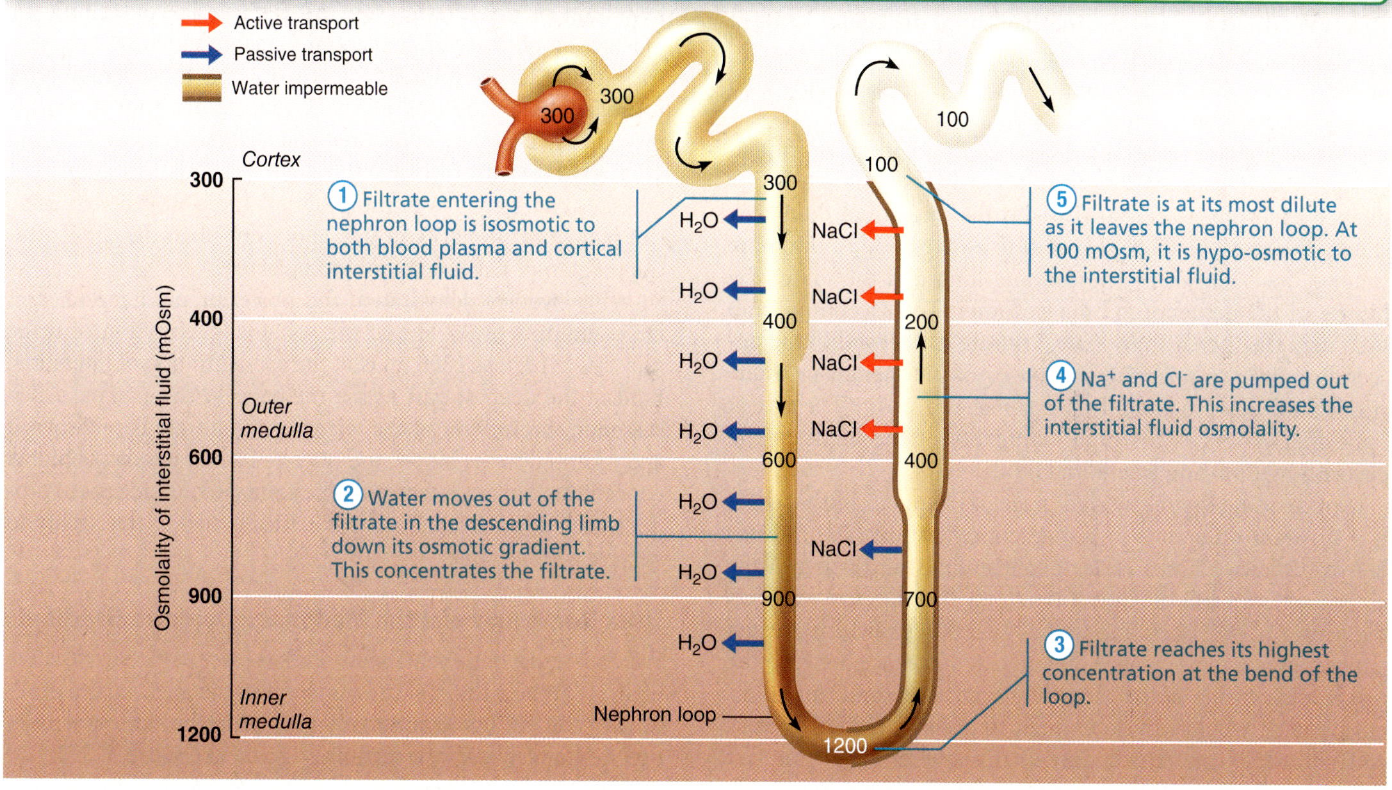

(b) Vasa recta preserve the gradient.

The entire length of the vasa recta is highly permeable to water and solutes. Due to countercurrent exchanges between each section of the vasa recta and its surrounding interstitial fluid, the blood within the vasa recta remains nearly isosmotic to the surrounding fluid. As a result, the vasa recta do not undo the osmotic gradient as they remove reabsorbed water and solutes.

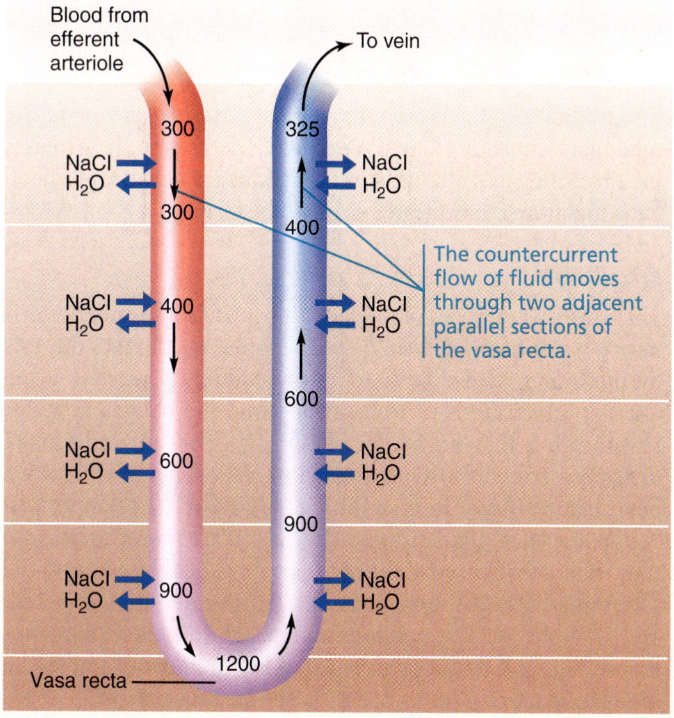

(c) Collecting ducts use the gradient.

Under the control of antidiuretic hormone, the collecting ducts determine the final concentration and volume of urine. This process is fully described in Figure 25.17.

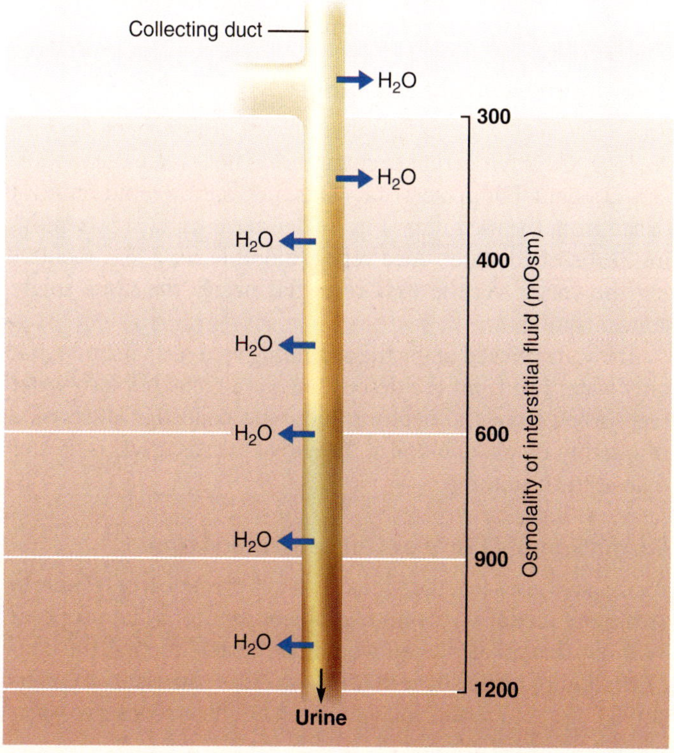

The Countercurrent Multiplier

Take some time to study the mechanism of the countercurrent multiplier in Figure 25.16a. The countercurrent multiplier depends on actively transporting solutes out of the ascending limb ("Start" of the positive feedback cycle).

Although the two limbs of the nephron loop are not in direct contact with each other, they are close enough to influence each other's exchanges with the interstitial fluid they share. The more NaCl the ascending limb extrudes, the more water diffuses out of the descending limb and the saltier the filtrate in the descending limb becomes. The ascending limb then uses the increasingly "salty" filtrate left behind in the descending limb to raise the osmolality of the medullary interstitial fluid even further. This establishes a positive feedback cycle that produces the high osmolality of the fluids in the descending limb and interstitial fluid.

Notice at the top of the right page of Figure 25.16 that there is a constant difference in filtrate concentration (200 mOsm) between the two limbs of the nephron loop, and between the ascending limb and the interstitial fluid. This difference reflects the power of the ascending limb's NaCl pumps, which are just powerful enough to create a 200 mOsm difference between the inside and outside of the ascending limb. A 200 mOsm gradient by itself would not be enough to allow excretion of very concentrated urine. The beauty of this system lies in the fact that, because of countercurrent flow, the nephron loop is able to "multiply" these small changes in solute concentration into a gradient change along the vertical length of the loop (both inside and outside) that is closer to 900 mOsm (1200 mOsm − 300 mOsm).

Notice also that while much of the Na^+ and Cl^- reabsorption in the ascending limb is active (via Na^+-K^+-$2Cl^-$ cotransporters in the thick ascending limb), some is passive (mostly in the thin portion of the ascending limb).

The Countercurrent Exchanger

The vasa recta act as countercurrent exchangers (Figure 25.16b). Countercurrent exchange does not create the medullary gradient, but preserves it (1) by preventing rapid removal of salt from the medullary interstitial space, and (2) by removing reabsorbed water. As a result, blood leaving and reentering the cortex via the vasa recta has nearly the same solute concentration.

The water picked up by the ascending vasa recta includes not only water lost from the descending vasa recta, but also water reabsorbed from the nephron loop and collecting duct. As a result, the volume of blood at the end of the vasa recta is greater than at the beginning.

Formation of Dilute or Concentrated Urine

As we have just seen, the kidneys go to a great deal of trouble to create the medullary osmotic gradient. But for what purpose? Without this gradient, you would not be able to raise the concentration of urine above 300 mOsm—the osmolality of interstitial fluid. As a result, you would not be able to conserve water when you are dehydrated.

Figure 25.17 shows the body's response to either overhydration or dehydration and ADH's role in controlling the production of dilute or concentrated urine. When we are overhydrated, ADH production decreases and the osmolality of urine falls as low as 100 mOsm. If aldosterone (not shown) is present, the DCT and collecting duct cells can remove Na^+ and selected other ions from the filtrate, making the urine that enters the renal pelvis even more dilute. The osmolality of urine can plunge as low as 50 mOsm, about one-sixth the concentration of glomerular filtrate or blood plasma.

When we are dehydrated, the posterior pituitary releases large amounts of ADH and the solute concentration of urine may rise as high as 1200 mOsm, the concentration of interstitial fluid in the deepest part of the medulla. With maximal ADH secretion, up to 99% of the water in the filtrate is reabsorbed and returned to the blood, and only half a liter per day of highly concentrated urine is excreted. The ability of our kidneys to produce such concentrated urine is critically tied to our ability to survive without water.

Urea Recycling and the Medullary Osmotic Gradient

We're not quite done yet. There's one last piece of the puzzle left—urea. We usually think of urea as simply a metabolic waste product, but conserving water is so important that the kidneys actually use urea to help form the medullary gradient (Figure 25.17).

1. Urea enters the filtrate by facilitated diffusion in the ascending thin limb of the nephron loop.
2. As the filtrate moves on, the cortical collecting duct usually reabsorbs water, leaving urea behind.
3. When filtrate reaches the portion of the collecting duct in the deep medullary region, urea, now highly concentrated, moves by facilitated diffusion out of the tubule into the interstitial fluid of the medulla. These movements of urea form a pool of urea that recycles back into the ascending thin limb of the nephron loop and contributes substantially to the high osmolality in the medulla.

Antidiuretic hormone enhances urea transport out of the medullary collecting duct. When ADH is present, it increases urea recycling and strengthens the medullary osmotic gradient, allowing more concentrated urine to be formed.

Diuretics

There are several types of **diuretics**, chemicals that enhance urinary output. Alcohol, essentially a sedative, encourages diuresis by inhibiting release of ADH. Other diuretics increase urine flow by inhibiting Na^+ reabsorption and the obligatory water reabsorption that normally follows. Examples include many drugs prescribed for hypertension or the edema of congestive heart failure. Most diuretics inhibit Na^+-associated symporters. "Loop diuretics" [like furosemide (Lasix)] are powerful because they inhibit formation of the medullary gradient by acting at the ascending limb of the nephron loop. Thiazides are less potent and act at the DCT. An *osmotic diuretic* is a substance that is not reabsorbed and that carries water out with it (for example, the high blood glucose levels of a diabetes mellitus patient).

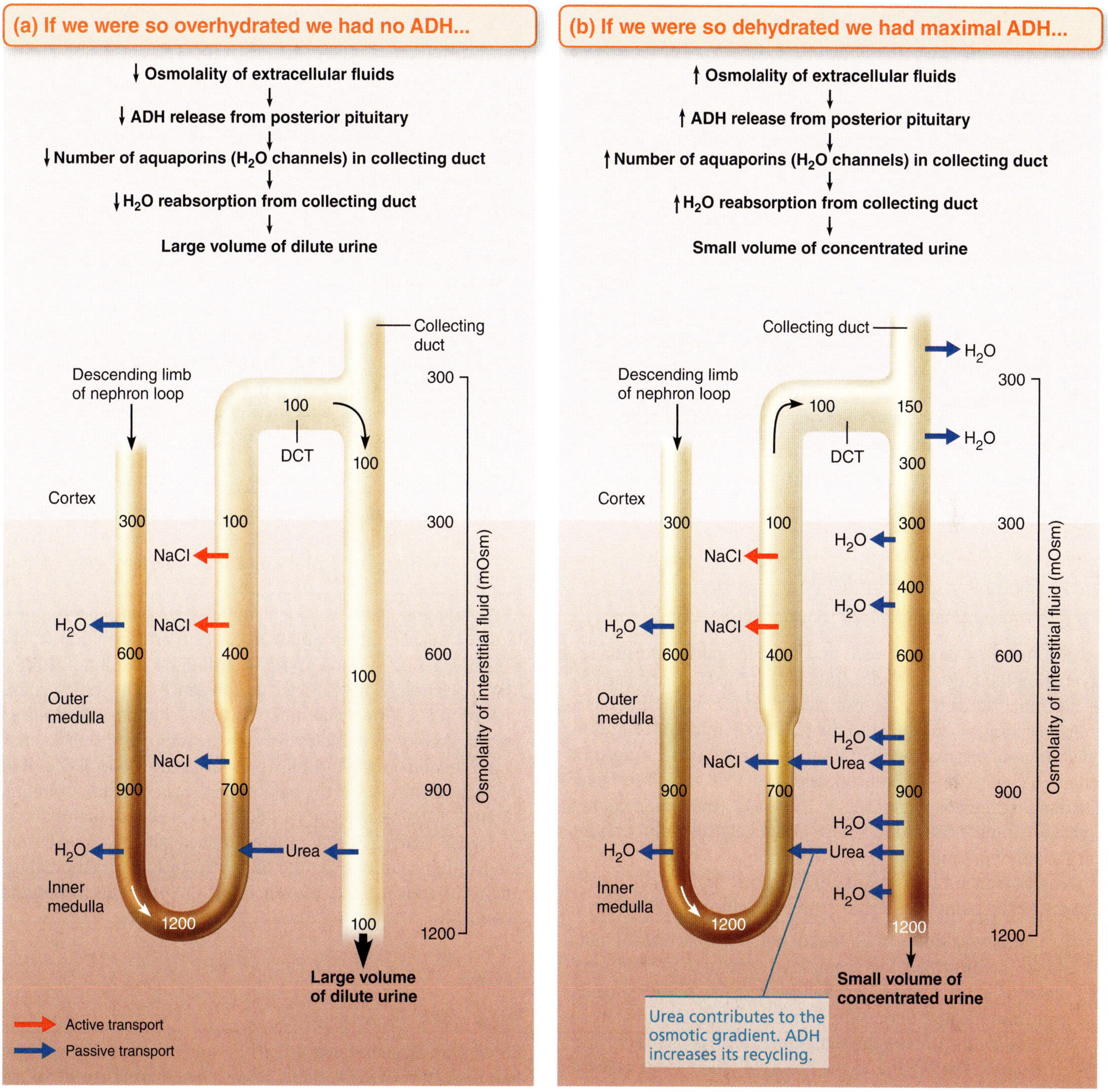

Figure 25.17 Mechanism for forming dilute or concentrated urine. Under the control of antidiuretic hormone (ADH), the collecting ducts fine-tune urine concentration using the medullary osmotic gradient.

Check Your Understanding

14. Describe the special characteristics of the descending and ascending limbs of the nephron loop that cause the formation of the medullary osmotic gradient.
15. Under what conditions is ADH released from the posterior pituitary? What effect does ADH have on the collecting ducts?

For answers, see Appendix H.

Clinical Evaluation of Kidney Function

✓ Define renal clearance and explain how this value summarizes the way a substance is handled by the kidney.

✓ Describe the normal physical and chemical properties of urine.

✓ List several abnormal urine components, and name the condition characterized by the presence of detectable amounts of each.

Since the time of the ancient Greek Hippocrates, physicians have examined their patients' urine for signs of disease. However, to fully understand renal function, we need to analyze *both blood and urine*. For example, renal function is often assessed by measuring levels of *nitrogenous wastes* in blood, whereas determination of renal clearance requires that both blood and urine be tested. Normal blood and urine values for various substances are found in Appendix F.

Renal Clearance

Renal clearance refers to the volume of plasma from which the kidneys clear (completely remove) a particular substance in a given time, usually 1 minute. Renal clearance tests are done to determine the GFR, which allows us to detect glomerular damage and follow the progress of renal disease.

The renal clearance rate (C) of any substance, in ml/min, is calculated from the equation

$$C = UV/P$$

where

U = concentration of the substance in urine (mg/ml)

V = flow rate of urine formation (ml/min)

P = concentration of the substance in plasma (mg/ml)

Because it is freely filtered and neither reabsorbed nor secreted by the kidneys, *inulin* (in′u-lin) is the standard used to determine the GFR. Inulin is a plant polysaccharide that has a renal clearance value equal to the GFR. When inulin is infused such that its plasma concentration is 1 mg/ml ($P = 1$ mg/ml), then generally $U = 125$ mg/ml, and $V = 1$ ml/min. Therefore, its renal clearance is $C = (125 \times 1)/1 = 125$ ml/min, meaning that in 1 minute the kidneys have cleared all the inulin present in 125 ml of plasma.

The clearance value tells us about the net handling of a substance by the kidneys. There are three possible cases:

- A clearance value less than that of inulin means that the substance is reabsorbed. For example, urea has a C of 70 ml/min, meaning that of the 125 ml of glomerular filtrate formed each minute, approximately 70 ml is completely cleared of urea, while the urea in the remaining 55 ml is recovered and returned to the plasma. If the C is zero (such as for glucose in healthy individuals), reabsorption is complete or the substance is not filtered.
- If the C is equal to that of inulin, there is no net reabsorption or secretion.
- If the C is greater than that of inulin, the tubule cells are secreting the substance into the filtrate. This is the case with most drug metabolites. Knowing a drug's renal clearance value is essential because if it is high, the drug dosage must also be high and administered frequently to maintain a therapeutic level.

Creatinine, which has a C of 140 ml/min, is freely filtered but also secreted in small amounts. It is often used nevertheless to give a "quick and dirty" estimate of GFR because it does not need to be intravenously infused into the patient as does inulin.

25

Homeostatic Imbalance 25.4

Chronic renal disease, defined as a GFR of less than 60 ml/min for at least three months, often develops silently and insidiously over many years. Filtrate formation decreases gradually, nitrogenous wastes accumulate in the blood, and blood pH drifts toward the acidic range. The leading cause of chronic renal disease is diabetes mellitus (44% of new cases), with hypertension a close second (28% of new cases). Other causes include repeated kidney infections, physical trauma, and chemical poisoning by heavy metals.

In **renal failure** (GFR $<$ 15 ml/min), filtrate formation decreases or stops completely. The clinical syndrome associated with renal failure is called **uremia** (literally "urine in the blood") and includes fatigue, anorexia, nausea, mental changes, and muscle cramps.

While uremia was once attributed to accumulation of nitrogenous wastes (particularly urea), we now know that urea is not especially toxic. Rather, this multiorgan failure is caused by the interplay of multiple factors, particularly ionic and hormonal imbalances (including anemia due to lack of erythropoietin), as well as metabolic abnormalities and accumulation of various toxic molecules that interfere with normal metabolism.

At this point, the treatment options are hemodialysis or a kidney transplant. **Hemodialysis** uses an "artificial kidney" apparatus, passing the patient's blood through a membrane tubing that is permeable only to selected substances. The tubing is immersed in a solution that differs slightly from normal cleansed plasma. As blood circulates through the tubing, substances such as nitrogenous wastes and K^+ present in the blood (but not in the bath) diffuse out of the blood into the surrounding solution. Meanwhile, substances to be added to the blood, mainly buffers for H^+ (and glucose for malnourished patients), move from the bathing solution into the blood. In this way, hemodialysis retains or adds needed substances, while removing wastes and excess ions. ✚

Urine

Physical Characteristics

Color and Transparency Freshly voided urine is clear and pale to deep yellow. Its yellow color is due to **urochrome** (u′ro-krōm), a pigment that results when the body destroys hemoglobin. The more concentrated the urine, the deeper the color.

An abnormal color (such as pink, brown, or a smoky tinge) may result from eating certain foods (beets, rhubarb) or from the presence of bile pigments or blood in the urine. Additionally, some commonly prescribed drugs and vitamin supplements alter the color of urine. Cloudy urine may indicate a urinary tract infection.

Odor Fresh urine is slightly aromatic, but if allowed to stand, it develops an ammonia odor as bacteria metabolize its urea solutes. Some drugs and vegetables alter the usual odor of urine, as do some diseases. For example, in uncontrolled diabetes mellitus the urine smells fruity because of its acetone content.

pH Urine is usually slightly acidic (around pH 6), but changes in body metabolism or diet may cause the pH to vary from about 4.5 to 8.0. A predominantly *acidic* diet that contains large amounts of protein and whole wheat products produces acidic urine. A vegetarian (*alkaline*) diet, prolonged vomiting, and bacterial infection of the urinary tract all cause the urine to become alkaline.

Specific Gravity The ratio of the mass of a substance to the mass of an equal volume of distilled water is its **specific gravity**. Because urine is water plus solutes, a given volume has a greater mass than the same volume of distilled water. The specific gravity of distilled water is 1.0 and that of urine ranges from 1.001 to 1.035, depending on its solute concentration.

Chemical Composition

Water accounts for about 95% of urine volume; the remaining 5% consists of solutes. The largest component of urine by weight, apart from water, is **urea**, which is derived from the normal breakdown of amino acids. Other **nitrogenous wastes** in urine include **uric acid** (an end product of nucleic acid metabolism) and **creatinine** (a metabolite of creatine phosphate, which is found in large amounts in skeletal muscle tissue where it stores energy to regenerate ATP).

Normal solute constituents of urine, in order of decreasing concentration, are urea, Na^+, K^+, PO_4^{3-}, SO_4^{2-}, creatinine, and uric acid. Much smaller but highly variable amounts of Ca^{2+}, Mg^{2+}, and HCO_3^- are also present.

Unusually high concentrations of any solute, or the presence of abnormal substances such as blood proteins, WBCs (pus), or bile pigments, may indicate pathology (Table 25.2). (Normal urine values are listed in Appendix F.)

☑ Check Your Understanding

16. What would you expect the normal clearance value for amino acids to be? Explain.
17. What are the three major nitrogenous wastes excreted in the urine?

For answers, see Appendix H.

Urine Transport, Storage, and Elimination

The kidneys form urine continuously and the ureters transport it to the bladder. It is usually stored in the bladder until its release through the urethra is convenient, a process called *micturition*.

Ureters

✓ Describe the general location, structure, and function of the ureters.

The **ureters** are slender tubes that convey urine from the kidneys to the bladder (Figure 25.1 and **Figure 25.18**). Each ureter begins at the level of L_2 as a continuation of the renal pelvis. From there, it descends behind the peritoneum and runs obliquely through the posterior bladder wall. This arrangement prevents backflow of urine because any increase in bladder pressure compresses and closes the distal ends of the ureters.

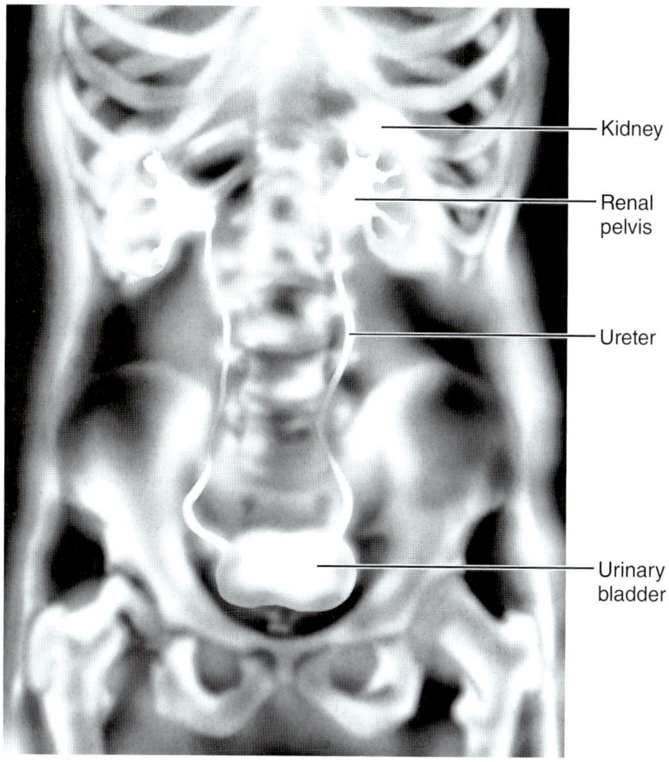

Figure 25.18 Pyelogram. This X-ray image was obtained using a contrast medium to show the ureters, kidneys, and urinary bladder.

Histologically, the ureter wall has three layers **(Figure 25.19)**. From the inside out:

- The *mucosa* contains a transitional epithelium that is continuous with the mucosae of the kidney pelvis superiorly and the bladder medially.
- The *muscularis* is composed chiefly of two smooth muscle sheets: the internal longitudinal layer and the external circular layer. An additional smooth muscle layer, the external longitudinal layer, appears in the lower third of the ureter.
- The *adventitia* covering the ureter's external surface is typical fibrous connective tissue.

The ureter plays an active role in transporting urine. Incoming urine distends the ureter and stimulates its muscularis to contract, propelling urine into the bladder. (Urine does *not* reach the bladder through gravity alone.) The strength and frequency of the peristaltic waves are adjusted to the rate of urine formation. Both sympathetic and parasympathetic fibers innervate each ureter, but neural control of peristalsis appears to be insignificant compared to the way ureteral smooth muscle responds to stretch.

Homeostatic Imbalance 25.5

On occasion, calcium, magnesium, or uric acid salts in urine may crystallize and precipitate in the renal pelvis, forming **renal calculi** (kal′ku-li; *calculus* = little stone), or kidney stones.

Table 25.2 Abnormal Urinary Constituents

SUBSTANCE	NAME OF CONDITION	POSSIBLE CAUSES
Glucose	Glycosuria	Diabetes mellitus
Proteins	Proteinuria, albuminuria	Nonpathological: excessive physical exertion, pregnancy Pathological (over 150 mg/day): heart failure, severe hypertension, glomerulonephritis, often initial sign of asymptomatic renal disease
Ketone bodies	Ketonuria	Excessive formation and accumulation of ketone bodies, as in starvation and untreated diabetes mellitus
Hemoglobin	Hemoglobinuria	Various: transfusion reaction, hemolytic anemia, severe burns, etc.
Bile pigments	Bilirubinuria	Liver disease (hepatitis, cirrhosis) or obstruction of bile ducts from liver or gallbladder
Erythrocytes	Hematuria	Bleeding urinary tract (due to trauma, kidney stones, infection, or cancer)
Leukocytes (pus)	Pyuria	Urinary tract infection

Most calculi are under 5 mm in diameter and pass through the urinary tract without causing problems. However, larger calculi can obstruct a ureter and block urine drainage. Increasing pressure in the kidney causes excruciating pain, which radiates from the flank to the anterior abdominal wall on the same side. Pain also occurs during peristalsis when the contracting ureter wall closes in on the sharp calculi.

Predisposing conditions are frequent bacterial infections of the urinary tract, urine retention, high blood levels of calcium, and alkaline urine. Surgical removal of calculi has been almost entirely replaced by *shock wave lithotripsy*, a noninvasive procedure that uses ultrasonic shock waves to shatter the calculi. The pulverized, sandlike remnants of the calculi are then painlessly eliminated in the urine. People with a history of kidney stones are encouraged to drink enough water to keep their urine dilute. +

25

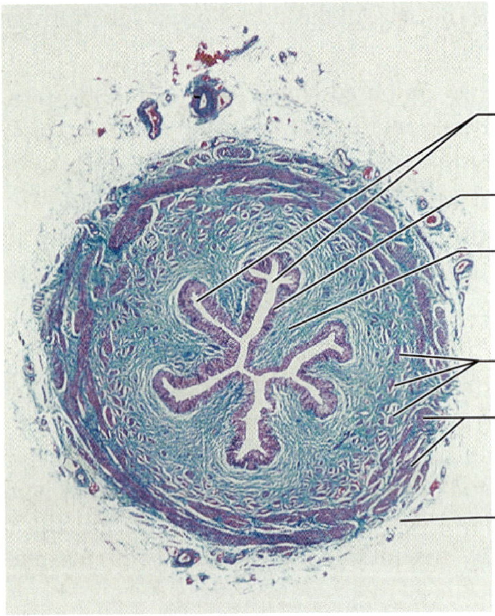

Figure 25.19 Cross-sectional view of the ureter wall (10×). The prominent mucosal folds seen in an empty ureter stretch and flatten to accommodate large pulses of urine.

Urinary Bladder

✓ Describe the general location, structure, and function of the urinary bladder.

The **urinary bladder** is a smooth, collapsible, muscular sac that stores urine temporarily.

Urinary Bladder Anatomy

The bladder is located retroperitoneally on the pelvic floor just posterior to the pubic symphysis. The prostate (part of the male reproductive system) lies inferior to the bladder neck, which empties into the urethra. In females, the bladder is anterior to the vagina and uterus (see Figure 27.12 on p. 1035).

The interior of the bladder has openings for both ureters and the urethra **(Figure 25.20)**. The smooth, triangular region of the bladder base outlined by these three openings is the **trigone** (tri′gōn; *trigon* = triangle), important clinically because infections tend to persist in this region.

The bladder wall has three layers: a mucosa containing transitional epithelium, a thick muscular layer, and a fibrous adventitia (except on its superior surface, where it is covered by the peritoneum). The muscular layer, called the **detrusor** (detru′sor; "to thrust out"), consists of intermingled smooth muscle fibers arranged in inner and outer longitudinal layers and a middle circular layer.

Urine Storage Capacity

The bladder is very distensible and uniquely suited for its function of urine storage. When empty, the bladder collapses into its basic pyramidal shape and its walls are thick and thrown into folds (*rugae*). As urine accumulates, the bladder expands, becomes pear shaped, and rises superiorly in the abdominal cavity. The muscular wall stretches and thins, and rugae disappear. These changes allow the bladder to store more urine without a significant rise in internal pressure.

A moderately full bladder is about 12 cm (5 inches) long and holds approximately 500 ml (1 pint) of urine, but it can hold nearly double that if necessary. When tense with urine, it can be palpated well above the pubic symphysis. The maximum

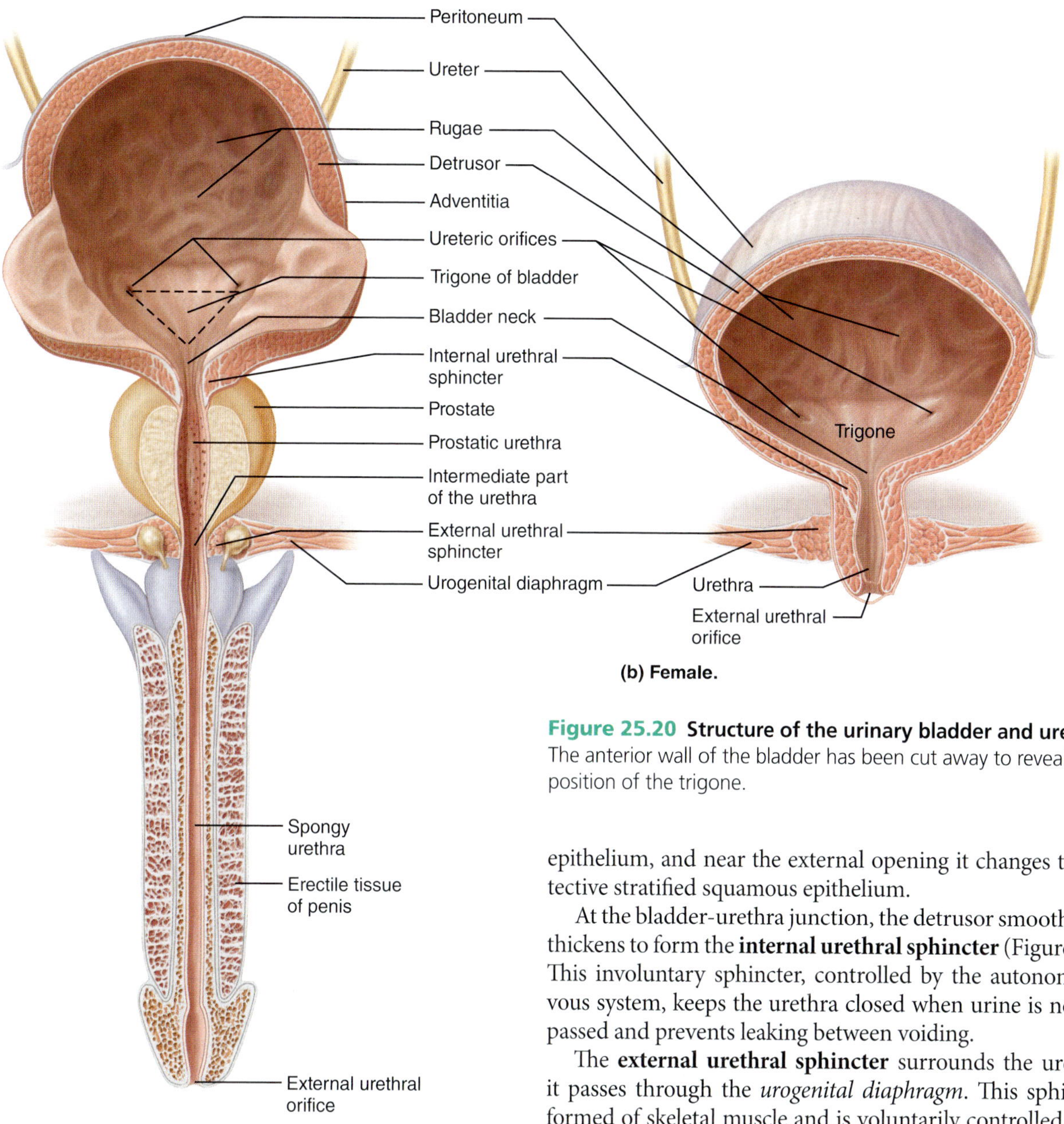

(a) **Male.** The long male urethra has three regions: prostatic, intermediate, and spongy.

(b) Female.

Figure 25.20 Structure of the urinary bladder and urethra. The anterior wall of the bladder has been cut away to reveal the position of the trigone.

capacity of the bladder is 800–1000 ml and when it is overdistended, it may burst.

Urethra

✓ Describe the general location, structure, and function of the urethra.

✓ Compare the course, length, and functions of the male urethra with those of the female.

The **urethra** is a thin-walled muscular tube that drains urine from the bladder and conveys it out of the body. The epithelium of its mucosal lining is mostly pseudostratified columnar epithelium. However, near the bladder it becomes transitional epithelium, and near the external opening it changes to a protective stratified squamous epithelium.

At the bladder-urethra junction, the detrusor smooth muscle thickens to form the **internal urethral sphincter** (Figure 25.20). This involuntary sphincter, controlled by the autonomic nervous system, keeps the urethra closed when urine is not being passed and prevents leaking between voiding.

The **external urethral sphincter** surrounds the urethra as it passes through the *urogenital diaphragm*. This sphincter is formed of skeletal muscle and is voluntarily controlled. The *levator ani* muscle of the pelvic floor also serves as a voluntary constrictor of the urethra (see Table 10.7, pp. 344–345).

The length and functions of the urethra differ in the two sexes. In females the urethra is only 3–4 cm (1.5 inches) long and fibrous connective tissue binds it tightly to the anterior vaginal wall. Its external opening, the **external urethral orifice**, lies anterior to the vaginal opening and posterior to the clitoris.

In males the urethra is approximately 20 cm (8 inches) long and has three regions.

- The **prostatic urethra**, about 2.5 cm (1 inch) long, runs within the prostate.
- The **intermediate part of the urethra** (or *membranous urethra*), which runs through the urogenital diaphragm, extends about 2 cm from the prostate to the beginning of the penis.
- The **spongy urethra**, about 15 cm long, passes through the penis and opens at its tip via the **external urethral orifice**.

The male urethra has a double function: It carries semen as well as urine out of the body. We discuss its reproductive function in Chapter 27.

Homeostatic Imbalance 25.6

Because the female's urethra is very short and its external orifice is close to the anal opening, improper toilet habits (wiping back to front after defecation) can easily carry fecal bacteria into the urethra. Actually, most *urinary tract infections* occur in sexually active women, because intercourse drives bacteria from the vagina and external genital region toward the bladder. The use of spermicides magnifies this problem, because the spermicide kills helpful bacteria, allowing infectious fecal bacteria to colonize the vagina. Overall, 40% of all women get urinary tract infections.

The urethral mucosa is continuous with that of the rest of the urinary tract, and an inflammation of the urethra (*urethritis*) can ascend the tract to cause bladder inflammation (*cystitis*) or even renal inflammations (*pyelitis* or *pyelonephritis*). Symptoms of urinary tract infection include dysuria (painful urination), urinary *urgency* and *frequency*, fever, and sometimes cloudy or blood-tinged urine. When the kidneys are involved, back pain and a severe headache often occur. Antibiotics easily cure most urinary tract infections. +

Micturition

✓ Define micturition and describe its neural control.

Micturition (mik″tu-rish′un; *mictur* = urinate), also called **urination** or *voiding*, is the act of emptying the urinary bladder. For micturition to occur, three things must happen simultaneously: (1) the detrusor must contract, (2) the internal urethral sphincter must open, and (3) the external urethral sphincter must open.

The detrusor and its internal urethral sphincter are composed of smooth muscle and are innervated by both the parasympathetic and sympathetic nervous systems, which have opposing actions. The external urethral sphincter, in contrast, is skeletal muscle, and therefore is innervated by the somatic nervous system.

25

How are the three events required for micturition coordinated? Micturition is most easily understood in infants where a spinal reflex coordinates the process. As urine accumulates, distension of the bladder activates stretch receptors in its walls. Impulses from the activated receptors travel via visceral afferent fibers to the sacral region of the spinal cord. Visceral afferent impulses, relayed by sets of interneurons, excite parasympathetic neurons and inhibit sympathetic neurons **(Figure 25.21)**. As a result, the detrusor contracts and the internal sphincter opens. Visceral afferent impulses also decrease the firing rate of somatic efferents that normally keep the external urethral sphincter closed. This allows the sphincter to relax so urine can flow.

Between ages 2 and 3, descending circuits from the brain have matured enough to begin to override reflexive urination. The pons has two centers that participate in control of micturition. The *pontine storage center* inhibits micturition, whereas the *pontine micturition center* promotes this reflex. Afferent impulses from bladder stretch receptors are relayed to the pons, as well as to higher brain centers that provide the conscious awareness of bladder fullness.

Lower bladder volumes primarily activate the pontine storage center, which inhibits urination by suppressing parasympathetic and enhancing sympathetic output to the bladder. When a person chooses not to void, reflex bladder contractions subside within a minute or so and urine continues to accumulate. Because the external sphincter is voluntarily controlled, we can choose to keep it closed and postpone bladder emptying temporarily. After additional urine has collected, the micturition reflex occurs again and, if urination is delayed again, is damped once more.

The urge to void gradually becomes greater and greater, and micturition usually occurs before urine volume exceeds 400 ml. After normal micturition, only about 10 ml of urine remains in the bladder.

Homeostatic Imbalance 25.7

After the toddler years, **incontinence** is usually a result of weakened pelvic muscles following childbirth or surgery, physical pressure during pregnancy, or nervous system problems. In *stress incontinence*, a sudden increase in intra-abdominal pressure (during laughing and coughing) forces urine through the external sphincter. This condition is common during pregnancy when the heavy uterus stretches the muscles of the pelvic floor and the urogenital diaphragm that support the external sphincter. In *overflow incontinence*, urine dribbles from the urethra whenever the bladder overfills.

In **urinary retention**, the bladder is unable to expel its contained urine. Urinary retention is common after general anesthesia (it takes a little time for the detrusor to regain its activity). Urinary retention in men often reflects hypertrophy of the prostate, which narrows the urethra, making it difficult to void. When urinary retention is prolonged, a slender drainage tube called a **catheter** (kath′ĕ-ter) must be inserted through the urethra to drain the urine and prevent bladder trauma from excessive stretching. +

☑ Check Your Understanding

18. A kidney stone blocking a ureter would interfere with urine flow to which organ? Why would the pain occur in waves?
19. What is the trigone of the bladder, and which landmarks define its borders?
20. Name the three regions of the male urethra.
21. How does the detrusor respond to increased firing of the parasympathetic fibers that innervate it? How does this affect the internal urethral sphincter?

For answers, see Appendix H.

Developmental Aspects of the Urinary System

✓ Trace the embryonic development of the urinary organs.

✓ List several changes in urinary system anatomy and physiology that occur with age.

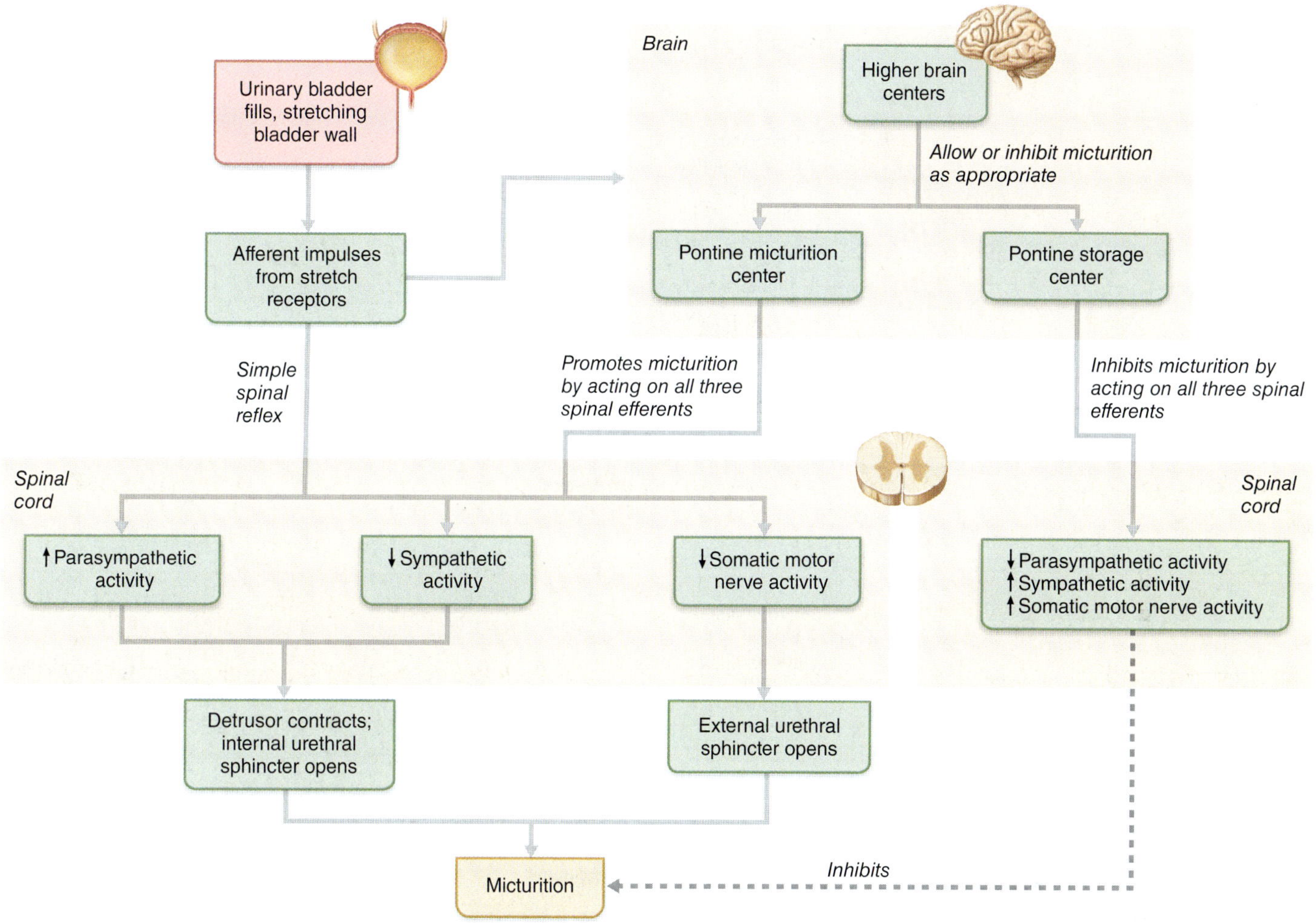

Figure 25.21 **Control of micturition.**

As the kidneys develop in a young embryo, it almost seems as if they are unable to "make up their mind" how to go about it. Three different sets of kidneys develop from the *urogenital ridges*, paired elevations of the intermediate mesoderm that give rise to both the urinary organs and reproductive organs **(Figure 25.22)**. Only the last set persists to become adult kidneys.

During the fourth week of development, the first tubule system, the **pronephros** (pro-nef′ros; "prekidney"), forms and then quickly degenerates as a second, lower set appears. Although the pronephros never functions and is gone by the sixth week, the **pronephric duct** that connects it to the cloaca persists and is used by the later-developing kidneys. (The cloaca is the terminal part of the gut that opens to the body exterior.)

As the second renal system, the **mesonephros** (mez″o-nef′ros; "middle kidney"), claims the pronephric duct, it comes to be called the **mesonephric duct** (Figure 25.22a, b). The mesonephric kidneys degenerate (with remnants incorporated into the male reproductive system) once the third set, the **metanephros** (met″ah-nef′ros; "after kidney"), makes its appearance (Figure 25.22b, c).

The metanephros starts to develop at about five weeks as hollow **ureteric buds** that push superiorly from the mesonephric duct into the urogenital ridge, inducing the mesoderm there to form nephrons. The distal ends of the ureteric buds form the renal pelves, calyces, and collecting ducts, and their unexpanded proximal parts, now called the **ureteric ducts**, become the ureters (Figure 25.22d).

Because the kidneys develop in the pelvis and then ascend to their final position, they receive their blood supply from successively higher sources. Although the lower blood vessels usually degenerate, they sometimes persist, and for this reason multiple renal arteries are common. The metanephric kidneys excrete urine by the third month of fetal life, and most of the amniotic fluid that surrounds a developing fetus is fetal urine. Nonetheless, the fetal kidneys do not work nearly as hard as they will after birth because exchange through the placenta allows the mother's urinary system to clear most of the undesirable substances from the fetal blood.

As the metanephros is developing, the cloaca subdivides to form the future rectum and anal canal and the **urogenital sinus**, into which the urinary and genital ducts empty. The urinary bladder and the urethra then develop from the urogenital sinus (Figure 25.22b–d).

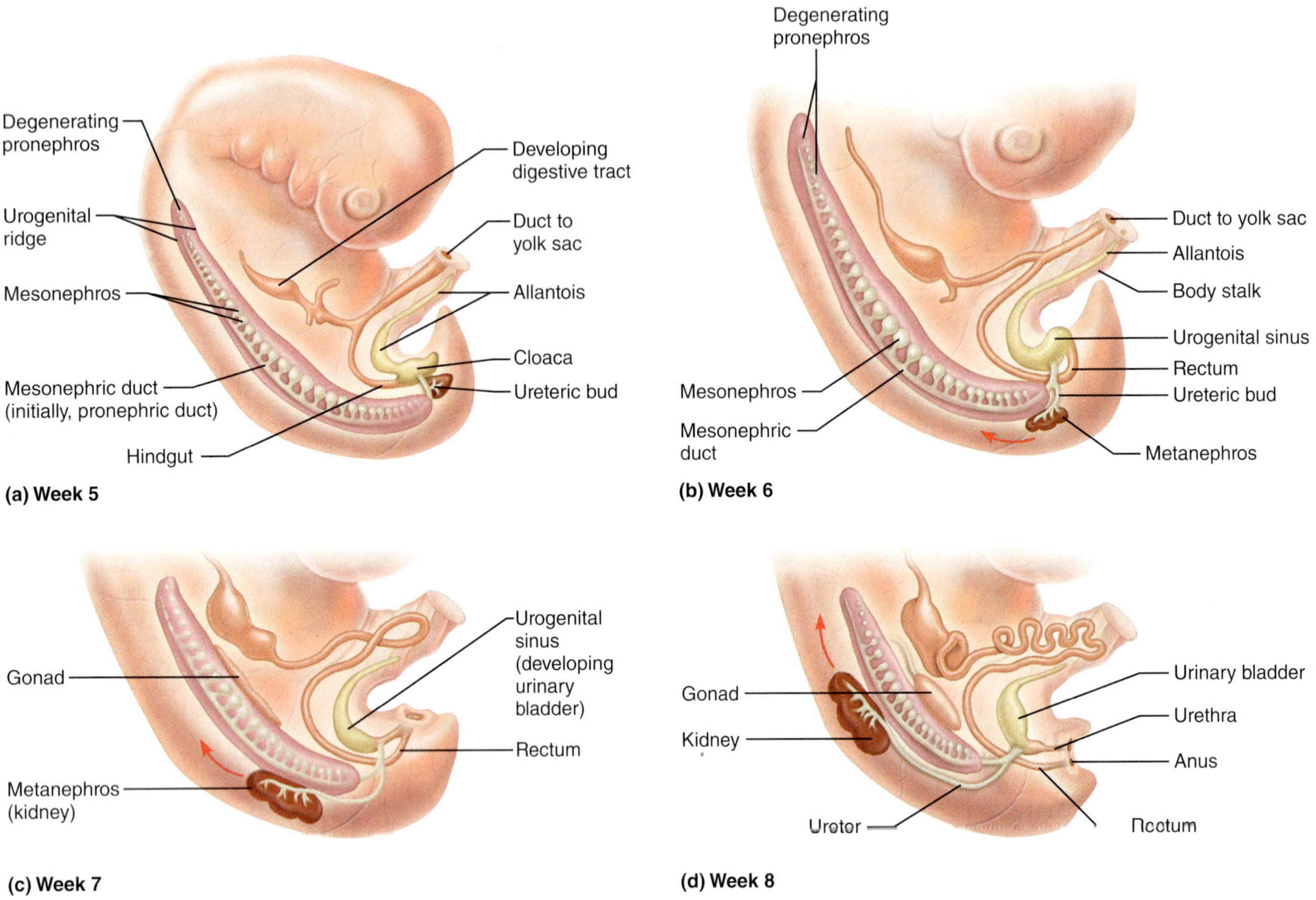

Figure 25.22 Development of the urinary system in the embryo. Red arrows indicate the direction of metanephros migration as it develops.

Homeostatic Imbalance 25.8

Three of the most common congenital abnormalities of the urinary system are horseshoe kidney, hypospadias, and polycystic kidney.

When ascending from the pelvis the kidneys are very close together, and in 1 out of 600 people they fuse across the midline, forming a single, U-shaped *horseshoe kidney*. This condition is usually asymptomatic, but it may be associated with other kidney abnormalities, such as obstructed drainage, that increase the risk of frequent kidney infections.

Hypospadias (hi″po-spa′de-as), found in male infants only, is the most common congenital abnormality of the urethra. It occurs when the urethral orifice is located on the ventral surface of the penis. This problem is corrected surgically when the child is around 12 months old.

Polycystic kidney disease (*PKD*) is a group of disorders characterized by the presence of many fluid-filled cysts in the kidneys. These interfere with renal function, ultimately leading to renal failure. These disorders can be grouped into two general forms:

- *Autosomal dominant PKD*, the less severe form, is much more common, affecting 1 in 500 people. The cysts develop so gradually that they produce no symptoms until about 40 years of age. Then both kidneys begin to enlarge as blister-like cysts containing fluid accumulate. The damage caused by these cysts progresses slowly, and many victims live without problems until their 60s. Ultimately, however, the kidneys become "knobby" and grossly enlarged, reaching a mass of up to 14 kg (30 lb) each.
- *Autosomal recessive PKD* is more severe and much less common, affecting 1 in 20,000 people. Almost half of newborns with recessive PKD die just after birth, and survivors generally develop renal failure in early childhood.

Mutations associated with PKD have been identified in two gene families that code for signaling proteins. These signaling proteins form a mechanoreceptor complex that is part of the primary cilium (see p. 91) that detects the flow of fluid past kidney cells. It is not yet clear how defects in these proteins lead to cyst formation. As yet, the only treatments are the usual treatments for kidney failure—renal dialysis or a kidney transplant. ✚

Because its bladder is very small and its kidneys are less able to concentrate urine for the first two months, a newborn baby voids 5 to 40 times daily, depending on fluid intake. By 2 months, infants void approximately 400 ml/day, and the amount steadily increases until adolescence, when adult urine output (about 1500 ml/day) is achieved.

Incontinence, the inability to control micturition, is normal in infants because their nervous systems have not matured enough to control the external urethral sphincter. Reflex voiding occurs each time a baby's bladder fills enough to activate the stretch receptors. Control of the voluntary urethral sphincter goes hand in hand with nervous system development. By 15 months, most toddlers know when they have voided. By 24 months, some children are ready to begin toilet training. Daytime control usually is achieved first. It is unrealistic to expect complete nighttime control before age 4.

From childhood through late middle age, most urinary system problems are infectious conditions. *Escherichia coli* (esh″ĕ-rik′e-ah ko′li) bacteria are normal residents of the digestive tract and generally cause no problems there, but these bacteria account for 80% of all urinary tract infections. *Sexually transmitted infections* can also inflame the urinary tract and clog some of its ducts. Childhood streptococcal infections such as strep throat and scarlet fever, if not treated promptly, may cause long-term inflammatory renal damage.

Only about 3% of elderly people have histologically normal kidneys, and kidney function declines with advancing age. The kidneys shrink as the nephrons decrease in size and number, and the tubule cells become less efficient. By age 80, the GFR is only half that of young adults, possibly due to atherosclerotic narrowing of the renal arteries. Diabetics are particularly at risk for renal disease, accounting for almost half of new cases.

The bladder of an aged person is shrunken, with less than half the capacity of a young adult (250 ml versus 600 ml). Loss of bladder tone causes an annoying increase in frequency of micturition. *Nocturia* (nok-tu′re-ah), the need to get up during the night to urinate, plagues almost two-thirds of this population. Many people eventually experience incontinence, which can usually be treated with exercise, medications, or surgery.

☑ Check Your Understanding

22. Name the three sets of embryonic kidneys in the order that they develop.
23. List two factors that might contribute to urinary retention in elderly men.

For answers, see Appendix H.

The ureters, urinary bladder, and urethra play important roles in transporting, storing, and eliminating urine from the body, but when the term "urinary system" is used, it is the kidneys that capture center stage. As summarized in *System Connections* in Chapter 26, other organ systems of the body contribute to the well-being of the urinary system in many ways. In turn, without continuous kidney function, the electrolyte and fluid balance of the blood is dangerously disturbed, and internal body fluids quickly become contaminated with nitrogenous wastes. No body cell can escape the harmful effects of such imbalances.

Now that we have described renal mechanisms, we are ready to integrate kidney function into the larger topic of fluid and electrolyte balance in the body—the focus of Chapter 26.

Chapter Summary

Kidney Anatomy (pp. 955–963)

Location and External Anatomy (pp. 955–956)

1. The paired kidneys are retroperitoneal in the superior lumbar region.
2. A fibrous capsule, a perirenal fat capsule, and renal fascia surround each kidney. The perirenal fat capsule helps hold the kidneys in position.

Internal Gross Anatomy (pp. 956–957)

3. A kidney has a superficial cortex, a deeper medulla consisting mainly of medullary pyramids, and a medial pelvis. Extensions of the pelvis (calyces) surround and collect urine draining from the apices of the medullary pyramids.

Blood and Nerve Supply (pp. 957–958)

4. The kidneys receive 25% of the total cardiac output per minute.
5. The vascular pathway through a kidney is as follows: renal artery → segmental arteries → interlobar arteries → arcuate arteries → cortical radiate arteries → afferent arterioles → glomeruli → efferent arterioles → peritubular capillary beds → cortical radiate veins → arcuate veins → interlobar veins → renal vein.
6. The nerve supply of the kidneys is derived from the renal plexus.

Nephrons (pp. 958–963)

7. Nephrons are the structural and functional units of the kidneys.
8. Each nephron consists of a glomerulus (a high-pressure capillary bed), a glomerular capsule, and a renal tubule that is continuous with the capsule. Subdivisions of the renal tubule (from the glomerular capsule) are the proximal convoluted tubule, nephron loop, and distal convoluted tubule. A second capillary bed, the low-pressure peritubular capillary bed, is closely associated with the renal tubule of each nephron.
9. The more numerous cortical nephrons are located almost entirely in the cortex; only a small part of their nephron loop penetrates into the medulla. Glomeruli of juxtamedullary

nephrons are located at the cortex-medulla junction, and their nephron loops dip deeply into the medulla. Instead of directly forming peritubular capillaries, the efferent arterioles of many juxtamedullary nephrons form unique bundles of straight vessels, called vasa recta, that serve tubule segments in the medulla. Juxtamedullary nephrons and the vasa recta play an important role in establishing the medullary osmotic gradient.

10. Collecting ducts receive urine from many nephrons and help concentrate urine. They form the medullary pyramids.
11. The juxtaglomerular complex is at the point of contact between the afferent arteriole and the most distal part of the ascending limb of the nephron loop. It consists of the granular cells, the macula densa, and extraglomerular mesangial cells.

iP Urinary System; Topic: Anatomy Review, pp. 1–20.

Kidney Physiology: Mechanisms of Urine Formation (pp. 963–977)

1. Functions of the nephrons include glomerular filtration, tubular reabsorption, and tubular secretion. Via these functional processes, the kidneys regulate the volume, composition, and pH of the blood, and eliminate nitrogenous metabolic wastes.

Urine Formation, Step 1: Glomerular Filtration (pp. 965–968)

2. The filtration membrane consists of the fenestrated glomerular endothelium, the intervening basement membrane, and the podocyte-containing visceral layer of the glomerular capsule. It permits free passage of substances smaller than (most) plasma proteins.
3. The glomeruli function as filters. High glomerular blood pressure (55 mm Hg) occurs because the glomeruli are fed and drained by arterioles, and the afferent arterioles are larger in diameter than the efferent arterioles.
4. About one-fifth of the plasma flowing through the kidneys is filtered from the glomeruli into the glomerular capsule.
5. Usually about 10 mm Hg, the net filtration pressure (NFP) is determined by the relationship between forces favoring filtration (glomerular hydrostatic pressure) and forces that oppose it (capsular hydrostatic pressure and blood colloid osmotic pressure).
6. The glomerular filtration rate (GFR) is directly proportional to the net filtration pressure and is about 125 ml/min (180 L/day).
7. Intrinsic renal control, or renal autoregulation, enables the kidneys to maintain a relatively constant renal blood flow and glomerular filtration rate. Intrinsic control involves a myogenic mechanism and a tubuloglomerular feedback mechanism mediated by the macula densa.
8. Extrinsic control of GFR, via nerves and hormones, maintains blood pressure. Strong sympathetic nervous system activation causes constriction of the afferent arterioles, which decreases filtrate formation.

iP Urinary System; Topic: Glomerular Filtration, pp. 1–15.

9. The renin-angiotensin-aldosterone mechanism raises systemic blood pressure by generating angiotensin II. Renin is released from granular cells in response to (1) direct sympathetic nervous system stimulation, (2) paracrines released by the macula densa, and (3) reduced stretch of granular cell membranes.

Urine Formation, Step 2: Tubular Reabsorption (pp. 968–972)

10. During tubular reabsorption, needed substances are removed from the filtrate by the tubule cells and returned to the peritubular capillary blood. The primary active transport of Na^+ by a Na^+-K^+ ATPase pump at the basolateral membrane accounts for Na^+ reabsorption and establishes the electrochemical gradient that drives the reabsorption of most other solutes and H_2O. Na^+ enters at the apical surface of the tubule cell via facilitated diffusion through channels or as part of a cotransport mechanism.
11. Passive tubular reabsorption is driven by electrochemical gradients established by active reabsorption of sodium ions. Water, many ions, and various other substances (for example, urea) are reabsorbed passively by diffusion via transcellular or paracellular pathways.
12. Secondary active tubular reabsorption occurs by cotransport with Na^+ via transport proteins. Transport of such substances is limited by the number of carriers available. Actively reabsorbed substances include glucose, amino acids, and some ions.
13. The proximal tubule cells are most active in reabsorption. Most of the nutrients, 65% of the water and sodium ions, and the bulk of actively transported ions are reabsorbed in the proximal convoluted tubules.
14. Reabsorption of additional sodium ions and water occurs in the distal tubules and collecting ducts and is hormonally controlled. Aldosterone increases the reabsorption of sodium; antidiuretic hormone (ADH) enhances water reabsorption by the collecting ducts.

Urine Formation, Step 3: Tubular Secretion (pp. 972–973)

15. Tubular secretion adds substances to the filtrate (from the blood or tubule cells). It is an active process that is important in eliminating drugs, certain wastes, and excess ions and in maintaining the acid-base balance of the blood.

Regulation of Urine Concentration and Volume (pp. 973–977)

16. The graduated hyperosmolality of the medullary fluids (largely due to the cycling of NaCl and urea) ensures that the filtrate reaching the distal convoluted tubule is dilute (hypo-osmolar). This allows urine with osmolalities ranging from 50 to 1200 mOsm to be formed.
    - The descending limb of the nephron loop is permeable to water, which leaves the filtrate and enters the medullary interstitial space. The filtrate and medullary fluid at the bend of the nephron loop are hyperosmolar.
    - The ascending limb is impermeable to water. Na^+ and Cl^- move out of the filtrate into the interstitial space, passively in the thin portion and actively in the thick portion. The filtrate becomes more dilute.
    - As filtrate flows through the collecting ducts in the inner medulla, urea diffuses into the interstitial space. From here, urea reenters the ascending thin limb and is recycled.
    - The blood flow in the vasa recta is sluggish, and the contained blood equilibrates with the medullary interstitial fluid. Hence, blood exiting the medulla in the vasa recta is nearly isotonic to blood plasma and the high solute concentration of the medulla is maintained.
17. In the absence of antidiuretic hormone, dilute urine is formed because the dilute filtrate reaching the collecting duct is simply allowed to pass from the kidneys.
18. When extracellular fluid osmolality rises, blood levels of antidiuretic hormone rise, and the collecting ducts become more permeable to water. Water moves out of the filtrate as it flows through the hyperosmotic medullary areas. Consequently, more concentrated urine is produced, and in smaller amounts.

iP Urinary System; Topics: Early Filtrate Processing, pp. 1–22; Late Filtrate Processing, pp. 1–13.

Clinical Evaluation of Kidney Function (pp. 977–979)

Renal Clearance (p. 978)

1. Renal clearance is the volume of plasma that is completely cleared of a particular substance per minute. Studies of renal clearance provide information about renal function or the course of renal disease.
2. Renal failure has serious consequences: The kidneys are unable to concentrate urine, acid-base and electrolyte imbalances occur, and nitrogenous wastes accumulate in the blood.

Urine (pp. 978–979)

3. Urine is typically clear, yellow, aromatic, and slightly acidic. Its specific gravity ranges from 1.001 to 1.035.
4. Urine is 95% water; solutes include nitrogenous wastes (urea, uric acid, and creatinine) and various ions (always sodium, potassium, sulfate, and phosphate).
5. Substances not normally found in urine include glucose, proteins, erythrocytes, leukocytes, hemoglobin, and bile pigments.

Urine Transport, Storage, and Elimination (pp. 979–982)

Ureters (pp. 979–980)

1. The ureters are slender tubes running retroperitoneally from each kidney to the bladder. They conduct urine by peristalsis from the renal pelvis to the urinary bladder.

Urinary Bladder (pp. 980–981)

2. The urinary bladder, which functions to store urine, is a distensible muscular sac that lies posterior to the pubic symphysis. It has two inlets (ureters) and one outlet (urethra) that outline the trigone. In males, the prostate surrounds the bladder outlet.
3. The bladder wall consists of a mucosa containing transitional epithelium; a three-layered detrusor; and an adventitia.

Urethra (pp. 981–982)

4. The urethra is a muscular tube that conveys urine from the bladder to the body exterior.
5. Where the urethra leaves the bladder, it is surrounded by an internal urethral sphincter, an involuntary smooth muscle sphincter. Where it passes through the urogenital diaphragm, the voluntary external urethral sphincter is formed by skeletal muscle.
6. In females the urethra is 3–4 cm long and conducts only urine. In males it is 20 cm long and conducts both urine and semen.

Micturition (p. 982)

7. Micturition is emptying of the bladder.
8. Accumulating urine stretches the bladder wall, which initiates the micturition reflex. In infants, this is a simple spinal reflex: Parasympathetic fibers are excited (and sympathetic fibers inhibited), causing the detrusor to contract and the internal urethral sphincter to open. In adults, pontine storage and micturition centers can override this simple reflex.
9. Because the external sphincter is voluntarily controlled, micturition can usually be delayed temporarily.

Developmental Aspects of the Urinary System (pp. 982–985)

1. Three sets of kidneys (pronephric, mesonephric, and metanephric) develop from the intermediate mesoderm. The metanephros excretes urine by the third month of development.
2. Common congenital abnormalities are horseshoe kidney, hypospadias, and polycystic kidney disease (PKD).
3. The kidneys of newborns are less able to concentrate urine; their bladder is small and voiding is frequent. Neuromuscular maturation generally allows toilet training for micturition to begin by 24 months of age.
4. The most common urinary system problems in children and young to middle-aged adults are bacterial infections.
5. With age, nephrons are lost, the filtration rate decreases, and tubule cells become less efficient at concentrating urine.
6. Bladder capacity and tone decrease with age, leading to frequent micturition and (often) incontinence. Urinary retention is a common problem of elderly men.

Review Questions

Multiple Choice/Matching

(Some questions have more than one correct answer. Select the best answer or answers from the choices given.)

1. The lowest blood concentration of nitrogenous waste occurs in the **(a)** hepatic vein, **(b)** inferior vena cava, **(c)** renal artery, **(d)** renal vein.
2. The glomerular capillaries differ from other capillary networks in the body because they **(a)** have a larger area of anastomosis, **(b)** are derived from and drain into arterioles, **(c)** are not made of endothelium, **(d)** are sites of filtrate formation.
3. Damage to the renal medulla would interfere *first* with the functioning of the **(a)** glomerular capsules, **(b)** distal convoluted tubules, **(c)** collecting ducts, **(d)** proximal convoluted tubules.
4. Which is reabsorbed by the proximal convoluted tubule cells? **(a)** Na^+, **(b)** K^+, **(c)** amino acids, **(d)** all of the above.
5. Glucose is not normally found in the urine because it **(a)** does not pass through the walls of the glomerulus, **(b)** is kept in the blood by colloid osmotic pressure, **(c)** is reabsorbed by the tubule cells, **(d)** is removed by the body cells before the blood reaches the kidney.
6. Filtration at the glomerulus is inversely related to **(a)** water reabsorption, **(b)** capsular hydrostatic pressure, **(c)** arterial blood pressure, **(d)** acidity of the urine.
7. Tubular reabsorption **(a)** of glucose and many other substances is a T_m-limited active transport process, **(b)** of chloride is always linked to the passive transport of Na^+, **(c)** is the movement of substances from the blood into the nephron, **(d)** of sodium occurs only in the proximal tubule.
8. If a freshly voided urine sample contains excessive amounts of urochrome, it has **(a)** an ammonia-like odor, **(b)** a pH below normal, **(c)** a dark yellow color, **(d)** a pH above normal.
9. Conditions such as diabetes mellitus and starvation are closely linked to **(a)** ketonuria, **(b)** pyuria, **(c)** albuminuria, **(d)** hematuria.
10. Which of the following is/are true about ADH? **(a)** It promotes obligatory water reabsorption, **(b)** it is secreted in response to an increase in extracellular fluid osmolality, **(c)** it causes insertion of aquaporins in the PCT, **(d)** it promotes Na^+ reabsorption.

Short Answer Essay Questions

11. What is the importance of the perirenal fat capsule that surrounds the kidney?
12. Trace the pathway a creatinine molecule takes from a glomerulus to the urethra. Name every microscopic or gross structure it passes through on its journey.
13. Explain the important differences between blood plasma and glomerular filtrate, and relate the differences to the structure of the filtration membrane.
14. Describe the mechanisms that contribute to renal autoregulation.
15. Describe the mechanisms of extrinsic regulation of GFR, and their physiological role.
16. Describe what is involved in active and passive tubular reabsorption.
17. Explain how the peritubular capillaries are adapted for receiving reabsorbed substances.
18. Explain the process and purpose of tubular secretion.
19. How does aldosterone modify the chemical composition of urine?
20. Explain why the filtrate becomes hypotonic as it flows through the ascending limb of the nephron loop. Also explain why the filtrate at the bend of the nephron loop (and the interstitial fluid of the deep portions of the medulla) is hypertonic.
21. How does urinary bladder anatomy support its storage function?
22. Define micturition and describe the micturition reflex.
23. Describe the changes that occur in kidney and bladder anatomy and physiology in old age.

Critical Thinking and Clinical Application Questions

1. Mrs. Bigda, a 60-year-old woman, was brought to the hospital by the police after falling to the pavement. She is found to have alcoholic hepatitis. She is put on a salt- and protein-restricted diet and diuretics are prescribed to manage her ascites (accumulated fluid in the peritoneal cavity). How will diuretics reduce this excess fluid? Name and describe the mechanisms of action of three types of diuretics. Why is her diet salt-restricted?
2. While repairing a frayed utility wire, Herbert, an experienced lineman, slips and falls to the ground. Medical examination reveals a fracture of his lower spine and transection of the lumbar region of the spinal cord. How will Herbert's micturition be controlled from this point on? Will he ever again feel the need to void? Will there be dribbling of urine between voidings? Explain the reasoning behind all your responses.
3. What is cystitis? Why do women suffer from cystitis more frequently than men?
4. Hattie, aged 55, is awakened by excruciating pain that radiates from her right abdomen to the loin and groin regions on the same side. The pain is not continuous but recurs at intervals of 3 to 4 minutes. Diagnose her problem, and cite factors that might favor its occurrence.
5. Why does use of a spermicide increase a woman's risk for urinary tract infection?
6. Why are renal failure patients undergoing dialysis at risk for anemia and osteoporosis? What medications or supplements could you give them to prevent these problems?

AT THE CLINIC

Related Clinical Terms

Acute glomerulonephritis (GN) (glo-mer″u-lo-nef-ri′tis) Inflammation of the glomeruli, leading to increased permeability of the filtration membrane. In some cases, circulating immune complexes (antibodies bound to foreign substances, such as streptococcal bacteria) become trapped in the glomerular basement membranes. In other cases, immune responses are mounted against one's own kidney tissues, leading to glomerular damage. In either case, the inflammatory response that follows damages the filtration membrane, allowing blood proteins and even blood cells to pass into the renal tubules and into the urine. As the osmotic pressure of blood drops, fluid seeps from the bloodstream into the tissue spaces, causing bodywide edema. Renal shutdown requiring dialysis may occur temporarily, but normal renal function usually returns within a few months. If permanent glomerular damage occurs, chronic GN and ultimately renal failure result.

Bladder cancer Bladder cancer, three times more common in men than in women, accounts for about 2% of all cancer deaths. It usually involves neoplasms of the bladder's lining epithelium and may be induced by carcinogens from the environment or the workplace that end up in urine. Smoking, exposure to industrial chemicals, and arsenic in drinking water also have been linked to bladder cancer. Blood in the urine is a common warning sign.

Cystocele (sis′to-sēl; *cyst* = a sac, the bladder; *cele* = hernia, rupture) Herniation of the urinary bladder into the vagina; a common result of tearing of the pelvic floor muscles during childbirth.

Cystoscopy (sis-tos′ko-pe; *cyst* = bladder; *scopy* = observation) Procedure in which a thin viewing tube is threaded into the bladder through the urethra to examine the bladder's mucosal surface.

Diabetes insipidus (in-sĭ′pĭ-dus; *insipid* = tasteless, bland) See Chapter 16, p. 600. Nephrogenic diabetes insipidus is due to lack of ADH receptors in the collecting duct.

Intravenous pyelogram (IVP) (pi′ĕ-lo-gram; *pyelo* = kidney pelvis; *gram* = written) An X ray of the kidneys and ureters obtained after intravenous injection of a contrast medium (as in Figure 25.18). Allows assessment for obstructions, viewing renal anatomy (pelvis and calyces), and determining rate of excretion of the contrast medium.

Nephrotoxin A substance (heavy metal, organic solvent, or bacterial toxin) that is toxic to the kidneys.

Nocturnal enuresis (NE) (en″u-re′sis) An inability to control urination at night during sleep; bed-wetting. In children over 6, called primary NE if control has never been achieved and secondary NE if control was achieved and then lost. Secondary NE often has psychological causes. Primary NE is more common and results from a combination of inadequate nocturnal ADH production, unusually sound sleep, or a small bladder capacity. Synthetic ADH often corrects the problem.

Related Clinical Terms *(continued)*

Renal infarct Area of dead, or necrotic, renal tissue due to blockage of the vascular supply to the kidney or hemorrhage. A common cause of localized renal infarct is an obstructed interlobar artery. Because interlobar arteries do not anastomose, their obstruction leads to ischemic necrosis of the portions of the kidney they supply.

Urinalysis Analysis of urine to diagnose health or disease. The most significant indicators of disease in urine are proteins, glucose, ketone bodies, blood, and pus.

Urologist (u-rol′o-jist) Physician who specializes in diseases of urinary structures in both sexes and in diseases of the reproductive tract of males.

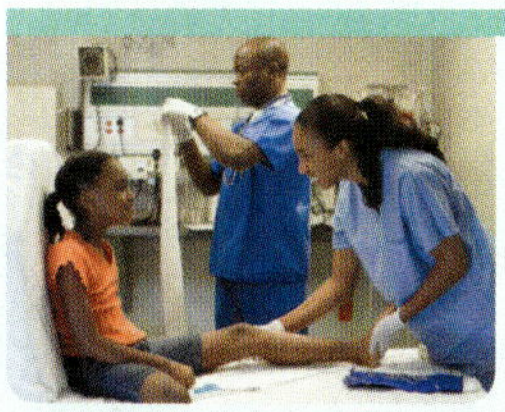

Case Study Urinary System

Let's return to Kyle Boulard, whom we met in the previous chapter. After two days in the hospital, Mr. Boulard has recovered from his acute diabetic crisis and his type 1 diabetes is once again under control. The last update on his chart before he is discharged includes the following:

- BP 150/95, HR 75, temperature 37.2°C
- Urine: pH 6.9, negative for glucose and ketones; 24-hour urine collection reveals 170 mg albumin in urine per day

Mr. Boulard is prescribed a thiazide diuretic and an angiotensin converting enzyme (ACE) inhibitor. He is counseled on the importance of keeping his diabetes under control, taking his medications regularly, and keeping his outpatient follow-up appointments.

1. What is albumin? Is it normally found in the urine? If not, what does its presence suggest?
2. Why were these medications prescribed for Mr. Boulard?
3. Where and how do thiazide diuretics act in the kidneys and how does this reduce blood pressure?

At his two-week appointment at the outpatient clinic, Mr. Boulard complains of fatigue, weakness, muscle cramps, and irregular heartbeats. A physical examination and lab tests produce the following observations:

- BP 133/90, HR 75
- Blood K^+ 2.9 mEq/L (normal 3.5–5.5 mEq/L); blood Na^+ 135 mEq/L (normal 135–145 mEq/L)
- Urine K^+ 55 mEq/L (normal <40 mEq/L); urine Na^+ 21 mEq/L (normal >20 mEq/L)

4. What is Mr. Boulard's main problem at this point?
5. Explain how the thiazide diuretic might have caused this problem.

When asked about his medications, Mr. Boulard admits that he did not fill his ACE inhibitor prescription because it was too expensive. He could only afford the thiazide medications along with his insulin.

6. How do ACE inhibitors reduce blood pressure?
7. Would taking ACE inhibitors and thiazides together have prevented Mr. Boulard's current symptoms? Explain.

(Answers in Appendix H)

26

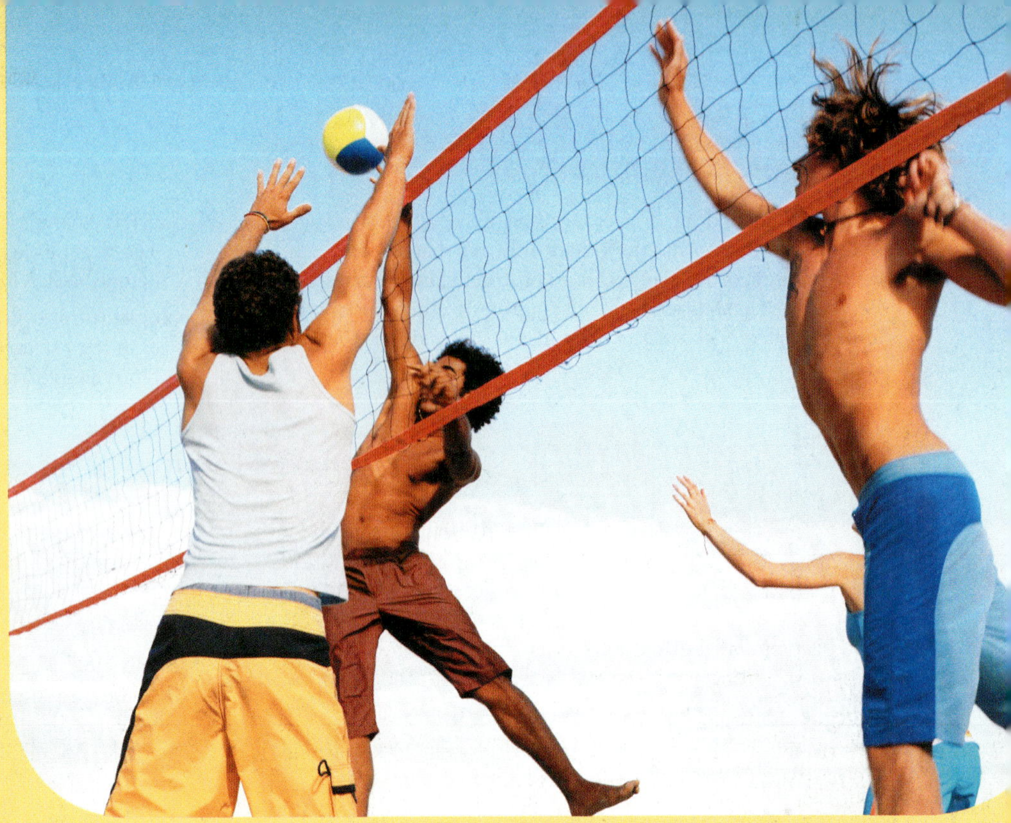

Fluid, Electrolyte, and Acid-Base Balance

Have you ever wondered why on some days you don't urinate for hours at a time, while on others it seems like you void every few minutes? Or why on occasion you cannot seem to quench your thirst? These situations reflect one of the body's most important functions: maintaining fluid, electrolyte, and acid-base balance.

Cell function depends not only on a continuous supply of nutrients and removal of metabolic wastes, but also on the physical and chemical homeostasis of the surrounding fluids. The French physiologist Claude Bernard recognized this truth with style in 1857 when he said, "It is the fixity of the internal environment which is the condition of free and independent life."

In this chapter, we first examine the composition and distribution of fluids in the internal environment and then consider the roles of various body organs and functions in establishing, regulating, and altering this balance.

Body Fluids

- ✓ List the factors that determine body water content and describe the effect of each factor.
- ✓ Indicate the relative fluid volume and solute composition of the fluid compartments of the body.
- ✓ Contrast the overall osmotic effects of electrolytes and nonelectrolytes.
- ✓ Describe factors that determine fluid shifts in the body.

Body Water Content

Not all bodies contain the same amount of water. Total body water is a function not only of age and body mass, but also of sex and the relative amount of body fat. Infants, with their low body fat and low bone mass, are 73% or more water. (This high level of hydration accounts for their "dewy" skin, like that of a freshly picked peach.) After infancy total body water declines throughout life, accounting for only about 45% of body mass in old age.

A healthy young man is about 60% water, and a healthy young woman about 50%. This difference between the sexes reflects the fact that females have relatively more body fat and less skeletal muscle than males. Of all body tissues, adipose tissue is *least* hydrated (containing up to 20% water)—even bone contains more water than does fat. By contrast, skeletal muscle is about 75% water, so people with greater muscle mass have proportionately more body water.

Fluid Compartments

Water occupies two main **fluid compartments** within the body **(Figure 26.1)**. Almost two-thirds by volume is in the **intracellular fluid (ICF) compartment**, which actually consists of trillions of tiny individual "compartments": the cells. In an adult male of average size (70 kg, or 154 lb), ICF accounts for about 25 L of the 40 L of body water.

The remaining one-third or so of body water is outside cells, in the **extracellular fluid (ECF) compartment**. The ECF constitutes the body's "internal environment" referred to by Claude Bernard and is the external environment of each cell. As Figure 26.1 shows, the ECF compartment is divisible into two subcompartments: (1) **plasma**, the fluid portion of blood, and (2) **interstitial fluid (IF)**, the fluid in the microscopic spaces between tissue cells. There are numerous other examples of ECF that are distinct from both plasma and interstitial fluid—lymph, cerebrospinal fluid, humors of the eye, synovial fluid, serous fluid, gastrointestinal secretions—but most of these are similar to IF and are usually considered part of it.

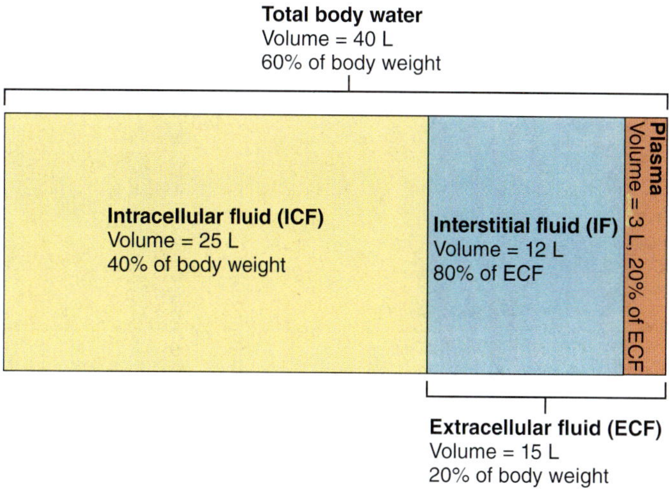

Figure 26.1 The major fluid compartments of the body. [Values are for a 70-kg (154-lb) male.]

Composition of Body Fluids

Water serves as the *universal solvent* in which a variety of solutes are dissolved. Solutes may be classified broadly as *electrolytes* and *nonelectrolytes*.

Electrolytes and Nonelectrolytes

Nonelectrolytes have bonds (usually covalent bonds) that prevent them from dissociating in solution. For this reason, no electrically charged species are created when nonelectrolytes dissolve in water. Most nonelectrolytes are organic molecules—glucose, lipids, creatinine, and urea, for example.

In contrast, **electrolytes** are chemical compounds that *do* dissociate into ions in water. (See Chapter 2 if necessary to review these concepts of chemistry.) Because ions are charged particles, they can conduct an electrical current—and so have the name *electrolyte*. Typically, electrolytes include inorganic salts, both inorganic and organic acids and bases, and some proteins.

Although all dissolved solutes contribute to the osmotic activity of a fluid, electrolytes have much greater osmotic power than nonelectrolytes because each electrolyte molecule dissociates into at least two ions. For example, a molecule of sodium chloride (NaCl) contributes twice as many solute particles as glucose (which remains undissociated), and a molecule of magnesium chloride ($MgCl_2$) contributes three times as many:

$NaCl \rightarrow Na^+ + Cl^-$ (electrolyte; two particles)

$MgCl_2 \rightarrow Mg^{2+} + 2Cl^-$ (electrolyte; three particles)

glucose → glucose (nonelectrolyte; one particle)

Regardless of the type of solute particle, water moves according to osmotic gradients—from an area of lesser osmolality to an area of greater osmolality. For this reason, electrolytes have the greatest ability to cause fluid shifts.

26

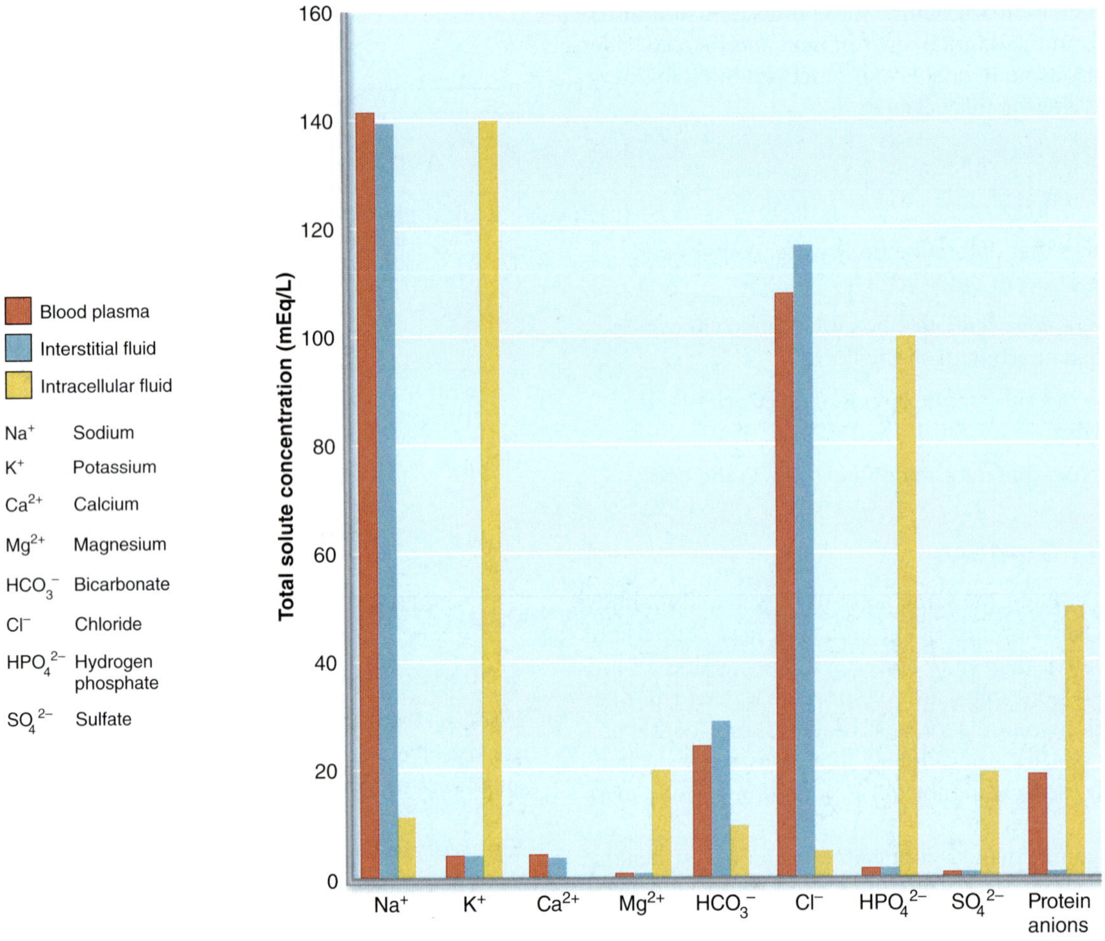

Figure 26.2 Electrolyte composition of blood plasma, interstitial fluid, and intracellular fluid. The very low intracellular Ca^{2+} concentration (10^{-7} *M*) does not include Ca^{2+} stores sequestered inside organelles. The high concentration of intracellular HPO_4^{2-} includes large amounts bound to intermediate metabolites, proteins, and lipids.

Electrolyte concentrations of body fluids are usually expressed in **milliequivalents per liter (mEq/L)**, a measure of the number of electrical charges in 1 liter of solution. We can compute the concentration of any ion in solution using the equation

$$\text{mEq/L} = \frac{\text{ion concentration (mg/L)}}{\text{atomic weight of ion (mg/mmol)}} \times \begin{array}{l}\text{no. of}\\ \text{electrical}\\ \text{charges on}\\ \text{one ion}\end{array}$$

To calculate the mEq/L of sodium or calcium ions in solution in plasma, we would determine the normal concentration of these ions in plasma, look up their atomic weights in the periodic table (see Appendix E), and plug these values into the equation:

$$Na^+: \quad \frac{3300\text{ mg/L}}{23\text{ mg/mmol}} \times 1 = 143\text{ mEq/L}$$

$$Ca^{2+}: \quad \frac{100\text{ mg/L}}{40\text{ mg/mmol}} \times 2 = 5\text{ mEq/L}$$

Notice that for ions with a single charge, 1 mEq is equal to 1 mmol, which, when dissolved in 1 kg of water, produces 1 mOsm (see p. 973). On the other hand, 1 mEq of ions with a double charge (like calcium) is equal to ½ mOsm. In either case, 1 mEq provides the same amount of charge.

Comparison of Extracellular and Intracellular Fluids

A quick glance at the bar graphs in **Figure 26.2** reveals that each fluid compartment has a distinctive pattern of electrolytes. Except for the relatively high protein content in plasma, however, the extracellular fluids are very similar. Their chief cation is sodium, and their major anion is chloride. However, plasma contains somewhat fewer chloride ions than interstitial fluid, because the nonpenetrating plasma proteins are normally anions and plasma is electrically neutral.

In contrast to extracellular fluids, the ICF contains only small amounts of Na^+ and Cl^-. Its most abundant cation is potassium, and its major anion is HPO_4^{2-}. Cells also contain substantial quantities of soluble proteins (about three times the amount found in plasma).

Notice that sodium and potassium ion concentrations in ECF and ICF are nearly opposite (Figure 26.2). The characteristic distribution of these ions on the two sides of cellular membranes reflects the activity of cellular ATP-dependent sodium-potassium pumps, which keep intracellular Na^+ concentrations low and K^+ concentrations high. Renal mechanisms can reinforce these ion distributions by secreting K^+ into the filtrate as Na^+ is reabsorbed from the filtrate.

Electrolytes are the most abundant solutes in body fluids and determine most of their chemical and physical reactions, but they do not constitute the *bulk* of dissolved solutes in these fluids. Proteins and some nonelectrolytes (phospholipids, cholesterol, and triglycerides) found in the ECF are large molecules. They account for about 90% of the mass of dissolved solutes in plasma, 60% in the IF, and 97% in the ICF.

Fluid Movement Among Compartments

Osmotic and hydrostatic pressures regulate the continuous exchange and mixing of body fluids. Although water moves freely between the compartments along osmotic gradients, solutes are unequally distributed because of their size, electrical charge, or dependence on transport proteins. Anything that changes the solute concentration in any compartment leads to net water flows.

Figure 26.3 summarizes the exchanges of gases, solutes, and water across the body's borders and between the three fluid compartments within the body. In general, substances must pass through both the plasma and IF to reach the ICF. In the lungs, gastrointestinal tract, and kidneys, exchanges between the "outside world" and the plasma occur almost continuously. These exchanges alter plasma composition and volume, with plasma serving as the "highway" for delivering substances throughout the body (see Chapter 17). Compensating adjustments between the plasma and the other two fluid compartments follow quickly so that balance is restored.

Let's review the movement of water and solutes across the boundaries between these compartments:

- **Exchanges between plasma and IF occur across capillary walls.** We described the pressures driving these fluid movements in *Focus on Bulk Flow Across Capillary Walls* (Figure 19.17 on pp. 718–719). To recap, the hydrostatic pressure of blood forces nearly protein-free plasma out of the blood into the interstitial space. This filtered fluid is then almost completely reabsorbed into the bloodstream in response to the colloid osmotic pressure of plasma proteins. Under normal circumstances, lymphatic vessels pick up the small net leakage that remains behind in the interstitial space and return it to the blood.
- **Exchanges between the IF and ICF occur across plasma membranes.** As described in Chapter 3, exchanges across the plasma membrane depend on its permeability properties. As a general rule, two-way osmotic flow of water is substantial. But ion fluxes are restricted and, in most cases, ions move selectively by active transport or through channels. Movements of nutrients, respiratory gases, and wastes are typically unidirectional. For example, glucose and oxygen move into the cells and metabolic wastes move out.

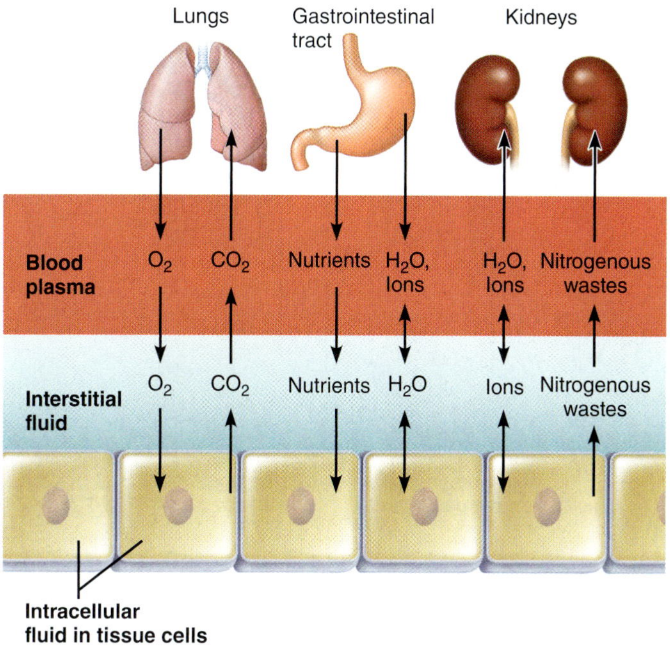

Figure 26.3 Exchange of gases, nutrients, water, and wastes between the three fluid compartments of the body.

Many factors can change ECF and ICF volumes. Because water moves freely between compartments, however, the osmolalities of all body fluids are equal (except during the first few minutes after a change occurs in one of the fluids). Increasing the ECF solute content (mainly the NaCl concentration) causes osmotic and volume changes in the ICF—namely, a shift of water out of the cells. Conversely, decreasing ECF osmolality causes water to move into the cells. Thus, ECF solute concentration determines ICF volume.

It is important for you to understand the concepts above, because they underlie all events that control fluid balance in the body.

Check Your Understanding

1. Which do you have more of, extracellular or intracellular fluid? Plasma or interstitial fluid?
2. What is the major cation in the ECF? In ICF? What are the intracellular anion counterparts of ECF's chloride ions?
3. If you eat salty pretzels without drinking, what happens to the volume of your extracellular fluid? Explain.

For answers, see Appendix H.

Water Balance and ECF Osmolality

✓ List the routes by which water enters and leaves the body.

✓ Describe feedback mechanisms that regulate water intake and hormonal controls of water output in urine.

✓ Explain the importance of obligatory water losses.

✓ Describe possible causes and consequences of dehydration, hypotonic hydration, and edema.

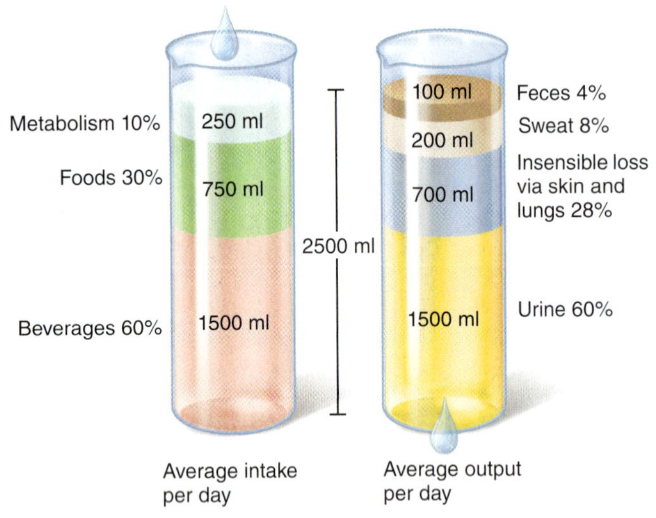

Figure 26.4 Major sources of water intake and output. When intake and output are in balance, the body is adequately hydrated.

For the body to remain properly hydrated, water intake must equal water output. *Water intake* varies widely from person to person and is strongly influenced by habit, but is typically about 2500 ml a day in adults **(Figure 26.4)**. Most water enters the body through ingested liquids and solid foods. Body water produced by cellular metabolism is called **metabolic water** or **water of oxidation**.

Water output occurs by several routes. Water that vaporizes out of the lungs in expired air or diffuses directly through the skin is called **insensible water loss**. Some is lost in obvious perspiration and in feces. The kidneys excrete the rest (about 60%) in urine.

Healthy people have a remarkable ability to maintain the osmolality of their body fluids within very narrow limits (280–300 mOsm). A rise in plasma osmolality triggers (1) thirst, which prompts us to drink water, and (2) release of antidiuretic hormone (ADH), which causes the kidneys to conserve water and excrete concentrated urine. On the other hand, a decline in osmolality inhibits both thirst and ADH release, and the latter prompts the kidneys to excrete large volumes of dilute urine.

In the body, water and Na^+ are closely tied together. In fact, Na^+ acts as a powerful "water magnet." However, the ADH and thirst mechanisms controlling osmolality regulate water *independently* of sodium. Later, we will describe mechanisms that regulate Na^+ and water *together* for the purpose of maintaining blood volume and pressure.

Regulation of Water Intake

The **thirst mechanism** is the driving force for water intake. It is governed by the hypothalamic *thirst center*, which is activated by various stimuli **(Figure 26.5)**:

- *Osmoreceptors.* Hypothalamic *osmoreceptors* detect ECF osmolality through changes in plasma membrane stretch that result from gaining or losing water. An increase in osmolality of only 1–2% activates these osmoreceptors.

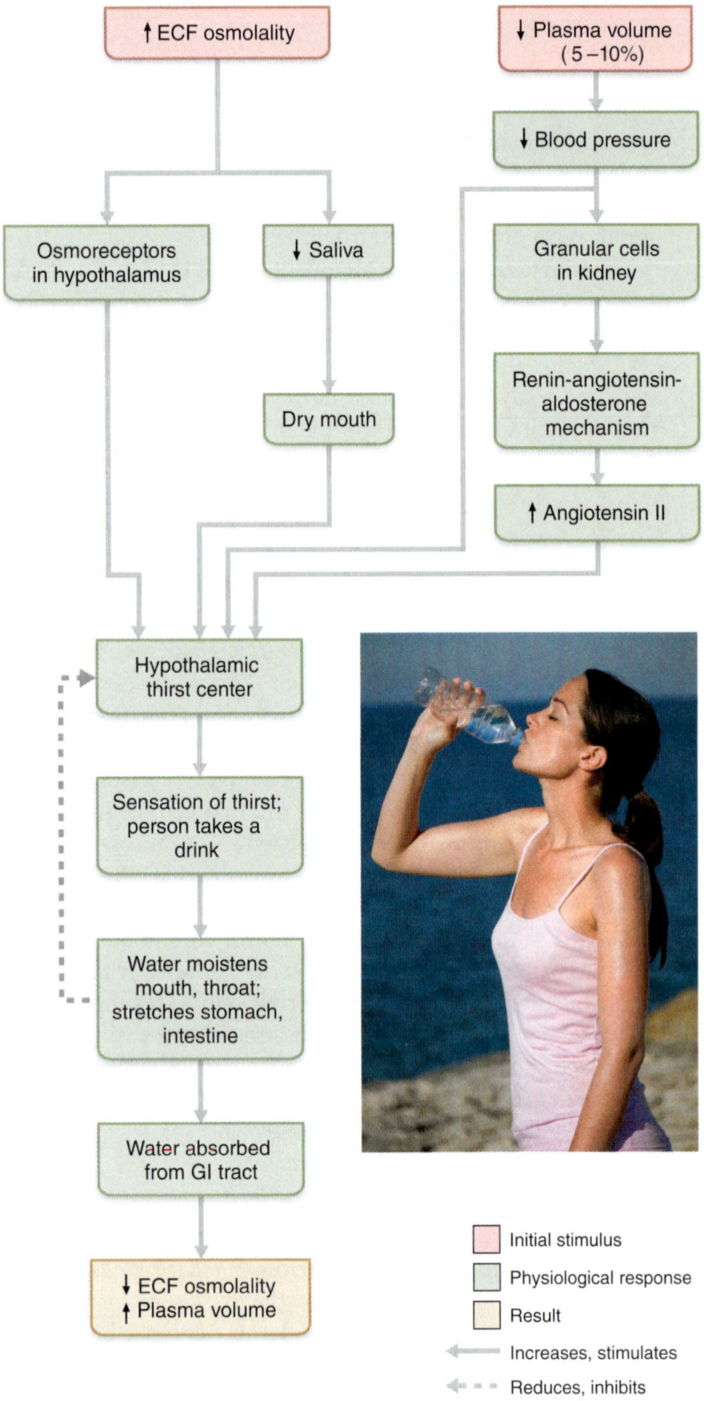

Figure 26.5 The thirst mechanism for regulating water intake. Only large volume changes (5–10% of plasma volume) activate the thirst mechanism. Osmolality changes are the normal stimuli.

- *Dry mouth.* When the blood's osmotic pressure increases, the salivary glands produce less saliva because the osmotic gradient drawing water from the blood into the salivary ducts is reduced.
- *A decrease in blood volume (or pressure).* A substantial decrease in blood volume or pressure (5–10%, as in hemor-

rhage) also triggers the thirst mechanism. These changes in volume or pressure are signaled by baroreceptors that directly activate the thirst center, and by angiotensin II as we described in Chapter 19.

Collectively, these events cause a subjective sensation of thirst, which motivates us to get a drink. This mechanism explains why some cocktail lounges provide free *salty* snacks to their patrons.

Curiously, thirst is quenched almost as soon as we begin drinking water, even though the water has yet to be absorbed into the blood. How does this happen? Incoming liquid moistens the mucosa of the mouth and throat and activates osmoreceptors and stretch receptors in the stomach and small intestine, providing feedback signals that inhibit the thirst center. Premature quenching of thirst prevents us from drinking more than we need and overdiluting our body fluids, and allows time for the osmotic changes to come into play as regulatory factors.

As effective as thirst is, it is not always a reliable indicator of need. This is particularly true during athletic events, when thirst can be satisfied long before sufficient liquids have been drunk to maintain the body in top form. Additionally, elderly or confused people may not recognize or heed thirst signals. In contrast, fluid-overloaded renal or cardiac patients may feel thirsty despite their condition.

Regulation of Water Output

Output of certain amounts of water is unavoidable. Such **obligatory water losses** help to explain why we cannot survive for long without drinking. Even the most heroic conservation efforts by the kidneys cannot compensate for zero water intake. Obligatory water loss includes the *insensible water losses* described above, water that accompanies undigested food residues in feces, and a minimum daily **sensible water loss** of 500 ml in urine.

Obligatory water loss in urine reflects the fact that human kidneys must normally flush 600 mmol per day of urine solutes (end products of metabolism and so forth) out of the body in water. The maximum concentration of urine is about 1200 mOsm, so at least 500 ml of water must be excreted.

Beyond obligatory water loss, the solute concentration and volume of urine excreted depend on fluid intake, diet, and water loss via other avenues. For example, if you perspire profusely on a hot day, you have to excrete much less urine than usual to maintain water balance. Normally, the kidneys begin to eliminate excess water about 30 minutes after it is ingested. This delay reflects the time required to inhibit ADH release. Diuresis reaches a peak about 1 hour after drinking and declines to its lowest level after 3 hours.

Influence of Antidiuretic Hormone (ADH)

The amount of water reabsorbed in the renal collecting ducts is proportional to ADH release. When ADH levels are low, most of the water reaching the collecting ducts is not reabsorbed because the lack of aquaporins in the apical membranes of the principal cells prevents the movement of water. Instead, the water simply flows on by. The result is dilute urine and a reduced volume of body fluids. When ADH levels are high, aquaporins are inserted in the principal cell apical membranes, nearly all of the filtered water is reabsorbed, and a small volume of concentrated urine is excreted.

Osmoreceptors of the hypothalamus sense the ECF solute concentration and trigger or inhibit ADH release from the posterior pituitary accordingly **(Figure 26.6)**. An increase in ECF osmolality prompts ADH release by stimulating the hypothalamic osmoreceptors. In contrast, a decrease in ECF osmolality inhibits ADH release and allows more water to be excreted in urine, restoring normal blood osmolality.

Large changes in blood volume or blood pressure also influence ADH secretion. A decrease in blood pressure increases ADH release both directly via baroreceptors in the atria and various blood vessels, and indirectly via the renin-angiotensin-aldosterone mechanism.

The key word here is "large" because changes in ECF osmolality are much more important as day-to-day stimulatory or inhibitory factors. Factors that trigger ADH release by reducing blood volume include excessive sweating, vomiting, or diarrhea; severe blood loss; traumatic burns; and prolonged fever. Under these conditions, high concentrations of ADH also act to constrict arterioles, directly increasing blood pressure—hence its other name: *vasopressin*. For a summary of how renal mechanisms involving ADH, aldosterone, and angiotensin II tie into overall controls of blood volume and blood pressure, see Figure 26.10 (p. 1002), but remember that the main thrust of ADH is to maintain ECF osmolality.

Disorders of Water Balance

Few people really appreciate the importance of water in keeping the body's "machinery" working at peak efficiency. The principal abnormalities of water balance are dehydration, hypotonic hydration, and edema—each presenting a special set of problems.

Dehydration

Clinically, **dehydration** is defined as fluid loss, either the loss of water or the loss of water and solutes together. For example, when water output exceeds intake over a period of time, the body becomes dehydrated. Dehydration is a common sequel to hemorrhage, severe burns, prolonged vomiting or diarrhea, profuse sweating, water deprivation, and diuretic abuse. Dehydration may also be caused by endocrine disturbances, such as diabetes mellitus or diabetes insipidus (see Chapter 16).

Early signs and symptoms of dehydration include a "cottony" or sticky oral mucosa, thirst, dry flushed skin, and decreased urine output (*oliguria*). Prolonged dehydration may lead to weight loss, fever, and mental confusion. Another serious consequence of water loss from plasma is inadequate blood volume to maintain normal circulation and ensuing *hypovolemic shock*.

Water and solutes can be lost together (as in hemorrhage), or more water than solutes can be lost (as in profuse sweating). If the body loses more water than solutes, water moves osmotically

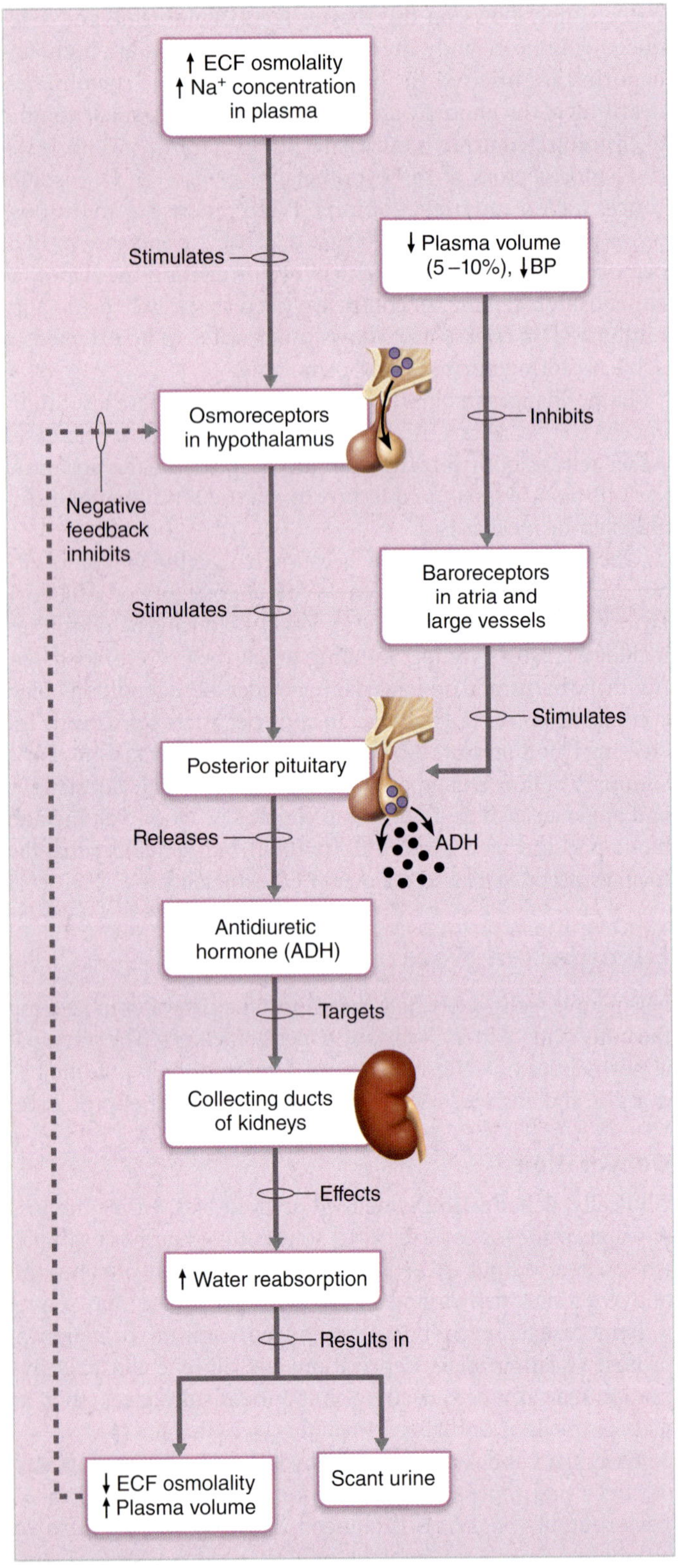

Figure 26.6 Mechanisms and consequences of ADH release. (Vasoconstrictor effects of ADH are not shown.)

from the cells into the ECF **(Figure 26.7a)**. This water movement equalizes the osmolality of the extracellular and intracellular fluids even though the total fluid volume has been reduced.

Hypotonic Hydration

Declining ECF osmolality sets several compensatory mechanisms into motion. ADH release is inhibited, and as a result, less water is reabsorbed and excess water is quickly flushed from the body in urine. But, when there is renal insufficiency or we drink an extraordinary amount of water very quickly, a type of cellular *overhydration* called **hypotonic hydration** may occur. In either case, the ECF is diluted—its sodium content is normal, but excess water is present. For this reason, the hallmark of hypotonic hydration is **hyponatremia** (low ECF Na^+ concentration), which promotes net osmosis into tissue cells, causing them to swell as they become abnormally hydrated (Figure 26.7b).

Hypotonic hydration leads to severe metabolic disturbances evidenced by nausea, vomiting, muscular cramping, and cerebral edema. It is particularly damaging to neurons. Uncorrected cerebral edema quickly leads to disorientation, convulsions, coma, and death. Indeed, several marathon runners have died of overhydration after drinking too much water. Sudden and severe hyponatremia is treated by administering intravenous hypertonic saline to reverse the osmotic gradient and "pull" water out of the cells.

Edema

Edema (ĕ-de′mah; "a swelling") is an atypical accumulation of fluid in the interstitial space, leading to tissue (but not cell) swelling. Unlike hypotonic hydration, which increases the amount of fluid in all compartments due to an imbalance between water intake and output, edema is an increase in volume of *only* the IF. It may be caused by any event that steps up the flow of fluid out of the blood or hinders its return.

Factors that accelerate fluid loss from the blood include increases in capillary hydrostatic pressure and permeability. Increased capillary hydrostatic pressure can result from incompetent venous valves, localized blood vessel blockage, congestive heart failure, or high blood volume. Whatever the cause, the abnormally high capillary hydrostatic pressure intensifies filtration at the capillary beds.

Increased capillary permeability is usually due to an ongoing inflammatory response. Recall from p. 767 that inflammatory chemicals cause local capillaries to become very porous, allowing large amounts of exudate (containing not only clotting proteins but also other plasma proteins, nutrients, and immune elements) to form.

Edema caused by hindered fluid return to the blood usually reflects an imbalance in the colloid osmotic pressures on the two sides of the capillary membranes. For example, **hypoproteinemia** (hi″po-pro″te-ĭ-ne′me-ah), a condition of unusually low levels of plasma proteins, results in tissue edema because protein-deficient plasma has an abnormally low colloid osmotic pressure. Fluids are forced out of the capillary beds at the arterial ends by blood pressure as usual, but fail to return to the blood at the venous ends. As a result, the interstitial spaces become congested with fluid. Hypoproteinemia may result from protein malnutrition, liver disease, or *glomerulonephritis* (in

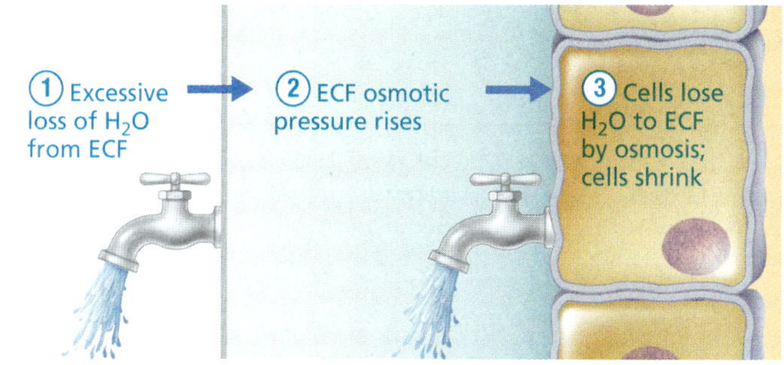

(a) Consequences of dehydration. If more water than solutes is lost, cells shrink.

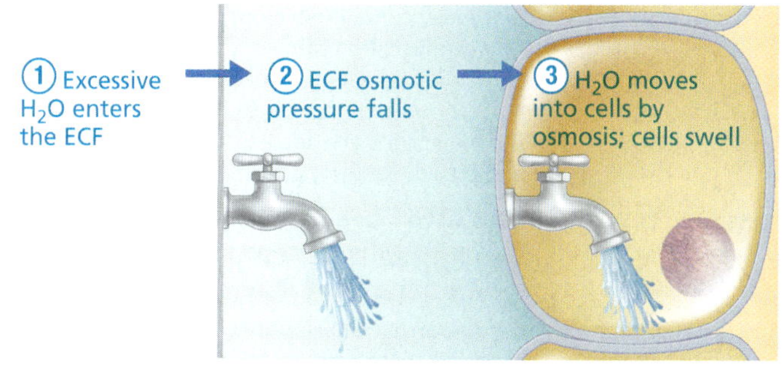

(b) Consequences of hypotonic hydration (water gain). If more water than solutes is gained, cells swell.

Figure 26.7 Disturbances in water balance.

which plasma proteins pass through "leaky" renal filtration membranes and are lost in urine).

Edema can also result when lymphatic vessels are blocked or have been surgically removed. The small amounts of plasma proteins that seep out of the bloodstream do not return to the blood as usual. As the leaked proteins accumulate in the IF, they exert an ever-increasing colloid osmotic pressure, which draws fluid from the blood and holds it in the interstitial space.

Edema can impair tissue function because excess fluid in the interstitial space increases the distance nutrients and oxygen must diffuse between the blood and the cells. However, the most serious problems resulting from rapid onset of edema affect the cardiovascular system. When fluid leaves the bloodstream and accumulates in the interstitial space, both blood volume and blood pressure decline and the efficiency of the circulation can be severely impaired.

Check Your Understanding

4. What change in plasma is most important for triggering thirst? Where is that change sensed?
5. ADH, by itself, cannot reduce an increase in osmolality in body fluids. Why not? What other mechanism is required?
6. For each of the following, state whether it might result in dehydration, hypotonic hydration, or edema: (a) decreased synthesis of plasma proteins due to liver failure; (b) copious sweating; (c) using ecstasy (MDMA), which promotes ADH secretion.

For answers, see Appendix H.

Electrolyte Balance

- ✓ Indicate routes of electrolyte entry and loss from the body.
- ✓ Describe the importance of sodium in the body's fluid and electrolyte balance, and indicate its relationship to normal cardiovascular system functioning.
- ✓ Describe mechanisms involved in regulating sodium balance, blood volume, and blood pressure.
- ✓ Explain how potassium, calcium, and anion balances in plasma are regulated.

Electrolytes include salts, acids, bases, and some proteins, but the term **electrolyte balance** usually refers to salt balance in the body. Salts are important in controlling fluid movements and provide minerals essential for excitability, secretory activity, and membrane permeability. Although many electrolytes are crucial for cellular activity, here we will specifically examine the regulation of sodium, potassium, and calcium. In the next section we will consider acids and bases, which are intimately involved in determining the pH of body fluids.

Salts enter the body in foods and fluids, and small amounts are generated during metabolic activity. For example, phosphates are liberated during catabolism of nucleic acids and bone matrix. Obtaining enough electrolytes is usually not a problem. Indeed, most of us have a far greater taste than need for salt. We shake table salt (NaCl) on our food even though natural foods contain ample amounts and processed foods contain exorbitant quantities. The taste for very salty foods is learned, but some liking for salt may be innate to ensure adequate intake of these two vital ions.

We lose salts from the body in perspiration, feces, urine, and vomit. Even though sweat is normally hypotonic, large amounts of salt can be lost on a hot day simply because more sweat is produced. Gastrointestinal disorders can also lead to large salt losses in feces or vomitus. Consequently, the flexibility of renal mechanisms that regulate the electrolyte balance of the blood is a critical asset. Table 26.1 summarizes several causes and consequences of electrolyte imbalance.

Homeostatic Imbalance 26.1

Severe electrolyte deficiencies may prompt a craving for salty or sour foods, such as smoked meats or pickled eggs. This is common in those with *Addison's disease*, a disorder entailing deficient mineralocorticoid hormone production by the adrenal cortex.

When minerals such as iron are deficient, a person may even eat substances not usually considered foods, like chalk, clay, starch, and burnt match tips. This appetite for abnormal substances is called *pica*. +

The Central Role of Sodium in Fluid and Electrolyte Balance

Sodium holds a central position in fluid and electrolyte balance and overall body homeostasis. Indeed, regulating the balance between sodium input and output is one of the most important

Table 26.1 Causes and Consequences of Electrolyte Imbalances

ION	ABNORMALITY (SERUM VALUE)	POSSIBLE CAUSES	CONSEQUENCES
Sodium	Hypernatremia (Na^+ excess: >145 mEq/L)	Dehydration; uncommon in healthy individuals; may occur in infants or the confused aged (individuals unable to indicate thirst) or may result from excessive intravenous NaCl administration	Thirst. CNS dehydration leads to confusion and lethargy progressing to coma; increased neuromuscular irritability evidenced by twitching and convulsions.
	Hyponatremia (Na^+ deficit: <135 mEq/L)	Solute loss, water retention, or both (e.g., excessive Na^+ loss through vomiting, diarrhea, burned skin, tubal drainage of stomach, or excessive use of diuretics); deficiency of aldosterone (Addison's disease); renal disease; excess ADH release; excess H_2O ingestion	Most common signs are those of neurologic dysfunction due to brain swelling. If sodium amounts are actually normal but water is excessive, the symptoms are the same as those of water excess: mental confusion; giddiness; coma if development occurs slowly; muscular twitching, irritability, and convulsions if the condition develops rapidly. In hyponatremia accompanied by water loss, the main signs are decreased blood volume and blood pressure (circulatory shock).
Potassium	Hyperkalemia (K^+ excess: >5.5 mEq/L)	Renal failure; deficit of aldosterone; rapid intravenous infusion of KCl; burns or severe tissue injuries that cause K^+ to leave cells	Nausea, vomiting, diarrhea; bradycardia; cardiac arrhythmias, depression, and arrest; skeletal muscle weakness; flaccid paralysis.
	Hypokalemia (K^+ deficit: <3.5 mEq/L)	Gastrointestinal tract disturbances (vomiting, diarrhea), gastrointestinal suction; Cushing's syndrome; inadequate dietary intake (starvation); hyperaldosteronism; diuretic therapy	Cardiac arrhythmias, flattened T wave; muscular weakness; metabolic alkalosis; mental confusion; nausea; vomiting.
Phosphate	Hyperphosphatemia (HPO_4^{2-} excess: >2.9 mEq/L)	Decreased urinary loss due to renal failure; hypoparathyroidism; major tissue trauma; increased intestinal absorption	Clinical symptoms arise because of reciprocal changes in Ca^{2+} levels rather than directly from changes in plasma phosphate concentrations.
	Hypophosphatemia (HPO_4^{2-} deficit: <1.6 mEq/L)	Decreased intestinal absorption; increased urinary output; hyperparathyroidism	
Chloride	Hyperchloremia (Cl^- excess: >105 mEq/L)	Dehydration; increased retention or intake; metabolic acidosis; hyperparathyroidism	No direct clinical symptoms; symptoms generally associated with the underlying cause, which is often related to pH abnormalities.
	Hypochloremia (Cl^- deficit: <95 mEq/L)	Metabolic alkalosis (e.g., due to vomiting or excessive ingestion of alkaline substances); aldosterone deficiency	
Calcium	Hypercalcemia (Ca^{2+} excess: >5.2 mEq/L or 10.5 mg%)*	Hyperparathyroidism; excessive vitamin D; prolonged immobilization; renal disease (decreased excretion); malignancy	Decreased neuromuscular excitability leading to cardiac arrhythmias and arrest, skeletal muscle weakness, confusion, stupor, and coma; kidney stones; nausea and vomiting.
	Hypocalcemia (Ca^{2+} deficit: <4.5 mEq/L or 9 mg%)*	Burns (calcium trapped in damaged tissues); hypoparathyroidism; vitamin D deficiency; renal tubular disease; renal failure; hyperphosphatemia; diarrhea; alkalosis	Increased neuromuscular excitability leading to tingling fingers, tremors, skeletal muscle cramps, tetany, convulsions; depressed excitability of the heart; osteomalacia; fractures.
Magnesium	Hypermagnesemia (Mg^{2+} excess: >2.2 mEq/L)	Rare; occurs in renal failure when Mg^{2+} is not excreted normally; excessive ingestion of Mg^{2+}-containing antacids	Lethargy; impaired CNS functioning, coma, respiratory depression; cardiac arrest.
	Hypomagnesemia (Mg^{2+} deficit: <1.4 mEq/L)	Alcoholism; chronic diarrhea, severe malnutrition; diuretic therapy	Tremors, increased neuromuscular excitability, tetany, convulsions.

*1 mg% = 1 mg/100 ml

26

renal functions. The salts $NaHCO_3$ and NaCl account for 90–95% of all solutes in the ECF, and they contribute about 280 mOsm of the total ECF solute concentration (300 mOsm).

At its normal plasma concentration of about 142 mEq/L, Na^+ is the single most abundant cation in the ECF and the only one exerting *significant* osmotic pressure. Additionally, cellular plasma membranes are relatively impermeable to Na^+ (some does manage to diffuse in and must be pumped out against its electrochemical gradient). These two qualities give sodium the primary role in controlling ECF volume and water distribution in the body.

Remember: *Water follows salt.* Because all body fluids are in osmotic equilibrium, a change in plasma Na^+ levels affects not only plasma volume and blood pressure, but also ICF and IF volumes. In addition, sodium ions continuously move back and forth between the ECF and body secretions. For example, about 8 L of Na^+-containing secretions (gastric, intestinal, and pancreatic juice, saliva, bile) are spewed into the digestive tract daily, only to be almost completely reabsorbed. Finally, renal acid-base control mechanisms (which we will discuss shortly) are coupled to Na^+ transport.

Sodium Concentration Versus Sodium Content

For ions other than Na^+, their concentration in body fluids is the only important variable. For Na^+, however, both the concentration and the total body content are important.

- **Concentration of Na^+.** The concentration of Na^+ in the ECF largely determines the osmolality of ECF fluids and influences electrical excitability of neurons and muscles. The concentration of Na^+ normally remains relatively stable because water immediately moves by osmosis into or out of the ICF, counteracting the change in Na^+ concentration. In the long term, the ADH and thirst mechanisms control the ECF Na^+ concentration by controlling water loss or gain.
- **Content of Na^+.** The total body content of Na^+ determines the ECF volume and therefore blood pressure. Na^+ content is regulated by the renin-angiotensin-aldosterone and atrial natriuretic peptide (ANP) hormone mechanisms that control Na^+ reabsorption and excretion (Na^+ balance). We will review these mechanisms in the next section.

It helps to think about these aspects of Na^+ balance as separate and distinct because they have different roles in homeostasis **(Table 26.2)**. Nevertheless, there is some overlap between them and their mechanisms are intertwined. For example, as ECF Na^+ content increases, ECF osmolality rises as well, which triggers the ADH and thirst mechanisms. This increases water retention and intake, simultaneously reducing the Na^+ concentration and increasing the ECF volume.

Regulation of Sodium Balance

Despite the crucial importance of sodium, receptors that specifically monitor the concentration or content of Na^+ in body fluids have yet to be found. Because regulation of the Na^+ balance is inseparably linked to blood volume and pressure, changes in these two variables trigger a variety of neural and hormonal controls that regulate total body Na^+ content.

Table 26.2 Sodium Concentration and Sodium Content

	ECF Na^+ CONCENTRATION	BODY Na^+ CONTENT
Homeostatic Importance	ECF osmolality	Blood volume and blood pressure
Sensors	Osmoreceptors	Baroreceptors
Regulation	ADH and thirst mechanisms	Renin-angiotensin-aldosterone and ANP hormone mechanisms*

*ADH and thirst are also required to maintain blood volume and for long-term control of blood pressure.

Influence of Aldosterone and Angiotensin II

The hormone **aldosterone** "has the most to say" about renal regulation of sodium ions. But whether aldosterone is present or not, some 65% of the Na^+ in the renal filtrate is reabsorbed in the proximal tubules of the kidneys and another 25% is reclaimed in the nephron loops (see Chapter 25).

When aldosterone concentrations are high, essentially *all* the remaining filtered Na^+ is actively reabsorbed in the distal convoluted tubules and collecting ducts. Consistent with aldosterone's central role in maintaining blood volume and blood pressure, water always follows Na^+. This water comes from either the intracellular fluid or, if ADH is present, from the filtrate in the collecting ducts. One way or another, aldosterone increases ECF volume.

When aldosterone release is inhibited, virtually no Na^+ reabsorption occurs beyond the distal convoluted tubule. Urinary excretion of large amounts of Na^+ *always* results in the excretion of large amounts of water as well, but the reverse is *not* true. Substantial amounts of nearly sodium-free urine can be eliminated as needed to achieve water balance.

The most important trigger for aldosterone release from the adrenal cortex is the renin-angiotensin-aldosterone mechanism mediated by the juxtaglomerular complex (JGC) of the renal tubules. In addition, elevated K^+ concentration in the ECF can directly stimulate adrenal cortical cells to release aldosterone **(Figure 26.8)**

The result of aldosterone release is increased reabsorption of Na^+ and increased secretion of K^+. Aldosterone brings about its effects slowly, over a period of hours to days. The principal effects of aldosterone are to decrease urinary output and increase blood volume.

Low blood volume and blood pressure (reflecting decreased body Na^+ content) trigger renin release from the granular cells of the JGC in three ways shown in Figure 26.10: (1) sympathetic stimulation, (2) decreased filtrate NaCl concentration, or (3) decreased stretch of the granular cells. Renin catalyzes the initial step in the reactions that produce angiotensin II. Angiotensin II

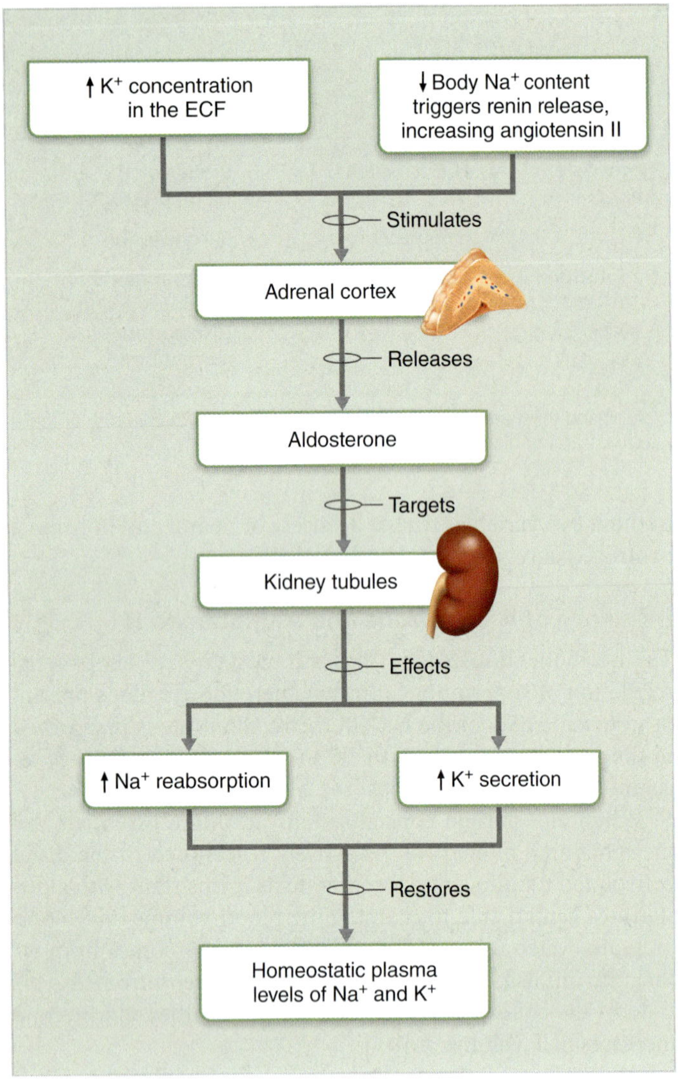

Figure 26.8 Mechanisms and consequences of aldosterone release.

26

prods the adrenal cortex to release aldosterone, and also directly increases Na^+ reabsorption by kidney tubules. In addition, it has a number of other actions described in Chapter 19 (pp. 709–710) that are all aimed at raising blood volume and blood pressure.

Homeostatic Imbalance 26.2

People with Addison's disease (hypoaldosteronism) lose tremendous amounts of NaCl and water to urine. They are perpetually teetering on the brink of hypovolemia, but as long as they ingest adequate amounts of salt and fluids, they can avoid problems with Na^+ balance. ✚

Influence of Atrial Natriuretic Peptide (ANP)

We can summarize the influence of **atrial natriuretic peptide (ANP)** in one sentence: It reduces blood pressure and blood volume by inhibiting nearly all events that promote vasoconstriction and Na^+ and water retention **(Figure 26.9)**. A hormone that is released by certain cells of the heart atria when they are stretched by the effects of elevated blood pressure, ANP has diuretic and natriuretic (salt-excreting) effects. It promotes excretion of Na^+ and water by the kidneys by inhibiting the ability of the collecting ducts to reabsorb Na^+ and by suppressing the release of ADH, renin, and aldosterone. Additionally, ANP acts both directly and indirectly (by inhibiting renin-induced generation of angiotensin II) to relax vascular smooth muscle, and in this way it causes vasodilation. Collectively, these effects reduce blood pressure.

Influence of Other Hormones

Female Sex Hormones The **estrogens** are chemically similar to aldosterone and, like aldosterone, enhance NaCl reabsorption by the renal tubules. Because water follows, many women retain fluid as their estrogen levels rise during the menstrual cycle. Estrogens are also largely responsible for the edema experienced by many pregnant women.

Progesterone appears to decrease Na^+ reabsorption by blocking the effect aldosterone has on the renal tubules. Thus, progesterone has a diuretic-like effect and promotes Na^+ and water loss.

Glucocorticoids **Glucocorticoids**, such as cortisol and hydrocortisol, enhance tubular reabsorption of Na^+, but they also promote an increased glomerular filtration rate that may mask their effects on the tubules. However, when their plasma levels are high, the glucocorticoids exhibit potent aldosterone-like effects and promote edema.

Cardiovascular Baroreceptors

Blood volume is carefully monitored and regulated to maintain blood pressure and cardiovascular function. Because Na^+ content determines fluid volume and fluid volume determines blood pressure, the baroreceptors indirectly monitor Na^+ content.

As blood volume (and with it, pressure) rises, baroreceptors in the heart and the large vessels of the neck and thorax (carotid arteries and aorta) alert the cardiovascular centers in the brain stem. Shortly after, sympathetic nervous system impulses to the kidneys decline, allowing the afferent arterioles to dilate. As the glomerular filtration rate rises, Na^+ output and water output increase. This phenomenon, part of the baroreceptor reflex described in Chapter 19 (pp. 706–707), reduces blood volume and blood pressure.

Drops in systemic blood pressure lead to reflex constriction of systemic arterioles including the afferent arterioles, which reduces filtrate formation and urinary output and increases systemic blood pressure **(Figure 26.10)**. The baroreceptors provide information on the "fullness" or volume of the circulation that is critical for maintaining cardiovascular homeostasis.

Regulation of Potassium Balance

Potassium, the chief intracellular cation, is required for normal neuromuscular functioning as well as for several essential metabolic activities. Even slight changes in K^+ concentration in the ECF have profound and potentially life-threatening effects on

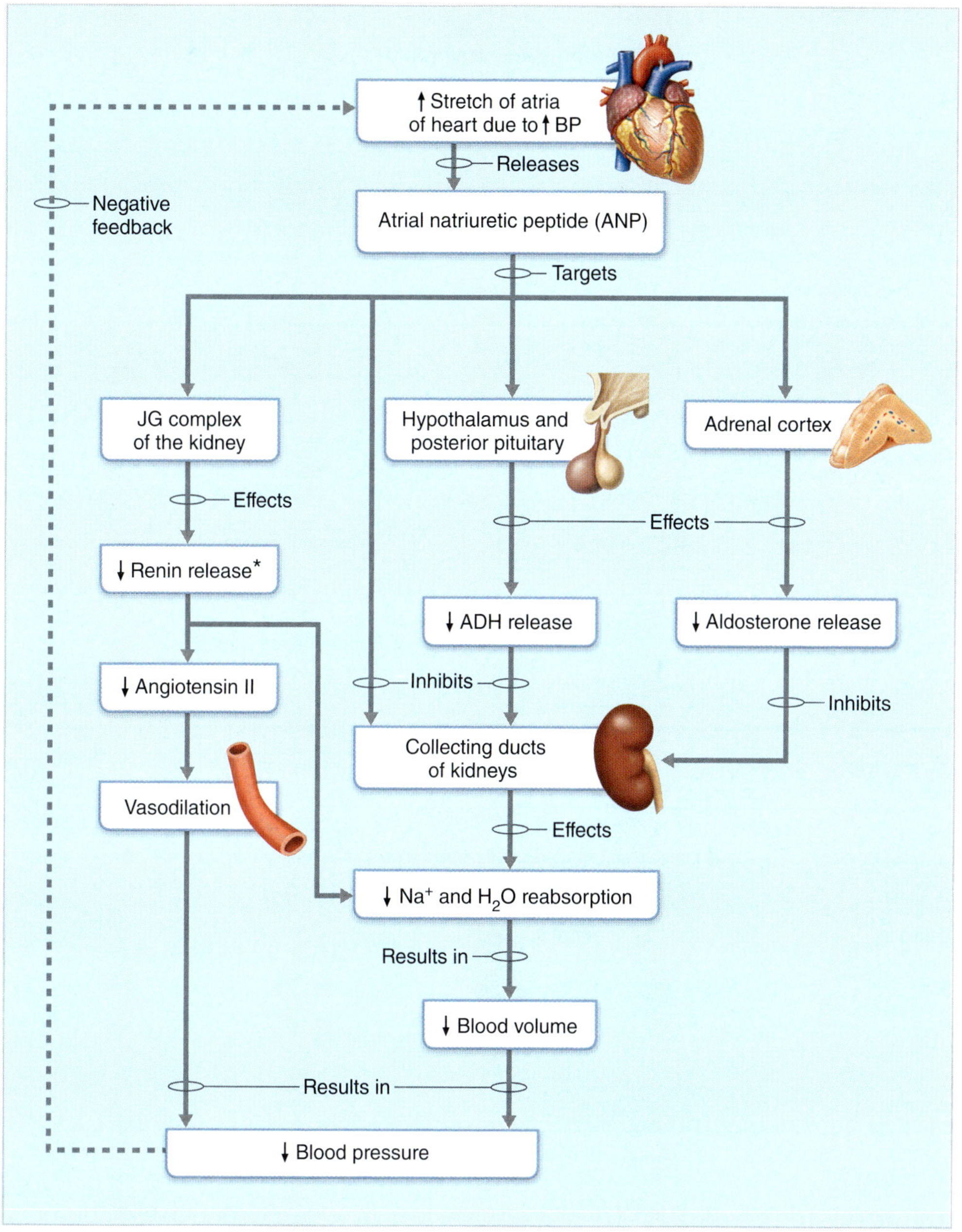

Figure 26.9 Mechanisms and consequences of ANP release.

*↓ Renin release also inhibits ADH and aldosterone release and hence the effects of those hormones.

26

neurons and muscle fibers because the relative ICF-ECF potassium concentration directly affects the resting membrane potential of these cells. K^+ excess in the ECF decreases their membrane potential, causing depolarization, often followed by reduced excitability. Too little K^+ in the ECF causes hyperpolarization and nonresponsiveness.

The heart is particularly sensitive to K^+ levels. Both too much and too little K^+ (hyperkalemia and hypokalemia, respectively) can disrupt electrical conduction in the heart, leading to sudden death (Table 26.1 and p. 684).

Potassium is also part of the body's buffer system, which resists changes in the pH of body fluids. Shifts of hydrogen ions (H^+) into and out of cells induce corresponding shifts of K^+ in the opposite direction to maintain cation balance. Consequently, ECF potassium levels rise with acidosis, as K^+ leaves and H^+ enters the cells, and fall with alkalosis, as K^+ enters the cells and H^+ leaves them to enter the ECF. Although these pH-driven shifts do not change the total amount of K^+ in the body, they can seriously interfere with the activity of excitable cells.

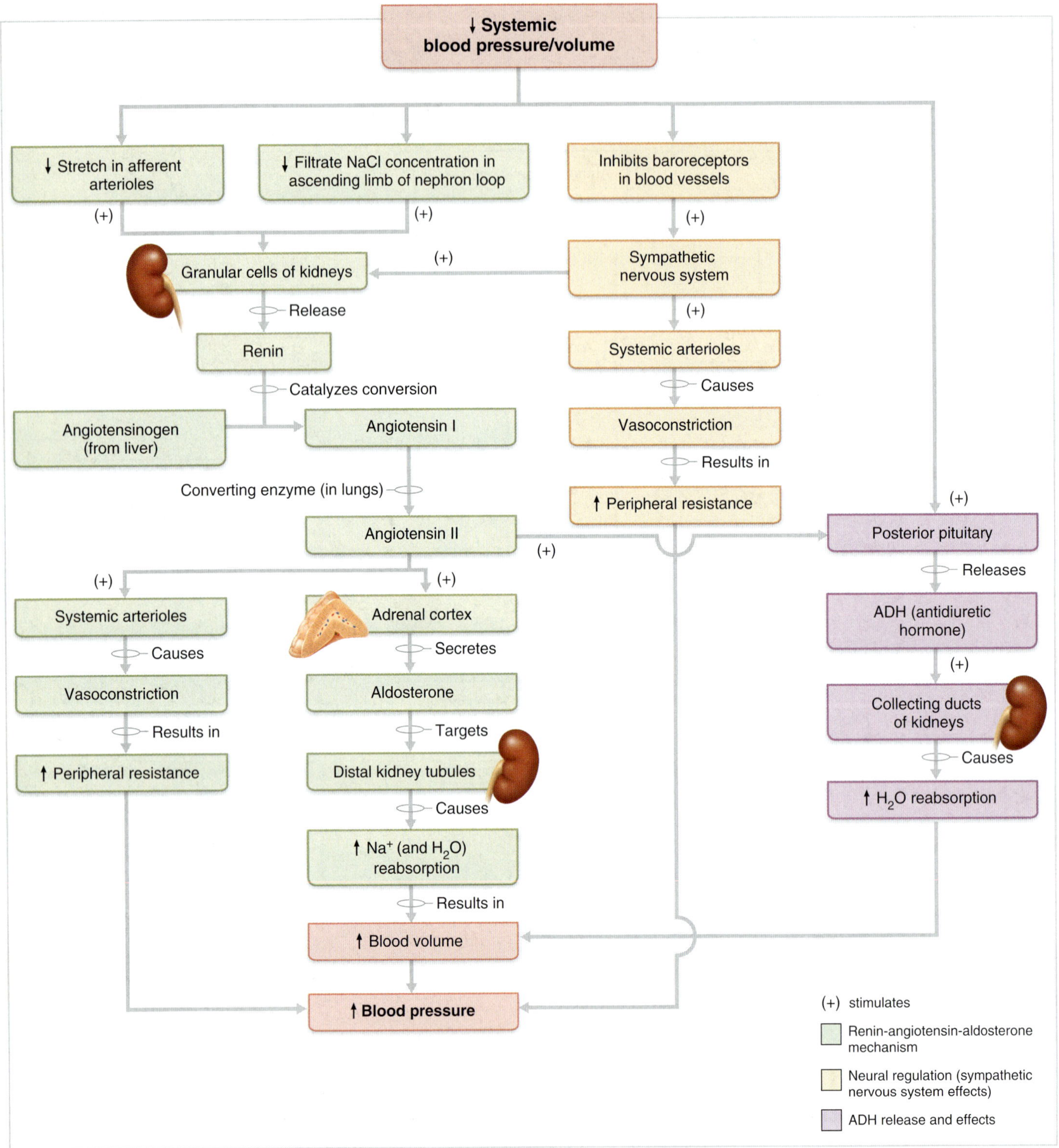

Figure 26.10 Mechanisms regulating sodium and water balance help maintain blood pressure homeostasis. The thirst mechanism, activated by angiotensin II and other factors, is not shown (see Figure 26.5).

Regulatory Site: The Collecting Duct

Like Na^+ balance, K^+ balance is maintained chiefly by renal mechanisms. However, there are important differences in the way this balance is achieved. The amount of Na^+ reabsorbed in the tubules is precisely tailored to need, and Na^+ is *never* secreted into the filtrate.

In contrast, the proximal tubules reabsorb about 60–80% of the filtered K^+, and the thick ascending limb of the nephron loop absorbs another 10–20% or so regardless of need, leaving about 10% at the beginning of the collecting ducts. The responsibility for K^+ balance falls chiefly on the collecting ducts. They achieve this balance mainly by changing the amount of K^+ *secreted* into the filtrate.

As a rule, K^+ levels in the ECF are sufficiently high that K^+ needs to be excreted, and the principal cells of the cortical collecting ducts secrete K^+ into the filtrate. (At times, the amount of K^+ excreted may actually exceed the amount filtered.) When ECF potassium concentrations are abnormally low, the renal principal cells conserve K^+ by reducing its secretion and excretion to a minimum. Note that these principal cells are the same cells that mediate aldosterone-induced reabsorption of Na^+ and ADH-stimulated reabsorption of water.

Additionally, *type A intercalated cells*, a unique population of collecting duct cells, can reabsorb some of the K^+ left in the filtrate (in conjunction with active secretion of H^+), thereby helping to reestablish K^+ (and pH) balance. However, keep in mind that the main thrust of renal regulation of K^+ is to *excrete* it. Because the kidneys have a limited ability to retain K^+, it may be lost in urine even in the face of a deficiency. Consequently, people who don't eat potassium-rich foods can eventually develop a severe deficiency.

Influence of Plasma Potassium Concentration

The single most important factor influencing K^+ secretion is the K^+ concentration in the ECF. A high-potassium diet increases the K^+ content of the ECF. This favors entry of K^+ into the principal cells of the cortical collecting duct and prompts them to secrete K^+ into the filtrate so that more of it is excreted. Conversely, a low-potassium diet or accelerated K^+ loss depresses its secretion (and promotes its limited reabsorption) by the collecting ducts.

Influence of Aldosterone

The second factor influencing K^+ secretion into the filtrate is aldosterone. As it stimulates the principal cells to reabsorb Na^+, aldosterone simultaneously enhances K^+ secretion (see Figure 26.8). Adrenal cortical cells are *directly* sensitive to the K^+ content of the ECF bathing them. When it increases even slightly, the adrenal cortex is strongly stimulated to release aldosterone, which increases K^+ secretion by the exchange process we just described. The result is that K^+ controls its own concentrations in the ECF via feedback regulation of aldosterone release.

Aldosterone is also secreted in response to the renin-angiotensin-aldosterone mechanism previously described. Given the opposing effects of aldosterone on plasma Na^+ and K^+, you might expect that Na^+- and volume-driven changes in aldosterone would disrupt K^+ balance. This generally does not occur because other compensatory mechanisms in the kidneys maintain plasma K^+.

Homeostatic Imbalance 26.3

To reduce their NaCl intake, many people have turned to salt substitutes, which are high in potassium. However, heavy consumption of these substitutes is safe only when aldosterone release in the body is normal. In the absence of aldosterone, hyperkalemia is swift and lethal regardless of K^+ intake (Table 26.1). Conversely, when a person has an adrenocortical tumor that pumps out tremendous amounts of aldosterone, ECF potassium levels fall so low that neurons all over the body hyperpolarize and paralysis occurs. ✚

Regulation of Calcium and Phosphate Balance

About 99% of the body's calcium is found in bones in the form of calcium phosphate salts, which make the skeleton rigid and strong. The bony skeleton provides a dynamic reservoir from which calcium and phosphate can be withdrawn or deposited to maintain the balance of these electrolytes in the ECF.

Homeostatic Imbalance 26.4

Ionic calcium in the ECF is important for normal blood clotting, cell membrane permeability, and secretory behavior, but its most important effect by far is on neuromuscular excitability. Hypocalcemia increases excitability and causes muscle tetany. Hypercalcemia is equally dangerous because it inhibits neurons and muscle cells and may cause life-threatening cardiac arrhythmias (Table 26.1). ✚

ECF calcium ion levels are closely regulated by **parathyroid hormone (PTH)**, and rarely deviate from normal limits. (The hormone calcitonin, produced by the thyroid, is often thought of as a calcium-lowering hormone, but, as we discussed in Chapter 16, its effects on blood calcium levels in humans are negligible.) Parathyroid hormone is released by the tiny parathyroid glands located on the posterior aspect of the thyroid gland in the neck. Declining plasma levels of Ca^{2+} directly stimulate the parathyroid glands to release PTH, which promotes an increase in calcium levels by targeting the following organs (see also Figure 16.13 on p. 611):

- **Bones.** PTH activates bone-digesting osteoclasts, which break down the bone matrix, releasing Ca^{2+} and HPO_4^{2-} to the blood.
- **Kidneys.** PTH increases Ca^{2+} reabsorption by the renal tubules while decreasing phosphate ion reabsorption. In this way, calcium conservation and phosphate excretion go hand in hand. The *mathematical product* of Ca^{2+} and HPO_4^{2-} concentrations ($[Ca^{2+}] \times [HPO_4^{2-}]$) in the ECF remains constant, preventing calcium-salt deposits in bones or soft body tissues.
- **Small intestine.** PTH enhances intestinal absorption of Ca^{2+} indirectly by stimulating the kidneys to transform vitamin D to its active form, which is necessary for the small intestine to absorb Ca^{2+}.

Most Ca^{2+} is reabsorbed passively in the PCT via diffusion through the paracellular route (a process driven by its electrochemical gradient). However, as with other ions, Ca^{2+} reabsorption is fine-tuned in the distal nephron. PTH-regulated Ca^{2+} channels control Ca^{2+} entry into DCT cells at the apical membrane, while Ca^{2+} pumps and antiporters export it at the basolateral membrane. Under normal circumstances about 98% of the filtered Ca^{2+} is reabsorbed owing to the action of PTH.

As a rule, 75% of the filtered phosphate ions (including $H_2PO_4^-$, HPO_4^{2-}, and PO_4^{3-}) are reabsorbed in the PCT by secondary active transport. Phosphate reabsorption is set by its transport maximum. Amounts over that maximum simply flow out in urine. PTH inhibits active transport of phosphate by decreasing its transport maximum.

When ECF calcium levels are within normal limits (9–11 mg/100 ml of blood) or higher, PTH secretion is inhibited. Consequently, release of Ca^{2+} from bone is inhibited, more Ca^{2+} is lost in feces and urine, and more phosphate is retained. Hormones other than PTH alter phosphate reabsorption. For example, insulin increases it while glucagon decreases it.

Regulation of Anions

Chloride is the major anion accompanying Na^+ in the ECF and, like sodium, Cl^- helps maintain the osmotic pressure of the blood. When blood pH is within normal limits or slightly alkaline, about 99% of filtered Cl^- is reabsorbed. In the PCT, it moves passively and simply follows sodium ions out of the filtrate and into the peritubular capillary blood. In most other tubule segments, Na^+ and Cl^- transport are coupled.

When acidosis occurs, less Cl^- accompanies Na^+ because HCO_3^- reabsorption is stepped up to restore blood pH to its normal range. Thus, the choice between Cl^- and HCO_3^- serves acid-base regulation. Most other anions, such as sulfates and nitrates, have transport maximums, and when their concentrations in the filtrate exceed the amount that can be reabsorbed, the excess spills into urine.

☑ Check Your Understanding

7. Jacob has Addison's disease (insufficient aldosterone release). How does this affect his plasma Na^+ and K^+ levels? How does this affect his blood pressure? Explain.
8. Renal handling of Na^+ can be summed up as "The kidneys reabsorb almost all of the Na^+ as filtrate passes through its tubules." Make a similar summary for K^+.
9. Which hormone is the major regulator of Ca^{2+} in the blood? What are the effects of hypercalcemia? Hypocalcemia?

For answers, see Appendix H.

26

Acid-Base Balance

✓ List important sources of acids in the body.

Because of their abundant hydrogen bonds, all functional proteins (enzymes, hemoglobin, cytochromes, and others) are influenced by H^+ concentration. It follows then that nearly all biochemical reactions are influenced by the pH of their fluid environment, and the **acid-base balance** of body fluids is closely regulated. (For a review of the basic principles of acid-base reactions and pH, see Chapter 2.)

Optimal pH varies from one body fluid to another, but not by much. The normal pH of arterial blood is 7.4, that of venous blood and IF is 7.35, and that of ICF averages 7.0. The lower pH in cells and venous blood reflects their greater amounts of acidic metabolites and carbon dioxide, which combines with water to form carbonic acid, H_2CO_3.

Whenever the pH of arterial blood rises above 7.45, a person is said to have **alkalosis** (al″kah-lo′sis) or **alkalemia**. A drop in arterial pH below 7.35 results in **acidosis** (as″ĭ-do′sis) or **acidemia**. Because pH 7.0 is neutral, chemically speaking 7.35 is not acidic. However, it is a higher-than-optimal H^+ concentration for most cells, so any arterial pH between 7.0 and 7.35 is called *physiological acidosis.*

Although small amounts of acidic substances enter the body via ingested foods, most hydrogen ions originate as metabolic by-products or end products. For example:

- Breakdown of phosphorus-containing proteins releases *phosphoric acid* into the ECF.
- Anaerobic respiration of glucose produces *lactic acid.*
- Fat metabolism yields other organic acids, such as fatty acids and *ketone bodies.*
- Loading and transport of carbon dioxide in the blood as HCO_3^- liberates hydrogen ions.

The H^+ concentration in blood is regulated sequentially by (1) chemical buffers, (2) brain stem respiratory centers, and (3) renal mechanisms. Chemical buffers, the first line of defense, act within a fraction of a second to resist pH changes. Within 1–3 minutes, changes in respiratory rate and depth occur to compensate for acidosis or alkalosis. The kidneys, the body's most potent acid-base regulatory system, ordinarily require hours to a day or more to alter blood pH.

Chemical Buffer Systems

✓ List the three major chemical buffer systems of the body and describe how they resist pH changes.

Recall that acids are *proton donors,* and that the acidity of a solution reflects only the *free* hydrogen ions, not those bound to anions. *Strong acids* dissociate completely and liberate all their H^+ in water **(Figure 26.11a)**. They can dramatically change a solution's pH. By contrast, *weak acids* dissociate only partially (Figure 26.11b). Accordingly, they have a much smaller effect on pH. However, weak acids are efficient at preventing pH changes, and this feature allows them to play important roles in chemical buffer systems.

Bases are *proton acceptors.* Strong bases are those that dissociate easily in water and quickly tie up H^+. Conversely, weak bases are less likely to accept protons.

A **chemical buffer** is a system of one or more compounds that resists changes in pH when a strong acid or base is added. They do this by binding to H^+ whenever the pH drops and releasing them when pH rises.

The three major chemical buffer systems in the body are the *bicarbonate, phosphate,* and *protein buffer systems.* Anything that causes a shift in H^+ concentration in one fluid compartment simultaneously causes a change in the others. As a result, the buffer systems actually buffer one another, so the *entire* buffer system resists any drifts in pH.

Bicarbonate Buffer System

The **bicarbonate buffer system** is a mixture of carbonic acid (H_2CO_3) and its salt, sodium bicarbonate ($NaHCO_3$, a weak base), in the same solution. Although it also buffers the ICF, it is the *only* important ECF buffer.

Carbonic acid, a weak acid, does not dissociate to any great extent in neutral or acidic solutions. When a strong acid such as HCl is added to this buffer system, the existing carbonic acid remains intact. However, the bicarbonate ions of the salt act as weak bases to tie up the H^+ released by the stronger acid (HCl), forming *more* carbonic acid:

$$\underset{\text{strong acid}}{HCl} + \underset{\text{weak base}}{NaHCO_3} \rightarrow \underset{\text{weak acid}}{H_2CO_3} + \underset{\text{salt}}{NaCl}$$

Because it is converted to the weak acid H_2CO_3, HCl lowers the pH of the solution only slightly.

When a strong base such as sodium hydroxide (NaOH) is added to the same buffer solution, a weak base such as sodium bicarbonate ($NaHCO_3$) does not dissociate further under the alkaline conditions. However, the added base forces the carbonic acid to dissociate further, donating more H^+ to tie up the OH^- released by the strong base:

$$\underset{\text{strong base}}{NaOH} + \underset{\text{weak acid}}{H_2CO_3} \rightarrow \underset{\text{weak base}}{NaHCO_3} + \underset{\text{water}}{H_2O}$$

The net result is that a weak base ($NaHCO_3$) replaces a strong base (NaOH), so the pH of the solution rises very little.

Although the bicarbonate salt in the example is sodium bicarbonate, other bicarbonate salts function in the same way because HCO_3^- is the important ion, not the cation it is paired with. In cells, where little Na^+ is present, potassium and magnesium bicarbonates are part of the bicarbonate buffer system.

The buffering power of this type of system is directly related to the concentrations of the buffering substances. If enough acid enters the blood so that all the available HCO_3^- ions, often referred to as the **alkaline reserve**, are tied up, the buffer system becomes ineffective and blood pH changes.

The bicarbonate ion concentration in the ECF is normally around 25 mEq/L and is closely regulated by the kidneys. The concentration of H_2CO_3 is just over 1 mEq/L but the supply of H_2CO_3 (which comes from the CO_2 released during cellular respiration) is almost limitless, so obtaining that member of the buffer pair is usually not a problem. The H_2CO_3 content of the blood is subject to respiratory controls.

Phosphate Buffer System

The operation of the **phosphate buffer system** is nearly identical to that of the bicarbonate buffer. The components of the phosphate system are the sodium salts of dihydrogen phosphate ($H_2PO_4^-$) and monohydrogen phosphate (HPO_4^{2-}). NaH_2PO_4 acts as a weak acid. Na_2HPO_4, with one less hydrogen atom, acts as a weak base.

Again, H^+ released by strong acids is tied up in weak acids:

$$\underset{\text{strong acid}}{HCl} + \underset{\text{weak base}}{Na_2HPO_4} \rightarrow \underset{\text{weak acid}}{NaH_2PO_4} + \underset{\text{salt}}{NaCl}$$

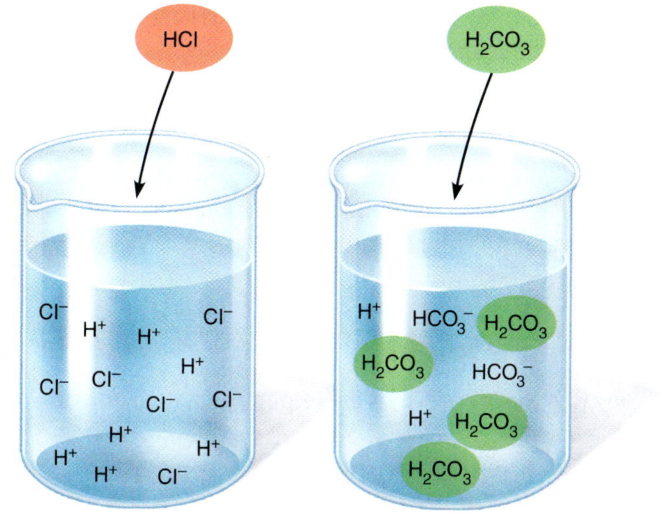

Figure 26.11 Dissociation of strong and weak acids in water. HCl: hydrochloric acid; H_2CO_3: carbonic acid. Undissociated molecules are shown in colored ovals.

and strong bases are converted to weak bases:

$$\underset{\text{strong base}}{NaOH} + \underset{\text{weak acid}}{NaH_2PO_4} \rightarrow \underset{\text{weak base}}{Na_2HPO_4} + \underset{\text{water}}{H_2O}$$

Because the phosphate buffer system is present in low concentrations in the ECF (approximately one-sixth that of the bicarbonate buffer system), it is relatively unimportant for buffering blood plasma. However, it is a very effective buffer in urine and in ICF, where phosphate concentrations are usually higher.

Protein Buffer System

Proteins in plasma and in cells are the body's **protein buffer system**. In fact, at least three-quarters of all the buffering power of body fluids resides in cells, and most of this reflects the powerful buffering activity of intracellular proteins.

As described in Chapter 2, proteins are polymers of amino acids. Some of the linked amino acids have exposed groups of atoms called *carboxyl groups* (—COOH), organic acid groups that release H^+ when the pH begins to rise:

$$R\text{—}COOH \rightarrow R\text{—}COO^- + H^+$$

(Note that R indicates the rest of the organic molecule, which contains many atoms.)

Other amino acids have exposed groups that can act as bases and accept H^+. For example, an exposed $\text{—}NH_2$ group can bind with a hydrogen ion, becoming $\text{—}NH_3^+$:

$$R\text{—}NH_2 + H^+ \rightarrow R\text{—}NH_3^+$$

Because this binding removes free hydrogen ions from the solution, it prevents the solution from becoming too acidic. Consequently, a single protein molecule can function reversibly as either an acid or a base depending on the pH of its environment. Molecules with this ability are called **amphoteric molecules** (am″fo-ter′ik).

26

Hemoglobin in red blood cells is an excellent example of a protein that functions as an intracellular buffer. As we explained in Chapter 22 (p. 829), CO_2 released from the tissues forms H_2CO_3, which dissociates to liberate H^+ and HCO_3^- in the blood. Meanwhile, hemoglobin is unloading oxygen, becoming reduced hemoglobin, which carries a negative charge. Because H^+ rapidly binds to the hemoglobin anions, pH changes are minimized. In this case, carbonic acid, a weak acid, is buffered by an even weaker acid, hemoglobin.

Respiratory Regulation of H^+

✓ Describe the influence of the respiratory system on acid-base balance.

The respiratory and renal systems together form the *physiological buffering systems* that control pH by regulating the amount of acid or base in the body. Although physiological buffer systems act more slowly than chemical buffer systems, they have many times the buffering power of all the body's chemical buffers combined.

As we described in Chapter 22, the respiratory system eliminates CO_2, an acid, from the blood while replenishing its supply of O_2. Carbon dioxide generated by cellular respiration enters erythrocytes in the circulation and is converted to bicarbonate ions for transport in the plasma:

$$CO_2 + H_2O \underset{}{\overset{\text{carbonic anhydrase}}{\rightleftharpoons}} \underset{\text{carbonic acid}}{H_2CO_3} \rightleftharpoons H^+ + \underset{\text{bicarbonate ion}}{HCO_3^-}$$

The first set of double arrows indicates a reversible equilibrium between dissolved carbon dioxide and water on the left and carbonic acid on the right. The second set indicates a reversible equilibrium between carbonic acid on the left and hydrogen and bicarbonate ions on the right. Because of these equilibria, an increase in any of these chemical species pushes the reaction in the opposite direction. Notice also that the right side of the equation is equivalent to the bicarbonate buffer system.

26

Healthy individuals expel CO_2 from the lungs at the same rate it is formed in the tissues. During carbon dioxide unloading, the reaction shifts to the left, and H^+ generated from carbonic acid is reincorporated into water. Because of the protein buffer system, H^+ produced by CO_2 transport is not allowed to accumulate and has little or no effect on blood pH.

If P_{CO_2} rises, it activates medullary chemoreceptors (via cerebral acidosis promoted by excessive accumulation of CO_2) that respond by increasing respiratory rate and depth (see Figure 22.25, p. 836). Additionally, a rising plasma H^+ concentration resulting from any metabolic process excites the respiratory center indirectly (via peripheral chemoreceptors) to stimulate deeper, more rapid respiration. As ventilation increases, more CO_2 is removed from the blood, pushing the reaction to the left and reducing the H^+ concentration.

When blood pH rises, the respiratory center is depressed. As respiratory rate drops and respiration becomes shallower, CO_2 accumulates, pushing the equilibrium to the right and causing the H^+ concentration to increase. Again blood pH is restored to the normal range. These respiratory system–mediated corrections of blood pH are accomplished within a minute or so.

Changes in alveolar ventilation can produce dramatic changes in blood pH—far more than is needed. For example, doubling alveolar ventilation can raise blood pH by about 0.2 pH unit. Likewise, cutting alveolar ventilation in half can lower blood pH by the same amount. Because normal arterial pH is 7.4, a change of 0.2 pH unit yields a blood pH of 7.6 or 7.2—both well beyond the normal limits. Respiratory controls of blood pH have a tremendous reserve capacity because alveolar ventilation can rise about 15-fold or fall (briefly) to zero.

Anything that impairs respiratory system functioning causes acid-base imbalances. For example, net carbon dioxide retention (hypoventilation) leads to acidosis. On the other hand, hyperventilation, which causes net elimination of CO_2, causes alkalosis. When respiratory system problems cause the pH imbalance, the resulting condition is either *respiratory acidosis* or *respiratory alkalosis* (see Table 26.3 on p. 1010).

☑ Check Your Understanding

10. Define acidemia and alkalemia.
11. To minimize a shift in pH brought about by adding a strong acid to a solution, would it be better if the solution contained a weak base or a strong base?
12. What are the body's three major chemical buffer systems? What is the most important buffer inside cells?
13. Joanne, a diabetic patient, is at the emergency department with acidosis due to the production of ketone bodies. Would you expect her ventilation to be increased or decreased? Why?

For answers, see Appendix H.

Renal Mechanisms of Acid-Base Balance

✓ Describe how the kidneys regulate hydrogen and bicarbonate ion concentrations in the blood.

The ultimate acid-base regulatory organs are the kidneys, which act slowly but surely to compensate for acid-base imbalances resulting from variations in diet or metabolism, or disease. Chemical buffers can tie up excess acids or bases temporarily, but they cannot eliminate them from the body. And while the lungs can dispose of the **volatile acid** carbonic acid by eliminating CO_2, only the kidneys can rid the body of other acids generated by cellular metabolism: phosphoric, uric, and lactic acids, and ketone bodies. These acids are referred to as **nonvolatile (fixed) acids**. Additionally, only the kidneys can regulate blood levels of alkaline substances and renew chemical buffers that are used up in regulating H^+ levels in the ECF.

The most important renal mechanisms for regulating acid-base balance of the blood involve (1) conserving (reabsorbing) or generating new HCO_3^-, and (2) excreting HCO_3^-. If we look back at the equation for the carbonic acid–bicarbonate buffer system, we can see that losing a HCO_3^- from the body produces the same net effect as gaining a H^+, because it pushes the equation to the right, increasing the H^+ level. By the same token, generating or reabsorbing HCO_3^- is the same as losing H^+ because it pushes the equation to the left, decreasing the H^+ level. For this reason,

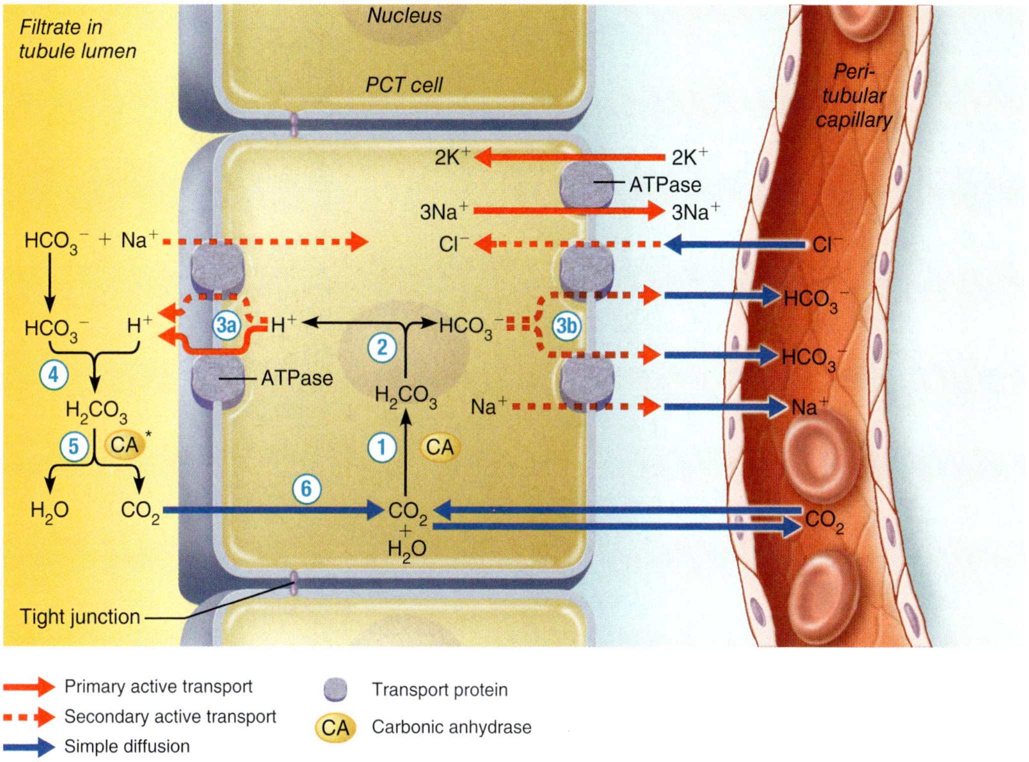

Figure 26.12 Reabsorption of filtered HCO_3^- is coupled to H^+ secretion.

*The breakdown of H_2CO_3 to CO_2 and H_2O in the tubule lumen is catalyzed by carbonic anhydrase only in the PCT.

to reabsorb bicarbonate, the kidney has to secrete H^+, and when it excretes excess HCO_3^-, H^+ is retained (not secreted).

Because the mechanisms for regulating acid-base balance depend on H^+ being secreted into the filtrate, we consider that process first. Secretion of H^+ occurs mainly in the PCT and in type A intercalated cells of the collecting duct. The H^+ secreted comes from the dissociation of carbonic acid, created from the combination of CO_2 and water within the tubule cells, a reaction catalyzed by *carbonic anhydrase* (**Figure 26.12** (1), (2)). As H^+ is secreted into the lumen of the PCT, Na^+ is reabsorbed from the filtrate, maintaining the electrical balance (Figure 26.12 (3a)).

The rate of H^+ secretion rises and falls with CO_2 levels in the ECF. The more CO_2 in the peritubular capillary blood, the faster the rate of H^+ secretion. Because blood CO_2 levels directly relate to blood pH, this system can respond to both rising and falling H^+ concentrations. Notice that secreted H^+ can combine with HCO_3^- in the filtrate, generating CO_2 and water (Figure 26.12 (4), (5)). In this case, H^+ is bound in water. The rising concentration of CO_2 in the filtrate creates a steep diffusion gradient for its entry into the tubule cell, where it promotes still more H^+ secretion (Figure 26.12 (6)).

Conserving Filtered Bicarbonate Ions: Bicarbonate Reabsorption

Bicarbonate ions (HCO_3^-) are an important part of the bicarbonate buffer system, the most important inorganic blood buffer. If this reservoir of base, the *alkaline reserve*, is to be maintained, the kidneys must do more than just eliminate enough hydrogen ions to counter rising blood H^+ levels. Depleted stores of HCO_3^- have to be replenished. This task is more complex than it seems because the tubule cells are almost completely impermeable to the HCO_3^- in the filtrate—they cannot reabsorb it.

However, the kidneys can conserve filtered HCO_3^- in a rather roundabout way. As you can see, dissociation of carbonic acid liberates HCO_3^- as well as H^+ (Figure 26.12 (2)). Although the tubule cells cannot reclaim HCO_3^- directly from the filtrate, they can and do shunt HCO_3^- generated within them (as a result of splitting H_2CO_3) into the peritubular capillary blood. HCO_3^- leaves the tubule cell either accompanied by Na^+ or in exchange for Cl^- (Figure 26.12 (3b)). H^+ is actively secreted, mostly by a Na^+-H^+ antiporter, but also by a H^+ ATPase (Figure 26.12 (3a)). In the filtrate, H^+ combines with filtered HCO_3^-, as we saw earlier (Figure 26.12 (4), (5)). For this reason, reabsorption of HCO_3^- depends on the active secretion of H^+.

In short, for each filtered HCO_3^- that "disappears" from the filtrate, a HCO_3^- generated within the tubule cells enters the blood—a one-for-one exchange. When large amounts of H^+ are secreted, correspondingly large amounts of HCO_3^- enter the peritubular blood. The net effect is to remove HCO_3^- almost completely from the filtrate.

Generating New Bicarbonate Ions

Two renal mechanisms commonly carried out by cells of the PCT and collecting ducts generate *new* HCO_3^- that can be added to plasma. Both mechanisms involve renal excretion of

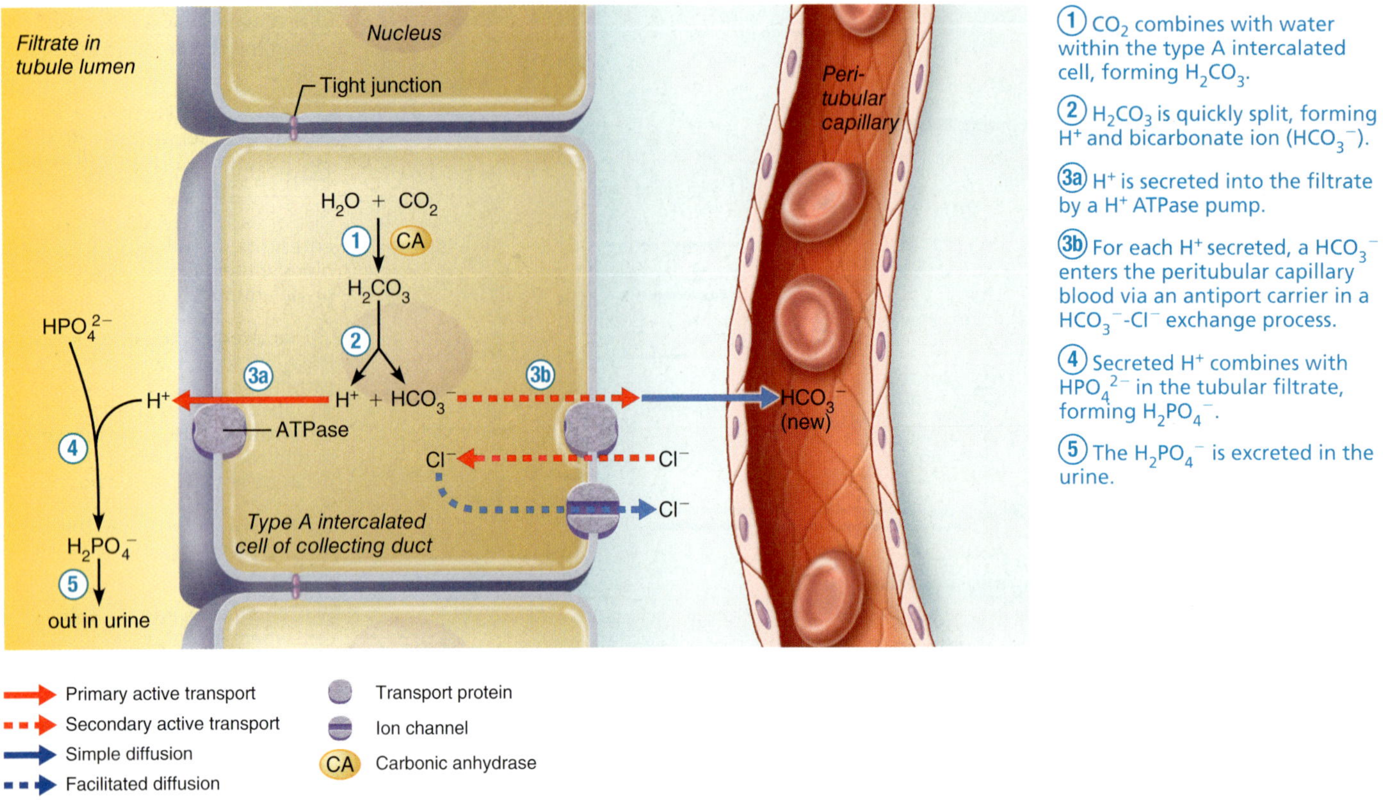

Figure 26.13 New HCO_3^- is generated via buffering of secreted H^+ by HPO_4^{2-} (monohydrogen phosphate).

acid, *via secretion and excretion* of either H^+ or ammonium ions in urine. Let's examine how these mechanisms differ.

As long as *filtered bicarbonate* is reclaimed, as we saw in Figure 26.12, the secreted H^+ is *not excreted or lost* from the body in urine. Instead, the H^+ is buffered by HCO_3^- in the filtrate and ultimately becomes part of water molecules (most of which are reabsorbed).

However, once the filtered HCO_3^- is "used up" (usually by the time the filtrate reaches the collecting ducts), any additional H^+ secreted is excreted in urine. More often than not, this is the case.

Reclaiming filtered HCO_3^- simply restores the bicarbonate concentration of plasma that exists at the time. However, metabolism of food normally releases new H^+ into the body. This additional H^+ uses up HCO_3^- and so must be balanced by generating *new* HCO_3^- (as opposed to filtered HCO_3^-) that moves into the blood to counteract acidosis. This process of alkalinizing the blood is the way the kidneys compensate for acidosis.

Via Excretion of Buffered H^+ Binding H^+ to buffers in the filtrate minimizes the H^+ concentration gradient, allowing the proton pumps of the type A intercalated cells to secrete the large numbers of H^+ that the body must get rid of to prevent acidosis. (H^+ secretion ceases when urine pH falls to 4.5 because the proton pumps cannot pump against this large gradient.) The most important urine buffer is the *phosphate buffer system*, specifically its weak base *monohydrogen phosphate* (HPO_4^{2-}).

The components of the phosphate buffer system filter freely into the tubules, and about 75% of the filtered phosphate is reabsorbed. However, their reabsorption is inhibited during acidosis. As a result, the buffer pair becomes more and more concentrated as the filtrate moves through the renal tubules.

As shown in **Figure 26.13** (3a), the type A intercalated cells secrete H^+ actively via a H^+ ATPase pump and via a K^+-H^+ antiporter (not illustrated). The secreted H^+ combines with HPO_4^{2-}, forming $H_2PO_4^-$ which then flows out in urine (Figure 26.13 (4) and (5)).

Bicarbonate ions generated in the cells during the same reaction move into the interstitial space via a $HCO_3^- - Cl^-$ antiport process and then move passively into the peritubular capillary blood (Figure 26.13 (3b)). Notice again that when H^+ is being excreted, "brand new" bicarbonate ions are added to the blood—over and above those reclaimed from the filtrate. As you can see, in response to acidosis, the kidneys generate new HCO_3^- and add it to the blood (alkalinizing the blood) while adding an equal amount of H^+ to the filtrate (acidifying the urine).

Via NH_4^+ Excretion The second and more important mechanism for excreting acid uses the ammonium ion (NH_4^+) produced by glutamine metabolism in PCT cells. Ammonium ions are weak acids that donate few H^+ at physiological pH.

As **Figure 26.14** step (1) shows, for each glutamine metabolized (deaminated, oxidized, and acidified by combining with H^+), two NH_4^+ and two HCO_3^- result. The HCO_3^- moves through the basolateral membrane into the blood (Figure 26.14 (2b)). The NH_4^+, in turn, is excreted and lost in urine (Figure 26.14 (2a), (3)). As with the phosphate buffer system, this buffering mechanism replenishes the alkaline reserve of the blood, because the newly made HCO_3^- enters the blood as NH_4^+ is secreted.

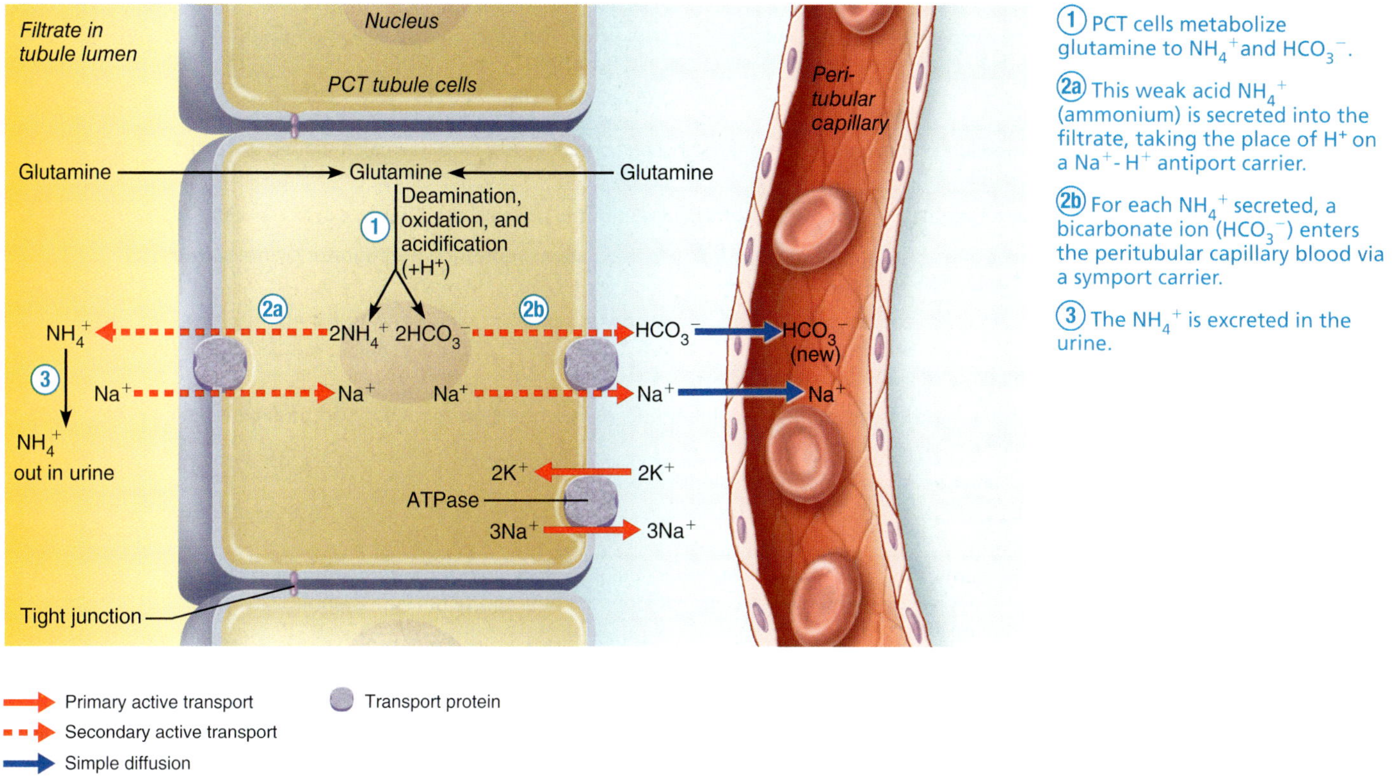

Figure 26.14 **New HCO_3^- is generated via glutamine metabolism and NH_4^+ secretion.**

Bicarbonate Ion Secretion

When the body is in alkalosis, another population of intercalated cells (type B) in the collecting ducts exhibit net HCO_3^- secretion (rather than net HCO_3^- reabsorption) while reclaiming H^+ to acidify the blood. Overall we can think of the type B cells as "flipped" type A cells, and we can visualize the HCO_3^- secretion process as the exact opposite of the HCO_3^- reabsorption process illustrated in Figure 26.12. However, the predominant process in the nephrons and collecting ducts is HCO_3^- reabsorption, and even during alkalosis, much more HCO_3^- is conserved than excreted.

☑ Check Your Understanding

14. Reabsorption of HCO_3^- is always tied to the secretion of which ion?
15. What is the most important urinary buffer of H^+?
16. List the two mechanisms by which tubule and collecting duct cells generate new HCO_3^-.

For answers, see Appendix H.

Abnormalities of Acid-Base Balance

✓ Distinguish between acidosis and alkalosis resulting from respiratory and metabolic factors. Describe the importance of respiratory and renal compensations to acid-base balance.

All cases of acidosis and alkalosis can be classed according to cause as *respiratory* or *metabolic* **(Table 26.3)**. *A Closer Look* on p. 1011 discusses methods for determining the cause of an acid-base disturbance and whether it is being compensated (whether the lungs or kidneys are taking steps to correct the imbalance).

Respiratory Acidosis and Alkalosis

Respiratory pH imbalances result from some failure of the respiratory system to perform its normal pH-balancing role. The partial pressure of carbon dioxide (P_{CO_2}) is the single most important indicator of the adequacy of respiratory function. When respiratory function is normal, the P_{CO_2} fluctuates between 35 and 45 mm Hg. Generally speaking, values above 45 mm Hg indicate respiratory acidosis, and values below 35 mm Hg signal respiratory alkalosis.

Respiratory acidosis is a common cause of acid-base imbalance. It most often occurs when a person breathes shallowly or when gas exchange is hampered by diseases such as pneumonia, cystic fibrosis, or emphysema. Under such conditions, CO_2 accumulates in the blood. Thus, respiratory acidosis is characterized by falling blood pH and rising P_{CO_2}.

Respiratory alkalosis results when carbon dioxide is eliminated from the body faster than it is produced. This is called **hyperventilation** (see p. 836), and results in the blood becoming more alkaline. While respiratory acidosis is frequently associated with respiratory system pathology, respiratory alkalosis is often due to stress or pain.

Metabolic Acidosis and Alkalosis

Metabolic pH imbalances include all abnormalities of acid-base imbalance *except* those caused by too much or too little carbon

Table 26.3 Causes and Consequences of Acid-Base Imbalances

CONDITION AND HALLMARK	POSSIBLE CAUSES; COMMENTS
Respiratory Acidosis (Hypoventilation)	
If uncompensated (uncorrected): P_{CO_2} >45 mm Hg; pH <7.35	**Impaired lung function** (e.g., chronic bronchitis, cystic fibrosis, emphysema): impaired gas exchange or alveolar ventilation **Impaired ventilatory movement:** paralyzed respiratory muscles, chest injury, extreme obesity **Narcotic or barbiturate overdose or injury to brain stem:** depression of respiratory centers, resulting in hypoventilation and respiratory arrest
Respiratory Alkalosis (Hyperventilation)	
If uncompensated: P_{CO_2} <35 mm Hg; pH >7.45	**Strong emotions:** pain, anxiety, fear, panic attack **Hypoxemia:** asthma, pneumonia, high altitude; represents effort to raise P_{O_2} at the expense of excessive CO_2 excretion **Brain tumor or injury:** abnormal respiratory controls
Metabolic Acidosis	
If uncompensated: HCO_3^- <22 mEq/L; pH <7.35	**Severe diarrhea:** bicarbonate-rich intestinal (and pancreatic) secretions rushed through digestive tract before their solutes can be reabsorbed; bicarbonate ions are replaced by renal mechanisms that generate new bicarbonate ions **Renal disease:** failure of kidneys to rid body of acids formed by normal metabolic processes **Untreated diabetes mellitus:** lack of insulin or inability of tissue cells to respond to insulin, resulting in inability to use glucose; fats are used as primary energy fuel, and ketoacidosis occurs **Starvation:** lack of dietary nutrients for cellular fuels; body proteins and fat reserves are used for energy—both yield acidic metabolites as they are broken down for energy **Excess alcohol ingestion:** results in excess acids in blood
Metabolic Alkalosis	
If uncompensated: HCO_3^- >26 mEq/L; pH >7.45	**Vomiting or gastric suctioning:** loss of stomach HCl requires that H^+ be withdrawn from blood to replace stomach acid; thus H^+ decreases and HCO_3^- increases proportionately **Selected diuretics:** cause K^+ depletion and H_2O loss. Low K^+ directly stimulates tubule cells to secrete H^+. Reduced blood volume elicits the renin-angiotensin-aldosterone mechanism, which stimulates Na^+ reabsorption and H^+ secretion. **Ingestion of excessive sodium bicarbonate (antacid):** bicarbonate moves easily into ECF, where it enhances natural alkaline reserve **Excess aldosterone** (e.g., adrenal tumors): promotes excessive reabsorption of Na^+, which pulls increased amount of H^+ into urine. Hypovolemia promotes the same relative effect because aldosterone secretion is increased to enhance Na^+ (and H_2O) reabsorption.

dioxide in the blood. Bicarbonate ion levels below or above the normal range of 22–26 mEq/L indicate a metabolic acid-base imbalance.

The second most common cause of acid-base imbalance, **metabolic acidosis**, is recognized by low blood pH and HCO_3^- levels. Typical causes are ingesting too much alcohol (which is metabolized to acetic acid) and excessive loss of HCO_3^-, as might result from persistent diarrhea. Other causes are accumulation of lactic acid during exercise or shock, the ketosis that occurs in diabetic crisis or starvation, and, infrequently, kidney failure.

Metabolic alkalosis, indicated by rising blood pH and HCO_3^- levels, is much less common than metabolic acidosis. Typical causes are vomiting the acidic contents of the stomach (or loss of those secretions through gastrointestinal suctioning) and intake of excess base (too many antacids, for example).

Effects of Acidosis and Alkalosis

The absolute blood pH limits for life are a low of 6.8 and a high of 7.8. When blood pH falls below 6.8, the central nervous system is so depressed that the person goes into coma and death soon follows. When blood pH rises above 7.8, the nervous system is overexcited, leading to such characteristic signs as muscle tetany, extreme nervousness, and convulsions. Death often results from respiratory arrest.

Respiratory and Renal Compensations

If one of the physiological buffer systems (lungs or kidneys) malfunctions and disrupts acid-base balance, the other system tries to compensate. The respiratory system attempts to compensate for metabolic acid-base imbalances, and the kidneys (although much slower) work to correct imbalances caused by

Sleuthing: Using Blood Values to Determine the Cause of Acidosis or Alkalosis

Students, particularly nursing students, are often given blood values and asked to determine (1) whether the **patient** is in **acidosis** or **alkalosis**, (2) the **cause** of the condition (respiratory or metabolic), and (3) whether the condition is being **compensated**. If you approach these questions systematically, they are not nearly as difficult as they may appear.

To analyze a person's acid-base balance, scrutinize the blood values in the following order:

1. *Note the pH.* This tells you whether the person is in acidosis (pH below 7.35) or alkalosis (pH above 7.45), but it does not tell you the cause.
2. *Check the P_{CO_2} to see if this is causing the acid-base imbalance.* Because the respiratory system is a fast-acting system, an excessively high or low P_{CO_2} may indicate that the respiratory system is either causing the condition or compensating for it. For example, if the pH indicates acidosis and
   - **a.** The P_{CO_2} is over 45 mm Hg, then the respiratory system is the cause of the problem and the condition is respiratory acidosis
   - **b.** The P_{CO_2} is below normal limits (below 35 mm Hg), then the respiratory system is *not the cause but is compensating*
   - **c.** The P_{CO_2} is within normal limits, then the condition is *neither caused nor compensated* by the respiratory system
3. *Check the bicarbonate level.* If step 2 proves that the respiratory system is not responsible for the imbalance, then the condition is metabolic and should be reflected in increased or decreased bicarbonate levels. HCO_3^- values below 22 mEq/L indicate metabolic acidosis, and values over 26 mEq/L indicate metabolic alkalosis. Notice that whereas P_{CO_2} levels vary inversely with blood pH (P_{CO_2} rises as blood pH falls), HCO_3^- levels vary directly with blood pH (increased HCO_3^- results in increased pH).

Beyond this bare-bones approach there is something else to consider when you are assessing acid-base problems. If an imbalance is fully compensated, the pH may be normal even while the patient is in trouble. Hence, when the pH is normal, carefully scrutinize the P_{CO_2} or HCO_3^- values for clues to what imbalance may be occurring.

Consider the following two examples of the three-step approach.

Problem 1

Blood values: pH 7.6; P_{CO_2} 24 mm Hg; HCO_3^- 23 mEq/L

Analysis:

1. The pH is elevated: alkalosis.
2. The P_{CO_2} is very low: the cause of the alkalosis.
3. The HCO_3^- value is within normal limits.

Conclusion: This is respiratory alkalosis not compensated by renal mechanisms, as might occur during short-term hyperventilation.

Problem 2

Blood values: pH 7.48; P_{CO_2} 46 mm Hg; HCO_3^- 33 mEq/L

Analysis:

1. The pH is elevated: alkalosis.
2. The P_{CO_2} is elevated: the cause of acidosis, not alkalosis. Thus, the respiratory system is compensating and is not the cause.
3. The HCO_3^- is elevated: the cause of the alkalosis.

Conclusion: This is metabolic alkalosis being compensated by respiratory acidosis (retention of CO_2 to restore blood pH to the normal range).

Use the accompanying simple chart to help you in your future sleuthing.

	Normal Range in Plasma		
Acid-Base Disturbance	**pH 7.35–7.45**	**P_{CO_2} 35–45 mm Hg**	**HCO_3^- 22–26 mEq/L**
Respiratory acidosis	↓	↑	↑ if compensating
Respiratory alkalosis	↑	↓	↓ if compensating
Metabolic acidosis	↓	↓ if compensating	↓
Metabolic alkalosis	↑	↑ if compensating	↑

respiratory disease. We can recognize these **respiratory** and **renal compensations** by the resulting changes in plasma P_{CO_2} and bicarbonate ion concentrations (see *A Closer Look*). Because the compensations act to restore normal blood pH, a patient may have a normal pH despite a significant medical problem.

Respiratory Compensations As a rule, changes in respiratory rate and depth are evident when the respiratory system is attempting to compensate for metabolic acid-base imbalances. In metabolic acidosis, respiratory rate and depth are usually elevated—an indication that high H^+ levels are stimulating the respiratory centers. Blood pH is low (below 7.35) and the HCO_3^- level is below 22 mEq/L. As the respiratory system "blows off" CO_2 to rid the blood of excess acid, the P_{CO_2} falls below 35 mm Hg. By contrast, in respiratory acidosis, the respiratory rate is often depressed and *is the immediate cause of the acidosis* (with some exceptions such as pneumonia or emphysema where gas exchange is impaired).

Respiratory compensation for metabolic alkalosis involves slow, shallow breathing, which allows CO_2 to accumulate in the blood. Evidence of metabolic alkalosis being compensated by respiratory mechanisms includes a pH over 7.45 (at least initially), elevated bicarbonate levels (over 26 mEq/L), and a P_{CO_2} above 45 mm Hg.

Renal Compensations When an acid-base imbalance is of respiratory origin, renal mechanisms are stepped up to compensate for the imbalance. For example, a hypoventilating individual will exhibit acidosis. When renal compensation is occurring, both the P_{CO_2} and the HCO_3^- levels are high. The high P_{CO_2} causes the acidosis, and the rising HCO_3^- level indicates that the kidneys are retaining bicarbonate to offset the acidosis.

Conversely, a person with renal-compensated respiratory alkalosis will have a high blood pH and a low P_{CO_2}. Bicarbonate ion levels begin to fall as the kidneys eliminate more HCO_3^- from the body by failing to reclaim it or by actively secreting it. Note that the kidneys cannot compensate for alkalosis or acidosis if that condition reflects a *renal* problem.

Check Your Understanding

17. Which two abnormalities in plasma are key features of an uncompensated metabolic alkalosis? An uncompensated respiratory acidosis?
18. How do the kidneys compensate for respiratory acidosis?

For answers, see Appendix H.

Developmental Aspects of Fluid, Electrolyte, and Acid-Base Balance

✓ Explain why infants and the aged are at greater risk for fluid and electrolyte imbalances than are young adults.

26

An embryo and a very young fetus are more than 90% water, but solids accumulate as fetal development continues, and at birth an infant is "only" 70–80% water. (The average value for adults is 50–60%.) Infants have proportionately more ECF than adults and, consequently, a much higher NaCl content in relation to K^+, Mg^{2+}, and PO_4^{3-} salts.

Distribution of body water begins to change about two months after birth and achieves the adult pattern by the time the child is 2 years old. Plasma electrolyte concentrations are similar in infants and adults, but K^+ and Ca^{2+} values are higher and Mg^{2+}, HCO_3^-, and total protein levels are lower in the first few days of life than at any other time. At puberty, sex differences in body water content become obvious as males develop relatively greater amounts of skeletal muscle.

Problems with fluid, electrolyte, and particularly acid-base balance are most common in infancy, reflecting the following conditions:

- *The very low residual volume of infant lungs* (approximately half that of adults relative to body weight). When respiration is altered, P_{CO_2} can shift rapidly and dramatically.
- *The high rate of fluid intake and output in infants* (about seven times higher than in adults). Infants may exchange fully half their ECF daily. Though infants have proportionately much more body water than adults, this does not protect them from excessive fluid shifts. Even slight alterations in fluid balance can cause serious problems. Further, although adults can live without water for about ten days, infants can survive for only three to four days.
- *The relatively high infant metabolic rate* (about twice that of adults). The higher metabolic rate yields much larger amounts of metabolic wastes and acids that the kidneys must excrete. This, along with buffer systems that are not yet fully effective, results in a tendency toward acidosis.
- *The high rate of insensible water loss in infants because of their larger surface area relative to body volume* (about three times that of adults). Infants lose substantial amounts of water through their skin.
- *The inefficiency of infant kidneys.* At birth, the kidneys are immature, only about half as proficient as adult kidneys at concentrating urine, and notably inefficient at ridding the body of acids.

All these factors put newborns at risk for dehydration and acidosis, at least until the end of the first month when the kidneys achieve reasonable efficiency. Bouts of vomiting or diarrhea greatly amplify the risk.

In old age, total body water often decreases (the loss is largely from the intracellular compartment) because muscle mass progressively declines and body fat rises. Few changes occur in the solute concentrations of body fluids, but the speed with which homeostasis is restored after being disrupted declines with age.

Elders may be unresponsive to thirst cues and thus are at risk for dehydration. Additionally, they are the most frequent prey of diseases that lead to severe fluid, electrolyte, or acid-base problems, such as congestive heart failure (and its attendant edema) and diabetes mellitus. Because most fluid, electrolyte, and acid-base imbalances occur when body water content is highest or lowest, the very young and the very old are the most frequent victims.

Check Your Understanding

19. Infants have a higher urine output than adults relative to their body weight. In addition to their relatively higher fluid intake, what are the reasons for this?

For answers, see Appendix H.

In this chapter we have examined the chemical and physiological mechanisms that provide the optimal internal environment for survival. The kidneys are the superstars among homeostatic organs in regulating water, electrolyte, and acid-base balance, but they do not and cannot act alone. Rather, their activity is made possible by a host of hormones and enhanced both by bloodborne buffers, which give the kidneys time to react, and by the respiratory system, which shoulders a substantial responsibility for acid-base balance of the blood.

Now that we have discussed the topics relevant to renal functioning, and once you read in *System Connections* how the urinary system interacts with other body systems, the topics in Chapters 25 and 26 should draw together in an understandable way.

Homeostatic Interrelationships Between the Urinary System and Other Body Systems

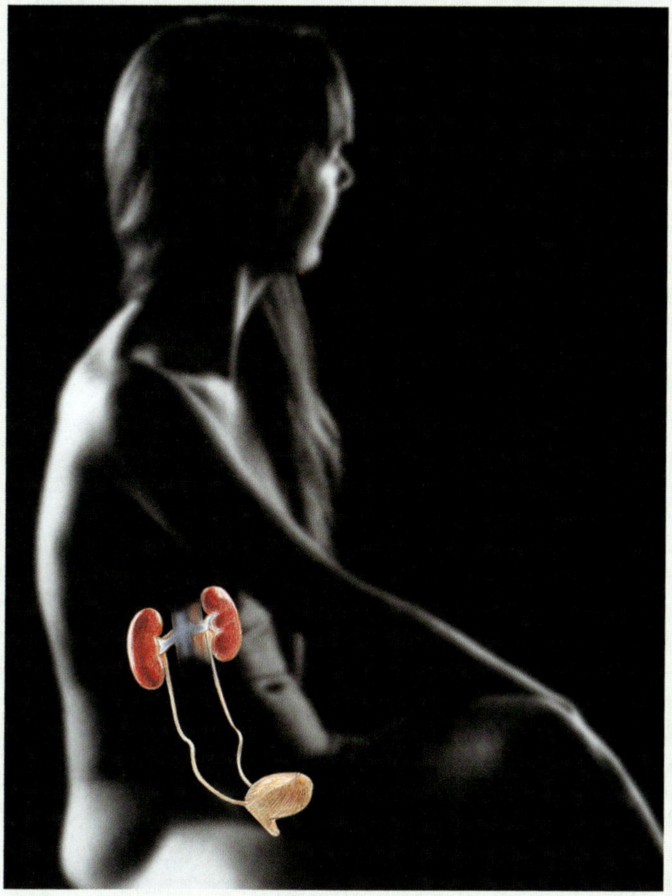

Integumentary System Chapter 5

- Kidneys dispose of nitrogenous wastes; maintain fluid, electrolyte, and acid-base balance of blood
- Skin provides external protective barrier; site of water loss (via perspiration); vitamin D synthesis site

Skeletal System Chapters 6–8

- Kidneys dispose of nitrogenous wastes; maintain fluid, electrolyte, and acid-base balance of blood
- Bones of rib cage provide some protection to kidneys; form major store of calcium and phosphate ions

Muscular System Chapters 9–10

- Kidneys dispose of nitrogenous wastes; maintain fluid, electrolyte, and acid-base balance of blood; renal regulation of K^+, Ca^{2+}, and Na^+ content in ECF crucial for muscle excitability and contractility
- Muscles of pelvic diaphragm and external urethral sphincter function in voluntary control of micturition; creatinine is a nitrogenous waste product of muscle metabolism that must be excreted by the kidneys

Nervous System Chapters 11–15

- Kidneys dispose of nitrogenous wastes; maintain fluid, electrolyte, and acid-base balance of blood; renal control of K^+, Ca^{2+}, and Na^+ in ECF essential for normal neural function
- Neural controls involved in micturition; sympathetic nervous system activity triggers the renin-angiotensin-aldosterone mechanism

Endocrine System Chapter 16

- Kidneys dispose of nitrogenous wastes; maintain fluid, electrolyte, and acid-base balance of blood; produce erythropoietin; renal regulation of Na^+ and water balance essential for blood pressure homeostasis and hormone transport in blood
- ADH, aldosterone, ANP, and other hormones help regulate renal reabsorption of water and electrolytes

Cardiovascular System Chapters 17–19

- Kidneys dispose of nitrogenous wastes; maintain fluid, electrolyte, and acid-base balance of blood; renal regulation of Na^+ and water balance essential for blood pressure homeostasis. K^+, Ca^{2+}, and Na^+ regulation maintains cardiac excitability
- Systemic arterial blood pressure is the driving force for glomerular filtration; heart secretes atrial natriuretic peptide; blood transports nutrients, oxygen, etc. to urinary organs

Lymphatic System/Immunity Chapters 20–21

- Kidneys dispose of nitrogenous wastes; maintain fluid, electrolyte, and acid-base balance of blood
- By returning leaked plasma fluid to cardiovascular system, lymphatic vessels help ensure normal systemic arterial pressure required for kidney function; immune cells protect urinary organs from infection and cancer

Respiratory System Chapter 22

- Kidneys dispose of nitrogenous wastes; maintain fluid, electrolyte, and long-term acid-base balance of blood
- Respiratory system provides oxygen required by kidney cells for their high metabolic activity; disposes of carbon dioxide; rapid acid-base balance of blood; lung capillary endothelial cells convert angiotensin I to angiotensin II

Digestive System Chapter 23

- Kidneys dispose of nitrogenous wastes; maintain fluid, electrolyte, and acid-base balance of blood; metabolize vitamin D to the active form needed for calcium absorption
- Digestive organs provide nutrients needed for kidney cell health; liver synthesizes urea and glutamine to transport waste nitrogen to the kidneys for excretion

Reproductive System Chapter 27

- Kidneys dispose of nitrogenous wastes; maintain fluid, electrolyte, and acid-base balance of blood

Chapter Summary

MAP™ For more chapter study tools, go to the Study Area of MasteringA&P at **www.masteringaandp.com**.
There you will find:

- Interactive Physiology iP
- A&PFlix A&PFlix
- Practice Anatomy Lab PAL
- PhysioEx PEx
- Videos, Practice Quizzes and Tests, MP3 Tutor Sessions, Case Studies, and much more!

Body Fluids (pp. 991–993)

Body Water Content (p. 991)

1. Water accounts for 45–75% of body weight, depending on age, sex, and amount of body fat.

Fluid Compartments (p. 991)

2. About two-thirds (25 L) of body water is found within cells in the intracellular fluid (ICF) compartment; the balance (15 L) is in the extracellular fluid (ECF) compartment. The ECF includes plasma and interstitial fluid.

Composition of Body Fluids (pp. 991–993)

3. Solutes dissolved in body fluids include electrolytes and nonelectrolytes. Electrolyte concentration is expressed in mEq/L.
4. Plasma contains more proteins than does interstitial fluid; otherwise, extracellular fluids are similar. The most abundant ECF electrolytes are sodium, chloride, and bicarbonate ions.
5. Intracellular fluids contain large amounts of protein anions and potassium, phosphate, and magnesium ions.

iP Fluid, Electrolyte, and Acid/Base Balance; Topic: Introduction to Body Fluids, pp. 1–8.

26

Fluid Movement Among Compartments (p. 993)

6. Substances usually pass through the plasma and interstitial fluid to reach the intracellular fluid.
7. Osmotic and hydrostatic pressure regulate fluid exchanges between compartments: (a) Hydrostatic pressure forces filtrate out of the capillaries and colloid osmotic pressure pulls filtrate back in. (b) Water moves freely between the ECF and the ICF by osmosis, but solute movements are restricted by size, charge, and dependence on transport proteins. (c) Water flows always follow changes in ECF osmolality.

iP Fluid, Electrolyte, and Acid/Base Balance; Topic: Introduction to Body Fluids, pp. 19–23.

Water Balance and ECF Osmolality (pp. 993–997)

1. Sources of body water are ingested foods and fluids and metabolic water.
2. Water leaves the body primarily via the lungs, skin, gastrointestinal tract, and kidneys.

Regulation of Water Intake (pp. 994–995)

3. Increased plasma osmolality triggers the thirst mechanism, mediated by hypothalamic osmoreceptors. Thirst, inhibited by distension of the gastrointestinal tract by ingested water and then by reduced osmolality, may be damped before body needs for water are met.

Regulation of Water Output (p. 995)

4. Obligatory water loss is unavoidable and includes insensible water losses from the lungs, the skin, and in feces, and about 500 ml of urine output daily.
5. Beyond obligatory water loss, the volume of urinary output depends on water intake and loss via other routes and reflects the influence of antidiuretic hormone on the renal collecting ducts.

Influence of Antidiuretic Hormone (ADH) (p. 995)

6. Antidiuretic hormone causes aquaporins (water channels) to be inserted in the cell membranes of the collecting ducts, so that most filtered water is reabsorbed. ADH release is triggered if ECF osmolality is high, or if a large drop in blood volume or pressure occurs.

Disorders of Water Balance (pp. 995-997)

7. Dehydration occurs when water loss exceeds water intake over time. It is evidenced by thirst, dry skin, and decreased urine output. A serious consequence is hypovolemic shock.
8. Hypotonic hydration occurs when body fluids are excessively diluted and entering water makes cells swell. The most serious consequence is cerebral edema.
9. Edema is an abnormal accumulation of fluid in the interstitial space (increased IF), which may impair blood circulation.

iP Fluid, Electrolyte, and Acid/Base Balance; Topic: Water Homeostasis, pp. 1–27.

Electrolyte Balance (pp. 997–1004)

1. Most electrolytes are obtained from ingested foods and fluids. Salts, particularly NaCl, are often ingested in excess of need.
2. Electrolytes are lost in perspiration, feces, and urine. The kidneys are most important in regulating electrolyte balance.

The Central Role of Sodium in Fluid and Electrolyte Balance (pp. 997–999)

3. Sodium salts are the most abundant solutes in ECF. They exert the bulk of ECF osmotic pressure and control water volume and distribution in the body.

Regulation of Sodium Balance (pp. 999–1000)

4. Sodium ion balance is linked to ECF volume and blood pressure regulation and involves both neural and hormonal controls.
5. Aldosterone promotes Na^+ reabsorption to maintain blood volume and blood pressure.
6. Declining blood pressure and falling filtrate NaCl concentration stimulate the granular cells to release renin. Renin, via angiotensin II, enhances systemic blood pressure, Na^+ reabsorption, and aldosterone release.
7. Atrial natriuretic peptide, released by certain atrial cells in response to rising blood pressure (or blood volume), causes systemic vasodilation and inhibits renin, aldosterone, and ADH release. Hence, it enhances Na^+ and water excretion, reducing blood volume and blood pressure.
8. Estrogens and glucocorticoids increase renal retention of sodium. Progesterone promotes enhanced sodium and water excretion in urine.

9. Cardiovascular system baroreceptors sense changing arterial blood pressure, prompting changes in sympathetic vasomotor activity. Rising arterial pressure leads to vasodilation and enhanced Na^+ and water loss in urine. Falling arterial pressure promotes vasoconstriction and conserves Na^+ and water.

Regulation of Potassium Balance (pp. 1000–1003)

10. The more proximal regions of the nephrons reabsorb about 90% of filtered potassium.
11. The main thrust of renal regulation of K^+ is to excrete it. Aldosterone and increased plasma K^+ content enhance potassium ion secretion by the principal cells of the collecting ducts. Type A intercalated cells of the collecting duct reabsorb small amounts of K^+ during K^+ deficit.

Regulation of Calcium and Phosphate Balance (pp. 1003–1004)

12. Calcium balance is regulated primarily by parathyroid hormone (PTH), which enhances blood Ca^{2+} levels by targeting the bones, kidneys, and intestine. PTH-regulated reabsorption occurs primarily in the DCT.
13. PTH decreases renal reabsorption of phosphate ions.

Regulation of Anions (p. 1004)

14. When blood pH is normal or slightly high, chloride is the major anion accompanying sodium reabsorption. In acidosis, bicarbonate replaces chloride.
15. Reabsorption of most other anions is regulated by their transport maximums (T_m).

iP Fluid, Electrolyte, and Acid/Base Balance; Topic: Electrolyte Homeostasis, pp. 1–38.

Acid-Base Balance (pp. 1004–1012)

1. The homeostatic pH range of arterial blood is 7.35 to 7.45. A higher pH represents alkalosis; a lower pH reflects acidosis.
2. Some acids enter the body in foods, but most are generated by breakdown of phosphorus-containing proteins, incomplete oxidation of fats or glucose, and the loading and transport of carbon dioxide in the blood.
3. Acid-base balance is achieved by chemical buffers, respiratory regulation, and in the long term by renal regulation of bicarbonate ion (hence, hydrogen ion) concentration of body fluids.

iP Fluid, Electrolyte, and Acid/Base Balance; Topic: Acid/Base Homeostasis, pp. 1–15.

Chemical Buffer Systems (pp. 1004–1006)

4. Acids are proton (H^+) donors; bases are proton acceptors. Acids that dissociate completely in solution are strong acids; those that dissociate incompletely are weak acids. Strong bases are more effective proton acceptors than are weak bases.
5. Chemical buffers are single or paired sets (a weak acid and its salt) of molecules that act rapidly to resist excessive shifts in pH by releasing or binding H^+.
6. Chemical buffers of the body include the bicarbonate, phosphate, and protein buffer systems.

iP Fluid, Electrolyte, and Acid/Base Balance; Topic: Acid/Base Homeostasis, pp. 16–26.

Respiratory Regulation of H^+ (p. 1006)

7. Respiratory regulation of acid-base balance of the blood utilizes the bicarbonate buffer system and the fact that CO_2 and H_2O are in reversible equilibrium with H_2CO_3.
8. Acidosis activates the respiratory center to increase respiratory rate and depth, which eliminates more CO_2 and causes blood pH to rise. Alkalosis depresses the respiratory center, resulting in CO_2 retention and a fall in blood pH.

iP Fluid, Electrolyte, and Acid/Base Balance; Topic: Acid/Base Homeostasis, pp. 27–28.

Renal Mechanisms of Acid-Base Balance (pp. 1006–1009)

9. The kidneys provide the major long-term mechanism for controlling acid-base balance by maintaining stable HCO_3^- levels in the ECF. Nonvolatile acids (organic acids other than carbonic acid) can be eliminated from the body only by the kidneys.
10. Secreted hydrogen ions come from the dissociation of carbonic acid generated within the tubule cells.
11. Tubule cells are impermeable to bicarbonate in the filtrate, but they can conserve filtered bicarbonate ions indirectly by absorbing HCO_3^- generated within them (by dissociation of carbonic acid to HCO_3^- and H^+). For each HCO_3^- (and Na^+) reabsorbed, one H^+ is secreted into the filtrate, where it combines with HCO_3^-.
12. To generate and add new HCO_3^- to plasma to counteract acidosis, either of two mechanisms may be used:
    - Secreted H^+, buffered by bases other than HCO_3^-, is excreted from the body in urine (the major urine buffer is the phosphate buffer system).
    - NH_4^+ (derived from glutamine catabolism) is excreted in urine.
13. To counteract alkalosis, bicarbonate ion is secreted into the filtrate and H^+ is reabsorbed.

iP Fluid, Electrolyte, and Acid/Base Balance; Topic: Acid/Base Homeostasis, pp. 29–37.

Abnormalities of Acid-Base Balance (pp. 1009–1012)

14. Acid-base imbalances can be classified as metabolic or respiratory based on their cause.
15. Respiratory acidosis results from carbon dioxide retention. Respiratory alkalosis occurs when carbon dioxide is eliminated faster than it is produced.
16. Metabolic acidosis occurs when nonvolatile acids (lactic acid, ketone bodies, and others) accumulate in the blood or when bicarbonate is lost from the body. Metabolic alkalosis occurs when bicarbonate levels are excessive.
17. Extremes of pH for life are 6.8 and 7.8.
18. Compensations occur when the respiratory system or kidneys counteract acid-base imbalances resulting from abnormal or inadequate functioning of the alternate system. Respiratory compensations involve changes in respiratory rate and depth. Renal compensations modify blood levels of HCO_3^-.

iP Fluid, Electrolyte, and Acid/Base Balance; Topic: Acid/Base Homeostasis, pp. 38–59.

Developmental Aspects of Fluid, Electrolyte, and Acid-Base Balance (p. 1012)

1. Infants have a higher risk of dehydration and acidosis because of their low lung residual volume, high rate of fluid intake and output, high metabolic rate, relatively large body surface area, and functionally immature kidneys at birth.
2. The elderly are at risk for dehydration because of their low percentage of body water and insensitivity to thirst cues. Diseases that promote fluid and acid-base imbalances (cardiovascular disease, diabetes mellitus, and others) are most common in the aged.

Review Questions

Multiple Choice/Matching

(Some questions have more than one correct answer. Select the best answer or answers from the choices given.)

1. Body water content is greatest in **(a)** infants, **(b)** young adults, **(c)** elderly adults.
2. Potassium, magnesium, and phosphate ions are the predominant electrolytes in **(a)** plasma, **(b)** interstitial fluid, **(c)** intracellular fluid.
3. Sodium balance is regulated primarily by control of amount(s) **(a)** ingested, **(b)** excreted in urine, **(c)** lost in perspiration, **(d)** lost in feces.
4. Water balance is regulated by control of amount(s) (use choices in question 3).

Answer questions 5 through 10 by choosing responses from the following:

(a) ammonium ions	**(f)** magnesium
(b) bicarbonate	**(g)** phosphate
(c) calcium	**(h)** potassium
(d) chloride	**(i)** sodium
(e) hydrogen ions	**(j)** water

5. Two main substances regulated by the influence of aldosterone on the kidney tubules.
6. Two substances regulated by parathyroid hormone.
7. Two substances secreted into the proximal convoluted tubules in exchange for sodium ions.
8. Part of an important chemical buffer system in plasma.
9. Two ions produced during catabolism of glutamine.
10. Substance regulated by ADH's effects on the renal tubules.
11. Which of the following factors will enhance ADH release? **(a)** increase in ECF volume, **(b)** decrease in ECF volume, **(c)** decrease in ECF osmolality, **(d)** increase in ECF osmolality.
12. The pH of blood varies directly with **(a)** HCO_3^-, **(b)** P_{CO_2}, **(c)** H^+, **(d)** none of the above.
13. In an individual with metabolic acidosis, a clue that the respiratory system is compensating is provided by **(a)** high blood bicarbonate levels, **(b)** low blood bicarbonate levels, **(c)** rapid, deep breathing, **(d)** slow, shallow breathing.

26

Short Answer Essay Questions

14. Name the body fluid compartments, noting their locations and the approximate fluid volume in each.
15. Describe the thirst mechanism, indicating how it is triggered and terminated.
16. Explain why and how ECF osmolality is maintained.
17. Explain why and how sodium balance, ECF volume, and blood pressure are jointly regulated.
18. Describe the role of the respiratory system in controlling acid-base balance.
19. Explain how the chemical buffer systems resist changes in pH.
20. Explain the relationship of the following to renal secretion and excretion of hydrogen ions: (a) plasma carbon dioxide levels, (b) phosphate, and (c) sodium bicarbonate reabsorption.
21. List several factors that place newborn babies at risk for acid-base imbalances.

Critical Thinking and Clinical Application Questions

1. Mr. Jessup, a 55-year-old man, is operated on for a cerebral tumor. About a month later, he appears at his physician's office complaining of excessive thirst. He claims to have been drinking about 20 liters of water daily for the past week and says he has been voiding nearly continuously. A urine sample is collected and its specific gravity is reported as 1.001. What is your diagnosis of Mr. Jessup's problem? What connection might exist between his previous surgery and his present problem?
2. For each of the following sets of blood values, name the acid-base imbalance (acidosis or alkalosis), determine its cause (metabolic or respiratory), decide whether the condition is being compensated, and cite at least one possible cause of the imbalance.
   Problem 1: pH 7.63; P_{CO_2} 19 mm Hg; HCO_3^- 19.5 mEq/L
   Problem 2: pH 7.22; P_{CO_2} 30 mm Hg; HCO_3^- 12.0 mEq/L
3. Explain how emphysema and congestive heart failure can lead to acid-base imbalance.
4. Mrs. Bush, a 70-year-old woman, is admitted to the hospital. Her history states that she has been suffering from diarrhea for three weeks. On admission, she complains of severe fatigue and muscle weakness. A blood chemistry study yields the following information: Na^+ 142 mEq/L; K^+ 1.5 mEq/L; Cl^- 92 mEq/L; P_{CO_2} 32 mm Hg. Which electrolytes are within normal limits? Which are so abnormal that the patient has a medical emergency? Which of the following represents the greatest danger to Mrs. Bush? (a) a fall due to her muscular weakness, (b) edema, (c) cardiac arrhythmia and cardiac arrest.
5. During a routine medical checkup, Candace, a 26-year-old physiotherapy student, is surprised to hear that her blood pressure is 180/110. She also has a rumbling systolic and diastolic abdominal bruit (murmur) that is loudest at the mid-epigastric area. Her physician suspects renal artery stenosis (narrowing). She orders an abdominal ultrasound and renal artery arteriography, which confirm that Candace has a small right kidney and the distal part of her right renal artery is narrowed by more than 70%. Her physician prescribes diuretics and calcium channel blockers as temporary measures, and refers Candace to a cardiovascular surgeon. Explain the connection between Candace's renal artery stenosis and her hypertension. Why is her right kidney smaller than her left? What would you expect Candace's blood levels of K^+, Na^+, aldosterone, angiotensin II, and renin to be?

AT THE CLINIC

Related Clinical Terms

Antacid An agent that counteracts acidity, such as sodium bicarbonate, aluminum hydroxide gel, and magnesium trisilicate. Commonly used to manage heartburn.

Hyperaldosteronism (Conn's disease) A condition of hypersecretion of aldosterone by adrenal cortical cells accompanied by excessive loss of potassium and generalized muscular weakness, hypernatremia, and hypertension. Usual cause is adrenal tumor; usual treatment is adrenal-suppressing drugs prior to tumor removal.

Renal tubular acidosis A metabolic acidosis resulting from impaired renal reabsorption of bicarbonate; the urine is alkaline.

Syndrome of inappropriate ADH secretion (SIADH) A group of disorders associated with excessive ADH secretion in the absence of appropriate (osmotic or nonosmotic) stimuli. Characterized by hypotonic hydration (hyponatremia, fluid retention, and weight gain) and concentrated urine. Usual causes are ectopic secretion of ADH by cancer cells (e.g., small cell lung cancers) and brain disorders or trauma affecting the ADH-secreting hypothalamic neurons. Temporary management involves restricting water intake.

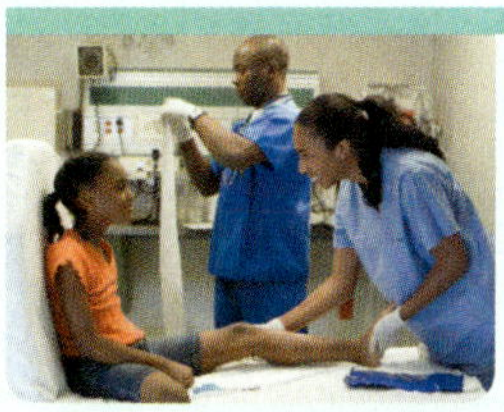

Case Study Urinary System

Mr. Heyden, a somewhat stocky 72-year-old man, is brought in to the emergency room (ER). The paramedics report that his left arm and the left side of his body trunk were pinned beneath some wreckage, and that when he was freed, his left hypogastric and lumbar areas appeared to be compressed and his left arm was blanched and without sensation. On admission, Mr. Heyden is alert, slightly cyanotic, and complaining of pain in his left side; he loses consciousness shortly thereafter. His vital signs are taken, blood is drawn for laboratory tests, and Mr. Heyden is catheterized and immediately scheduled for a CT scan of his left abdominal region.

Analyze the information that was subsequently recorded on Mr. Heyden's chart:

- Vital signs: Temperature 39°C (102°F); BP 90/50 mm Hg and falling; heart rate 116 beats/min and thready; 30 respirations/min

1. Given the values above and his attendant cyanosis, what would you guess is Mr. Heyden's immediate problem? Explain your reasoning.

- CT scan reveals a ruptured spleen and a large hematoma in the upper left abdominal quadrant. Splenic repair surgery is scheduled but unsuccessful; the spleen is removed.

2. Rupture of the spleen results in massive hemorrhage. Explain this observation. Which organs (if any) will compensate for the removal of Mr. Heyden's spleen?

- Hematology: Most blood tests yield normal results. However, renin, aldosterone, and ADH levels are elevated.

3. Explain the cause and consequence of each of the hematology findings.

- Urinalysis: Some granular casts (particulate cell debris) are noted, and the urine is brownish-red in color; other values are normal, but urine output is very low. An order is given to force fluids.

4. (a) What might account for the low volume of urine output? (Name at least two possibilities.) (b) What might explain the casts and abnormal color of his urine? Can you see any possible relationship between his crush injury and these findings?

The next day, Mr. Heyden is awake and alert. He says that he now has feeling in his arm, but he still complains of pain. However, the pain site appears to have moved from the left upper quadrant to his lumbar region. His urine output is still low. He is scheduled once again for a CT scan, this time of his lumbar region. The order to force fluids is renewed and some additional and more specific blood tests are ordered. We will visit Mr. Heyden again shortly, but in the meantime think about what these new findings may indicate.

(Answers in Appendix H)

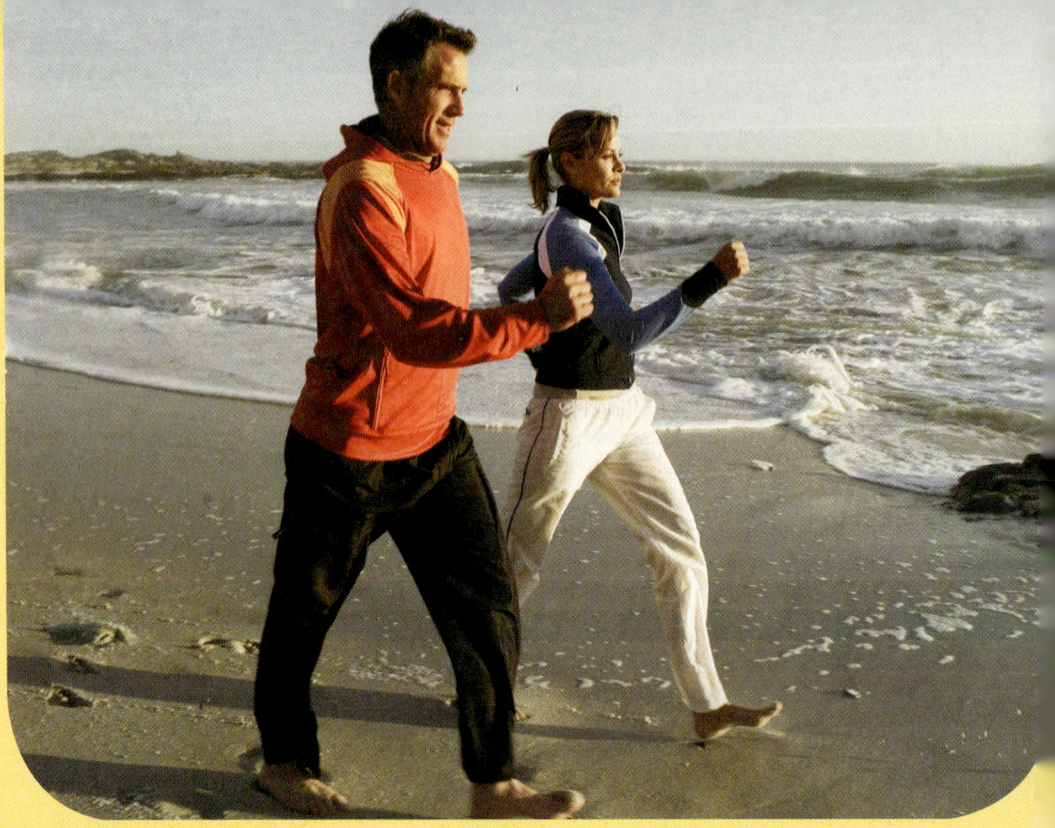

27 The Reproductive System

Most organ systems function almost continuously to maintain the well-being of the individual. The **reproductive system**, however, appears to "slumber" until puberty. The **primary sex organs**, or **gonads** (go′nadz; "seeds"), are the testes in males and the ovaries in females. The gonads produce sex cells, or **gametes** (gam′ēts; "spouses"), and secrete a variety of steroid hormones commonly called **sex hormones**. The remaining reproductive structures—ducts, glands, and external genitalia (jen-ĭ-ta′le-ah)—are the **accessory reproductive organs**. Although male and female

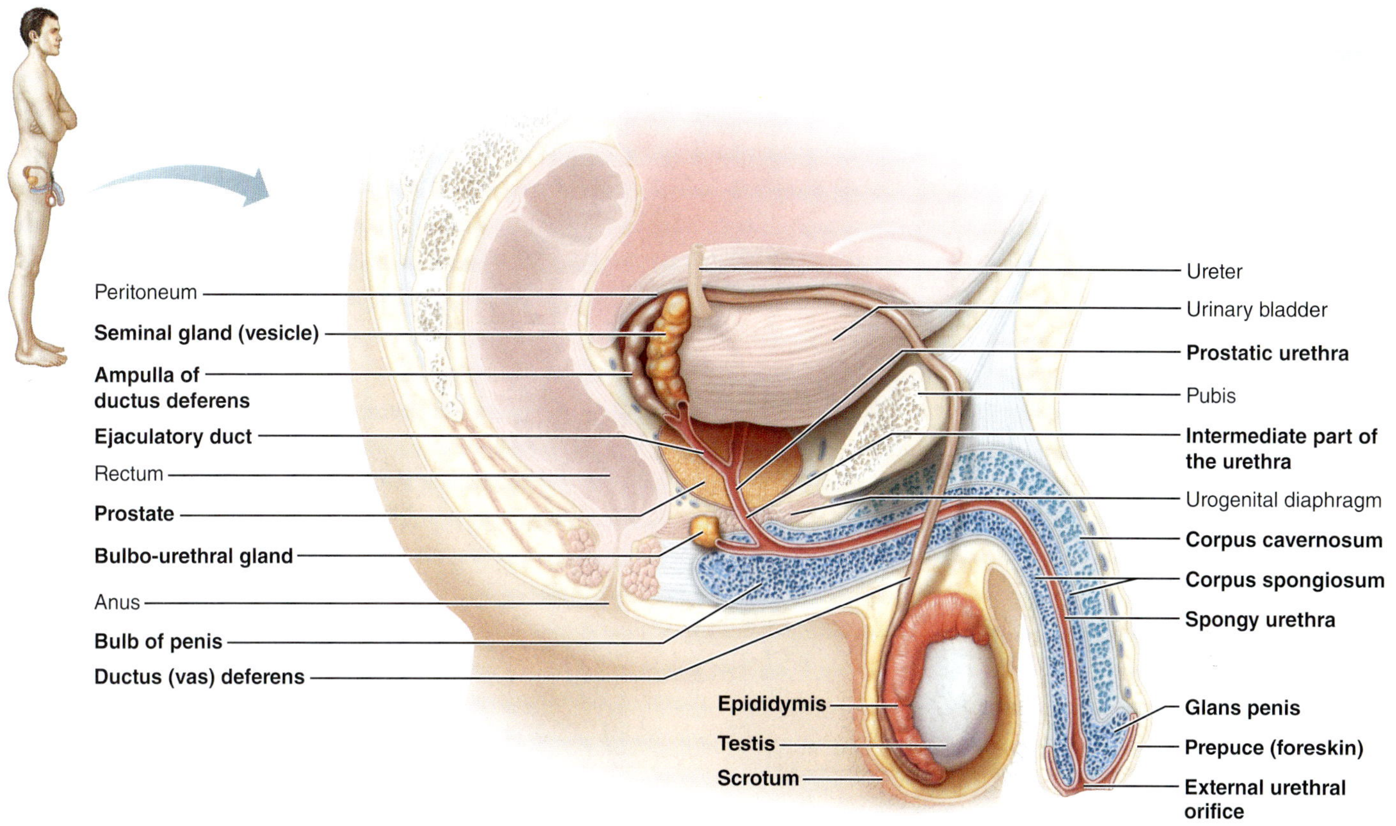

Figure 27.1 Reproductive organs of the male, sagittal view. A portion of the pubis of the hip bone has been left to show the relationship of the ductus deferens to the bony pelvis. (For related images, see *A Brief Atlas of the Human Body*, Figures 72 and 73.)

reproductive organs are quite different, their common purpose is to produce offspring.

The male's reproductive role is to manufacture male gametes called *sperm* and deliver them to the female reproductive tract, where fertilization can occur. The complementary role of the female is to produce female gametes, called *ova* or *eggs*. As a result of appropriately timed intercourse, a sperm and an egg may fuse to form a fertilized egg, or *zygote*. The zygote is the first cell of a new individual, from which all body cells will arise.

The male and female reproductive systems are equal partners in events leading up to fertilization, but once fertilization has occurred, the female partner's uterus provides the protective environment where the embryo develops until birth. Sex hormones—androgens in males and estrogens and progesterone in females—play vital roles both in the development and function of the reproductive organs and in sexual behavior and drives. These hormones also influence the growth and development of many other organs and tissues of the body.

Anatomy of the Male Reproductive System

✓ Describe the structure and function of the testes, and explain the importance of their location in the scrotum.

The sperm-producing **testes** (tes′tez; "witnesses"), or **male gonads**, lie within the *scrotum*. From the testes, the sperm are delivered to the body exterior through a system of ducts including (in order) the *epididymis*, the *ductus deferens*, the *ejaculatory duct*, and finally the *urethra*, which opens to the outside at the tip of the *penis*. The accessory sex glands, which empty their secretions into the ducts during ejaculation, are the *seminal glands*, *prostate*, and *bulbo-urethral glands*. Take a moment to trace the duct system in **Figure 27.1**, and identify the testis and accessory glands before continuing.

The Scrotum

The **scrotum** (skro′tum; "pouch") is a sac of skin and superficial fascia that hangs outside the abdominopelvic cavity at the root of the penis (Figure 27.1 and **Figure 27.2**). It is covered with sparse hairs, and contains paired oval testes. A midline *septum* divides the scrotum, providing a compartment for each testis.

This seems a rather vulnerable location for a man's testes, which contain his entire ability to father offspring. However, because viable sperm cannot be produced in abundance at core body temperature (37°C), the superficial location of the scrotum, which provides a temperature about 3°C lower, is an essential adaptation.

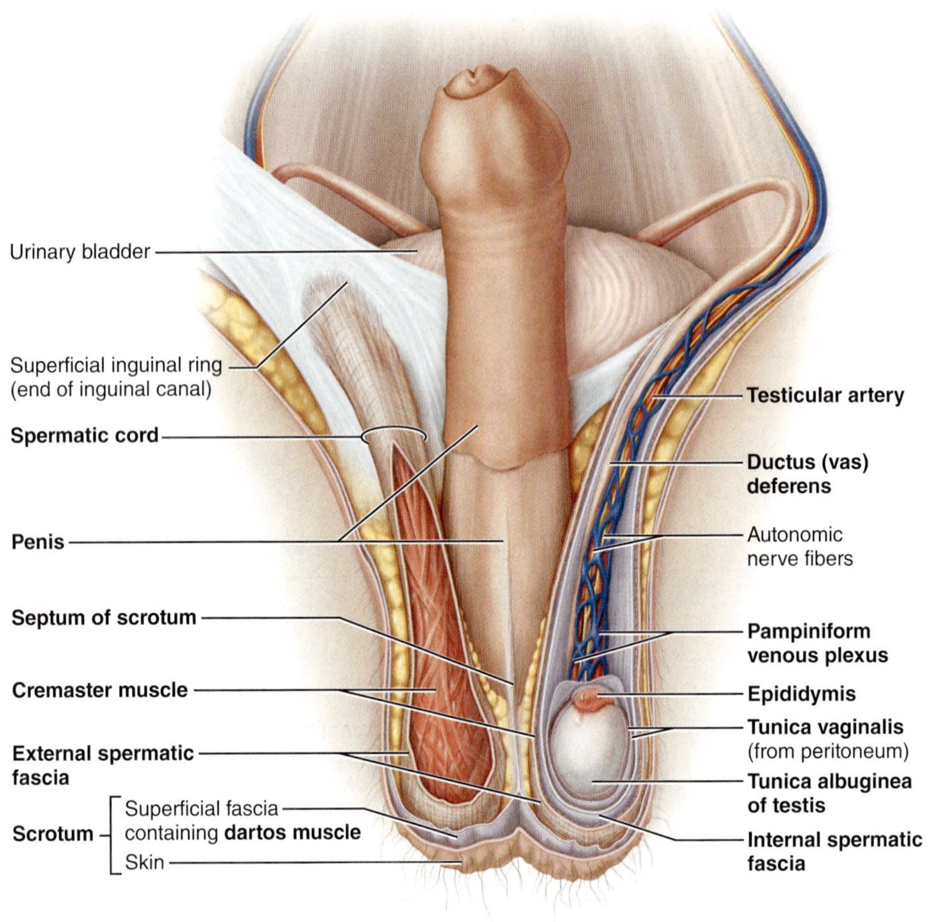

Figure 27.2 Relationships of the testis to the scrotum and spermatic cord. The scrotum has been opened and its anterior portion removed.

Furthermore, the scrotum is affected by temperature changes. When it is cold, the testes are pulled closer to the pelvic floor and the warmth of the body wall, and the scrotum becomes shorter and heavily wrinkled, decreasing its surface area and increasing its thickness to reduce heat loss. When it is warm, the scrotal skin is flaccid and loose to increase the surface area for cooling (sweating) and the testes hang lower, away from the body trunk.

These changes in scrotal surface area help maintain a fairly constant intrascrotal temperature and reflect the activity of two sets of muscles that respond to ambient temperature. The **dartos muscle** (dar′tos; "skinned"), a layer of smooth muscle in the superficial fascia, wrinkles the scrotal skin. The **cremaster muscles** (kre-mas′ter; "a suspender"), bands of skeletal muscle that arise from the internal oblique muscles of the trunk, elevate the testes.

The Testes

Each plum-sized testis is approximately 4 cm (1.5 inches) long by 2.5 cm (1 inch) wide and is surrounded by two tunics. The outer tunic is the two-layered **tunica vaginalis** (vaj″ĭ-nal′is), derived from an outpocketing of the peritoneum (Figure 27.2 and **Figure 27.3a**). Deep to this serous layer is the **tunica albuginea** (al″bu-jin′e-ah; "white coat"), the fibrous capsule of the testis.

Septa extending inward from the tunica albuginea divide the testis into about 250 wedge-shaped *lobules* (Figure 27.3). Each contains one to four tightly coiled **seminiferous tubules** (sem″ĭ-nif′er-us; "sperm-carrying"), the actual "sperm factories" consisting of a thick stratified epithelium surrounding a central fluid-containing lumen. The epithelium consists of spheroid *spermatogenic* ("sperm-forming") *cells*, embedded in substantially larger columnar cells called *sustentocytes*. The sustentocytes are supporting cells that play several roles in sperm formation as described shortly.

Surrounding each seminiferous tubule are three to five layers of smooth muscle–like **myoid cells** (Figure 27.3c). By contracting rhythmically, myoid cells may help to squeeze sperm and testicular fluids through the tubules and out of the testes.

The seminiferous tubules of each lobule converge to form a **straight tubule** that conveys sperm into the **rete testis** (re′te), a tubular network on the posterior side of the testis. From the rete testis, sperm leave the testis through the *efferent ductules* and

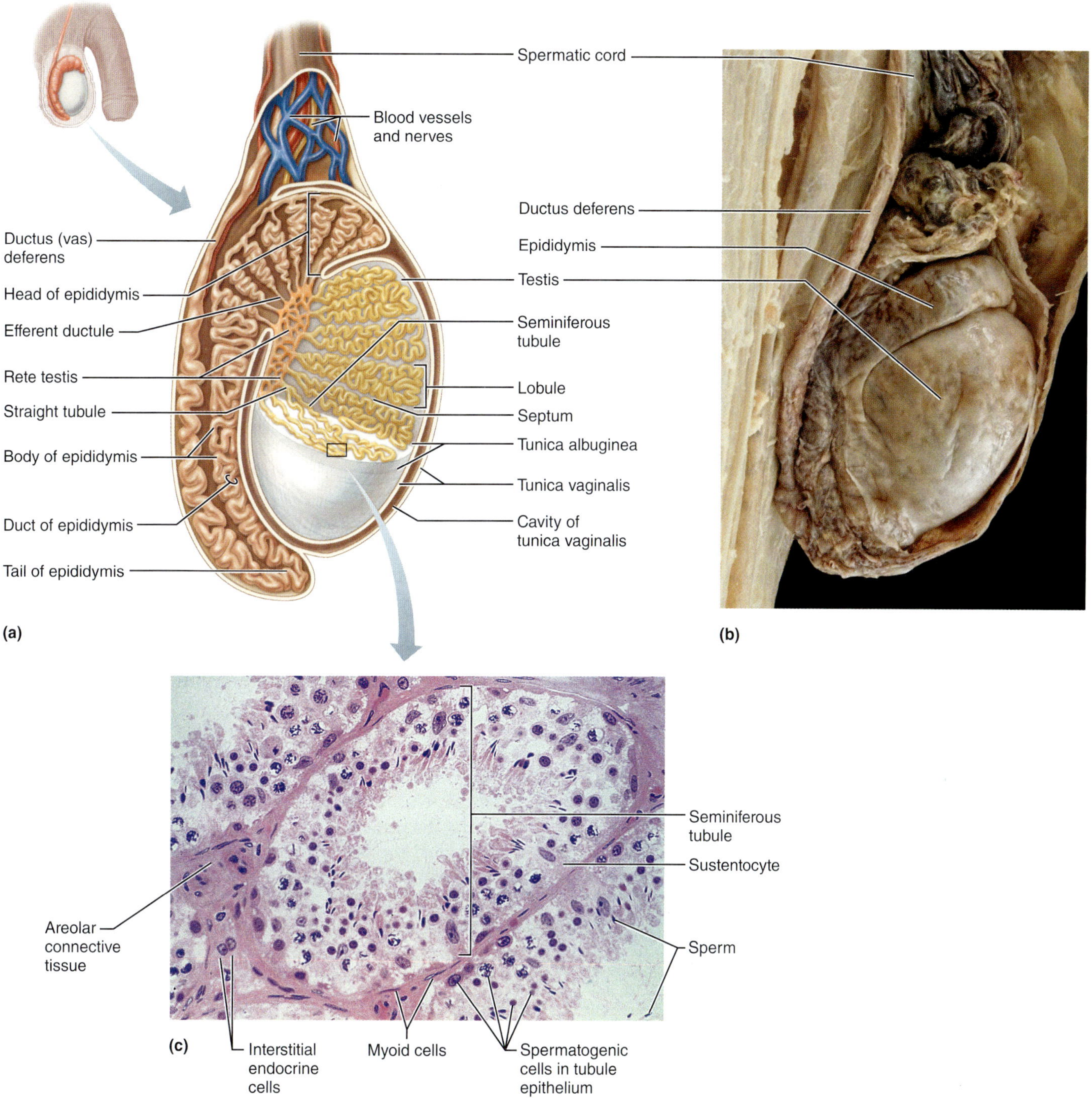

Figure 27.3 Structure of the testis. (a) Partial sagittal section through the testis and epididymis. The anterior aspect is to the right. (For a related image, see *A Brief Atlas of the Human Body*, Figure 73). **(b)** External view of a testis from a cadaver; same orientation as in (a). **(c)** Seminiferous tubule in cross section (270×). Note the spermatogenic (sperm-forming) cells in the tubule epithelium and the interstitial endocrine cells in the connective tissue between the tubules.

enter the *epididymis* (ep″ĭ-did′ĭ-mis), which hugs the external testis surface posteriorly. The immature sperm pass through the head, the body, and then move into the tail of the epididymis, where they are stored until ejaculation.

Lying in the soft connective tissue surrounding the seminiferous tubules are the **interstitial endocrine cells**, also called *Leydig cells* (Figure 27.3c). These cells produce androgens (most importantly *testosterone*), which they secrete into the surrounding interstitial fluid. Thus, completely different cell populations carry out the sperm-producing and hormone-producing functions of the testis.

The long **testicular arteries**, which branch from the abdominal aorta superior to the pelvis (see *gonadal arteries* in Figure 19.24c, p. 732), supply the testes. The **testicular veins** draining the testes arise from a network called the **pampiniform venous plexus** (pam-pin′ĭ-form; "tendril-shaped") that surrounds the portion of each testicular artery within the scrotum like a climbing vine (see Figure 27.2). The cooler venous blood in each pampiniform plexus absorbs heat from the arterial blood, cooling it before it enters the testes. In this way, these plexuses help to keep the testes at their cool homeostatic temperature.

Both divisions of the autonomic nervous system serve the testes, and when the testes are hit forcefully, associated sensory nerves transmit impulses that result in agonizing pain and nausea. A connective tissue sheath encloses nerve fibers, blood vessels, and lymphatics. Collectively these structures make up the **spermatic cord**, which passes through the inguinal canal (see Figure 27.2).

Homeostatic Imbalance 27.1

Although *testicular cancer* is relatively rare (affecting one of every 50,000 males), it is the most common cancer in young men ages 15 to 35. A history of mumps or orchitis (inflammation of the testis) and substantial maternal exposure to environmental toxins before birth increase the risk, but the most important risk factor for this cancer is *cryptorchidism* (nondescent of the testes, see p. 1057).

Every male should examine his testes regularly. The most common sign of testicular cancer is a painless solid mass in the testis. If detected early, testicular cancer has an impressive cure rate. Over 90% of cases are cured by surgical removal of the cancerous testis (*orchiectomy*) alone or in combination with radiation therapy or chemotherapy. +

Check Your Understanding

1. What are the two major functions of the testes?
2. Which of the tubular structures shown in Figure 27.3a are the sperm "factories"?
3. Muscle activity and the pampiniform venous plexus help to keep the temperature of the testes at homeostatic levels. How do they do that?

For answers, see Appendix H.

The Male Perineum

The male **perineum** (per″ĭ-ne′um; "around the anus") suspends the scrotum and contains the root of the penis, and the anus. More specifically, it is the diamond-shaped region located between the pubic symphysis anteriorly, the coccyx posteriorly, and the ischial tuberosities laterally **(Figure 27.4).** The floor of the perineum is formed by muscles described in Chapter 10 (pp. 344–345).

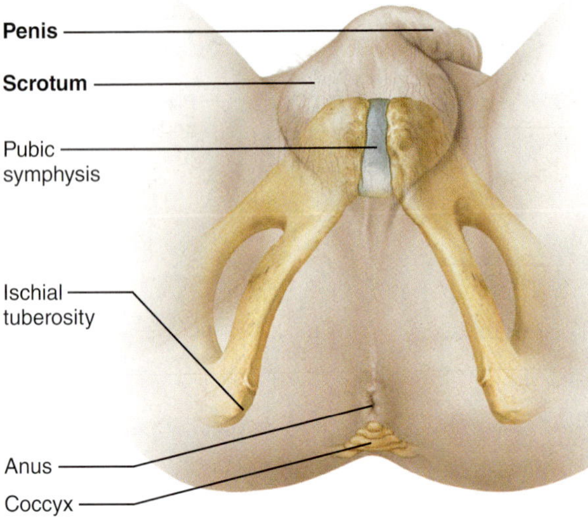

Figure 27.4 The male perineum, inferior view.

The Penis

✓ Describe the location, structure, and function of the accessory reproductive organs of the male.

The **penis** ("tail") is a copulatory organ, designed to deliver sperm into the female reproductive tract (Figure 27.1 and **Figure 27.5**). The penis and scrotum, which hang suspended from the perineum, make up the external reproductive structures, or **external genitalia**, of the male.

The penis consists of an attached root and a free *body* or *shaft* that ends in an enlarged tip, the **glans penis**. The skin covering the penis is loose, and when it slides distally it forms a cuff called the **prepuce** (pre′pūs), or **foreskin**, around the glans. Frequently, the foreskin is surgically removed shortly after birth, a procedure called *circumcision* ("cutting around"). Interestingly, over 60% of newborn boys in the United States are circumcised, compared to 15% in other parts of the world. Circumcision is charged by some as being medically unnecessary, but its proponents cite studies showing a 60% reduction in risk of acquiring HIV (the virus that causes AIDS), as well as significantly reduced risks for other reproductive system infections.

To understand penile anatomy, it is important to know that its dorsal and ventral surfaces are named in reference to the erect penis. Internally, the penis contains the spongy urethra and three long cylindrical bodies (*corpora*) of erectile tissue, each covered by a sheath of dense fibrous connective tissue. This *erectile tissue* is a spongy network of connective tissue and smooth muscle riddled with vascular spaces. During sexual excitement, the vascular spaces fill with blood, causing the penis to enlarge and become rigid. This event, called *erection*, enables the penis to serve as a penetrating organ.

The midventral erectile body, the **corpus spongiosum** (spon″je-o′sum; "spongy body") surrounds the urethra. It expands distally to form the glans and proximally to form the

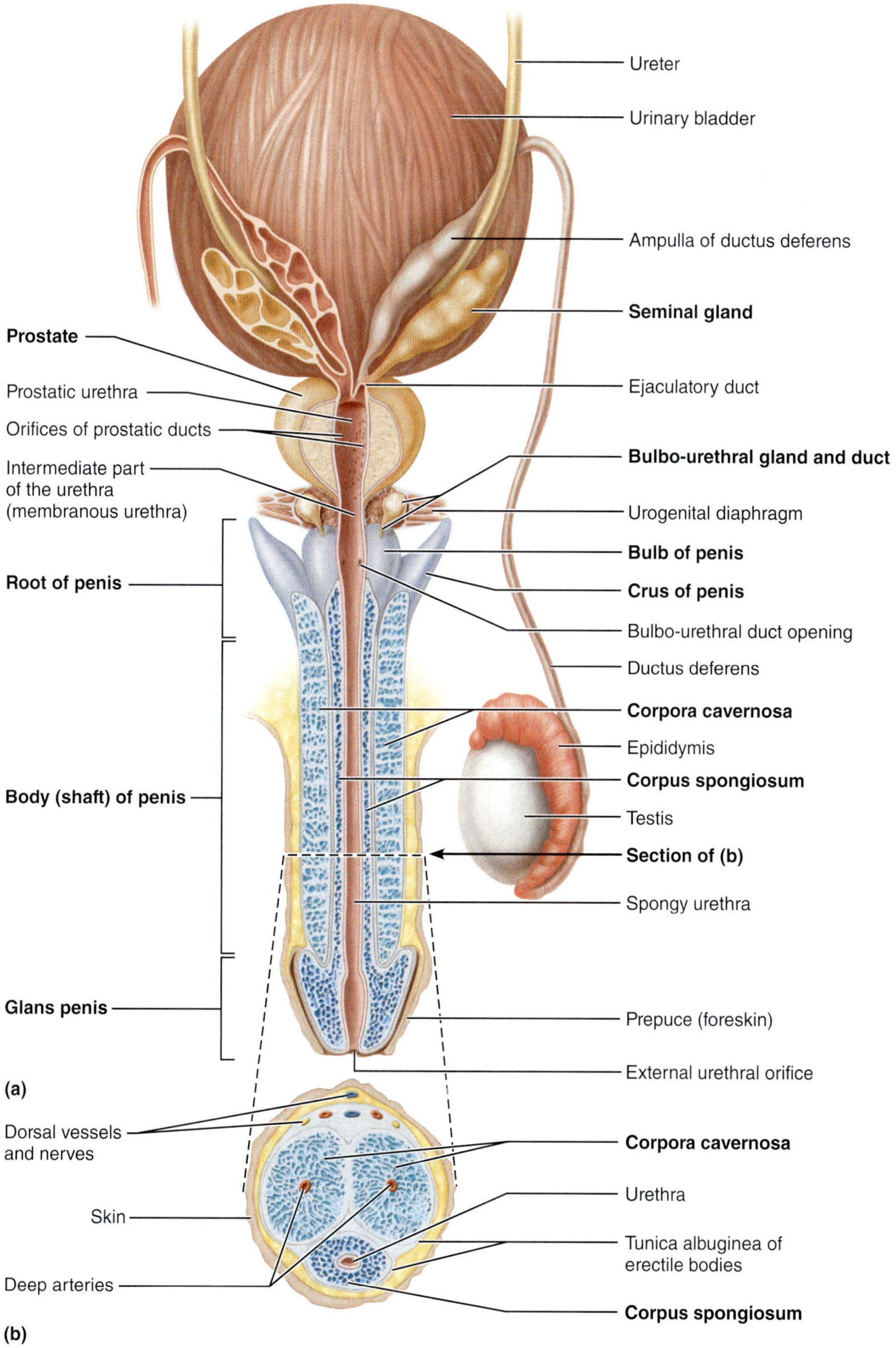

Figure 27.5 Male reproductive structures. (a) Posterior view showing longitudinal (frontal) section of the penis. **(b)** Transverse section of the penis, dorsal aspect at top.

part of the root called the **bulb of the penis**. The sheetlike bulbospongiosus muscle covers the bulb externally and secures it to the urogenital diaphragm.

The paired dorsal erectile bodies, called the **corpora cavernosa** (kor′por-ah kă-ver-no′sah; "cavernous bodies"), make up most of the penis and are bound by the fibrous tunica albuginea. Their proximal ends form the **crura of the penis** (kroo′rah; "legs"; singular: crus). Each crus is surrounded by an ischiocavernosus muscle and anchors to the pubic arch of the bony pelvis.

The Male Duct System

As we mentioned earlier, sperm travel from the testes to the body exterior through a system of ducts. In order (proximal to distal), the **accessory ducts** are the epididymis, ductus deferens, ejaculatory duct, and urethra.

The Epididymis

The cup-shaped **epididymis** (*epi* = beside; *didym* = the testes) is about 3.8 cm (1.5 inches) long (Figures 27.1 and 27.3a, b). Its *head*, which contains the efferent ductules, caps the superior aspect of the testis. Its *body* and *tail* are on the posterolateral area of the testis.

Most of the epididymis consists of the highly coiled **duct of the epididymis**, which has an uncoiled length of about 6 m (20 feet). Some pseudostratified epithelial cells of the duct mucosa exhibit long, nonmotile microvilli (*stereocilia*). The huge surface area of these stereocilia allows them to absorb excess testicular fluid and to pass nutrients to the many sperm stored temporarily in the lumen.

The immature, nearly nonmotile sperm that leave the testis are moved slowly along the duct of the epididymis through fluid that contains several kinds of antimicrobial proteins, including defensins. As they move along its tortuous course (a trip that takes about 20 days), the sperm gain the ability to swim.

Sperm are ejaculated from the epididymis, not the testes as many believe. When a male is sexually stimulated and ejaculates, the smooth muscle in the ducts of the epididymis contracts, expelling sperm into the next segment of the duct system, the *ductus deferens*.

Sperm can be stored in the epididymis for several months. If they are held longer, epithelial cells of the epididymis eventually phagocytize them. This is not a problem for the man, as sperm are generated continuously.

The Ductus Deferens and Ejaculatory Duct

The **ductus deferens** (duk′tus def′er-ens; "carrying away"), or *vas deferens*, is about 45 cm (18 inches) long. It runs upward as part of the spermatic cord from the epididymis through the inguinal canal into the pelvic cavity (Figure 27.1). Easily palpated as it passes anterior to the pubic bone, it then loops medially over the ureter and descends along the posterior bladder wall. Its terminus expands to form the **ampulla** of the ductus deferens and then joins with the duct of the seminal gland to form the short **ejaculatory duct**. Each ejaculatory duct enters the prostate, and there it empties into the urethra.

27

Like that of the epididymis, the mucosa of the ductus deferens is pseudostratified epithelium. However, its muscular layer is extremely thick and the duct feels like a hard wire when squeezed between the fingertips. During ejaculation, the smooth muscle in its walls creates strong peristaltic waves that rapidly squeeze the sperm forward along the tract and into the urethra.

As Figure 27.3 illustrates, part of the ductus deferens lies in the scrotal sac. Some men opt to take full responsibility for birth control by having a **vasectomy** (vah-sek′to-me; "cutting the vas"). In this relatively minor operation, the physician makes a small incision into the scrotum and then cuts through and ligates (ties off) each ductus deferens. Sperm are still produced, but they can no longer reach the body exterior. Eventually, they deteriorate and are phagocytized. Vasectomy is simple and provides highly effective birth control (close to 100%). For those wishing to reverse that procedure, the success rate is about 50%.

The Urethra

The **urethra** is the terminal portion of the male duct system (Figures 27.1 and 27.5). It conveys both urine and semen (at different times), so it serves both the urinary and reproductive systems. Its three regions are:

- *Prostatic urethra*, the portion surrounded by the prostate
- *Intermediate part of the urethra* (or membranous urethra) in the urogenital diaphragm
- *Spongy urethra*, which runs through the penis and opens to the outside at the *external urethral orifice*

The spongy urethra is about 15 cm (6 inches) long and accounts for 75% of urethral length. Its mucosa contains scattered *urethral glands* that secrete lubricating mucus into the lumen just before ejaculation.

☑ Check Your Understanding

4. What is the function of the erectile tissue of the penis?
5. Name the organs of the male duct system in order, from the epididymis to the body exterior.
6. What are two functions of the stereocilia on the epididymal epithelium?
7. Which accessory organ of the male duct system runs from the scrotum into the abdominal cavity?

For answers, see Appendix H.

The Male Accessory Glands

✓ Discuss the sources and functions of semen.

The **accessory glands** include the paired seminal glands and bulbo-urethral glands and the single prostate (Figures 27.1 and 27.5). Together these glands produce the bulk of *semen* (sperm plus accessory gland secretions).

The Seminal Glands

The **seminal glands** (sem′ĭ-nul), or **seminal vesicles**, lie on the posterior bladder surface. Each of these fairly large, hollow glands is about the shape and length (5–7 cm) of a little finger. However, because a seminal gland is pouched, coiled, and folded back on itself, its uncoiled length is actually about 15 cm. Its fibrous capsule encloses a thick layer of smooth muscle that contracts during ejaculation to empty the gland.

The seminal gland mucosa is a secretory pseudostratified columnar epithelium. Stored within the mucosa's honeycomb of crypts and blind alleys is a yellowish viscous alkaline fluid containing fructose sugar, citric acid, a coagulating enzyme (vesiculase), and prostaglandins, as well as other substances that enhance sperm motility or fertilizing ability. The yellow color of seminal fluid is due to a yellow pigment that fluoresces under UV light, a capability that allows investigators to recognize a sperm trail or residue in instances of sexual attack.

As noted, the duct of each seminal gland joins that of the ductus deferens on the same side to form the ejaculatory duct. Sperm and seminal fluid mix in the ejaculatory duct and enter the prostatic urethra together during ejaculation. Seminal gland secretion accounts for some 70% of the volume of semen.

The Prostate

The **prostate** (pros′tāt) is a single doughnut-shaped gland about the size of a peach pit (Figures 27.1 and 27.5). It encircles the urethra just inferior to the bladder. Enclosed by a thick connective tissue capsule, it is made up of 20 to 30 compound tubuloalveolar glands embedded in a mass (stroma) of smooth muscle and dense connective tissue.

During ejaculation, prostatic smooth muscle contracts, squeezing the prostatic secretion into the prostatic urethra via several ducts. This fluid plays a role in activating sperm and accounts for up to one-third of the semen volume. It is a milky, slightly acid fluid that contains citrate (a nutrient source), several enzymes (including fibrinolysin, hyaluronidase, and acid phosphatase), and prostate-specific antigen (PSA).

Prostate Disorders

Disorders that bedevil the prostate range from inflammations caused by bacteria, immune cells, or unknown factors, to benign overgrowth of the gland, to prostate cancer. As a result, the prostate has gained a reputation as a health destroyer (perhaps reflected in the common mispronounciation "prostrate"). Let's take a look.

Prostatitis The term **prostatitis** (pros″tah-ti′tis) refers to a number of inflammatory disorders with a variety of causes.

- Acute bacterial prostatitis is usually due to a bacterial infection (most commonly *E. coli*) in the prostate. Symptoms may include a few to several of the following: fever, chills, muscle and joint pain, frequency, urgency, or painful urination, and back pain. Treatment usually includes antibiotics (for up to four weeks) and pain relief.
- Chronic bacterial prostatitis tends to be caused by the same bacteria as the acute type and has many of the same symptoms. However, it is harder to diagnose, and tends to recur as bacteria in the prostate invade the bladder over and over. Treatment is difficult and long (three to four months) because the antibacterial drugs penetrate poorly into the chronically inflamed prostate.
- Chronic prostatitis/pelvic pain syndrome is the most common and least understood type of prostatitis. It has two manifestations. Those with the inflammatory type have several of the urinary tract infection symptoms, as well as pains in the external genitalia and lower back. Leukocytes, but not bacteria, are present in the urine.

  The noninflammatory type has symptoms that mimic the inflammatory type, but neither leukocytes nor bacteria appear in the urine. Its treatment is largely symptomatic.

Benign Prostatic Hyperplasia Hypertrophy of the prostate, which is called **benign prostatic hyperplasia (BPH)** and affects nearly every elderly male. Its precise cause is unknown, but it may be associated with age-related changes in hormone levels. It distorts the urethra, and the more the man strains to urinate, the more the valvelike prostatic mass blocks the opening, enhancing the risk of bladder infections (cystitis) and kidney damage.

Traditional treatment has been surgical. Newer options include:

- Using microwaves or drugs to shrink the prostate
- Inserting and inflating a small balloon to compress the prostate tissue away from the prostatic urethra
- Inserting a catheter containing a tiny needle to incinerate excess prostate tissue with bursts of radio-frequency radiation

Finasteride, which ratchets down production of dihydrotestosterone, the hormone linked to male pattern balding and prostate enlargement, is helpful in some cases. Additionally, several drugs are available that relax the smooth muscles at the bladder outlet, aiding bladder emptying.

Prostate Cancer **Prostate cancer** is the second most common cause of cancer death in men (after lung cancer), accounting for an estimated 218,000 new cases and 32,000 deaths per year. It is twice as common in blacks as in whites. Risk factors include fatty diet and genetic predisposition. XMRV, a retrovirus closely related to a virus that causes various cancers in mice, has been implicated in an aggressive form of prostate cancer.

Screening for prostate cancer typically involves digital examination by a health professional (palpating the prostate through the anterior rectal wall), assessment of serum PSA levels, and/or transrectal ultrasound imaging. Although it is a normal component of blood at levels below 2.5 ng/ml, PSA is a tumor marker and its rising serum level follows BPH as well as the clinical disease course of prostate cancer. Screening procedures are followed by biopsies of suspicious prostate areas, if deemed necessary, and metastases (most commonly to the pelvic lymph nodes and the skeleton) are detected by bone or MRI scans.

When possible, prostate cancer is treated surgically, alone or in conjunction with radiotherapy. Because prostate cancer is typically androgen dependent, alternative therapies for metastasized cancers involve castration or drugs that block androgen receptors (flutamide), or inhibit gonadotropin release, such as LHRH (luteinizing hormone–releasing hormone) analogues. LHRH is another term for GnRH (gonadotropin-releasing hormone, see p. 1033). Deprived of the stimulatory effects of androgens, the prostatic tissue regresses and urinary symptoms typically decline. Cryosurgery, chemotherapy, high-intensity focused ultrasound, and proton beam therapy are now in clinical trials to assess their benefits.

However, many prostate cancers are slow growing and may never represent a threat, particularly if the patient is elderly. In such cases, regular tests to monitor the tumor for any changes may be all that is necessary.

The Bulbo-Urethral Glands

The **bulbo-urethral glands** (bul″bo-u-re′thral) are pea-sized glands located inferior to the prostate in the urogenital diaphragm (Figures 27.1 and 27.5). They produce a thick, clear mucus, some of which drains into the spongy urethra and lubricates the glans penis when a man becomes sexually excited. Additionally, the mucus neutralizes traces of acidic urine and lubricates the urethra just prior to ejaculation.

Semen

Semen (se′men) is a milky white, somewhat sticky mixture of sperm, testicular fluid, and accessory gland secretions. The liquid provides a transport medium and nutrients and contains chemicals that protect and activate the sperm and facilitate their movement. Mature sperm cells are streamlined cellular "missiles" containing little cytoplasm or stored nutrients. Catabolism of the fructose in seminal gland secretions provides nearly all the fuel needed for sperm ATP synthesis.

Semen contains several substances that play many roles:

- Prostaglandins decrease the viscosity of mucus guarding the entry (cervix) of the uterus and stimulate reverse peristalsis in the uterus, facilitating sperm movement through the female reproductive tract.
- The hormone relaxin and certain enzymes in semen enhance sperm motility.
- Contained ATP provides energy.
- Certain ingredients suppress the immune response in the female's reproductive tract.
- Antibiotic chemicals destroy some bacteria.
- Clotting factors in semen coagulate it just after it is ejaculated. Coagulation causes the sperm to stick to the walls of the vagina and prevents the initially immobile sperm from draining out of the vagina. Soon after semen coagulates, fibrinolysin liquefies the sticky mass and the sperm swim out and begin their journey through the female duct system.

Semen, as a whole, is alkaline (pH 7.2–8.0), which helps neutralize the acid environment of the male's urethra and the female's vagina, protecting the delicate sperm and enhancing their motility. Sperm are sluggish under acidic conditions (below pH 6).

27

The amount of semen propelled out of the male duct system during ejaculation is relatively small, only 2–5 ml and only 10% sperm, but there are between 20 and 150 million sperm per milliliter.

Check Your Understanding

8. Adolph, a 68-year-old gentleman, has trouble urinating and is scheduled for a rectal exam. What is his most probable condition and what is the purpose of the rectal exam?
9. Which glandular accessory organ produces the largest proportion of semen?
10. What is semen?

For answers, see Appendix H.

Physiology of the Male Reproductive System

Male Sexual Response

✓ Describe the phases of the male sexual response.

Although there is more to it, the chief phases of the male sexual response are (1) *erection* of the penis, which allows it to penetrate the female vagina, and (2) *ejaculation*, which expels semen into the vagina.

Erection

Erection, enlargement and stiffening of the penis, results from engorgement of the erectile bodies with blood. When a man is not sexually aroused, arterioles supplying the erectile tissue are constricted and the penis is flaccid. However, sexual excitement triggers a parasympathetic reflex that promotes release of nitric oxide (NO) locally. NO relaxes smooth muscle in the penile blood vessel walls, dilating these arterioles, and the erectile bodies fill with blood. Expansion of the corpora cavernosa of the penis compresses their drainage veins, retarding blood outflow and maintaining engorgement. The corpus spongiosum expands but not nearly as much as the cavernosa. Its main job is to keep the urethra open during ejaculation. It is important that the erect penis not kink or buckle during intercourse. The longitudinal and circular arrangement of collagen fibers surrounding the penis prevents this problem.

Erection of the penis is one of the rare examples of parasympathetic control of arterioles. Another parasympathetic effect is stimulation of the bulbo-urethral glands, the secretion of which lubricates the glans penis.

A variety of sexual stimuli can initiate erection—touch, mechanical stimulation of the penis, and erotic sights, sounds, and smells. The CNS responds by activating parasympathetic neurons that innervate the internal pudendal arteries serving the penis. Sometimes erection is induced solely by emotional or higher mental activity (the thought of a sexual encounter). Emotions and thoughts can also inhibit erection, causing vasoconstriction and a return to the flaccid penile state.

Ejaculation

Ejaculation (*ejac* = to shoot forth) is the propulsion of semen from the male duct system. Although erection is under parasympathetic control, ejaculation is under sympathetic control. When impulses provoking erection reach a critical level, a spinal reflex is initiated, and a massive discharge of nerve impulses occurs over the sympathetic nerves serving the genital organs (largely at the level of L_1 and L_2). As a result,

1. The bladder sphincter muscle constricts, preventing expulsion of urine or reflux of semen into the bladder.

2. The reproductive ducts and accessory glands contract, emptying their contents into the urethra.
3. Semen in the urethra triggers a spinal reflex through somatic motor neurons. The bulbospongiosus muscles of the penis undergo a rapid series of contractions, propelling semen from the urethra at a speed of up to 500 cm/s (200 inches/s, close to 11 mi/h). These rhythmic contractions are accompanied by intense pleasure and many systemic changes, such as generalized muscle contraction, rapid heartbeat, and elevated blood pressure.

The entire ejaculatory event is called **climax** or **orgasm**. Orgasm is quickly followed by **resolution**, a period of muscular and psychological relaxation. Activity of sympathetic nerve fibers constricts the *internal pudendal arteries* (and penile arterioles), reducing blood flow into the penis, and activates small muscles that squeeze the cavernous bodies, forcing blood from the penis into the general circulation. Although the erection may persist a little longer, the penis soon becomes flaccid again. After ejaculation, there is a *latent*, or *refractory*, *period*, ranging from minutes to hours, during which a man is unable to achieve another orgasm. The latent period lengthens with age.

Check Your Understanding

11. What is erection and which division of the ANS regulates it?
12. What occurs during resolution and what brings it about?

For answers, see Appendix H.

Homeostatic Imbalance 27.2

Erectile dysfunction (ED), the inability to attain an erection when desired, usually occurs when the parasympathetic nerves serving the penis do not release enough NO. Approximately 50% of American men over age 40 (about 32 million) have some degree of erectile dysfunction. Psychological factors, alcohol, or certain drugs (antihypertensives, antidepressants, and others) can cause temporary ED.

When chronic, ED is largely the result of problems with hormones (diabetes mellitus), blood vessels (arteriosclerosis, varicose veins), or the nervous system (stroke, penile nerve damage, multiple sclerosis). In men with varicose veins, incompetent valves that fail to retain blood in the penis during the erection phase may be the major cause.

Until recently, most ED remedies entailed using a vacuum pump to suck blood into the penis, or implanting a device into the penis to make it rigid. Viagra and similar drugs (e.g., Cialis and Levitra) potentiate the effect of the existing NO, a remedy that most men can live with. These drugs are taken orally, work within minutes to an hour to produce a sustained blood flow to the penis, and have essentially no significant side effects in healthy males. However, to avoid a fatal result, those with preexisting heart disease or diabetes mellitus must heed the warning that these drugs reduce systemic blood pressure. ✚

Spermatogenesis

✓ Define meiosis. Compare and contrast it to mitosis.

✓ Outline the events of spermatogenesis.

Spermatogenesis (sper″mah-to-jen′ĕ-sis; "sperm formation") is the sequence of events in the seminiferous tubules of the testes that produces male gametes—*sperm* or *spermatozoa*. The process begins around the age of 14 years (and often earlier) in males, and continues throughout life. Every day, a healthy adult male makes about 400 million sperm. It seems that nature has made sure that the human species will not be endangered for lack of sperm!

Before we describe spermatogenesis, let's define some terms. First, having two sets of chromosomes, one from each parent, is a key factor in the human life cycle. The normal chromosome number in most body cells is the **diploid chromosomal number** (dip′loid) of the organism, symbolized as **$2n$**. In humans, the diploid chromosomal number is 46, and diploid cells contain 23 pairs of similar chromosomes called **homologous chromosomes** (ho-mol′ŏ-gus), or homologues. One member of each pair is from the male parent (the *paternal chromosome*), and the other is from the female parent (the *maternal chromosome*).

Generally speaking, the two homologues of each chromosome pair look alike and carry genes that code for the same traits, though not necessarily for identical expression of those traits. (Consider, for example, the homologous genes controlling the expression of freckles. The paternal gene might code for an ample sprinkling of freckles and the maternal gene for no freckles.) In Chapter 29, we will consider how our mom's and dad's genes interact to produce our visible traits.

The number of chromosomes in human gametes is 23, referred to as the **haploid chromosomal number** (hap′loid), or **n**. Gametes contain only one member of each homologous pair. When sperm and egg fuse, they form a fertilized egg that reestablishes the typical diploid chromosomal number of human cells ($2n$).

Gamete formation in both sexes involves **meiosis** (mi-o′sis; "a lessening"), a unique kind of nuclear division that, for the most part, occurs only in the gonads. Recall that *mitosis* (the process by which most body cells divide) distributes replicated chromosomes equally between the two daughter cells. Consequently, each daughter cell receives a full set of chromosomes identical to that of the mother cell. Meiosis, on the other hand, consists of two consecutive nuclear divisions that follow one round of DNA replication. Its product is four daughter cells instead of two, each with *half* as many chromosomes as typical (diploid) body cells.

In other words, meiosis reduces the diploid chromosomal number by half (from $2n$ to n) in gametes. Additionally, meiosis introduces genetic variation because each of the haploid daughter cells has only some of the genes of each parent, as explained shortly.

Meiosis Compared to Mitosis

The two nuclear divisions of meiosis, called *meiosis I* and *meiosis II*, are divided into phases for convenience. These phases have the same names as those of mitosis (prophase, metaphase, anaphase, and telophase), but some events of meiosis I are quite different from those of mitosis. **Figure 27.6** compares mitosis and meiosis.

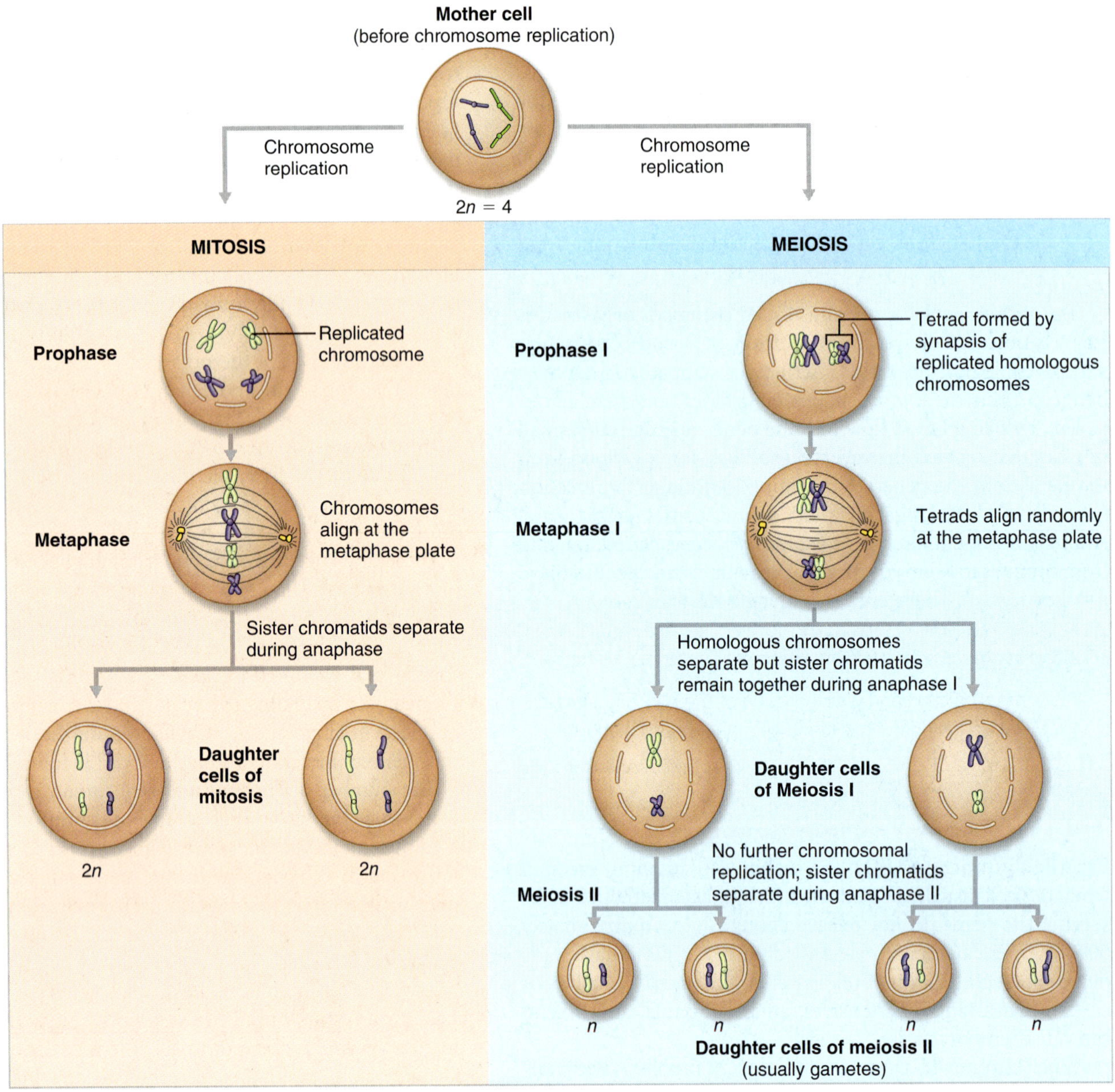

	MITOSIS	MEIOSIS
Number of divisions	One, consisting of prophase, metaphase, anaphase, and telophase.	Two, each consisting of prophase, metaphase, anaphase, and telophase. DNA replication does not occur between the two nuclear divisions.
Synapsis of homologous chromosomes	Does not occur.	Occurs during prophase I; tetrads form, allowing crossovers.
Daughter cell number and genetic composition	Two. Each diploid (2*n*) cell is identical to the mother cell.	Four. Each haploid (*n*) cell contains half as many chromosomes as the mother cell and is genetically different from the mother cell.
Roles in the body	For development of multicellular adult from zygote. Produces cells for growth and tissue repair as multicellular adult develops. Ensures genetic makeup of all body cells is constant.	Produces cells for reproduction (gametes). Introduces genetic variability in the gametes and reduces chromosomal number by half so that when fertilization occurs, the normal diploid chromosomal number is restored (in humans, $2n = 46$).

Figure 27.6 Comparison of mitosis and meiosis in a mother cell with a diploid number (2*n*) of 4. (Not all the phases of mitosis and meiosis are shown, and only one possible alignment of the tetrads at metaphase I is illustrated.)

Recall that prior to mitosis all the chromosomes are replicated. Then the identical copies remain together as *sister chromatids* connected by a centromere throughout prophase and during metaphase. At anaphase, the centromeres split and the sister chromatids separate from each other so that each daughter cell inherits a copy of *every* chromosome possessed by the mother cell (Figure 27.6, left side). Let's look at how meiosis differs (Figure 27.6, right side).

Meiosis I Meiosis I is sometimes called the **reduction division of meiosis** because it reduces the chromosome number from *2n* to *n*. As in mitosis, chromosomes replicate before meiosis begins and in prophase the chromosomes coil and condense, the nuclear envelope and nucleolus break down and disappear, and a spindle forms.

But prophase I of meiosis includes an event never seen in mitosis (nor in meiosis II for that matter): The replicated chromosomes seek out their homologous partners and pair up with them. This alignment takes place at discrete spots along the entire length of the homologues—more like buttoning together than zipping. This process, called **synapsis**, forms little groups of four chromatids called **tetrads** (Figure 27.6 and **Figure 27.7**).

During synapsis, a second unique event, called crossover, occurs. **Crossovers**, also called **chiasmata** (singular: chiasma), form within each tetrad as the free ends of one maternal and one paternal chromatid wrap around each other at one or more points. Crossover allows the paired maternal and paternal chromosomes to exchange genetic material (see Figure 29.3, p. 1098). Prophase I accounts for about 90% of the total period of meiosis. By its end, the tetrads are attached to the spindle and are moving toward the spindle equator.

During metaphase I, the tetrads line up *randomly* at the spindle equator, so that either the paternal or maternal chromosome can be on a given side of the equator (Figure 27.6). During anaphase I, the sister chromatids representing each homologue behave as a unit—almost as if replication had not occurred—and the *homologous chromosomes*, each still composed of two joined sister chromatids (a dyad), are distributed to opposite ends of the cell.

As a result, when meiosis I ends, each daughter cell has:

- *Two* copies of one member of each homologous pair (either the paternal or maternal) and none of the other
- A *haploid* chromosomal number (because the still-united sister chromatids are considered a single chromosome), but twice the amount of DNA in each chromosome

Meiosis II The second meiotic division, meiosis II, mirrors mitosis in every way, except that the chromosomes are *not* replicated before it begins. Instead, the sister chromatids in the two daughter cells of meiosis I are simply parceled out among four cells. Meiosis II is sometimes called the **equational division of meiosis** because the chromatids are distributed equally to the daughter cells (as in mitosis) (Figure 27.7).

In short, meiosis accomplishes two important tasks: (1) It reduces the chromosomal number by half, and (2) it introduces genetic variability. The random alignment of the homologous pairs during meiosis I (see Figure 27.6) provides tremendous variability in the resulting gametes by scrambling genetic characteristics of the two parents in different combinations. Crossover also increases variability—during late prophase I, the homologues break at crossover points and exchange chromosomal segments (Figure 27.7). (We will describe this process in Chapter 29.) As a result, it is likely that no two gametes are exactly alike, and all are different from the original mother cells.

Spermatogenesis: Summary of Events in the Seminiferous Tubules

A histological section of an adult testis shows that most cells making up the epithelial walls of the seminiferous tubules are in various stages of cell division **(Figure 27.8a)**. These cells, collectively called **spermatogenic cells** (*spermatogenic* = sperm forming), give rise to sperm in the following series of divisions and cellular transformations (Figure 27.8b, c).

Mitosis of Spermatogonia: Forming Spermatocytes The outermost tubule cells, which are in direct contact with the epithelial basal lamina, are stem cells called **spermatogonia** (sper″mah-to-go′ne-ah; "sperm seed"). The spermatogonia divide more or less continuously by *mitosis* and, until puberty, all their daughter cells become spermatogonia.

Spermatogenesis begins during puberty, and from then on, each mitotic division of a spermatogonium results in two distinctive daughter cells—types A and B. The **type A daughter cell** remains at the basal lamina to maintain the pool of dividing germ cells. The **type B daughter cell** gets pushed toward the lumen, where it becomes a **primary spermatocyte** destined to produce four sperm. (To keep these cell types straight, remember that just as the letter A is always at the beginning of our alphabet, a type A cell is always at the tubule basal lamina ready to begin a new generation of gametes.)

Meiosis: Spermatocytes to Spermatids Each primary spermatocyte generated during the first phase undergoes meiosis I, forming two smaller haploid cells called **secondary spermatocytes** (Figure 27.8b, c). The secondary spermatocytes continue on rapidly into meiosis II. Their daughter cells, called **spermatids** (sper′mah-tidz), are small round cells, with large spherical nuclei, seen closer to the lumen of the tubule. Midway through spermatogenesis, the developing sperm "turn off" nearly all their genes and compact their DNA into dense pellets.

Spermiogenesis: Spermatids to Sperm Each spermatid has the correct chromosomal number for fertilization (*n*), but is nonmotile. It still must undergo a streamlining process called **spermiogenesis**, during which it elongates, sheds its excess cytoplasmic baggage, and forms a tail. Follow the details of this process in **Figure 27.9a** ①–⑦ on p. 1032.

Each resulting sperm, or **spermatozoon** (sper″mah-to-zo′on; "animal seed"), has a head, midpiece, and tail, which correspond roughly to *genetic*, *metabolic*, and *locomotor regions*, respectively (Figure 27.9a ⑦). Sperm "pack" lightly.

The **head** of a sperm consists almost entirely of its flattened nucleus, which contains the compacted DNA. A helmetlike **acrosome** (ak′ro-sōm; "tip piece") adheres to the top of the

(Text continues on p. 1032.)

27

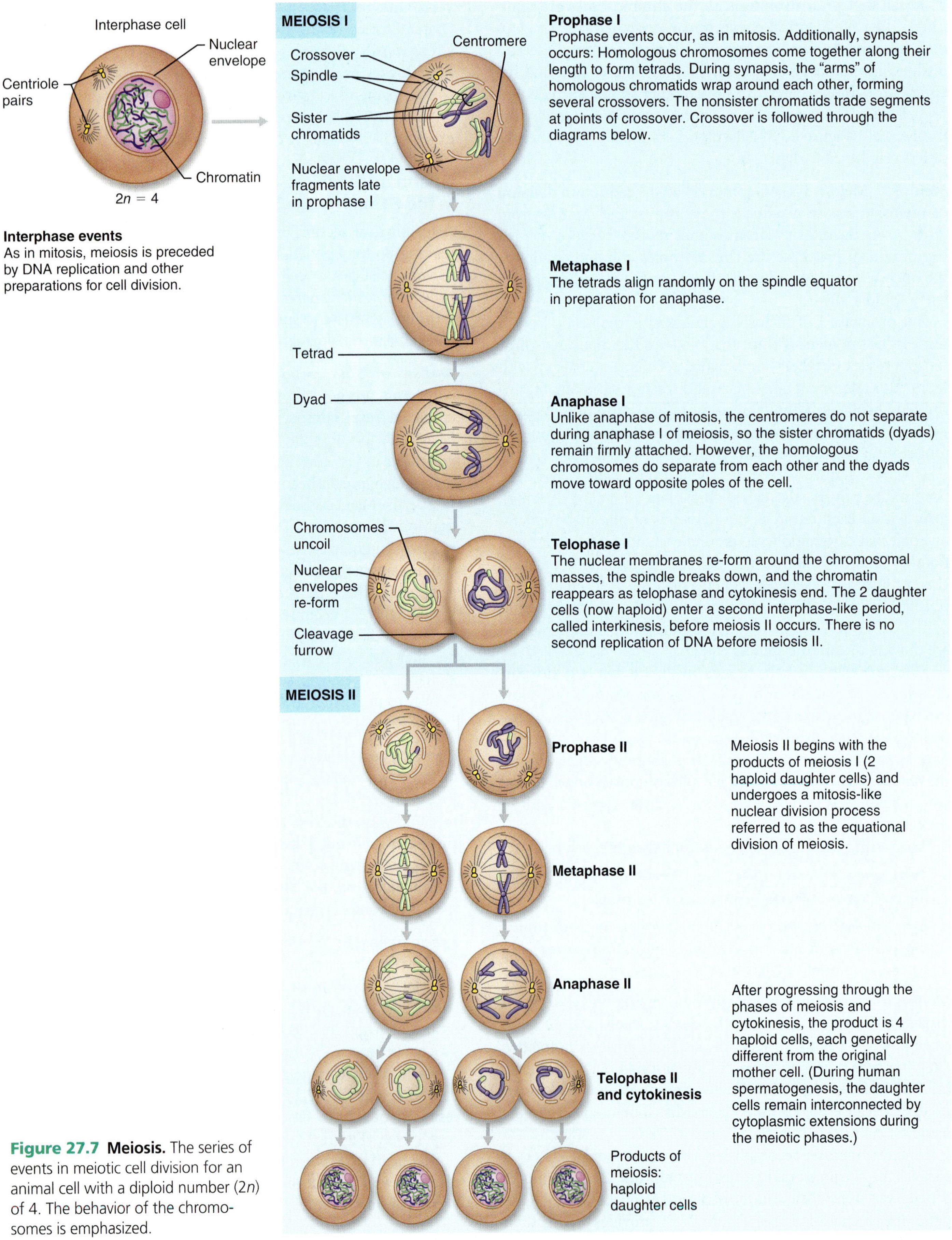

Figure 27.7 Meiosis. The series of events in meiotic cell division for an animal cell with a diploid number ($2n$) of 4. The behavior of the chromosomes is emphasized.

Figure 27.8 Spermatogenesis. (Note: The process of spermatogenesis encompasses the phases through the production of sperm. Conversion of the haploid spermatids to sperm cells is specifically called spermiogenesis.)

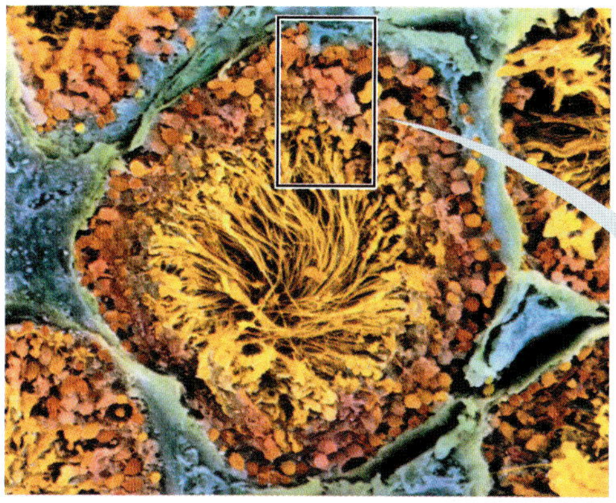

(a) Scanning electron micrograph of a cross-sectional view of a seminiferous tubule (165×)

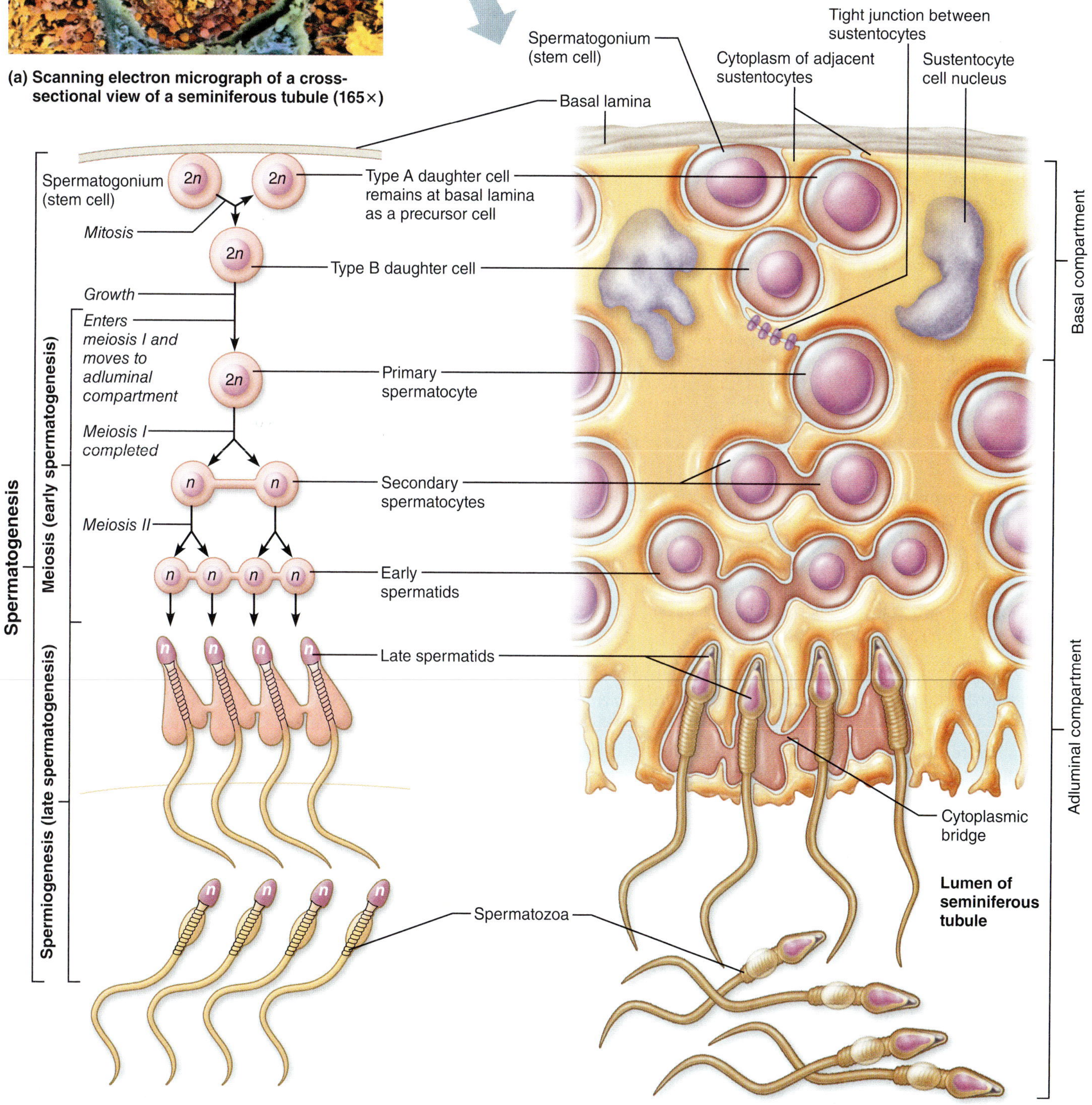

(b) Events of spermatogenesis, showing the relative position of various spermatogenic cells

(c) A portion of the seminiferous tublule wall, showing the spermatogenic cells surrounded by sustentocytes (colored gold)

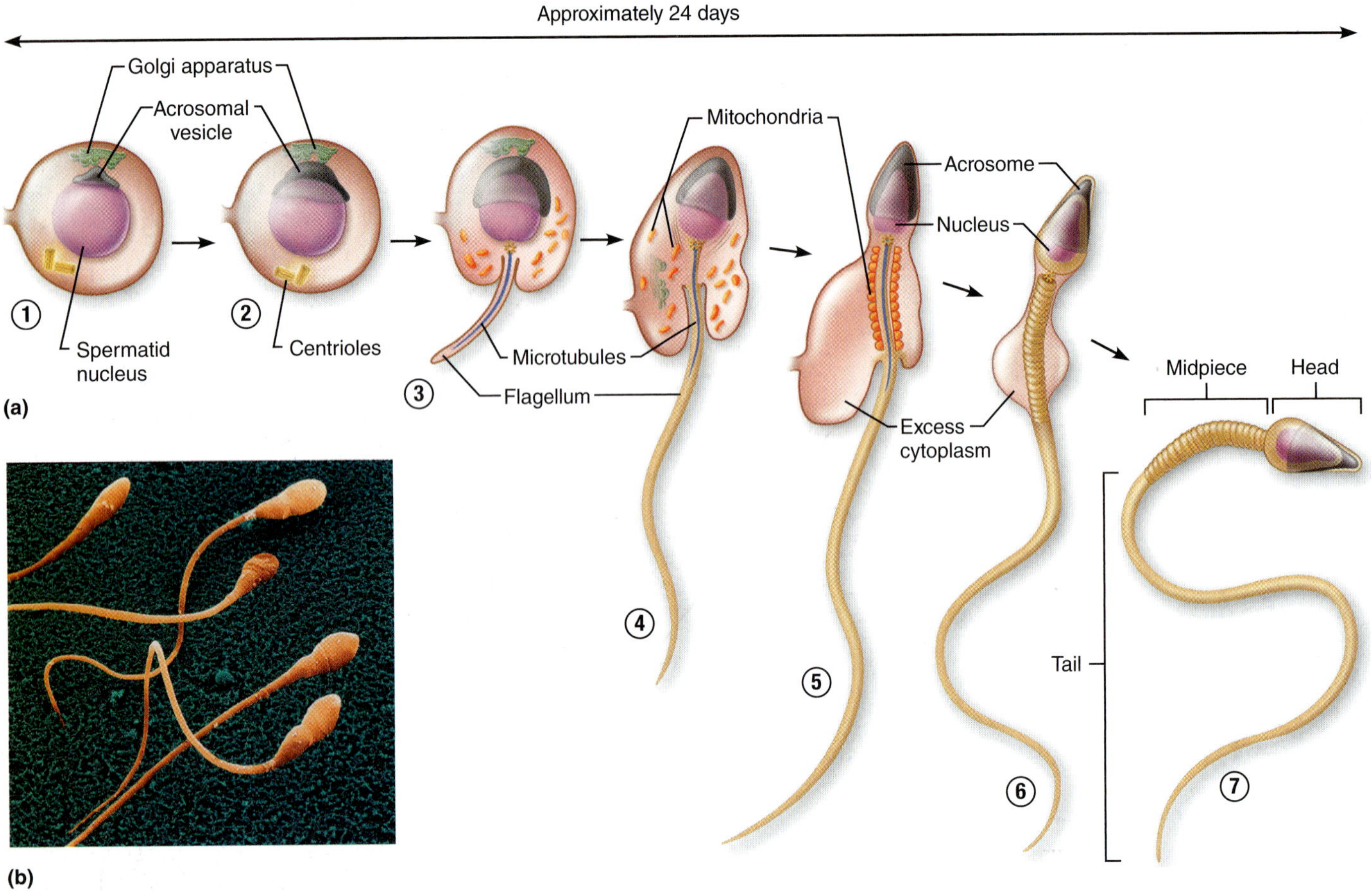

Figure 27.9 Spermiogenesis: transformation of a spermatid into a functional sperm. (a) During the stepwise process of spermiogenesis: ① the Golgi apparatus packages the acrosomal enzymes, ② the acrosome forms at the anterior end of the nucleus and the centrioles gather at the opposite end of the nucleus, ③ microtubules elaborate to form the flagellum, ④ mitochondria multiply and take up position around the proximal portion of the flagellum, and ⑤ excess cytoplasm sloughs off. ⑥ Structure of an immature sperm that has just been released from a sustentocyte. ⑦ Structure of a fully mature sperm. **(b)** Scanning electron micrograph of mature sperm (900×).

nucleus (Figure 27.9a ⑤ and ⑥). Like a lysosome produced by the Golgi apparatus, the acrosome contains hydrolytic enzymes that, in this case, enable the sperm to penetrate and enter an egg.

The sperm **midpiece** contains mitochondria spiraled tightly around the microtubules of the tail. The long **tail** is a typical flagellum produced by one centriole (actually a basal body) near the nucleus. The mitochondria provide the metabolic energy (ATP) needed for the whiplike movements of the tail that will propel the sperm along its way in the female reproductive tract.

Role of the Sustentocytes Throughout spermatogenesis, descendants of the same spermatogonium remain closely attached to one another by cytoplasmic bridges (see Figure 27.8c). They are also surrounded by and connected to nonreplicating supporting cells called **sustentocytes** or *Sertoli cells*, which extend from the basal lamina to the tubule lumen.

27

The sustentocytes, bound to each other laterally by tight junctions, divide the seminiferous tubule into two compartments. The **basal compartment** extends from the basal lamina to their tight junctions and contains spermatogonia and the earliest primary spermatocytes. The **adluminal compartment** lies internal to the tight junctions and includes the meiotically active cells and the tubule lumen (see Figure 27.8c).

The tight junctions between the sustentocytes form the **blood testis barrier**. This barrier prevents the membrane antigens of differentiating sperm from escaping through the basal lamina into the bloodstream where they would activate the immune system. Because no sperm are formed until puberty, they are absent when the immune system is being programmed to recognize a person's own tissues early in life. The spermatogonia, which are recognized as "self," are outside the barrier and for this reason can be influenced by bloodborne chemical messengers that prompt spermatogenesis. Following mitosis of the spermatogonia, the tight junctions of the sustentocytes open to allow type B daughter cells to pass into the adluminal compartment—much as locks in a canal open to allow a boat to pass.

In the adluminal compartment, spermatocytes and spermatids are nearly enclosed in recesses in the sustentocytes (see Figure 27.8), anchored there by a particular glycoprotein on the spermatogenic cell.

The sustentocytes:

- Provide nutrients and essential signals to the dividing cells, even telling them to live or die
- Move the cells along to the lumen
- Secrete **testicular fluid** (rich in androgens and metabolic acids) that provides the transport medium for sperm in the lumen
- Phagocytize faulty germ cells and the excess cytoplasm sloughed off as the spermatids transform into sperm
- Produce chemical mediators (inhibin and androgen-binding protein) that help regulate spermatogenesis

Given hospitable conditions, spermatogenesis—from formation of a primary spermatocyte to release of immature sperm into the lumen—takes 64 to 72 days. Sperm in the lumen are unable to "swim" and are incapable of fertilizing an egg. The pressure of the testicular fluid pushes them through the tubular system of the testes into the epididymis, where they gain increased motility and fertilizing power.

Homeostatic Imbalance 27.3

Roughly one in seven American couples seek treatment for infertility, mostly because of problems with sperm quality or quantity. According to some studies, a gradual decline in male fertility has been occurring in the past 50 years.

Some believe the main culprit is *xenobiotics*, alien molecules that have invaded our lives in a variety of forms—environmental toxins, PVCs, phthalates (oily solvents that make plastics flexible), pesticides and herbicides, and especially compounds with estrogenic effects. These estrogen-like compounds, which block the action of male sex hormones as they program sexual development, are now found in our meat supply as well as in the air.

Common antibiotics such as tetracycline may suppress sperm formation, and radiation, lead, marijuana, lack of selenium, and excessive alcohol can cause abnormal (two-headed, multiple-tailed, etc.) sperm to be produced. Male infertility may also be caused by the lack of a specific type of Ca^{2+} channel (Ca^{2+} is needed for normal sperm motility), anatomical obstructions, hormonal imbalances, and oxidative stress (which fragments sperm DNA). Thermal-related events that inhibit sperm maturation include fever and overusing hot tubs. +

Check Your Understanding

13. What is the final outcome of meiosis?
14. Describe the major structural and functional regions of a sperm.
15. What is the role of sustentocytes? Of interstitial endocrine cells?

For answers, see Appendix H.

Hormonal Regulation of Male Reproductive Function

✓ Discuss hormonal regulation of testicular function and the physiological effects of testosterone on male reproductive anatomy.

Hormonal interactions between the hypothalamus, anterior pituitary gland, and gonads, a relationship called the **hypothalamic-pituitary-gonadal (HPG) axis**, regulate the production of gametes and sex hormones. Let's take a look.

The Hypothalamic-Pituitary-Gonadal (HPG) Axis

The sequence of regulatory events involving the HPG axis, shown schematically in **Figure 27.10**, is as follows:

1. The hypothalamus releases **gonadotropin-releasing hormone (GnRH)**, which reaches the anterior pituitary cells via the blood of the hypophyseal portal system. GnRH controls the release of the two anterior pituitary gonadotropins: **follicle-stimulating hormone (FSH)** and **luteinizing hormone (LH)**, both named for their effects on the female gonad.
2. GnRH binds to pituitary cells (gonadotropic cells), prompting them to secrete FSH and LH into the blood.
3. FSH stimulates spermatogenesis indirectly by stimulating the sustentocytes to release **androgen-binding protein (ABP)**. ABP keeps the concentration of **testosterone** in the vicinity of the spermatogenic cells high, which in turn stimulates spermatogenesis. In this way, FSH enhances testosterone's stimulatory effects.
4. LH binds to the interstitial endocrine cells in the soft connective tissue surrounding the seminiferous tubules, prodding them to secrete testosterone (and a small amount of estrogen). Locally, rising testosterone levels serve as the final trigger for spermatogenesis.
5. Testosterone entering the bloodstream exerts a number of effects at other body sites. It stimulates maturation of sex organs, development and maintenance of secondary sex characteristics, and libido (sex drive).
6. Rising levels of testosterone feed back to inhibit hypothalamic release of GnRH and act directly on the anterior pituitary to inhibit gonadotropin release.
7. **Inhibin** (in-hib′in), a protein hormone produced by the sustentocytes, serves as a "barometer" of the normalcy of spermatogenesis. When the sperm count is high, more inhibin is released, inhibiting anterior pituitary release of FSH and hypothalamic release of GnRH. (The inhibitory effect of testosterone and inhibin on the hypothalamus is not illustrated in Figure 27.10.) When the sperm count falls below 20 million/ml, inhibin secretion declines steeply.

As you can see, the amount of testosterone and sperm produced by the adult testes reflects a balance among the three interacting sets of hormones that make up the HPG axis:

- GnRH, which indirectly stimulates the testes via its effect on FSH and LH release
- Gonadotropins (FSH and LH), which directly stimulate the testes
- Gonadal hormones (testosterone and inhibin), which exert negative feedback controls on the hypothalamus and anterior pituitary

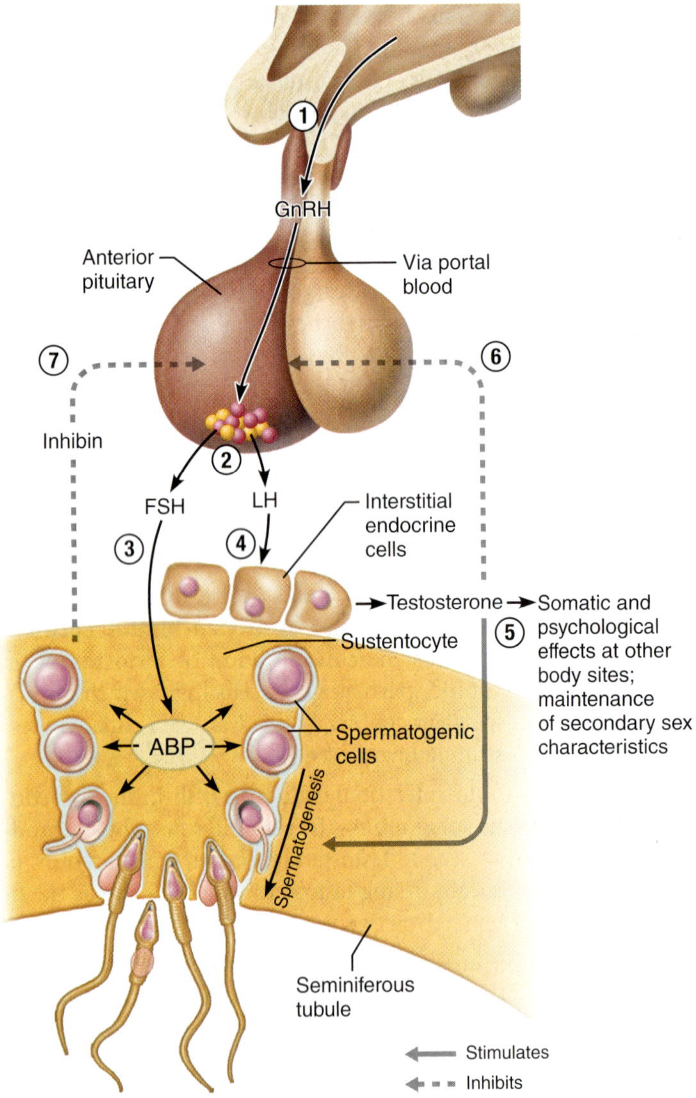

Figure 27.10 Hormonal regulation of testicular function, the hypothalamic-pituitary-gonadal (HPG) axis. (Only one sustentocyte is depicted to show its structural relationship to the spermatogenic cells it encloses. However, it would be flanked by sustentocytes on each side.)

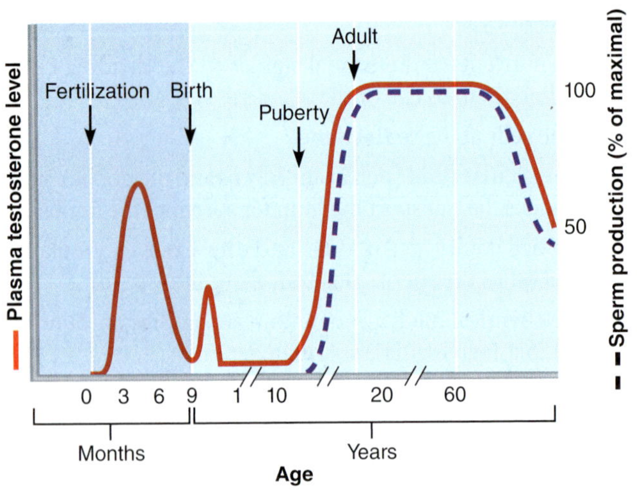

Figure 27.11 Plasma testosterone and sperm production levels versus age in male humans.

Once this balance is established during puberty (a process that takes about three years), the amount of testosterone and sperm produced remains fairly stable throughout life.

Because input from other brain areas also influences the hypothalamus, the whole axis is under CNS control. In the absence of GnRH and gonadotropins, the testes atrophy, and sperm and testosterone production cease.

Development of male reproductive structures (discussed later in the chapter) depends on prenatal secretion of male hormones, and for a few months before birth, a male infant has plasma gonadotropin and testosterone levels nearly two-thirds those of an adult male **(Figure 27.11)**. Soon after birth, blood levels of these hormones recede and they remain low throughout childhood. As puberty nears, higher levels of testosterone are required to suppress hypothalamic release of GnRH. So, as more GnRH is released, the testes secrete more testosterone, but the threshold for hypothalamic inhibition keeps rising until the adult pattern of hormone interaction is achieved, as evidenced by the presence of mature sperm in the semen.

Mechanism and Effects of Testosterone Activity

Like all steroid hormones, testosterone is synthesized from cholesterol and exerts its effects by activating specific genes, which results in enhanced synthesis of certain proteins in the target cells. (See Chapter 16 for mechanisms of steroid hormone action.)

In some target cells, testosterone must be transformed into another steroid to exert its effects. In the prostate, testosterone is converted to *dihydrotestosterone* (*DHT*) before it can bind in the nucleus, and in certain neurons of the brain, testosterone is converted to *estradiol* (es″trah-di′ol), a female sex hormone, to bring about its stimulatory effects. These transformations often occur in a single enzymatic step because testosterone and the other gonadal hormones are structurally similar.

As puberty ensues, testosterone not only prompts spermatogenesis but also has multiple anabolic effects throughout the body (see Table 27.1, p. 1052). It targets accessory reproductive organs—ducts, glands, and the penis—causing them to grow to adult size and function. In adult males, normal plasma levels of testosterone maintain these organs. When the hormone is deficient or absent, all accessory organs atrophy, semen volume declines markedly, and erection and ejaculation are impaired. Thus, a man becomes both sterile and unable to carry out sexual intercourse. Testosterone replacement therapy can remedy this situation.

Male secondary sex characteristics—that is, features induced in *nonreproductive* organs by the male sex hormones (mainly testosterone)—develop at puberty. These include the appearance of pubic, axillary, and facial hair, enhanced hair growth on the chest or other body areas in some men, and a deepening voice as the larynx enlarges. The skin thickens and becomes oilier (which predisposes young men to acne), bones

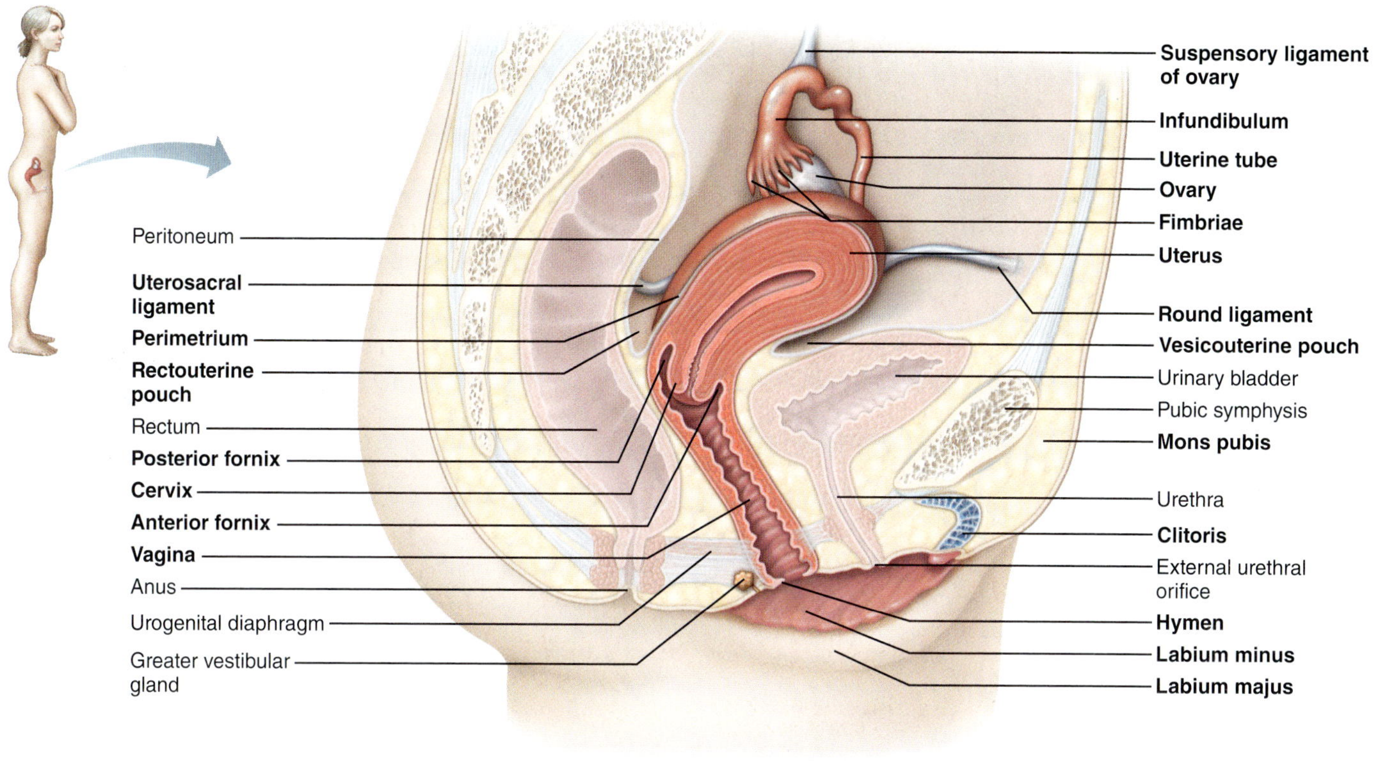

Figure 27.12 Internal organs of the female reproductive system, midsagittal section. (For a related image, see *A Brief Atlas of the Human Body*, Figure 74.)

grow and increase in density, and skeletal muscles increase in size and mass. The last two effects are often referred to as the *somatic effects* of testosterone (*soma* = body). Testosterone also boosts basal metabolic rate and influences behavior. It is the basis of the male libido, whether heterosexual or homosexual. As noted later (p. 1053), the adrenal androgen DHEA appears to be more important than testosterone in creating or driving the *female* libido.

In embryos, testosterone masculinizes the brain. Testosterone also appears to continue to shape certain regions of the male brain well into adult life, as indicated by the differences in males' and females' brain areas involved in sexual arousal (for example, the amygdala).

The testes are not the only source of androgens. The adrenal glands of both sexes also release them. However, the relatively small amounts of adrenal androgens are insufficient to support normal testosterone-mediated functions, so we can assume that it is the testosterone production by the testes that supports male reproductive function.

☑ Check Your Understanding

16. What is the HPG axis?
17. How does FSH indirectly stimulate spermatogenesis?
18. What are three secondary sex characteristics promoted by testosterone?

For answers, see Appendix H.

Anatomy of the Female Reproductive System

The reproductive role of the female is far more complex than that of a male. Not only must she produce gametes, but her body must prepare to nurture a developing fetus for approximately nine months. **Ovaries**, the **female gonads**, are the primary reproductive organs of a female, and like the male testes, ovaries serve a dual purpose: They produce the female gametes (ova) and sex hormones, **estrogen** and **progesterone** (pro-ges′tě-rōn). Estrogen includes *estradiol*, *estrone*, and *estriol*, but estradiol is the most abundant and is most responsible for estrogenic effects in humans.

As illustrated in **Figure 27.12**, a female's **internal genitalia**—her ovaries and duct system—are mostly located in the pelvic cavity. The female's accessory ducts, from the vicinity of the ovary to the body exterior, are the *uterine tubes*, the *uterus*, and the *vagina*. They transport or otherwise serve the needs of the reproductive cells and a developing fetus. The external sex organs of females are referred to as **external genitalia**.

The Ovaries

✓ Describe the location, structure, and function of the ovaries.

The paired ovaries flank the uterus on each side (Figure 27.12). Shaped like an almond and about twice as large, each ovary is

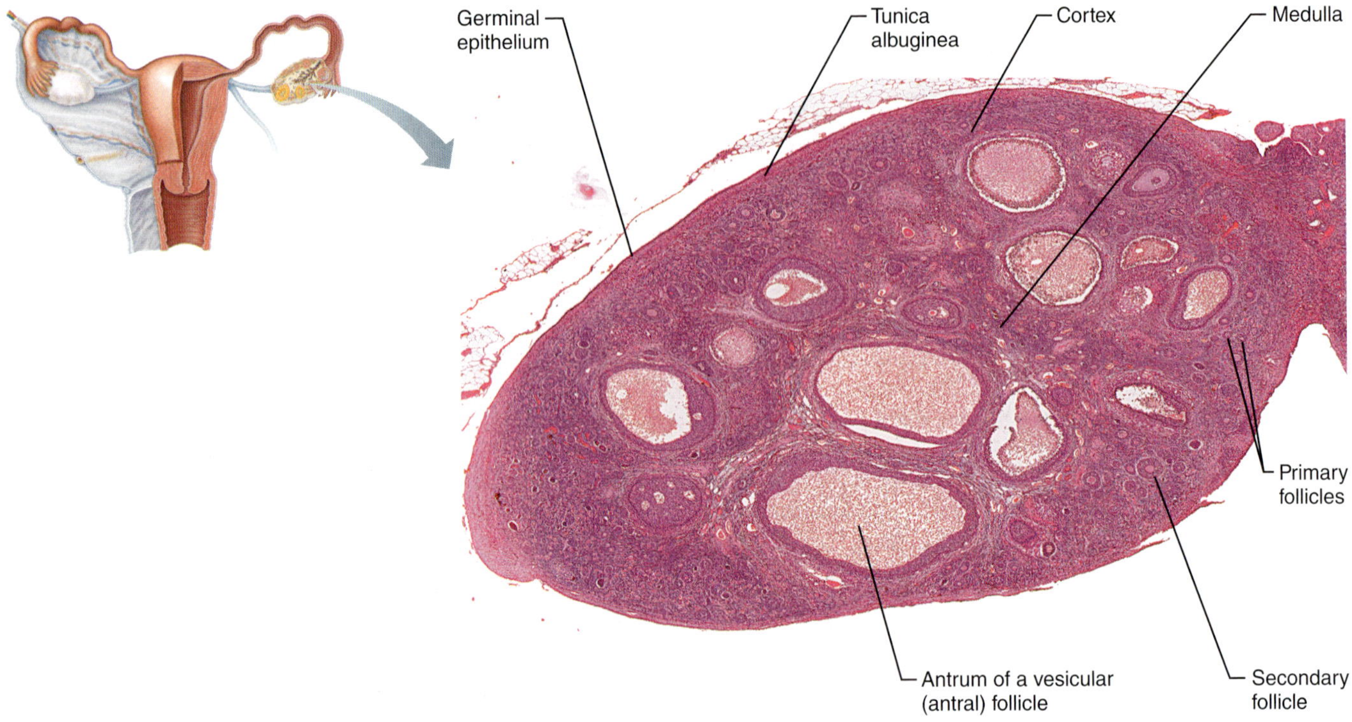

Figure 27.13 Photomicrograph of a mammalian ovary showing follicles in different developmental phases. Note that most follicles are in the cortex (3×).

held in place by several ligaments in the fork of the iliac blood vessels within the peritoneal cavity. The **ovarian ligament** anchors the ovary medially to the uterus; the **suspensory ligament** anchors it laterally to the pelvic wall; and the **mesovarium** (mez″o-va′re-um) suspends it in between (see Figures 27.12 and 27.14). The suspensory ligament and mesovarium are part of the **broad ligament**, a peritoneal fold that "tents" over the uterus and supports the uterine tubes, uterus, and vagina. The broad ligament encloses the ovarian ligaments.

The ovaries are served by the **ovarian arteries**, branches of the abdominal aorta (see Figure 19.24c), and by the *ovarian branch of the uterine arteries.* The ovarian blood vessels reach the ovaries by traveling through the suspensory ligaments and mesovaria (see Figure 27.14).

Like each testis, each ovary is surrounded externally by a fibrous **tunica albuginea (Figure 27.13)**, which is in turn covered externally by a layer of cuboidal epithelial cells called the *germinal epithelium*, actually a continuation of the peritoneum. The ovary has an outer *cortex*, which houses the forming gametes, and an inner *medulla* containing the largest blood vessels and nerves, but the relative extent of each region is poorly defined.

27

Embedded in the highly vascular connective tissue of the ovary cortex are many tiny saclike structures called **ovarian follicles**. Each follicle consists of an immature egg, called an **oocyte** (o′o-sīt; *oo* = egg), encased by one or more layers of very different cells. The surrounding cells are called **follicle cells** if a single layer is present, and **granulosa cells** when more than one layer is present.

Follicles at different stages of maturation are distinguished by their structure, which ranges from *primordial follicles* with a single layer of follicle cells surrounding the oocyte to more mature follicles with several layers of granulosa cells. The fully mature **vesicular follicle**, also called an **antral**, or **tertiary**, **follicle**, is identified by its central fluid-filled cavity called an **antrum** (Figure 27.13). When mature, the follicle extends from the deepest part of the ovarian cortex and bulges from the surface of the ovary, and its oocyte "sits proudly" on a stalk of granulosa cells at one side of the antrum.

Each month in women of childbearing age, one of the ripening follicles ejects its oocyte from the ovary, an event called *ovulation* (see Figure 27.20, ⑤). After ovulation, the ruptured follicle is transformed into a very different looking glandular structure called the **corpus luteum** (lu′te-um; "yellow body"; plural: corpora lutea), which eventually degenerates (not shown in Figure 27.13). As a rule, most of these structures can be seen within the same ovary. In older women, the surfaces of the ovaries are scarred and pitted, revealing that many oocytes have been released.

☑ Check Your Understanding

19. Briefly, what are the internal genitalia of a woman?
20. What two roles do the ovaries assume?
21. What name is given to the fluid-filled cavity of a mature follicle?

For answers, see Appendix H.

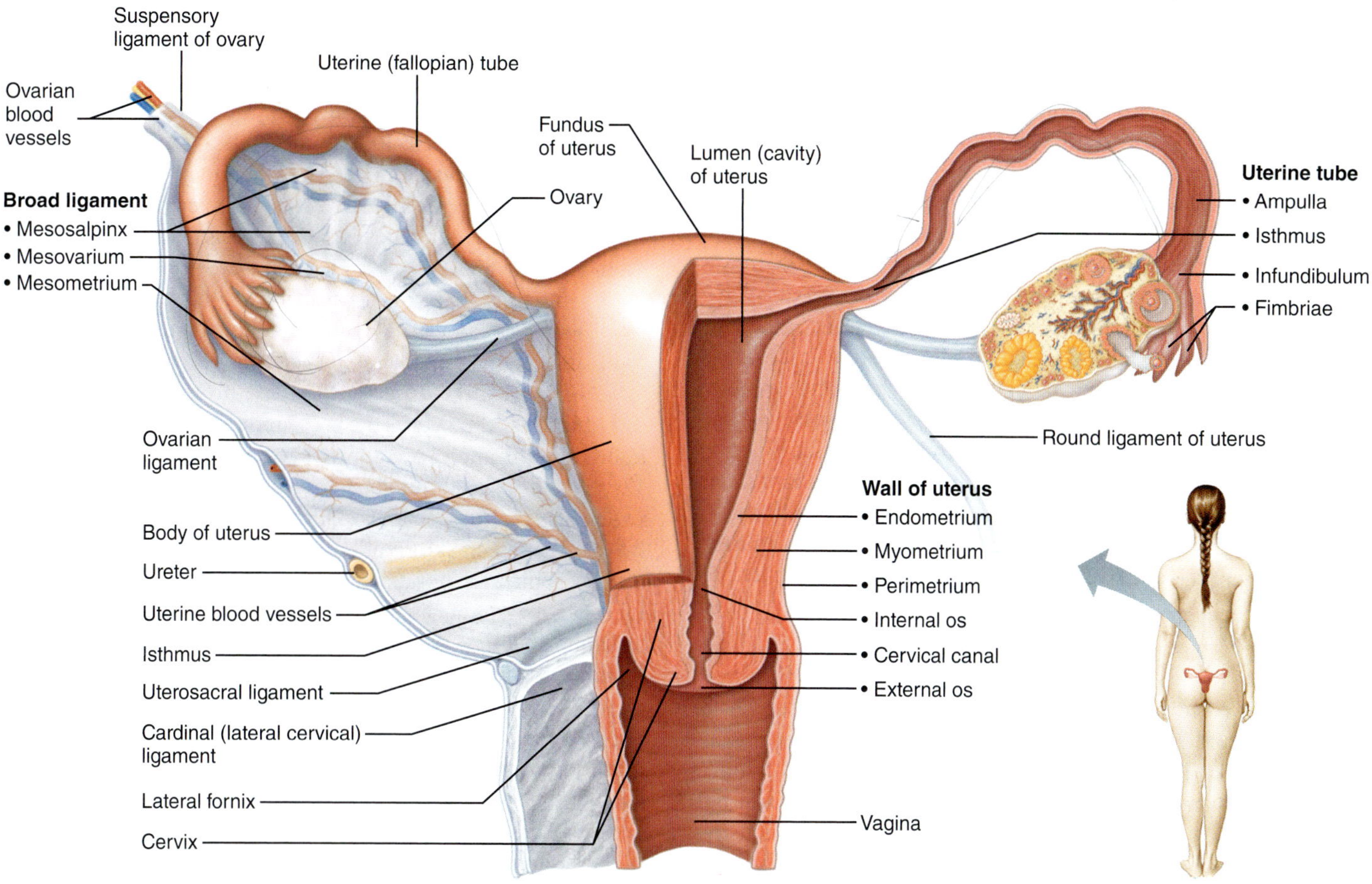

Figure 27.14 Internal reproductive organs of a female, posterior view. The posterior walls of the vagina, uterus, and uterine tubes, and the broad ligament (a peritoneal fold) have been removed on the right side to reveal the shape of the lumen of these organs. (For a related image, see *A Brief Atlas of the Human Body*, Figure 75.)

The Female Duct System

✓ Describe the location, structure, and function of each of the organs of the female reproductive duct system.

Unlike the male duct system, which is continuous with the tubules of the testes, the female duct system has little or no actual contact with the ovaries. An ovulated oocyte is cast into the peritoneal cavity, and some oocytes are lost there.

The Uterine Tubes

The **uterine tubes** (u′ter-in), also called **fallopian tubes** or **oviducts**, form the initial part of the female duct system (Figure 27.12 and Figure 27.14). They receive the ovulated oocyte and are the site where fertilization generally occurs. Each uterine tube is about 10 cm (4 inches) long and extends medially from the region of an ovary to empty into the superolateral region of the uterus via a constricted region called the **isthmus** (is′mus). The distal end of each uterine tube expands as it curves around the ovary, forming the **ampulla**. The ampulla ends in the **infundibulum** (in″fun-dib′u-lum), an open, funnel-shaped structure bearing ciliated, fingerlike projections called *fimbriae* (fim′bre-e; "fringe") that drape over the ovary.

Around the time of ovulation, the uterine tube performs a complex "dance" to capture oocytes. It bends to drape over the ovary while the fimbriae stiffen and sweep the ovarian surface. The beating cilia on the fimbriae create currents in the peritoneal fluid that tend to carry an oocyte into the uterine tube, where it begins its journey toward the uterus.

The uterine tube contains sheets of smooth muscle, and its thick, highly folded mucosa contains both ciliated and nonciliated cells. The oocyte is carried toward the uterus by a combination of muscular peristalsis and the beating cilia. Nonciliated cells of the mucosa have dense microvilli and produce a secretion that keeps the oocyte (and sperm, if present) moist and nourished.

Externally, the uterine tubes are covered by peritoneum and supported along their length by a short mesentery (part of the broad ligament) called the **mesosalpinx** (mez″o-sal′pinks; "mesentery of the trumpet"; *salpin* = trumpet), a reference to the trumpet-shaped uterine tube it supports (Figure 27.14).

Homeostatic Imbalance 27.4

The fact that the uterine tubes are not continuous with the ovaries places women at risk for *ectopic pregnancy*, in which an oocyte fertilized in the peritoneal cavity or distal portion of the uterine tube begins developing there. Because the tube lacks adequate mass and vascularization to support a full-term pregnancy, ectopic pregnancies tend to naturally abort, often with substantial bleeding.

Another potential problem is infection spreading into the peritoneal cavity from other parts of the reproductive tract. Sexually transmitted microorganisms, including gonorrhea bacteria, sometimes infect the peritoneal cavity in this way, causing an extremely severe inflammation called **pelvic inflammatory disease (PID)**. Unless treated promptly with broad-spectrum antibiotics, PID can cause scarring of the narrow uterine tubes and of the ovaries, resulting in sterility. Scarring and closure of the uterine tubes, which have an internal diameter as small as the width of a human hair in some regions, is one of the major causes of female infertility. ✚

The Uterus

The **uterus** (Latin for "womb") is located in the pelvis, anterior to the rectum and posterosuperior to the bladder (Figures 27.12 and 27.14). It is a hollow, thick-walled, muscular organ that receives, retains, and nourishes a fertilized ovum. In a fertile woman who has never been pregnant, the uterus is about the size and shape of an inverted pear, but it is usually larger in women who have borne children. Normally, the uterus flexes anteriorly to some extent where it joins the vagina (see Figure 27.12), causing the uterus as a whole to be inclined forward, or *anteverted*. However, the organ is frequently turned backward, or *retroverted*, in older women.

The major portion of the uterus is referred to as the **body** (Figures 27.12 and 27.14). The rounded region superior to the entrance of the uterine tubes is the **fundus**, and the slightly narrowed region between the body and the cervix is the *isthmus*. The **cervix** of the uterus is its narrow neck, or outlet, which projects into the vagina inferiorly.

The cavity of the cervix, called the **cervical canal**, communicates with the vagina via the *external os* (*os* = mouth) and with the cavity of the uterine body via the *internal os*. The mucosa of the cervical canal contains *cervical glands* that secrete a mucus that fills the cervical canal and covers the external os, presumably to block the spread of bacteria from the vagina into the uterus. Cervical mucus also blocks sperm entry except at midcycle, when it becomes less viscous and allows sperm to pass through.

27

Homeostatic Imbalance 27.5

Cancer of the cervix strikes about 450,000 women worldwide each year, killing about half. It is most common among women between the ages of 30 and 50. Risk factors include frequent cervical inflammations, sexually transmitted infections (including genital warts), and multiple pregnancies. The cancer cells arise from the epithelium covering the cervical tip.

In a *Papanicolaou (Pap) smear*, or cervical smear test, some of these cells are scraped away and then examined for abnormalities. A Pap smear is the most effective way to detect this slow-growing cancer, and American Cancer Society guidelines advise women to have one yearly until age 65, at which time this monitoring can be stopped if there have been no abnormal results in the past 10 years. However, the Federal Government Source for Women's Health recommends a Pap smear be conducted every two years in women ages 21 to 30, and yearly over age 30. If results for three years in a row are negative, the physician may suggest doing the tests farther apart and discontinuing them after age 65.

When results are inconclusive, a test for the sexually transmitted human papillomavirus (HPV), the cause of most cervical cancers, can be done from the same Pap sample or a blood sample.

Gardasil, a three-dose vaccine that protects against HPV-induced cervical cancer, is the latest addition to the official childhood immunization schedule. It is recommended for all 11- and 12-year-old girls, although it may be administered to girls as young as 9. In unexposed girls, the vaccine specifically blocks two cancer-causing kinds of HPV as well as two additional types of HPV which are not associated with cervical cancer. All four types of the virus are associated with genital warts and mild Pap test abnormalities. Whether this vaccine will become a requirement for school is presently decided on a state-to-state basis. ✚

Supports of the Uterus The uterus is supported laterally by the **mesometrium** ("mesentery of the uterus") portion of the broad ligament (Figure 27.14). More inferiorly, the **cardinal (lateral cervical) ligaments** extend from the cervix and superior vagina to the lateral walls of the pelvis, and the paired **uterosacral ligaments** secure the uterus to the sacrum posteriorly. The uterus is bound to the anterior body wall by the fibrous **round ligaments**, which run through the inguinal canals to anchor in the subcutaneous tissue of the labia majora. These ligaments allow the uterus a good deal of mobility, and its position changes as the rectum and bladder fill and empty.

Homeostatic Imbalance 27.6

Despite its many anchoring ligaments, the uterus is principally supported by the muscles of the pelvic floor, namely those of the urogenital and pelvic diaphragms (Table 10.7). These muscles stretch and sometimes tear during childbirth. Subsequently, the unsupported uterus may sink inferiorly, until the tip of the cervix protrudes through the external vaginal opening. This condition is called **prolapse of the uterus.** ✚

The undulating course of the peritoneum produces several cul-de-sacs, or blind-ended peritoneal pouches. The most important of these are the *vesicouterine pouch* (ves″i-ko-u′ter-in) between the bladder and uterus, and the *rectouterine pouch* between the rectum and uterus (see Figure 27.12).

The Uterine Wall The wall of the uterus is composed of three layers (Figure 27.14):

- **Perimetrium**, the incomplete outermost serous layer.
- **Myometrium** (mi″o-me′tre-um; "muscle of the uterus"), the bulky middle layer, composed of interlacing bundles of smooth muscle. The myometrium contracts rhythmically during childbirth to expel the baby from the mother's body.

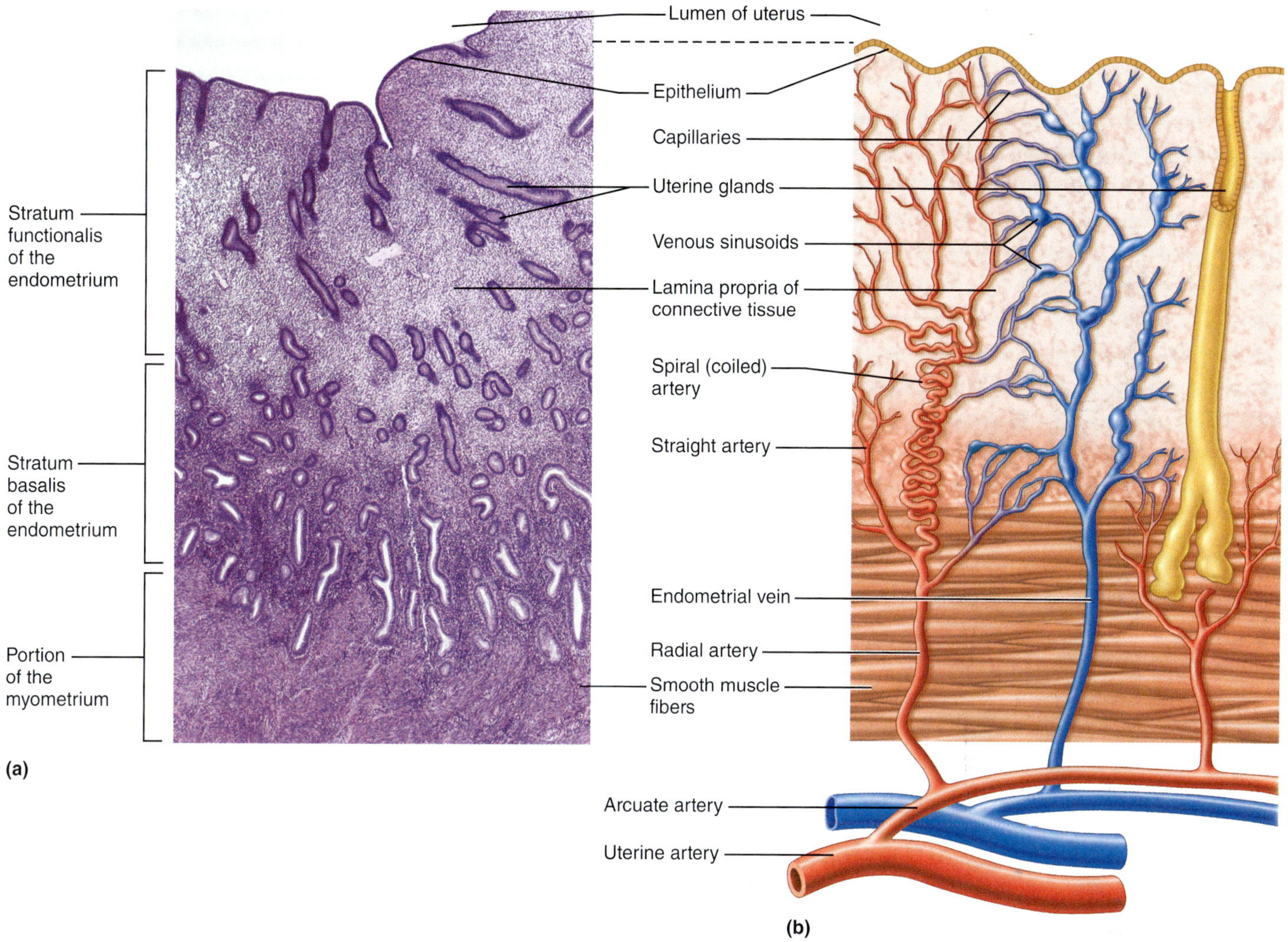

Figure 27.15 The endometrium and its blood supply. (a) Photomicrograph of the endometrium, longitudinal section, showing its functionalis and basalis regions (28×). **(b)** Diagrammatic view of the endometrium, showing the straight arteries that serve the stratum basalis and the spiral arteries that serve the stratum functionalis. The thin-walled veins and venous sinusoids are also illustrated.

- **Endometrium**, the mucosal lining of the uterine cavity **(Figure 27.15)**. It is a simple columnar epithelium underlain by a thick lamina propria. If fertilization occurs, the young embryo burrows into the endometrium (implants) and resides there for the rest of its development.

The endometrium has two chief *strata* (layers). The **stratum functionalis** (fungk-shun-a′lis), or **functional layer**, undergoes cyclic changes in response to blood levels of ovarian hormones and is shed during menstruation (approximately every 28 days). The thinner, deeper **stratum basalis** (ba-să′lis), or **basal layer**, forms a new functionalis after menstruation ends. It is unresponsive to ovarian hormones. The endometrium has numerous *uterine glands* that change in length as endometrial thickness changes during the menstrual cycle (see Figure 27.22).

The vascular supply of the uterus is key to understanding the cyclic changes of the uterine endometrium, which we will discuss later in the chapter. The **uterine arteries** arise from the *internal iliacs* in the pelvis, ascend along the sides of the uterus, and send branches into the uterine wall (Figures 27.14 and 27.15b). These branches break up into several **arcuate arteries** (ar′ku-āt) within the myometrium. The arcuate arteries send **radial arteries** into the endometrium, where they in turn give off **straight arteries** to the stratum basalis and **spiral (coiled) arteries** to the stratum functionalis. The spiral arteries repeatedly degenerate and regenerate, and it is their spasms that actually cause the functionalis layer to be shed during menstruation. Veins in the endometrium are thin walled and form an extensive network with occasional sinusoidal enlargements.

27

The Vagina

The **vagina** ("sheath") is a thin-walled tube, 8–10 cm (3–4 inches) long. It lies between the bladder and the rectum and extends from the cervix to the body exterior (see Figure 27.12). The urethra parallels its course anteriorly. Often called the

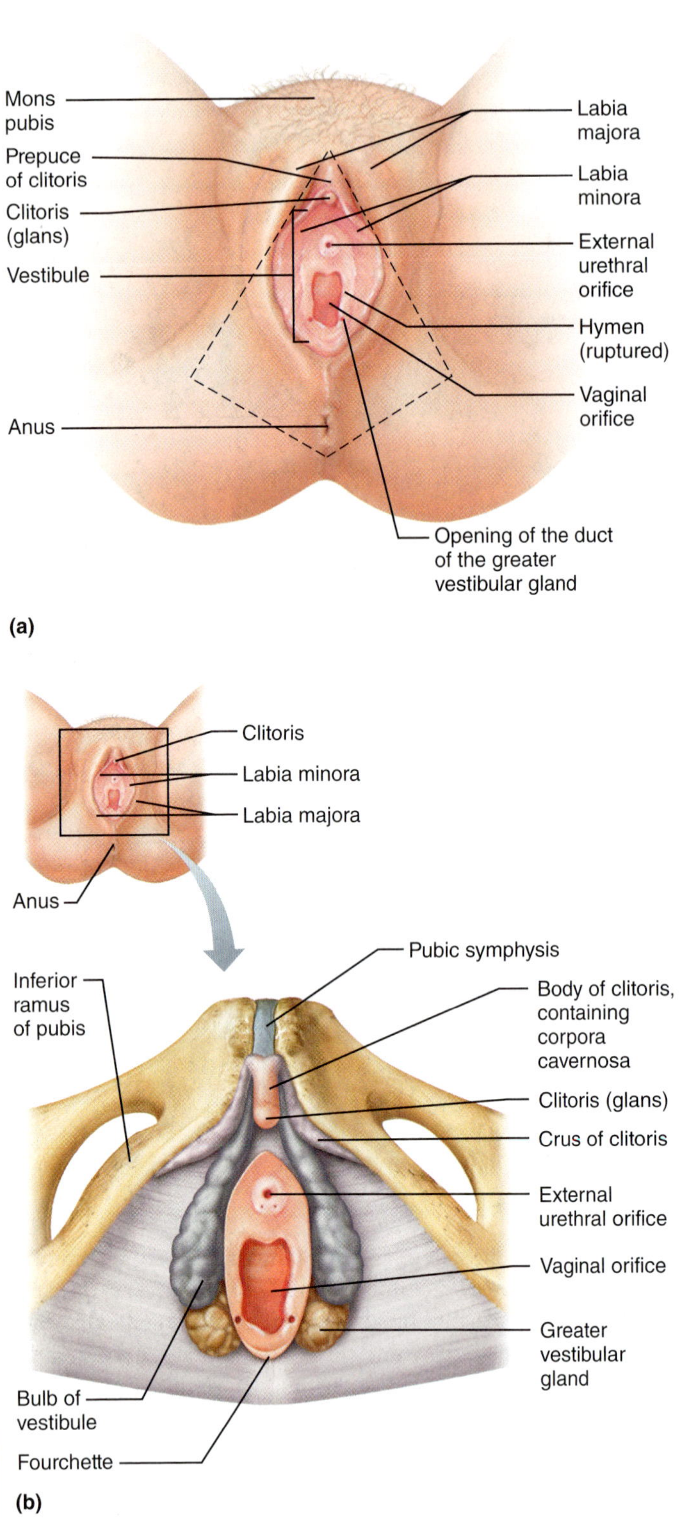

Figure 27.16 The external genitalia (vulva) of the female. **(a)** Superficial structures. The region enclosed by dashed lines is the perineum. **(b)** Deep structures. The labia majora and associated skin have been removed to show the underlying erectile bodies. For the associated superficial muscles, see Figure 10.13 on p. 345.

birth canal, the vagina provides a passageway for delivery of an infant and for menstrual flow. Because it receives the penis (and semen) during sexual intercourse, it is the *female organ of copulation*.

The distensible wall of the vagina consists of three coats: an outer fibroelastic *adventitia*, a smooth muscle *muscularis*, and an inner *mucosa* marked by transverse ridges or rugae, which stimulate the penis during intercourse. The mucosa is a stratified squamous epithelium adapted to stand up to friction. *Dendritic cells* in the mucosa act as antigen-presenting cells and are thought to provide the route of HIV transmission from an infected male to the female during sexual intercourse. (Chapter 21 describes AIDS, the immune deficiency disease caused by the HIV virus.)

The vaginal mucosa has no glands. Instead, it is lubricated by the cervical mucous glands and the mucosal transudate that "weeps" from the vaginal walls. Its epithelial cells release large amounts of glycogen, which resident bacteria metabolize anaerobically to lactic acid. Consequently, the pH of a woman's vagina is normally quite *acidic*. This acidity helps keep the vagina healthy and free of infection, but it is also hostile to sperm. Although vaginal fluid of adult females is acidic, it tends to be alkaline in adolescents, predisposing sexually active teenagers to sexually transmitted infections.

In virgins (those who have never participated in sexual intercourse), the mucosa near the distal **vaginal orifice** forms an incomplete partition called the **hymen** (hi′men) **(Figure 27.16a)**. The hymen is very vascular and may bleed when it stretches or ruptures during the first coitus (sexual intercourse). However, its durability varies. In some females, it is ruptured by sports, inserting tampons, or pelvic examinations. Occasionally, it is so tough that it must be breached surgically if intercourse is to occur.

The upper end of the vaginal canal loosely surrounds the cervix of the uterus, producing a vaginal recess called the **vaginal fornix**. The posterior part of this recess, the *posterior fornix*, is much deeper than the *lateral* and *anterior fornices* (see Figures 27.12 and 27.14). Generally, the lumen of the vagina is quite small and, except where the cervix holds it open, its posterior and anterior walls touch each other. The vagina stretches considerably during copulation and childbirth, but its lateral distension is limited by the ischial spines and the sacrospinous ligaments.

Homeostatic Imbalance 27.7

The uterus tilts away from the vagina. For this reason, attempts by untrained persons to induce an abortion by entering the uterus with a surgical instrument may puncture the posterior wall of the vagina. This causes hemorrhage and—if the instrument is unsterile—peritonitis. +

Check Your Understanding

22. Why are women more at risk for PID than men?
23. Oocytes are ovulated into the peritoneal cavity and yet women do get pregnant. What action of the uterine tubes helps to direct the oocytes into the woman's duct system?

27

24. What portion of the female duct system is the usual site of fertilization? Which is the "incubator" for fetal development?

For answers, see Appendix H.

The External Genitalia

✓ Describe the anatomy of the female external genitalia.

The female reproductive structures that lie external to the vagina are called the *external genitalia* (Figure 27.16). Also called the **vulva** (vul′vah; "covering") or **pudendum** ("shameful"), these structures include the mons pubis, labia, clitoris, and structures associated with the vestibule.

The **mons pubis** (mons pu′bis; "mountain on the pubis") is a fatty, rounded area overlying the pubic symphysis. After puberty, this area is covered with pubic hair. Running posteriorly from the mons pubis are two elongated, hair-covered fatty skin folds, the **labia majora** (la′be-ah mah-jor′ah; "larger lips"). These are the counterpart, or homologue, of the male scrotum (that is, they derive from the same embryonic tissue). The labia majora enclose the **labia minora** (mi-nor′ah; "smaller"), two thin, hair-free skin folds, homologous to the ventral penis.

The labia minora enclose a recess called the vestibule ("entrance hall"), which contains the external openings of the urethra and the vagina. Flanking the vaginal opening are the pea-size **greater vestibular glands**, homologous to the bulbo-urethral glands of males (Figure 27.16b). These glands release mucus into the vestibule and help to keep it moist and lubricated, facilitating intercourse. At the extreme posterior end of the vestibule the labia minora come together to form a ridge called the **fourchette**.

Just anterior to the vestibule is the **clitoris** (klit′o-ris; "hill"), a small, protruding structure composed largely of erectile tissue, which is homologous to the penis of the male. Its exposed portion is called the **glans of the clitoris**. It is hooded by a skin fold called the **prepuce of the clitoris**, formed by the junction of the labia minora folds.

The clitoris is richly innervated with sensory nerve endings sensitive to touch. It becomes swollen with blood and erect during tactile stimulation, contributing to a female's sexual arousal. Like the penis, the **body of the clitoris** has dorsal erectile columns (corpora cavernosa) attached proximally by crura, but it lacks a corpus spongiosum that conveys a urethra.

In males the urethra carries both urine and semen and runs through the penis, but the female urinary and reproductive tracts are completely separate. Instead, the **bulbs of the vestibule** (Figure 27.16b), which lie along each side of the vaginal orifice and deep to the bulbospongiosus muscles, are the homologues of the single penile bulb and corpus spongiosum of the male. During sexual stimulation the bulbs of the vestibule engorge with blood. This may help the vagina grip the penis and also squeezes the urethral orifice shut, which prevents semen (and bacteria) from traveling superiorly into the bladder during intercourse.

The Female Perineum

The female **perineum** is a diamond-shaped region located between the pubic arch anteriorly, the coccyx posteriorly, and the ischial tuberosities laterally (Figure 27.16a). The soft tissues of the perineum overlie the muscles of the pelvic outlet, and the posterior ends of the labia majora overlie the *central tendon*, into which most muscles supporting the pelvic floor insert (see Table 10.7).

☑ Check Your Understanding

25. What is the female homologue of the bulbo-urethral glands of males?
26. Cite similarities and differences between the penis and clitoris.

For answers, see Appendix H.

The Mammary Glands

✓ Discuss the structure and function of the mammary glands.

The **mammary glands** are present in both sexes, but they normally function only in females **(Figure 27.17)**. The biological role of the mammary glands is to produce milk to nourish a newborn baby, so they are important only when reproduction has already been accomplished.

Developmentally, mammary glands are modified sweat glands that are really part of the *skin*, or *integumentary system*. Each mammary gland is contained within a rounded skin-covered breast within the hypodermis (superficial fascia), anterior to the pectoral muscles of the thorax. Slightly below the center of each breast is a ring of pigmented skin, the **areola** (ah-re′o-lah), which surrounds a central protruding **nipple**. Large sebaceous glands in the areola make it slightly bumpy and produce sebum that reduces chapping and cracking of the skin of the nipple. Autonomic nervous system controls of smooth muscle fibers in the areola and nipple cause the nipple to become erect when stimulated by tactile or sexual stimuli, or cold temperatures.

Internally, each mammary gland consists of 15 to 25 **lobes** that radiate around and open at the nipple. The lobes are padded and separated from each other by fibrous connective tissue and fat. The interlobar connective tissue forms **suspensory ligaments** that attach the breast to the underlying muscle fascia and the overlying dermis. As suggested by their name, the suspensory ligaments provide natural support for the breasts, like a built-in brassiere.

Within the lobes are smaller units called **lobules**, which contain glandular **alveoli** that produce milk when a woman is lactating. These compound alveolar glands pass the milk into the **lactiferous ducts** (lak-tif′er-us), which open to the outside at the nipple. Just deep to the areola, each duct has a dilated region called a **lactiferous sinus** where milk accumulates during nursing. We describe the process and regulation of lactation in Chapter 28.

The description of mammary glands that we have just given applies only to nursing women or women in the last trimester of pregnancy. In nonpregnant women, the glandular structure

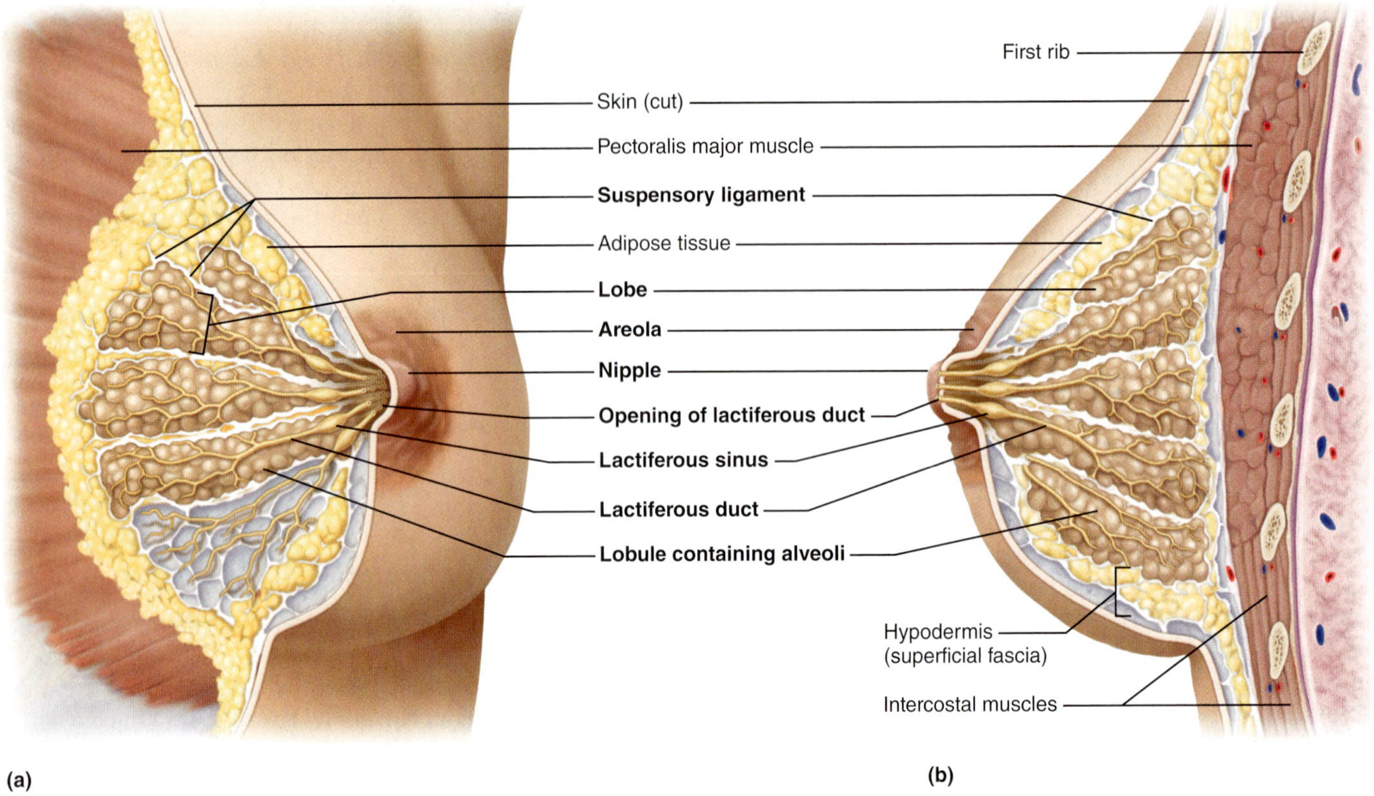

Figure 27.17 Structure of lactating mammary glands. (a) Anterior view of a partially dissected breast. **(b)** Sagittal section of a breast.

of the breast is largely undeveloped and the duct system is rudimentary. For this reason, breast size is largely due to the amount of fat deposits.

Breast Cancer

Except for nonmelanoma skin cancer, invasive breast cancer is the most common malignancy and the second most common cause of cancer death of U.S. women. Thirteen percent of women in the general population (132 out of 1000 individuals) will develop this condition—approximately 207,000 cases of invasive breast cancer and an additional 54,000 cases of noninvasive breast cancer annually.

Breast cancer usually arises from the epithelial cells of the smallest ducts, not from the alveoli. A small cluster of cancer cells grows into a lump in the breast from which cells eventually metastasize.

Known risk factors for developing breast cancer include: early onset menstruation and late menopause, no pregnancies or first pregnancy later in life and no or short periods of breast feeding, and family history of breast cancer (especially in a sister or mother).

27

Some 10% of breast cancers stem from hereditary defects and half of these can be traced to dangerous mutations in a pair of genes, dubbed *BRCA1* (breast cancer 1) and *BRCA2*. Of those who carry the altered genes, 50–80% develop breast cancer, and have a greater risk of ovarian cancer as well. However, more than 70% of women who develop breast cancer have no known risk factors for the disease.

Diagnosis Breast cancer is often signaled by a change in skin texture, skin puckering, or leakage from the nipple. Since most breast lumps are discovered by women themselves in routine monthly breast exams, this simple examination should be a priority in every woman's life.

The American Cancer Society has recommended **mammography**—X-ray examination that detects breast cancers too small to feel (less than 1 cm)—every year for women over 40 years old **(Figure 27.18)**. However, some authorities suggest that yearly is too frequent, and the U.S. Prevention Services Task Force on Breast Cancer Screening recommends delaying mammography screening until age 50.

Diagnostic MRI scans seem to be preferable for at-risk women who carry a mutated *BRCA* gene. Besides heightened monitoring, many women with the BRCA mutation are opting to have their breasts and/or ovaries surgically removed as a preventive measure.

Treatment Once diagnosed, breast cancer is treated in various ways depending on specific characteristics of the lesion. Current therapies include (1) radiation therapy, (2) chemotherapy, and (3) surgery, often followed by radiation or chemotherapy to destroy stray cancer cells. Drug therapies for estrogen-responsive cancers include:

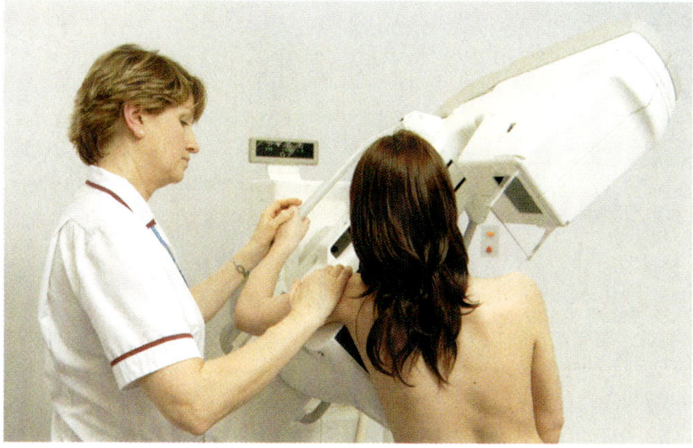

(a) Mammogram procedure

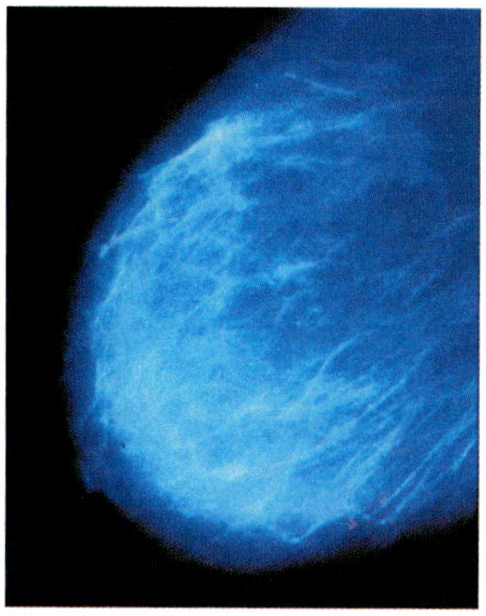

(b) Film of normal breast

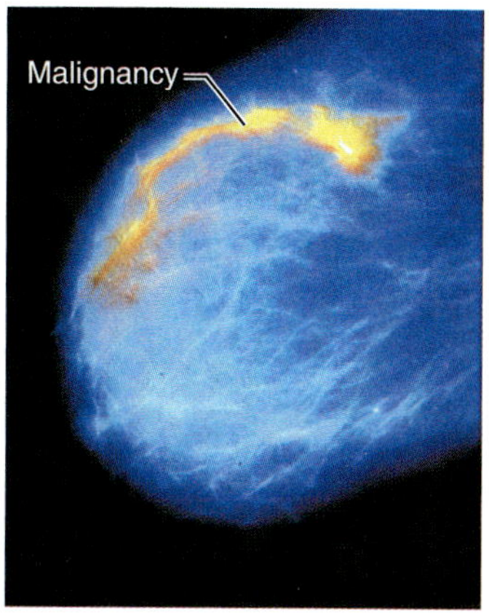

(c) Film of breast with tumor

Figure 27.18 **Mammograms.**

- Trastuzumab (Herceptin), a drug containing bioengineered antibodies that jam estrogen receptors to control aggressively growing cancer cells
- Tamoxifen, an antiestrogen compound that blocks estrogen's effects and significantly improves the outcome for premenopausal women with early- or late-stage breast cancer
- Letrozole (Femara), which disables the enzyme needed to make estrogen and reduces breast cancer recurrence in women (particularly postmenopausal women) who have exhausted the usefulness of tamoxifen

Until the 1970s, the standard treatment was **radical mastectomy** (mas-tek′to-me; "breast cutting")—removal of the entire affected breast, plus all underlying muscles, fascia, and associated lymph nodes. Most physicians now recommend less extensive surgeries such as **lumpectomy**, which excises only the cancerous lump, or **simple mastectomy**, which removes only the breast tissue (and perhaps some of the axillary lymph nodes).

Many mastectomy patients opt for breast reconstruction to replace the excised tissue. Tissue "flaps," containing muscle, fat, and skin taken from the patient's abdomen or back, are used for "sculpting" a natural-looking breast.

Check Your Understanding

27. Developmentally, mammary glands are modifications of certain skin glands. Which type?
28. From what cell types does breast cancer usually arise?

For answers, see Appendix H.

Physiology of the Female Reproductive System

Gamete production in males begins at puberty and continues throughout life, but the situation is quite different in females. It has been assumed that a female's total supply of eggs is already determined by the time she is born, and the time span during which she releases them extends only from puberty to menopause (about age 51). However, studies done in adult mice show that egg stem cells are alive and generating little "egglets" throughout life. More recent reports indicate that human egg stem cells can arise from epithelial cells of the ovary surface. These findings might seem to overturn the assumption that the number of oocytes is limited—an idea that has been part of the bedrock of biology. However, it is still too early to retire the "no new eggs" doctrine based on these preliminary data.

Oogenesis

✓ Describe the process of oogenesis and compare it to spermatogenesis.

Meiosis, the specialized nuclear division that occurs in the testes to produce sperm, also occurs in the ovaries. In this case, it produces female sex cells in a process called **oogenesis** (o″o-gen′e-sis; "the beginning of an egg"). The process of oogenesis takes years to complete **(Figure 27.19)**.

First, in the fetal period the **oogonia**, the diploid stem cells of the ovaries, multiply rapidly by mitosis. Gradually, **primordial follicles** appear as the oogonia transform into **primary oocytes** and become surrounded by a single layer of flattened cells called *follicle cells.* The primary oocytes begin the first meiotic division, but become "stalled" late in prophase I and do not complete it.

By birth, a female is presumed to have her lifetime supply of primary oocytes. Of the original 7 million oocytes, approximately 1 million escape programmed death and are already in place in the cortical region of the immature ovary. By puberty, an endowment of perhaps 300,000 oocytes remain. Over time, quiescent primordial follicles are recruited into a growing pool of primary follicles. This recruitment process begins during fetal life and continues throughout life until the supply of primordial follicles is depleted, a time called *menopause* (see p. 1058).

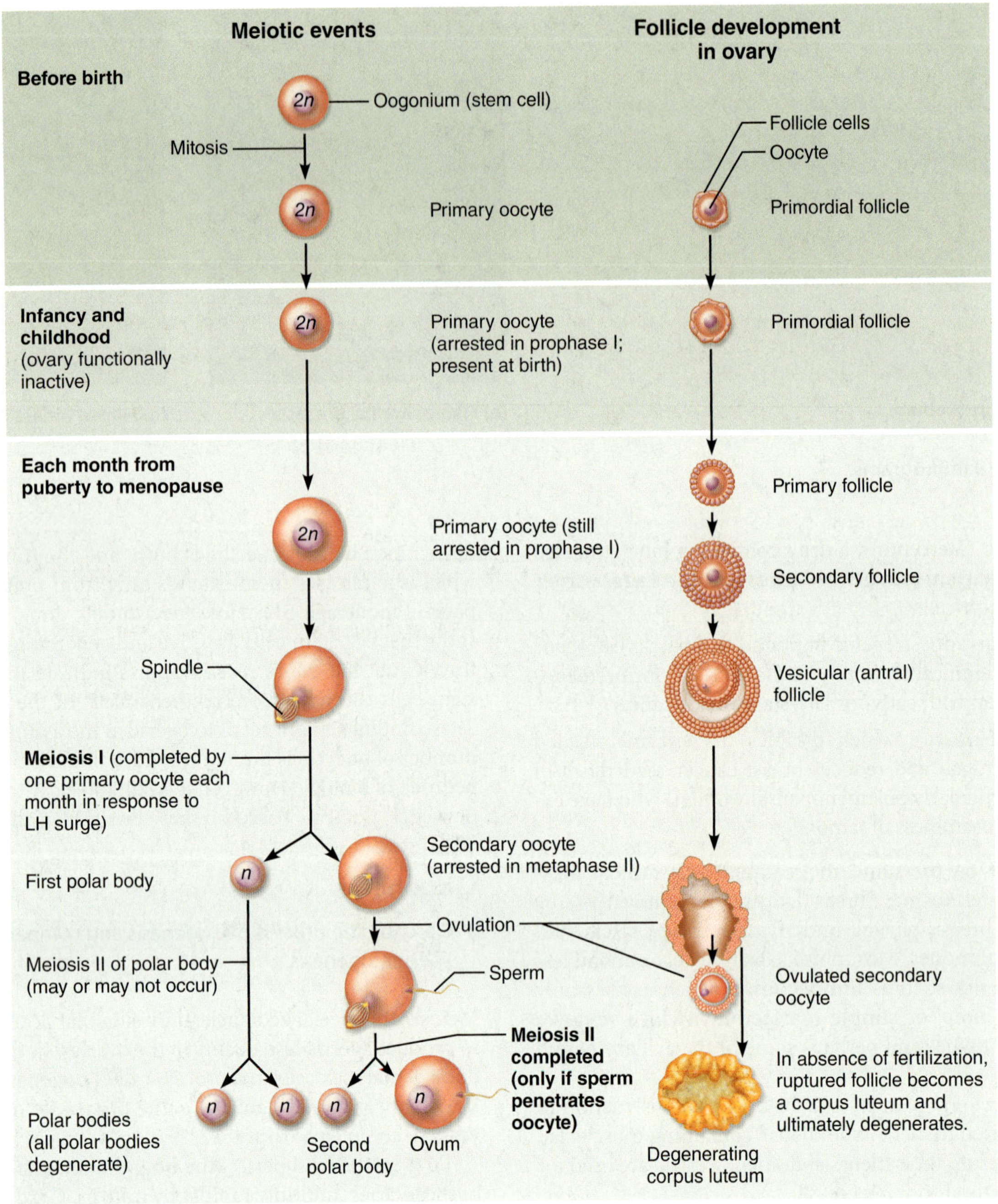

Figure 27.19 Events of oogenesis. Left, flowchart of meiotic events. Right, correlation with follicle development and ovulation in the ovary. At various stages, unsuccessful oocytes undergo atresia (not shown). Corresponding illustrations of meiotic events and follicle development lie opposite each other.

27

Oogenesis After Puberty

Before puberty, all of the primordial follicles that are recruited undergo atresia (apoptosis, or programmed cell death). Beginning at puberty, FSH rescues a small number of growing follicles from that fate each month. In each cycle, one of the rescued follicles is "selected" to become the *dominant follicle* and continue meiosis I, ultimately producing two haploid cells (each with 23 replicated chromosomes) that are quite dissimilar in size. The smaller cell is called the **first polar body**. The larger cell, which contains nearly all the cytoplasm of the primary oocyte, is the **secondary oocyte**. Those maturing follicles not selected undergo atresia.

The events of this first maturation division ensure that the polar body receives almost no cytoplasm or organelles. Notice in Figure 27.19 (left) that a spindle forms at the very edge of the oocyte. A little "nipple" also appears at that edge, and the polar body chromosomes are cast into it.

The first polar body may continue its development and undergo meiosis II, producing two even smaller polar bodies.

However, in humans, the secondary oocyte arrests in metaphase II, and it is this cell (not a functional ovum) that is ovulated. If a sperm does not penetrate an ovulated secondary oocyte, the oocyte deteriorates. But, if a sperm penetration does occur, the oocyte quickly completes meiosis II, yielding one large **ovum** and a tiny **second polar body** (Figure 27.19). The union of the egg and sperm nuclei, described in Chapter 28, constitutes fertilization.

Comparison of Oogenesis and Spermatogenesis

What you should realize now is that the potential end products of oogenesis are three tiny polar bodies, nearly devoid of cytoplasm, and one large ovum. All of these cells are haploid, but only the ovum is a *functional gamete*. This is quite different from spermatogenesis, where the product is four viable gametes—spermatozoa.

The unequal cytoplasmic divisions that occur during oogenesis ensure that a fertilized egg has ample nutrients for its six- to seven-day journey to the uterus. Lacking nutrient-containing cytoplasm, the polar bodies degenerate and die. Since the reproductive life of a woman is at most about 40 years (from about age 11 to 51) and typically only one ovulation occurs each month, fewer than 500 oocytes out of her estimated pubertal potential of 300,000 are ever released during a woman's lifetime.

Perhaps the most striking difference between male and female meiosis is the error rate. As many as 20% of oocytes but only 3–4% of sperm have the wrong number of chromosomes, a situation that often results from failure of the homologues to separate during meiosis I. It appears that faced with meiotic disruption, meiosis in males grinds to a halt but in females it marches on.

☑ Check Your Understanding

29. How do the haploid cells arising from oogenesis differ structurally and functionally from those arising from spermatogenesis?

For answers, see Appendix H.

The Ovarian Cycle

✓ Describe ovarian cycle phases, and relate them to events of oogenesis.

The monthly series of events associated with the maturation of an egg is called the **ovarian cycle**. The ovarian cycle is best described in terms of two consecutive phases. The **follicular phase** is the period when the dominant follicle is selected and begins to secrete large amounts of estrogen. It generally lasts from the first to the fourteenth day of the ovarian cycle, at which point ovulation typically occurs. The **luteal phase** is the period of corpus luteum activity, days 14–28. The so-called typical ovarian cycle repeats at intervals of 28 days, with *ovulation* occurring midcycle.

However, only 10–15% of women naturally have 28-day cycles, and cycles as long as 40 days or as short as 21 days are fairly common. In such cases, the length of the follicular phase and timing of ovulation vary, but the luteal phase remains constant: It is always 14 days from the time of ovulation to the end of the cycle.

Follicular Phase of the Ovarian Cycle

Maturation of a primordial follicle involves preantral and antral phases and several events. The first phase, the gonadotropin-independent *preantral phase*, is when intrafollicular paracrines such as cytokines and growth factors control oocyte and follicle development. Phase 2 is the *antral phase*, directed by FSH and LH. During this phase, the activated follicles grow tremendously and the primary occyte in the dominant follicle resumes meiosis I.

Let's look at events of these phases shown in **Figure 27.20**.

- **A primordial follicle becomes a primary follicle.** When a primordial follicle (1) is activated (this occurs almost a year before its possible ovulation) the squamouslike cells surrounding the primary oocyte grow, becoming cuboidal cells, and the oocyte enlarges. The follicle is now called a primary (1°) follicle (2).
- **A primary follicle becomes a secondary follicle.** Next, the follicular cells proliferate, forming a stratified epithelium around the oocyte. As soon as more than one cell layer is present, the follicle is called a **secondary (2°) follicle** (3a) and the follicle cells take on the name *granulosa cells*. The granulosa cells are connected to the developing oocyte by gap junctions, through which ions, metabolites, and signaling molecules can pass. From this point on, bidirectional "conversations" occur between the oocyte and granulosa cells, so they guide one another's development. One of the signals passing from the granulosa cells "tells" the oocyte to grow. Other signals dictate asymmetry (polarity) in the future egg. The oocyte grows tremendously during this stage and FSH receptors begin to appear on the granulosa cells.
- **A secondary follicle becomes a late secondary follicle.** Late in stage (3), a layer of connective tissue and epithelial cells condenses around the follicle, forming the **theca folliculi** (the′kah fah-lik′u-li; "box around the follicle"). As the follicle grows, the thecal and granulosa cells cooperate to produce estrogens. In response to LH the inner thecal cells produce androgens, which the granulosa cells convert to estrogens. At the same time, the oocyte secretes a glycoprotein-rich substance that forms a thick transparent extracellular layer or membrane, called the **zona pellucida** (pĕ-lu′sid-ah), that encapsulates it (see Figure 27.20, (4)).

  At the end of stage (3), clear liquid begins to accumulate between the granulosa cells, producing the **late secondary follicle** (3b).
- **A late secondary follicle becomes a vesicular (antral) follicle.** The late secondary follicle ushers in events of the antral phase encompassing events from (3b) to (4). In this phase, the follicle reaches the critical preovulatory stage and all granulosa cells bear FSH receptors. When six to seven layers of granulosa cell layers are present, the fluid between the granulosa cells coalesces to form a large fluid-filled cavity called

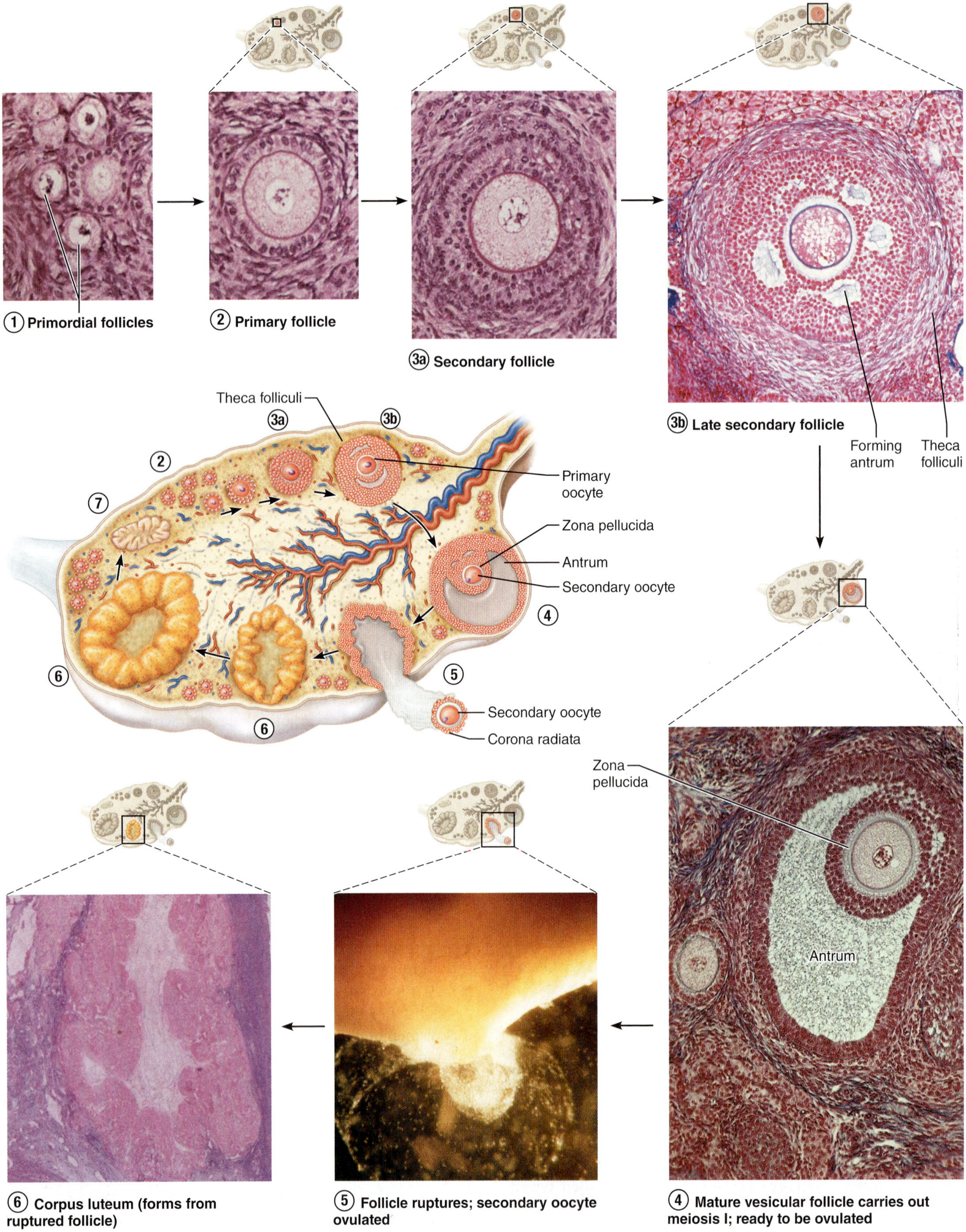

Figure 27.20 Schematic and microscopic views of the ovarian cycle: development and fate of ovarian follicles. The numbers on the diagram indicate the sequence of stages in follicle development, not the movement of a developing follicle within the ovary. During stage ⑦ (no photomicrograph), the corpus luteum degenerates into the corpus albicans. No primordial follicle (①) is shown in the central schematic view.

the **antrum** ("cave"), an event that distinguishes the early **vesicular follicle** from the late secondary follicle and all prior follicles (*preantral follicles*).

The antrum continues to expand with fluid until it isolates the oocyte, along with its surrounding capsule of granulosa cells called a **corona radiata** ("radiating crown"), so the oocyte is "sitting proudly" on a stalk on one side of the follicle. When a follicle is full size (about 2.5 cm, or 1 inch, in diameter), it bulges from the external ovarian surface like an "angry boil." This usually occurs by day 14.

As one of the final events of follicle maturation, the primary oocyte completes meiosis I to form the secondary oocyte and first polar body (see Figure 27.19). Once this has occurred, the stage is set for ovulation. At this point, the granulosa cells send another important signal to the oocyte that says, in effect, "Wait, do not complete meiosis yet!" It is estimated that follicle growth from the primordial stage to this stage takes about a year. So each follicle that ovulates actually began to grow some 10–12 ovarian cycles earlier.

Ovulation

Ovulation (stage ⑤ in Figure 27.20) occurs when the ballooning ovary wall ruptures and expels the secondary oocyte, still surrounded by its corona radiata, into the peritoneal cavity. Some women experience a twinge of pain in the lower abdomen when ovulation occurs. The precise cause of this pain, called *mittelschmerz* (mit′el-shmārts; German for "middle pain"), is not known, but possible reasons include intense stretching of the ovarian wall during ovulation and irritation of the peritoneum by blood or fluid released from the ruptured follicle.

In the ovaries of an adult female, there are always several follicles at different stages of maturation. As a rule, one follicle outstrips the others and is at the peak stage of maturation when the hormonal (LH) stimulus is given for ovulation. FSH is a survival factor for antral follicles and plays a role in selecting the so-called *dominant follicle*, but how this follicle is selected, or selects itself, is still uncertain. It is probably the one that adds the most gonadotropin receptors and so attains the greatest FSH sensitivity the quickest. The others degenerate (undergo apoptosis) and are reabsorbed.

In 1–2% of all ovulations, more than one oocyte is ovulated. This phenomenon, which increases with age, can result in multiple births. Since, in such cases, different oocytes are fertilized by different sperm, the siblings are *fraternal*, or nonidentical, twins. *Identical twins* result from the fertilization of a single oocyte by a single sperm, followed by separation of the fertilized egg's daughter cells during early development. Additionally, it now appears that in some women oocytes may be released at times unrelated to hormone levels. This timing may help to explain why a rhythm method of contraception sometimes fails and why some fraternal twins have different conception dates.

Luteal Phase of the Ovarian Cycle

After ovulation, the ruptured follicle collapses and the antrum fills with clotted blood. This *corpus hemorrhagicum* is eventually absorbed. The remaining granulosa cells enlarge, and along with the internal thecal cells they form a new, quite different endocrine structure, the *corpus luteum* ("yellow body") (Figure 27.20, stage ⑥). It settles right into its role and begins to secrete progesterone and some estrogen.

If pregnancy does not occur, the corpus luteum starts degenerating in about 10 days and its hormonal output ends. In this case, all that ultimately remains is a scar called the *corpus albicans* (al′bĭ-kans; "white body") as shown in Figure 27.20, ⑦. The last two or three days of the luteal phase, when the endometrium is just beginning to erode, is sometimes called the *luteolytic* or *ischemic phase*.

On the other hand, if the oocyte is fertilized and pregnancy ensues, the corpus luteum persists until the placenta is ready to take over its hormone-producing duties in about three months.

☑ Check Your Understanding

30. How do identical twins differ developmentally from fraternal twins?
31. What occurs in the luteal phase of the ovarian cycle?

For answers, see Appendix H.

Hormonal Regulation of the Ovarian Cycle

✓ Describe the regulation of the ovarian and uterine cycles.

Ovarian events are much more complicated than those occurring in the testes, but the hormonal controls set into motion at puberty are similar in both sexes. Gonadotropin-releasing hormone (GnRH), pituitary gonadotropins, and, in this case, ovarian estrogen and progesterone interact to produce the cyclic events occurring in the ovaries.

However, in females another hormone plays an important role in stimulating the hypothalamus to release GnRH. The onset of puberty in females is linked to the amount of adipose tissue, and the messenger from fatty tissue to the hypothalamus is leptin. If blood levels of lipids and leptin (better known for its role in energy production and appetite) are low, puberty is delayed.

Establishing the Ovarian Cycle

During childhood, the ovaries grow and continuously secrete small amounts of estrogens, which inhibit hypothalamic release of GnRH. Provided that leptin levels are adequate, the hypothalamus becomes less sensitive to estrogen as puberty nears and begins to release GnRH in a rhythmic pulselike manner. GnRH, in turn, stimulates the anterior pituitary to release FSH and LH, which prompt the ovaries to secrete hormones (primarily estrogens).

Gonadotropin levels continue to increase for about four years. During this time, pubertal girls are still not ovulating and cannot become pregnant. Eventually, the adult cyclic pattern is achieved, and hormonal interactions stabilize. These events are heralded by the young woman's first menstrual period, referred to as **menarche** (mĕ-nar′ke; *men* = month, *arche* = first). Usually, it is not until the third year postmenarche that the cycles become regular and all are ovulatory.

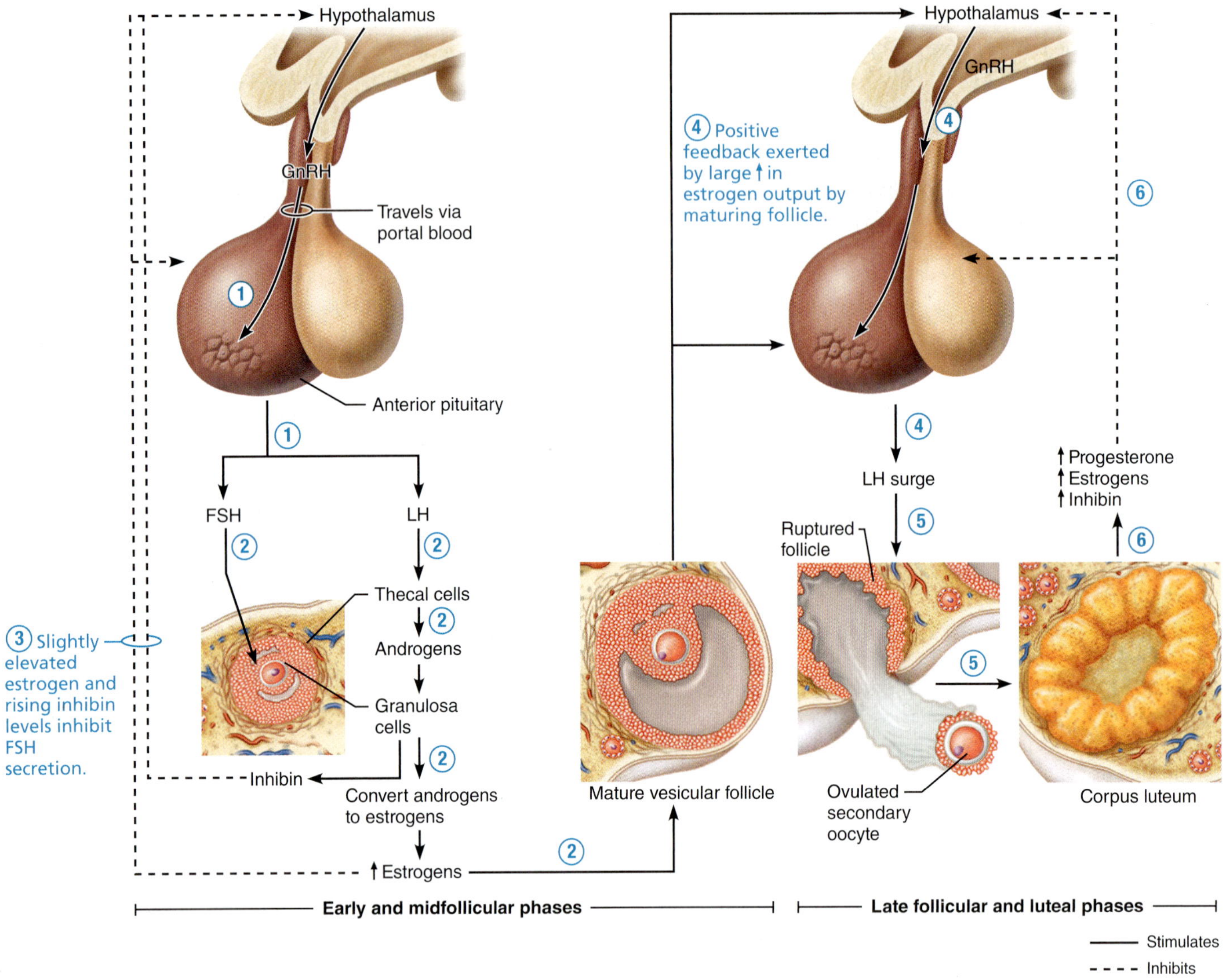

Figure 27.21 Regulation of the ovarian cycle. Numbers refer to events listed in the text. Note that all feedback signals exerted by ovarian hormones are negative except one—that exerted by estrogens immediately before ovulation. Events that follow step (6) (negative feedback inhibition of the hypothalamus and anterior pituitary by progesterone and estrogens) are not depicted, but involve a gradual deterioration of the corpus luteum and, therefore, a decline in ovarian hormone production. Ovarian hormones reach their lowest blood levels around day 28.

Hormonal Interactions During the Ovarian Cycle

Next, let's look at how the waxing and waning of anterior pituitary gonadotropins (FSH and LH) and ovarian hormones and the negative and positive feedback interactions regulate ovarian function. **Figure 27.21** shows these events in a 28-day cycle.

(1) **GnRH stimulates FSH and LH secretion.** GnRH secreted by the hypothalamus stimulates the anterior pituitary to produce and release follicle-stimulating hormone (FSH) and luteinizing hormone (LH).

(2) **FSH and LH stimulate follicles to grow, mature, and secrete sex hormones.** FSH exerts its main effects on the granulosa cells of late secondary and vesicular follicles, causing them to release estrogens, whereas LH (at least initially) prods the thecal cells to release androgens (actually the steroid hormone androstenedione). These hormones diffuse through the basement membrane, where the granulosa cells convert them to estrogens. Only tiny amounts of ovarian androgens enter the blood, because they are almost completely converted to estrogens within the ovaries.

(3) **Negative feedback inhibits gonadotropin release.** As estrogen levels in the plasma rise, they exert *negative feedback* on the hypothalamus and anterior pituitary, inhibiting release of FSH and LH. Within the ovary, estrogen enhances output of estrogens by intensifying the effect of FSH on

follicle maturation. *Inhibin*, released by the granulosa cells, also exerts negative feedback controls on FSH release during this period. Only the dominant follicle survives this dip in FSH—the other developing follicles fail to develop further, and they deteriorate.

(4) **Positive feedback stimulates gonadotropin release.** Although the initial small rise in bloodborne estrogen inhibits the hypothalamic-pituitary-gonadal axis, the high estrogen level produced by the dominant follicle has the opposite effect. Once estrogen reaches a critical blood concentration, it briefly exerts *positive feedback* on the brain and anterior pituitary.

(5) **LH surge triggers ovulation and formation of the corpus luteum.** The high estrogen level sets a cascade of events into motion. There is a sudden burstlike release of accumulated LH (and, to a lesser extent, FSH) by the anterior pituitary about midcycle (also see Figure 27.22a).

The LH surge rouses the primary oocyte of the dominant follicle from its resting state and it completes its first meiotic division, forming a secondary oocyte that continues on to metaphase II. Around day 14, LH—aided by intraovarian paracrine factors—stimulates many events that lead to ovulation: It increases local vascular permeability and triggers an inflammatory response that promotes release of metalloproteinase enzymes that weaken the ovary wall. As a result, blood stops flowing through the protruding part of the follicle wall. Within minutes, that region of the follicle wall thins, bulges, and ruptures, forming a hole or *stigma*. The oocyte, still surrounded by its corona radiata, exits, accomplishing ovulation. The role (if any) of FSH in this process is unknown.

Shortly after ovulation, estrogen levels decline. This probably reflects the damage to the dominant estrogen-secreting follicle during ovulation.

The LH surge also transforms the ruptured follicle into a corpus luteum (which gives LH its name, "luteinizing" hormone). LH stimulates this newly formed endocrine structure to produce large amounts of progesterone and some estrogen almost immediately after it is formed. Progesterone helps maintain the stratum functionalis and is essential for maintaining pregnancy should conception occur.

(6) **Negative feedback inhibits LH and FSH release.** Rising progesterone and estrogen blood levels exert a powerful negative feedback effect on the hypothalamus and the anterior pituitary release of LH and FSH. Inhibin, released by the corpus luteum and granulosa cells, enhances this inhibitory effect. Declining gonadotropin levels inhibit the maturation of new vesicular follicles and prevent additional LH surges that might cause additional oocytes to be ovulated.

In cycles in which fertilization does not occur, the stimulus for luteal activity ends when LH blood levels fall and the corpus luteum degenerates. As goes the corpus luteum, so go the levels of ovarian hormones, and blood estrogen and progesterone levels drop sharply. The marked decline in ovarian hormones at the end of the cycle (days 26–28) ends their blockade of FSH and LH secretion, and the cycle starts anew.

We have just described ovarian events as if we are following one follicle through the 28-day cycle, but this is not really the case. What is happening is that the increase of FSH at the beginning of each cycle allows several vesicular follicles to continue to mature. Then, with the midcycle LH surge, one (or more) vesicular follicles undergo ovulation. However, the ovulated oocyte would actually have been activated up to 12 months before, not 14 days before.

The Uterine (Menstrual) Cycle

Although the uterus is where an embryo implants and develops, it is receptive to implantation for only a short period each month. Not surprisingly, this brief interval is exactly the time when a developing embryo would normally begin implanting, six to seven days after ovulation. The **uterine**, or **menstrual** (men′stroo-al), **cycle** is a series of cyclic changes that the uterine endometrium goes through each month as it responds to the waxing and waning of ovarian hormones in the blood. These endometrial changes are coordinated with the phases of the ovarian cycle, which are dictated by gonadotropins released by the anterior pituitary.

Changes in ovarian steroid hormone levels drive the events of the uterine cycle **(Figure 27.22d)** as follows:

1. **Days 1–5: Menstrual phase.** In this phase, **menstruation** (men″stroo-a′shun) or **menses**, the uterus sheds all but the deepest part of its endometrium. (Note in Figure 27.22a and c that at the beginning of this stage, ovarian hormones are at their lowest normal levels and gonadotropins are beginning to rise.) The thick, hormone-dependent functional layer of the endometrium detaches from the uterine wall, a process accompanied by bleeding for 3–5 days. The detached tissue and blood pass out through the vagina as the menstrual flow. By day 5, the growing ovarian follicles start to produce more estrogen (Figure 27.22c).
2. **Days 6–14: Proliferative (preovulatory) phase.** In this phase, the endometrium rebuilds itself: Under the influence of rising blood levels of estrogens, the basal layer of the endometrium generates a new functional layer. As this new layer thickens, its glands enlarge and its spiral arteries increase in number (also see Figure 27.15). Consequently, the endometrium once again becomes velvety, thick, and well vascularized. During this phase, estrogens also induce the endometrial cells to synthesize progesterone receptors, readying them for interaction with progesterone.

   Normally, cervical mucus is thick and sticky, but rising estrogen levels cause it to thin and form channels that facilitate sperm passage into the uterus. *Ovulation*, which takes less than five minutes, occurs in the ovary at the end of the proliferative stage (day 14) in response to the sudden release of LH from the anterior pituitary. As we saw earlier, LH also converts the ruptured follicle to a corpus luteum.

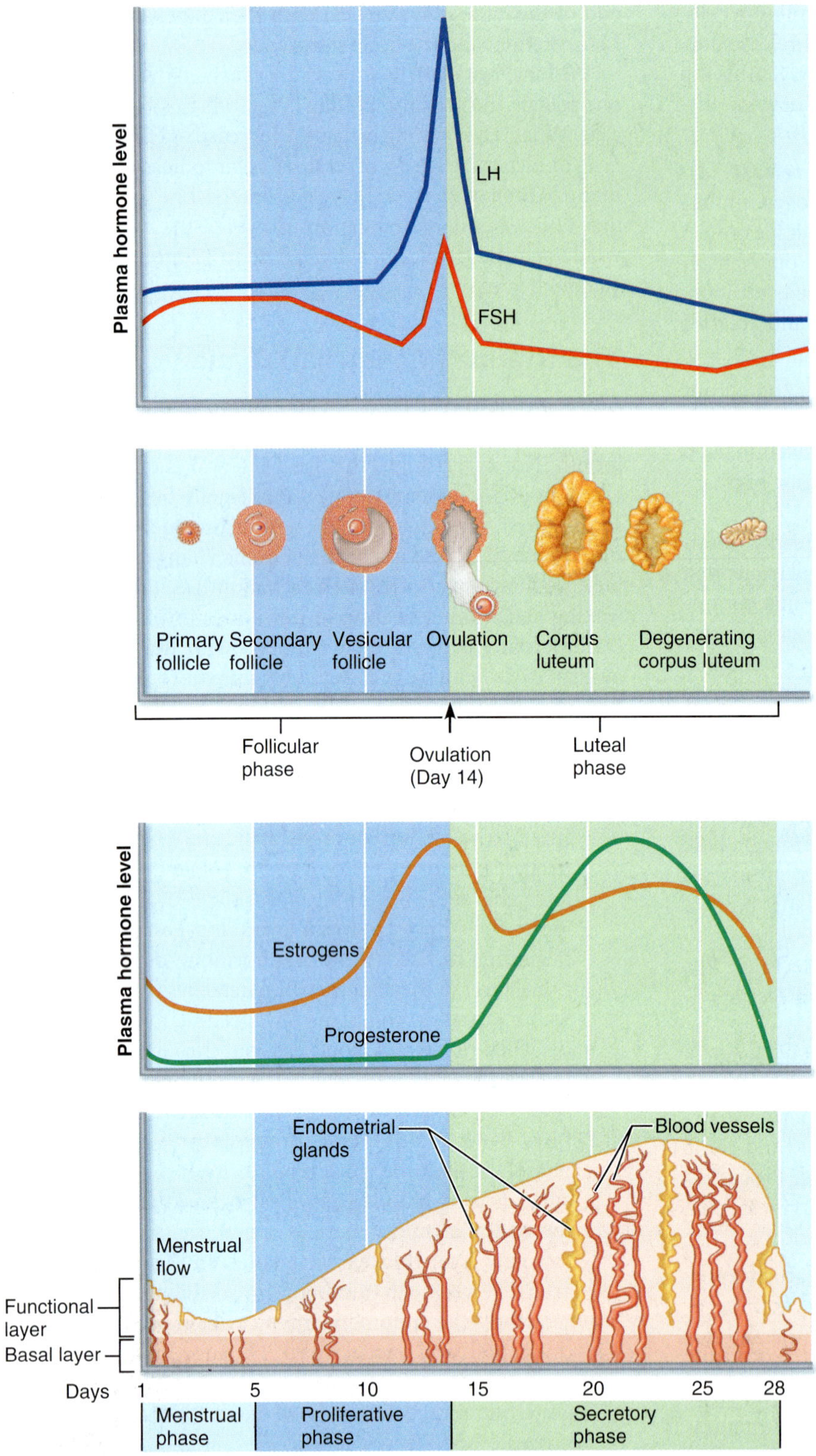

(a) Fluctuation of gonadotropin levels: Fluctuating levels of pituitary gonadotropins (follicle-stimulating hormone and luteinizing hormone) in the blood regulate the events of the ovarian cycle.

(b) Ovarian cycle: Structural changes in the ovarian follicles during the ovarian cycle are correlated with (d) changes in the endometrium of the uterus during the uterine cycle.

(c) Fluctuation of ovarian hormone levels: Fluctuating levels of ovarian hormones (estrogens and progesterone) cause the endometrial changes of the uterine cycle. The high estrogen levels are also responsible for the LH/FSH surge in (a).

(d) The three phases of the uterine cycle:
- Menstrual: The functional layer of the endometrium is shed.
- Proliferative: The functional layer of the endometrium is rebuilt.
- Secretory: Begins immediately after ovulation. Enrichment of the blood supply and glandular secretion of nutrients prepare the endometrium to receive an embryo.

Both the menstrual and proliferative phases occur before ovulation, and together they correspond to the follicular phase of the ovarian cycle. The secretory phase corresponds in time to the luteal phase of the ovarian cycle.

27

Figure 27.22 Correlation of anterior pituitary and ovarian hormones with structural changes of the ovary and uterus. The time bar at the bottom of the figure, reading Days 1 to 28, applies to all four parts of this figure. (For a related image, see *A Brief Atlas of the Human Body*, Plate 53.)

3. **Days 15–28: Secretory (postovulatory) phase.** This 14-day phase is the most constant timewise. During the secretory phase the endometrium prepares for an embryo to implant. Rising levels of progesterone from the corpus luteum act on the estrogen-primed endometrium, causing the spiral arteries to elaborate and converting the functional layer to a secretory mucosa. The endometrial glands enlarge, coil, and begin secreting nutrients into the uterine cavity that will sustain the embryo until it has implanted in the blood-rich endometrial lining.

   As progesterone levels rise, the cervical mucus becomes viscous again, forming the *cervical plug*, which helps to block entry of sperm and pathogens or other foreign materials. Progesterone also plays an important role in keeping the uterus "private" in the event an embryo has begun to implant. Rising progesterone (and estrogen) levels inhibit LH release by the anterior pituitary.

   As noted earlier, if fertilization has not occurred, the corpus luteum degenerates toward the end of the secretory phase as LH blood levels decline. Progesterone levels fall, depriving the endometrium of hormonal support, and the spiral arteries kink and go into spasms. Denied oxygen and nutrients, the ischemic endometrial cells die and the glands regress, setting the stage for menstruation to begin on day 28. The spiral arteries constrict one final time and then suddenly relax and open wide. As blood gushes into the weakened capillary beds, they fragment, causing the functional layer to slough off. The uterine cycle starts over again on this first day of menstrual flow.

Figure 27.22b and d also illustrate how the ovarian and uterine cycles fit together. Notice that the menstrual and proliferative phases overlap the follicular phase and ovulation in the ovarian cycle, and that the uterine secretory phase corresponds to the ovarian luteal phase.

Homeostatic Imbalance 27.8

Extremely strenuous physical activity can delay menarche in girls and disrupt the normal menstrual cycle in adult women, even causing *amenorrhea* (a-men″o-re′ah), cessation of menstruation. Female athletes have little body fat, and adipose cells help convert adrenal androgens to estrogens and are the source of leptin which, as noted above, plays a critical permissive role in the onset of puberty in females. Leptin informs the hypothalamus whether energy stores are sufficient to support the high energy demands of reproduction. If not, the reproductive cycles are shut down.

Amenorrhea is usually reversible when the woman discontinues athletic training, but it has a worrisome consequence in young, healthy adult women: dramatic losses in bone mass normally seen only in osteoporosis of old age. Once estrogen levels drop and the menstrual cycle stops (regardless of cause), bone loss begins. +

Check Your Understanding

32. Which hormone plays an important role in "letting the brain know" that puberty may occur in girls?
33. Which hormone(s) prompt follicle growth? Which hormone prompts ovulation?
34. Which gonadal hormone exerts positive feedback on the anterior pituitary that results in a burstlike release of LH?

For answers, see Appendix H.

Effects of Estrogens and Progesterone

✓ Discuss the physiological effects of estrogens and progesterone.

With a name meaning "generators of sexual activity," estrogens are analogous to testosterone, the male steroid. As estrogen levels rise during puberty, they (1) promote oogenesis and follicle growth in the ovary and (2) exert anabolic effects on the female reproductive tract **(Table 27.1)**. Consequently, the uterine tubes, uterus, and vagina enlarge and become functional—more ready to support a pregnancy. The uterine tubes and uterus exhibit enhanced motility; the vaginal mucosa thickens; and the external genitalia mature.

Estrogens also support the growth spurt at puberty that makes girls grow much more quickly than boys between the ages of 11 and 12. But this growth is short-lived because rising estrogen levels also cause the epiphyses of long bones to close sooner, and females reach their full height between the ages of 13 and 15. In contrast, the aggressive growth of males continues until ages 15 to 19, at which point rising estrogen levels cause epiphyseal closure.

The estrogen-induced secondary sex characteristics of females include:

- Breast development
- Increasing deposition of subcutaneous fat, especially in the hips and breasts
- Development of a wider and lighter pelvis (adaptations for childbirth)

Estrogens also have several metabolic effects, including maintaining low total blood cholesterol levels (and high HDL levels) and facilitating calcium uptake, which helps sustain the density of the skeleton. These metabolic effects begin under estrogen's influence during puberty, but they are not true secondary sex characteristics.

Progesterone works with estrogen to establish and then help regulate the uterine cycle and promotes changes in cervical mucus (see Table 27.1). Its other effects are exhibited largely during pregnancy, when it inhibits uterine motility and takes up where estrogen leaves off in preparing the breasts for lactation. Indeed, progesterone is named for these important roles (*pro* = for, *gestation* = pregnancy). However, the source of progesterone and estrogen during most of pregnancy is the placenta, not the ovaries.

Female Sexual Response

✓ Describe the phases of the female sexual response.

The **female sexual response** is similar to that of males in most respects. During sexual excitement, the clitoris, vaginal mucosa, bulbs of the vestibule, and breasts engorge with blood and the

Table 27.1 Summary of Hormonal Effects of Gonadal Estrogens, Progesterone, and Testosterone

SOURCE, STIMULUS, EFFECTS	ESTROGENS (MOSTLY ESTRADIOL)	PROGESTERONE	TESTOSTERONE
Major source	Ovary: developing follicles and corpus luteum.	Ovary: mainly the corpus luteum.	Testes: interstitial endocrine cells.
Stimulus for release	FSH (and LH).	LH.	LH and declining levels of inhibin produced by the sustentocytes.
Feedback effects exerted	Both negative and positive feedback exerted on anterior pituitary release of gonadotropins.	Negative feedback exerted on anterior pituitary release of gonadotropins.	Negative feedback suppresses release of LH by the anterior pituitary and release of GnRH by the hypothalamus.
Effects on reproductive organs	Stimulate growth and maturation of reproductive organs and breasts at puberty and maintain their adult size and function. Promote the proliferative phase of the uterine cycle. Stimulate production of watery cervical mucus and activity of fimbriae and uterine tube cilia.	Cooperates with estrogen in stimulating growth of breasts. Promotes the secretory phase of the uterine cycle. Stimulates production of viscous cervical mucus. Progesterone surge after ovulation enhances beating of cilia in the uterine tube, promoting meeting of sperm and oocyte.	Stimulates formation of male reproductive ducts, glands, and external genitalia. Promotes descent of the testes. Stimulates growth and maturation of the internal and external genitalia at puberty; maintains their adult size and function.
	Promote oogenesis and ovulation by stimulating formation of FSH and LH receptors on follicle cells. Stimulate capacitation of sperm in the female reproductive tract.	During pregnancy, quiets the myometrium and acts with estrogen to cause mammary glands to achieve their mature milk-producing state.	Required for normal spermatogenesis via effects promoted by ABP, which keeps its concentration high near spermatogenic cells. Suppresses mammary gland development.
	During pregnancy stimulate growth of the uterus and enlargement of the external genitalia and mammary glands.		
Promotion of secondary sex characteristics and somatic effects	Promote long bone growth and feminization of the skeleton (particularly the pelvis); inhibit bone reabsorption and then stimulate epiphyseal closure. Promote hydration of the skin and female pattern of fat deposit.		Stimulates the growth spurt at puberty; promotes increased skeletal and muscle mass during adolescence. Promotes growth of the larynx and vocal cords and deepening of the voice. Enhances sebum secretion and hair growth, especially on the face, axillae, genital region, and chest.
	During pregnancy act with relaxin (placental hormone) to induce softening and relaxation of the pelvic ligaments and pubic symphysis.		
Metabolic effects	Generally anabolic. Stimulate Na^+ reabsorption by the renal tubules, hence inhibit diuresis. Enhance HDL (and reduce LDL) blood levels (cardiovascular sparing effect).	Promotes diuresis (antiestrogenic effect). Increases body temperature.	Generally anabolic. Stimulates hematopoiesis. Enhances the basal metabolic rate.
Neural effects	Along with DHEA (an androgen produced by the adrenal cortex) are partially responsible for female libido (sex drive).		Responsible for libido in males; promotes aggressiveness.

nipples become erect. Increased activity of the vestibular glands and "sweating" of the vaginal walls lubricate the vestibule and facilitate entry of the penis. These events, though more widespread, are analogous to the *erection* phase in men. Touch and psychological stimuli promote sexual excitement, which is mediated along the same autonomic nerve pathways as in males.

The final phase of the female sexual response, *orgasm*, is not accompanied by ejaculation. However, muscle tension increases throughout the body, pulse rate and blood pressure rise, and the uterus contracts rhythmically. As in males, orgasm is accompanied by a sensation of intense pleasure followed by relaxation. But unlike what is seen in males, a refractory period does not follow orgasm, so females may experience multiple orgasms during a single sexual experience. Female orgasm is not required for conception. Indeed, some women never experience orgasm, yet are perfectly able to conceive.

Although the female libido was formerly believed to be prompted by testosterone, new studies indicate that dehydroepiandrosterone (DHEA), an androgen produced by the adrenal cortex, is in fact the male sex hormone associated with desire in females.

Check Your Understanding

35. Which gonadal hormone causes the secondary sex characteristics to appear in a young woman?
36. Which gonadal hormone promotes epiphyseal closure in both males and females?

For answers, see Appendix H.

Sexually Transmitted Infections

✓ Indicate the infectious agents and modes of transmission of gonorrhea, syphilis, chlamydia, trichomoniasis, genital warts, and genital herpes.

Sexually transmitted infections (STIs), also called *sexually transmitted diseases* (*STDs*) or *venereal diseases* (*VDs*), are infectious diseases spread through sexual contact. The United States has the highest rates of infection among developed countries. Over 12 million people in the U.S., a quarter of them adolescents, get STIs each year. Latex condoms can help prevent the spread of STIs, and their use is strongly encouraged.

As a group, STIs are the single most important cause of reproductive disorders. Until recently, the bacterial infections gonorrhea and syphilis were the most common STIs, but now viral diseases have taken center stage. AIDS, the most notorious STI, is caused by HIV, the virus that cripples the immune system (see Chapter 21). Here we focus on other important bacterial and viral STIs: gonorrhea, syphilis, chlamydia, trichomoniasis, genital warts, and genital herpes.

Gonorrhea

The causative agent of **gonorrhea** (gon″o-re′ah) is *Neisseria gonorrhoeae*, which invades the mucosae of the reproductive and urinary tracts. These bacteria are spread by contact with genital, anal, and pharyngeal mucosal surfaces. Commonly called "the clap," gonorrhea occurs most frequently in adolescents and young adults.

In men, the most common symptom of gonorrhea is *urethritis*, inflammation of the urethra accompanied by painful urination and discharge of pus from the penis (penile "drip"). Symptoms vary in women, ranging from none (about 20% of cases) to abdominal discomfort, vaginal discharge, abnormal uterine bleeding, and occasionally, urethral symptoms similar to those seen in males.

In men, untreated gonorrhea can cause urethral constriction and inflammation of the entire male duct system. In women, it causes pelvic inflammatory disease and sterility. With the advent of antibiotics these complications have declined, and cases of gonorrhea in the United States have dropped to the lowest rate ever recorded. However, antibiotic-resistant strains are becoming increasingly prevalent. Currently, ceftriaxone is the antibiotic used most often to treat gonorrhea.

Syphilis

Syphilis (sif′ĭ-lis), caused by the corkscrew-shaped bacterium *Treponema pallidum*, is usually transmitted sexually, but it can be contracted congenitally from an infected mother. Fetuses infected with syphilis are usually stillborn or die shortly after birth.

The bacterium easily penetrates intact mucosae and abraded skin. Within a few hours of exposure, an asymptomatic body-wide infection is in progress. After an incubation period of two to three weeks, a red, painless primary lesion called a *chancre* (shang′ker) appears at the site of bacterial invasion. In males, this is typically the penis, but in females the lesion often goes undetected within the vagina or on the cervix. The chancre ulcerates and becomes crusty, and then it heals spontaneously and disappears within a few weeks.

If syphilis is untreated, its secondary signs appear several weeks later. A pink skin rash all over the body is one of the first symptoms. Fever and joint pain are common. These signs and symptoms disappear spontaneously in three to twelve weeks. Then the disease enters the *latent period* and is detectable only by a blood test. The latent stage may last a person's lifetime (or the immune system may kill the bacteria), or it may be followed by *tertiary syphilis*.

Tertiary syphilis is characterized by *gummas* (gum′ahs), destructive lesions of the CNS, blood vessels, bones, and skin. Penicillin is still the treatment of choice for all stages of syphilis, but the number of recorded cases continues to increase in the U.S.

Chlamydia

Chlamydia (klah-mid′e-ah; *chlamys* = cloak) is a largely undiagnosed, silent epidemic that is currently on the rise in college-age people. It infects perhaps 4–5 million people yearly, making it the most common bacterial sexually transmitted infection in the United States.

Chlamydia is responsible for 25–50% of all diagnosed cases of pelvic inflammatory disease (and, consequently, at least a one-in-four chance of ectopic pregnancy). Each year more than 150,000 infants are born to infected mothers. About 20% of men and 30% of women infected with gonorrhea are also infected by *Chlamydia trachomatis*, the causative agent of chlamydia.

Chlamydia is a bacterium with a viruslike dependence on host cells. Its incubation period within the body cells is about one week. Symptoms include urethritis (involving painful, frequent urination and a thick penile discharge); vaginal discharge; abdominal, rectal, or testicular pain; painful intercourse; and irregular menses. In men, it can cause arthritis as well as widespread urogenital tract infection. In women, 80% of whom suffer *no* symptoms from the infection, it is a major cause of sterility. Newborns infected in the birth canal tend to develop conjunctivitis (specifically, *trachoma*, a painful eye infection that leads to corneal scarring if untreated (often the case in nonindustrialized countries) and respiratory tract inflammations including pneumonia.

Chlamydia can be diagnosed by cell culture techniques and is easily treated with tetracycline. In 2010, reported cases of chlamydia in the United States reached a record high of 1.2 million cases.

Trichomoniasis

Trichomoniasis is the most common *curable* STI in sexually active young women in the United States. Accounting for about 7.4 million new cases of STI per year, this parasitic infection is easily and inexpensively treated. Trichomoniasis is indicated by a yellow-green vaginal discharge with a strong odor. However, many of its victims exhibit no symptoms.

Genital Warts

Genital warts due to the *human papillomavirus* (*HPV*)—actually a group of about 60 viruses—is the second most common STI in the United States. About 6.2 million new cases of genital warts develop in Americans each year, and it appears that HPV infection increases the risk for cancers in infected body regions. Indeed, the virus is linked to 80% of all cases of invasive cervical cancer. Importantly, most of the strains that cause genital warts do not cause cervical cancer.

Treatment is difficult and controversial, and the warts tend to reappear. Some clinicians prefer to leave the warts untreated unless they become widespread, whereas others recommend their removal by cryosurgery or laser therapy, and/or treatment with alpha interferon.

Genital Herpes

The cause of **genital herpes** is the *herpes simplex virus 2*, and these viruses are among the most difficult human pathogens to control. They remain silent for weeks or years and then suddenly flare up, causing a burst of blisterlike lesions. The virus is transmitted via infectious secretions or direct skin-to-skin contact when the virus is shedding. The painful lesions that appear on the reproductive organs of infected adults are usually more of a nuisance than a threat. However, congenital herpes infections can cause severe malformations of a fetus.

Most people who have genital herpes do not know it, and it has been estimated that one-quarter to one-half of all adult Americans harbor the herpes simplex virus 2. Only about 15% of that population displays signs of infection.

The antiviral drug *acyclovir*, which helps the lesions heal faster and reduces the frequency of flare-ups, is the treatment of choice. However, once contracted, genital herpes never leaves. It just goes into periodic remissions.

Check Your Understanding

37. Which pathogen is most associated with cervical cancer?
38. What is the most common bacterial STI in the United States?

For answers, see Appendix H.

Developmental Aspects of the Reproductive System

So far, we have described the reproductive organs as they exist and operate in adults. Now we are ready to look at events that cause us to become reproductive individuals. These events begin long before birth and end, at least in women, in late middle age.

Embryological and Fetal Events

✓ Discuss the determination of genetic sex and prenatal development of male and female structures.

Determination of Genetic Sex

Aristotle believed that the "heat" of lovemaking determined maleness. Not so! Genetic sex is determined at the instant the genes of a sperm combine with those of an ovum, and the determining factor is the **sex chromosomes** each gamete contains. Of the 46 chromosomes in the fertilized egg, two (one pair) are sex chromosomes. The other 44 are called **autosomes**.

Two types of sex chromosomes, quite different in size, exist in humans: the large **X chromosome** and the much smaller **Y chromosome**. The body cells of females have two X chromosomes and are designated XX, and the ovum resulting from normal meiosis in a female always contains an X chromosome. Males have one X chromosome and one Y in each body cell (XY). Approximately half of the sperm produced by normal meiosis in males contain an X and the other half a Y.

If the fertilizing sperm delivers an X chromosome, the fertilized egg and its daughter cells will contain the female (XX) composition, and the embryo will develop ovaries. If the sperm bears a Y chromosome, the offspring will be male (XY) and will develop testes. A single gene on the Y chromosome—the ***SRY*** (for **s**ex-determining **r**egion of the **Y** chromosome) **gene**—is the master switch that initiates testes development and hence maleness. Thus, the father's gamete determines the genetic sex of the offspring. All subsequent events of sexual differentiation depend on which gonads form during embryonic life.

However, some of the genes present in autosomes are necessary for a male to become a functional male. Mutation of the *SRY* gene can result in XY individuals with the male chromosome but female sex characteristics.

Homeostatic Imbalance 27.9

When meiosis distributes the sex chromosomes to the gametes improperly, an event called **nondisjunction**, abnormal combinations of sex chromosomes occur in the zygote (fertilized egg) and cause striking abnormalities in sexual and reproductive system development.

For example, females with a single X chromosome (XO), a condition called *Turner's syndrome*, never develop ovaries. As a rule, females carrying four or more X chromosomes are mentally retarded and have underdeveloped ovaries and limited fertility.

Klinefelter's syndrome, which affects one out of 500 live male births, is the most common sex chromosome abnormality.

Affected individuals usually have a single Y chromosome, two or more X chromosomes, and are sterile males. Although XXY males are normal (or only slightly below normal) intellectually, the incidence of mental retardation increases as the number of X chromosomes rises. Males with no X chromosome (YO) die during embryonic development. ✚

Sexual Differentiation of the Reproductive System

The gonads of both males and females begin their development during week 5 of gestation as masses of mesoderm called the **gonadal ridges** **(Figure 27.23)**. These ridges bulge from the dorsal abdominal wall just medial to the mesonephros (a transient kidney system, see p. 983). The **paramesonephric**, or **Müllerian, ducts** (future female ducts) develop lateral to the **mesonephric (Wolffian) ducts** (future male ducts), and both sets of ducts empty into a common chamber called the *cloaca*. At this stage of development, the embryo is said to be in the **sexually indifferent stage**, because the gonadal ridge tissue can develop into either male or female gonads and both duct systems are present.

Shortly after the gonadal ridges appear, **primordial germ cells** migrate to them from a different region of the embryo, the hindgut, presumably guided by a gradient of chemical signals (chemokines). There they seed the developing gonads with stem cells destined to become spermatogonia or oogonia. Once these cells are in residence, the gonadal ridges form testes or ovaries, depending on the genetic makeup of the embryo.

The process of forming the testes begins in week 7 in male embryos. Seminiferous tubules form in the internal part of the gonadal ridges and join the mesonephric duct via the efferent ductules. Further development of the mesonephric duct produces the duct system of the male. The paramesonephric ducts degenerate.

In female embryos the process of gonad formation begins about a week later. The outer, or cortical, part of each immature ovary forms follicles, and the paramesonephric ducts differentiate into the structures of the female duct system (the uterine tubes and uterus). The mesonephric ducts degenerate.

Like the gonads, the external genitalia arise from the same structures in both sexes **(Figure 27.24)**. During the sexually indifferent stage, all embryos exhibit a small external projection called the **genital tubercle**. The urogenital sinus, which develops from subdivision of the cloaca (future urethra and bladder), lies deep to the tubercle. The **urethral groove**, the external opening of the urogenital sinus, is on the tubercle's inferior surface and is flanked laterally by the **urethral folds** and then the **labioscrotal swellings**.

During week 8, the external genitalia begin to develop rapidly. In males, the genital tubercle enlarges, forming the penis. The urethral folds fuse in the midline, forming the spongy urethra in the penis. Only the tips of the folds remain unfused to form the *urethral orifice* at the tip of the penis. The labioscrotal swellings also fuse medially to form the scrotum.

In females, the genital tubercle gives rise to the clitoris and the urethral groove persists as the vestibule. The unfused urethral folds become the labia minora, and the unfused labioscrotal folds become the labia majora.

Differentiation of accessory structures and the external genitalia into male or female structures depends on whether testosterone is present. When testes form, they quickly begin to release testosterone, which continues until four to five days after birth and which causes the development of male accessory ducts and external genitalia. In the absence of testosterone, the female ducts and external genitalia develop.

Homeostatic Imbalance 27.10

Any interference with the normal pattern of sex hormone production in the embryo results in abnormalities. For example:

- If the embryonic testes do not produce testosterone, a genetic male develops female accessory structures and external genitalia.
- If a genetic female is exposed to testosterone (as might happen if the mother has an androgen-producing tumor of her adrenal gland), the embryo has ovaries but develops the male ducts and glands, as well as a penis and an empty scrotum.

It appears that the female pattern of reproductive structures has an intrinsic ability to develop (it is the default condition). In the absence of testosterone it proceeds to do so, regardless of the embryo's genetic makeup.

Individuals with external genitalia that do not "match" their gonads are called *pseudohermaphrodites* (soo-do-her-maf′ro-dīts). (True *hermaphrodites* who possess both ovarian and testicular tissue are rare.) Many pseudohermaphrodites have sought sex-change operations to match their outer selves (external genitalia) with their inner selves (gonads). ✚

Descent of the Gonads

About two months before birth, the testes begin their descent toward the scrotum, dragging their supplying blood vessels and nerves along behind them. They finally exit from the pelvic cavity via the inguinal canals and enter the scrotum. Testosterone made by the fetus's testes stimulates this migration. The migration is mechanically guided by a strong fibrous cord called the **gubernaculum** ("governor"), which extends from the testis to the floor of the scrotal sac.

Initially the gubernaculum is a column of soft connective tissue, but it becomes increasingly fibrous as it continues to grow. By the seventh month of fetal development, it stops growing and its inferior part fills the inguinal canal. The gubernaculum's cessation of growth, coupled with the rapid growth of the fetal body, helps to pull the testes into the scrotum.

The *tunica vaginalis* covering of the testis is derived from a fingerlike outpocketing of the parietal peritoneum, the *vaginal process*. The accompanying blood vessels, nerves, and fascial layers form part of the *spermatic cord*, which helps suspend the testis within the scrotum.

Like the testes, the ovaries descend during fetal development, but in this case only to the pelvic brim, where the tentlike broad ligament stops their progress. Each ovary is guided in its descent by a gubernaculum (anchored in the labium majus) that later divides, becoming the ovarian and round ligaments that help support the internal genitalia in the pelvis.

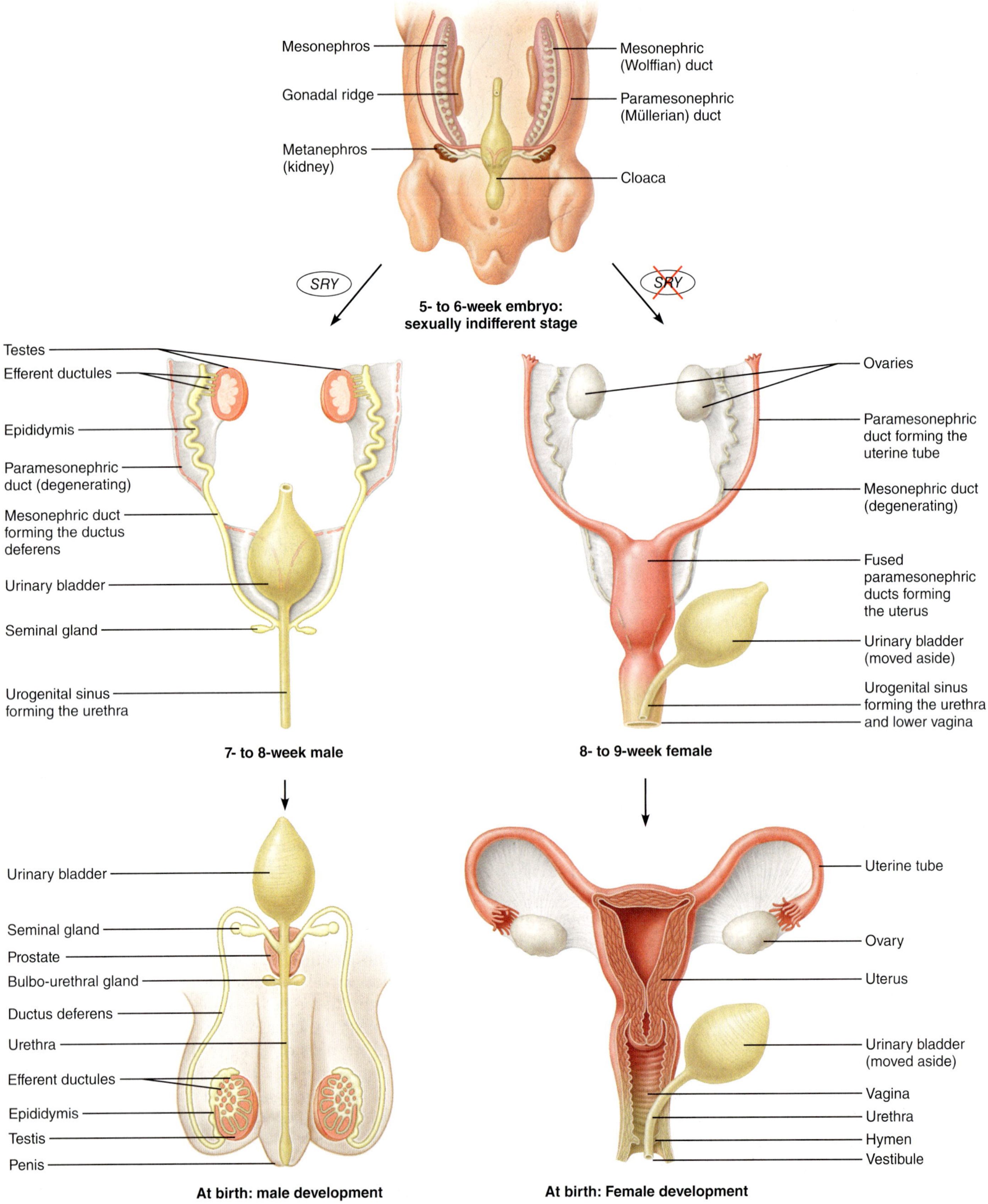

Figure 27.23 Development of the internal reproductive organs. (*SRY* = sex-determining region of the Y chromosome.)

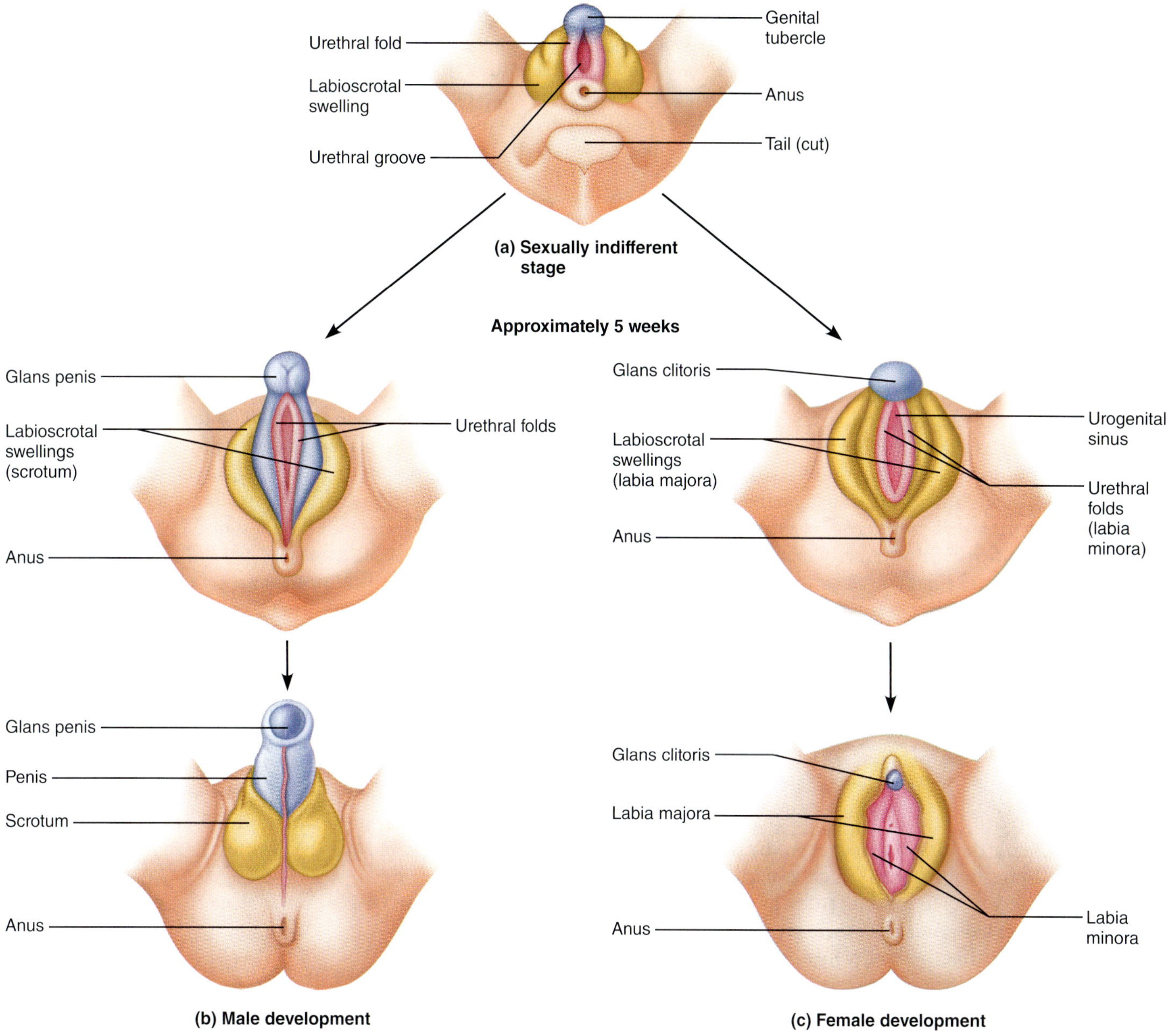

Figure 27.24 Development of homologous structures of the external genitalia in both sexes. The two pictures at the bottom of the figure show the fully developed perineal region.

Homeostatic Imbalance 27.11

Failure of the testes to make their normal descent leads to *cryptorchidism* (*crypt* = hidden, concealed; *orchi* = testicle). Because cryptorchidism causes sterility and increases the risk of testicular cancer, surgery is usually performed during early childhood to rectify this problem. +

Check Your Understanding

39. If a fertilized egg contains X and Y sex chromosomes, a baby girl will develop, right?
40. What is the sexually indifferent stage of development?
41. Which structure guides the descent of the testis into the scrotum?

For answers, see Appendix H.

Puberty

✓ Describe the significant events of puberty and menopause.

FSH and LH levels, elevated at birth, fall to low levels within a few months and remain low throughout the prepubertal years. Between the ages of 10 and 15 years, a host of interacting hormones bring on the changes of puberty.

Puberty is the period of life when the reproductive organs grow to adult size and become functional. As puberty nears, these changes occur in response to rising levels of gonadal hormones (testosterone in males and estrogen in females). Earlier we described secondary sex characteristics and regulatory events of puberty. But it is important to remember that puberty represents the earliest time that reproduction is possible.

The events of puberty occur in the same sequence in all individuals, but the age at which they occur varies widely.

In males, secretion of adrenal androgens, particularly dehydroepiandrosterone (DHEA), begins to rise several years before the testosterone surge of puberty and initiates facial, pubic, and axillary hair growth and other pubertal events. The major event that signals puberty's onset in males is enlargement of the testes and scrotum between the ages of 8 and 14. The penis grows over the next two years, and sexual maturation is evidenced by the presence of mature sperm in the semen (see Figure 27.11). In the meantime, the young man has unexpected erections and occasional nocturnal emissions ("wet dreams") as his hormones surge and the hormonal control axis struggles to achieve a normal balance.

In females, the first sign of puberty is budding breasts between the ages of 8 and 13, followed by the appearance of axillary and pubic hair. Menarche usually occurs about two years later. Dependable ovulation and fertility await the maturation of the hormonal controls, which takes nearly two more years.

Epiphyseal plate closure and termination of skeletal growth in height occurs in response to rising estrogen levels late in puberty in both boys and girls.

Menopause

Most women reach the peak of their reproductive abilities in their late 20s. After that, ovarian function declines gradually, presumably because the ovaries become less and less responsive to gonadotropin signals. At age 30, there are still some 100,000 oocytes in the ovaries but the quality (hence fertility) has begun to decline. By age 50, there are probably 1000 eggs left (the pantry is nearly bare).

As estrogen production declines, many ovarian cycles become anovulatory, while in others 2 to 4 oocytes per month are ovulated, a sign of declining control. Increasingly frequent multiple ovulations explain why twins and triplets are more common in women who have deferred childbearing until their late 30s. In the perimenopausal period, menstrual periods become erratic and increasingly shorter. Eventually, ovulation and menstruation cease entirely. This normally occurs between the ages of 46 and 54, an event called *menopause*. **Menopause** is considered to have occurred when a whole year has passed without menstruation.

Although the ovaries continue to produce estrogen for a while after menopause, they finally stop functioning as endocrine organs. Without sufficient estrogen the reproductive organs and breasts begin to atrophy, the vagina becomes dry, and vaginal infections become increasingly common. Other sequels due to lack of estrogen include irritability and depression (in some women); intense vasodilation of the skin's blood vessels, which causes uncomfortable, sweat-drenching "hot flashes"; gradually thinning skin; and loss of bone mass. Slowly rising total blood cholesterol levels and falling HDL levels place postmenopausal women at risk for cardiovascular disorders. At one time physicians prescribed low-dose estrogen-progesterone preparations to help women through this period and prevent skeletal and cardiovascular complications. This seemed like a great idea and by 2002, approximately 14 million American women were taking some form of estrogen-containing hormone replacement therapy (HRT). Then, the Women's Health Initiative (WHI) abruptly ended a clinical trial of 16,000 postmenopausal women, reporting that those who took a popular progesterone-estrogen medication had an increased risk of 51% in heart disease, 24% in invasive breast cancer, 31% in stroke, and a doubled risk of dementia compared to those taking placebos.

The backlash of this information (aired in the popular press) is still spreading through physicians' offices and research labs. It is restricting funding and the ability to find new volunteers for future studies, and has dampened enthusiasm for HRT in both the medical community and postmenopausal women. However, newer data suggest that the smallest dose of HRT for the shortest time is OK to reduce symptoms in women who do not have existing breast cancer or mutated *BRCA* gene(s).

There is no equivalent of menopause in males, and healthy men are able to father offspring well into their eighth decade of life thanks to their small but enduring population of stem cells (spermatogonia). However, aging men do exhibit a steady decline in testosterone secretion and experience a longer latent period after orgasm, a condition sometimes called *andropause*, and testosterone replacement therapy is currently being prescribed for more older men. Additionally, there is a noticeable difference in sperm motility with aging. Sperm of a young man can make it up the uterine tubes in 20–50 minutes, whereas those of a 75-year-old take 2½ days for the same trip.

☑ Check Your Understanding

42. What are the early signs of puberty's onset in boys?
43. What is the definition of menopause?

For answers, see Appendix H.

The reproductive system is unique among organ systems in at least two ways: (1) It is nonfunctional during the first 10–15 years of life, and (2) it is capable of interacting with the complementary system of another person—indeed, it *must* do so to carry out its biological function of pregnancy and birth. To be sure, having a baby is not always what the interacting partners have in mind, and we humans have devised a variety of techniques for preventing this outcome (see *A Closer Look* on pp. 1090–1091).

The major goal of the reproductive system is ensuring the healthy function of its own organs so that conditions are optimal for producing offspring. However, as illustrated in *System Connections*, gonadal hormones do influence other body organs, and the reproductive system depends on other body systems for oxygen and nutrients and to carry away and dispose of its wastes.

Now that we know how the reproductive system prepares itself for childbearing, we are ready to consider the events of pregnancy and prenatal development of a new living being, the topics of Chapter 28.

Homeostatic Interrelationships Between the Reproductive System and Other Body Systems

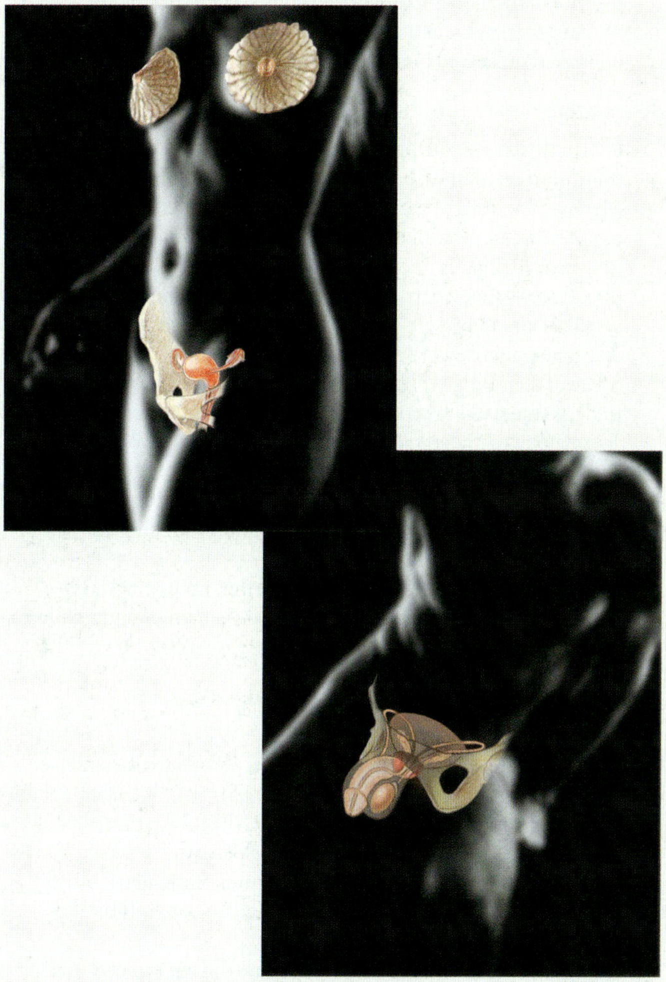

Integumentary System Chapter 5

- Androgens activate oil glands that lubricate skin and hair; gonadal hormones stimulate characteristic fat distribution and appearance of pubic and axillary hair; estrogen increases skin hydration, and during pregnancy it enhances facial skin pigmentation
- Skin protects all body organs by external enclosure; mammary gland secretions (milk) nourish the infant

Skeletal System Chapters 6–8

- Androgens masculinize the skeleton and increase bone density; estrogen feminizes the skeleton and maintains bone mass in females
- The bony pelvis encloses some reproductive organs; if narrow, the bony pelvis may hinder vaginal delivery of an infant

Muscular System Chapters 9–10

- Androgens promote increased muscle mass
- Abdominal muscles active during childbirth; muscles of the pelvic floor support reproductive organs and aid erection of penis/clitoris

Nervous System Chapters 11–15

- Sex hormones masculinize or feminize the brain and influence sex drive
- Hypothalamus regulates timing of puberty; neural reflexes regulate events of sexual response

Endocrine System Chapter 16

- Gonadal hormones exert feedback effects on hypothalamic-pituitary axis; placental hormones promote maternal hypermetabolism
- Gonadotropins (and GnRH) help regulate function of gonads; leptin signals the hypothalamus about the body's state of energy availability (in fat stores)

Cardiovascular System Chapters 17–19

- Estrogens lower blood cholesterol levels and promote cardiovascular health in premenopausal women; pregnancy increases workload of the cardiovascular system
- Cardiovascular system transports needed substances to organs of reproductive system; local vasodilation involved in erection; blood transports sex hormones

Lymphatic System/Immunity Chapters 20–21

- Developing embryo/fetus escapes immune surveillance (not rejected)
- Lymphatic vessels drain leaked tissue fluids; transport sex hormones; immune cells protect reproductive organs from disease; IgA is present in breast milk

Respiratory System Chapter 22

- Pregnancy impairs descent of the diaphragm, promotes dyspnea
- Respiratory system provides oxygen; disposes of carbon dioxide; tidal volume increases during pregnancy while residual volume declines

Digestive System Chapter 23

- Developing fetus crowds digestive organs; heartburn, constipation common during pregnancy
- Digestive system provides nutrients needed for health

Urinary System Chapters 25–26

- Hypertrophy of the prostate inhibits urination; compression of bladder during pregnancy leads to urinary frequency and urgency
- Kidneys dispose of nitrogenous wastes and maintain acid-base balance of blood of mother and fetus; semen discharged through the urethra of the male

Chapter Summary

MAP™ For more chapter study tools, go to the Study Area of MasteringA&P at www.masteringaandp.com.

There you will find:

- Interactive Physiology iP
- A&PFlix A&PFlix
- Practice Anatomy Lab PAL
- PhysioEx PEx
- Videos, Practice Quizzes and Tests, MP3 Tutor Sessions, Case Studies, and much more!

1. The function of the reproductive system is to produce offspring. The gonads produce gametes (sperm or ova) and sex hormones. All other reproductive organs are accessory organs.

Anatomy of the Male Reproductive System (pp. 1019–1026)

The Scrotum (pp. 1019–1020)

1. The scrotum contains the testes. It provides a temperature slightly lower than that of body temperature, as required to produce viable sperm.

The Testes (pp. 1020–1022)

2. Each testis is covered externally by a tunica albuginea that extends internally to divide the testis into many lobules. Each lobule contains sperm-producing seminiferous tubules and interstitial endocrine cells that produce androgens.

The Male Perineum and the Penis (pp. 1022–1023)

3. The male perineum which suspends the scrotum and penis, is the region encompassed by the pubic symphysis, ischial tuberosities, and coccyx.
4. The penis is largely erectile tissue (corpus spongiosum and corpora cavernosa). Engorgement of the erectile tissue with blood causes the penis to become rigid, an event called erection.

The Male Duct System (p. 1024)

5. The epididymis hugs the external surface of the testis and serves as a site for sperm maturation and storage.
6. The ductus (vas) deferens, extending from the epididymis to the ejaculatory duct, propels sperm into the urethra by peristalsis during ejaculation. Its terminus fuses with the duct of the seminal gland, forming the ejaculatory duct, which empties into the urethra within the prostate.
7. The urethra extends from the urinary bladder to the tip of the penis. It conducts semen and urine to the body exterior.

The Male Accessory Glands (pp. 1024–1026)

8. The accessory glands produce the bulk of the semen, which contains fructose from the seminal glands, an activating fluid from the prostate, and mucus from the bulbo-urethral glands.

Semen (p. 1026)

9. Semen is an alkaline fluid that dilutes and transports sperm. Important chemicals in semen are nutrients, prostaglandins, and antibiotic chemicals.

Physiology of the Male Reproductive System (pp. 1026–1035)

Male Sexual Response (pp. 1026–1027)

1. Parasympathetic reflexes control erection.
2. Ejaculation is expulsion of semen from the male duct system, promoted by the sympathetic nervous system. Ejaculation is part of male orgasm, which also includes pleasurable sensations and increased pulse and blood pressure.

Spermatogenesis (pp. 1027–1033)

3. Spermatogenesis, the production of male gametes in the seminiferous tubules, begins at puberty.
4. Meiosis, the basis of gamete production, consists of two consecutive nuclear divisions without DNA replication in between. Meiosis reduces the chromosomal number by half and introduces genetic variability. Events unique to meiosis include synapsis and crossover of homologous chromosomes.
5. Spermatogonia divide by mitosis to maintain the germ cell line. Some of their progeny become primary spermatocytes, which undergo meiosis I to produce secondary spermatocytes. Secondary spermatocytes undergo meiosis II, each producing two haploid (n) spermatids.
6. Spermiogenesis converts spermatids to functional sperm, stripping away superfluous cytoplasm and producing an acrosome and a flagellum (tail).
7. Sustentocytes form the blood testis barrier, nourish spermatogenic cells, move them toward the lumen of the tubules, and secrete fluid for sperm transport.

Hormonal Regulation of Male Reproductive Function (pp. 1033–1035)

8. GnRH, produced by the hypothalamus, stimulates the anterior pituitary gland to release FSH and LH. FSH causes sustentocytes to produce androgen-binding protein (ABP). LH stimulates interstitial endocrine cells to release testosterone, which binds to ABP, stimulating spermatogenesis. Testosterone and inhibin (produced by sustentocytes) feed back to inhibit the hypothalamus and anterior pituitary.
9. Maturation of hormonal controls occurs during puberty and takes about three years.
10. Testosterone stimulates maturation of the male reproductive organs and triggers the development of the secondary sex characteristics of the male. It exerts anabolic effects on the skeleton and skeletal muscles, stimulates spermatogenesis, and is responsible for male sex drive.

Anatomy of the Female Reproductive System (pp. 1035–1043)

1. The female reproductive system produces gametes and sex hormones and houses a developing infant until birth.

The Ovaries (pp. 1035–1036)

2. The ovaries flank the uterus laterally and are held in position by the ovarian and suspensory ligaments and mesovaria.
3. Within each ovary are oocyte-containing follicles at different stages of development and possibly a corpus luteum.

The Female Duct System (pp. 1037–1041)

4. The uterine tube, supported by the mesosalpinx, extends from near the ovary to the uterus. Its fimbriae and ciliated distal end along with peristalsis create currents that help move an ovulated oocyte into the uterine tube.
5. The uterus has fundus, body, and cervical regions. It is supported by the broad, cardinal, uterosacral, and round ligaments.

6. The uterine wall is composed of the outer perimetrium, the myometrium, and the inner endometrium. The endometrium consists of a functional layer (stratum functionalis), which sloughs off periodically unless an embryo has implanted, and an underlying basal layer (stratum basalis), which rebuilds the functional layer.
7. The vagina extends from the uterus to the exterior. It is the copulatory organ and allows passage of the menstrual flow or a baby.

The External Genitalia and Female Perineum (p. 1041)

8. The female external genitalia (vulva) include the mons pubis, labia majora and minora, clitoris, and the urethral and vaginal orifices. The labia majora house the mucus-secreting greater vestibular glands.

The Mammary Glands (pp. 1041–1043)

9. The mammary glands lie over the pectoral muscles of the chest and are surrounded by adipose and fibrous connective tissue. Each mammary gland consists of many lobules, which contain milk-producing alveoli.

Physiology of the Female Reproductive System (pp. 1043–1053)

Oogenesis (pp. 1043–1045)

1. Oogenesis, the production of eggs, begins in the fetus. Oogonia, the diploid stem cells of female gametes, are converted to primary oocytes before birth. The infant female's ovaries contain about 1 million primary oocytes arrested in prophase of meiosis I.
2. At puberty, meiosis resumes. Each month, one primary oocyte completes meiosis I, producing a large secondary oocyte and a tiny first polar body. Meiosis II of the secondary oocyte produces a functional ovum and a second polar body, but does not occur in humans unless a sperm penetrates the secondary oocyte.
3. The ovum contains most of the primary oocyte's cytoplasm. The polar bodies are nonfunctional and degenerate.

The Ovarian Cycle (pp. 1045–1047)

4. During the follicular phase (days 1–14), several primary follicles begin to mature. Generally, only one follicle per month completes the maturation process, becoming the dominant follicle. Late in this phase, the oocyte in the dominant follicle completes meiosis I. Ovulation occurs about day 14, releasing the secondary oocyte into the peritoneal cavity. Other developing follicles deteriorate.
5. In the luteal phase (days 15–28), the ruptured follicle is converted to a corpus luteum, which produces progesterone and estrogen for the remainder of the cycle. If fertilization does not occur, the corpus luteum degenerates after about 10 days.

Hormonal Regulation of the Ovarian Cycle (pp. 1047–1049)

6. Beginning at puberty, the hormones of the hypothalamus, anterior pituitary, and ovaries interact to establish and regulate the ovarian cycle. Establishment of the mature cyclic pattern, indicated by menarche, takes about four years. Leptin serves a permissive role in puberty's onset, stimulating the hypothalamus when adipose tissue is sufficient for the energy requirements of reproduction.
7. The hormonal events of each ovarian cycle are as follows: (1) GnRH stimulates the anterior pituitary to release FSH and LH, which stimulate follicle maturation and estrogen production. (2) When blood estrogen reaches a certain level, positive feedback exerted on the hypothalamic-pituitary-gonadal axis causes a sudden release of LH that stimulates the primary oocyte to continue meiosis and triggers ovulation. LH then causes conversion of the ruptured follicle to a corpus luteum and stimulates its secretory activity. (3) Rising levels of progesterone and estrogen inhibit the hypothalamic-pituitary-gonadal (HPG) axis, the corpus luteum deteriorates, ovarian hormones drop to their lowest levels, and the cycle begins anew.

The Uterine (Menstrual) Cycle (pp. 1049–1051)

8. Varying levels of ovarian hormones in the blood trigger events of the uterine cycle.
9. During the menstrual phase of the uterine cycle (days 1–5), the functional layer sloughs off in menses. During the proliferative phase (days 6–14), rising estrogen levels stimulate its regeneration, making the uterus receptive to implantation about one week after ovulation. During the secretory phase (days 15–28), the uterine glands secrete nutrients, and endometrial vascularity increases further.
10. Falling levels of ovarian hormones during the last few days of the ovarian cycle cause the spiral arteries to become spastic and cut off the blood supply of the functional layer, and the uterine cycle begins again with menstruation.

Effects of Estrogens and Progesterone (p. 1051)

11. Estrogen promotes oogenesis. At puberty, it stimulates the growth of the reproductive organs and the growth spurt and promotes the appearance of the secondary sex characteristics.
12. Progesterone cooperates with estrogen in breast maturation and regulation of the uterine cycle.

Female Sexual Response (pp. 1051–1053)

13. The female sexual response is similar to that of males. Orgasm in females is not accompanied by ejaculation.

Sexually Transmitted Infections (pp. 1053–1054)

1. Sexually transmitted infections (STIs) are infectious diseases spread via sexual contact. Gonorrhea, syphilis, and chlamydia are bacterial diseases. Syphilis has broader consequences than most other sexually transmitted bacterial diseases since it can infect organs throughout the body. Trichomoniasis is a parasitic infection. Genital herpes and genital warts are viral infections; genital warts, caused by the HPV virus, are implicated in cervical cancer.

Developmental Aspects of the Reproductive System (pp. 1054–1058)

Embryological and Fetal Events (pp. 1054–1057)

1. Genetic sex is determined by the sex chromosomes: an X from the mother, an X or a Y from the father. If the fertilized egg contains XX, it is a female and develops ovaries; if it contains XY, it is a male and develops testes.
2. Gonads of both sexes arise from the mesodermal gonadal ridges. The mesonephric ducts produce the male accessory ducts and glands. The paramesonephric ducts produce the female duct system.
3. The external genitalia arise from the genital tubercle and associated structures. The development of male accessory structures and external genitalia depends on the presence of testosterone produced by the embryonic testes. In its absence, female structures develop.
4. The testes descend into the scrotum from the abdominal cavity.

Puberty (pp. 1057–1058)

5. Puberty is the interval when reproductive organs mature and become functional. It begins in males with penile and scrotal growth and in females with breast development.

Menopause (p. 1058)

6. During menopause, ovulation and menstruation cease. Hot flashes and mood changes may occur. Postmenopausal events include atrophy of the reproductive organs, bone mass loss, and increasing risk for cardiovascular disease. Men experience andropause with milder signs and symptoms of testosterone deficit.

Review Questions

Multiple Choice/Matching

(Some questions have more than one correct answer. Select the best answer or answers from the choices given.)

1. The structures that draw an ovulated oocyte into the female duct system are **(a)** cilia, **(b)** fimbriae, **(c)** microvilli, **(d)** stereocilia.
2. The usual site of embryo implantation is **(a)** the uterine tube, **(b)** the peritoneal cavity, **(c)** the vagina, **(d)** the uterus.
3. The male homologue of the female clitoris is **(a)** the penis, **(b)** the scrotum, **(c)** the penile urethra, **(d)** the testis.
4. Which of the following is correct relative to female anatomy? **(a)** the vaginal orifice is the most dorsal of the three openings in the perineum, **(b)** the urethra is between the vaginal orifice and the anus, **(c)** the anus is between the vaginal orifice and the urethra, **(d)** the urethra is the more ventral of the two orifices in the vulva.
5. Secondary sex characteristics are **(a)** present in the embryo, **(b)** a result of male or female sex hormones increasing in amount at puberty, **(c)** the testis in the male and the ovary in the female, **(d)** not subject to withdrawal once established.
6. Which of the following produces the male sex hormones? **(a)** seminal glands, **(b)** corpus luteum, **(c)** developing follicles of the testes, **(d)** interstitial endocrine cells.
7. Which will occur as a result of nondescent of the testes? **(a)** male sex hormones will not be circulated in the body, **(b)** sperm will have no means of exit from the body, **(c)** inadequate blood supply will retard the development of the testes, **(d)** viable sperm will not be produced.
8. The normal diploid number of human chromosomes is **(a)** 48, **(b)** 47, **(c)** 46, **(d)** 23, **(e)** 24.
9. Relative to differences between mitosis and meiosis, choose the statements that apply *only* to events of meiosis. **(a)** tetrads present, **(b)** produces two daughter cells, **(c)** produces four daughter cells, **(d)** occurs throughout life, **(e)** reduces the chromosomal number by half, **(f)** synapsis and crossover of homologues occur.
10. Match the key choices with the descriptive phrases below.

Key:

(a) androgen-binding protein	**(e)** inhibin
(b) estrogens	**(f)** LH
(c) FSH	**(g)** progesterone
(d) GnRH	**(h)** testosterone

____ (1) Hormones that directly regulate the ovarian cycle
____ (2) Chemicals in males that inhibit the hypothalamic-pituitary-testicular axis
____ (3) Hormone that makes the cervical mucus viscous
____ (4) Potentiates the activity of testosterone on spermatogenic cells
____ (5) In females, exerts feedback inhibition on the hypothalamus and anterior pituitary
____ (6) Stimulates the secretion of testosterone

11. The menstrual cycle can be divided into three continuous phases. Starting from the first day of the cycle, their consecutive order is **(a)** menstrual, proliferative, secretory, **(b)** menstrual, secretory, proliferative, **(c)** secretory, menstrual, proliferative, **(d)** proliferative, menstrual, secretory, **(e)** secretory, proliferative, menstrual.
12. Spermatozoa are to seminiferous tubules as oocytes are to **(a)** fimbriae, **(b)** corpus albicans, **(c)** ovarian follicles, **(d)** corpora lutea.
13. Which of the following does not add a secretion that makes a major contribution to semen? **(a)** prostate, **(b)** bulbo-urethral glands, **(c)** testes, **(d)** ductus deferens.
14. The corpus luteum is formed at the site of **(a)** fertilization, **(b)** ovulation, **(c)** menstruation, **(d)** implantation.
15. The sex of a child is determined by **(a)** the sex chromosome contained in the sperm, **(b)** the sex chromosome contained in the oocyte, **(c)** the number of sperm fertilizing the oocyte, **(d)** the position of the fetus in the uterus.
16. FSH is to estrogen as estrogen is to **(a)** progesterone, **(b)** LH, **(c)** FSH, **(d)** testosterone.
17. A drug that "reminds the pituitary" to produce gonadotropins might be useful as **(a)** a contraceptive, **(b)** a diuretic, **(c)** a fertility drug, **(d)** an abortion stimulant.

Short Answer Essay Questions

18. Why is the term *urogenital system* more applicable to males than to females?
19. Describe the major structural (and functional) regions of a sperm.
20. Oogenesis in the female results in one functional gamete—the egg, or ovum. What other cells are produced? What is the significance of this rather wasteful type of gamete production—that is, production of a single functional gamete instead of four, as seen in males?
21. Describe the events and possible consequences of menopause.
22. Define menarche. What does it indicate?
23. Trace the pathway of a sperm from the male testes to the uterine tube of a female.
24. In menstruation, the stratum functionalis is shed from the endometrium. Explain the hormonal and physical factors responsible for this shedding. (Hint: See Figure 27.22.)
25. Both the epithelium of the vagina and the cervical glands of the uterus help prevent the invasion and spread of vaginal pathogens. Explain how each of these mechanisms works.
26. Some anatomy students were saying that the bulbo-urethral glands of males act like city workers who come around and clear parked cars from the street before a parade. What did they mean by this analogy?
27. A man swam in a cold lake for an hour and then noticed that his scrotum was shrunken and wrinkled. His first thought was that he had lost his testicles. What had really happened?

Critical Thinking and Clinical Application Questions

1. Gina Marciano, a 44-year-old mother of eight children, visited her physician complaining of a "bearing down" sensation in her pelvis, low backache, and urinary incontinence. A vaginal examination showed that the external os of her cervix was just inside the vaginal orifice and her perineum exhibited large

keloids (masses of scar tissue). Her history revealed that she was a member of a commune located in the nearby mountains that shunned hospital births (if at all possible). What do you think Gina's problem is and what caused it? (Be anatomically specific.)

2. Harry, a sexually active adolescent, appeared in the emergency room complaining of a penile "drip" and pain during urination. An account of his recent sexual behavior was requested and recorded. (a) What do you think Harry's problem is? (b) What is the causative agent of this disorder? (c) How is the condition treated, and what may happen if it isn't treated?
3. A 36-year-old mother of four is considering tubal ligation to ensure that her family gets no larger. She asks the physician if she will become "menopausal" after the surgery. (a) How would you answer her question and explain away her concerns? (b) Explain what a tubal ligation is.
4. Mr. Scanlon, a 76-year-old gentleman, is interested in a much younger woman. Concerned because of his age, he asks his urologist if he will be able to father a child. What questions would a physician ask of this man, and what diagnostic tests would be ordered?
5. Lucy had both her left ovary and her right uterine tube removed surgically at age 17 because of a cyst and a tumor in these organs. Now, at age 32, she remains healthy and is expecting her second child. How could Lucy conceive a child with just one ovary and one uterine tube, widely separated on opposite sides of the pelvis like this?

AT THE CLINIC

Related Clinical Terms

Dysmenorrhea (dis″men-ō-re′ah; *dys* = bad, *meno* = menses, a month) Painful menstruation; may reflect abnormally high prostaglandin activity during menses.

Endometrial cancer Cancer that arises from the uterine endometrium (usually from uterine glands). Most important sign is vaginal bleeding, which allows early detection. Risk factors include obesity and HRT.

Endometriosis (en″do-me″tre-o′sis) An inflammatory condition in which endometrial tissue occurs and grows atypically in the pelvic cavity. Characterized by abnormal uterine or rectal bleeding, dysmenorrhea, and pelvic pain. May cause sterility.

Gynecology (gi″nĕ-kol′o-je; *gyneco* = woman, *ology* = study of) Specialized branch of medicine that deals with the diagnosis and treatment of female reproductive system disorders.

Gynecomastia (gi″nĕ-ko-mas′te-ah) Development of breast tissue in the male; a consequence of adrenal cortex hypersecretion of estrogens, certain drugs (cimetidine, spironolactone, and some chemotherapeutic agents), and marijuana use.

Hysterectomy (his″tĕ-rek′to-me; *hyster* = uterus, *ectomy* = cut out) Surgical removal of the uterus.

Inguinal hernia Protrusion of part of the intestine into the scrotum or through a separation in the abdominal muscles in the groin region. Since the inguinal canals represent weak points in the abdominal wall, inguinal hernia may be caused by heavy lifting or other activities that increase intra-abdominal pressure.

Laparoscopy (lap″ah-ros′ko-pe; *lapar* = the flank, *scopy* = observation) Examination of the abdominopelvic cavity with a laparoscope, a viewing device at the end of a thin tube inserted through the anterior abdominal wall. Laparoscopy is often used to assess the condition of a woman's pelvic reproductive organs.

Oophorectomy (o″of-o-rek′to-me; *oophor* = ovary) Surgical removal of the ovary.

Orchitis (or-ki′tis; *orcho* = testis) Inflammation of the testes, sometimes caused by the mumps virus.

Ovarian cancer Malignancy that typically arises from the cells in the germinal epithelial covering of the ovary. The fifth most common reproductive system cancer, its incidence increases with age. Called the "disease that whispers" because early symptoms are nondescript and easily mistaken for other disorders (back pain, abdominal discomfort, nausea, bloating, and flatulence). Diagnosis may involve palpating a mass during a physical exam, visualizing it with an ultrasound probe, or conducting blood tests for a protein marker for ovarian cancer (CA-125). However, medical assessment is often delayed until after metastasis has occurred; five-year survival rate is 90% if the condition is diagnosed before metastasis.

Ovarian cysts The most common disorders of the ovary; some are tumors. Types include (1) *simple follicle retention cysts* in which single or clustered follicles become enlarged with a clear fluid; (2) *dermoid cysts*, which are filled with a thick yellow fluid and contain partially developed hair, teeth, bone, etc.; and (3) *chocolate cysts* filled with dark gelatinous material, which are the result of endometriosis of the ovary. None of these is malignant, but the latter two may become so.

Polycystic ovary syndrome (PCOS) The most common endocrinopathy in women and the most common cause of anovulatory infertility. Affects 5–10% of women; characterized by signs of androgen excess, increased cardiovascular risk (evidenced by high blood pressure, decreased HDL cholesterol levels, and high triglycerides); and linked to extreme obesity and some degree of insulin resistance. Treated with insulin-sensitizing drugs.

Salpingitis (sal″pin-ji′tis; *salpingo* = uterine tube) Inflammation of the uterine tubes.

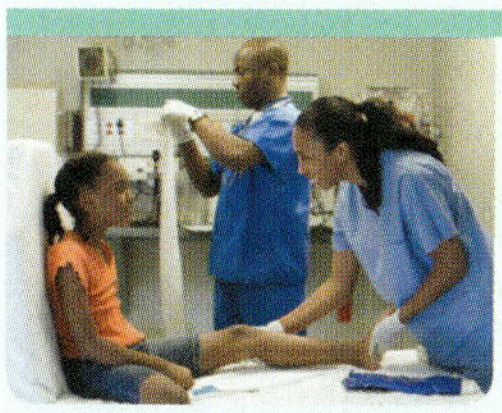

Case Study Reproductive System

We are back to look in on Mr. Heyden today. Since we last saw him (Chapter 26), he has had an X ray to determine the cause of his back pain, and his blood test results have come in. According to the note recorded at radiology: X irradiation of skeleton displays numerous carcinomatous metastases in his skull and lumbar vertebrae. The hematology note of interest here reads: PSA levels abnormally high.

1. What is carcinoma? What do you suppose is the primary source of the secondary carcinoma lesions in his skull and spine?
2. On what basis did you come to this conclusion?
3. What other tests might be of some diagnostic help here?
4. What type of therapy do you predict Mr. Heyden will be given to treat his carcinoma? Why?

(Answers in Appendix H)

28

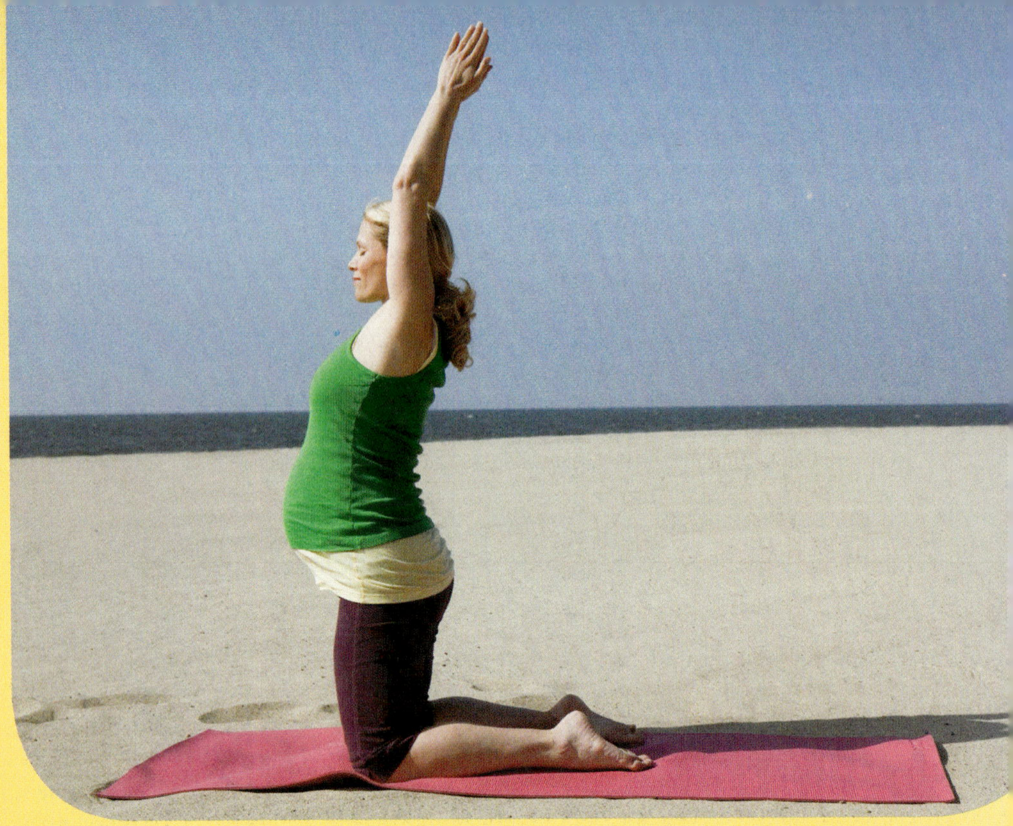

Pregnancy and Human Development

The birth of a baby is such a familiar event that we tend to lose sight of the wonder of this accomplishment: How does a single cell, the fertilized egg, grow to become a complex human being consisting of trillions of cells? The details of this process can fill a good-sized book. Our intention here is simply to outline the important events of gestation and to consider briefly the events occurring immediately after birth.

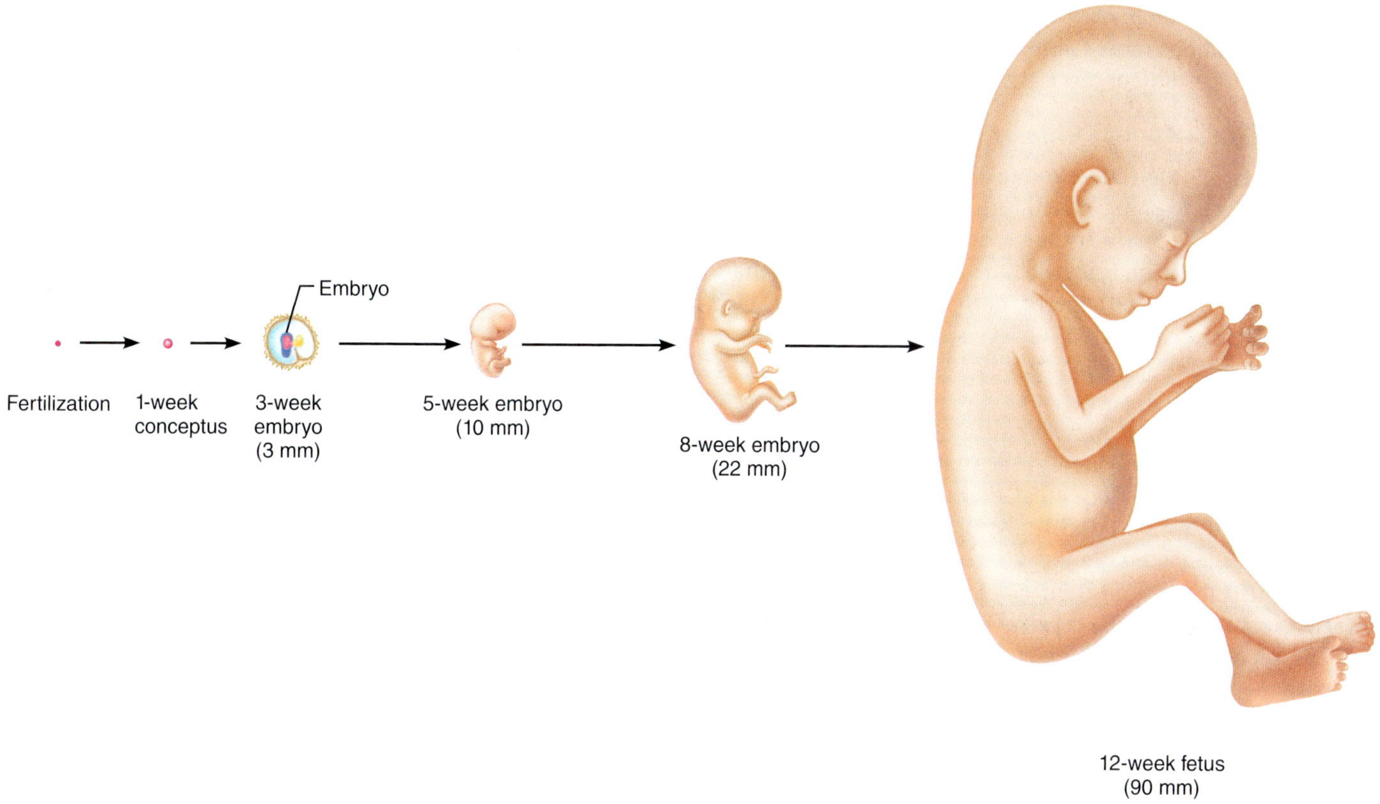

Figure 28.1 Diagrams showing the approximate size of a human conceptus from fertilization to the early fetal stage. The embryonic stage is from fertilization through week 8; the fetal stage begins in week 9. (Measurements are crown to rump length.)

Let's get started by defining some terms. The term **pregnancy** refers to events that occur from the time of fertilization (conception) until the infant is born. The pregnant woman's developing offspring is called the **conceptus** (kon-sep′tus; "that which is conceived"). Development occurs during the **gestation period** (*gestare* = to carry), which extends by convention from the last menstrual period (a date the woman is likely to remember) until birth, approximately 280 days. So, at the moment of fertilization, the mother is officially (but illogically) two weeks pregnant!

From fertilization through week 8, the *embryonic period*, the conceptus is called an **embryo**, and from week 9 through birth, the *fetal period*, the conceptus is called a **fetus** ("the young in the womb"). At birth, it is an infant. **Figure 28.1** shows the changing size and shape of the conceptus as it progresses from fertilization to the early fetal stage.

From Egg to Zygote

✓ Describe the importance of sperm capacitation.

✓ Explain the mechanism of the slow block to polyspermy.

✓ Define fertilization.

Before fertilization can occur, sperm must reach the ovulated secondary oocyte. The oocyte is viable for 12 to 24 hours after it is cast out of the ovary. The chance of pregnancy drops to almost zero the next day. Most sperm retain their fertilizing power for 24 to 48 hours after ejaculation. Consequently, for successful fertilization to occur, coitus must occur no more than two days before ovulation and no later than 24 hours after. At this point the oocyte is approximately one-third of the way down the length of the uterine tube.

Accomplishing Fertilization

Fertilization occurs when a sperm's chromosomes combine with those of an egg (actually a secondary oocyte) to form a fertilized egg, or **zygote** (zi′gōt; "yoked together"), the first cell of the new individual. Let's look at the events leading to fertilization.

28

Sperm Transport and Capacitation

During copulation, a man expels millions of sperm with considerable force into his partner's vaginal canal. Despite this "head start," most sperm don't reach the oocyte, even though it is only about 12 cm (5 inches) away. Millions of sperm leak from the vagina almost immediately after being deposited there. Of those remaining, millions more are destroyed by the vagina's acidic environment. Millions more fail to make it through the cervix, unless the thick "curtain" of cervical mucus has been made fluid by estrogens.

Sperm that do reach the uterus, propelled by their whiplike tail movements, are then subjected to forceful uterine contractions that act in a washing machine–like manner to disperse them throughout the uterine cavity, where thousands more are destroyed by resident phagocytes. Only a few thousand (and sometimes fewer than 100) sperm, out of the millions in the male ejaculate, are conducted by reverse peristalsis into the uterine tube, where the oocyte may be moving leisurely toward the uterus.

These difficulties aside, there is still another hurdle to overcome. Sperm freshly deposited in the vagina are incapable of penetrating an oocyte. They must first be **capacitated** over the next 2 to 10 hours. Specifically, their motility must be enhanced and their membranes must become fragile so that the hydrolytic enzymes in their acrosomes can be released. As sperm swim through the cervical mucus, uterus, and uterine tubes, secretions of the female tract remove some of their protective membrane proteins, and the cholesterol that keeps their acrosomal membranes "tough" and stable is depleted. Even though the sperm may reach the oocyte within a few minutes, they must "wait around" (so to speak) for capacitation to occur.

This elaborate mechanism prevents the spilling of acrosomal enzymes. But consider the alternative. Fragile acrosomal membranes could rupture prematurely in the male reproductive tract, causing some degree of autolysis (self-digestion) of the male reproductive organs.

How do sperm navigate to find a released oocyte in the uterine tube? This question is an area of active research. It now appears that they "sniff" their way to the oocyte. Sperm bear proteins called *olfactory receptors* that respond to chemical stimuli. It is presumed that the oocyte or its surrounding cells release signaling molecules that direct the sperm.

Acrosomal Reaction and Sperm Penetration

The ovulated oocyte is encapsulated by the corona radiata and by the deeper zona pellucida, a transparent layer of glycoprotein-rich extracellular matrix secreted by the oocyte. Both must be breached before the oocyte can be penetrated. Once in the immediate vicinity of the oocyte, a sperm weaves its way through the cells of the corona radiata. This journey is assisted by a cell-surface hyaluronidase on the sperm that digests the intercellular cement between the granulosa cells in the local area, causing them to fall away from the oocyte (*Focus on Sperm Penetration and the Cortical Reaction,* **Figure 28.2** ①, p. 1068).

28

After breaching the corona, the sperm head binds to a ZP3 glycoprotein of the zona pellucida, which functions as a sperm receptor. This binding opens calcium channels, which leads to a rise in Ca^{2+} inside the sperm that triggers the acrosomal (ak″ro-so′mal) reaction (Figure 28.2 ②). The **acrosomal reaction** involves the release of acrosomal enzymes (hyaluronidase, acrosin, proteases, and others) that digest holes through the zona pellucida. Hundreds of acrosomes must undergo exocytosis to digest holes in the zona pellucida. This is one case that does not bear out the adage, "The early bird catches the worm." A sperm that comes along later, after hundreds of sperm have undergone acrosomal reactions to expose the oocyte membrane, is in the best position to be *the* fertilizing sperm.

Once a path is cleared, the sperm's whiplike tail gyrates, forcing the sperm's head to rock and move toward the oocyte membrane. There the sperm's postacrosomal "collar," the rear portion of the acrosomal membrane, binds to the oocyte's plasma membrane receptors (Figure 28.2 ③). This binding event has two consequences. (a) It causes the oocyte to form microvilli that surround the sperm head, and the sperm and oocyte membranes to fuse (Figure 28.2 ④), and then (b) like a snake crawling out of its skin, the cytoplasmic contents of the sperm enter the oocyte, leaving the sperm's plasma membrane behind (Figure 28.2 ⑤). The gametes fuse together with such perfect contact that the contents of both cells are combined within a single membrane—all without spilling a drop.

Block to Polyspermy

Polyspermy (entry of several sperm into an egg) occurs in some animals, but in humans only one sperm is allowed to penetrate the oocyte, ensuring **monospermy**, the one-sperm-per-oocyte condition. Once the sperm head has entered the oocyte, waves of Ca^{2+} are released by the oocyte's endoplasmic reticulum into its cytoplasm, which activates the oocyte to prepare for the second meiotic division. These calcium surges also cause the **cortical reaction** (Figure 28.2 ⑤), in which granules located just inside the plasma membrane spill their enzymes into the extracellular space beneath the zona pellucida. These enzymes, called *zonal inhibiting proteins* (*ZIPs*), destroy the sperm receptors, preventing any more sperm from entering.

Additionally, the spilled material binds water, and as the material swells and hardens, it detaches all sperm still bound to receptors on the oocyte membrane, completing the so-called *slow block to polyspermy*. In the rare cases of polyspermy that do occur, the embryos contain too much genetic material and die.

Completion of Meiosis II and Fertilization

As the sperm's cytoplasmic contents enter the oocyte, the sperm loses its plasma membrane. The centrosome from its midpiece elaborates microtubules which the sperm uses to locomote its DNA-rich nucleus toward the oocyte nucleus. On the way, its nucleus swells to about five times its normal size to form the **male pronucleus** (pro-nu′kle-us; *pro* = before). Meanwhile the secondary oocyte, activated from its semidormant state by the calcium surges, completes meiosis II, forming the ovum nucleus and the second polar body (**Figure 28.3a** ① and ②, p. 1070).

This accomplished, the ovum nucleus swells, becoming the **female pronucleus**, and the two pronuclei approach each other.

As a mitotic spindle develops between them (Figure 28.3a ③), the pronuclei membranes rupture, releasing their chromosomes together into the immediate vicinity of the newly formed spindle.

The true moment of fertilization occurs as the maternal and paternal chromosomes combine and produce the diploid *zygote*, or fertilized egg (Figure 28.3a ④). Some sources define the term fertilization simply as the act of oocyte penetration by the sperm. However, unless the chromosomes in the male and female pronuclei are actually combined, the zygote is never formed in humans. Almost as soon as the male and female pronuclei come together, their chromosomes replicate. The zygote, the first cell of a new individual, is now ready to undergo the first mitotic division of the conceptus.

Check Your Understanding

1. What has to happen before ejaculated sperm can penetrate an oocyte?
2. What is the cortical reaction and what does it accomplish?

For answers, see Appendix H.

Events of Embryonic Development: Zygote to Blastocyst Implantation

Early embryonic development begins with fertilization and continues as the embryo travels through the uterine tube, floats free in the cavity of the uterus, and finally implants in the uterine wall. Significant events of this early embryonic period are *cleavage,* which produces a structure called a blastocyst, and *implantation* of the blastocyst.

Cleavage and Blastocyst Formation

✓ Describe the process and product of cleavage.

Cleavage is a period of fairly rapid mitotic divisions of the zygote without intervening growth (**Figure 28.4**, p. 1071). The goal of this first phase of development is to produce small cells with a high surface-to-volume ratio, which enhances their uptake of nutrients and oxygen and the disposal of wastes. It also provides a large number of cells to serve as building blocks for constructing the embryo. Consider, for a moment, the difficulty of trying to construct a building from one huge block of granite. If you now consider how much easier it would be if instead you could use hundreds of bricks, you will quickly grasp the importance of cleavage.

Some 36 hours after fertilization, the first cleavage division of the zygote has produced two identical cells called *blastomeres.* These divide to produce four cells (Figure 28.4b), then eight, and so on. By 72 hours after fertilization, a loose collection of cells that form a berry-shaped cluster of 16 or more cells called the **morula** (mor′u-lah; "little mulberry") has been formed (Figure 28.4c). All the while, transport of the embryo toward the uterus continues.

By day 4 or 5 after fertilization, the embryo consists of about 100 cells, has begun accumulating fluid within an internal cavity, and floats free in the uterus (Figure 28.4d). The zona pellucida now starts to break down and the inner structure, now called a blastocyst, "hatches" from it. The **blastocyst** (blas′to-sist) is a fluid-filled hollow sphere composed of a single layer of large, flattened cells called **trophoblast cells** (tro′fo-blast) and a small cluster of 20 to 30 rounded cells, called the **inner cell mass**, located at one side (Figure 28.4e).

Soon after the blastocyst forms, trophoblast cells begin to display L-selectin adhesion molecules on their surface. They take part in placenta formation, as suggested by the literal translation of "trophoblast" (nourishment generator). They also secrete and display several factors with immunosuppressive effects that protect the trophoblast (and the developing embryo) from attack by the mother's cells.

The inner cell mass becomes the *embryonic disc*, which forms the embryo proper, and three of the four extraembryonic membranes. (The fourth membrane, the chorion, is a trophoblast derivative.)

Check Your Understanding

3. Why is the multicellular blastocyst only slightly larger than the single-celled zygote?
4. What is the function of the trophoblast cells?

For answers, see Appendix H.

Implantation

✓ Describe implantation.

While the blastocyst floats in the uterine cavity for two to three days, it is nourished by the glycoprotein-rich uterine secretions, which also contain steroids and various nutrients including iron and fat-soluble vitamins. Then, some six to seven days after ovulation, given a properly prepared endometrium, **implantation** begins. The receptivity of the endometrium to implantation—the so-called *window of implantation*—is opened by the surging levels of ovarian hormones (estrogens and progesterone) in the blood. If the mucosa is properly prepared, integrin and selectin proteins on the trophoblast cells bind respectively to the extracellular matrix components (collagen, fibronectin, laminin, and others) of the endometrial cells and to selectin-binding carbohydrates on the inner uterine wall, and the blastocyst implants high in the uterus. If the endometrium is not yet optimally mature, the blastocyst detaches and floats to a lower level, implanting when it finds a site with the proper receptors and chemical signals.

(Text continues on p. 1070.)

FOCUS Sperm Penetration and the Cortical Reaction

Figure 28.2 Sperm use acrosomal enzymes and receptors to approach, bind, and enter the oocyte. The cortical reaction prevents further sperm entry, ensuring that only two copies of each chromosome are present in the fertilized ovum.

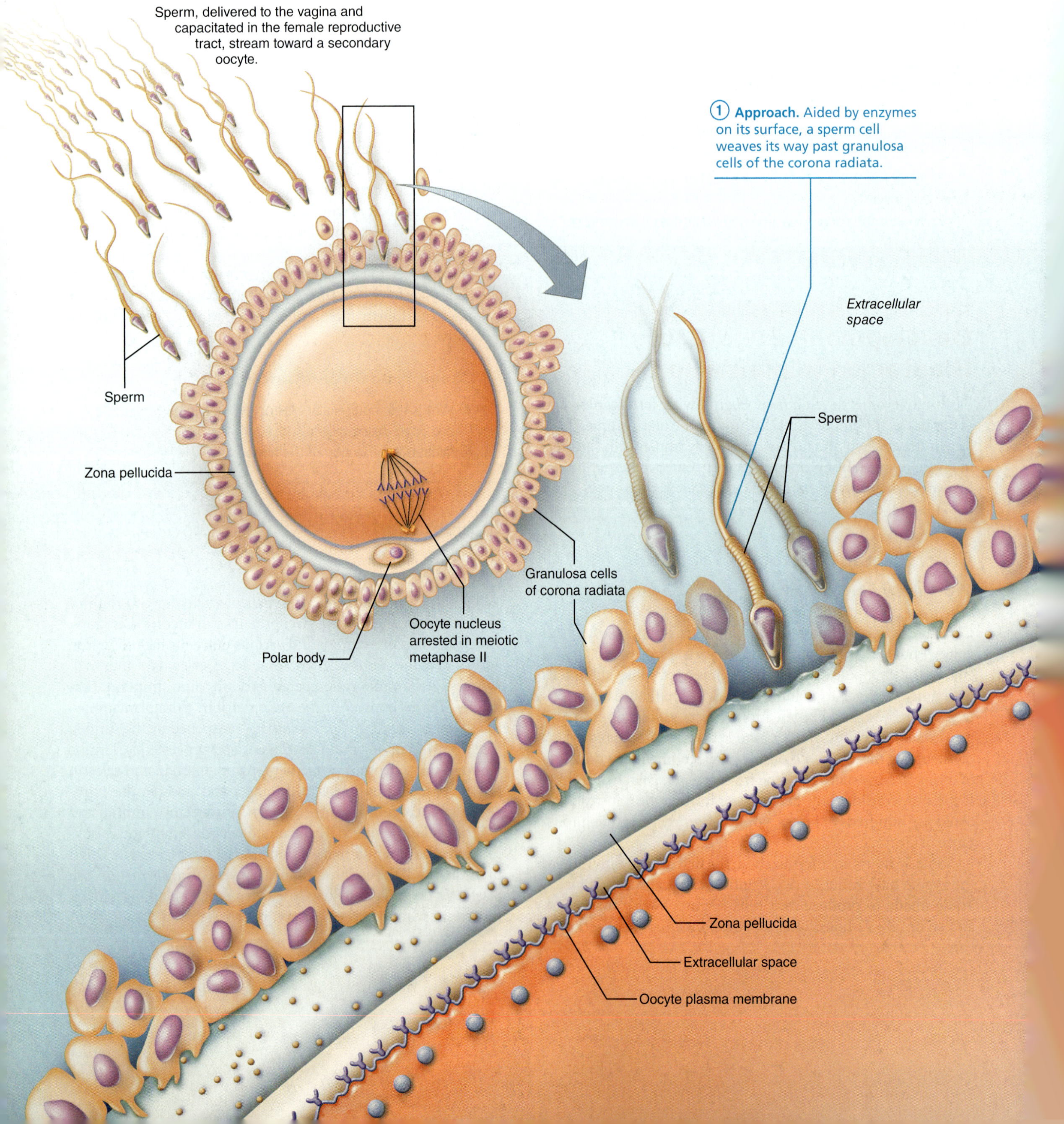

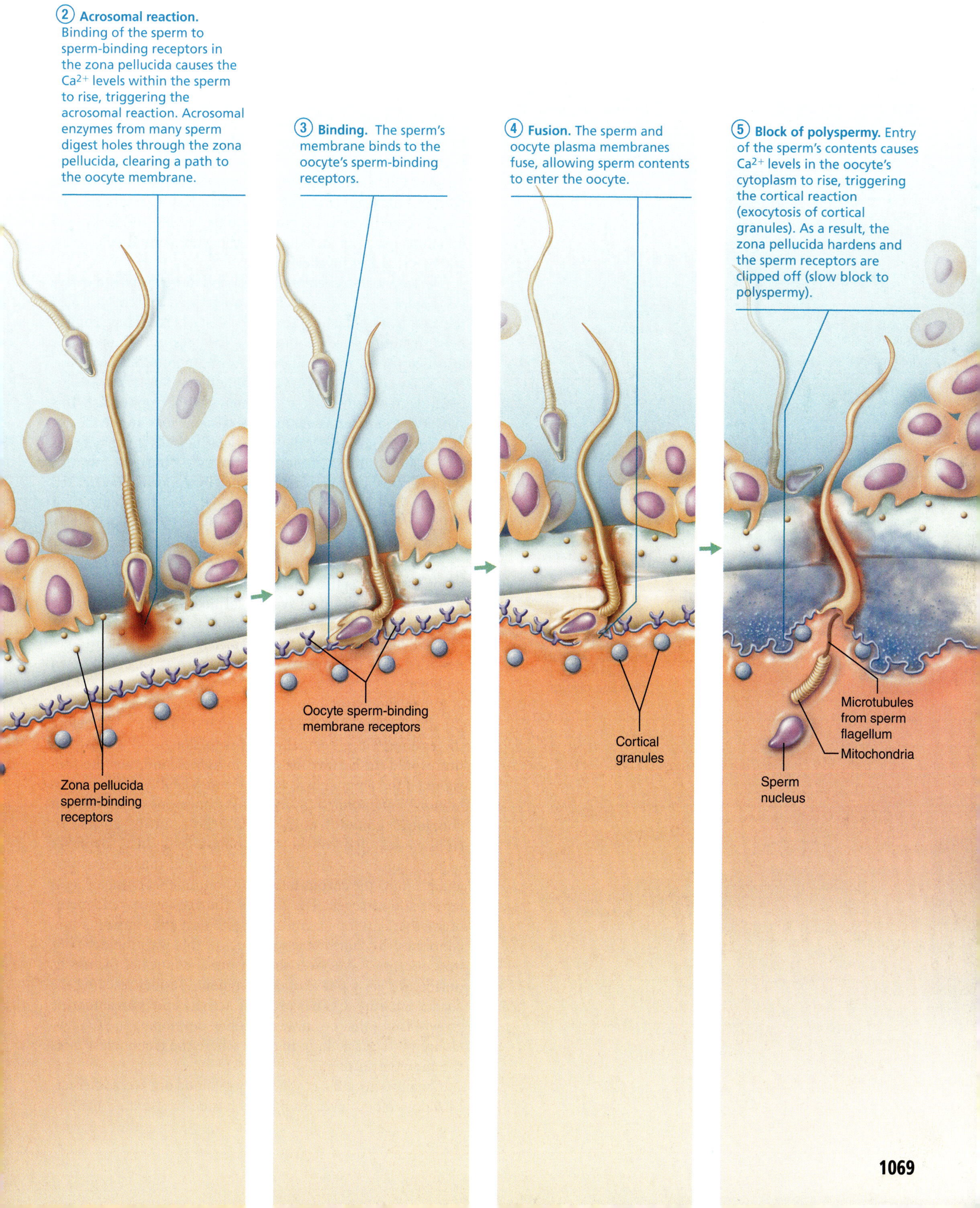

② Acrosomal reaction. Binding of the sperm to sperm-binding receptors in the zona pellucida causes the Ca^{2+} levels within the sperm to rise, triggering the acrosomal reaction. Acrosomal enzymes from many sperm digest holes through the zona pellucida, clearing a path to the oocyte membrane.
③ Binding. The sperm's membrane binds to the oocyte's sperm-binding receptors.
④ Fusion. The sperm and oocyte plasma membranes fuse, allowing sperm contents to enter the oocyte.
⑤ Block of polyspermy. Entry of the sperm's contents causes Ca^{2+} levels in the oocyte's cytoplasm to rise, triggering the cortical reaction (exocytosis of cortical granules). As a result, the zona pellucida hardens and the sperm receptors are clipped off (slow block to polyspermy).
Zona pellucida sperm-binding receptors
Oocyte sperm-binding membrane receptors
Cortical granules
Microtubules from sperm flagellum
Mitochondria
Sperm nucleus

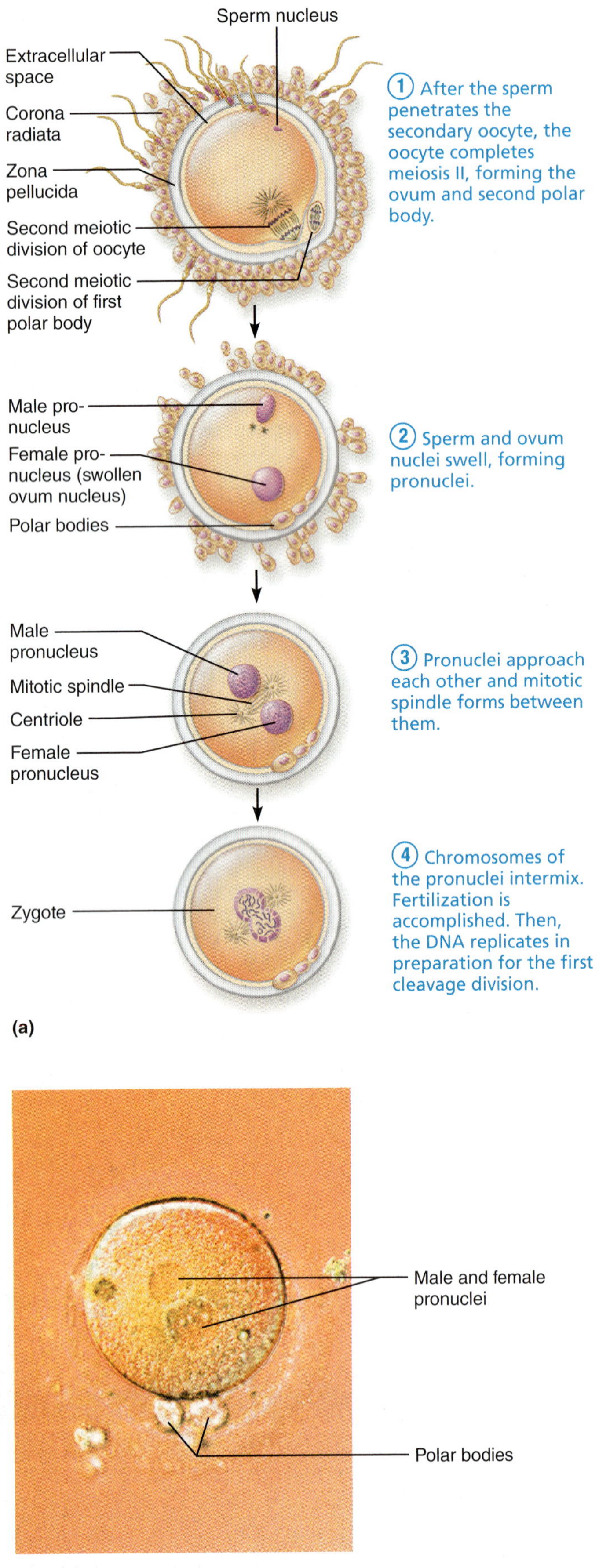

Figure 28.3 Events of fertilization. (a) Events from sperm penetration to zygote formation. **(b)** Micrograph of an oocyte in which the male and female pronuclei are beginning to fuse to accomplish fertilization and form the zygote. Occurs in time between steps (3) and (4) of (a).

The trophoblast cells overlying the inner cell mass adhere to the endometrium **(Figure 28.5a, b)** and secrete digestive enzymes and growth factors against the endometrial surface. The endometrium quickly thickens at the point of contact and takes on characteristics of an acute inflammatory response—the uterine blood vessels become more permeable and leaky, and inflammatory cells including lymphocytes, natural killer cells, and macrophages invade the area.

The trophoblast then proliferates and forms two distinct layers (Figure 28.5c). The cells in the inner layer, collectively called the **cytotrophoblast** (si″to-tro′fo-blast) or **cellular trophoblast**, retain their cell boundaries. The cells in the outer layer lose their plasma membranes and form a multinuclear cytoplasmic mass called the **syncytiotrophoblast** (sin-sit″e-o-tro′fo-blast; *syn* = together, *cyt* = cell) or **syncytial trophoblast**. This syncytial region sends out long protrusions that invade the endometrium and rapidly digest the uterine cells it contacts. As the endometrium is eroded, the blastocyst burrows into this thick, velvety lining and is surrounded by a pool of blood leaked from degraded endometrial blood vessels. Shortly, proliferation of the endometrial cells covers and seals off the implanted blastocyst from the uterine cavity (Figure 28.5d).

In cases where implantation fails to occur, a receptive uterus becomes nonreceptive once again. It is estimated that a minimum of two-thirds of all zygotes formed fail to implant by the end of the first week or spontaneously abort. Moreover, an estimated 30% of implanted embryos later miscarry due to genetic defects of the embryo, uterine malformation, or unknown problems.

When successful, implantation takes about five days and is usually completed by the 12th day after ovulation—just before the endometrium normally begins to slough off. Menstruation would flush away the embryo as well and must be prevented if the pregnancy is to continue. Viability of the corpus luteum is maintained by an LH-like hormone called **human chorionic gonadotropin (hCG)** (ko″re-on′ik go-nad″o-trōp′in) secreted by the trophoblast cells. hCG bypasses hypothalamic-pituitary-ovarian controls at this critical time and prompts the corpus luteum to continue secreting progesterone and estrogen. The *chorion*, the extraembryonic membrane that develops from the trophoblast after implantation, continues this hormonal stimulus. In this way, the developing conceptus takes over the hormonal control of the uterus during this early phase of development. Besides rescuing the corpus luteum, hCG has protease activity and is an autocrine growth factor that promotes placental development. hCG levels are particularly high in areas where the trophoblast faces the endometrium.

Usually detectable in the mother's blood one week after fertilization, blood levels of hCG continue to rise until the end

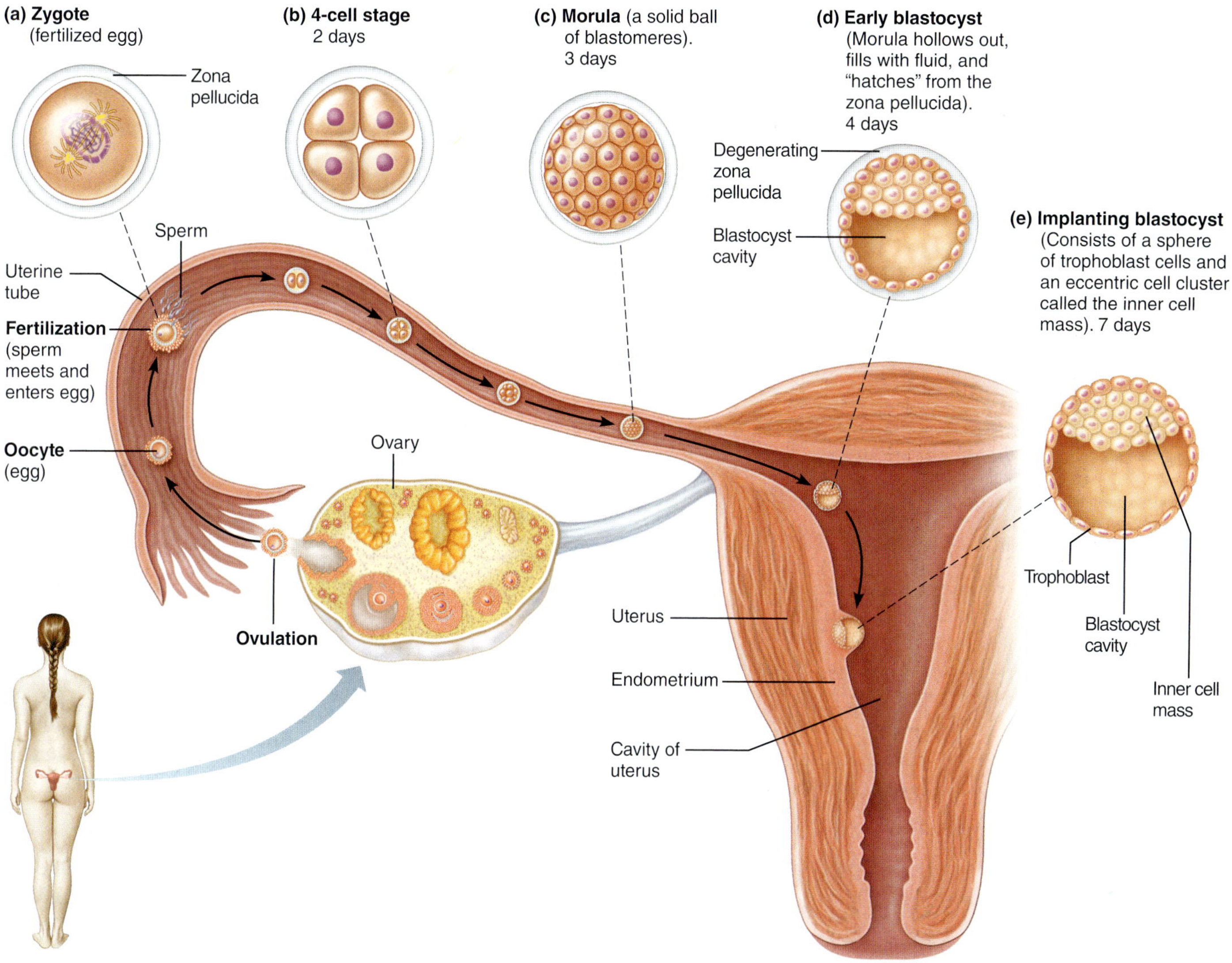

Figure 28.4 Cleavage: From zygote to blastocyst. The zygote begins to divide about 24 hours after fertilization, and continues the more rapid mitotic divisions of cleavage as it travels down the uterine tube. Three to four days after ovulation, the embryo reaches the uterus and floats freely for two to three days, nourished by secretions of the endometrial glands. Because there is little time for growth between successive cleavage divisions, the resulting blastocyst is only slightly larger than the zygote. At the late blastocyst stage, the embryo implants into the endometrium; this begins at about day 7 after ovulation.

of the second month. Then, blood levels decline sharply to reach a low value by 4 months, a situation that persists for the remainder of gestation **(Figure 28.6)**. Between the second and third month, the placenta (which we describe next) assumes the role of progesterone and estrogen production for the remainder of the pregnancy. The corpus luteum then degenerates and the ovaries remain inactive until after birth. All pregnancy tests used today are antibody tests that detect hCG in a woman's blood or urine.

Initially, the implanted embryo obtains its nutrition by digesting the endometrial cells, but by the second month, the placenta is providing nutrients and oxygen to the embryo and carrying away embryonic metabolic wastes. Since placenta formation is a continuation of the events of implantation, we will consider it next, although we will be getting a little ahead of ourselves as far as embryonic development is concerned.

☑ Check Your Understanding

5. Which portion of the trophoblast accomplishes implantation?
6. Marie, wondering if she is pregnant, buys an over-the-counter pregnancy test to assess this possibility. How will the blastocyst, if present, "make itself known"?

For answers, see Appendix H.

28

Placentation

✓ Describe placenta formation, and list placental functions.

Placentation (plas″en-ta′shun) refers to the formation of a **placenta** ("flat cake"), a temporary organ that originates from both embryonic and maternal (endometrial) tissues. Cells from the original inner cell mass give rise to a layer of extraembryonic mesoderm that

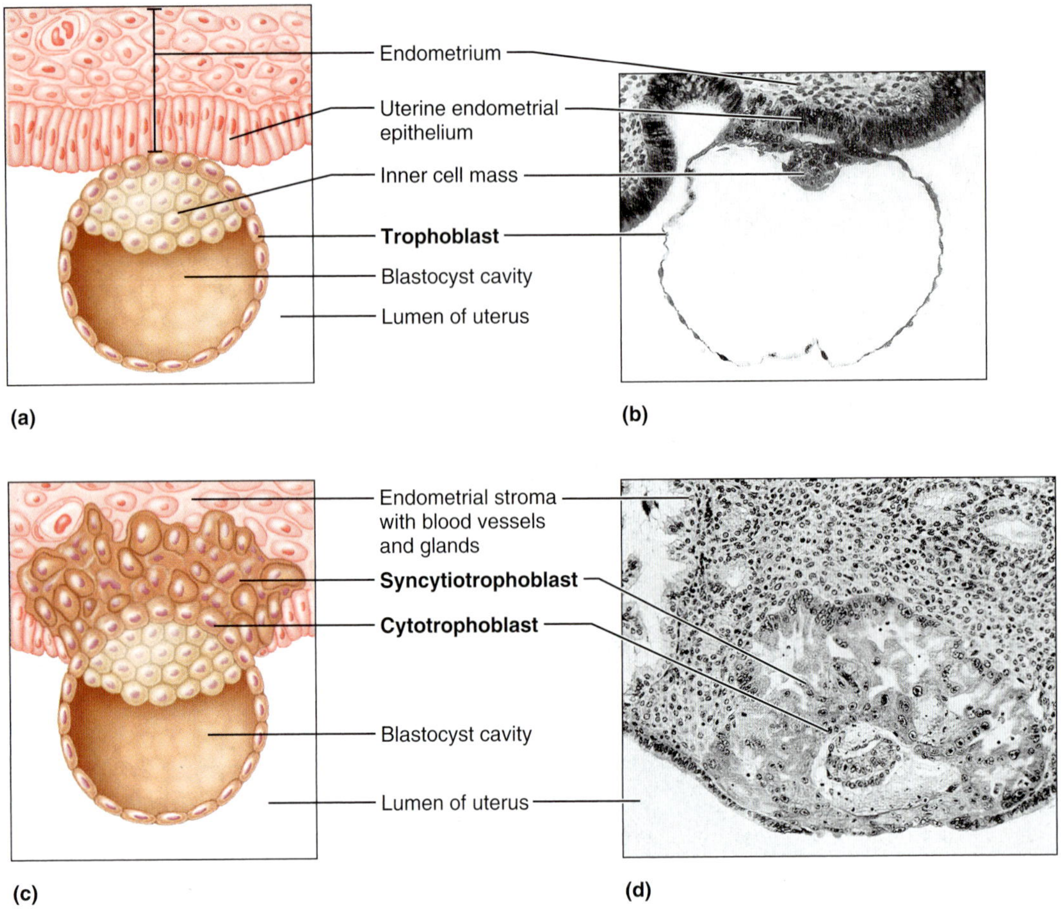

Figure 28.5 Implantation of the blastocyst. **(a)** Diagrammatic view of a blastocyst that has just adhered to the uterine endometrium and **(b)** microscopic view. **(c)** Slightly later stage of an implanting embryo (approximately seven days after ovulation), depicting the cytotrophoblast and syncytiotrophoblast of the eroding trophoblast. **(d)** Light micrograph of an implanted blastocyst (approximately 12 days after ovulation).

Source: (b) R. O'Rahilly and R. Muller, *Human Embryology and Teratology*, Wiley–Liss, 3rd Edition, 2001. This material is reproduced with permission of Wiley–Liss, Inc., a subsidiary of John Wiley & Sons, Inc.

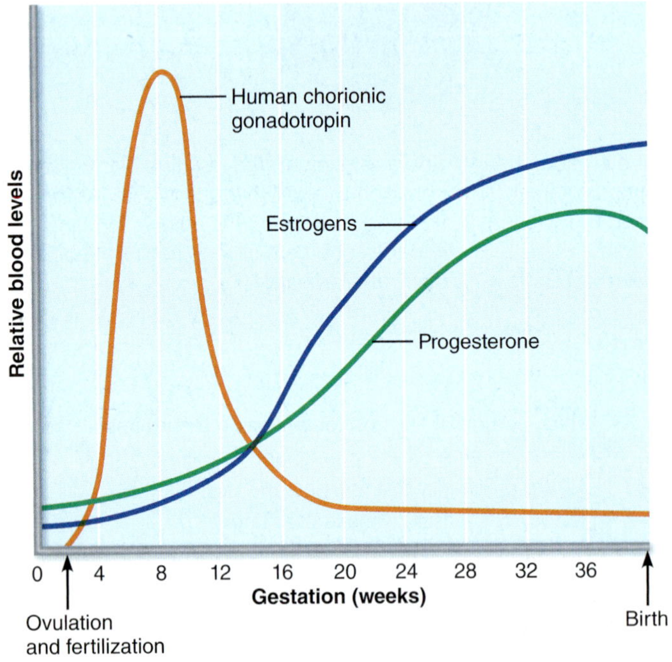

Figure 28.6 Hormonal changes during pregnancy. The relative changes in maternal blood levels of three hormones that maintain pregnancy are depicted, rather than actual blood concentrations.

lines the inner surface of the trophoblast **(Figure 28.7b)**. Together these become the **chorion**. The chorion develops fingerlike **chorionic villi**, which become especially elaborate where they are in contact with maternal blood (Figure 28.7c).

Soon the mesodermal cores of the chorionic villi are invaded by newly forming blood vessels, which extend to the embryo as the umbilical arteries and vein. The continuing erosion produces large, blood-filled **lacunae**, or **intervillous spaces**, in the stratum functionalis of the endometrium (see Figure 27.15, p. 1039). The villi come to lie in these spaces totally immersed in maternal blood, which is continouously refreshed by extravascularized maternal blood (Figure 28.7d). The part of the endometrium that lies beneath the embryo becomes the **decidua basalis** (de-sid′u-ah), and that surrounding the uterine cavity face of the implanted embryo forms the **decidua capsularis** (Figure 28.7d and e). Together, the chorionic villi and the decidua basalis form the disc-shaped placenta.

The placenta detaches and sloughs off after the infant is born, so the name of the maternal portion—*decidua* ("that which falls off")—is appropriate. During development, the decidua capsularis expands to accommodate the fetus, which eventually fills and stretches the uterine cavity. As the developing fetus grows, the villi in the decidua capsularis are compressed and degenerate, while those in the decidua basalis increase in number and branch even more profusely.

The placenta is usually fully functional as a nutritive, respiratory, excretory, and endocrine organ by the end of the third

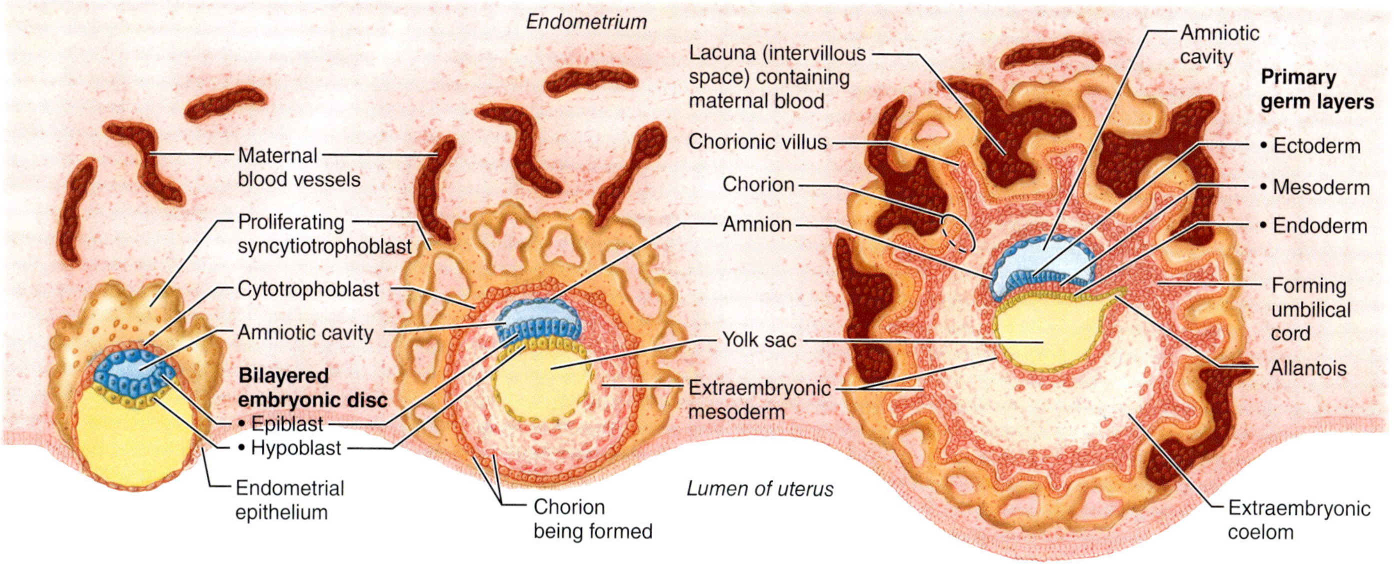

(a) Implanting 7½-day blastocyst. The syncytiotrophoblast is eroding the endometrium. Cells of the embryonic disc are now separated from the amnion by a fluid-filled space.

(b) 12-day blastocyst. Implantation is complete. Extraembryonic mesoderm is forming a discrete layer beneath the cytotrophoblast.

(c) 16-day embryo. Cytotrophoblast and associated mesoderm have become the chorion, and chorionic villi are elaborating. The embryo exhibits all three germ layers, a yolk sac, and an allantois, which forms the basis of the umbilical cord.

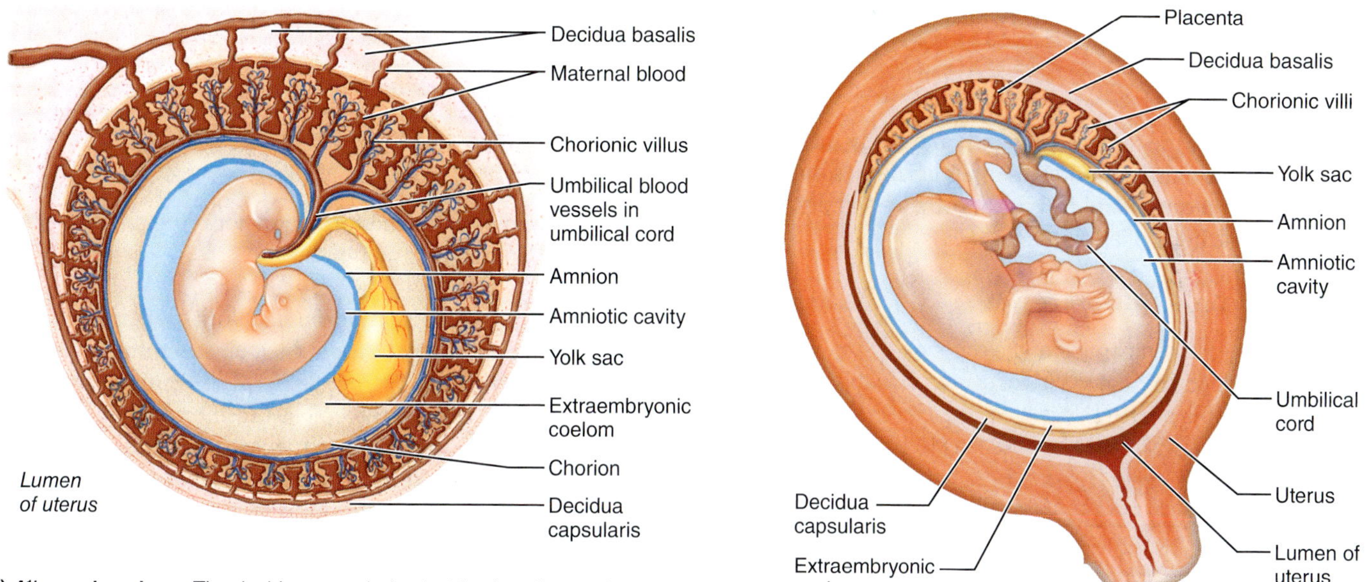

(d) 4½ -week embryo. The decidua capsularis, decidua basalis, amnion, and yolk sac are well formed. The chorionic villi lie in blood-filled intervillous spaces within the endometrium. The embryo is nourished via the umbilical vessels that connect it (through the umbilical cord) to the placenta.

(e) 13-week fetus.

Figure 28.7 Events of placentation, early embryonic development, and extraembryonic membrane formation.

month of pregnancy. However, well before this time, oxygen and nutrients are diffusing from maternal to embryonic blood, and embryonic metabolic wastes are passing in the opposite direction. The barriers to free passage of substances between the two blood supplies are embryonic barriers—the membranes of the chorionic villi and the endothelium of embryonic capillaries. Although the maternal and embryonic blood supplies are very close, they normally do not intermix **(Figure 28.8)**.

The placenta secretes hCG from the beginning, but the ability of its syncytiotrophoblast cells (the "hormone manufacturers") to produce the estrogens and progesterone of pregnancy matures much more slowly. If, for some reason, placental hormones are inadequate when hCG levels wane, the endometrium degenerates and the pregnancy is aborted. Throughout pregnancy, blood levels of estrogens and progesterone continue to increase (see Figure 28.6). They encourage growth and further

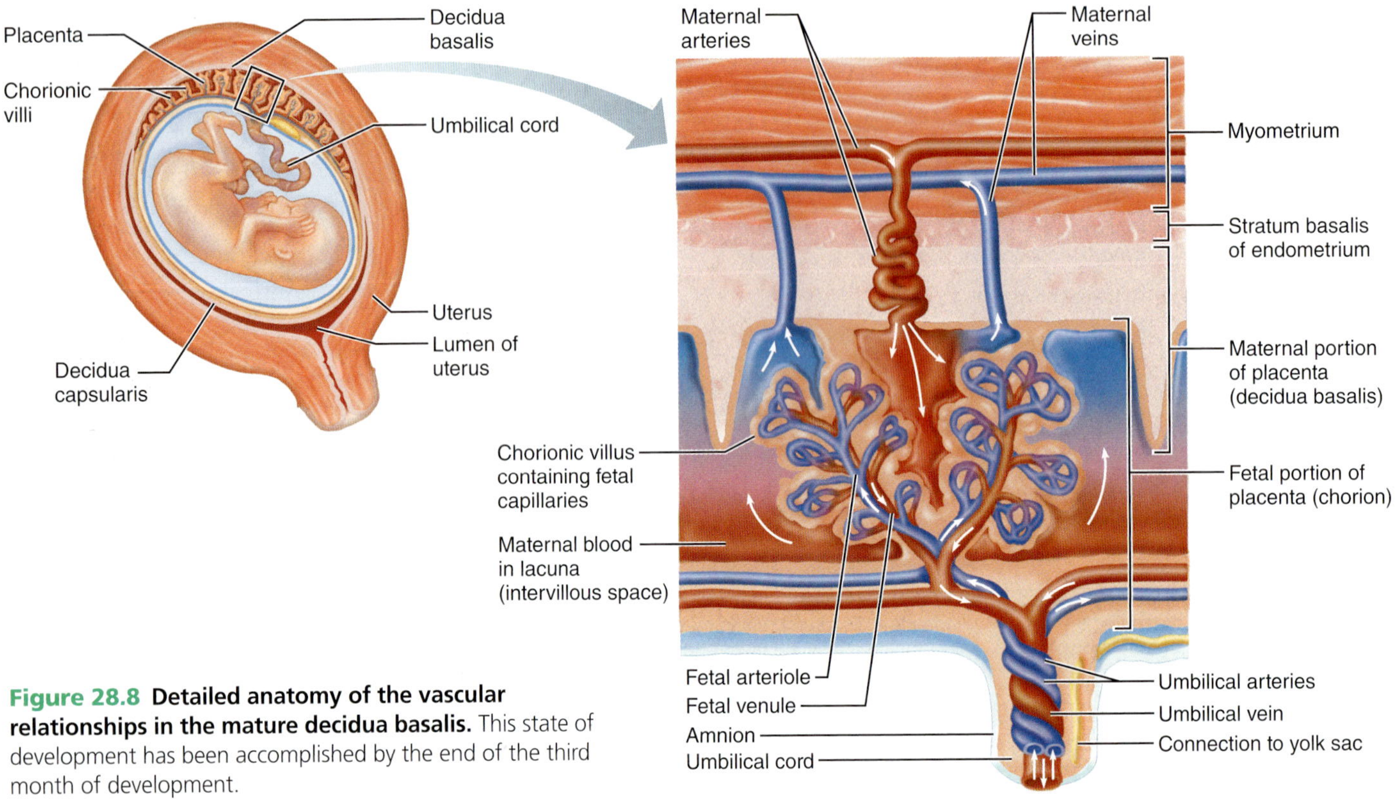

Figure 28.8 Detailed anatomy of the vascular relationships in the mature decidua basalis. This state of development has been accomplished by the end of the third month of development.

differentiation of the mammary glands and ready them for lactation. The placenta also produces other hormones, such as *human placental lactogen* and *relaxin*. Shortly we will describe the effects of these hormones on the mother.

Check Your Understanding

7. What is the composition of the chorion?
8. What endometrial decidua cooperates with the chorionic villi to form the placenta?
9. Generally speaking, when does the placenta become fully functional?

For answers, see Appendix H.

Events of Embryonic Development: Gastrula to Fetus

28

Having followed placental development into the fetal stage, we will now backtrack and consider development of the embryo during and after implantation, referring again to Figure 28.7. Even while implantation is occurring, the blastocyst is being converted to a **gastrula** (gas′troo-lah), in which the three primary germ layers form, and the extraembryonic membranes develop. Before becoming three-layered, the inner cell mass first subdivides into two layers—the upper *epiblast* and the lower *hypoblast* (Figure 28.7a, b). The subdivided inner cell mass is now called the **embryonic disc**.

Formation and Roles of the Extraembryonic Membranes

✓ Name and describe the formation, location, and function of the extraembryonic membranes.

The **extraembryonic membranes** that form during the first two to three weeks of development include the amnion, yolk sac, allantois, and chorion (Figure 28.7c). The **amnion** (am′ne-on) develops when cells of the epiblast fashion themselves into a transparent membranous sac. This sac, the amnion, becomes filled with **amniotic fluid**. Later, as the embryonic disc curves to form the tubular body, the amnion curves with it. Eventually, the sac extends all the way around the embryo, broken only by the umbilical cord (Figure 28.7d).

Sometimes called the "bag of waters," the amnion provides a buoyant environment that protects the developing embryo against physical trauma, and helps maintain a constant homeostatic temperature. The fluid also prevents the rapidly growing embryonic parts from adhering and fusing together and allows the embryo considerable freedom of movement. Initially, the fluid is derived from the maternal blood, but as the fetal kidneys become functional later in development, fetal urine contributes to amniotic fluid volume.

The **yolk sac** forms from cells of the primitive gut, which arrange themselves into a sac that hangs from the ventral surface of the embryo (Figure 28.7b–d). The amnion and yolk sac resemble two balloons touching one another with the embryonic disc at the point of contact. In many species, the yolk sac is the main source of nutrition for the embryo, but human

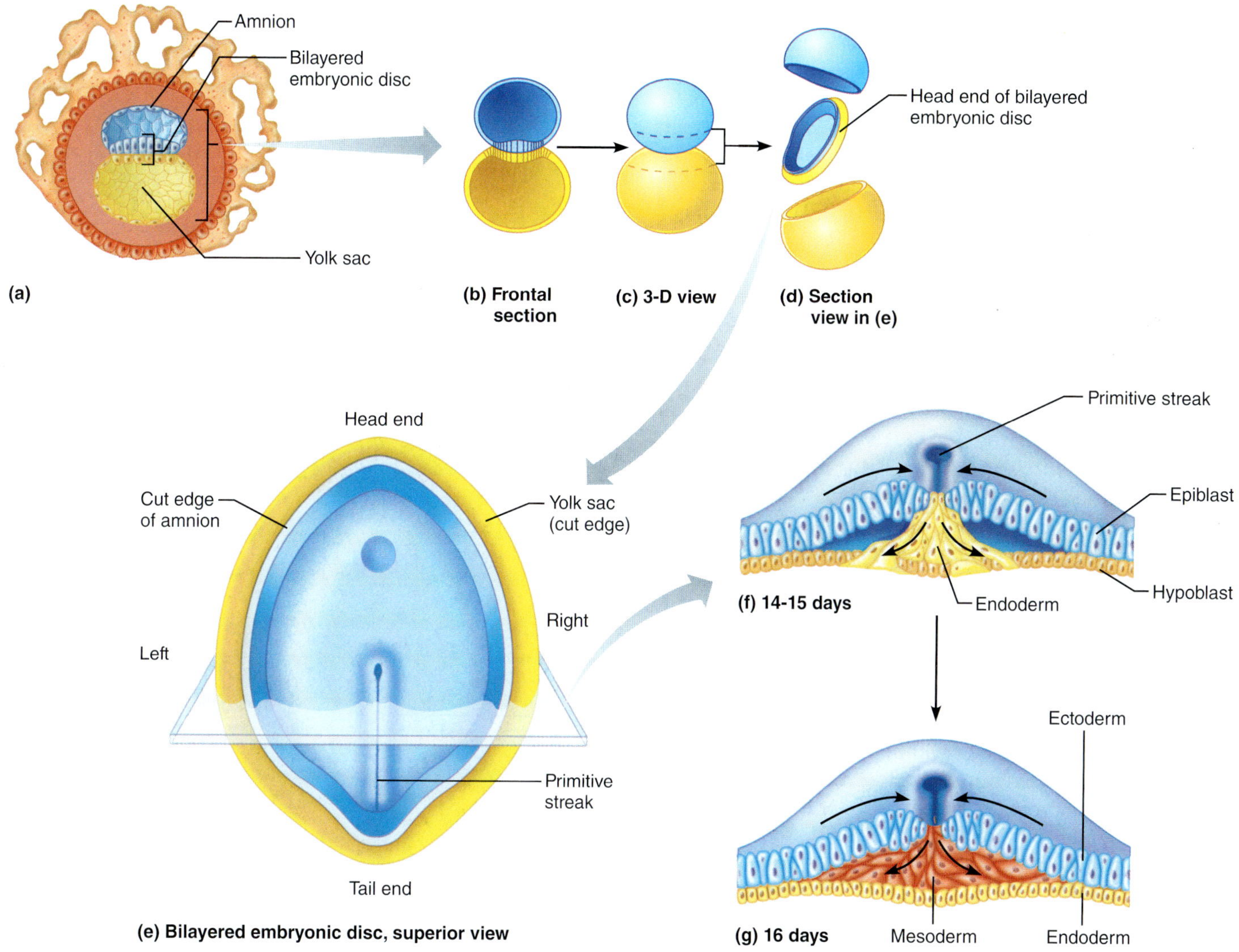

Figure 28.9 Formation of the three primary germ layers. (a–d) Orienting diagrams. **(e)** Surface view of an embryonic disc, amnion and yolk sac removed. **(f, g)** Cross sections of the embryonic disc, showing the germ layers resulting from cell migration. The first epiblast cells that migrate medially into the primitive streak **(f)** become endoderm. Those that follow **(g)** become mesoderm. The epiblast surface is now called ectoderm.

eggs contain very little yolk and nutritive functions have been taken over by the placenta. Nevertheless, the yolk sac is important in humans because it (1) forms part of the gut (digestive tube), and (2) is the source of the earliest blood cells and blood vessels.

The **allantois** (ah-lan′to-is) forms as a small outpocketing of embryonic tissue at the caudal end of the yolk sac (Figure 28.7c). In animals that develop in shelled eggs, the allantois is a disposal site for solid metabolic wastes (excreta). In humans, the allantois is the structural base for the **umbilical cord** that links the embryo to the placenta, and ultimately it becomes part of the urinary bladder. The fully formed umbilical cord contains a core of embryonic connective tissue (Wharton's jelly), the umbilical arteries and vein, and is covered externally by amniotic membrane.

We have already described the *chorion*, which helps to form the placenta (Figure 28.7c). As the outermost membrane, the chorion encloses the embryonic body and all other membranes.

☑ Check Your Understanding

10. What is the function of the amnion?
11. Which extraembryonic membrane provides a path for the embryonic blood vessels to reach the placenta?

For answers, see Appendix H.

Gastrulation: Germ Layer Formation

✓ Describe gastrulation and its consequence.

During week 3, the two-layered embryonic disc transforms into a three-layered *embryo* in which the **primary germ layers**—*ectoderm, mesoderm,* and *endoderm*—are present (Figure 28.7c). This process, called **gastrulation** (gas″troo-la′shun), involves cellular rearrangements and migrations.

Figure 28.9 focuses on the changes that take place in the days between Figure 28.7b (12-day embryo) and Figure 28.7c

(16-day embryo). Gastrulation begins when a groove with raised edges called the **primitive streak** appears on the dorsal surface of the embryonic disc and establishes the longitudinal axis of the embryo (Figure 28.9e). Surface (epiblast) cells of the embryonic disc then migrate medially across other cells and enter the primitive streak. The first cells to enter the groove displace the hypoblast cells of the yolk sac and form the most inferior germ layer, the **endoderm** (Figure 28.9f). Those that follow push laterally between the cells at the upper and lower surfaces, forming the **mesoderm** (Figure 28.9g). As soon as the mesoderm is formed, the mesodermal cells immediately beneath the early primitive streak aggregate, forming a rod of mesodermal cells called the **notochord** (no′to-kord), the first axial support of the embryo (see Figure 28.12a). The cells that remain on the embryo's dorsal surface are the **ectoderm**. At this point, the embryo is about 2 mm long.

The three primary germ layers serve as the *primitive tissues* from which all body organs derive. Ectoderm ("outer skin") fashions structures of the nervous system and the skin epidermis. Endoderm ("inner skin") forms the epithelial linings of the digestive, respiratory, and urogenital systems, and associated glands. Mesoderm ("middle skin") forms virtually everything else.

Both ectoderm and endoderm consist mostly of cells that are securely joined to each other and are *epithelia*. Mesoderm, by contrast, is a *mesenchyme* [literally, "poured into the middle (of the embryo)"], an embryonic tissue with star-shaped cells that are free to migrate widely within the embryo. Figure 28.13 (p. 1079) lists the germ layer derivatives. Some of the details of the differentiation processes are described next.

Organogenesis: Differentiation of the Germ Layers

- ✓ Define organogenesis and indicate the important roles of the three primary germ layers in this process.
- ✓ Describe unique features of the fetal circulation.

Gastrulation lays down the basic structural framework of the embryo. It also sets the stage for the rearrangements that occur during **organogenesis** (or″gah-no-jen′ĕ-sis), formation of body organs and organ systems. By the end of the embryonic period at 8 weeks, when the embryo is about 22 mm (slightly less than 1 inch) long from head to buttocks (referred to as the *crown-rump measurement*), all the adult organ systems are recognizable. It is truly amazing how much organogenesis occurs in such a short time in such a small amount of living matter.

28

As **Figure 28.10** shows, the embryo starts off as a flat plate, but as it grows, it folds to achieve a cylindrical body shape which lifts off the yolk sac and protrudes into the amniotic cavity. In the simplest sense, this process resembles three stacked sheets of paper folding laterally into a tube (Figure 28.10a, b). At the same time, the folding occurs from both ends (the head and tail regions) and progresses toward the central part of the embryonic body, where the yolk sac and umbilical vessels protrude. As the endoderm undercuts and its edges come together and fuse, it encloses part of the yolk sac (Figure 28.10d).

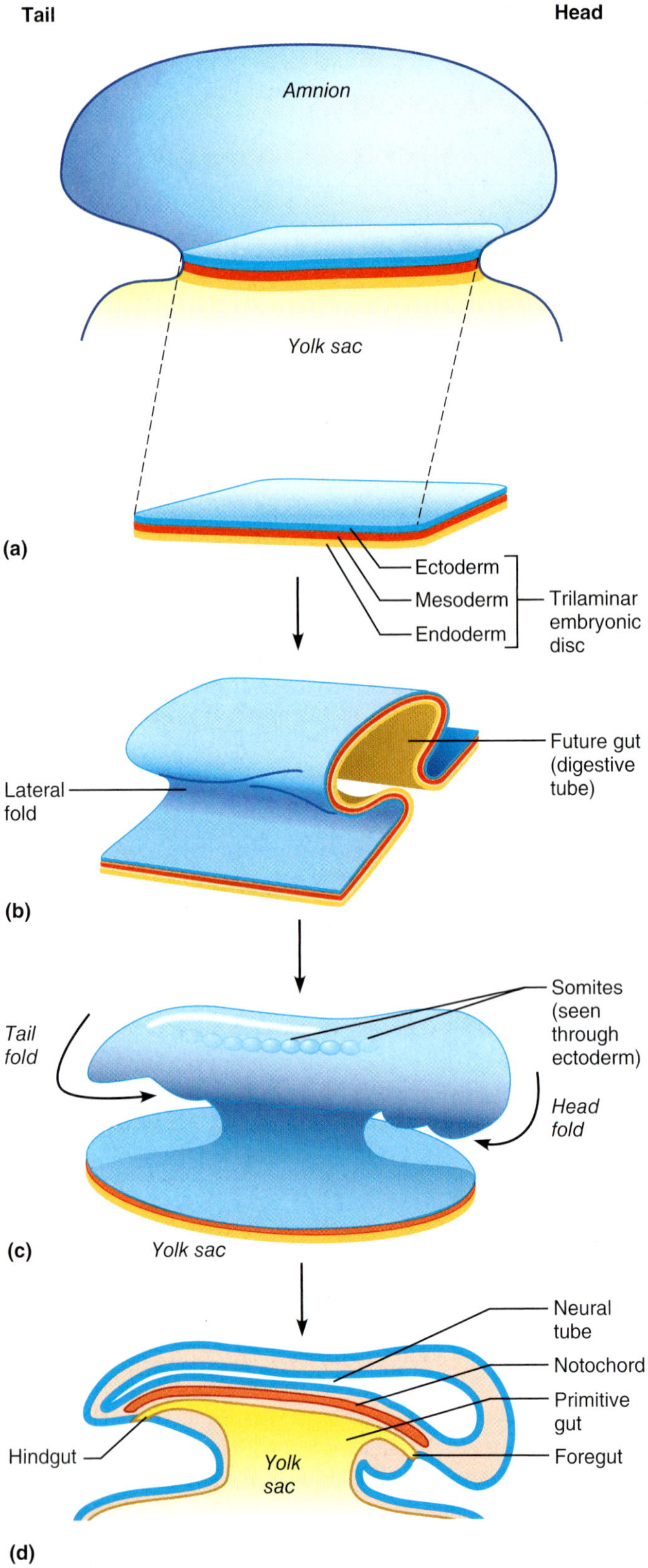

Figure 28.10 Folding of the embryonic body, lateral views. **(a)** Model of the flat three-layered embryo as three sheets of paper. **(b, c)** Folding begins with lateral folds, then head and tail folds appear. **(d)** A 24-day embryo in sagittal section. Notice the primitive gut, which derives from the yolk sac, and the notochord and neural tube dorsally.

Specialization of the Endoderm

The tube of endoderm formed by the folding process described is called the **primitive gut**. It becomes the epithelial lining (mucosa) of the gastrointestinal tract **(Figure 28.11)**. The organs of the GI tract (pharynx, esophagus, etc.) quickly become apparent, and then the oral and anal openings perforate. The mucosal lining of the respiratory tract forms as an outpocketing from the *foregut* (pharyngeal endoderm), and glands arise as endodermal outpocketings at various points further along the tract. For example, the epithelium of the thyroid, parathyroids, and thymus forms from the pharyngeal endoderm.

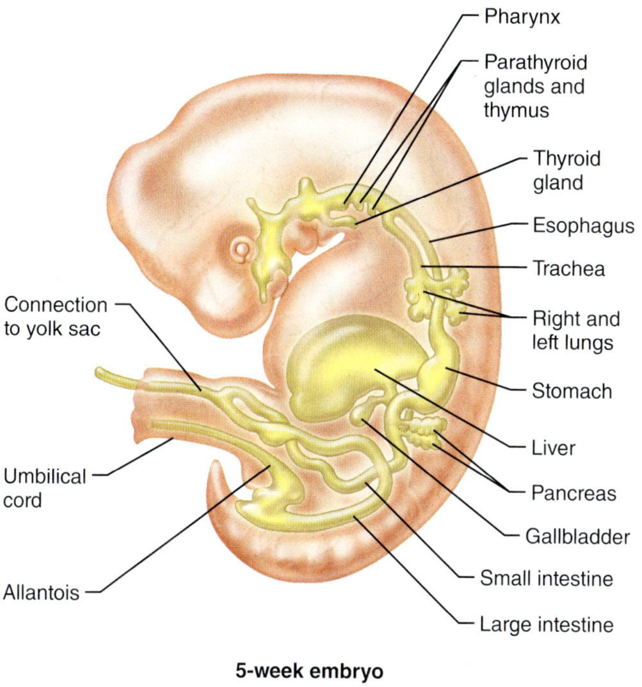

Figure 28.11 Endodermal differentiation. Endoderm forms the epithelial linings of the digestive and respiratory tracts and associated glands.

Specialization of the Ectoderm

The first major event in organogenesis is **neurulation**, the differentiation of ectoderm that produces the brain and spinal cord **(Figure 28.12)**. This process is *induced* (stimulated to happen) by chemical signals from the *notochord*, the rod of mesoderm that defines the body axis, mentioned earlier. The ectoderm overlying the notochord thickens, forming the **neural plate** (Figure 28.12a). Then the ectoderm starts to fold inward as a **neural groove**. As the neural groove deepens it forms prominent **neural folds** (Figure 28.12b). By day 22, the superior margins of the neural folds fuse, forming a **neural tube**, which soon pinches off from the ectodermal layer and becomes covered by surface ectoderm (Figure 28.12c).

As we described in Chapter 12, the anterior end of the neural tube becomes the brain and the rest becomes the spinal cord. The associated **neural crest cells** (Figure 28.12c) migrate widely and give rise to the cranial, spinal, and sympathetic ganglia (and associated nerves), to the chromaffin cells of the adrenal medulla, to pigment cells of the skin, and contribute to some connective tissues.

By the end of the first month of development, the three primary brain vesicles (fore-, mid-, and hindbrain) are apparent. By the end of the second month, all brain flexures are evident, the cerebral hemispheres cover the top of the brain stem (see Figure 12.2), and brain waves can be recorded. Most of the remaining ectoderm forming the surface layer of the embryonic body differentiates into the epidermis of the skin. Other ectodermal derivatives are indicated in Figure 28.13.

Specialization of the Mesoderm

The first evidence of mesodermal differentiation is the appearance of the notochord in the embryonic disc (see Figure 28.12a). The notochord is eventually replaced by the vertebral column, but its remnants persist in the springy *nucleus pulposus* of the intervertebral discs. Shortly thereafter, three mesodermal aggregates appear on either side of the notochord (Figure 28.12b, c). The largest of these, the *somites* (so′mīts), are paired mesodermal blocks that hug the notochord on either side. All 40 pairs of somites are present by the end of week 4. Flanking the somites laterally are small clusters of segmented mesoderm called *intermediate mesoderm* and then double sheets of *lateral plate mesoderm*.

Each **somite** has three functional parts—*sclerotome, dermatome*, and *myotome* (Figure 28.12d). Cells of the **sclerotome** (skle′ro-tōm; "hard piece") migrate medially, gather around the notochord and neural tube, and produce the vertebra and rib at the associated level. **Dermatome** ("skin piece") cells help form the dermis of the skin in the dorsal part of the body. The **myotome** (mi′o-tōm; "muscle piece") cells develop in conjunction with the vertebrae. They form the skeletal muscles of the neck, body trunk, and, via their **limb buds**, the muscles of the limbs.

Cells of the **intermediate mesoderm** form the gonads and kidneys. The **lateral plate mesoderm** consists of paired mesodermal plates: the *somatic mesoderm* and the more inferior *splanchnic mesoderm*. Cells of the superior plates help to form (1) the skin dermis; (2) the parietal serosa that lines the ventral body cavity; and (3) most tissues of the limbs. The more inferior plates provide the mesenchymal cells that form the heart and blood vessels and most connective tissues of the body, as well as nearly the entire wall of the digestive and respiratory organs. The lateral mesodermal layers cooperate to form the serosae of the **coelom** (se′lom), or ventral body cavity. The mesodermal derivatives are summarized in **Figure 28.13**.

By the end of the embryonic period, the bones have begun to ossify and the skeletal muscles are well formed and contracting spontaneously. Metanephric kidneys are developing, gonads are formed, and the lungs and digestive organs are attaining their final shape and body position. Blood delivery to and from the placenta via the umbilical vessels is constant and efficient. The heart and the liver are competing for space and form a conspicuous bulge on the ventral surface of the embryo's body. All this by the end of eight weeks in an embryo about 2.5 cm (1 inch) long from crown to rump!

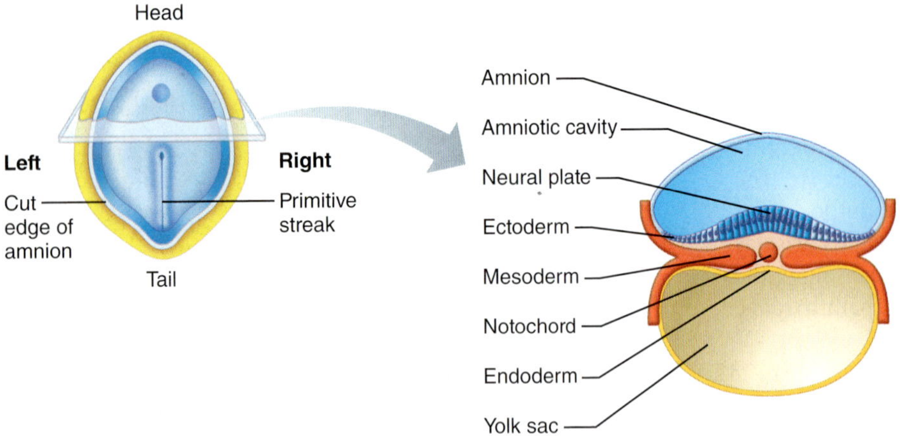

(a) 17 days. The flat three-layered embryo has completed gastrulation. Notochord and neural plate are present.

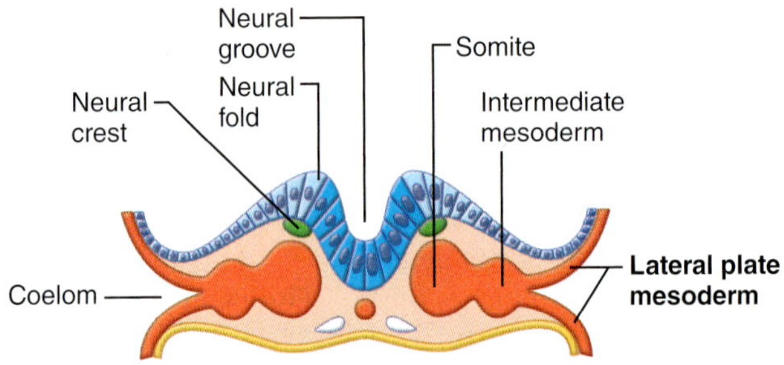

(b) 20 days. The neural folds form by folding of the neural plate, which then deepens, producing the neural groove. Three mesodermal aggregates form on each side of the notochord (somite, intermediate mesoderm, and lateral plate mesoderm).

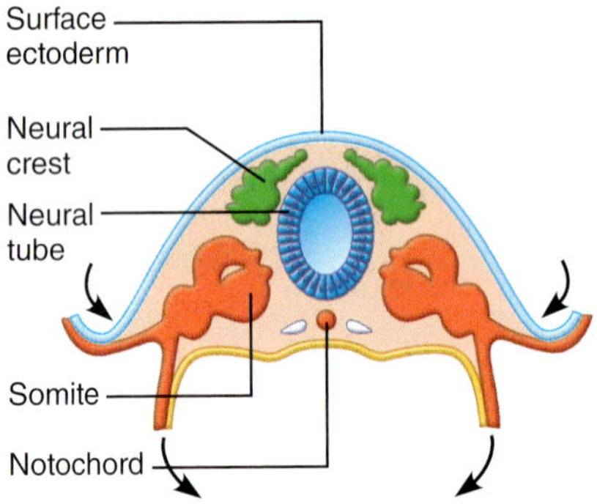

(c) 22 days. The neural folds have closed, forming the neural tube which has detached from the surface ectoderm and lies between the surface ectoderm and the notochord. Embryonic body is beginning to undercut.

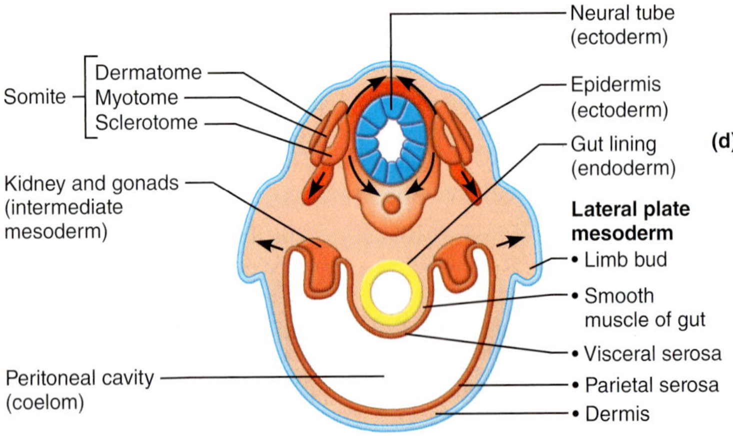

(d) End of week 4. Embryo undercutting is complete. Somites have subdivided into sclerotome, myotome, and dermatome, which form the vertebrae, skeletal muscles, and dermis respectively. Body coelom present.

Figure 28.12 Neurulation and early mesodermal differentiation.

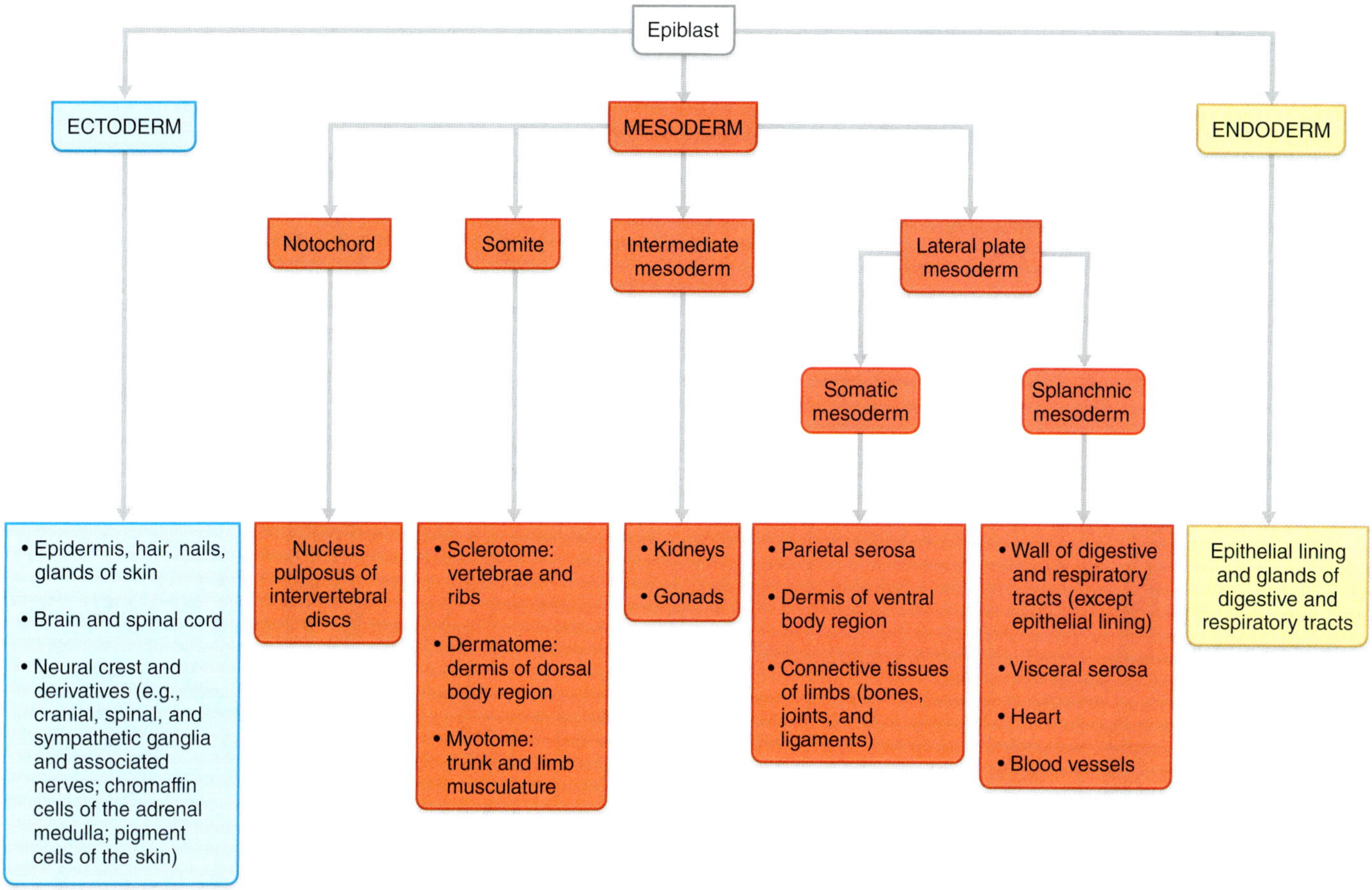

Figure 28.13 **Flowchart showing major derivatives of the embryonic germ layers.**

Development of the Fetal Circulation Embryonic development of the cardiovascular system lays the groundwork for the fetal circulatory pattern, which is converted to the adult pattern at birth. The first blood cells arise in the yolk sac. Before week 3 of development, tiny spaces appear in the splanchnic mesoderm. These are quickly lined by endothelial cells, covered with mesenchyme, and linked together into rapidly spreading vascular networks, destined to form the heart, blood vessels, and lymphatics. By the end of week 3, the embryo has a system of paired blood vessels, and the two vessels forming the heart have fused and bent into an S shape. By 3½ weeks, the miniature heart is pumping blood for an embryo less than a quarter inch long.

Unique cardiovascular modifications seen only during prenatal development include the **umbilical arteries** and **vein** and three *vascular shunts* **(Figure 28.14)**. All of these structures are occluded at birth. As you read about these vessels, keep in mind that the blood is flowing from and to the fetal heart. The large umbilical vein carries freshly oxygenated blood returning from the placenta into the embryonic body, where it is conveyed to the liver. There, some of the returning blood percolates through the liver sinusoids and out the hepatic veins. Most of the blood coursing through the umbilical vein, however, enters the **ductus venosus** (duk′tus ve-no′sus), a venous shunt that bypasses the liver sinusoids. Both the hepatic veins and the ductus venosus empty into the inferior vena cava where the placental blood mixes with deoxygenated blood returning from the lower parts of the fetus's body. The vena cava in turn conveys this "mixed load" of blood directly to the right atrium of the heart.

After birth, the liver plays an important role in nutrient processing, but during embryonic life the mother's liver performs these functions. Consequently, blood flow through the fetal liver during development is important only to ensure that the liver cells remain healthy.

Blood entering and leaving the heart encounters two more shunt systems, each serving to bypass the nonfunctional lungs. Some of the blood entering the right atrium flows directly into the left atrium via the **foramen ovale** ("oval hole"), an opening in the interatrial septum loosely closed by a flap of tissue. Blood that enters the right ventricle is pumped out into the pulmonary trunk. However, the second shunt, the **ductus arteriosus**, transfers most of that blood directly into the aorta, again bypassing the pulmonary circuit. (The lungs *do* receive adequate blood to maintain their growth.) Blood enters the two pulmonary bypass shunts because the heart chamber or vessel on the other side of each shunt is a lower-pressure area, owing to the low volume of venous return from the lungs. Blood flowing distally through

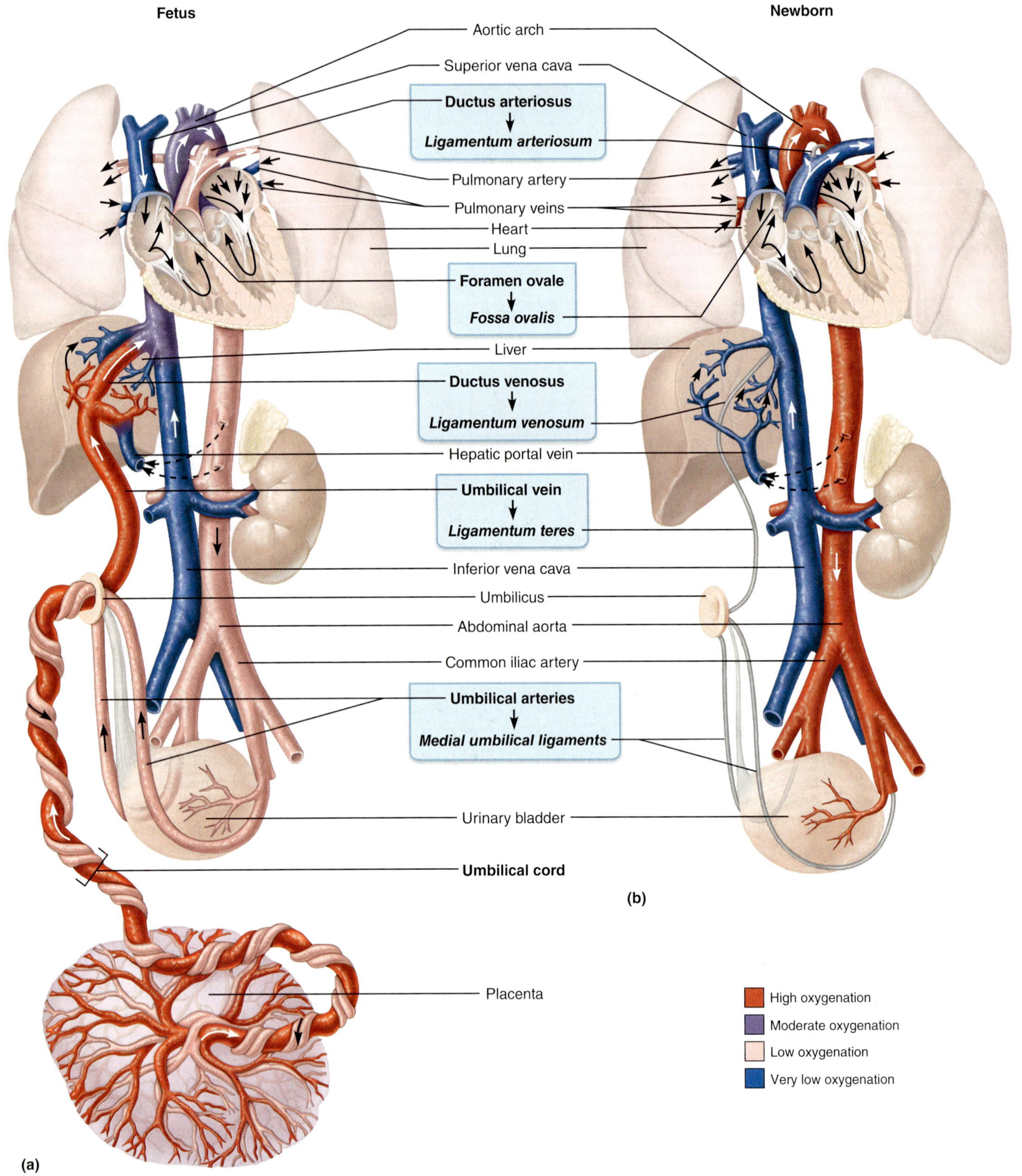

Figure 28.14 Circulation in fetus and newborn. Arrows on blood vessels indicate direction of blood flow. Arrows in color screens go from the fetal structure to what it becomes after birth. **(a)** Special adaptations for embryonic and fetal life. The umbilical vein carries oxygen- and nutrient-rich blood from the placenta to the fetus. The umbilical arteries carry waste-laden blood from the fetus to the placenta. The ductus arteriosus and foramen ovale bypass the nonfunctional lungs. Note that blood passing through the foramen ovale comes mostly from the inferior vena cava. The ductus venosus allows blood to partially bypass the liver. **(b)** Changes in the cardiovascular system at birth. The umbilical vessels as well as the liver and lung bypasses are occluded.

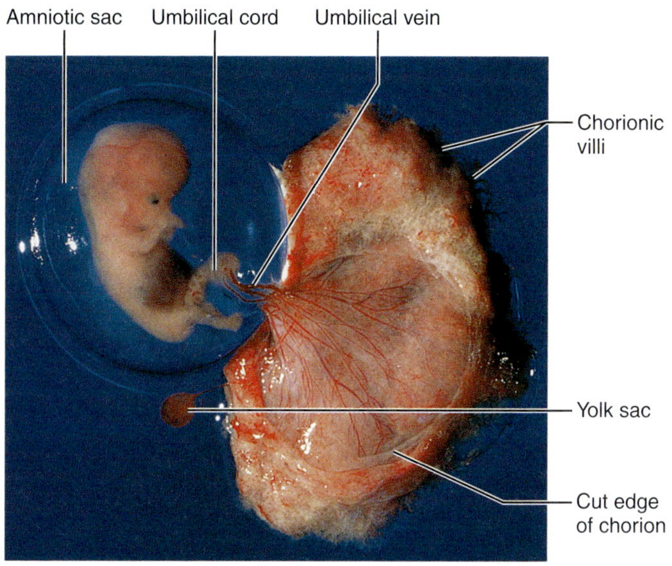

(a) Embryo at week 7, about 17 mm long.

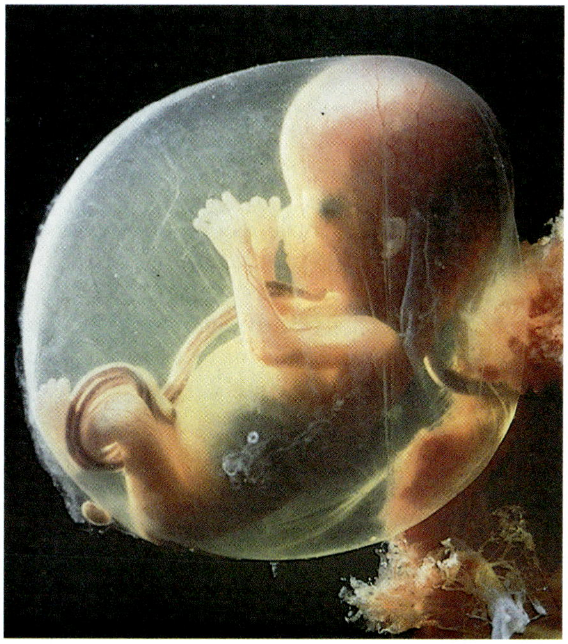

(b) Fetus in month 3, about 6 cm long.

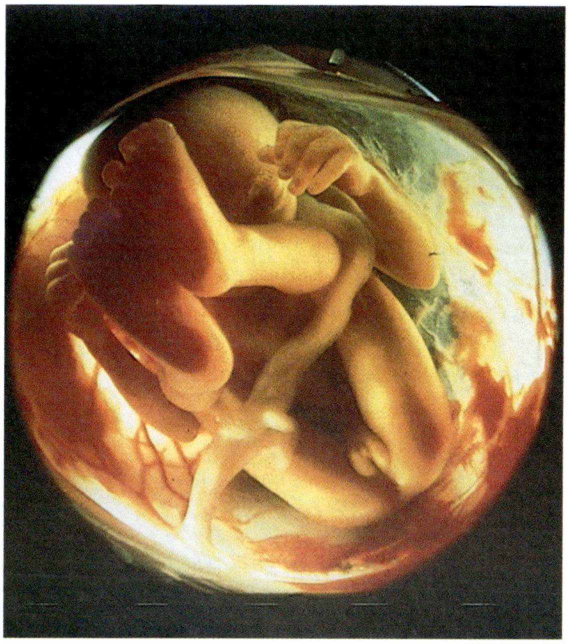

(c) Fetus late in month 5, about 19 cm long.

Figure 28.15 Photographs of a developing fetus. By birth, the fetus is typically 36 cm long from crown to rump.

the aorta eventually reaches the umbilical arteries, which are branches of the internal iliac arteries serving the pelvis. From here the largely deoxygenated blood, laden with metabolic wastes, is delivered back to the capillaries in the chorionic villi of the placenta. The changes in the circulatory plan that occur at birth are illustrated in Figure 28.14b.

Check Your Understanding

12. The early embryo is flat like a three-layered pancake. What event must occur before organogenesis can get going in earnest?
13. What germ layer gives rise to essentially all body tissues except nervous tissue, the epidermis, and mucosae?

For answers, see Appendix H

Events of Fetal Development

✓ Indicate the duration of the fetal period, and note the major events of fetal development.

During the fetal period, the developing fetus grows from a crown-to-rump length of about 22 mm (slightly less than 1 inch) and a weight of approximately 2 g (0.06 ounce) to about 360 mm (14 inches) and 3.2 kg (7 lb) or more. (Total body length at birth is about 550 mm, or 22 inches.) As you might expect with such tremendous growth, the changes in fetal appearance are quite dramatic (**Figure 28.15**). The fetal period is a time of

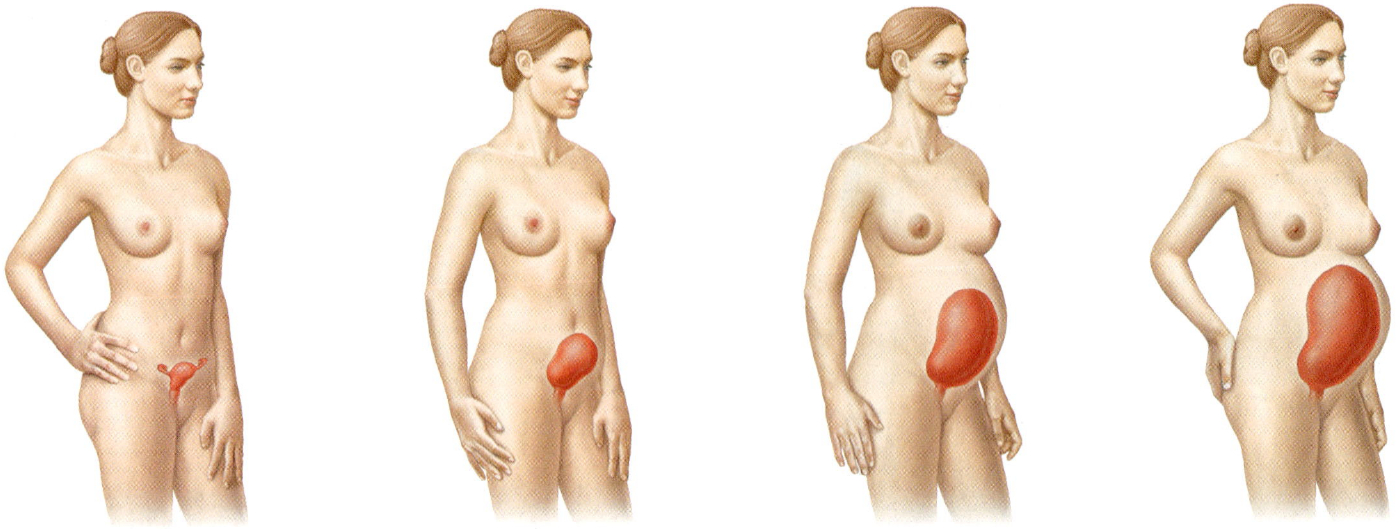

(a) Before conception
(Uterus the size of a fist and resides in the pelvis.)

(b) 4 months
(Fundus of the uterus is halfway between the pubic symphysis and the umbilicus.)

(c) 7 months
(Fundus is well above the umbilicus.)

(d) 9 months
(Fundus reaches the xiphoid process.)

Figure 28.16 Relative size of the uterus before conception and during pregnancy.

rapid growth of the body structures that were established in the embryo. During the first half of this period, cells are still differentiating into specific cell types to form the body's distinctive tissues and are completing the fine details of body structure. The main events of the fetal period—weeks 9 through 38—are listed chronologically in **Table 28.1** on p. 1084. The greatest amount of growth occurs in the first 8 weeks of life, when the embryo grows from one cell to a fetus of 1 inch.

Check Your Understanding

14. When does the fetal period begin?

For answers, see Appendix H.

Effects of Pregnancy on the Mother

- Describe functional changes in maternal reproductive organs and in the cardiovascular, respiratory, and urinary systems during pregnancy.
- Indicate the effects of pregnancy on maternal metabolism and posture.

28

The mean duration of pregnancy is 38 weeks from the time of ovulation to birth. Pregnancy can be a difficult time for the mother because profound adaptations occur in several body systems. Not only are there anatomical changes, but striking changes in her metabolism and physiology occur to support the pregnancy and prepare her body for delivery and lactation.

Anatomical Changes

As pregnancy progresses, the female reproductive organs become increasingly vascular and engorged with blood, and the vagina develops a purplish hue (*Chadwick's sign*). The enhanced vascularity increases vaginal sensitivity and sexual intensity, and some women achieve orgasm for the first time when they are pregnant. Prodded by rising levels of estrogen and progesterone, the breasts enlarge and engorge with blood, and their areolae darken. Some women develop increased pigmentation of facial skin of the nose and cheeks, a condition called *chloasma* (klo-az′mah; "to be green") or the "mask of pregnancy."

The degree of uterine enlargement during pregnancy is remarkable. Starting as a fist-sized organ, the uterus fills most of the pelvic cavity by 16 weeks **(Figure 28.16a, b)**. Though the fetus is only about 140 mm long (crown-to-rump) at this time, the placenta is fully formed, uterine muscle is hypertrophied, and amniotic fluid volume is increasing.

As pregnancy continues, the uterus pushes higher into the abdominal cavity, exerting pressure on both abdominal and pelvic organs (Figure 28.16c). As birth nears, the uterus reaches the level of the xiphoid process and occupies most of the abdominal cavity (Figure 28.16d). The crowded abdominal organs press superiorly against the diaphragm, which intrudes on the thoracic cavity. As a result, the ribs flare, causing the thorax to widen.

The increasing bulkiness of the anterior abdomen changes the woman's center of gravity, and many women develop *lordosis* (accentuated lumbar curvature) and backaches during the last few months of pregnancy. Placental production of the hormone **relaxin** causes pelvic ligaments and the pubic symphysis to relax, widen, and become more flexible. This increased flexibility eases birth passage, but it may result in a waddling gait in the meantime. Considerable weight gain occurs during a normal pregnancy. Because some women are over- or underweight before pregnancy begins, it is almost impossible to state the ideal or desirable weight gain. However, summing up the weight increases resulting from fetal and placental growth, increased size of the maternal reproductive organs and breasts, and greater blood volume during pregnancy, a weight gain of approximately 13 kg (about 28 lb) usually occurs.

Good nutrition is necessary all through pregnancy if the developing fetus is to have all the building materials (especially proteins, calcium, and iron) needed to form its tissues. Additionally, multivitamins containing folic acid reduce the risk of having a baby with neurological problems, including such birth defects as spina bifida and anencephaly, as well as spontaneous preterm birth. (Indeed, a recent study on preconceptual folic acid supplementation for a year or more resulted in a reduction of spontaneous preterm birth by 50–70%.) However, a pregnant woman needs only 300 additional calories daily to sustain proper fetal growth. The emphasis should be on eating high-quality food, not just more food.

Not surprisingly, effects of the fetal environment may not show up until decades later. Below-normal birth weight, for instance, places females at risk for type 2 diabetes and increases the general risk of cardiovascular disease later in life for both men and women.

Metabolic Changes

As the placenta enlarges, it secretes increasing amounts of **human placental lactogen (hPL)**, also called **human chorionic somatomammotropin (hCS)**. hPL works cooperatively with estrogens and progesterone to stimulate maturation of the breasts for lactation, promotes growth of the fetus, and exerts a glucose-sparing effect in the mother. Consequently, maternal cells metabolize more fatty acids and less glucose than usual, sparing glucose for use by the fetus. Gestational diabetes mellitus occurs in about 10% of pregnancies, but over half of those women go on to develop type 2 diabetes later in life.

Plasma levels of parathyroid hormone and activated vitamin D rise, so that pregnant women tend to be in positive calcium balance throughout pregnancy. This state ensures that the developing fetus will have adequate calcium to mineralize its bones.

Physiological Changes

Physiological changes take place in many systems during pregnancy. A few of these changes are described next.

Gastrointestinal System

The nausea and vomiting (commonly called morning sickness) suffered by many women during the first few months of pregnancy are believed to be related to elevated levels of hCG, estrogens, and progesterone. (Nausea is also a side effect of many birth control pills.) *Heartburn*, due to reflux of stomach acid into the esophagus, is common because the esophagus is displaced and the stomach is crowded by the growing uterus. *Constipation* occurs because motility of the digestive tract declines during pregnancy.

Homeostatic Imbalance 28.1

Because many potentially harmful substances can cross placental barriers and enter the fetal blood, a pregnant woman should be aware of what she is taking into her body, particularly during the embryonic period when the body's foundations are laid down. **Teratogens** (ter′ah-to-jenz; *terato* = monster), factors that may cause severe congenital abnormalities or even fetal death, include alcohol, nicotine, many drugs (anticoagulants, sedatives, antihypertensives, and some antibiotics), and maternal infections, particularly German measles. For example, when a woman drinks alcohol, her fetus becomes inebriated as well. However, the fetal consequences may be much more lasting and result in the *fetal alcohol syndrome* (*FAS*) typified by microcephaly (small head), mental retardation, and abnormal growth. Nicotine hinders oxygen delivery to the fetus, impairing normal growth and development. The sedative **thalidomide** (thah-lid′o-mīd) was used by thousands of pregnant women in the 1960s to alleviate morning sickness. When taken during the period of limb bud differentiation (days 26–56), it sometimes resulted in tragically deformed infants with short flipperlike legs and arms. ✚

Urinary System

The kidneys produce more urine during pregnancy because of the mother's increased metabolic rate and the additional burden of disposing of fetal metabolic wastes. As the growing uterus compresses the bladder, urination becomes more frequent, more urgent, and sometimes uncontrollable (*stress incontinence*).

Respiratory System

The nasal mucosa responds to estrogens by becoming edematous and congested. Thus, nasal stuffiness and occasional nosebleeds may occur. Tidal volume increases markedly during pregnancy, while respiratory rate is relatively unchanged and residual volume declines. The increase in tidal volume is due to the mother's greater need for oxygen during pregnancy and the fact that progesterone enhances the sensitivity of the medullary respiratory center to CO_2. Many women exhibit *dyspnea* (disp-ne′ah), or difficult breathing, during the later stages of pregnancy.

Cardiovascular System

The most dramatic physiological changes occur in the cardiovascular system. Total body water rises, and blood volume may increase as much as 40% by the 32nd week to accommodate the additional needs of the fetus. The rise in blood volume also safeguards against blood loss during birth. Mean blood pressure typically decreases during midpregnancy, but then rises to normal levels during the third trimester. Cardiac output increases by 35–40% at various stages of pregnancy. This helps propel the greater circulatory volume around the body. The uterus presses on the pelvic blood vessels, which may impair venous return from the lower limbs, resulting in *varicose veins* and leg edema.

Table 28.1 Developmental Events of the Fetal Period

TIME		CHANGES AND ACCOMPLISHMENTS
8 weeks (end of embryonic period)	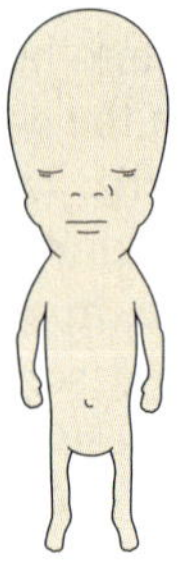 8 weeks	Head nearly as large as body; all major brain regions present; first brain waves in brain stem Liver disproportionately large and begins to form blood cells Limbs present; digits are initially webbed, but fingers and toes are free by the end of this interval Ossification just begun; weak, spontaneous muscle contractions occur Cardiovascular system fully functional (heart has been pumping blood since the fourth week) All body systems present in at least rudimentary form Approximate crown-to-rump length: 22 mm (0.9 inch); weight: 2 grams (0.06 ounce)
9–12 weeks (month 3)	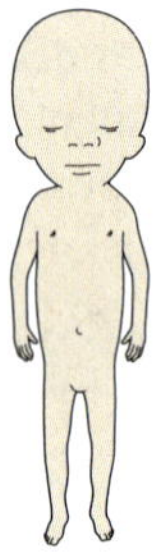 12 weeks	Head still dominant, but body elongating; brain continues to enlarge, shows its general structural features; cervical and lumbar enlargements apparent in spinal cord; retina of eye is present Skin epidermis and dermis obvious; facial features present in crude form Liver prominent and bile being secreted; palate is fusing; most glands of endodermal origin are developed; walls of hollow visceral organs gaining smooth muscle Blood cell formation begins in bone marrow Notochord degenerating and ossification accelerating; limbs well molded Sex readily detected from the genitals Approximate crown-to-rump length at end of interval: 90 mm
13–16 weeks (month 4)	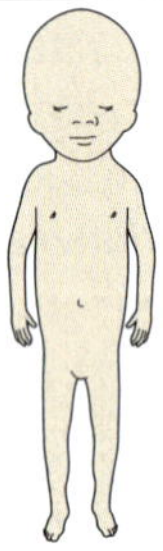 16 weeks	Cerebellum becoming prominent; general sensory organs differentiated; eyes and ears assume characteristic position and shape; blinking of eyes and sucking motions of lips occur Face looks human and growth of the body beginning to outpace that of the head Glands developed in GI tract; meconium is collecting Kidneys attain typical structure Most bones are now distinct and joint cavities are apparent Approximate crown-to-rump length at end of interval: 140 mm
17–20 weeks (month 5)		Vernix caseosa (fatty secretions of sebaceous glands) covers body; lanugo (silklike hair) covers skin Fetal position (body flexed anteriorly) assumed because of space restrictions Limbs reach near-final proportions Quickening occurs (mother feels spontaneous muscular activity of fetus) Approximate crown-to-rump length at end of interval: 190 mm
21–30 weeks (months 6 and 7)		Period of substantial increase in weight (may survive if born prematurely at 27–28 weeks, but hypothalamic temperature regulation and lung production of surfactant are still inadequate) Myelination of spinal cord begins; eyes are open Distal limb bones are beginning to ossify Skin is wrinkled and red; fingernails and toenails are present; tooth enamel is forming on deciduous teeth Body is lean and well proportioned Bone marrow becomes sole site of blood cell formation Testes reach scrotum in seventh month (in males) Approximate crown-to-rump length at end of interval: 280 mm
30–40 weeks (term) (months 8 and 9)	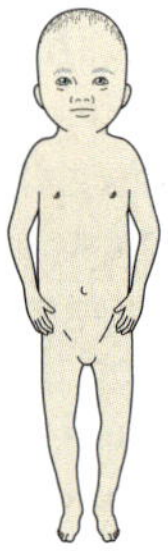 At birth	Skin whitish pink; fat laid down in subcutaneous tissue (hypodermis) Approximate crown-to-rump length at end of interval: 360 mm (14 inches); weight: 3.2 kg (7 lb)

Homeostatic Imbalance 28.2

A dangerous complication of pregnancy called **preeclampsia** results in an insufficient placental blood supply, which can starve a fetus of oxygen. The pregnant woman becomes edematous and hypertensive, and proteinuria occurs. This condition, which affects one in 10 pregnancies, is believed to be due to immunological abnormalities in some cases, because its occurrence seems to be positively correlated with the number of fetal cells that enter the maternal circulation. +

Check Your Understanding

15. What causes the difficult breathing that some women experience during pregnancy? What causes the waddling gait seen in some?
16. What is the cause of morning sickness?
17. What is the role of the hormone hPL?

For answers, see Appendix H.

Parturition (Birth)

✓ Explain how labor is initiated, and describe the three stages of labor.

Parturition (par″tu-rish′un; "bringing forth young") is the culmination of pregnancy—giving birth to the baby. It usually occurs within 15 days of the calculated due date (280 days from the last menstrual period). The series of events that expel the infant from the uterus are collectively called **labor**.

Initiation of Labor

Several events and hormones interlock to trigger labor. During the last few weeks of pregnancy, estrogens reach their highest levels in the mother's blood. Studies indicate that the fetus determines its own birth date. Rising levels of fetal adrenocortical hormones (especially cortisol) late in pregnancy are believed to stimulate the placenta to release such large amounts of estrogens. In addition, increased production of *surfactant protein A* (*SP-A*) by the fetal lungs in the weeks before delivery appears to trigger an inflammatory response in the cervix that stimulates its softening in preparation for labor.

The rise in estrogens has three important consequences. (1) It stimulates the myometrial cells of the uterus to form abundant oxytocin receptors **(Figure 28.17)**. (2) It promotes formation of gap junctions between the uterine smooth muscle cells. (3) It antagonizes progesterone's quieting influence on uterine muscle. As a result, the myometrium becomes increasingly irritable, and weak, irregular uterine contractions begin to occur. These contractions, called *Braxton Hicks contractions*, have caused many women to go to the hospital, only to be told that they were in **false labor** and sent home.

As birth nears, two more chemical signals cooperate to convert these false labor pains into the real thing. Certain fetal cells begin to produce **oxytocin** (ok″sĭ-to′sin), which causes the placenta to release **prostaglandins** (pros″tah-glan′dinz) (Figure 28.17) which, like estrogens, stimulate the synthesis of more gap junctions in uterine smooth muscle. Both hormones are powerful uterine muscle stimulants, and since the myometrium is now highly sensitive to oxytocin, contractions become more frequent and more vigorous. While elevated levels of oxytocin and prostaglandins sustain labor once it begins, many studies indicate that it is the prostaglandins (acting as paracrines) that actually trigger the rhythmic expulsive contractions of true labor, and play a major role in the thinning and softening of the cervix just before and during labor. At this point, the increasing cervical distension activates the mother's hypothalamus, which signals for oxytocin release by the posterior pituitary.

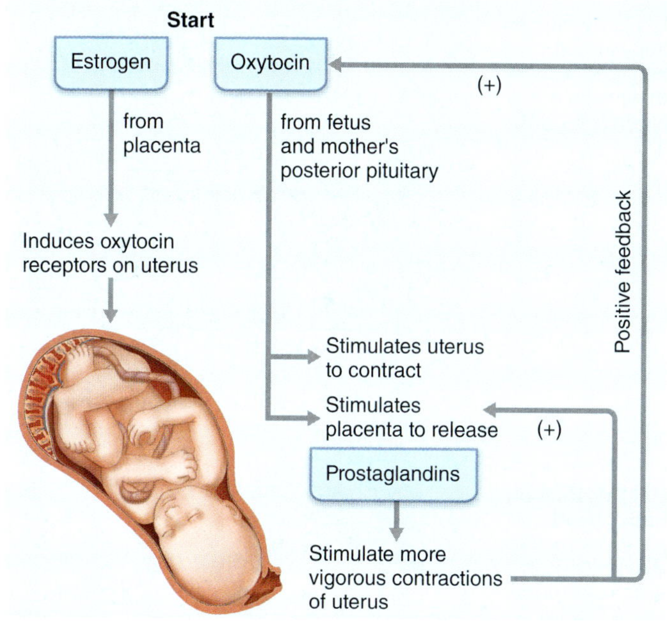

Figure 28.17 Hormonal induction of labor.

Once the hypothalamus is involved, several *positive feedback mechanisms* involving prostaglandins and oxytocin are propelled into action—greater distension of the cervix causes the release of more oxytocin, which causes greater contractile force, and so on (Figure 28.17). These expulsive contractions are aided by the fact that *fetal fibronectin*, a natural "stickum" (adhesive protein) that binds the fetal and maternal tissues of the placenta together throughout pregnancy, changes to a lubricant just before true labor begins.

As mentioned earlier, prostaglandins are essential for initiating labor in humans, and interfering with their production will hinder onset of labor. For example, antiprostaglandin drugs such as ibuprofen can inhibit the early stages of labor and such drugs are used occasionally to prevent preterm births.

Stages of Labor

Labor includes the dilation, expulsion, and placental stages illustrated in **Figure 28.18**.

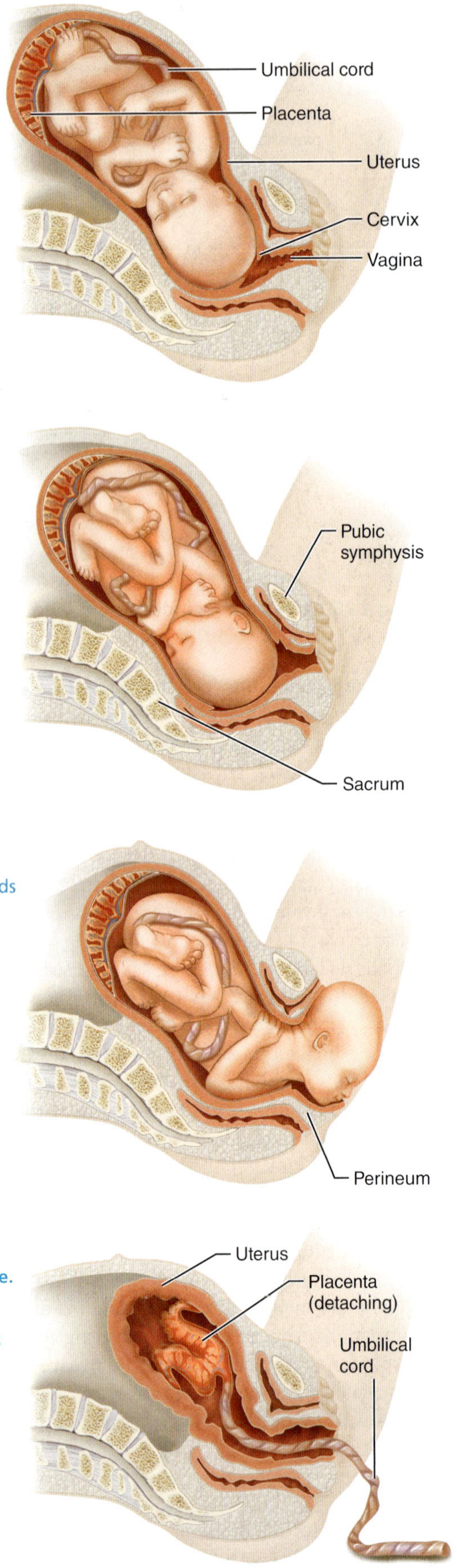

(1a) Early dilation. Baby's head engaged; widest dimension is along left-right axis.

(1b) Late dilation. Baby's head rotates so widest dimension is in anteroposterior axis (of pelvic outlet). Dilation nearly complete.

(2) Expulsion. Baby's head extends as it is delivered.

(3) Placental stage. After baby is delivered, the placenta detaches and is removed.

Figure 28.18 Parturition.

(1) **Dilation stage.** The **dilation stage** is the time from labor's onset until the cervix is fully dilated by the baby's head (about 10 cm in diameter). As labor starts, weak but regular contractions begin in the upper part of the uterus and move toward the vagina. At first, only the superior uterine muscle is active; contractions are 15–30 minutes apart, and last for 10–30 seconds. As labor progresses, the contractions become more vigorous and rapid, and the lower part of the uterus gets involved. As the infant's head is forced against the cervix with each contraction, the cervix softens and thins (*effaces*), and dilates. Eventually the amnion ruptures, releasing the amniotic fluid, an event commonly called "breaking the water."

The dilation stage is the longest part of labor, lasting 6–12 hours or more. Several events happen during this phase. *Engagement* occurs when the infant's head enters the true pelvis. As descent continues through the birth canal, the baby's head rotates so that its greatest dimension is in the anteroposterior line, which allows it to navigate the narrow dimensions of the pelvic outlet (Figure 28.18 (1b)).

(2) **Expulsion stage.** The **expulsion stage** lasts from full dilation to delivery of the infant, or actual childbirth. By the time the cervix is fully dilated, strong contractions occur every 2–3 minutes and last about 1 minute. In this stage, a mother undergoing labor without local anesthesia has an increasing urge to push or bear down with the abdominal muscles. Although this phase may last 2 hours, it is typically 50 minutes in a first birth and around 20 minutes in subsequent births.

Crowning occurs when the largest dimension of the baby's head distends the vulva. At this point, an *episiotomy* (e-piz″e-ot′o-me) may be done to reduce tissue tearing. An episiotomy is an incision made to widen the vaginal orifice. The baby's neck extends as the head exits from the perineum, and once the head has been delivered, the rest of the baby's body is delivered much more easily. After birth, the umbilical cord is clamped and cut.

When the infant is in the usual *vertex*, or head-first, *presentation*, the skull (its largest diameter) acts as a wedge to dilate the cervix. The head-first presentation also allows the baby to be suctioned free of mucus and to breathe even before it has completely exited from the birth canal. In *breech* (buttock-first) and other nonvertex presentations, these advantages are lost and delivery is much more difficult, often requiring the use of forceps, or a C-section (see below).

Homeostatic Imbalance 28.3

If a woman has a deformed or malelike pelvis, labor may be prolonged and difficult. This condition is called *dystocia* (dis-to′se-ah; *dys* = difficult; *toc* = birth). Besides extreme maternal fatigue, another possible consequence of dystocia is fetal brain damage, resulting in cerebral palsy or epilepsy. To prevent these outcomes, a *cesarean* (*C-*) *section* (se-sa′re-an) is performed in many such cases. A C-section is delivery of the infant through an incision made through the abdominal and uterine walls. +

(3) **Placental stage.** The **placental stage**, or the delivery of the placenta and its attached fetal membranes, which are collectively called the **afterbirth**, is usually accomplished within 30 minutes after birth of the infant. The strong uterine contractions that continue after birth compress uterine blood vessels, limit bleeding, and shear the placenta off the uterine wall (cause placental detachment). It is very important that all placental fragments be removed to prevent continued uterine bleeding after birth (*postpartum bleeding*).

Check Your Understanding

18. What is a breech presentation?
19. What chemical is most responsible for triggering true labor?
20. Why does a baby turn as it travels through the birth canal?

For answers, see Appendix H.

Adjustments of the Infant to Extrauterine Life

✓ Outline the events leading to the first breath of a newborn.

✓ Describe changes that occur in the fetal circulation after birth.

The **neonatal period** is the four-week period immediately after birth. Here we will be concerned with the events of just the first few hours after birth in a normal infant. As you might suspect, birth represents quite a shock to the infant. Exposed to physical trauma during the birth process, it is suddenly cast out of its watery, warm environment and its placental life supports are severed. Now it must do for itself all that the mother had been doing for it—respire, obtain nutrients, excrete, and maintain its body temperature.

At 1 and 5 minutes after birth, the infant's physical status is assessed based on five signs: heart rate, respiration, color, muscle tone, and reflexes (tested by response to catheter in nostril). Each observation is given a score of 0 to 2, and the total is called the **Apgar score**. An Apgar score of 8 to 10 indicates a healthy baby. Lower scores reveal problems in one or more of the physiological functions assessed.

Taking the First Breath and Transition

The crucial first requirement is to breathe. Vasoconstriction of the umbilical arteries, initiated when they are stretched during birth, leads to loss of placental support. Once carbon dioxide is no longer removed by the placenta, it accumulates in the baby's blood, causing central acidosis. This excites respiratory control centers in the baby's brain and triggers the first inspiration. The first breath requires a tremendous effort—the airways are tiny, and the lungs are collapsed. However, once the lungs have been inflated in full-term babies, surfactant in alveolar fluid reduces surface tension in the alveoli, and breathing is easier. The rate of respiration is rapid (about 45 respirations/min) during the first two weeks and then gradually declines.

Keeping the lungs inflated is much more difficult for premature infants (those weighing less than 2500 g, or about 5.5 lb, at birth) because surfactant production occurs during the last months of prenatal life. Consequently, preemies are usually put on respiratory assistance (a ventilator) until their lungs are mature enough to function on their own.

For 6–8 hours after birth, infants pass through an unstable **transitional period** marked by alternating periods of increased activity and sleep. During the activity periods, vital signs are irregular and the baby gags frequently as it regurgitates mucus and debris. After this, the infant stabilizes, with waking periods (dictated by hunger) occurring every 3–4 hours.

Occlusion of Special Fetal Blood Vessels and Vascular Shunts

After birth the special umbilical blood vessels and fetal shunts are no longer necessary (see Figure 28.14b). The umbilical arteries and vein constrict and become fibrosed. The proximal parts of the umbilical arteries persist as the *superior vesical arteries* that supply the urinary bladder, and their distal parts become the **medial umbilical ligaments**. The remnant of the umbilical vein becomes the **round ligament of the liver**, or **ligamentum teres**, that attaches the umbilicus to the liver. The ductus venosus collapses as blood stops flowing through the umbilical vein and is eventually converted to the **ligamentum venosum** on the liver's undersurface.

As the pulmonary circulation becomes functional, pressure in the left side of the heart increases and that in the right side of the heart decreases, causing the pulmonary shunts to close. The flap of the foramen ovale is pushed to the shut position, and its edges fuse to the septal wall. Ultimately, only a slight depression, the **fossa ovalis**, marks its position. The ductus arteriosus constricts and is converted to the cordlike **ligamentum arteriosum**, connecting the aorta and pulmonary trunk.

Except for the foramen ovale, all of the special circulatory adaptations of the fetus are functionally occluded within 30 minutes after birth. Closure of the foramen ovale is usually complete within the year. As we described in Chapter 18, failure of the ductus arteriosus or foramen ovale to close leads to congenital heart defects.

Check Your Understanding

21. What two modifications of the fetal circulation allow most blood to bypass parts of the heart?
22. What happens to the special fetal circulatory modifications after birth?

For answers, see Appendix H.

Lactation

✓ Explain how the breasts are prepared for lactation.

Lactation is production of milk by the hormone-prepared mammary glands. Rising levels of (placental) estrogens, progesterone, and human placental lactogen toward the end of

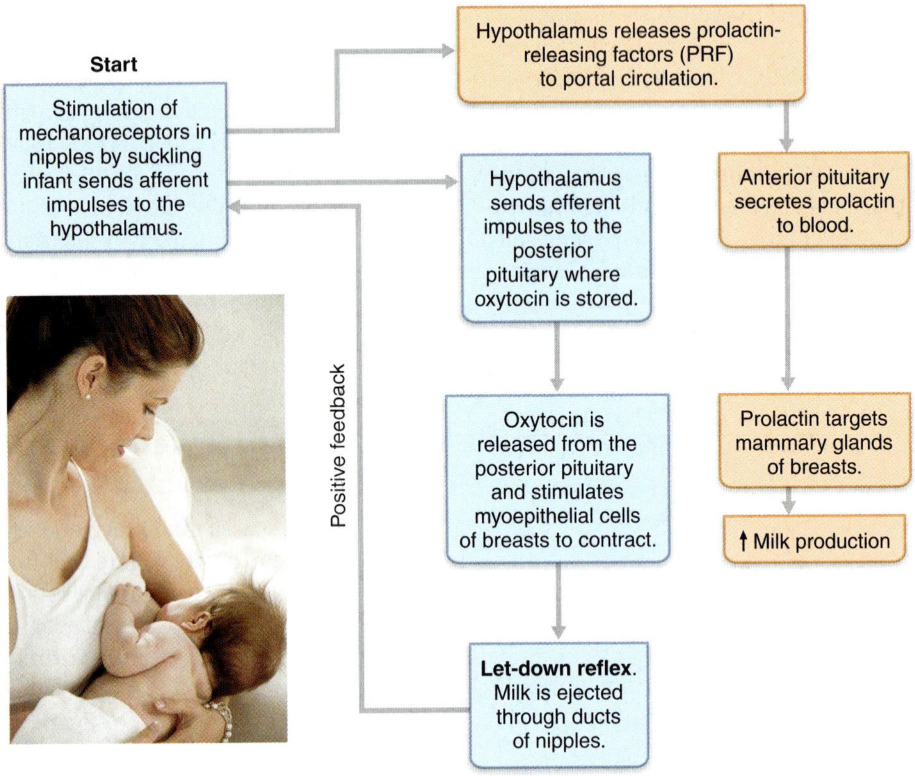

Figure 28.19 Milk production and the positive feedback mechanism of the milk let-down reflex.

pregnancy stimulate the hypothalamus to release prolactin-releasing factors (PRFs). The anterior pituitary gland responds by secreting **prolactin**. (This mechanism is described below.) After a delay of two to three days following birth, true milk production begins.

During the initial delay (and during late gestation), the mammary glands secrete a yellowish fluid called **colostrum** (ko-los′trum). It has less lactose than milk and almost no fat, but it contains more protein, vitamin A, and minerals than true milk. Like milk, colostrum is rich in IgA antibodies. Since these antibodies are resistant to digestion in the stomach, they may help to protect the infant's digestive tract against bacterial infection. Additionally, these IgA antibodies are absorbed by endocytosis and subsequently enter the bloodstream to provide even broader immunity.

After birth, prolactin release gradually wanes, and continual milk production depends on mechanical stimulation of the nipples, normally provided by the suckling infant. Mechanoreceptors in the nipple send afferent nerve impulses to the hypothalamus, stimulating secretion of PRF. This results in a burstlike release of prolactin, which stimulates milk production for the next feeding.

The same afferent impulses also prompt hypothalamic release of oxytocin from the posterior pituitary via a *positive feedback mechanism*. Oxytocin causes the **let-down reflex**, the actual ejection of milk from the alveoli of the mammary glands **(Figure 28.19)**. Let-down occurs when oxytocin binds to myoepithelial cells surrounding the glands, after which milk is ejected from *both* breasts, not just the suckled one. During nursing, oxytocin also stimulates the recently emptied uterus to contract, helping it to return to (nearly) its prepregnant size.

Breast milk has advantages for the infant:

- *Its fats and iron are better absorbed and its amino acids are metabolized more efficiently* than those of cow's milk.
- *It has a host of beneficial chemicals*, including IgA, complement, lysozyme, interferon, and lactoperoxidase, that protect infants from life-threatening infections. Mother's milk also contains interleukins and prostaglandins that prevent overzealous inflammatory responses, and a glycoprotein that deters the ulcer-causing bacterium (*Helicobacter pylori*) from attaching to the stomach mucosa.
- *Its natural laxative effect helps to cleanse the bowels of* **meconium** (mĕ-ko′ne-um), a tarry green-black paste containing sloughed-off epithelial cells, bile, and other substances. Since meconium, and later feces, provides the route for eliminating bilirubin from the body, clearing meconium as quickly as possible helps to prevent *physiological jaundice* (see the Related Clinical Terms section). Breast milk also encourages bacteria (the source of vitamin K and some B vitamins) to colonize the large intestine.

When nursing is discontinued, the stimulus for prolactin release and milk production ends, and the mammary glands stop producing milk. Women who nurse their infants for six months or more lose a significant amount of calcium from their bones, but those on sound diets usually replace lost bone calcium after weaning the infant.

While prolactin levels are high, the normal hypothalamic-pituitary controls of the ovarian cycle are damped, probably because stimulation of the hypothalamus by suckling causes it to release beta endorphin, a peptide hormone that inhibits hypothalamic release of GnRH and, consequently, the release of gonadotropins by the pituitary. Because of this inhibition of ovarian function, nursing has been called natural birth control. Nonetheless, there is a good deal of "slippage" in these controls, and most women begin to ovulate even while continuing to nurse their infants.

Check Your Understanding

23. What hormone causes the let-down reflex?

For answers, see Appendix H.

Assisted Reproductive Technology and Reproductive Cloning

✓ Describe some techniques of ART including IVF, ZIFT, and GIFT.

So far we have been describing how babies are made. But if a couple lacks that capability for some reason, what recourse do they have? Hormone therapy may increase sperm or egg production in cases where that is the problem, and surgery can open blocked uterine tubes. Recently, an artificial ovary, which allows eggs to mature outside the body, has been developed that preserves a woman's fertility if she needs to undergo treatment for cancer.

Beyond that are *assisted reproductive technology* (*ART*) procedures that entail surgically removing oocytes from a woman's ovaries following hormone stimulation, fertilizing the oocytes, and then returning them to the woman's body. These procedures, now performed worldwide in major medical centers, have produced thousands of infants, but they are expensive, emotionally draining, and painful for the oocyte donor. Unused oocytes, sperm, and embryos can be frozen for later attempts at accomplishing pregnancy.

In the most common ART process, *in vitro fertilization* (*IVF*), harvested oocytes are incubated with sperm in culture dishes (*in vitro*) for several days to allow fertilization to occur. In cases where the quality or number of sperm is low, the oocytes are injected with sperm. Embryos reaching the two-cell or blastocyst stage are then carefully transferred into the woman's uterus in the hope that implantation will occur.

In *zygote intrafallopian transfer* (*ZIFT*), oocytes fertilized in vitro are immediately transferred to the woman's uterine (fallopian) tubes. The goal is to have development to the blastocyst stage occur followed by normal implantation in the uterus.

In *gamete intrafallopian transfer* (*GIFT*), no in vitro procedures are used. Instead, sperm and harvested oocytes are transferred together into the woman's uterine tubes in the hope that fertilization will take place there.

Although there is a great deal of hubbub in the scientific community about using cloning as another possible avenue to produce offspring, humans have proved notoriously difficult to create and sustain past very early (blastocyst) development. Cloning entails insertion of a somatic cell nucleus into an oocyte from which the nucleus is removed and then an incubation period to dedifferentiate the inserted nucleus. This technique has proved more successful in creating stem cells for therapeutic use in treating selected diseases than for reproductive cloning to produce whole and healthy human offspring. Furthermore, human reproductive cloning is currently fraught with legal, moral, ethical, and political roadblocks.

In this chapter, we have focused on changes that occur during human development in utero. But having a baby is not always what the interacting partners have in mind, and we humans have devised a variety of techniques for preventing this outcome (see *A Closer Look* on p. 1090).

We must admit that the description of embryonic development here has fallen short because we have barely touched upon the phenomenon of differentiation. How does an unspecialized cell that can become *anything* in the body develop into a specific *something* (a heart cell, for example)? And what paces the developmental sequence, so that if a particular process fails to occur at a precise time, it never occurs at all? Scientists are beginning to believe that there are master switches in the genes. In Chapter 29, the final chapter of this book, we describe a small part of the "how" as we examine the interaction of genes and other components that determine who we finally become.

Contraception: To Be or Not To Be

In a society such as ours, where many women opt for professional careers or work for economic reasons, **contraception** (*contra* = against, *cept* = taking), commonly called **birth control**, is often seen as a necessity.

The key to birth control is **dependability**. As the red arrows in the accompanying flowchart show, the birth control techniques currently available have many sites of action for **blocking reproduction**. Generally speaking, birth control methods can be categorized into three groups based on how each prevents pregnancy—behavioral methods, barrier methods, or hormonal methods. Let's examine a few of them more closely.

Behavioral methods (coitus interruptus, the rhythm method, and abstinence) consist of altering behavior to prevent pregnancy. *Coitus interruptus*, or withdrawal of the penis just before ejaculation, is unreliable because control of ejaculation is never ensured.

Rhythm or *temporary abstinence methods* involve avoiding intercourse during periods of ovulation or fertility. This may be accomplished by recording daily basal body temperatures (body temperature drops slightly immediately prior to ovulation and then rises slightly after ovulation). This technique requires accurate record keeping for several cycles before it can be used with confidence, but has a high success rate for those willing to take the time necessary. With a failure rate of 10–20%, it is obvious that some people are willing and some are not.

Barrier methods include diaphragms, cervical caps, male and female condoms, and spermicides. These techniques prevent the sperm and egg from meeting and implanting. They are quite effective, especially when used in combination—for example, condoms and spermicides. But many people avoid them because they can reduce the spontaneity of sexual encounters.

Hormonal methods include a broad variety of hormone-containing contraceptive products (the pill, IUD, patches, vaginal ring, and implanted or injected agents). These methods are highly effective, with a failure rate of less than 1%, and have a low risk of adverse effects in most women.

The most-used contraceptive product in the United States is the *oral contraceptive pill* (*OCP*) or simply "the pill," first

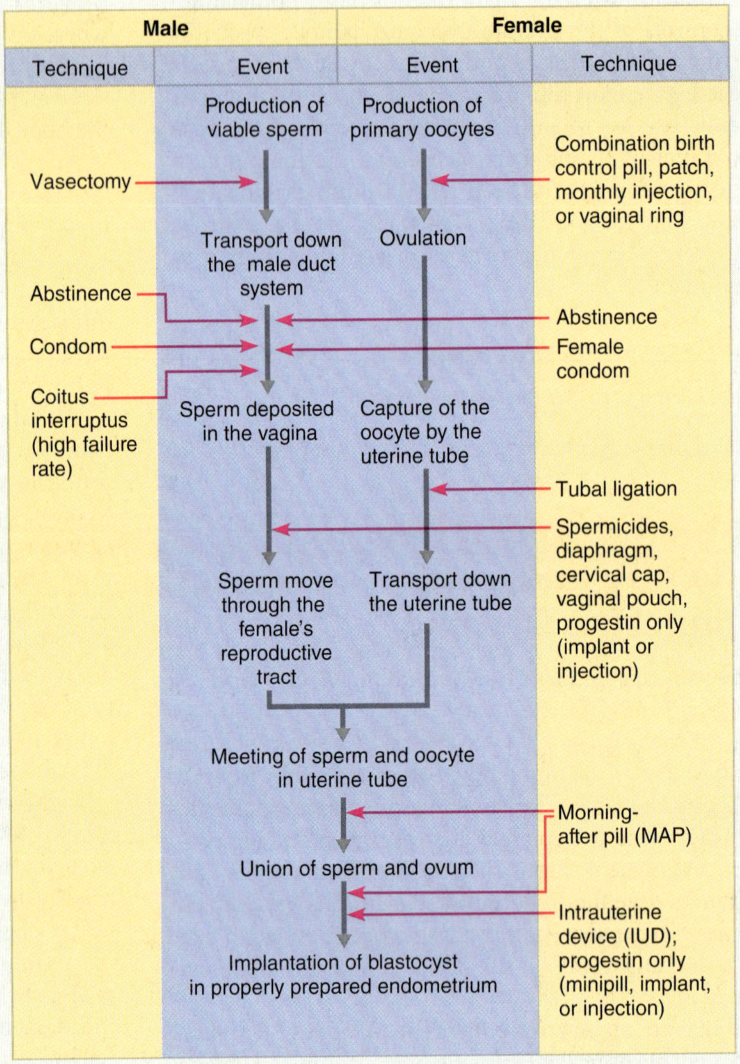

Mechanisms of contraception. Techniques or products that interfere with events from production of gametes to implantation are indicated by red arrows at the site of interference and act to prevent the next step from occurring.

marketed in 1960. Supplied in 28-tablet packets, the first 20 or 21 tablets contain minute amounts of estrogens and progestins (progesterone-like hormones) which are taken daily; the hormones contained may be of fixed or of varying combinations. The last seven tablets are hormone free—are placebos or are iron pills. The pill tricks the hypothalamic-pituitary-gonadal axis and "lulls it to sleep," because the relatively constant blood levels of ovarian hormones make it appear that the woman is pregnant (both estrogen and progesterone are produced throughout pregnancy). Ovarian follicles do not develop, ovulation ceases, and menstrual flow is much reduced. However, since hormonal balance is one of the most precisely controlled body functions, some women cannot tolerate these changes—they become nauseated and/or hypertensive. The pill has adverse cardiovascular effects in a small number of users and there is still debate about whether it increases the risk of uterine, ovarian, or (particularly) breast cancer. Presently, well over 50 million women use the pill.

Other delivery methods using the combination hormone approach include two slow-release products—a flexible ring that is inserted into the vagina, and a transdermal (skin) patch. Failure rates and side effects of the vaginal ring and skin patch are comparable to those of the pill. Combination birth control pills with substantially higher hormone concentrations used for *postcoital contraception* have a 75% effectiveness. Taken within three days of unprotected intercourse, these *morning-after pills* (*MAPs*), or *emergency contraceptive pills* (ECPs) as they are also called, "mess up" normal hormonal signals enough to prevent a fertilized egg from implanting or prevent fertilization altogether.

Other hormonal approaches to contraception use progestin-only products that thicken the cervical mucus enough to block sperm entry into the uterus, decrease the frequency of ovulation, and make the endometrium inhospitable to implantion. These include match-size silicone rods implanted just under the skin that release progestin over a five-year period (Norplant), and an injectable form that lasts for three months (Depo Provera). New intrauterine devices (IUDs) that are inserted into the uterus provide sustained local delivery of synthetic progesterone to the endometrium and are particularly recommended for women who have given birth and are nursing or those in monogamous relationships. The failure rates of progestin treatments are even less than that of the "pill."

Sterilization techniques permanently prevent gamete release. *Tubal ligation* or vasectomy (cutting or cauterizing the uterine tubes or ductus deferentia, respectively) are nearly foolproof and are the choice of approximately 33% of couples of childbearing age in the United States. Both procedures can be done in the physician's office. However, these techniques are usually permanent, making them unpopular with individuals who still plan to have children but want to select the time.

This summary doesn't even begin to touch on the experimental birth control drugs now awaiting clinical trials, and other methods are sure to be developed in the near future. In the final analysis, however, the only 100% effective means of birth control is the age-old one—total abstinence.

Chapter Summary

For more chapter study tools, go to the Study Area of MasteringA&P at **www.masteringaandp.com**. There you will find:

- Interactive Physiology iP
- A&PFlix
- Practice Anatomy Lab PAL
- PhysioEx PEx
- Videos, Practice Quizzes and Tests, MP3 Tutor Sessions, Case Studies, and much more!

1. The gestation period of approximately 280 days extends from the woman's last menstrual period to birth. The conceptus undergoes embryonic development for 8 weeks after fertilization, and fetal development from week 9 to birth.

From Egg to Zygote (pp. 1065–1067)

Accomplishing Fertilization (pp. 1065–1067)

1. An oocyte is fertilizable for up to 24 hours; most sperm are viable within the female reproductive tract for one to two days.
2. Sperm must survive the hostile environment of the vagina and become capacitated (capable of reaching and fertilizing the oocyte).
3. Hundreds of sperm must release their acrosomal enzymes to break down the egg's corona radiata and zona pellucida.
4. When one sperm binds to receptors on the egg, it triggers the slow block to polyspermy (release of cortical granules).
5. Following sperm penetration, the secondary oocyte completes meiosis II. Then the ovum and sperm pronuclei fuse (fertilization), forming a zygote.

Events of Embryonic Development: Zygote to Blastocyst Implantation (pp. 1067–1074)

Cleavage and Blastocyst Formation (p. 1067)

1. Early development consists of cleavage, a rapid series of mitotic divisions without intervening growth, that begins with the zygote and ends with a blastocyst. The blastocyst consists of the trophoblast and an inner cell mass. Cleavage produces a large number of cells with a favorable surface-to-volume ratio.

Implantation (pp. 1067, 1070–1071)

2. The trophoblast adheres to, digests, and implants in the endometrium. Implantation is completed when the blastocyst is entirely surrounded by endometrial tissue, about 12 days after ovulation.
3. hCG released by the blastocyst maintains hormone production by the corpus luteum, preventing menses. hCG levels decline after four months.

Placentation (pp. 1071–1074)

4. The placenta acts as the respiratory, nutritive, and excretory organ of the fetus and produces the hormones of pregnancy. It is formed from embryonic (chorionic villi) and maternal (endometrial decidua) tissues. The chorion develops when the trophoblast becomes associated with extraembryonic mesoderm. Typically, the placenta is functional as an endocrine organ by the third month.

Events of Embryonic Development: Gastrula to Fetus (pp. 1074–1081)

Formation and Roles of the Extraembryonic Membranes (pp. 1074–1075)

1. The fluid-filled amnion forms from cells of the superior surface (epiblast) of the embryonic disc. It protects the embryo from physical trauma and adhesion formation, provides a constant temperature, and allows fetal movements.
2. The yolk sac forms from the hypoblast of the embryonic disc; it is the source of early blood cells.
3. The allantois, a caudal outpocketing adjacent to the yolk sac, forms the structural basis of the umbilical cord.
4. The chorion is the outermost membrane and takes part in placentation.

Gastrulation: Germ Layer Formation (pp. 1075–1076)

5. Gastrulation involves cellular migrations that ultimately transform the inner cell mass into a three-layered embryo

(gastrula) containing ectoderm, mesoderm, and endoderm. Cells that move through the midline primitive streak become endoderm if they form the most inferior layer of the embryonic disc and mesoderm if they ultimately occupy the middle layer. Cells remaining on the superior surface become ectoderm.

Organogenesis: Differentiation of the Germ Layers (pp. 1076–1081)

6. Endoderm forms the mucosa of the digestive and respiratory systems, and the epithelial cells of all associated glands (thyroid, parathyroids, thymus, liver, pancreas). It becomes a continuous tube when the embryonic body undercuts and fuses ventrally.
7. Ectoderm forms the nervous system and the epidermis of the skin and its derivatives. The first event of organogenesis is neurulation, which produces the brain and spinal cord. By the eighth week, all major brain regions are formed.
8. Mesoderm forms all other organ systems and tissues. It segregates early into (1) a dorsal superior notochord, (2) paired somites that form the vertebrae, skeletal trunk muscles, and part of the dermis, and (3) paired masses of intermediate and lateral plate mesoderm. The intermediate mesoderm forms the kidneys and gonads. The lateral plate mesoderm forms the dermis of skin; parietal serosa; bones and muscles of the limbs; the cardiovascular system; and the visceral serosae.
9. The fetal cardiovascular system is formed in the embryonic period. The umbilical vein delivers nutrient- and oxygen-rich blood to the embryo; the paired umbilical arteries return oxygen-poor, waste-laden blood to the placenta. The ductus venosus allows most of the blood to bypass the liver; the foramen ovale and ductus arteriosus are pulmonary shunts.

Events of Fetal Development (pp. 1081–1082)

1. All organ systems are laid down during the embryonic period; growth and tissue/organ specialization are the major events of the fetal period.
2. During the fetal period, fetal length increases from about 22 mm to 360 mm, and weight increases from less than an ounce to 7 pounds or more.

Effects of Pregnancy on the Mother (pp. 1082–1085)

Anatomical Changes (pp. 1082–1083)

1. Maternal reproductive organs and breasts become increasingly vascularized during pregnancy, and the breasts enlarge.
2. The uterus eventually occupies nearly the entire abdominopelvic cavity. Abdominal organs are pushed superiorly and encroach on the thoracic cavity, causing the ribs to flare.
3. The increased abdominal mass changes the woman's center of gravity; lordosis and backache are common. A waddling gait occurs as pelvic ligaments and joints are loosened by placental relaxin.
4. A typical weight gain during pregnancy in a woman of normal weight is 28 pounds.

28

Metabolic Changes (p. 1083)

5. Human placental lactogen has anabolic effects and promotes glucose sparing in the mother.

Physiological Changes (pp. 1083–1085)

6. Many women suffer morning sickness, heartburn, and constipation during pregnancy.
7. The kidneys produce more urine, and pressure on the bladder may cause frequency, urgency, and stress incontinence.
8. Respiratory tidal volume increases, but residual volume decreases. The respiratory rate remains relatively unchanged. Dyspnea is common.
9. Total body water and blood volume increase dramatically and cardiac output rises. Blood pressure declines in midpregnancy and then rises to normal levels during the third trimester.

Parturition (Birth) (pp. 1085–1087)

1. Parturition encompasses a series of events called labor.

Initiation of Labor (p. 1085)

2. When estrogen levels are sufficiently high, they induce oxytocin receptors on the myometrial cells and inhibit progesterone's quieting effect on uterine muscle. Weak, irregular contractions begin.
3. Fetal cells produce oxytocin, which stimulates prostaglandin production by the placenta. Both hormones stimulate contraction of uterine muscle. Increasing distension of the cervix activates the hypothalamus, causing oxytocin release from the mother's posterior pituitary; this sets up a positive feedback loop resulting in true labor.

Stages of Labor (pp. 1085–1087)

4. The dilation stage is from the onset of rhythmic, strong contractions until the cervix is fully dilated. The head of the fetus rotates as it descends through the pelvic outlet.
5. The expulsion stage extends from full cervical dilation until birth of the infant.
6. The placental stage is the delivery of the afterbirth (the placenta and attached fetal membranes).

Adjustments of the Infant to Extrauterine Life (p. 1087)

1. The infant's Apgar score is recorded immediately after birth.

Taking the First Breath and Transition (p. 1087)

2. After the umbilical cord is clamped, carbon dioxide accumulates in the infant's blood, causing respiratory centers in the brain to trigger the first inspiration.
3. Once the lungs are inflated, breathing is eased by the presence of surfactant, which decreases the surface tension of the alveolar fluid.
4. During transition, the first 8 hours after birth, the infant is physiologically unstable and adjusting. After stabilizing, the infant wakes approximately every 3–4 hours in response to hunger.

Occlusion of Special Fetal Blood Vessels and Vascular Shunts (p. 1087)

5. Inflation of the lungs causes pressure changes in the circulation; as a result, the umbilical arteries and vein, ductus venosus, and ductus arteriosus collapse, and the foramen ovale closes. The occluded blood vessels are converted to fibrous cords; the site of the foramen ovale becomes the fossa ovalis.

Lactation (pp. 1087–1089)

1. The breasts are prepared for lactation during pregnancy by high blood levels of estrogen, progesterone, and human placental lactogen.
2. Colostrum, a premilk fluid, is a fat-poor fluid that contains more protein, vitamin A, and minerals than true milk. It is produced toward the end of pregnancy and for the first two to three days after birth.

3. True milk is produced around day 3 in response to suckling, which stimulates the hypothalamus to prompt anterior pituitary release of prolactin and posterior pituitary release of oxytocin. Prolactin stimulates milk production. Oxytocin triggers milk let-down. Continued breast-feeding is required for continued milk production.
4. At first, ovulation and menses are absent or irregular during nursing, but in most women the ovarian cycle is eventually reestablished while still nursing.

Assisted Reproductive Technology and Reproductive Cloning (pp. 1089–1091)

1. Assisted reproductive technology (ART) procedures assist infertile couples to bear children. Among the most-used techniques are IVF, ZIFT, and GIFT. IVF and ZIFT attempt to fertilize harvested oocytes in vitro and then return the embryo or zygote to the woman's body. GIFT utilizes in vivo methods—sperm and oocytes are transferred together to the woman's uterine tubes.
2. Reproductive cloning in humans has proved difficult to achieve and the practice has met several roadblocks.

Review Questions

Multiple Choice/Matching

(Some questions have more than one correct answer. Select the best answer or answers from the choices given.)

1. Indicate whether each of the following statements is describing **(a)** cleavage or **(b)** gastrulation.
   ____ **(1)** period during which a morula forms
   ____ **(2)** period when vast amounts of cell migration occur
   ____ **(3)** period when the three embryonic germ layers appear
   ____ **(4)** period during which the blastocyst is formed
2. Most systems are operational in the fetus by four to six months. Which system is the exception to this generalization, affecting premature infants? **(a)** the circulatory system, **(b)** the respiratory system, **(c)** the urinary system, **(d)** the digestive system.
3. The zygote contains chromosomes from **(a)** the mother only, **(b)** the father only, **(c)** both the mother and father, but half from each, **(d)** each parent and synthesizes others.
4. The outer layer of the blastocyst, which later attaches to the uterus, is the **(a)** decidua, **(b)** trophoblast, **(c)** amnion, **(d)** inner cell mass.
5. The fetal membrane that forms the basis of the umbilical cord is the **(a)** allantois, **(b)** amnion, **(c)** chorion, **(d)** yolk sac.
6. In the fetus, the ductus arteriosus carries blood from **(a)** the pulmonary artery to the pulmonary vein, **(b)** the liver to the inferior vena cava, **(c)** the right ventricle to the left ventricle, **(d)** the pulmonary trunk to the aorta.
7. Which of the following changes occur in the baby's cardiovascular system after birth? **(a)** Umbilical arteries and vein become fibrosed, **(b)** pulmonary circulation begins to function, and pressure in the left side of the heart increases, **(c)** the ductus venosus becomes obliterated, as does the ductus arteriosus, **(d)** all of these.
8. Following delivery of the infant, the delivery of the afterbirth includes the **(a)** placenta only, **(b)** placenta and decidua, **(c)** placenta and attached (torn) fetal membranes, **(d)** chorionic villi.
9. The umbilical vein carries **(a)** waste products to the placenta, **(b)** oxygen and food to the fetus, **(c)** oxygen and food to the placenta, **(d)** oxygen and waste products to the fetus.
10. The germ layer from which the skeletal muscles, heart, and skeleton are derived is the **(a)** ectoderm, **(b)** endoderm, **(c)** mesoderm.
11. Which of the following cannot pass through placental barriers? **(a)** blood cells, **(b)** glucose, **(c)** amino acids, **(d)** gases, **(e)** antibodies.
12. The most important hormone in initiating and maintaining lactation after birth is **(a)** estrogen, **(b)** FSH, **(c)** prolactin, **(d)** oxytocin.
13. The initial stage of labor, during which the neck of the uterus is stretched, is the **(a)** dilation stage, **(b)** expulsion stage, **(c)** placental stage.
14. Match each adult structure in column B with the embryonic structure it derives from in column A.

Column A	Column B
____ **(1)** notochord	**(a)** kidney
____ **(2)** ectoderm (not neural tube)	**(b)** peritoneal cavity
	(c) pancreas, liver
____ **(3)** intermediate mesoderm	**(d)** parietal serosa, dermis
____ **(4)** lateral plate mesoderm	**(e)** nucleus pulposus
____ **(5)** sclerotome	**(f)** hair and epidermis
____ **(6)** coelom	**(g)** brain
____ **(7)** neural tube	**(h)** ribs and vertebrae
____ **(8)** endoderm	

Short Answer Essay Questions

15. What is the function of hCG and why is it not important after the first trimester of pregnancy?
16. Fertilization involves much more than a mere restoration of the diploid chromosome number. (a) What does the process of fertilization entail on the part of both the egg and sperm? (b) What are the effects of fertilization?
17. Cleavage is an embryonic event that mainly involves mitotic divisions. How does cleavage differ from mitosis occurring during life after birth, and what are its important functions?
18. The life span of the ovarian corpus luteum is extended for nearly three months after implantation, but otherwise it deteriorates. (a) Explain why this is so. (b) Explain why it is important that the corpus luteum remain functional following implantation.
19. The placenta is a marvelous, but temporary, organ. Starting with a description of its formation, show how it is an intimate part of both fetal and maternal anatomy and physiology during the gestation period.
20. Why is it that only one sperm out of the hundreds (or thousands) available enters the oocyte?
21. What is the function of gastrulation?
22. Cite two problems with a breech presentation.
23. What factors are believed to bring about uterine contractions at the termination of pregnancy?
24. Explain how the flat embryonic disc takes on the cylindrical shape of a tadpole.

Critical Thinking and Clinical Application Questions

1. Jennie, a freshman in your dormitory, tells you she just discovered that she is three months pregnant. She recently bragged that since she came to college she has been drinking alcohol heavily and experimenting with every kind of recreational drug she could find. From the following, select the advice you would give her, and explain why it is the best choice. (a) She must stop taking drugs, but they could not have affected her fetus during these first few months of her pregnancy. (b) Harmful substances usually cannot pass from mother to embryo, so she can keep using drugs. (c) There could be defects in the fetus, so she should stop using drugs and visit a doctor as soon as possible. (d) If she has not taken any drugs in the last week, she is okay.
2. During Mrs. Jones's labor, the obstetrician decided that it was necessary to perform an episiotomy. What is an episiotomy, and why is it done?
3. A woman in substantial pain called her doctor and explained (between sobs) that she was about to have her baby "right here." The doctor calmed her and asked how she had come to that conclusion. She said that her water had broken and that her husband could see the baby's head. (a) Was she right? If so, what stage of labor was she in? (b) Do you think that she had time to make it to the hospital 60 miles away? Why or why not?
4. Mary is a heavy smoker and has ignored a friend's advice to stop smoking during her pregnancy. On the basis of what you know about the effect of smoking on physiology, describe how Mary's smoking might affect her fetus.
5. While Mortimer was cramming for his anatomy test, he read that some parts of the mesoderm become segmented. He suddenly realized that he could not remember what segmentation is. Define segmentation, and give two examples of segmented structures in the embryo.
6. Assume a sperm has penetrated a polar body and their nuclei fuse. Why would it be unlikely for the resulting cell to develop into a healthy embryo?

AT THE CLINIC

Related Clinical Terms

Abortion (*abort* = born prematurely) Termination of a pregnancy that is in progress; may be spontaneous or induced.

Ectopic pregnancy (ek-top′ik; *ecto* = outside) A pregnancy in which the embryo implants in any site other than the uterus; most often the site is a uterine tube (tubal pregnancy). Since the uterine tube (as well as most other ectopic sites) is unable to establish a placenta or accommodate growth, the uterine tube ruptures unless the condition is diagnosed early, or the pregnancy spontaneously aborts.

Hydatid (hydatidiform) mole (hi′dah-tid; *hydat* = watery) Developmental abnormality of the placenta; the conceptus degenerates and the chorionic villi convert into a mass of vesicles that resemble tapioca. Signs include vaginal bleeding, which contains some of the grapelike vesicles.

Physiological jaundice (jawn′dis) Jaundice sometimes occurring in normal newborns within three to four days after birth. Fetal erythrocytes are short-lived, and they break down rapidly after birth; the infant's liver may be unable to process the bilirubin (breakdown product of hemoglobin pigment) fast enough to prevent its accumulation in blood and subsequent deposit in body tissues.

Abruptio placenta (ah-brup′she-o; *abrupt* = broken away from) Premature separation of the placenta from the uterine wall; if this occurs before labor, it can result in fetal death due to anoxia.

Placenta previa (pre′ve-ah) Placental formation adjacent to or across the internal os of the uterus. Represents a problem because as the uterus and cervix stretch, separation of the placenta may occur. Additionally, the placenta precedes the infant during labor.

Ultrasonography (ul″trah-son-og′rah-fe) Noninvasive technique that uses sound waves to visualize the position and size of the fetus and placenta (see *A Closer Look*, Chapter 1).

Case Study Pregnancy

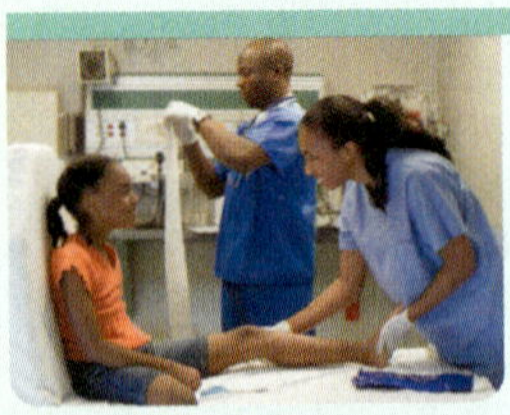

When paramedics arrived on the crash scene on Route 91, they found Maria Rodriguez, a 34-year-old female, lying on the edge of the road. Mrs. Rodriguez was responsive, but had deep lacerations on both legs and her right arm. Her clothes were heavily stained with blood, despite the efforts of another passenger to slow the bleeding by applying compression. On initial examination, Mrs. Rodriguez's blood pressure was 100/70 with a heart rate of 88. The paramedics started an IV of normal saline, stabilized her, and controlled the bleeding during transport to the hospital. Mrs. Rodriguez was released from the hospital three days later and scheduled for a follow-up visit in one week. At her follow-up appointment, she complained of fatigue and reported that her period was overdue by one week. Hospital blood tests revealed that Mrs. Rodriguez was mildly anemic—and pregnant. While she was excited, she was also very concerned that the blood loss she suffered may have harmed her baby.

1. What hormone did the hospital detect in Mrs. Rodriguez's blood to determine that she was pregnant?
2. Where is the hormone made that you identified in question 1? What function does it play during the early stages of a pregnancy?
3. Mrs. Rodriguez's doctors explained that the blood loss she suffered as a result of the accident occurred approximately 10–12 days after her most recent ovulation. Explain why this may help ease Mrs. Rodriguez's fears about harm to her baby.
4. Describe the major developmental events and stages of embryonic development that have occurred during the time prior to Mrs. Rodriguez's accident.
5. Mrs. Rodriguez is currently in the third week of pregnancy. Describe the important embryonic developmental event that occurs during this time.

(Answers in Appendix H)

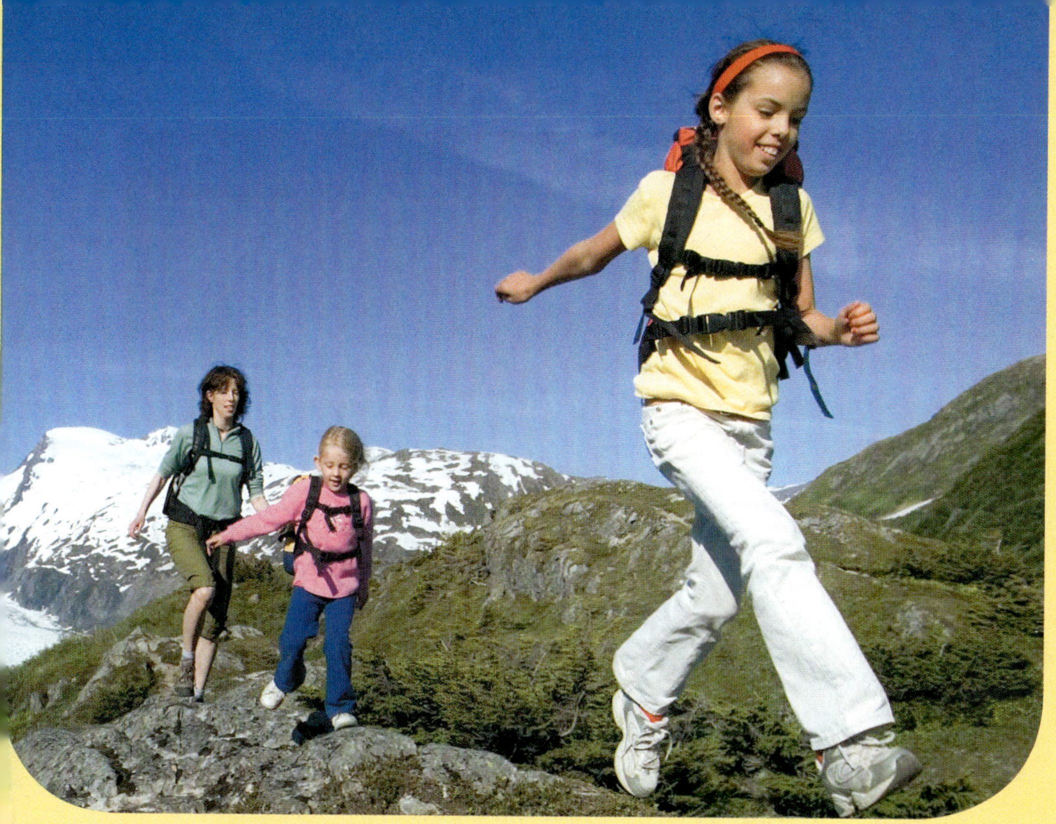

29

Heredity

The wondrous growth and development of a new individual is guided by the gene-bearing chromosomes it receives from its parents in egg and sperm. As we described in Chapter 3, individual *genes*, or DNA segments, contain the "recipes" or genetic blueprints for proteins. Many of these proteins are enzymes that dictate the synthesis of virtually all the body's molecules. Consequently, genes are ultimately expressed in your hair color, sex, blood type, and so on.

Genes, however, do not act as free agents. As you will see, a gene's ability to prompt the development of a specific trait is enhanced or inhibited by interactions with other genes, as well as by environmental factors.

The science of genetics, which studies the mechanism of heredity (*genes* = give birth to), is relatively young, but our understanding of how human genes act and interact has advanced considerably since Gregor Mendel first proposed the basic principles of heredity in the mid-1800s. Mendel studied characteristics that vary in an either-or fashion, which is easier to understand than the more-or-less fashion in which many human traits vary.

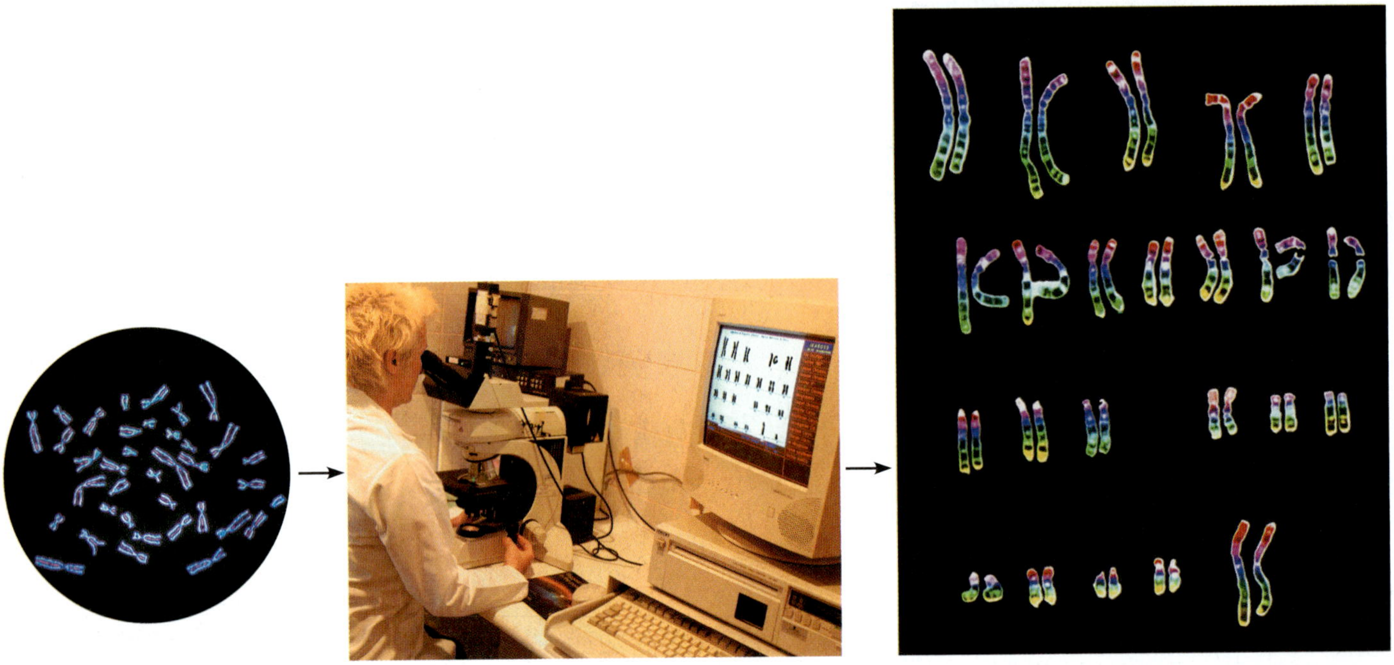

(1) The slide is viewed with a microscope, and the chromosomes are photographed.

(2) The photograph is entered into a computer, and the chromosomes are electronically rearranged into homologous pairs according to size and structure.

(3) The resulting display is the karyotype, which is examined for chromosome number and structure.

Figure 29.1 Preparing a karyotype. After lymphocytes are stimulated to divide and grow in culture for several days, they are treated with a drug that arrests mitosis in metaphase, a stage when the chromosomes are easily identified. The cells are harvested, treated with a solution that makes their chromosomes spread out, photographed, and then subjected to computer analysis and arrangement of the chromosomes into homologous pairs. The patterns of stained bands in the karyotype help to identify specific chromosomes and parts of chromosomes.

However, the urge to understand human inheritance is powerful. The *Human Genome Project*, which scanned and determined the human DNA sequence, is enabling geneticists to manipulate and engineer human genes to examine their expression. This research has tremendous promise for more sophisticated genetic screening, and for drug development to treat or cure disease. Although we touch upon some of these newer topics, we will concentrate on the principles of heredity discovered by Mendel more than a century ago.

The Vocabulary of Genetics

✓ Define allele.

✓ Differentiate between genotype and phenotype.

The nuclei of all human cells except gametes contain the diploid number of chromosomes (46), consisting of 23 pairs of homologous chromosomes. Recall that *homologous chromosomes* are pairs of chromosomes—one from the father (sperm) and one from the mother (egg)—that look similar and carry genes for the same traits, but do not necessarily bring about the same expressions of those traits. Two of the 46 chromosomes are **sex chromosomes** (X and Y), which determine genetic sex (male = XY; female = XX). The other 44 are the 22 pairs of **autosomes** that guide the expression of most other traits.

The complete human **karyotype** (kar′e-o-tīp), or diploid chromosomal complement displayed in homologous pairs, is illustrated in Figure 29.1 (3). The diploid **genome** (je′nōm), or genetic (DNA) makeup, represents two sets of genetic instructions—one from the egg and the other from the sperm.

Gene Pairs (Alleles)

Because chromosomes are paired, it follows that the genes in them are paired as well. Consequently, each of us receives *two* genes, one from each parent (for the most part), that interact to dictate each trait. Matched genes, which are at the same *locus* (location) on homologous chromosomes, are called **alleles** (ah-lēlz′) of each other. Alleles may code for the same or for alternative forms of a given trait. For example, of the alleles that dictate whether or not you have loose thumb ligaments, one allele might code for tight ligaments and the other for loose ligaments (the double-jointed thumb condition). When the two alleles controlling a trait are the same, a person is said to be **homozygous** (ho-mo-zi′gus) for that trait. When the two alleles are different, the individual is **heterozygous** (het″er-o-zi′gus) for the trait.

Sometimes, one allele masks or suppresses the expression of its partner. Such an allele is said to be **dominant**, whereas the allele that is masked is said to be **recessive**. By convention, a dominant allele is represented by a capital letter (for example, *J*),

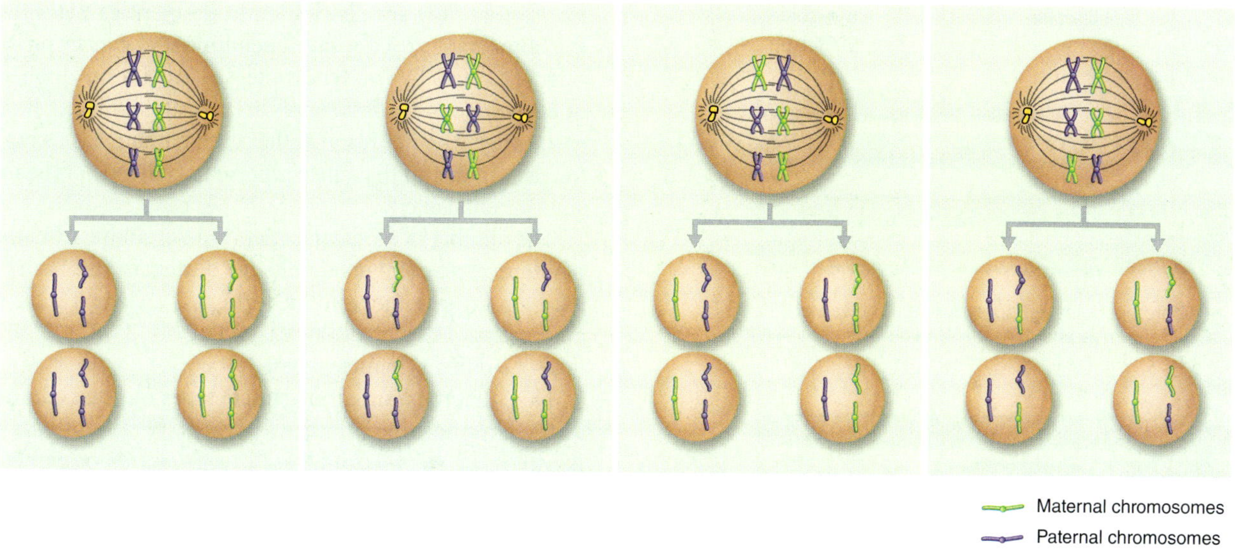

Figure 29.2 Gamete variability resulting from independent assortment. During metaphase of meiosis I, the tetrads of homologous chromosomes align independently of other tetrads. The large circles depict the possible alignments in a mother cell having a diploid number of 6. The small circles show the gametes arising from each alignment. Some gametes contain all maternal or all paternal chromosomes; others have various combinations of maternal and paternal chromosomes.

and a recessive allele by the lowercase form of the same letter (*j*). Dominant alleles are expressed, or make themselves "known," when they are present in either single or double dose. For recessive alleles to be expressed, they must be present in double dose, that is, the homozygous condition. Returning to our thumb example, a person whose genetic makeup includes either the gene pair *JJ* (the homozygous dominant condition) or the gene pair *Jj* (the heterozygous condition) will have double-jointed thumbs. The combination *jj* (the homozygous recessive condition) is needed to produce tight thumb ligaments.

Genotype and Phenotype

A person's genetic makeup is referred to as his or her **genotype** (jen′o-tīp). The way that genotype is expressed in the body is called one's **phenotype** (fe′no-tīp). For example, the double-jointed condition is the phenotype produced by a genotype of *JJ* or *Jj*.

Check Your Understanding

1. When a geneticist orders a karyotype, why are cells in metaphase studied instead of those in interphase?
2. What term refers to chromosomes other than our sex chromosomes?
3. Is an allele represented by a capital letter presumed to be dominant or recessive?
4. Harold is homozygous for the dominant alleles *HH*, *CC*, and *LL*, and heterozygous for *Bb* and *Kk*. He is blond and blue-eyed and has a very hairy chest. Which of these descriptions refer to his phenotype?

For answers, see Appendix H.

Sexual Sources of Genetic Variation

✓ Describe events that lead to genetic variability of gametes.

Before we examine how genes interact, let us consider why (with the possible exception of identical siblings) each of us is one of a kind, with a unique genotype and phenotype. This variability reflects three events that occur before we are even a twinkle in our parents' eyes: independent assortment of chromosomes, crossover of homologues, and random fertilization of eggs by sperm.

Chromosome Segregation and Independent Assortment

As we described in Chapter 27, each pair of homologous chromosomes synapses during meiosis I, forming a tetrad. This happens during both spermatogenesis and oogenesis. Because chance determines how the tetrads align (line up) on the meiosis I metaphase spindle, maternal and paternal chromosomes are randomly distributed to daughter nuclei.

As illustrated in **Figure 29.2**, this simple event leads to an amazing amount of variation in gametes. The cell in our example has a diploid number of 6, and so three tetrads form. As you can see, the possible combinations of alignments of the three tetrads result in eight gamete possibilities. Because the way each tetrad aligns is random, and because many cells are undergoing meiosis simultaneously, each alignment and each type of gamete occurs with the same frequency as all others.

Two important points about metaphase of meiosis I: (1) The two alleles determining each trait are **segregated**, which

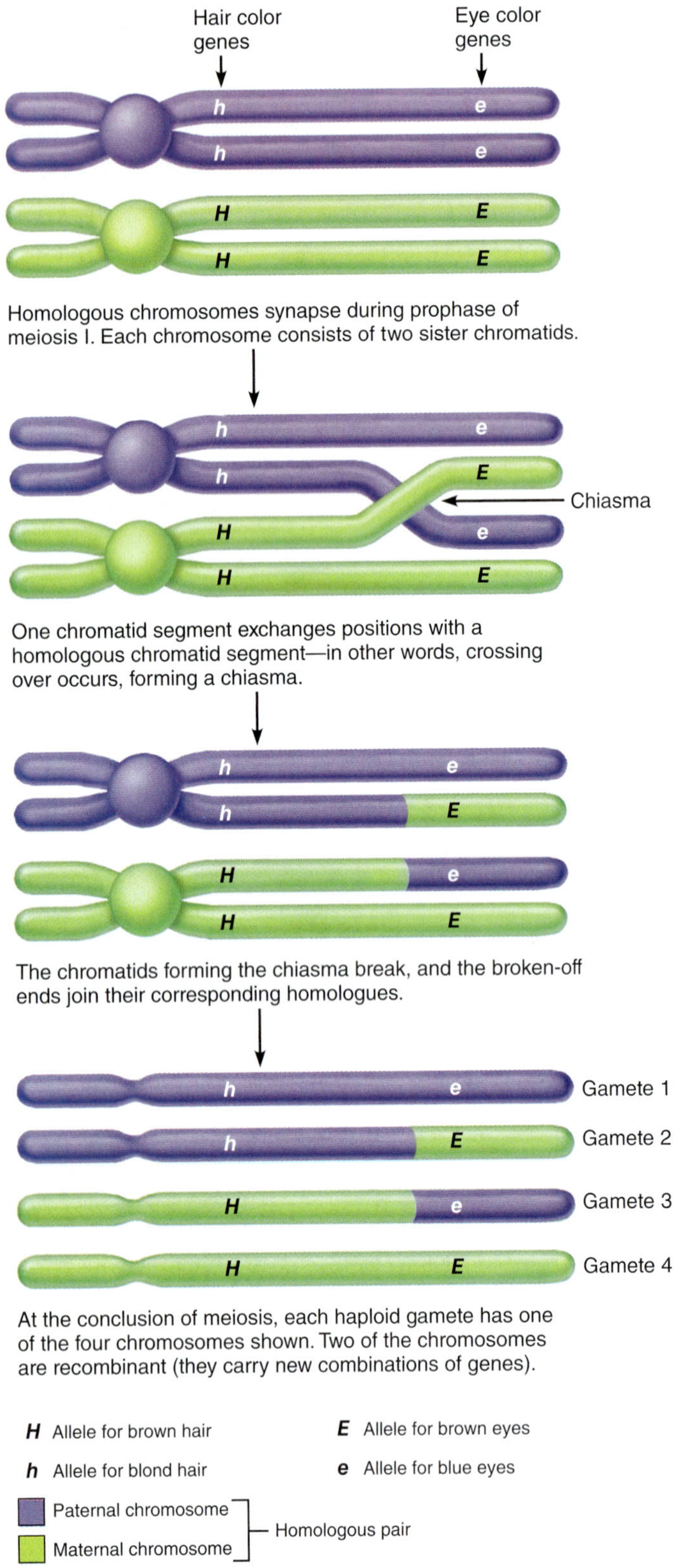

Figure 29.3 Crossover and genetic recombination. These meiosis I events increase genetic variability in the gametes formed. For simplicity, only two chromatids are shown taking part in crossover. Multiple crossovers result in more complex patterns.

means that they are distributed to different gametes. Errors in this important process have been linked to cancer progression, infertility, and Down syndrome. (2) Alleles on different pairs of homologous chromosomes are distributed independently of each other. The net result is that each gamete has a single allele for each trait, and that allele represents only one of the four possible parental alleles.

The number of different gamete types resulting from this **independent assortment** of homologues during meiosis I can be calculated for any genome from the formula 2^n, where n is the number of homologous pairs. In our example, $2^n = 2^3$ ($2 \times 2 \times 2$), for a total of 8 different gamete types.

Note that the number of gamete types increases dramatically as the chromosome number increases. A cell with six pairs of homologues would produce 2^6, or 64, kinds of gametes. In a man's testes, the number of gamete types that can be produced on the basis of independent assortment alone is 2^{23}, or about 8.5 million—an incredible variety. The number of different gamete types produced simultaneously in a woman's ovaries is substantially less because her ovaries complete at most 500 reduction divisions in her lifetime. Still, each ovulated oocyte will most likely be novel genetically because of independent assortment.

Crossover of Homologues and Gene Recombination

Additional gamete variation results from the crossing over and exchange of chromosomal parts during meiosis I. Genes are arranged linearly along a chromosome's length, and genes on the same chromosome are said to be **linked** because they are transmitted as a unit to daughter cells during mitosis. However, as we described in Chapter 27, chromosomes can break and precisely exchange gene segments with their homologous counterparts during meiosis. This exchange gives rise to **recombinant chromosomes** that have mixed contributions from each parent.

In the hypothetical example shown in **Figure 29.3**, the genes for hair and eye color are linked. The paternal chromosome contains alleles coding for blond hair and blue eyes, and the maternal alleles code for brown hair and brown eyes. In the **crossover**, or **chiasma**, shown, the break occurs between these linked genes, resulting in one gamete with alleles for blond hair and brown eyes and another with alleles for brown hair and blue eyes. As a result of the crossover, two of the four chromatids present in the tetrad end up with a mixed set of alleles—some maternal and some paternal. This means that when the chromatids segregate, each gamete will receive a unique combination of parental genes.

Because humans have 23 tetrads, with crossovers going on in all of them during meiosis I, the variability resulting from this factor alone is tremendous.

Random Fertilization

At any point in time, gametogenesis is turning out gametes with all variations possible from independent assortment and random crossovers. Fertilization compounds this variety because a single human egg will be fertilized by a single sperm on a totally haphazard, or random, basis. If we consider variation resulting only from independent assortment and random fertilization, any offspring represents one out of the close to 72 trillion (8.5 million × 8.5 million) zygotes possible. The additional variation introduced by crossovers increases this number exponentially. Perhaps now you can understand why brothers and sisters are so different, and marvel at how they can also be so alike in many ways.

Check Your Understanding

5. We said that genetic variability is introduced by independent assortment. Just what is assorting independently?
6. How does crossover increase genetic variability?

For answers, see Appendix H.

Types of Inheritance

A few human phenotypes can be traced to a single gene pair (as we will describe shortly), but most such traits are very limited in nature, or reflect variation in a single enzyme. Most human traits are determined by multiple alleles or by the interaction of several gene pairs.

Dominant-Recessive Inheritance

✓ Compare and contrast dominant-recessive inheritance with incomplete dominance and codominance.

Dominant-recessive inheritance reflects the interaction of dominant and recessive alleles. A simple diagram, called the **Punnett square**, is used to figure out, for a single trait, the possible gene combinations that would result from the mating of parents of known genotypes (**Figure 29.4**). In the example shown, both parents can roll their tongue into a U because both are heterozygous for the dominant allele (*T*) that confers this ability. In other words, each parent has the genotype *Tt*. The alleles of one parent are written along one side of the Punnett square, and the alleles for the other parent are shown along an adjacent side. The alleles are then combined down and across to determine the possible gene combinations (genotypes) and their expected frequency in the offspring of these two parents.

As the completed Punnett square shows, the probability of these parents producing a homozygous dominant child (*TT*) is 25% (1 out of 4); of producing a heterozygous child (*Tt*), 50% (2 out of 4); and of producing a homozygous recessive child, 25% (1 out of 4). The *TT* and *Tt* offspring will be tongue rollers. Only the *tt* offspring will not be able to roll their tongues.

The Punnett square predicts only the *probability* of a particular genotype (and phenotype). The larger the number of offspring, the greater the likelihood that the ratios will conform to the predicted values—just as the chances of getting heads half the time and tails half the time increase with the number of tosses of a coin. If we toss only twice, we may well get heads both times. Likewise, if the couple in our example had only two children, it would not be surprising if both children had the genotype *Tt*.

What are the chances of having two children of the same genotype? To determine the probability of two events happening in succession, we must multiply the probabilities of the separate

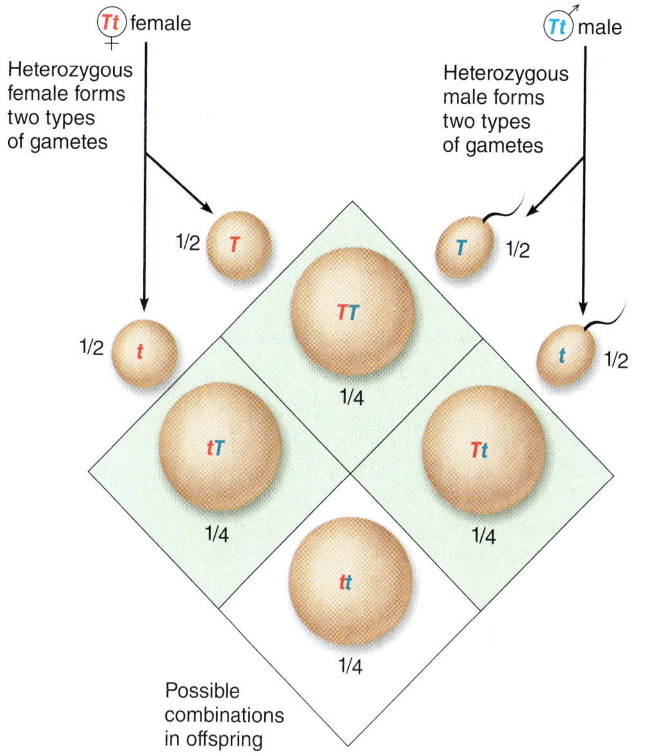

Figure 29.4 Genotype and phenotype probabilities resulting from a mating of two heterozygous parents. The Punnett square shows all possible combinations of a set of alleles in the zygote. In this example, the *T* allele is dominant and determines tongue-rolling ability; the *t* allele is recessive.

events happening. The probability of getting heads in one coin toss is 1/2, so the probability of getting two heads in a row is 1/2 × 1/2 = 1/4. Remember that the production of each child, like each coin toss in a series, is an *independent event* that does not influence the production of any other child by the same couple. If you get heads on the first toss, the chance of getting heads the second time is still 1/2. Likewise, if our couple's first child is a *tt*, they still have a 1/4 chance of getting a *tt* the next time.

Dominant Traits

Human traits dictated by dominant alleles include widow's peaks, dimples, and freckles.

Disorders caused by dominant genes are uncommon because *lethal dominant genes* are almost always expressed and result in the death of the embryo, fetus, or child. However, in some dominant disorders the person is less impaired or at least survives long enough to reproduce. One example is *Huntington's disease*, a fatal nervous system disease involving degeneration of the basal nuclei. It involves a *delayed-action gene* that is expressed when the affected individual is about 40. Offspring of a parent with Huntington's disease have a 50% chance of inheriting the lethal gene. (The parent is heterozygous, because the dominant homozygous condition is lethal to the fetus.) Many informed offspring of such parents are opting not to become parents themselves.

These and some other dominant gene–determined traits are listed in **Table 29.1**.

Table 29.1 Traits Determined by Simple Dominant-Recessive Inheritance

PHENOTYPE DUE TO EXPRESSION OF:	
DOMINANT GENES (*ZZ* OR *Zz*)	RECESSIVE GENES (*zz*)
Tongue roller	Inability to roll tongue into a U shape
Astigmatism	Normal vision
Freckles	Absence of freckles
Dimples in cheeks	Absence of dimples
PTC* taster	PTC nontaster
Widow's peak	Straight hairline
Double-jointed thumb	Tight thumb ligaments
Syndactyly (webbed digits)	Normal digits
Achondroplasia (heterozygous: dwarfism; homozygous: lethal)	Normal endochondral ossification
Huntington's disease	Absence of Huntington's disease
Normal skin pigmentation	Albinism
Absence of Tay-Sachs disease	Tay-Sachs disease
Absence of cystic fibrosis	Cystic fibrosis

*PTC is phenylthiocarbamide, a harmless bitter chemical.

Recessive Traits

Some examples of recessive inheritance are the more desirable genetic condition. For example, normal vision is dictated by recessive alleles, whereas astigmatism is prescribed by dominant alleles. However, many if not most genetic disorders are inherited as simple recessive traits. These include conditions as different as *albinism* (lack of skin pigmentation); *cystic fibrosis*, a condition of excessively thick mucus production that impairs lung and pancreatic functioning; and *Tay-Sachs disease*, a disorder of brain lipid metabolism, caused by an enzyme deficit that shows itself a few months after birth.

Recessive genetic disorders are more frequent than those caused by dominant alleles because those who carry a *single* recessive allele for a recessive genetic disorder do not themselves express the disease. However, they can pass the gene on to offspring and so are called carriers of the disorder. Conversely, as we explained above, few individuals with dominant genetic disorders get a chance to pass on the detrimental gene.

29

Incomplete Dominance

In dominant-recessive inheritance, one allele variant completely masks the other. Some traits, however, exhibit **incomplete dominance**. In such instances, the heterozygote has a phenotype intermediate between those of homozygous dominant and homozygous recessive individuals. Incomplete dominance is uncommon in humans.

Perhaps the best human example is inheritance of the *sickling gene* (*s*), which causes a substitution of one amino acid in the beta chain of hemoglobin. Hemoglobin molecules containing the abnormal beta chains crystallize when blood

Table 29.2 ABO Blood Groups

BLOOD GROUP (PHENOTYPE)	GENOTYPE	FREQUENCY (% OF U.S. POPULATION) WHITE	BLACK	ASIAN
O	*ii*	45	49	40
A	I^AI^A or I^Ai	40	27	28
B	I^BI^B or I^Bi	11	20	27
AB	I^AI^B	4	4	5

oxygen levels are low, causing the erythrocytes to assume a sickle shape (see Figure 17.8b, p. 639). Individuals with a double dose of the sickling allele (*ss*) have **sickle-cell anemia**, and any condition that lowers their blood oxygen level, such as respiratory difficulty or excessive exercise, can precipitate a *sickle-cell crisis*. The deformed erythrocytes jam up and fragment in small capillaries, causing intense pain.

Individuals heterozygous for the sickling gene (*Ss*) have **sickle-cell trait**. They make both normal and sickling hemoglobin, and as a rule, these individuals are healthy. However, they can suffer a crisis if there is prolonged reduction in blood oxygen levels, as might happen when traveling in high-altitude areas, and they can transmit the sickling gene to their offspring.

Multiple-Allele Inheritance

Although we inherit only two alleles for each gene, some genes exhibit more than two allele forms, leading to a phenomenon called **multiple-allele inheritance**. For example, three alleles determine the ABO blood types in humans: I^A, I^B, and *i*. Each of us receives two of these. The I^A and I^B alleles are *codominant*, and both are expressed when present, resulting in the AB blood type. The *i* allele is recessive to the other two. Genotypes determining the four possible ABO blood groups are shown in **Table 29.2**.

Check Your Understanding

7. Why are there so few genetic disorders caused by dominant genes?
8. How does incomplete dominance differ from codominance?

For answers, see Appendix H.

Sex-Linked Inheritance

✓ Describe the mechanism of sex-linked inheritance.

Inherited traits determined by genes on the sex chromosomes are said to be **sex-linked**. The X and Y sex chromosomes are not homologous in the true sense. The Y, which contains the gene (or genes) that determines maleness, is much smaller than the X chromosome **(Figure 29.5)**. The X bears over 2500 genes, and a disproportionately large number of them code for proteins important to brain function. Because the Y carries only 78 genes as of the last count, it lacks many of the genes present on the X. For example, genes coding for certain clotting factors, cone pigments, and even

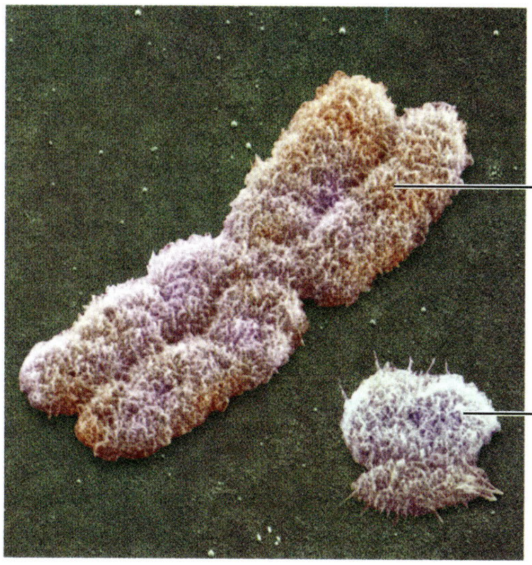

Figure 29.5 Human sex chromosomes (14,100×)

testosterone receptors are present on X but not on Y. A gene found only on the X chromosome is said to be **X-linked**.

Only relatively short regions at either end of the Y chromosome (corresponding to about 5% of the Y's DNA) code for nonsexual characteristics corresponding to those on the X. Those regions are the only areas that can participate in crossovers with the X.

When a male inherits an X-linked recessive allele—for example, for hemophilia or for red-green color blindness—its expression is never masked or damped, because there is no corresponding allele on his Y chromosome. Consequently, the recessive gene is always expressed, even when present only in single dose. In contrast, females must have two X-linked recessive alleles to express such a disorder, and as a result, very few females exhibit any X-linked conditions.

X-linked traits are typically passed from mother to son, never from father to son, because males receive no X chromosome from their father. Of course, the mother can also pass the recessive allele to her daughter, but unless the daughter receives another such allele from her father, she will not express the trait.

Polygene Inheritance

✓ Explain how polygene inheritance differs from that resulting from the action of a single pair of alleles.

So far, we have considered only traits inherited by mechanisms of classical Mendelian genetics, which are fairly easy to understand, and such traits typically have two, or perhaps three, alternate forms. However, many phenotypes depend on several gene pairs at different locations acting in tandem. Such **polygene inheritance** results in *continuous*, or *quantitative*, phenotypic variation between two extremes and explains many human characteristics. Examples of polygene traits in humans include skin color, height, metabolic rate, and intelligence.

Skin color, for instance, is controlled by three separately inherited genes, each existing in two allelic forms: *A*, *a*; *B*, *b*; *C*, *c*. The *A*, *B*, and *C* alleles confer dark skin pigment, and their effects are additive. The *a*, *b*, and *c* alleles confer pale skin tone. An individual with an *AABBCC* genotype would be about as dark-skinned as a human can get, while an *aabbcc* person would be very fair. However, when individuals heterozygous for at least one of these gene pairs mate, a broad range of pigmentation is possible in their offspring. Such polygene inheritance results in a distribution of genotypes and phenotypes that, when plotted, yields a bell-shaped curve (Figure 29.6).

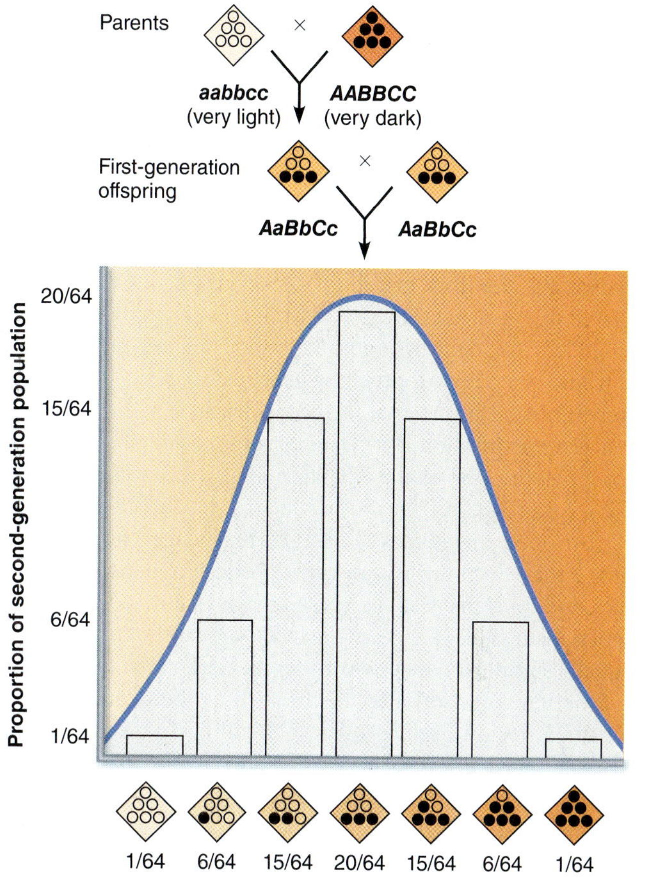

Figure 29.6 Simplified model for polygene inheritance of skin color based on three gene pairs. Alleles for dark skin are incompletely dominant over those for light skin. Each dominant gene (*A*, *B*, *C*) contributes 1 "unit" of darkness (indicated by a dark dot) to the phenotypes.

Here the parents are homozygotes at opposite ends of the phenotype range. Each child inherits 3 "units" of darkness (is a heterozygote) and has intermediate pigmentation. When they grow up, if they mate with people with the same alleles, their offspring (second generation) may have a wide variation in pigmentation, as shown by the plotted distribution of skin colors.

Check Your Understanding

9. Why does a male always express an X-linked recessive allele?
10. How can you explain why parents of average height can produce very tall or very short offspring?

For answers, see Appendix H.

29

Environmental Factors in Gene Expression

✓ Provide examples illustrating how gene expression may be modified by environmental factors.

In many situations environmental factors override or at least influence gene expression. Our genotype (discounting mutations) is as unchanging as the Rock of Gibraltar, but our phenotype is more like clay. If this were not the case, we would never get a tan, women bodybuilders would never be able to develop bulging muscles, and there would be no hope for treating genetic disorders.

Sometimes, such maternal factors as drugs or pathogens alter normal gene expression during embryonic development. Take, for example, the case of the "thalidomide babies" (discussed on p. 1083). As a result of their mothers taking that sedative, the embryos developed phenotypes (flipperlike appendages) not directed by their genes. Such environmentally produced phenotypes that mimic conditions that may be caused by genetic mutations (permanent transmissible changes in the DNA) are called **phenocopies**.

Equally significant are environmental factors that may influence genetic expression after birth, such as the effect of poor infant nutrition on brain growth, general body development, and height. In this way, a person with "tall genes" can be stunted by insufficient nutrition. Furthermore, part of a gene's environment consists of the influence of other genes. For example, hormonal deficits during childhood can lead to abnormal skeletal growth and proportions, as in cretinism, a type of dwarfism resulting from hypothyroidism.

☑ Check Your Understanding

11. Which of the following factors may alter gene expression? Other genes, measles in a pregnant woman, lack of key nutrients in the diet.

For answers, see Appendix H.

Nontraditional Inheritance

Mendel's writings underlie mainstream thinking about heredity, but some genetic outcomes do not fit his rules. Among these nontraditional types of inheritance are influences due to RNA-only genes, to chemical groups attached to DNA or histone proteins, and to *extranuclear inheritance* conferred by mitochondrial DNA.

29

Beyond DNA: Regulation of Gene Expression

✓ Describe how RNA-only genes and epigenetic marks affect gene expression.

Our genome is a biochemical system of awesome complexity, with three basic levels of controls. The protein-coding genes that we have been describing to this point only make up the first level and account for less than 2% of the DNA of a human cell. This is the part of the genome traditionally considered to be a "blueprint" for protein structure.

Since the 1960s, scientists have been finding second and third layers of information important in directing development elsewhere—in the noncoding DNA and even totally outside the DNA sequences. So what are these other regulatory systems?

Small RNAs

The second layer appears to be the product of the abundant "RNA-only genes," formerly believed to be "junk," that are found in the vast oceans of non-protein-coding DNA. They form a parallel regulatory system that generates single-stranded microRNAs (miRNAs) and short interfering RNAs (siRNAs) (see p. 105). These small RNA molecules are "control freaks" that can act directly on DNA, other RNAs, or proteins. They also can tame or inactivate aggressive (jumping) genes, called *transposons*, that tend to replicate themselves and then insert the copies into distant DNA sites, disabling or hyperactivating those genes.

Small RNAs control timing of programmed cell death during development and can also prevent translation of another gene. Mutations in these RNA-only areas have already been linked to several conditions including prostate and lung cancers and schizophrenia.

It takes relatively few genes to build a human being. Our complexity is the result of the small RNAs that control the expression of genes especially during growth and differentiation. Nucleotide sequences of these RNA-specifying DNA areas are now worked out and biochemical companies are investing heavily in gene therapy research. They are especially hot on synthesizing RNA-interfering drugs to silence or shut down particular genes to treat age-related macular degeneration, Parkinson's disease, cancer, and a host of other disorders.

Epigenetic Marks

Epigenetic marks form the third layer of gene controls. This continually changing information is stored in the proteins and chemical groups that bind to the DNA and in the way chromatin is packaged in the cell. Within cells, chemical tags such as methyl and acetyl groups bound to DNA segments and to histones determine whether the DNA is available for transcription (acetylation) or silenced (methylation). Epigenetic marks also account for the inactivation (by methylation) of one of the female's X chromosomes in the early embryo.

Epigenetic marks or lack of them may predispose a cell for transformation from normal to cancerous, and even slight deviations in the epigenetic marks on specific chromosomes can result in devastating human illness.

Epigenetic marks also underlie the phenomenon called genomic imprinting. For most genes, the maternal and paternal genes turn on or off at the same time. This balance is upset during gametogenesis when certain genes in both sperm and eggs are modified by the addition of a methyl ($—CH_3$) group, a process called **genomic imprinting**. Genomic imprinting somehow tags the genes as paternal or maternal and confers important functional differences in the embryo. The developing embryo "reads" these tags, and then either expresses the mother's gene while the father's version remains idle or vice versa. In each generation, the old imprints are "erased" when new gametes are produced and all the chromosomes are newly imprinted according to the sex of the parents.

Mutations of imprinted genes may lead to pathology. For example, victims of Prader-Willi syndrome are mildly to moderately retarded, short, and grossly obese. Children with Angelman syndrome are severely retarded, unable to speak coherently, laugh uncontrollably, and exhibit jerky, lurching movements as if tied to a puppeteer's strings. The symptoms of these two disorders are very different, but the genetic cause is the same—deletion of a particular region of chromosome 15. If the defective chromosome comes from the father, the result is Prader-Willi syndrome; the mother's defective chromosome confers Angelman syndrome. Thus, it seems that the same allele can have different effects depending on which parent it comes from.

In short, protein-coding genes are not the only instructions to which cells refer. RNA matters, and so do the tiny chemical tags that attach to the chromatin.

Extranuclear (Mitochondrial) Inheritance

✓ Describe the basis of extranuclear (mitochondria-based) genetic disorders.

Although we have focused on the chromosomal basis of inheritance, remember that not all genes are in the cell's nucleus. Some 37 genes (referred to as mtDNA) are in mitochondria. Mitochondrial genes are transmitted to the offspring almost exclusively by the mother because the ovum donates essentially all the cytoplasm in the fertilized egg. Additionally, sperm mitochondrial DNA is selectively destroyed by elimination factors in both the sperm and egg.

A growing list of disorders, all rare, is now being linked to errors (mutations) in mitochondrial genes. Most involve problems with oxidative phosphorylation within the mitochondria, but a few lead to unusual degenerative muscle disorders or neurological problems. Some researchers suggest that Alzheimer's and Parkinson's disease may be among them.

☑ Check Your Understanding

12. What process labels genes as paternal or maternal?
13. What is the source of the genes that confer extranuclear inheritance?

For answers, see Appendix H.

Genetic Screening, Counseling, and Therapy

✓ List and explain several techniques used to determine or predict genetic diseases.

✓ Describe briefly some approaches of gene therapy.

Genetic screening and *genetic counseling* provide information and options for prospective parents not even dreamed of 100 years ago. Newborn infants are routinely screened for a number of anatomical disorders (congenital hip dysplasia, imperforate anus, and others), and testing for phenylketonuria (PKU) and other metabolic diseases is mandated by law in many states. These tests alert the new parents that treatment is necessary to ensure the well-being of their infant. Anatomical defects are usually treated surgically, and PKU is managed by strict dietary measures that exclude most phenylalanine-containing foods.

Adult children of parents with Huntington's disease are obvious candidates for these services, but many other genetic conditions also place babies at risk. For example, a woman pregnant at age 35 may wish to know if her baby has trisomy-21, or Down syndrome (see Related Clinical Terms, p. 1107), a chromosome abnormality with a high incidence in children of older mothers.

Depending on the condition being investigated, screening can occur before conception by carrier recognition, or during fetal testing.

Carrier Recognition

There are two major avenues for identifying carriers of detrimental genes: pedigrees and blood tests. A **pedigree** traces a genetic trait through several generations and helps predict the future. For prospective parents, a genetic counselor collects phenotype information on as many family members as possible and uses it to construct the pedigree (often called the family tree). By working backward from current individuals and applying the rules of dominant-recessive inheritance, a counselor can deduce the genotypes of the parents and figure out the genotypes of the other individuals in their parents' generation.

Simple blood tests are used to screen for the sickling gene in heterozygotes, and sophisticated *blood chemistry tests* and *DNA probes* can detect the presence of other unexpressed recessive genes. At present, carriers of the Tay-Sachs and cystic fibrosis genes can be identified with such tests.

Fetal Testing

Fetal testing is used when there is a known risk of a genetic disorder. The most common type of fetal testing is **amniocentesis** (am″ne-o-sen-te′sis), in which a wide-bore needle is inserted into the amniotic sac through the mother's abdominal wall, and about 10 ml of fluid is withdrawn (**Figure 29.7a**). Because there is a chance of injuring the fetus before ample amniotic fluid is present, this procedure is not normally done before the 14th week of pregnancy. Using ultrasound to visualize the position of the fetus and the amniotic sac has dramatically reduced the risk of this procedure.

The fluid is checked for enzymes and other chemicals that serve as markers for specific diseases, but most tests are done on the sloughed-off fetal cells in the fluid. These cells are cultured in laboratory dishes over a period of several weeks. Then the cells are examined for DNA markers of genetic disease and karyotyped to check for chromosomal abnormalities (see Figure 29.1).

Chorionic villus sampling (CVS) suctions off bits of the chorionic villi from the placenta for examination (Figure 29.7b). A small tube is inserted through the vagina and cervical canal and guided by ultrasound to an area where a piece of placental tissue can be removed. CVS allows testing at 8 weeks but waiting until after the 10th week is usually recommended. Karyotyping

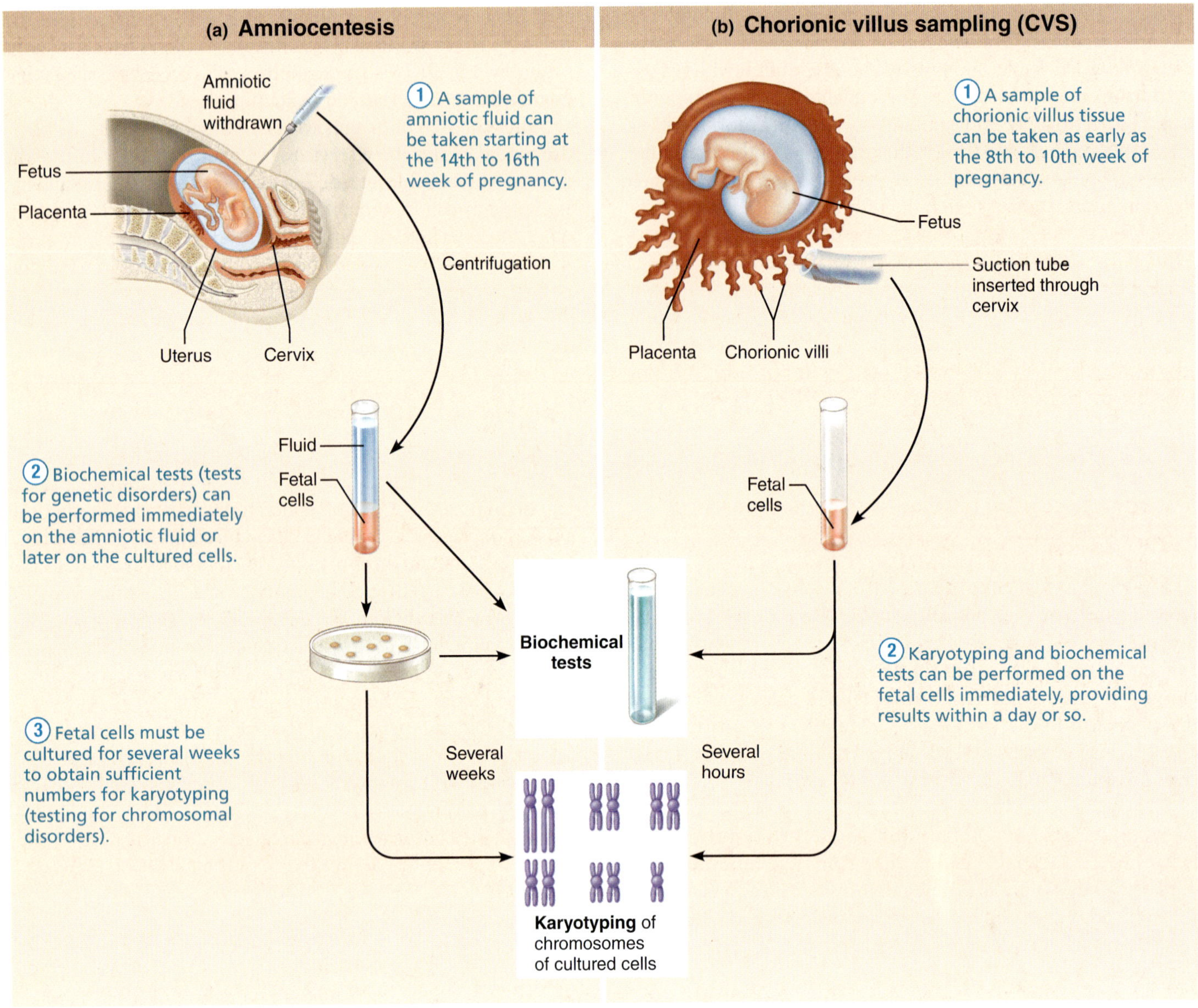

Figure 29.7 Fetal testing—amniocentesis and chorionic villus sampling.

can be done almost immediately on the rapidly dividing chorionic cells, much earlier than in amniocentesis.

Both of these procedures are invasive, and they carry with them an inherent risk to both fetus and mother. (For example, increased fetal risk of finger and toe defects is linked to CVS.) These tests are routinely ordered for pregnant women over 35 (because of the higher risk of Down syndrome), but they are performed on younger women when the probability of finding a severe fetal disorder is greater than the probability of doing harm during the procedure. If a serious genetic or congenital defect is detected in the developing fetus, the parents must decide whether or not to continue the pregnancy.

Human Gene Therapy

As indicated earlier, the Human Genome Project has opened an exciting world to scientists investigating gene expression. Advances in diagnosing human genetic diseases have been followed quickly by new applications of "gene therapy" to alleviate or even cure the disorders, particularly in cases traced to a single defective gene or protein. Indeed, genetic engineering has the potential to replace a defective gene with a normal version.

One approach (used successfully in treatment of severe combined immunodeficiency disorders) is to "infect" the defective cells with a virus into which a functional gene has been inserted. Another is to inject the "corrected" DNA directly into the patient's cells. Such therapies have had mixed results in treating cystic fibrosis and muscular dystrophy. However, genetic engineering processes are prohibitively expensive and raise some thorny ethical, religious, and societal questions: Who will pay? Who determines who will be treated with the new therapies? Are we playing God?

Check Your Understanding

14. Which fetal testing procedure depends on analyzing amniotic fluid?
15. What noninvasive imaging procedure is used to determine some aspects of fetal development? (You many want to check *A Closer Look* in Chapter 1, pp. 16–17, for this.)

For answers, see Appendix H.

In this chapter, we have explored some of the basic principles of genetics, the manner in which genes are expressed, and the means by which gene expression can be modified. Considering the precision required to make perfect copies of genes and chromosomes, and the incredible mechanical events of meiotic division, it is amazing that genetic defects are as rare as they are. Perhaps, after reading this chapter, you have a greater sense of wonder that you turned out as well as you did.

Chapter Summary

For more chapter study tools, go to the Study Area of MasteringA&P at **www.masteringaandp.com**.
There you will find:
- Interactive Physiology iP
- A&PFlix A&PFlix
- Practice Anatomy Lab PAL
- PhysioEx PEx
- Videos, Practice Quizzes and Tests, MP3 Tutor Sessions, Case Studies, and much more!

1. Genetics is the study of heredity and mechanisms of gene transmission.

The Vocabulary of Genetics (pp. 1096–1097)

1. A complete diploid set of chromosomes is called the karyotype of an organism; the complete genetic complement is the genome. A person's genome consists of two sets of instructions, one from each parent.

Gene Pairs (Alleles) (pp. 1096–1097)

2. Genes coding for the same trait and found at the same locus on homologous chromosomes are called alleles.
3. Alleles may be the same or different in expression. When the allele pair is identical, the person is homozygous for that trait; when the alleles differ, the person is heterozygous.

Genotype and Phenotype (p. 1097)

4. The actual genetic makeup of cells is the genotype; phenotype is the manner in which those genes are expressed.

Sexual Sources of Genetic Variation (pp. 1097–1099)

Chromosome Segregation and Independent Assortment (pp. 1097–1098)

1. During meiosis I of gametogenesis, tetrads align randomly on the metaphase plate, and chromatids are randomly distributed to the daughter cells. This is called independent assortment of the homologues. Each gamete receives only one allele of each gene pair.
2. Each different metaphase I alignment produces a different assortment of parental chromosomes in the gametes, and all combinations of maternal and paternal chromosomes are equally possible.

Crossover of Homologues and Gene Recombination (p. 1098)

3. During meiosis I, all four chromatids of each tetrad cross over at one or more points and exchange corresponding gene segments. The recombinant chromosomes contain new gene combinations, adding to the variability arising from independent assortment.

Random Fertilization (pp. 1098–1099)

4. The third source of genetic variation is random fertilization of eggs by sperm.

Types of Inheritance (pp. 1099–1101)

Dominant-Recessive Inheritance (pp. 1099–1100)

1. Dominant genes are expressed when present in single or double dose; recessive genes must be present in double dose to be expressed.
2. For traits following the dominant-recessive pattern, the laws of probability predict the outcome of a large number of matings.
3. Genetic disorders more often reflect the homozygous recessive condition than the homozygous dominant or heterozygous condition because dominant genes are expressed and, if they are lethal genes, the pregnancy usually results in miscarriage. Genetic disorders caused by dominant alleles include achondroplasia and Huntington's disease; recessive disorders include cystic fibrosis and Tay-Sachs disease.
4. Carriers are heterozygotes who carry a deleterious recessive gene (but do not express the trait) and have the potential of passing it on to offspring.

Incomplete Dominance (p. 1100)

5. In incomplete dominance, the heterozygote exhibits a phenotype intermediate between those of the homozygous dominant and recessive individuals. Inheritance of sickle-cell trait is an example of incomplete dominance.

Multiple-Allele Inheritance (p. 1100)

6. Multiple-allele inheritance involves genes that exist in more than two allelic forms in a population. Only two of the alleles are inherited, but on a random basis. Inheritance of ABO blood types is an example of multiple-allele inheritance in which the I^A and I^B alleles are codominant.

Sex-Linked Inheritance (pp. 1100–1101)

7. Traits determined by genes on the X and Y chromosomes are said to be sex-linked. The small Y chromosome lacks most genes present on the X chromosome. Recessive genes located only on the X chromosome are expressed in single dose in males. Examples of such X-linked conditions, passed from mother to son, include hemophilia and red-green color blindness.

Polygene Inheritance (p. 1101)

8. Polygene inheritance occurs when several gene pairs interact to produce phenotypes that vary quantitatively over a broad range. Height, intelligence, and skin pigmentation are examples.

Environmental Factors in Gene Expression (p. 1102)

1. Environmental factors may influence the expression of genotype.
2. Maternal factors that cross the placenta may alter expression of fetal genes. Environmentally provoked phenotypes that mimic genetically determined ones are called phenocopies. Nutritional deficits or hormonal imbalances may alter anticipated growth and development during childhood.

Nontraditional Inheritance (pp. 1102–1103)

Beyond DNA: Regulation of Gene Expression (pp. 1102–1103)

1. Control of gene expression occurs at three levels: protein-coding genes, RNA-only genes, and epigenetic marks. The latter two account for many cases of inherited disease that fail to follow traditional genetics.
2. The products of the RNA-only genes (siRNA and miRNA) may silence genes or prevent their expression and appear to play a role in directing apoptosis during development.
3. Epigenetic marks involve attachment of small chemical groups (methyl or acetyl) to DNA or histone proteins. In general, methylation prevents access to the DNA whereas acetylation provides access to the DNA. Genomic imprinting, which involves methylation of certain genes during gametogenesis, confers different effects and phenotypes on maternal and paternal genes. It is reversible, and occurs anew each generation.

Extranuclear (Mitochondrial) Inheritance (p. 1103)

4. Cytoplasmic (mitochondrial) genes pass to offspring via the ovum and help to determine certain characteristics. Deletions or mutations in mitochondrial genes are responsible for some problems with oxidative phosphorylation and some rare genetic diseases.

Genetic Screening, Counseling, and Therapy (pp. 1103–1105)

Carrier Recognition (p. 1103)

1. The likelihood of an individual carrying a deleterious recessive gene may be assessed by constructing a pedigree. Some of these genes can be deduced by various blood tests and DNA probes.

Fetal Testing (pp. 1103–1104)

2. Amniocentesis is fetal testing based on aspirated samples of amniotic fluid. Fetal cells in the fluid are cultured for several weeks, then examined for chromosomal defects (karyotyped) or for DNA markers of genetic disease. Amniocentesis cannot be performed until the 14th week of pregnancy.
3. Chorionic villus sampling is fetal testing based on a sample of the chorion. This tissue is rapidly mitotic, so karyotyping can be done almost immediately. Samples may be obtained by the 8th week.

Human Gene Therapy (pp. 1104–1105)

4. The Human Genome Project has allowed research on diagnosis of genetic disease and on its treatment to surge forward. Thus far, gene therapy has been particularly useful for correcting single-gene disorders. The most common approach involves transferring a corrected gene via a virus to the affected cells to restore normal function.

Review Questions

Multiple Choice/Matching

(Some questions have more than one correct answer. Select the best answer or answers from the choices given.)

1. Match one of the following terms (a–i) with each of the descriptions below:

Key: (a) alleles (b) autosomes (c) dominant allele (d) genotype (e) heterozygote (f) homozygote (g) phenotype (h) recessive allele (i) sex chromosomes

____ (1) genetic makeup
____ (2) how genetic makeup is expressed
____ (3) chromosomes that dictate most body characteristics
____ (4) alternate forms of the same gene
____ (5) an individual bearing two alleles that are the same for a particular trait
____ (6) an allele that is expressed whether in single or double dose
____ (7) an individual bearing two alleles that differ for a particular trait
____ (8) an allele that must be present in double dose to be expressed

2. Match the following types of inheritance (a–f) with the descriptions below:

Key: (a) dominant-recessive (b) incomplete dominance (c) multiple-allele (d) polygene (e) sex-linked (f) extranuclear

____ (1) only sons show the trait
____ (2) homozygotes and heterozygotes have the same phenotype
____ (3) heterozygotes exhibit a phenotype intermediate between those of the homozygotes
____ (4) phenotypes of offspring may be more varied than those of the parents
____ (5) inheritance of ABO blood types
____ (6) inheritance of stature
____ (7) reflects activity of mitochondrial DNA

Short Answer Essay Questions

3. Describe the important mechanisms that lead to genetic variations in gametes.
4. The ability to taste PTC (phenylthiocarbamide) depends on the presence of a dominant gene *T*; nontasters are homozygous for the recessive gene *t*. This is a situation of classical dominant-recessive inheritance. (a) Consider a mating between heterozygous parents producing three offspring. What proportion of the offspring are likely to be tasters? What is the chance that all three offspring will be tasters? Nontasters? What is the chance that two will be tasters and one will be a nontaster? (b) Consider a mating between *Tt* and *tt* parents. What is the anticipated percentage of tasters? Nontasters? What proportion can be expected to be homozygous recessive? Heterozygous? Homozygous dominant?
5. Most albino children are born to normally pigmented parents. Albinos are homozygous for the recessive gene (*aa*). What can you conclude about the genotypes of the nonalbino parents?

29

6. A woman with blood type A has two children. One has type O blood and the other has type B blood. What is the genotype of the mother? What are the genotype and phenotype of the father? What is the genotype of each child?
7. In skin color inheritance, what will be the relative range of pigmentation in offspring arising from the following parental matches? (a) *AABBCC* × *aabbcc*, (b) *AABBCC* × *AaBbCc*, (c) *Aabbcc* × *aabbcc*.
8. Compare and contrast amniocentesis and chorionic villus sampling as to the time at which they can be performed and the techniques used to obtain information on the fetus's genetic status.

Critical Thinking and Clinical Application Questions

1. A color-blind man marries a woman with normal vision. The woman's father was also color-blind. (a) What is the chance that their first child will be a color-blind son? A color-blind daughter? (b) If they have four children, what is the chance that two will be color-blind sons? (Be careful on this one.)
2. Brian is a college student. His genetics assignment is to do a family pedigree for dimples in the cheeks. Absence of dimples is recessive; presence of dimples reflects a dominant allele. Brian has dimples, as do his three brothers. His mother and maternal grandmother are dimple free, but his father and all other grandparents have dimples. Construct a pedigree spanning three generations for Brian's family. Show the phenotype and genotype for each person.
3. Mr. and Mrs. Lehman have sought genetic counseling. Mrs. Lehman is concerned because she is unexpectedly pregnant and her husband's brother died of Tay-Sachs disease. She can recall no incidence of Tay-Sachs disease in her own family. Do you think biochemical testing should be recommended to detect the deleterious gene in Mrs. Lehman? Explain your answer.
4. The Browns are both carriers of the recessive allele that causes the metabolic disorder called phenylketonuria. What is the probability of each of the following occurring? (a) All three children will have the disorder. (b) None of their three children will have the disorder. (c) One or more of their children will have the disorder. (d) At least one of their children will be phenotypically normal.

AT THE CLINIC

Related Clinical Terms

Deletion Chromosomal aberration in which part of a chromosome is lost.

Down syndrome Formerly called mongolism, this condition usually reflects the presence of an extra autosome (trisomy of chromosome 21). The child has slightly slanted eyes, flattened facial features, a large tongue, and a tendency toward short stature and stubby fingers. Some, but not all, affected people are mentally retarded. Down syndrome individuals have mitochondrial defects, which have been associated with neurodegeneration in other disorders. A distinctive feature of Down syndrome is early onset of Alzheimer's disease. The most important risk factor appears to be advanced maternal (or paternal) age.

Mutation (*mutare* = change) A permanent structural change in a gene. The mutation may or may not affect function, depending on the precise site and nature of the alteration.

Nondisjunction Abnormal segregation of chromosomes during meiosis, resulting in gametes receiving two or no copies of a particular parental chromosome. It is more common in female meiosis than in male meiosis. If the abnormal gamete participates in fertilization, the resulting zygote will have an abnormal chromosomal complement (monosomy or trisomy) for that particular chromosome (as in Down syndrome).

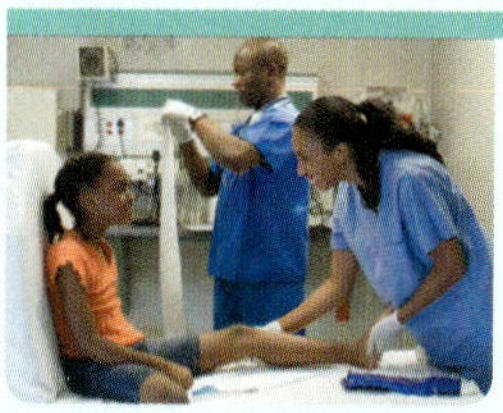

Case Study Heredity

We will now return to the case of Maria Rodriguez, whom we met in Chapter 28. Recall that Mrs. Rodriguez had found out that she was pregnant and was concerned about the health of her baby. Mrs. Rodriguez went on to have a normal pregnancy without complications. During Mrs. Rodriguez's treatment in the hospital, she discovered that her blood is type O. During one of her regular visits to her doctor, Mrs. Rodriguez asked what type of blood her baby will have, given that her husband's blood type is type A. Her doctor explained to Mrs. Rodriguez that she would need to know more about the blood type of Mr. Rodriguez's parents.

1. Describe the difference between genotype and phenotype. What are the phenotypes and genotypes of Mr. and Mrs. Rodriguez?
2. Describe the type of inheritance that is represented by blood type.
3. Mr. Rodriguez's mother has O blood type and his father has A blood type. Explain how this information helps you understand Mr. Rodriguez's genotype.
4. What is the probability that Mrs. Rodriguez's baby will have O blood type? A? B? AB?

(Answers in Appendix H)

29

The Metric System

MEASUREMENT	UNIT AND ABBREVIATION	METRIC EQUIVALENT	METRIC TO ENGLISH CONVERSION FACTOR	ENGLISH TO METRIC CONVERSION FACTOR
Length	1 kilometer (km)	= 1000 (10^3) meters	1 km = 0.62 mile	1 mile = 1.61 km
	1 meter (m)	= 100 (10^2) centimeters = 1000 millimeters	1 m = 1.09 yards 1 m = 3.28 feet 1 m = 39.37 inches	1 yard = 0.914 m 1 foot = 0.305 m
	1 centimeter (cm)	= 0.01 (10^{-2}) meter	1 cm = 0.394 inch	1 foot = 30.5 cm 1 inch = 2.54 cm
	1 millimeter (mm)	= 0.001 (10^{-3}) meter	1 mm = 0.039 inch	
	1 micrometer (µm) [formerly micron (µ)]	= 0.000001 (10^{-6}) meter		
	1 nanometer (nm)	= 0.000000001 (10^{-9}) meter		
	1 angstrom (Å)	= 0.0000000001 (10^{-10}) meter		
Area	1 square meter (m^2)	= 10,000 square centimeters	1 m^2 = 1.1960 square yards 1 m^2 = 10.764 square feet	1 square yard = 0.8361 m^2 1 square foot = 0.0929 m^2
	1 square centimeter (cm^2)	= 100 square millimeters	1 cm^2 = 0.155 square inch	1 square inch = 6.4516 cm^2
Mass	1 metric ton (t)	= 1000 kilograms	1 t = 1.103 ton	1 ton = 0.907 t
	1 kilogram (kg)	= 1000 grams	1 kg = 2.205 pounds	1 pound = 0.4536 kg
	1 gram (g)	= 1000 milligrams	1 g = 0.0353 ounce 1 g = 15.432 grains	1 ounce = 28.35 g
	1 milligram (mg)	= 0.001 gram	1 mg = approx. 0.015 grain	
	1 microgram (µg)	= 0.000001 gram		
Volume (solids)	1 cubic meter (m^3)	= 1,000,000 cubic centimeters	1 m^3 = 1.3080 cubic yards 1 m^3 = 35.315 cubic feet	1 cubic yard = 0.7646 m^3 1 cubic foot = 0.0283 m^3
	1 cubic centimeter (cm^3 or cc)	= 0.000001 cubic meter = 1 milliliter	1 cm^3 = 0.0610 cubic inch	1 cubic inch = 16.387 cm^3
	1 cubic millimeter (mm^3)	= 0.000000001 cubic meter		
Volume (liquids and gases)	1 kiloliter (kl or kL)	= 1000 liters	1 kL = 264.17 gallons	1 gallon = 3.785 L
	1 liter (l or L)	= 1000 milliliters	1 L = 0.264 gallon 1 L = 1.057 quarts	1 quart = 0.946 L
	1 milliliter (ml or mL)	= 0.001 liter = 1 cubic centimeter	1 ml = 0.034 fluid ounce 1 ml = approx. $\frac{1}{5}$ teaspoon 1 ml = approx. 15–16 drops (gtt)	1 quart = 946 ml 1 pint = 473 ml 1 fluid ounce = 29.57 ml 1 teaspoon = approx. 5 ml
	1 microliter (µl or µL)	= 0.000001 liter		
Time	1 second (s)	= $\frac{1}{60}$ minute		
	1 millisecond (ms)	= 0.001 second		
Temperature	Degrees Celsius (°C)		°F = $\frac{9}{5}$(°C) + 32	°C = $\frac{5}{9}$(°F − 32)

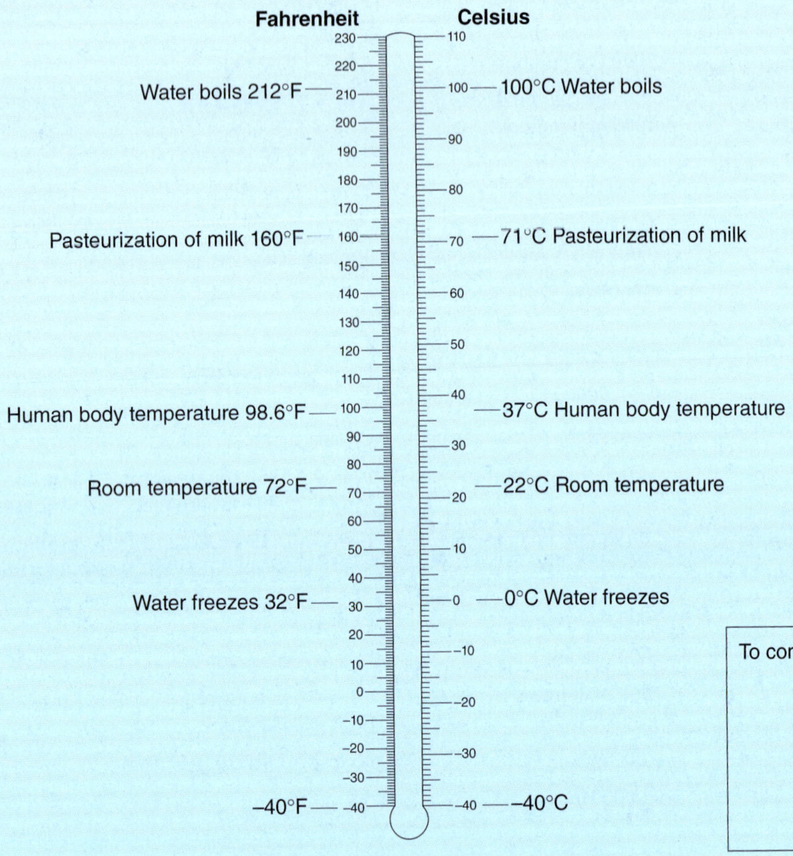

Fahrenheit and Celsius scales compared

To convert temperature scales:

$$°C = \frac{5(°F - 32)}{9}$$

$$°F = \frac{9(°C)}{5} + 32$$

$$K = °C + 273$$

Functional Groups in Organic Molecules

Functional group	General formula	Name of compounds	Example	Where else found
Hydroxyl —OH (or HO—)	—O—H	Alcohols	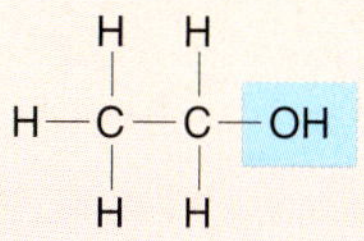 Ethanol	Sugars; water-soluble vitamins
Carbonyl >CO	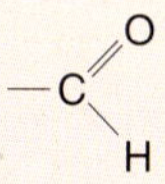	Aldehydes	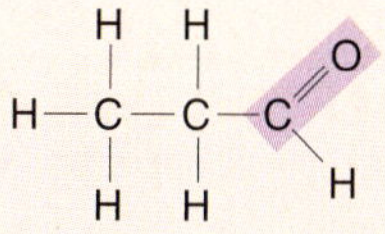 Propanal	Some sugars; formaldehyde (a preservative)
	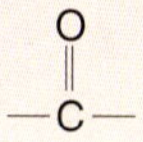	Ketones	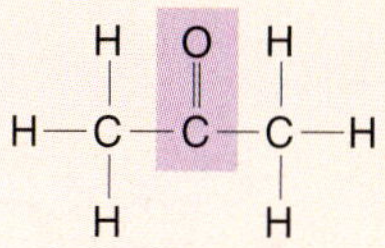 Acetone	Some sugars; "ketone bodies" in urine (from fat breakdown)
Carboxyl —COOH	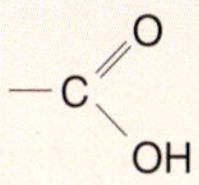	Carboxylic acids	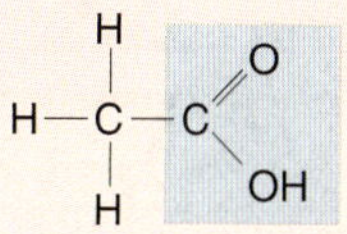 Acetic acid	Amino acids; proteins; some vitamins; fatty acids
Amino $—NH_2$ (or H_2N—)	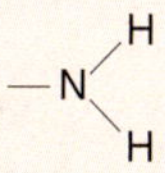	Amines	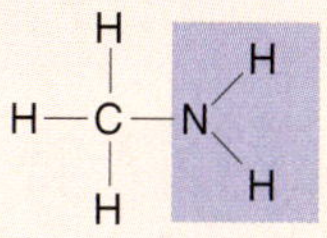 Methylamine	Amino acids; proteins; urea in urine (from protein breakdown)

The Amino Acids

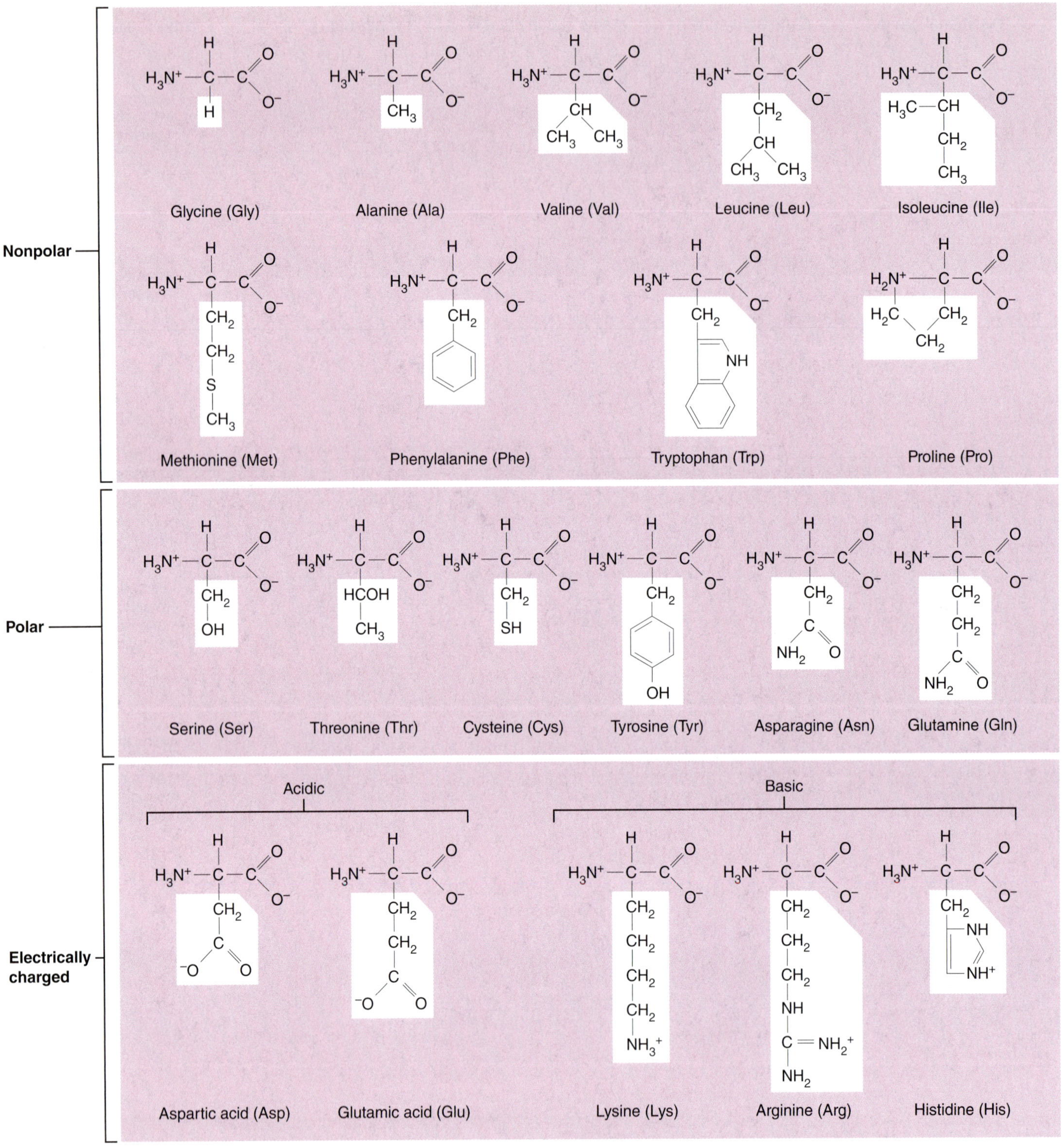

Two Important Metabolic Pathways

(1) Glucose enters the cell and is phosphorylated by the enzyme hexokinase, which catalyzes the transfer of a phosphate group, indicated as P, from ATP to the number six carbon of the sugar, producing glucose-6-phosphate. The electrical charge of the phosphate group traps the sugar in the cell because the plasma membrane is impermeable to ions. Phosphorylation of glucose also makes the molecule more chemically reactive. Although glycolysis is supposed to *produce* ATP, ATP is actually consumed in step 1—an energy investment that will be repaid with dividends later in glycolysis.

(2) Glucose-6-phosphate is rearranged and converted to its isomer, fructose-6-phosphate. Isomers, remember, have the same number and types of atoms but in different structural arrangements.

(3) In this step, still another molecule of ATP is used to add a second phosphate group to the sugar, producing fructose-1,6-bisphosphate. So far, the ATP ledger shows a debit of –2. With phosphate groups on its opposite ends, the sugar is now ready to be split in half.

(4) This is the reaction from which glycolysis gets its name. An enzyme cleaves the sugar molecule into two different 3-carbon sugars: glyceraldehyde 3-phosphate and dihydroxyacetone phosphate. These two sugars are isomers of one another.

(5) An isomerase enzyme interconverts the 3-carbon sugars, and if left alone in a test tube, the reaction reaches equilibrium. This does not happen in the cell, however, because the next enzyme in glycolysis uses only glyceraldehyde phosphate as its substrate and not dihydroxyacetone phosphate. This pulls the equilibrium between the two 3-carbon sugars in the direction of glyceraldehyde phosphate, which is removed as fast as it forms. Thus, the net result of steps 4 and 5 is cleavage of a 6-carbon sugar into two molecules of glyceraldehyde phosphate; each will progress through the remaining steps of glycolysis.

(6) An enzyme now catalyzes two sequential reactions while it holds glyceraldehyde phosphate in its active site. First, the sugar is oxidized by the transfer of H from the number one carbon of the sugar to NAD^+, forming NADH + H^+. Here we see in metabolic context the oxidation-reduction reaction described in Chapter 24. This reaction releases substantial amounts of energy, and the enzyme capitalizes on this by coupling the reaction to the creation of a high-energy phosphate bond at the number one carbon of the oxidized substrate. The source of the phosphate is inorganic phosphate (P_i) always present in the cytosol. The enzyme releases NADH + H^+ and 1,3-bisphosphoglyceric acid as products. Notice in the figure that the new phosphate bond is symbolized with a squiggle (~), which indicates that the bond is at least as energetic as the high-energy phosphate bonds of ATP.

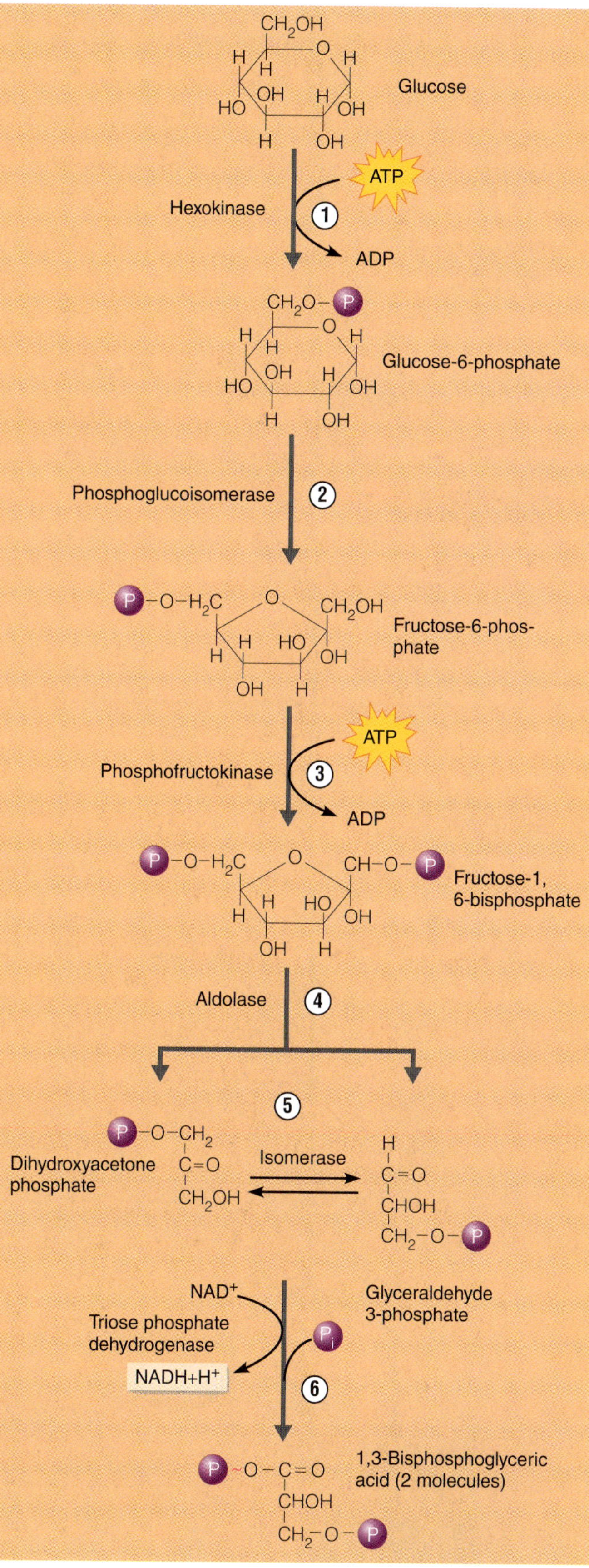

THE TEN STEPS OF GLYCOLYSIS Each of the ten steps of glycolysis is catalyzed by a specific enzyme found dissolved in the cytoplasm. All steps are reversible. An abbreviated version of the three major phases of glycolysis appears in the lower right-hand corner of the next page.

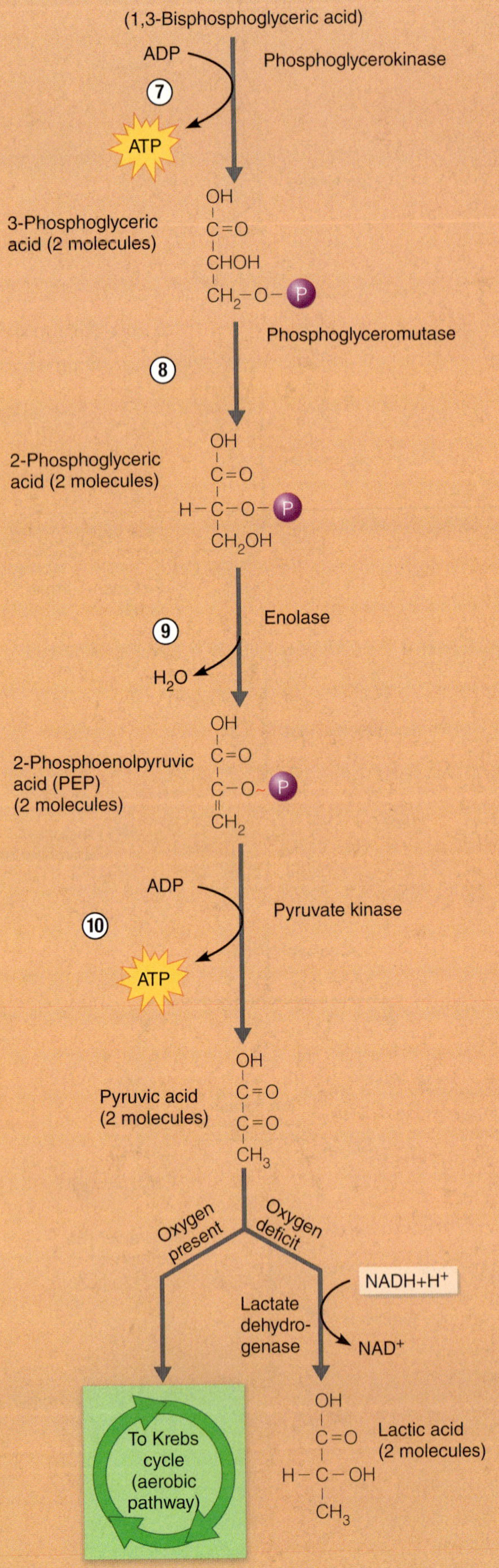

(7) Finally, glycolysis produces ATP. The phosphate group, with its high-energy bond, is transferred from 1,3-bisphosphoglyceric acid to ADP. For each glucose molecule that began glycolysis, step 7 produces two molecules of ATP, because every product after the sugar-splitting step (step 4) is doubled. Of course, two ATPs were invested to get sugar ready for splitting. The ATP ledger now stands at zero. By the end of step 7, glucose has been converted to two molecules of 3-phosphoglyceric acid. This compound is not a sugar. The sugar was oxidized to an organic acid back in step 6, and now the energy made available by that oxidation has been used to make ATP.

(8) Next, an enzyme relocates the remaining phosphate group of 3-phosphoglyceric acid to form 2-phosphoglyceric acid. This prepares the substrate for the next reaction.

(9) An enzyme forms a double bond in the substrate by removing a water molecule from 2-phosphoglyceric acid to form phosphoenolpyruvic acid, or PEP. This results in the electrons of the substrate being rearranged in such a way that the remaining phosphate bond becomes very unstable; it has been upgraded to high-energy status.

(10) The last reaction of glycolysis produces another molecule of ATP by transferring the phosphate group from PEP to ADP. Because this step occurs twice for each glucose molecule, the ATP ledger now shows a net gain of two ATPs. Steps 7 and 10 each produce two ATPs for a total credit of four, but a debt of two ATPs was incurred from steps 1 and 3. Glycolysis has repaid the ATP investment with 100% interest. In the meantime, glucose has been broken down and oxidized to two molecules of pyruvic acid, the compound produced from PEP in step 10.

Summary

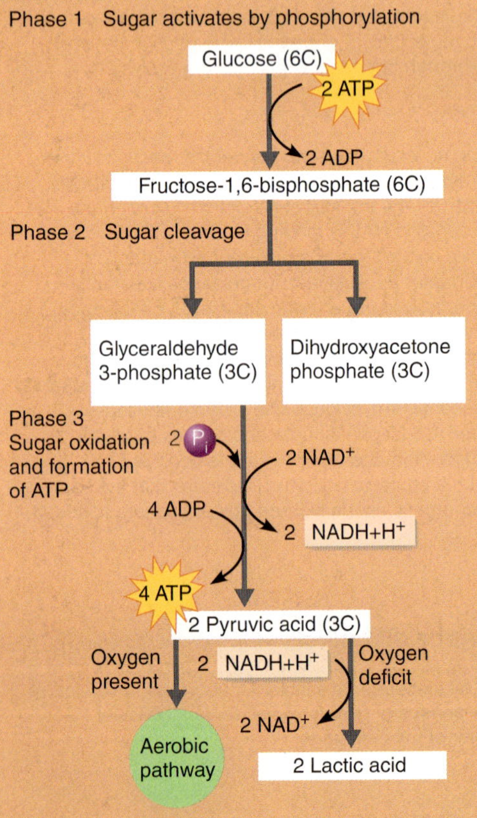

① Two-carbon acetyl CoA is combined with oxaloacetic acid, a 4-carbon compound. The unstable bond between the acetyl group and CoA is broken as oxaloacetic acid binds and CoA is freed to prime another 2-carbon fragment derived from pyruvic acid. The product is the 6-carbon citric acid, for which the cycle is named.

② A molecule of water is removed, and another is added back. The net result is the conversion of citric acid to its isomer, isocitric acid.

③ The substrate loses a CO_2 molecule, and the remaining 5-carbon compound is oxidized, forming an α-ketoglutaric acid and reducing NAD^+.

④ This step is catalyzed by a multienzyme complex very similar to the one that converts pyruvic acid to acetyl CoA. CO_2 is lost; the remaining 4-carbon compound is oxidized by the transfer of electrons to NAD^+ to form $NADH+H^+$ and is then attached to CoA by an unstable bond. The product is succinyl CoA.

⑤ Substrate-level phosphorylation occurs in this step. CoA is displaced by a phosphate group, which is then transferred to GDP to form guanosine triphosphate (GTP). GTP is similar to ATP, which is formed when GTP donates a phosphate group to ADP. The products of this step are succinic acid and ATP.

⑥ In another oxidative step, two hydrogens are removed from succinic acid (forming fumaric acid) and transferred to FAD to form $FADH_2$. The function of this coenzyme is similar to that of $NADH+H^+$, but $FADH_2$ stores less energy. The enzyme that catalyzes this oxidation-reduction reaction is the only enzyme of the cycle that is embedded in the mitochondrial membrane. All other enzymes of the citric acid cycle are dissolved in the mitochondrial matrix.

⑦ Bonds in the substrate are rearranged in this step by the addition of a water molecule. The product is malic acid.

⑧ The last oxidative step reduces another NAD^+ and regenerates oxaloacetic acid, which accepts a 2-carbon fragment from acetyl CoA for another turn of the cycle.

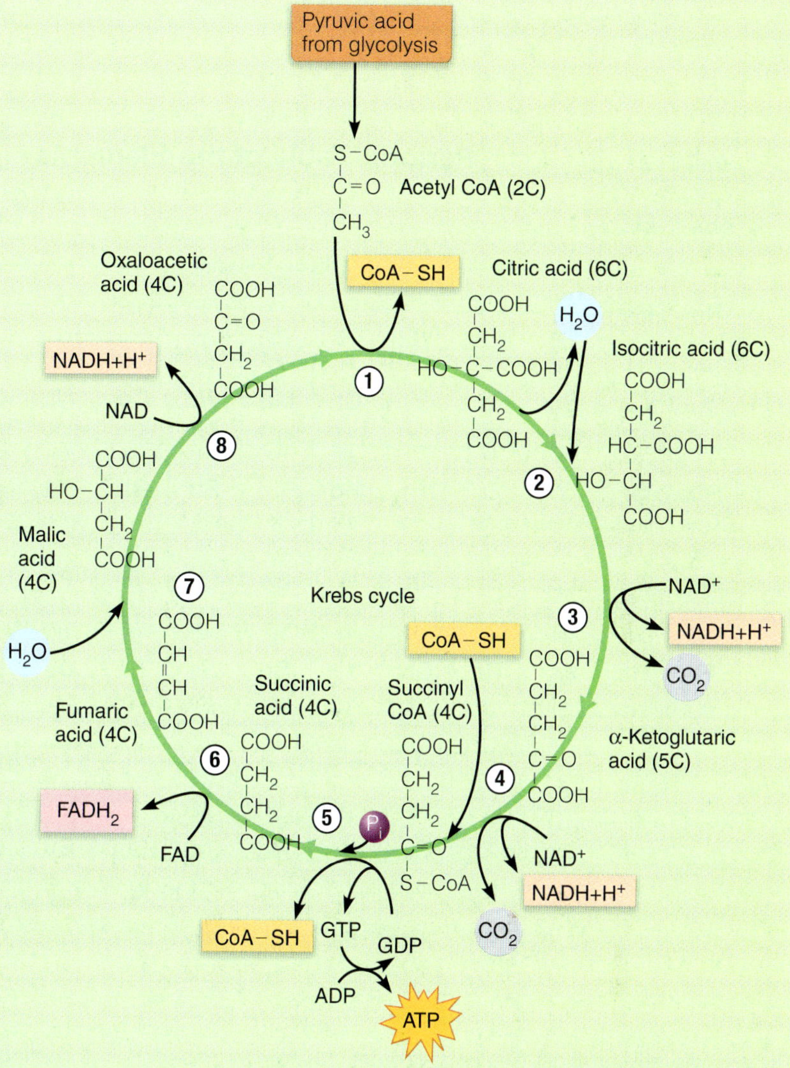

KREBS CYCLE (CITRIC ACID CYCLE) All but one of the steps (step 6) occur in the mitochondrial matrix. The preparation of pyruvic acid (by oxidation, decarboxylation, and reaction with coenzyme A) to enter the cycle as acetyl CoA is shown above the cycle. Acetyl CoA is picked up by oxaloacetic acid to form citric acid; and as it passes through the cycle, it is oxidized four more times [forming three molecules of reduced NAD ($NADH + H^+$) and one of reduced FAD ($FADH_2$)] and decarboxylated twice (releasing 2 CO_2). Energy is captured in the bonds of GTP, which then acts in a coupled reaction with ADP to generate one molecule of ATP by substrate-level phosphorylation.

Periodic Table of the Elements

Representative (main group) elements | Transition metals | Representative (main group) elements

Period	IA	IIA	IIIB	IVB	VB	VIB	VIIB	VIIIB	VIIIB	VIIIB	IB	IIB	IIIA	IVA	VA	VIA	VIIA	VIIIA
1	1 H 1.0079																	2 He 4.003
2	3 Li 6.941	4 Be 9.012											5 B 10.811	6 C 12.011	7 N 14.007	8 O 15.999	9 F 18.998	10 Ne 20.180
3	11 Na 22.990	12 Mg 24.305											13 Al 26.982	14 Si 28.086	15 P 30.974	16 S 32.065	17 Cl 35.453	18 Ar 39.948
4	19 K 39.098	20 Ca 40.078	21 Sc 44.956	22 Ti 47.867	23 V 50.942	24 Cr 51.996	25 Mn 54.938	26 Fe 55.845	27 Co 58.933	28 Ni 58.69	29 Cu 63.546	30 Zn 65.38	31 Ga 69.723	32 Ge 72.64	33 As 74.922	34 Se 78.96	35 Br 79.904	36 Kr 83.8
5	37 Rb 85.468	38 Sr 87.62	39 Y 88.906	40 Zr 91.224	41 Nb 92.906	42 Mo 95.96	43 Tc 98	44 Ru 101.07	45 Rh 102.906	46 Pd 106.42	47 Ag 107.868	48 Cd 112.411	49 In 114.82	50 Sn 118.71	51 Sb 121.76	52 Te 127.60	53 I 126.905	54 Xe 131.29
6	55 Cs 132.905	56 Ba 137.327	57 La 138.906	72 Hf 178.49	73 Ta 180.948	74 W 183.84	75 Re 186.207	76 Os 190.23	77 Ir 192.22	78 Pt 195.08	79 Au 196.967	80 Hg 200.59	81 Tl 204.383	82 Pb 207.2	83 Bi 208.980	84 Po 209	85 At 210	86 Rn 222
7	87 Fr 223	88 Ra 226	89 Ac 227	104 Rf 267	105 Db 268	106 Sg 271	107 Bh 272	108 Hs 270	109 Mt 276	110 Ds 281	111 Rg 280	112 Cn 285	113 Uut 284	114 Uuq 289	115 Uup 288	116 Uuh 293	117 Uus 292	118 Uuo 294

Rare earth elements

Lanthanides	58 Ce 140.116	59 Pr 140.908	60 Nd 144.24	61 Pm 145	62 Sm 150.36	63 Eu 151.964	64 Gd 157.25	65 Tb 158.925	66 Dy 162.5	67 Ho 164.93	68 Er 167.26	69 Tm 168.934	70 Yb 173.054	71 Lu 174.967
Actinides	90 Th 232.038	91 Pa 231.036	92 U 238.029	93 Np 237.048	94 Pu 244	95 Am 243	96 Cm 247	97 Bk 247	98 Cf 251	99 Es 252	100 Fm 257	101 Md 258	102 No 259	103 Lr 262

The periodic table arranges elements according to atomic number and atomic weight into horizontal rows called periods and 18 vertical columns called groups or families. The elements in the groups are classified as being in either A or B classes.

Elements of each group of the A series have similar chemical and physical properties. This reflects the fact that members of a particular group have the same number of valence shell electrons, which is indicated by the roman numeral of the group. For example, group IA elements have one valence shell electron, group IIA elements have two, and group VA elements have five. In contrast, as you progress across a period from left to right, the properties of the elements change in discrete steps, varying gradually from the very metallic properties of groups IA and IIA elements to the nonmetallic properties seen in group VIIA (chlorine and others), and finally to the inert elements (noble gases) in group VIIIA. This change reflects the continual increase in the number of valence shell electrons seen in elements (from left to right) within a period.

Class B elements are referred to as transition elements. All transition elements are metals, and in most cases they have one or two valence shell electrons. (In these elements, some electrons occupy more distant electron shells before the deeper shells are filled.)

In this periodic table, the colors are used to convey information about the phase (solid, liquid, or gas) in which a pure element exists under standard conditions (25 degrees Celsius and 1 atmosphere of pressure). If the element's symbol is solid black, then the element exists as a solid. If its symbol is red, then it exists as a gas. If its symbol is dark blue, then it is a liquid. If the element's symbol is green, the element does not exist in nature and must be created by some type of nuclear reaction.

*Atomic weights of the elements per IUPAC Commission on Isotopic Abundances and Atomic Weights, 2007.

Appendix F Reference Values for Selected Blood and Urine Studies

The reference values listed for the selected blood and urine studies are common ranges for adults, but specific "normals" are established by the laboratory performing the analysis. The values may be affected by a wide range of circumstances, including testing methods and equipment used, client age, body mass, sex, diet, activity level, medications, and extent of disease processes.

Reference values are identified in both standard or conventional units and in the system of international (SI) units. SI units (given in parentheses) are measurements of amount per volume and are used in most countries and scientific journals. SI units are often given as moles or millimoles per liter. Most clinical laboratories and textbooks in the United States use conventional or standard units, which measure mass per volume. These values are given as grams, milligrams, or milliequivalents per deciliter or liter. It is anticipated that the United States will eventually use SI units exclusively.

For enzymes, 1 international unit (IU) represents an arbitrary but defined amount of activity, whereas 1 katal (kat) is the amount of enzyme required to consume 1 mol of substrate per second.

Sample types in column 1 are serum (S), plasma (P), arterial whole blood (A), and whole blood (WB).

TEST (SAMPLE)	REFERENCE VALUES: CONVENTIONAL (SI)	PHYSIOLOGICAL INDICATION AND CLINICAL IMPLICATIONS
Blood Chemistry Studies		
Ammonia (P)	15–120 μg/dl (9–70 μmol/L)	Liver and renal function. Increased values in liver disease, renal failure, newborn hemolytic disease, heart failure, cor pulmonale. Decreased values in hypertension.
Amylase (S)	56–190 IU/L (0.4–2.1 μkat/L)	Pancreatic function. Increased values in pancreatitis, mumps, obstruction of pancreatic duct, ketoacidosis. Decreased values in kidney disease, pancreatic damage or cancer, toxemia of pregnancy.
Aspartate aminotransferase (AST, or SGOT) (S)	≤40 IU/L (≤0.7 μkat/L)	Cellular damage. Increased after myocardial infarction, acute liver disease, drug toxicity, muscle trauma. Decreased in pyridoxine (vitamin B_6) deficiency.
Bilirubin (S)	Total: 0.1–1.0 mg/dl (1.7–17.1 μmol/L) Direct: <0.4 mg/dl (<6.8 μmol/L) Indirect: 0.1–1.0 mg/dl (1.7–17.1 μmol/L) Newborn: <13.0 mg/dl (<222 μmol/L)	Liver function and red cell breakdown. Increased levels of direct in liver disease and biliary obstruction. Increased levels of indirect in hemolysis of red blood cells.
Blood urea nitrogen (S)	7–26 mg/dl (2.5–9.3 mmol/L)	Kidney function. Increased values in renal disease, dehydration, urinary obstruction, congestive heart failure, myocardial infarction, burns. Decreased values in liver failure, overhydration, impaired protein absorption, pregnancy.
Cholesterol	<200 mg/dl (<5.2 mmol/L)	Metabolism—fat utilization. Increased values in diabetes mellitus, pregnancy, use of oral contraceptives or anabolic steroids.
High-density lipoprotein (HDL) cholesterol (S)	20–30% of total >40 mg/dl (>1.0 mmol/L)	Increased levels in liver disease, aerobic exercise. Decreased levels in atherosclerotic heart disease, malnutrition.
Low-density lipoprotein (LDL) cholesterol (S)	60–70% of total <130 mg/dl (<3.4 mmol/L)	Increased values in hyperlipidemia, atherosclerotic heart disease. Decreased values in fat malabsorption and malnutrition.
Very low density lipoprotein cholesterol (VLDL) (S)	10–15% of total	Same as LDL.
Creatine kinase (CK) (S)	Female: ≤190 U/L (≤3.2 μkat/L) Male: ≤235 U/L (≤3.9 μkat/L)	Cellular damage. Increased values in myocardial infarction, muscular dystrophy, hypothyroidism, pulmonary infarction, cerebrovascular accident (CVA), shock, tissue damage, and trauma.
Creatinine (S)	0.5–1.2 mg/dl (44–106 μmol/L)	Renal function. Increased values in renal disease and acromegaly. Decreased in muscular dystrophy.

TEST (SAMPLE)	REFERENCE VALUES: CONVENTIONAL (SI)	PHYSIOLOGICAL INDICATION AND CLINICAL IMPLICATIONS
Blood Chemistry Studies *(continued)*		
Gases (A)		
Bicarbonate	22–26 mEq/L (22–26 mmol/L)	Acid-base balance. Increased values in metabolic alkalosis and respiratory acidosis. Decreased values in metabolic acidosis and respiratory alkalosis.
Carbon dioxide content	Arterial: 19–24 mEq/L (19–24 mmol/L) Venous: 22–30 mEq/L (22–30 mmol/L)	
Carbon dioxide partial pressure (P_{CO_2})	Arterial: 35–45 mm Hg Venous: 45 mm Hg	
Oxygen (O_2) saturation	95–98% (same)	Values increased slightly in hyperventilation. Decreased values (hypoxia) in pulmonary disease, hypoventilation, high altitude.
Oxygen partial pressure (P_{O_2})	80–105 mm Hg	
pH	7.35–7.45 (same)	Increased values in metabolic and respiratory alkalosis. Decreased values in metabolic and respiratory acidosis.
Glucose (S)	70–120 mg/dl (3.9–6.7 mmol/L)	Metabolic function. Increased values in diabetes mellitus, Cushing's syndrome, liver disease, acute stress, and acromegaly. Decreased levels in Addison's disease, insulinomas.
Immunoglobulins (S)		
IgG	560–1800 mg/dl (5.6–18 g/L)	Immune response. Increased levels in chronic infections, rheumatic fever, liver disease, rheumatoid arthritis. Decreased levels in amyloidosis, leukemia, and preeclampsia.
IgE	<43.2 μg/dl (<432 μg/L)	Allergic responses. Increased values in allergic responses. Decreased values in agammaglobulinemia.
IgA	85–563 mg/dl (0.85–5.6 g/L)	Immune integrity. Increased values in liver disease, rheumatic fever, chronic infection, inflammatory bowel disease. Decreased values in immunodeficiency disorders and immunosuppression.
IgM	55–375 mg/dl (0.5–3.8 g/L)	Immune integrity. Increased in autoimmune disease (e.g., rheumatoid arthritis), acute infections. Decreased in amyloidosis and leukemia.
IgD	0.5–14 mg/dl (5–140 mg/L)	Immune integrity. Increased values in myelomas.
Ketone bodies (S or P)	Negative Toxic level >20 mg/dl (0.2 g/L)	Fatty acid catabolism. Increased values (ketosis, ketoacidosis) in starvation, low-carbohydrate diet, uncontrolled diabetes mellitus, aspirin overdose.
Lactate dehydrogenase (LDH) (S)	105–333 U/L (1.7–5.6 μkat/L)	Tissue damage of organs or striated muscle. Increased in myocardial infarction, pulmonary infarction, liver disease, cerebrovascular accident, infectious mononucleosis, muscular dystrophy, fractures.
Lactic acid (lactate) (P)	9–16 mg/dl (1.0–1.8 mmol/L)	Anaerobic tissue metabolism. Increased values in congestive heart failure, shock, hemorrhage, strenuous exercise.
Osmolality (S)	280–300 mOsm/kg H_2O (280–300 mmol/kg H_2O)	Fluid and electrolyte balance. Increased levels in hypernatremia, dehydration, kidney disease, alcohol ingestion. Decreased levels in hyponatremia, overhydration, and syndrome of inappropriate ADH secretion (SIADH).
Phosphate (S) (phosphorus)	2.5–4.5 mg/dl (0.8–1.5 mmol/L)	Parathyroid function; bone disease. Increased levels in hypoparathyroidism, renal failure, bone metastasis, hypocalcemia. Decreased values in hyperparathyroidism, hypercalcemia, alcoholism, vitamin D deficiency, ketoacidosis, osteomalacia.
Potassium (S)	3.5–5.5 mEq/L (3.5–5.5 mmol/L)	Fluid and electrolyte balance. Increased levels in renal disease, Addison's disease, ketoacidosis, burns, and crush injuries. Decreased levels in vomiting, diarrhea, Cushing's syndrome, alkalosis, diuretics.

TEST (SAMPLE)	REFERENCE VALUES: CONVENTIONAL (SI)	PHYSIOLOGICAL INDICATION AND CLINICAL IMPLICATIONS
Blood Chemistry Studies *(continued)*		
Protein (S)		
Total	6.0–8.5 g/dl (60–85 g/L)	Osmotic pressure; immune system integrity. Increased values in multiple myeloma, dehydration, myxedema. Decreased values in protein malnutrition, burns, diarrhea, renal failure, liver failure.
Albumin	3.2–5.0 g/dl (32–50 g/L)	Osmotic pressure. Increased levels in dehydration. Decreased levels in liver disease, malnutrition, Crohn's disease, nephrotic syndrome, systemic lupus erythematosus.
Sodium (S)	135–145 mEq/L (135–145 mmol/L)	Fluid and electrolyte balance. Increased values in dehydration, diabetes insipidus, Cushing's syndrome. Decreased values in vomiting, diarrhea, burns, Addison's disease, myxedema, congestive heart failure, overhydration, syndrome of inappropriate ADH secretion (SIADH).
Triglycerides	10–150 mg/dl (0.1–1.5 g/L)	Increased values in diabetes mellitus, liver disease, nephrotic syndrome, pregnancy.
Uric acid (S)	Female: 2.0–7.3 mg/dl (119–434 μmol/L) Male: 2.1–8.5 mg/dl (125–506 μmol/L)	Renal function. Increased in lead poisoning, impaired renal function, gout, alcoholism, hematologic cancers. Decreased in Wilson's disease.
Hematology Studies		
Hemoglobin (S)	Female: 12–16 g/dl (120–160 g/L) Male: 13–18 g/dl (130–180 g/L)	Oxygenation status. Increased values in dehydration, polycythemia, congestive heart failure, chronic obstructive pulmonary disease, high altitudes. Decreased levels in anemia, hemorrhage, bone marrow cancer, renal disease, systemic lupus erythematosus, nutritional deficiency.
Hematocrit (WB)	Female: 37–47% (same) Male: 42–52% (same)	Oxygenation status. Increased levels in polycythemia, dehydration, congestive heart failure, shock, surgery. Decreased levels in anemia, hemorrhage, bone marrow disease, malnutrition, cirrhosis, rheumatoid arthritis.
Partial thromboplastin time (activated) (PTT or aPTT)	20–36 s (same)	Clotting mechanisms. Increased values in clotting factor deficiencies, cirrhosis, vitamin K deficiency, disseminated intravascular coagulation (DIC). Decreased values in early DIC, extensive cancer.
Platelet count (WB)	150,000–400,000/μl (150–400 × 10^9/L)	Clotting mechanisms. Increased values in polycythemia, cancers, rheumatoid arthritis, trauma. Decreased values in liver disease, hemolytic uremic syndrome, disseminated intravascular coagulation (DIC), idiopathic thrombocytopenic purpura (ITP), systemic lupus erythematosus (SLE).
Prothrombin time (PT) (WB)	11–12.5 s (same) 1.5–2 × control (evaluating anticoagulant treatment)	Clotting mechanisms. Increased values in liver disease, vitamin K deficiency, salicylate intoxication. Decreased values in disseminated intravascular coagulation (DIC).
Red blood cell count (RBC) (WB)	Female: 4.2–5.4 million/μl (4.2–5.4 × 10^{12}/L) Male: 4.7–6.1 million/μl (4.7–6.1 × 10^{12}/L)	Oxygenation status. Increased values in high altitudes, polycythemia, hemoconcentration, cor pulmonale. Decreased values in hemorrhage, hemolysis, anemias, chronic illness, nutritional deficiencies, leukemia, overhydration.
Reticulocyte count (WB)	0.5–2.0% (same)	Bone marrow function. Increased values in hemolytic anemia, sickle-cell anemia, leukemia, pregnancy. Decreased values in pernicious anemia, folic acid deficiency, cirrhosis, chronic infection, bone marrow depression or failure.
White blood cell count (WBC) (WB)		
Total (males)	4800–10,800/μl (4.8–10.8 × 10^9/L)	Immune system integrity. Increased values in infection, trauma, stress, tissue necrosis, inflammation. Decreased values in bone marrow depression or failure, drug toxicity, overwhelming infection, malnutrition.

➤

TEST (SAMPLE)	REFERENCE VALUES: CONVENTIONAL (SI)	PHYSIOLOGICAL INDICATION AND CLINICAL IMPLICATIONS
Hematology Studies *(continued)*		
White blood cell count, differential (WB)		
Neutrophils	50–70% (same)	Immune system integrity. Increased values in acute bacterial infections, stress, Cushing's syndrome, inflammatory disorders, ketoacidosis, gout. Decreased levels in aplastic anemia, bone marrow suppression, and overwhelming bacterial infections.
Lymphocytes	25–40% (same)	Immune system integrity. Increased values in viral infections (e.g., mumps, rubella, infectious mononucleosis, hepatitis), lymphocytic leukemia, certain bacterial infections. Decreased levels in leukemia, immunodeficiency, lupus erythematosus, bone marrow depressive drugs.
Eosinophils	1–4% (same)	Immune system integrity. Increased levels in allergic reactions, parasitic infections, leukemia. Decreased levels in excess adrenocorticosteroid production.
Monocytes	3–8% (same)	Immune system integrity. Increased levels in certain infections (e.g., tuberculosis, malaria), inflammatory disorders.
Basophils	0.5–1.0% (same)	Immune system integrity. Increased levels in myeloproliferative disorders, leukemia. Decreased levels in allergic reactions, hyperthyroidism, stress.
Urine Tests		
Amylase (24 h)	<6000 Somogyi units/24 h 0–500 U/24 h (0–8.3 μkat/24 h)	Pancreatic function. Increased values in pancreatic disease or obstruction, inflammation of the salivary glands, and cholecystitis.
Bilirubin (random)	Negative (same)	Liver function. Increased values in liver disease, extrahepatic obstruction (gallstones, tumor, inflammation).
Blood (hemoglobin) (random)	Negative (same)	Urinary system function. Increased values in cystitis, renal disease, hemolytic anemia, transfusion reaction, prostatitis, burns.
Osmolality (random or fasting)	Random: 50–1200 mOsm/kg H_2O (50–1200 mmol/kg H_2O) Fluid restriction: ≥850 mOsm/kg H_2O (≥850 mmol/kg H_2O)	Fluid and electrolyte balance, renal function, and endocrine function. Increased levels in hypernatremia, syndrome of inappropriate ADH secretion (SIADH), congestive heart failure, metabolic acidosis. Decreased levels in diabetes insipidus, water intoxication, pyelonephritis, renal tubular necrosis, aldosteronism.
Phosphate (24 h)	0.9–1.3g/24 hr (same)	Parathyroid function. Increased levels in hyperparathyroidism, osteomalacia, certain renal diseases, vitamin D deficiency. Decreased levels in hypoparathyroidism.
Potassium (24 h)	25–120 mEq/24 h (25–120 mmol/24 h)	Fluid and electrolyte balance. Increased values in renal tubular necrosis, metabolic acidosis, dehydration, aldosteronism, Cushing's syndrome. Decreased values in Addison's disease, malabsorption, acute renal failure.
Protein (random)	<8 mg/dl (<80 mg/L)	Renal function. Increased levels in nephrotic syndrome, renal trauma, hyperthyroidism, diabetic nephropathy, systemic lupus erythematosus.
Sodium (24 h)	40–220 mEq/24 h (40–220 mmol/24 h)	Fluid and electrolyte balance. Increased values in dehydration, ketoacidosis, syndrome of inappropriate ADH secretion (SIADH), adrenocortical insufficiency. Decreased levels in congestive heart failure, renal failure, diarrhea, aldosteronism.
Uric acid (24 h)	250–750 mg/24 h (1.5–4.5 mmol/24 h)	Renal function and metabolism. Increased in gout, leukemia, liver disease, ulcerative colitis. Decreased in renal disease, alcoholism, lead toxicity, folic acid deficiency.

TEST (SAMPLE)	REFERENCE VALUES: CONVENTIONAL (SI)	PHYSIOLOGICAL INDICATION AND CLINICAL IMPLICATIONS
Urine Tests *(continued)*		
Urinalysis (random)		
Color	Straw, yellow, amber	Fluid balance and renal function. Darker in dehydration. Lighter in overhydration, diabetes insipidus. Color varies with disease states, diet, and medications.
Odor	Aromatic	Metabolic function, infection. Abnormal odors in infection, ketonuria, rectal fistula, hepatic failure, phenylketonuria.
Specific gravity	1.001–1.035	An indirect measurement of urine concentration (osmolality). Same physiological indications and clinical implications as osmolality.
pH	4.5–8.0	A crude indicator of acid-base balance. Decreased by acidic diet (proteins). Increased by a vegetarian diet, prolonged vomiting, and bacterial infection of the urinary tract.
Urobilinogen (24 h)	0.2–1.0 mg/dl (2–10 mg/L)	Liver function. Increased in hemolytic anemias, hepatitis, cirrhosis, biliary disease. Decreased in common bile duct obstruction.
Volume (24 h)	800–2000 ml/24 h (0.8–2.0 L/24 h)	Fluid and electrolyte balance, renal function. Increased values in diabetes insipidus, diabetes mellitus, renal disease. Decreased values in dehydration, syndrome of inappropriate ADH secretion (SIADH), renal disease.

Figure G.1 **Each upper limb is innervated by five major nerves arising from the brachial plexus.**

The nerves from the **anterior division of the brachial plexus** innervate the muscles in the anterior compartments: the flexor muscles of the arm, forearm, and hand. These nerves continue distally to supply cutaneous innervation to the forearm and hand.

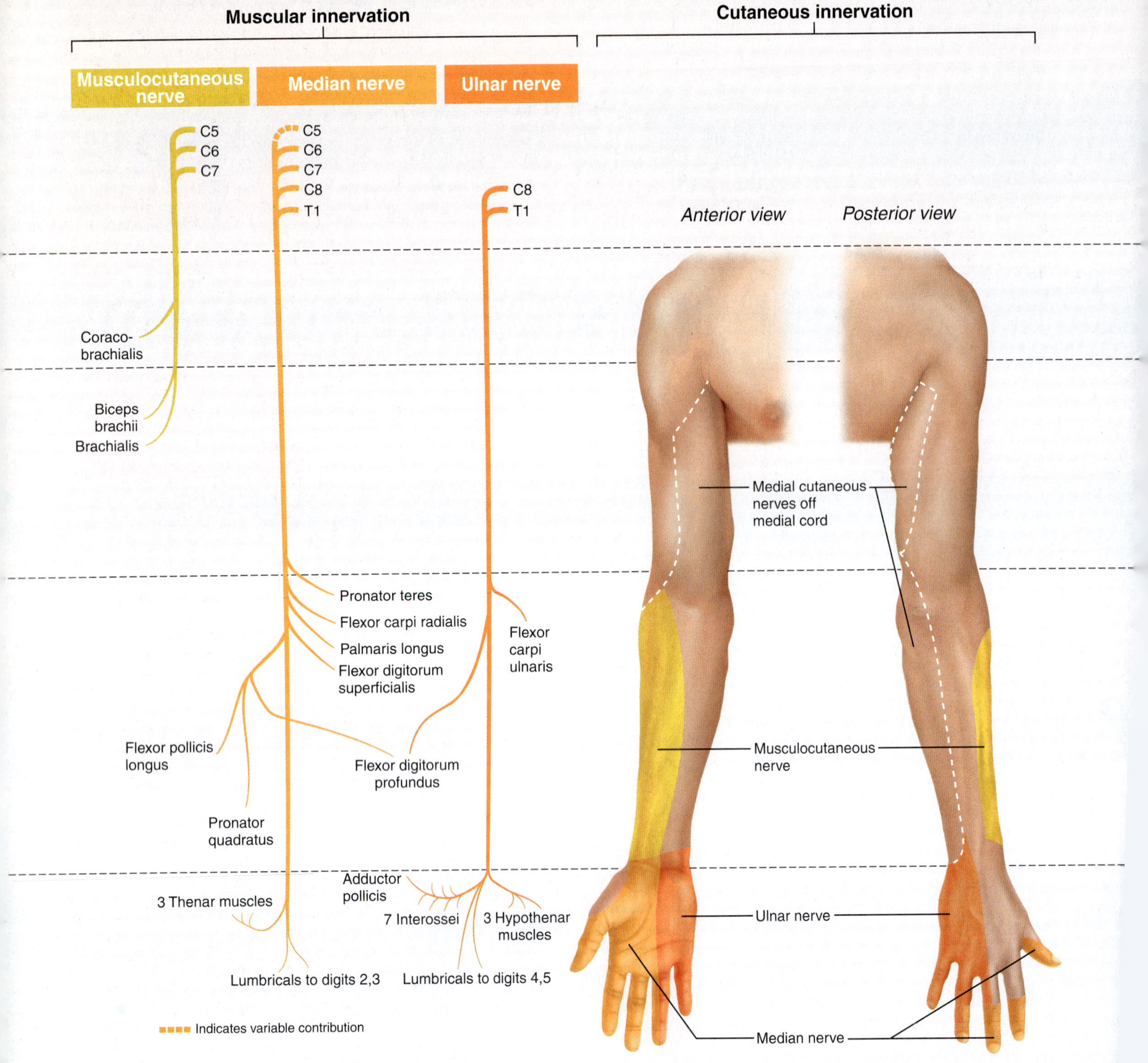

The nerves from the **posterior division of the brachial plexus** innervate the muscles in the posterior compartments: the extensor muscles of the upper limb. These nerves continue distally to supply cutaneous innervation to much of the posterior arm, forearm, and hand.

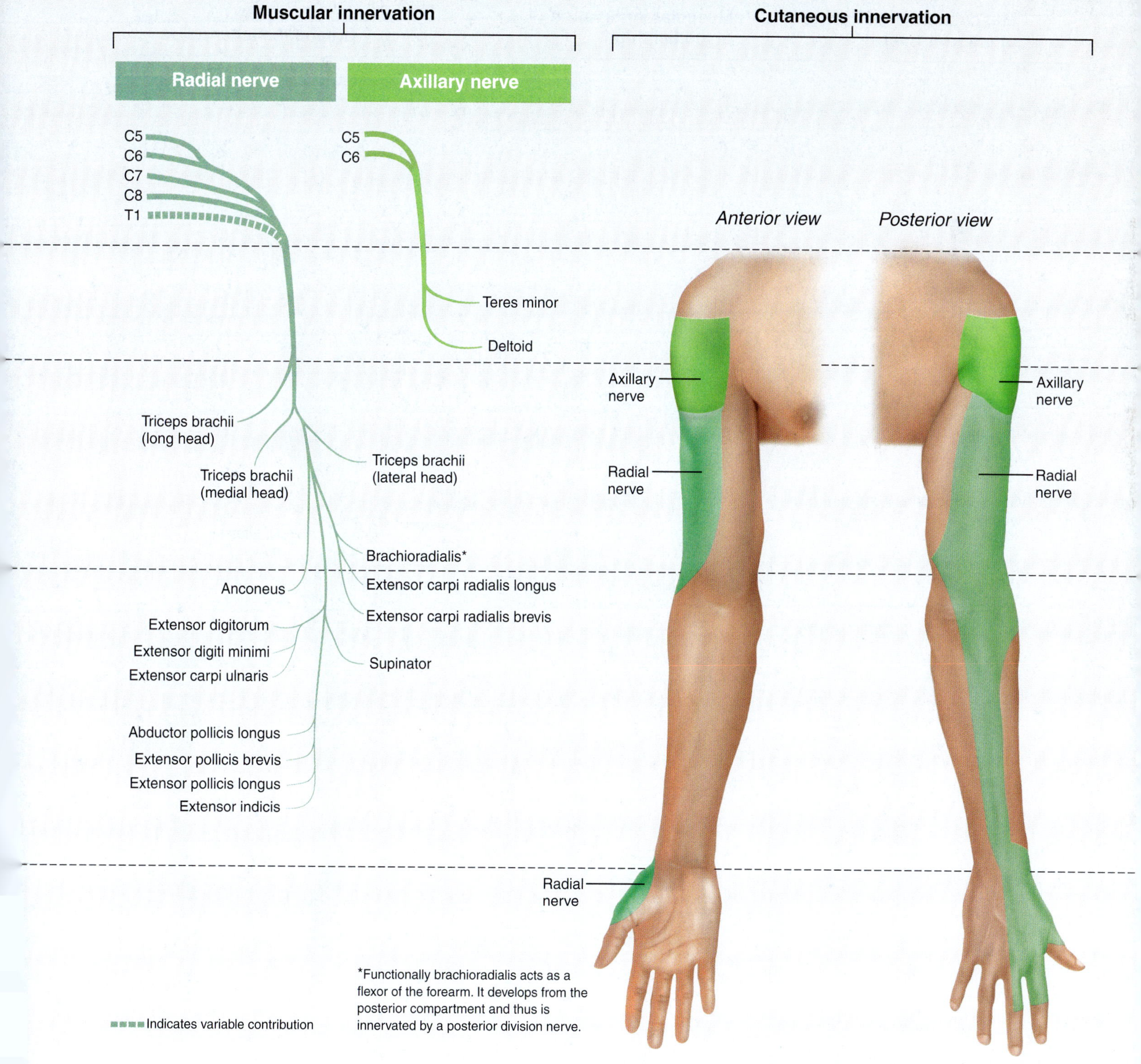

*Functionally brachioradialis acts as a flexor of the forearm. It develops from the posterior compartment and thus is innervated by a posterior division nerve.

Figure G.2 **Each lower limb is innervated by nerves arising from the lumbar and sacral plexuses, together called the lumbosacral plexus.**

The nerves from the **lumbar plexus** innervate the muscles in the anterior and medial compartments of the thigh, and supply cutaneous innervation to anterior and medial portions of the thigh and leg.

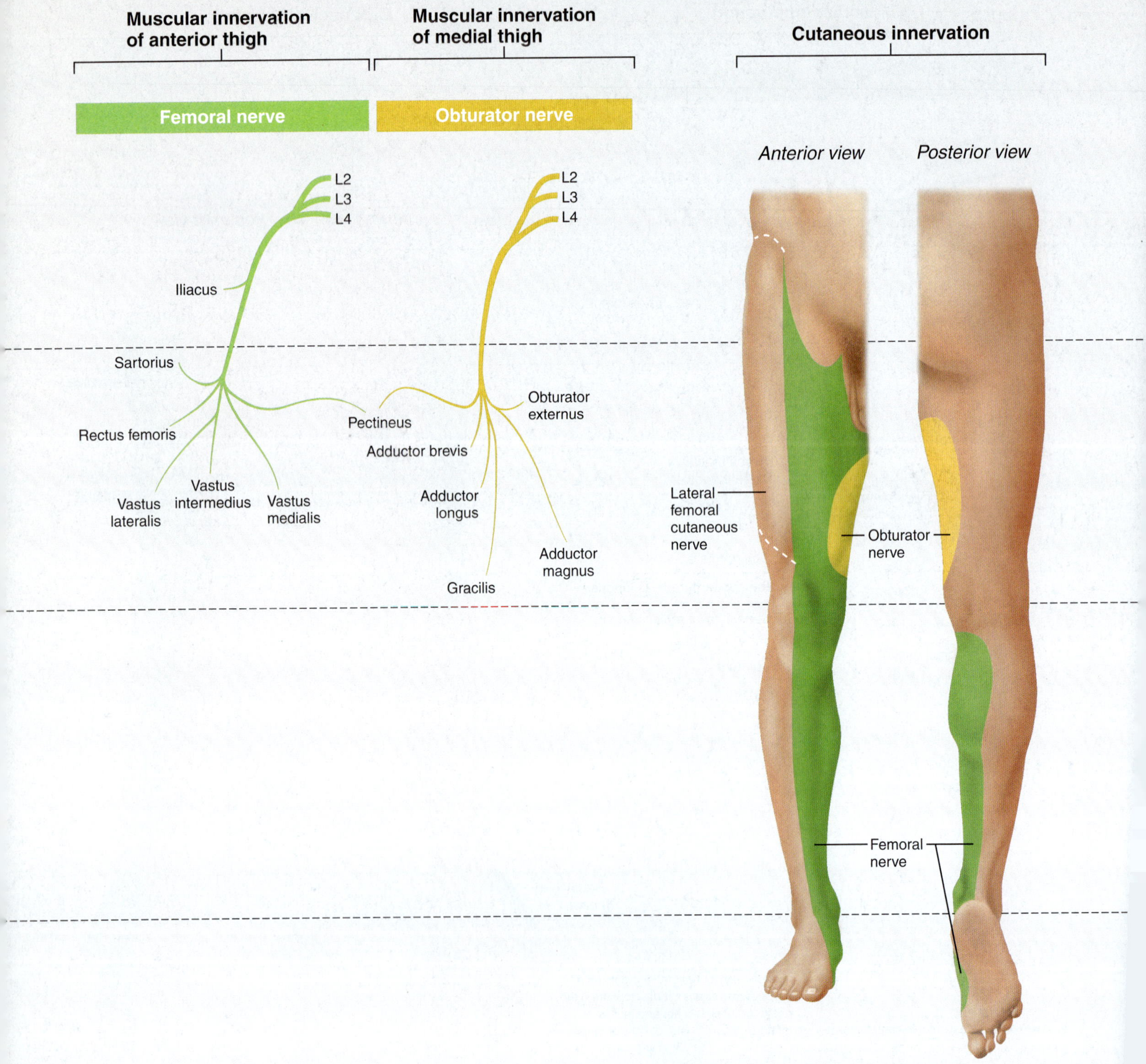

The nerves from the **sacral plexus** innervate the muscles in the posterior compartments of the thigh and all of the muscles in the leg, and supply cutaneous innervation to the lateral and posterior portions of the leg and to the foot.

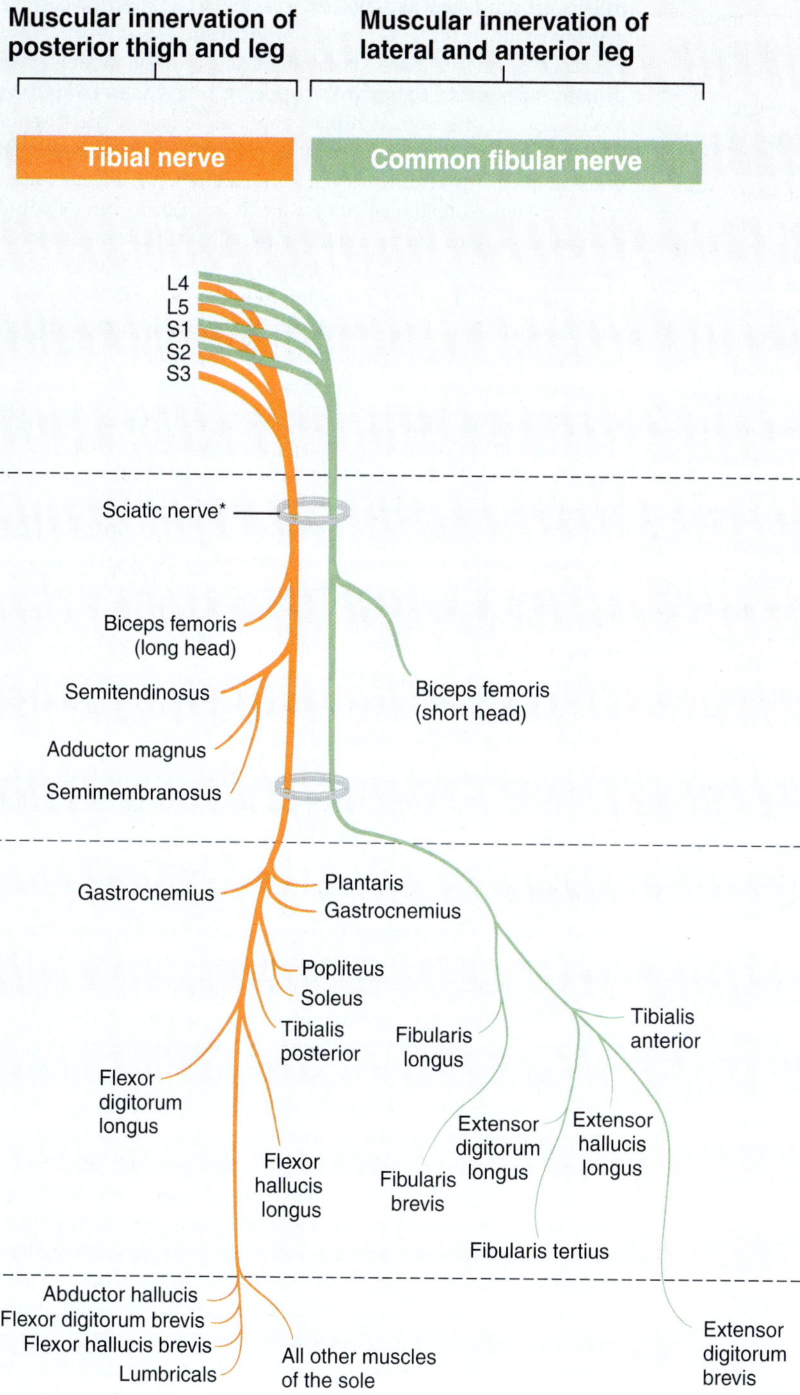

*Sciatic nerve formed by tibial and common fibular nerves wrapped by common sheath.

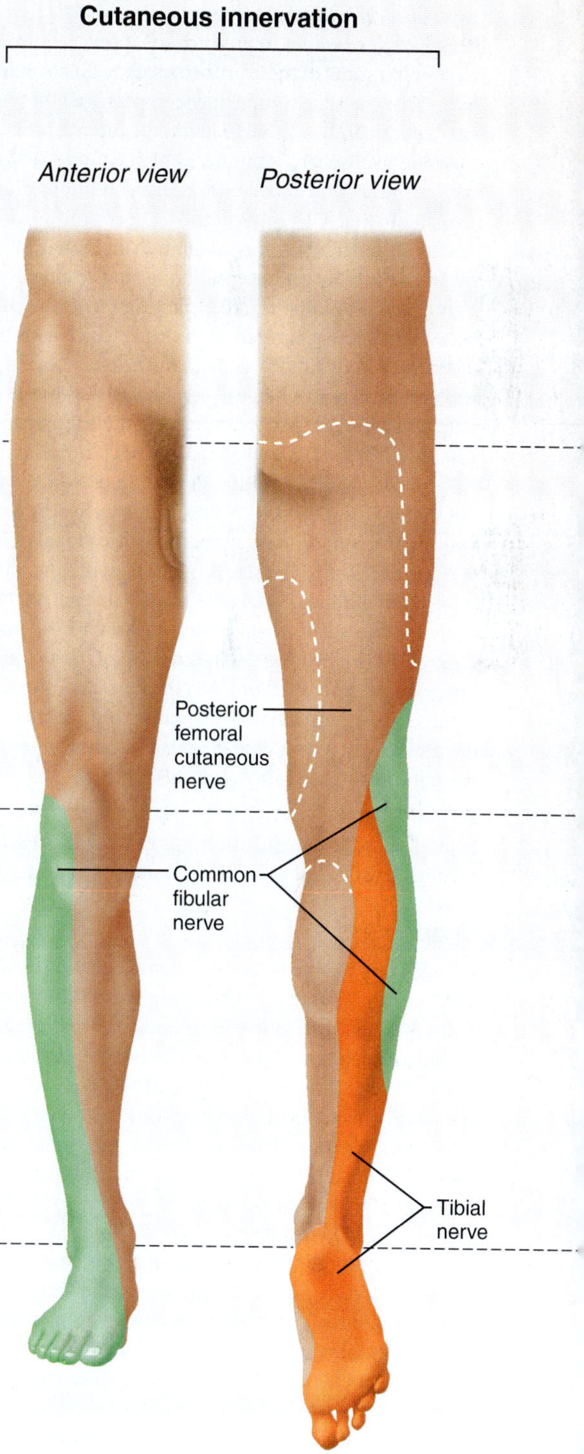

Appendix H Answers to Check Your Understanding, Multiple Choice, Matching Questions, and Case Study

Chapter 1

Check Your Understanding 1. The operation or function of a structure is promoted or prevented by its anatomy. For example, oxygen and carbon dioxide are exchanged across the very thin membranes of the lungs but not across the skin. **2.** Muscle shortening is a topic of physiology. The body location of the lungs is an anatomy topic. **3.** Cytologists study the cellular level of organization. **4.** The order in the structural hierarchy is cell, tissue, organ, and organism. **5.** Bones and cartilages are part of the skeletal system. The nasal cavity, lungs, and trachea are respiratory system organs. **6.** Living organisms can maintain their boundaries, move, respond to environmental changes, digest nutrients, carry out metabolism, dispose of wastes, reproduce, and grow. While inanimate objects may exhibit some of these properties, they do not exhibit all of them. **7.** Metabolism is the term that encompasses all the chemical reactions that occur in body cells. **8.** In flight, the cabin must be pressurized because the atmosphere is thinner at high altitudes and the amount of oxygen entering the blood under such conditions may be insufficient to maintain life. **9.** Negative feedback mechanisms allow us to adjust to conditions outside the normal temperature range by causing heat to be lost from the body (in hot conditions) and retained or generated by the body (in cold conditions). **10.** Thirst is part of a negative feedback control system because it prods us to drink, which ends the thirst stimulus and returns body fluid volume to the normal range. **11.** This is a positive feedback mechanism because it enhances the change (formation of a platelet plug) set into motion by the stimulus (damage to the blood vessel). The response ends when the platelet plug has plugged the hole in the blood vessel. **12.** The position in which a person is standing erect with feet slightly separated and palms facing anteriorly. Knowing the anatomical position is important because directional terms refer to the body as if it is in this position. **13.** Axillary region is the armpit. Acromial area is the tip of the shoulder. **14.** A frontal (coronal) section would separate the brain into anterior and posterior parts. **15.** He may have appendicitis if the pain is in the lower right quadrant of his abdomen. **16.** Of these organs, only the spinal cord is in the dorsal body cavity. **17.** As mobile organs (heart, lungs, digestive organs) work, friction is greatly reduced by the presence of serous fluid. Serous fluid allows the surrounding serous membranes to glide easily over one another.

Review Questions 1. c; **2.** a; **3.** e; **4.** a, d; **5.** (a) wrist (b) hip bone (c) nose (d) toes (e) scalp; **6.** neither c nor d would be visible in the median section; **7.** (a) dorsal (b) ventral (c) dorsal (d) ventral; **8.** b; **9.** b; **10.** c

Chapter 2

Check Your Understanding 1. Foods contain chemical energy. **2.** Electrical energy is the energy used by nerve cells to transmit messages in the body. **3.** Potential energy (PE) is available when we are still. PE is converted to kinetic (working) energy when we exercise. **4.** Besides hydrogen and nitrogen, carbon and oxygen help to make up the bulk of living matter. **5.** This element has 82 protons in its nucleus and 82 electrons in its orbitals (electron cloud). **6.** Atomic mass indicates the sum of the protons and neutrons in a given atom's nucleus. Atomic weight indicates the average mass of all the isotopes of a given element. **7.** A molecule is 2 or more atoms held together by chemical bonds. **8.** A compound is formed when two or more different kinds of atoms chemically bond together, as in NaCl. Oxygen gas is 2 oxygen atoms (the same kind of atom) bonded together. **9.** Blood is a mixture because its components are not changed by their combination and they can be separated by physical means. **10.** Hydrogen bonds (linking H of one water molecule to O of another) form between water molecules. **11.** Argon's valence shell is full:)2e)8e)8e. Hence it is nonreactive. **12.** Electrons would spend more time in the vicinity of the more electronegative atom in XY, whereas electrons in XX would orbit both X atoms to an equal extent. **13.** Fats are digested in the small intestine by decomposition reactions. **14.** Biochemical reactions in the body tend to be irreversible because (a) one or more of the products is removed from the reaction site or (b) the product is needed more than the reactants, so the cell would not provide energy to reverse the reaction. **15.** Decomposition reactions in which foods are broken down for energy are oxidation-reduction (redox) reactions. **16.** Water is an excellent solvent because of its polarity. As a dipole, it can orient itself to the end of other molecules, causing them to dissociate or go into solution. **17.** Electrolytes are substances like salts that will conduct an electrical current in aqueous solution. **18.** H^+ is responsible for acidity. **19.** It is better to add a weak base, which will act to buffer the strong acid. **20.** Monomers of carbohydrates are called monosaccharides or simple sugars. Glucose is blood sugar. **21.** The animal form of stored carbohydrate is glycogen. **22.** Triglycerides, the major source of stored energy in the body, are composed of three fatty acid chains and a glycerol molecule and are found in fat tissue. Phospholipids consist of two fatty acid chains and a charged P-containing group. They are found in all cell membranes and form the basis of those membranes. **23.** Hydrolysis reactions break down polymers or macromolecules to their monomers by adding water to each bond joining monomers. **24.** An "amino acid" has an amine group (NH_2) and a COOH group that has acidic properties. **25.** The primary structure of proteins is the stringlike chain of amino acids. **26.** The secondary structures of proteins are the alpha helix and the beta-pleated sheet. **27.** Molecular chaperones prevent inaccurate or inappropriate folding in the 3-D structure of a protein. **28.** Enzymes hold the substrate(s) in a desirable position to interact. **29.** DNA contains deoxyribose sugar and the bases A, T, G, C. RNA contains ribose sugar and the bases A, U, G, C. **30.** DNA dictates protein structure by its base sequence and reproduces itself before a cell divides to ensure that the genetic information in the daughter cells is identical. **31.** ATP stores energy in smaller packets that are more readily released and transferred (during ATP hydrolysis) than the energy stored in glucose. Hence the use of ATP as an energy source keeps energy waste to a minimum. **32.** When ATP releases energy, it loses a phosphate group and becomes ADP (also energy rich).

Review Questions 1. d; **2.** d; **3.** b; **4.** a; **5.** b; **6.** a; **7.** a; **8.** b; **9.** d; **10.** a; **11.** b; **12.** a, c; **13.** (1)a, (2)c; **14.** c; **15.** d; **16.** e; **17.** d; **18.** d; **19.** a; **20.** b; **21.** b; **22.** c

Chapter 3

Check Your Understanding 1. The cell is the structural and functional unit of life. The activity of an organism depends on the activities of its cells. The activities of cells depend on their form and relative numbers of subcellular structures. Continuity of life has a cellular basis. **2.** It is the cell concept that includes structures and functions common to all cells. **3.** All cellular membranes consist of a double layer of phospholipids in which proteins are embedded. **4.** Hydrophobic regions (tails of phospholipid molecules) orient toward each other while the hydrophilic regions (phospholipid heads) orient to the aqueous fluid inside and outside the cell. **5.** The sugar residues of the glycocalyx provide recognizable biological markers for cells to recognize each other. **6.** The heart has desmosomes (anchoring junctions) that secure cardiac cells together as the heart works and gap junctions (communicating junctions) that allow ions to flow from cardiac cell to cardiac cell. **7.** Diffusion is driven by kinetic energy of the molecules. **8.** The relative concentration of the substance in different areas determines the direction of diffusion. Diffusion occurs from regions of high concentration to regions of low concentration. **9.** In channel-mediated diffusion, the diffusing substance moves through a membrane channel. In carrier-mediated diffusion, the diffusing substance attaches to a membrane (protein) carrier that moves it across the membrane. **10.** Phosphorylation of the Na^+-K^+ pump causes the pump protein to change shape so that it "pumps" Na^+ across the membrane. K^+ binding to the pump protein triggers the release of phosphate and the pump protein returns to its original shape. **11.** The plasma membrane expands as a result of exocytosis. **12.** Phagocytic cells engulf debris, and a smoker's lungs would be laden with carbon particles and other debris from smoke inhalation. **13.** Cholesterol is taken in by receptor-mediated endocytosis. **14.** Diffusion of ions, mainly the diffusion of K^+ from the cell through leakage channels, establishes the resting membrane potential. **15.** In a polarized membrane, the inside is negative relative to its outside. **16.** Signaling chemicals that bind to membrane receptors are called ligands. G protein–linked receptors direct intracellular events by promoting formation of second messengers. **17.** Mitochondria are the major sites of ATP synthesis. **18.** Ribosomes are the sites of protein synthesis. The rough ER provides a site for ribosome attachment, and its cisterns package in vesicles the proteins made on the ribosomes for transport to the Golgi apparatus. The Golgi apparatus modifies and packages the proteins it receives for various destinations within or outside the cell. **19.** The lysosomal enzymes digest foreign substances engulfed by the cell, nonuseful or deteriorating organelles, or even the cell itself to prevent the buildup of cellular debris. The enzymes in peroxisomes detoxify harmful chemicals and neutralize free radicals. **20.** Both microfilaments and microtubules are involved in organelle movements within the cell and/or movements of the cell as a whole. **21.** Intermediate filaments are the most important cytoskeletal elements in maintaining cell shape. **22.** The major function of microvilli is to increase the cell's surface area for absorption of substances. **23.** If a cell loses its nucleus, it is doomed to die because it will be unable to make proteins, which include the enzymes needed for all metabolic reactions. **24.** Nucleoli are the site of synthesis of ribosomal subunits. **25.** Histone proteins provide the means to pack DNA in a compact, orderly way, and they play a role in gene regulation. **26.** The base sequence of the corresponding strand will be GCTTAC. **27.** DNA is synthesized during the S phase. **28.** Nuclear envelope breaks up, spindle forms, nucleoli disappear, and the chromosomes coil and condense. **29.** Codons are three-base sequences in mRNA, each of which specifies an amino acid. Anticodons are three-base sequences in tRNA that are complementary to the codons specifying the amino acid they transport to the ribosome during protein synthesis. **30.** The A site is the entry site for tRNA at the ribosome. The P site is where the tRNA carrying the growing polypeptide is located. The E site is the tRNA exit site from the ribosome. **31.** DNA provides the coded instructions (is the template) for protein synthesis via the mRNA synthesized on it. **32.** Ubiquitin attaches to misfolded, damaged, or unneeded proteins, tagging them for destruction by proteasomes. **33.** Blood plasma is extracellular fluid that transports nutrients, gases, hormones, and other substances throughout the body. Interstitial fluid is an important transport and dissolving medium. **34.** Apoptosis is a process of programmed cell death which rids the body of cells that are stressed, damaged, old, or no longer needed. **35.** The wear-and-tear theory of aging attributes aging to little chemical insults and free radicals, which have cumulative detrimental effects.

Review Questions 1. d; **2.** a, c; **3.** b; **4.** b; **5.** e; **6.** c; **7.** d; **8.** a; **9.** d; **10.** a; **11.** b; **12.** d; **13.** c; **14.** b; **15.** d; **16.** a; **17.** b; **18.** d; **19.** c

Chapter 4

Check Your Understanding 1. Fixing tissue preserves it and prevents it from deteriorating. **2.** Heavy metal salts are used to stain tissues viewed by electron microscopes. **3.** Epithelial tissue lines body cavities and covers the body's external surface; thus polarity with one free (apical) surface is a requirement. **4.** Epithelial tissue can regenerate and its cells are joined by lateral contacts. **5.** Simple epithelia are "built" to provide for efficient absorption and filtration across their thin epithelial barriers. **6.** Pseudostratified epithelia appear to be stratified because their cells' nuclei lie at different distances from the basement membrane. However, all cells rest on the basement membrane. **7.** Transitional epithelium is found in the urinary bladder and other hollow urinary organs. The ability of this epithelium to thin allows the urinary organs to handle (store or transport) a larger urine volume when necessary. **8.** All unicellular exocrine glands secrete the protein mucin (which becomes mucus on mixing with water). **9.** These exocrine glands are classified by duct structure and secretory mode. **10.** Holocrine glands have the highest rate of cell division. The secretory cells fragment and are lost in the secretion; thus the secretory cells must be continuously replaced. **11.** Connective tissue functions to bind, support, protect, and insulate body organs. In addition, blood acts to transport substances throughout the body. **12.** Reticular, collagen, and elastic fibers are found in the various connective tissues. **13.** Areolar connective tissue, because of its loose weblike nature, is capable of serving as a fluid reservoir. **14.** Dense regular connective tissue is damaged when you lacerate a tendon. **15.** Hyaline cartilage forms the growth plates. **16.** Cardiac muscle cells have striations and are branching cells. **17.** Skeletal muscle tissue is voluntary and is the muscle tissue injured when you "pull a muscle" while exercising. **18.** With extended processes, a neuron can conduct electrical signals a great distance within the body. **19.** A mucous membrane consists of both connective tissue and epithelium. It lines body cavities open to the exterior. **20.** The serous membranes called pleurae line the thorax walls and cover the lungs. **21.** The three main steps of tissue repair are inflammation, organization, and regeneration and fibrosis (which is a permanent repair). **22.** More severe injuries damage and destroy more tissue, requiring greater replacement with scar tissue. **23.** The three embryonic germ layers are the ectoderm, mesoderm, and endoderm. **24.** Ectoderm gives rise to the nervous system. **25.** Epithelium and blood-forming tissue remain highly mitotic all through life.

Review Questions 1. (1)a, (2)c, (3)d, (4)b; **2.** c, e; **3.** (1)b, (2)f, (3)a, (4)d, (5)g, (6)d; **4.** b; **5.** c; **6.** b

Chapter 5

Check Your Understanding 1. Since the sole of the foot has thick skin, the layers from most superficial to deepest would be the stratum corneum, stratum lucidum, stratum granulosum, stratum spinosum, and stratum basale. **2.** The stratum basale undergoes almost continuous mitosis to replace cells lost by abrasion. **3.** The skin is subjected to a lot of abrasion and physical trauma. The desmosomes, which are connecting junctions, help to hold the cells together during such stress. **4.** The stratum basale, which abuts the dermis where the blood supply is, has the best nourished cells. **5.** The papillary layer of the dermis gives rise to fingerprint patterns. **6.** Fatty tissue in the hypodermis gives it insulating and shock-absorbing properties. **7.** Because there is no bleeding, the cut has penetrated into the avascular epidermis only. **8.** The third pigment contributing to skin color is hemoglobin, the pigment contained in red blood cells found in blood vessels of the dermis. **9.** Cyanosis is a bluish cast of the skin that indicates that hemoglobin in the red blood cells in the dermal capillaries is poorly oxygenated. **10.** Jaundice or a yellow cast to the skin due to the deposit of yellow bile pigments in body tissues may indicate a liver disorder. **11.** The regions of a hair from outside in are the cuticle, cortex, and medulla. **12.** There are no nerves in a hair, so cutting hair is painless. **13.** The arrector pili muscles pull the hair (normally slanted) to the upright position (when cold or scared). **14.** The hair papilla contains a knot of capillaries that supplies nutrients to cells of the hair bulb. **15.** The lunule of the nail is white because the thick nail matrix that underlies it blocks the rosy color of the dermal blood supply from showing through. **16.** Nails are hard because the keratin they contain is the hard keratin variety. **17.** Sebaceous (oil) glands and apocrine glands are associated with the hair follicles. **18.** His sympathetic nervous system activated his eccrine sweat glands and caused heat-induced sweating in order to cool the body. **19.** Heat-induced sweating occurs all over the body when we are overheated. A cold sweat is emotionally induced sweating that begins on the palms, soles, and armpits and then spreads to other body areas. Both types of sweating are produced by the eccrine sweat glands, but activity of apocrine sweat glands is also likely during a cold sweat. **20.** The palms of the hands and soles of the feet are thick skin areas. It would be dangerous to have oily soles, and oily palms would decrease the ability of the hands to hang onto things. **21.** The low pH of skin secretions (acid mantle) inhibits division of bacteria, and many bacteria are killed by bactericidal substances in sebum or by natural antibiotics called defensins. Damaged skin secretes cathelicidins that are effective against a certain strain of strep bacteria. **22.** The epidermal dendritic cells play a role in body immunity. **23.** Sunlight causes the skin to produce a precursor of vitamin D from cholesterol. Vitamin D is essential for bone synthesis. **24.** The skin carries out chemical conversions that supplement some of the protective conversions carried out by the liver, convert some chemicals into carcinogens, activate some steroid hormones, and synthesize the vitamin D precursor. **25.** Basal cell carcinoma develops from the youngest epidermal cells. **26.** The ABCD rule helps one to recognize signs of melanoma. **27.** First- and second-degree burns can heal uneventfully by regeneration of epidermal cells as long as infection does not occur. Third-degree burns destroy the entire depth of skin and regeneration is not possible. Infection and loss of body fluid and proteins are problematic. **28.** Burns to the face are serious because damage to the respiratory passageways can occur in such burns. **29.** Vernix caseosa is a product of the sebaceous glands. **30.** Loss of subcutaneous fat, common in the elderly, leads to cold intolerance seen in this group of people. **31.** UV radiation degrades collagen and leads to loss of skin elasticity and water-holding capacity.

Review Questions 1. a; **2.** c; **3.** d; **4.** d; **5.** b; **6.** b; **7.** c; **8.** c; **9.** b; **10.** a; **11.** d; **12.** b

Case Study 1. The skin separates and protects the internal environment of the body from potentially dangerous elements in the external environment. Mrs. DeStephano's chart indicates epidermal abrasions, which represent the loss of this barrier. Epidermal loss will also cost Mrs. DeStephano the acid mantle of her skin, protection against UV radiation, and dendritic cells, which protect against invasion by microorganisms. **2.** Macrophages found in the dermis can act as a backup system against bacterial and viral invasion when the epidermis is damaged. **3.** Suturing brings the edges of wounds close together and promotes faster healing because smaller amounts of granulation tissue need to be formed. This is termed healing by first intention. **4.** Cyanosis signals a decrease in the amount of oxygen carried by hemoglobin in the blood. Respiratory system and/or cardiovascular system impairments can lead to cyanosis.

Chapter 6

Check Your Understanding 1. Hyaline cartilage is the most plentiful in the adult body. **2.** The epiglottis and external ear cartilages are flexible elastic cartilage. **3.** Interstitial growth is growth from within. **4.** The components of the axial skeleton are the skull, the vertebral column, and the thoracic cage. **5.** The major function of the axial skeleton is to establish the long axis of the body and to protect structures that it encloses. The general function of the appendicular skeleton is to allow us mobility for propulsion and manipulation of our environment. **6.** The ribs and skull bones are flat bones. **7.** Skeletal muscles use bones as levers to cause movement of the body and its parts. **8.** Bone matrix stores minerals and growth factors. **9.** Bone marrow cavities serve as sites for blood cell formation and fat storage. **10.** Crests, tubercles, and spines are bony projections. **11.** Compact bone looks fairly solid and homogeneous whereas spongy bone has an open network of bone spicules. **12.** Endosteum lines the internal canals and covers the trabeculae. **13.** Bone's inorganic component (bone salts) makes it hard. **14.** The osteoclast fits this description. **15.** Bones begin as fibrous membranes or hyaline cartilages. **16.** The cartilage model grows, then breaks down and is replaced by bone. **17.** The primary ossification center in a long bone is in the center of the shaft. The secondary ossification centers are in the epiphyses (bone ends). **18.** The chondrocytes are enlarging and their lacunae are breaking down and leaving holes in the cartilage matrix. **19.** If bone-destroying cells (osteoclasts) are more active than bone-forming cells (osteoblasts), bone mass will decrease. **20.** The hormonal stimulus maintains homeostatic blood calcium levels. **21.** In an open fracture, the bone ends are exposed to the external environment. In a closed fracture, the bone ends do not penetrate the external boundary of the skin. **22.** Bone growth increases bone mass, as during childhood or when exceptional stress is placed on the bones. Bone remodeling follows bone growth to maintain the proper proportions of the bone considering stresses placed upon it. **23.** Paget's disease is characterized by excessive deposit of weak, poorly mineralized bone. **24.** Sufficient vitamin D, calcium, and weight-bearing exercise all help to maintain healthy bone density. **25.** Adult rickets is called osteomalacia. **26.** At birth, most bones are well formed and ossified except for their epiphyses. **27.** The skull bones do not appear to lose mass with aging.

Review Questions 1. e; **2.** b; **3.** c; **4.** d; **5.** e; **6.** b; **7.** c; **8.** b; **9.** d, e; **10.** c; **11.** b; **12.** c; **13.** a; **14.** b

Case Study 1. Mrs. DeStephano's broken leg has a transverse fracture of the open variety because the broken ends of the bone are protruding through the skin. **2.** The laceration of the skin caused by the broken end of the bone creates a breach in the protective barrier created by the skin, providing an entry point for bacteria and other microorganisms. In addition, the protruding ends of the bone have now been exposed to the nonsterile external environment. This could result in the development of osteomyelitis, a bacterial infection, which can be treated with antibiotics. **3.** Reduction of a fracture is the clinical term for "setting the bone." Mrs. DeStephano's physician chose internal reduction, in which surgery is performed and the broken ends of the bone are secured together by pins or wires. A cast was applied to keep the aligned ends of the bone immobile until healing of the fracture has occurred. **4.** Healing of Mrs. DeStephano's fracture will begin as bony callus formation fills the break in the bone with bony tissue. This process begins 3–4 weeks after the break occurs and is completed within 2–3 months. **5.** Nutrient arteries supply blood to the bone tissue. In order for Mrs. DeStephano's break to heal normally, the bony tissue must be supplied with oxygen (to generate ATP for energy) and nutrients in order to rebuild the bone. Damage to a nutrient artery will decrease the delivery of these building materials and could slow the process of healing. **6.** For a fracture that is slow to heal, new techniques that promote healing include electrical stimulation, which promotes the deposition of new bone tissue; ultrasound treatments, known to speed healing; and possibly the addition of bone substitutes to the fractured area. **7.** At age 45, Mrs. DeStephano will most likely not regenerate her knee cartilage. (Cartilage growth typically ends during adolescence.) Cartilage damage that occurs during adulthood is slow to heal, due to the avascular nature of cartilage, and is usually irreparable. Surgical removal of cartilage fragments to allow improved movement of the joint is the usual treatment for this type of damage.

Chapter 7

Check Your Understanding 1. The three main parts of the axial skeleton are the skull, vertebral column, and thoracic cage. **2.** The axial skeleton is more important in protecting internal organs. **3.** The frontal, parietal, temporal, sphenoid, and ethmoid bones are all cranial bones. **4.** The ethmoid bone forms the crista galli. **5.** The temporal bones house the external ear canals. **6.** The parietal bones abut each other at the sagittal suture. The occipital bone abuts the parietal bones at the lambdoid suture. **7.** The zygomatic bones are the cheekbones. **8.** Eating or talking, because the only freely movable joints of the skull are the temporomandibular joints of the jaw. **9.** The maxillae are the keystone bones of the facial skeleton. **10.** The sphenoid, ethmoid, frontal, and maxillary bones contain paranasal sinuses. **11.** The cribriform plates of the ethmoid bone form the roof of the nasal cavity. **12.** The maxillae form the bulk of the orbit floor. The eye is housed in the orbit. **13.** The five major regions of the vertebral column are the cervical, thoracic, lumbar, sacral, and coccygeal regions. **14.** The cervical and lumbar regions are concave posteriorly. **15.** The fibrocartilage discs contribute to the flexibility of the vertebral column. **16.** There are 7 cervical and 12 thoracic vertebrae. **17.** The dens is the axis on which the atlas rotates. If it's broken, movements of the atlas would be less controllable. **18.** A lumbar vertebra is heavier and its massive body is kidney shaped. Its spinous processes are short and project directly back. A thoracic vertebral body is generally heart shaped, its spinous process is long, sharp, and points downward, and its transverse processes have facets for articulating with the ribs. **19.** A true rib connects to the sternum by its own costal cartilage. A false rib connects to the sternum via costal cartilages of other ribs or not at all. **20.** The sternal angle is a ridge across the front of the sternum where the manubrium joins the sternal body. It acts as a hinge allowing the sternum to swing anteriorly when we inhale. Because it is aligned with the second rib, it is a handy cue for finding that rib and then counting the ribs during a physical exam. **21.** The thoracic vertebrae also contribute to the thoracic cage. **22.** Each pectoral girdle is formed by a scapula and a clavicle. **23.** The pectoral girdle attaches to the sternal manubrium of the axial skeleton via the medial end of its clavicle. **24.** A consequence of its flexibility is that it is easily dislocated. **25.** Together the ulna and humerus form the elbow joint. **26.** The ulna and the radius each have a styloid process distally. **27.** Carpals are found in the proximal region of the palm. They are short bones. **28.** The third bone of the os coxae is the ischium. **29.** The pelvic girdle receives the weight of the upper body (trunk, head, and upper limbs) and transmits that weight to the lower limbs. **30.** The female pelvis is wider and has a shorter sacrum and a more movable coccyx. **31.** The tibia is the second largest bone in the body. **32.** The medial malleolus is located on the distalmost medial aspect of the tibia. **33.** The lateral condyles are not sites of muscle attachment, they are articular surfaces. **34.** Because of their springiness, the foot arches save energy during locomotion. **35.** The two largest tarsals are the talus and the calcaneus, which forms the heel. **36.** The enlargement of the facial skeleton between ages 6 and 13 is due to the enlargement of the nose and paranasal sinuses and the development of the permanent teeth. **37.** The lumbar curvature develops when the baby begins to walk.

Review Questions 1. (1)b, g; (2)h; (3)d; (4)d, f; (5)e; (6)c; (7)a, b, d, h; (8)i; **2.** (1)g, (2)f, (3)b, (4)a, (5)b, (6)c, (7)d, (8)e; **3.** (1)b, (2)c, (3)e, (4)a, (5)h, (6)e, (7)f

Case Study 1. The hemispherical socket at the point where her femur attaches is called the *acetabulum*. **2.** The structure on the femur that forms the "ball" that fits into the "socket" named in question 1 is called the *head* of the femur. **3.** The three bones in the pelvic girdle that fuse together at a point within the structure identified in question 1 are the *ilium, ischium*, and *pubis*. **4.** If you were asked to rest your hands on your hips, your hands would be resting on the *iliac crests*. **5.** The structures on the femur where the large muscles of the buttocks and thigh attach are the *greater trochanter* and *lesser trochanter*. **6.** The structure of the pelvis that the sciatic nerve passes through as it travels into the upper thigh is the *greater sciatic notch* of the *ilium*.

Chapter 8

Check Your Understanding 1. Joint and articulation are synonyms. **2.** The synarthroses are the least mobile of the joint types. **3.** Symphyses and synchondroses are cartilaginous joints. **4.** In general, the more stable a joint, the less mobile it is. **5.** The fibrous layer and the synovial membrane make up the wall of the articular capsule. **6.** Bursae and tendon sheaths help to reduce friction during joint movement. **7.** The muscle tendons that cross the joint are typically the most important factor in stabilizing synovial joints. **8.** Weeping lubrication helps keep the joint cartilages nourished and "lubricates" the joint surfaces. **9.** John's hip joint was flexed and his knees extended and his thumb was in opposition (to his index finger). **10.** The hinge and pivot joints are uniaxial joints. **11.** The knee and temporomandibular joints have menisci. The elbow and knee act mainly as a uniaxial hinge. The shoulder depends largely on muscle tendons for stability. **12.** Arthritis means inflammation of the joint. **13.** RA typically produces pain, swelling, and joint deformations that tend to be bilateral and crippling. OA patients tend to have pain, particularly on arising, which is relieved by gentle exercise, and enlarged bone ends (due to spurs) in affected joints. Affected joints may exhibit crepitus. **14.** Lyme disease is caused by spirochete bacteria and transmitted by a tick bite. **15.** Regular exercise strengthens joints and keeps them well nourished.

Review Questions 1. (1)c, (2)a, (3)a, (4)b, (5)c, (6)b, (7)b, (8)a, (9)c; **2.** b; **3.** d; **4.** d; **5.** b; **6.** d; **7.** d

Case Study 1. The hip joint would be structurally classified as a *synovial joint* and functionally classified as a *diarthrotic* (freely movable) joint. **2.** The six distinguishing features that define a synovial joint are: (1) articular cartilage, (2) joint (synovial) cavity, (3) articular capsule, (4) synovial fluid, (5) reinforcing ligaments, (6) nerves and blood vessels. **3.** The joint space in a synovial joint is normally filled with *synovial fluid*. **4.** The acetabular labrum is a piece of fibrocartilage that attaches to and extends the rim of the acetabulum. The diameter of the labrum is less than the diameter of the head of the femur, and this helps stabilize the joint to prevent it from dislocating. **5.** Mrs. Tanner's hip was bent (flexed) and her thigh was pulled toward the midline of her body (adducted) and turned in toward this midline (medially rotated). **6.** Mrs. Tanner suffered a posterior dislocation of the hip. When the head of the femur comes away from the acetabulum and then turns posteriorly, it causes the femur to rotate counterclockwise. This can be determined from the fact that her thigh was adducted and medially rotated. **7.** The hip movements include flexion, extension, abduction, adduction, rotation, and circumduction of the thigh.

Chapter 9

Check Your Understanding 1. Striated means "with stripes." **2.** He should respond "smooth muscle," which fits the description. **3.** "Epimysium" literally translates to "outside the muscle" and this connective tissue sheath is the outermost muscle sheath, enclosing the entire muscle. **4.** The thin myofilaments have binding sites for calcium on the troponin molecules forming part of those filaments. **5.** In a resting muscle fiber, the SR would have the highest concentration of calcium ions. The mitochondrion provides the ATP needed for muscle activity. **6.** The components of the neuromuscular junction are the axon terminal, the synaptic cleft, and the junctional folds of the sarcolemma. **7.** The final trigger for contraction is a certain concentration of calcium ions in the cytosol. The initial trigger is depolarization of the sarcolemma. **8.** There are always some myosin cross bridges bound to the actin myofilament during the contraction phase. Thus, backward sliding of the actin filaments is prevented. **9.** Without ATP, rigor would occur because the myosin heads could not detach. **10.** A motor unit is an axon of a motor neuron and all the muscle fibers it innervates. **11.** During the latent period, events of excitation-contraction coupling are occurring. **12.** Immediately after Jay grabs the bar, his biceps muscles are contracting isometrically. As his body moves upward toward the bar, they are contracting isotonically and concentrically. As he lowers his body toward the mat, the biceps are contracting isotonically and eccentrically. **13.** Eric was breathing heavily because it takes some time for his heart rate and overall metabolism to return to the resting state after exercise. Moreover, he had likely incurred an oxygen debt that required he take in extra oxygen for the restorative process, the so-called EPOC. Although jogging is primarily an aerobic exercise, there is always some anaerobic respiration that occurs as well—the amount depends on exercise intensity. As fatigue occurs, potassium ions accumulate in the T tubules, and lactic acid and phosphate ions accumulate in the muscle cells. **14.** Factors that influence muscle contractile force include muscle fiber size, the number of muscle fibers stimulated, the frequency of stimulation, and the degree of muscle stretch. Factors that influence velocity of contraction include muscle fiber type, load, and the number of motor units contracting. **15.** Fast glycolytic fibers would provide for short periods of intense strength needed to lift and move furniture. **16.** To increase muscle size and strength, anaerobic exercise is best. Muscle endurance is enhanced by aerobic exercise. **17.** Both skeletal and smooth muscle fibers are elongated cells, but unlike smooth muscle cells, which are spindle shaped, uninucleate, and nonstriated, skeletal muscle cells are very large cigar-shaped, multinucleate, striated cells. **18.** Calcium binds to troponin on the thin filaments in skeletal muscle cells. In smooth muscle cells, it binds to a cytoplasmic protein called calmodulin. **19.** Hollow organs that have smooth muscle cells helping to form their walls often must temporarily store the organ's contents (urine, food residues, etc.), an ability ensured by the stress-relaxation response. **20.** During development of skeletal muscle fibers, the myoblast cells join together, forming multinucleate myotubes. **21.** The connective tissue in muscles increases with age, causing the muscles to get stringier. **22.** Regular exercise and strength training help to defer the loss in strength and muscle wasting that tends to occur with age, and improve neuromuscular function.

Review Questions 1. c; **2.** b; **3.** (1)b, (2)a, (3)b, (4)a, (5)b, (6)a; **4.** c; **5.** a; **6.** a; **7.** d; **8.** a; **9.** (1)a, (2)a, c, (3)b, (4)c, (5)b, (6)b; **10.** a; **11.** c; **12.** c; **13.** c; **14.** b

Case Study 1. The first reaction to tissue injury is the initiation of the inflammatory response. The inflammatory chemicals increase the permeability of the capillaries in the injured area, allowing white blood cells, fluid, and other substances to reach the injured area. The next step in healing involves the formation of granulation tissue, in which the vascular supply for the injured area is regenerated and collagen fibers that knit the torn edges of the tissue together are formed. Skeletal muscle does not regenerate well, so the damaged areas of Mrs. DeStephano's muscle tissue will probably be repaired primarily by the formation of fibrous tissue, creating scar tissue. **2.** Healing is aided by good circulation of blood within the injured area. Vascular damage compromises healing because the supply of oxygen and nutrients to the tissue is reduced. **3.** Under normal circumstances, skeletal muscles receive electrical signals from the nervous system continuously. These signals help to maintain muscle tone and readiness. Severing of the sciatic nerve removes this continuous nervous input to the muscles and will lead to muscle atrophy. Immobility of muscles will lead to a replacement of contractile muscle tissue with noncontractile fibrous connective tissue. Distal to the point of transection, the muscle will begin to decrease in size within 3–7 days of becoming immobile. This process can be delayed by electrically stimulating the tissues. Passive range-of-motion exercises also help prevent loss of muscle tone and joint range, and improve circulation in the injured areas. **4.** Mrs. DeStephano's physician wants to supply her damaged tissues with the necessary building materials to encourage healing. A high-protein diet will provide plenty of amino acids to rebuild or replace damaged proteins, carbohydrates will provide the fuel molecules needed to generate the required ATP, and vitamin C is important for the regeneration of connective tissue.

Chapter 10

Check Your Understanding 1. The term "prime mover" refers to the muscle that bears the most responsibility for causing a particular movement. **2.** The iliacus overlies the iliac bone; the adductor brevis is a small (size) muscle that adducts (movement caused) the thigh; and the quadriceps (4 heads) femoris muscle follows the course of the femur. **3.** Of the muscles illustrated in Figure 10.2, the one with the parallel arrangement (sartorius) could shorten to the greatest degree. The stocky bipennate (rectus femoris) and multipennate (deltoid) muscles would be most powerful because they pack in the most fibers. **4.** Third-class levers are the fastest levers. **5.** A lever that operates at a mechanical advantage allows the muscle to exert less force than the load being moved. **6.** John was using the frontal belly of his epicranius to raise his eyebrows and the orbicularis oculi muscles to wink at Sarah. **7.** To make a sad clown's face you would contract your platysma, depressor anguli oris, and depressor labii inferioris muscles. **8.** The deltoid has a broad origin. When only its anterior fibers contract, it flexes and medially rotates the humerus. When only its posterior fibers contract, it extends and laterally rotates the humerus. **9.** The opponens pollicis does not have an insertion on the bones of the thumb.

Review Questions 1. c; **2.** c; **3.** (1)e, (2)c, (3)g, (4)f, (5)d; **4.** a; **5.** c; **6.** d; **7.** c; **8.** c; **9.** b; **10.** d; **11.** b; **12.** a; **13.** c; **14.** d; **15.** a, b; **16.** a

Case Study 1. A prime mover is a muscle that has primary or major responsibility for producing a specific movement. A synergist is a muscle that supports or helps the action of a prime mover by adding extra force, or providing stability so that the prime mover can perform its action. **2.** An antagonist is a muscle that opposes, resists, or reverses a particular movement. By mimicking the action of an antagonist, the therapist can test the strength of the agonist muscle and compare it with the same muscle in the other limb. **3.** Ideally, the therapist would assess each muscle individually. In reality, these assessments usually measure the function of a group of muscles because multiple muscles are often involved in similar actions. (a) This assessment focuses on the thigh adductors (magnus, longus, brevis), pectineus, and gracilis. Specifically, the adductor magnus is innervated by the damaged sciatic nerve. (b) This assessment addresses Mrs. Tanner's ability to dorsiflex her foot. Dorsiflexion involves all of the muscles in the anterior compartment of the lower leg: the tibialis anterior, extensor digitorum longus, fibularis (peroneus) tertius, and extensor hallucis longus. (c) This assessment addresses the function of the muscles of the posterior compartment of the thigh. The hamstrings (biceps femoris, semitendinosus, semimembranosus) are the prime movers involved in knee flexion. **4.** To assess these muscles, the therapist would apply resistance to the natural action of these muscles. (a) The extensor hallucis longus inserts on the distal phalanx of the great toe. The therapist can apply resistance to the top of the toe and ask Mrs. Tanner to extend the toe. (b) The fibularis longus is involved in eversion of the foot and plantar flexion. The therapist can apply resistance to the lateral aspect of the foot and ask Mrs. Tanner to evert (turn out) her ankle. In addition, resistance can be applied to the bottom of the foot and Mrs. Tanner asked to push against that resistance. (c) The gastrocnemius, along with the soleus, is a powerful plantar flexor. The therapist can (1) ask Mrs. Tanner to raise her body up on her toes using her right foot, or (2) apply pressure to the bottom of the foot and ask Mrs. Tanner to push against that resistance.

Chapter 11

Check Your Understanding 1. Integration involves processing and interpreting sensory information, and making a decision about motor output. Integration occurs primarily in the CNS. **2.** (a) This "full stomach" feeling would be relayed by the sensory (afferent) division of the PNS (via its visceral afferent fibers). (b) The somatic nervous system, which is part of the motor (efferent) division of the PNS, controls movement of skeletal muscle. (c) The autonomic nervous system, which is part of the motor (efferent) division of the PNS, controls the heart rate. **3.** Astrocytes control the extracellular environment around neuron cell bodies in the CNS, whereas satellite cells perform this function in the PNS. **4.** Oligodendrocytes and Schwann cells form myelin sheaths in the CNS and PNS, respectively.

5. A nerve fiber is a long axon, an extension of the cell. In connective tissue, fibers are extracellular proteins that provide support. In muscle tissue, a muscle fiber is a muscle cell. **6.** A nucleus within the brain is a cluster of cell bodies, whereas the nucleus within each neuron is a large organelle that acts as the control center of the cell. **7.** In the CNS, a myelin sheath is formed by oligodendrocytes that wrap their plasma membranes around the axon. The myelin sheath protects and electrically insulates axons and increases the speed of transmission of nerve impulses. **8.** Burning a finger will first activate unipolar (pseudounipolar) neurons that are sensory (afferent) neurons. The impulse to move your finger away from the heat will be carried by multipolar neurons that are motor (efferent) neurons. **9.** The concentration gradient and the electrical gradient—together called the electrochemical gradient—determine the direction in which ions flow through an open membrane channel. **10.** There is more leakage of K^+ than of any other cations. **11.** Action potentials are larger than graded potentials and travel further. Graded potentials generally initiate action potentials. **12.** An action potential is regenerated anew at each membrane patch. **13.** Conduction of action potentials is faster in myelinated axons because myelin allows the axon membrane between myelin sheath gaps to change its voltage rapidly, and allows current to flow only at the widely spaced gaps. **14.** If a second stimulus occurs before the end of the absolute refractory period, no AP can occur because sodium channels are still inactivated. **15.** At an electrical synapse, neurons are joined by gap junctions. **16.** Voltage-gated ion (Ca^{2+}) channels are found in the presynaptic axon terminal and open when an action potential reaches the axon terminal. Chemically gated ion channels are found in the postsynaptic membrane and open when neurotransmitter binds to the receptor protein. **17.** IPSPs result from the flow of either K^+ or Cl^- through chemically gated channels. EPSPs result from the flow of both Na^+ and K^+ through chemically gated channels. **18.** Temporal summation is summation in time of graded potentials occurring in quick succession at the postsynaptic membrane. It can result from EPSPs arising from just one synapse. Spatial summation is summation in space—a postsynaptic neuron is stimulated by a large number of terminals at the same time. **19.** ACh interacts with more than one specific receptor type, and this explains how it can excite at some synapses and inhibit at others. **20.** cAMP is called a second messenger because it relays the message between the first messenger (the original chemical messenger) outside of the cell and effector molecules that will ultimately bring about the desired response within the cell. **21.** Reverberating circuits and parallel after-discharge circuits both result in prolonged output. **22.** The pattern of neural processing is serial processing. The response is a reflex arc. **23.** The pattern of neural processing is parallel processing. **24.** The growing tip of an axon is called a growth cone. Neurotropins are chemicals that signal the growth cone.

Review Questions 1. b; **2.** (1)d, (2)b, (3)f, (4)c, (5)a; **3.** b; **4.** c; **5.** a; **6.** c; **7.** b; **8.** d; **9.** c; **10.** c; **11.** a; **12.** (1)d, (2)b, (3)a, (4)c

Case Study 1. The electrical signals generated by neurons are called *action potentials.* An action potential is a change in membrane potential that involves depolarization and repolarization phases. **2.** An inhibitory postsynaptic potential (IPSP) is a signal that makes it less likely that a postsynaptic neuron will be able to generate an action potential. This effect is usually produced when the signal causes the membrane potential of the postsynaptic neuron to become more negative, moving away from the axon's threshold potential. **3.** GABA falls into the amino acid class of neurotransmitters. This same class includes glycine, glutamate, and aspartate. **4.** To enhance the actions of GABA at a synapse, a drug could either (1) act presynaptically to increase the release of GABA at the synapse, (2) decrease the reuptake of GABA after it has been released, or (3) act postsynaptically to either increase the binding strength of GABA at its receptors, or increase the number of receptors. **5.** An influx of Cl^- into the postsynaptic cell causes the membrane potential to become more negative (hyperpolarize). When hyperpolarized, the cell is farther from its threshold potential and so is less likely to produce an action potential.

Chapter 12

Check Your Understanding 1. The third ventricle is surrounded by the diencephalon. **2.** The cerebral hemispheres and the cerebellum have an outside layer of gray matter in addition to central gray matter and its surrounding white matter. **3.** Convolutions increase surface area of the cortex, which allows more neurons to occupy the limited space within the skull. **4.** The central sulcus separates primary motor areas from somatosensory areas. **5.** Motor functions on the left side of the body are controlled by the right hemisphere of the brain because motor tracts from the right hemisphere cross over (in the medulla oblongata) to the left side of the spinal cord to go to the left side of the body. **6.** Commissural fibers (which form commissures) allow the cerebral hemispheres to "talk to each other." **7.** The caudate nucleus, putamen, and globus pallidus together form the basal nuclei. **8.** Virtually all inputs ascending to the cerebral cortex synapse in the thalamus en route. **9.** The hypothalamus oversees the autonomic nervous system. **10.** The pyramids of the medulla are the corticospinal (pyramidal) tracts, the large voluntary motor tracts descending from the motor cortex. The result of decussation (crossing over) is that each side of the motor cortex controls the opposite side of the body. **11.** The cerebral peduncles and the colliculi are associated with the midbrain. **12.** There are many possible answers to this question—here are a few: Structurally, the cerebellum and cerebrum are similar in that they both have a thin outer cortex of gray matter, internal white matter, and deep gray matter nuclei. Also, both have body maps (homunculi) and large fiber tracts connecting them to the brain stem. Both receive sensory input and influence motor output. A major difference is that the cerebellum is almost entirely concerned with motor output, whereas the cerebrum has much broader responsibilities. Also, while a cerebral hemisphere controls the opposite side of the body, a cerebellar hemisphere controls the same side of the body. **13.** The hypothalamus is part of the limbic system and also an autonomic (visceral) control center. **14.** Taylor is increasing the amount of sensory stimuli she receives, which will be relayed to the reticular activating system, which, in turn, will increase activation of the cerebral cortex. **15.** Delta waves are typically seen in deep sleep in normal adults. **16.** Drowsiness (or lethargy) and stupor are stages of consciousness between alertness and coma. **17.** Most skeletal muscles are actively inhibited during REM sleep. **18.** Transfer of memory from STM to LTM is enhanced by (1) rehearsal, (2) association (tying "new" information to "old" information), and (3) a heightened emotional state (for example, alert, motivated, surprised, or aroused). **19.** The basal nuclei and premotor cortex are involved in procedural (skills) memory, but not in declarative memory. **20.** CSF, formed by the choroid plexuses as a filtrate of blood plasma, is a watery "broth" similar in composition to plasma. It protects the brain and spinal cord from blows and other trauma, helps nourish the brain, and carries chemical signals from one part of the brain to another. **21.** A TIA is a temporary loss of blood supply to brain tissue, and it differs from a stroke in that the resultant impairment is fully reversible. **22.** Mrs. Lee might have Parkinson's disease. **23.** The nerves serving the limbs arise in the cervical and lumbar enlargements of the spinal cord. **24.** In the spinothalamic pathway, the cell bodies of first-order sensory neurons are outside the spinal cord in a ganglion, cell bodies of second-order sensory neurons are in the dorsal horn of the spinal cord, and cell bodies of third-order sensory neurons are in the thalamus. (See also Figure 12.31b.) **25.** A loss of motor function is called paralysis. Lower limb paralysis could be caused by a spinal cord injury in the thoracic region (between T_1 and L_1). If the spinal cord is transected, the result is paraplegia. If the cord is only bruised, he may regain function in the limbs. An MRI scan (or CT scan) of the spinal cord would be helpful. **26.** Alar plate neuroblasts become interneurons, whereas basal plate neuroblasts become motor (efferent) neurons. **27.** Premature babies have trouble regulating body temperature because the hypothalamus is immature. **28.** Reversible causes of dementia include prescription drug effects, low blood pressure, poor nutrition, hormone imbalances, depression, and dehydration.

Review Questions 1. a; **2.** d; **3.** c; **4.** a; **5.** (1)d, (2)f, (3)e, (4)g, (5)b, (6)f, (7)i, (8)a; **6.** b; **7.** c; **8.** a; **9.** (1)a, (2)b, (3)a, (4)a, (5)b, (6)a, (7)b, (8)b, (9)a; **10.** d; **11.** (1)d, (2)e, (3)c and d, (4)a; **12.** c

Case Study 1. The four regions of the brain are the cerebral hemispheres, diencephalon, brain stem, and cerebellum. A cerebral hemisphere is involved in this case. Motor functions and language are both located in this cerebral hemisphere and have been affected by the injury. **2.** The left side of the brain has been affected in this case. The motor dysfunction on the right side of the body is the primary piece of evidence used to determine this. In addition, the brain areas serving speech are usually located in the left side. **3.** The motor dysfunction on the right side of the body suggests that the injury has affected the primary motor cortex and possibly the premotor cortex of the left cerebral hemisphere. In addition to the problems with motor function, Mrs. Bryans experienced difficulty with language. Two areas of the brain associated with language, Broca's and Wernicke's area, are usually located in the left cerebral cortex. The type of aphasia described suggests damage to Broca's area. **4.** From the surface of the brain to the skull, the three membranes that make up the meninges include the pia mater, arachnoid mater, and dura mater. **5.** The subarachnoid hemorrhage involves bleeding into the region below (*sub* = below) the arachnoid mater. The subdural hematoma involves blood collecting between the dura mater and the arachnoid mater.

Chapter 13

Check Your Understanding 1. In addition to nerves, the PNS also consists of sensory receptors, motor endings, and ganglia. **2.** Nociceptors respond to painful stimuli. They are exteroceptors that are nonencapsulated (free nerve endings). **3.** The three levels of sensory integration are receptor level, circuit level, and perceptual level. **4.** Phasic receptors adapt, whereas tonic receptors exhibit little or no adaptation. Pain receptors are tonic so that we are reminded to protect the injured body part. **5.** Hot and cold are conveyed by different sensory receptors that are parts of separate "labeled lines." Cool and cold are two different intensities of the same stimulus, detected by frequency coding—the frequency of APs would be higher for a cold than a cool stimulus. Action potentials arising in the fingers and foot arrive at different locations in the somatosensory cortex via their own "labeled lines" and in this way the cortex can determine their origin. **6.** Ganglia are collections of neuron cell bodies in the PNS. **7.** Nerves also contain connective tissue, blood vessels, lymphatic vessels, and the myelin surrounding the axons. **8.** Schwann cells, macrophages, and the neurons themselves were all important in healing the nerve. **9.** The oculomotor (III), trochlear (IV), and abducens (VI) nerves control eye movements. Sticking out your tongue involves the hypoglossal nerve (XII). The vagus nerve (X) influences heart rate and digestive activity. The accessory nerve (XI) innervates the trapezius muscle, which is involved in shoulder shrugging. **10.** Roots lie medial to spinal nerves, whereas rami lie lateral to spinal nerves. Dorsal roots are purely sensory, whereas dorsal rami carry both motor and sensory fibers. **11.** The spinal nerve roots were C_3–C_5, the spinal nerve was the phrenic nerve, the plexus was the cervical plexus. The phrenic nerve is the sole motor nerve supply to the diaphragm, the primary muscle for respiration. **12.** Varicosities are the series of knoblike swellings that are the axon endings of autonomic motor neurons. You would find them on axon endings serving smooth muscle or glands. **13.** The cerebellum and basal nuclei, which form the precommand level of motor control, plan and coordinate complex motor activities. **14.** The five components of a reflex arc are receptor, sensory neuron, integration center, motor neuron, and effector. **15.** The stretch reflex is important for maintaining muscle tone and adjusting it reflexively by causing muscle contraction in response to increased muscle length (stretch). It maintains posture. The flexor or withdrawal reflex is initiated by a painful stimulus and causes automatic withdrawal of the painful body part from the stimulus. It is protective. **16.** This response is called Babinski's sign and it indicates damage to the corticospinal tract or primary motor cortex. **17.** The vertebral column, spinal nerves, and dermatomes are all examples of segmentation in the adult.

Review Questions 1. b; **2.** c; **3.** d; **4.** c; **5.** e; **6.** c; **7.** (1)d, (2)c, (3)f, (4)b, (5)e, (6)a; **8.** (1)f, (2)i, (3)b, (4)g, h, (5)e, (6)i, (7)c, (8)k, (9)l, (10)c, d, f, k; **9.** (1)b 6; (2)d 8; (3)c 2; (4)c 5; (5)a 4; (6)a 3, 9; (7)a 7; (8)a 7; (9)d 1; (10)a 3, 4, 7, 9; **10.** (1)a, 1 and 5; (2)a, 3 and 5; (3)a, 4; (4)a, 2; (5)c, 2; (6)b, 2; **11.** c

Case Study 1. Cerebrospinal fluid (CSF) is leaking out of Mr. Hancock's right ear. The fracture must have torn both the dura mater and arachnoid mater. In addition, the tympanic membrane must have ruptured. Antibiotics were administered to prevent infection by bacteria that might enter through the ruptured meninges, causing meningitis. Elevating the head of the bed decreases the CSF pressure in the skull. (This allows the torn meninges to heal spontaneously in the majority of cases.) **2.** The observations on Mr. Hancock's chart indicate: (a) Either damage to CN VIII (the vestibulocochlear nerve, which transmits afferent impulses for the sense of hearing) or destruction of the cochlea (the sensory organ for hearing). (b) Damage to CN V_3 (the mandibular division of the trigeminal nerve), which runs through the foramen ovale. This nerve conveys sensory information from the lower part of the face. (c) Damage to CN V_2 (the maxillary division of the trigeminal nerve), which runs through the foramen rotundum. This nerve conveys sensory information from the skin of the upper lip, lower eyelid, and cheek. (d) Damage to CN VI (the abducens nerve), which innervates the lateral rectus muscle of the eye. Because this muscle is responsible for pulling the eye laterally (abduction), loss of tone in this muscle at rest will cause the eye to turn inward. Diplopia will worsen when looking to the right because the eye cannot abduct. **3.** The facial nerve (cranial nerve VII) is the primary motor nerve associated with facial expression. The facial nerve also contains parasympathetic fibers that control secretion of tears from the lacrimal glands. Damage to this nerve explains both the motor symptoms and the dryness of his eye.

Chapter 14

Check Your Understanding 1. The effectors of the autonomic nervous system are cardiac muscle, smooth muscle, and glands. **2.** The somatic motor system relays instructions to muscles more quickly because it involves only one motor neuron, whereas the ANS uses a two-neuron chain. Moreover, axons of somatic motor neurons are typically heavily myelinated, whereas preganglionic autonomic axons are lightly myelinated and postganglionic axons are nonmyelinated. **3.** While you relax in the sun on the beach, the parasympathetic branch of the ANS would probably predominate. When you perceive danger (as in a shark), the sympathetic branch of the ANS predominates. **4.** "Short preganglionic fibers," "origin from thoracolumbar region of spinal cord," "collateral ganglia," and "innervates adrenal medulla" are all characteristic of the sympathetic nervous system. Terminal ganglia are found in the parasympathetic nervous system. **5.** The major differences are (1) the ANS has visceral afferents rather than somatic afferents, (2) the ANS has a two-neuron efferent chain, whereas the somatic nervous system (SNS) has one, and (3) the effectors of the ANS are smooth muscles, cardiac muscle, and glands, whereas the effectors of the SNS are skeletal muscles. **6.** The parasympathetic nervous system increases digestive activity and decreases heart rate. The sympathetic nervous system increases blood pressure, dilates bronchioles, stimulates the adrenal medulla to release its hormones, and causes ejaculation. **7.** You would find nicotinic receptors on skeletal muscle and the hormone-producing cells of the adrenal medulla, but not on smooth muscle or glands. Virtually all types of receptors (including nicotinic receptors) are also found in the CNS (see Table 11.3 on p. 415). **8.** The main integration center of the ANS is the hypothalamus, although the most direct influence is through the brain stem reticular formation and the reflex centers in the pons and medulla oblongata. **9.** Jackson's doctor may have prescribed a beta-blocker because Jackson has hypertension. (Chronic stress is a factor in causing hypertension.) The beta-blocker will decrease blood pressure by blocking beta-adrenergic receptors in the heart, thereby decreasing heart rate and force of contraction, and by decreasing renin release from the kidneys. **10.** The neural crest gives rise to both autonomic ganglia and the adrenal medulla.

Review Questions 1. d; **2.** (1)S, (2)P, (3)P, (4)S, (5)S, (6)P, (7)P, (8)S, (9)P, (10)S, (11)P, (12)S; **3.** b; **4.** c; **5.** a

Case Study 1. The location of Jimmy's lacerations and bruises and his inability to rise led the paramedics to suspect a head, neck, or back injury. They immobilized his head and torso to prevent any further damage to the brain and spinal cord. **2.** The worsening neurological signs indicate a probable intracranial hemorrhage. The blood escaping from the ruptured blood vessel(s) will begin to compress Jimmy's brain and increase his intracranial pressure. Jimmy's surgery will involve repair of the damaged vessel(s) and removal of the mass of clotted blood pressing on his brain. **3.** Loss of motor and sensory function below the level of the nipples indicates a lesion at T_4. See Figure 13.13. **4.** Jimmy is suffering from spinal shock, which occurs as a result of injury to the spinal cord. Spinal shock is a temporary condition in which all reflex and motor activities caudal to the level of spinal cord injury are lost, so Jimmy's muscles are paralyzed. His blood pressure is low due to the loss of sympathetic tone in his vasculature. **5.** Jimmy's exaggerated reflexes are caused by damaged upper motor neuron axons in the spinal cord. These upper motor neurons normally inhibit spinal reflexes. He is incontinent because there are no longer pathways to support voluntary control of bowel and bladder emptying. **6.** This condition is called autonomic dysreflexia (or autonomic hyperreflexia). This is a condition in which a normal stimulus triggers a massive activation of autonomic neurons. **7.** Extremely high arterial blood pressure can cause a rupture of the cerebral blood vessels (as well as other blood vessels in the body) and put Jimmy's life at risk.

Chapter 15

Check Your Understanding 1. Tears (lacrimal fluid) are a dilute saline secretion that contains mucus, antibodies, and lysozyme. They are secreted by the lacrimal glands. **2.** The blind spot of the eye is the optic disc. It is the part of the retina where the optic nerve exits the eye and it is "blind" because it is a region of the retina that lacks photoreceptors. **3.** An increase in intraocular pressure is called glaucoma and is due to an accumulation of aqueous humor, usually because of impaired drainage of the fluid. **4.** Light passes through the cornea, aqueous humor, lens, vitreous humor, ganglion cells and bipolar cells before it reaches the photoreceptors. **5.** The ciliary muscles and sphincter pupillae relax for distant vision. (If you said the medial rectus muscles also relax, this is true, but remember that the rectus muscles are extrinsic eye muscles, not intrinsic.) **6.** The near point moves farther away as you age because the lens becomes less flexible (presbyopia), so that it is unable to assume the more rounded shape required for near vision. **7.** The following are characteristics of cones: "vision in bright light," "color vision," and "higher acuity." The following are characteristics of rods: "only one type of visual pigment," "most abundant in the periphery of the retina," "many feed into one ganglion cell," and "higher sensitivity." **8.** Breakdown of the retinal-opsin combination is called bleaching of the pigment. It occurs with exposure to light. **9.** A tumor in the right visual cortex would affect the left visual field. A tumor compressing the right optic nerve would affect both the left and right visual fields from the right eye only. **10.** The five taste modalities are sweet, sour, bitter, salty, and umami. The fungiform, vallate, and foliate papillae contain taste buds. **11.** The cilia and hairs of these receptor cells greatly increase the surface area for sensory receptors. **12.** The tympanic membrane separates the external from the middle ear. The oval and round windows separate the middle from the inner ear. **13.** The basilar membrane allows us to differentiate sounds of different pitch. **14.** You would not be able to locate the origin of a sound if the brain stem did not receive input from both ears. **15.** The following apply to a macula: "contains otholiths," "responds to linear acceleration or deceleration," and "inside a saccule." The following apply to a crista ampullaris: "inside a semicircular canal," "has a cupula," "responds to rotational acceleration and deceleration." **16.** The "fullness" in Mohammed's ears is likely due to an accumulation of fluid in the middle ear as a result of his upper respiratory infection ("cold") spreading into his ear. He has a form of conduction deafness. **17.** With age, the lens discolors and loses its clarity and the dilator pupillae muscles become less efficient, decreasing the amount of light that reaches the retinas at night.

Review Questions 1. c; **2.** d; **3.** a; **4.** b; **5.** c; **6.** c; **7.** b; **8.** a; **9.** b; **10.** b; **11.** b; **12.** d; **13.** d; **14.** a; **15.** d; **16.** c; **17.** d; **18.** b; **19.** b; **20.** c; **21.** d; **22.** b; **23.** b; **24.** e; **25.** b; **26.** c; **27.** c; **28.** c; **29.** c

Case Study 1. The ear is divided into three major areas: external ear, middle ear, and internal ear. The portion of the internal ear, or labyrinth, associated with balance and equilibrium is the part of the ear affected in Mr. Rhen's BPPV. **2.** Maintaining balance and equilibrium requires multiple sources of sensory input. The three main sources of sensory input are the vestibular apparatus of the ear, visual input, and input from the proprioceptors of the skin, muscles, and joints. **3.** The two functional divisions are the vestibule and semicircular canals. The vestibule's sensory receptors are the maculae, which sense linear (straight line) acceleration and deceleration. The semicircular canals' receptors are the cristae ampullares, which detect rotational acceleration and deceleration. **4.** Mr. Rhen's vertigo is brought on by rotational movements of the head, suggesting that the cristae ampullares of the semicircular canals are affected. **5.** The added mass of the displaced otoliths pushes on a cupula of a semicircular canal when the head is rotated during the Dix-Hallpike maneuver. The otoliths either stick to the gelatinous cupula, or swirl through the canals during head movement and drift against the cupula like snow. In both cases, the bending of the cupula is prolonged and vertigo persists. As a result, vestibular nystagmus is observed when it would ordinarily be absent.

Chapter 16

Check Your Understanding 1. The endocrine system is more closely associated with growth and development, and its responses tend to be long-lasting, whereas nervous system responses tend to be rapid and discrete. **2.** The thyroid and parathyroid glands are found in the neck. **3.** Hormones are released into the blood and transported throughout the body, whereas paracrines act locally, generally within the same tissue. **4.** The two major chemical classes of hormones are amino acid–based hormones and steroids. Steroids are all lipid soluble. Thyroid hormones are the only amino acid–based hormones that are lipid soluble. **5.** Water-soluble hormones act on receptors in the plasma membrane coupled most often via regulatory molecules called G proteins to intracellular second messengers. Lipid-soluble hormones act on intracellular receptors, directly activating genes and stimulating synthesis of specific proteins. **6.** Hormone release can be triggered by humoral, neural, or hormonal stimuli. **7.** The hypothalamus communicates with the anterior pituitary via hormones released into a special portal system of blood vessels. In contrast, it communicates with the posterior pituitary via action potentials traveling down axons that connect the hypothalamus to the posterior pituitary. **8.** Drinking alcoholic beverages inhibits ADH secretion from the posterior pituitary and causes copious urine output and dehydration. The dehydration causes the hangover effects. **9.** LH and FSH are tropic hormones that act on the gonads, TSH is a tropic hormone that acts on the thyroid, and ACTH is a tropic hormone that acts on the adrenal cortex. (If you said growth hormone, that's also a good answer, as GH causing the liver to release IGFs might also be considered a tropic effect.) **10.** Thyroid hormone increases basal metabolic rate (and heat production) in the body. Parathyroid hormone increases blood Ca^{2+} levels in a variety of ways. Calcitonin at high (pharmacological) levels has a Ca^{2+}-lowering, bone-sparing effect. (At normal blood levels its effects in humans are negligible.) **11.** Thyroid follicular cells release thyroid hormone, parathyroid cells in the parathyroid gland release parathyroid hormone, and parafollicular (C) cells in the thyroid gland release calcitonin. **12.** Glucocorticoids are stress hormones that, among many effects, increase blood glucose. Mineralocorticoids increase blood Na^+ (and blood pressure) and decrease blood K^+. Gonadocorticoids are male and female sex hormones that are thought to have a variety of effects (for example, contribute to onset of puberty, sex drive in women, pubic and axillary hair development in women). **13.** Melatonin is used by some individuals as a sleep aid, particularly to counter jet lag. **14.** When we say Sharon is diabetic, this means that she has insufficient insulin action in her body. The most likely explanation for Sharon's behavior is that she has taken too much insulin and is experiencing hypoglycemia. You could help her by making sure she immediately ingests a sugary snack or drink. **15.** Diabetes mellitus is due to a lack of insulin production or action, whereas diabetes insipidus is due to a lack of ADH. Both conditions are characterized by production of copious amounts of urine. You would find glucose in the urine of a patient with diabetes mellitus, but not in the urine of a patient with diabetes insipidus. **16.** The gonadal hormones are steroid hormones. A major endocrine gland that also secretes steroid hormones is the adrenal cortex. **17.** The heart produces atrial natriuretic peptide (ANP). ANP decreases blood volume and blood pressure by increasing the kidneys' production of salty urine. **18.** Vitamin D_3, produced in inactive form by the skin, increases intestinal absorption of calcium. **19.** The decline in growth hormone with age contributes to muscle atrophy. The decline in estrogen contributes to osteoporosis in women.

Review Questions 1. b; **2.** a; **3.** c; **4.** d; **5.** (1)c, (2)a and b, (3)f, (4)d, (5)e, (6)g, (7)a, (8)h, (9)b and e, (10)a; **6.** d; **7.** c; **8.** b; **9.** d; **10.** b; **11.** d; **12.** b; **13.** c; **14.** d

Case Study 1. Rationale for orders: As Mr. Gutteman is unconscious, the level of damage to his brain is unclear. Monitoring his responses and vital signs every hour will provide information for his care providers about the extent of his injuries. Turning him every 4 hours and providing careful skin care will prevent decubitus ulcers (bedsores) as well as stimulating his proprioceptive pathways. **2.** Mr. Gutteman's condition is termed diabetes insipidus, a condition in which insufficient quantities of antidiuretic hormone (ADH) are produced or released. Diabetes insipidus patients excrete large volumes of urine but do not have glucose or ketones present in the urine. The head trauma could have damaged Mr. Gutteman's hypothalamus, which produces the hormone, or injured his posterior pituitary gland, which releases ADH into the bloodstream. **3.** Diabetes insipidus is not life threatening for most individuals with normal thirst mechanisms, as they will be thirsty and drink to replenish the lost fluid. However, Mr. Gutteman is comatose, so his fluid output must be monitored closely so that the volume lost can be replaced by IV line. His subsequent recovery may be complicated if he has suffered damage to his hypothalamus, which houses the thirst center neurons.

Chapter 17

Check Your Understanding 1. The hematocrit is the percentage of blood that is occupied by erythrocytes. It is normally about 45%. **2.** Blood can prevent blood loss by forming clots when a blood vessel is damaged. Blood can prevent infection because it contains antimicrobial proteins and white blood cells. **3.** Plasma proteins are not used as fuel for body cells because their presence in blood is required to perform many key functions. **4.** Each hemoglobin molecule can transport four O_2. The heme portion of the hemoglobin binds the O_2. **5.** The kidneys' synthesis of erythropoietin is compromised in advanced kidney disease, so RBC production decreases, causing anemia. **6.** Monocytes become macrophages in tissues. Neutrophils are also voracious phagocytes.
7. "Thrombopoietin" is derived from the same word as "thrombocyte." It is the hormone that promotes platelet formation. **8.** Amos's red bone marrow is spewing out many abnormal white blood cells, which are crowding out the production of normal bone marrow elements. The lack of normal white blood cells allows the infections, the lack of platelets fails to stop bleeding, and the lack of erythrocytes is anemia. **9.** The three steps of hemostasis are vascular spasm, platelet plug formation, and coagulation. **10.** Fibrinogen is water soluble, whereas fibrin is not. Prothrombin is an inactive precursor, whereas thrombin acts as an enzyme. Most factors are inactive in blood before activation and become enzymes upon activation. (There are exceptions, such as fibrinogen and calcium.)
11. Thrombocytopenia (platelet deficiency) results in failure to plug the countless small tears in blood vessels, and so manifests as small purple spots. Hemophilia A results from the absence of clotting factor VIII.
12. Nigel has anti-A antibodies in his blood and type B agglutinogens on his RBCs. He can donate blood to an AB recipient, but he should not receive blood from an AB donor because his anti-A antibodies will cause a transfusion reaction. **13.** If Emily has a bacterial meningitis, a differential WBC count would likely reveal an increase in neutrophils because neutrophils are a major body defense against bacteria. **14.** Hemoglobin F has a higher affinity (binding strength) for oxygen than adult hemoglobin does. It has 2 α and 2 γ chains rather than 2 α and 2 β chains.

Review Questions 1. c; **2.** c; **3.** d; **4.** b; **5.** d; **6.** a; **7.** a; **8.** b; **9.** c; **10.** d

Case Study 1. Saline infusion temporarily replaces the lost blood volume, thereby helping to restore Mr. Malone's circulation. **2.** The PBRCs contain oxygen-carrying hemoglobin. While the saline replaces lost blood volume, it cannot replace the hemoglobin in the lost RBCs. (In acute trauma, the rule of thumb is to use no more than 2 liters of normal saline before starting PRBCs, so that the hematocrit does not drop below 30%.) **3.** O negative blood cells bear neither the A nor the B nor the Rh agglutinogens (antigens). People with O negative blood are sometimes called "universal donors" because their cells lack the antigens responsible for most major transfusion reactions. **4.** Mr. Malone's blood would have anti-B antibodies (agglutinins) so he would not be able to receive B or AB blood. He can safely receive A and O blood. **5.** If doctors had transfused type B or AB blood into Mr. Malone's circulation, his anti-B antibodies would have "attacked" these foreign cells and caused them to agglutinate. This transfusion reaction can be dangerous because the agglutinated cells can clog small vessels. In addition the transfused cells would begin to hemolyze (rupture) or would be destroyed by phagocytes.

Chapter 18

Check Your Understanding 1. The mediastinum is the medial cavity of the thorax within which the heart, great vessels, and trachea are found. **2.** The layers of the heart wall are the endocardium, the myocardium, and the epicardium. The epicardium is also called the visceral layer of the serous pericardium. This is surrounded by the parietal layer of the serous pericardium and the fibrous pericardium. **3.** The serous fluid decreases friction caused by movement of the layers against one another. **4.** The papillary muscles and chordae tendineae keep the AV valve flaps from everting into the atria as the ventricles contract. **5.** The right side of the heart acts as the pulmonary pump, whereas the left acts as the systemic pump. **6.** (a) True. The left ventricle wall is thicker than the right. (b) True. The left ventricle pumps blood at much higher pressure than the right ventricle because the left ventricle supplies the whole body, whereas the right ventricle supplies only the lungs. (c) False. Each ventricle pumps the same amount of blood with each beat. If this were not true, blood would back up in either the systemic or pulmonary circulation (because the two ventricles are in series). **7.** The branches of the right coronary artery are the right marginal artery and the posterior interventricular artery. **8.** (a) The refractory period is almost as long as the contraction in cardiac muscle. (b) The source of Ca^{2+} for the contraction is only SR in skeletal muscle. (c) The AP exhibits a plateau phase in cardiac muscle. (d) Both skeletal muscle and cardiac muscle have troponin. (e) Only skeletal muscle has triads. **9.** Cardiac muscle cannot go into tetany because the absolute refractory period is almost as long as the contraction. **10.** The subendocardial conducting network excites ventricular muscle fibers. The depolarization wave travels upward from the apex toward the atria, and from endocardium to epicardium. **11.** (a) The QRS wave occurs during ventricular depolarization. (b) The T wave of the ECG occurs during ventricular repolarization. (c) The P-R interval of the ECG occurs during atrial depolarization and the conduction of the action potential through the rest of the intrinsic conduction system. **12.** The second heart sound is associated with the closing of the semilunar valves. **13.** The murmur of mitral insufficiency occurs during ventricular systole (because this is when the valve should be closed, and the murmur is due to blood leaking through the incompletely closed valve into the atrium). **14.** The periods when all four valves are closed are the isovolumetric contraction phase and the isovolumetric relaxation phase. **15.** Exercise activates the sympathetic nervous system. Sympathetic nervous system activity increases heart rate. It also directly increases ventricular contractility, thereby increasing Josh's stroke volume. **16.** If the heart is beating very rapidly, the amount of time for ventricular filling between contractions is decreased. This decreases the end diastolic volume, decreases the stroke volume, and therefore decreases the cardiac output. **17.** The foramen ovale and the ductus arteriosus both allow blood to bypass the fetal lungs. **18.** Elderly athletes may be hampered by sclerosis and thickening of heart valve flaps, a decline in cardiac reserve, fibrosis of cardiac muscle, and atherosclerosis.

Review Questions 1. a; **2.** c; **3.** b; **4.** c; **5.** b; **6.** b; **7.** c; **8.** d; **9.** b

Case Study 1. The weak and thready pulse indicates a drop in stroke volume (SV). The pulse is felt as blood is ejected from the heart during ventricular contraction (systole). The weak and thready pulse suggests that less blood is being ejected during each contraction (a lower SV). **2.** An increase in heart rate leads to an increase in cardiac output (recall $CO = HR \times SV$). Mr. Ayers's CO is abnormally low (as shown by his decreasing blood pressure). This is probably due to a decrease in SV. The increase in HR is an attempt to compensate for the decrease in SV in order to maintain CO as close to normal as possible. **3.** In cardiac tamponade, the fluid around the heart compresses the heart and prevents it from fully expanding as it relaxes (diastole). As a result of this restriction, less blood will flow into the heart (ventricular filling). With less blood flowing into the ventricles, the degree of stretch of the heart muscle (preload) will also be reduced. These events lead to a reduction in SV. **4.** Heart sounds are produced by the closing of heart valves during a normal cardiac cycle. When EDV is reduced, there is both reduced SV and reduced force of contraction, leading to slower, quieter valve closure. **5.** The enlarged mediastinum and pericardial effusions suggest that the bleeding is restricted within these compartments. The tear would most likely be located in the proximal portion of the ascending aorta (the part closest to the heart). This part of the aorta is located within the pericardium. The tear then proceeded distally but was contained within the aortic wall, causing the back pain. An uncontained tear in the aortic arch or descending aorta would lead to bleeding in the thoracic and/or abdominal cavities, which was not observed in this case. **6.** In the face of reduced SV, blood returning to the heart backs up, leading to a rise in venous pressure. This is a key sign of tamponade.

Chapter 19

Check Your Understanding 1. The sympathetic nervous system innervates blood vessels. The sympathetic nerves innervate the tunica media. The effector cells in the tunica media are smooth muscle cells. **2.** When vascular smooth muscle contracts, the diameter of the blood vessel becomes smaller. This is called vasoconstriction. **3.** Elastic arteries play a major role in dampening the pulsatile pressure of heart contractions. Dilation or constriction of arterioles determines blood flow to individual capillary beds. Muscular arteries have the thickest tunica media relative to their lumen size. **4.** If you were doing calf raises, your capillary bed would be in the condition depicted in part (a). The true capillaries would be flushed with blood to ensure that the working calf muscles could receive the needed nutrients and dispose of their metabolic wastes. **5.** Valves prevent blood from flowing backwards in veins. They are formed from folds of the tunica intima. **6.** In the systemic circuit, veins contain more blood than arteries (see Figure 19.5). **7.** The three factors that determine resistance are blood viscosity, vessel length, and vessel diameter. Vessel diameter is physiologically most important. **8.** The rate of flow will decrease 81-fold from its original flow ($3 \times 3 \times 3 \times 3 = 81$). **9.** When you first stand up, mean arterial pressure (MAP) temporarily decreases and this is sensed by aortic and carotid baroreceptors. Medullary cardiac and vasomotor center reflexes increase sympathetic and decrease parasympathetic outflow to the heart. Heart rate and contractility increase, increasing cardiac output, and therefore MAP. Further, sympathetic constriction of arterioles increases peripheral resistance, also increasing MAP. (In addition, increased constriction of veins increases venous return, which increases end diastolic volume, increasing stroke volume, and therefore cardiac output and MAP.) See also Figure 19.9 (bottom). **10.** The kidneys help maintain MAP by influencing blood volume. In renal artery obstruction, the blood pressure in the kidney is lower than in the rest of the body (because it is downstream of the obstruction). Low renal blood pressure triggers both direct and indirect renal mechanisms to increase blood pressure by increasing blood volume. This can cause hypertension (called "secondary hypertension" because it is secondary to a defined cause—in this case the renal artery obstruction). **11.** In a bicycle race, autoregulation by intrinsic metabolic controls causes arteriolar smooth muscle in your legs to relax, dilating the vessels and supplying more O_2 and nutrients to the exercising muscles. **12.** Extrinsic mechanisms, primarily the sympathetic nervous system, prevent blood pressure from plummeting by constricting arterioles elsewhere (such as gut, kidneys). In addition, cardiac output increases, which also helps maintain MAP. **13.** (a) An increase in interstitial fluid osmotic pressure (OP_{if}) would tend to pull more fluid out of capillaries (causing localized swelling, or edema). (b) An increase of OP_{if} to 10 mm Hg would increase the outward pressure on both the arteriole and venule ends of the capillary. The NFP at the venous end would become 1 mm Hg (27 mm Hg − 26 mm Hg). (c) Fluid would flow out of the venous end of the capillary rather than in. **14.** Bob is in vascular shock due to anaphylaxis, a systemic allergic reaction to his medication. His blood pressure is low because of widespread vasodilation triggered by the massive release of histamine. Bob's rapid heart rate is a result of the baroreceptor reflex triggered by his low blood pressure. This activates the sympathetic nervous system, increasing heart rate, in an attempt to restore blood pressure. **15.** The external carotid arteries supply most of the tissues of the head except for the brain and orbits. **16.** The cerebral arterial circle (circle of Willis) is the arterial anastomosis at the base of the cerebrum. **17.** The four unpaired arteries that emerge from the abdominal aorta are the celiac trunk, the superior and inferior mesenteric arteries, and the median sacral artery. **18.** You would palpate the popliteal artery behind the knee, the posterior tibial artery behind the medial malleolus of the tibia, and the dorsalis pedis artery on the foot. (See also Figure 19.12.) **19.** The vertebral arteries help supply the brain, but the vertebral veins do not drain much blood from the brain. **20.** The internal jugular veins drain the dural venous sinuses. Each internal jugular vein joins a subclavian vein to form a brachiocephalic vein. **21.** A portal system is a system where two capillary beds occur in series. In other words, in a portal system, a capillary bed is drained by a vein that leads into a second capillary bed. The function of the hepatic portal system is to transport venous blood from the digestive organs to the liver for processing before it enters the rest of the systemic circulation. This plays an important role in defense against absorbed toxins or microorganisms and also allows direct delivery of absorbed nutrients to the liver for processing. **22.** The leg veins that often become varicosed are the great and small saphenous veins. **23.** Three differences between arteries and veins are (1) arteries run deep while veins are both deep and superficial, (2) venous pathways are more interconnected than arterial pathways, and (3) the brain and digestive systems have unique venous drainage systems, whereas their arterial supply patterns are not substantially different from those of other organs. **24.** The foramen ovale and the ductus arteriosus both bypass the fetal lungs. The ductus venosus bypasses the fetal liver. **25.** Varicose veins, atherosclerosis, and hypertension are associated with aging.

Review Questions 1. d; **2.** b; **3.** d; **4.** c; **5.** e; **6.** d; **7.** c; **8.** b; **9.** b; **10.** a; **11.** (1)b, e, g; (2)c; (3)i; (4)f, h; (5)d; **12.** b; **13.** c; **14.** d

Case Study 1. The tissues in Mr. Hutchinson's right leg were deprived of oxygen and nutrients for at least one-half hour. When tissues are deprived of oxygen, tissue metabolism decreases and eventually ceases, so these tissues may have died due to anoxia. **2.** Mr. Hutchinson's vital signs (low BP; rapid, thready pulse) indicate that he is facing a life-threatening problem that must be stabilized before other, less vital problems can be addressed. As for surgery, he may be scheduled for open reduction of his crushed bone, depending upon the condition of the tissues in his crushed right leg. If tissue death has occurred in his leg, he may undergo amputation of that limb. **3.** Mr. Hutchinson's rapid, thready pulse and falling blood pressure are indications of hypovolemic shock, a type of shock resulting from decreased blood volume. Because his blood volume is low, his heart rate is elevated to increase cardiac output in an effort to maintain the blood supply to his vital organs. Mr. Hutchinson's blood volume must be increased as quickly as possible with blood transfusions or intravenous saline. This will stabilize his condition and allow his physicians to continue with his surgery.

Chapter 20

Check Your Understanding 1. Lymph is the fluid inside lymphatic vessels. It enters lymphatic vessels from interstitial fluid. Interstitial fluid, in turn, is a filtrate of blood plasma. **2.** The right lymphatic duct receives lymph from the right upper arm and the right side of the head and thorax. The thoracic duct drains lymph from the rest of the body. **3.** Lymph movement is driven by the contraction of adjacent skeletal muscles, pressure changes in the thorax during breathing, the pulsations of nearby arteries, and contraction of smooth muscle in the lymphatic vessel walls. (Valves in lymphatic vessels prevent backflow of lymph.) **4.** Lymphoid follicles are solid, spherical bodies consisting of tightly packed reticular fibers and lymphoid cells, often with a lighter-staining central region. They are regions where B cells predominate. **5.** Having fewer efferents causes lymph to accumulate in lymph nodes, allowing more time for its cleansing. **6.** MALT (mucosa-associated lymphoid tissue) is lymphoid tissue found in the mucosa of the digestive, respiratory, and genitourinary tracts. It includes tonsils, Peyer's patches, and the appendix. **7.** The spleen cleanses the blood, stores breakdown products of RBCs, stores platelets and monocytes, and is thought to be a site of erythrocyte production in the fetus. **8.** The thymus develops first.

Review Questions 1. c; **2.** c; **3.** a, d; **4.** c; **5.** a; **6.** b; **7.** a; **8.** b; **9.** d

Case Study 1. The red streaks radiating from Mr. Hutchinson's finger indicate that his lymphatic vessels are inflamed. This inflammation may be caused by a bacterial infection. If Mr. Hutchinson's arm had exhibited edema without any accompanying red streaks, the problem would likely have been impaired lymph transport from his arm back to his trunk, due to injury or blockage of his lymphatic vessels. **2.** Mr. Hutchinson's arm was placed in a sling to immobilize it, slowing the drainage of lymph from the infected area in an attempt to limit the spread of the infection. **3.** Mr. Hutchinson's low lymphocyte count indicates that his body's ability to fight infection by bacteria or viruses is impaired. The antibiotics and additional staff protection will protect Mr. Hutchinson until his lymphocyte count increases again. Gloving and gowning also protect the staff caring for Mr. Hutchinson from any body infection he might have. **4.** Mr. Hutchinson's recovery may be problematic, as he probably already has an ongoing bacterial infection and his ability to raise a defense to this infection is impaired.

Chapter 21

Check Your Understanding 1. The innate defense system is always ready to respond immediately, whereas it takes considerable time to mount the adaptive defense system. The innate defenses consist of surface barriers and internal defenses, whereas the adaptive defenses consist of humoral and cellular immunity, which rely on B and T lymphocytes. **2.** Surface barriers (the skin and mucous membranes) constitute the first line of defense. **3.** Opsonization is the process of making pathogens more susceptible to phagocytosis by decorating their surface with molecules that phagocytes can bind. Antibodies and complement proteins are examples of molecules that act as opsonins. **4.** Our own cells are killed by NK cells when they have been infected by viruses or when they have become cancerous. **5.** Redness, heat, swelling, and pain are the cardinal signs of inflammation. Redness and local heat are both caused by vasodilation of arterioles, which increases the flow of blood (warmed by the body core) to the affected area. The swelling (edema) is due to the release of histamine and other chemical mediators of inflammation, which increase capillary permeability. This increased permeability allows proteins to leak into the interstitial fluid (IF), increasing the IF osmotic pressure and drawing more fluid out of blood vessels and into the tissues, thereby causing swelling. The pain is due to two things: (1) the actions of certain chemical mediators (kinins and prostaglandins) on nerve endings, and (2) the swelling, which can compress free nerve endings. **6.** Three key characteristics of adaptive immunity are that it is specific, it is systemic, and it has memory. **7.** A complete antigen has both immunogenicity and reactivity, whereas a hapten has reactivity but not immunogenicity. **8.** Self-antigens, particularly MHC proteins, mark a cell as self. **9.** Development of immunocompetence of a B or T cell is signaled by the appearance on its surface of specific and unique receptors for an antigen. In the case of a B cell, this receptor is a membrane-bound antibody. (In T cells, it is simply called the T cell receptor.) **10.** The T cell that would survive is (c), one that recognizes MHC but not self-antigen. **11.** Dendritic cells, macrophages, and B cells can all act as APCs. Dendritic cells are most important for T cell activation. **12.** In clonal selection, the antigen does the selecting. What is being selected is a particular clone of B or T cells that has antigen receptors corresponding to that antigen. **13.** The secondary response to an antigen is faster than the primary response because the immune system has already been "primed" and has memory cells that are specific for that particular antigen. **14.** Vaccinations protect by providing the initial encounter to an antigen—the primary response to that antigen. As a result, when the pathogen for that illness is encountered again, the pathogen elicits the much faster, more powerful secondary response, which is generally effective enough to prevent clinical illness. **15.** IgG antibody is most abundant in blood. IgM is secreted first in a primary immune response. IgA is most abundant in secretions. **16.** Antibodies can bring about destruction of pathogen via "PLAN"—**p**hagocytosis, **l**ysis (via complement), **a**gglutination, or **n**eutralization. **17.** Class II MHC proteins display exogenous antigens. Class II MHC proteins are recognized by CD4 T cells (which usually become helper T cells). APCs display class II MHC proteins. **18.** Binding of antigens in the absence of co-stimulators causes the lymphocyte to develop anergy—a state of permanent unresponsiveness to that antigen. **19.** Helper T cells are central to both humoral and cellular immunity because they are required for activation of both cytotoxic T cells and most B cells. **20.** The cytotoxic T cell releases perforins and granzymes onto the identified target cell. Perforins form a pore in the target cell membrane, and granzymes enter through this pore, activating enzymes that trigger apoptosis (cell suicide). **21.** MHC proteins and blood type antigens (ABO, etc.) are carefully matched before an organ transplant. **22.** HIV is particularly hard for the immune system to defeat because (1) it destroys helper T cells, which are key players in adaptive immunity and (2) it has a high mutation rate and so it rapidly becomes resistant to drugs. **23.** Binding of an allergen onto specific IgE antibodies attached to mast cells triggers the mast cells to release histamine.

Review Questions 1. c; **2.** a; **3.** d; **4.** d, e; **5.** a; **6.** d; **7.** b; **8.** c; **9.** d; **10.** d; **11.** d; **12.** (1)b, g; (2)d, i; (3)a, e; (4)a, e, f, h; (5)e, h; (6)c, f, g

Case Study 1. The two kidneys transplanted in this case represent allografts. **2.** A major histocompatibility complex (MHC) protein is a type of cell surface protein that the human body uses to recognize *self* and to help coordinate the recognition of *nonself*, or foreign, antigens. These proteins are involved in the display of antigens to T cells. **3.** Class I MHC proteins are found on virtually all of the body's cells, while class II MHCs are found only on antigen-presenting cells (APCs). Class I MHCs display antigens for recognition by CD8 T cells (including cytotoxic T cells). Class II MHCs display antigens for recognition by CD4 T cells (including helper T cells). **4.** A foreign MHC protein will provoke an immune response, so the donor's and recipient's MHCs must match as closely as possible to minimize such an attack. Tissue typing dramatically reduces the risk of organ rejection due to attack by the recipient's immune system. **5.** In this case, the donor and recipients were not genetically identical. Even with very careful tissue typing and compatibility testing, there will still be some differences that the recipients' immune systems will recognize as foreign. To reduce the risk of organ rejection, the recipients are given drugs to suppress their immune systems.

Chapter 22

Check Your Understanding 1. The structures that air passes by are the nasal cavity (nares, nasal vestibule, nasal conchae), nasopharynx (with pharyngeal tonsil), oropharynx (with palatine tonsil), laryngopharynx, and larynx (with epiglottis, vestibular fold, and vocal fold). **2.** The epiglottis seals the larynx when we swallow. **3.** The incomplete, C-shaped cartilage rings of the trachea allow it to expand and contract and yet keep it from collapsing. **4.** The many tiny alveoli together have a large surface area. This and the thinness of their respiratory membranes make them ideal for gas exchange. **5.** The peanut was most likely in the right main bronchus because it is wider and more vertical than the left. **6.** The two circulations of the lungs are the pulmonary circulation, which delivers deoxygenated blood to the lungs for oxygenation and returns oxygenated blood to the heart, and the bronchial circulation, which provides systemic (oxygenated) blood to lung tissue. **7.** The driving force for pulmonary ventilation is a pressure gradient created by changes in the thoracic volume. **8.** The intrapulmonary pressure decreases during inspiration because of the increase in thoracic cavity volume brought about by the muscles of inspiration. **9.** The partial vacuum (negative pressure) inside the pleural cavity is caused by the opposing forces acting on the visceral and parietal pleurae. The visceral pleurae are pulled inward by the lungs' natural tendency to recoil and the surface tension of the alveolar fluid. The parietal pleurae are pulled outward by the elasticity of the chest wall. If air enters the pleural cavity, the lung on that side will collapse. This condition is called pneumothorax. **10.** Airway resistance is low because (1) the diameters of most airways are relatively large, (2) for smaller airways there are many in parallel, making their combined diameter large, and (3) air has a low viscosity. **11.** A lack of surfactant increases surface tension in the alveoli and causes them to collapse between breaths. (In other words, it markedly decreases lung compliance.) **12.** Slow, deep breaths ventilate the alveoli more effectively because a smaller fraction of the tidal volume of each breath is spent moving air into and out of the dead space. **13.** In a sealed container, the air and water would be at equilibrium. Therefore, the partial pressures of CO_2 and O_2 (P_{CO_2} and P_{O_2}) will be the same in the water as in the air: 100 mm Hg each. More CO_2 than O_2 molecules will be dissolved in the water (even though they are at the same partial pressure) because CO_2 is much more soluble than O_2 in water. **14.** The difference in P_{O_2} between inspired air and alveolar air can be explained by (1) the gas exchange occurring in the lungs (O_2 continuously diffuses out of the alveoli into the blood), (2) the humidification of inspired air (which adds water molecules that dilute the O_2 molecules), and (3) the mixing of newly inspired air with gases already present in the alveoli. **15.** The arterioles leading into the O_2-enriched alveoli would be dilated. This response allows matching of blood flow to availability of oxygen. **16.** Both CO_2 and H^+ increase O_2 unloading by binding to Hb. This is called the Bohr effect. **17.** About 70% of CO_2 is transported as bicarbonate ion (HCO_3^-) in plasma. Just over 20% is transported bound to hemoglobin in the RBCs, and 7–10% is dissolved in plasma. **18.** As blood CO_2 increases, blood pH decreases. This is because CO_2 combines with water to form carbonic acid. (However, the change in pH in blood for a given increase in CO_2 is minimized by other buffer systems.) **19.** The ventral respiratory group of the medulla (VRG) is thought to be the rhythm-generating area. **20.** CO_2 in blood normally provides the most powerful stimulus to breathe. Central chemoreceptors are most important in this response (see Figure 22.25). **21.** The injured soccer player's P_{CO_2} is low. (Recall that normal $P_{CO_2} = 40$ mm Hg.) The low P_{CO_2} reveals that this is hyperventilation and not hyperpnea (which is not accompanied by changes in blood CO_2 levels). **22.** Long-term adjustments to altitude include an increase in erythropoiesis, resulting in a higher hematocrit; an increase in BPG, which decreases Hb affinity for oxygen; and an increase in minute respiratory volume. **23.** The obstruction in asthma is reversible, and acute exacerbations are typically followed by symptom-free periods. In contrast, the obstruction in chronic bronchitis is generally not reversible. **24.** The underlying defect in cystic fibrosis is an abnormality in a protein (CFTR protein) that acts as a membrane channel for chloride ions. **25.** Vital capacity declines with age because the thoracic wall becomes more rigid and the lungs lose their elasticity.

Review Questions 1. b; **2.** a and c; **3.** c; **4.** c; **5.** b; **6.** d; **7.** d; **8.** b; **9.** c, d; **10.** c; **11.** b; **12.** b; **13.** b; **14.** c; **15.** b; **16.** b

Case Study 1. Spinal cord injury from a fracture at the level of the C_2 vertebra would interrupt the normal transmission of signals from the brain stem down the phrenic nerve to the diaphragm, and Barbara would be unable to breathe due to paralysis of the diaphragm. **2.** Barbara's head, neck, and torso should have been immobilized to prevent further damage to the spinal cord. In addition, she required assistance to breathe, so her airway was probably intubated to permit ventilation of her lungs. **3.** Cyanosis is a decrease in the degree of oxygen saturation of hemoglobin. As Barbara's respiratory efforts cease, her alveolar P_{O_2} will fall, so there is less oxygen to load onto hemoglobin. In her peripheral tissues, what little oxygen hemoglobin carries will be consumed, leaving these tissues with a bluish tinge. **4.** Injury to the spinal cord at the level of the C_2 vertebra will cause quadriplegia (paralysis of all four limbs). **5.** Atelectasis is the collapse of a lung. Because it is the right thorax that is compressed, only her right lung is affected. Because the lungs are in separate pleural cavities, only the right lung collapsed. **6.** Barbara's fractured ribs probably punctured her lung tissue and allowed air within the lung to enter the pleural cavity. **7.** The atelectasis will be reversed by inserting a chest tube and removing the air from the pleural cavity. This will allow her lung to heal and reinflate.

Chapter 23

Check Your Understanding 1. The esophagus is found in the thorax. Three alimentary canal organs found in the abdominal cavity include the stomach, small intestine, and large intestine. **2.** The usual site of ingestion in a healthy person is the mouth. **3.** The process of absorption moves nutrients into the body. **4.** Reflexes associated with the GI tract promote muscle contraction and secretion of digestive juices or hormones. **5.** The term "gut brain" refers to the enteric nervous system or web of neurons closely associated with the digestive organs. **6.** The visceral peritoneum is the outermost layer of the digestive organ; the parietal peritoneum is the serous membrane covering the wall of the abdominal cavity. **7.** The pancreas is retroperitoneal. **8.** The hepatic portal circulation is the venous portion of the splanchnic circulation. **9.** From deep to superficial the layers of the alimentary canal are the mucosa, submucosa, muscularis externa, and serosa. **10.** He should temporarily refrain from eating because the parasympathetic nervous system oversees digestive activities. **11.** The oral vestibule is the region between the cheek and the teeth. The oral cavity proper is the area enclosed by the teeth. **12.** The palate forms the roof of the mouth. The hard palate supported by bone is anterior to the soft palate (no bony support). **13.** The tongue is important for speech, particularly for uttering consonants, and taste. **14.** The serous portion of saliva is rich in salivary amylase, an enzyme that chemically breaks down starch. Additionally, the serous portion of saliva helps to hydrate the foodstuffs and helps provide protection against microorganisms. **15.** Antimicrobial substances found in saliva include lysozyme, defensins, and IgA antibodies. **16.** Tina's "show and tell" tooth is a primary tooth, also called a deciduous tooth. **17.** Enamel is harder than bone. Pulp consists of nervous tissue and blood vessels. **18.** The molars are grinding teeth. **19.** The pharynx is part of the digestive and respiratory systems. **20.** The esophageal mucularis externa undergoes a transformation along its length from skeletal muscle superiorly to smooth muscle near the stomach. **21.** The esophagus is merely a chute for food passage and is subjected to a good deal of abrasion, which a stratified squamous epithelium can withstand. The stomach mucosa is a secretory mucosa served well by a simple columnar epithelium. **22.** The tongue mixes the chewed food with saliva, compacts the food into a bolus, and initiates swallowing. **23.** During swallowing the larynx rises and the epiglottis covers its lumen so that foodstuffs are diverted into the esophagus posteriorly. **24.** The stomach has three layers of smooth muscle—longitudinal, circular, and oblique. Addition of the oblique layer allows the stomach to pummel food in addition to its peristaltic movements. **25.** The chief cells produce pepsinogen, which is the inactive enzyme pepsin, and the parietal cells secrete HCl needed to activate pepsinogen. **26.** The mucosal barrier consists of the thick alkaline mucus secreted by the mucous cells, the fact that the epithelial cells of the mucosa are joined by tight junctions, and the quick replacement of dead or dying cells by stem cells. **27.** The three phases of gastric secretion are the cephalic, gastric, and intestinal phases. **28.** The presence of food in the duodenum inhibits gastric activity by triggering the enterogastric reflex and the secretion of enterogastrones (hormones). **29.** Venous blood leaving the stomach during a meal becomes more alkaline due to the alkaline tide occurring during HCl secretion. **30.** All of these modifications increase the surface area of the small intestine. The circular folds force the chyme to spiral through the lumen. **31.** Brush border enzymes are enzymes associated with the microvilli of the small intestine mucosal cells. **32.** A lacteal is a blind-ended lymphatic capillary that picks up lymph (fluid and proteins leaked from the blood stream), which is then returned to the blood. **33.** IgA, HCl, defensins, and lysozyme protect the intestinal cells from bacterial damage. **34.** A portal triad is a region at the corner of a hepatic lobule that contains a branch of the hepatic portal vein, a branch of the hepatic artery, and a bile duct. **35.** The enterohepatic circulation is an important recycling mechanism for retaining bile salts needed for fat absorption. **36.** Stellate macrophages rid the blood of bacteria and dead cells. **37.** Zymogen granules contain inactive digestive enzymes. **38.** Pancreatic acini produce the exocrine products of the pancreas (digestive enzymes and bicarbonate-rich juice). The islets produce pancreatic hormones, most importantly insulin and glucagon. **39.** Fluid in the pancreatic duct is bicarbonate-rich, enzyme-rich pancreatic juice. Fluid in the cystic and bile ducts is bile. **40.** CCK is secreted in response to the entry of chyme rich in protein and fat into the duodenum. It causes the pancreatic acini to secrete digestive enzymes, stimulates the gallbladder to contract, and relaxes the hepatopancreatic sphincter. **41.** Distension of stomach walls enhances stomach secretory activity. Distension of the walls of the small intestine reduces stomach secretory activity (to give the small intestine time to carry out its digestive and absorptive activities). **42.** Segmentation is more important for moving food along the small intestine. **43.** MMC is the migrating motor complex, a pattern of peristalsis seen in the small intestine that moves the last remnants of a meal plus bacteria and other debris into the large intestine. MMC is important to prevent the overgrowth of bacteria in the small intestine. **44.** Mass movements and haustral contractions are unique to the large intestine. Mass movements are long, slow, powerful contractions that move over large areas of the colon three or four times a day, forcing the contents toward the rectum. Haustral contractions are a special type of segmentation. **45.** Activation of stretch receptors in the rectal wall initiates the defecation reflex. **46.** Enteric bacteria synthesize B vitamins and some of the vitamin K the liver needs to synthesize clotting proteins. **47.** All food digestion depends on hydrolysis reactions. **48.** Amylase is to starch as lipase is to fats. **49.** Bile salts emulsify fats so that they can be acted on efficiently by lipase enzymes, and form micelles that aid fat absorption. **50.** The digestive system mucosa develops from the endoderm. **51.** The thick viscous mucus produced in cystic fibrosis patients clogs pancreatic ducts and prevents the delivery of pancreatic fluid to the duodenum, thus inhibiting fat digestion and absorption. **52.** Colon and stomach cancers are dangerous because they have few early signs and symptoms.

Review Questions 1. c; **2.** d; **3.** d; **4.** b; **5.** b; **6.** a; **7.** d; **8.** d; **9.** b; **10.** c; **11.** c; **12.** a; **13.** d; **14.** d; **15.** b; **16.** c; **17.** a

Case Study 1. Mr. Gutteman's statement about the effects of milk on his digestive tract suggests that he may be deficient in lactase, a brush border enzyme that breaks down lactose (milk sugar). **2.** His responses to the questions reduced the possibility that he has gastric ulcers. Mr. Gutteman's diarrhea may be due to gluten-sensitive enteropathy. To verify this diagnosis, Mr. Gutteman should be screened for specific IgA antibodies in his blood. If these screening tests are positive, a biopsy of the intestinal mucosa would be performed. Observation of damaged intestinal villi and microvilli would confirm the diagnosis. A positive diagnosis of gluten-sensitive enteropathy would lead to a lifelong dietary restriction of all grains except rice and corn. Grains should not be restricted prior to the biopsy.

Chapter 24

Check Your Understanding 1. The six major nutrients are carbohydrates, proteins, fats, water, minerals, and vitamins. **2.** Cellulose provides fiber, which helps in elimination. **3.** Triglycerides are used for ATP synthesis, body insulation and protective padding, and to help the body absorb fat-soluble vitamins. Cholesterol is the basis of our steroid hormones and bile salts, and stabilizes cellular membranes. **4.** Beans (legumes) and grains (wheat) are good sources of protein, but neither is a complete one. However, together they provide all the essential amino acids. **5.** Vitamins serve as the basis for coenzymes, which work with enzymes to accomplish metabolic reactions. **6.** Vitamin B_{12} needs intrinsic factor to be absorbed by the intestine. **7.** Iodine is essential for thyroxine synthesis. Calcium in the form of bone salts is needed to make bones hard. Iron is needed to make functional hemoglobin. **8.** A redox reaction is a combination of an oxidation and a reduction reaction. As one substance is oxidized, another is reduced. **9.** Some of the energy released during catabolism is captured in the bonds of ATP, which provides the energy needed to carry out the constructive activities of anabolism. **10.** The energy released during the oxidation of food fuels is used to pump protons across the inner mitochondrial membrane. **11.** In substrate-level phosphorylation, high-energy phosphate groups are transferred directly from phosphorylated intermediates to ADP to form ATP. In oxidative phosphorylation, electron transport proteins forming part of the mitochondrial cristae use energy released during oxidation of glucose to create a steep gradient for protons across the crista membrane. Then as protons flow back through the membrane, gradient energy is captured to attach phosphate to ADP. **12.** If oxygen is not available, glycolysis will stop because the supply of NAD^+ is limited and glycolysis can continue only if the reduced coenzymes ($NADH + H^+$) formed during glycolysis are relieved of their extra hydrogen. **13.** Oxidation (via removal of H) is common in the Krebs cycle; it is indicated by the reduction of a coenzyme (either NAD^+ or FAD). Decarboxylations are also common, and are indicated by the removal of CO_2 from the cycle. **14.** Glycogenolysis is the reaction in which glycogen is broken down to its glucose units. **15.** Carbo loading forces the skeletal muscles to store more glycogen than they ordinarily would. **16.** Glycerol, a breakdown product of fat metabolism, enters the glycolytic pathway. **17.** Acetyl CoA is the central molecule of fat metabolism. **18.** The products of beta oxidation are acetyl CoA (acetic acid + coenzyme A), $NADH^+ + H^+$, and $FADH_2$. **19.** The liver uses keto acids drained off the Krebs cycle and amino groups (from other nonessential amino acids) as substrates to make the nonessential amino acids that the body needs. **20.** The ammonia removed from amino acids is combined with carbon dioxide to form urea, which is then eliminated by the kidneys. **21.** The three organs or tissues that regulate the directions of interconversions in the nutrient pools are the liver, skeletal muscles, and adipose tissues. **22.** Anabolic reactions and energy storage typify the absorptive state. Catabolic reactions (to increase blood sugar levels) such as lipolysis and glycogenolysis, and glucose sparing occur in the postabsorptive state. **23.** The main antagonist of glucagon is insulin. **24.** A rise in amino acid levels in blood increases both insulin and glucagon release. **25.** High HDLs would be preferable because the cholesterol these particles transport are destined for the liver and elimination from the body. **26.** A total cholesterol level of 200 mg/dl of blood or lower is recommended. **27.** Trans fats are oils that have been hydrogenated (with H atoms). They are unhealthy because they cause LDLs to increase and HDLs to decrease, exactly the opposite of what is desirable. **28.** Among short-term stimuli influencing feeding behavior are neural signals from the digestive tract, nutrient signals related to energy stores, and GI tract hormones (CCK, insulin, glucagon, and ghrelin). **29.** Leptin is the most important long-term regulator of feeding behavior. **30.** Of the factors listed, breathing and kidney function contribute to BMR. **31.** Samantha has a larger relative body surface area and therefore has a higher BMR. **32.** The body's core is the organs within the skull and the thoracic and abdominal cavities. **33.** Cindy's body temperature is rising as heat-promoting mechanisms (shivering, chills) are activated. Something (an infection?) has caused the hypothalamic thermostat to be set to a higher level (fever) temporarily. **34.** In conduction, heat is transferred directly from one object to another (a hot surface to your palm). In convection, air warmed by body heat is continually removed (warm air rises) and replaced by cooler air (cool air falls), which in turn will absorb heat radiating from the body. **35.** Metabolic rate falls in old age because muscle mass declines and physical activity tends to be reduced. **36.** Elderly nutrition can be influenced and impaired by alcohol, certain antibiotics that interfere with food absorption, other drugs that may cause electrolyte imbalances, and use of mineral oil.

Review Questions 1. a; **2.** c; **3.** b; **4.** d; **5.** b; **6.** c; **7.** a; **8.** d; **9.** d; **10.** a; **11.** b; **12.** d; **13.** c; **14.** d; **15.** a

Case Study 1. Blood pH: Low (normal: 7.35–7.45); Blood glucose: High (normal: 70–120 mg/dl); Blood ketone bodies: High (normally negative); Urine pH: Low (normal: 4.5–8.0) **2.** Ketone bodies have an acetone smell that can be detected in the urine and the breath. Mr. Boulard is producing abnormal amounts of ketone bodies, which are accumulating in his blood. These substances are being excreted into the urine and diffusing out of the lungs and into the exhaled air. **3.** Ketogenesis, or the production of ketone bodies, is a process that occurs primarily in hepatocytes (liver cells) when carbohydrates are unavailable as an energy source. In this case, the hepatocytes metabolize fats. The fatty acids produced from fat breakdown (lipolysis) are converted to acetyl CoA by beta oxidation. In the absence of glucose, these acetyl CoA molecules cannot enter the Krebs cycle, and hepatocytes convert them into ketone bodies. **4.** Mr. Boulard's elevated blood glucose and his acidotic state indicate diabetes mellitus. In both type 1 and type 2 diabetes, the absence of insulin's actions means that the cells are unable to efficiently take up and utilize glucose from the blood. As a result, blood glucose levels are high, yet the cells are forced to switch to an alternative energy source such as lipids, which results in the production of ketone bodies in a diabetic patient. The stress of alcohol-induced dehydration can trigger ketoacidosis by causing the release of stress hormones that make diabetes worse. **5.** The pH of Mr. Boulard's blood and urine is abnormally low because ketone bodies are acidic (keto acids). As the concentration of ketone bodies in the blood rises, the blood pH falls (acidosis). The kidneys correct the blood pH by moving ketone bodies into the urine, making acidic urine.

Chapter 25

Check Your Understanding 1. The lower part of his rib cage and the perirenal fat capsule protect his kidneys from blows. **2.** The layers of supportive tissue around each kidney are the fibrous capsule, the perirenal fat capsule, and the renal fascia. The parietal peritoneum overlies the anterior renal fascia. **3.** The renal pelvis, which has extensions called calyces, is continuous with the ureter. **4.** Filtrate is formed in the glomerular capsule and then passes through the proximal convoluted tubule (PCT), the descending and ascending limbs of the nephron loop, and the distal convoluted tubule (DCT). **5.** The structural differences are (1) juxtamedullary nephrons have long nephron loops (with long thin segments) and renal corpuscles that are near the cortex-medulla junction, whereas cortical nephrons have short nephron loops and renal corpuscles that lie more superficially in the cortex; (2) efferent arterioles of juxtamedullary nephrons supply vasa recta, while efferent arterioles of cortical nephrons supply peritubular capillaries. **6.** The glomerular capillaries are fenestrated capillaries. (See Figure 19.3 on p. 697 to refresh your memory of capillary types.) Their function is to filter large amounts of plasma into the glomerular capsule. **7.** Intrinsic controls serve to maintain a nearly constant GFR in spite of changes in systemic blood pressure. Extrinsic controls serve to maintain systemic blood pressure. **8.** Net filtration pressure is 5 mm Hg [50 mm Hg − (25 mm Hg + 20 mm Hg)]. **9.** Hydrostatic pressure in the glomerular capillaries (HP_{gc}) is regulated by intrinsic and extrinsic controls of GFR. **10.** The majority of reabsorption occurs in the proximal convoluted tubule. **11.** In primary active transport, the energy for the process is provided directly by the cleavage of ATP. In secondary active transport, the energy for the process is provided by the Na^+ concentration gradient. As Na^+ moves down its own concentration gradient established by the active pumping of Na^+ occurring elsewhere in the cell, it drives the movement of another substance (e.g., glucose) against its concentration gradient. **12.** The reabsorption of Na^+ by primary active transport drives reabsorption of amino acids and glucose by secondary active transport. It also drives passive reabsorption of chloride, and reabsorption of water by osmosis. The reabsorption of water leaves behind other solutes, which become more concentrated and can therefore be reabsorbed by diffusion. **13.** H^+, K^+, NH_4^+, creatinine, urea, and uric acid are all substances that are secreted into the kidney tubules. **14.** The descending limb of the nephron loop is permeable to water and impermeable to NaCl. The ascending limb is impermeable to water and permeable to NaCl. **15.** ADH is released from the posterior pituitary in response to hyperosmotic extracellular fluid (as sensed by hypothalamic osmoreceptors). ADH causes insertion of aquaporins into the apical membrane of the principal cells of the collecting ducts. **16.** The normal renal clearance value for amino acids is zero. You would expect this because amino acids are valuable as nutrients and as the building blocks for protein synthesis, so it would not be good to lose them in the urine. **17.** The three major nitrogenous wastes excreted in urine are urea, creatinine, and uric acid. **18.** A kidney stone blocking the ureter would interfere with urine flow to the bladder. The pain would occur in waves that coincide with the peristaltic contractions of the smooth muscle of the ureter. **19.** The trigone is a smooth triangular region at the base of the bladder. Its borders are defined by the openings for the ureters and the urethra. **20.** The prostatic urethra, the intermediate part of the urethra, and the spongy urethra are the three regions of the male urethra. **21.** The detrusor contracts in response to increased firing of parasympathetic nerves. The internal urethral sphincter opens. **22.** The three sets of embryonic kidneys in the order that they develop are the pronephros, mesonephros, and metanephros. **23.** Both loss of bladder tone with age and an increase in size of the prostate can contribute to urinary retention in elderly men.

Review Questions 1. d; **2.** b; **3.** c; **4.** d; **5.** c; **6.** b; **7.** a; **8.** c; **9.** a; **10.** b

Case Study 1. Albumin is the smallest and most abundant plasma protein. More than trace amounts of albumin are not normally found in urine, so its presence indicates damage to the filtration membrane of the nephron. **2.** These medications were prescribed to treat Mr. Boulard's hypertension. Both diabetes and hypertension can cause kidney damage, and hypertension is a major cause of other cardiovascular diseases such as heart failure and stroke. Albuminuria indicates that Mr. Boulard already has damage to his kidneys, so it is important to protect his kidneys from further damage. **3.** Thiazide diuretics increase urine output by inhibiting Na^+ reabsorption in the DCT. This decreases blood volume, which decreases blood pressure. **4.** While Mr. Boulard still has hypertension, his main problem is that his blood K^+ is low. He is losing too much K^+ in his urine. This is the underlying cause of his irregular heartbeat, which could turn into a fatal arrhythmia if his hypokalemia is not corrected. **5.** Thiazide diuretics increase Na^+ excretion and decrease blood pressure. To compensate for these thiazide effects, Mr. Boulard's renin-angiotensin-aldosterone mechanism is activated. Aldosterone increases Na^+ reabsorption and K^+ secretion, resulting in hypokalemia (low blood K^+). **6.** ACE inhibitors decrease blood pressure by blocking the action of angiotensin converting enzyme and so reducing the amount of circulating angiotensin II. Because angiotensin II increases blood pressure in a number of ways, including by increasing aldosterone release and causing vasoconstriction (see Figure 19.10 on p. 708), ACE inhibitors are very effective at lowering blood pressure. (ACE inhibitors also help minimize kidney damage in diabetes.) **7.** Yes. The ACE inhibitors would have prevented the formation of excess angiotensin II and the resulting release of aldosterone. This would have lessened excess secretion of K^+.

Chapter 26

Check Your Understanding 1. You have more intracellular than extracellular fluid and more interstitial fluid than plasma. **2.** Na^+ is the major cation in the ECF and K^+ is the major cation in the ICF. The intracellular counterparts to extracellular Cl^- are HPO_4^{2-} and protein anions. **3.** If you eat salty pretzels, your extracellular fluid volume will expand even if you don't ingest fluids. This is because water will flow by osmosis from the intracellular fluid to the extracellular fluid. **4.** An increase in osmolality of the plasma is most important for triggering thirst. This change is sensed by osmoreceptors in the hypothalamus. **5.** ADH cannot add water—it can only conserve what is already there. In order to reduce an increase in osmolality of body fluids, the thirst mechanism is required. **6.** (a) A loss of plasma proteins causes edema. (b) Copious sweating causes dehydration. (c) Using ecstasy (together with drinking lots of fluids) could cause hypotonic hydration because it promotes ADH secretion, which interferes with the body's ability to get rid of extra water. **7.** Insufficient aldosterone would cause Jacob's plasma Na^+ to be decreased and his plasma K^+ to be elevated. The decrease in plasma Na^+ would cause a decrease in blood pressure, because plasma Na^+ is directly related to blood volume, which is a major determinant of blood pressure. **8.** The kidneys' handling of K^+ can be summed up as "The kidneys reabsorb most of the filtered K^+ in the proximal parts of the kidney's tubules and then secrete just the right amount in the distal parts (collecting duct)." **9.** The major regulator of calcium in the blood is parathyroid hormone. Hypercalcemia decreases excitability of neurons and muscle cells and may cause life-threatening cardiac arrhythmias. Hypocalcemia increases excitability and causes muscle tetany. **10.** Acidemia is an arterial pH below 7.35 and alkalemia is a pH above 7.45. **11.** A weak base would be better at minimizing the shift in pH caused by adding a strong acid to a solution because its ability to loosely tie up H^+ allows it to act as a buffer. **12.** The three major chemical buffer systems of the body are the bicarbonate buffer system, the phosphate buffer system, and the protein buffer system. The most important intracellular buffer is the protein buffer system. **13.** Joanne's ventilation would be increased. The acidosis caused by the accumulated ketone bodies will stimulate the peripheral chemoreceptors, and this will cause more CO_2 to be "blown off" in an attempt to restore pH to normal. **14.** Reabsorption of HCO_3^- is always linked with secretion of H^+. **15.** The most important urine buffer of H^+ is the phosphate buffer system. **16.** The tubule and collecting duct cells generate new HCO_3^- either by excreting ammonium ion (NH_4^+) or by excreting buffered H^+ ions. **17.** Key features of an uncompensated metabolic alkalosis are an increase in blood pH and an increase in blood HCO_3^-. Key features of an uncompensated respiratory acidosis are a decrease in blood pH and an increase in blood P_{CO_2}. **18.** The kidneys compensate for respiratory acidosis by excreting more H^+ and generating new HCO_3^- to buffer the acidosis. **19.** Infants' immature kidneys are not as proficient at concentrating urine. In addition, they have a high metabolic rate, so they produce more metabolic water and also have larger amounts of metabolic wastes and acids that need to be excreted with water.

Review Questions 1. a; **2.** c; **3.** b; **4.** a and b; **5.** h, i; **6.** c, g; **7.** a, e; **8.** b; **9.** a, b; **10.** j; **11.** b, d; **12.** a; **13.** c

Case Study 1. Mr. Heyden's vital signs suggest that he is in hypovolemic shock, which is probably due to an internal hemorrhage. **2.** The spleen is a highly vascular organ due to its role as a blood-filtering organ. The macrophages in Mr. Heyden's liver and bone marrow will help compensate for the loss of his spleen. **3.** Elevation of renin, aldosterone, and antidiuretic hormone indicate that Mr. Heyden's body is trying to compensate for his falling blood pressure and blood loss. Renin: released when renal blood flow is diminished and blood pressure falls. The angiotensin-aldosterone response is initiated by renin. The formation of angiotensin II leads to vasoconstriction, which will increase blood pressure, and to the release of aldosterone. Aldosterone: increases Na^+ reabsorption by the kidney. The movement of this reabsorbed Na^+ into the bloodstream will promote the movement of water from the interstitial fluid, resulting in an increase in blood volume. Antidiuretic hormone (ADH): released when the hypothalamic osmoreceptors sense an increase in osmolality. ADH has two consequences: It is a potent vasoconstrictor and will increase blood pressure, and it promotes water retention by the kidney, increasing blood volume. **4.** (a) Mr. Heyden's urine production may be decreased for several reasons. The severe drop in his blood pressure would reduce renal blood flow, thus reducing glomerular blood pressure and decreasing his glomerular filtration rate. The elevation in his ADH levels can reduce urine output due to increased water reabsorption by the kidney. He may also have damage to the kidney due to his crush injury in the left lumbar region. (b) The presence of casts and a brownish-red color in his urine are probably due to damaged cells and blood. If he has suffered kidney damage due to being crushed, he may have nephron damage that would include disruption of the filtration membrane, allowing red blood cells to pass into the filtrate and therefore the urine. He may also have damaged renal tubules and peritubular capillaries, allowing entry of blood and damaged renal tubule epithelial cells into the filtrate.

Chapter 27

Check Your Understanding 1. The testes produce the male gametes (sperm) and testosterone. **2.** The sperm factories are the seminiferous tubules. **3.** When the ambient temperature is cold, the associated muscles contract, bringing the testes close to the warm body wall. When body temperature is high, the associated muscles relax, allowing the testes to hang away from the body wall. The pampiniform venous plexus absorbs heat from the arterial blood before it enters the testes. **4.** The erectile tissue of the penis allows the penis to become stiff so that it may more efficiently enter the female vagina to deliver sperm. **5.** The organs of the male duct system in order from the epididymis to the body exterior are the ductus deferens, ejaculatory duct, prostatic urethra, intermediate part of the urethra, and spongy urethra. **6.** These stereocilia pass nutrients to the sperm and absorb excess testicular fluid. **7.** The ductus deferens runs from the scrotum into the abdominal cavity. **8.** Adolph probably has a hypertrophied prostate, a condition which can be felt through the anterior wall of the rectum. **9.** The seminal glands produce the bulk of seminal fluid. **10.** Semen is sperm plus the secretions of the male accessory glands. **11.** Erection is the stiffening of the penis that occurs when blood in the cavernous tissue is prevented from leaving the penis. It is caused by the parasympathetic division of the autonomic nervous system. **12.** Resolution is a period of muscular and psychological relaxation that follows orgasm. It results as the sympathetic nervous system causes constriction of the internal pudendal arteries, reducing blood flow to the penis, and activates small muscles that force blood out of the penis. **13.** Meiosis reduces the chromosomal count from $2n$ to n and introduces variability. **14.** The sperm head is the compacted DNA-containing nucleus. The acrosome that caps the head is a lysosome-like sac of enzymes. The midpiece contains the energy-producing mitochondria. The tail, a flagellum fashioned by a centriole, is the propulsive structure. **15.** Sustentocytes provide nutrients and essential development signals to the developing sperm and form the blood testis barrier that prevents sperm antigens from escaping into the blood. Interstitial endocrine cells secrete testosterone. **16.** The HPG axis is the hormonal interrelationship between the hypothalamus, anterior pituitary, and gonads that regulates the production of gametes and sex hormones (e.g., sperm production and testosterone in the male). **17.** Follicle-stimulating hormone indirectly stimulates spermatogenesis by prompting the sustentocytes to secrete androgen-binding protein. Androgen-binding protein keeps the concentration of testosterone high in the vicinity of the spermatogenic cells, which directly stimulates spermatogenesis. **18.** Secondary sex characteristics of males include appearance of pubic, axillary, and facial hair, deepening of the voice, increased oiliness of the skin, and increased size (length and mass) of the bones and skeletal muscles. **19.** The female's internal genitalia include the ovaries and duct system (uterine tubes, uterus, and vagina). **20.** The ovaries produce the female gametes and secrete female sex hormones (estrogens and progesterone). **21.** The antrum is the fluid-filled cavity of a mature follicle. **22.** Women are more at risk for PID than men because the duct system of women is incomplete—there is no physical connection between the ovary and the uterine tubes, which are open to the pelvic cavity. In men, the duct system is continuous from the testes to the body exterior. **23.** The waving action of the fimbriae and currents created by the beating cilia help to direct the ovulated oocytes into the uterine tube. **24.** The usual site of fertilization is the uterine tube. The uterus serves as the incubator for fetal development. **25.** The greater vestibular glands are the female homologue of the male bulbo-urethral glands. **26.** Both the penis and clitoris are hooded by a skin fold and are largely erectile tissue. However, the clitoris lacks a corpus spongiosum containing a urethra, so the urinary and reproductive systems are completely separate in females. **27.** Developmentally, the mammary glands are modified sweat glands. **28.** Breast cancer usually arises from the epithelial cells of the small ducts. **29.** The products of meiosis in females are 3 polar bodies (tiny haploid cells with essentially no cytoplasm) and 1 haploid ovum (functional gamete). Meiosis in males yields 4 functional gametes, the haploid sperm. **30.** Identical twins develop from separation of a very young embryo (the result of fertilization by a single sperm) into two parts. Fraternal twins develop when different oocytes are fertilized by different sperm. **31.** In the luteal phase, the ovulated follicle develops into a corpus luteum, which then secretes progesterone (and some estrogen). **32.** Leptin is important in advising the brain of the girl's readiness (relative to energy stores) for puberty. **33.** FSH prompts follicle growth and LH prompts ovulation. **34.** Estrogen exerts positive feedback on the anterior pituitary that leads to a burstlike release of LH. **35.** Estrogen is responsible for the secondary sex characteristics of females. **36.** Estrogen promotes epiphyseal closure in both males and females. **37.** The human papillomavirus (HPV) is most associated with cervical cancer. **38.** Chlamydia is the most common bacterial sexually transmitted infection in the U.S. **39.** No. If the sex chromosomes are XY, a male baby will develop. **40.** The sexually indifferent stage of development is the early period when the presumptive reproductive structures can produce either male or female organs. **41.** The gubernaculum guides the descent of the testis into the scrotum. **42.** Early signs of puberty's onset in boys are enlargement of the testes and scrotum. **43.** Menopause has happened when menstruation has not occurred for a year.

Review Questions 1. a and b; **2.** d; **3.** a; **4.** d; **5.** b; **6.** d; **7.** d; **8.** c; **9.** a, c, e, f; **10.** (1)c, f; (2)e, h; (3)g; (4)a; (5)b, e, and g; (6)f; **11.** a; **12.** c; **13.** d; **14.** b; **15.** a; **16.** b; **17.** c

Case Study 1. Carcinoma is the term for cancer originating from epithelial tissue. The primary source of Mr. Heyden's cancer is likely to be the prostate. **2.** Elevation of PSA levels suggests carcinoma of the prostate. (In addition, Mr. Heyden's age places him in a group that is at relatively higher risk for this type of cancer.) **3.** Digital examination of Mr. Heyden's prostate should detect the presence of carcinoma in this tissue. In addition, transrectal ultrasound imaging may be used in screening, and biopsies of prostate tissue follow positive results of tests. **4.** Mr. Heyden's carcinoma has advanced to the point of metastasis. He will probably undergo a treatment that reduces the levels of androgens in his body, as androgens promote growth of the prostate-derived tissue. These treatments could include castration or administration of drugs that block the production and/or effects of androgens.

Chapter 28

Check Your Understanding 1. Before they can penetrate an oocyte, sperm must be capacitated, and an oocyte's zona pellucida must be eroded by the acrosomal enzymes of many sperm. **2.** The cortical reaction, or slow block to polyspermy, involves the release of enzymes from cortical granules to the oocyte exterior, which accomplishes destruction of the oocyte's sperm receptors and also the detachment of any sperm still bound to receptors. These events ensure monospermy. **3.** The blastocyst is only slightly larger than the zygote because, although cell division has been going on (cleavage divisions), there is essentially no time for growth between divisions, so the resulting cells get smaller and smaller. The result is a large number of cells with a high surface-to-volume ratio. **4.** The trophoblast cells contribute to the formation of the placenta. **5.** The syncytiotrophoblast actually accomplishes implantation. **6.** The blastocyst secretes the hormone human chorionic gonadotropin, which is detectable in the urine. **7.** The chorion develops from the trophoblast and a layer of extraembryonic mesoderm. **8.** The decidua basalis cooperates with the chorionic villi to form the placenta. **9.** The placenta is usually fully functional by the end of the third month of pregnancy. **10.** The amnion helps to maintain a constant temperature for the developing fetus, protects it from physical trauma, and prevents adhesion of fetal parts. **11.** The allantois provides the basis of the umbilical cord, which provides a pathway for the embryonic blood vessels to reach the placenta. **12.** Before organogenesis can occur in earnest, the embryonic body must fold and undercut to form a tubular embryo. **13.** The mesoderm gives rise to essentially all body tissues except neural and epidermal tissue and mucosae. **14.** The fetal period begins at the end of 8 weeks. **15.** Difficult breathing during late pregnancy is due to the fact that the uterus is pressing against and crowding the diaphragm (and hence the lungs). The waddling gait is due to the relaxing effect of relaxin on the pelvic ligaments and the pubic symphysis. **16.** While the exact cause of morning sickness is unknown, it is thought to be due to the rising levels of female sex hormones and hCG in the mother's blood, which sometimes takes a while to get used to. **17.** The hormone hPL works with estrogen and progesterone to stimulate breast maturation in the pregnant woman, promotes fetal growth, and exerts a glucose-sparing effect on the mother. **18.** Breech presentation is a buttock-first presentation of the baby during labor. **19.** Prostaglandins are most responsible for triggering true labor. **20.** The descent of the baby's head (the largest part of its body) follows the widest dimensions of the bony pelvis. **21.** The foramen ovale and ductus arteriosus allow most of the blood to bypass the heart. **22.** For the most part, the special fetal circulatory modifications are occluded at birth or shortly thereafter. **23.** Oxytocin causes the let-down reflex.

Review Questions 1. (1)a, (2)b, (3)b, (4)a; **2.** b; **3.** c; **4.** b; **5.** a; **6.** d; **7.** d; **8.** c; **9.** b; **10.** c; **11.** a; **12.** c; **13.** a; **14.** (1)e, (2)f, (3)a, (4)d, (5)h, (6)b, (7)g, (8)c

Case Study 1. A hospital pregnancy test works by detecting human chorionic gonadotropin (hCG) in the blood. Home pregnancy test kits detect this hormone in urine. **2.** Human chorionic gonadotropin is a hormone produced by the trophoblast cells that helps to maintain the viability of the corpus luteum. The corpus luteum is essential during early pregnancy because it is responsible for the production of estrogen and progesterone. These two hormones are required to maintain the uterus during the early stages of a pregnancy. **3.** While any amount of trauma can be cause for concern with a pregnancy, Mrs. Rodriguez's accident occurred prior to the formation of the placenta. If her accident had occurred a few weeks later, her blood loss may have had an impact on the oxygenation of her developing fetus. **4.** First, the egg that Mrs. Rodriguez released during her most recent ovulation is fertilized to form the zygote. Over the next week, embryonic development features many rapid rounds of cell division as the embryo moves through the uterine tube. Cleavage is the very early period of rapid cell division. By 72 hours after fertilization, the embryo is a ball of 16 or more cells called the morula. Around day 4, a fluid-filled cavity appears, which signals the formation of the blastocyst. Approximately one week after fertilization, the embryo has made its way into the uterus and begins the process of implantation. **5.** At this time, Mrs. Rodriguez's embryo transforms into a three-layered structure as the result of a process called gastrulation. This process involves the rearrangement and migration of cells as the three primary germ layers (ectoderm, mesoderm, and endoderm) are formed. These three layers serve as the primitive tissues from which all of the body organs will be formed as development continues.

Chapter 29

Check Your Understanding 1. Chromosomes are not visible during interphase. The DNA-containing material is in the form of dispersed strands of chromatin. As mitosis begins, the chromatin coils and condenses, becoming visible as chromosomes. Chromosomes continue to condense throughout prophase and are most visible during metaphase. **2.** Chromosomes other than sex chromosomes are called autosomes. **3.** An allele represented by a capital letter is presumed to be a dominant allele. **4.** Descriptions of his phenotype are blond, blue-eyed, and hairy chest. **5.** The alleles on different pairs of homologous chromosomes are segregated independently of each other to different gametes. **6.** It causes separations of linked genes on the same chromosome, producing gametes with variable genomes. **7.** Dominant genes are expressed. Thus if the dominant gene is lethal, the carrier will probably not live very long or will die during development. **8.** In incomplete dominance, the heterozygote has a phenotype intermediate between that of the dominant and recessive alleles [for example, for the sickling gene, the dominant homozygote (SS) has no evidence of sickling; the heterozygote (Ss) has sickle-cell trait; and the homozygote for the recessive gene (ss) has sickle-cell anemia]. In codominance, both dominant alleles are expressed (as in ABO blood types). **9.** A male always expresses an X-linked recessive allele because, unlike a female, he does not have a second X containing homologous alleles to blunt or counteract the effect. The Y chromosome lacks most of the genes carried on the X chromosome. **10.** Height is an example of a trait conferred by polygene inheritance in which several genes on different chromosomes contribute to the trait. Such traits show a distribution of phenotypes that yields a bell-shaped curve. **11.** Other genes, measles in a pregnant woman, and lack of key dietary nutrients all may alter gene expression. **12.** Genomic imprinting labels genes as maternal or paternal. **13.** Maternal mitochondrial DNA confers extranuclear inheritance. **14.** Amniocentesis analyzes chemicals and cells in amniotic fluid. **15.** Ultrasound imaging is used to determine some aspects of fetal development (fetal age for example) and is noninvasive.

Review Questions 1. (1)d, (2)g, (3)b, (4)a, (5)f, (6)c, (7)e, (8)h; **2.** (1)e, (2)a, (3)b, (4)d, (5)c, (6)d, (7)f

Case Study 1. A person's genotype is a description of the alleles that they carry. Phenotype refers to the way that those genes are expressed and show up as traits in the body. Mrs. Rodriguez's genotype is *ii* and her phenotype is O. Mr. Rodriguez's genotype is either I^AI^A or I^Ai. Either one of these genotypes would result in his phenotype, which is represented by his A blood type. **2.** Blood type is determined by multiple-allele inheritance. Three alleles (I^A, I^B, i) represent the three different blood types (A, B, O). The alleles for A and B blood type are codominant, which means that they are both expressed when combined together. The result of this combination would be the AB blood type. The allele for O blood type is recessive to both the A and B blood type alleles. **3.** Mr. Rodriguez's genotype can be either I^AI^A or I^Ai. We now know that Mr. Rodriguez's mother had O blood type, and that means that she carries two copies of the O blood type allele (*ii*). She must have passed on one of these alleles to Mr. Rodriguez. This means that Mr. Rodriguez's father must have passed on the allele for the A blood type. Mr. Rodriguez's genotype *must* be I^Ai. **4.** We know that Mrs. Rodriguez's genotype is *ii* and Mr. Rodriguez's genotype is I^Ai. The results of a Punnett square reveal that there is a 50% chance that Mrs. Rodriguez's baby will have the O blood type and a 50% chance that the baby will have the A blood type. The B and AB blood type require that one of the parents is carrying the B allele (I^B). Neither Mr. Rodriguez nor Mrs. Rodriguez carries this allele, so there should be a 0% chance of the baby having the B or AB blood type.

Glossary

Pronunciation Key

′ = Primary accent

″ = Secondary accent

Pronounce:

a, fa, āt	as in	fate	o, no, ōt	as in	note
ă, hă, at		hat	ŏ, frŏ, og		frog
ah		father	oo		soon
ar		tar	or		for
e, stre, ēt		street	ow		plow
ĕ, hĕ, en		hen	oy		boy
er		her	sh		she
ew		new	u, mu, ūt		mute
g		go	ŭ, sŭ, un		sun
i, bi, īt		bite	z		zebra
ĭ, hĭ, im		him	zh		measure
ng		ring			

Abduct (ab-dukt′) To move away from the midline of the body.

Absolute refractory period Period following stimulation during which no additional action potential can be evoked.

Absorption Process by which the products of digestion pass through the alimentary tube mucosa into the blood or lymph.

Accessory digestive organs Organs that contribute to the digestive process but are not part of the alimentary canal; include the tongue, teeth, salivary glands, pancreas, liver.

Accommodation The process of increasing the refractive power of the lens of the eye; focusing.

Acetabulum (as″ĕ-tab′u-lum) Cuplike cavity on lateral surface of the hip bone that receives the femur.

Acetylcholine (ACh) (as″ĕ-til-ko′lēn) Chemical transmitter substance released by some nerve endings.

Acetylcholinesterase (AChE) (as″ĕ-til-ko″lin-es′ter-ās) Enzyme present at the neuromuscular junction and synapses that degrades acetylcholine and terminates its action.

Achilles tendon *See* Calcaneal tendon.

Acid A substance that releases hydrogen ions when in solution (compare with Base); a proton donor.

Acid-base balance Situation in which the pH of the blood is maintained between 7.35 and 7.45.

Acidosis (as″ĭ-do′sis) State of abnormally high hydrogen ion concentration in the extracellular fluid.

Actin (ak′tin) A contractile protein of muscle.

Action potential A large transient depolarization event, including polarity reversal, that is conducted along the membrane of a muscle cell or a nerve fiber.

Activation energy The amount of energy required to push a reactant to the level necessary for action.

Active immunity Immunity produced by an encounter with an antigen; provides immunological memory.

Active site Region on the surface of a functional (globular) protein where it binds and interacts chemically with other molecules of complementary shape and charge.

Active (transport) processes (1) Membrane transport processes for which ATP is required, e.g., solute pumping and endocytosis. (2) "Active transport" also refers specifically to solute pumping.

Adaptation (1) Any change in structure or response to suit a new environment; (2) decline in the transmission of a sensory nerve when a receptor is stimulated continuously and without change in stimulus strength.

Adduct (a-dukt′) To move toward the midline of the body.

Adenine (A) (ad′ĕ-nēn) One of the two major purines found in both RNA and DNA; also found in various free nucleotides of importance to the body, such as ATP.

Adenohypophysis (ad″ĕ-no-hi-pof′ĭ-sis) Anterior pituitary; the glandular part of the pituitary gland.

Adenoids (ad′en-noids) Pharyngeal tonsil.

Adenosine triphosphate (ATP) (ah-den′o-sēn tri″fos′fāt) Organic molecule that stores and releases chemical energy for use in body cells.

Adipocyte (ad′ĭ-po-sīt) An adipose, or fat, cell.

Adipose tissue (ad′ĭ-pōs) Areolar connective tissue modified to store nutrients; a connective tissue consisting chiefly of fat cells.

Adrenal glands (uh-drē′nul) Hormone-producing glands located superior to the kidneys; each consists of medulla and cortex areas.

Adrenergic fibers (ad″ren-er′jik) Nerve fibers that release norepinephrine.

Adrenocorticotropic hormone (ACTH) (ah-dre″no-kor″tĭ-ko-trop′ik) Anterior pituitary hormone that influences the activity of the adrenal cortex.

Adventitia (ad″ven-tish′e-ah) Outermost layer or covering of some organs.

Aerobic (a′er-ōb″ik) Oxygen-requiring.

Aerobic endurance The length of time a muscle can continue to contract using aerobic pathways.

Aerobic respiration Respiration in which oxygen is consumed and glucose is broken down entirely; water, carbon dioxide, and large amounts of ATP are the final products.

Afferent (af′er-ent) Carrying to or toward a center.

Afferent (sensory) nerve Nerve that contains processes of sensory neurons and carries nerve impulses to the central nervous system.

Agglutination (ah-gloo″tĭ-na′shun) Clumping of (foreign) cells; induced by cross-linking of antigen-antibody complexes.

Agonist (ag′o-nist) Muscle that bears the major responsibility for effecting a particular movement; a prime mover.

AIDS Acquired immune deficiency syndrome; caused by human immunodeficiency virus (HIV); symptoms include severe weight loss, night sweats, swollen lymph nodes, opportunistic infections.

Albumin (al-bu′min) The most abundant plasma protein.

Aldosterone (al-dos′ter-ōn) Hormone produced by the adrenal cortex that regulates Na^+ reabsorption and K^+ secretion by the kidneys.

Alimentary canal (al″ĭ-men′tar-e) The continuous hollow tube extending from the mouth to the anus; its walls are constructed by the oral cavity, pharynx, esophagus, stomach, and small and large intestines.

Alkalosis (al″kah-lo′sis) State of abnormally low hydrogen ion concentration in the extracellular fluid.

Allantois (ah″lan′to-is) Embryonic membrane; its blood vessels develop into blood vessels of the umbilical cord.

Alleles Genes coding for the same trait and found at the same locus on homologous chromosomes.

Allergy A type of hypersensitivity (overzealous immune response to an otherwise harmless antigen) that involves IgE antibodies and histamine release.

Alopecia (al″o-pe′she-ah) Baldness.

Alpha (α)-helix The most common type of secondary structure of the amino acid chain in proteins; resembles the coils of a telephone cord.

Alveolar (acinar) gland (al-ve′o-lar) A gland whose secretory cells form small, flasklike sacs.

Alveolar ventilation rate (AVR) An index of respiratory efficiency; measures volume of fresh air that flows in and out of alveoli.

Alveolus (al-ve′o-lus) (1) One of the microscopic air sacs of the lungs; (2) tiny milk-producing glandular sac in the breast; (3) tooth socket.

Alzheimer's disease (AD) (altz′hi-merz) Degenerative brain disease resulting in progressive loss of memory and motor control, and increasing dementia.

Amino acid (ah-me′no) Organic compound containing nitrogen, carbon, hydrogen, and oxygen; building block of protein.

Ammonia (NH_3) Common waste product of protein breakdown in the body; a colorless volatile gas, very soluble in water and capable of forming a weak base; a proton acceptor.

Amniocentesis A common form of fetal testing in which a small sample of fluid is removed from the amniotic cavity.

Amnion (am′ne-on) Fetal membrane that forms a fluid-filled sac around the embryo.

Amoeboid motion (ah-me′boyd) The flowing movement of the cytoplasm of a phagocyte.

Amphiarthrosis (am″fe-ar-thro′sis) A slightly movable joint.

Ampulla (am-pul′lah) A localized dilation of a canal or duct.

Amylase Digestive system enzyme that breaks down starchy foods.

Anabolism (ah-nab′o-lizm) Energy-requiring building phase of metabolism in which simpler substances are combined to form more complex substances.

Anaerobic (an-a′er-ōb-ik) Not requiring oxygen.

Anaerobic glycolysis (gli-kol′ĭ-sis) Energy-yielding conversion of glucose to lactic acid in various tissues, notably muscle, when sufficient oxygen is not available.

Anaerobic threshold The point at which muscle metabolism converts to anaerobic glycolysis.

Anaphase Third stage of mitosis, meiosis I, and meiosis II in which daughter chromosomes move toward each pole of a cell.

Anastomosis (ah-nas″to-mo′sis) A union or joining of nerves, blood vessels, or lymphatics.

Anatomy Study of the structure of living organisms.

Androgen (an′dro-jen) A hormone such as testosterone that controls male secondary sex characteristics.

Anemia (ah-ne′me-ah) Reduced oxygen-carrying ability of blood resulting from too few erythrocytes or abnormal hemoglobin.

Aneurysm (an′u-rizm) Blood-filled sac in an artery wall caused by dilation or weakening of the wall.

Angina pectoris (an′jĭ-nah pek′tor-is) Severe suffocating chest pain caused by brief lack of oxygen supply to heart muscle.

Angiotensin II (an″je-o-ten′sin) A potent vasoconstrictor activated by renin; also triggers release of aldosterone.

Anion (an′i-on) An ion carrying one or more negative charges and therefore attracted to a positive pole.

Anoxia (ah-nŏk′se-ah) Deficiency of oxygen.

Antagonist (an-tag′o-nist) (1) Muscle that reverses, or opposes, the action of another muscle. (2) Hormone that opposes the action of another hormone.

Anterior pituitary *See* Adenohypophysis.

Antibody A protein molecule that is released by a plasma cell (a daughter cell of an activated B lymphocyte) and that binds specifically to an antigen; an immunoglobulin.

Anticodon (an″ti-ko′don) The three-base sequence complementary to the messenger RNA (mRNA) codon.

Antidiuretic hormone (ADH, also called vasopressin) (an″ti-di″yer-eh′tik) Hormone produced by the hypothalamus and released by the posterior pituitary; stimulates the kidneys to reabsorb more water, reducing urine volume.

Antigen (Ag) (an′tĭ-jen) A substance or part of a substance (living or nonliving) that is recognized as foreign by the immune system, activates the immune system, and reacts with immune cells or their products.

Antigen-presenting cell (APC) A specialized cell (dendritic cell, macrophage, or B cell) that captures, processes, and presents antigens on its surface to T lymphocytes.

Anucleate cell (a-nu′kle-āt) A cell without a nucleus.

Anus (a′nus) Distal end of digestive tract; outlet of rectum.

Aorta (a-or′tah) Major systemic artery; arises from the left ventricle of the heart.

Aortic body Receptor in the aortic arch sensitive to changing oxygen, carbon dioxide, and pH levels of the blood.

Apgar score Evaluation of an infant's physical status at 1 and 5 minutes after birth by assessing five criteria: heart rate, respiration, color, muscle tone, and reflexes.

Apnea Breathing cessation.

Apocrine sweat gland (ap′o-krin) The less numerous type of sweat gland; produces a secretion containing water, salts, proteins, and fatty acids.

Apoenzyme (ap′ō-en-zīm) The protein portion of an enzyme.

Aponeurosis (ap″o-nu-ro′sis) Fibrous or membranous sheet connecting a muscle and the part it moves.

Apoptosis A process of controlled cellular suicide; eliminates cells that are unneeded, stressed, or aged.

Appendicitis (ă-pen′dĭ-sī-′tis) Inflammation of the appendix (wormlike sac attached to the cecum of the large intestine).

Appendicular Relating to the limbs; one of the two major divisions of the body.

Appositional growth Growth accomplished by the addition of new layers onto those previously formed.

Aquaporins (ă″kwă-por′ins) Transmembrane proteins that form water channels.

Aqueous humor (a′kwe-us) Watery fluid in the anterior segment of the eye.

Arachnoid (ah-rak′noid) Weblike; specifically, the weblike arachnoid mater, the middle layer of the three meninges.

Areola (ah-re′o-lah) Circular, pigmented area surrounding the nipple; any small space in a tissue.

Areolar connective tissue A type of loose connective tissue.

Arrector pili (ah-rek′tor pi′li) Tiny, smooth muscles attached to hair follicles; contraction causes the hair to stand upright.

Arrhythmia (a-rith′me-ah) Irregular heart rhythm, often caused by defects in the intrinsic conduction system.

Arteries Blood vessels that conduct blood away from the heart and into the circulation.

Arteriole (ar-tēr′e-ōl) A minute artery.

Arteriosclerosis (ar-tē-r′e-o-skler-o′sis) Any of a number of proliferative and degenerative changes in the arteries leading to their decreased elasticity.

Arthritis Inflammation of the joints.

Arthroscopic surgery (ar-thro-skop′ik) Procedure enabling a surgeon to repair the interior of a joint through a small incision.

Articular capsule Double-layered capsule composed of an outer fibrous layer lined by synovial membrane; encloses the joint cavity of a synovial joint.

Articular cartilage Hyaline cartilage covering bone ends at movable joints.

Articulation (joint) The junction of two or more bones.

Association areas Functional areas of the cerebral cortex that act mainly to integrate diverse information for purposeful action.

Astigmatism (ah-stig′mah-tizm) A condition in which unequal curvatures in different parts of the cornea or lens of the eye lead to blurred vision.

Astrocyte (as′tro-sīt) A type of CNS supporting cell; assists in exchanges between blood capillaries and neurons.

Atelectasis (at″ĕ-lik′tah-sis) Lung collapse.

Atherosclerosis (a″ther-o″skler-o′sis) Changes in the walls of large arteries consisting of lipid deposits on the artery walls; one form of arteriosclerosis.

Atmospheric pressure Force that air exerts on the surface of the body (760 mm Hg at sea level).

Atom Smallest particle of an elemental substance that exhibits the properties of that element; composed of protons, neutrons, and electrons.

Atomic number The number of protons in an atom.

Atomic symbol The one- or two-letter symbol used to indicate an element; usually the first letter(s) of the element's name.

Atomic weight The average of the mass numbers of all the isotopes of an element.

ATP (adenosine triphosphate) (ah-den′o-sēn tri″fos′fāt) Organic molecule that stores and releases chemical energy for use in body cells.

Atria (a′tre-ah) The two superior receiving chambers of the heart.

Atrial natriuretic peptide (ANP) (a′tre-al na″tre-u-ret′ik) A hormone released by certain cells of the heart atria that reduces blood pressure and blood volume by inhibiting nearly all events that promote vasoconstriction and Na^+ and water retention.

Atrioventricular (AV) bundle (a″tre-o-ven-trĭ′kyoo-ler) Bundle of specialized fibers that conduct impulses from the AV node to the right and left ventricles; also called bundle of His.

Atrioventricular (AV) node Specialized mass of conducting cells located at the atrioventricular junction in the heart.

Atrioventricular (AV) valve Valve that prevents backflow into the atrium when the connected ventricle is contracting.

Atrophy (at′ro-fe) Reduction in size or wasting away of an organ or cell resulting from disease or lack of use.

Auditory ossicles (ah′sih-kulz) The three tiny bones serving as transmitters of vibrations and located within the middle ear: the malleus, incus, and stapes.

Auditory tube *See* Pharyngotympanic tube.

Autoimmunity Production of antibodies or effector T cells that attack a person's own tissue.

Autolysis (aw″tol′ĭ-sis) Process of autodigestion (self-digestion) of cells, especially dead or degenerate cells.

Autonomic ganglion Collection of sympathetic or parasympathetic postganglionic neuronal cell bodies.

Autonomic nervous system (ANS) Efferent division of the peripheral nervous system that innervates cardiac and smooth muscles and glands; also called the involuntary or visceral motor system.

Autonomic (visceral) reflexes Reflexes that activate smooth or cardiac muscle and/or glands.

Autoregulation The automatic local adjustment of blood flow to a particular body area in response to its current requirements.

Autosomes Chromosomes number 1 to 22; do not include the sex chromosomes.

Avogadro's number (av″o-gad′rōz) The number of molecules in one mole of any substance, 6.02×10^{23}.

Axial Relating to the head, neck, and trunk; one of the two major divisions of the body.

Axolemma (ak″so-lem′ah) The plasma membrane of an axon.

Axon Neuron process that carries impulses away from the nerve cell body; efferent process; the conducting portion of a nerve cell.

Axon terminals (terminal boutons) The bulbous distal endings of the terminal branches of an axon.

B cells Also called B lymphocytes; oversee humoral immunity; their descendants differentiate into antibody-producing plasma cells.

Baroreceptor (bayr″o-re-sep′tor) A sensory nerve ending in the wall of the carotid sinus or aortic arch sensitive to vessel stretching.

Basal body (ba′sal) An organelle structurally identical to a centriole and forming the base of a cilium or flagellum.

Basal ganglia *See* Basal nuclei.

Basal lamina (lam′ĭ-nah) Noncellular, adhesive supporting sheet consisting largely of glycoproteins secreted by epithelial cells.

Basal metabolic rate (BMR) Rate at which energy is expended (heat produced) by the body per unit time under controlled (basal) conditions: 12 hours after a meal, at rest.

Basal nuclei (basal ganglia) Specific gray matter areas located deep within the white matter of the cerebral hemispheres.

Basal surface The surface near the base or interior of a structure; nearest the lower side or bottom of a structure.

Base A substance capable of binding with hydrogen ions; a proton acceptor.

Basement membrane Extracellular material consisting of a basal lamina secreted by epithelial cells and a reticular lamina secreted by underlying connective tissue cells.

Basophil (ba′zo-fil) White blood cell whose granules stain purplish-black and nucleus purple with basic dye.

Benign (be-nīn′) Not malignant.

Bile Greenish-yellow or brownish fluid produced in and secreted by the liver, stored in the gallbladder, and released into the small intestine.

Bilirubin (bil″i-roo′bin) Yellow pigment of bile.

Bipolar neuron Neuron with axon and dendrite that extend from opposite sides of the cell body.

Blastocyst (blas′to-sist) Stage of early embryonic development; the product of cleavage.

Blood pressure (BP) Force exerted by blood against a unit area of the blood vessel walls; differences in blood pressure between different areas of the circulation provide the driving force for blood circulation.

Blood brain barrier Mechanism that inhibits passage of materials from the blood into brain tissues; reflects relative impermeability of brain capillaries.

Bolus (bo′lus) A rounded mass of food prepared by the mouth for swallowing; any soft round mass.

Bone marrow Fat- or blood-forming tissue found within bone cavities; called yellow and red bone marrow, respectively.

Bone (osseous tissue) (os′e-us) A connective tissue that forms the bony skeleton.

Bone remodeling Process involving bone formation and destruction in response to hormonal and mechanical factors.

Bone resorption The removal of osseous tissue; part of the continuous bone remodeling process.

Bowman's capsule (bo-manz) *See* Glomerular capsule.

Boyle's law States that when the temperature is constant, the pressure of a gas varies inversely with its volume.

Bradycardia (brad″e-kar′de-ah) A heart rate below 60 beats per minute.

Brain death State of irreversible coma, even though life-support measures may have restored other body organs.

Brain stem Collectively the midbrain, pons, and medulla of the brain.

Brain ventricle Fluid-filled cavity of the brain.

Branchial groove (brang′ke-al) An indentation of the surface ectoderm in the embryo; the external acoustic meatus develops from it.

Bronchioles Smaller ($<$1 mm in diameter) branching air passageways inside the lungs.

Bronchus (brong′kus) One of the two large branches of the trachea that lead to the lungs.

Buffer Chemical substance or system that minimizes changes in pH by releasing or binding hydrogen ions.

Burn Tissue damage inflicted by intense heat, electricity, radiation, or certain chemicals, all of which denature cell proteins and kill cells in the affected areas.

Bursa (ber′sa) A fibrous sac lined with synovial membrane and containing synovial fluid; occurs between bones and muscle tendons (or other structures), where it acts to decrease friction during movement.

Bursitis Inflammation of a bursa.

Calcaneal tendon (kal-ka′ne-al) Tendon that attaches the calf muscles to the heelbone (calcaneus); also called the Achilles tendon.

Calcitonin (kal″sih-to′nin) Hormone released by the thyroid. Lowers blood calcium levels only when present at high (therapeutic) levels.

Calculus (kal′ku-lus) A stone formed within various body parts.

Callus (kal′lus) (1) Localized thickening of skin epidermis resulting from physical trauma; (2) repair tissue (fibrous or bony) formed at a fracture site.

Calorie (cal) Amount of energy needed to raise the temperature of 1 gram of water 1° Celsius. Energy exchanges associated with biochemical reactions are usually reported in kilocalories (1 kcal = 1000 cal), also called large calories (Cal).

Calyx (ka′liks) A cuplike extension of the pelvis of the kidney.

Canaliculus (kan″ah-lik′u-lus) Extremely small tubular passage or channel.

Cancer A malignant, invasive cellular neoplasm that has the capability of spreading throughout the body or body parts.

Capillaries (kap′il-layr″ēs) The smallest of the blood vessels and the sites of exchange between the blood and tissue cells.

Carbohydrate (kar″bo-hi′drāt) Organic compound composed of carbon, hydrogen, and oxygen; includes starches, sugars, cellulose.

Carbonic acid–bicarbonate buffer system Chemical system that helps maintain pH homeostasis of the blood.

Carbonic anhydrase (kar-bon′ik an-hi′drās) Enzyme that facilitates the combination of carbon dioxide with water to form carbonic acid.

Carcinogen (kar″sĭ′no-jin) Cancer-causing agent.

Cardiac cycle Sequence of events encompassing one complete contraction and relaxation of the atria and ventricles of the heart.

Cardiac muscle Specialized muscle of the heart.

Cardiac output (CO) Amount of blood pumped out of a ventricle in one minute.

Cardiac reserve The difference between resting and maximal cardiac output.

Cardiogenic shock Pump failure; the heart is so inefficient that it cannot sustain adequate circulation.

Cardiovascular system Organ system that distributes the blood to deliver nutrients and remove wastes.

Carotene (kar′o-tēn) Yellow to orange pigment that accumulates in the stratum corneum epidermal layer and in fatty tissue of the hypodermis.

Carotid body (kar-rot′id) A receptor in the common carotid artery sensitive to changing oxygen, carbon dioxide, and pH levels of the blood.

Carotid sinus (si′nus) A dilation of a common carotid artery; involved in regulation of systemic blood pressure.

Carrier A transmembrane protein that changes shape to envelop and transport a polar substance across the cell membrane.

Cartilage (kar′tĭ-lij) White, semiopaque connective tissue.

Cartilage bone (endochondral bone) Bone formed by using hyaline cartilage structures as models for ossification.

Cartilaginous joints (kar″ti-laj′ĭ-nus) Bones united by cartilage; no joint cavity is present.

Catabolism (ka-tab′o-lizm) Process in which living cells break down substances into simpler substances.

Catalyst (kat′ah-list) Substance that increases the rate of a chemical reaction without itself becoming chemically changed or part of the product.

Cataract Clouding of the eye's lens; often congenital or age-related.

Catecholamines (kat″ĕ-kol′ah-mēnz) Epinephrine, norepinephrine, and dopamine; a class of amines that act as chemical transmitters.

Cation (kat′i-on) An ion with a positive charge.

Caudal (kaw′dul) Literally, toward the tail; in humans, the inferior portion of the anatomy.

Cecum (se′kum) The blind-ended pouch at the beginning of the large intestine.

Cell Structural unit of all living things.

Cell differentiation The development of specific and distinctive features in cells, from a single cell (the fertilized egg) to all the specialized cells of adulthood.

Cell cycle Series of changes a cell goes through from the time it is formed until it reproduces itself.

Cell membrane *See* Plasma membrane.

Cellular immunity Immunity conferred by activated T cells, which directly kill infected or cancerous body cells or cells of foreign grafts and release chemicals that regulate the immune response. Also called cell-mediated immunity.

Cellular respiration Metabolic processes in which ATP is produced.

Cellulose (sel′u-lōs) A fibrous carbohydrate that is the main structural component of plant tissues.

Central (Haversian) canal (hah-ver′zhan) The canal in the center of each osteon that contains minute blood vessels and nerve fibers that serve the needs of the osteocytes.

Central nervous system (CNS) Brain and spinal cord.

Centriole (sen′tre-ol) Minute body found near the nucleus of the cell; active in cell division.

Centrosome (cell center) A region near the nucleus which contains paired organelles called centrioles.

Cerebellum (ser″ĕ-bel′um) Brain region most involved in producing smooth, coordinated skeletal muscle activity.

Cerebral aqueduct (ser′ĕ-bral, sĕ-re′bral) The slender cavity of the midbrain that connects the third and fourth ventricles.

Cerebral arterial circle (*circle of Willis*) An arterial anastomosis at the base of the brain.

Cerebral cortex The outer gray matter region of the cerebral hemispheres.

Cerebral dominance Designates the hemisphere that is dominant for language.

Cerebral palsy Neuromuscular disability in which voluntary muscles are poorly controlled or paralyzed as a result of brain damage.

Cerebral white matter Consists largely of myelinated fibers bundled into large tracts; provides for communication between cerebral areas and lower CNS centers.

Cerebrospinal fluid (CSF) (ser″ĕ-bro-spi′nal) Plasmalike fluid that fills the cavities of the CNS and surrounds the CNS externally; protects the brain and spinal cord.

Cerebrovascular accident (CVA) (ser″ĕ-bro-vas′ku-lar) Condition in which brain tissue is deprived of a blood supply, as in blockage of a cerebral blood vessel; a stroke.

Cerebrum (ser′ĕ-brum) The cerebral hemispheres (including the cerebral cortex, white matter, and basal nuclei).

Cervical vertebrae The seven vertebrae of the vertebral column located in the neck.

Cervix Lower outlet of the uterus extending into the vagina.

Channel A transmembrane protein that forms an aqueous pore, allowing substances to move from one side of the membrane to the other.

Chemical bond An energy relationship holding atoms together; involves the interaction of electrons.

Chemical energy Energy stored in the bonds of chemical substances.

Chemical equilibrium A state of apparent repose created by two reactions proceeding in opposite directions at equal speed.

Chemical reaction Process in which molecules are formed, changed, or broken down.

Chemoreceptor (ke″mo-re-sep′ter) Receptor sensitive to various chemicals in solution.

Chemotaxis (ke″mo-tak′sis) Movement of a cell, organism, or part of an organism toward or away from a chemical substance.

Cholecystokinin (CCK) (ko″le-sis″to-ki′nin) An intestinal hormone that stimulates gallbladder contraction and pancreatic juice release.

Cholesterol (ko-les′ter-ol″) Steroid found in animal fats as well as in most body tissues; made by the liver.

Cholinergic fibers (ko″lin-er′jik) Nerve endings that, upon stimulation, release acetylcholine.

Chondroblast (kon′dro-blast) Actively mitotic cell of cartilage.

Chondrocyte (kon′dro-sīt) Mature cell of cartilage.

Chorion (kor′e-on) Outermost fetal membrane; helps form the placenta.

Chorionic villus sampling (ko″re-on′ik vil′us) Fetal testing procedure in which bits of the chorionic villi from the placenta are snipped off and the cells karyotyped. This procedure can be done as early as 8 weeks into the pregnancy.

Choroid (ko′roid) The vascular middle layer of the eye.

Choroid plexus (ko′roid plex′sus) A capillary knot that protrudes into a brain ventricle; produces cerebrospinal fluid.

Chromatin (kro′mah-tin) Structures in the nucleus that carry the hereditary factors (genes).

Chromosomes (kro′mo-somz) Barlike bodies of tightly coiled chromatin; visible during cell division.

Chronic obstructive pulmonary disease (COPD) Collective term for progressive, obstructive respiratory disorders; includes emphysema, chronic bronchitis.

Chyme (kīm) Semifluid, creamy mass consisting of partially digested food and gastric juice.

Cilia (sil′e-ah) Tiny, hairlike projections on cell surfaces that move in a wavelike manner.

Circumduction (ser″kum-duk′shun) Movement of a body part so that it outlines a cone in space.

Cirrhosis (sĭ-ro′sis) Chronic disease of the liver, characterized by an overgrowth of connective tissue, or fibrosis.

Cisterna chyli (sis-ter′nah ki′li) An enlarged sac at the base of the thoracic duct; the origin of the thoracic duct.

Cisternae (sis-ter′ne) Any cavity or enclosed space serving as a reservoir.

Cleavage An early embryonic phase consisting of rapid mitotic cell divisions without intervening growth periods; product is a blastocyst.

Clonal selection (klo′nul) Process during which a B cell or T cell becomes activated by binding with an antigen.

Clone Descendants of a single cell.

Coagulation Process in which blood is transformed from a liquid to a gel; blood clotting.

Cochlea (kok′le-ah) Snail-shaped chamber of the bony labyrinth that houses the receptor for hearing [the spiral organ (organ of Corti)].

Codon (ko′don) The three-base sequence on a messenger RNA molecule that provides the genetic information used in protein synthesis; code for a given amino acid.

Coenzyme (ko-en′zīm) Nonprotein substance associated with and activating an enzyme, typically a vitamin.

Cofactor Metal ion or organic molecule that is required for enzyme activity.

Collagen fiber The most abundant of the three fibers found in the matrix of connective tissue.

Colloid (kol′oid) (1) A mixture in which the solute particles (usually proteins) do not settle out readily. (2) Substance in the thyroid gland containing thyroglobulin protein.

Colloid osmotic pressure (kol′oid ahz-mah′tik) Pressure created in a fluid by large nondiffusible molecules, such as plasma proteins that are prevented from moving through a (capillary) membrane. Such substances tend to draw water to them.

Colon Regions of the large intestine; includes ascending, transverse, descending, and sigmoid portions.

Combination (synthesis) reaction Chemical reaction in which larger, more complex atoms or molecules are formed from simpler ones.

Complement A group of bloodborne proteins, which, when activated, enhance the inflammatory and immune responses and may lead to cell lysis.

Complementarity of structure and function The relationship between a structure and its function; i.e., structure determines function.

Complementary base Refers to how a given nitrogenous base of DNA or RNA bonds to another nitrogenous base. For example, adenine (A) is the complementary base of thymine (T). The result is base pairing.

Complete blood count (CBC) Clinical test that includes counts of all formed elements, a hematocrit, and measurements of erythrocyte size and hemoglobin content.

Compound Substance composed of two or more different elements, the atoms of which are chemically united.

Concentration gradient The difference in the concentration of a particular substance between two different areas.

Conducting zone Includes all respiratory passageways that provide conduits for air to reach the sites of gas exchange (the respiratory zone).

Conductivity Ability to transmit an electrical impulse.

Cones One of the two types of photoreceptor cells in the retina of the eye; provide for color vision.

Congenital (kun-jeh′nih-tul) Existing at birth.

Congestive heart failure (CHF) Condition in which the pumping efficiency of the heart is depressed so that circulation is inadequate to meet tissue needs.

Conjunctiva (kon″junk-ti′vah) Thin, protective mucous membrane lining the eyelids and covering the anterior surface of the eye itself.

Connective tissue A primary tissue; form and function vary extensively. Functions include support, storage, and protection.

Consciousness The ability to perceive, communicate, remember, understand, appreciate, and initiate voluntary movements.

Contraception The prevention of conception; birth control.

Contractility Muscle cell's ability to move by shortening.

Contraction To shorten or develop tension, an ability highly developed in muscle cells.

Contralateral Relating to the opposite side.

Cornea (kor′ne-ah) Transparent anterior portion of the eyeball; part of the fibrous layer.

Corona radiata (kor-o′nah ra-de-ah′tah) (1) Arrangement of elongated follicle cells around a mature ovum; (2) crownlike arrangement of nerve fibers radiating from the internal capsule of the brain to every part of the cerebral cortex.

Coronary circulation The functional blood supply of the heart; shortest circulation in the body.

Cortex (kor′teks) Outer surface layer of an organ.

Corticosteroids (kor″tĭ-ko-stě′roidz) Steroid hormones released by the adrenal cortex.

Cortisol (hydrocortisone) (kor′tih-sol) Glucocorticoid produced by the adrenal cortex.

Covalent bond (ko-va′lent) Chemical bond created by electron sharing between atoms.

Cranial nerves The 12 nerve pairs that arise from the brain.

Craniosacral division Another name for the parasympathetic division of the autonomic nervous system.

Cranium (cranial bones) (kra′ne-um) Bony protective encasement of the brain and organs of hearing and equilibrium.

Creatine kinase (kre′ah-tin) Enzyme that catalyzes the transfer of phosphate from creatine phosphate to ADP, forming creatine and ATP; important in muscle contraction.

Creatine phosphate (CP) (fos-fāt) Compound that serves as an alternative energy source for muscle tissue.

Creatinine (kre-at′ĭ-nin) A nitrogenous waste molecule which is not reabsorbed by the kidney; this characteristic makes it useful for measurement of the GFR and glomerular function.

Crista ampullaris Sensory receptor organ for rotational acceleration and deceleration housed within the ampulla of each semicircular canal of the inner ear.

Cross section A cut running horizontally from right to left, dividing the body or an organ into superior and inferior parts.

Cutaneous (ku-ta′ne-us) Pertaining to the skin.

Cutaneous sensory receptors Receptors located throughout the skin that respond to stimuli arising outside the body; part of the nervous system.

Cyclic AMP Intracellular second messenger that mediates the effects of the first (extracellular) messenger (hormone or neurotransmitter); formed from ATP by a plasma membrane enzyme (adenylate cyclase).

Cystic fibrosis (CF) Genetic disorder in which secretion of overly viscous mucus clogs the respiratory passages, predisposes to fatal respiratory infections.

Cytochromes (si′to-krōmz) Brightly colored iron-containing proteins that form part of the inner mitochondrial membrane and function as electron carriers in oxidative phosphorylation.

Cytokines Small proteins that act as chemical messengers between various parts of the immune system.

Cytokinesis (si″to-kĭ-ne′sis) The division of cytoplasm that occurs after the cell nucleus has divided.

Cytoplasm (si′to-plazm) The cellular material surrounding the nucleus and enclosed by the plasma membrane.

Cytosine (C) (si′to-sēn) Nitrogen-containing base that is part of a nucleotide structure.

Cytoskeleton Literally, cell skeleton. An elaborate series of rods running through the cystol, supporting cellular structures and providing the machinery to generate various cell movements.

Cytosol Viscous, semitransparent fluid substance of cytoplasm in which other elements are suspended.

Cytotoxic T cell (T_C cell) Effector T cell that directly kills foreign cells, cancer cells, or virus-infected body cells by inducing apoptosis (cell suicide).

Deamination (de″am-ih-na′shun) Removal of an amine group from an organic compound.

Decomposition reaction Chemical reaction in which a molecule is broken down into smaller molecules or its constituent atoms.

Defecation (def″ih-ka′shun) Elimination of the contents of the bowels (feces).

Deglutition (deg″loo-tish′un) Swallowing.

Dehydration (de″hi-dra′shun) Condition of excessive water loss.

Dehydration synthesis Process by which a large molecule is synthesized by removing water and covalently bonding smaller molecules together.

Dendrite (den′drīt) Branching neuron process that serves as a receptive, or input, region; transmits an electrical signal toward the cell body.

Dendritic cells Protective cells that phagocytize antigens, migrate to lymph nodes, and present the antigen to T cells, causing them to activate and mount an immune response; those in the skin are sometimes called Langerhans cells.

Depolarization (de-po″ler-ah-za′shun) Loss of a state of polarity; loss or reduction of negative membrane potential.

Dermatome (der′mah-tōm) Portion of somite mesoderm that forms the dermis of the skin; also the area of skin innervated by the cutaneous branches of a single spinal nerve.

Dermis Layer of skin deep to the epidermis; composed mostly of dense irregular connective tissue.

Desmosome (dez′muh-sōm) Cell junction composed of thickened plasma membranes joined by filaments.

Diabetes insipidus (di″ah-be′tēz in-sih′pih-dus) Disease characterized by passage of a large quantity of dilute urine plus intense thirst and dehydration caused by inadequate release of antidiuretic hormone (ADH).

Diabetes mellitus (DM) (meh-li′tus) Disease caused by deficient insulin release or by insulin resistance, leading to inability of the body cells to use carbohydrates.

Dialysis (di-al′ah-sis) Diffusion of solute(s) through a semipermeable membrane.

Diapedesis (di″ah-pĕ-de′sis) Passage of white blood cells through intact vessel walls into tissue.

Diaphragm (di′ah-fram) (1) Any partition or wall separating one area from another; (2) a muscle that separates the thoracic cavity from the lower abdominopelvic cavity.

Diaphysis (di-af′ĭ-sis) Elongated shaft of a long bone.

Diarthrosis (di″ar-thro′sis) Freely movable joint.

Diastole (di-as′to-le) Period of the cardiac cycle when either the ventricles or the atria are relaxing.

Diastolic pressure (di-as-tah′lik) Arterial blood pressure reached during or as a result of diastole; lowest level of any given cardiac cycle.

Diencephalon (interbrain) (di″en-seh′fuh-lon) That part of the forebrain between the cerebral hemispheres and the midbrain including the thalamus, the epithalamus, and the hypothalamus.

Differential white blood cell count Diagnostic test to determine relative proportion of individual leukocyte types.

Diffusion (dĭ-fu′zhun) The spreading of particles in a gas or solution with a movement toward uniform distribution of particles; driven by kinetic energy.

Digestion A series of catabolic steps in which complex food molecules are broken down to their building blocks by enzymes.

Digestive system System that processes food into absorbable units and eliminates indigestible wastes.

Dipeptide A combination of two amino acids united by means of a peptide bond.

Diploë (dip′lo-e) The internal layer of spongy bone in flat bones.

Diploid chromosomal number The chromosomal number characteristic of an organism, symbolized as $2n$; twice the chromosomal number (n) of the gamete; in humans, $2n = 46$.

Diplopia (dĭ-plo′pe-ah) Double vision.

Dipole (polar molecule) Nonsymmetrical molecules that contain electrically unbalanced atoms.

Disaccharide (di-sak′ah-rīd″, di-sak′ah-rid) Literally, double sugar; e.g., sucrose, lactose.

Dislocation (luxation) Occurs when bones are forced out of their normal alignment at a joint.

Displacement (exchange) reaction Chemical reaction in which bonds are both made and broken; atoms become combined with different atoms.

Distal (dis′tul) Away from the attached end of a limb or the origin of a structure.

Diuretics (di″u-ret′iks) Chemicals that enhance urinary output.

Diverticulum (di″ver-tik′u-lum) A pouch or sac in the walls of a hollow organ or structure.

DNA (deoxyribonucleic acid) (de-ok″sĭ-ri″bo-nu-kla′ik) A nucleic acid found in all living cells; it carries the organism's hereditary information.

DNA replication Process that occurs before cell division; ensures that all daughter cells have identical genes.

Dominant traits Occurs when one allele masks or suppresses the expression of its partner.

Dominant-recessive inheritance Reflects the interaction of dominant and recessive alleles.

Dorsal (dor′sul) Pertaining to the back; posterior.

Dorsal root ganglion Peripheral collection of cell bodies of first-order afferent neurons whose central axons enter the spinal cord.

Double helix The secondary structure assumed by two strands of DNA, held together throughout their length by hydrogen bonds between bases on opposite strands.

Duct (dukt) A canal or passageway; a tubular structure that provides an exit for the secretions of a gland, or for conducting any fluid.

Ductus (vas) deferens Extends from the epididymis to the urethra; propels sperm into the urethra by peristalsis during ejaculation.

Duodenum (du″o-de′num) First part of the small intestine.

Dura mater (du′rah ma′ter) Outermost and toughest of the three membranes (meninges) covering the brain and spinal cord.

Dynamic equilibrium Sense that reports on angular (rotatory) acceleration or deceleration of the head in space.

Dyskinesia (dis-kĭ-ne′ze-ah) Disorders of muscle tone, posture, or involuntary movements.

Dyspnea (disp-ne′ah) Difficult or labored breathing; air hunger.

Eccrine glands (ek′rin) Sweat glands abundant on the palms, soles of feet, and the forehead.

Ectoderm (ek′to-derm) Embryonic germ layer; forms the epidermis of the skin and its derivatives, and nervous tissues.

Edema (ĕ-de′mah) Abnormal increase in the amount of interstitial fluid; causes swelling.

Effector (ef-ek′ter) Organ, gland, or muscle capable of being activated by nerve endings.

Efferent (ef′er-ent) Carrying away or away from, especially a nerve fiber that carries impulses away from the central nervous system.

Elastic cartilage Cartilage with abundant elastic fibers; more flexible than hyaline cartilage.

Elastic fiber Fiber formed from the protein elastin, which gives a rubbery and resilient quality to the matrix of connective tissue.

Electrical energy Energy formed by the movement of charged particles across cell membranes.

Electrocardiogram (ECG or **EKG)** (e-lek″tro-car′de-o-gram″) Graphic record of the electrical activity of the heart.

Electrochemical gradient The combined difference in concentration and charge; influences the distribution and direction of diffusion of ions.

Electroencephalogram (EEG) (e-lek″tro-en-sef′ah-lo-gram″) Graphic record of the electrical activity of nerve cells in the brain.

Electrolyte (e-lek′tro-līt) Chemical substances, such as salts, acids, and bases, that ionize and dissociate in water and are capable of conducting an electrical current.

Electrolyte balance Refers to the balance between input and output of salts (sodium, potassium, calcium, magnesium) in the body.

Electromagnetic radiation Emitted photons (wave packets) of energy, e.g., light, X ray, infrared.

Electron Negatively charged subatomic particle; orbits the atom's nucleus.

Electron shells (energy levels) Regions of space that consecutively surround the nucleus of an atom.

Element One of a limited number of unique varieties of matter that composes substances of all kinds; e.g., carbon, hydrogen, oxygen.

Embolism (em′bo-lizm) Obstruction of a blood vessel by an embolus (blood clot, fatty mass, bubble of air, or other debris) floating in the blood.

Embryo (em′bre-o) Developmental stage extending from fertilization to the end of the eighth week.

Emesis Reflexive emptying of the stomach through the esophagus and pharynx; also known as vomiting.

Encephalitis (en″seh-fuh-lī-′tis) Inflammation of the brain.

Endergonic reaction Chemical reaction that absorbs energy, e.g., an anabolic reaction.

Endocardium (en″do-kar′de-um) Endothelial membrane that lines the interior of the heart.

Endochondral ossification (en″do-kon′dral) Embryonic formation of bone by the replacement of calcified cartilage; most skeletal bones are formed by this process.

Endocrine glands (en′do-krin) Ductless glands that empty their hormonal products directly into the blood.

Endocrine system Body system that includes internal organs that secrete hormones.

Endocytosis (en″do-si-to′sis) Means by which fairly large extracellular molecules or particles enter cells, e.g., phagocytosis, pinocytosis, receptor-mediated endocytosis.

Endoderm (en′do-derm) Embryonic germ layer; forms the lining of the digestive tube and its associated structures.

Endogenous (en-doj′ĕ-nŭs) Originating or produced within the organism or one of its parts.

Endometrium (en″do-me′tre-um) Mucous membrane lining of the uterus.

Endomysium (en″do-mis′e-um) Thin connective tissue surrounding each muscle cell.

Endoplasmic reticulum (ER) (en″do-plaz′mik rĕ-tik′u-lum) Membranous network of tubular or saclike channels in the cytoplasm of a cell.

Endosteum (en-dos′te-um) Connective tissue membrane covering internal bone surfaces.

Endothelium (en″do-the′le-um) Single layer of simple squamous cells that line the walls of the heart, blood vessels, and lymphatic vessels.

Energy The capacity to do work; may be stored (potential energy) or in action (kinetic energy).

Energy intake Energy liberated during food oxidation.

Energy output Sum of energy lost as heat, as work, and as fat or glycogen storage.

Enzyme (en′zīm) A protein that acts as a biological catalyst to speed up a chemical reaction.

Eosinophil (e″o-sin′o-fil) Granular white blood cell whose granules readily take up an acid stain called eosin.

Ependymal cell (ĕ-pen′dĭ-mul) A type of CNS supporting cell; lines the central cavities of the brain and spinal cord.

Epidermis (ep″ĭ-der′mis) Superficial layer of the skin; composed of keratinized stratified squamous epithelium.

Epididymis (ep″ĭ-dĭ′dĭ-mis) That portion of the male duct system in which sperm mature. Empties into the ductus (or vas) deferens.

Epidural space Area between the bony vertebrae and the dura mater of the spinal cord.

Epiglottis (ep″ĭ-glot′is) Elastic cartilage at the back of the throat; covers the opening of the larynx during swallowing.

Epileptic seizures Abnormal electrical discharges of groups of brain neurons, during which no other messages can get through.

Epimysium (ep″ĭ-mis′e-um) Sheath of fibrous connective tissue surrounding a muscle.

Epinephrine (ep″ĭ-nef′rin) Chief hormone produced by the adrenal medulla. Also called adrenaline.

Epiphyseal plate (e″pĭ-fis′e-ul) Plate of hyaline cartilage at the junction of the diaphysis and epiphysis that provides for growth in length of a long bone.

Epiphysis (e-pif′ĭ-sis) The end of a long bone, attached to the shaft.

Epithalamus Most dorsal portion of the diencephalon; forms the roof of the third ventricle with the pineal gland extending from its posterior border.

Epithelium (epithelial tissue) (ep″ĭ-the′le-ul) Pertaining to a primary tissue that covers the body surface, lines its internal cavities, and forms glands.

Erythrocytes (e-rith′ro-sīts) Red blood cells.

Erythropoiesis (ĕ-rith″ro-poi-e′sis) Process of erythrocyte formation.

Erythropoietin (EPO) (ĕ-rith″ro-poi′ĕ-tin) Hormone that stimulates production of red blood cells.

Esophagus (ĕ-sof′ah-gus) Muscular tube extending from the laryngopharynx through the diaphragm to join the stomach; collapses when not involved in food propulsion.

Estrogens (es′tro-jenz) Hormones that stimulate female secondary sex characteristics; female sex hormones.

Eupnea (ūp-ne′ah) Normal respiratory rate and rhythm.

Excess postexercise oxygen consumption (EPOC) The volume of oxygen required after exercise to replenish stores of O_2, ATP, creatine phosphate, and glycogen and oxidize the lactic acid formed during exercise. Also called oxygen debt.

Exchange (displacement) reaction Chemical reaction in which bonds are both made and broken; atoms become combined with different atoms.

Excitability (responsiveness) Ability to respond to stimuli.

Excitation-contraction (E-C) coupling Sequence of events by which transmission of an action potential along the sarcolemma leads to the sliding of myofilaments.

Excitatory postsynaptic potential (EPSP) Depolarizing graded potential in a postsynaptic neuron.

Excretion (ek-skre′shun) Elimination of waste products from the body.

Exergonic reaction Chemical reaction that releases energy, e.g., a catabolic or oxidative reaction.

Exocrine glands (ek′so-krin) Glands that have ducts through which their secretions are carried to a particular site.

Exocytosis (ek″so-si-to′sis) Mechanism by which substances are moved from the cell interior to the extracellular space as a secretory vesicle fuses with the plasma membrane.

Exons Amino acid–specifying informational sequences (separated by introns) in the genes of higher organisms.

Extension Movement that increases the angle of a joint, e.g., straightening a flexed knee.

Exteroceptor (ek″ster-o-sep′tor) Sensory receptor that responds to stimuli from the external world.

Extracellular fluid (ECF) Internal fluid located outside cells; includes interstitial fluid, blood plasma, and cerebrospinal fluid.

Extracellular matrix Nonliving material in connective tissue consisting of ground substance and fibers that separates the living cells.

Extrasystole (ek″strah-sis′to-le) Premature heart contraction.

Extrinsic (ek-strin′sik) Of external origin.

Extrinsic eye muscles The six skeletal muscles that attach to and move each eye.

Facilitated diffusion Passive transport process used by certain large or charged molecules (e.g., glucose, Na^+) that are unable to pass through the plasma membrane unaided. Involves movement through channels or movement facilitated by a membrane carrier.

Fallopian tube (fah-lō′pe-un) *See* Uterine tube.

Fascia (fash′e-ah) Layers of fibrous tissue covering and separating muscle.

Fascicle (fas′ĭ-kl) Bundle of nerve or muscle fibers bound together by connective tissue.

Fatty acids Linear chains of carbon and hydrogen atoms (hydrocarbon chains) with an organic acid group at one end. A constituent of fat.

Feces (fe′sēz) Material discharged from the bowel; composed of food residue, secretions, bacteria.

Fenestrated (fen′es-tra-tid) Pierced with one or more small openings.

Fertilization Fusion of the sperm and egg nuclei.

Fetus Developmental stage extending from the ninth week of development to birth.

Fiber A slender threadlike structure or filament. *See also* Nerve fiber, Muscle fiber.

Fibrillation Condition of rapid and irregular or out-of-phase heart contractions.

Fibrin (fi′brin) Fibrous insoluble protein formed during blood clotting.

Fibrinogen (fi-brin′o-jin) A soluble blood protein that is converted to insoluble fibrin during blood clotting.

Fibrinolysis Process that removes unneeded blood clots when healing has occurred.

Fibroblast (fi′bro-blast) Young, actively mitotic cell that forms the fibers of connective tissue.

Fibrocartilage The most compressible type of cartilage; resistant to stretch. Forms vertebral discs and knee joint cartilages.

Fibrocyte (fi′bro-sīt) Mature fibroblast; maintains the matrix of fibrous types of connective tissue.

Fibrosis Proliferation of fibrous connective tissue called scar tissue.

Fibrous joints Bones joined by fibrous tissue; no joint cavity is present.

Filtrate A plasma-derived fluid that is processed by the renal tubules to form urine.

Filtration Passage of a solvent and dissolved substances through a membrane or filter.

First-degree burn A burn in which only the epidermis is damaged.

Fissure (fih′sher) (1) A groove or cleft; (2) the deepest depressions or inward folds on the brain.

Fixator (fix′a-ter) Muscle that immobilizes one or more bones, allowing other muscles to act from a stable base.

Flagellum (flah-jel′lum) Long, whiplike cellular extension containing microtubules; propels sperm and some single-celled eukaryotes.

Flexion (flek′shun) Movement that decreases the angle of the joint, e.g., bending the knee from a straight to an angled position.

Flexor (withdrawal) reflex Reflex initiated by a painful stimulus (actual or perceived); causes automatic withdrawal of the threatened body part from the stimulus.

Fluid mosaic model A depiction of the structure of the membranes of a cell as phospholipid bilayers in which proteins are dispersed.

Follicle (fah′lih-kul) (1) Ovarian structure consisting of a developing egg surrounded by one or more layers of follicle cells; (2) colloid-containing structure of the thyroid gland; (3) B cell–rich region in lymphoid tissue.

Follicle-stimulating hormone (FSH) Hormone produced by the anterior pituitary that stimulates ovarian follicle production in females and sperm production in males.

Fontanelles (fon″tah-nelz′) Fibrous membranes at the angles of cranial bones that accommodate brain growth in the fetus and infant.

Foramen (fo-ra′men) Hole or opening in a bone or between body cavities.

Forebrain (prosencephalon) Anterior portion of the brain consisting of the telencephalon and the diencephalon.

Formed elements Cellular portion of blood.

Fossa (fos′ah) A depression, often an articular surface.

Fovea (fo′ve-ah) A pit.

Fracture A break in a bone.

Free radicals Highly reactive chemicals with unpaired electrons that can scramble the structure of proteins, lipids, and nucleic acids.

Frontal (coronal) plane Longitudinal (vertical) plane that divides the body or an organ into anterior and posterior parts.

Fulcrum The fixed point on which a lever moves when a force is applied.

Fundus (fun′dus) Base of an organ; part farthest from the opening of the organ. For example, the posterior wall of the eye.

G protein Protein that relays signals between extracellular first messengers (hormones or neurotransmitters) and intracellular second messengers (such as cyclic AMP) via an effector enzyme.

Gallbladder Sac beneath the right lobe of the liver used for bile storage.

Gallstones (biliary calculi) Crystallized cholesterol that obstructs the flow of bile from the gallbladder.

Gamete (gam′ēt) Sex or germ cell.

Gametogenesis (gam″eh-to-jen′eh-sis) Formation of *gametes.*

Ganglion (gang′gle-on) Collection of nerve cell bodies outside the CNS.

Gap junction A passageway between two adjacent cells; formed by transmembrane proteins called connexons.

Gastrin Hormone secreted in the stomach; regulates gastric juice secretion by stimulating HCl production.

Gastroenteritis Inflammation of the gastrointestinal tract.

Gastrulation (gas″troo-la′shun) Developmental process that produces the three primary germ layers (ectoderm, mesoderm, and endoderm).

Gene One of the biological units of heredity located in chromatin; transmits hereditary information.

Genetic code Refers to the rules by which the base sequence of a DNA gene is translated into protein structures (amino acid sequences).

Genitalia (jen″ĭ-ta′le-ă) The internal and external reproductive organs.

Genome The complete set of chromosomes derived from one parent (the haploid genome); or the two sets of chromosomes, i.e., one set from the egg, the other from the sperm (the diploid genome).

Genotype (jen′o-tīp) One's genetic makeup or genes.

Germ layers Three cellular layers (ectoderm, mesoderm, and endoderm) that represent the initial specialization of cells in the embryonic body and from which all body tissues arise.

Gestation period (jes-ta′shun) The period of pregnancy; about 280 days for humans.

Gland Organ specialized to secrete or excrete substances for further use in the body or for elimination.

Glaucoma (glaw-ko′mah) Condition in which intraocular pressure increases to levels that cause compression of the retina and optic nerve; results in blindness unless detected early.

Glial cells (gle′al) *See* Neuroglia.

Glomerular capsule (glo-mer′yoo-ler) Double-walled cup at end of a renal tubule; encloses a glomerulus. Also called Bowman's capsule.

Glomerular filtration rate (GFR) Rate of filtrate formation by the kidneys.

Glomerulus (glo-mer′u-lus) (1) Cluster of capillaries forming part of the nephron; forms filtrate; (2) odor-specific processing unit in olfactory bulb.

Glottis (glah′tis) Opening between the vocal cords in the larynx.

Glucagon (gloo′kah-gon) Hormone formed by alpha cells of pancreatic islets; raises the glucose level of blood.

Glucocorticoids (gloo″ko-kor′tĭ-koidz) Adrenal cortex hormones that increase blood glucose levels and aid the body in resisting long-term stressors.

Gluconeogenesis (gloo″ko-ne″o-jen′ĕ-sis) Formation of glucose from noncarbohydrate molecules.

Glucose (gloo′kōs) Principal blood sugar; a hexose.

Glycerol (glis′er-ol) A modified simple sugar (a sugar alcohol); a building block of fats.

Glycocalyx (cell coat) (gli″ko-kal′iks) A layer of externally facing glycoproteins on a cell's plasma membrane; its components determine blood type and are involved in the cellular interactions of fertilization, embryonic development, and immunity, and act as an adhesive between cells.

Glycogen (gli′ko-jin) Main carbohydrate stored in animal cells; a polysaccharide.

Glycogenesis (gli″ko-jen′ĕ-sis) Formation of glycogen from glucose.

Glycogenolysis (gli″ko-jĕ-nol′ĭ-sis) Breakdown of glycogen to glucose.

Glycolipid (gli″ko-lip′id) A lipid with one or more covalently attached sugars.

Glycolysis (gli-kol′ĭ-sis) Breakdown of glucose to pyruvic acid—an anaerobic process.

Goblet cells Individual cells (unicellular glands) that produce mucus.

Golgi apparatus (gol′je) Membranous system close to the cell nucleus that packages protein secretions for export, packages enzymes into lysosomes for cellular use, and modifies proteins destined to become part of cellular membranes.

Gonad (go′nad) Primary reproductive organ; i.e., the testis of the male or the ovary of the female.

Gonadocorticoids (gon″ah-do-kor′tĭ-koidz) Sex hormones, primarily androgens, secreted by the adrenal cortex.

Gonadotropins (gon″ah-do-trōp′inz) Gonad-stimulating hormones produced by the anterior pituitary.

Graded muscle responses Variations in the degree of muscle contraction by changing either the frequency or strength of the stimulus.

Graded potential A local change in membrane potential that varies directly with the strength of the stimulus, declines with distance.

Graves' disease Disorder resulting from hyperactive thyroid gland.

Gray matter Gray area of the central nervous system; contains neuronal cell bodies and their dendrites.

Growth hormone (GH) Hormone that stimulates growth in general; produced in the anterior pituitary; also called somatotropin.

Guanine (G) (gwan′ēn) One of two major purines occurring in all nucleic acids.

Gustation (gus-ta′shun) Taste.

Gyrus (ji′rus) An outward fold of the surface of the cerebral cortex.

Hair follicle Structure with outer and inner root sheaths extending from the epidermal surface into the dermis and from which new hair develops.

Hapten (hap′ten) An incomplete antigen; has reactivity but not immunogenicity.

Haversian system (hah-ver′zhen) *See* Osteon.

Heart attack (coronary) *See* Myocardial infarction.

Heart block Impaired transmission of impulses from atrium to ventricle resulting in abnormally slow heart rhythms.

Heart murmur Abnormal heart sound (usually resulting from valve problems).

Heimlich maneuver Procedure in which the air in a person's own lungs is used to expel an obstructing piece of food.

Helper T cell (T_H cell) Type of T lymphocyte that orchestrates cellular immunity by direct contact with other immune cells and by releasing chemicals called cytokines; also helps to mediate the humoral response by interacting with B cells.

Hematocrit (he-mat′o-krit) The percentage of total blood volume occupied by erythrocytes.

Hematoma (he″mah-to′mah) Mass of clotted blood that forms at an injured site.

Hematopoiesis (hem″ah-to-poi-e′sis) Blood cell formation; hemopoiesis.

Hematopoietic stem cell (hem″ah-to-poi-et′ik) Bone marrow cell that gives rise to all the formed elements of blood; hemocytoblast.

Heme (hēm) Iron-containing pigment that is essential to oxygen transport by hemoglobin.

Hemoglobin (he′muh-glo-bin) Oxygen-transporting protein of erythrocytes.

Hemolysis (he-mah′lĕ-sis) Rupture of erythrocytes.

Hemophilia (he″mo-fil′e-ah) A term loosely applied to several different hereditary bleeding disorders that exhibit similar signs and symptoms.

Hemopoiesis (he″mo-poi-e′sis) *See* Hematopoiesis.

Hemorrhage (hem′or-ij) Loss of blood from the vessels by flow through ruptured walls; bleeding.

Hemostasis (he″mo-sta′sis) Stoppage of bleeding.

Heparin Natural anticoagulant secreted into blood plasma.

Hepatic portal system (hĕ-pat′ik) Circulation in which the hepatic portal vein carries dissolved nutrients to the liver tissues for processing.

Hepatitis (hep″ah-ti′tis) Inflammation of the liver.

Hernia (her′ne-ah) Abnormal protrusion of an organ or a body part through the containing wall of its cavity.

Heterozygous (het″er-o-zi′gus) Having different allelic genes at a given locus or (by extension) many loci.

Hilton's law Any nerve serving a muscle that produces movement at a joint also innervates the joint and the skin over the joint.

Hilum (hi′lum) The indented region of an organ from which blood and/or lymphatic vessels and nerves enter and exit.

Hippocampus Limbic system structure that plays a role in converting new information into long-term memories.

Histamine (his′tuh-mēn) A chemical messenger (neurotransmitter or paracrine); causes vasodilation and increased capillary permeability; in stomach causes acid secretion.

Histology (his-tol′o-je) Branch of anatomy dealing with the microscopic structure of tissues.

HIV (human immunodeficiency virus) Virus that destroys helper T cells, thus depressing adaptive immunity; symptomatic AIDS gradually appears when lymph nodes can no longer contain the virus.

Holocrine glands (hol′o-krin) Glands that accumulate their secretions within their cells; secretions are discharged only upon rupture and death of the cell.

Homeostasis (ho″me-o-sta′sis) A state of body equilibrium or stable internal environment of the body.

Homologous (ho-mol′ŏ-gus) Parts or organs corresponding in structure but not necessarily in function.

Homozygous (ho-mo-zi′gus) Having identical genes at one or more loci.

Hormones Steroidal or amino acid–based molecules released to the blood that act as chemical messengers to regulate specific body functions.

Humoral immunity (hu′mer-ul) Immunity conferred by antibodies present in blood plasma and other body fluids.

Huntington's disease Hereditary disorder leading to degeneration of the basal nuclei and the cerebral cortex.

Hyaline cartilage (hi′ah-līn) The most abundant cartilage type in the body; provides firm support with some pliability.

Hydrochloric acid (HCl) (hi″dro-klor′ik) Acid that aids protein digestion in the stomach; produced by parietal cells.

Hydrogen bond Weak bond in which a hydrogen atom forms a bridge between two electron-hungry atoms. An important intramolecular bond.

Hydrogen ion (H^+) A hydrogen atom minus its electron and therefore carrying a positive charge (i.e., a proton).

Hydrolysis (hi″drah′lă-sis) Process in which water is used to split a substance into smaller particles.

Hydrophilic (hi″dro-fil′ik) Refers to molecules, or portions of molecules, that interact with water and charged particles.

Hydrophobic (hi″dro-fo′bik) Refers to molecules, or portions of molecules, that interact only with nonpolar molecules.

Hydrostatic pressure (hi″dro-stă′tic) Pressure of fluid in a system.

Hydroxyl ion (OH^-) (hi-drok′sil) An ion liberated when a hydroxide (a common inorganic base) is dissolved in water.

Hyperalgesia Pain amplification.

Hypercapnia (hi″per-kap′ne-ah) High carbon dioxide levels in the blood.

Hyperemia An increase in blood flow into a tissue or organ; congested with blood.

Hyperglycemic (hi″per-gli-se′mik) Term used to describe hormones such as glucagon that elevate blood glucose level.

Hyperopia (hi″per-o′pe-ah) A condition in which visual images are routinely focused behind rather than on the retina; commonly known as farsightedness.

Hyperplasia (hi″per-pla′ze-ah) Accelerated growth, e.g., in anemia, the bone marrow produces red blood cells at a faster rate.

Hyperpnea (hi″perp-ne′ah) An increase in ventilation in response to metabolic need (e.g., during exercise).

Hyperpolarization An increase in membrane potential in which the membrane becomes more negative than resting membrane potential.

Hypersensitivity Overzealous immune response to an otherwise harmless antigen.

Hypertension (hi″per-ten′shun) High blood pressure.

Hypertonic (hi″per-ton′ik) Excessive, above normal, tone or tension.

Hypertonic solution A solution that has a higher concentration of nonpenetrating solutes than the reference cell; having greater osmotic pressure than the reference solution (blood plasma or interstitial fluid).

Hypertrophy (hi-per′trah-fe) Increase in size of a tissue or organ independent of the body's general growth.

Hyperventilation An increase in the depth and rate of breathing that is in excess of the body's need for removal of carbon dioxide.

Hypocapnia Low carbon dioxide levels in the blood.

Hypodermis (superficial fascia) Subcutaneous tissue just deep to the skin; consists of adipose plus some areolar connective tissue.

Hypoglycemic (hi″po-gli-se′mik) Term used to describe hormones such as insulin that decrease blood glucose level.

Hyponatremia Abnormally low concentrations of sodium ions in extracellular fluid.

Hypoproteinemia (hi″po-pro″te-ĭ-ne′me-ah) A condition of unusually low levels of plasma proteins causing a reduction in colloid osmotic pressure; results in tissue edema.

Hypotension Low blood pressure.

Hypothalamic-hypophyseal tract (hi″po-thah-lam′ik hi″po-fiz′-e-al) Nerve bundles that run through the infundibulum and connect the posterior pituitary to the hypothalamus.

Hypothalamus (hi″po-thal′ah-mus) Region of the diencephalon forming the floor of the third ventricle of the brain.

Hypotonic (hi″po-ton′ik) Below normal tone or tension.

Hypotonic solution A solution that is more dilute (containing fewer nonpenetrating solutes) than the reference cell. Cells placed in hypotonic solutions plump up rapidly as water rushes into them.

Hypoventilation A decrease in the depth and rate of breathing; characterized by an increase in blood carbon dioxide.

Hypovolemic shock (hi″po-vo-le′mik) Most common form of shock; results from extreme blood loss.

Hypoxia (hi-pok′se-ah) Condition in which inadequate oxygen is available to tissues.

Ileocecal valve (il″e-o-se′kal) Site where the small intestine joins the large intestine.

Ileum (il′e-um) Terminal part of the small intestine; between the jejunum and the cecum of the large intestine.

Immune system A functional system whose components attack foreign substances or prevent their entry into the body.

Immunity (im″ūn′ĭ-te) Ability of the body to resist many agents (both living and nonliving) that can cause disease; resistance to disease.

Immunocompetence Ability of the body's immune cells to recognize (by binding) specific antigens; reflects the presence of plasma membrane–bound receptors.

Immunodeficiency Any congenital or acquired condition causing a deficiency in the production or function of immune cells or certain molecules (complement, antibodies, etc.) required for normal immunity.

In vitro (in ve′tro) In a test tube, glass, or artificial environment.

In vivo (in ve′vo) In the living body.

Incompetent valve Valve which does not close properly.

Incontinence Inability to control micturition or defecation voluntarily.

Infarct (in′farkt) Region of dead, deteriorating tissue resulting from a lack of blood supply.

Infectious mononucleosis Highly contagious viral disease; marked by excessive agranulocytes.

Inferior (caudal) Pertaining to a position toward the lower or tail end of the long axis of the body.

Inferior vena cava Vein that returns blood from body areas below the diaphragm.

Inflammation (in″flah-ma′shun) An innate (nonspecific) defensive response of the body to tissue injury; includes dilation of blood vessels and an increase in vessel permeability; indicated by redness, heat, swelling, and pain.

Infundibulum (in″fun-dib′u-lum) (1) A stalk of tissue that connects the pituitary gland to the hypothalamus; (2) the distal end of the uterine (fallopian) tube.

Inguinal (ing′wĭ-nal) Pertaining to the groin region.

Inhibitory postsynaptic potential (IPSP) A graded potential in a postsynaptic neuron that inhibits action potential generation; usually hyperpolarizing.

Inner cell mass Accumulation of cells in the blastocyst from which the embryo develops.

Innervation (in″er-va′shun) Supply of nerves to a body part.

Inorganic compound Chemical substances that do not contain carbon, including water, salts, and many acids and bases.

Insertion Movable attachment of a muscle.

Insula Lobe of the cerebral cortex that is buried in the lateral sulcus beneath portions of the parietal, frontal, and temporal lobes.

Insulin A hormone that enhances the carrier-mediated diffusion of glucose into tissue cells, thus lowering blood glucose levels.

Insulin resistance State in which a greater than normal amount of insulin is required to maintain normal glucose blood levels.

Integration The process by which the nervous system processes and interprets sensory input and makes decisions about what should be done at each moment.

Integumentary system (in-teg″u-men′tar-e) Skin and its derivatives; provides the external protective covering of the body.

Intercalated discs (in-ter′kah-la″ted) Specialized connections between myocardial cells containing gap junctions and desmosomes.

Interferons (IFNs) (in-ter-fēr′ons) Proteins released from virus-infected (and other) cells that protect uninfected cells from viral takeover. Also inhibit some cancers.

Internal capsule Band of projection fibers that runs between the basal nuclei and the thalamus.

Internal respiration Exchange of gases between blood and tissue fluid and between tissue fluid and cells.

Interneuron (association neuron) Nerve cell located between motor and sensory neurons that shuttles signals through CNS pathways where integration occurs.

Interoceptor (in″ter-o-sep′tor) Sensory receptor in the viscera that is sensitive to changes and stimuli within the body's internal environment; also called visceroceptor.

Interphase One of two major periods in the cell life cycle; includes the period from cell formation to cell division.

Interstitial endocrine cells Cells located in the loose connective tissue surrounding the seminiferous tubules; they produce androgens (most importantly testosterone), which are secreted into the surrounding interstitial fluid.

Interstitial fluid (IF) (in″ter-stish′al) Fluid between the cells.

Interstitial lamellae Incomplete lamellae that lie between intact osteons, filling the gaps between forming osteons, or representing the remnants of an osteon that has been cut through by bone remodeling.

Intervertebral discs (in″ter-ver′teh-brul) Discs of fibrocartilage between vertebrae.

Intracapsular ligament Ligament located within and separate from the articular capsule of a synovial joint.

Intracellular fluid (ICF) (in″trah-sel′u-ler) Fluid within a cell.

Intrinsic factor Substance produced by the stomach that is required for vitamin B_{12} absorption.

Intron Noncoding segment or portion of DNA that ranges from 60 to 100,000 nucleotides long.

Involuntary muscle Muscle that cannot ordinarily be controlled voluntarily (e.g., smooth and cardiac muscle).

Involuntary nervous system The autonomic nervous system.

Ion (ī′on) Atom or molecule with a positive or negative electric charge.

Ionic bond (ī-ah′nik) Chemical bond formed by electron transfer between atoms.

Ipsilateral (ip″sih-lă′ter-ul) Situated on the same side.

Ischemia (is-ke′me-ah) Local decrease in blood supply.

Isograft Tissue graft donated by an identical twin.

Isomer (i′so-mer) One of two or more substances that has the same molecular formula but with its atoms arranged differently.

Isometric contraction (i″so-mĕ′trik) Contraction in which the muscle does not shorten (the load is too heavy) but its internal tension increases.

Isotonic contraction (i″so-tah′nik) Contraction in which muscle tension remains constant at a given load, and the muscle shortens.

Isotonic solution A solution with a concentration of nonpenetrating solutes equal to that found in the reference cell.

Isotopes (i′so-tōps) Different atomic forms of the same element, which vary only in the number of neutrons they contain; the heavier species tend to be radioactive.

Jejunum (jĕ-joo′num) The part of the small intestine between the duodenum and the ileum.

Joint (articulation) The junction of two or more bones.

Joint kinesthetic receptor (kin″es-thet′ik) Receptor that provides information on joint position and motion.

Juxtaglomerular complex (JGC) (juks″tah-glo-mer′u-lar) Cells of the distal part of the ascending limb of the nephron loop and afferent arteriole located close to the glomerulus; involved in blood pressure regulation (via release of the hormone renin) and autoregulation of GFR.

Karyotype (kar′e-o-tīp) The diploid chromosomal complement, typically shown as homologous chromosome pairs arranged from longest to shortest (X and Y are arranged by size rather than paired).

Keratin (ker′ah-tin) Fibrous protein found in the epidermis, hair, and nails that makes those structures hard and water resistant; precursor is keratohyaline.

Ketones (ketone bodies) (ke′tōnz) Fatty acid metabolites; strong organic acids.

Ketosis (kē-tō′sis) Excess levels of ketone bodies in blood. Called ketoacidosis if blood pH is low.

Killer T cell *See* Cytotoxic T cell.

Kilocalories (kcal) *See* Calorie.

Kinetic energy (ki-net′ik) The energy of motion or movement, e.g., the constant movement of atoms, or the push given to a swinging door that sets it into motion.

Krebs cycle Aerobic metabolic pathway occurring within mitochondria, in which food metabolites are oxidized and CO_2 is liberated, and coenzymes are reduced. Also called the citric acid cycle.

Labia (la′be-ah) Lips; singular: labium.

Labor Collective term for the series of events that expel the fetus from the uterus.

Labyrinth (lab′ĭ-rinth″) Bony cavities and membranes of the inner ear.

Lacrimal (lak′ri-mal) Pertaining to tears.

Lactation (lak-ta′shun) Production and secretion of milk.

Lacteal (lak′te-al) Special lymphatic capillaries of the small intestine that take up lipids.

Lactic acid (lak′tik) Product of anaerobic metabolism, especially in muscle.

Lacuna (lah-ku′nah) A small space, cavity, or depression; lacunae in bone or cartilage are occupied by cells.

Lamella (lah-mel′ah) A layer, such as of bone matrix in an osteon of compact bone.

Lamina (lam′ĭ-nah) (1) A thin layer or flat plate; (2) the portion of a vertebra between the transverse process and the spinous process.

Large intestine Portion of the digestive tract extending from the ileocecal valve to the anus; includes the cecum, appendix, colon, rectum, and anal canal.

Larynx (lar′ingks) Cartilaginous organ located between the trachea and the pharynx; voice box.

Latent period Period of time between stimulation and the onset of muscle contraction.

Lateral Away from the midline of the body.

Leptin Hormone released by fat cells that signals satiety.

Leukemia Refers to a group of cancerous conditions of white blood cells.

Leukocytes (loo′ko-sīts) White blood cells; formed elements involved in body protection that take part in inflammatory and immune responses.

Leukocytosis An increase in the number of leukocytes (white blood cells); usually the result of a microbiological attack on the body.

Leukopenia (loo″ko-pe′ne-ah) Abnormally low white blood cell count.

Leukopoiesis The production of white blood cells.

Lever system Consists of a lever (bone), effort (muscle action), resistance (weight of object to be moved), and fulcrum (joint).

Ligament (lig′ah-ment) Band of regular fibrous tissue that connects bones.

Ligands Signaling chemicals that bind specifically to membrane receptors.

Limbic system (lim′bik) Functional brain system involved in emotional response and memory formation.

Lipid (lih′pid) Organic compound formed of carbon, hydrogen, and oxygen; examples are fats and cholesterol.

Lipolysis (lĭ-pol′ĭ-sis) The breakdown of stored fats into glycerol and fatty acids.

Liver Lobed accessory organ that overlies the stomach; produces bile to help digest fat, and serves other metabolic and regulatory functions.

Lumbar (lum′bar) Portion of the back between the thorax and the pelvis.

Lumbar vertebrae The five vertebrae of the lumbar region of the vertebral column, commonly called the small of the back.

Lumen (loo′min) Cavity inside a tube, blood vessel, or hollow organ.

Luteinizing hormone (LH) (lu′te-in-īz″ing) Anterior pituitary hormone that aids maturation of cells in the ovary and triggers ovulation in females. In males, causes the interstitial endocrine cells of the testis to produce testosterone.

Lymph (limf) Protein-containing fluid transported by lymphatic vessels.

Lymph node Small lymphoid organ that filters lymph; contains macrophages and lymphocytes.

Lymphatic system (lim-fat′ik) System consisting of lymphatic vessels, lymph nodes, and lymph; drains excess tissue fluid from the extracellular space. The nodes provide sites for immune surveillance.

Lymphatics General term used to designate the lymphatic vessels that collect and transport lymph.

Lymphocyte Agranular white blood cell that arises from bone marrow and becomes functionally mature in the lymphoid organs of the body.

Lysosomes (li′so-sōmz) Organelles that originate from the Golgi apparatus and contain strong digestive enzymes.

Lysozyme (li′so-zīm) Enzyme in sweat, saliva, and tears that is capable of destroying certain kinds of bacteria.

Macromolecules Large, complex molecules containing from 100 to over 10,000 subunits.

Macrophage (mak′ro-fāj″) Protective cell type common in connective tissue, lymphoid tissue, and many body organs; phagocytizes tissue cells, bacteria, and other foreign debris; presents antigens to T cells in the immune response.

Macula (mak′u-lah) (1) Receptor for linear acceleration, deceleration, and gravity, located within the vestibule of the inner ear; (2) a colored area or spot.

Malignant (muh-lig′nent) Life threatening; pertains to neoplasms that spread and lead to death, such as cancer.

Malignant melanoma (mel″ah-no′mah) Cancer of the melanocytes; can begin wherever there is pigment.

Mammary glands (mam′mer-e) Milk-producing glands of the breast.

Mandible (man′dĭ-bl) Lower jawbone; U shaped, largest bone of the face.

Mass number Sum of the number of protons and neutrons in the nucleus of an atom.

Mast cells Immune cells that function to detect foreign substances in the tissue spaces and initiate local inflammatory responses against them; typically found clustered deep to an epithelium or along blood vessels.

Mastication (mas″tĭ-ka′shun) Chewing.

Meatus (me-a′tus) External opening of a canal.

Mechanical advantage (power lever) Condition that occurs when the load is close to the fulcrum and the effort is applied far from the fulcrum; allows a small effort exerted over a relatively large distance to move a large load over a small distance.

Mechanical disadvantage (speed lever) Condition that occurs when the load is far from the fulcrum and the effort is applied near the fulcrum; the effort applied must be greater than the load to be moved.

Mechanical energy The energy directly involved in moving matter; e.g., in bicycle riding, the legs provide the mechanical energy that moves the pedals.

Mechanoreceptor (meh″kĕ-no-re-sep′tor) Receptor sensitive to mechanical pressure such as touch, sound, or exerted by muscle contraction.

Medial (me′de-ahl) Toward the midline of the body.

Median (midsagittal) plane Specific sagittal plane that lies exactly in the midline.

Mediastinum (me″de-ah-sti′num) The medial cavity of the thorax containing the heart, great vessels, and trachea.

Medulla (mĕ-dul′ah) Central portion of certain organs.

Medulla oblongata (mĕ-dul′ah ob″long-gah′tah) Inferiormost part of the brain stem.

Medullary cavity Central cavity of a long bone. Contains yellow or red (bone) marrow.

Meiosis (mi-o′sis) Nuclear division process that reduces the chromosomal number by half and results in the formation of four haploid (*n*) cells; occurs only in certain reproductive organs.

Melanin (mel′ah-nin) Dark pigment formed by cells called melanocytes; imparts color to skin and hair.

Melatonin (mel″ah-to′nin) A hormone secreted by the pineal gland; secretion peaks at night and helps set sleep-wake cycles; also a powerful antioxidant.

Membrane potential Voltage across the plasma membrane.

Membrane receptors A large, diverse group of integral proteins and glycoproteins that serve as binding sites for signaling molecules.

Memory cells Members of T cell and B cell clones that provide for immunological memory.

Menarche (mĕ-nar′ke) Establishment of menstrual function; the first menstrual period.

Meninges (mĕ-nin′jēz) Protective coverings of the central nervous system; from the most external to the most internal, the dura mater, arachnoid mater, and pia mater.

Meningitis (mĕ-nin-ji′tis) Inflammation of the meninges.

Menopause Period of life when, prompted by hormonal changes, ovulation and menstruation cease.

Menstruation (men″stroo-a′shun) The periodic, cyclic discharge of blood, secretions, tissue, and mucus from the mature female uterus in the absence of pregnancy.

Merocrine glands (mer′o-krin) Glands that produce secretions intermittently; secretions do not accumulate in the gland.

Mesencephalon (mes″en-sef′ah-lon) One of the three primary vesicles of the developing brain; becomes the midbrain.

Mesenchyme (meh′zin-kīm) Common embryonic tissue from which all connective tissues arise.

Mesenteries (mes″en-ter′ēz) Double-layered extensions of the peritoneum that support most organs in the abdominal cavity.

Mesoderm (mez′o-derm) Primary germ layer that forms the skeleton and muscles of the body.

Mesothelium (mez″o-the′le-um) The epithelium found in serous membranes lining the ventral body cavity and covering its organs.

Messenger RNA (mRNA) Long nucleotide strands that reflect the exact nucleotide sequences of the genetically active DNA and carry the DNA's message.

Metabolic rate (mĕt″ah-bol′ik) Energy expended by the body per unit time.

Metabolic water (water of oxidation) Water produced from cellular metabolism (about 10% of our body's water).

Metabolism (mĕ-tab′o-lizm) Sum total of the chemical reactions occurring in the body cells.

Metaphase Second stage of mitosis.

Metastasis (mĕ-tas′tah-sis) The spread of cancer from one body part or organ into another not directly connected to it.

Metencephalon (afterbrain) A secondary brain vesicle; anterior portion of the rhombencephalon of the developing brain; becomes the pons and the cerebellum.

MHC (major histocompatibility complex) proteins Molecules on the outer surface of the plasma membrane of all cells; help the immune system distinguish self from nonself. T cells recognize antigens only when combined with these proteins.

Microfilaments (mi″kro-fil′ah-ments) Thin strands of the contractile protein actin.

Microglial cells (mi-kro′gle-al) A type of CNS supporting cell; can transform into phagocytes in areas of neural damage or inflammation.

Microtubules (mi″kro-tu′būlz) One of three types of rods in the cytoskeleton of a cell; hollow tubes made of spherical protein that determine the cell shape as well as the distribution of cellular organelles.

Microvilli (mi″kro-vil′i) Tiny projections on the free surfaces of some epithelial cells; increase surface area for absorption.

Micturition (mik″tu-rish′un) Urination, or voiding; emptying the bladder.

Midbrain (mesencephalon) Region of the brain stem between the diencephalon and the pons.

Midsagittal (median) plane Specific sagittal plane that lies exactly in the midline.

Milliequivalents per liter (mEq/L) The units used to measure electrolyte concentrations of body fluids; a measure of the number of electrical charges in 1 liter of solution.

Mineralocorticoid (min″er-al″ō-kor′tih-koyd) Steroid hormone of the adrenal cortex that regulates Na^+ and K^+ metabolism and fluid balance.

Minerals Inorganic chemical compounds found in nature; salts.

Mitochondria (mi″to-kon′dre-ah) Cytoplasmic organelles responsible for ATP generation for cellular activities.

Mitosis Process during which the chromosomes are redistributed to two daughter nuclei; nuclear division. Consists of prophase, metaphase, anaphase, and telophase.

Mitotic (M) phase One of two major periods in the cell life cycle; involves the division of the nucleus (mitosis) and the division of the cytoplasm (cytokinesis).

Mitral (bicuspid) valve (mi′tral) The left atrioventricular valve.

Mixed nerves Nerves containing the processes of motor and sensory neurons; their impulses travel to and from the central nervous system.

Molar (mo′lar) (1) A solution concentration determined by mass of solute—1 liter of solution contains an amount of solute equal to its molecular weight in grams. (2) Broad back teeth that grind and crush.

Molarity (mo-lar′ĭ-te) A way to express the concentration of a solution; moles per liter of solution.

Mole (mōl) A mole of any element or compound is equal to its atomic weight or its molecular weight (sum of atomic weights) measured in grams.

Molecule Particle consisting of two or more atoms joined together by chemical bonds.

Monoclonal antibodies (mon″o-klo′nal) Pure preparations of identical antibodies that exhibit specificity for a single antigen.

Monocyte (mon′o-sīt) Large single-nucleus white blood cell; agranular leukocyte.

Monosaccharide (mon″o-sak′ah-rīd) Literally, one sugar; building block of carbohydrates; e.g., glucose.

Morula (mor′u-lah) The mulberry-like solid mass of blastomeres resulting from cleavage in the early conceptus.

Motor areas Functional areas in the cerebral cortex that control voluntary motor functions.

Motor (efferent) nerves Nerves that carry impulses leaving the brain and spinal cord, and destined for effectors.

Motor unit A motor neuron and all the muscle cells it stimulates.

Mucous membranes (mucosae) Membranes that form the linings of body cavities open to the exterior (digestive, respiratory, urinary, and reproductive tracts).

Mucus (myoo′kus) A sticky, thick fluid secreted by mucous glands and mucous membranes; keeps the free surface of membranes moist.

Multinucleate cell (mul″tĭ-nu′kle-āt) Cell with more than one nucleus, e.g., skeletal muscle cells, osteoclasts.

Multiple sclerosis (MS) Demyelinating disorder of the CNS; causes hardened patches (sclerosis) in the brain and spinal cord.

Multipolar neurons Neurons with three or more processes; most common neuron type in the CNS.

Muscarinic receptors (mus″kah-rin′ik) Acetylcholine-binding receptors of the autonomic nervous system's target organs; named for activation by the mushroom poison muscarine.

Muscle fiber A muscle cell.

Muscle spindle Encapsulated receptor found in skeletal muscle that is sensitive to stretch.

Muscle tension The force exerted by a contracting muscle on some object.

Muscle tone Low levels of contractile activity in relaxed muscle; keeps the muscle healthy and ready to act.

Muscle twitch The response of a muscle to a single brief threshold stimulus.

Muscular dystrophy A group of inherited muscle-destroying diseases.

Muscular system The organ system consisting of the skeletal muscles of the body and their connective tissue attachments.

Myelencephalon (spinal brain) A secondary brain vesicle; lower part of the developing hindbrain, especially the medulla oblongata.

Myelin sheath (mi′ĕ-lin) Fatty insulating sheath that surrounds all but the smallest nerve fibers.

Myoblasts Embryonic mesoderm cells from which all muscle fibers develop.

Myocardial infarction (MI) (mi″o-kar′de-al in-fark′shun) Condition characterized by dead tissue areas in the myocardium; caused by interruption of blood supply to the area. Commonly called heart attack.

Myocardium (mi″o-kar′de-um) Layer of the heart wall composed of cardiac muscle.

Myofibril (mi″o-fi′bril) Rodlike bundle of contractile filaments (myofilaments) found in muscle fibers (cells).

Myofilament (mi″o-fil′ah-ment) Filament that constitutes myofibrils. Of two types: actin and myosin.

Myoglobin (mi″o-glo′bin) Oxygen-binding pigment in muscle.

Myogram A graphic recording of mechanical contractile activity produced by an apparatus that measures muscle contraction.

Myometrium (mi″o-me′tre-um) Thick uterine musculature.

Myopia (mi-o′pe-ah) A condition in which visual images are focused in front of rather than on the retina; nearsightedness.

Myosin (mi′o-sin) One of the principal contractile proteins found in muscle.

Myxedema (mik″sĕ-de′mah) Condition resulting from underactive thyroid gland.

Nares (na′rez) Nostrils.

Natural killer (NK) cell Defensive cell (a type of lymphocyte) that can kill cancer cells and virus-infected body cells before the adaptive immune system is activated.

Necrosis (nĕ-kro′sis) Death or disintegration of a cell or tissues caused by disease or injury.

Negative feedback mechanisms The most common homeostatic control mechanism. The net effect is that the output of the system shuts off the original stimulus or reduces its intensity.

Neonatal period The four-week period immediately after birth.

Neoplasm (ne′o-plazm) An abnormal mass of proliferating cells. Benign neoplasms remain localized; malignant neoplasms are cancers, which can spread to other organs.

Nephron (nef′ron) Structural and functional unit of the kidney; consists of the renal corpuscle and renal tubule.

Nerve A bundle of axons in the peripheral nervous system.

Nerve fiber Axon of a neuron.

Nerve growth factor (NGF) Protein that promotes survival and development of neurons; secreted by their target cells and many other cell types.

Nerve impulse A self-propagating wave of depolarization; also called an action potential.

Nerve plexuses Interlacing nerve networks that occur in the cervical, brachial, lumbar, and sacral regions and primarily serve the limbs.

Nervous system Fast-acting control system that triggers muscle contraction or gland secretion.

Neural tube Fetal structure that gives rise to the brain, spinal cord, and associated neural structures; formed from ectoderm by day 23 of embryonic development.

Neuroglia (nu-rog′le-ah) Nonexcitable cells of neural tissue that support, protect, and insulate the neurons; glial cells.

Neurohypophysis (nu″ro-hi-pof′ĭ-sis) Posterior pituitary plus infundibulum; portion of the pituitary gland derived from the brain.

Neuromuscular junction Region where a motor neuron comes into close contact with a skeletal muscle cell.

Neuron (nerve cell) (nu′ron) Cell of the nervous system specialized to generate and transmit electrical signals (action potentials and graded potentials).

Neuron cell body The biosynthetic center of a neuron; also called the perikaryon, or soma.

Neuronal pools Functional groups of neurons that process and integrate information.

Neuropeptides (nu″ro-pep′tīds) A class of neurotransmitters including beta endorphins and enkephalins (which act as euphorics and reduce perception of pain) and gut-brain peptides.

Neurotransmitter Chemical messenger released by neurons that may, upon binding to receptors of neurons or effector cells, stimulate or inhibit those neurons or effector cells.

Neutral fats Consist of fatty acid chains and glycerol; also called triglycerides or triacylglycerols. Commonly known as oils when liquid.

Neutralization reaction Displacement reaction in which mixing an acid and a base forms water and a salt.

Neutron (nu′tron) Uncharged subatomic particle; found in the atomic nucleus.

Neutrophil (nu′tro-fil) Most abundant type of white blood cell.

Nicotinic receptors (nik″o-tin′ik) Acetylcholine-binding receptors of all autonomic ganglionic neurons and skeletal muscle neuromuscular junctions; named for activation by nicotine.

Nitric oxide (NO) A gaseous chemical messenger; diverse functions include participation in memory formation in the brain, and causing vasodilation throughout the body.

Nociceptor (no″se-sep′tor) Receptor sensitive to potentially damaging stimuli that result in pain.

Nondisjunction Failure of sister chromatids to separate during mitosis or failure of homologous pairs to separate during meiosis; results in abnormal numbers of chromosomes in the resulting daughter cells.

Nonmyelinated fibers (non-mi′ĕ-lĭ-nāt″ed) Axons lacking a myelin sheath and therefore conducting impulses quite slowly.

Nonpolar molecules Electrically balanced molecules.

Nonvolatile (fixed) acid Acid generated by cellular metabolism that must be eliminated by the kidneys.

Norepinephrine (NE) (nor″ep-ĭ-nef′rin) A catecholamine neurotransmitter and adrenal medullary hormone, associated with sympathetic nervous system activation.

Nuclear envelope The double membrane barrier of a cell nucleus.

Nucleic acid (nu-kle′ik) Class of organic molecules that includes DNA and RNA.

Nucleoli (nu-kle′o-li) Dense spherical bodies in the cell nucleus involved with ribosomal RNA (rRNA) synthesis and ribosomal subunit assembly.

Nucleosome (nu′kle-o-sōm) Fundamental unit of chromatin; consists of a strand of DNA wound around a cluster of eight histone proteins.

Nucleotide (nu′kle-o-tīd) Building block of nucleic acids; consists of a sugar, a nitrogen-containing base, and a phosphate group.

Nucleus (nu′kle-is) (1) Control center of a cell; contains genetic material; (2) clusters of nerve cell bodies in the CNS.

Nutrients Chemical substances taken in via the diet that are used for energy and cell building.

Oblique section A cut made diagonally between the horizontal and vertical plane of the body or an organ.

Occlusion (ah-kloo′zhun) Closure or obstruction.

Octet rule (rule of eights) (ok-tet′) The tendency of atoms to interact in such a way that they have eight electrons in their valence shell.

Olfaction (ol-fak′shun) Smell.

Oligodendrocyte (ol″ĭ-go-den′dro-sīt) A type of CNS supporting cell that composes myelin sheaths.

Oocyte (o′o-sīt) Immature female gamete.

Oogenesis (o″o-jen′ĕ-sis) Process of ovum (female gamete) formation.

Ophthalmic (of-thal′mik) Pertaining to the eye.

Optic (op′tik) Pertaining to the eye or vision.

Optic chiasma (op′tik ki-az′muh) The partial crossover of fibers of the optic nerves.

Organ A part of the body formed of two or more tissues and adapted to carry out a specific function; e.g., the stomach.

Organ system A group of organs that work together to perform a vital body function; e.g., the nervous system.

Organelles (or″gah-nelz′) Small cellular structures (ribosomes, mitochondria, and others) that perform specific metabolic functions for the cell as a whole.

Organic compound Any compound composed of atoms (some of which are carbon) held together by covalent (shared electron) bonds.

Organic Pertaining to carbon-containing molecules, such as proteins, fats, and carbohydrates.

Organism The living animal (or plant), which represents the sum total of all its organ systems working together to maintain life.

Origin Attachment of a muscle that remains relatively fixed during muscular contraction.

Osmolality The number of solute particles dissolved in 1 kilogram (1000 g) of water; reflects the solution's ability to cause osmosis.

Osmolarity (oz″mo-lar′ĭ-te) The number of solute particles present in 1 liter of a solution.

Osmoreceptor (oz″mo-re-sep′tor) Structure sensitive to osmotic pressure or concentration of a solution.

Osmosis (oz-mo′sis) Diffusion of a solvent through a membrane from a dilute solution into a more concentrated one.

Osmotic pressure A measure of the tendency of water to move into a more concentrated solution.

Ossicles *See* Auditory ossicles.

Ossification (os″ĭ-fi-ka′shun) *See* Osteogenesis.

Osteoblasts (os′te-o-blasts) Bone-forming cells.

Osteoclasts (os′te-o-klasts) Large cells that resorb or break down bone matrix.

Osteocyte (os′te-o-sīt) Mature bone cell.

Osteogenesis (os″te-o-jen′e-sis) The process of bone formation; also called ossification.

Osteoid (os′te-oid) Unmineralized bone matrix.

Osteomalacia (os″te-o-mah-la′she-ah) Disorder in which bones are inadequately mineralized; soft bones.

Osteon (os′te-on) System of interconnecting canals in the microscopic structure of adult compact bone; unit of bone; also called Haversian system.

Osteoporosis (os″te-o-po-ro′sis) Decreased density and strength of bone resulting from a gradual decrease in rate of bone formation.

Ovarian cycle (o-vayr′e-an) Monthly cycle of follicle development, ovulation, and corpus luteum formation in an ovary.

Ovary (o′var-e) Female reproductive organ in which ova (eggs) are produced; female gonad.

Ovulation (ov″u-la′shun) Ejection of an immature egg (oocyte) from the ovary.

Ovum (o′vum) Female gamete; egg.

Oxidases Enzymes that catalyze the transfer of oxygen in oxidation-reduction reactions.

Oxidation (oks′ĭ-da″shun) Process of substances combining with oxygen or the removal of hydrogen.

Oxidation-reduction (redox) reaction A reaction that couples the oxidation (loss of electrons) of one substance with the reduction (gain of electrons) of another substance.

Oxidative phosphorylation (ok′sĭ-da″tiv fos″for-ĭ-la′shun) Process of ATP synthesis during which an inorganic phosphate group is attached to ADP; occurs via the electron transport chain within the mitochondria.

Oxyhemoglobin (ok″sĭ-he″mo-glo′bin) Oxygen-bound form of hemoglobin.

Oxytocin (ok″sĭ-to′sin) Hormone synthesized in the hypothalamus and secreted by the posterior pituitary; stimulates contraction of the uterus during childbirth and the ejection of milk during nursing.

Paget's disease (paj′ets) Disorder characterized by excessive bone breakdown and abnormal bone formation.

Palate (pal′at) Roof of the mouth.

Pancreas (pan′kre-us) Gland located behind the stomach, between the spleen and the duodenum; produces both endocrine and exocrine secretions.

Pancreatic juice (pan″kre-at′ik) Bicarbonate-rich secretion of the pancreas containing enzymes for digestion of all food categories.

Papilla (pah-pil′ah) Small, nipple-like projection; e.g., dermal papillae are projections of dermal tissue into the epidermis.

Paracrine (par′ah-krin) A chemical messenger that acts locally within the same tissue and is rapidly destroyed. Examples are prostaglandins and nitric oxide.

Parasagittal planes All sagittal planes offset from the midline.

Parasympathetic division The division of the autonomic nervous system that oversees digestion, elimination, and glandular function; the resting and digesting subdivision.

Parasympathetic tone Normal (background) level of parasympathetic output; sustains normal gastrointestinal and urinary tract activity, lowers heart rate.

Parathyroid glands (par″ah-thi′roid) Small endocrine glands located on the posterior aspect of the thyroid gland.

Parathyroid hormone (PTH) Hormone released by the parathyroid glands that regulates blood calcium level.

Parietal (pah-ri′ĕ-tal) Pertaining to the walls of a cavity.

Parietal serosa The part of the double-layered membrane that lines the walls of the ventral body cavity.

Parkinson's disease Neurodegenerative disorder of the basal nuclei due to insufficient secretion of the neurotransmitter dopamine; symptoms include tremor and rigid movement.

Partial pressure The pressure exerted by a single component of a mixture of gases.

Parturition (par″tu-rish′un) Culmination of pregnancy; giving birth.

Passive immunity Short-lived immunity resulting from the introduction of "borrowed antibodies" obtained from an immune animal or human donor; immunological memory is not established.

Passive (transport) processes Membrane transport processes that do not require cellular energy (ATP), e.g., diffusion, which is driven by kinetic energy.

Pathogen (path′o-jen) Disease-causing organism.

Pectoral (pek′tor-al) Pertaining to the chest.

Pectoral (shoulder) girdle Bones that attach the upper limbs to the axial skeleton; includes the clavicle and scapula.

Pedigree Traces a particular genetic trait through several generations and helps predict the genotype of future offspring.

Pelvic girdle (hip girdle) Consists of the paired coxal bones and sacrum that attach the lower limbs to the axial skeleton.

Pelvis (pel′vis) (1) Basin-shaped bony structure composed of the pelvic girdle, sacrum, and coccyx; (2) funnel-shaped tube within the kidney continuous with the ureter.

Penis (pe′nis) Male organ of copulation and urination.

Pepsin Enzyme capable of digesting proteins in an acid pH.

Peptide bond (pep′tīd) Bond joining the amine group of one amino acid to the acid carboxyl group of a second amino acid with the loss of a water molecule.

Perforating canals Canals that run at right angles to the long axis of the bone, connecting the vascular and nerve supplies of the periosteum to those of the central canals and medullary cavity; also called Volkmann's canals.

Pericardium (per″ĭ-kar′de-um) Double-layered sac enclosing the heart and forming its superficial layer; has fibrous and serous layers.

Perichondrium (per″ĭ-kon′dre-um) Fibrous, connective-tissue membrane covering the external surface of cartilaginous structures.

Perimysium (per″ĭ-mis′e-um) Connective tissue that bundles muscle fibers into fascicles.

Perineum (per″ĭ-ne′um) That region of the body spanning the region between the ischial tuberosities and extending from the pubic arch to the coccyx.

Periosteum (per″e-os′te-um) Double-layered connective tissue that covers and nourishes the bone.

Peripheral congestion Condition caused by failure of the right side of the heart; results in edema in the extremities.

Peripheral nervous system (PNS) Portion of the nervous system consisting of nerves and ganglia that lie outside of the brain and spinal cord.

Peripheral resistance A measure of the amount of friction encountered by blood as it flows through the blood vessels.

Peristalsis (per″ĭ-stal′sis) Progressive, wavelike contractions that move foodstuffs through the alimentary tube organs (or that move other substances through other hollow body organs).

Peritoneum (per″ĭ-to-ne′um) Serous membrane lining the interior of the abdominal cavity and covering the surfaces of abdominal organs.

Peritonitis (per″ĭ-to-ni′tis) Inflammation of the peritoneum.

Permeability That property of membranes that permits passage of molecules and ions.

Peroxisomes (pĕ-roks′ĭ-sōmz) Membranous sacs in cytoplasm containing powerful oxidase enzymes that use molecular oxygen to detoxify harmful or toxic substances, such as free radicals.

Peyer's patches (pi′erz) Lymphoid organs located in the small intestine; also called aggregated lymphoid nodules.

pH unit (pe-āch) The measure of the relative acidity or alkalinity of a solution.

Phagocytosis (fag″o-si-to′sis) Engulfing of foreign solids by (phagocytic) cells.

Phagosome (fag′o-sōm) Vesicle formed as a result of phagocytosis.

Pharmacological dose A drug dose that is dramatically higher than normal levels of that substance (e.g., hormone) in the body.

Pharyngotympanic tube Tube that connects the middle ear and the pharynx. Also called auditory tube, eustachian tube.

Pharynx (fayr′inks) Muscular tube extending from the region posterior to the nasal cavities to the esophagus.

Phenotype (fe′no-tīp) Observable expression of the genotype.

Phospholipid (fos″fo-lip′id) Modified lipid, contains phosphorus.

Phosphorylation A chemical reaction in which a phosphate molecule is added to a molecule; for example, phosphorylation of ADP yields ATP.

Photoreceptor (fo″to-re-sep′tor) Specialized receptor cells that respond to light energy; rods and cones.

Physiological acidosis (as″ĭ-do′sis) Arterial pH lower than 7.35 resulting from any cause.

Physiological dose A drug dose that replicates normal levels of that substance (e.g., hormone) in the body. (*Compare with* Pharmacological dose.)

Physiology (fiz″e-ol′o-je) Study of the function of living organisms.

Pineal gland (body) (pin′e-al) A hormone-secreting part of the diencephalon of the brain thought to be involved in setting the biological clock and influencing reproductive function.

Pinocytosis (pe″no-si-to′sis) Engulfing of extracellular fluid by cells.

Pituitary gland (pĭ-tu′ih-tayr″e) Neuroendocrine gland located beneath the brain that serves a variety of functions including regulation of gonads, thyroid, adrenal cortex, lactation, and water balance.

Placenta (plah-sen′tah) Temporary organ formed from both fetal and maternal tissues that provides nutrients and oxygen to the developing fetus, carries away fetal metabolic wastes, and produces the hormones of pregnancy.

Plasma (plaz′mah) The nonliving fluid component of blood within which formed elements and various solutes are suspended and circulated.

Plasma cells Members of a B cell clone; effector B cells specialized to produce and release antibodies.

Plasma membrane Membrane, composed of phospholipids, cholesterol, and proteins, that encloses cell contents; outer limiting cell membrane.

Platelet (plāt′let) Cell fragment found in blood; involved in clotting.

Pleurae (ploo′re) Two layers of serous membrane that line the thoracic cavity and cover the external surface of the lung.

Pleural cavity (ploo′ral) A potential space between the two layers of pleura; contains a thin film of serous fluid.

Plexus (plek′sus) A network of converging and diverging nerve fibers, blood vessels, or lymphatics.

Polar molecules Nonsymmetrical molecules that contain electrically unbalanced atoms.

Polarized State of a plasma membrane of an unstimulated neuron or muscle cell in which the inside of the cell is relatively negative in comparison to the outside; the resting state.

Polycythemia (pol″e-si-the′me-ah) An abnormally high number of erythrocytes.

Polymer A substance of high molecular weight with long, chainlike molecules consisting of many similar (repeated) units.

Polypeptide (pol″e-pep′tīd) A chain of amino acids.

Polyps Benign mucosal tumors.

Polysaccharide (pol″e-sak′ah-rīd) Literally, many sugars, a polymer of linked monosaccharides; e.g., starch, glycogen.

Pons (1) Any bridgelike structure or part; (2) the part of the brain stem connecting the medulla with the midbrain, providing linkage between upper and lower levels of the central nervous system.

Pore The surface opening of the duct of a sweat gland.

Positive feedback mechanisms Feedback that tends to cause the level of a variable to change in the same direction as an initial change.

Posterior pituitary Neural part of pituitary gland; part of the neurohypophysis.

Postganglionic neuron (post″gan″gle-ah′nik) Autonomic motor neuron that has its cell body in a peripheral ganglion and projects its axon to an effector.

Potential energy Stored or inactive energy.

Preganglionic neuron Autonomic motor neuron that has its cell body in the central nervous system and projects its axon to a peripheral ganglion.

Presbyopia (pres″be-o′pe-ah) A condition that results in the loss of near focusing ability; typical onset is around age 40.

Pressure gradient Difference in pressure (hydrostatic or osmotic) that drives movement of fluid.

Primary active transport A type of active transport in which the energy needed to drive the transport process is provided directly by hydrolysis of ATP.

Prime mover Muscle that bears the major responsibility for effecting a particular movement; an agonist.

Process (1) Prominence or projection; (2) series of actions for a specific purpose.

Progesterone (pro-jes′ter-ōn) Hormone partly responsible for preparing the uterus for the fertilized ovum.

Prolactin (PRL) (pro-lak′tin) Adenohypophyseal hormone that stimulates the breasts to produce milk.

Pronation (pro-na′shun) Inward rotation of the forearm causing the radius to cross diagonally over the ulna—palms face posteriorly.

Prophase The first stage of mitosis, consisting of coiling of the chromosomes accompanied by migration of the two daughter centrioles toward the poles of the cell, and nuclear membrane breakdown.

Proprioceptor (pro″pre-o-sep′tor) Receptor located in a joint, muscle, or tendon; concerned with locomotion, posture, and muscle tone.

Prostaglandin (pros″tah-glan′din) A lipid-based chemical messenger synthesized by most tissue cells; acts locally as a paracrine.

Prostate Accessory reproductive gland; produces one-third of semen volume, including fluids that activate sperm.

Protein (pro′tēn) Organic compound composed of carbon, oxygen, hydrogen, and nitrogen; types include enzymes, structural components; 10–30% of cell mass.

Prothrombin time Diagnostic test to determine status of hemostasis system.

Proton (pro′ton) Subatomic particle that bears a positive charge; located in the atomic nucleus.

Proton acceptor A substance that takes up hydrogen ions in detectable amounts. Commonly referred to as a base.

Proton donor A substance that releases hydrogen ions in detectable amounts; an acid.

Proximal (prok′si-mul) Toward the attached end of a limb or the origin of a structure.

Pseudounipolar neuron (soo″do-u″nĭ-po′lar) Another term for unipolar neuron.

Puberty Period of life when reproductive maturity is achieved.

Pulmonary (pul′muh-nayr-e) Pertaining to the lungs.

Pulmonary arteries Vessels that deliver blood to the lungs to be oxygenated.

Pulmonary circuit System of blood vessels that serves gas exchange in the lungs; i.e., pulmonary arteries, capillaries, and veins.

Pulmonary edema (ĕ-de′muh) Leakage of fluid into the air sacs and tissue of the lungs.

Pulmonary veins Vessels that deliver freshly oxygenated blood from the respiratory zones of the lungs to the heart.

Pulmonary ventilation Breathing; consists of inspiration and expiration.

Pulse Rhythmic expansion and recoil of arteries resulting from heart contraction; can be felt from outside the body.

Pupil Opening in the center of the iris through which light enters the eye.

Pus Fluid product of inflammation composed of white blood cells, the debris of dead cells, and a thin fluid.

Pyloric sphincter (pi-lor′ik sfink′ter) Valve of the distal end of the stomach that controls food entry into the duodenum.

Pyramidal (corticospinal) tracts Major motor pathways concerned with voluntary movement; descend from pyramidal cells in the frontal lobes of each cerebral hemisphere.

Pyruvic acid An intermediate compound in the metabolism of carbohydrates.

Radioactivity The process of spontaneous decay seen in some of the heavier isotopes, during which particles or energy is emitted from the atomic nucleus; results in the atom becoming more stable.

Radioisotope (ra″de-o-i′so-tōp) Isotope that exhibits radioactive behavior.

Ramus (ra′mus) Branch of a nerve, artery, vein, or bone.

Rapid eye movement (REM) sleep Stage of sleep in which rapid eye movements, an alert EEG pattern, and dreaming occur.

Reactant A substance taking part in a chemical reaction.

Receptor (re-sep′tor) (1) A cell or nerve ending of a sensory neuron specialized to respond to particular types of stimuli; (2) protein that binds specifically with other molecules, e.g., neurotransmitters, hormones, paracrines, antigens.

Receptor-mediated endocytosis The type of endocytosis in which engulfed particles attach to receptors before endocytosis occurs.

Receptor potential A graded potential that occurs at a sensory receptor membrane.

Recessive traits A trait due to a particular allele that does not manifest itself in the presence of other alleles that generate traits dominant to it; must be present in double dose to be expressed.

Reduction Chemical reaction in which electrons and energy are gained by a molecule (often accompanied by gain of hydrogen ions) or oxygen is lost.

Referred pain Pain felt at a site other than the area of origin.

Reflex Automatic reaction to stimuli.

Refraction The bending of a light ray when it meets a different surface at an oblique rather than right angle.

Regeneration Replacement of destroyed tissue with the same kind of tissue.

Regulatory T cells (T_{Reg} cells) Population of T cells (usually expressing CD4) that suppress the immune response.

Relative refractory period Follows the absolute refractory period; interval when a threshold for action potential stimulation is markedly elevated.

Renal (re′nal) Pertaining to the kidney.

Renal autoregulation Process the kidney uses to maintain a nearly constant glomerular filtration rate despite fluctuations in systemic blood pressure.

Renal clearance The volume of plasma from which a particular substance is completely removed in a given time, usually 1 minute; provides information about renal function.

Renin (re′nin) Enzyme released by the kidneys that raises blood pressure by initiating the renin-angiotensin-aldosterone mechanism.

Rennin Stomach-secreted enzyme that acts on milk protein; not produced in adults.

Repolarization Movement of the membrane potential to the initial resting (polarized) state.

Reproductive system Organ system that functions to produce offspring.

Resistance exercise High-intensity exercise in which the muscles are pitted against high resistance or immovable forces and, as a result, muscle cells increase in size.

Respiration The processes involved in supplying the body with oxygen and disposing of carbon dioxide.

Respiratory system Organ system that carries out gas exchange; includes the nose, pharynx, larynx, trachea, bronchi, lungs.

Resting membrane potential The voltage that exists across the plasma membrane during the resting state of an excitable cell; ranges from −90 to −20 millivolts depending on cell type.

Reticular activating system (RAS) (re-tik′u-lar) Diffuse brain stem neural network that receives a wide variety of sensory input and maintains wakefulness of the cerebral cortex.

Reticular connective tissue Connective tissue with a fine network of reticular fibers that form the internal supporting framework of lymphoid organs.

Reticular formation Functional system that spans the brain stem; involved in regulating sensory input to the cerebral cortex, cortical arousal, and control of motor behavior.

Reticular lamina A layer of extracellular material containing a fine network of collagen protein fibers; together with the basal lamina it is a major component of the basement membrane.

Reticulocyte (rĕ-tik′u-lo-sīt) Immature erythrocyte.

Retina (ret′ĭ-nah) Inner layer of the eyeball; contains photoreceptors (rods, cones).

Rhombencephalon (hindbrain) (romb″en-sef′ah-lon) Caudal portion of the developing brain; constricts to form the metencephalon and myelencephalon; includes the pons, cerebellum, and medulla oblongata.

Ribosomal RNA (rRNA) A constituent of ribosome; exists within the ribosomes of cytoplasm and assists in protein synthesis.

Ribosomes (ri′bo-sōmz) Cytoplasmic organelles at which proteins are synthesized.

RNA (ribonucleic acid) (ri′bo-nu-kle′ik) Nucleic acid that contains ribose and the bases A, G, C, and U. Carries out DNA's instructions for protein synthesis.

Rods One of the two types of photosensitive cells in the retina.

Rotation The turning of a bone around its own long axis.

Rugae (ru′ge) Elevations or ridges, as in stomach mucosa.

Rule of nines Method of computing the extent of burns by dividing the body into a number of areas, each accounting for 9% (or a multiple thereof) of the total body area.

S (synthetic) phase The part of the interphase period of the cell cycle in which DNA replicates itself, ensuring that the two future cells will receive identical copies of genetic material.

Sagittal plane (saj′ĭ-tal) A longitudinal (vertical) plane that divides the body or any of its parts into right and left portions.

Saliva Secretion of the salivary glands; cleanses and moistens the mouth and begins chemical digestion of starchy foods.

Saltatory conduction Transmission of an action potential along a myelinated fiber in which the nerve impulse appears to leap from gap to gap.

Sarcolemma The plasma membrane of a muscle fiber.

Sarcomere (sar′ko-mēr) The smallest contractile unit of muscle; extends from one Z disc to the next.

Sarcoplasm The nonfibrillar cytoplasm of a muscle fiber.

Sarcoplasmic reticulum (SR) (sar″ko-plaz′mik rĕ-tik′u-lum) Specialized endoplasmic reticulum of muscle cells.

Schwann cell A type of supporting cell in the PNS; forms myelin sheaths and is vital to peripheral nerve fiber regeneration.

Sclera (skle′rah) White opaque portion of the fibrous layer of the eyeball.

Scrotum (skro′tum) External sac enclosing the testes.

Sebaceous glands (oil glands) (se-ba′shus) Epidermal glands that produce an oily secretion called sebum.

Sebum (se′bum) Oily secretion of sebaceous glands.

Second-degree burn A burn in which the epidermis and the upper region of the dermis are damaged.

Second messenger Intracellular molecule generated by the binding of a chemical (hormone or neurotransmitter) to a receptor protein; mediates intracellular responses to the chemical messenger.

Secondary sex characteristics Anatomical features, not directly involved in the reproductive process, that develop under the influence of sex hormones, e.g., male or female pattern of muscle development, bone growth, body hair distribution.

Secretion (se-kre′shun) (1) The passage of material formed by a cell to its exterior; (2) cell product that is transported to the exterior of a cell.

Secretory vesicles (granules) Vesicles that migrate to the plasma membrane of a cell and discharge their contents from the cell by exocytosis.

Section A cut through the body (or an organ) that is made along a particular plane; a thin slice of tissue prepared for microscopic study.

Segregation During meiosis, the distribution of the members of the allele pair to different gametes.

Selectively permeable membrane A membrane that allows certain substances to pass while restricting the movement of others; also called differentially permeable membrane.

Semen (se′men) Fluid mixture containing sperm and secretions of the male accessory reproductive glands.

Semilunar valves (sĕ″me-loo′ner) Valves that prevent blood return to the ventricles after contraction; aortic and pulmonary valves.

Seminiferous tubules (sem″ĭ-nif′er-us) Highly convoluted tubes within the testes; form sperm.

Sense organs Localized collections of many types of cells working together to accomplish a specific receptive process.

Sensory (afferent) nerves Nerves that contain processes of sensory neurons and carry impulses to the central nervous system.

Sensory areas Functional areas of the cerebral cortex that provide for conscious awareness of sensation.

Sensory receptor A cell or part of a cell (e.g., receptive endings of sensory neurons) specialized to respond to a stimulus.

Serosa (serous membrane) (se-ro′sah) The moist membrane found in closed ventral body cavities.

Serous fluid (sēr′us) Clear, watery fluid secreted by cells of a serous membrane.

Serum (sēr′um) Amber-colored fluid that exudes from clotted blood as the clot shrinks; plasma without clotting factors.

Sesamoid bones (ses′ah-moid) Short bones embedded in tendons, variable in size and number, many of which influence the action of muscles; largest is the patella (kneecap).

Severe combined immunodeficiency syndromes (SCIDs) Congenital conditions resulting in little or no protection against disease-causing organisms of any type.

Sex chromosomes The chromosomes, X and Y, that determine genetic sex (XX = female; XY = male); the 23rd pair of chromosomes.

Sex-linked inheritance Inherited traits determined by genes on the sex chromosomes, e.g., X-linked genes are passed from mother to son, Y-linked genes are passed from father to son.

Sexually transmitted infection (STI) Any infectious disease spread through sexual contact.

Signal sequence A short peptide segment present in a protein being synthesized that causes the associated ribosome to attach to the membrane of rough ER.

Simple diffusion The unassisted transport across a plasma membrane of a lipid-soluble or very small particle.

Sinoatrial (SA) node (si″no-a′tre-al) Specialized myocardial cells in the wall of the right atrium; pacemaker of the heart.

Sinus (si′nus) (1) Mucous-membrane-lined, air-filled cavity in certain cranial bones; (2) dilated channel for the passage of blood or lymph.

Skeletal muscle Muscle composed of cylindrical multinucleate cells with obvious striations; the muscle(s) attached to the body's skeleton; voluntary muscle.

Skeletal system System of protection and support composed primarily of bone and cartilage.

Skull Bony protective encasement of the brain and the organs of hearing and equilibrium; includes cranial and facial bones.

Small intestine Convoluted tube extending from the pyloric sphincter to the ileocecal valve where it joins the large intestine; the site where digestion is completed and virtually all absorption occurs.

Smooth muscle Spindle-shaped cells with one centrally located nucleus and no externally visible striations (bands). Found mainly in the walls of hollow organs.

Sodium-potassium (Na^+-K^+) pump A primary active transport system that simultaneously drives Na^+ out of the cell against a steep gradient and pumps K^+ back in. Also called Na^+-K^+ ATPase.

Sol-gel transformation Reversible change of a colloid from a fluid (sol) to a more solid (gel) state.

Solute (sol′yoot) The substance that is dissolved in a solution.

Solute pump Enzyme-like protein carrier that mediates active transport of solutes such as amino acids and ions uphill against their concentration gradients.

Somatic nervous system (so-mă′tik) Division of the peripheral nervous system that provides the motor innervation of skeletal muscles; also called the voluntary nervous system.

Somatic reflexes Reflexes that activate skeletal muscle.

Somatosensory system That part of the sensory system dealing with reception in the body wall and limbs; receives inputs from exteroceptors, proprioceptors, and interoceptors.

Somite (so′mīt) A mesodermal segment of the body of an embryo that contributes to the formation of skeletal muscles, vertebrae, and dermis of skin.

Spatial discrimination The ability of neurons to identify the site or pattern of stimulation.

Special senses The senses of taste, smell, vision, hearing, and equilibrium.

Specific gravity Term used to compare the weight of a substance to the weight of an equal volume of distilled water.

Sperm (spermatozoon) Male gamete.

Spermatogenesis (sper″mah-to-jen′ĕ-sis) The process of sperm (male gamete) formation; involves meiosis.

Sphincter (sfink′ter) A circular muscle surrounding an opening; acts as a valve.

Spinal cord The bundle of nervous tissue that runs from the brain to the first to third lumbar vertebrae and provides a conduction pathway to and from the brain.

Spinal nerves The 31 nerve pairs that arise from the spinal cord.

Splanchnic circulation (splangk′nik) The blood vessels serving the digestive system.

Spleen Largest lymphoid organ; provides for lymphocyte proliferation, immune surveillance and response, and blood-cleansing functions.

Spongy bone Internal layer of skeletal bone. Also called cancellous bone.

Sprain Ligaments reinforcing a joint are stretched or torn.

Static equilibrium Sense of head position in space with respect to gravity.

Stenosis (stĕ-no′sis) Abnormal constriction or narrowing.

Steroids (stĕ′roidz) Group of chemical substances including certain hormones and cholesterol; they are fat soluble and contain little oxygen.

Stimulus (stim′u-lus) An excitant or irritant; a change in the environment that evokes a response.

Stomach Temporary reservoir in the gastrointestinal tract where chemical breakdown of proteins begins and food is converted into chyme.

Stressor Any stimulus that directly or indirectly causes the hypothalamus to initiate stress-reducing responses, such as the fight-or-flight response.

Stroke *See* Cerebrovascular accident.

Stroke volume (SV) Amount of blood pumped out of a ventricle during one contraction.

Stroma (stro′mah) The basic internal structural framework of an organ.

Structural (fibrous) proteins Consist of extended, strandlike polypeptide chains forming a strong, ropelike structure that is linear, insoluble in water, and very stable; e.g., collagen.

Subcutaneous (sub″kyu-ta′ne-us) Beneath the skin.

Subendocardial conducting network Modified ventricular muscle fibers of the conduction system of the heart. Also called Purkinje fibers.

Substrate A reactant on which an enzyme acts to cause a chemical action to proceed.

Sudoriferous gland (su″do-rif′er-us) Epidermal gland that produces sweat.

Sulcus (sul′kus) A furrow on the brain, less deep than a fissure.

Summation Accumulation of effects, especially those of muscular, sensory, or mental stimuli.

Superficial Located close to or on the body surface.

Superior Toward the head or upper body regions.

Superior vena cava Vein that returns blood from body regions superior to the diaphragm.

Supination (soo″pĭ-na′shun) The outward rotation of the forearm causing palms to face anteriorly.

Surfactant (ser-fak′tant) Secretion produced by certain cells of the alveoli that reduces the surface tension of water molecules, thus preventing the collapse of the alveoli after each expiration.

Suspension Heterogeneous mixtures with large, often visible solutes that tend to settle out.

Suture (soo′cher) An immovable fibrous joint; with one exception, all bones of the skull are united by sutures.

Sweat gland *See* Sudoriferous gland.

Sympathetic division The division of the autonomic nervous system that prepares the body for activity or to cope with some stressor (danger, excitement, etc.); the fight, fright, and flight subdivision.

Sympathetic (vasomotor) tone State of partial vasoconstriction of the blood vessels maintained by sympathetic fibers.

Symphysis (sim′fih-sis) A joint in which the bones are connected by fibrocartilage.

Synapse (sin′aps) Functional junction or point of close contact between two neurons or between a neuron and an effector cell.

Synapsis (sĭ-nap′sis) Pairing of homologous chromosomes during the first meiotic division.

Synaptic cleft (sĭ-nap′tik) Fluid-filled space at a synapse.

Synaptic delay Time required for a signal to cross a synapse between two neurons.

Synaptic vesicles Small membranous sacs containing neurotransmitter.

Synarthrosis (sin″ar-thro′sis) Immovable joint.

Synchondrosis (sin″kon-dro′sis) A joint in which the bones are united by hyaline cartilage.

Syndesmosis (sin″des-mo′sis) A joint in which the bones are united by a ligament or a sheet of fibrous tissue.

Synergist (sin′er-jist) (1) Muscle that aids the action of a prime mover by effecting the same movement or by stabilizing joints across which the prime mover acts, preventing undesirable movements. (2) Hormone that amplifies the effect of another hormone at a target cell.

Synostosis (sin″os-to′sis) A completely ossified joint; a fused joint.

Synovial fluid Fluid secreted by the synovial membrane; lubricates joint surfaces and nourishes articular cartilages.

Synovial joint Freely movable joint exhibiting a joint cavity; also called a diarthrosis.

Synthesis (combination) reaction A chemical reaction in which larger, more complex atoms or molecules are formed from simpler ones.

Systemic (sis-tem′ik) Pertaining to the whole body.

Systemic circuit System of blood vessels that serves gas exchange in the body tissues.

Systole (sis′to-le) Period when either the ventricles or the atria are contracting.

Systolic pressure (sis-tah′lik) Pressure exerted by blood on the blood vessel walls during ventricular contractions.

T cells Lymphocytes that mediate cellular immunity; include helper, cytotoxic, regulatory, and memory cells. Also called T lymphocytes.

T tubule (transverse tubule) Extension of the muscle cell plasma membrane (sarcolemma) that protrudes deeply into the muscle cell.

Tachycardia (tak″e-kar′de-ah) A heart rate over 100 beats per minute.

Taste buds Sensory receptor organs that house gustatory cells, which respond to dissolved food chemicals.

Telencephalon (endbrain) (tel″en-seh′fuh-lon) Anterior subdivision of the primary forebrain that develops into olfactory lobes, cerebral cortex, and basal nuclei.

Telophase The final phase of mitosis; begins when migration of chromosomes to the poles of the cell has been completed and ends with the formation of two daughter nuclei.

Tendon (ten′dun) Cord of dense fibrous tissue attaching muscle to bone.

Tendon organ Proprioceptor located in tendon; monitors muscle tension to prevent tearing and help smooth onset and termination of muscle contraction.

Tendonitis Inflammation of tendon sheaths, typically caused by overuse.

Terminal branches Branching ends of an axon that allow it to form many axon terminals; terminal arborization.

Testis (tes′tis) Male primary reproductive organ that produces sperm; male gonad.

Testosterone (tes-tos′tĕ-rōn) Male sex hormone produced by the testes; during puberty promotes virilization, and is necessary for normal sperm production.

Tetanus (tet′ah-nus) (1) A smooth, sustained muscle contraction resulting from high-frequency stimulation; (2) an infectious disease caused by an anaerobic bacterium.

Thalamus (thal′ah-mus) A mass of gray matter in the diencephalon of the brain.

Thermogenesis (ther″mo-jen′ĕ-sis) Heat production.

Thermoreceptor (ther″mo-re-sep′ter) Receptor sensitive to temperature changes.

Third-degree burn A burn that involves the entire thickness of the skin; also called a full-thickness burn. Usually requires skin grafting.

Thoracic cage (bony thorax) Bones and costal cartilages that form the framework of the thorax; includes sternum, ribs, and thoracic vertebrae.

Thoracic duct Large duct that receives lymph drained from the entire lower body, the left upper extremity, and the left side of the head and thorax.

Thoracic vertebrae The 12 vertebrae that are in the middle part of the vertebral column and articulate with the ribs.

Thorax (tho′raks) That portion of the body trunk above the diaphragm and below the neck.

Threshold stimulus Weakest stimulus capable of producing a response in an excitable tissue.

Thrombin (throm′bin) Enzyme that induces clotting by converting fibrinogen to fibrin.

Thrombocyte (throm′bo-sīt) Platelet; cell fragment that participates in blood coagulation.

Thrombocytopenia (throm″bo-si″to-pe′ne-ah) A reduction in the number of platelets circulating in the blood.

Thrombus (throm′bus) A clot that develops and persists in an unbroken blood vessel.

Thymine (T) (thi′mēn) Single-ring base (a pyrimidine) in DNA.

Thymus (thi′mus) Lymphoid organ and endocrine gland active in immune response; site of maturation of T lymphocytes.

Thyroid gland (thi′roid) One of the largest of the body's endocrine glands; straddles the anterior trachea.

Thyroid hormone (TH) The major hormone secreted by thyroid follicles; stimulates enzymes concerned with glucose oxidation.

Thyroid-stimulating hormone (TSH) Anterior pituitary hormone that regulates secretion of thyroid hormones.

Thyroxine (T_4) (thi-rok′sin) Iodine-containing hormone secreted by the thyroid gland; accelerates cellular metabolic rate in most body tissues.

Tight junction Area where plasma membranes of adjacent cells are tightly bound together, forming an impermeable barrier.

Tissue A group of similar cells and their intercellular substance specialized to perform a specific function; primary tissue types of the body are epithelial, connective, muscle, and nervous tissue.

Tissue perfusion Blood flow through body tissues or organs.

Tonicity (to-nis′ĭ-te) A measure of the ability of a solution to cause a change in cell shape or tone by promoting osmotic flows of water.

Tonsils A ring of lymphoid tissue around the entrance to the pharynx. *See also* Adenoids.

Trabecula (trah-bek′u-lah) (1) Any of the fibrous bands extending from the capsule into the interior of an organ; (2) strut or thin plate of bone in spongy bone.

Trachea (tra′ke-ah) Windpipe; cartilage-reinforced tube extending from larynx to bronchi.

Tract A collection of axons in the central nervous system having the same origin, termination, and function.

Transcription One of the two major steps in the transfer of genetic code information from a DNA base sequence to the complementary base sequence of an mRNA molecule.

Transduction (trans-duk′shun) The conversion of the energy of a stimulus into an electrical event.

Transepithelial transport (trans-ep″ĭ-the′le-al) Movement of substances through, rather than between, adjacent epithelial cells connected by tight junctions, such as absorption of nutrients in the small intestine.

Transfer RNA (tRNA) Short-chain RNA molecules that transfer amino acids to the ribosome.

Transfusion reaction Agglutination and destruction of red blood cells following transfusion of incompatible blood.

Translation One of the two major steps in the transfer of genetic code information, in which the information carried by mRNA is decoded and used to assemble polypeptides.

Transverse (horizontal) plane A plane running from right to left, dividing the body or an organ into superior and inferior parts.

Tricuspid valve (tri-kus′pid) The right atrioventricular valve.

Triglycerides (tri-glis′er-īdz) Fats and oils composed of fatty acids and glycerol; are the body's most concentrated source of energy fuel; also known as neutral fats.

Triiodothyronine (T_3) (tri″i-o″do-thi′ro-nēn) Thyroid hormone; secretion and function similar to those of thyroxine (T_4).

Trophoblast (tro′fo-blast) Outer sphere of cells of the blastocyst.

Tropic hormone (tropin) (trōp′ik) A hormone that regulates the secretory action of another endocrine organ.

Trypsin Proteolytic enzyme secreted by the pancreas.

Tubular reabsorption The movement of filtrate components from the renal tubules into the blood.

Tubular secretion The movement of substances (such as drugs, urea, excess ions) from blood into filtrate.

Tumor An abnormal growth of cells; a swelling; may be cancerous.

Tunica (too′nĭ-kah) A covering or tissue coat; membrane layer.

Tympanic membrane (tim-pan′ik) Eardrum.

Ulcer (ul′ser) Lesion or erosion of the mucous membrane, such as gastric ulcer of stomach.

Umbilical cord (um-bĭ′lĭ-kul) Structure bearing arteries and veins connecting the placenta and the fetus.

Umbilicus (um-bĭ′lĭ-kus) Navel; marks site where umbilical cord was attached in fetal stage.

Unipolar neuron Neuron in which embryological fusion of the two processes leaves only one process extending from the cell body.

Uracil (U) (u′rah-sil) A smaller, single-ring base (a pyrimidine) found in RNA.

Urea (u-re′ah) Main nitrogen-containing waste excreted in urine.

Ureter (u-re′ter) Tube that carries urine from kidney to bladder.

Urethra (u-re′thrah) Canal through which urine passes from the bladder to outside the body.

Uric acid The nitrogenous waste product of nucleic acid metabolism; component of urine.

Urinary bladder A smooth, collapsible, muscular sac that stores urine temporarily.

Urinary system System primarily responsible for water, electrolyte, and acid-base balance and removal of nitrogenous wastes.

Uterine tube (u′ter-in) Tube through which the ovum is transported to the uterus. Also called fallopian tube.

Uterus (u′ter-us) Hollow, thick-walled organ that receives, retains, and nourishes fertilized egg; site where embryo/fetus develops.

Uvula (u′vu-lah) Tissue tag hanging from soft palate.

Vaccine Preparation that provides artificially acquired active immunity.

Vagina Thin-walled tube extending from the cervix to the body exterior; often called the birth canal.

Valence shell (va′lens) Outermost electron shell (energy level) of an atom that contains electrons.

Varicosities Knoblike swellings of certain autonomic axons containing mitochondria and synaptic vesicles.

Vas (vaz′) A duct; vessel.

Vasa recta (va′sah rek′tah) Capillary branches that supply nephron loops in the medulla region of the kidney.

Vascular Pertaining to blood vessels or richly supplied with blood vessels.

Vascular spasm Immediate response to blood vessel injury; results in constriction.

Vasoconstriction (vas″o-kon-strik′shun) Narrowing of blood vessels.

Vasodilation (vas″o-di-la′shun) Relaxation of the smooth muscles of the blood vessels, producing dilation.

Vasomotion (vas″o-mo′shun) Intermittent contraction or relaxation of the precapillary sphincters, resulting in a staggered blood flow when tissue needs are not extreme.

Vasomotor center (vas″o-mo′ter) Brain area concerned with regulation of blood vessel resistance.

Vasomotor fibers Sympathetic nerve fibers that cause the contraction of smooth muscle in the walls of blood vessels, thereby regulating blood vessel diameter.

Veins (vānz″) Blood vessels that return blood toward the heart from the circulation.

Ventral Pertaining to the front; anterior.

Ventricles (1) Paired, inferiorly located heart chambers that function as the major blood pumps; (2) cavities in the brain.

Venule (ven′ūl) A small vein.

Vertebral column (spine) (ver′tĕ-brul) Formed of a number of individual bones called vertebrae and two composite bones (sacrum and coccyx).

Vesicle (vĕ′sĭ-kul) A small liquid-filled sac or bladder.

Vesicular transport Transport of large particles and macromolecules into or out of a cell or between its compartments in membrane-bound sacs.

Vesicular follicle Mature ovarian follicle.

Vestibule An enlarged area at the beginning of a canal, i.e., inner ear, nose, larynx.

Villus (vil′us) One of the fingerlike projections of the small intestinal mucosa that tremendously increase its surface area for absorption.

Visceral (vis′er-al) Pertaining to an internal organ of the body or the inner part of a structure.

Visceral muscle Type of smooth muscle; its cells contract as a unit and rhythmically, are electrically coupled by gap junctions, and often exhibit spontaneous action potentials. Also called unitary smooth muscle.

Visceral organs (viscera) A group of internal organs housed in the ventral body cavity.

Visceral serosa (se-ro′sah) The part of the double-layered membrane that lines the outer surfaces of organs within the ventral body cavity.

Viscosity (vis′kos′ĭ-te) A measurement of thickness (stickiness) of a fluid.

Visual field The field of view seen when the head is still.

Vital capacity (VC) The volume of air that can be expelled from the lungs by forcible expiration after the deepest inspiration; total exchangeable air.

Vital signs Includes pulse, blood pressure, respiratory rate, and body temperature measurements.

Vitamins Organic compounds required by the body in minute amounts.

Vocal folds Mucosal folds that function in voice production (speech); also called the true vocal cords.

Volatile acid An acid that can be eliminated by the lungs; carbonic acid is converted to CO_2, which diffuses into the alveoli.

Volkmann's canals *See* Perforating canals.

Voluntary muscle Muscle under strict nervous control; skeletal muscle.

Voluntary nervous system The somatic nervous system.

Vulva (vul′vuh) Female external genitalia.

Wallerian degeneration (wal-er′ē-an) A process of disintegration of an axon that occurs when it is crushed or severed and cannot receive nutrients from the cell body.

White matter White substance of the central nervous system; myelinated nerve fibers.

Xenograft Tissue graft taken from another animal species.

Yolk sac (yōk) One of the extraembryonic membranes; involved in early blood cell formation.

Zygote (zi′gōt) Fertilized egg.

Photo and Illustration Credits

Photo Credits

Chapter 1
Chapter Opener: Blend Images/Alamy. 1.1: GoGo Images/Jupiter Images. 1.3: Pearson Science. 1.8.1: Jenny Thomas, Pearson Science. 1.8.2: Scott Camazine/Photo Researchers. 1.8.3: James Cavallini/Photo Researchers. 1.8.4: CNRI/Science Photo Library/Photo Researchers. 1.12a: Custom Medical Stock Photo, Inc. A Closer Look: a: Clinique Ste Catherine/CNRI/Science Photo Library/Photo Researchers. b: Zephyr/Photo Researchers. c: Willaim Klunk, Chet Mathis, University of Pittsburgh, PET Amyloid Imaging Group.

Chapter 2
Chapter Opener: Prisma, SuperStock. 2.4.1: Stockbyte/Getty Images. 2.4.2: Algecireño/Shutterstock. 2.4.3: Henry Hong – CSB, Imagineering © Pearson. 2.10b: Herman Eisenbeiss/Photo Researchers. 2.22c: Computer Graphics Laboratory, University of California, San Francisco.

Chapter 3
Chapter Opener: John Middlebrook/Cal Sport Media/Newscom. 3.9a-c: David M. Philips/Photo Researchers. 3.14b: Dr. Birgit H. Satir. 3.17b: Professors P. Motta & T. Naguro/SPL/Photo Researchers. 3.18b: CNR/Photo Researchers. 3.19b: P. Motta & T. Naguro/SPL/Photo Researchers. 3.21: Dr. Gopal Murti/Photo Researchers. 3.23a: Mary Osborn, Max Planck Institute. 3.23b: Frank Solomon and J. Dinsmore, Massachusetts Institute of Technology. 3.23c: Mark S. Ladinsky and J. Richard McIntosh, University of Colorado. 3.25b: Don W. Fawcett/Photo Researchers. 3.26.1: OMIKRON/Science Source/Photo Researchers. 3.26.2 and 3: W. L. Dentler/Biological Photo Service. 3.28: Don W. Fawcett/Photo Researchers. 3.29b.1: From L. Orci and A. Perrelet, *Freeze-Etch Histology*. (Heidelberg: Springer-Verlag, 1975) © 1975 Springer-Verlag. 3.29b.2: From A. C. Faberge, *Cell Tiss. Res.* 151 (1974):403. © 1974 Springer-Verlag. 3.29b.3: U. Aebi et al. *Nature* 323 (1996):560–564, Figure 1a. Used by permission. 3.30.1: Dr. Victoria E. Foe. 3.30.2: GF Bahr, Armed Forces Institute of Pathology. 3.33.1–6: Conly Rieder. 3.38b: Barbara Hamkalo.

Chapter 4
Chapter Opener: Fuse/Jupiter Images. 4.3a: William Karkow, Pearson Science. 4.3b, f: Allen Bell, University of New England; Pearson Science. 4.3c, d: Ed Reschke/Photolibrary. 4.3e: Nina Zanetti, Pearson Science. 4.4a: SPL/Photo Researchers, Inc. 4.8a, g: PAL 3.0, Pearson Science. 4.8b, f, h: Nina Zanetti, Pearson Science. 4.8c: Allen Bell, University of New England; Pearson Science. 4.8d, e, k: Lisa Lee, Pearson Science. 4.8i, j: Allen Bell, University of New England; Pearson Science. 4.9a: PAL 3.0, Pearson Science. 4.9b: Ed Reschke/Photolibrary. 4.9c, 4.10: Biophoto Associates/Photo Researchers. A Closer Look: David Musher/Photo Researchers.

Chapter 5
Chapter Opener: Jupiter Images. 5.2a: Ed Reschke/Photolibrary. 5.3: Ed Reschke/Photolibrary. 5.4a: Clouds Hill Imaging/Photo Researchers. 5.4c: John Wilson White, Pearson Science. 5.5b: Manfred Kage/Photo Researchers. 5.5d: Manfred Kage/Photolibrary. 5.7: Lisa Lee, Pearson Science. 5.8a: Biophoto Associates/Photo Researchers. 5.8b: P. Marazzi/SPL/Photo Researchers. 5.8c: Zeva Oelbaum/Photolibrary. 5.10a: Scott Camazine/Photo Researchers. 5.10b: Dr. M.A. Ansary/Photo Researchers.

Chapter 6
Chapter Opener: Belinda Images/SuperStock. 6.3.1: Donald Gregory Clever. 6.3.2: Steve Gschmeissner/Photo Researchers. 6.7c.1: Andrew Syred/Photo Researchers. 6.7c.2: Ed Reschke/Photolibrary. 6.10: Lisa Lee, Pearson Science. 6.14a: PCN Photography/Alamy. 6.16: P. Motta, Department of Anatomy, University "La Sapienza," Rome/Science Photo Library/Photo Researchers. 6.17: Scott Camazine/Photo Researchers. Table 6.2.1: Lester Bergman/Corbis. Table 6.2.2: ISM/Centers for Disease Control and Prevention (CDC). Table 6.2.3: SIU/Photolibrary. Table 6.2.4: Frank Gaillard - Radiopaedia.org, Imagineering © Pearson. Table 6.2.5: William T. C. Yuh. Table 6.2.6: Charles Stewart.

Chapter 7
Chapter Opener: Exactostock/SuperStock. 7.5b, d: PAL 3.0, Pearson Science. 7.6b: PAL 3.0, Pearson Science. 7.7b: Michael Wiley - Univ. of Toronto, Imagineering © Pearson. 7.8: PAL 3.0, Pearson Science. 7.9a, b: PAL 3.0, Pearson Science. 7.10: Michael Wiley - Univ. of Toronto, Imagineering © Pearson. 7.11c: PAL 3.0, Pearson Science. 7.12a: PAL 3.0, Pearson Science. 7.17a: NMSB/Custom Medical Stock Photo. 7.17b: Nordic Photos/SuperStock. 7.17c: Steve Gorton/Dorling Kindersley. 7.18d: Neil Borden/Photo Researchers. 7.23b: Dissection by Shawn Miller, photography by Mark Nielsen and Alexa Doig. 7.24c: Pearson Science. 7.31c, d: Ralph T. Hutchings. 7.33c: PAL 3.0, Pearson Science. 7.33d: Michael Wiley - Univ. of Toronto, Imagineering © Pearson. 7.33e: Biophoto Associates/Science Source/Photo Researchers. 7.35b: Elaine N. Marieb. 7.37: Center For Cranialfacial Anomalies, University of California, San Francisco. 7.38: Reik/age fotostock. Table 7.4.2-5: From *A Stereoscopic Atlas of Human Anatomy* by David L. Bassett.

Chapter 8
Chapter Opener: Imagesource/Photolibrary. 8.5a–f: John Wilson White, Pearson Science. 8.6a–f: John Wilson White, Pearson Science. 8.8f: PAL 3.0, Pearson Science. 8.10b: Mark Neilsen, University of Utah; Pearson Science. 8.10e: VideoSurgery/Photo Researchers. 8.11c: From *A Stereoscopic Atlas of Human Anatomy* by David L. Bassett. 8.12b: From *A Stereoscopic Atlas of Human Anatomy* by David L. Bassett. 8.14: Elaine Marieb. 8.15: SIU/Photolibrary. A Closer Look: 1: Lawrence Livermore National Laboratory/Photo Researchers. 2: Elaine N. Marieb.

Chapter 9
Chapter Opener: altrendo images/Jupiter Images. 9.1b: Lisa Lee, Pearson Science. 9.2a: Marian Rice. 9.4: John Heuser. 9.6.1: Don W. Fawcett/Photo Researchers. 9.6.2: Biophoto Associates/Photo Researchers. 9.13b: Eric Graves/Photo Researchers. A Closer Look: Corbis/SuperStock. Table 9.3.4: Eric Graves/Photo Researchers. Table 9.3.5: Marian Rice. Table 9.3.6: SPL/Photo Researchers.

Chapter 10
Chapter Opener: Aaron Packard/Jupiter Images. 10.7a: David Bassett. 10.9b: Creative Digital Visions, Pearson Science. 10.10c: Dissection by Shawn Miller, photography by Mark Nielsen and Alexa Doig. 10.11c: From *A Stereoscopic Atlas of Human Anatomy* by David L. Bassett. 10.14b: Dissection by Dr. Olga Malakhova and photography by Winston Charles Poulton of University of Florida College of Medicine, Gainesville/Pearson Science. 10.14d, e: Dissection by Shawn Miller, photography by Mark Nielsen and Alexa Doig. 10.15d: Dissection by Shawn Miller, photography by Mark Nielsen and Alexa Doig. 10.21b: David Bassett.

Chapter 11
Chapter Opener: Imagesource/Photlibrary. 11.4b: Manfred Kage/Photolibrary. 11.5b: Don W. Fawcett/ Photo Researchers. 11.16b: Oliver Meckes/Ottawa/Photo Researchers. 11.25: Tibor Harkany, Science Magagzine. A Closer Look: Brookhaven National Laboratory/Jupiter Images.

Chapter 12
Chapter Opener: Exactostock/SuperStock. 12.4a: From *A Stereoscopic Atlas of Human Anatomy*

by David L. Bassett. 12.4b: A. Glauberman/Photo Researchers. 12.5: Volker Steger/Photolibrary. 12.8a: Ralph T. Hutchings. 12.8b: From *A Stereoscopic Atlas of Human Anatomy* by David L. Bassett. 12.9b: PAL 3.0, Pearson Science. 12.10b: David Bassett. 12.12: PAL 3.0, Pearson Science. 12.15a: Ralph T. Hutchings. 12.15c: David L. Bassett. 12.18a: Hank Morgan/Photo Researchers. 12.23b: From *A Stereoscopic Atlas of Human Anatomy* by David L. Bassett. 12.25: Ansary/Custom Medical Stock Photo/Newscom. 12.26b, c, d: PAL 3.0, Pearson Science. 12.35: Biophoto Associates/Science Source/Photo Researchers.

Chapter 13
Chapter Opener: Dominique Douieb/Jupiter Images. 13.4: Thomas Deerinck, NCMIR/Photo Researchers. 13.10d: Dissection by Dr. Olga Malakhova and photography by Winston Charles Poulton of University of Florida College of Medicine, Gainesville/Pearson Science. 13.12c: Dissection by Dr. Olga Malakhova and photography by Winston Charles Poulton of University of Florida College of Medicine, Gainesville/Pearson Science. Table 13.2.8: William Thompson, Pearson Science.

Chapter 14
Chapter Opener: Paul Kennedy/SuperStock.

Chapter 15
Chapter Opener: agefotostock/SuperStock. 15.1a: Richard Tauber, Pearson Science. 15.4b: From *A Stereoscopic Atlas of Human Anatomy* by David L Bassett. 15.6c: Lisa Lee, Pearson Science. 15.7: Dr. Charles Klettke, Pearson Science. 15.9: SPL/Photo Researchers. 15.11: Keith Leighton/Alamy. 15.19b: Stephen Spector/Pearson Science. 15.22c: PAL 3.0, Pearson Science. 15.27d: P. Motta/Department of Anatomy/University "La Sapienza," Rome/Science Photo Library/Photo Researchers. 15.31: Science Vol. 279 March 1998, p. 1870, Karen P. Steele. 15.35b: I. M. Hunter-Duvar, Department of Otolaryngology, The Hospital for Sick Children, Toronto.

Chapter 16
Chapter Opener: Khoroshunova Olga Underwater/Alamy. 16.7: Getty Images. 16.9b: Michael Wiley - Univ. of Toronto, Imagineering © Pearson. 16.11a: John Paul Kay/Photolibrary. 16.11b: Photo Researchers. 16.12b: PAL 3.0, Pearson Science 16.14b: Lisa Lee, Pearson Science. 16.16a: Charles B. Wilson, Neurological Surgery, University of California Medical Center, San Francisco. 16.16b: Charles B. Wilson, Neurological Surgery, University of California Medical Center, San Francisco. 16.18: Lisa Lee, Pearson Science. A Closer Look: Saturn Stills/SPL/Photo Researchers.

Chapter 17
Chapter Opener: Robert Harding Picture Library Ltd/Alamy. 17.2: Ed Reshke/Peter Arnold. 17.8a: Cheryl Power/Photo Researchers. 17.8b: Omikron/Photo Researchers. 17.10a–e: PAL 3.0, Pearson Science. 17.15: Meckes/Ottawa/Photo Researchers. 17.16.1–4: Jack Scanlon, Holyoke Community College.

Chapter 18
Chapter Opener: Thomas Schloemann/Photolibrary. 18.5a: A. & F. Michler/Photolibrary. 18.5c, f: David Bassett. 18.6b: PAL 3.0, Pearson Science. 18.6c: Lennart Nilsson, The Body Victorious, New York: Dell, © Boehringer Ingelheim International GmbH. 18.6d: David L. Bassett. 18.12a: Manfred Cage/Photolibrary. 18.20: John Wilson White, Pearson Science. 18.22: Eric Gevaert/Shutterstock.

Chapter 19
Chapter Opener: Erik Isakson/Jupiter Images. 19.1a: Ed Reschke/Photolibrary. 19.13: Asia Images Group/Getty Images. 19.22c: CNRI/Science Photo Library/Photo Researchers. A Closer Look: 1: Sheila Terry/Science Photo Library/Photo Researchers. 2: GJLP/Photo Researchers.

Chapter 20
Chapter Opener: giovanni mereghetti/SuperStock. 20.3: Francis Leroy, Biocosmos/Science Photo Library/Photo Researchers. 20.4b: Biophoto Associates/Photo Researchers. 20.6c: Mark Neilsen, Pearson Science. 20.6d: Victor Eroschenko, Pearson Science. 20.7: Lisa Lee, Pearson Science. 20.8: Biophoto Associates/Photo Researchers. 20.9: Biophoto Associates/Science Source/Photo Researchers.

Chapter 21
Chapter Opener: Jules Frazier/Jupiter Images. 21.2: Lennart Nilsson/Scanpix Sweden AB. 21.10: David Scharf/Photo Researchers. 21.14b: Dr. Lawrence W. Haynes. 21.19b: Andrejs Liepins/Science Photo Library/Photo Researchers.

Chapter 22
Chapter Opener: David Madison/Jupiter Images. 22.2a: Jenny Thomas, Pearson Science. 22.3a: From *A Stereoscopic Atlas of Human Anatomy* by David L. Bassett. 22.4c, d: From *A Stereoscopic Atlas of Human Anatomy* by David L. Bassett. 22.6b: Nina Zanetti/Pearson Science. 22.6c: Science Photo Library/Photo Researchers. 22.8b: Lisa Lee, Pearson Science. 22.9b: MOTTA & MACCHIARELLI/ANATOMY DEPT/UNIV. LA SAPIENZA/SPL/Photo Researchers. 22.10b: From *A Stereoscopic Atlas of Human Anatomy* by David L. Bassett.

Chapter 23
Chapter Opener: Score/Jupiter Images. 23.9b: SPL/Photo Researchers. 23.12a: Biophoto Associates/Photo Researchers. 23.12b: Lisa Lee, Pearson Science. 23.14b: From *A Stereoscopic Atlas of Human Anatomy* by David L. Bassett. 23.16a: CNRI / Photo Researchers. 23.16b: Oliver Meckes/Ottawa/Photo Researchers. 23.22c: Steve Gschmeissner/Photo Researchers. 23.23: Secchi-Lecaque-Roussel-UCLAF/CNRI/Science Photo Library/Photo Researchers. 23.24a, b: From *A Stereoscopic Atlas of Human Anatomy* by David L. Bassett. 23.25b: From *A Stereoscopic Atlas of Human Anatomy* by David L. Bassett. 23.26b: Lisa Lee, Pearson Science. 23.30a: From *A Stereoscopic Atlas of Human Anatomy* by David L. Bassett.

Chapter 24
Chapter Opener: moodboard/SuperStock. 24.10: Andreas Engel and Daniel J. Müller. 24.25: Blend Images/SuperStock. A Closer Look: Ilene MacDonald/Alamy.

Chapter 25
Chapter Opener: Ingram Publishing/SuperStock. 25.2b: Richard Tauber, Pearson Science. 25.3a: Karen Krabbenhoft, University of Wisconsin-Madison School of Medicine and Public Health/Pearson Science. 25.6a: Lisa Lee, Pearson Science. 25.6b: Tom Fink, East Carolina University, Department of Biology/Pearson Science. 25.7b: Steve Gschmeissner/Photo Researchers. 25.10b: P. Motta and M. Castellucci/Science Photo Library/Photo Researchers. 25.18: National Institute of Health. 25.19: Biophoto Associates/Photo Researchers.

Chapter 26
Chapter Opener: Stockbyte/Jupiter Images. 26.5: hartphotography/Shutterstock.

Chapter 27
Chapter Opener: Stockbyte/Jupiter Images. 27.3b: PAL 3.0, Pearson Science. 27.3c: Ed Reschke. 27.8a: Prof. P.M. Motta/Univ. "La Sapienza," Rome/Photo Researchers. 27.9b: Juergen Berger/Photo Researchers. 27.13: Lisa Lee, Pearson Science. 27.15a: PAL 3.0, Pearson Science. 27.18b, c: Leonard Lessin/Photolibrary. 27.20.1–3a: Science Pictures Ltd./Photo Researchers. 27.20.3.b: Biophoto Associates/Photo Researchers. 27.20.4: Ed Reschke/Photolibrary. 27.20.5: C. Edelman/La Vilette/Photo Researchers. 27.20.6: Lester V. Bergman/Corbis.

Chapter 28
Chapter Opener: Reggie Casagrande/Jupiter Images. 28.3b: CC Studios/Science Photo Library/Photo Researchers. 28.5b: R. O'Rahilly and R. Muller, *Human Embryology and Teratology*. This material is reproduced with permission of Wiley-Liss, Inc., a subsidiary of John Wiley & Sons, Inc. 28.5d: Allen C. Enders, University of California, Davis/Carnegie Collection. 28.15a: From *A Stereoscopic Atlas of Human Anatomy* by David L. Bassett. 28.15b, c: From Lennart Nilsson/Albert Bonniers Forlag. 28.19: Comstock Images/Getty Images.

Chapter 29
Chapter Opener: Michael DeYoung/Photolibrary. 29.1.1: Alfred Pasieka/Photolibrary 29.1.2: Hop Americain / Photo Researchers. 29.1.3: L.Williatt, East Anglian Regional Genetics/SPL/Photo Researchers. 29.5: Andrew Syred/Photo Researchers.

Illustration Credits
All illustrations by Imagineering STA Media Services unless otherwise noted.

Chapter 1
1.3: Vincent Perez/Wendy Hiller Gee. 1.7: Imagineering STA Media Services/Precision Graphics.

Chapter 3
3.2, 3.3, 3.20, 3.27: Imagineering STA Media Services/Precision Graphics. 3.24: Campbell, Neil A., *Biology*, 4th Edition, © 1996, p. 128. Reprinted by permission of Pearson Education, Inc., Upper Saddle River, NJ. 3.37: Electronic Publishing Services, Inc./Imagineering STA Media Services.

Chapter 4
4.6: Matthews, Christopher K.; VanHolde, Kensal E.; Ahern, Kevin G., *Biochemistry*, 3rd Edition, © 2000. Adapted by permission of Pearson Education, Inc. Upper Saddle River, NJ.

Chapter 5
5.1, 5.2, 5.7: Electronic Publishing Services, Inc. System Connections: Vincent Perez/Wendy Hiller Gee.

Chapter 6
6.8: Imagineering STA Media Services/Precision Graphics. System Connections: Vincent Perez/Wendy Hiller Gee.

Chapter 8
8.7: Electronic Publishing Services, Inc./Imagineering STA Media Services.

Chapter 9
9.1, 9.2: Imagineering STA Media Services/Precision Graphics. 9.9, 9.25–9.27, 9.29: Electronic Publishing Services, Inc. System Connections: Vincent Perez/ Wendy Hiller Gee.

Chapter 10
10.1: Electronic Publishing Services, Inc./ Imagineering STA Media Services.

Chapter 11
11.2, 11.24: Electronic Publishing Services, Inc. 11.3, 11.5: Imagineering STA Media Services/ Precision Graphics.

Chapter 12
12.1–12.3, 12.6, 12.7, 12.11, 12.13–12.17, 12.21, 12.22, 12.24, 12.28b, 12.29–12.33: Electronic Publishing Services, Inc.

Chapter 13
13.1, 13.4–13.6, 13.14, 13.15, 13.19, 13.20: Electronic Publishing Services, Inc. 13.16, 13.T02.6: Imagineering STA Media Services/Precision Graphics.

Chapter 14
14.1–14.4, 14.6–14.8: Electronic Publishing Services, Inc. System Connections: Vincent Perez/Wendy Hiller Gee.

Chapter 15
15.1–15.6, 15.8, 15.15, 15.16, 15.18, 15.20, 15.22, 15.23, 15.25–15.27, 15.30, 15.32–15.35: Electronic Publishing Services, Inc. 15.24: Electronic Publishing Services, Inc./Precision Graphics.

Chapter 16
16.1: Electronic Publishing Services, Inc. 16.5: Electronic Publishing Services, Inc./Imagineering STA Media Services. 16.9: Imagineering STA Media Services/Precision Graphics. System Connections: Vincent Perez/Wendy Hiller Gee.

Chapter 18
18.2: Electronic Publishing Services, Inc./Precision Graphics. 18.3–18.6, 18.12, 18.15: Electronic Publishing Services, Inc. 18.7: Imagineering STA Media Services/Precision Graphics. 18.9: Electronic Publishing Services, Inc./Imagineering STA Media Services.

Chapter 19
19.1, 19.4, 19.21–19.30: Electronic Publishing Services, Inc. 19.17: Electronic Publishing Services, Inc./ Imagineering STA Media Services. System Connections: Vincent Perez/Wendy Hiller Gee.

Chapter 20
System Connections: Vencent Perez/Wendy Hiller Gee.

Chapter 21
21.16: Johnson, Michael D., *Human Biology: Concepts and Current Issues,* 2nd Edition, © 2002. Reprinted by permission of Pearson Education, Inc., Upper Saddle River, NJ.

Chapter 22
22.1: Electronic Publishing Services, Inc./Precision Graphics. 22.3, 22.4, 22.7–22.10, 22.20, 22.26: Electronic Publishing Services, Inc. System Connections: Vincent Perez/Wendy Hiller Gee.

Chapter 23
23.1, 23.6–23.9, 23.14, 23.15, 23.21, 23.22, 23.29–23.31: Electronic Publishing Services, Inc. 23.25: Electronic Publishing Services, Inc./Precision Graphics. 23.28: Imagineering STA Media Services/ Precision Graphics. System Connections: Vincent Perez/Wendy Hiller Gee.

Chapter 24
24.8: Electronic Publishing Services, Inc.

Chapter 25
25.1, 25.5, 25.8, 25.10, 25.11, 25.16, 25.20: Electronic Publishing Services, Inc. 25.12: Imagineering STA Media Services/Precision Graphics.

Chapter 26
26.10: Imagineering STA Media Services/Precision Graphics. System Connections: Vincent Perez/ Wendy Hiller Gee.

Chapter 27
27.1–27.3, 27.12–12.14: Electronic Publishing Services, Inc. System Connections: Vincent Perez/ Wendy Hiller Gee.

Chapter 28
28.2, 28.4, 28.13: Electronic Publishing Services, Inc.

Index

NOTE: Page numbers in **boldface** indicate a definition. A *t* following a page number indicates tabular material, an *f* indicates an illustration, and a *b* indicates boxed material.

Word Roots, Prefixes, Suffixes, and Combining Forms

Prefixes and Combining Forms

a-, an- *absence, lack* acardia, lack of a heart; anaerobic, in the absence of oxygen
ab- *departing from, away from* abnormal, departing from normal
acou- *hearing* acoustics, the science of sound
ac-, acro- *extreme or extremity, peak* acrodermatitis, inflammation of the skin of the extremities
ad- *to, toward* adorbital, toward the orbit
aden-, adeno- *gland* adeniform, resembling a gland in shape
adren- *toward the kidney* adrenal gland, adjacent to the kidney
aero- *air* aerobic respiration, oxygen-requiring metabolism
af- *toward* afferent neurons, which carry impulses to the central nervous system
agon- *contest* agonistic and antagonistic muscles, which oppose each other
alb- *white* corpus albicans of the ovary, a white scar tissue
aliment- *nourish* alimentary canal, or digestive tract
allel- *of one another* alleles, alternative expressions of a gene
amphi- *on both sides, of both kinds* amphibian, an organism capable of living in water and on land
ana- *apart, up, again* anaphase of mitosis, when the chromosomes separate
anastomos- *come together* arteriovenous anastomosis, a connection between an artery and a vein
aneurysm *a widening* aortic aneurysm, a weak spot that causes enlargement of the blood vessel
angi- *vessel* angiitis, inflammation of a lymph vessel or blood vessel
angin- *choked* angina pectoris, a choked feeling in the chest due to dysfunction of the heart
ant-, anti- *opposed to, preventing, inhibiting* anticoagulant, a substance that prevents blood coagulation
ante- *preceding, before* antecubital, in front of the elbow
aort- *great artery* aorta
ap-, api- *tip, extremity* apex of the heart
append- *hang to* appendicular skeleton
aqua-, aque- *water* aqueous solutions
arbor *tree* arbor vitae of the cerebellum, the treelike pattern of white matter
areola- *open space* areolar connective tissue, a loose connective tissue
arrect- *upright* arrector pili muscles of the skin, which make the hairs stand erect
arthr-, arthro- *joint* arthropathy, any joint disease
artic- *joint* articular surfaces of bones, the points of connection
atri- *vestibule* atria, upper chambers of the heart
auscult- *listen* auscultatory method for measuring blood pressure
aut-, auto- *self* autogenous, self-generated
ax-, axi-, axo- *axis, axle* axial skeleton, axis of vertebral column
azyg- *unpaired* azygous vein, an unpaired vessel
baro- *pressure* baroreceptors for monitoring blood pressure
basal *base* basal lamina of epithelial basement membrane
bi- *two* bicuspid, having two cusps
bili- *bile* bilirubin, a bile pigment
bio- *life* biology, the study of life and living organisms
blast- *bud, germ* blastocyte, undifferentiated embryonic cell
brachi- *arm* brachial plexus of peripheral nervous system supplies the arm
brady- *slow* bradycardia, abnormally slow heart rate
brev- *short* fibularis brevis, a short leg muscle
broncho- *bronchus* bronchospasm, spasmodic contraction of bronchial muscle
bucco- *cheek* buccolabial, pertaining to the cheek and lip
calor- *heat* calories, a measure of energy
capill- *hair* blood and lymph capillaries
caput- *head* decapitate, remove the head
carcin- *cancer* carcinogen, a cancer-causing agent
cardi-, cardio- *heart* cardiotoxic, harmful to the heart
carneo- *flesh* trabeculae carneae, ridges of muscle in the ventricles of the heart
carot- *(1) carrot, (2) stupor* (1) carotene, an orange pigment, (2) carotid arteries in the neck, blockage of which causes fainting
cata- *down* catabolism, chemical breakdown
caud- *tail* caudal (directional term)
cec- *blind* cecum of large intestine, a blind-ended pouch
cele- *abdominal* celiac artery, in the abdomen
cephal- *head* cephalometer, an instrument for measuring the head
cerebro- *brain, especially the cerebrum* cerebrospinal, pertaining to the brain and spinal cord
cervic-, cervix *neck* cervix of the uterus
chiasm- *crossing* optic chiasma, where optic nerves cross
chole- *bile* cholesterol, cholecystokinin, a bile-secreting hormone
chondr- *cartilage* chondrogenic, giving rise to cartilage
chrom- *colored* chromosome, so named because they stain darkly
cili- *small hair* ciliated epithelium
circum- *around* circumnuclear, surrounding the nucleus
clavic- *key* clavicle, a "skeleton key"
co-, con- *together* concentric, common center, together in the center
coccy- *cuckoo* coccyx, which is beak-shaped
cochlea *snail shell* the cochlea of the inner ear, which is coiled like a snail shell
coel- *hollow* coelom, the ventral body cavity
commis- *united* gray commissure of the spinal cord connects the two columns of gray matter
concha *shell* nasal conchae, coiled shelves of bone in the nasal cavity
contra- *against, opposite* contraceptive, agent preventing conception

corn-, cornu- *horn* stratum corneum, outer layer of the skin composed of (horny) cells
corona *crown* coronal suture of the skull
corp- *body* corpse; corpus luteum, hormone-secreting body in the ovary
cort- *bark* cortex, the outer layer of the brain, kidney, adrenal glands, and lymph nodes
cost- *rib* intercostal, between the ribs
crani- *skull* craniotomy, a skull operation
crypt- *hidden* cryptomenorrhea, a condition in which menstrual symptoms are experienced but no external loss of blood occurs
cusp- *pointed* bicuspid, tricuspid valves of the heart
cutic- *skin* cuticle of the nail
cyan- *blue* cyanosis, blue color of the skin due to lack of oxygen
cyst- *sac, bladder* cystitis, inflammation of the urinary bladder
cyt- *cell* cytology, the study of cells
de- *undoing, reversal, loss, removal* deactivation, becoming inactive
decid- *falling off* deciduous (milk) teeth
delta *triangular* deltoid muscle, roughly triangular in shape
den-, dent- *tooth* dentin of the tooth
dendr- *tree, branch* dendrites, branches of a neuron
derm- *skin* dermis, deep layer of the skin
desm- *bond* desmosome, which binds adjacent epithelial cells
di- *twice, double* dimorphism, having two forms
dia- *through, between* diaphragm, the wall through or between two areas
dialys- *separate, break apart* kidney dialysis, in which waste products are removed from the blood
diastol- *stand apart* cardiac diastole, between successive contractions of the heart
diure- *urinate* diuretic, a drug that increases urine output
dors- *the back* dorsal, dorsum, dorsiflexion
duc-, duct *lead, draw* ductus deferens, tube which carries sperm from the epididymis into the urethra during ejaculation
dura *hard* dura mater, tough outer meninx
dys- *difficult, faulty, painful* dyspepsia, disturbed digestion
ec-, ex-, ecto- *out, outside, away from* excrete, to remove materials from the body
ectop- *displaced* ectopic pregnancy; ectopic focus for initiation of heart contraction
edem- *swelling* edema, accumulation of water in body tissues
ef- *away* efferent nerve fibers, which carry impulses away from the central nervous system
ejac- *to shoot forth* ejaculation of semen
embol- *wedge* embolus, an obstructive object traveling in the bloodstream
en-, em- *in, inside* encysted, enclosed in a cyst or capsule
enceph- *brain* encephalitis, inflammation of the brain
endo- *within, inner* endocytosis, taking particles into a cell
entero- *intestine* enterologist, one who specializes in the study of intestinal disorders
epi- *over, above* epidermis, outer layer of skin
erythr- *red* erythema, redness of the skin; erythrocyte, red blood cell
eso- *within* esophagus
eu- *well* euesthesia, a normal state of the senses
excret- *separate* excretory system
exo- *outside, outer layer* exophthalmos, an abnormal protrusion of the eye from the orbit
extra- *outside, beyond* extracellular, outside the body cells of an organism
extrins- *from the outside* extrinsic regulation of the heart
fasci-, fascia- *bundle, band* superficial and deep fascia
fenestr- *window* fenestrated capillaries
ferr- *iron* transferrin, ferritin, both iron-storage proteins
flagell- *whip* flagellum, the tail of a sperm cell
flat- *blow, blown* flatulence
folli- *bag, bellows* hair follicle
fontan- *fountain* fontanelles of the fetal skull
foram- *opening* foramen magnum of the skull
foss- *ditch* fossa ovalis of the heart; mandibular fossa of the skull
gam-, gamet- *married, spouse* gametes, the sex cells
gangli- *swelling, or knot* dorsal root ganglia of the spinal nerves
gastr- *stomach* gastrin, a hormone that influences gastric acid secretion
gene *beginning, origin* genetics
germin- *grow* germinal epithelium of the gonads
gero-, geront- *old man* gerontology, the study of aging
gest- *carried* gestation, the period from conception to birth
glauc- *gray* glaucoma, which causes gradual blindness
glom- *ball* glomeruli, clusters of capillaries in the kidneys
glosso- *tongue* glossopathy, any disease of the tongue
gluco-, glyco- gluconeogenesis, the production of glucose from noncarbohydrate molecules
glute- *buttock* gluteus maximus, largest muscle of the buttock
gnost- *knowing* the gnostic sense, a sense of awareness of self
gompho- *nail* gomphosis, the term applied to the joint between tooth and jaw
gon-, gono- *seed, offspring* gonads, the sex organs
gust- *taste* gustatory sense, the sense of taste
hapt- *fasten, grasp* hapten, a partial antigen
hema-, hemato-, hemo- *blood* hematocyst, a cyst containing blood
hemi- *half* hemiglossal, pertaining to one-half of the tongue
hepat- *liver* hepatitis, inflammation of the liver
hetero- *different or other* heterosexuality, sexual desire for a person of the opposite sex
hiat- *gap* the hiatus of the diaphragm, the opening through which the esophagus passes
hippo- *horse* hippocampus of the brain, shaped like a seahorse
hirsut- *hairy* hirsutism, excessive body hair
hist- *tissue* histology, the study of tissues
holo- *whole* holocrine glands, whose secretions are whole cells
hom-, homo- *same* homeoplasia, formation of tissue similar to normal tissue; homocentric, having the same center
hormon- *to excite* hormones
humor- *a fluid* humoral immunity, which involves antibodies circulating in the blood
hyal- *glass, clear* hyaline cartilage, which has no visible fibers
hydr-, hydro- *water* dehydration, loss of body water
hyper- *excess* hypertension, excessive tension
hypno- *sleep* hypnosis, a sleeplike state
hypo- *below, deficient* hypodermic, beneath the skin; hypokalemia, deficiency of potassium
hyster-, hystero- *uterus, womb* hysterectomy, removal of the uterus; hysterodynia, pain in the womb
ile- *intestine* ileum, the last portion of the small intestine
im- *not* impermeable, not permitting passage, not permeable
inter- *between* intercellular, between the cells
intercal- *insert* intercalated discs, the end membranes between adjacent cardiac muscle cells
intra- *within, inside* intracellular, inside the cell
iso- *equal, same* isothermal, equal, or same, temperature
jugul- *throat* jugular veins, prominent vessels in the neck
juxta- *near, close to* juxtaglomerular complex, a cell cluster next to a glomerulus in the kidneys
karyo- *kernel, nucleus* karyotype, the assemblage of the nuclear chromosomes
kera- *horn* keratin, the water-repellent protein of the skin
kilo- *thousand* kilocalories, equal to 1000 calories
kin-, kines- *move* kinetic energy, the energy of motion

labi-, labri- *lip* labial frenulum, the membrane which joins the lip to the gum
lact- *milk* lactose, milk sugar
lacun- *space, cavity, lake* lacunae, the spaces occupied by cells of cartilage and bone tissue
lamell- *small plate* concentric lamellae, rings of bone matrix in compact bone
lamina *layer, sheet* basal lamina, part of the epithelial basement membrane
lat- *wide* latissimus dorsi, a broad muscle of the back
laten- *hidden* latent period of a muscle twitch
later- *side* lateral (directional term)
leuko- *white* leukocyte, white blood cell
leva- *raise, elevate* levator labii superioris, muscle that elevates upper lip
lingua- *tongue* lingual tonsil, adjacent to the tongue
lip-, lipo- *fat, lipid* lipophage, a cell that has taken up fat in its cytoplasm
lith- *stone* cholelithiasis, gallstones
luci- *clear* stratum lucidum, clear layer of the epidermis
lumen *light* lumen, center of a hollow structure
lut- *yellow* corpus luteum, a yellow, hormone-secreting structure in the ovary
lymph *water* lymphatic circulation, return of clear fluid to the bloodstream
macro- *large* macromolecule, large molecule
macula *spot* macula lutea, yellow spot on the retina
magn- *large* foramen magnum, largest opening of the skull
mal- *bad, abnormal* malfunction, abnormal functioning of an organ
mamm- *breast* mammary gland, breast
mast- *breast* mastectomy, removal of a mammary gland
mater *mother* dura mater, pia mater, membranes that envelop the brain
meat- *passage* external acoustic meatus, the ear canal
medi- *middle* medial (directional term)
medull- *marrow* medulla, the middle portion of the kidney, adrenal gland, and lymph node
mega- *large* megakaryocyte, large precursor cell of platelets
meio- *less* meiosis, nuclear division that halves the chromosome number
melan- *black* melanocytes, which secrete the black pigment melanin
men-, menstru- *month* menses, the cyclic menstrual flow
meningo- *membrane* meningitis, inflammation of the membranes of the brain
mer-, mero-, *a part* merocrine glands, the secretions of which do not include the cell
meso- *middle* mesoderm, middle germ layer
meta- *beyond, between, transition* metatarsus, the part of the foot between the tarsus and the phalanges
metro- *uterus* endometrium, the lining of the uterus
micro- *small* microscope, an instrument used to make small objects appear larger
mictur- *urinate* micturition, the act of voiding the bladder
mito- *thread, filament* mitochondria, small, filament-like structures located in cells
mnem- *memory* amnesia
mono- *single* monospasm, spasm of a single limb
morpho- *form* morphology, the study of form and structure or organisms
multi- *many* multinuclear, having several nuclei
mur- *wall* intramural ganglion, a nerve junction within an organ
muta- *change* mutation, change in the base sequence of DNA
myelo- *spinal cord, marrow* myeloblasts, cells of the bone marrow
myo- *muscle* myocardium, heart muscle
nano- *dwarf* nanometer, one-billionth of a meter
narco- *numbness* narcotic, a drug producing stupor or numbed sensations
natri- *sodium* atrial natriuretic peptide, a sodium-regulating hormone
necro- *death* necrosis, tissue death
neo- *new* neoplasm, an abnormal growth
nephro- *kidney* nephritis, inflammation of the kidney
neuro- *nerve* neurophysiology, the physiology of the nervous system
noci- *harmful* nociceptors, receptors for pain
nom- *name* innominate artery; innominate bone
noto- *back* notochord, the embryonic structure that precedes the vertebral column
nucle- *pit, kernel, little nut* nucleus
nutri- *feed, nourish* nutrition
ob- *before, against* obstruction, impeding or blocking up
oculo- *eye* monocular, pertaining to one eye
odonto- *teeth* orthodontist, one who specializes in proper positioning of the teeth in relation to each other
olfact- *smell* olfactory nerves
oligo- *few* oligodendrocytes, neuroglial cells with few branches
onco- *a mass* oncology, study of cancer
oo- *egg* oocyte, precursor of female gamete
ophthalmo- *eye* ophthalmology, the study of the eyes and related disease
orb- *circular* orbicularis oculi, muscle that encircles the eye
orchi- *testis* cryptorchidism, failure of the testes to descend into the scrotum
org- *living* organism
ortho- *straight, direct* orthopedic, correction of deformities of the musculoskeletal system
osm- *smell* anosmia, loss of sense of smell
osmo- *pushing* osmosis
osteo- *bone* osteodermia, bony formations in the skin
oto- *ear* otoscope, a device for examining the ear
ov-, ovi- *egg* ovum; oviduct
oxy- *oxygen* oxygenation, the saturation of a substance with oxygen
pan- *all, universal* panacea, a cure-all
papill- *nipple* dermal papillae, projections of the dermis into the epidermal area
para- *beside, near* paranuclear, beside the nucleus
pect-, pectus *breast* pectoralis major, a large chest muscle
pelv- *a basin* pelvic girdle, which cradles the pelvic organs
peni- *a tail* penis; penile arteriole
penna- *feather* unipennate, bipennate muscles, whose fascicles have a feathered appearance
pent- *five* pentose, a 5-carbon sugar
pep-, peps-, pept- *digest* pepsin, a digestive enzyme of the stomach; peptic ulcer
per-, permea- *through* permeate; permeable
peri- *around* perianal, situated around the anus
phago- *eat* phagocyte, a cell that engulfs and digests particles or cells
pheno- *show, appear* phenotype, the physical appearance of an individual
phleb- *vein* phlebitis, inflammation of the veins
pia *tender* pia mater, delicate inner membrane around the brain and spinal cord
pili *hair* arrector pili muscles of the skin, which make the hairs stand erect
pin-, pino- *drink* pinocytosis, the engulfing of small particles by a cell
platy- *flat, broad* platysma, broad, flat muscle of the neck
pleur- *side, rib* pleural serosa, the membrane that lines the thoracic cavity and covers the lungs
plex-, plexus *net, network* brachial plexus, the network of nerves that supplies the arm
pneumo- *air, wind* pneumothorax, air in the thoracic cavity
pod- *foot* podiatry, the treatment of foot disorders
poly- *multiple* polymorphism, multiple forms
post- *after, behind* posterior, places behind (a specific) part
pre-, pro- *before, ahead of* prenatal, before birth
procto- *rectum, anus* proctoscope, an instrument for examining the rectum
pron- *bent forward* prone, pronate

propri- *one's own* proprioception, awareness of body parts and movement
pseudo- *false* pseudotumor, a false tumor
psycho- *mind, psyche* psychogram, a chart of personality traits
ptos- *fall* renal ptosis, a condition in which the kidneys drift below their normal position
pub- *of the pubis* puberty
pulmo- *lung* pulmonary artery, which brings blood to the lungs
pyo- *pus* pyocyst, a cyst that contains pus
pyro- *fire* pyrogen, a substance that induces fever
quad-, quadr- *four-sided* quadratus lumborum, a muscle with a square shape
re- *back, again* reinfect
rect- *straight* rectus abdominis, rectum
ren- *kidney* renal; renin, an enzyme secreted by the kidney
retin-, retic- *net, network* endoplasmic reticulum, a network of membranous sacs within a cell
retro- *backward, behind* retrogression, to move backward in development
rheum- *watery flow, change, flux* rheumatoid arthritis; rheumatic fever
rhin-, rhino- *nose* rhinitis, inflammation of the nose
ruga- *fold, wrinkle* rugae, the folds of the stomach, gallbladder, and urinary bladder
sagitt- *arrow* sagittal (directional term)
salta- *leap* saltatory conduction, the rapid conduction of impulses along myelinated neurons
sanguin- *blood* consanguineous, indicative of a genetic relationship between individuals
sarco- *flesh* sarcomere, unit of contraction in skeletal muscle
saphen- *visible, clear* great saphenous vein, superficial vein of the thigh and leg
sclero- *hard* sclerodermatitis, inflammatory thickening and hardening of the skin
seb- *grease* sebum, the oil of the skin
semen *seed, sperm* semen, the discharge of the male reproductive system
semi- *half* semicircular, having the form of half a circle
sens- *feeling* sensation, sensory
septi- *rotten* sepsis, infection; antiseptic
septum *fence* nasal septum
sero- *serum* serological tests, which assess blood conditions
serrat- *saw* serratus anterior, a muscle of the chest wall that has a jagged edge
sin-, sino- *a hollow* sinuses of the skull
soma- *body* somatic nervous system
somn- *sleep* insomnia, inability to sleep
sphin- *squeeze* sphincter
splanchn- *organ* splanchnic nerve, autonomic supply to abdominal viscera
spondyl- *vertebra* ankylosing spondylitis, rheumatoid arthritis affecting the spine
squam- *scale, flat* squamous epithelium, squamous suture of the skull
steno- *narrow* stenocoriasis, narrowing of the pupil
strat- *layer* strata of the epidermis; stratified epithelium
stria- *furrow, streak* striations of skeletal and cardiac muscle tissue
stroma *spread out* stroma, the connective tissue framework of some organs
sub- *beneath, under* sublingual, beneath the tongue
sucr- *sweet* sucrose, table sugar
sudor- *sweat* sudoriferous glands, the sweat glands
super- *above, upon* superior, quality or state of being above other parts
supra- *above, upon* supracondylar, above a condyle
sym-, syn- *together, with* synapse, the region of communication between two neurons
synerg- *work together* synergism
systol- *contraction* systole, contraction of the heart
tachy- *rapid* tachycardia, abnormally rapid heartbeat
tact- *touch* tactile sense
telo- *the end* telophase, the end of mitosis
templ-, tempo- *time* temporal summation of nerve impulses
tens- *stretched* muscle tension
terti- *third* fibularis tertius, one of three fibularis muscles
tetan- *rigid, tense* tetanus of muscles
therm- *heat* thermometer, an instrument used to measure heat
thromb- *clot* thrombocyte, thrombus
thyro- *a shield* thyroid gland
tissu- *woven* tissue
tono- *tension* tonicity, hypertonic
tox- *poison* toxicology, study of poisons
trab- *beam, timber* trabeculae, spicules of bone in spongy bone tissue
trans- *across, through* transpleural, through the pleura
trapez- *table* trapezius, the four-sided muscle of the upper back
tri- *three* trifurcation, division into three branches
trop- *turn, change* tropic hormones, whose targets are endocrine glands
troph- *nourish* trophoblast, from which develops the fetal portion of the placenta
tuber- *swelling* tuberosity, a bump on a bone
tunic- *covering* tunica albuginea, the covering of the testis
tympan- *drum* tympanic membrane, the eardrum
ultra- *beyond* ultraviolet radiation, beyond the band of visible light
vacc- *cow* vaccine
vagin- *a sheath* vagina
vagus *wanderer* the vagus nerve, which starts at the brain and travels into the abdominopelvic cavity
valen- *strength* valence shells of atoms
venter, ventr- *abdomen, belly* ventral (directional term), ventricle
vent- *the wind* pulmonary ventilation
vert- *turn* vertebral column
vestibul- *a porch* vestibule, the anterior entryway to the mouth and nose
vibr- *shake, quiver* vibrissae, hairs of the nasal vestibule
villus *shaggy hair* microvilli, which have the appearance of hair in light microscopy
viscero- *organ, viscera* visceroinhibitory, inhibiting the movements of the viscera
viscos- *sticky* viscosity, resistance to flow
vita- *life* vitamin
vitre- *glass* vitreous humor, the clear jelly of the eye
viv- *live* in vivo
vulv- *a covering* vulva, the female external genitalia
zyg- *a yoke, twin* zygote

Suffixes

-able *able to, capable of* viable, ability to live or exist
-ac *referring to* cardiac, referring to the heart
-algia *pain in a certain part* neuralgia, pain along the course of a nerve
-apsi *juncture* synapse, where two neurons communicate
-ary *associated with, relating to* coronary, associated with the heart
-asthen *weakness* myasthenia gravis, a disease involving paralysis
-bryo *swollen* embryo
-cide *destroy or kill* germicide, an agent that kills germs
-cipit *head* occipital
-clast *break* osteoclast, a cell that dissolves bone matrix
-crine *separate* endocrine organs, which secrete hormones into the blood
-dips *thirst, dry* polydipsia, excessive thirst associated with diabetes
-ectomy *cutting out, surgical removal* appendectomy, cutting out of the appendix
-ell, -elle *small* organelle
-emia *condition of the blood* anemia, deficiency of red blood cells
-esthesi *sensation* anesthesia, lack of sensation

-ferent *carry* efferent nerves, nerves carrying impulses away from the CNS
-form, -forma *shape* cribriform plate of the ethmoid bone
-fuge *driving out* vermifuge, a substance that expels worms of the intestine
-gen *an agent that initiates* pathogen, any agent that produces disease
-glea, -glia *glue* neuroglia, the connective tissue of the nervous system
-gram *data that are systematically recorded, a record* electrocardiogram, a recording showing action of the heart
-graph *an instrument used for recording data or writing* electrocardiograph, an instrument used to make an electrocardiogram
-ia *condition* insomnia, condition of not being able to sleep
-iatrics *medical specialty* geriatrics, the branch of medicine dealing with disease associated with old age
-ism *condition* hyperthyroidism
-itis *inflammation* gastritis, inflammation of the stomach
-lemma *sheath, husk* sarcolemma, the plasma membrane of a muscle cell
-logy *the study of* pathology, the study of changes in structure and function brought on by disease
-lysis *loosening or breaking down* hydrolysis, chemical decomposition of a compound into other compounds as a result of taking up water
-malacia *soft* osteomalacia, a process leading to bone softening
-mania *obsession, compulsion* erotomania, exaggeration of the sexual passions
-nata *birth* prenatal development
-nom *govern* autonomic nervous system
-odyn *pain* coccygodynia, pain in the region of the coccyx
-oid *like, resembling* cuboid, shaped as a cube
-oma *tumor* lymphoma, a tumor of the lymphatic tissues
-opia *of the eye* myopia, nearsightedness
-ory *referring to, of* auditory, referring to hearing
-pathy *disease* osteopathy, any disease of the bone
-phasia *speech* aphasia, lack of ability to speak
-phil, -philo *like, love* hydrophilic, water-attracting molecules
-phobia *fear* acrophobia, fear of heights
-phragm *partition* diaphragm, which separates the thoracic and abdominal cavities
-phylax *guard, preserve* prophylaxis, to guard in advance, as in preventive treatment
-plas *grow* neoplasia, an abnormal growth
-plasm *form, shape* cytoplasm
-plasty *reconstruction of a part, plastic surgery* rhinoplasty, reconstruction of the nose through surgery
-plegia *paralysis* paraplegia, paralysis of the lower half of the body or lower limbs
-rrhagia *abnormal or excessive discharge* metrorrhagia, uterine hemorrhage
-rrhea *flow or discharge* diarrhea, abnormal emptying of the bowels
-scope *instrument used for examination* stethoscope, instrument used to listen to sounds of parts of the body
-some *body* chromosome
-sorb *suck in* absorb
-stalsis *compression, constriction* peristalsis, muscular contractions that propel food along the digestive tract
-stasis *arrest, fixation* hemostasis, arrest of bleeding
-stitia *come to stand* interstitial fluid, between the cells
-stomy *establishment of an artificial opening* enterostomy, the formation of an artificial opening into the intestine through the abdominal wall
-tegm *cover* integument
-tomy *to cut* appendectomy, surgical removal of the appendix
-trud *thrust* protrude, detrusor muscle
-ty *condition of, state* immunity, condition of being resistant to infection or disease
-uria *urine* polyuria, passage of an excessive amount of urine
-zyme *ferment* enzyme